D1759459

WID

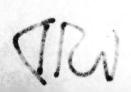

FOWLER'S

ZOO AND WILD ANIMAL MEDICINE

R. Eric Miller, DVM, DACZM
Senior Vice President for Zoological Operations
Director, WildCare Institute
Saint Louis Zoo
Forest Park
St. Louis, Missouri;
Adjunct Associate Professor of Veterinary Medicine and Surgery
College of Veterinary Medicine
University of Missouri
Columbia, Missouri

Murray E. Fowler, DVM, DACZM, DACVIM, DABVT
Professor Emeritus, Zoological Medicine
School of Veterinary Medicine
University of California, Davis
Davis, California

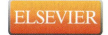

SIH
636.0889 FOW

ELSEVIER
SAUNDERS

3251 Riverport Lane
St. Louis, Missouri 63043

FOWLER'S ZOO AND WILD ANIMAL MEDICINE   ISBN: 978-1-4557-7397-8
Copyright © 2015, 2012, 2008, 2003, 1999, 1993, 1986, 1978 by Saunders, an imprint of Elsevier Inc.

No part of this publication may be reproduced or transmitted in any form or by any means, electronic or mechanical, including photocopying, recording, or any information storage and retrieval system, without permission in writing from the publisher. Details on how to seek permission, further information about the Publisher's permissions policies and our arrangements with organizations such as the Copyright Clearance Center and the Copyright Licensing Agency, can be found at our website: www.elsevier.com/permissions.

This book and the individual contributions contained in it are protected under copyright by the Publisher (other than as may be noted herein).

Notices

Knowledge and best practice in this field are constantly changing. As new research and experience broaden our understanding, changes in research methods, professional practices, or medical treatment may become necessary.

Practitioners and researchers must always rely on their own experience and knowledge in evaluating and using any information, methods, compounds, or experiments described herein. In using such information or methods they should be mindful of their own safety and the safety of others, including parties for whom they have a professional responsibility.

With respect to any drug or pharmaceutical products identified, readers are advised to check the most current information provided (i) on procedures featured or (ii) by the manufacturer of each product to be administered, to verify the recommended dose or formula, the method and duration of administration, and contraindications. It is the responsibility of practitioners, relying on their own experience and knowledge of their patients, to make diagnoses, to determine dosages and the best treatment for each individual patient, and to take all appropriate safety precautions.

To the fullest extent of the law, neither the Publisher nor the authors, contributors, or editors, assume any liability for any injury and/or damage to persons or property as a matter of products liability, negligence or otherwise, or from any use or operation of any methods, products, instructions, or ideas contained in the material herein.

Library of Congress Cataloging-in-Publication Data
Fowler's zoo and wild animal medicine / [edited by] R. Eric Miller, Murray Fowler.—8.
    p. ; cm.
  Zoo and wild animal medicine
  Preceded by Fowler's zoo and wild animal medicine / R. Eric Miller, Murray Fowler. c2012.
  Includes bibliographical references and index.
  ISBN 978-1-4557-7397-8 (hardcover)
  I. Miller, R. Eric, editor. II. Fowler, Murray E., editor. III. Title: Zoo and wild animal medicine.
  [DNLM: 1. Animals, Zoo.   2. Animals, Wild.   3. Veterinary Medicine. SF 996]
  SF996
    636.089—dc23
                                                                    2014008396

Senior Vice President, Content: Loren Wilson
Content Strategy Director: Penny Rudolph
Content Development Specialist: Brandi Graham
Publishing Services Manager: Catherine Jackson
Senior Project Manager: Rachel E. McMullen
Designer: Margaret Reid

Printed in the United States of America

Last digit is the print number: 9 8 7 6 5 4 3 2

Working together
to grow libraries in
developing countries

www.elsevier.com • www.bookaid.org

Contributors

Mary Agnew, PhD
Program Coordinator
AZA Wildlife Contraception Center
Saint Louis Zoo
St. Louis, Missouri
Contraception

Roberto F. Aguilar, DVM, DECZM
(Zoo Health Management)
Senior Practicing Veterinarian in Wildlife
Health
Veterinary Teaching Hospital
Massey University
Palmerston North, New Zealand
Xenarthra

Jack L. Allen, DVM, DACZM
Senior Veterinarian
Veterinary Services
San Diego Zoo Safari Park
Escondido, California
Equidae

Cheryl Asa, BA, MS, PhD
Adjunct Professor
Department of Biology
Saint Louis University
Saint Louis, Missouri
Director of Research
AZA Wildlife Contraception Center
Research Department
Saint Louis Zoo
Saint Louis, Missouri
Contraception

Kay A. Backues, DVM, DACZM
Director of Animal Health
Veterinary Health Department
Tulsa Zoo
Tulsa, Oklahoma
Adjunct Professor
Lab Animal and Exotic Pet Medicine
Tulsa Community College
Tulsa, Oklahoma
Adjunct Professor
Zoo-Exotic Medicine Service
Oklahoma State University
Stillwater, Oklahoma
Anseriformes

Eric J. Baitchman, DVM, DACZM
Director of Veterinary Services
Zoo New England
Boston, Massachusetts
Caudata (Urodela): Tailed Amphibians

Ray L. Ball, DVM
Senior Veterinarian/Director of Medical
Sciences
Tampa's Lowry Park Zoo
Tampa, Florida
*Recent Updates for Antemortem Tuberculosis
Diagnostics in Zoo Animals*

Katrin Baumgautner, DrMedVet
Specialist in Zoo and Wildlife Medicine
Specialist in animal welfare
Zoo Nuremberg
Nuremberg, Germany
Avian Deflighting Techniques

Hugues Beaufrère, DVM, PhD,
DABVP(Avian), DECZM(Avian)
Avian and Exotic Veterinarian
Health Sciences Center, Clinical Studies
Ontario Veterinary College
University of Guelph
Guelph, Ontario, Canada
*Gruiformes (Cranes, Limpkins, Rails,
Gallinules, Coots, Bustards)*

R. Avery Bennett, DVM, DACVS
Lauderdale Veterinary Specialists
Fort Lauderdale, Florida
Avian Deflighting Techniques

Mads F. Bertelsen, DVM, DVSc,
DACZM, DECZM (Zoo Health
Management)
Associate Veterinarian
Center for Zoo and Wild Animal Health
Copenhagen Zoo
Frederiksberg, Denmark
Giraffidae

Tiffany Blackett, BVetMed, MRCVS
Northamptonshire, United Kingdom
Wildpro Multimedia

Rosemary J. Booth, BVSc
Director
Wild Animals Solutions
Gold Coast
Queensland, Australia
Caprimulgiformes (Nightjars and Allies)

Debra Bourne, MA, VetMB, PhD,
MRCVS
Senior Veterinary Editor
Wildlife Information Network
East Midland Zoological Society,
Atherstone,
Kent, Great Britain
Wildpro Multimedia

P. Walter Bravo, DVM, MS, PhD
Carrera Profesional de Medicina
Veterinaria, Canchis
Universidad Nacional San Antonio Abad
Cusco, Peru
Camelidae

Elizabeth L. Buckles, DVM, PhD,
DACVP
Clinical Associate Professor
Department of Biomedical Sciences
College of Veterinary Medicine
Cornell University
Ithaca, New York
Chiroptera (Bats)

Peter E. Buss, BVSc, MMedVet (fer)
Veterinary Senior Manager
Veterinary Wildlife Services
Kruger National Park
South African National Parks
Mpumalanga, South Africa
Tubulidentata (Aardvark)
Rhinoceridae (Rhinoceroses)

Paul P. Calle, VMD, DACZM
Chief Veterinarian & Director
Zoological Health Program
Wildlife Conservation Society
Bronx, New York
New World and Old World Monkeys

Norin Chai, DVM, MSc, MSc Vet, PhD
Head Vet, Deputy Director
Ménagerie du Jardin des Plantes
Département des Jardins Botaniques et
Zoologiques
Muséum national d'Histoire naturelle
Paris, France
Anurans

Jason Shih-Chien Chin, DVM, MS
Director
Taipei Zoo
President
Taiwan Aquarium and Zoo Association
Taipei, Taiwan
Pholidota

Leigh Ann Clayton, DVM, DABVP
(Avian)
Director
Department of Animal Health
National Aquarium
Baltimore, Maryland
Caecilians

iii

Darin M. Collins, DVM
Director of Animal Health Programs
Animal Health Department
Woodland Park Zoo
Seattle, Washington
Ursidae

Juan Cornejo, PhD
Bird Curator
Loro Parque Fundacion
Santa Cruz De Tenerife Area, Spain
Psittaciformes

Jennifer D'Agostino, DVM, DACZM
Director of Veterinary Services
Oklahoma City Zoo
Oklahoma City, Oklahoma
Insectivores (Insectivora, Macroscelidea, Scandentia)

Martine de Wit, DVM, DABVP (Avian)
Florida Fish and Wildlife Conservation Commission
Fish and Wildlife Research Institute
Marine Mammal Pathobiology Laboratory
St. Petersburg, Florida
Sirenia

Sharon L. Deem, DVM, PhD, DACZM
Adjunct Associate Professor
Biology
University of Missouri-Saint Louis
Director
Institute for Conservation Medicine
Saint Louis Zoo
St. Louis, Missouri
Conservation Medicine to One Health: The Role of Zoologic Veterinarians

Gregory M. Dennis, MSc, JD†
Member
Leongatha Law, LLC d/b/a Veterinary Law Center
Independence, Missouri
A Legal Overview for Zoological Medicine Veterinarians

Ryan S. DeVoe, DVM, MSpVM, DACZM, DABVP
Senior Veterinarian
North Carolina Zoological Park,
Asheboro, North Carolina
Lacertilia (Lizards, Skinks, Geckos) and Amphisbaenids (Worm Lizards)

Christopher Dold, DVM
Vice President of Veterinary Services
Zoological Department
SeaWorld Parks & Entertainment
Orlando, Florida
Cetacea (Whales, Dolphins, Porpoises)

Genevieve Dumonceaux, DVM
Clinical Veterinarian
Animal Health
Palm Beach Zoo
West Palm Beach, Florida
Trogoniformes

Mary Duncan, BVMS, PhD, DACVP, MRCVS
Staff Pathologist
Saint Louis Zoo
St. Louis, Missouri
Gout in Exotic Animals

Jesus Fernandez-Moran, DVM, PhD
President, European Association for Aquatic Mammals
Fundación Parques Reunidos
Casa de campo
Zoo Madrid-Parques, Reunidos
Madrid, Spain
Mustelidae

Edmund Flach, MA, VetMB, MSc, DZooMed, DECZM (Zoo Health Management), MRCVS
European Veterinary Specialist in Zoological Medicine (Zoo Health Management)
Zoo and Wildlife Pathologist
Zoological Society of London
London, United Kingdom
Tragulidae, Moschidae, and Cervidae

Joseph P. Flanagan, DVM
Director of Veterinary Services
Houston Zoo, Inc.
Houston, Texas
Chelonians (Turtles, Tortoises)

Gregory J. Fleming, DVM, DACZM†
Veterinarian
Department of Animal Health
Walt Disney Parks and Resorts
Bay Lake, Florida
Crocodilians (Crocodiles, Alligators, Caiman, Gharial)

Deidre K. Fontenot, DVM
Veterinarian
Department in Animal Health
Disney's Animals, Science and Environment
Lake Buena Vista, Florida
Crocodilians (Crocodiles, Alligators, Caiman, Gharial)

Kathryn C. Gamble, DVM, MS, DACZM, DECZM (ZHM)
Dr Lester E Fisher Director of Veterinary Medicine
Veterinary Services
Lincoln Park Zoo
Chicago, Illinois
Coraciiformes (Kingfishers, Motmots, Bee-Eaters, Hoopoes, Hornbills)

Hanno Gerritsmann, DTzT
Veterinarian
Research Institute of Wildlife Ecology
Department of Integrative Biology and Evolution
University of Veterinary Medicine Vienna
Vienna, Austria
Update on Remote Delivery and Restraint Equipment

Jennifer E. Graham, DVM, DABVP (Avian/Exotic Companion Mammal), DACZM
Assistant Professor of Zoological Companion Animal Medicine
Department of Clinical Sciences
Tufts Cummings School of Veterinary Medicine
North Grafton, Massachusetts
Lagomorpha (Pikas, Rabbits, and Hares)

Zoltan S. Gyimesi, DVM
Associate Veterinarian
Louisville Zoological Garden
Louisville, Kentucky
Columbiformes

J. Jill Heatley, DVM, MS
Associate Professor
Veterinary Small Animal Clinical Sciences
Department of College of Veterinary Medicine and Biomedical Sciences
Texas A&M University
College Station, Texas
Psittaciformes

Timothy A. Herman, BSc, MSc
Herpetologist
Department of Herpetology
Toledo Zoological Society
Toledo, Ohio
Caudata (Urodela): Tailed Amphibians

Sonia Hernandez, BA, DVM, PhD, DACVIM
Assistant Professor
Graduate and Externship Coordinator
College of Veterinary Medicine
The University of Georgia
Athens, Georgia
Tapiridae

Thomas Bernd Hildebrandt, DrMedVet, HonFRCVS, DECZM (Zoo Health Management)
Professorial Fellow
Zoology
University of Melbourne
Melbourne, Victoria, Australia
Head, Professor
Reproduction Management
Leibniz Institute for Zoo and Wildlife Research
Berlin, Germany
Use of Ultrasonography in Wildlife Species

†Deceased.

Clayton D. Hilton, MS, DVM
Vice-President of Animal Care &
 Conservation
Birmingham Zoo, Inc.
Birmingham, Alabama
Canidae

Peter Holz, BVSc, DVSc, MACVSc,
 DACZM
Veterinarian
Tidbinbilla Nature Reserve
Tharwa, A.C.T., Australia
Monotremata (Echidna, Platypus)

Richard M. Jakob-Hoff, BVMS (Hons),
 MANZCVS (Wildlife Medicine)
Senior Veterinarian, Conservation and
 Research
New Zealand Centre for Conservation
 Medicine
Auckland Zoo
Auckland, New Zealand
Sphenodontia: The Biology and Veterinary
 Care of Tuatara

Donald L. Janssen, DVM, DACZM
Corporate Director, Animal Health
San Diego Zoo Global
San Diego, California
Equidae
Guidelines for the Management of Zoonotic
 Diseases

Janis Ott Joslin, BA, DVM
Professor, Zoo and Wildlife Medicine
College of Veterinary Medicine
Western University of Health Sciences
Pomona, California
New World and Old World Monkeys

Jacques Kaandorp
Safaripark Beekse Bergen
Hilvarenbeek, The Netherlands
The EAZWV and AAZV Infectious Diseases
 Notebooks

Cornelia J. Ketz-Riley, DrMedVet, DVM,
 DACZM
Clinical Assistant Professor, Service Head
Avian, Exotic, and Zoo Medicine Service
Department of Clinical Sciences
Center for Veterinary Health Sciences
Stillwater, Oklahoma
Trochiliformes (Hummingbirds)

George V. Kollias, DVM, PhD
J. Hyman Professor of Wildlife Medicine
Section of Zoological Medicine
Department of Clinical Sciences
College of Veterinary Medicine
Cornell University
Ithaca, New York
Mustelidae

Maya S. Kummrow, DrMedVet, DVSc,
 FTA Wildtiere (ZB Zootiere),
 DACZM, DECZM (Zoo Health
 Management)
Head of Veterinary Service, Vice Zoological
 Director
Zoo Wuppertal
Wuppertal, North Rhine-Westfalia,
 Germany
Ratites or Struthioniformes: Struthiones,
 Rheae, Cassuarii, Apteryges (Ostriches,
 Rheas, Emus, Cassowaries, and Kiwis),
 and Tinamiformes (Tinamous)

Claude Lacasse, DVM, MANZCVS
 (Wildlife Medicine)
Veterinary Services Manager
Australia Zoo Wildlife Hospital
Beerwah, Queensland, Australia
Falconiformes (Falcons, Hawks, Eagles, Kites,
 Harriers, Buzzards, Ospreys, Caracaras,
 Secretary Birds, and Old World and New
 World Vultures)

Nadine Lamberski, DVM, DACZM
Associate Director
Veterinary Services
San Diego Zoo Safari Park
Escondido, California
Felidae

Alex Lecu, DVM
Paris Zoo
Paris, France
Recent Updates for Antemortem Tuberculosis
 Diagnostics in Zoo Animals

Brad A. Lock, DVM, DACZM
Curator
Herpetology
Zoo Atlanta
Atlanta, Georgia
Ophidia (Snakes)

Linda J. Lowenstine, DVM, PhD,
 DACVP
Professor Emeritus
Department of Pathology, Immunology and
 Microbiology
School of Veterinary Medicine, University
 of California, Davis
Davis, California
Update on Iron Overload in Zoologic Species

Robert A. MacLean, BA, DVM
Senior Veterinarian
Audubon Nature Institute
New Orleans, Louisiana
Adjunct Professor
Louisiana State University School of
 Veterinary Medicine
Baton Rouge, Louisiana
Gruiformes (Cranes, Limpkins, Rails,
 Gallinules, Coots, Bustards)

Mariano Makara, Dr.med.vet. DECVDI
Faculty of Veterinary Science
The University of Sydney
Sydney, Australia
The Use of Computed Tomography and
 Magnetic Resonance Imaging in Zoo
 Animals

Nicholas J. Masters, MA, VetMB,
 MRCVS
Head of Veterinary Services
Veterinary Department
Zoological Society of London
London, United Kingdom
Tragulidae, Moschidae, and Cervidae

Stephanie McCain, DVM, DACZM
Veterinarian
Birmingham Zoo
Birmingham, Alabama
Charadriiformes

Tracey McNamara, DVM, DACVP
Professor of Pathology
College of Veterinary Medicine
Western University of Health Sciences
Pomona, California
Updates on West Nile Virus

Thomas P. Meehan, DVM
Adjunct Assistant Professor
Department of Veterinary Clinical
 Medicine
College of Veterinary Medicine
University of Illinois
Urbana, Illinois;
Vice President of Veterinary Services
Chicago Zoological Society
Brookfield, Illinois
AAZV Guidelines for Zoo and Aquarium
 Veterinary Medical Programs and
 Veterinary Hospitals

Leith C.R. Meyer, BSc (Hon), BVSc,
 PhD
Paraclinical Science
University of Pretoria, Faculty of
 Veterinary Science, Onderstepoort
Pretoria, Gauteng, South Africa
Tubulidentata (Aardvark)

David S. Miller, DVM, PhD, DACZM
Miller Veterinary Services
Loveland, Colorado
A Legal Overview for Zoological Medicine
 Veterinarians

Michele A. Miller, DVM, MS, PhD, MPH
Conservation Veterinarian
Faculty of Medicine and Health Sciences
Rare Species Conservatory Foundation
Loxahatchee, Florida
Affiliate Professor
Department of Clinical Sciences
Colorado State University College of
 Veterinary Medicine
Fort Collins, Colorado
Rhinoceridae (Rhinoceroses)

R. Eric Miller, DVM, DACZM
Senior Vice President for Zoological Operations
Director, WildCare Institute
Saint Louis Zoo
Forest Park
St. Louis, Missouri;
Adjunct Associate Professor of Veterinary
    Medicine and Surgery
College of Veterinary Medicine
University of Missouri
Columbia, Missouri
*The Journal of Zoo and Wildlife Medicine
    (JZWM)*

Teresa Y. Morishita, DVM, PhD, DACPV
Associate Dean for Academic Affairs
Professor of Poultry Medicine and Food
    Safety
College of Veterinary Medicine
Western University of Health Sciences
Pomona, California
Galliformes

Haylee Westin Murphy, DVM
Director of Veterinary Services
Veterinary Services
Zoo Atlanta
Atlanta, Georgia
Great Apes

**Natalie D. Mylniczenko, MS, DVM,
    DACZM**
Staff Veterinarian
Disney's Animals, Science & Environment
Walt Disney World
Lake Buena Vista, Florida
Caecilians

Julia E. Napier, DVM
Senior Veterinarian
Zoo Hospital
Omaha's Henry Doorly Zoo & Aquarium
Omaha, Nebraska
Hyrocoidea (Hyraxes)

Donald L. Neiffer, VMD, DACZM
Veterinary Operations Manager
Disney's Animal Programs
Department of Animal Health
Orlando, Florida
Trogoniformes

Terry M. Norton, DVM, DACZM
Director and Veterinarian
Georgia Sea Turtle Center
Jekyll Island, Georgia
Wildlife Veterinarian
St. Catherine's Island Foundation
Midway, Georgia
Ciconiiformes (Herons, Ibises, Spoonbills, Storks)

Luis R. Padilla, DVM, DACZM
Staff Veterinarian
Department of Animal Health
St. Louis Zoo
St. Louis, Missouri
*Gaviiformes, Podicipediformes, and
    Procellariiformes (Loons, Grebes,
    Petrels, and Albatrosses)*
Canidae

**Romain Pizzi, BVSc, MSc, DZooMed,
    MACVSc (Surg) FRES, FRGS,
    MRCVS**
Royal College of Veterinary Surgeons
    Recognized Specialist in Zoo & Wildlife
    Medicine
Special Lecturer in Zoo & Wildlife
    Medicine
School of Veterinary Medicine and Science
University of Nottingham
Sutton Bonington, Leicestershire, United
    Kingdom;
Veterinary Surgeon
Royal Zoological Society of Scotland
Edinburgh Zoo
Edinburgh, Scotland;
Head of the Veterinary Service
Scottish SPCA National Wildlife Rescue
    Centre
Fishcross, Clackmannanshire, Scotland;
Chairman of the Board of Trustees
Wildlife Surgery International
United Kingdom
Minimally Invasive Surgery Techniques

Julia B. Ponder, DVM
Executive Director
The Raptor Center
College of Veterinary Medicine
University of Minnesota
St. Paul, Minnesota
Strigiformes

Edward Ramsay, DVM, DACZM
Professor
Department of Small Animal Clinical
    Sciences
University of Tennessee
Knoxville, Tennessee
Procyonids and Viverids

**Sharon Redrobe, BSc (Hons), BVetMed,
    CertLAS, DZooMed, MRCVS**
Royal College of Veterinary Surgeons
Recognized Specialist in Zoological
    Medicine
Honorary Associate Professor of Zoo, Wild
    and Exotic Animal Medicine
Honorary Associate Professor
School of Veterinary Medicine and Science
University of Nottingham
Nottingham, United Kingdom
Zoological Director
Life Sciences
Twycross Zoo
Atherstone, Warwickshire, United
    Kingdom
*Pelecaniformes (Pelicans, Tropicbirds,
    Cormorants, Frigatebirds, Anhingas,
    Gannets)*

Carlos R. Sanchez, DVM, MSc
Zoo Veterinarian
Chicago, Illinois
Trochiliformes (Hummingbirds)
Apodiformes and Coliiformes

Joseph Saragusty, DVM, PhD
Scientist
Department of Reproduction Management
Leibniz Institute for Zoo and wildlife
    Research
Berlin, Germany
Use of Ultrasonography in Wildlife Species

Joseph A. Smith, DVM
Director of Animal Health
Fort Wayne Children's Zoo,
Fort Wayne, Indiana
Passeriformes (Songbirds, Perching Birds)

Gabrielle Stalder, DVM, DrMedVet
Research Institute of Wildlife Ecology
Department of Integrative Biology and
    Evolution
University of Veterinary Medicine
Vienna, Austria
Hippopotamidae (Hippopotamus)

Iga M. Stasiak, DVM, DVSc
Pathobiology
Ontario Veterinary College, University of
    Guelph
Guelph, Ontario, Canada
Wildlife Health Center
Toronto Zoo
Scarborough, Ontario, Canada
Update on Iron Overload in Zoologic Species

**Hanspeter W. Steinmetz, DrMedVet,
    MSc, DACZM**
Director of Animal Care and Science
Knies Kinderzoo
Gebr Knie, Schweizer-National-Circus AG
Rapperswil, Switzerland
*The Use of Computed Tomography and
    Magnetic Resonance Imaging in Zoo
    Animals*

William Kirk Suedmeyer, DVM, DACZM
Director
Animal Health
Kansas City Zoo
Kansas City, Missouri
Adjunct Assistant Professor
Zoological Medicine
College of Veterinary Medicine
University of Missouri-Columbia
Columbia, Missouri
Hyaenidae

Mariella Superina, DrMedVet, PhD
Assistant Researcher
Instituto de Medicina y Biología
    Experimental de Cuyo (IMBECU)
CCT CONICET Mendoza
Mendoza, Argentina
Xenarthra

Meg Sutherland-Smith, DVM, DACZM
Associate Director
Veterinary Services
San Diego Zoo
San Diego, California
Suidae and Tayassuidae (Wild Pigs, Peccaries)

John M. Sykes IV, DVM, DACZM
Associate Veterinarian
Zoological Health
Wildlife Conservation Society
Bronx, New York
Piciformes (Honeyguides, Barbets, Woodpeckers, Toucans)

J. Andrew Teare, MSc, DVM
International Species Information System
Eagan, Minnesota
ISIS, MedARKS, ZIMS, and Global Sharing of Medical Information by Zoologic Institutions

Maryanne E. Tocidlowski, DVM, DACZM
Associate Veterinarian
Veterinary Services
Houston Zoo, Inc.
Houston, Texas
Musophagiformes

Eric Hsienshao Tsao, PhD
Associate Researcher
Taipei Zoo,
Taipei, Taiwan
Pholidota

William George Van Bonn, DVM
Adjunct Clinical Assistant Professor
Clinical Medicine
College of Veterinary Medicine
University of Illinois
Urbana-Champaign, Illinois
Research Associate
Wildlife Health Center
University of California, Davis
Davis, California
Vice President for Animal Health
Animal Health
John G. Shedd Aquarium
Chicago, Illinois
Pinnipedia

Larry Vogelnest, BVSc, MVS, MACVSc, PSM
Senior Veterinarian
Taronga Wildlife Hospital
Taronga Zoo
Taronga Conservation Society Australia
Sydney, New South Wales, Australia
Marsupialia (Marsupials)

Roberta S. Wallace, DVM
Adjunct Assistant Professor
Department of Surgical Sciences
School of Veterinary Medicine
University of Wisconsin
Madison, Wisconsin
Senior Staff Veterinarian
Milwaukee County Zoo
Milwaukee, Wisconsin
Sphenisciformes (Penguins)

Michael T. Walsh, DVM
Co-director Aquatic Animal Health Program, Clinical Associate Professor
Large Animal Clinical Sciences
College of Veterinary Medicine
University of Florida
Gainesville, Florida
Sirenia

Chris Walzer, DrMedVet, DECZM (Wildl. Pop. Health)
Professor
Chair Conservation Medicine
FIWI - Research Institute of Wildlife Ecology
University of Veterinary Medicine
Vienna, Austria
Hippopotamidae (Hippopotamus)
Update on Remote Delivery and Restraint Equipment

Martha A. Weber, DVM, DACZM
Staff Veterinarian
St. Louis, Missouri
Sheep, Goats, and Goat-Like Animals

Jim Wellehan, DVM, PhD, DACZM, DACVM (Virology, Bacteriology/ Mycology)
Assistant Professor
College of Veterinary Medicine
University of Florida
Gainesville, Florida
Ophidia (Snakes)

Christian J. Wenker, DrMedVet
Zoo Veterinarian
Zoo Basel
Basel, Switzerland
Phoenicopteriformes

Douglas P. Whiteside, DVM, DVSc, DACZM
Clinical Associate Professor
Department of Ecosystem and Public Health
University of Calgary Faculty of Veterinary Medicine
Calgary, Alberta, Canada
Senior Staff Veterinarian
Calgary Zoo Animal Health Centre
Calgary, Alberta, Canada
Ciconiiformes (Herons, Ibises, Spoonbills, Storks)
Cuculiformes (Cuckoos, Roadrunners)

Ellen Wiedner, VMD, DACVIM (Large Animal)
Clinical Assistant Professor
Zoo and Wildlife Medicine
College of Veterinary Medicine
University of Florida
Gainesville, Florida
Proboscidea

Michelle M. Willette, BS, DVM
Staff Veterinarian
The Raptor Center
College of Veterinary Medicine
University of Minnesota
St. Paul, Minnesota
Strigiformes

Cathy V. Williams, DVM
Senior Veterinarian
Duke Lemur Center
Duke University
Durham, North Carolina
Adjunct Assistant Professor of Zoological Medicine
Department of Clinical Sciences
College of Veterinary Medicine
North Carolina State University
Raleigh, North Carolina
Prosimians

Barbara A. Wolfe, DVM, PhD, DACZM
Associate Professor-Clinical
Veterinary Preventive Medicine
Ohio State University
Columbus, Ohio
Chief Science Officer
Columbus Zoo and Aquarium and the Wilds
Columbus, Ohio
Bovidae (Except Sheep and Goats) and Antilocapridae

Fabia S. Wyss, DrMedVet
Assistant Veterinarian
Clinic for Zoo Animals, Exotic Pets and Wildlife
University of Zurich
Zurich, Switzerland
Phoenicopteriformes

Enrique Yarto-Jaramillo, DVM, MSc
Exotic Pets and Zoo Animal Clinician
Centro Veterinario México
Mexico City, Mexico
Adjunct Veterinarian
Clinical Department
ZooLeón, Zoológico de Morelia & Zoológico de Culiacán
Mexico City, Mexico
President
Instituto Mexicano de Fauna Silvestre y Animales de Compañía (IMFAC, SC)
Mexico City, Mexico
Rodentia

Dawn M. Zimmerman, DVM, MS
Regional Veterinary Manager
Mountain Gorilla Veterinary Project
Musanze, Rwanda
Tapiridae

Preface

The first two editions of *Zoo and Wild Animal Medicine* (ZAWAM) covered the world's animal groups in a comprehensive fashion, as did the 5th edition published in 2003. The 3rd, 4th, 6th, and 7th editions reflected a Current Veterinary Therapy format focusing on specific topics of current interest. This edition returns to the overall taxa format and it is hoped that it will provide an updated reference for zoo and wildlife veterinarians around the world. It has been designed to offer a timely format with guidance to where more detailed information can be found.

To ensure a "fresh" approach to this edition, each Senior Author has been changed from the ZAWAM 5. Many of the authors were chosen in their roles as Veterinary Advisors to the taxa that they review as it was felt that this provided a central overview to problems of that animal group. In some cases, authors generously donated their time to research species which are rarely held in captivity or studied in the wild.

The problems of zoo animals and wildlife are worldwide, and as before, this edition reflects a diverse, international authorship. Senior authors represent 15 countries: Austria, Australia, Brazil, Canada, Denmark, France, Germany, Mexico, New Zealand, South Africa, Switzerland, Taiwan, The Netherlands, The United Kingdom, and the United States of America.

ACKNOWLEDGMENTS

As with previous issues, the authors freely shared their information and time for the benefit of the wild animals and the people who care for them. Therefore, our special thanks to those authors who contributed to this edition of *Zoo and Wild Animal Medicine*, as all of the royalties support wild animal health research, with none going to the authors or editors.

One Editor (REM) would like to thank the Saint Louis Zoo for its support throughout this process, and his administrative assistant, Amy Brauss, who carefully helped keep that Editor and the process on track. We also thank the production staff at Elsevier who blended the styles of so many authors into one cohesive text. Last, but certainly not least, our heartfelt thanks goes out to our wives, Mary Jean and Audrey, who supported us in many ways during our months of editing.

Contents

†Deceased.

CHAPTER 1

Anurans

Norin Chai

BIOLOGY

More than 6200 species of anurans have been currently recorded,[1] and these live on all continents except Antarctica. Although the larvae are aquatic, anurans have successfully expanded their habitats into numerous and markedly different ecologic types, in the Arctic Circle, in deserts, in tropical rain forests, and practically everywhere in between. Actually, 54 families are proposed; however, anuran taxonomy is still a matter of dispute. Table 1-1 lists some relevant families. The goliath frog (*Conraua goliath*), the largest anuran, is able to grow up to 33 cm and weigh up to 3 kg. The smallest known frog is *Paedophryne amauensis* (Microhylidae); with its 7.7 mm length, it is also the world's smallest known vertebrate. In captivity, average life spans are typically 4 to 15 years. The goliath frog may live up to 21 years in captivity.

In a strict sense, the term "toads" represent frogs belonging to the family Bufonidae. In a larger sense, "toad" is used for any terrestrial frog having "warty"—dry skin and parotid glands—voluminous glandular masses behind the eyes. Other frogs have smooth, moist skin without warts and (most of the time) lack parotid glands. The terms "frog" and "toad" are not clear. For instance, the European Fire-bellied Toad (*Bombina bombina*) is a warty, semi-aquatic "toad" with no parotids behind the eyes.

Anurans are the best represented in zoos, compared with other amphibians. Some, such as *Xenopus laevis* and *Silurana tropicalis*, have been model species for research for many years. With the Amphibian Crisis, publicized by the EAZA in 2008 with the "Year of Amphibians," wild anurans are now the focus of major global ecologic concerns, including pollution, climate changes, habitat destruction, and nonnative species translocation. Campaigns all around the world (for example, the Amphibian ARK) of awareness and information on amphibians, have led to a huge amount of information available online on the husbandry of many anuran species. Consequently, veterinarians are consulted more frequently for information on health and disease.

ANATOMY AND PHYSIOLOGY

All adult anurans are without a tail (the "tail" of tailed frogs [*Ascaphus* sp.] is, in fact, an extension of the male cloacae, used as a copulatory organ). Highly specialized in the hopping mode of locomotion, their long hind legs have given rise to their alternative name *salientias* (jumpers). However, considerable specialization exists in this regard. Some arboreal frogs may move by quadrapedal walking or climbing. Burrowing frogs dig head first with hind legs adapted for excavation. Eyes are voluminous; vision plays a great role in nutritional behavior. Prey movement triggers the feeding response. A nictitating membrane is present. Posterior to each eye, the circular tympanic membrane represents the ear externally. A large tongue is attached anteriorly and is folded back into the oral cavity such that its distal, bifid end lies posteriorly. The tongue is extended to catch insects. A single row of small teeth lies around the margin of the upper jaw.

The coelomic cavity is not divided. The intestinal tract is relatively short and follows the normal vertebrate plan. The liver serves as an important erythropoietic center and plays an important role in immune function, the synthesis of nitrogenous compounds, antioxidation reactions, and the metabolism of various endogenous and exogenous substances. The gall bladder is intimately associated with the liver, with a bile duct connecting it to the duodenum. In some species, it joins the pancreatic duct before it enters the intestinal tract. The cloaca is present posteriorly. However, due to the absence of a tail, it appears to be located somewhat dorsally.

Anurans are ectothermic and environmental temperature may really modulate their life history, influencing body temperature, evaporative water loss, digestion, and oxygen uptake, as well as the velocity of muscle contraction, locomotion, and vocalization. Anurans will compensate daily thermal fluctuation by modifying their behavior and metabolic changes, for instance, by oriented aerobic depression of several organs.[9] Therefore, it is important to keep the animals within the preferred optimal temperature zone (POTZ). Some species (mostly temperate) hibernate and estivate. Anurans that hibernate in colder climatic conditions accumulate more energy before winter and even after emerging and before breeding. Fats are the preferred substrates of aerobic metabolism if oxygen is not limiting, and are the main source of at least 80% of the energy used during hibernation.[9] The skin not only has a protective and sensory capacities but also plays critical roles in thermoregulation, fluid balance, respiration, transport of essential ions, respiration, and sex recognition.

The cutaneous gland (in the dermis) secretions may be irritating, toxic, and even potentially lethal, like the steroid alkaloid toxins of the poison frogs (*Dendrobates* and *Phyllobates*). One of the natural defenses of the skin is production of antimicrobial peptides in granular glands.[14] Discharge of the granular glands is initiated by the stimulation of sympathetic nerves. Antimicrobial peptides produced in the skin are an important defense against skin pathogens and may affect survival of populations. The skin has low resistance for water evaporation, and most anurans are vulnerable to rapid water loss. In terrestrial species, mucous or waxy substances are produced by a variety of glands to reduce evaporative water loss. All anurans may absorb water through the ventral pelvic skin and also reabsorb water in the kidney and from the urinary bladder.

Amphibian lymph consists of all the components of blood, with the exception of erythrocytes. In anurans, the lymphatic system is highly developed and has a major role in fluid exchange and blood volume regulation. It is composed of pulsatile lymph hearts (that beat independently of the heart), an elaborate series of lymph vessels, and subcutaneous lymph sacs. Lymph flow is unidirectional; one-way valves are present between the sacs. Lymph heart failure should be in the differentials for subcutaneous and coelomic cavitary accumulations of fluid.

In anurans, the primary nitrogenous waste may be ammonia, urea, or uric acid. Aquatic species excrete a higher concentration of ammonia, whereas many terrestrial anurans have evolved metabolic adaptations to excrete urea and even uric acid. Dehydrated animals will decrease their glomerular filtration rate, thereby accumulating ammonia in body tissues, which may lead to azotemia. Anurans seem to be quite resistant to high plasma urea levels. Urea is less toxic than ammonia and may be stored in body tissues until water may

TABLE 1-1

Selected Families of Anurans

Family	Number of Species, Representative Species	Geographic Location and Comments
Bombinatoridae	10 species Bombina frogs (*Bombina* sp.)	Eurasia Specialized glands in their skin secrete a toxin, which may cause irritation; often display the unken reflex when disturbed
Pipidae	33 species Clawed frogs (*Xenopus* sp., *Silurana* sp.) Surinam toads (*Pipa* sp.)	South America (genus *Pipa*) and sub-Saharan Africa (four other genera) Tongueless frogs, lack vocal cords, exclusively aquatic, and often found in animal facilities
Hemiphractidae	100 species Marsupial frogs (*Gastrotheca* sp., *Flectonotus* sp.)	Central and South Americas Marsupial female frogs possess a dorsal pouch, where fertilized eggs are kept; *Gastrotheca riobambae* is well represented in zoos
Bufonidae	571 species True toads (*Bufo* sp.) Common toad (*Bufo bufo*)	Widespread on every continent except Australia and Antarctica Terrestrial, toothless, dry warty skin, a pair of parotid glands; all males have the Bidder organ (potentially active ovary)
Dendrobatidae	177 species Poison dart frogs (*Dendrobates* sp., *Phyllobates* sp.)	Nicaragua to the Amazon Basin of Bolivia and to southeastern Brazil Small, very colorful frogs, famous for their toxic skin production; very popular with hobbyists and zoos; *Phyllobates terribilis* secrete one of the most dangerous venoms in the world
Hylidae	926 species Known as "tree frogs" (*Hyla* sp., *Litoria* sp., *Phyllomedusa* sp., *Agalychnis* sp.), even though some hylids are terrestrial or semi-aquatic	America, Eurasia to Australo-Papuan region; extreme northern Africa Most are arboreal and have forward-facing eyes and have adhesive pads at the extremity of each finger; monkey frogs (*Phyllomedusa bicolor*) have parotid glands and were the origin of the prototypical antimicrobial peptide family, the dermaseptins; white tree frog (*Litoria caerulea*) is a very popular pet frog
Ranidae "True frogs"	355 species Common frog (*Rana* sp.)	Worldwide except Antarctica Ranids species are commonly pet frogs; many wild populations are subjects of research work; also used in research facilities
Leptodactylidae	189 species Argentine horned frog (*Ceratophrys ornata*), Smokey Jungle frog (*Leptodactylus pentadactylus*)	Southern United States, Mexico, northern Antilles, south to Brazil Argentine horned frog, also called "Pacman frogs," and Smokey Jungle Frog are very popular pets
Microhylidae	519 species Tomato frogs (*Dyscophus* sp.)	North and South America, sub-Saharan Africa, India to northern Australia Very colorful species of frogs; popular pets; Madagascar tomato frog (*D. antongilii*) endangered as a result of deforestation and overcollecting for the pet trade

be replenished. However, the limit after which toxic effects appear is not clear. Still, urea will be excreted rapidly on rehydration.

Larval stages maintain gills for respiration, whereas adults primarily respire via the lungs and the buccopharyngeal cavity. In addition, all anurans show some degree of cutaneous oxygen respiration.[12]

The heart has three chambers, with two atria and one ventricle. All anurans show a complete interatrial septum, limiting the mixing of oxygenated and unoxygenated blood that still occurs in the single ventricle. The heart is seen contracting on the midline just caudal to the animal's shoulders. A renal portal venous blood system exists.

SPECIAL HOUSING REQUIREMENTS

Housing requirements for anurans will definitively depend on their specific needs and their natural habitat. However, several key points should always be monitored. Providing an appropriate temperature gradient and a mosaic of thermal zones allows these animals to self-regulate their body temperature (heat lamps may desiccate the animals and should be avoided). Unlike reptiles, most sick amphibians recuperate better in a cooler rather than a warmer environment. Anurans that are kept above or below their POTZ may show signs of inappetence, weight loss, agitation changes in skin color, immunosuppression, and bacterial overgrowth.

Monitoring hygrometry prevents evaporative water loss. Tadpoles and aquatic species need dechlorinated water. Water quality parameters (ammonia, pH, and chlorine) should be routinely evaluated with home aquarium test kits. Poor water circulations, overcrowding, or both commonly lead to water quality problems. Waste material and uneaten foods should be removed. Dilute chlorine bleach is a simple and good general disinfectant. Review of husbandry and zoological records is part of the diagnostic process. Most diseases come from a lack of understanding of specific management requirements.

FEEDING

In general, natural feeding is opportunistic. Although most tadpoles are herbivorous or omnivorous, all adult anurans are carnivorous, consuming a wide variety of live invertebrates and also mice, rat pups, fish, or any small vertebrates for the large ones. Terrestrial anurans only target moving prey. Many aquatic amphibians are more likely to target food by scent and may consume inert food. Most anurans are voracious feeders and tend to eat anything that fits into their mouth. Gastric overload and impaction, as well as ingestion of non-food items are fairly common.

Frequency of feeding depends on the primary energy and nutritional requirements of the species, their seasonal activity, and breeding cycle. For energetic species such as *Dendrobates* sp., insects should remain in the enclosure between feedings so that the animals are fed *ad libitum*. In this case, having an insect farm is essential. In more sedentary species, which are prone to obesity, feeding rates should be adjusted accordingly. For instance, an adult *Ceratophrys* sp. is fed every 10 to 15 days (with various insects, neonatal or suckling mice, and dead adult mice [to prevent bites]). Digestion, assimilation, and metabolic rates generally increase with increased temperature, and feeding increases to a peak and then declines as temperatures become too high.

Amphibians cannot synthesize carotinoids, including vitamin A.[23] Nutritional disorders caused by unbalanced vitamin A supplementation have been observed.[15,23] Analysis of longstanding husbandry practices showed that ultraviolet B (UVB) exposure and dietary calcium-to-phosphorus ratio were deficient compared with wild conditions—likely causing chronic underlying metabolic bone disease.[2,21]

The key point for feeding anurans in captivity is to provide few invertebrates of different species and of different sizes. In our zoo, we have our own insect and rodent farms: grasshoppers, crickets, locusts, mealworms, and mice. In our opinion, it would be hazardous to supplement the diet of the frogs and toads directly. It is better to prevent single-item food sources and give a balanced diet to the prey. A huge amount on feeding information of many species may be found in the hobbyist and professional literature.[23]

RESTRAINT, ANESTHESIA, AND ANALGESIA

Most anurans are docile; however, large ones may bite. Once a *Ceratophrys* sp. has bitten, it never opens the mouth (to prevent the prey from escaping!). Smooth nets, plastic bags, or gloves may be used for moving animals. Wrapping with wet paper towel is a good technique to restrain an animal for a quick examination or for medication administration. Wearing moistened, powder-free gloves prevents the transfer of microorganisms from the hands of the clinician and also provides protection against secreted toxins. In all cases, manual restraint is used for short and nonpainful procedures. For a longer clinical examination, it is better to place the animal in a transparent container only used for this purpose.

General anesthesia may be required for biopsies, blood sampling, and surgical procedures such as gastrotomy and laparoscopic or exploratory surgery. Surgery and other invasive procedures are often perceived as painful. Thus, anurans should always be given analgesic drugs. Analgesia potentiates the effects of anesthetic drugs and reduces recovery time.[10] We have been using meloxicam empirically for several years at a dosage of 0.2 milligrams per kilogram (mg/kg). A recent study recommends systemic administration of meloxicam at a dosage of 0.1 mg/kg once daily.[17] In general, anurans do not require fasting prior to anesthesia. Their larynx remains tightly closed even under general anesthesia, and the chance of aspiration is very low. However, it is better not to feed large frogs and toads 24 to 48 hours before anesthesia. The righting reflex is used as a primary indicator to determine the stage of anesthesia. Loss of this reflex suggests a light stage of anesthesia. A surgical plane is indicated by the loss of the withdrawal reflex. Anesthetized amphibians usually become apneic; abdominal and gular respirations may cease. Heart rate is a useful tool for anesthesia monitoring. Putting the frog in dorsal recumbency may help perform direct visualization. In our opinion, electrocardiography (ECG) leads are traumatic, and the use of alcohol may be deleterious. The drug of choice for sedation or anesthesia is tricaine methanesulfonate (MS-222), which has also demonstrated analgesic potential (Figure 1-1). Table 1-2 presents only those protocols that have been used and evaluated by us. More protocols may be found elsewhere.[6] Aquatic animals should have their head out of water during recovery.

SURGERY

Amphibians are generally good candidates for surgery. They are quite resistant to blood loss. Biopsies and skin surgery follow the same techniques used in other vertebrates. For biopsies, only a small surface of the skin may be taken, as it is not very extensible. When the surgery is too extensive (neoplasia or abscess), we may perform chemical cauterization with metacresolsulfonic acid and formaldehyde 36% (Lotagen TM, Schering-Plough Animal Health). Lotagen has an astringent action on healthy mucous membrane and promotes granulation and epithelialization. We frequently use these compounds with good results. Coelomic exploratory and gastrointestinal surgeries are common procedures.

TABLE 1-2

Protocols for Anesthesia and Analgesia in Anurans

Drug	Dosage and Route	Comments
Tricaine methanesulfonate (MS-222)	Tadpoles and aquatic frogs 0.25 to 0.5 g/L (Bath) Adult frogs and toads 1 g/L (Bath) (see Figure 1-1)	Buffer 2 g of MS-222 with 40 mL of Na_2HPO_4 (0.5 mL/L). Induction times are variable. After induction, place the frog into a shallow amount of nonanesthetic water or on a wet towel. Recovery is generally achieved 30 to 90 minutes after the anesthetic is removed.
Isoflurane	5% in oxygen (inhalation or bubbling in bath) (see Figure 1-1)	Gentle stimulation encourages continued respiration. Effective but slow induction.
	2 to 3 mL/L (Bath)	Isoflurane is sprayed directly into the water.
	0.01 to 0.06 mL/g (topical)	Apply directly OR dilute 3 mL of liquid isoflurane in 1.5 mL of water, and 3.5 mL of K-Y Jelly. Shake until a uniform gel. This gel is applied at dosages of 0.025 to 0.035 mL/g.
Lidocaine / Prilocaine	0.5 mL /150 g (topical)	Short induction for 30 minutes of surgical plane.
Medetomidin (M) / Ketamin (K) / Meloxicam (Mel) / Butorphanol (But)	M 0.5 mg/kg + K 50 mg/kg + Mel 0.2 mg/kg + But 25 mg/kg (IM)	Effective protocol in *Xenopus laevis* for heart surgery (n = 12, unpublished data). Reversed with atipamezole hydrochloride at equal volume to medetomidine IM.
Butorphanol	25 mg/kg (IM)	Unpublished data.
Meloxicam	0.1 to 0.2 mg/kg (IM or ICe)	

g/L, Gram per liter; *IM*, intramuscular; *mg/kg*, milligram per kilogram; *mL/g*, milliliter per gram; *mL/L*, milliliter per liter.

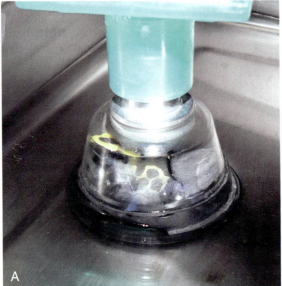

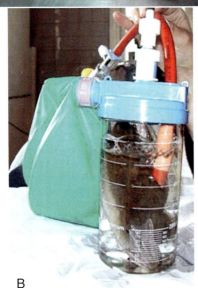

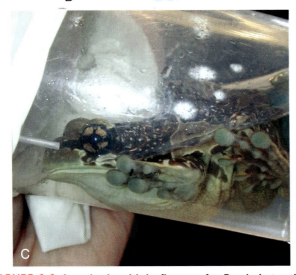

FIGURE 1-1 **Anesthesia with isoflurane of a *Dendrobates tinctorius*. A,** Hygrometry must be maintained high to prevent desiccation. **B,** Isoflurane bubbling in bath with a *Xenopus laevis*. **C,** Bath with MS222 of a *Trachycephalus resinifictrix*. (Courtesy of Norin Chai.)

Presurgical preparations include hydration of the animal in a shallow water bath and prophylactic antimicrobial therapy (either by bath or injection). Preparation of the skin is accomplished by gently tapping the skin with cotton-tipped applicators and povidone-iodine solution diluted with sterile saline ($\frac{1}{10}$). Incisions should be made with one bold, clean stroke. When performing a laparotomy, the surgeon must take care of macroscopic glands, lymph hearts, and blood vessels, especially the midventral vein. The abdominal membrane is punctured and dissected smoothly. Everting-type suture patterns, with simple interrupted sutures using nonabsorbable material, are recommended for skin closure (Figure 1-2). Surgical tissue glues may also be used in conjunction with sutures for skin closure. Insufflation is needed in laparoscopy to improve the visibility of all organs. Management of cloacal prolapse sometimes requires surgery (Table 1-3). Veterinarians are sometime asked to surgically withdraw eggs for research purposes (Figure 1-3). Postoperative infections are rare in healthy animals.[24]

CLINICAL TECHNIQUES

Clinical signs are generally nonpathognomonic. Thorough physical examination (evaluation of locomotion, responsiveness to stimulation and novel environmental factors, behavior, respiratory rate, body condition, hydration status, abdominal palpation, etc.) should be followed by several clinical tests. Magnification and a good light source may be extremely helpful for close examination, especially in ophthalmology (Figure 1-4). In dermatology, skin scraping and smears (which are less traumatic) are easy and useful clinical techniques. Use of Wright-Giemsa or acid-fast staining provides cellular definition. With bloating, aspiration and analysis of fluid (e.g., total protein, cell count, and cytologic examination) should be performed in most cases and will help exclude some infectious causes of effusion such as bacterial septicemia (Figure 1-5). Fluid samples with low total protein and low cell counts and samples that lack cytologic evidence of an infectious agent are more likely to be associated with organ dysfunction or physiologic and environmental factors. Fresh feces should be collected for fecal examination and culture. In anorexic animals, force-feeding may be necessary before obtaining a fecal sample.

In ectotherms, about 50% of the blood may be removed at one time. The smallest frog from which 0.2 milliliter (mL) may be sampled weighs 4 grams (g) and that from which 0.5 mL whole blood may be removed weighs 10 g. The blood volume of a *Xenopus laevis* is 13.4% of the body weight. However, we generally consider a frog's blood volume to be 10%. Ten percent may be withdrawn safely from healthy frogs and 5% from ill frogs. In large specimens, blood sampling may be done from the ventral vein. In our experience, cardiocentesis is the easiest method to use in the majority of amphibians (Figure 1-5). An appropriately sized needle (generally 25- to 27-gauge) is inserted into the apex, and blood is taken from the ventricle. The aspiration is slow with a heparinized syringe.

It is wise to make only two attempts. Lithium heparin is the preferred anticoagulant, because EDTA lyses the red blood cells. Individual species exhibit dramatic hematologic variations, depending on the sex, local environment, season, and metamorphic state. Interpretation on hematologic and plasma biochemistry values on a single animal is questionable. It may be more relevant to repeat blood work or to compare with a clinically normal animal of the same age and sex living in the same environment. Thus, we have chosen not to give here physiologic and hematologic values of anurans species. These values may be obtained elsewhere.[6,23] However, evaluation of a blood smear may help the clinician appreciate cellular changes (the assessment of the differential white blood cell count, cellular morphology, incidence of toxic changes, inclusion bodies, bacteremia). In anurans, the neutrophil-to-lymphocyte ratio seems to positively correlate with corticosterone during all periods. This ratio is useful to gauge the stress level of anurans.[18] Lymph and blood plasma are isotonic and similar in composition. They are frequently accepted as being equivalent. As lymph may be extracted more easily with less

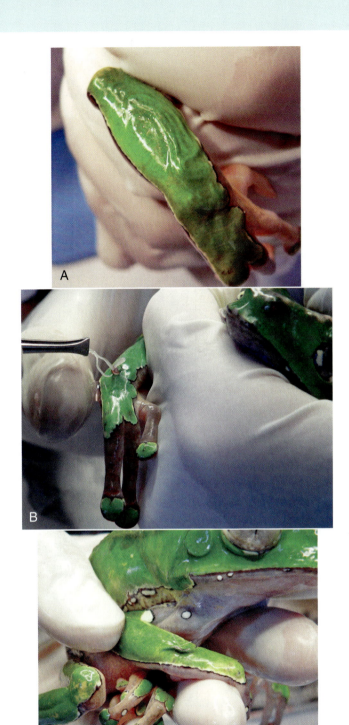

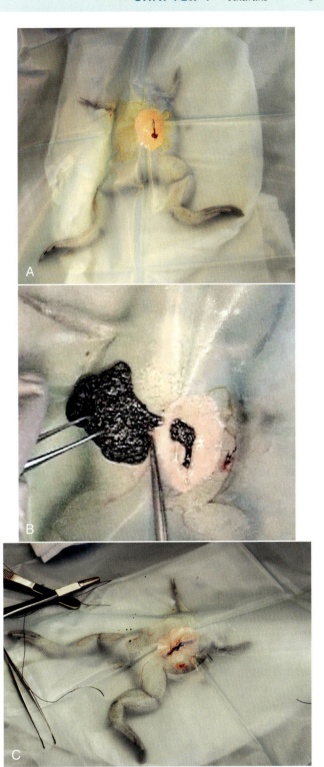

FIGURE 1-2 A, Removing the filarial nematodes in a *Phyllomedusa bicolor* under light anesthesia. **B,** After incision, the parasites were taken out very gently with an ophthalmic hemostatic grip. **C,** The skin was closed with a single suture point. (Courtesy of Norin Chai.)

FIGURE 1-3 Withdrawing eggs surgically in a *Xenopus laevis*. A, One bold stroke is made, leaving a clean incision. Eggs (a small amount or the entire grape) are withdrawn by smooth dissection. **B,** No coagulation is needed. **C,** Everting-type suture to close the skin. (Courtesy of Norin Chai.)

risk of serious injury, lymph work for biochemistry values could be an interesting alternative to blood work. A paper describes a safe technique developed in tree frog (*Litoria caerulea*).[20] Radiography is mainly used to detect suspected foreign body and skeletal disease. Ultrasonography is more useful for detailed evaluation of soft tissue structures. Using clinically normal individuals for comparison is helpful when ultrasound results appear unfamiliar. In many cases, use of a water-filled plastic bag or a plastic container improves imaging and minimizes direct contact.

DISEASES

Infectious and Parasitic Diseases

Selected bacterial infections, viral infections, fungal infections, and parasitic diseases of anurans are summarized in Tables 1-4, 1-5, 1-6, and 1-7, respectively. Bacterial diseases are important causes of morbidity and mortality, common consequences of other problems such

TABLE 1-3

Selected Noninfectious Diseases Presented by Clinical Signs or Syndromes

Disease or Syndrome	Etiology	Signs	Management
Anorexia (without wasting disease)	Poor husbandry Behavioral, seasonal Toxins Ocular disease	Anorexia	Review husbandry (temperature and light cycle) Imaging, diagnostic Screening for any other infectious and parasitic diseases
Anorexia with weight loss, weakness, poor condition	Malnutrition/starvation Inadequate levels or imbalanced ratios of some essential nutrients in preys Liver degeneration: hypervitaminosis A (Rich diets such as rodents and liver; oversupplementation with vitamin A), parasitic, environmental toxins	Anorexia, cachexia, anemia	Review husbandry Change types and sizes of food and timing of feedings Reduce vitamin A supplementation Supportive care Imaging, diagnostic Parasitic screening Screening for any other systemic disease
Anorexia with enlarged abdomen (with or without ascites)	Gastric overload with food, affecting respiration and circulation Gastrointestinal foreign bodies Abscess, coelemic mass, organomegaly	Anorexia Abnormal stool, diarrhea or lack Regurgitation, Overdistension of the stomach, "Mass" on physical exam and abdominal palpation	Imaging, diagnostic Evaluation of fluid Lubricants (impactions): mineral oil, cat laxative by gavage, mineral oil Limit volume of food Removal of foreign bodies (endoscopy) Surgery
Ascites, edema, and anasarca	Heart failure, lymph heart failure, kidney disease, liver disease, hypocalcemia, osmotic imbalances Retained ova	Accumulation of fluid in body cavities and tissues	Husbandry review, water quality Imaging, diagnostic Aspiration of fluid Treat underlying disease
Bloat	Intragastric fermentation Air swallowing (aquatic)	Congestion of skin legs, abnormal distress movement	Removal of air (stomach tube or transabdominal aspiration)
Chemical toxicity	Pesticide, cleaning agents or disinfectants (including bleach, iodine), metal, nitrite, nitrate, ammonia	Great variability, poor growth, deformities, neurologic signs, lethargy, and death	Review husbandry Test water Vigorous rinsing after cleaning Supportive care
Cloacal prolapse	Excessive local irritation Tenesmus Parasites Foreign bodies Enteritis, peritonitis Retained ova, recent egg laying, neoplasia	Prolapse of the cloaca, rectum, colon, stomach, bladder, oviduct, fat pads	Keep in water Clean the organ with sterile saline or 0.75% chlorhexidine before reduction Purse string suture Colopexy Treat underlying cause
Conjunctivitis	Trauma, Dehydration Hypovitaminosis A	Anorexia Conjunctivitis Dehydration may involve adherences of the eyelids	Hydration Supportive care Antimicrobials for injuries Screening for any other systemic disease

Condition	Etiology	Clinical signs	Treatment
Corneal lipidosis (lipid keratopathy) (see Figure 1-4)	Idiopathic Diet high in cholesterol	Corneal opacities spread to cover 100% of the cornea Painful	Limit high–cholesterol items Reduce total caloric intake) No treatment known
Gas bubble disease in aquatic species and larvae	Air leaks in water filtration, supersaturation of water with air-pressurized system	Skin hyperemia, abnormal swimming, bubbles in skin and tissue	Condition corrects itself once water quality is restored Check pumps and lines
Metabolic bone disease (MBD)	Imbalanced ratios of calcium and phosphorus Failure to ingest or adequately process vitamin D3 Elevated levels of vitamin A Young animals mostly	Abnormal posture and locomotion, tetany, anasarca, vertebral and mandibular deformities, fractures	Radiology Supplementation with calcium and vitamin D3 UVB light Use defluoridated water.
Neurologic signs	Trauma, deficiency of B vitamins, vitamin E deficiency, toxins	Musculoskeletal abnormalities, hindlimb paresis and paralysis, scoliosis	Radiography Husbandry review Vitamins B and E Appropriate antimicrobials Supportive care
Orthopedic disorders (See also MBD)	Trauma Nutritional deficiency Congenital defects	Fractures	Splint fractures and external fixation may be attempted.
Rostral abrasions, and other traumatic injuries	Rough shipment, inadequate husbandry, inter- and intraspecies aggression, stressed frogs in glass tanks	Rostral nasal abrasions, sometimes deeper wounds Conjunctivitis Corneal edema Secondary infections	Correct husbandry Correct water quality Reduce disturbance Use of antimicrobial topical and systemic agents Cauterization
Short tongue syndrome (captive postmetamorphic toads)	Hypovitaminosis A inducing squamous metaplasia of the tongue	Wasting, and reduced ability to capture live prey with the tongue	Vitamin A (oral, or bath), force feeding Supportive care
Skin discoloration	Behavioral or seasonal Thermal stress Toxic insult Clotting disorder Early bacterial infection Gas bubble disease	Nonspecific pigmentation Petechiation or ecchymosis	Clean water Vitamins B and K Parasite screening (chromomycosis, algae, trematods) Screening for other systemic disease
Tadpoles: Poor condition	Oxalate toxicity due to overfeeding spinach and kale	Renal calculi and edema	Husbandry review Avoid oxalate-rich diets, vary the diet
Tadpoles: Fail to metamorphose and abnormal grow Spindly leg syndrome in young froglets	Deficient diet or excess goitrogens (cabbage, spinach) Various chemical, nutritional, genetic, environmental, and parasitic causes (metacercariae of the *trematode Ribeiroia* sp. during specific developmental stages)	Absent, fused, or supernumerary digit, limb, and eyes Curved tails Hypoplasia of forelimb, musculature, and bones	Husbandry and diet review, water quality Iodine supplementation and thyroxine Treatment against the adult life stage of strematode with repeated administration of praziquantel
Tachypnea	Thermal stress Behavioral stress Poor water quality	Abnormal distress movement	Check water quality Correct husbandry Supportive care

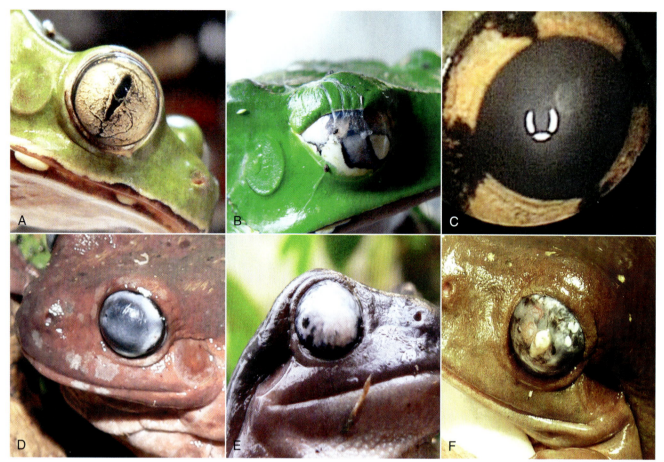

FIGURE 1-4 Some ophthalmic features. A, Abnormal corneal vascularization in a *Phyllomedusa*; fluorescein staining will reveal an ulcer. **B,** Adherences of the eyelids caused by dehydration in a *Phyllomedusa*. **C,** Funduscopic examinations (no tapetum is present) in a *Trachycephalus*. We may also see a local lens opacification. **D–F,** Dramatic evolution of lipid keratopathy in a Litoria. (Courtesy of Norin Chai.)

as traumatic injury in unsanitary captive situations, and may be secondary to viral infections and mycotic skin infections. Most bacterial environmental agents become pathogens in stressed animals. The majority of pathogenic bacteria are gram-negative organisms, yet gram-positive bacteria may also produce significant disease. *Red leg syndrome* is so named because of hyperemia of the ventral skin of the thighs and abdomen of septicemic anurans. Bacterial dermosepticemia is an important concern. Historically, this syndrome has been associated with *Aeromonas hydrophila*, but many other infectious agents produce similar integumentary signs. Only atypical mycobacteria have been isolated in anurans.[8] Widely accepted treatments do not exist. However, a recent paper proposes a propagation method of saving valuable strains from an epizootic infection in Western clawed frogs (*Silurana tropicalis*).[7] Reports of chlamydiosis among both wild and captive populations of anurans have been published.[5] Clinically healthy anurans may carry agents of zoonotic concerns (*Salmonella*, *Leptospira*). Knowledge of anuran viral diseases has increased. In the past, overdiagnosed bacterial diseases (when they are secondary infections) and postmortem misinterpretation may likely contribute to underdiagnosis of viral diseases. The most significant and well-studied anurans viruses are Ranaviruses (Iridoviridae).[11] Fungal organisms are relatively common pathogens in anurans. In general, infections are acquired from the environment, as these agents are ubiquitous. The chytrid fungus *Batrachochytrium dendrobatidis* (Bd), associated with the decline of the amphibian population around the world, is one of the most well-described pathogens of anurans.[19] In addition to treatments that have been described previously, chloramphenicol has been shown to be

effective: 24-hour bath with 20 milligrams per liter (mg/L), changed daily for 2 to 4 weeks. A huge variety of parasites occur in captive and wild anurans.[23] As a rule, treatment must depend on the type of organisms identified and the parasites load quantified. The topic is wide; Table 1-7 lists only a few selected agents. As a rule, along with optimal husbandry practices, quarantine and health screening of newly imported or collected animals are paramount.

Noninfectious Diseases

Noninfectious medical problems are commonly encountered in captive anuran species. Selected noninfectious diseases, categorized by clinical signs or syndromes, are listed in Table 1-7. Rostral abrasions are very common in captive anurans. These are often seen after rough shipment or in excitable or stressed animals. Anurans are sensitive to environmental toxins and UV radiation. Exposures have been linked to impaired growth, development, immune function, and reproduction.[4,13] Care must be taken when using disinfectants, as they may be associated with toxicity and acute death. Dilute chlorine is the disinfectant of choice but must be removed with copious rinsing from the environment after use. As mentioned before, nutritional disorders are not uncommon. Moreover, they may have subtle effects and only be diagnosed in advanced cases. A good growth may be achieved in spite of nutritionally unbalanced diets, but asymptomatic poor health and increasing susceptibility to concurrent diseases will result eventually. Noninfectious causes of dermal masses are relatively rare. In all cases, aspiration or biopsy for histology (with acid-fast staining) must be performed. Various neoplastic diseases are reported to occur in amphibians.[22]

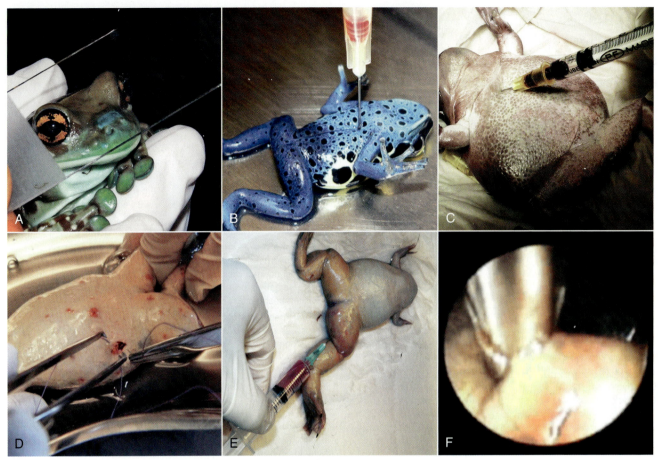

FIGURE 1-5 Some clinical techniques. Impression smears on a rostral abrasion in a *Trachycephalus* (**A**); for blood sampling, the needle is introduced either through the sternum in a *Dendrobates* (**B**) or under the sternum in a *Litoria* (**C**). Skin biopsy in a *Xenopus* (**D**). Fluid ponction of a hindlimb swelling in a *Xenopus*; the aspect suggests an inflammatory cause (**E),** and the etiology was a sarcoma. Liver biopsy by endoscopy in a *Lepidobatrachus* (**F**). (Courtesy of Norin Chai.)

Deformities in the wild populations of anurans have been described for more than a decade. Recent papers have included interesting reviews on the subject.[3,16] One reinforces the hypothesis of selective predation on tadpoles by dragonfly nymphs and other aquatic predators.[3]

Therapeutics

Again, before any treatment, a complete review of husbandry is paramount. Resolving environment defects is part of the therapeutic process. Anurans have a low metabolic rate but a high *turnover* of their body fluids. The weight is very variable, depending on the state of hydration. The clinician should not hesitate to reweigh the animal. Sick anurans have a metabolic rate higher than that of the healthy subjects. Administration of medications in anurans remains mainly empirical.[6] Intramuscular (IM) injection is done when sufficient muscle mass is present, in the forelimbs and hindlimbs as well. The significance of the renal portal system on drug kinetics and toxicity is not clearly demonstrated. Subcutaneous injections are rarely done in practice. Intralymphatic injections are quite effective and are usually done in the back dorsal quadrant, but the location may vary among species. Topical application reduces the need for handling the animal and is especially useful for small patients. Baths are commonly used, less stressful, and also effective. Fluid therapy may be accomplished while placing the animal in the classical "amphibian Ringer solution" (6.6 g sodium chloride [NaCl], 0.15 g calcium chloride [$CaCl^2$], 0.15 g potassium chloride [KCl], and 0.2 g sodium bicarbonate [$NaHCO_3$] per liter of fresh dechlorinated water). If amphibian Ringer solution is not available, a solution comprising four parts lactated Ringer solution to one part 5% dextrose may be used. In debilitated adult anurans, high-energy, critical-care cat food may be used for force-feeding. These may be given initially at 1% of body weight once a day, diluted 50 : 50 with chlorine-free fresh water, and then gradually increased to 2% of body weight. Weighing the animal regularly is paramount.

Reproduction

Males produce territorial and courtship vocalizations. The thumbs present hypertrophies in males (nuptial pads) to help them hold the female during amplexus. If sexual dimorphisms are not obvious, sexing may also be achieved by using ultrasonography (Figure 1-6). The ovaries vary in size, depending on the stage of the reproductive cycle, and may be massive, occupying a large part of the pleuroperitoneal cavity. The small, ovoid testes of the male are much less apparent, being confined to their relatively dorsal position and thus covered by other viscera. Stored nutrients in the fat bodies are primarily used to nourish the developing gametes. Thus, they vary greatly with the stage of the reproductive cycle. Except in the genus *Ascaphus*, fertilization is external in Anurans. Eggs are usually laid in water or moist locations. Anurans generally have an aquatic tadpole or larval stage and undergo metamorphosis to produce the radically different adult form. However, some members of the Pipidae produce eggs that develop directly into juvenile frogs. Some species of *Nectophrynoides* (Bufonidae) are viviparous. In *Gastrotheca* sp. (Hylidae), the juvenile frogs develop directly in pouches in the female's skin. In *Rhinoderma darwinii* (Rhinodermatidae), the tadpoles complete their development in the vocal sacs of the male. Every

TABLE 1-4

Selected Bacterial Diseases

Bacteria	Species Affected	Signs	Management
Red leg syndrome (bacterial dermosepticemia): *Aeromonas, Pseudomonas,* Enterobacteria (*Citrobacter, Proteus Salmonella*), *Streptococcus, Staphylococcus*	Most species	Generalized systemic bacterial disease with cutaneous erythema, swelling, edema (generalized or localized to extremities), coelomic effusions, skin erosions, ulcers, sloughing, necrosis, anorexia, sudden death	Difficult diagnostic (many commensals bacterial) Body fluids sampled Smears and fast staining Biopsy for histology, bacteriology and sensitivity Review husbandry Reduce stress Targeted antibiotics concurrent with an antifungal drug Supportive care
Flavobacterium (Flavobacteriosis): *Flavobacterium oderans, Flavobacterium indologenes, Flavobacterium meningosepticum*	Widely present in aquatic environments Leopard frog and Wyoming toad (*Bufo hemiophrys baxteri*)	Nonspecific effusions in the lymphatic sacs, hydrocoelom, lingual or corneal edema, meningitis, incoordination, petechiation, visceral congestion	Diagnostic with bacterial culture and molecular analysis Antibiotic therapy based on antimicrobial sensitivity testing using premortem bacterial culture
Mycobacteriosis: *M. chelonae* subsp. *abscessus, M. gordonae, M. fortuitum, M. marinum, M. avium, M. xenopi, M. szulgai, M. liflandii*	Mostly described in African clawed frogs (*Xenopus* sp.; *Silurana* [*Xenopus*] *tropicalis*) Also observed in various species	Chronic granulomatous infection All tissues may be involved No pathognomonic clinical signs	Histology, acid-fast staining Culture on liquid and solid media, molecular diagnostic methods No widely accepted treatments
Chlamydiosis: *Chlamydophila psittaci, Chlamydophila pneumoniae, Chlamydia suis, Chlamydophila abortus*	Various wild and captive anurans, including the clawed frog (*Xenopus* sp.), Gunther's triangle frog (*Ceratobatrachus guentheri*), the giant barred frog (*Mixophyes iteratus*)	Systemic infection with pyogranulomatous aspect, pneumonia, petechiation, sloughing of skin, ulcers, cutaneous depigmentation, hydrocoelom, lethargy, anemia, pancytopenia, hepatitis, splenitis, and high mortality rate	Differentiate from red leg syndrome and ranaviral infections by cell culture, histology, immunofluorescence, immunohistochemistry, electron microscopy, PCR testing Liver is the organ of choice for histological Oral administration of tetracycline-class antibiotics
Nonhemolytic group B *Streptococcus*	American bullfrog (*Rana catesbeiana*)	Necrotizing hepatitis, splenitis and nephritis	*Streptococcus* also may be cultured from healthy frogs
Brucella inopinata–like bacterium	Big-eyed tree frog (*Leptopelis vermiculatus*)	Subcutaneous abscesses	Surgical debridement Fluoroquinolone Facultative zoonotic pathogens

TABLE 1-5

Selected Viral Diseases

Virus	Species Affected	Signs	Management
Ranaviruses: Iridoviridae family Frog virus 3 (FV-3) (ranavirus type I) and FV-3–like Bohle iridovirus (BIV) *Rana esculenta* virus (REIV)	Anurans worldwide but mostly pre- or perimetamorphic life stages are most susceptible FV-3 seen in Ranids and Hylids BIV, virulent pathogen of the burrowing frog (Lymnodynastes) May infect other species REIV, seen in edible frogs (*Pelophylax kl. esculentus*)	Sudden death Lethargy, anorexia, abnormal body posture, erratic swimming, necrotizing and ulcerative dermatitis, erythematous skin particularly around the mouth or base of the hindlimbs, systemic hemorrhages and necrosis, gastrointestinal ulceration	Differentiate from red leg syndrome and chlamydiosis by cell culture, histology, immunofluorescence, immunohistochemistry, electron microscopy Polymerase chain reaction (PCR) testing Supportive care and control of secondary bacterial infection Acyclovir may have a potential clinical use in controlling the disease
Frog erythrocytic viruses: Iridoviridae family	In erythrocytes of bullfrogs (*Rana catesbeiana*), green frogs (*R. clamitans*), mink frogs (*R. septentrionalis*), marine toad (*Bufo marinus*)	No clinical signs recorded No gross or histologic findings have been reported Possible anemia	May be transmitted mechanically by the mosquito (*Culex territans*) or midge (*Forcipomyia fairfaxensis*) FEV inclusions are large acidophilic inclusions

TABLE 1-5

Selected Viral Diseases—cont'd

Virus	Species Affected	Signs	Management
Herpesviruses: Ranid herpesvirus-1 (RaHV-1 or Lucke herpesvirus) Herpesvirus of *Rana dalmatina* (HVRD)	RaHV-1 seen in Leopard frog (*Rana pipiens*) only HVRD seen in Spring frog (*Rana dalmatina*)	RaHV-1–induced renal carcinoma Possible metastasis to other organs HVRD may induce cutaneous, vesicles, epidermal hyperplasia	Intranuclear inclusions Lucke herpesvirus replicates only at temperatures below 12°C Diagnosis of RaHV-1 is through light and electron microscopy
Adenoviruses: Frog adenovirus 1 (FrAdV-1) *Crotalus calicivirus* type 1 (Cro-1)	FrAdV-1 isolated from Leopard frog (Rana pipiens) Cro-1 isolated from a horned frog (Ceratophrys ornata)	FrAdV-1 induces kidney tumors No clinical signs recorded for Cro-1	FrAdV-1 has also been isolated in healthy wild frogs
Parvovirus–like viruses	Spring peepers (*Pseudacris crucifer*)	Degeneration, atrophy, and necrosis of the tongue and limb musculature	Lesions with eosinophilic intranuclear inclusion bodies
Retroviruses	Various species, including experimental hybrid Asian frogs and toads	Pancreatic carcinomas with C-type retrovirus	Pathogenesis is not actually clear An endogenous virus has been sequenced from *Xenopus laevis*
Caliciviruses	Isolated in two horned frog (*C. ornata*)	Both animals had pneumonia	For some authors, the cause and effect are not established

TABLE 1-6

Selected Fungal Diseases

Fungi	Species Affected	Signs	Management
Chytridiomycosis (*Batrachochytrium dendrobatidis*)	Various The number of species of anurans is increasing constantly Many species have been shown experimentally to be highly susceptible to the diseases Tadpoles are usually infected subclinically	Clinical signs result in the alteration of the skin and opportunistic secondary infections. Skin lesions (hyperemia, dysecdysis, hyperplasia, small skin ulcers or necrosis of digits/feet), dehydration. Loss of righting reflex, lethargy, abnormal behavior, death. Often no gross lesions evident.	Cytology of stained or unstained skin smears for the detection of zoosporangia Histopathology Molecular methods (high sensitivity and specificity) Treatment with itraconazole, chloramphenicol, and supportive care
Zygomycoses (*Mucor* sp. and *Rhizopus* sp.)	Reported in Wyoming toad (*Bufo baxteri*), giant toad (*Bufo marinus*), Colorado River toad (*Bufo alvarius*), White's tree frog (*Pelodryas caerulea*)	Lethargy, and multifocal hyperemic nodules with visible fungal growth particularly on the ventral integument Systemic infection with nodules and granulomas in a variety of internal organs Progressive weight loss Death	Cytology on smears, histology, culture To date, no successful treatment Zygomycetes are found in soil and decaying material
Chromomycosis (*Phialophora* sp., *Fonsecaea* sp., *Rhinocladiella* sp., *Cladosporium* sp.)	Various wild and captive anurans	Progressive weight loss, anorexia Two clinical forms Cutaneous: swelling, dermal nodules and ulcers Systemic: granulomas in kidney, lungs, liver, spleen	Cytology on smears, histology (pigmented hyphae), culture and identification No treatment to date
Saprolegniasis (*Saprolegnia* sp. and related fungi: *Achlya*, *Leptolegnia*)	Aquatic frogs and tadpoles	Erythematous or ulcerated skin with fluffy or cottonlike texture Mild inflammatory response Death may result from osmoregulatory impairment	Histology, culture of the water mold Molecular testing Improve husbandry Bath treatment with benzalkonium chloride, copper sulfate, potassium permanganate
Mesomycetozoans (*Amphibiothecum* sp. (formerly *Dermosporidium* sp.), *Amphibiocystidium* sp., and *Ichthyophonus* sp.)	Various anurans, including bufonids, ranids, and hylids	Dermal nodules filled with spores typically located in the ventral dermis In general healing within 4 to 8 weeks Myositis associated with Ichthyophonus-like fungi was reported	Standard supportive care However, ichthyophoniasis may lead to death, especially in adult frogs by debilitation and emaciation Implication of amphibian leech (*Placobdella picta*) in *Ichthyophonus* sp. transmission

TABLE 1-7

Selected Parasitic Diseases

Parasitic disease	Etiology	Location	Signs and comments
Amebiasis	*Entamoeba ranarum*	Colon, a renal form in *B. marinum*, hepatic abscessation	Anorexia, weight loss, gastrointestinal disorders, edema and coelomic fluid Treatment with metronidazole
Trypanosomes *Trypanosoma* sp.	*T. inopinatum,* *T. rotatorium,* *T. pipientis*	Blood	Hemorrhage, swollen lymph glands, anemia, and death
Coccidiosis	*Eimeria* and *Isospora*	Gastrointestinal tract, kidneys	Weight loss, diarrhea, dehydration, nephritis Most in young or stress animals
Microsporidiosis	*Microsporidium* sp., *Pleistophora myotrophica, Alloglugea* sp.	Striated muscles	Wasting, poor body condition Vertical transmission seen with *M. schuetzi*
Myxozoan infection	*Chloromyxum* sp., *Myxidium immersum, Myxobolus hylae*	Kidney, gallbladder, reproductive organs, intestines	No established treatment for anurans
Rhabdia infection	*Rhabdia* sp.	Lungs, some may encyst in other organs, inducing granulomas	Most common lungworms in anurans Isolate infected animals. Treatment with ivermectin orlevamisole baths.
Capillarioid nematode	*Pseudocapillaroides xenopi*	Epidermis of *Xenopus* sp.	Weight loss, sloughing of the epidermis, erythema, ulcers, and death
Trematodes	Encysted metacercariae generally involved	Lungs, urinary bladder, kidney, gastrointestinal tract, and skin	Disease is associated with high numbers of trematodes encysting or migrating through host tissues.
Filarial nematodes (see Figure 1-2)	*Dracunculus* *Foleyella*	Subcutis and also coelomic cavity and tissues for *Foleyella*	Remove the worms through a skin incision Look for microfilaria in the blood
Acanthocephala	*Acanthocephalus ranae*	Stomach and intestine	Can cause perforation, coelomitis, and death No treatment known
External parasites	Most leeches Larvae of trombiculid mites ("chiggers") *Amblyomma* ticks	Skin with focal congestion and hemorrhage	Treatment for external leeches: hypertonic saline bath Treatment for chiggers: long-term oral or topical ivermectin

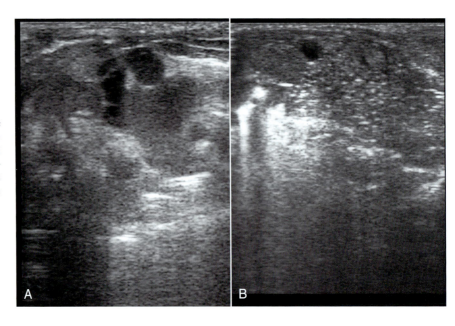

FIGURE 1-6 Sexing two *Bufo paracnemis* by ultrasonography. Male (**A**) and female (**B**). In the female, the irregularly shaped ovaries are generally conspicuous, "speckled" structures containing developing follicles that are usually visible. (Courtesy of Norin Chai.)

species has its reproductive strategies and biology. To stimulate reproduction, environmental conditions have to be arranged to simulate changes in natural habits: raining, cooling, heating, varying photoperiod, and varying amounts of food. Optimal reproduction of one species in captivity is linked to extensive knowledge of its natural biology.

REFERENCES

1. AmphibiaWeb: Information on amphibian biology and conservation, California, Berkeley. http://amphibiaweb.org. Accessed January 25, 2013.
2. Antwis R, Browne RK: Ultraviolet radiation and vitamin D3 in amphibian health, behaviour, diet and conservation. *Comparat Biochem Physiol* Part A, 154(2):184–190, 2009.
3. Ballengée B, Sessions SK: Explanation for missing limbs in deformed amphibians. *J Exp Zool (Mol Dev Evol)* 312B:665–666, 2009.
4. Blaustein AR, Romansic JM, Kiesecker JM, Hatch AC: 2003. Ultraviolet radiation, toxic chemicals, and amphibian population declines. *Divers Distrib* 9:123–140, 2003.
5. Blumer C, Zimmermann DR, Weilenmann R, et al: Chlamydiae in free-ranging and captive frogs in Switzerland. *Vet Pathol* 44:144–150, 2007.
6. Carpenter JW, Mashima TY, Rupiper DJ, editors: *Exotic animal formulary*, ed 3, Philadelphia, PA, 2005, Saunders.
7. Chai N, Bronchain O, Panteix G, et al: A Propagation method of saving valuable strains from a *Mycobacterium liflandii* infection in Western clawed frogs (*Silurana tropicalis*). *J Zoo Wildl Med* 43(1):15–19, 2012.
8. Chai N: Mycobacteriosis in amphibians. In Fowler M, Miller R, editors: *Zoo and wild animal medicine*, ed 7, St. Louis, MO, 2012, WB Saunders.
9. Chen W, Zhang LX, Lu X: Higher pre-hibernation energy storage in anurans from cold environments: a case study on a temperate frog *Rana chensinensis* along a broad latitudinal and altitudinal gradients. *Annales Zoologici Fennici* 48(4):214–220, 2011.
10. Craig WS: Analgesia in amphibians: preclinical studies and clinical applications. *Vet Clin North Am Exot Anim Pract* 14(1):33–34, 2011.
11. Crawshaw G: Amphibian viral diseases. In Fowler M, Miller R, editors: *Zoo and wild animal medicine*, ed 7, St. Louis, MO, 2012, WB Saunders.
12. Gargaglioni LH, Milsom WK: Control of breathing in anuran amphibians. *Comparat Biochem Physiol* Part A, 147:665–684, 2007.
13. Hayes TB, Case P, Chui S, et al: Pesticide mixtures, endocrine disruption, and amphibian declines: are we underestimating the impact? *Environ Health Perspect* 114(Suppl 1):40–50, 2006.
14. Jackwaya RJ, Pukalaa TL, Donnellanb SC, et al: Skin peptide and cDNA profiling of Australian anurans: genus and species identification and evolutionary trends. *Peptides* 32:161–172, 2011.
15. Li H, Vaughan MJ, Browne RK: A complex enrichment diet improves growth and health in the endangered Wyoming toad (*Bufo baxteri*). *Zoo Biol* 28(3):197–213, 2009.
16. Lunde KB, Pieter TJJ: A practical guide for the study of malformed amphibians and their causes. *J Herpetol* 46(4):429–441, 2012.
17. Minter LJ, Clarke EO, Gjeltema JL, et al: Effects of intramuscular meloxicam administration on prostaglandin E2 synthesis in the North American bullfrog (*Rana catesbeiana*). *J Zoo Wildl Med* 42(4):680–685, 2011.
18. Narayan EAB, Hero JMA: Urinary corticosterone responses and haematological stress indicators in the endangered Fijian ground frog (*Platymantis vitiana*) during transportation and captivity. *Austral J Zool* 59(2):79–85, 2011.
19. Pessier AP: Diagnosis and control of amphibian chytridiomycosis. In Fowler M, Miller R, editors: *Zoo and wild animal medicine*, ed 7, St. Louis, MO, 2012, WB Saunders.
20. Reynolds SJ, Christian KA, Tracy CR: Application of a method for obtaining lymph from anuran amphibians. *J Herpetol* 43(1):148–153, 2009.
21. Shaw S, Bishop JP, Harvey C, et al: Fluorosis as a probable factor in metabolic bone disease in captive New Zealand native frogs (*Leiopelma* species). *J Zoo Wildl Med* 43(3):549–565, 2012.
22. Stacy BA, Parker JM: Amphibian oncology. *Vet Clin Exot Anim* 7:673–695, 2004.
23. Wright KM: Overview of amphibian medicine. In Mader DR, editor: *Reptile medicine and surgery*, ed 2, St. Louis, MO, 2006, Saunders.
24. Wright KM: Surgical techniques. In Wright KM, Whitaker BR, editors: *Amphibian medicine and captive husbandry*, Malabar, FL, 2001, Publishing Co.

CHAPTER 2

Caudata (Urodela): Tailed Amphibians

Eric J. Baitchman and Timothy A. Herman

BIOLOGY

Taxonomy

The order Caudata comprises 10 families of salamanders, the tailed amphibians (Table 2-1).[4] The earliest fossil record for this group dates back to the Jurassic period, over 150 million years ago. Their present distribution is primarily Holarctic, limited to the northern hemisphere regions of North and Central Americas, Europe, Asia, and northern Africa, with relatively few species occurring below the equator in South America. The largest family within the order is, by far, the Plethodontidae, a diverse group of lungless salamanders, containing nearly 70% of all species of Caudata.

Unique Anatomy

As the name implies, the unifying anatomic feature of this order is the presence of a tail. The plethodontid salamanders exhibit tail autotomy as a defensive mechanism, and many have a visible constriction at the cleavage site near the base of the tail.[55] Generally, Caudata species have four limbs, except for the Sirenidae, which have small forelimbs and no hindlimbs. The Amphiumidae have four

TABLE 2-1

Families of Caudata

Family Name	Common Name	Species
Ambystomatidae	Mole salamanders	34
Amphiumidae	Amphiumas	3
Cryptobranchidae	Giant salamanders	3
Dicamptodontidae	Pacific giant salamanders	4
Hynobiidae	Asian salamanders	59
Plethodontidae	Lungless salamanders	435
Proteidae	Mud puppies, olms, and water dogs	6
Rhyacotritonidae	Torrent salamanders	4
Salamandridae	True salamanders and newts	98
Sirenidae	Sirens	4

small vestigial limbs with only one, two, or three digits per limb, varying by species.

The larvae of salamanders and their relatives are distinguished from anuran tadpoles by the presence of external gills. As larvae undergo metamorphosis, the gills regress. Some fully aquatic species such as the axolotl (*Ambystoma mexicanum*), the Sirenidae, and the Proteidae, are neotenic, or pedomorphic, retaining the juvenile gills through adulthood.

Lungs are reduced in the torrent salamander family, Rhyacotritonidae, and in the Central Asian salamander, *Ranodon sibiricus*, and lungs are completely absent in the Plethodontidae and in the clawed salamanders, *Onychodactylus* spp. All other members of Caudata, including fully aquatic and neotenic species, do possess lungs.[21]

Sexual dimorphism varies greatly among species, and visible differences between sexes may be subtle. Females may be larger and have wider coelomic cavities compared with males in some species, whereas males may be drastically larger in others with competitive mating systems. Many male European newts (i.e., *Triturus* spp., *Ommatotriton* spp.) display ornate dorsal crests during the breeding season. A variety of male secondary sexual characteristics have evolved in the Plethodontidae, including mental glands, tail glands, cirri, and hypertrophied jaw muscles, which may become exaggerated seasonally during breeding. Some newts develop darkly colored keratinized nuptial pads, or excrescences, along the forelimbs or hindlimbs to aid in gripping females. Some male salamanders and newts also develop swollen vents from enlargement of seasonally responsive cloacal glands for the production of spermatophores.[21]

The hyobranchial apparatus is dramatically adapted to rapidly project the tongue and associated skeletal elements out of the mouth as a ballistic feeding mechanism in several genera of the Plethodontidae. In *Hydromantes*, tongue protraction is driven by dorsolaterally positioned subarcualis rectus muscles that extend from the floor of the mouth caudally past the forelimbs. The tongue is retracted by the rectus cervicis profundus muscles originating on the posterior pelvis and continuously running along the ventral abdomen to the tongue pad and are coiled near the heart between feeding events. Such essential feeding structures should be considered during any invasive procedure on these lungless salamanders.

Special Physiology

Mechanisms of respiratory exchange in Amphibia are remarkable for the taxa as a whole and may occur via four routes: branchial, buccopharyngeal, cutaneous, or pulmonary. The Caudata are unique in the extent to which different families have adapted to different primary routes. Branchial respiration is present in all amphibians as larvae, whereas only some neotenic salamander species retain this means of respiration as a primary route through adulthood.

Cutaneous respiration is also employed by all amphibians to various degrees, although to a greater extent in caudates than in anurans. In anurans, cutaneous respiration occurs primarily as a means of carbon dioxide exchange, with the majority of oxygen exchange occurring in the lungs.[21,31] Most caudates, by comparison, take up most of their oxygen through cutaneous respiration, even in species that possess lungs.[58] Respiratory capillaries are concentrated in the skin in taxa that rely on the cutaneous route as the primary site for gas exchange, as in the lungless Plethodontidae and aquatic Cryptobrachidae. The cryptobranchids also use modified skinfolds to increase surface area and vascularization to enhance respiratory exchange underwater.[31]

SPECIAL HOUSING REQUIREMENTS

Most salamanders come from habitats with relatively stable thermal environments. These temperatures, by and large, are substantially lower than the preferred temperatures of many frogs, with normal activity and feeding in most caudates typically occurring between 10° C and 18° C. Depending on the species in question, surface activity and even reproduction may occur at temperatures near freezing. Air conditioning and water chillers are required to maintain desired temperatures in most facilities. Thermoregulation in most species is limited to selecting refugia of the appropriate temperature.[21] Providing a thermal gradient within the enclosure is optimal, allowing the animal to choose its preferred body temperature. Humidity levels which limit water loss are a critical component of refugia selection by terrestrial salamanders and may be a more important criterion than temperature.[58]

In the case of all caudates, it is important to completely secure the enclosure to prevent escapes. Many species are highly adapted for climbing smooth or slippery surfaces and wedging into very small crevices. These traits translate to scaling glass or smooth plastic with ease and exploiting any gap around the lid, drain cover, or intake filter of a pump. Foam weather stripping, silicone sealant, or duct tape should be used to seal gaps around lids, and fiberglass screening to prevent salamanders from entering the plumbing. Large aquatic salamanders such as cryptobranchids, amphiumas, and sirens are powerful swimmers and may leap to knock off an unsecured tank lid. In the case of smaller species and juveniles, plastic shoeboxes, food storage containers, or plastic deli cups with tight fitting lids with minimal modification are sufficient to securely house small salamanders.

Organic substrates should be thoroughly soaked in clean water and the enclosure established prior to introducing salamanders. As in a new aquarium, a cycle of bacterial and fungal colonization and sequential establishment occurs on these substrates when they become wet, with associated byproducts of nitrogen decomposition. Substrates should be regularly rinsed and allowed to "cycle" until any stagnant or foul smelling odors dissipate. The addition of springtails (order Collembola) to the substrate may also facilitate the decomposition of waste and serve as a supplemental food source for smaller salamanders.

Most salamanders exhibit a nocturnal or crepuscular activity pattern and seek refuge under stones, logs, leaves, or woody debris or in burrows or rock crevices when not active. As such, suitable refugia should always be provided in a captive setting to mimic these environments. All cage furnishings, particularly large rocks, should be stably secured to prevent shifting, which could crush salamanders.

FEEDING

Most salamanders are eager and enthusiastic feeders so long as the appropriate food items are provided. A salamander that frequently refuses food is likely suffering from compromised health or an inadequate environment. Unlike most frog species, many salamanders use olfactory cues in conjunction with movement to detect food. As a result, some species (typically aquatic taxa) will feed on nonliving foods, including frozen thawed insect larvae and even commercially available pelleted foods. Many aquatic salamanders and larvae use a lateral line system, similar to that of fish, to detect movement of prey underwater. By and large, live moving food items are more readily detected and eaten by all salamanders. Many caudates have occasionally been documented to eat other salamanders, and the risk of consumption of smaller taxa or conspecifics should be considered in husbandry.

A broad diversity of invertebrates comprises the staple diet of most salamander species. Earthworms and nightcrawlers (*Lumbricus terrestris* and others) are an excellent food source for many terrestrial and aquatic taxa, although the "red wiggler" (*Eisenia foetida*) sold for bait and composting may be refused because of its production of yellow defensive secretions. Smaller worm species that may be used for larval and adult salamander food include California blackworms (*Lumbriculus variegatus*), tubifex worms (*Tubifex* spp.), whiteworms (*Enchytraeus albidus*), Grindal worms (*Enchytraeus buchholzi*), and microworms (*Panagrellus* spp.). Insects provide the staple diet of most terrestrial salamanders. In captivity, the most readily available and useful feeder insects include the domestic cricket (*Acheta domestica*), wax moth larvae (*Galleria mellonella*), house fly larvae (*Musca domestica*), fruit flies (*Drosophila melanogaster* and *D. hydei*), bean beetles (*Callosobruchus maculatus*), terrestrial isopods (woodlice), and springtails. Aquatic insect larvae form an important dietary component of many salamander larvae, although their availability is limited in captivity. Fly larvae such as bloodworms (family Chironomidae) and glassworms (family Chaoboridae) are occasionally available at pet stores, live or frozen as food for tropical fish. Mosquito larvae (family Culicidae) and other aquatic insect larvae may be locally collected for salamander food.

The large aquatic taxa (cryptobranchids, *Necturus*, *Amphiuma*, and *Siren*) all include crustaceans, fish, and opportunistically other vertebrates in their diet. Fish, crayfish, and large earthworms may be regularly fed to the large aquatic species and occasionally rodents, although only as a component of a broader varied diet. Feeding exclusively fish may result in nutritional deficiencies, and frequent feedings of rodents will quickly result in obesity in many species. The sourcing of live aquatic foods from a "clean" source may be difficult, and this route of transmission should be investigated if disease and parasite issues persist in a captive collection. Crayfish, in particular, have been shown to be a vector for chytrid and may pose a significant infection risk to captive salamanders.[36]

The frequency of feeding salamanders should match the metabolic needs of the animals. Because of the cool temperatures at which most species are kept, weekly or twice weekly feedings are sufficient to maintain most of them. During seasonal cooling periods, these feedings may be reduced further or eliminated entirely, depending on the activity level of the salamanders.

Besides obesity, most nutritional problems in salamanders may be avoided by providing a diverse diet. Occasional supplementation with a quality vitamin or mineral supplement designed for amphibians seems sufficient to maintain good dietary health.

RESTRAINT AND HANDLING

As with handling any amphibian, care should be taken to avoid damage to the delicate skin and mucous layer. Rinsed, nonpowdered, disposable gloves should be worn when handling the animals (Figure 2-1). Clean, moistened plastic sandwich bags or sealable bags may provide an effective and safe restraint for procedures such as radiography or to administer injections. Soft, nonabrasive aquarium nets are suitable for capture of aquatic species, taking care not to damage the delicate gills of neotenic species.

Some species of salamander will attempt to spin or roll on their long axis when in hand, and along with the slippery mucous secretions from the skin, this behavior may make it very difficult to appropriately restrain the animal. Chemical restraint may be required to safely perform more than cursory examinations or treatments in some species. Restraining an animal by the tail should be avoided,

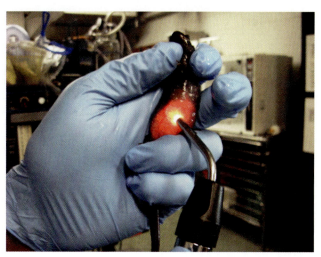

FIGURE 2-1 Restraint of a salamander for examination. Transillumination is a useful aid for coelomic evaluation and identification of blood vessel pathways.

as it may induce autotomy, especially if the animal begins a defensive rolling behavior.

SURGERY AND ANESTHESIA

Indications for surgery are the same as with any other amphibian, and safe anesthesia practices are well established. Surgical cases have been reported for biopsies, endoscopies, gastric foreign bodies, mass removal, radiotelemetry implantation, and limb amputation in both clinical and research settings. Amputated limbs may regenerate in salamanders and newts, and amputation sites may be left open for normal regeneration, with topical care to prevent infection. Closure of the amputation site with a skin flap may cause abnormal regeneration or may prevent it completely.[3] Intracoelomic surgery is best approached through a paramedian incision to avoid the ventral abdominal vein present on the midline. Skin closure is recommended with an everting pattern. Because of the aquatic environment of many species, use of nonabsorbable monofilament suture in an interrupted pattern is recommended to avoid premature dissolution of absorbable materials and potential dehiscence.[2,59] Cyanoacrylate tissue adhesive is waterproof and may be used for primary closure or for additional protection.[3,59]

Anesthesia of amphibians has been summarized elsewhere.[6] Special considerations for this order are particularly for the neotenic species, which may have shorter induction times compared with metamorphic adults, and for hellbenders, which require much lower induction doses compared with other amphibians.[11] Tricaine methanesulfonate, benzocaine, and eugenol immersion baths, as well as injectable propofol, have all proven effective in salamander species.[17,38,59] In the author's experience, topical isoflurane baths have not provided a surgical plane of anesthesia in salamanders at doses described for anurans.

Analgesia is provided as for other amphibians.[6] Amphibians have served as models in analgesic research, revealing that the relative analgesic potency of mu, delta, and kappa opioid agonists are correlated with that seen in mammalian models.[49] A specific study using Eastern red-spotted newts (*Notophthalmus viridescens*) corroborated other findings seen with opioid use in amphibians, that they require higher doses, have prolonged time to onset, and longer duration of action than in mammals. Given the delayed onset of action, early administration is recommended for opioid use, well ahead of anticipated need for analgesia.[33]

Table 2-2 lists anesthetic and analgesic agents that have been used in Caudata species.

DIAGNOSTICS

Diagnostic sample collection and imaging may be performed similar to appropriate clinical investigations in any species. As for fish and other amphibians, water quality parameters should be measured as part of the basic workup, especially in aquatic species. The use of brief sedation should be considered when physical restraint is stressful to the animal or insufficient for completion of diagnostic procedures. Lighted magnification (such as with an otoscope head) is a useful aid in performing examinations. Transillumination is also useful for examination of the coelom, especially in less pigmented species; however, even in darkly pigmented species, it is usually possible to distinguish between fluid, air, or soft tissue coelomic distensions by this method. Transillumination is particularly useful as an aid in identifying the pathways of major blood vessels such as the ventral abdominal vein (see Figure 2-1).

Blood collection is performed with small-gauge needles, 25-gauge to 27-gauge, and 1-milliliter (mL) syringes for most species.

Heparinization of the syringe aids in preservation of small, slowly collected samples. The preferred site for most species is the ventral tail vein, approached perpendicularly on the ventral midline along the proximal third of the tail.[2] The needle is advanced until contact with bone is made. A flash of blood indicates the appropriate location, and rotation of the syringe on its axis may better introduce the bevel of the needle into the vascular lumen for slow-flowing samples. One source suggests guidelines for selecting the tail vein in animals weighing greater than 10 grams (g) and using cardiac puncture in animals weighing between 4 and 10 g.[50] The heart in salamander species is accessed just anterior to the thoracic girdle, almost in the caudal cervical region.[50] The ventral abdominal vein may also be used in larger species. Anesthesia may be helpful for blood collection and is particularly recommended for cardiac puncture.

Published reference ranges for selected species are listed in Tables 2-3 and 2-4.[15,19,47,59]

TABLE 2-2

Anesthetic and Analgesic Agents for Caudata

Agent	Dosage	Notes
Tricaine methanesulfonate (MS-222)	Larvae: 0.2 g/L Adults: 1 g/L Hellbenders: 0.25g/L	Solutions must be buffered to pH 7.0
Eugenol	450 mg/L	Surgical anesthesia in *Ambystoma tigrinum*
Benzocaine	Larvae: 0.05–0.1 g/L Adults: 0.2–0.3 g/L	Paedomorphic adults induce faster than metamorphic adults
Propofol	35 mg/kg intracoelomic	Surgical anesthesia in *Ambystoma tigrinum*; prolonged induction
Buprenorphine	50 mg/kg, subcutaneously	>4 hr duration in *Notophthalmus viridescens*
Butorphanol	0.5 mg/L bath	Given as a continuous 72-hr bath in *Notophthalmus viridescens*

TABLE 2-4

Serum Biochemical Parameters of Selected Caudata Species

Parameter	*Ambystoma mexicanum*	*Cryptobranchus alleganiesis*[a]	*Andrias japonicus*[b]
Glucose (mg/dL)	20–30	11–25	31
Urea nitrogen (mg/dL)	2	1.4–7.6	12.0
Total protein (g/dL)	—	2.8–4.6	3.8
Albumin (g/dL)	—	1.0–1.9	—
Globulin (g/dL)	—	1.8–2.7	—
AST (Units/L)	—	95–205	—
Calcium (mg/dL)	7.0–10.0	7.8–13	9.0
Phosphorus (mg/dL)	2.0–5.0	6.2–14.5	7.0
Sodium (mEq/L)	—	101–113	—
Potassium (mEq/L)	—	3.2–11.4	—
Chloride (mEq/L)	—	75–80	—
CPK (Units/L)	—	760–8869	—
Uric acid (mg/dL)	—	0.5–4.1	<0.3

[a]The range equals averages between sexes and four different localities, n = 84.
[b]n = 1.
AST, Aspartate aminotransferase; *CPK*, creatine phosphokinase; *g/dL*, gram per deciliter; *mEq/L*, milliequivalents per liter; *mg/dL*, milligram per deciliter; *Units/L*, units per liter.

TABLE 2-3

Hematologic Parameters of Selected Caudata Species

Parameter	*Ambystoma mexicanum* (Metamorphosed)	*Ambystoma mexicanum* (Immature)	*Plethodon cinereus*	*Notophthalmus viridescens*	*Cryptobranchus alleganiesis*	*Cynops pyrrhogaster*
PCV (%)	30.00	27.7	—	—	31–47	40.0
Hemoglobin (g/dL)	7.6	7.5	—	—	10.7–8.32	—
MCV (fL)	—	8000–12,000	—	—	7425	—
Leukocytes (×10³/μL)	2.5	2–3	—	—	2.6–6.4	1.8
Heterophils (%)	20–30	20–40	21.7	24.3	32–54	2.8
Lymphocytes (%)	40–60	30–50	65	63.5	28–58	3.0
Eosinophils (%)	2–10	0–10	3.6	6.2	0.5–19	4.0
Monocytes (%)	—	0.2	0.8	2.8	0–1.3	6.0
Basophils (%)	—	0–10	8.8	3.2	3–19.5	57.0

g/dL, Grams per deciliter; *MCV*, mean corpuscular volume; *PCV*, packed cell volume.

INFECTIOUS DISEASES

Globally, the most important infectious diseases of amphibians are chytridiomycosis, caused by the chytrid fungus *Batrachochytrium dendrobatidis* (Bd), and ranavirus infections. Both diseases are reportable to the World Organization for Animal Health (OIE) under the Aquatic Animal Health Code.[45] Both are prevalent in the tailed amphibians, although they have distinctly different characteristics in caudates than they do in anurans.

Chytridiomycosis

Salamanders in the wild seem to be relatively resistant to disease caused by Bd infection compared with the decimating effect this disease has on many anuran species. Very few reports have implicated chytridiomycosis as a cause for population decline in caudate species, including fire salamanders (*Salamandra salamandra*) in Spain and neotropical salamanders in Panama.[11,34] A novel chytrid species, *Batrachochytrium salamandrivorans* (Bs), has been described causing ulcerative skin disease and a brief period of anorexia followed by mortality in fire salamanders.[35] This presentation is unique compared to chytridiomycosis caused by Bd in anurans, which is typically not erosive, but is characterized by epidermal hyperplasia and hyperkeratosis. Additionally, Bs does not appear to be pathogenic to anurans thus far.[35] *Batrachochytrium salamandrivorans* has not yet been found in other caudate species, while Bd has been detected in numerous caudate populations across the globe without any obvious link to disease or population declines, even within communities of aquatic salamanders, where prevalence appears to be fairly high.[9,14,18,26,48,57] Experimental Bd infection of salamanders also reveals resistance to disease and, in many cases, the ability to clear infections without treatment.[18,24,54] Typically, disease is absent, with no clinical signs beyond some increased skin shedding. Ambystomid and plethodontid salamanders have been described as having dark, melanized spots on the skin coinciding with focal clusters of Bd. These spots are cleared with the shedding skin.[18,51,57] On histopathologic examination of infected animals, minimal hyperkeratosis is present compared with the pronounced hyperkeratotic lesions observed in anurans.[18,53] Experimental infections that have produced mortality are achieved by manipulating the laboratory environment to favor cool and moist conditions that are optimal for Bd growth and reproduction.[53,57] Survival and clearance of infection are improved under drier conditions, and it may be that seasonal changes or summer estivation, especially with terrestrial salamanders, may be responsible for the stability of the wild populations coexisting with chytrid.[57]

Other Bd resistance mechanisms in salamanders include chytrid-inhibiting peptides or commensal bacteria that are naturally found on salamander skin. The red-backed salamander, *Plethodon cinereus*, carries *Janthinobacterium lividum*, a bacterium that produces an antifungal metabolite called *violacein*, which is shown to provide resistance to Bd infection.[7,13] Attempts have been made to use this beneficial flora of *P. cinereus* to provide resistance to other species, including anurans. However, benefit is realized only when augmenting *J. lividum* in species where it might already occur and has only minimal and transient effect when attempts are made to inoculate amphibians that would not naturally carry these bacteria.[8,29]

Itraconazole is the recommended treatment agent in most amphibians and has been successfully used with multiple caudate species using the typically described protocol of 0.01% itraconazole immersion baths for 5 to 10 minutes daily for 10 consecutive days.[32,51,52]

Ranavirus

Ranaviruses in the family *Iridoviridae* have caused significant mortality in wild salamander populations in North America.[27] Several distinct *Ranavirus* species have been associated with mass mortality events. The two primary viruses described are (1) frog virus 3 (FV3), the type-virus for the genus, and (2) *Ambystoma tigrinum* virus (ATV), although distinct FV3-like and ATV-like viruses have also been identified in outbreaks.[10,20,46] FV3 has a wide distribution and may infect a broad number of amphibian species.[43] However, mass mortality events attributed to FV3 are most commonly associated with ambystomid larvae in eastern North America, particularly larvae of the spotted salamander, *Ambystoma maculatum*.[20] ATV, thus far, has only been found in western North America, where it apparently has high virulence in all tiger salamander subspecies (*Ambystoma tigrinum* spp.) causing mass mortality rates of greater than 90% in both larvae and adults.[40,43] It is unclear what precipitates ranavirus outbreaks, whether it is environmental conditions, introduction of novel viruses to a population, or immunosuppression from toxins or other stressors. Although mortality rates may be very high during outbreaks, the prevalence may be high in unaffected caudates and other sympatric amphibians that may serve as reservoirs for the virus.[22,28,32,48]

Outbreaks in captivity may be associated with high density of animals and stressful conditions. A group of red-tailed knobby newts (*Tylototriton kweichowensis*) recently imported to the European pet trade and concurrently infected with high burdens of *Rhabdias* lung worms, suffered high mortality from FV3 infection.[39] Mass mortality was also seen in farmed Chinese giant salamanders (*Andrias davidianus*) in China, where 350 of 570 animals died with ranavirus infections after introduction of recently collected animals.[25]

Clinical signs and lesions of ranavirus disease in caudates are not specific, but the description of lesions in published reports seems consistent across all species. Clinical signs in larvae include lethargy, circling, buoyancy problems, and death.[20] Adults may show lethargy, anorexia, bloody stools, vomiting, thick mucous secretions from the skin, and death.[10,25] Gross lesions in both larvae and adults include cutaneous hemorrhage, vesicles, ulceration, subcutaneous edema, fluid-filled hemorrhagic intestines, pale, swollen, and ecchymotic serosal surfaces.[10,20,25,39] Histopathologic examination reveals cellular degeneration and necrosis in the kidneys, liver, intestinal epithelium, spleen, and lymphoid tissues; intradermal and submucosal edema progressing to ulceration; and intralesional basophilic intracytoplasmic inclusions, which coincide with the foci of virions consistent with *Iridoviridae* seen on electron microscopy.[10,20,25]

No specific treatment for ranaviral infections exists, besides supportive care to protect against dehydration and secondary bacterial infections. Elevated temperatures may increase survival. Most *A. tigrinum* larvae survived infection at 26°C, whereas most or all died at lower temperatures.[44]

Antiviral Immunity

Ranaviral infections have been used to study antiviral immunity in salamanders, with the axolotl serving as the principal study model. Caudates appear to have weak immune systems compared with those of anurans, as evidenced by lack of red and white pulp compartmentalization in the spleen; production of only two immunoglobulin types; lack of detectable humeral responses to soluble antigens; and chronic rejection of skin allografts.[43] It is not known whether the relatively poor adaptive responses in caudates might make them more susceptible to virulent pathogens. It may be that caudates rely more heavily on innate immune responses such as antimicrobial peptides, phagocytic and cytotoxic cells, and complement.[16]

Other Infectious Diseases

Many other diseases may be the same as in anurans (see Chapter 1). Few are actually *infectious*, that is, having the potential to be transmitted to other animals. Rather, they tend to be secondary, opportunistic pathogens such as gram-negative bacteria, water molds, or mycobacteria, which gain entry through wounds, skin defects, or immunosuppression. Maintenance of a healthy environment through hygiene, proper nutrition, and species-appropriate husbandry may avoid most of these types of infections.

PARASITIC DISEASES

No parasites are unique to caudates that are not found in other amphibian orders.[15] Many different parasites have been reported in the literature in salamander species, although with little or unknown clinical significance. Rhabditiform nematodes of the lungs (*Rhabdias* spp.) or intestines (*Strongyloides* spp.) are among the most clinically significant and common in captivity because of their direct life cycle. Treatment is with fenbendazole (50–100 mg/kg orally, repeated in 10 days) or with several other common antinematode medications.[1,59]

Trombiculid mites of the genus *Hannemania* are common ectoparasites, particularly of plethodontid salamanders.[5,12,59] Mite larvae penetrate the skin and embed in the dermis, where they feed on the host's tissues, creating inflammatory reactions. Infection sites are often on the feet, although infection and occlusion of the nasolabial groove, which may interfere with olfactory functions necessary for finding food, mates, or territory, have also been reported.[5,12] Treatment is with ivermectin (0.2 to 0.4 mg/kg orally or topically, repeated weekly; or 10 milligrams per liter [mg/L] immersion bath for 30–60 minutes).[59]

Two species within the fungus-like protozoal class Mesomycetozoea cause morbidity and mortality in North America. An *Ichthyophonus* sp. appears enzootic in red-spotted newts, causing myositis, visible whitish spores encysted beneath the skin, and swelling of axial musculature that may lead to ulcerations. Secondary infections gaining entry through ulcerated lesions is suspected to be the proximate cause of mortality in these newts.[30,37,42] *Ichthyophonus*-like infection has also been reported in spotted salamanders.[56] A second mesomycetozoan species, *Amphibiocystidium viridescens*, appears widely distributed at low prevalence in red-spotted newts. Infection causes whitish cysts of various shapes, primarily in the subcutaneous tissues on ventral surfaces as well as in the liver.[41] No treatment is reported for mesomycetozoan infections.

Dermal nodules caused by encysted trematode metacercariae, usually *Clinostomum* sp., are commonly seen in wild salamanders or newts and may be seen in wild-collected animals in captivity.[27] Treatment is not usually necessary, although in cases where associated inflammation is present or when removal is desired, extraction is usually easily performed through a tiny stab incision in to the cyst and extrication of the larva with fine forceps or the tip of a needle.

NONINFECTIOUS DISEASES

Traumatic injury from conspecifics or environmental conditions are relatively common. Wounds should be monitored and treated, if necessary, for secondary infection with gram-negative bacteria or with *Saprolegnia* sp. in aquatic species. Traumatic or surgical amputation in salamander species may result in limb regeneration. Healing begins immediately following amputation in axolotls, with migrating epidermis completely covering the wound surface within hours. Within 1 to 3 days, a well-formed epidermis is present.[23] Limb regrowth is completed in as little as 30 days in an axolotl, 40 days in a newt, and up to a year or more in adult terrestrial *Ambystoma* species (Figure 2-2).[60] Surgically closing the amputation site with a

skin flap will actually prevent limb regeneration.[3] Therefore, the amputation site should be left open and kept clean, treating infection only if necessary.

Nutritional diseases are common in captive amphibians. Metabolic bone disease caused by deficiencies of calcium or vitamin D_3 may be seen.[59] A growing variety of conditions attributable to hypovitaminosis A are beginning to be recognized in anurans. Although nothing has yet been reported in caudates with regard to vitamin A deficiency, it may be prudent to ensure provision of both vitamin and mineral supplements as recommended for anurans. Salamanders develop obesity if overfed.

A wide range of neoplasias have been reported in salamanders. A comprehensive review is provided in the book by Wright and Whitaker.[59]

REPRODUCTION

Reproduction in most caudates is triggered by seasonal fluctuation in temperature, photoperiod, and rainfall. Many temperate salamanders move into rock crevices, burrows, caves, springs, or other underground refugia during winter months thereby avoiding subfreezing temperatures. In some cases, these temperatures are only a few degrees above freezing, and such cold temperatures may be essential triggers for breeding. Replicating these cool, dark, and sometimes dry conditions, followed by a period of gradual warming, increasing photoperiod, and simulated spring rains will induce reproductive behavior in many species. Courtship and spermatophore deposition is promoted by rainfall and increased humidity in some salamanders. In some species, mating takes place in a season different from that of oviposition, with sperm or fertilized eggs retained until environmental conditions are favorable for larval development. Individual females may skip one or more years between reproductive events to replenish depleted energy stores following oviposition.

Salamanders primarily use chemical and olfactory cues for communication during reproduction. Pheromonal components left behind in skin secretions and feces likely convey information relating to dominance, sexual receptivity, and territorial boundaries. In an enclosed captive setting or closed aquatic system, these cues may become amplified and interfere with normal social behavior. A flow-through water system, frequent water changes, and periodic rinsing of all cage furnishings may ameliorate this situation.

Although courtship and mating may occur successfully in captivity, often eggs are retained by females. The causes of this condition are variable and may include improper environmental cycling, improper mating opportunities or conditioning, lack of suitable oviposition sites, nutritional deficiencies, or stress from disturbance by keepers or cagemates.

Eggs of the species that do not exhibit parental care may be hatched in the breeding tank after the adults are removed or transferred to a separate system with similar water chemistry and temperature. Parental care is exhibited by many caudates, providing both physical and microbial defense of the eggs.[58] If the eggs are abandoned or show signs of fungal contamination, they may be carefully removed from the enclosure to be reared apart from the adults. Eggs are typically adhered to a substrate and should not be detached, unless absolutely necessary, to avoid physical damage. Terrestrial eggs may be maintained on damp perlite in a sealed plastic container with one or two small air holes punched in the lid for ventilation. The water level in the container should never come in contact with the eggs, as this may lead to rapid swelling and premature rupture of the egg capsule. The addition of itraconazole at 10 mg/L to the water used to dampen the perlite has been used successfully with several genera of plethodontids to inhibit fungal growth. Aquatic eggs may be transferred to clean plastic deli cups containing a few centimeters of fresh water matching the temperature and chemistry of the breeding enclosure. Separating the eggs into multiple cups limits the probability of a total loss from fungal or bacterial infection. Fungal growth in aquatic eggs has been successfully controlled by

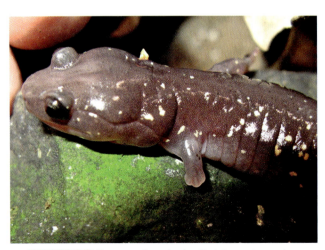

FIGURE 2-2 Regeneration of a forelimb in a salamander.

using either itraconazole or methylene blue treatments. Time to hatching is contingent on temperature.

Upon hatching, many larvae and neonates have substantial yolk reserves and will not take food for weeks or months until these reserves are exhausted and development has concordantly progressed. The first foods offered to juveniles are contingent on the size of the animal and may include brine shrimp nauplii or small whiteworms for tiny aquatic larvae and springtails for small hatchlings of direct developing species and recent metamorphs. The duration of the larval period is highly variable between species and may range from a few weeks to several years. The timing of metamorphosis may be influenced by temperature and availability of food.

ACKNOWLEDGMENTS

We are deeply grateful to Brandi Baitchman and Maria Herman for their support (and tolerance) of our endeavors.

REFERENCES

1. A Manual for Control of Infectious Diseases in Amphibian Survival Assurance Colonies and Reintroduction Programs. In Pessier AP, Medelson JR, editors: *Apple Valley, MN, IUCN/SSC Conservation Breeding Specialist Group*, 2010. <http://www.amphibianark.org/pdf/Amphibian_Disease_Manual.pdf>. Accessed 10/16/2013.
2. Allender MC, Fry MM: Amphibian hematology. *Vet Clin North Am Exot Anim Pract* 11(3):463–480, vi, 2008.
3. Altizer AM, Stewart SG, Albertson BK, et al: Skin flaps inhibit both the current of injury at the amputation surface and regeneration of that limb in newts. *J Experiment Zool* 293(5):467–477, 2002.
4. AmphibiaWeb: Information on amphibian biology and conservation. [web application]. 2013; <http://amphibiaweb.org/>. Accessed April 18, 2013.
5. Anthony CD, Joseph RM, III, Simons RR: Differential parasitism by sex on plethodontid salamanders and histological evidence for structural damage to the nasolabial groove. *Am Midland Naturalist* 132(2):302–307, 1994.
6. Baitchman EJ, Stetter MD: Amphibians. In West G, Heard D, Caulkett N, editors: *Zoo Animal and Wildlife Immobilization and Anesthesia*, ed 2, Ames, IA, 2013, Wiley-Blackwell.
7. Becker MH, Brucker RM, Schwantes CR, et al: The bacterially produced metabolite violacein is associated with survival of amphibians infected with a lethal fungus. *Appl Environment Microbiol* 75(21):6635–6638, 2009.
8. Becker MH, Harris RN, Minbiole KP, et al: Towards a better understanding of the use of probiotics for preventing chytridiomycosis in Panamanian golden frogs. *EcoHealth* 8(4):501–506, 2011.
9. Bodinof CM, Briggler JT, Duncan MC, et al: Historic occurrence of the amphibian chytrid fungus *Batrachochytrium dendrobatidis* in hellbender *Cryptobranchus alleganiensis* populations from Missouri. *Dis Aquat Organisms* 96(1):1–7, 2011.
10. Bollinger TK, Mao J, Schock D, et al: Pathology, isolation, and preliminary molecular characterization of a novel iridovirus from tiger salamanders in Saskatchewan. *J Wildl Dis* 35(3):413–429, 1999.
11. Bosch J, Martínez-Solano I: Chytrid fungus infection related to unusual mortalities of *Salamandra salamandra* and *Bufo bufo* in the Peñalara Natural Park, Spain. *Oryx* 40(01):84, 2006.
12. Brown JD, Keel MK, Yabsley MJ, et al: Clinical challenge. *J Zoo Wildl Med* 37(4):571–573, 2006.
13. Brucker RM, Harris RN, Schwantes CR, et al: Amphibian chemical defense: antifungal metabolites of the microsymbiont *Janthinobacterium lividum* on the salamander *Plethodon cinereus*. *J Chem Ecol* 34(11):1422–1429, 2008.
14. Chatfield MW, Moler P, Richards-Zawacki CL: The amphibian chytrid fungus, *Batrachochytrium dendrobatidis*, in fully aquatic salamanders from Southeastern North America. *PLoS ONE* 7(9):e44821, 2012.
15. Cooper JE: Urodela (Caudata, Urodela): Salamanders, Sirens. In Fowler ME, Miller RE, editors: *Zoo and wild animal medicine*, ed 5, St. Louis, MO, 2003, Saunders, pp 33–40.
16. Cotter JD, Storfer A, Page RB, et al: Transcriptional response of Mexican axolotls to *Ambystoma tigrinum* virus (ATV) infection. *BMC Genomics* 9:493, 2008.
17. Crook AC, Whiteman HH: An evaluation of MS-222 and benzocaine as anesthetics for metamorphic and paedomorphic tiger salamanders (*Ambystoma tigrinum nebulosum*). *Am Midland Naturalist* 155(2):417–421, 2006.
18. Davidson EW, Parris M, Collins JP, et al: Pathogenicity and transmission of chytridiomycosis in tiger salamanders (*Ambystoma tigrinum*). *Copeia* 3:601–607, 2003.
19. Davis AK, Durso AM: White blood cell differentials of northern cricket frogs (*Acris crepitans*) with a compilation of published values from other amphibians. *Herpetologica* 65(3):260–267, 2009.
20. Docherty D, Meteyer C, Wang J, et al: Diagnostic and molecular evaluation of three iridovirus-associated salamander mortality events. *J Wildl Dis* 39(3):556–566, 2003.
21. Duellman WE, Trueb L: *Biology of amphibians*, Baltimore, MD, 1994, Johns Hopkins University Press.
22. Duffus AL, Pauli BD, Wozney K, et al: Frog virus 3-like infections in aquatic amphibian communities. *J Wildl Dis* 44(1):109–120, 2008.
23. Endo T, Bryant SV, Gardiner DM: A stepwise model system for limb regeneration. *Dev Biol* 270(1):135–145, 2004.
24. Gahl MK, Longcore JE, Houlahan JE: Varying responses of northeastern North American amphibians to the chytrid pathogen *Batrachochytrium dendrobatidis*. *Conservat Biol J Soc Conservat Biol* 26(1):135–141, 2012.
25. Geng Y, Wang KY, Zhou ZY, et al: First report of a ranavirus associated with morbidity and mortality in farmed Chinese giant salamanders (*Andrias davidianus*). *J Comparat Pathol* 145(1):95–102, 2011.
26. Goka K, Yokoyama J, Une Y, et al: Amphibian chytridiomycosis in Japan: distribution, haplotypes and possible route of entry into Japan. *Mol Ecol* 18(23):4757–4774, 2009.
27. Green DE, Converse KA, Schrader AK: Epizootiology of sixty-four amphibian morbidity and mortality events in the USA, 1996–2001. *Ann N Y Acad Sci* 969(1):323–339, 2002.
28. Greer AL, Brunner JL, Collins JP: Spatial and temporal patterns of *Ambystoma tigrinum* virus (ATV) prevalence in tiger salamanders *Ambystoma tigrinum nebulosum*. *Dis Aquat Organisms* 85(1):1–6, 2009.
29. Harris RN, Brucker RM, Walke JB, et al: Skin microbes on frogs prevent morbidity and mortality caused by a lethal skin fungus. *ISME J* 3(7):818–824, 2009.
30. Herman RL: Ichthyophonus-like infection in newts (*Notophthalmus viridescens rafinesque*). *J Wildl Dis* 20(1):55–56, 1984.
31. Hillman SS, Withers PC, Drewes RC, et al: *Ecological and environmental physiology of amphibians*, New York, 2009, Oxford University Press, Inc.
32. Junge RE: Hellbender medicine. In Miller RE, Fowler ME, editors: *Zoo and wild animal medicine: current therapy*, vol 7, St. Louis, MO, 2012, Saunders.
33. Koeller CA: Comparison of buprenorphine and butorphanol analgesia in the eastern red-spotted newt (*Notophthalmus viridescens*). *J Am Assoc Lab Anim Sci: JAALAS* 48(2):171–175, 2009.
34. Lips KR, Brem F, Brenes R, et al: Emerging infectious disease and the loss of biodiversity in a neotropical amphibian community. *Proc Nat Acad Sci U S A* 103(9):3165–3170, 2006.
35. Martel A, Spitzen-van der Sluijs A, Blooi M, et al: *Batrachochytrium salamandrivorans* sp. nov. causes lethal chytridiomycosis in amphibians. *Proc Nat Acad Sci U S A* 110(38):15325–15329, published ahead of print September 3, 2013.
36. McMahon TA, Brannelly LA, Chatfield MW, et al: Chytrid fungus *Batrachochytrium dendrobatidis* has nonamphibian hosts and releases chemicals that cause pathology in the absence of infection. *Proc Nat Acad Sci U S A* 110(1):210–215, 2013.
37. Mikaelian I, Ouellet M, Pauli B, et al: Ichthyophonus-like infection in wild amphibians from Quebec, Canada. *Dis Aquat Organisms* 40(3):195–201, 2000.
38. Mitchell MA, Riggs SM, Singleton CB, et al: Evaluating the clinical and cardiopulmonary effects of clove oil and propofol in tiger salamanders (*Ambystoma tigrinum*). *J Exot Pet Med* 18(1):50–56, 2009.
39. Pasmans F, Blahak S, Martel A, et al: Ranavirus-associated mass mortality in imported red tailed knobby newts (*Tylototriton kweichowensis*): a case report. *Vet J* 176(2):257–259, 2008.

40. Picco AM, Brunner JL, Collins JP: Susceptibility of the endangered California tiger salamander, *Ambystoma californiense*, to ranavirus infection. *J Wildl Dis* 43(2):286–290, 2007.
41. Raffel TR, Bommarito T, Barry DS, et al: Widespread infection of the Eastern red-spotted newt (*Notophthalmus viridescens*) by a new species of Amphibiocystidium, a genus of fungus-like mesomycetozoan parasites not previously reported in North America. *Parasitol* 135(2):203–215, 2008.
42. Raffel TR, Dillard JR, Hudson PJ: Field evidence for leech-borne transmission of amphibian *Ichthyophonus* sp. *J Parasitol* 92(6):1256–1264, 2006.
43. Robert J, George E, De Jesus Andino F, et al: Waterborne infectivity of the Ranavirus frog virus 3 in *Xenopus laevis*. *Virology* 417(2):410–417, 2011.
44. Rojas S, Richards K, Jancovich JK, et al: Influence of temperature on Ranavirus infection in larval salamanders *Ambystoma tigrinum*. *Dis Aquat Organisms* 63(2–3):95–100, 2005.
45. Schloegel LM, Daszak P, Cunningham AA, et al: Two amphibian diseases, chytridiomycosis and ranaviral disease, are now globally notifiable to the World Organization for Animal Health (OIE): an assessment. *Dis Aquat Organisms* 92(2–3):101–108, 2010.
46. Schock DM, Bollinger TK, Gregory Chinchar V, et al: Experimental evidence that amphibian ranaviruses are multi-host pathogens. *Copeia* 2008(1):133–143, 2008.
47. Solís ME, Bandeff JM, Huang Y: Hematology and serum chemistry of Ozark and eastern hellbenders (*Cryptobranchus alleganiensis*). *Herpetologica* 63(3):285–292, 2007.
48. Souza MJ, Gray MJ, Coclough P, et al: Prevalence of infection by *Batrachochytrium dendrobatidis* and Ranavirus in eastern hellbenders (*Cryptobranchus alleganiensis alleganiensis*) in eastern Tennessee. *J Wildl Dis* 48(3):560–566, 2012.
49. Stevens CW: Analgesia in amphibians: preclinical studies and clinical applications. *Vet Clin North Am Exot Anim Pract* 14(1):33–44, 2011.
50. Survey USG: Collection of blood samples from adult amphibians. 2001; <http://www.nwhc.usgs.gov/publications/amphibian_research_procedures/blood_samples.jsp>. Accessed February 2, 2013.
51. Tamukai K, Une Y, Tominaga A, et al: Treatment of spontaneous chytridiomycosis in captive amphibians using itraconazole. *J Vet Med Sci / Jap Soc Vet Sci* 73(2):155–159, 2011.
52. Une Y, Matsui K, Tamukai K, et al: Eradication of the chytrid fungus *Batrachochytrium dendrobatidis* in the Japanese giant salamander *Andrias japonicus*. *Dis Aquat Organisms* 98(3):243–247, 2012.
53. Vazquez VM, Rothermel BB, Pessier AP: Experimental infection of North American plethodontid salamanders with the fungus *Batrachochytrium dendrobatidis*. *Dis Aquat Organisms* 84(1):1–7, 2009.
54. Venesky MD, Parris MJ, Altig R: Pathogenicity of *Batrachochytrium dendrobatidis* in larval ambystomid salamanders. *Herpetol Conservation Biol* 5(5):174–182, 2010.
55. Wake DB, Dresner IG: Functional morphology and evolution of tail autotomy in salamanders. *J Morphol* 122(4):265–305, 1967.
56. Ware JL, Viverette C, Kleopfer JD, et al: Infection of spotted salamanders (*Ambystoma maculatum*) with *Ichthyophonus*-like organisms in Virginia. *J Wildl Dis* 44(1):174–176, 2008.
57. Weinstein SB: An aquatic disease on a terrestrial salamander: individual and population level effects of the amphibian chytrid fungus, *Batrachochytrium dendrobatidis*, on *Batrachoseps attenuatus* (Plethodontidae). *Copeia* 2009(4):653–660, 2009.
58. Wells KD: *The ecology and behavior of amphibians*, Chicago, IL, 2007, The University of Chicago Press.
59. Wright KM, Whitaker BR: *Amphibian medicine and captive husbandry*, 2001, Krieger.
60. Young HE, Bailey CF, Dalley BK: Gross morphological analysis of limb regeneration in postmetamorphic adult Ambystoma. *Anatomic Rec* 206(3):295–306, 1983.

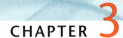

CHAPTER 3

Caecilians

Leigh Ann Clayton and Natalie D. Mylniczenko

GENERAL BIOLOGY

Caecilians (Table 3-1) are elongate, limbless amphibians and may be confused with snakes, eels, or worms because of this morphology. Extant caecilians are genetically most closely related to salamanders.[3] They are in the order Gymnophiona and are currently classified into 10 families comprising 192 species; Caeciliidae (42 species), Chikilidae (1 species), Dermophiidae (14 species), Herpelidae (9 species), Ichtyophiidae (53 species), Indotyphlidae (21 species), Rhinatrematidae (11 species), Scolecomorphidae (6 species), Siphonopidae (22 species), and Typhonectidae (13 species).[1] They inhabit tropical climates in Southeast Asia, India, Africa, Mexico, and South America and may be found in subterranean (fossorial), semi-aquatic, and aquatic environments. Most are nocturnal. In one survey of captive animals, the most common species reported were *Dermophis mexicanus*, *Geotrypetes seraphini*, *Ichthyophis kohtaoensis*, *Schistometopum thomense*, and *Typhlonectes natans*.[12] Longevity in captivity appears to be approximately 11 years according to medical records available to one author (NDM); anecdotally life span may be up to 20 years.

UNIQUE ANATOMY

Caecilians have cylindrical bodies with annular rings and typically range in length from 90 to 1600 mm.[28] Dermal scales are covered by skin. The integument is vascular and permeable to water. In many species, specialized skin glands produce toxins, which may cause mucous membrane irritation[13] and hemolysis (*in vitro*).[21] Mucus from *Typhlonectes* sp. may be toxic to fish, although fish have also been kept successfully with the species.[28] *Schistometopum* sp. may have caused mortality in *Feylinia* sp. housed in the same enclosure.[7] Caecilians do not have vestigial limbs or shoulder or pelvic girdles, and the ribs do not support the body.[14] Caecilians lack functional bone marrow, and hematopoiesis occurs in the liver, kidney, spleen, and thymus.[38]

Most have a functioning right lung and a vestigial left lung,[18] although two lungless species have been described.[29,33] A tracheal

TABLE 3-1

Biologic Information on Caecilians, Order Gymnophiona

Scientific Name	Common Name	Family Name	Total Length (mm)	Body Width (mm)	Distribution	Color	Environment	Reproduction	Larvae
Dermophis mexicanus	Mexican caecilian	Caeciliidae	600	20	Southern Mexico	Dorsal: gray-brown ventrum: yellow-ivory	Fossorial	Viviparous	Aquatic larvae
Geotrypetes seraphini	Gaboon caecilian	Caeciliidae	309	12	Southwest Nigeria, Cameroon	Violet to lavender	Fossorial	Viviparous	Direct development
Gymnopis multiplicata	Varagua caecilian	Caeciliidae	397	13	Panama, Costa Rica, Nicaragua, Honduras	Dark gray	Fossorial	Viviparous	Direct development
Ichthyophis kohtaoensis	Koh Tao Island caecilian	Ichthyophiidae	500	12	Thailand	Lavender brown, cream stripe laterally	Fossorial	Oviparous	Terrestrial eggs, aquatic larvae
Schistometopum thomense	Island caecilian	Caeciliidae	283	14	Sao Tome (Gulf of Guinea)	Bright yellow	Fossorial	Viviparous	Direct development
Typhlonectes compressicauda	Cayenne caecilian	Caeciliidae	523	25	Brazil, French Guiana, Guyana, Peru, Venezuela	Dark gray	Aquatic	Viviparous	Direct development, aquatic larvae
Typhlonectes natans	Rio Cauca caecilian	Caeciliidae	508	15	Columbia, Venezuela	Dark gray	Aquatic	Viviparous	Direct development, aquatic larvae

lung is described in *Typhlonectes natans* and a review of the upper respiratory anatomy is available.[18] The respiratory cycle is a single, long exhalation with a series of short inhalations through buccopharyngeal pumping.[2,5,18] This pattern prevents the mixing of inspiratory and expiratory airflow, unlike in the majority of amphibians.[5,18] Respiration may occur by pulmonic, buccopharyngeal, and cutaneous mechanisms, and the normal respiratory rate of *T. natans* is 4 to 7 breaths per hour.[5,18] Overall, oxygen uptake appears to rely on pulmonic respiration, whereas carbon dioxide elimination is via cutaneous respiration in the species studied.[5,38] In *T. natans*, respiratory rate approximately doubled in response to aerial hypoxia; aquatic hypoxia had no effect on respiration rate.[5] Aquatic hypercapnia nearly tripled respiratory rate, whereas aerial hypercapnia had minimal effect on respiratory rate.[5] Large gills are transiently present in larval caecilians immediately after birth but regress within 48 hours. The metabolic rate in caecilians appears lower than the rate in other amphibian orders.[23]

As is common with other amphibians, terrestrial caecilians appear to be uricotelic and aquatic caecilians ammonotelic.[23] Many species have a bilobate bladder. A renal portal system is believed to exist.

Caecilian locomotion varies with species and substrate, but all species studied may utilize concertina movement.[6] Hydrostatic pressure generated between the skin and the muscle layer are important for burrowing.[6,14] Some species, primarily in the larval stage, have lateral lines with ampullary organs that detect water movement and weak electric fields.[15,22,25] The tentacle (a chemosensory and tactile organ) protrudes from an opening between each eye and nostril and is attached to the tear duct and the vomeronasal (Jacobson's) organ. Innervation is via the trigeminal nerve, and the tentacle serves as the major means of environmental perception, as ocular development is poor. Rod-type structures and visual pigments are present in the retina; no cone photoreceptors have been identified.[10] Caecilians appear to sense light intensity but not images. The eyes are covered by skin or bone in most species. Prey is detected via olfaction and grasped in the jaws; bicuspid teeth help retain prey and break prey into smaller pieces.[15,28] Most species lack outer and middle ear cavities and audition is limited to detection of low frequency vibrations. Vocalizations are rare and may be heard as squeaks or clicks.[22]

SPECIAL HOUSING REQUIREMENTS

Glass aquaria are most appropriate as enclosures and should have tight-fitting lids for all species. Full-spectrum lighting may be provided on a diurnal light cycle. Fossorial caecilians (*Siphonops* sp., *Pseudosiphonops* sp., and *Ichthyophis kohtaoensis*) live in rich soils with forest litter. In general, 70% to 80% humidity is usually recommended for terrestrial caecilians, but a thorough review of natural habitat is appropriate, as some species may be adapted to dryer environments. Soil substrates should be organically rich and pH balanced (neutral). Soil depth should be 3 to 10 cm and kept moist (except with dry soil species), but not wet, to allow for tunnel formation. Soil should be lightly compacted. Some animals require moisture gradients within the soil, and aquaria may be tilted so that the bottom layers have standing water and the top layers are drier. Soil and leaf litter should be sterilized to prevent introduction of infectious agents or arthropods. Vermiculite is a potential foreign body and should be avoided in the substrate. Peat moss and manure are acidic and may cause skin irritation and should therefore also be avoided. Soil should be replaced every few months. *Scolecomorphus* sp. do not burrow and need flat surfaces with hiding spots. Enclosures for semi-aquatic species such as *Geotrypetes seraphini* and *Siphonops annulatus* should have standing water. Water for semi-aquatic and fully aquatic species such as *Typhlonectes* sp. and *Potomotyphlus* sp. should be maintained following freshwater fish water chemistry parameters, and aquariums should have appropriate life support systems, including filtration (mechanical and biologic) and aeration. Dissolved oxygen should be greater than 80% to maintain the biologic filter.[31] Undergravel filters may be used, but tubing

components must be small enough to prevent animal access. A 10% to 20% water change with aged or dechlorinated water should be done every 1 to 2 weeks. Aquatic caecilians depend on breathing air for adequate respiration, and aquariums should provide ready access to the air–water interface; shallow water is generally appropriate. This is particularly important with neonatal larvae. Aquatic species should be provided with terrestrial areas to allow for the full range of natural behavior. The website AmphibiaWeb (amphibiaweb.org) is a routinely updated centralized source of research information and may be consulted for species-specific natural history information.

FEEDING

All caecilians are carnivorous. Free-ranging diet includes annelids (earthworms), platyhelminths, arthropods (amphipods, crayfish, orthopterans, lepidopteran larvae, coleopteran larvae, hemipteran larvae, termites, ant eggs), frog eggs, tadpoles, and anoline lizards.[7,13,16,25,26,28] One African species (*Boulengerula* sp.) eats only termites,[8] but most species are less selective.

Successful captive diets include earthworms, turtle gel diets, mealworms, waxworms, tadpoles, chopped fish (e.g., smelt, goldfish), mussels, neonatal mice (pinkies), *Tubifex* sp., shrimp, tadpoles and frog eggs, and beef or pig heart.

RESTRAINT AND HANDLING

Manual restraint should be limited to reduce disruption of the protective mucus layer, skin, or both. Standard protocols for handling amphibians should be followed, but additional focus on atraumatic capture and restraint such as utilizing clear containers appears warranted with these species during capture and physical examinations.[37] For example, clear plastic "bag" nets or simple plastic bags may be used to remove aquatic animals from enclosures and facilitate examinations.[40] Damp flannel cloth pre-coated with a water-soluble gel or a moistened foam rubber sponge may be useful for further immobilization.[37] Alternatively, the animal may be allowed to crawl into a syringe case or smooth clear tube such as those used for snake restraint and be held in place. Medication was successfully administered to *Dermophis* sp. by restraining in a wet hand, opening the mouth, and medicating with a metal avian gavage tube. Gentle technique is critical; iatrogenic jaw fractures have been anecdotally reported.

Immobilization is achieved with buffered MS-222 (tricaine methane sulfonate) at 1 to 3 grams per liter (g/L) for induction followed by 100 to 200 milligrams per liter (mg/L) for maintenance.[30] Unbuffered solutions should not be used as the solution is acidic and may cause skin irritation and escape behavior.[40] Other sedative and anesthetic drugs have not been reported in the veterinary literature.

SURGERY

Standard surgical protocols described for other amphibians are applicable to caecilians.[24,39] In aquatic caecilians, dermatitis and subsequent osmotic imbalance appears to be a major complicating factor that may increase morbidity.[12,24] Clinicians should address preexisting dermatitis prior to surgery and proactively minimize skin disruption during handling.

Persistent cloacal prolapse in *T. natans* was noted to cause morbidity and mortality in one review.[12] Osmotic imbalance secondary to dermatitis was suspected to be responsible for mortality after management via reinsertion (n = 1) and anastomosis and resection (n = 1).[12] One case of coelomic exploratory surgery in *Typhlonectes* sp. has been published.[24] The animal did not recover from surgery, and the case authors speculate that sepsis and fluid overload secondary to preexisting dermatitis complicated recovery.[24] One author (NDM), successfully completed coelomic exploratory in a *T. natans*. The animal survived for 5 days, and the incision site appeared to be healing normally, but preexisting renal disease led to mortality. Successful surgical debridement and management of a severe tail wound has been reported.[17]

OTHER PHARMACEUTICALS

No pharmaceutical studies exist in the veterinary literature to guide management decisions; medication administration is largely based on extrapolation from other species. The metabolic rate of caecilians appears to be lower than that of anurans and caudates,[23] although the clinical implication of this has not been explored.

Successful treatment of sepsis was noted in one published health review, and injectable antibiotics appear to be tolerated and effective.[12] A comprehensive list of bacterial species cultured from caecilians is available and may help guide empirical antibiotic choice pending diagnostic results.[13] Gram-negative bacteria were most commonly isolated but gram-positive organisms, particularly from cutaneous lesions, were also identified.[12] Levamisole 200 to 300 mg/L immersion bath for over 12 hours caused flaccid paralysis in two of six *T. natans*, but lower dosages or shorter exposure times were not associated with negative side effects.[12] Levamisole, but not ivermectin, intramuscularly caused significant agitation, according to one report.[12] Praziquantel may cause an injection site reaction. Pain medications have not been reported in the literature but may be effective and expedite recovery, per the experience of one author (NDM).

Itraconazole at 0.01% as a 30-minute bath in the primary aquarium every 5 days for four treatments was used for possible *Batrachochytrium dendrobatidis* (Bd) infection in Kaup's caecilians (*Potymotyphlus kaupii*).[4] Negative side effects were not reported, but efficacy was not evaluated.[4] In another report, maintaining water temperature at 32.2°C (90°F) for 72 hours eliminated infection as evaluated by TaqMan PCR in nonclinical *Typhlonectes* sp.[19]

PHYSICAL EXAMINATION AND DIAGNOSTICS

Standard protocols for amphibian physical examinations may be employed with caecilians.[40] Careful evaluation of the skin and general body condition is important, particularly in aquatic animals. Animals that appear overweight should be carefully evaluated for possible excessive fluid accumulation. In aquatic and semi-aquatic species, water quality information must be evaluated as part of any medical evaluation and should include parameters such as temperature, pH, ammonia, nitrites, nitrates, and dissolved oxygen. In terrestrial animals, attention should be paid to substrate to ensure it is not excessively acidic.[12]

Available information on diagnostic tests specific to this order is limited, although standard workups may be conducted. Fecal examination should be routinely performed, particularly in newly acquired, wild-caught animals. Direct smears, rectal washes, flotations, gram stains, and acid fast stains may all be used. Nonpathogenic organisms from food sources include *Monocystis* sp. (from earthworms) and mite nymphs (from rodents). Impression smears (touch preparations) or skin scraping cytology and cultures should be performed on skin lesions. Fine-needle aspirations or biopsies should be obtained from masses. If abnormal fluid accumulation is present, fluid samples may be aspirated and appropriate cytology and culture performed. Blood (Table 3-2) may be obtained under anesthesia by cardiocentesis using a Doppler probe. Lithium heparin is the anticoagulant of choice in amphibians. A complete blood cell count, serum chemistries, and blood cultures should be performed if the opportunity arises; details on blood cell morphology have been reviewed.[36] Radiography may be performed with the use of a closed plastic box or shallow water bath without general anesthesia. In young animals, the caudal vertebrae are less radiodense than cranial vertebrae,[34] and this should be taken into account when evaluating radiographs. Ultrasonography may be performed by immersing the animal in a water bath with the probe outside the bath directed toward the animal. Full necropsies with appropriate ancillary testing should be completed following death of animals.

DISEASES

General

Clinical signs of illness may include bobbing in and out of water, spending time on the soil surface rather than burrowing, displaying erratic swimming, failure to submerge, bouts of lethargy, red mucosa around the vent (vascular blush), shedding mucous strips with increased frequency, skin ulceration, inappetence, reduced appetite, or sudden death. Generally treatment begins with isolation of the sick individual in a species-appropriate hospital tank. Treatment of aquatic animals involves correcting any abnormal water quality parameters, particularly if the animals cannot be moved to appropriate water. For weak aquatic animals, water levels should be shallow, and an area of moist terrestrial space should be provided to reduce the risk of drowning. Treatment should be pursued as with other

TABLE 3-2

Reported Hematologic and Serum Chemistry Parameters in Caecilians

	Boulengerula taitanus[21]	Typhlonectes compressicauda[21]	T. natans	Dermophis mexicanus
Hct%	40	37.6	—	45
Hb (g/dL)	10.3	11.3	—	12
RBC 10⁶/mL	0.68	—	—	0.22
MCV mm³	588	—	—	2045
WBC 10³/mL	—	—	—	0.28
Heterophils 10³/mL	—	—	—	0.157
Lymphocytes 10³/mL	—	—	—	0.095
Monocytes 10³/mL	—	—	—	0.011
Basophils 10³/mL	—	—	—	0.017
Ca (mg/dL)	—	—	9.8	9.8
P (mg/dL)	—	—	4.1	4.1
Uric acid (mg/dL)	—	—	—	<0.3
Total protein (g/dL)	—	—	—	6.5

Ca, Calcium; *mg/dL*, milligram per deciliter; *Hb*, hemoglobin; *Hct*, hematocrit; *MCV*, mean corpuscular value; *mg/dL*, milligram per deciliter; *P*, phosphorus; *RBC*, red blood cell; *WBC*, white blood cell.

amphibians. General supportive care may include intracoelomic fluids, nutritional support, prevention of secondary infections, osmotic support with electrolyte baths,[35] and artificial mucous (slime) products marketed for fish. A review of captive caecilian morbidity and mortality is available.[12]

Infectious Diseases

Primary or secondary bacterial infection appears to be a common source of morbidity and mortality in caecilians.[12] Most identified bacteria were gram-negative environmental organisms, although gram-positive organisms have also been described, particularly associated with cutaneous lesions.[12] Renal, respiratory, and gastrointestinal (GI) disease have been reported with various bacterial and protozoal etiologies, but no specific trends among species have been reported. Vesicular or ulcerative dermatitis is common in caecilians, and bacteria and fungi are commonly associated with lesions.[12] Water molds (e.g., *Saprolegnia* sp.) were the most commonly identified fungi in aquatic caecilians.[12] Aquatic caecilians often die soon after dermatitis is identified and mortality appears to be related to osmotic imbalances in these cases.[13,24] Dermatitis was frequently associated with suboptimal husbandry.[12]

Chytridiomycosis has not been identified as a major pathogen of wild caecilians. It was identified in 53 of 85 apparently healthy animals of four species (*Geotrypetes seraphini, Herpele squalostoma, Idiocranium* cf. *russeli, Crotaphatrema lamottei*) surveyed via quantitative polymerase chain reaction (qPCR) in Cameroon (Thomas Doherty-Bone, personal communication). Caecilians in captivity may also be infected. In one group of confiscated *Typhlonectes* sp., infection was diagnosed during routine quarantine testing via TaqMan PCR in 13 of 24 animals and was not associated with clinical disease.[19] In another case, a *T. natans* housed in a zoologic collection developed abnormal behavior, severe skin sloughing, and increased mucus production. The animal subsequently died, and histologic findings supported chytridiomycosis as the cause of death. No abnormalities were identified, except multifocal epidermal hyperplasia, hyperkeratosis, and cystlike structures consistent with chytrid zoospores within keratinocytes. Another *T. natans* housed with this animal subsequently tested positive for *Batrachochytrium dendrobatidis* (Bd) via TaqMan PCR (Dr. Sarah M. Churgin, personal communication).

Parasitic migration by nematodes has resulted in skin lesions that manifest as white plaques.[28] It is assumed that parasitic migrations occur in immunocompromised animals; often these are recently wild-caught individuals. In one review, nematodes were the most frequently identified parasites in captive caecilians but were not associated with disease.[12]

Viral disease has not yet been described in caecilians.

Noninfectious Diseases

Poor Water Quality

High ammonia levels may cause neuropathies and sudden death. Low chronic levels may cause dermatitis and skin sloughing, dementia, respiratory distress, and kidney disease. High nitrite levels cause methemoglobinemia. Nitrate levels of 2.5 to 100 mg/L have been shown to cause anorexia, disequilibrium, paralysis, and death in amphibians in the wild because of conversion to nitrites within the GI tract.[20] Inappropriate pH may cause excess mucus production, hyperemia, and skin irritation; it also disrupts normal acid–base status. Alkalinity over 100 mg/L may cause death in young animals and result in the formation of white plaques that look like rubber cement on the skin. Chlorine levels of 0.5 parts per million (ppm) may be irritating to the amphibian skin. High copper levels (10 milligrams per deciliter [mg/dL]) have been associated with sudden death. Environmental temperatures below 21°C (70°F) predispose to fungal or mold infections (e.g., *Saprolegnia* sp.). Dermatitis is most often caused by poor water quality; rapid changes in temperature, pH, and salinity; or trauma from cagemate aggression, sharp enclosure objects, or inappropriate handling.[12] Gas bubble disease occurs when dissolved gases (oxygen and nitrogen) supersaturate in an aquatic system and may form bubbles in all organs of the body (noticeable as bubbles on the skin) that may cause lethal emboli.

Trauma

Inappropriate furniture or overcrowding may lead to wounds and stress. Aquarium heaters may cause thermal burns because caecilians wrap around these devices. Escaping from the enclosure may lead to dehydration, sepsis, shock, and vesicular dermatitis. Renal disease may be a sequela of dehydration.[12] Healthy animals in appropriate environments may heal wounds readily, but compromised animals or large wounds may need treatment.[17] In aquatic animals, secondary water mold infection may lead to increased morbidity and mortality.[12]

Other Conditions

Renal failure appears to be an important cause of mortality in *T. natans*.[12] Renal tubular disease has been most frequently identified, although one case of renal carcinoma and four cases of cystic kidney have also been noted.[12] Liver disease has been reported as well, although its etiology and significance are not clear.[12] Floating may occur and may be caused by GI dilatation (bloat) secondary to enteritis or dietary intolerance and emphysema secondary to respiratory disease; dilation is harder to diagnose in terrestrial species. Presumed nutritional secondary hyperparathyroidism has been observed in *Dermophis* sp.[12] Cloacal prolapse has been reported and may be self-limiting (particularly when associated with handling) or warrant treatment. Almost all caecilians rely on pulmonary respiration, and drowning is possible in both fossorial and aquatic species. Dysecdysis may occur in fossorial animals and result in constriction. Heat stress may cause death.

Toxins

Methylene blue and malachite green have been reported anecdotally by hobbyists to be highly fatal to caecilians. However, no references exist to substantiate these reports, and these two compounds have been successfully used topically and as baths with no side effects.

See the sections on pharmaceutical and water quality for more information on other toxicities.

REPRODUCTION

External sex characteristics are not easily recognizable but are present in some species.[9,13,25] The male has a complex erectile phallodeum, and a detailed review of this structure is available.[9] Internal fertilization is reported to occur in all species.[27] Copulation appears to last 30 minutes to a few hours, although detailed reports are lacking.[9] Oviductal, but not cloacal, sperm storage for up to a few weeks has been reported, and oviduct anatomy has been reviewed.[8,27] Most species are viviparous, although oviparity with larvae and direct development has also been reported.[9] In live bearers, the gestation period varies; nearly 12 months in *Dermophis* sp. and 11 months in *Typhlonectes* sp.[11,25] Some live-bearer larvae receive nutrition from oviductal secretions ("uterine milk") or feeding on the uterine wall, and reviews of caecilian reproductive strategies are available.[9,27] Parental care, including nest guarding and maternal dermatophagy (neonates feeding on maternal skin), has been reported in a number of species.[9,27,32] Larval caecilians do not undergo metamorphosis and post-hatch or newly born animals resemble adults. They use branchial respiration en ovo or in the oviduct.[38] *Typhlonectes natans* neonates have large gills immediately caudal to the head, which are shed by 48 hours after birth. Adult size and sexual maturity generally occur at 1 to 3 years.

PREVENTIVE MEDICINE

Standard amphibian quarantine protocols are appropriate for caecilians. Quarantine should be a minimum of 30 days with three negative fecal examinations. Although not thoroughly researched or reported on extensively, preliminary reports indicated caecilians may carry *Bd*, so appropriate testing is warranted. Water quality should be examined weekly and soil changed regularly with intervals, depending on population size and organic waste production. Furniture should be cleaned, disinfected, and copiously rinsed with water.

Meticulous attention to basic husbandry is important at all stages of captive care. Animals should be evaluated daily or twice daily to ensure abnormalities are identified early. Many species are secretive, so attention to subtle changes in feeding or other behaviors is clinically relevant. This is particularly important in dermatitis and sepsis cases, where early treatment appears to be associated with improved survival.[12] Water quality should be routinely evaluated, just as for a properly managed fish system. Tight-fitting lids should be present on enclosures to eliminate escape and exposure to inappropriate environments. Institutions that maintained a high level of care appear to have improved longevity.[12]

ACKNOWLEDGMENTS

The authors wish to thank Dr. Allan Pessier of the Institute for Conservation Research, San Diego Zoo Global, and Dr. Carlos E. Rodriguez of Disney's Animals, Science, and the Environment for their assistance with the information on chytridiomycosis.

BIBLIOGRAPHY

Churgin SM: Personal communication, The Phoenix Zoo, 455 North Galvin Parkway, Phoenix, AZ, 85008, USA, 2013.

Doherty-Bone T: Personal communication, School of Geography, University of Leeds, Leeds, UK; and Department of Life Sciences, Natural History Museum, London, London, UK. Manuscript in press: <http://www.int-res.com/prepress/d02557.html>. Accessed February 9, 2013. Subsequently published: Doherty-Bone TM, Gonwouo NL, Hirschfeld M, et al: *Batrachochytrium dendrobatidis* in amphibians of Cameroon, including first records for caecilians. *Dis Aquat Org* 102:187–194, 2013.

REFERENCES

1. AmphibiaWeb: *Information on amphibian biology and conservation.* [web application], Berkeley, CA, 2013, AmphibiaWeb. Available at: <http://amphibiaweb.org/>. Accessed January 19, 2013.
2. Carrier DR, Wake MH: Mechanisms of lung ventilation in the caecilian, *Dermophis mexicanus. J Morphol* 226:289–295, 1995.
3. Carroll RL: The conquest of land and the radiation of amphibians. In *Vertebrate paleontology and evolution*, New York, 1988, WH Freeman and Company, pp 180–184.
4. Forzán MJ, Gunn H, Scott P: Chytridiomycosis in an aquarium collection of frogs: diagnosis, treatment, and control. *J Zoo Wildl Med* 39(3):406–411, 2008.
5. Gardner MN, Smits AW, Smatresk NJ: The ventilatory responses of the caecilian *Typhlonectes natans* to hypoxia and hypercapnia. *Physiol Biochem Zool* 73(1):23–29, 2000.
6. Herrel A, Measey GJ: The kinematics of locomotion in caecilians: effects of substrate and body shape. *J Exp Zool* 313A(5):301–309, 2010.
7. Hofer D: Caecilians in the wild and captivity: observations from 20 years of amateur research. *Tentaculata: a Newsletter for Caecilian Researchers* 4, 1999.
8. Kuehnel S, Kupfer A: Sperm storage in caecilian amphibians. *Front Zool* 9:12, 2012.
9. Kühnel S, Reinhard S, Kupfer A: Evolutionary reproductive morphology of amphibians: an overview. *Bonn Zool Bull* 57(2):119–126, 2010.
10. Mohum SM, Davies WL, Bowmaker JK, et al: Identification and characterization of visual pigments in caecilians (Amphibia: Gymnophiona), an order of limbless vertebrates with rudimentary eyes. *J Exp Biol* 213(Pt 20):3586–3592, 2010.
11. Murphy JB, Quinn H, Campbell JA: Observations on the breeding habits of the aquatic caecilian. *Copeia* 1:66–69, 1977.
12. Mylniczenko ND: A medical health survey of diseases in captive caecilian amphibians. *J Herp Med Surg* 16(4):120–128, 2006.
13. O'Reilly J, Fenolio D, Ready M: Limbless amphibians: caecilians. *Vivarium* 7(1):26–54, 1995.
14. O'Reilly JC, Ritter DA, Carrier DR: Hydrostatic locomotion in a limbless tetrapod. *Nature* 386:269–272, 1997.
15. O'Reilly JC: Keeping caecilians in captivity. *Advanc Herpetoculture* 1:39–45, 1996.
16. Pinheiro SR: Class amphibia (amphibians): frogs, toads. In Fowler ME, Cubas ZS, editors: *Biology, medicine, and surgery of South American wild animals*, Ames, IA, 2001, Iowa State University Press, pp 4–5.
17. Poll CP: Wound management in amphibians: etiology and treatment of cutaneous lesions. *J Exotic Pet Med* 8(1):20–35, 2009.
18. Prabha KC, Bernard DG, Gardner M, et al: Ventilatory mechanics and the effects of water depth on breathing pattern in the aquatic caecilians *Typhlonectes natans. J Exp Biol* 203(2):263–272, 2000.
19. Raphael BL, Pramuk J: Treatment of chytrid infection in *Typhlonectes* spp. using elevated water temperatures. In *Proceedings of Integrated Research Challenges in Environmental Biology on Amphibian Declines and Chytridiomycosis*, Tempe, AZ, 2007.
20. Rouse JD, Bishop CA, Struger J: Nitrogen pollution: an assessment of its threat to amphibian survival. *Environ Health Perspect* 107(10):799–803, 1999.
21. Schwartz EN, Schwartz CA, Sebben A: Occurrence of hemolytic activity in the skin secretion of the caecilian *Siphonops paulensis. Nat Toxins* 6(5):179–182, 1998.
22. Stebbins RC, Cohen NW: *Ears and hearing. A natural history of amphibians*, Princeton, NJ, 1997, Princeton University Press, pp 147–156.
23. Stiffler DF, Talbot CR: Exchanges of oxygen, carbon dioxide, nitrogen and water in the caecilian *Dermophis mexicanus. J Comp Physiol Bull* 170(7):505–509, 2000.
24. Sykes JM, Reel D, Henry GA, et al: Whole body edema and mineralized fat necrosis in an aquatic caecilian, *Typhlonectes* sp. *J Herp Med Surg* 16(2):53–57, 2006.
25. Taylor EH: *The caecilians of the world: a taxonomic review*, Lawrence, KS, 1968, University of Kansas Press.
26. Verdade VK, Schiesari LC, Bertoluci JA: Diet of juvenile aquatic caecilians, *Typhlonectes compressicauda. J Herp* 34(2):291–293, 2000.
27. Wake MH, Dickie R: Oviduct structure and function and reproductive modes in amphibians. *J Exp Zoo* 282(4–5):477–506, 1998.
28. Wake MH: Caecilians (Amphibia: Gymnophiona) in captivity. In Murphy JB, Adler K, Collins JT, editors: *Captive management and conservation of amphibians and reptiles*, Ithaca, NY, 1994, Society for the Study of Amphibians and Reptiles, pp 223–228.
29. Wake MH, Donnelly MA: A new lungless caecilian (Amphibia: Gymnophiona) from Guyana. *Proc R Soc B* 277(1683):915–922, 2010.
30. Whitaker BR, Wright KM, Barnett SL: Basic husbandry and clinical assessment of the amphibian patient. *Exotic Anim Pract Clin North Am* 2(2):265–290, 1999.
31. Whitaker BR: Water quality. In Wright KM, Whitaker BR, editors: *Amphibian medicine and captive husbandry*, Malabar, FL, 2001, Krieger Publishing, pp 147–156.
32. Wilkinson M, Kupfer A, Marques-Porto R, et al: One hundred million years of skin feeding? Extended parental care in a neotropical caecilian (Amphibia: Gymnophiona). *Biol Lett* 4(4):358–361, 2008.
33. Wilkinson M, Nussbaum RA: Comparative morphology and evolution of the lungless caecilian *Atretochoana eiselti. Biol J Linn Soc* 62:39–109, 1997.
34. Wright KM, Whitaker BR: Nutritional disorders. In Wright KM, Whitaker BR, editors: *Amphibian medicine and captive husbandry*, Malabar, FL, 2001, Krieger Publishing, pp 73–88.
35. Wright KM, Whitaker BR: Pharmacotherapeutics. In Wright KM, Whitaker BR, editors: *Amphibian medicine and captive husbandry*, Malabar, FL, 2001, Krieger Publishing, pp 309–331.
36. Wright KM: Amphibian hematology. In Wright KM, Whitaker BR, editors: *Amphibian medicine and captive husbandry*, Malabar, FL, 2001, Krieger Publishing, pp 129–140.

37. Wright KM: Amphibian husbandry and medicine. In Mader DR, editor: *Reptile medicine and surgery*, Philadelphia, PA, 1996, WB Saunders, pp 436–458.

38. Wright KM: Anatomy for the clinician. In Wright KM, Whitaker BR, editors: *Amphibian medicine and captive husbandry*, Malabar, FL, 2001, Krieger Publishing, pp 15–30.

39. Wright KM: Surgical techniques. In Wright KM, Whitaker BR, editors: *Amphibian medicine and captive husbandry*, Malabar, FL, 2001, Krieger Publishing, pp 273–282.

40. Wright KM: Restraint techniques and euthanasia. In Wright KM, Whitaker BR, editors: *Amphibian medicine and captive husbandry*, Malabar, FL, 2001, Krieger Publishing, pp 111–121.

CHAPTER 4

Chelonians (Turtles, Tortoises)

Joseph P. Flanagan

BIOLOGY

Currently, 322 living species of tortoises and freshwater and marine turtles are in existence (Table 4-1). They are found in diverse habitats on all continents except Antarctica and in all oceans except the Arctic. The largest concentrations of turtle species occur in North America, more than in any other temperate region of the world. Ninety-eight species of chelonians are endangered or critically endangered because of habitat degradation, human encroachment, and harvesting for food, medicines, and the pet trade. Of the chelonians with known threat status in 2010, 53% of the species are considered threatened, making chelonians the most highly endangered of any of the major vertebrate groups.[8]

Unique Anatomy

Chelonians range in size from the 100-gram (g) speckled tortoise (*Homopus signatus*) to the leatherback turtles (*Dermochelys coriacae*) weighing more than 800 kilograms (kg). Turtles and tortoises may be instantly recognized by the presence of a shell comprising the carapace (dorsal) and the plastron (ventral), which are joined laterally at the bridge. In most species, keratinized epithelium overlies a rigid bony structure that provides protection. The extent of shell coverage, flexibility, degree of mineralization, fenestration, hinging, and epithelial coverage vary. Most species have keratinized epithelium covering a thin dermis layer consisting of collagen fibers, melanophores, vessels, and nerves, beneath which is dermal bone.[4] Most terrestrial species have firm, dense shells such as those of gopher tortoises (*Gopherus polyphemus*). Loss of bone in the central portions of the carapace and plastron of the pancake tortoise (*Malacochersus tornieri*) is normal and allows the species to wedge itself into rock crevices, where it may inflate itself to escape predation. Shells may be flexible at the bridges, which allows the hinged plastron of some species (*Terrepene* spp., *Cuora* spp., *Kinosternon* spp.) to seal tight against the carapace, whereas tortoises in the genus *Kinyxs* have hinged carapaces for protection. Certain aquatic species such as snapping turtles and certain species of the genus *Kinosternon* have reduced plastrons providing minimal rigid protection of the limbs. Vertebrae are incorporated into the carapace from the first thoracic vertebra caudally to the coccygeal vertebra. Sea turtles are unable to retract their heads and necks fully under their shells. Retraction of the head and neck may be in a horizontal plane as in the Pleurodiran species (side-necked and snake-necked turtles), or in a vertical plane by direct caudal retraction as is done in Cryptodiran species (typical of all land tortoises and most freshwater species of the northern hemisphere).

Chelonian limbs are highly variable between species groups. Sea turtles and the freshwater pig-nosed turtle (*Carettochelys*) have flattened limbs that are highly adapted to an aquatic existence but that serve very poorly for walking on land. Most freshwater turtle species have varying degrees of interdigital webbing to facilitate swimming but retain the ability to walk on land. Some aquatic species such as snapping turtles are not good swimmers but "walk" on the bottom substrate during normal locomotion. Fully terrestrial species (Testudinadae) may have flattened forelimbs for burrowing and tend to have elephantine hindlimbs adapted for walking on land.

The renal-portal system directs blood from the caudal region of the body through the kidneys or may divert it into the central circulation. Blood is shunted through the kidneys in times of water deprivation; however, pharmacokinetic studies have shown no significant difference in drug metabolism if injections are given in the caudal region versus the cranial limbs.[3]

Special Physiology

All chelonians are considered ectothermic, although leatherback sea turtles are somewhat homeothermic. Preferred optimal temperatures differ according to species and should be considered in housing chelonians. Temperatures in the natural environment change according to diurnal and seasonal cycles. Captive animals should not be subjected to constant temperatures but should be provided with a diurnal fluctuation and a thermal gradient. Most turtles and tortoises depend on behavioral adaptations such as basking in the sun, seeking shade, or entering water or burrows to elevate, maintain, or decrease body temperatures. Immune function is enhanced when animals may achieve their preferred optimal temperature. For highly aquatic species, maintaining appropriate water temperature ranges is critical for behavioral reasons and for physiologic functions such as digestion.

Chelonians may demonstrate episodic breathing and may shunt blood to or away from the lungs via vascular and intracardiac shunting mechanisms. Additionally, species adept at breath-holding demonstrate adaptations such as tolerance of hypoxia, large lung volume, rapid and extensive air exchange during ventilation, and physiologic buffering by bone, blood, and pericardial fluid of lactic acid and hydrogen ions built up during anaerobic metabolism. In aquatic species, gas exchange may also occur through the integument, pharynx, or cloacal tissues. Soft-shelled turtles may obtain up to 70% of their oxygen during submergence through their leathery shell.[9]

The kidneys of turtles have fewer nephrons than those of mammals and no loop of Henle, which creates an inability to concentrate urine. Nitrogenous waste is excreted as ammonia, urea, or uric acid. Proportions vary according to the biology of the species. Marine turtles and highly aquatic freshwater turtles may excrete up to 25% of their nitrogenous waste as ammonia. Other aquatic turtles may excrete primarily urea. Tortoises excrete most nitrogenous waste as relatively insoluble uric acid to prevent water loss. Water may be held in the urinary bladder and resorbed into general circulation. The ability of tortoises to store water in this manner enhances survival in xeric habitats and during times of drought. When handling tortoises in the wild, care must be taken to prevent the animals from urinating because this could result in significant losses of fluids that the animal might not be able to replace.

FEEDING

The diverse species of chelonians demonstrate great diversity in diet and feeding habits. They may be omnivores, eating a broad spectrum of foods to constitute a complete diet, or they may be specialist feeders and have a strict, narrow spectrum of food items that they will accept. They may be herbivores, omnivores, or carnivores. Many have feeding strategies that change during different life stages.

TABLE 4-1

Biologic Information for Families of Chelonia

Family (Number of Species)	Common Name	Weight (Adult)	Habitat	Geographic Distribution
Carettochelyidae (1)	Fly river (pig-nosed) turtle	15 kg	Rivers	Australia and New Guinea
Chelidae (54)	Snake-necked turtles	0.25 to 20 kg	Rivers and lakes	Australia, New Guinea, Eastern South America
Cheloniidae (6)	Sea turtles	80 to 500 kg	Oceans	Worldwide
Chelydridae (4)	Snapping turtles	90 kg	Lakes, slow moving streams	Central, Eastern North America, Eastern Mexico, Western Columbia
Dermatemydidae (1)	Central American river turtle	30 kg	Rivers	Central America
Dermochelyidae (1)	Leatherback turtle	350 to 800 kg	Oceans	Worldwide
Emydidae (51)	Emydid turtles: terrapins, box turtles, sliders, and cooters	0.25 to 50 kg	Lakes, rivers, streams, and brackish water	Americas, Europe, North Africa, Middle East
Geoemydidae (69)	Asian box and freshwater turtles, and neotropical wood turtles	0.1 kg to 50 kg	Freshwater and terrestrial habitats	Asia, Mexico to northern South America
Kinosternidae (25)	Mud and musk turtles	0.15 to 2 kg	Freshwater; mud banks	Americas
Pelomedusidae (19)	Afro-American sidenecks	Up to 90 kg	Freshwater lakes, streams	South America and Africa
Platysternidae (1)	Bigheaded turtles	Up to 0.5 kg	Mountain streams	Asia
Podocnemididae (8)	South American and Malagasy sidenecks	Up to 75 kg	Rivers	South America and Madagascar
Testudinidae (59)	Tortoises	0.1 to 250 kg	Semi-arid, arid, mountain, and forest	Americas, Europe, Africa, and Asia
Trionychidae (31)	Softshell turtles	0.25 to 300 kg	Rivers and lakes	North America, Africa, and Asia

Wild-caught animals may be very difficult to acclimate to novel food items, and some may never willingly transition to captive foods. It is important to be familiar with the natural history of certain "specialized feeders" to provide familiar and acceptable food items while transferring animals to a balanced captive diet. Tortoises are herbivores that tend to graze on grasses and annual forbs but have very little natural exposure to fruits. Freshwater turtles are primarily omnivorous, consuming fish, crustaceans, snails, aquatic grasses, fallen fruits, and many other food items. Some are more carnivorous as juveniles but become more herbivorous with age. Complete rations have been formulated specifically for different groups of animals, and some may be used successfully for all life stages. Like other aquatic turtles, sea turtles may be omnivorous, carnivorous, or herbivorous. Green sea turtles feed on sea grasses and algae. Loggerhead and Ridley sea turtles prefer a diet of molluscs and crustaceans, whereas hawksbills specialize on sponges and leatherback sea turtles consume primarily jellyfish. Captive sea turtles will eat fish, crustaceans, and molluscs and may be acclimated to balanced diets in pellet or gelatin form. Obesity is not uncommon in captive turtles. One should remember that in nature, chelonians may spend a considerable amount of time foraging as a daily activity and such activity may provide benefits for well-being beyond simple nutrition. In general, hatchling chelonians of all species should be fed daily. Frequency of feeding may be reduced with age, but most species should be fed at least twice per week as adults.

RESTRAINT AND HANDLING

Most chelonia are relatively easily restrained. A potential risk exists for handlers from bites, scratches from claws, or cuts from projections of scales or points on the shell. Green sea turtles may flap their front flippers forcefully enough to fracture their humerus and may easily injure handlers while struggling. It is generally most safe to lift larger animals, placing one hand on the anterior carapace over the neck and the other hand on the caudal carapace over the tail.

This minimizes the potential for bites or scratches. For species that may be lifted easily, care must be taken not to flip them upside down rapidly. This may cause immediate changes in hemodynamics that may cause distress to the animal, may impair ventilation because of compression of the lungs under the weight of coelomic viscera, or result in intestinal or uterine torsion. Aggressive animals may require diversion, immobilization, or blocking of the head to safely examine them. Materials such as rolls of tape or padded sticks or polyvinyl chloride pipes serve well as bite blocks placed in the mouth and secured with tape around the head. For small species, pushing the head under the carapace in a natural position and maintaining it there manually or with padding covered and taped to the shell allows nonpainful procedures on other portions of the body to proceed in safety. Many tortoises will not struggle if their eyes are covered or the heads are in the confines of their shells. Conversely, when chelonians are regressed completely into their shells, extricating limbs or the head without harming the animal is challenging. Some animals will extend their limbs when securely balanced on a pedestal, allowing for visual examination of the appendages and potentially permitting restraint of a limb or the head and neck. Using a small metal spatula, usually, even the tightest hinged plastron of a box turtle or the armored front leg of a tortoise may be breeched. Gentle, steady traction on the closed plastron or leg is usually rewarded by relaxation of the defense mechanisms. In extreme cases, chemical immobilization must be used to examine or treat the animal.

SURGERY AND ANESTHESIA

General anesthesia may be induced and maintained with parenteral agents given through intravenous or intramuscular routes (Table 4-2). Gas anesthetics may be used to induce and maintain anesthesia, but induction under voluntary respiration may be prolonged when animals hold their breath. Direct intubation of the glottis may be accomplished in the awake chelonian through use of an oral speculum. The glottis is located at the base of the tongue and is closed

TABLE 4-2

Sedative, Anesthetic, Analgesic, and Restraint Agents Used in Chelonians

Generic (Trade) Name	Dose and Route	Comment
Atipamezole (Antisedan)	5× dose of medetomidine, 10× dose of dexmedetomidine	α-adrenergic reversal for medetomidine and dexmedetomidine
Bupivacaine	1 to 2 mg/kg local infiltration 4 mg/kg maximum dose	Local anesthetic
Buprenorphine	0.075 mg/kg SC	Effect lasts 24 or more hours
Butorphanol (Torbugesic)	0.2 mg/kg IM	Tranquilizer
Dexmedetomidine (Dexdomitor)	0.03 to 0.075 mg/kg	Anesthesia Use in combination with ketamine Reverse with atipamezole
Diazepam (Valium)	0.2 to 1.0 mg/kg IM	Use with ketamine for relaxation
Isoflurane (IsoFlo)	3% to 5%	Use face mask, chamber, or endotracheal tube Long induction time
Ketamine HCl (Multiple)	5 to 25 mg/kg IV or 20 to 60 mg/kg IM	Highly variable response to IM dosing Use lower doses IV or in combination with α-adrenergic and higher dose IM or when given alone
Lidocaine (0.05-2%) (Multiple)	Up to 2 mg/kg total dose, 1 mL 2%/20 kg for epithecal	Local infiltration or epithecal
Medetomidine (Dormitor; Zaloprim)	0.1 to 0.15 mg/kg IV or IM	Use with ketamine, 5 mg/kg Reverse with atipamezole
Meloxicam	0.1 to 0.5 mg/kg PO, IM, or 0.22 mg/kg IV	Analgesia Study in red-eared sliders Better absorption IM versus PO Rapid elimination after IV administration
Morphine	1.5 to 6.5 mg/kg SC	Analgesia Higher dose has more rapid onset (2 hours versus 4), both last over 8 hours
Propofol (Deprivan)	5 to 10 mg/kg IV	Restraint for 30 to 60 minutes May cause respiratory depression requiring intubation and positive-pressure ventilation
Tiletamine/zolazapam (Telazol)	5 to 10 mg/kg IV or IM	Prolonged recovery, generally insufficient as sole anesthetic Reverse with flumazenil 1 mg/20 mg zolezepam IM or IV
Tramadol	10 mg/kg PO 10 mg/kg SC	Analgesia Lasts 9 to 96 hours Analgesia Lasts 12 to 48 hours
Xylazine (Rompun)	0.1 to 1.25 mg/kg IV or IM	Variable results, not recommended Reverse with yohimbine 0.125 mg/kg IM

IM, Intramuscularly; *IV*, intravenously, *PO*, per os.

unless the animal is taking a breath. An appropriate sized endotracheal tube may be gently forced into the glottis and the animal induced using positive pressure ventilation until an acceptable level of anesthesia is achieved. The trachea bifurcates into paired bronchi in the cranial one third of the cervical area and has complete cartilagenous rings. Care should be taken to prevent unilateral bronchial intubation. Anesthetic agents are metabolized more slowly under low body temperatures, so special attention should be given to maintaining the anesthetized chelonian at or near its preferred optimal temperature range. The turtle's ability to withstand prolonged anoxia may cause reduced ventilation, resulting in reduced exchange of anesthetic gases. Whenever possible, animals under anesthesia should be intubated and provided with assisted ventilation. Recovery after gas anesthesia may be prolonged because ventilation is not induced by hypercapnea and decreases during hyperoxia. The use of room air rather than oxygen will speed anesthetic recovery.[7] The use of local anesthetic (lidocaine 2% or bupivacaine 0.5%) may be used as adjunct to general anesthesia. Epithecal anesthesia (2%

lidocaine at 1 mL/20 kg) may be used alone or in conjunction with general anesthesia for surgeries of the cloaca and tail (Figures 4-1 and 4-2).[6]

Surgical procedures should be performed under appropriate anesthesia and aseptic conditions. Intracoelomic surgery such as ovariectomy, salpingotomy for removing retained eggs, or enterotomy for removing a foreign body may be achieved by accessing the coelom through the prefemoral fossa. Incision size may be kept to a minimum by using rigid endoscopy to retract the ovarian tissue, oviduct, or intestine and bring it to the skin incision. Intracoelomic access may be limited via this route, however, and surgical objectives may require cutting through the plastron. In brief, the shell is cut to make a beveled edge by using a drill or a saw while attempting to keep a portion of the cut shell attached by preserving the periosteum. Care is taken to identify the coelomic blood vessels before incising them. With the shell out of the way, surgery may proceed as for any routine abdominal procedure. After the primary surgical objectives are met, closure of the coelom is accomplished by replacing the shell

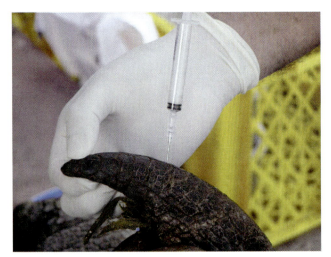

FIGURE 4-1 Needle insertion for epithecal injection in a giant tortoise.

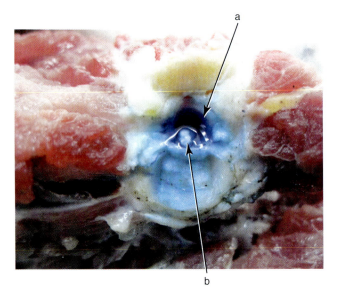

FIGURE 4-2 Cross-section of caudal vertebra showing epithecal space *(a)* and spinal cord *(b)*. (Photo courtesy of Steve Divers.)

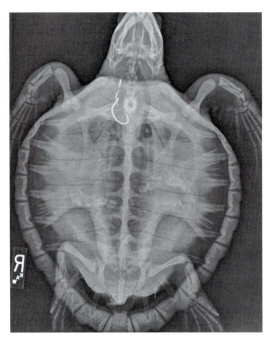

FIGURE 4-3 Radiograph of a Kemp's ridley sea turtle with esophageal foreign body. The hook was removed via caudal cervical esophagotomy.

with the use of the beveled edge to help position and stabilize the flap during closure. The flap is affixed to the plastron using materials such as bone cement, acrylic, screws, and cerclage wire, in combination or alone. As with any orthopedic manipulation, complete healing of the shell may take months. Plastrotomy is not advised in species having dynamic movement of the plastron during normal respiration or diving (e.g., sea turtles), as the surgery site will be in constant motion, impeding or preventing the healing process. Fish hooks are commonly ingested by sea turtles and frequently lodge in the lower esophagus near the base of the heart. These may generally be accessed through a ventral cervical incision, retracting the esophagus cranially to access the site where the hook has lodged (Figure 4-3).

Orthopedic procedures are similar to those for other animals. The density of long bones is generally greater than for mammals, and external splints may be challenging to maintain. Limbs may be taped inside shell openings for crude but effective means of immobilizing fractures of extremities. Shell fracture is a common presentation of animals hit by automobiles or speedboats. The fracture site is frequently grossly contaminated with dirt or water, with contamination of the lungs or coelomic cavity being a potential risk. The wound

should be cleaned and the fragments stabilized by using support bars or cerclage wire, which will allow treatment of the fracture site as an open wound. Large defects with loss of shell fragments may be treated with vacuum-assisted closure. Healing time may take up to a year for bony bridging and reepithelialization.

CLINICAL PROCEDURES

Physical Examination

It may be daunting to try to perform a physical examination on a chelonian that is completely and firmly withdrawn into its shell, but the foundation of diagnosis lies with a good physical examination in combination with the history and signalment of the patient. Ideally, the patient should be examined in its primary enclosure, where it may be observed swimming or ambulating. In aquatic species, buoyancy, limb use, respiratory pattern, and environmental awareness have to be assessed. Once "in hand," the animal should be weighed. Healthy chelonians often seem slightly heavier than expected when picked up. If an animal feels light, it may be malnourished or dehydrated. It is possible to overpower most smaller individuals, but patience and gentle, firm handling will often yield excellent results. Visual examination of the head, neck, limbs, and tail should help assess symmetry, skin condition, presence or absence of scars, ectoparasites, excess skin, overgrown nails, and presence and density of epibionts (algae and other commensal organisms) on the carapace. Presence of an abundance of epibionts may indicate chronicity of a problem. Thick algae on the carapace of a basking species may indicate that it has not hauled out to thermoregulate, and high numbers of barnacles on sea turtles may indicate prolonged lethargy or reduced activity, as healthy turtles tend to have cleaner shells. Evaluation of the gastrointestinal (GI) system starts with the oral cavity (often easily done with more aggressive species!) for abnormal mucosa or foreign bodies (fish hooks are common in some species). The cloaca is examined for swelling, foreign bodies, or trauma. Evaluation of the respiratory system is done through examination of the nares, choana, and glottis. This is followed by listening to respiration and auscultating the lung over the dorsum of the carapace. Percussion of both right and left lungs should sound the same. Neurologic evaluation includes observation of posture, carriage of head, symmetry of muscle mass, tone, and strength. Reflexes may be evaluated using tactile stimuli such as a toe pinch. Eyes should be clear and symmetrical, with no discharge or swelling of adnexa. The tympanum, located just caudal and ventral to the eye should be flat and bilaterally symmetrical. Abdominal palpation performed in the prefemoral fossae may reveal the presence of coelomic masses, ova, bladder stones, and ascites.

Blood samples should be drawn into tubes or syringes containing the anticoagulants sodium or lithium heparin. Ethylenediaminetetraacetic acid (EDTA) should not be used because it causes hemolysis, which precludes obtaining accurate hematocrits and electrolyte determination. In addition, blood smears do not stain optimally with EDTA compared with heparin. Several sites are easily accessible for blood collection. Venipuncture of the jugular is the most reliable site for uncontaminated peripheral blood samples. The jugular vein is easily visualized in most species when the head and neck are held in extension. Extending the head and neck may be challenging in strong or aggressive species and may require tranquilization to prevent injury. Sample contamination with lymph is common to most venipuncture sites other than the jugular vein. The dorsal coccygeal vein requires the least overall restraint and is located just dorsal to the dorsal aspect of the vertebral body on the tail. The needle is introduced into the dorsal skin at a 45- to 90-degree angle to the vertebra. Vascular access to the axillary branch of the brachial vein in the forelimb may be achieved by extending the animal's front leg and inserting a needle through the skin distal to the carpus and between the carpal flexor tendons aiming toward the posterior side of the carpal joint. The subcarapacal sinus is located just under the carapace immediately caudal to the last cervical and cranial to the first thoracic vertebrae. The venipuncture site may be accessed by pushing the head down and into the shell then palpating the bony prominence of the vertebra where it meets the carapace. The needle is inserted on the midline just caudal to the juncture of the skin with the carapace, aiming toward the carapace just cranial to the vertebral prominence. In sea turtles, the dorsal cervical sinus (supravertebral), located one third the distance from the carapace to the base of the skull, affords a reliable site for uncontaminated blood collection with minimal restraint. The head is directed forward and down, and an appropriate length needle (up to $3\frac{1}{2}$ inches in large animals) is introduced lateral to midline on either side. Raising the turtle's body relative to the head enhances filling of the sinus. Ultrasonography may be used to locate the vein if difficulty is encountered.

The occipital sinus may also be used for blood collection, but this requires that the head be restrained firmly in an extended position and tilted down at a 45-degree angle to the spine. A needle is introduced just caudal to the occiputus, perpendicular to the spine. Lymphatic contamination sometimes is encountered at this site.

Diagnostics

Hematology

Complete blood cell counts generally are performed using manual cell-counting techniques, although automated methods have been used for red blood cell (RBC) counts. Hemoglobin determination is accomplished by serometer, hemoglobinometer, or automated methods. Microhematocrit centrifugation is the standard for packed cell volume (PCV) determination. RBCs are nucleated and range in number from 0.154 to 0.980 × $10^6/\mu$L, depending on species and time of year. RBCs have long life spans, with the mean in box turtles being 600 to 800 days. Peak reticulocyte response to blood loss takes up to 5 weeks to achieve. Because turtles have a total blood volume of 5% to 8% of total body weight and the standard procedure is to limit blood collection to 10% of the total, restricting sample size to 0.5% to 0.8% of the body weight (0.5 to 0.8 mL for a 100-g animal) is appropriate. Drawing blood frequently over a short period or in excess of recommended volumes may cause iatrogenic anemia, which corrects slowly.

White blood cell (WBC) differentiation is best performed on smears that have been made immediately after collection. Heparin is the preferred anticoagulant because of less distortion of WBC

morphology. Blood smears made in the field do not stain well if staining is delayed more than a few days, even when they are fixed soon after being made. For best results, smears should be stained within a few hours of being made. Total WBC counts may be determined by the direct method (Natt-Herricks) or indirectly (phloxin B solution or estimation from smear). The most reliable results are obtained by consistent processing and analysis. All methods require some level of technical skill to achieve accuracy, and methods may not be comparable directly one with another within or between laboratories. It is ideal to use one laboratory and one or two technicians with similar training and skills, as significant variation may occur between laboratories because of the interpretations of the technicians handling the samples.

The chelonian leukocyte response is less predictable than in mammals or birds. Normal (reference) values are hard to establish because of variations by species, season, nutritional status, type of stain, venipuncture site, handling of sample, age, sex, and anticoagulant used. Twofold changes in a parameter constitute a significant change. The best use of hematologic values is to monitor a patient's response to therapy. Blood values change seasonally, especially with species that undergo brumation (hibernation). For example, total RBC counts are highest before brumation and lowest immediately thereafter. Other parameters change as well and should be considered relative to the environmental conditions and sample handling and processing. Heterophil counts increase during summer and decrease during brumation. Increased counts may indicate inflammation or bacterial disease. "Toxic" heterophils display cytoplasmic basophilia, abnormal granulation, and a lobed nucleus and are present in cases of inflammation. Eosinophilia may be seen in parasitic disease. Basophilia may be present in parasitic infection as well as in viral disease processes. Lymphocyte counts are low to absent in the winter and are low in cases of malnutrition and in diseases secondary to stress and immunosuppression. Lymphocytosis is seen in wound healing, parasitic disease, and viral infections. Monocyte numbers increase in granulomatous inflammation. Reference ranges for selected chelonian species are available elsewhere.[1]

Biochemistry

Biochemistries may be determined on plasma or serum. Whole blood should be cooled or centrifuged within 15 minutes of collection to prevent changes from RBC metabolism such as loss of potassium into the plasma. The anticoagulant EDTA causes changes in potassium and calcium directly and in other parameters through the effects of hemolysis.

Serum biochemical parameters are similarly affected by the factors that affect hematology values. Blood samples yield a higher volume of plasma compared with serum, so biochemical assays are routinely run on plasma. Often, blood samples are obtained with a varying degree of lymph contamination. Values of glucose, calcium, phosphorous, sodium, urea, and enzymes in lymph are comparable with those in plasma. Lymph is lower in total protein and potassium compared with plasma. Assessment of renal function in chelonians is more difficult because of the physiologic differences between freshwater, saltwater, and terrestrial species. Blood urea nitrogen (BUN) and creatinine are generally poor indicators of renal disease. Values are generally low (<40 milligrams per deciliter [mg/dL]) in terrestrial and freshwater species and higher in marine species (~100 mg/dL) and terrestrial species during dry season when they are conserving water. A low value in marine species may be an indicator of prolonged anorexia. Plasma uric acid levels in chelonians are generally lower than 5 mg/dL. Elevations may be seen in cases of bacteremia, septicemia, nephrocalcinosis, and nephrotoxicity but may also represent gout or the recent ingestion of a high-protein diet. Sodium levels range from 120 to 150 milliequivalents per liter (mEq/L) in tortoises and freshwater turtles and from 150 to 170 mEq/L in sea turtles. Hyponatremia may result from GI or renal disease, oversupplementation of fluids low in sodium, disease of the salt gland, or maintenance of saltwater species in fresh water. Hypernatremia may occur in dehydration or excessive dietary intake. Potassium levels normally range from 2 to 6 mEq/L. They are elevated because of hemolysis and reduced renal secretion and are low because of reduced intake or excess GI loss. Normal blood pH ranges from 7.5 to 7.7 at temperatures of 23° C to 25° C. Increasing temperature will reduce blood pH, and prolonged anesthesia will increase it. Blood calcium levels range from 8 to 11 mg/dL. Levels may increase two to four times because of follicular development. Levels less than 8 may be caused by anorexia, dietary deficiencies of calcium or vitamin D3, hypoalbuminemia, alkalosis, or hypoparathyroidism. Normal phosphorous levels range from 1 to 5 mg/dL. Low levels are caused by starvation or nutritional deficiency. Hyperphosphatemia results from excessive dietary phosphorous, hypervitaminosis D, renal disease, or severe tissue trauma or may be falsely elevated because of leakage from RBCs when not separated quickly enough from serum or plasma.

Aspartate aminotransferase (AST) and lactate dehydrogenase (LDH) activities are high in chelonian liver tissue but are not specific for this organ. AST is found in many tissues. Levels above 250 international units per liter (IU/L) suggest liver or muscle damage, septicemia, or toxicity. LDH levels above 1000 IU/L may be associated with hemolysis or with damage to the liver, heart, and skeletal muscle. Elevation of LDH and AST in the absence of elevation of creatinine kinase (CK) is indicative of liver disease. Plasma protein levels range from 3 to 7 g/dL. Low levels are seen in chronic malnutrition, protein-losing enteropathies, and maldigestion and in chronic liver and kidney disease. Elevated levels are most commonly seen during folliculogenesis but may also be seen in dehydration or may be caused by hyperglobulinemia associated with infectious disease. Plasma glucose normally ranges from 60 to 100 mg/dL. Low levels may be caused by starvation, malnutrition, hepatobiliary disease and septicemia. Elevated levels are most likely iatrogenic and caused by excess glucose administration or the administration of glucocorticoids. CK is a muscle-specific enzyme. Elevations occur with muscle injury from trauma, struggling, systemic infection, or administration of intramuscular injection of fluids or irritating drugs such as enrofloxacin. Reference ranges for selected chelonian species are available elsewhere.[1]

Other Tests

Serologic testing (enzyme-linked immunosorbent assay [ELISA]) for *Mycoplasma* spp. is performed readily on small quantities of plasma or serum. At the time of sampling, nasal flushes should be performed and frozen for polymerase chain reaction (PCR) testing or culture, to be run if the titer is positive.

Fresh or formalin-fixed feces may be used for fecal centrifugation or flotation and for direct examination for detection of enteric parasites and ova. Immunofluorescent antibody testing also may be performed for detection of *Cryptosporidium* spp. Fresh feces, feces in neutral media, and feces frozen in tryptose soy broth or neutral media are appropriate for enteric culture. Fresh or frozen feces also may be examined routinely under transmission electron microscopy for viral particles. If enteric clostridial infections are suspected, frozen feces may be used for assaying for clostridial toxins. Urinalysis may be performed on voided urine. The kidney cannot concentrate, and urine passes from the kidney, through the urodeum, into the bladder, so it cannot be considered sterile. Standard urine dipsticks appear to be useful but have not been validated on reptile urine. Urine pH tends to be alkaline in herbivorous species and acidic in carnivorous species. Urine protein levels should be zero to trace. Glucose should be negative. Hemoglobin, myoglobin, or RBCs may produce a positive reaction on the blood test of the strip. Any positive reading should be followed up with a urine sediment evaluation. Ketones may be detected from animals coming out of brumation or hibernation, but abnormal urine color may result in a false-positive test. Urine sediment evaluation may reveal crystals, casts, bacteria, fungi, protozoans, and helminth eggs. Interpretation of findings should be made relative to the animal's clinical presentation, keeping in mind that urine passes through the common urodeum and is likely contaminated with products from the genital and GI systems.

Gross postmortem evaluation with histopathologic examination should be done on any animal that has died.

Imaging

The old adage "A picture is worth a thousand words" holds true with respect to recording visual observations. Digital photographs are useful in recording the appearance of animals at presentation and for tracking change over time. Radiography is useful for diagnosing a variety of conditions. Three whole-body views commonly are obtained for general surveys: anteroposterior, dorsoventral, and lateral (Figures 4-4, 4-5, and 4-6). The anteroposterior and lateral

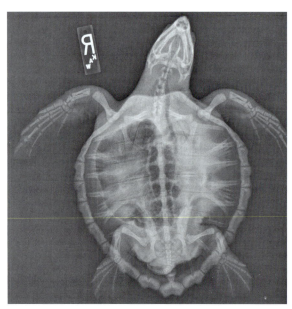

FIGURE 4-4 Dorsoventral radiograph of a Kemp's ridley sea turtle showing opacity in the left lung field.

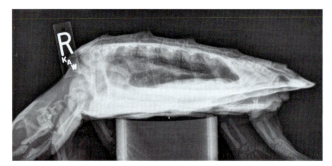

FIGURE 4-5 Horizontal beam lateral view of Kemp's ridley sea turtle.

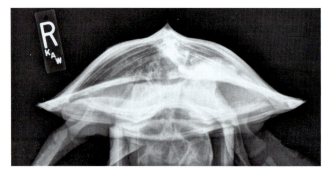

FIGURE 4-6 Horizontal beam anteroposterior view of Kemp's ridley sea turtle showing opacity in left lung field.

views are best obtained by maintaining the animal in a normal posture (rather than turning the animal on its side or upending it) with the x-ray tube being moved relative to the animal to obtain the desired view. The anteroposterior view is best for screening for potential pneumonia and the dorsoventral view for surveying the GI and reproductive systems. Contrast radiography is performed by administration of the appropriate media via gavage or intravenously. In leopard tortoises, transit time for barium sulfate from the stomach to the large intestine is 5 to 8 hours, with emptying of the large intestine occurring in 144 to 166 hours, whereas transit time in Galapagos giant tortoises may be 2 to 4 weeks.

Ultrasonography of the coelom commonly is performed to assess the cardiac, hepatic, renal, and reproductive systems. The prefemoral fossae provide a window to the coelom and are adequate for most studies. With animals that are too small for the ultrasound probe to fit into this space, the body of the animal may be placed into water, and scanning may be done with water providing conductivity so that the probe may be offset with resulting magnification of the images.

Magnetic resonance imaging (MRI) and computed tomography (CT) are modalities that are useful for imaging internal lesions after initial screening with radiography and ultrasonography.

Rigid endoscopy may be used for directly visualizing the viscera and taking biopsies and may be used for sex determination of young animals. Flexible endoscopy also provides nonsurgical access to the GI and respiratory tracts for evaluation and biopsy.

TREATMENT MODALITIES

Parenteral treatments may be administered intramuscularly, subcutaneously, intracoelomically, or intravenously. The pectoral muscle mass is the preferred site of intramuscular (IM) injection in most species. It may be accessed from the cranial direction and is ventral to the thoracic limb. Intracoelomic injections may be given from the cranial aspect between the bridge and the thoracic limb, directing the needle parallel to the bridge, and caudally toward the coelomic cavity. Injections may also be given into the prefemoral fossa, but it is easy to inject into the urinary bladder at this site. Intraosseous catheterization may be performed using the bones of the bridges of the shell.

Many treatments may be administered per os, on food, or with a ball-ended feeding tube. To avoid excessive restraint on the head and neck, many chelonians may be encouraged to open their mouths in a defensive posture. The lubricated feeding tube may be placed in the mouth quickly, and usually the animal, in an attempt to reject the metal object, will advance its head, and the feeding tube may be advanced gently down the esophagus without the head being tightly restrained.

For repeated gavage treatments or for enteral nutrition, use of an indwelling pharyngostomy tube is indicated. The animal is anesthetized, and the left side of the neck is prepared surgically. A closed hemostat is placed into the mouth and past the pharynx into the esophagus. An incision is made over the point of the hemostat, through the skin, and into the esophagus. A rubber feeding tube of appropriate size for the animal is grasped by the hemostats and pulled into the esophagus. The tube then is advanced to the level of the stomach, is secured with sutures at the neck, and then is taped to the carapace, leaving enough length for extension of the neck. Taping of the left leg into the shell to prevent it from dislodging the tube may be necessary. Pharyngostomy tubes may be left in place for months. Aquatic turtles may have access to water with the tube in place. In the case of anorexic animals, the tube should be left in place until the animal is eating consistently.[5]

Treatment of pneumonia may be enhanced by using pulmonic catheters for direct administration of antimicrobials or removal of mucous or purulent material. To place the catheter, a small hole is made in the carapace, and a catheter with stylet is introduced into the lung. Samples for culture may be obtained through the catheter before introducing medication. The catheter is capped with an injection port and taped to the carapace. In the case of aquatic animals, silicon or cyanoacrylic may be used to seal the hole to prevent entry of water.[5]

DISEASES

The relative prevalence of disease in captive chelonia is related to husbandry, housing, and movements of animals among collections (Tables 4-3 to 4-5). Environments that are stable, with the provision of adequate nutrition and few or no additions of new animals, afford little opportunity for infectious disease to gain a foothold. At the other end of the spectrum are some animal dealers and collections with numerous additions of animals from diverse sources, fluctuations in environmental conditions, and marginal nutrition. Under those extremes, without proper quarantine programs, infectious diseases are not uncommon. Additionally, individual animals are more likely to be affected by potential pathogens when good husbandry practices are not followed. In free-ranging animals, change in habitat, vegetative cover, water clarity, temperature, food resources or predators from change associated with invasive species, and the introduction of novel potential pathogens are important determinants of disease status. The presence of a potential pathogen is not synonymous with disease and should be evaluated relative to the condition of the animal and the potential impact on a group of animals, captive or free-ranging.

Diseases of concern in captive collections include infectious, parasitic, nutritional, metabolic, and traumatic. Infectious diseases may be controlled or prevented by screening animals before adding them to a collection, by quarantining all incoming animals, and by maintaining good environmental conditions and hygiene. During quarantine routine physical examination, fecal centrifugation or flotation, and direct examination, screening for pertinent infectious diseases, survey radiography, complete blood cell count and chemistries, and banking of plasma for further testing, if necessary, should all be performed. Treatment for parasites should be provided, as indicated (Tables 4-6 and 4-7). Animals showing signs of illness, in quarantine and in the collection, should be isolated until resolution of the problem. Because some diseases may be spread via fomites or other secondary methods, all quarantined or ill animals should be serviced after healthy ones or preferably by separate staff.

Routine screening tests may sometimes yield positive results for potential pathogens. Decisions regarding the significance of the finding should not depend solely on the test results but should take into consideration such factors as the test status of potential contact animals, predictive value of the test for the species in question, value of the animal (genetic, conservation), morbidity or mortality potential of the disease being tested, and treatment possibilities. As chelonian-specific testing modalities are developed, more diseases will be elucidated. Pathogens may be encountered in species or individuals where they were not previously recognized or encountered. A condition of "zero risk" is unlikely to be achieved with respect to disease transmission. Relative risks and potentially mitigating actions need to be evaluated and weighed against the conservation, education, or display potential of the action considered. This holds true for translocations of free-ranging animals as well.

REPRODUCTION

All chelonia lay shelled eggs on land, usually in a nest cavity dug with the hindlimbs. The texture of the eggs ranges from leathery to hard. Clutch size may range from one in small tortoises and turtles, to greater than 100 in sea turtles and some freshwater turtles. Clutch size and potentially the number of clutches per season are influenced by nutritional status. In desert tortoises, the number of eggs laid is reduced rather than a size reduction of the eggs laid during a poor nutritional state.[2] Incubation time may vary from 45 to 360 days, depending on the species. A few species have been shown to undergo diapause prior to embryonic development, potentially extending incubation time by months, even within the same species. Most species of turtles have temperature-dependent sex

TABLE 4-3

Selected Infectious Diseases of Chelonians

Disease (Agent)	Epizootiology and Affected Species	Signs	Diagnosis	Management
Adenovirus (Siadenovirus)	Sulawesi tortoise (*Indotestudo forsteni*)	Anorexia, lethargy, mucosal ulcerations and palatine erosions of the oral cavity, nasal and ocular discharge, and diarrhea	Consensus PCR and sequencing	Quarantine, isolation, potential treatment with cidofovir
Herpesviral infection of tortoises, freshwater turtles, and sea turtles (gray-patch disease; lung, eye, and trachea disease; fibropapillomatosis) (Herpesvirus)	Animal-to-animal and contaminated environment. Documented in freshwater turtles, tortoises, and sea turtles	Nasal discharge, weight loss, necrotizing bronchitis, hepatitis, conjunctivitis, stomatitis, tracheitis, pneumonia, dermatitis, fibropapillomatous tumors, and death	Histopathology: intranuclear inclusions in a variety of tissues; plasma neutralization and plasma ELISA; isolation of virus in viral culture	Isolate infected animals. Supportive care is required. Excise tumors
Iridovirus, Ranavirus (Iridovirus)	Tortoises (*Testudo and Gopherus*), Eastern box turtles (*Terrapene carolina*)	Necrotic stomatitis, esophagitis, rhinitis, pneumonia, abscess, splenitis, vasculitis, and death	Hepatic foci and basophilic intracytoplasmic inclusions. Consensus PCR and sequencing	Isolate affected animals. Supportive care. No specific treatment is available
Salmonellosis (*Salmonella* spp.)	All species are susceptible. Found commonly in asymptomatic animals. May cause disease when new serotypes are encountered or with concomitant stressors	Enteritis and sepsis	Blood culture and cloacal culture	Appropriate systemic antibiotic and supportive treatment are required
Septicemic cutaneous ulcerative disease (Bacteria, including *Citrobacter freundii* and *Pseudomonas* spp.)	Animals in contaminated environment or with chronic environmental stressors. Aquatic turtles and many species are susceptible	Cutaneous ulceration, sloughing skin, septicemia, dehydration, and death	Clinical signs; blood culture; and cutaneous culture	Provide antibiotic therapy; increase environmental temperature; increase salinity of the water temporarily; use medicated baths; and give supportive care
Upper respiratory disease (*Mycoplasma* spp.)	Animal to animal contact, possibly fomites. Tortoises (*Gopherus and Testudo*). Serosurveys indicate exposure in other groups of chelonia	Nasal and ocular discharge, pneumonia, weight loss, unthriftiness, and death	PCR of nasal flush, rising serological titers, and culture	Isolate seropositive animals. May attempt treatment with systemic antibiotics. Supportive care is required

ELISA, Enzyme-linked immunosorbent assay; *PCR*, polymerase chain reaction.

determination, that is, the sex of the embryo is determined by the temperatures to which the eggs are exposed during certain stages of incubation. With exception, females are produced at higher temperatures and males at lower temperatures. Age at reproduction varies by species. Large, slow-growing tortoises may require 15 to 20 years to reach sexual maturity. Faster growth may result in breeding at an earlier age, and slow growth may delay reproduction for years. Research has shown that in desert tortoises (*Gopherus agassizii*), reaching adult size and weight is not a predictor of successful reproduction in females.

During folliculogenesis, plasma calcium levels exceeding 25 mg/dL, globulin levels greater than 8.0, and cholesterol levels greater than 200 are not uncommon. Folliculogenesis may be diagnosed directly by ultrasonography or indirectly via plasma biochemicals. If oviductal eggs are detected by palpation or appear to be calcified via ultrasonography, radiography may be used to count the number of eggs present. If females do not have a secure place to deposit their eggs, they may retain them for an extended period. One method for recovering eggs to lower the likelihood of damage is to place the animal in a shallow pool of water after administering oxytocin (10 IU/kg intramuscularly or intracoelomically, or 7.5 IU oxytocin/kg mixed with 1.5 mg/kg prostaglandin F2α [Feldmans M, personal communication]). The eggs will be deposited in the water and then float so that the animal is less likely to crush them than if they were deposited on land in a less than optimal site. Also, when there are multiple animals in an exhibit, exhibit mates are less likely to damage the eggs. Several species have been observed not to deposit all the eggs present in the oviduct in one clutch. Retention of shelled eggs in an otherwise healthy animal is not cause for concern. If the animal becomes anorexic or lethargic or otherwise seems systemically affected, more aggressive intervention consisting of subcutaneous or intracoelomic administration of fluids, calcium gluconate (100 mg/kg), and repeated oxytocin or oxytocin with prostaglandin is indicated. Surgical extraction of the eggs occasionally is required. Rarely,

TABLE 4-4

Selected Noninfectious and Nutritional Diseases of Chelonians

Disorder	Cause	Signs	Treatment
Drowning	Fishing nets; getting caught in drains or on obstacles in enclosures	Dyspnea or apnea, raspy respirations, coma, and death	Treat for shock; keep on a head-down incline; intubate and apply PPV; oxygenate; and give antibiotics.
Foreign body ingestion	Unusual items in environment mistaken for food items and ingested (plastic bags, coins, or fish hooks)	Weight loss and lethargy; diagnosis with radiography and endoscopy	Remove foreign body via endoscopy, laparoscopy, stomach flushing, or surgery
Hyperthermia	Not able to thermoregulate downward	Hyperactivity, then depression and subsequent organ failure	Cool animal to ambient temperature with water baths, provide intracoelomic fluids, treat for shock, and administer antibiotics
Hypervitaminosis A	Iatrogenic, administration of too high a dose of vitamin A parenterally, or chronic dietary oversupplementation	Flaking and sloughing skin	Treat sloughed skin locally and prevent infection until skin is healed
Hypothermia; cold stunned	Sea turtles (rapid change in water temperatures); captive or terrestrial (sudden suboptimal temperatures with no basking areas available)	Coma, flaccidity, depressed respirations, and bradycardia	Warm animal to optimal temperatures slowly over days to weeks Give supportive treatment with fluids, steroids, antibiotics, antifungals, and parenteral nutrition
Hypovitaminosis A	Deficiency of vitamin A in diet	Squamous metaplasia blepharoedema, nasal discharge, and pneumonia	Give vitamin A parenterally once or twice, followed by addition of vitamin A to diet
Metabolic bone disease	Low calcium diet, inadequate exposure to ultraviolet radiation, chronic low environmental temperatures, and renal failure	Soft shells, abnormal shell formation, inability to raise body off of ground, and hypocalcemic tetany	Increase dietary calcium without increasing phosphorus; provide a source of ultraviolet radiation; administer calcium gluconate parenterally; increase environmental temperatures; address cause of renal failure; and treat symptomatically
Pneumonia	Bacteria, fungus, or protozoa; chronically low environmental temperatures Fungal pneumonia may be seen subsequent to prolonged antibiotic use	Mucopurulent tracheal discharge, radiographic lesions in lungs, and floating asymmetrically in water	Parenteral antimicrobial therapy, intrapulmonic therapy, and supportive care are required Prolonged treatment usually is required
Scute abnormalities	Genetic and incubation factors	Asymmetry of scutes sometimes results in significant deformities during growth	Supportive and palliative care are required
Shell rot	Bacteria, possible emboli, or fungus; environmental contamination; suboptimal environmental and nutritional conditions; and sequelae to sepsis, inability to bask at preferred temperature	Soft spots in shell, hyperemia, fibrinonecrotic debris	Provide systemic antimicrobial therapy and antimicrobial baths Do not debride over-vigorously too often Prolonged treatment usually is required.
Shell trauma	External force	Shell broken or displaced	Surgically debride and cleanse; repair with external fixation (acrylics, wires, and tape)

PPV, Positive pressure ventilation.

an egg may be too large to pass. However, some softening of the posterior portions of the shell may occur, allowing an apparently oversized egg to pass. In most cases, failure to lay eggs is attributable to concurrent nutritional, infectious, or husbandry problems.

Assessing reproductive status of free-ranging females successfully is accomplished by ultrasonography. Although the numbers of eggs cannot be determined accurately, for field studies that occur other than just during egg laying (5% to 10% of the year), ultrasonography provides a way to assess ovarian activity without exposing the ovary to multiple radiographic events. The presence of mature ovarian follicles does not ensure that ovulation will occur because some females are capable of resorbing preovulatory follicles.

The primary reproductive problem in males is a prolapsed phallus. Occasionally, during attempted breeding, an injury may occur or the time of engorgement or extrusion out of the cloaca may be extended. Retraction of the phallus becomes impossible because of damage to musculature or directly to the phallus. If intervention occurs early enough, the organ may be cleansed and manually replaced into the cloaca, and a purse string suture may be placed around the cloaca for 5 to 7 days. Attempts to reduce engorgement by using hyperosmotic agents, topical steroids, and cooling may be helpful. If the phallus cannot be reduced promptly and kept in place, it will reprolapse readily and may require amputation, which may be done under general or epithecal anesthesia.

TABLE 4-5

Selected Parasitic Diseases of Chelonia

Disease	Etiologic Life Cycle	Location in Host	Diagnosis	Clinical Signs	Management
Acariasis (ticks)	Nymphs and adults on chelonians They drop off to lay eggs	Axillary, inguinal, neck, and shell	Visual	Usually minor May cause dermatitis	Use resmethrin and pyrethrins Spray is approved for use in chelonians USDA is concerned about imported tortoises because of presence of *Cowdria ruminatum* in some ticks.
Amebiasis	Direct	Colon, liver, and portal vessels	Direct fecal and histopathologic examinations	Weight loss, enteritis, and death	Keep terrestrial and aquatic separate Treat with metronidazole, paromomycin, or iodochlorhydroxyquin
Coccidiosis	Direct; may be intermediate host	Intestine, renal, and intranuclear	Fecal and histopathologic examination	Renal failure, enteritis, weight loss, and death	Treatment of renal coccidia with toltrazuril may be attempted Treat enteric coccidea with sulfonamides
Cryptosporidium spp.	Direct	Mucosa of stomach and intestine	Fecal, gastric wash IFA and direct plasma EIA	Usually none; may be associated with chronic weight loss	No treatments are proven; toltrazuril has been used.
Hexamitiasis	Direct	Kidney and gall bladder	Cloacal wash	Weight loss and depression	Isolate ill animals and treat with metronidazole, paromomycin, or iodochlorhydroxyquin
Nematodes	Direct and/or intermediate host	Gastrointestinal tract, vascular microfilaria, and lungs	Fecal flotation, direct, lung wash, and blood smear	Weight loss, enteritis, gastrointestinal blockage, pneumonia	Administer parasiticade and give supportive therapy Do not use Ivermectin!
Trematodes	Amphibians, crustaceans are intermediate hosts	Liver, gall bladder, lungs, and vascular system	Direct visualization, lung washes, and sedimentation fecal exams	Pneumonia, granulomatous inflammation, and enteritis	Treat with albendazole, Praziquantel Freeze intermediate hosts before feeding

EIA, Enzyme immunoassay; *IFA,* immunofluorescent antibody; *USDA,* U.S. Department of Agriculture.

TABLE 4-6

Antimicrobials Recommended for Chelonians

Generic Name	Dosage (mg/kg)	Route	Interval (Hours)	Duration
Amikacin	2.5–5	IM	48–72	5–10 Tx
Ampicillin	20–50	IM	12–24	7–14 days
Carbenicillin	200–400	IM	48	5–7 Tx
Ceftazidime	20–40	IM	48–72	5–14 Tx
Ceftiofur sodium	2.2–4	IM	24	7–21 days
Chloramphenicol	25–50	IM or PO	24	7–14 days
Clarithromycin	15	PO	48–72	5–7 days
Doxycycline	50 once, then 25	IM	72	5–7 Tx
Enrofloxacin	2.5–10	IM or PO	24–96	7–21 days Do not use IM in Galapagos tortoises
Fluconazole	5	PO	24	10–40 Tx
Gentamicin	5–10	IM	48–72	5 Tx
Ketoconazole	15–30	PO	24	7–21 days
Metronidazole	20–50	PO	24	5–14 days
Oxytetracycline	5–10 mg/kg	IM	24	5–10 days
Trimethoprim- sulfamethoxazole	30	PO	24	7–10 days

IM, Intramuscular; *PO,* by mouth; *Tx,* treatment(s).

TABLE 4-7

Parasiticides Recommended for Chelonians

Generic Name (Trade Name)	Dosage (mg/kg)	Route	Frequency and Duration	Comments
Albendazole (Valbazen)	50	PO	Repeat in 2 weeks	Flukes and nematodes
Fenbendazole (Panacur)	25–50	PO	1–3 days; repeat in 10–14 days	Leukopenia at higher doses
Levamisole (Levasol)	5–10	SQ or intracoelomic	Every 14 days for two treatments	Nematodes
Metronidazole (Flagyl)	100	PO	Every 14 days for three treatments	Protozoa
Paromomycin (Humatin)	35–100	PO	Every 24 hours for up to 4 weeks	Amebae and cryptosporidia
Permethrin (Provent-a-mite)	1 second/ square foot	Topical spray	Axillary and inguinal regions 1–5 seconds	Immediate kill of ticks Rinse aquatic turtles before placing in water Approved for use by USDA for imported chelonians
Praziquantel (Droncit)	8 or 25 TID for 1 day	SQ, IM, or PO	Repeat in 2 weeks	For tapeworms and flukes Sprirorchidiasis in sea turtles
Sulfadimethoxine (Sulmet)	90 once, then 45	PO	Every 24 hours for 5–7 days	Coccidia
Toltrazuril (Baycox)	15	PO	Every 3 weeks	For intranuclear coccidia; not available in the United States

IM, Intramuscular; *PO*, by mouth; *SQ*, subcutaneous; *USDA*, U.S. Department of Agriculture.

CONSIDERATIONS FOR FREE-RANGING CHELONIANS

The long-term survival of many species of turtles and tortoises is precarious. Field studies and attempts at protection and enhancement of survival have been in progress for years and are increasing in number. Well-meaning attempts to bolster populations via translocations or introductions of animals have been undertaken in the past, with little attention paid to health considerations. The International Union for the Conservation of Nature, Species Survival Commission Reintroduction Specialist Group and the Veterinary Advisory Group have specific guidelines for the quarantine and health assessment of individuals before their release into the wild. For the safety of recipient populations, any animals bred or reared in captivity and intended for release should be raised in strict quarantine away from other animals. In addition, providing health screening for free-ranging populations is recommended to establish baseline levels of individual health parameters and group exposure to diseases and chemical contaminants and to assess reproductive and nutritional status. Longitudinal studies through such efforts may provide an indication of the long-term health of a population independent of whether they are involved in reintroduction or translocation projects.

BIBLIOGRAPHY

Barten SL: Shell damage. In Mader DR, editor: *Reptile medicine and surgery*, ed 2, St. Louis, MO, 2006, Elsevier.

Berry KH, Christopher MM: Guidelines for the field evaluation of desert tortoise health and disease. *J Wildl Dis* 37(3):427–450, 2001.

Boyer TH, Boyer DM: Turtles, tortoises, and terrapins. In Mader DR, editor: *Reptile medicine and surgery*, ed 2, St. Louis, MO, 2006, Elsevier.

Campbell TW: Clinical pathology of reptiles. In Mader DR, editor: *Reptile medicine and surgery*, ed 2, St. Louis, MO, 2006, Elsevier.

Campbell TW, Ellis CK: *Avian and exotic animal hematology and cytology*, ed 2, Ames, IA, 2007, Blackwell.

Christopher TE, Henen BR, Smith EM, et al: Does a high plane of nutrition decrease age of reproduction in desert tortoises (Gopherus agassizzi)? In *Proceedings of the second symposium of the Comparative Nutrition Society*, Banff, Alberta, 1998.

Divers SJ: Reptile diagnostic endoscopy and endosurgery. *Vet Clin North Am Exot Anim Pract* 13(2):217–242, 2010.

Duncan A: Reptile and amphibian analgesia. In Miller RE, Fowler ME, editors: *Zoo and wild animal medicine, current therapy*, ed 7, St. Louis, MO, 2012, Elsevier.

Fitzgerald KT, Vera R: Reported toxicities in reptiles. In Mader DR, editor: *Reptile medicine and surgery*, ed 2, St. Louis, MO, 2006, Elsevier.

Flanagan JP: Vets and conservation: helping to restore the balance. *Vet Rec* 2011. doi: 10.1136/vr.d194.

Garner MM, Gardiner C, Linn M, et al: Seven new cases of intranuclear coccidiosis in tortoises: an emerging disease? In *Proceedings of the American Association of Zoo Veterinarians and American Association of Wildlife Veterinarians*, Omaha, NB, 1998.

Hatt JM: Raising giant tortoises. In Fowler ME, Miller RE, editors: *Zoo and wild animal medicine, current therapy*, ed 6, St. Louis, MO, 2008, Elsevier.

Holz P: Renal anatomy and physiology. In Mader DR, editor: *Reptile medicine and surgery*, ed 2, St. Louis, MO, 2006, Elsevier.

Innis CJ, Boyer TH: Chelonian reproductive disorders. *Vet Clin North Am Exot Anim Pract* 5(3):555–578, 2002.

International Union for Conservation of Nature and Natural Resources Species Survival Commission: *Guidelines for re-introductions*, Gland, Switzerland, 1995, IUCN Press.

Jacobson ER: *Infectious diseases and pathology of reptiles*, Boca Raton, 2007, CRC Press.

Jacobson ER, Berry KH, Wellehan JFX, et al: Serologic and molecular evidence for testunidid herpesvirus 2 infection in wild Agassiz's desert tortoises, Gopherus agassizii. *J Wildlife Dis* 48:747, 2012.

Kimble SJA, Williams RA: Temporal variance in hematologic and plasma biochemical reference intervals for free-ranging eastern box turtles (*Terrapene carolina carolina*). *J Wildlife Dis* 48:799, 2012.

Knafo SJ, Divers S, Rivera S, et al: Sterilisation of hybrid Galapagos tortoises (*Geochelone nigra*) for island restoration. Part 1: endoscopic oophorectomy of females under ketamine-medetomidine anaesthesia. *Vet Rec* 2011.

Kuchling G: How to minimize risk and optimize information gain in assessing reproductive condition and fecundity of live female chelonians. *Chelonian Conserv Biol* 3(1):118–123, 1998.

Ladyman JM, Kuchling G, Burford D, et al: Skin disease affecting the conservation of the western swamp tortoise (*Pseudemydura umbrina*). *Aust Vet J* 76(11):743–745, 1998.

Martinez-Jimenez D, Hernandez-Divers SJ: Emergency care of reptiles. *Vet Clin North Am Exot Anim Pract* 10(2):557–585, 2007.

McArthur S, Barrows M: Nutrition. In McArthur S, Wilkinson R, Meyer J, editors: *Medicine and surgery of tortoises and turtles*, Ames, IA, 2004, Blackwell Publishing Ltd.

Mosley C: Pain and nociception in reptiles. *Vet Clin North Am Exot Anim Pract* 14(1):45–60, 2011.

Muro J, Cuenca R, Pastor J, et al: Effects of lithium heparin and tripotassium EDTA on hematologic values of Hermann's tortoises (*Testudo hermanni*). *J Zoo Wildl Med* 29(1):40–44, 1998.

Murray MJ: Cardiopulmonary anatomy and physiology. In Mader DR, editor: *Reptile medicine and surgery*, ed 2, St. Louis, MO, 2006, Elsevier.

Norton TM, Walsh MT: Sea turtle rehabilitation. In Miller RE, Fowler ME, editors: *Zoo and wild animal medicine, current therapy*, ed 7, St. Louis, MO, 2012, Elsevier.

Origgi FC: Herpesvirus in tortoises. In Mader DR, editor: *Reptile medicine and surgery*, ed 2, St. Louis, MO, 2006, Elsevier.

Origgi FC, Jacobson ER: Diseases of the respiratory tract of chelonians. *Vet Clin North Am Exot Anim Pract* 3(2):537–549, 2000.

Ritchie B: Virology. In Mader DR, editor: *Reptile medicine and surgery*, ed 2, St. Louis, MO, 2006, Elsevier.

Rivera S, Divers SJ, Knafo SE, et al: Sterilisation of hybrid Galapagos tortoises (*Geochelone nigra*) for island restoration. Part 2: phallectomy of males under intrathecal anaesthesia with lidocaine. *Vet Rec* 2011.

Schumacher J: Respiratory medicine of reptiles. *Vet Clin North Am Exot Anim Pract* 13(2):207–224, 2011.

Schumacher J: Fungal diseases of reptiles. *Vet Clin North Am Exot Anim Pract* 6(2):327–335, 2003.

Sykes JM: Updates and practical approaches to reproductive disorders in reptiles. *Vet Clin North Am Exot Anim Pract* 13(3):349–373, 2010.

Turtle Taxonomy Working Group [Van Dijk PP, Iverson JB, et al]: Turtles of the world, 2011 update: annotated checklist of taxonomy, synonymy, distribution, and conservation status. In Rhodin AGJ, Pritchard PCH, van Dijk PP, et al, editors: *Conservation biology of freshwater turtles and tortoises: a compilation project of the IUCN/SSC Tortoise and Freshwater Turtle Specialist Group*, Chelonian Research Monographs No.5, pp. 000.165-000.242, doi:10.3854/crm.5.000.checklist.v4.2011. http://www.iucn-tftsg.org/cbftt/.

Westhouse RA, Jacobson ER, Harris RK, et al: Respiratory and pharyngoesophageal iridovirus infection in a gopher tortoise (*Gopherus polyphemus*). *J Wildlife Dis* 32(4):682–686, 1996.

Wyneken J: The anatomy of sea turtles. U.S. Department of Commerce NOAA Technical Memorandum NMFS-SEFSC-470, 2001.

Wyneken J, Godfrey MH, Bels V, editors: *Biology of turtles*, Boca Raton, FL, 2008, CRC Press.

Zwart P: Renal pathology in reptiles. *Vet Clin North Am Exot Anim Pract* 9(1):129–159, 2006.

REFERENCES

1. Gibbons PM, Klaphake E, Carpenter JW: Reptiles. In Carpenter JW, editor: *Exotic animal formulary*, ed 4, St. Louis, MO, 2013, Elsevier.
2. Henen BT, Oftedal OT: The importance of dietary nitrogen to the reproductive output of female desert tortoises (Gopherus agassizii). In *Proceedings of the second symposium of the Comparative Nutrition Society*, Banff, Alberta, 1998, pp 83–88.
3. Hunt CJG: Herpesvirus outbreak in a group of Mediterranean tortoises (*Testudo* spp). *Vet Clin North Am Exot Anim Pract* 9(3):568–574, 2006.
4. Jacobson ER, Berry KH: *Mycoplasma testudineum* in free-ranging desert tortoises, (*Gopherus agassizii*). *J Wildlife Dis* 48:1063, 2012.
5. Mitchell MA: Therapeutics. In Mader DR, editor: *Reptile medicine and surgery*, ed 2, St. Louis, MO, 2006, Elsevier.
6. Rivera S, Wellehan JF, McManamon R, et al: Systemic adenovirus infection in Sulawesi tortoises (*Indotestudo forsteni*) caused by a novel siadenovirus. *J Vet Diagn Invest* 21(4):415–426, 2009.
7. Schumacher J, Yellen T: Anesthesia and analgesia. In Mader DR, editor: *Reptile medicine and surgery*, ed 2, St. Louis, MO, 2006, Elsevier.
8. Wellehan JFX: Virology of nonavian reptiles: an update. In Miller RE, Fowler ME, editors: *Zoo and wild animal medicine, current therapy*, ed 7, St. Louis, MO, 2012, Elsevier.
9. Wyneken J, Mader DR, Weber ES, Merigo C: Medical care of sea turtles. In Mader DR, editor: *Reptile medicine and surgery*, ed 2, St. Louis, MO, 2006, Elsevier.

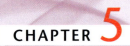

CHAPTER 5

Crocodilians (Crocodiles, Alligators, Caiman, Gharial)

Gregory J. Fleming[†] and Deidre K. Fontenot

Many of the 26 living crocodilian species are now endangered and are in need of both in situ and ex situ conservation programs. Because of this, crocodilians are more commonly being held in captive situations in conservation facilities, including zoos. Crocodilians are often long-lived display animals popular with zoo guests and require the skilled attention of veterinary and husbandry teams alike.

[†]Deceased.

ANATOMY AND PHYSIOLOGIC CONSIDERATIONS

Respiratory System

Crocodilians spend much of their time with their bodies entirely submerged with the exception of their eyes and nares. Each nostril acts as a water-proof valve that is closed with a muscular flap (composed of skeletal muscle) during submersion. In gharials

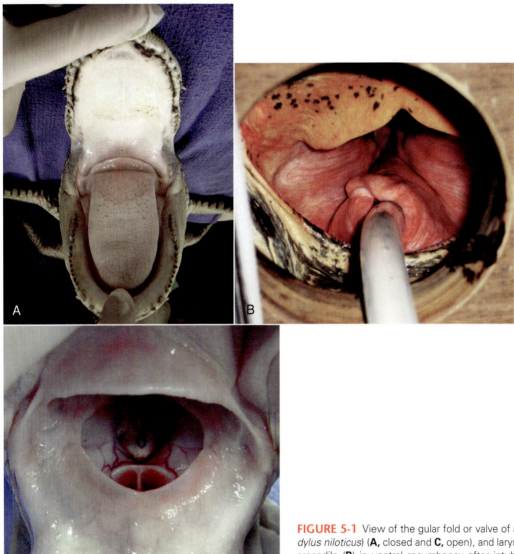

FIGURE 5-1 View of the gular fold or valve of a juvenile Nile crocodile (*Crocodylus niloticus*) (**A**, closed and **C**, open), and laryngeal view in an adult male Nile crocodile (**B**) in ventral recumbency after intubation during anesthetic procedure. Note the oral speculum wrapped with tape to secure the mouth open and the endotracheal tube in place.

(*Gavialis gangeticus*), the nasal opening has developed into a large protuberance, which acts as a vocal resonator.[26] Closing the nares may be obtunded by immobilizing agents that relax the muscles of the nostril allowing water into the respiratory tract.[6] An additional respiratory valve is formed by the soft palate and gular fold in crocodilians.[20] The elongated soft palate (palatine flap) presses down against the dorsal flap of the tongue forming the gular valve. This seal allows the crocodilian to open its mouth underwater without water rushing into the internal nares and the glottis. The gular valve has to be displaced to visualize the glottis for endotracheal intubation (Figure 5-1). The glottis has two folds, and in most crocodilians, the trachea bends to the left (not in alligators) before bifurcation to allow for large pieces of prey to be swallowed.[8,14] The lungs are well developed, and the vessel walls are thicker than in mammals to compensate for extra pressure during diving events. The primary respiratory muscle groups are the intercostal muscles and two transverse membranes, the postpulmonary membrane and the posthepatic membrane, both of which comprise primarily fibrous tissue with a muscular component.[8] The postpulmonary membrane separates the lungs from the liver, and the posthepatic membrane is attached to a sheet of muscle that enters at the os pubis. These two membranes act as a diaphragm. They, along with other coelomic partitions, also make endoscopic visualization of coelomic organs difficult (Figure 5-2). Ventilation is achieved by expanding the intercostal muscles, and then membranes pull the liver in a caudal direction creating a negative pressure around the lungs. The lungs expand, and the air is drawn into the nostrils and into the lungs. The glottic valve is then closed, holding the air in the lungs. Once the glottic valve relaxes, air in the lungs is expelled passively via the elastic recoil of the intercostal muscles and the postpulmonary or posthepatic membranes and lung tissue.[8] It is important to note that if the thoracic cavity is compressed, the animal cannot breathe. This may take place during restraint, as it is common to see multiple people sitting on the back of a crocodilian.

Cardiovascular System

Crocodiles are the only reptiles that possess four-chambered hearts.[16, 18] The heart functions like that of mammals; however, a number of anatomic differences allow for adaptation for an aquatic lifestyle. The three main differences are (1) a right aorta, which supplies the lungs, and a left aorta, which bypasses the lungs; (2) connective tissue extensions into the pulmonary outflow tract of the right ventricle, which restrict blood flow to the lungs (during diving) and allow a left to right shunt; and (3) the foramen of

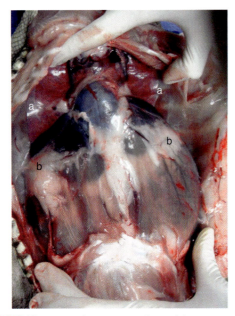

FIGURE 5-2 The post-pulmonary membrane (a) separates the lungs from the liver and the post-hepatic membrane (b) is attached to a sheet of muscle which enters at the os pubis. These two membranes act as a diaphragm.

Panizza, an opening between the left and right aortic arches allowing pressure equalization during diastole. All work together to ensure supply of blood to the coronary and cephalic circulation during a complete shutdown of the left side of the heart, which might occur during prolonged dives.[1,16,18]

The foramen of Panizza is a small opening located between the interventricular septum at the confluence of the left and right aortic arches.[16] This opening acts as a pressure valve allowing blood to flow between the venous and arterial systems. This flow from high pressure to low pressure results in venous admixture. When the animal is breathing, left ventricular pressure is greater, allowing a small amount of oxygenated blood to flow through the foramen of Panizza into the venous blood supply. When the crocodilian submerges, air held in the lungs restricts blood flow through the pulmonary capillary beds, resulting in pulmonary hypertension which increases right ventricular and pulmonary arterial pressures. As a result, blood flows from right to left through the foramen of Panizza.[16] Deoxygenated blood is diverted away from the lungs through the left aortic arch to organs that are not sensitive to low levels of oxygen (e.g., liver and stomach).[8] Oxygenated blood is diverted to oxygen-sensitive organs (i.e., the heart and the brain). A combination of blood shunting and anaerobic metabolism may allow an inactive crocodilian to stay submerged for 5 to 6 hours.[14] This right-to-left shunt through the foramen of Panizza may have clinical implications during anesthesia when the crocodilian does not have ventilatory support or is apneic. Shunting of blood away from the lungs will delay inhalant anesthetic uptake and removal. This emphasizes the importance of assisted ventilation during any immobilization event.

Blood Volume

Blood volume in crocodilians appears to be less than that in mammals, with a total blood volume of between 3.5% and 5.5%.[1,14,16,18] Thus, the maximum blood volume to remove from a crocodile will be about 0.03% to 0.05% by weight.

Renal Portal System

Crocodilians possess a renal portal system composed of the renal portal vein arising from the epigastric and external iliac veins.[16]

These vessels drain blood from the dorsal body wall, the cloaca, the sex organs, and the bladder. Drugs injected into the caudal half of the body, base of the tail and hindlimbs, may be cleared by the kidneys prior to reaching the systemic circulation. In other reptile species such as the red-eared slider, studies have showed a significant hepatic first-pass effect following hindlimb drug administration.[10] A study comparing forelimb and hindlimb injections of buprenorphine in red-eared sliders resulted in a 70% decrease in the bioavailability of buprenorphine when injected in the hindlimb.[13] Additionally, it appears that opioids are highly susceptible to significant hepatic extraction in reptiles.[8] Thus, care should be taken when administering nephrotoxic drugs in the hindlimbs, and when possible, anesthetic drugs should be injected in the forelimbs until further research is completed on crocodilian vascular anatomy.[17] However, the author of this chapter routinely uses the tail base and the hindlimbs for intramuscular drug delivery for safety reasons, with no complications and desired effects.

Eyes

Crocodilians have three eyelids: the upper, the lower, and the third eyelid, the nictitating membrane, which is translucent and protects the eye during diving. The eye may also be retracted into the socket via a skeletal muscle during feeding, and the retina has a tapedum lucidum to assist with night vision.[14]

Ears

Bilateral ear openings, just caudal to the eyes on the top of the skull, are covered by a flap that closes during diving. Once past this flap, the tympanic membrane may be visualized; however, the opening is very small and it may difficult to open in an unanesthetized crocodilian. The eustachian tubes leave the inner ear and enter the pharynx just caudal of the internal nares.[3] Inner ear infections are not common but may result in neurologic clinical signs such as spinning or rolling.

Skin

The skin of crocodilians contains both scales and scutes but no sweat glands. The dorsal scutes over the head and back contain bony plates, called *osteoderms*, which make darting or injecting challenging (Figure 5-3). Glandular secretions may occur from paired gular glands on the ventral mandible and some in the lips and cloaca in Nile crocodiles (*Crocodylus niloticus*), whereas Chinese alligators (*Alligator sinensis*) have rudimentary dorsal glands beneath the second to fifteenth rows of scales on the dorsum (Figure 5-4).[14]

Teeth

Crocodilians possess pointed conical teeth that are replaced over a crocodilian's lifetime. This may occur as fast as every 3 to 4 months in juvenile American alligators and starts from back to front in alternate teeth in young animals and reverses in older animals. It appears that a certain number of replacements are available, as very old crocodilians with no teeth have been reported.[4] Additionally, the two first positioned mandibular incisors may grow long enough to penetrate the upper maxilla in front of the nostrils. This is a normal anatomic development and does not cause any problem.

HUSBANDRY

Crocodilians are poikilothermic, regulating their body temperatures by using external environmental heat sources. They also operate at a preferred optimal body temperature (POBT) similar to mammalian internal body temperatures. For captive crocodilians, a good range for environmental temperatures is 25°C to 35°C.[5,8] Given a selection of temperatures, including a hot spot, crocodilians are able to select the POBT for their metabolic needs. Seasonal temperature fluctuations may result in a decrease or cessation of food consumption during winter months. It is common for species such as American alligators (*Alligator mississippiensis*) and Nile crocodiles, in both the wild and outdoor holding in captivity (Florida), to stop feeding for

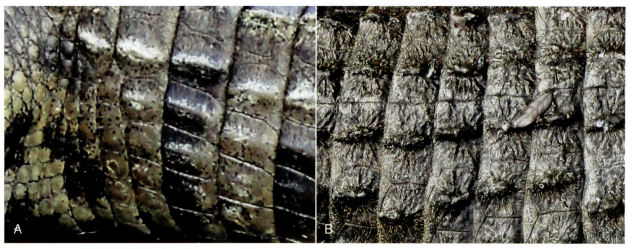

FIGURES 5-3 The skin of crocodilians contains both scales and scutes (**A**) with the dorsal scutes over the head and back containing bony plates called *osteoderms* (**B**).

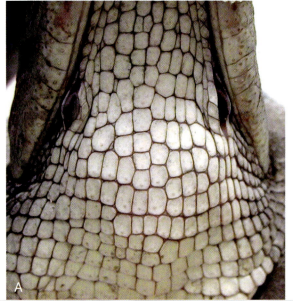

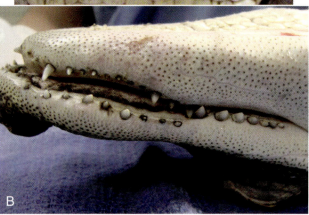

FIGURE 5-4 Paired gular gland on the ventral mandible (**A**) and some in the lips of Nile crocodiles (**B**). (From Lane TJ: Crocodilians. In Mader DR (ed): *Reptile medicine and surgery*. Philadelphia, PA, 1996, WB Saunders, pp. 78–94.)

4 to 5 months during the winter months. Even crocodilians held indoors in heated enclosures may have reduced appetite during the winter months with decreasing temperatures and light cycles. Anorexia with temperatures in the POBT of 26°C to 32°C should be considered abnormal and warrants physical examination and diagnostic workup.

Temperatures below and above POBT interfere with digestion and immune function. American alligators take twice as long to digest food at 20°C than 28°C, whereas smooth-sided caimans digest food three times faster at 30°C than 15°C.[8] Experimental infection of American alligators kept at 30°C demonstrated the greatest white blood cell (WBC) response to infection and survival of the infection, whereas alligators held above the POBT at 35°C succumbed to infection in 3 weeks.[8] These investigations indicate that it is important to routinely evaluate captive crocodilian enclosures for a proper thermoenvironment to ensure good health. Thermoregulation has an important role during anesthetic events. Crocodilians under general anesthesia should be kept at temperatures near their POBT or around 29.5°C.[8] Environmental temperatures below POBT decrease metabolism and thereby prolong clearance of injectable drugs, which results in delayed recoveries of up to days in length. Induction may also be prolonged because of slowed absorption and circulation times. For example, large Nile crocodiles induced with the neuromuscular blocker gallamine took twice as long to become recumbent at 14°C (40 minutes) than at 26°C (20 minutes).[6]

ENCLOSURE DESIGN

Water quality parameters for crocodilians should rival water quality in any aquarium system used for fish. Mechanical, biologic, and chemical filtration should be employed with routine testing of water quality parameters. Crocodilians may be able to handle poor water conditions for short periods, but this should not be the standard of care. In any crocodilian enclosure, clean water in the POBT with a dry, basking area is critical. The ability to dry off reduces the amount of superficial pathogens, through desiccation, and will also aid in achieving POBT through thermoregulation.

Most zoologic institutions have pairs or smaller groups of crocodilians living in one enclosure. However, in the case of housing numerous individuals in one enclosure, dominance and intraspecies aggression must be considered. In some species such as Chinese alligators, individual housing may be needed because of temperament issues. In group housing, a dominance order focusing on the

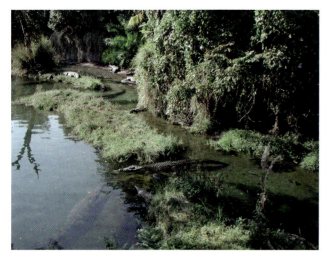

FIGURE 5-5 Exhibit pool for a large bachelor group (>20) Nile crocodiles at Disney's Animal Kingdom.

prime feeding and basking areas will be established. In these cases, additional enclosure furniture such as trees or rocks may be used to "break up" sight lines. When designing exhibit pools, a number of smaller outpockets is recommended while limiting narrow passages to assist in reducing territorial establishments and restricting the movements of other animals in the enclosure (Figure 5-5).

Pica and consumption of rocks or other objects is a common behavior of crocodilians. In necropsies preformed on wild Nile crocodilians, gastroliths, small rocks, up to 5 centimeters (cm) in size, is a normal finding (Hofmyer M, personal communication, 2011). Often, captive crocodiles may consume inappropriate objects to satisfy this behavior. Gastroliths are usually nonpathogenic and are often found during routine examination or during radiography. Small rocks do not cause medical issues and may be an incidental finding. Larger rocks less than 20 cm, pieces of PVC pipe, life support system components, coins, and metal foreign bodies may be of greater concern and require removal. In the case of metal objects such as coins, heavy metal toxicity, for example, zinc or lead toxicity, should be investigated. Removal of larger or irregular objects may be accomplished under general anesthesia with endoscopy. Small objects or coins may be removed simply via gastric lavage. Stomach lavage may be completed under general anesthesia, with the crocodilian intubated. In large crocodilians, a 1.5-meter (m) long, 7-cm diameter PVC pipe may be fashioned with an equine stomach tube taped to the PVC pipe. This set up may then be lubricated and inserted via the esophagus into the stomach. The pipe is typically palpable externally on the left side of the crocodile, and the smell coming out of the pipe should be acidic and typical of crocodilian ingesta. Flushing large amounts of water down the equine stomach tube with the animal's head angled down may displace smaller stomach content by allowing it to drain out through the PVC pipe. In a second technique, a homemade scoop with a long handle may be inserted into the stomach and used to scoop out stomach contents.

NUTRITION

In the wild, crocodilians are opportunistic carnivorous feeders, ranging from juveniles consuming small invertebrates and fish to large adults eating whole ruminants. In captivity, diets often consist of small to medium vertebrates and sometimes larger prey items. Prey items should be of high quality and not decomposed and are usually defrosted prior to feeding. Defrosting may be accomplished by placing the frozen item in a fridge 24 hours prior to feeding, which allows the food item to thaw but does not allow bacterial colonization and decomposition to start. Alternatively, in the case of smaller prey items such as mice, the frozen animal may be placed in a bucket of warm to hot water and defrosted in less than 30 minutes and then fed to the crocodilians. This does not allow for decomposition to set in and provides a warmed food item.

Whole Prey

Whole prey items (including organ tissue) from crickets to large vertebrates are the most common food source for crocodilians. Whole prey items are easy to manage, as they may be stored for months in a freezer. Frozen prey items should not be stored for longer than 3 months because of the nutritional breakdown of antioxidants such as vitamin E and other vitamins and minerals (Valdes E, personal communication, 2013). Many species of white fish (e.g., herring) have enteric thiaminase, which breaks down vitamin B_1. Thiaminase is not inactivated by freezing and thus continues to break down vitamin B in frozen fish. The longer the fish is frozen, the less vitamin B is available, which may result in hypovitaminosis B that leads to immune suppression and neurologic disease. Crocodilians fed a fish diet (caimans and gharials) may need to be supplemented with vitamins or other whole prey items, and frozen fish stocks should be rotated on a monthly schedule to reduce the buildup of thiaminase in frozen fish. Supplements such as calcium and mineral powders used to dust insects prior to feeding should be stored in a freezer. Refrigeration or freezing provides a more stable environment; however, supplements should be kept for no longer than 6 months. Studies have shown that storage of supplements in environments with fluctuating temperatures results in a fast degeneration of vitamins and minerals (Valdes E, personal communication, 2013).

Prepared Food Items

Prey items that have been skinned or have had the organ tissue removed are not considered whole prey items. In some institutions, feeding nutria (*Myocastor coypu*) that were skinned and the organs removed resulted in clinical signs of tooth loss, mandibular swelling, and reduced tooth replacement. Hypovitaminosis A and E, as well as high whole blood lead levels from lead shot found in the carcasses of the nutria, were noted in these reports. Crocodilians recovered with proper diet (pelleted and commercial meat product) and treatments with vitamin E and A supplements (retinyl palmitate and alpha-tocopherol (Heard D, personal communication, 2011).

Commercial Pelleted Diet

Alligator farms have been feeding pelleted diets for many years and zoos may offer similar diets as well. Pelleted diets are accepted by most species of crocodilians with reports of gharials being the exception. When feeding pelleted diets, it is easy to overfeed and cause obesity. Pelleted diets are concentrated nutritionally because of low water content. Whole prey items contain about one third of the caloric density (per kilogram, of food based on a dry-matter basis [DMB]) compared with a pelleted diet. For example, if a crocodilian is normally fed a diet of whole prey items (i.e., 9 kg per week), the animal would only need to be fed one third of 9 kg (3 kg of pellets) a week to achieve the same caloric intake. If the same weight amount in pellets were fed as whole prey, the crocodilians would be receiving a 200% increase in diet, which would result in obesity (Valdes E, personal communication, 2013).

Feeding guidelines may be highly variable and influenced by such factors as species, nutritional ecology, individual health status, nutritional goals (growth, maintenance, or weight loss), training plans, and environmental temperatures. As a general guideline for adult crocodilians, at mean feeding temperatures of 26°C to 37°C, the chapter author recommends feeding at a rate of 3.25 kilocalories per kilogram (kcal/kg) body weight (BW) (i.e., 600–1000 kcal/day for an adult Nile or American crocodile) providing protein at 60% to 65% on a DMB with energy at 5.5 to 5.82 kcal/g diet DMB, calcium at 1.93% to 2.4% DMB, and phosphorus at 1.39% to 1.92% DMB. An example diet for a monthly schedule with one diet item per week would include chicken (bones, skin, and no feathers), whole quail, crocodilian biscuit or pellet, whole tilapia, whole rabbits, whole rats, and herring. Juvenile diets are similar in composition (protein at 50% DMB, energy 6 to 6.1 kcal/g diet DMB, calcium at 1.38% to 2.4% DMB, and phosphorus at 1.28% to 1.38% DMB) but offer higher feeding rates at 8% BW per week (197 kcal/week, 840 kcal/month, average 28 kcal/day) or 19.3 kcal/kg BW with amount fed reevaluated frequently on the basis of the body condition score (BCS) and growth goals. Juvenile diets may also include smaller items such as prawns, lake smelt, mouse pinky or fuzzy, aquatic gel diets, insects (crickets or mealworms dusted with mineral supplements), and trout pellets (Valdes E, personal communication, 2013).

INFECTIOUS AND NONINFECTIOUS DISEASES

Crocodilians may be susceptible to a variety of bacterial, viral, parasitic, and fungal diseases; however, captive crocodilians held in zoologic institutions appear to have minimal infectious disease if held in appropriate social and environmental settings. Table 5-1 provides an overview of common infectious diseases in captive and wild crocodilian species.[11,12,14]

Noninfectious diseases related to nutritional issues appear to be more common in captive settings but are slowly becoming less evident with the development of nutritionally balanced commercial pelleted diets. Trauma is the most common noninfectious condition recently seen in institutions holding larger groups in an exhibit situation. Benefit and risk assessments are recommend for surgical intervention versus conservative medical care (empirical antibiotics and analgesics) and involve open dialogue between medical and husbandry team members. Factors in this risk assessment should include individual health status, loss of function of affected site of trauma, damage or exposure of vital structures at site, active blood loss, or all of these factors.

Other anecdotal reports of noninfectious diseases include gastric lymphoma in an adult male Nile crocodile (Terrell S, personal communication, 2013), although other neoplasms are likely. Gastric foreign bodies and gastrointestinal ileus outside of POBT should be a concern as well and have been discussed earlier in this chapter.

PREVENTIVE MEDICINE

As with all captive zoologic species, crocodilians should have a preventive health program. Most zoologic institutions may have only a few crocodilians with relatively few health problems, but this should not preclude having wellness programs similar to those for other taxa. Routine examinations may not be indicated on an annual basis, but baseline physical examination and blood work performed on a normal individual may prove advantageous when medical issues arise. With the development of behavioral husbandry techniques, routine examinations pose limited risk and stress to the crocodilian and to the veterinary and husbandry teams, making them a more viable option. Once training programs are developed as a regular husbandry practice, crocodilians will move into an examination crate on command. The entire process becomes simple for husbandry staff and the animals, reduces risks, and enhances the benefits of routine wellness examinations. Suggestions for preventive health programs are noted below.

For juvenile crocodilians, examinations are recommended annually for the first 3 to 4 years under physical restraint. This should include physical examination, transponder placement, weighing, and blood collection for a minimum database of complete blood cell count (CBC) and serum or plasma chemistry. If volume permits, serum trace minerals, fatty acids profile, and eastern equine encephalitis (EEE) and West Nile virus (WNV) serum or plasma titers (if animals are held outside) should be considered. Radiography should be considered and include the whole body to evaluate the skeleton for skeletal issues and the stomach for foreign bodies.

TABLE 5-1

Common Infectious Diseases of Captive and Wild Crocodilian Species

Disease	Etiology	Epizootiology	Signs	Diagnosis	Management
BACTERIAL DISEASE					
Salmonella	*Salmonella enteritidus* and *S. typhimurium* (many additional serovars)	Universal disease in farms and zoologic institutions	Hatchling enteritis and septicemia Adult carrier state	Culture and histopathology	Hatchlings: treat on the basis of culture Adult carriers: monitor and advise staff
Mycoplasma	*M. alligatoris, M. drocodyli*	Primarily in farming operations or other high density populations	Polyarthritis, pneumonia, and fatalities	Mycoplasma culture or PCR from synovial fluid, lung tissue, and feces	Screen with commercial ELISA test Treatment with tetracyclines not 100% efficacious
Chlamydia	*Chlamydia* sp., similar to *C. psittaci*	Hatchling disease in farming operations, associated with adenovirus hepatitis infections	Two forms: blepharoconjunctivitis and acute hepatitis	Swab or culture of eye and histology of liver	Treatment with tetracycline (1 g per 1 kg of dry feed)
Dermatophilosis	*Dermatophilus* sp.	Filamentous environmental pathogen, found in poor sanitary conditions	Brown discoloration of ventral scutes	Ventral lesions with cytology or histology or culture	Treatment with tetracycline (1 g per 1 kg of dry feed), or topical copper sulfate, hygienic conditions
VIRAL DISEASE					
Pox virus	*Parapox* sp.	Juvenile crocodilians with skin lesions	White to brown crust in oral cavity and ventral scutes	Histology with Bollinger bodies and Borrel bodies	Self-limiting, surgical removal of any large lesions

TABLE 5-1

Common Infectious Diseases of Captive and Wild Crocodilian Species—cont'd

Disease	Etiology	Epizootiology	Signs	Diagnosis	Management
Adenoviral hepatitis	*Adenovirus* sp.	Hatchlings under 5 months of age, vertical and horizontal transmission	Hepatitis	Virus may be found in liver, lung, pancreas, and intestines	No treatment, supportive care for secondary bacterial infections
Eastern equine encephalitis	EEE	Titers in healthy crocodilians, mosquito vector	No clinical signs typically	Winter reservoir for the virus	Monitor titers for spikes in EEE
West Nile virus	WNV	Titers in wild and captive crocodilians Mosquito vector and horizontal transmission	No clinical signs, neurologic disease, and lymphohistiocytic proliferative syndrome in farmed crocodilians	Single titers do not have a relationship to clinical disease	Monitor titers Does not cause mortalities
FUNGAL DISEASE					
	Numerous species including *Mucor* sp., *Aspergillus* sp., *Fusarium* sp., *Cladosporium* sp.	Dermatitis, gastric, oral, and respiratory mycosis	Related to poor sanitation and environmental conditions	Culture and histopathology	Sanitary conditions, topical and systemic antifungal treatment Poor prognosis for systemic mycosis
PARASITIC DISEASE					
Coccidiosis	*Eimeria* and *Isospora* Many are species specific	Fecal oral transmission, morbidity is variable, often seen in farming conditions	Intestinal coccidiosis with secondary bacterial infection, may result in intestinal blockage	Direct saline fecal examination or identification Histopathology	Screen incoming crocodilians Treat with sulfa derivative drugs (i.e., sulfachloropyrazine, sulfadiazine, and toltarazuril; Hutz 188)
Hepatozoonosis	Hemogregarines	Blood parasites transmitted by arthropods	Asexual schizonts may be found in the liver while gametes found in the blood Sexual reproduction takes place in the arthropod	Blood smears Usually none pathogenic unless immune suppression or chronic disease is present	Impossible to control in outdoor setting
Ascarids	Over 40 species identified	Intermediate host involved	Usually no clinical signs, stomach ulcers, mucosal lesions of gastrointestinal tract	Fecal examination	Pelleted diet and indoor housing eliminate ascarids Fenbendazole successful Freezing food for 72 hours may eliminate larvae
Trematodes	Over 80 species identified	Intermediate host required Internal (digenetic) and external species	Limited pathology with the exception of concurrent infection with other diseases	Direct visualization of parasite both antemortem and postmortem	Usually not treated in farming conditions due to limited pathology. Reduce feeding fresh water fish from the same habitat
Pentastomes	*Sebekia* sp. *Alofia* sp. *Liperia* sp.	Intermediate host Inhabit the upper respiratory tract and lungs Some species of pentastomides are zoonotic (*Armillifer* sp. in snakes)	May cause morbidity or mortality in young crocodilians Secondary infections at attachment sites	Eggs may be seen in feces Direct examination via endoscopy	Endoscopic removal

From Jacobson ER: Immobilization, blood sampling, necropsy techniques, and diseases of crocodilians: A review. *J Zoo Anim Med* 15:38, 1984; Klenk K, Snow J, Morgan K, et al: Alligators as West Nile virus amplifiers. *Emerg Infect Dis* [serial on the Internet], December 2004. Available at http://wwwnc.cdc.gov/eid/article/10/12/04-0264.htm. Accessed; Lane TJ: Crocodilians. In Mader DR (ed): *Reptile medicine and surgery*. Philadelphia, PA, 1996, WB Saunders, pp. 78-94.

Adult Crocodilian

Examinations are recommended every 2 to 3 years, with an established behavioral husbandry training program. This should include physical examination, transponder confirmation, weighing, blood collection for CBC, serum or plasma chemistry, trace minerals, fatty acids profile, EEE and WNV titers, whole blood lead and plasma or serum zinc serum levels. Radiography of the stomach may be helpful if a history of eating foreign bodies exists.

BEHAVIORAL CONDITIONING

Since the early 1990s, a significant increase has occurred in the use of operant conditioning techniques to train animals for husbandry purposes. As with other taxa, training techniques may easily facilitate basic husbandry and medical management of crocodilians with great success.[15] Crocodilians may be trained to voluntarily enter a crate and accept various veterinary procedures such as ultrasonography, radiography, blood collection, weighing, physical examinations, and medication administration. This is especially relevant when dealing with larger, potentially dangerous crocodilians.

To create a well thought out behavioral plan for your crocodilian, many facilities use the "SPIDER" framework taught in several courses given by the American Zoo and Aquarium Association (AZA). The "SPIDER" framework includes setting goals (S), planning (P), implementation (I), documenting (D), evaluating (E), and readjusting(R). More information on this process may be found at www.animaltraining.org. This process may be implemented at most institutions with an appropriately sized crate and a training plan. Most crocodilians may be trained in a few weeks to enter a crate and accept minor veterinary procedures (i.e., physical examination and blood collection). Crate training also facilitates establishing routine weighing, animal identification (ID) with transponder placement and identification, and transportation without immobilization or sedation. At Disney's Animal Kingdom, a bachelor group of 26 adult Nile crocodiles is managed with a crate training system. The crocodiles have become accustomed to the crate as a part of their husbandry process and often line up to enter the crate when the training cues commence. Routine physical examinations with weighing and blood sampling are possible on all 26 crocodilians within a week. Injured crocodiles with conspecific trauma have been motivated enough to shift into the crate for radiography and medical treatment within hours of observation of the trauma. The crate may also be used for inducing general anesthesia through intravenous (IV) or intramuscular (IM) injection. Behavioral modification has changed the way crocodiles are managed in captivity and may be implemented by any individual or organization with little expense.

ANESTHESIA AND RESTRAINT

Restraint Techniques

All crocodilians are capable of inflicting serious damage by ether biting or lashing out with their strong, muscular tails. For this reason, a number of restraint techniques have been developed for wild as well as captive crocodilians.[8] With the development of behavioral conditioning, the need for physical restraint is greatly reduced, and a safer environment is ensured for both the handler and the crocodilian. The disadvantage of prolonged physical restraint and struggling is the development of marked lactic acidemia with pH levels dropping to 6.6 to 6.8 (normal range 7.2 ± 0.2). Crocodilians, like other reptiles, take a prolonged period of time to recover from lactic acidemia, and this issue has been implicated in postrestraint fatalities.[24] Captured crocodilians may become unconscious and drown if not allowed to rest after prolonged physical restraint events.[21] When possible, for prolonged procedures, behavioral conditioning or anesthesia should be the choice versus physical restraint.

When handing an anesthetized crocodilian, the eyes should be covered with a damp towel, and the jaw should be taped shut, or taped open with an oral speculum, to facilitate intubation and ventilation under anesthesia (Figure 5-6A). Care must be taken to avoid taping the nostrils shut and to avoid pulling on the legs. Large crocodilians may weigh up to 500 kg, and pulling on legs to move them or lift them has resulted in fractures, luxations, or both.[8] To lift a crocodilian onto a tarp or out of shallow water, use of 1.5-m strips of flat, commercial grade crane straps should be placed to use as slings under the chest and hindlimbs. By using slings, the animals may easily be picked up and moved without pulling their legs.[6,8] With large crocodilians, an aluminum extension ladder may be placed under the crocodilian to support the entire body and the tail. Broom handles may be placed through the ladder and used as handles to lift and move the animals (see Figure 5-6B).

Injection Sites and Venous Access

Obtaining IV access has several goals: to obtain diagnostic samples, to administer therapeutic or immobilizing agents, and to establish venous access for emergency or supportive care. A number of access points are available in restrained crocodilians (Table 5-2; Figure 5-7).

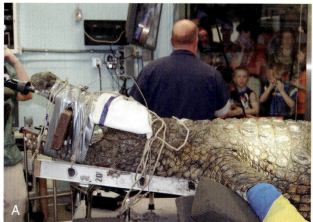

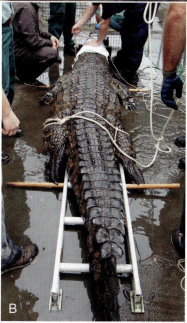

FIGURE 5-6 Suggested equipment for anesthesia of a Nile crocodile (*Crocodylus niloticus*), including damp towel as eye cover, jaw taped open with an oral speculum to facilitate intubation and ventilation under anesthesia (**A**), and aluminum extension ladder under the crocodilian to support the entire body and tail with broom handles through the ladder as handles to lift and move the animal (**B**).

If IV access cannot be obtained for anesthesia, the alternative is an IM injection. The goal in anesthetic drug delivery is to get close enough to the animal to administer the anesthetic safely; however, with large crocodilians, this may be a challenge. Darting or pole syringe techniques may be a satisfactory method of delivering injectable antibiotics or immobilizing agents to crocodilians; however, their use has several major disadvantages in these animals: (1) It is difficult to get an accurate shot while the crocodilian is in the water; (2) it is difficult to determine if the dart has fully discharged; (3) the osteoderms covering most of the dorsal surfaces of crocodilians may deflect the dart; and (4) once the animal is darted, if unrestrained, it may submerge, become immobilized, and drown. Darting should only be attempted in a captive in controlled situation (i.e., a dry enclosure). In field situations, traps and snares are commonly used to capture crocodilians.[6,8,21,24] The pole syringe is an option that may allow for injections of unrestrained crocodilians in a shallow pool or partially restrained crocodilians in a net, snare, or cage trap. The main disadvantage of a pole syringe is that the injector must be within 2 to 2.5 m of the crocodilian, and injection volumes are limited to 10 to 15 milliliters (mL). If the anesthetic agent is not administered fast enough, the pole syringe may be damaged, and a partial injection may result.[6,8,21,24] Of course, injection by hand syringe is the most controlled route of administration and, with behavioral conditioning, is more popular than the dart and pole syringe techniques.

Anesthetic Protocols

In formulating an anesthetic protocol for a crocodilian, consideration should be given to species, individual health status, procedural goals, and immobilizing conditions, including enclosure size, ambient temperature, and staffing. In general, the anesthesia plan generally includes induction with an injection of an anesthetic agent, IV or IM, intubation, and positive pressure ventilation with or without an inhalant gas anesthesia, maintenance with a continuous rate infusion or total IV anesthesia, or all of these. Below are two of the chapter author's most common techniques for anesthetizing crocodilians; however, these drugs and doses have not been tested on all crocodilian species, and some species differences are to be expected. Other anesthetic regimens have been reported in the primary and secondary literature, and some are included in Table 5-3.[8]

1. *Adult crocodilian IM induction regimen:* Medetomidine 100 microgram per kilogram (mcg/kg) and ketamine 10 mg/kg IM, intubation, and isoflurane at 2% to 3% at 1 to 2 L/min via an endotracheal tube (circle system), with forced ventilation at 3 to 4 breaths per minute should be used. While isoflurane reaches desired state of anesthesia, medetomidine may be reversed with atipamezole at five times the medetomidine dose.

2. *Juvenile crocodilian (manually restrained) or adult crocodilian (behavioral conditioned or restrained) IV induction regimen:* Propofol 3 to 5 mg/kg IV into the caudal or ventral tail vein, with a lateral or ventral approach. An IV extension set is recommended as part of the set up to maintain access through the entire procedure. Additional propofol may have to be titrated to effect. Maintenance with isoflurane at 2% to 3% at 300 to 500 mL/kg/min via an endotracheal tube (non-rebreathing system) with positive pressure ventilation at 3 to 4 breaths per minute.

Physiologic monitoring of crocodilians under anesthesia may include the use of the stethoscope, pulse oximeter, Doppler blood flow transducer, electrocardiography (ECG), ultrasonography, and arterial blood gas (ABG) analysis. Anesthetic depth is evaluated by using the withdrawal reflex of limbs, increasing or decreasing cardiac rates, righting response, and bite and corneal reflexes.[6,8,21,24] ECG

TABLE 5-2

Recommended Intravenous and Intramuscular Access Points in Restrained Crocodilians for Blood Collection and Injection Administration

	Advantage	Disadvantage	Comments
INTRAMUSCULAR INJECTION			
Base of tail, lateral aspect, caudal to hind leg for 7–10 scales	Large muscle group; no underlying organs; away from the head	Possible first pass through liver and kidneys	Anesthetic injections in this location are common and successful
Hindlimb	Smaller scales than tail; injection site is away from the head	Smaller area to inject with a dart or pole syringe; possible first pass through liver and kidneys	Difficult to dart legs; easy for hand injection
Forelimb	Small scales; no chance of first pass through liver and kidneys	Small area to inject with dart or pole syringe; close to the head	Good for hand injection once anesthetized
INTRAVENOUS INJECTION			
Internal jugular (occipital sinus)	Dorsal to the vertebral column; best accessed by flexing the head down and inserting needle between the atlas and axis	Becomes difficult in larger crocodilians Possible to pith the spinal cord	Injection of propofol in this area has resulted in mortalities
Ventral coccygeal vein	Ventral midline of the tail Vein lies just ventral to the spine	Becomes difficult in large crocodilians as the needle must be below the level of the body Possible first pass through liver and kidneys	Common site for blood draw and injection of intravenous drugs and anesthetic agents
Lateral coccygeal vein	Vein lies just ventral to the lateral aspect of the spinous process of the vertebrae	More convenient to utilize this intravenous site in larger crocodilians, as the tail can sit in normal position for the procedure	Insert needle at 45 degrees beneath the lateral aspect of the spinous process Common site for blood draw and injection of intravenous drugs and anesthetic agents

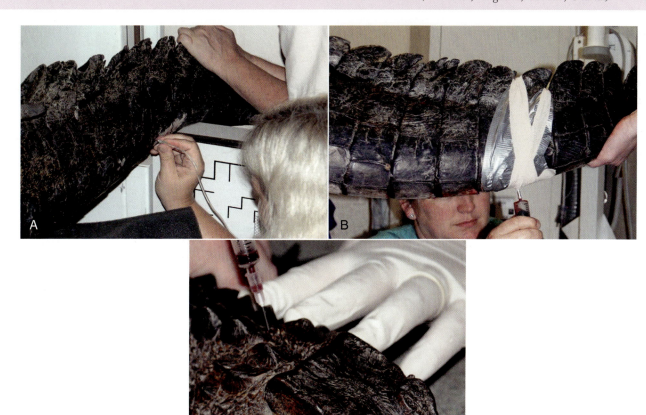

FIGURE 5-7 Intravenous blood collection and drug administration accessing the coccygeal vein laterally or ventrally (**A** and **B**) and the occipital sinus (internal jugular) dorsally (**C**).

and reference values have been described for the American alligator.[8] ECG leads are attached to 2.5-cm needles passed through the skin in a three-of-four lead format. Although pulse oximetry may be used to assess heart rate, it does not appear to accurately calculate oxygen saturation in reptiles.[17] Crocodilian skin thickness and pigmentation may further hamper measurement with the transmission probe, whereas a reflectance probe in the cloaca may improve the signal achieved. ABG measurements in crocodilians may be difficult to interpret because numerous variables such as temperature, feeding, sample site (arterial, venous, or a combination of both) may influence the results. American alligators have the ability to reduce the affinity of hemoglobin to reduce blood oxygen affinity at certain pH levels. This allows for more oxygen to be released from hemoglobin under certain conditions such as acidemia, increasing the total amount of oxygen available to tissues.[6,8,21,24]

The Doppler blood flow transducer appears to be a very reliable method of obtaining heart rate.[8,19] The probe is placed over the heart or a large blood vessel such as the ventral coccygeal, brachial, or femoral artery. Blood flow in the optic arteries may be detected by placing the probe against the globe, with the eye lid or the third eye lid closed. Alternatively, a dorsally directed probe placed in the cloaca may detect arterial blood flow. In the case of large crocodilians (>100 kg), ultrasonography may be used to visualize pulses or cardiac contractions.

PHYSIOLOGIC REFERENCE RANGES

Obtaining heart and respiratory rates may be challenging in awake crocodilians. In one study, juvenile American alligators and smooth-sided caimans (*Caiman sclerops*) were implanted with monitoring equipment and isolated from human contact for 12 to 20 hours before measuring cardiac and respiratory rates. Normal respiratory and heart rates at 22°C were 0.6 and 11.6 beats per minute (beats/min), and 1.6 and 14.2 beats/min, respectively. Following visual contact with humans, both heart and respiratory rates doubled to 30 beats/min and 6 breaths per minute.[8] Consequently, most restrained crocodilians are likely to be tachycardic and tachypneic. In general, heart and respiratory rates vary inversely with the size of the animal but are affected by environmental temperatures as well. In a study of Nile crocodiles, heart rates were observed to increase as temperatures increased from 1 to 8 beats/min at 10°C up to 24 to 40 beats/min at 28°C. Prolonged exposure to high temperatures above 40°C will likely cause irreversible cardiac damage. Heart rates as high as 55 beats/min at 29°C have been recorded in Nile crocodiles caught in traps.[8]

ANALGESIA

Information on the use of analgesics in reptiles, specifically crocodilians, is growing, and multiple analgesics are now available for use

TABLE 5-3

Suggested Anesthetic and Analgesic Agents for Use in Crocodilians

Drug	Dosage	Species	Remarks
ANALGESIA			
Morphine	0.8 mg/kg IM	C. porosus	
Meperidine	1–2 mg/kg IM	C. porosus	
Meloxicam	0.1–0.2 mg/kg IM or PO SID for 5–7 days	Most species	
Tramadol	5 mg/kg PO q3–5 days	Most species	May cause sedation
Ketoprofen	2 mg/kg IM q24–48h	Most species	
Butorphanol	0.2–0.4 mg/kg IM q24h	Most species	May cause sedation but not analgesia
ANESTHESIA			
Ketamine and medetomidine	10 mg/kg and 0.1 mg/kg IM	Most species	
Ketamine and xylazine	7.5–10 mg/kg nd 1–2 mg/kg IM	Most species	
Tiletamine or zolazepam	5–15 mg/kg IM	Most species	May result in prolonged recovery
Propofol	3–10 mg/kg IV	Most species	Titrate from low dose to effect for intubation; may result in transient apnea
Midazolam	0.5 mg/kg IM	Most species	Usually used in combination with other anesthetic drugs
ANTAGONISTS			
Atipamezole	Five times dose of medetomidine IM	Most species	
Yohimbine	0.1 mg/kg IM	Most species	
Flumazenil	10–20 times dose of benzodiazepine IV or IM	Most species	
Naltrexone	100 times the dose of opioid	Most species	
Neostigmine	0.03–0.06 mg/kg IM	C. niloticus	
INHALANTS			
Isoflurane	1–5%	Most species	2%-3% for maintenance
Sevoflurane	1–5%	Most species	5%-6% for maintenance
Halothane	1–5%	Most species	Not recommended because of hepatotoxicity or cardiotoxicity
PARALYTICS			
Gallamine	1–2 mg/kg IM	C. niloticus	No analgesic effects
Succinylcholine	0.33–5 mg/kg IM	Most species	No analgesic effects

From references 2, 7, 8, 9, 13, 22, 23, and 25.

in crocodilians (see Table 5-3).[2,7,8,9,13,22,23,25] The use of butorphanol as an analgesic in reptiles has been widespread; however, multiple studies on the use of butorphanol in other reptilian species such as green iguanas and red-eared sliders have revealed that butorphanol at higher doses may result in sedation but does not itself cause analgesia.[2,7,17,22] Until further analgesic trials with butorphanol in crocodilians are completed, the author of this chapter does not advocate its use as an analgesic.

The use of opioids such as morphine at (0.8 mg/kg) and meperidine (2 mg/kg) in juvenile salt water crocodiles has showed evidence of analgesia as measured with thermal antinociception.[8] Higher doses of morphine (1.5 and 6.5 mg/kg IM) in red-eared sliders resulted in analgesia but also long-lasting respiratory depression.[8,22] Using the same methodology, morphine at 10 and 20 mg/kg IM in bearded dragons resulted in analgesia, which was, however, delayed until 8 hours after administration.[22] Other opioid-based drugs such as tramadol, 5 mg/kg orally (PO) every 3 to 5 days, induces analgesia via both opioid and nonopioid pathways in red-eared sliders.[2,8] This author has used tramadol, at 5 mg/kg PO, in numerous reptilian species, including Nile crocodiles, with good anecdotal success; however, in some reptiles, a dose of 5 mg/kg every 3 days resulted in sedation.

Use of nonsteroidal anti-inflammatories such as meloxicam (0.2 mg/kg, PO, IM, IV) has been reported in reptiles, and IV or PO administration resulted in the same bioavailability.[8,9,25] This author has used meloxicam (0.1 mg/kg orally once a day for 14 days) in two adult Nile crocodiles with traumatic foot amputations. On the

day following treatment, both crocodiles showed marked improvement in ambulation, with no evidence of lameness. A single dose of ketoprofen at 2 mg/kg, IV and IM, in green iguanas demonstrated that the terminal half-life was greater than that of dogs, suggesting that dosing intervals for ketoprofen in reptiles should be longer than in mammals (i.e., <24 hours).[23]

ACKNOWLEDGMENTS

We offer our special acknowledgment to Dr. Diedre Fontenot, who completed Dr. Fleming's chapter after his death.

This chapter is dedicated to the memory of Greg Fleming, whose unfortunate death preceded the completion of his chapter. With his passion and knowledge, Greg was a driving force in zoologic medicine, especially in his area of special interest, reptile medicine. We believe that this chapter reflects Greg's drive and expertise, and it is with sadness, but also in celebration of a life fully lived, that we dedicate this chapter to him.

REFERENCES

1. Axlesson MA, Franklin CE: From anatomy to angioscopy: 164 years of crocodilian cardiovascular research, recent advances and speculations. *Comparat Biochem Physiol* 118A:51–62, 1997.

2. Baker BB, Sladky KK, Johnson SM: Evaluation of the analgesic effects of oral and subcutaneous tramadol administration in red-eared slider turtles. *J Am Vet Med Assoc* 238:220–227, 2011.

3. Colbert EH: Eustachian tubes of the crocodilian. *Copeia* 12–14, 1946.

4. Edmund AG: *Sequence and rate of tooth replacement in the Crocodilia*, Contribution No.56, Life Science Division, 1962, Royal Ontario Museum, University of Toronto, pp 42.

5. Fleming GJ, Isaza R, Spire MF, Heard DJ: Evaluation of reptile enclosures using digital thermography. *J Herpetol Med Surg* 13(1):38–42, 2007.

6. Fleming GJ: Capture and chemical immobilization of the Nile crocodile (*Crocodylus niloticus*) in South Africa. In *Proceedings of the 1996 Association of Reptile and Amphibian veterinarians*, Tampa, FL, 1996, pp 63–66.

7. Fleming GJ, Robertson S: Use of thermal threshold test response to evaluate the antinociceptive effects of butorphanol in juvenile Green iguanas (*Iguana iguana*). In *Proceedings of the American Association of Zoo Veterinarians*, Tampa, FL, 2006, pp 279.

8. Fleming G: Crocodilians (crocodiles, alligators, caimans, gharial). In West G, Heard D, Caulkett N, editors: *Zoo animal and wildlife immobilization and anesthesia*, Oxford, UK, 2007, Blackwell Publishing Ltd., pp 223–231.

9. Hernandez-Divers SJ, Papich M, McBride M, Stedman N: Pharmacokinetics of meloxicam following oral and intravenous administration in the green iguana (*Iguana iguana*). *Am J Vet Res* 71(11):1277–1283, 2010.

10. Holz P: The anatomy and perfusion of the renal portal system in the red-eared slider (*Trachemys scripta elegans*). *J Zoo Wildl Med* 28(4):378–385, 1997.

11. Jacobson ER: Immobilization, blood sampling, necropsy techniques, and diseases of crocodilians: A review. *J Zoo Anim Med* 15:38, 1984.

12. Klenk K, Snow J, Morgan K, et al: Alligators as West Nile virus amplifiers. *Emerg Infect Dis* [serial on the Internet], December 2004. Available at: http://wwwnc.cdc.gov/eid/article/10/12/04-0264.htm. Accessed.

13. Kummrow MS, Tseng F, Hesse L, et al: Pharmacokinetics of buprenorphine after single-dose subcutaneous administration in red-eared sliders (*Trachemys scripta elegans*). *J Zoo Wildl Med* 39:590, 2008.

14. Lane TJ: Crocodilians. In Mader DR, editor: *Reptile medicine and surgery*, Philadelphia, PA, 1996, WB Saunders, pp 78–94.

15. Lang JW: Crocodilian behavior: implications for management. In Webb GJW, Manolis SC, Whitehead PJ, editors: *Wildlife management: crocodiles and alligators*. Clipping Norton, Australia, Surrey Beatty and Sons Printing, 1987, pp 273–294.

16. Millichamp NJ: Surgical techniques in reptiles. In Jacobson ER, Kollias GV, editors: *Contemporary issues in small animal practice: exotic animals*, New York, 1988, Churchill Livingstone, pp 49.

17. Mosley C: Pain and nociception in reptiles. *Vet Clin North Am Exot Anim Pract* 14:45–60, 2011; Mosley CAE, Dyson D, Smith D: Minimum alveolar concentration of isoflurane in Green iguanas and the effect of butorphanol on minimum alveolar concentration. *J Am Vet Med Assoc* 222(11):1559–1564, 2003.

18. Murphy MJ: Cardiology and circulation. In Mader DR, editor: *Reptile medicine and surgery*, Philadelphia, PA, 1996, WB Saunders, pp 95–103.

19. Neilson L: Chemical immobilization of free-ranging terrestrial mammals. In Thurmon JC, Tranquilli WJ, Benson GJ, editors: *Lumb and Jones veterinary anesthesia*, ed 3, Baltimore, MA, 1996, Williams and Wilkins, pp 737.

20. Putterill JF, Soley JT: Morphology of the gular valve of the Nile crocodile, *Crocodylus niloticus*. *J Morph* 267(8):924–939, 2006.

21. Seymore RS, Webb GJW, Bennett AF, et al: Effect of capture on the physiology of *Crocodylus porosus*. In Webb GJW, Manolis SC, Whitehead PJ, editors: *Wildlife management: Crocodiles and alligators*, Clipping Norton, Australia, 1987, Surrey Beatty and Sons Printing, pp 253–257.

22. Sladky KK, Kinney ME, Johnson SM: Analgesic efficacy of butorphanol and morphine in bearded dragons and corn snakes. *J Am Vet Med Assoc* 233:267–273, 2008.

23. Tuttle AD, Papich M, Lewbart GA, et al: Pharmacokinetics of ketoprofen in the green iguana (*Iguana iguana*) following single intravenous and intramuscular injections. *J Zoo Wildl Med* 37:567, 2006.

24. Webb JW, Messel H: Crocodile capture techniques. *J Wildl Manage* 41(3):572–575, 1977.

25. Whiteside DP, Black SR: *The use of meloxicam in exotic felids at the Calgary Zoo*. The proceedings of the American Association of Zoo Veterinarians, San Diego, CA, 2004, pp 346–349.

26. Whitaker N, Basu D: The gharial (*Galvialis gangeticus*): A review. *Copeia* 531–548, 1983.

CHAPTER 6

Sphenodontia: The Biology and Veterinary Care of Tuatara

Richard M. Jakob-Hoff

GENERAL BIOLOGY

Taxonomy and Status

The tuatara is the only extant member of the order Sphenodontia. Previously found throughout New Zealand, tuatara are now restricted to approximately 35 offshore islands.[8] Rats (*Rattus norvegicus, R. rattus, R. exulans*) are considered the primary threat as predators of tuatara eggs and juveniles and competitors for food.[4] A recent taxonomic review concluded that all populations comprised a single species, *Sphenodon punctatus*.[9]

Anatomy and Physiology

Superficially similar to lizards, tuatara have a number of anatomic and physiologic features that, collectively, place them in their own order: (1) unique dentition,[10] (2) absence of an external auditory aperture,[15] (3) absence of a male intromittant copulatory organ,[4,7] (4) abdominal ribs (gastralia) reinforced by uncinate processes,[7,19] (5) a parietal eye,[7,15] and (6) activity at a low body temperature range between 2 and 22°C with maximal level of activity at 17°C.[14,17]

Growth and Development

Nelson N. (personal communication, 2013) has gathered verifiable evidence of tuatara conservatively estimated to be 91 years old. Adult male weights vary between 400 and 1000 grams (g) with a snout–vent length (SVL) of 200 to 290 millimeters (mm), and females weigh 200 to 500 g with an SVL of 180 to 240 mm.[7]

Reproduction

Sexual maturity occurs at 13 to15 years of age.[4,7] Females reproduce, on average, once every four years,[4] with mating occurring in late summer (January to March) and ovulation in April.[5] Significant seasonal variation is seen in sex steroids in both sexes corresponding to courtship and mating behavior. Both sexes may engage in aggressive interactions during the breeding season, and severe biting may result in facial wounds, fractured mandibles, and detached tails.[4] Radiography in September to October provides a reasonable estimate of the proportion of gravid females with shelled eggs (Figure 6-1). Up to 19 soft-shelled eggs are laid 10 to 50 centimeters (cm) deep in sunny areas.[6] Depending on the temperature, incubation may take 11 to 16 months,[4] with predominantly females produced at 20°C and males at 23°C.[13] After hatching, remnants of the midventral yolk sac persist for a few days.[7]

SPECIAL HOUSING REQUIREMENTS

Captive housing and husbandry have been well described elsewhere.[1,2,14] Housing features critical to the good health of the tuatara are (1) a minimum of 5 square meters (m²) per adult animal,[14] (2) porous soil substrate to allow for natural burrow construction and egg laying, (3) adequate insulation of artificial burrows to protect from excessive heat, cold, and moisture, (4) a variety of low-growing shrubs, rocks, hollow logs, and other cage furniture to provide visual screens between animals, refuges, shade, and opportunities for sun basking and exercise, (5) ambient temperature of 4°C to 15°C in winter and 10°C to 25°C in summer,[1] with the animals being given a choice of thermal gradients, (6) relative humidity maintained within the range 85% to 95%,[1,14] (7) basking opportunities providing 100 to 250 microwatts per square centimeter (µw/cm²) of ultraviolet B (UVB) (290–315 nanometer [nm], lower exposure in winter, higher in summer) and warmth for two hours in the morning and in the afternoon (Gibson R, personal communication, 2013), and (8) open ponds to enable the animals to soak in shallow water. This frequently stimulates defecation and helps prevent dysecdysis in the annual molt.

FEEDING

Captive diets should mimic the wild diet[7,14,18] as far as possible and include a variety of live invertebrates such as crickets, locusts, mealworm larvae, beetles (*Tenebrio* sp.), moths, earthworms, snails, woodlice, and occasionally in summer, small bird eggs or newly hatched chicks. At the Auckland Zoo, invertebrates are dusted with a high-calcium multi-vitamin and mineral powder (Miner-All, Sticky-Tongue Farms, Sun City, CA).

RESTRAINT AND HANDLING

Physical Restraint

Unnecessary handling of tuatara should be avoided as they are easily stressed. Where physical restraint is required, the animal is grasped around the neck, shoulders, and pelvis from above and held or placed on a solid surface. Alternatively, the animal may be supported on the forearm of the handler, who maintains a light grip on the animal's neck (Figure 6-2). In general, the lighter the restraint, the less inclined the animal will be to struggle. Autotomy may occur if the tail is held. A blindfold made from a nonadhesive stretch-fabric bandage may be applied and is particularly useful for radiography.

Chemical Restraint

Injectable induction agents used at the Auckland Zoo have included ketamine hydrochloride (Parnell Technologies Pty Ltd.), 70 milligrams per kilogram (mg/kg), intravenously (IV), producing deep sedation but prolonged recovery time; medetomidine (Domitor, Pfizer Animal Health) 0.095 mg/kg combined with ketamine 4.75 mg/kg, IV, also produced deep sedation but recovery time was shortened with the reversal agent atipamezole (Antisedan, Pfizer Animal Health) at 0.47 mg/kg, IV; alfaxalone (Alfaxan, Jurox NZ Ltd.) 4 to 9 mg/kg, intramuscularly (IM), resulted in prolonged recovery at the higher dose rate. The inhalant agents sevoflurane (SevoFlo, Abbott Laboratories) or isoflurane (Isoflurane-Vet, Merial

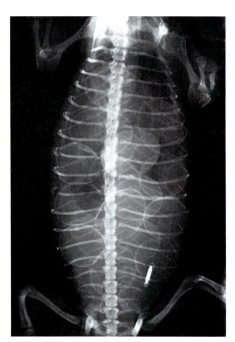

FIGURE 6-1 Radiograph of a gravid tuatara. (Photo Courtesy of the Auckland Zoo.)

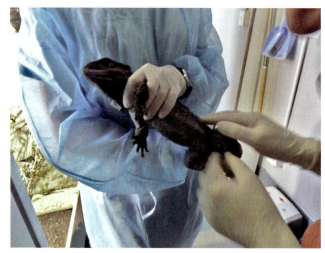

FIGURE 6-2 Tuatara physical restraint. (Photo Courtesy of the Auckland Zoo.)

NZ Ltd.) are used to achieve full anesthesia, initially administered via facemask and subsequently via an uncuffed endotracheal tube of 2 to 3 millimeters (mm) in diameter attached to an Ayres T-piece circuit. These inhalants have also been effectively used without a prior injectable agent, in which case recovery time was reduced. Apnea during anesthesia is common and intermittent positive pressure ventilation (IPPV) at 2 to 12 breaths per minute (bpm) is generally needed to establish and maintain a stable depth of anesthesia. Wells et al. (1990) recorded mean tidal volume of 60 milliliters (mL) or 11% of body volume in one 557-gram (g) male. During anesthesia, heart rates of 22 to 49 have been recorded by using a Doppler probe or stethoscope applied with lubricant over the heart located in the ventral midline between the thoracic limbs. Depth of anesthesia may be gauged by using the pedal withdrawal reflex.[3] Regional analgesia using bupivacaine or lignocaine may be a useful adjunct for performance of minor surgical procedures. Meloxicam 0.1 to 0.2 mg/kg orally (PO) once a day (SID) with or without butorphanol at 0.05 mg/kg, IM, SID are effective analgesics.

SURGERY

The general principles and approach to surgery in reptiles as described in Mader et al. (2006)[11] are also applicable to the tuatara. Maximum body temperature during and following surgery should not exceed 25°C and suture removal should be delayed for 12 to 16 weeks.[3]

DISEASES

The following is largely drawn from unpublished records from the New Zealand Department of Conservation's native species mortality database (*Huia*) and the medical and necropsy records of the Auckland Zoo.

Mycoses

Over a 20 year period 42 out of 74 (57%) tuatara at the Auckland Zoo were affected by dermatitis. In the majority of cases, this presented as a very mild superficial brown discoloration of single or small clusters of scales, mostly on the ventral skin. Although the specific etiology has not been identified, the condition is frequently associated with periods of cool, wet weather and resolves when animals are provided with drier, less exposed environments and treated with topical antiseptic solutions. More severe cases range from multiple raised, exudative plaques or more extensive, necrotizing ulcerative dermatitis occasionally progressing to fatal systemic mycoses. Skin biopsies have almost invariably demonstrated intralesional fungi and mixed bacteria with associated mononuclear inflammatory cells. Fungal isolates from different cases have included *Penicillium* spp., *Zygomycete*-like organisms, and *Chrysosporium* spp. Systemic therapy, based on culture and sensitivity results, has included itraconazole or fluconazole at 5 mg/kg, PO, once a day (SID), ceftazidime at 20 mg/kg, IM, q72h, enrofloxacin 5 to 10 mg/kg, subcutaneously (SQ) (diluted 1:3 v/v with 0.9% saline), q48h, and meloxicam 0.1 to 0.2 mg/kg, PO, SID. Terbinafine hydrochloride (Lamisil Cream, Novartis Australasia Pty Ltd.) has been used topically in some cases. Treatment has been maintained for 1 to 4 months. Avoiding prolonged exposure to extremes of cold and wet in winter and provision of adequate UVB exposure appear to be important preventive measures.

Parasites

Free-living tuatara are commonly hosts to ectoparasites and endoparasites (including the host-specific tick *Amblyomma sphenodonti*, the hemoparasite *Hepatozoon* tuatarae,[9] and the nematode *Hatterianema hollandei* [Heterakidae]),[12] but no clinical impacts from these parasites have been recorded to date. In captive animals, heavy burdens of intestinal nematodes have been treated with oxfendazole (Panacur 100, MSD Animal Health) 50 mg/kg, PO, repeated three times at two-week intervals.

Metabolic Conditions

Hypocalcemia (0.69 millimoles per liter [mmol/L]) during winter in a gravid captive tuatara with signs of weakness and poor muscle tone has been described.[16] This animal responded rapidly to parenteral calcium borogluconate. Juvenile tuatara, like other captive reptiles, are also prone to metabolic bone disease which may manifest with mandibular, spinal, and limb deformities; folding fractures; and muscular weakness classically associated with this condition. It is readily prevented through appropriate diet and husbandry, as described above.

Trauma

Tail loss and other injuries are relatively common in captive and wild animals.[7] Bite wounds, usually inflicted by males during the breeding season, may become infected and develop into localized abscesses requiring debridement, the use of Penrose drain, and systemic antimicrobial treatment based on culture sensitivities. Open wound management, following debridement, has included the topical application of DuoDerm paste (ConvaTec, E.R. Squibb & Sons) or a mixture of Intrasite gel (Smith & Nephew) and silver sulfadiazine (Flamizine, Smith & Nephew). Where dressings have been applied, the use of nanocrystalline silver-impregnated Acticoat (Smith & Nephew) under an adhesive Hypafix dressing (Smith & Nephew) reinforced with tissue glue (Tissumend II SC, Veterinary Product Labs, Phoenix, AZ) has been particularly effective in maintaining a clean, moist, healing environment while allowing animals to remain in an enclosure with natural substrate.

ACKNOWLEDGMENTS

I am indebted to Hannah Barton, Richard Gibson, Brett Gartrell, and Nicola Nelson for their assistance during the preparation of this chapter.

REFERENCES

1. Blanchard B: *Tuatara captive management plan and husbandry manual.* Threatened Species Occasional Publication 21, Wellington, New Zealand, 2002, Department of Conservation.
2. Boardman WSJ, Sibley MD: The captive management, diseases and veterinary care of tuatara. In *Proceedings of the American Association of Zoo Veterinarians*, 1991, pp 156–163.
3. Boardman W, Blanchard B: Biology, captive management and medical care of tuatara. In Mader DR, editor: *Reptile medicine and surgery*, ed 2, St. Louis, MO, 2006, Saunders.
4. Cree A, Daugherty C: Tuatara sheds its fossil image. *New Scientist* 22–26, 1990.
5. Cree A, Guillette LJ, Jr, Cockrem JF, et al: Absence of daily cycles in plasma sex steroids in male and female tuatara (*Sphenodon punctatus*) and the effects of acute capture stress on females. *Gen Comparat Endocrinol* 79:103–113, 1990.
6. Cree A, Daugherty CH, Schafer SF, Brown D: Nesting and clutch size of tuatara (*Sphenodon guntheri*) on North Brother Island, Cook Strait. *Tuatara* 31:9–16, 1991.
7. Dawbin WH: The tuatara in its natural habitat. *Endeavour* 21(81):16–24, 1962.
8. Hay JM, Sarre SD, Lambert DM, et al: Genetic diversity and taxonomy: A reassessment of species designation in tuatara (Sphenodon: Reptilia). *Conservation Genetics* 11:1063–1081, 2010.
9. Herbert JDK, Godfrey SS, Bull CM, Menz RI: Developmental stages and molecular phylogeny of *Hepatozoon tuatarae*, a parasite infecting the New Zealand tuatara, *Sphenodon punctatus*, and the tick, *Amblyomma sphenodonti*. *Int J Parasitol* 40(11):13111315, 2010.
10. Keiser JA: *Microstructure of dental hard tissues and bone in the tuatara dentary,* Sphenodon punctatus (Diapsida: Lepidosauria: Rhynchocephalia) *in comparative dental morphology: Selected papers of the 14th International Symposium on Dental Morphology*, Greifswald, Germany, August 27–30, 2008.
11. Mader DR, Bennett RA, Funk RS, et al: Surgery. In Mader DR, editor: *Reptile medicine and surgery*, ed 2, St. Louis, MO, 2006, Saunders.

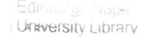Edinburgh Napier University Library

12. McKenna PB: An annotated checklist of ecto- and endoparasites of New Zealand reptiles. *Surveillance* 30(3):18–25, 2003.
13. Nelson NJ, Moore JA, Pillai S, Keall SN: Thermosensitive period for sex determination in tuatara. *Herpetol Conservation Biol* 5(2):324–329, 2010.
14. Newman DG, Crook IG, Moran LR: Some recommendations on the captive maintenance of tuataras. *Int Zoo Yearbook* 19:68–74, 1979.
15. Robb J: *Patterns of progress: The Tuatara*, Durham, England, 1977, Meadowfield Press Ltd., pp 1–64.
16. Sanderson A, Blanchard B: Vitamin D₃ levels in wild and captive tuatara (*Sphenodon punctatus*): A case study on the management of hypocalcae-mia in pregnancy. In *Proceedings of the American Association of Zoo Veterinarians*, 1977, pp 375–377.
17. Thompson MB, Daugherty CH: Metabolism of tuatara, *Sphenodon punctatus*. *Comparative Biochemistry and Physiology Part A: Molecular & Integrative Physiology* 119(2):519–522, 1998.
18. Walls GY: Feeding ecology of the tuatara (*Sphenodon punctatus*) on Stephens Island, Cook Strait. *N Z J Ecol* 4:89–97, 1981.
19. Wells RMG, Tetsns V, Housley GD, et al: Effect of temperature on control of breathing in the cryophilic rhynchocephalian reptile, *Sphenodon punctatus*. *Camp Biochem Physiol* 96A(2):333–340, 1990.

CHAPTER 7

Lacertilia (Lizards, Skinks, Geckos) and Amphisbaenids (Worm Lizards)

Ryan S. DeVoe

BIOLOGY AND TAXONOMY

The suborders Sauria/Lacertilia and Serpentes are found within the order Squamata, which contains between 6500 and 7000 species, depending on current taxonomic understanding. Approximately 5500 of the Squamates are assigned to the suborder Sauria/Lacertilia and are commonly referred to as *lizards*. A number of clades exist within the suborder Sauria/Lacertilia, including Iguania, Gekkota, Scincomorpha, Anguimorpha, and Amphisbaenia. These clades are further broken down into families, of which the Iguanidae, Agamidae, Varanidae, Scincidae, Chameleonidae, and Gekkonidae contain the vast number of species. The family Scincidae contains the largest number of species (approximately 20% of all lizard species), whereas other families such as the Helodermatidae contain only two species.

Lizards are extremely successful reptiles and inhabit myriad habitats worldwide, ranging from desert to aquatic, temperate to tropical, fossorial to arboreal. Lizards have evolved to effectively take advantage of all these different habitats. The only continent on which lizards do not naturally occur is Antarctica. As would be expected with such a large and varied taxa, dramatic variations in anatomy, physiology, dietary strategy, and reproduction exist among species. Animals within the Sauria/Lacertilia range in size from the Komodo dragon (*Varanus komodiensis*), which may reach lengths over 3 meters (m) and weights exceeding 100 kilograms (kg) to some species such as the dwarf chameleons (*Brookesia* sp.) and geckos (*Spaerodactylus* sp.), which may not exceed 2 centimeters (cm) in length.

Lizards are very popular as exhibit animals in zoos, aquaria, museums, and private collections. When properly managed, many lizard species are spectacular on display, hardy, and long-lived. Some species such as bearded dragons (*Pogona vitticeps*) and leopard geckos (*Eublepharius macularis*) have gained great popularity as pets and are propagated in large numbers to supply the pet trade. Relatively large amounts of information regarding the husbandry, reproduction, and medical care of these common species is available and may be judiciously extrapolated for use with similar species.

ANATOMY AND PHYSIOLOGY

Much variation exists in the anatomy and physiology in the Sauria/Lacertilia suborder; however, most lizards share a basic body form, and all others are variations on that theme. Most lizards have four well-developed legs and a tail.

The dentition of most lizards is classified as either *acrodont* (agamids, chameleons) or *pleurodont* (iguanids). Acrodont teeth are fused to the biting edge of the mandibles and the maxillae. Pleurodont teeth are attached to the periosteum on the medial surface of the mandibles and maxillae. Clinically, this is significant, as pleurodont teeth will regenerate if lost or broken, whereas acrodont teeth will not.[20]

Some lizards such as monitors and tegus have long, forked tongues, which are very similar to those seen in snakes and used for tracking prey. True chameleons have very long tongues (over a full body length) with a sticky, fleshy tip that is used for capturing prey. The tongue is supported and propelled or retracted by specialized lingual muscles, the hyobranchial apparatus, and elastic collagen tissue. Most other lizards have fleshy, mobile tongues that are also used to prehend food and as chemosensory organs, but they are much less specialized than those in the taxa previously mentioned. In some species such as the common green iguana (*Iguana iguana*) the rostral portion of the tongue is dramatically different in color and appearance compared with the caudal portion, and the line of demarcation between the two regions is obvious, leading many clinicians to assume the presence of pathology, when this is, in fact, normal anatomy.

Renal anatomy varies according to species, and exact location may be very significant to the clinician. In iguanids and some other species, the kidneys are found dorsally within the pelvic canal. In the normal animal, they are not palpable except via digital examination of the cloaca in a large enough specimen. In other species such as monitor lizards, the kidneys are found further cranial, well clear of the pelvic canal. Renal biopsies are relatively common procedures in lizards, so it is important to have a general idea of where the kidneys are normally located.[16]

Some lizard species have urinary bladders that communicate via a short, relatively wide urethra with the ventral aspect of the urodeum. The ureters deliver urine into the dorsolateral walls of the urodeum and do not connect directly to the urinary bladder when present. Many lizards (monitors, bearded dragons) do not possess urinary bladders and store urine in the colon, when necessary. Postrenal modification of urine in the bladder or the colon is possible, and the bladder serves as an important fluid storage organ in species from arid regions.

All lizards have three-chambered hearts and are capable of shunting blood past the lungs to varying degrees. Much has been made of the clinical significance of the renal portal system, which allows for perfusion of the renal tubules when glomerular filtration is diminished, as might occur when the animal is conserving water. In the few studies that have been performed, administration of medications in the caudal portion of the body and passage through the renal portal system do not seem to affect drug pharmacokinetics in a clinically significant manner. Despite this fact, many clinicians still preferentially administer drugs, especially potentially nephrotoxic drugs, into the cranial portion of the body.[16]

Some species (iguanas, geckos) are capable of tail autotomy, which is used as a predator avoidance strategy. Tails capable of autotomy reflexively fracture along specific planes and are cast with little to no hemorrhage. The tails will continue to wiggle vigorously after being cast, and ideally distract the predator, allowing the lizard to escape. The veterinary clinician should recognize which species are capable of casting their tails, as some will do so in response to even careful handling or simply to severe stress. Other lizard species have prehensile tails (chameleons, certain skinks), which aid in living an arboreal lifestyle.[20]

For many years, the members of the family Helodermatidae were the only lizards identified as venomous. In recent years, venom and associated glands or delivery systems have been identified in a number of lizard species, including monitors and agamas. Most notable is the Komodo dragon, which historically was thought to incapacitate prey by inducing septic shock via transfer of oral bacteria to bite wounds. It has been shown that it is a potent venom produced by the lizard, not bacterial toxins, that can dramatically impact blood pressure and hemostasis, incapacitating the prey following a bite. The venom delivery system in lizards differs from those in snakes in the location of the venom glands (along the mandible in heloderms) and the presence of many ducts that release venom at the base of teeth versus the single ducts and hypodermic-like fangs of snakes.[11]

The gastrointestinal (GI) tract is fairly simple in most species of lizard. A simple stomach and relatively short, unconvoluted intestinal tract are commonly found. Some herbivorous species such as green iguanas are hind-gut fermenters and have well-developed cecae and large sacculated colons.[6]

SPECIAL HOUSING REQUIREMENTS

Much of a captive lizard's health depends on provision of a proper environment. It is critical that configuration of the captive environment reflect the natural history of the animal. Temperature, light, humidity, and ventilation, as well as the size, spacial orientation, substrate, and cage furniture, are all extremely important parameters that need to be considered when creating the optimal lizard habitat. Many species will survive and even reproduce in spartan accommodations consisting of little more than a plastic box with newspaper substrate, a water bowl, and a hide box. However, a more recent trend is toward the provision of more naturalistic accommodations for all captive reptiles, including lizards. The animals are more visually pleasing when accommodated in naturalistic environments, and they also are more likely to exhibit a wider variety of behaviors that one might not see if the animals were provided with a less stimulating environment.

Lizards, like most nonavian reptiles, are ectothermic and behaviorally thermoregulate by movements within their environment. Ectothermic animals vary their body temperatures according to the prevailing metabolic need, so to function properly, they require access to a thermal gradient within their preferred temperature zone. Gradients are also important with other parameters such as light and humidity.

Minimum acceptable size for a lizard enclosure varies according to species with regard to not only the size of the lizard but also the activity level and flight distance. Bigger is typically better in most cases. The size of the enclosure should allow the animal to move about freely and accommodate creation of multiple comfortable resting spots for the animal. Obviously, the orientation of the cage should reflect the habits of the lizard. Arboreal species should be provided with a vertically oriented enclosure with appropriate climbing structures. Terrestrial and burrowing species should be given a horizontally oriented habitat with plenty of appropriate substrate. It is important that the lizard be able to choose its own appropriate environmental temperatures, humidity, and light exposure while feeling safe and secure. Many lizards will choose security over proper temperature, so basking spots need to be secure enough for the animals to use them properly. In a similar fashion, some lizards will choose thermal needs over the need for exposure to ultraviolet B (UVB) rays. Therefore, if possible, the artificial light and heat source should be combined.

Substrate may vary, including artificial materials such as newspaper and indoor–outdoor carpeting.

An overriding concern with any captive lizard enclosure is hygiene. Regardless of how beautiful and functional the habitat is otherwise, it if it cannot be properly serviced, it is useless and potentially harmful to its inhabitants.

PHYSICAL RESTRAINT AND HANDLING

Prior to the capture and physical restraint of a lizard, a basic plan should be in place to minimize handling time, and all necessary equipment should be assembled prior to getting the animal in hand, if possible. Also, care should be taken to provide secondary containment, if possible, in case the animal evades capture and escapes the primary enclosure.

Lizards are capable of inflicting damage on a handler through bites, scratches, and tail lashes. The size and conformation of the species determines the risk involved. A house gecko (*Hemidactylus* sp.) bite may be essentially ignored, but a bite from a species such as a crocodile monitor (*Varanus salvadorii*) may warrant a trip to the emergency room and may even result in permanent disability.

It is important to know the species' behavioral profile when planning a capture-and-restraint episode. For instance, it is helpful to know that many monitor species will initially defend themselves by delivering surprisingly accurate tail lashes. If that does not deter the person attempting the capture, they will quickly resort to biting and scratching.

Most lizards may be safely restrained by gaining control of the head and neck with one hand and the pelvic area with the other. With large and aggressive animals, the judicious use of towels and leather gloves may help facilitate capture and restraint and provide an extra measure of safety. Very large lizards such as Komodo dragons, water monitors, and crocodile monitors may require multiple personnel or chemical restraint to work with safely.

On the other end of the spectrum are very small or fragile species that pose no threat to the handler but are easily injured if extreme care is not employed. Certain gecko species have extremely thin and delicate skin, which may be torn as they struggle to escape restraint. Some species with tail autotomy will drop their tails, even if the handler is not actually touching it. There is also the possibility of other injuries associated with attempted or successful escapes from handlers, including fractures, crushing wounds, and so on. When working with these very small, delicate species, it is often easiest to perform most of the examination with the animal inside a clear container or anesthetized. A strategy that may be used with small geckos or other lizards is to induce anesthesia with an isoflurane or sevoflurane-soaked cotton ball in a sealable plastic bag. Most of a physical examination may be performed with the animal in the bag, and if venipuncture is required, the tail may be accessed by cutting the corner off the bag to exteriorize the tail. Care should be taken to work quickly with this method, as gas anesthetic levels created are quite high and could result in an overdose.

Frequent handling of some species of lizard (and many other taxa for that matter) may result in significant stress, which may affect the general health of the animal. True chameleons are notorious for this, so in most situations, handling should be kept to a bare minimum. Some captive animals may seem very docile, bonded to their keepers and not at all perturbed by handling; however, these individuals are the exception to the rule.

FEEDING

The nutritional requirements of the animals with the sub-order Lacertilia are incredibly varied. Lizards may be carnivores, insectivores, herbivores, or omnivores. Additionally, many species have very specific nutritional needs, being adapted to exploit particular resources in the wild. For instance, the caimen lizard (*Draecena guianensis*), a large and attractive species from South America, feeds exclusively on snails in the wild. Other specialized feeders include the horned lizards, which prey exclusively on ants and termites, and marine iguanas, which feed on marine vegetation. These specialized feeders create challenges in situations of captivity. Sometimes the preferred food item may be replaced with items more readily available with good results. However, in most situations, the animals will do poorly and refuse to accept anything but the preferred foodstuff.

A difficult issue to address in captivity is that with the exception of the specialized feeders, most wild animals are probably consuming a large variety of food items that are not readily available in captivity. Most captive animals receive very little variation in their diets, which may lead to unrecognized deficiencies.

Obesity is a common nutritional disorder in captive lizards. Captive animals expend much less energy than their wild counterparts, and well-meaning lizard keepers tend to enjoy interacting with their animals by feeding them. The consequences of obesity in lizards and reptiles in general are thought to mirror those seen in mammals, and clinical experience would suggest that this is true. Orthopedic disease, cardiovascular disease, and GI and reproductive dysfunctions all seem related to obesity in captive lizards. Care should be taken to limit caloric intake and maximize physical activity in captive animals to avoid the development of obesity. Data from wild animals may be used to guide weight management in captivity.[9] It is important to remember that most wild animals appear too thin to the average keeper!

ANESTHESIA AND ANALGESIA

Chemical immobilization may be required when an animal is potentially dangerous to the handlers or the procedure requires an immobile patient or is likely to induce pain. Many options exist for anesthesia in lizards (Table 7-1), and the choice of a plan for anesthesia should be based on the species, the animal's condition, and the reason for the procedure rather than adopting a "one size fits all" approach. Preanesthesia evaluation and planning are critical pieces of the puzzle, as it is unwise to attempt to anesthetize an animal with severe physiologic derangement unless absolutely necessary. Lizards, like most other reptiles, are sometimes capable of withstanding changes in fluid and electrolyte balance, circulation, and so on that would quickly result in the death of most mammals. Even though these animals may withstand these insults to a point, anesthesia may be the proverbial "straw that broke the camel's back" and result in the death of an animal that may have been able to recover if given proper support.

TABLE 7-1

Selected Sedative or Anesthetic and Analgesic Agents Used in Lizards

Generic Name	Trade Name	Dose (mg/kg)	Reversal Agent
Diazepam	Valium	0.2–1.0	Flumazenil
Midazolam	Versed	0.5–2.0	Flumazenil
Butorphanol	Torbugesic	0.4–2.0	Narcan
Ketamine	Ketaset	5.0–20.0	—
Tiletamine/ zolazepam	Telazol	4.0–6.0	Flumazenil for zolazepam
Medetomidine	Dormitor	0.06–0.15	Atipamezol
Propofol	Propofol	3.0–5.0	—
Alfaxolone	Alfaxan	6–15	—
Morphine	—	1.5–10	Narcan
Meloxicam	Metacam	0.1–0.5 q24h	—
Ketoprofen	Ketofen	2 q24h	—

Propofol is a common choice for induction of anesthesia in lizard species as long as intravenous or intraosseous access is possible. Use of propofol in lizard species is typically associated with very rapid onset of effect and recovery. Propofol may be used as a sole anesthetic agent through continuous rate infusion or delivery of repeated boluses.[1] In recent years, alfaxolone has become available in some countries and is in the process of evaluation for distribution in the United States. Alfaxolone has properties very similar to propofol with regard to induction, recovery, and minimal effect on cardiopulmonary status in lizards but has the very important added benefit of being effective when administered intramuscularly. When more widely available, alfaxalone will likely become the preferred anesthesia induction agent in most reptiles, including lizards.[2,31]

Ketamine is still a viable choice of injectable anesthetic for lizards, especially large and dangerous animals that may require remote drug delivery. However, induction and recovery times with ketamine may be quite unpredictable and prolonged. The effect of ketamine may be enhanced by addition of an α-2 agonist or benzodiazepine (diazepam or midazolam). Tiletamine-zolazepam may also be used effectively and usually results in rapid inductions, but recovery time may be extended.

Isoflurane and sevoflurane are frequently used for induction and maintenance of anesthesia in lizard species. Induction using inhalants may be difficult and prolonged, as lizards as well as other reptiles are capable of shunting blood away from their lungs and hold their breath for extremely long periods without any adverse effect. Rapid anesthesia induction for very short procedures such as venipuncture in diminutive species may be accomplished by placing the animal in an airtight container with a cotton ball soaked in isoflurane or sevoflurane. The resultant percentage of agent to which the animal is exposed is extremely high, so the animal should be monitored very closely and removed from the container as soon as adequate anesthesia is achieved. Small lizards may easily be euthanized via this method simply by leaving them in the container for an extended period.

Monitoring the physiologic parameters of lizard patients during anesthesia is important; however, critical limits to measured parameters are unknown in most cases. Nonetheless, it is probably best to try to maintain parameters such as heart rate, respiratory rate, and temperature as stable and close to what would be seen in a healthy, awake animal as possible. Much of the currently available monitoring equipment may be used with the larger lizard species. However, some lizards are so small that even a fingertip Doppler probe is too big for them. Caution should be used to not overinterpret the measurements delivered by equipment that has not been validated for use with the species in question. For instance, oscillometric blood pressure measurement via cuff on a hindlimb does not work well or correlate with direct arterial pressure measurements in the green iguana.[3]

In recent years, a number of studies have investigated the effectiveness of certain analgesics in lizard species, although most of the information available regarding the use and dosage of the majority of drugs is anecdotal. Morphine has proven to provide analgesia in bearded dragons,[33] and clinical impressions suggest that it is effective in other species at similar doses. Butorphanol has been evaluated by different researchers in the green iguana, with different conclusions regarding efficacy. However, in these studies, the observed result could be explained by differences in methodology. Other opioid medications that target the same receptors as morphine should theoretically be efficacious; however, they have not been evaluated, and dosing would be empirical at best. Nonsteroidal anti-inflammatory medications such as meloxicam and ketoprofen are frequently used in lizard species, and some pharmacokinetic data exist to guide usage.[7,35]

DIAGNOSTICS AND LABORATORY SAMPLE COLLECTION

It is critical to understand that the most useful diagnostic in any case is a thorough history and physical examination. A careful, systematic physical examination with an understanding of normal anatomy, conformation, and behavior is one of the first steps in proper case management. Appropriate use of light and magnification may aid an examination infinitely, especially in small specimens. In small species with thin skin, transillumination with a cool light may yield tremendously useful information.

Imaging using the various available modalities may be useful in the medical management of lizards.[32] Radiography is very commonly used, as it is available to most practitioners. The imaging of skeletal structures is fairly straightforward but may be difficult in very small specimens unless high detail systems are available. Lizard species with osteoderms or heavy scales may be difficult to radiograph, as their dermal structures do not allow for proper imaging of internal structures. Identification of soft tissue structures is possible with proper knowledge of normal anatomy. Techniques employing positive and negative contrast media may be useful in certain instances. The application of ultrasonography in the evaluation of lizard cases is becoming increasingly common as appropriate equipment becomes more readily available and clinicians gain confidence with the modality.[34] Since lizards may vary so dramatically in size, probes with various footprint sizes and shapes are necessary to accommodate the possible range of species. Small transducer probes capable of emitting frequencies in the 10- to 12-megahertz (MHz) range are extremely useful in small species. With very small specimens, a standoff, which may be purchased or simply manufactured by filling a latex glove with water, is extremely useful and allows for more complete imaging of the patient's anatomy. Coupling of the transducer probe with the sometimes heavily scaled skin of a lizard patient may create challenges. Gel may be effectively employed as a coupling agent, but often this leaves air bubbles under and around the scales creating artifacts that make evaluation difficult. Performing the examination with the lizard's body submerged in a tub of water may be an effective method of creating adequate transducer coupling. Combined with knowledge of the normal anatomy of the species, ultrasonography may be a very effective and useful tool for evaluation of soft tissue structures and facilitate collection of diagnostic samples via aspiration. Computed tomography (CT) and magnetic resonance imaging (MRI) are also used occasionally with lizards and may dramatically aid a diagnostic investigation if applied correctly. Many veterinary facilities house CT scanners that are capable to creating useful images, even in very small patients. Software that creates three-dimensional reconstructions of CT images is available. These reconstructions are especially useful, as they allow the clinician to visualize the anatomy of the region or structure in question

thoroughly from all angles. When evaluating soft tissue change, MRI is superior to CT, so in cases specifically evaluating the central nervous system or coelomic organs for mass lesions, MRI is the preferable modality.[32]

Because of lizards' stoic nature and ability to withstand significant insult without resultant changes in hematology or plasma biochemistry parameters, it is often necessary to directly visualize and collect biopsies of diseased tissue to make a diagnosis. Minimally invasive surgical techniques with endoscopy are frequently employed to assess lizards and collect samples.[8] These techniques are useful even in extremely small patients, as telescopes in the 2- to 3-millimeter (mm) range are available. Coelomic structures, as well as those in the GI, respiratory, and reproductive tracts, are all accessible via endoscopy. In addition to collection of diagnostic samples, endoscopy is also frequently used to determine sex in monomorphic species and to perform certain surgical procedures.

Collection of blood for hematology and plasma biochemistry analysis is a routine procedure in the evaluation of lizard patients.[29] It is generally accepted that an amount of blood of between 0.5% and 0.8% of body weight in grams may be collected safely in most lizard patients. Proper handling of the sample is important to obtain the most accurate information possible. Lithium heparin is the most commonly used anticoagulant in reptile species; however, ethylenediaminetetraacetic acid (EDTA) is considered the anticoagulant of choice in some species such as the green iguana and Chinese water dragon. Heparin may create clumping of leukocytes and thrombocytes and cause a blue cast to blood films, which makes evaluation difficult. Therefore, it is recommended that blood films be made prior to placement of the sample in the anticoagulant or very soon thereafter. A number of reference ranges have been published for various species (Tables 7-2 and 7-3), but it is important to understand that these values rarely represent true "normal reference ranges." Nonetheless, these reports may serve as a starting point for evaluation of clinical cases. Diagnostic blood samples from lizards are usually collected from the ventral coccygeal vein, but other options include the ventral abdominal vein, the jugular vein, and the cranial vena cava.[28] Samples for blood gas analysis may be collected from the lingual veins, as the blood in these vessels approximates arterial samples.

Many lizards are presented in severely debilitated states and suffering from chronic disease. In these cases, multiple organs are often involved in the process, and septicemia is frequently encountered. Aseptic collection of a blood sample for culture is warranted in these severely chronic cases and may provide information critical for successful treatment. Blood samples should be cultured for both aerobic and anaerobic bacterial isolates.

SURGERY

The first step to performing successful surgery on lizard patients is a sound understanding of normal anatomy. Some literature exists to guide veterinary clinicians, but nothing replaces first-hand experience. The interested clinician should take every opportunity to perform postmortem examinations on as many species as possible to gain experience. If no other options exist, it may be necessary to extrapolate from information known about similar species. Other requirements for lizard surgery include appropriate equipment, which is usually based on the size of the patient. With tiny patients, microsurgical instruments, magnification and light, and hemostatic implements such as radiosurgery and hemostatic clips are especially important.

A number of conditions commonly encountered in lizard species require surgical intervention. Surgery of the female reproductive tract is frequently necessary to address problems ranging from preovulatory follicular stasis to egg-binding or dystocia. Ovariectomy or ovariosalpingectomy is often performed as a preventive measure in captive lizards that are not intended for breeding because of the frequency of reproductive tract disease. Complete removal of all ovarian tissue is paramount, especially when the oviducts are

TABLE 7-2

Reference Ranges for Hematologic Parameters of Selected Lizard Species

Parameters	Tegu Lizard	Caimen Lizard	Egyptian Spiny-Tailed Lizard	Frilled Lizard	Mexican Beaded Lizard	Green Iguana	Prehensile-Tailed Skink	Crested Gecko	Gila Monster
Erythrocytes (×10⁶/μL)	0.8 ± 0.2		0.7 ± 0.2	0.9 ± 0.4	1.85 ± 2.62	1.4 ± 5.8	1.45		0.50 ± 0.13
PCV (%)	35 ± 7.5	32 ± 5.8	26 ± 6.3	40 ± 8.9	32 ± 5.9	38 ± 52	35	Male 36.2 ± 4.8 Female 30.6 ± 4.6	37 ± 8
Hemoglobin (g/dL)	9.1 ± 0.3		4.6 ± 1.4	9.5 ± 3.7	9.7 ± 1.4	11.7 ± 18.6	9.6		7.4 ± 0.9
MCV (fL)	424.7 ± 156.4		324.2 ± 61.6	519.2 ± 213.6	326.7 ± 182.3		263		812 ± 370
MCH (pg)	184.7 ± 76.7		86.6 ± 11.7	±	144.1 ± 56.0		69		±
MCHC (g/dL)	38.6 ± 0		23.4 ± 4.7	34.8 ± 20.0	31.7 ± 4.8		28		20.9 ± 5.3
Leukocytes (×10³/μL)	17.7 ± 13.2	10.6 ± 7.2	12.6 ± 7.9	17.9 ± 14.2	5.5 ± 4.5	1.7 ± 15	12.4	15.4 ± 7.1	4.72 ± 0.84
Heterophils (×10³/μL)	6.4 ± 3.8	3.6 ± 3.4	9.1 ± 6.8	9.0 ± 7.2	2.0 ± 1.6	5%–55%	4.4	3%–39%	2.17 ± 0.61
Lymphocytes (×10³/μL)	9.1 ± 8.0	1.9 ± 1.0	1.9 ± 1.3	6.5 ± 6.4	2.2 ± 2.4	33%–61%	2.7	10.7 ± 5.1	1.54 ± 0.8
Eosinophils (×10³/μL)	0.3 ± 0.2	0.8 ± 0.5	0.1 ± 0.0	0.3 ± 0.2	0.3 ± 0.4	0%–1%	0.6	0%–2%	0 ± 0
Monocytes (×10³/μL)	1.4 ± 1.1	1.9 ± 2.5	1.8 ± 1.7	0.9 ± 1.0	0.3 ± 0.4	12%–35%	0.1	6%–33%	0.07 ± 0.08
Basophils (×10³/μL)	0.6 ± 0.6	3.0 ± 2.1	0.7 ± 1.1	0.4 ± 0.4	0.8 ± 1.1	5%–11%	1.0	0%–12%	0.57 ± 0.23

Values in Mean ± SD (standard deviation), unless otherwise indicated.
fL, Femtoliter; *g/dL*, gram per deciliter; *μL*, microliter; *MCH*, mean corpuscular hemoglobin; *MCHC*, mean corpuscular hemoglobin concentration; *MCV*, mean corpuscular volume; *pg*, picogram.

removed. If ovarian remnants are left behind, the tissue may regenerate and ovulation may resume, resulting in peritonitis.

The surgical approach to the coelomic cavity in lizards may be made either on the ventral midline or on the paramedian. Both approaches are appropriate, as long as care is taken to avoid disruption of the ventral abdominal vein. If the ventral abdominal vein is transected, it may be ligated without any apparent ill effect. Incisions should be made between scales, when possible. Skin closure should be made in an everting pattern such as horizontal mattress or skin staples, as the edges of incisions into scaled skin tend to invert. Incisions heal relatively slowly in lizards and reptiles in general, and if no complications occur, sutures may be removed in 4 to 6 weeks.

Amputation of injured or infected limbs or tails is occasionally necessary. If a tail amputation is indicated, it is important to know if the species is capable of autotomy. If so, the skin should be left open if tail regrowth is desired. If the skin is closed, the tail will not regrow. In species that do not have caudal autotomy, the skin should be closed to expedite healing. Lizards may do well with limb amputations, but attention should be paid to avoid leaving a stump that may become traumatized. In most cases, this means amputating at the coxofemoral or scapulohumeral joint.

Abscesses in lizards should be treated as surgical cases, if possible. Complete surgical removal of the abscess and its capsule is necessary, as otherwise it is likely to re-form. In cases in which the abscess cannot be completely resected, it should be debrided as thoroughly as possible and treated topically repeatedly until resolved. Cytology or histopathology and culture and sensitivity should be performed on the resected capsule of the abscess to identify the causative agent, if possible.

NONINFECTIOUS DISEASES

Traumatic injuries from aggressive interactions (including breeding) between conspecifics are fairly commonly. Ideally, social groups are configured and monitored in an effort to avoid serious problems. Wound and fracture care is similar to what would be employed in a mammal, but the fact that healing time will, in most cases, be longer should be kept in mind.

Despite advances in knowledge regarding the captive husbandry and nutrition of lizards, nutritional secondary hyperparathyroidism (NSHP) remains a relatively common diagnosis in captive lizards. Hypovitaminosis A resulting in lesions affecting epithelial tissues is seen with some frequency in lizards and has been linked to the use of beta carotene in lieu of vitamin A in commercial vitamin supplements. Obesity is a problem in many captive lizards, especially carnivorous lizards. Overfeeding of high-fat prey items and lack of adequate exercise seems to be at the root of most cases of obesity.

Dystocia is relatively common in lizards and often is the direct result of improper husbandry. All efforts should be made to provide optimal environmental conditions, including an appropriate nesting site, for gravid female lizards. In many species, the female will retain a fully formed clutch of eggs if nesting conditions are not to its liking. Many cases may be managed conservatively and are not true

TABLE 7-3

Reference Ranges for Plasma Biochemical Parameters of Selected Lizard Species

Parameter	Green Iguana (*Iguana iguana*)	Prehensile-Tailed Skink (*Corucia zebrata*)	Tegu Lizard (*Tupinambis teguixin*)	Mexican Beaded Lizard (*Heloderma horridum*)	Crested Gecko (*Rhacodactylus ciliatus*)	Gila Monster (*Heloderma supectum*)
T. Protein (g/dL)	5.0	6.5	6.3 ± 1.3	6.8 ± 1.2	Male: 6.0 ± 0.6 Female: 6.6 ± 0.8	6.3 ± 0.5
Albumin (g/dL)	1.0–1.6		3.5 ± 0.6	3.6 ± 1.1	Male: 2.7 ± 0.2 Female: 2.9 ± 0.3	±
Globulin (g/dL)			2.7 ± 1.2	3.6 ± 1.0	3.5 ± 0.6	±
Calcium (mg/dL)	11.4	13.2	3.0 ± 0.2 (µmol/L)	3.5 ± 1.5 (µmol/L)	Male: 11.7–14.4 Female: 15.6–20.0	12.2 ± 0.8
T. Bilirubin (mg/dL)	0.4–1.0		5 ± 3 (µmol/L)	3 ± 3 (µmol/L)		±
Phosphorus (mg/dL)	6.8	3.7	1.8 ± 0.7 (µmol/L)	1.7 ± 1.2 (µmol/L)	Male: 4.0 ± 0.9 Female: 9.6 ± 4.3	3.4 ± 1.8
Sodium (MEq/L)	158		160 ± 5	152 ± 5	134n150	144 ± 3
Potassium (MEq/L)	3.0		2.6 ± 1.3	4.0 ± 1.1	1.1–6.5	3.9 ± 0.5
Chloride (MEq/L)	117		122 ± 6	115 ± 8		±
Creatinine (mg/dL)	0.1–0.7		27 ± 9 (µmol/L)	35 ± 18 (µmol/L)		±
BUN (mg/dL)	6–15		±	±		±
Cholesterol (mg/dl)	246	144	±	±		±
Glucose (mg/dL)	150	100	±	±	106.6 ± 33.1	48.3 ± 24.2
Uric acid (mg/dL)	1.5	1.6	±	±	0.8–11.5	16.8 ± 4.2
LDH (IU/L)			635 ± 541	119 ± 98		±
ALP (IU/L)			168 ± 90	57 ± 56		±
Ionized calcium (µmol/L)						1.26 ± 0.10
Creatine kinase (IU/L)					58–3905	600 ± 457
Aspartate aminotransferase (IU/L)					9–127	42 ± 13
Bile acids (µmol/L)					<35–89	16.2 ± 13.3

Values in Mean ± SD (standard deviation) unless otherwise indicated.
ALP, Alkaline phosphatase; *BUN*, blood urea nitrogen; *g/dL*, gram per deciliter; *IU/L*, international unit per liter; LDH, lactate dehydrogenase; *MEq/L*, megaequivalent per liter; *mg/dL*, milligram per deciliter; µmol/L, micromole per liter.

emergencies. In some cases where the animal is actively straining, an obvious obstruction exists, or both, emergency salpingotomy with or without salpingectomy may be indicated.

Neoplasia

As lizards live longer in captivity because of the advances in the understanding of husbandry requirements, neoplastic disease will likely become a more frequent occurrence. Various neoplastic conditions affecting all organ systems have been reported in lizard species. The practice of oncology in lizards is the same as it is in other species. Excellent reviews of reptile oncology are presented elsewhere.[27]

The incidence of certain specific neoplastic conditions in some species is high enough to warrant mention. Bearded dragons appear to be predisposed to developing squamous cell carcinomas, with over 90% of documented cases occurring in proximity to a mucocutaneous junction in one study.[14] In addition, gastric neuroendocrine carcinomas, peripheral nerve sheet tumors, and myelocytic leukemia appear to occur with some frequency.[27]

INFECTIOUS DISEASES

A wide variety of infectious agents have been found in association with diseases in lizards. It is important to understand that in many of these cases, the conditions of captivity may play a pivotal role in the disease process. A thorough understanding of organisms that pose a threat to a particular species is paramount in development of an effective preventive medicine and quarantine program.

Bacterial Diseases

Most bacterial infections in lizards are caused by gram-negative bacteria, although gram-positive infections also do occur. When empirically selecting an antibiotic for treatment of an apparent bacterial infection in a lizard, it makes sense to choose a drug with an effective gram-negative spectrum, but ideally antibiotic treatment should be based on culture and sensitivity. Many bacterial isolates from sick lizards are usually part of the normal microbial flora but have opportunistically caused disease secondary to trauma, poor hygiene, or possible immunosuppression. Organisms that are commonly encountered include *Pseudomonas* sp., *Klebsiella* sp., *Aeromonas* sp., *Proteus* sp., and *Salmonella* sp. Anaerobic bacteria such as *Clostridium* sp., *Bacteroides* sp., and *Fusobacterium* sp. are also encountered with some frequency. In some cases, bacteria that are part of the normal flora of one species, if transmitted to another, may cause disease. For instance, *Devriesea agamarum* may cause dermatitis and septicemia in *Uromastyx* sp., but bearded dragons (*P. vitticeps*) seem to be asymptomatic carriers.[5] Doses for various antibiotics have been published for lizards,[12] and some of the more commonly used medications are presented in Table 7-4. Pharmacokinetic data are sorely lacking for most drugs with regard to lizard species, so the clinician is encouraged to be appropriately cautious when implementing treatments.

Fungal Diseases

Infection with various saprophytic fungi occurs occasionally in captive lizards and is often thought to be associated with poor hygiene, immunosuppression, or both. In contrast, infection with the *Chrysosporium* anamorph of *Nannizziopsis vriesii* (CANV) has been reported to infect a variety of reptile species, including a number of species of lizards, and has been shown to be a primary pathogen in veiled chameleons (*Chamaeleo calyptratus*). Infection with CANV may result in severe and frequently fatal dermatitis. Diagnosis may be made with fungal culture or histopathology, and successful treatment has been described in lizard species.[15]

Viral Diseases

More and more viral pathogens are being identified in lizards as diagnostics become cheaper and more readily available. Herpesviruses have been found associated with stomatitis in plated lizards (*Gerrhosaurus* sp.) and green tree monitors (*Varanus prasinus*).[37,38] In green tree monitors, the stomatitis is proliferative in nature and may lead to the development of squamous cell carcinoma. Another varanid herpesvirus that was associated with hepatitis and enteritis in an unidentified varanid species has been identified.[17] Papillomatosis in green lizards (*Lacerta viridis*) is associated with infection with an agent similar to the sea turtle fibropapilloma-associated herpesvirus.[22]

Infection with a paramyxovirus has been associated with proliferative pneumonia and death in caimen lizards (*Draecena guianensis*).[19] Evidence of paramyxoviral exposure has been illustrated in both free-ranging lizards and those from a large captive collection.[13,23-25] A paramyxovirus isolate that displayed cytopathic effect in cell culture was recovered from the cloaca of an apparently healthy flathead knob-scaled lizard (*Xenosaurus platyceps*).[24]

Adenoviruses from the genus Atadenovirus have been recovered from a number of lizard species. Pathology varies and has included hepatitis, enteritis, splenitis, nephritis, pneumonia, and encephalopathy.[30,36] In bearded dragons, adenoviral infections are well-known causes of morbidity and mortality as a result of hepatic necrosis, especially in juveniles. Typically, affected lizards suffer from concurrent infections with coccidia and nematode parasites.[18]

Other reports of specific viral infections in lizards occur intermittently, and in many cases, the clinical significance of the isolates is unknown. Numerous rhabdoviruses and reoviruses have been sequenced from lizards; however, the behavior of most of these isolates within the lizard host has not been described.[26,39] In one case, reovirus infection was associated with mortality in a group of uromastyx lizards (*Uromastyx hardwickii*).[10]

Parasitic Diseases

Internal and external parasites are frequently encountered in captive lizard patients. Wild-caught animals may almost be guaranteed to harbor at least one parasitic organism. Parasitic infections may be challenging to address, so it is important to understand the behavior of the organism and its potential impact on the host to devise a sensible treatment plan. Table 7-5 lists parasiticides commonly used in lizards.

Fecal flotation, direct microscopic examination, or both are commonly employed to screen lizards for infections with endoparasites. Collection of an adequate fecal sample for analysis may be difficult, as some lizards do not defecate daily. Many times, in the absence of a fecal sample, clinicians will perform a cloacal or rectal wash and examine the recovered fluid for presence of parasites. In the author's experience, this is an insensitive screening tool, and negative results should be viewed with caution.

Ectoparasites

Mites and ticks are commonly seen infesting captive lizards, especially animals recently captured from the wild. The common snake mite (*Ophionyssus* spp.) may be seen on lizards as well as snakes. Other mite species from the families Trombiculidae and Pterygosomatidae are also commonly seen parasitizing lizards. Both hard (ixodid) and soft (argasid) ticks may infest lizards. Acariform

TABLE 7-4

Antimicrobial Agents Recommended for Lizards

Generic Name	Dosage (mg/kg)	Route of Administration	Interval (hr)
Amikacin	5 (LD) then 2.5	IM	72
Ampicillin	5–10	IM, SC	24
Ceftazidime	20	IM	24–48
Enrofloxacin	5–10	IM, SC, PO	24–48
Metronidazole	25–50	PO	24–48
Piperacillin	100–200	IM	24–48
Trimethoprim/ sulfadiazine	15–30	IM, SC, PO	24–48
Itraconazole	5	PO	24
Voriconazole	10	PO	24

IM, Intramuscular; *PO*, oral; *SC*, subcutaneous; LD, loading dose.

TABLE 7-5

Parasiticides Recommended for Lizards

Generic Name	Dosage (mg/kg)	Route of Administration	Comments
Albendazole	50	PO	Nematodes, trematodes, cestodes
Fenbendazole	50–100 25–50	PO q14d PO q24 hr × 3–5 days	Nematodes, flagellates, giardia
Ivermectin	0.2–0.4	PO, SC q14d	Nematodes, ectoparasites
Metronidazole	50–100	PO q14d	Protozoa
Oxfendazole	66	PO q14-28 days	Nematodes
Praziquantel	8–10	IM, PO	Cestodes, trematodes
Sulfadimethoxine	50	PO q24 hr × 3 days, then EOD	Coccidia
Toltrazuril	5–15	PO q24 hr × 3 days	Coccidia

EOD, Every other day; *IM*, intramuscular; *PO*, oral; *SC*, subcutaneous.

parasites have the potential to transmit bloodborne pathogens, although this has not been well documented to this point in lizards. Typically, the pathology associated with acariasis in lizards is limited to dermatitis, which may be severe, and potentially anemia.[4]

Endoparasites

Metazoan parasites are commonly encountered in lizard species. Oxyurids are frequently encountered in commonly kept species such as green iguanas (*Iguana iguana*) and bearded dragons (*P. vitticeps*) and rarely cause clinical disease. Ascarids from the genus *Hexametra* as well as others are known to infect the stomach and the intestinal tract of various lizard species. *Rhabdias* and *Strongyloides* spp. are known to infect lizards and may cause pathology in the respiratory tract and the intestinal tract, respectively. Filarid nematodes are commonly seen in wild-collected animals and may encyst in the subcutis or body cavities and cause pathology locally. Filarids in the genus *Folyella* are most commonly encountered in certain agamids and chameleons. Pentastomids in the genus *Raillietiella* have been associated with disease in lizards.[21] Generally, most host-adapted metazoan parasites are tolerated reasonably well by lizards unless parasite numbers become too high or the host becomes compromised for other reasons.

Protozoan parasites are extremely common in captive lizards. Carriage of *Isospora*, *Eimeria*, or both species is common and typically not associated with significant disease. An exception is *I. amphiboluri*, which is an important pathogen of captive bearded dragons. This coccidian has been associated with significant morbidity and mortality in young animals. Co-infections of bearded dragons with *I. amphiboluri*, adenovirus, and dependovirus have been reported as well. Cryptosporidiosis is an extremely important disease in captive lizards and has historically caused significant losses in many lizard collections. *Cryptosporidium saurophilum* has been recognized as the causative agent of cryptosporidiosis in lizards and appears to have a predilection for the intestinal tract.[40] However, gastric cryptosporidiosis similar to what is observed in snakes is occasionally seen in lizard species.[21] It is very likely that many additional *Cryptosporidium* species are capable of causing disease in reptiles. Molecular diagnostics are available for the detection of *Cryptosporidium* in biologic samples. Oocysts may also be detected on a fecal float or direct microscopic examination by a skilled individual. Acid-fast stains and others such as auramine stain may highlight cryptosporidial organisms and aid in microscopic identification. Amebiasis is another important protozoal disease of lizards. Organisms in the genus *Entamoeba* are the causative agents of amebiasis, *E. invadans* being the most frequently implicated. Severe, hemorrhagic enteritis and systemic spread of infection with abscessation of various organs are possible with clinical amoebiasis.[21] Outbreaks of amebiasis may be explosive in susceptible collections. Treatment with appropriate medications is possible but needs to be instituted early in the course of the disease to be effective.

Microsporidium infections are also documented as a relatively common cause of disease in bearded dragons. The organism infects multiple organs, including the brain, liver, lungs, and GI tract and results in variable and nonspecific clinical signs.[21]

PREVENTIVE MEDICINE

A quarantine program is strongly recommended for all lizard collections to avoid the introduction of disease into the established population, if at all possible. Quarantine programs should ideally be based on the species and the history of the collection. All appropriate diagnostic screening for infectious disease should be conducted prior to introduction of any new animal to the established collection. Under no circumstances should a sick animal be introduced to the collection. Routine physical examinations and review of husbandry parameters are recommended on a regular basis. Collection of blood for a complete blood cell count (CBC) and chemistry panel when the animal is in good health is desirable for future comparison should the animal become ill. Surgical sterilization of female lizards

that are not intended for breeding should be seriously considered to avoid reproductive tract disease as the animal ages. No routine vaccinations are recommended; however, screening and treatment for endoparasites should be performed at regular intervals. Necropsy of all collection animals that die is paramount for understanding the effectiveness of the husbandry and consequently the general health of the collection.

REFERENCES

1. Bennett RA, Schumacher JP, Hedjazi-Haring K, et al: Cardiopulmonary and anesthetic effects of propofol administered intraosseously to green iguanas. *J Am Vet Med Assoc* 212:93–98, 1998.
2. Bertelsen MF, Sauer CD: Alfaxalone anaesthesia in the green iguana (*Iguana iguana*). *Vet Anaesth Analg* 38:461–466, 2011.
3. Chinnadurai SK, De Voe RS, Koenig A, et al: Comparison of an implantable telemetry device and an oscillometric monitor for measurement of blood pressure in anaesthetized and unrestrained green iguanas (*Iguana iguana*). *Vet Anaesth Analg* 37:434–439, 2010.
4. Chinnadurai SK, De Voe RS: Selected infectious diseases of reptiles. *Vet Clin Exot Anim* 12:583–596, 2009.
5. Devloo R, Martel A, Hellebuyck T, et al: Bearded dragons (*Pogona vitticeps*) asymptomatically infected with *Devriesea agamarum* are a source of persistent clinical infection in captive colonies of dab lizards (*Uromastyx sp.*). *Vet Micro* 150:297–301, 2011.
6. Diaz-Figueroa O, Mitchell MA: Gastrointestinal anatomy and physiology. In Mader DR, editor: *Reptile medicine and surgery*, ed 2, St. Louis, MO, 2006, Elsevier, pp 145–162.
7. Divers SJ, Papich M, McBride M, et al: Pharmacokinetics of meloxicam following intravenous and oral administration in green iguanas (*Iguana iguana*). *Am J Vet Res* 71(11):1277–1283, 2010.
8. Divers SJ: Reptile diagnostic endoscopy and endosurgery. *Vet Clin Exot Anim* 13:217–242, 2010.
9. Donoghue S: Nutrition. In Mader DR, editor: *Reptile medicine and surgery*, ed 2, St. Louis, MO, 2006, Elsevier, pp 251–298.
10. Drury SEN, Gough RE, Welchman D: Isolation and identification of a reovirus from a lizard, *Uromastyx hardwickii*, in the United Kingdom. *Vet Rec* 151(21):637–638, 2002.
11. Fry BG, Wroe S, Teeuwisse W, et al: A central role for venom in predation by *Varanus komodoensis* (Komodo Dragon) and the extinct giant *Varanus (Megalania) priscus*. *Proc Nat Acad Sci United States* 106(22):8969–8974, 2009.
12. Gibbons PM, Klaphake E, Carpenter JW: Reptiles. In Carpenter JW, editor: *Exotic animal forumulary*, ed 4, St. Louis, MO, 2013, Elsevier, pp 83–182.
13. Gravendyck M, Ammermann P, Marschang RE, Kaleta EF: Paramyxoviral and reoviral infections of iguanas on Honduran islands. *J Wildl Dis* 34:33–38, 1998.
14. Hannon DE, Garner MM, Reavill DR: Squamous cell carcinomas in inland bearded dragons (*Pogona vitticeps*). *J Herp Med Surg* 21(4):101–106, 2011.
15. Hellebuyck T, Baert K, Pasmans F, et al: Cutaneous hyalohyphomycosis in a girdled lizard (*Cordylus giganteus*) caused by the *Chrysosporium* anamorph of *Nannizziopsis vriesii* and successful treatment with voriconazole. *Vet Dermatol* 21:429–433, 2010.
16. Holz P: Renal anatomy and physiology. In Mader DR, editor: *Reptile medicine and surgery*, ed 2, St. Louis, MO, 2006, Elsevier, pp 135–144.
17. Hughes-Hanks JM, Schommer SK, Mitchell WJ, Shaw DP: Hepatitis and enteritis caused by a novel herpesvirus in two monitor lizards (*Varanus* spp.). *J Vet Diag Invest* 22:295–299, 2010.
18. Hyndman T, Shilton CM: Molecular detection of two adenoviruses associated with disease in Australian lizards. *Aust Vet J* 89(6):232–235, 2011.
19. Jacobson ER, Origgi F, Pessier AP, et al: Paramyxovirus infection in caiman lizards (*Draecena guianensis*). *J Vet Diag Invest* 31:143–151, 2001.
20. Jacobson ER: Overview of reptile biology, anatomy and histology. In Jacobson ER, editor: *Infectious diseases and pathology of reptiles*, Boca Raton, FL, 2007, CRC Press, pp 1–130.

21. Jacobson ER: Parasites and parasitic diseases of reptiles. In Jacobson ER, editor: *Infectious diseases and pathology of reptiles*, Boca Raton, FL, 2007, CRC Press, pp 571–666.

22. Literak I, Robesova B, Majlathova V, et al: Herpesvirus-associated papillomatosis in a green lizard. *J Wildl Dis* 46(1):257–261, 2010.

23. Lloyd C, Manvell R, Drury S, Sainsbury AW: Seroprevalence and significance of paramyxovirus titres in a zoological collection of lizards. *Vet Rec* 156:578–580, 2005.

24. Marschang RE, Donahoe S, Manvell R, Lemos-Espinal J: Paramyxovirus and reovirus infections in wild caught Mexican lizards (*Xenosaurus* and *Ambronia* spp.). *J Zoo Wildl Med* 33:317–321, 2002.

25. Marschang RE, Papp T, Frost JW: Comparison of paramyxovirus isolates from snakes, lizards and a tortoise. *Virus Res* 144:272–279, 2009.

26. Marschang RE, Papp T: Isolation and partial characterization of three reoviruses from lizards. *J Herp Med Surg* 19(1):13–15, 2009.

27. Mauldin GN, Done LB: Oncology. In Mader DR, editor: *Reptile medicine and surgery*, ed 2, St. Louis, MO, 2006, Elsevier, pp 299–322.

28. Mayer J, Knoll J, Wrubel KM, Mitchell MA: Characterizing the hematologic and plasma chemistry profiles of captive crested geckos (*Rhacodactylus ciliatus*). *J Herp Med Surg* 21(2–3):68–75, 2011.

29. Nardini G, Leopardi S, Bielli M: Clinical hematology in reptilian species. *Vet Clin Exot Anim* 16:1–30, 2013.

30. Papp T, Fledelius B, Schmidt V, et al: PCR-sequence characterization of new adenoviruses found in reptiles and the first successful isolation of a lizard adenovirus. *Vet Micro* 134:233–240, 2008.

31. Scheelings TF, Baker RT, Hammersley G, et al: A preliminary investigation into the chemical restraint with alfaxalone of selected Australian squamate species. *J Herp Med Surg* 2–3:63–67, 2011.

32. Silverman S: Diagnostic imaging. In Mader DR, editor: *Reptile medicine and surgery*, ed 2, St. Louis, MO, 2006, Elsevier, pp 471–489.

33. Sladky KK, Kinney ME, Johnson SM: Analgesic efficacy of butorphanol and morphine in bearded dragons and corn snakes. *J Am Vet Med Assoc* 233(2):267–273, 2008.

34. Stetter MD: Ultrasonography. In Mader DR, editor: *Reptile medicine and surgery*, ed 2, St. Louis, MO, 2006, Elsevier, pp 665–674.

35. Tuttle AD, Papich M, Lewbart GA, et al: Pharmacokinetics of ketoprofen in the green iguana (*Iguana iguana*) following single intravenous and intramuscular injections. *J Zoo Wildl Med* 37(4):567–570, 2006.

36. Wellehan JFX, Johnson AJ, Harrach B, et al: Detection and analysis of six lizard adenoviruses by consensus primer PCR provides further evidence of a reptilian origin for the Atadenoviruses. *J of Virol* 78(23):13366–13369, 2004.

37. Wellehan JFX, Johnson AJ, Latimer KS, et al: Varanid herpesvirus 1: A novel herpesvirus associated with proliferative stomatitis in green tree monitors (*Varanus prasinus*). *Vet Micro* 105:83–92, 2004.

38. Wellehan JFX, Nichols DK, Li L, Kapur V: Three novel herpesviruses associated with stomatitis in Sudan plated lizards (*Gerrhosaurus major*) and a black-lined plated lizard (*Gerrhosaurus nigrolineatus*). *J Zoo Wildl Med* 35(1):50–54, 2004.

39. Wellehan JFX, Pessier AP, Archer LL, et al: Initial sequence characterization of the rhabdoviruses of squamate reptiles, including a novel rhabdovirus from a caiman lizard (*Dracaena guianensis*). *Vet Micro* 158:274–279, 2012.

40. Xiao L, Ryan UM, Graczyk TK, et al: Genetic diversity of *Cryptosporidium* spp. in captive reptiles. *Appl Environment Microbiol* 70(2):891–899, 2004.

CHAPTER 8

Ophidia (Snakes)

Brad A. Lock and Jim Wellehan

BIOLOGY

Taxonomy and Geographic Distribution

Snakes are in the class Reptilia and the order Squamata, in the clade Toxicofera, infraorder Serpentes (snakes). More than 2900 extant species of snakes exist within three major clades: Scolecophidia, Alethinophidia, and Caenophidia.[25,29]

Scolecophidians are fossorial, blind snakes with three families in the group: Anomalepdidae (15 species [sp.]), Typhlopidae (210+ sp.), and Leptotyphlopidae (90+ sp.). Scolecophidians are oviparous and retain pelvic remnants. The Anomalepdidae (early blind snakes) live in the forested regions of Central and South Americas. The Leptotyphlopidae (Thread snakes) inhabit the semi-desert to forested regions of the tropics and subtropics of Africa, the Americas, and Southwest Asia. Thread snakes lack the left lung, the tracheal lung, and the left oviduct. The Typhlopidae (blind snakes) exist in areas ranging from the semi-desert to the rain forest regions throughout the tropics. The left lung is vestigial, and the left oviduct is absent.

Ten families exist and comprise the Alethinophidian clade: Anomochilidae (2 sp.), Uropeltidae (45+ sp.), Cylindrophiidae (8 sp.), Aniliidae (1 sp.), Xenopeltidae (2 sp.), Loxocemidae (1 sp.), Boidae (40+ sp.), Pythonidae (25+ sp.), Bolyeriidae (2 sp.), and Tropidophiidae (23 sp.). Most of Alethinophidians have well developed, bilateral ovaries and retain both pelvic vestiges and hindlimb remnants as well as a left lung. Anomochilidae (false blind snakes) are fossorial and range from the Malay Peninsula, Sumatra, and Borneo. Uropeltidae (shield tail snakes) are fossorial species from Sri Lanka and India and possess no pelvic or hindlimb vestiges. Cylindrophiidae (pipe snakes) are fossorial snakes found in the forests of Sri Lanka, Southeast Asia, and the East Indies. The single member of the Aniliidae (false coral snake) is found in northern South America. Xenopeltidae (sunbeam snakes) are semi-fossorial species from the scrub and montane forests of Southeast Asia. Sunbeam snakes lack pelvic and hindlimb remnants. Loxocemidae (Mesoamerican python) is also semi-fossorial and inhabits the forested regions from Mexico to Costa Rica. The Boidae (boas) are a wide ranging group occupying fossorial, ground-dwelling, and arboreal habitats from the Americas, Central Africa, South Asia, Madagascar, the West Indies, and the Pacific Islands. Pythonidae (pythons) are restricted to the Old World and occupy diverse habitats in Africa, Asia, and Australia. Bolyeriidae (split jaw boas) possess a divided maxilla that has both anterior and posterior components, and this group is restricted to the island of Mauritius and its northern islets. Bolyeriids do not have pelvic or hindlimb remnants. Tropidophiidae (dwarf boas) do not have the left lung but are similar, anatomically, to boas and colubrids. This group is found in terrestrial and in semi-arboreal to arboreal niches in Malaysia, the Caribbean, and Central and South Americas.

The Caenophidian clade is represented by five families: Acrochordidae (3 sp.), Atractaspididae (57+ sp.), Colubridae (1660+ sp.), Elapidae (195 sp.), and Viperidae (121+ sp.). Caenophidians are known as *advanced snakes*, and most of them have no hindlimb vestiges or left lung, but many species possess a well-developed tracheal lung. In the vipers, the oviducts are well developed bilaterally. Acrochodidae (file and wart snakes) are highly aquatic and range from South Asia to Australia. Viperidae (vipers and pit vipers) are all venomous and occupy all habitat niches worldwide except Papua-Australia, the oceanic islands, and Antarctica. Atractaspididae (stiletto or mole vipers) are venomous and occupy grassland and forested habitats from sub-Saharan Africa and the Arabian Peninsula. The Colubridae (king snakes, water snakes, bull snakes, etc.) make up the largest and most diverse group of snakes found throughout the world except Antarctica. Both venomous and nonvenomous species are found within this family, and they occupy a wide array of habitat types. The Elapidae (cobras, mambas, kraits) are venomous snakes that occupy a range of habitats throughout the Americas, Africa, Australia, Asia, and the Pacific Islands.

In squamate evolution, the earliest divergence is the geckos, followed by the divergence of the skinks, night lizards, plated lizards, and girdled lizards. The next groups to branch off are the teiids, lacertids, and amphisbaenids, and the remaining group, comprising snakes, iguanids, agamids, chameleons, monitors, helodermatids, and anguids, is known collectively as the *Toxicofera*, named for the commonality of the presence of venom glands. Snakes diverge in the middle of the squamates, and if snakes are removed, lizards are not a monophyletic group. Snakes are a group of lizards, and a pine snake is a better model for a bearded dragon than a blue-tongued skink.[25,39]

Unique Anatomy and Physiology

With few and minor exceptions, the anatomy of the snake is consistent across species, and thus a general understanding of organ location can be developed.[18] In general, the typical snake can be separated into three sections. The proximal one third of the snake contains the esophagus, trachea, parathyroid glands, thymus, thyroid, and the heart. The second third has the lung(s), continuation of the esophagus, liver, stomach, spleen, pancreas, gallbladder, proximal small intestine, and the air sac. The caudal third is the site for the caudal small bowel, gonads, adrenal glands, kidneys, cecum, colon, and cloaca. This system of thirds is often useful when attempting to identify an area of interest, when looking at a diagnostic image, or when deciding on a surgical approach.

Snakes periodically shed their skins in one piece. This process is known as *ecdysis*, and the frequency is regulated by the thyroid gland. The integument of the snake is composed of two main types, scales and interscalar skin, both of which originate from the epidermis. Scales of both types (smaller scales on the dorsum and sides and larger ventral scales) are relatively inelastic and are composed of β-keratin, whereas the interscalar region composed of α-keratin is thin and highly elastic.[21] The shed skin in snakes should generally come off in a single piece; however, larger and heavy-bodied species often shed in a few pieces. The entire process of ecdysis takes approximately 14 days to completion. Snakes do not have eyelids and instead have clear epidermis, the spectacle or brille, protecting the cornea. This spectacle is shed during ecdysis like the rest of the epidermis. Retained spectacles are a common finding with shedding or dysecdysis problems and have been associated with secondary infections of the cornea and adnexa of the eye.

Normal snake skin is dry and warm and slightly cool to the touch when the animals are kept under proper husbandry conditions. Snake skin is dry because of the relative paucity of glands in the integument in most species. The well-known facial pit organs of vipers and many boas and pythons are extremely complex structures. These pits are true eyes and not just thermal receptors, which function not by photochemical reaction but on the basis of infrared and electromechanical radiation.[10] Trigeminal innervations of the pit differ among groups of snakes possessing them, but both have innervations to the optic tectum of the brain and thus can form a usable image from this information.[10]

The skeletal system of snakes has a number of unique and interesting anatomic features. The skull is highly kinetic and does not have a rigid mandibular symphysis. The two rami of the mandible have a ligamentous connection. Snakes do not dislocate their jaws, as is commonly believed, but instead have an extra bone, the quadrate bone, connecting the lower jaw to the skull. This extra joint allows the snake to open the jaws approximately 180 degrees. These two anatomic features of the skull allow snakes to ingest extremely large prey items. Although snakes have retained ancestral cervical musculature, no cervical vertebrae are present (a snake has no neck).[4,33] Almost all snakes possess pelvic remnants, but only the Alethinophidians have hindlimb vestiges, called *spurs*, which are often used to stimulate the female during copulation.

The tongue is used in olfaction and is extended from an opening rostrally, called the *filtrum*. The tongue picks up chemical particles and then is returned to the mouth and contacts the Jacobson organ in the roof of the oral cavity. The Jacobson organ has direct connections to the olfactory nerves and serves to differentiate odors. Venom glands are modified salivary glands and combined with the highly evolved and derived venom delivery system used primarily for acquisition of prey and only secondarily for defense.

Snakes only possess an inner ear structure, and the stapes bone is in direct contact with the quadrate bone and transmits vibrations allowing for the detection of low-frequency sounds (<600 hertz [Hz]).[41] Thus, it has been a widely held belief that snakes only "hear" or respond to vibrations. Recent work has demonstrated that snakes do "hear" and respond behaviorally, to airborne sounds of various frequencies. They are able to perceive both airborne and ground-borne (known as *somatic hearing*) vibrations.[40,41]

The glottis in snakes is located on the floor of the buccal cavity, and the trachea has incomplete rings. Snakes possess one or two lungs, with the more primitive groups—boas and pythons—having two, whereas the more advanced groups have only one lung (the right lung). When two lungs are present, the right one is the primary lung, and the left is reduced. Gas exchange occurs in the cranial compartment of the lung(s), and the caudal segment or air sac serves to store air and is used in defensive "puffing" displays.

The cloaca is comprised of the coprodeum, the urodeum, and the proctodeum (CUP). The coprodeum is positioned dorsally and receives fecal material from the colon. The urodeum is located ventrally and receives urine and urate material from the ureters and ova and offspring from the oviducts. The proctodeum is the common collection chamber for the urodeum and coprodeum.

The liver starts just caudal to the heart and ends at the cranial portion of the stomach. A gallbladder is present. However, the gallbladder is not associated with the liver but is positioned more caudally in the coelomic cavity, often near the pancreas and the spleen. The pancreas, spleen, and gallbladder can form a triad in some species, but in the majority of snakes, a combined spleno-pancreas is present. The gonads are located just cranial to the kidneys and are positioned asymmetrically, with the right organ being cranial to the left. The ovary can be extremely elongated, especially during the reproductive cycle. The kidneys are highly lobulated and usually dark in color. Male snakes have paired copulatory organs, called *hemipenes*, invaginated into the base of the tail. Female snakes can be oviparous (egg-laying) or viviparous (live bearing). Rattlesnakes in the past few years have been shown to display maternal care of offspring by remaining near the young until after the young have gone through a first shed. Female rattlesnakes have been seen to provide a refuge to the young. Rattlesnake neonates have been observed to seek out the mother when threatened, and mother rattlesnakes have been seen to actively move the young away from perceived danger.

SPECIAL HOUSING REQUIREMENTS

Temperature provision is an important husbandry parameter in the overall health and well-being of captive snakes. Snakes are ectothermic and depend on environmental temperature to regulate their core body temperature. A temperature mosaic (top to bottom, side to side, and front to back) should be established on the basis of the biology of the particular species being housed, using external infrared heat sources that create basking zones. In many species, a night time drop-in temperature is safe and necessary to maintain good health. Humidity within an enclosure is important to monitor in captivity. Environmental controls (HVAC) used to maintain building temperatures can cause enclosures to become excessively dry. Snakes maintained in environments with low humidity may be predisposed to chronic dehydration, dysecdysis, and chronic renal problems. In contrast, excessive humidity is associated with development of many forms of dermatitis. For enclosures not intended for public view, the author (BL) prefers the use of a humidity chamber to increase humidity. A simple humidity chamber can be created by placing moist sphagnum moss into a plastic container of the appropriate size, with an entrance hole for the snake. Ultraviolet (UV) lighting is generally not considered critical to the health of captive snakes. Recently, however, a study showed that certain snakes increase their circulating 25 hydroxyvitamin D_3 concentration when exposed to UVB radiation.[1] UVA and rich visible light, provided by full spectrum lighting, may be important to snakes for regulating behavior and for stimulating reproduction and feeding response. Venomous snakes should be housed in enclosures equipped with a locking mechanism, and the snake must be visible from outside. Large signs should be placed on the enclosure that indicate the presence of a venomous snake inside. An emergency snake bite protocol should be developed in conjunction with a local hospital.

FEEDING

Many species of snakes have specialized diets of one or just a few prey items. Snakes are true carnivores, and no snake has been documented to be herbivorous. If possible, prey items should come from a commercial source. Although no guarantee exists, this will usually reduce the chances of parasite transmission compared with collecting road-killed or wild-captured prey. Freezing prey items for a few days prior to offering them as food to the snake will also help reduce parasite transmission. All mammalian and avian prey should be fed prekilled. The vast majority of captive snakes will either take prekilled prey immediately or quickly learn to accept prekilled food items. Live prey items, especially rodents, may cause extensive trauma to snakes if left alone in the enclosure.

Frequency of feeding can be based on a number of factors. In general, juvenile snakes may be fed more often (every 5 to 10 days) compared with adult snakes (every 1 to 2 weeks). Clinically healthy snakes may also be fasted periodically for 4 to 8 weeks without harm. The reproductive status of both male and female snakes may alter the frequency of feeding as well. When cycling a female for the breeding season, more frequent feedings are often done to increase weight prior to the fasting period associated with the gravid state. Male snakes will often refuse food during the breeding season and may become anorexic for weeks or months. Snake species that consume fishes and amphibians will generally eat more often, and two to three times a week may be appropriate.

RESTRAINT AND HANDLING

Restraint of nonvenomous snakes can be accomplished by gently grasping the head of the snake immediately behind the mandible. The body of the snake is then supported by one or more handlers (one handler for each 3 to 4 feet of snake) to protect the spine.

Venomous snakes should only be manipulated and restrained by trained professionals. These animals should be manipulated by using hooks and tongs and then restrained with the use of a clear plastic tube. The snake is encouraged to enter the tube to the midpoint level, at which time the snake's body and the tube are grasped to prevent further advancement. This technique allows for safe management of the snake for physical examination, blood collection from the ventral coccygeal vein, and administration of parenteral or gas anesthetic agents.

ANESTHESIA AND ANALGESIA

Anesthesia and analgesia (Tables 8-1 and 8-2) in snakes are used to facilitate surgery and other painful or invasive procedures and enhance the quality or safety of diagnostic sampling while minimizing stress and discomfort. Dissociative anesthetics, propofol, local anesthetics, and inhalant anesthetics are the most commonly used anesthetics in snakes.

The inhalant anesthetics (isoflurane, sevoflurane, and nitrous oxide) may be used to provide general anesthesia in snakes, isoflurane being the most common. The induction times and

TABLE 8-1

Select Anesthetic Protocols for Snakes*

Snake	Premedication	Induction
Small	None	Propofol (5–10 mg/kg, IV) Direct intubation followed by ventilation with isoflurane or sevoflurane Tube induction with isoflurane or sevoflurane
Large	Tiletamine/zolazepam (5–10 mg/kg, IM), or None	Propofol (2–7 mg/kg, IV) Direct intubation followed by ventilation with isoflurane or sevoflurane
Venomous	None	Restraint in a tube followed by propofol (5–10 mg/kg, IV) Tube or chamber induction with isoflurane or sevoflurane

*Maintenance for each is isoflurane or sevoflurane via endotracheal tube with or without nitrous oxide.

TABLE 8-2

Selected Anesthetic and Analgesic Drugs and Dosages Used in Snakes

Generic Name	Dosage (mg/kg)	Reversal Agent
Propofol	3–10	
Midazolam	0.2–2	Flumazenil
Butorphanol	20 (Monitor for respiratory depression)	
Tiletamine/zolazepam	2–10	Flumazenil for zolazepam
	Mac %	
Isoflurane	1.5–2.1	
Sevoflurane	2.5	
Nitrous oxide	220	

cardiorespiratory parameters of isoflurane and sevoflurane in snakes are very similar.[6] Although no controlled studies have been performed in snakes, nitrous oxide used as a supplemental agent during induction in monitor lizards reduced the minimum alveolar concentration (MAC) by 25%.[5] Apart from this reduction in the primary agent, which may improve cardiopulmonary function, the use of nitrous oxide likely provides improved analgesia, but this has not been critically evaluated in snakes. The primary benefit of the inhalant anesthetics over injectable agents is more direct control over the anesthetic during the procedure. At a surgical plane of anesthesia, most snakes will become apneic for long periods and should be intubated and provided with positive pressure ventilation six times per minute. Recovery should be on room air in a warmed, dark environment.

Propofol is an alkylphenol in lipid suspension that may be used singularly to provide surgical induction of anesthesia. Propofol must be administered parenterally (intravenous [IV], intraosseous, intracardiac routes) and has rapid induction (1 to 5 minutes) and recovery (30 to 45 minutes) times in most cases.[20] Ventilation is generally needed following propofol use. A recent study evaluating the histologic effects of intracardiac administration in snakes showed that lesions in cardiac tissues were mild and resolved after 14 days.[20]

Alfaxalone is a neuroactive steroid molecule with properties of general anesthesia.[27] The effects of alfaxalone in a range of reptile species have been reported and include rapid induction with good muscle relaxation when given by the IV route but prolonged induction when given by the IM route. Recently, alfaxalone was evaluated in five snake species.[27] Heavy sedation was achieved in 13 of 15 individuals tested at a dose of 9 milligrams per kilogram (mg/kg) IV alfaxalone (10 milligrams per milliliter [mg/mL]) and all 13 were easily intubated. The authors suggest that alfaxalone may be preferable to propofol as an injectable induction agent because of less cardiorespiratory depression, shorter induction times, and shorter total duration of anesthesia.

The potent dissociative, tiletamine, combined with the benzodiazepine, zolazepam, continues to have some use in snake anesthesia. The onset of effects is faster than with ketamine, but variable effects are seen in snakes even at high doses (88 mg/kg).[6] Despite the long duration of action and variable effects, the author sometimes uses low doses for sedation of large, aggressive snakes prior to handling or intubation.

Compared with other classes of reptiles, very little is known about analgesia in snakes. Snakes seem to differ from the other lizards that have been investigated (primarily green iguanas and bearded dragons) and chelonians in that they show antinociceptive effects in response to the opioid butorphanol but not to morphine. In corn snakes, a butorphanol dose of 20 mg/kg significantly increased thermal withdrawal latencies 8 hours after subcutaneous (SQ) administration, whereas a lower dose of 2 mg/kg had no effect.[29] The effective dose of 20 mg/kg is much higher than in other reptile species. Further investigation of snakes and other squamates is needed.

SURGERY

Any presurgical workup for a snake should include the following: a complete physical examination, complete blood cell count (CBC), and plasma biochemistry. These will help assess the anesthetic risk and determine the suitability of the snake for surgery. Supplemental heat should be provided in all cases during the procedure.

The coeliotomy is the most common surgical procedure performed by the author in snakes. Coeliotomy is performed to gain access for clinical evaluation and biopsy of internal organs and masses and to correct dystocia. Because a snake's ventrum contacts the substrate and a large abdominal vein runs along the ventral midline, surgical approaches should not be made through the ventral scutes. Approaches to the coelomic cavity of a snake should be made between the second and third rows of lateral scales to prevent contamination of the incision by the substrate. Coeliotomy closure

should be performed in two layers: the body wall and the skin. The skin is considered the holding layer and should be closed by using an everting suture pattern such as a horizontal mattress suture. An absorbable synthetic suture should be used to close the body wall, whereas nonabsorbable suture can be used to close the skin. In one study, polyglyconate and poliglecaprone were the least reactive of the materials.[19] Sutures can be removed 4 to 8 weeks after surgery.

Indications for gastrointestinal (GI) surgery in snakes include removal of foreign bodies, management of intestinal prolapse or intussusception, excision of masses or granulomas, and relief of impaction that generally involves the colon. Clinical signs associated with GI surgical diseases include weight loss, anorexia, abdominal distention, and vomiting or regurgitation. The basic principles of GI surgery in mammals apply to snakes. Special care should be taken when manipulating the thin-walled intestine of the snake. When closing incisions in the GI tract, it is generally considered best to get serosa-to-serosa contact.[16] A two-layer closure is ideal to close the bowel, but this is often not possible in small snakes. If any concern regarding the integrity of the closure exists, a serosal patch should be applied. Any nearby organ that has a serosal surface such as an adjacent segment of bowel, the liver, and so on may be taken and tacked in place over the closed surgical site. The two serosal surfaces will rapidly adhere to each other, thus creating a seal. Once the bowel is closed, the coelomic cavity should be irrigated with warm, sterile saline. Broad-spectrum antimicrobials are indicated if contamination is suspected.

Dystocia in snakes is generally postfollicular, and clinical signs include anorexia, regurgitation, straining, and cloacal discharge. Salpingotomy is indicated in patients that are reproductively valuable, where noninvasive techniques have failed, or if radiographic evidence indicates that natural passage is not possible. The surgical approach is a standard coeliotomy approach. When performing a salpingotomy in a snake, the incision should be made into a relatively avascular region of the oviduct. In snakes, it is often necessary to make more than one incision to access all eggs or fetuses, as these are commonly adhered to the friable oviduct. Once the procedure is complete, the incision in the oviduct should be closed by using a simple-continuous pattern with absorbable suture.

Subspectacular abscesses are commonly seen and may occur as a result of ascending infections from the oral cavity. Because of the presence of the spectacle, topical treatment is unrewarding. Treatment requires excision of the spectacle to gain direct access to the subspectacular space. This procedure should be performed with the animal under general anesthesia. A small triangular wedge is excised from the ventral aspect of the spectacle to allow for drainage of purulent material. Samples for cytology and culture may be obtained from the site by using a sterile swab. The corneal surface is then irrigated with normal saline or ophthalmic solution to remove any material. A topical ophthalmic antibiotic is instilled three to four times per day to manage the infection. Systemic antimicrobials, based on culture and sensitivity, may be warranted in cases of panophthalmitis. Over time the spectacle will regenerate, but the original incision site must remain open until the infection is under control.

DIAGNOSTIC SAMPLING AND PHYSICAL EXAMINATION

In snakes, clinical signs of disease are often nonspecific (anorexia, lethargy), thus it is important to be able to use a variety of different diagnostic techniques and modalities to arrive at a diagnosis.

The physical examination in the snake should always begin by observation from a distance without restraining the animal. Special attention should be given to tongue usage, respiration, and locomotion. The physical examination should be performed thoroughly and consistently. The spectacles should be clear, with no indication of retained epidermis or subspectacular disease. The nares should be clear and free of discharge and retained shed. The oral cavity should be evaluated by using a soft, pliable speculum. The mucous

TABLE 8-3

Statistical Analysis of Summer and Winter Hematologic Data of Captive *Boa Constrictor Amarali* (mean and standard deviation).

Parameter	Winter	Summer	Mean	Standard Deviation
RBC (/μL)	404,375 (a)	520,298.0 (b)	462,336	81,970
PCV (%)	23.2	21.7	22.5	1.07
Hemoglobin (mg/dl)	7.4	7.2	7.3	0.16
WBC (/μL)	5904 (a)	10,126 (b)	8015	2,985
Lymphocytes (/μL)	2141 (a)	5825 (b)	3982	2,605
Azurophils (/μL)	2021	1983	2000	27.1
Heterophils (/μL)	1238	1206	1221	23.9
Monocytes (/μL)	2069 (a)	93.5 (b)	219	178
Thrombocytes (/μL)	6758 (a)	12,365 (b)	9561	3,965

Different letters indicate significant differences ($p < 0.05$) between seasons.
μL, Microliter; *PCV*, packed cell volume; *RBC*, red blood cell; *WBC*, white blood cell.
From Machado CC, Silva LF, Ramos PR, et al: Seasonal influence on hematologic values and hemoglobin electrophoresis in Brazilian *Boa constrictor amarali. J Zoo Wildl Med* 37(4):487-491, 2006.

membranes should be pale to pink, without the presence of thick, ropey mucus. The glottis should be free of discharge, and the tongue should be inspected for function. The integument should be inspected closely for ectoparasites, traumatic injuries, and inflammation (dermatitis). The spine and ribs should be palpated; the spine is prominent in snakes with muscle wasting. The epaxial muscles should be well developed. Palpation should be performed to assess the coelomic cavity for abnormal masses present, and these should then be further evaluated by using appropriate diagnostic tests. Doppler ultrasonography may be used to determine heart rate and rhythm.

Blood samples should be collected from the heart, the jugular veins, or the ventral coccygeal vein. Cardiocentesis is the most reliable venipuncture technique for snakes weighing more than 200 grams (g). Placing the snakes in dorsal recumbency facilitates visualization of the beating heart one fourth to one third the distance from the snout. The jugular veins are located cranial to the heart where the lateral and ventral scales meet. The snake should be placed in dorsal recumbency for the procedure. A 1- to 1.5-inch, 22-gauge needle attached to a 1- to 3-mL syringe should be inserted approximately nine ventral scales cranial to the heart on the medial aspect of the ribs. The ventral coccygeal vein is located ventral to the caudal vertebral bodies. A 1- to 1.5-inch, 22- to 25-gauge needle on a 1- to 3-mL syringe may be used to collect the sample. Using gravity can be very useful to collect the sample; tipping the snake up with the tail lower the head often causes pooling of blood in the tail. In male snakes, caution should be used to avoid the hemipenes in the tail base.

GI lavage and pulmonary lavage may be performed to collect samples from snakes that are regurgitating or showing signs of pneumonia. A red rubber tube may be used to collect the sample. The tube should be premeasured to ensure correct placement into the stomach or lungs or through the cloaca into the colon. Physiologic saline (5 to 10 mL/kg, 3% to 5% body weight in milliliters) may be used to perform the lavage. Centrifugation of samples is often used to concentrate organisms before submission.

Computed tomography (CT) has demonstrated usefulness in the diagnosis and monitoring of treatment for pneumonia in snakes, and a few papers have described normal CT anatomy.[3,24] Ultrasonography may be used for survey imaging and as a guide for collection of diagnostic samples. Ultrasound-guided fine-needle aspiration of identified masses and fluid areas is often rewarding. Ultrasonography is well suited for monitoring the reproductive cycle of snakes, and this can be valuable in endangered species. Endoscopy, which is

highly effective in snakes because of the elongated shape and dispensability, may be used to visually evaluate organs and collect diagnostic samples for culture, cytology, and histopathology.

Hematology

Blood cell counts and plasma biochemical values in snakes are affected by environmental conditions, reproductive status, season, location, and nutrition.[2,7,8,15,26,34] Reference material for hematologic and plasma biochemistry in snakes is sparse and variable, making interpretation of a given sample difficult. Given this, it may be most efficient and effective to establish in-house reference ranges for groups or individual snakes. If this is done over a few years in different seasons and conditions, the significance of subsequent changes detected will be more easily interpretable.

Blood volumes in reptiles vary from 5% to 8% of their total body weight. Of this amount, up to 10% may be safely collected for analysis without harm to the patient. Blood samples may be stored in EDTA (ethylenediaminetetraacetic acid) or lithium heparin microtainers. CBC may be performed on samples stored in either anticoagulant. Recently, it has been shown that mixing of the blood sample with 22% albumin (1 drop albumin to 5 drops of blood) will reduce white blood cell (WBC) damage during the smear process.[30] Reference ranges for select snake species under different conditions are presented in Tables 8-3 through 8-10.

DISEASES

Bacterial Diseases

The phyla Proteobacteria and Firmicutes contain the "classic" gram-negative and gram-positive bacteria, respectively. Many of these organisms are an important part of normal flora, and context is important when clinically interpreting culture results. The most significant member of Proteobacteria in snakes is *Salmonella enterica* arizonae. *S. enterica* arizonae isolates with flagellar antigens z4 and z23 have been documented to cause significant disease in snake collections at multiple facilities. Flagellar typing of isolates from collections is therefore important. *Salmonella* sp. also represents zoonotic risks. Postprandially, Firmicutes increase as a portion of GI flora in pythons. Some of the more clinically relevant taxa include *Streptococcus* sp. and *Clostridium* sp.

The phyla Actinobacterium, Chlamydiae, and Tenericutes contain some of the more challenging bacteria encountered clinically. They tend to be less likely to grow and be identified by classical

Text continued on p. 69

TABLE 8-4

Hematology and Plasma Biochemistry Reference Values for Apparently Healthy, Free-Ranging, Giant Garter Snake (*Thamnophis gigas*) and Valley Garter Snake (*Thamnophis sirtalis fitchi*).

Parameter	N (*T. gigas*)	N (*fitchi*)	Median (*T. gigas*)	Median (*T. fitchi*)	Range (*T. gigas*)	Range (*T. fitchi*)
WBC (×10–3/µL)	46	35	11.5 (a)	6.6 (b)	2.5–18.6	3.1–13.7
RBC (×10–6/µL)	46	36	0.8	0.9	0.2–1.4	0.5–1.3
PCV (%)	46	37	31	29.5	17–45	18.5–42
Heterophils (×10–3/µL)	45	37	0.99 (a)	0.59 (b)	0.35–2.18	0.23–3.70
Lymphocytes (×10–3/µL)	46	37	7.9 (a)	4.27 (b)	1.27–14.97	1.66–15.10
Basophils (×10–3/µL)	45	37	0.33	0.29	0.09–0.83	0.65–0.86
Azurophils (×10–3/µL)	44	36	1.75	0.73	0.37–4.4	0.19–1.94
Plasma protein (g/dL)	45	35	5	5.5	4.2–6.7	4.0–8.3
AST (IU/L)	44	34	22	16	8–74	8–48
Bile acids (µmol/L)	45	34	35	35	0–35	35–47
Creatinine kinase (IU/L)	42	35	439	387	20–1666	17–1428
Uric acid (mg/dL)	44	33	5.7	5.1	1.2–13.1	1.7–16.0
Glucose (mg/dL)	43	33	81	89	44–154	53–167
Calcium (mg/dL)	45	33	15.2	15.7	12.9–20.0	11.7–16.6
Phosphorus (mg/dL)	43	34	3.8	3.6	1.9–6.3	1.8–7.6
Total protein (g/dL)	44	35	5	5.2	3.9–6.1	4.1–7.9
Albumin (g/dL)	45	36	1.2	1.2	1.0–1.7	1.0–2.1
Globulin (g/dL)	43	36	3.6	4.0	2.7–4.7	0–7.0
Potassium (mmol/dL)	44	36	5.2	4.4	2.7–8.8	1.8–7.0
Sodium (mmol/dL)	44	35	159	157	147–170	136–166

Different letters indicate significant differences ($p < 0.05$) between species.

g/dL, Gram per deciliter; *IU/L*, international unit per liter; *mg/dL*, milligram per deciliter; *µL*, microliter; *µmol/L*, micromole per liter; *mmol/dL*, millimole per deciliter; *PCV*, packed cell volume; *RBC*, red blood cell; *WBC*, white blood cell.

From Wack RF, Hansen E, Small M, et al: Hematology and plasma biochemistry values for the giant garter snake (*Thamnophis gigas*) and valley garter snake (*Thamnophis sirtalis fitchi*) in the Central valley of California. *J Wildl Dis* 48(2):307-313, 2012.

TABLE 8-5

Median Hematology and Plasma Biochemistry Values for Parameters That Differed Significantly among Giant Garter Snakes (*Thamnophis gigas*) Captured at Different Sites within the Central Valley of California (*p* < 0.05).

Parameter	Site A	Site B	Site C	Site D
Heterophil (×10–3/µL)	0.93	2.01	0.88	1.06
Basophil (×10–3/µL)	0.47	0.37	0.38	0.23
Azurophil (×10–3/µL)	1.92	3.70	2.26	1.27
Calcium (mg/dL)	14.5	16.0	16.0	16.0
Phosphorous (mg/dL)	3.6	4.5	5.6	4.8
Albumin (g/dL)	1.2	1.3	1.5	1.4
Globulin (g/dL)	3.9	3.9	3.6	3.3
Potassium (mmol/L)	5.4	4.1	5.2	5.5
Sodium (mmol/L)	154	161	153	163

g/dL, Gram per deciliter; *mg/dL*, milligram per deciliter; *µL*, microliter; *mmol/dL*, millimole per deciliter.
From Wack RF, Hansen E, Small M, et al: Hematology and plasma biochemistry values for the giant garter snake (*Thamnophis gigas*) and valley garter snake (*Thamnophis sirtalis fitchi*) in the Central valley of California. *J Wildl Dis* 48(2):307-313, 2012.

TABLE 8-6

Median Hematology and Plasma Biochemistry Values for Parameters That Differed Significantly among Valley Garter Snakes (*Thamnophis sirtalis fitchi*) Captured at Different Sites within the Central Valley of California (*p* < 0.05).

Parameter	Site A	Site B	Site C	Site D
Hemoglobin (g/dL)	10.9	8.1	8.1	9.7
PCV (%)	33	30	25	30
Plasma protein (g/L)	6.6	5.5	4.4	5.9
Calcium (mg/dL)	16.0	15.6	13.8	16.0
Phosphorous (mg/dL)	2.6	4.1	3.5	4.5
Albumin (g/dL)	1.4	1.2	1.0	1.3
Globulin (g/dL)	5.2	3.8	3.4	4.3
Potassium (mmol/L)				
Sodium (mmol/L)				

g/dL, Gram per deciliter; *g/L*, gram per liter; *mg/dL*, milligram per deciliter; *mmol/dL*, millimole per deciliter; *PCV*, packed cell volume.
From Wack RF, Hansen E, Small M, et al: Hematology and plasma biochemistry values for the giant garter snake (*Thamnophis gigas*) and valley garter snake (*Thamnophis sirtalis fitchi*) in the Central valley of California. *J Wildl Dis* 48(2):307-313, 2012.

TABLE 8-7

Statistical Analysis between Captive and Wild-Caught Hematologic Data in King Cobras (*Ophiophagus hannah*) (Mean +/– Standard Deviation)

Parameter	April	December	September
	Wild-Caught		**Captive-Bred**
PCV (%)	19.3 +/– 5.8 (a)	20.3 +/– 5.6 (a)	32.7 +/– 4.8 (b)
Hemoglobin (g/dL)	6.0 +/– 1.7 (a)	6.5 +/– 1.6 (a)	10.0 +/– 1.4 (b)
RBC (×10–6/µL)	0.60 +/– 0.2 (a)	0.55 +/– 0.19 (a)	1.0 +/– 0.13 (b)
WBC (×10–3/µL)	13.53 +/– 3.63	13.01 +/– 0.77	17.27 +/– 4.70
Azurophils (×10–3/µL)	3.27 +/– 0.59	4.65 +/– 3.99	2.15 +/– 1.73
Heterophils (×10–3/µL)	1.76 +/– 1.17	2.79 +/– 2.68	1.39 +/– 1.02
Basophils (×10–3/µL)	0 +/– 0	0.02 +/– 0.06	0.05 +/– 0.09
Eosinophils (×10–3/µL)	0.01 +/– 0.01	0.02 +/– 0.02	0.02 +/– 0.02
Lymphocytes (×10–3/µL)	8.50 +/– 3.21 (a)	9.97 +/– 3.22 (a)	13.63 +/– 3.14 (b)
Monocytes (×10–3/µL)	0 +/– 0	0 +/– 0	0.01 +/– 0.01
Azurophils (%)	26.0 +/– 9.0 (a)	21.6 +/– 13.3 (a)	11.7 +/– 7.2 (b)
Heterophils (%)	13.2 +/– 7.1 (a)	15.0 +/– 9.6 (a)	7.7 +/– 4.5 (b)
Basophils (%)	0 +/– 0	0.1 +/– 0.4	0.3 +/– 0.5
Eosinophils (%)	0 +/– 0	0.1 +/– 0.4	0 +/– 0
Lymphocytes (%)	60.8 +/– 11.1 (a)	58.4 +/– 16.8 (a)	80.1 +/– 8.3 (b)
Monocytes (%)	0 +/– 0	0 +/– 0	0.07 +/– 0.03
Plasma protein (g/dL)	7.0 +/– 1.6 (a)	9.3 +/– 1.9 (b)	6.6 +/– 0.9 (a)

Different letters indicate significant differences (*p* < 0.05) between conditions.
g/dL, Gram per deciliter; *µL*, microliter; *PCV*, packed cell volume; *RBC*, red blood cell; *WBC*, white blood cell.
From Salakij C, Salakij J, Apibal S, et al: Hematology, morphology, cytochemical staining, and ultrastructural characteristics of blood cells in king cobras (*Ophiophagus hannah*). *Vet Clin Pathol* 31(3):116-126, 2002.

TABLE 8-8

Hematologic Measures for Apparently Healthy, Free-Ranging, Southwest Carpet Pythons (*Morelia spilota imbricata*) Looking at a Number of Different Conditions (Mean +/− Standard Deviation)

Factor	Category	Hb (g/L)	PCV	RBC (×10–12/L)	WBC (×10–9/L)	Heterophils (×10–9/L)	Lymphocytes	Basophils	Monophils
Study site	Coastal	60.6 +/− 16.3	0.209 +/− 0.05	0.6 +/− 0.15 (a)	14.9 +/− 6.85	7.05 +/− 0.75	3.11 +/− 2.31	0.309 +/− 0.326	4.28 +/− 2.39
	Jarrah forest	74.3 +/− 9.62	0.227 +/− 0.038	0.672 +/− 0.102	14.9 +/− 6.23	6.62 +/− 4.02	2.94 +/− 2.51	0.345 +/− 0.240	4.87 +/− 2.69
Sex	Female	68.7 +/− 16.7	0.203 +/− 0.053	0.581 +/− 0.159	15.8 +/− 8.08	7.28 +/− 5.49	3.45 +/− 2.64	0.238 +/− 0.186	4.45 +/− 2.83
	Male	72.7 +/− 13.0	0.225 +/− 0.039	0.649 +/− 0.128	14.2 +/− 5.29	6.66 +/− 3.68	2.76 +/− 2.10	0.393 +/− 0.354	4.44 +/− 2.21
Season	Summer	80.2 +/− 10.0	0.241 +/− 0.031	0.681 +/− 0.117	13.2 +/− 5.86	6.65 +/− 4.11	2.85 +/− 2.20	0.233 +/− 0.282	4.23 +/− 2.03
	Autumn	63.7 +/− 18.0	0.190 +/− 0.062	0.536 +/− 0.169	13.8 +/− 7.14	6.07 +/− 3.68	2.98 +/− 2.33	0.345 +/− 0.278	4.38 +/− 3.29
	Winter	65.0 +/− 12.2	0.195 +/− 0.042	0.618 +/− 0.133	15.2 +/− 9.02	6.54 +/− 5.77	2.51 +/− 2.49	0.207 +/− 0.234	4.81 +/− 3.00
	Spring	69.7 +/− 13.4	0.210 +/− 0.046	0.617 +/− 0.138	18.2 +/− 6.93	8.06 +/− 4.85	3.62 +/− 2.51	0.478 +/− 0.315	4.85 +/− 2.48
State	Anesthetized	72.0 +/− 15.7	0.211 +/− 0.047	0.623 +/− 0.154	14.4 +/− 6.15	7.23 +/− 4.65	3.15 +/− 2.26	0.368 +/− 0.319(a)	4.19 +/− 2.39
	Conscious	69.8 +/− 13.7	0.220 +/− 0.048	0.617 +/− 0.136	15.5 +/− 7.20	6.56 +/− 4.41	2.94 +/− 2.50	0.270 +/− 0.267	4.78 +/− 2.58
Radiotransmitter	Pre	76.5 +/− 17.1(a)	0.232 +/− 0.051(a)	0.669 +/− 0.174 (b)	14.9 +/− 6.94	6.40 +/− 3.76	3.09 +/− 2.19	0.232 +/− 0.246(a)	4.57 +/− 2.76
	Post	66.6 +/− 12.6	0.199 +/− 0.042	0.575 +/− 0.107	13.8 +/− 7.40	6.76 +/− 5.01	2.54 +/− 2.38	0.286 +/− 0.286	4.13 +/− 2.29
	Removal	68.1 +/− 11.3	0.199 +/− 0.036	0.600 +/− 0.119	16.1 +/− 5.11	8.02 +/− 5.18	3.56 +/− 2.61	0.521 +/− 0.314	4.59 +/− 2.25
Time in captivity	0–30 days	71.0 +/− 14.3	0.215 +/− 0.045	0.610 +/− 0.137	14.4 +/− 6.71	7.12 +/− 4.95	2.94 +/− 2.39	0.266 +/− 0.214	4.12 +/− 2.25
	30–60 days	69.1 +/− 17.5	0.212 +/− 0.058	0.624 +/− 0.179	16.4 +/− 6.79	5.84 +/− 3.87	3.34 +/− 2.50	0.366 +/− 0.375	5.11 +/− 2.93
	>60 days	76.7 +/− 9.14	0.220 +/− 0.025	0.683 +/− 0.075	13.7 +/− 5.70	8.57 +/− 2.85	3.00 +/− 1.92	0.553 +/− 0.414	4.72 +/− 2.44

Different letters indicate significant differences ($p < 0.05$) between conditions.

Hb, Hemoglobin; *g/L*, gram per liter; *PCV*, packed cell volume; *RBC*, red blood cell; *WBC*, white blood cell.

From Bryant GL, Fleming PA, Twomey L, et al: Factors affecting hematology and plasma biochemistry in the Southwest carpet python (*Morelia spilota imbricata*). *J Wild Dis* 48(2):282-291, 2012.

TABLE 8-9

Plasma Biochemical Measures for Apparently Healthy, Free-Ranging, Southwest Carpet Pythons (*Morelia spilota imbricata*) Looking at a Number of Different Conditions (Mean +/− Standard Deviation)

Factor	Category	CK (Unit/L)	AST (Unit/L)	Uric acid (mmol/L)	Total protein (g/L)	Albumin (g/L)	Globulin (g/L)	Albumin/Globulin ratio	Ca (mmol/L)	P (mmol/L)
Study site	Coastal	1,630 +/− 889	61.7 +/− 34.0	0.295 +/− 0.238	71.6 +/− 12.8	17.9 +/− 3.75	54.0 +/− 11.4	0.340 +/− 0.076	3.21 +/− 0.359	1.06 +/− 0.295
	Forest	1,910 +/− 1,200	88.6 +/− 84.1	0.185 +/− 0.069	76.6 +/− 13.4	21.0 +/− 3.25	55.7 +/− 11.7	0.387 +/− 0.077	3.26 +/− 0.788	1.21 +/− 0.437
Sex	Female	1,740 +/− 1,190	66.6 +/− 61.2	0.315 +/− 0.266	72.9 +/− 14.0	19.2 +/− 4.18	54.2 +/− 12.2	0.363 +/− 0.086	3.33 +/− 0.526	1.18 +/− 0.388
	Male	1,710 +/− 841	73.0 +/− 56.7	0.221 +/− 0.140	73.4 +/− 12.6	18.6 +/− 3.60	54.8 +/− 10.9	0.349 +/− 0.073	3.14 +/− 0.519	1.05 +/− 0.310
Season	Summer	2,050 +/− 1,260	104 +/− 72.0	0.211 +/− 0.136	73.7 +/− 11.5	21.1 +/− 2.85(a)	52.6 +/− 9.55	0.409 +/− 0.062(a)	3.37 +/− 0.309	1.32 +/− 0.395(a)
	Autumn	1,860 +/− 907	61.7 +/− 33.3	0.284 +/− 0.213	72.8 +/− 13.3	19.4 +/− 4.10	53.4 +/− 10.9	0.370 +/− 0.080	3.13 +/− 0.841	1.13 +/− 0.279
	Winter	1,410 +/− 776	45.2 +/− 23.4	0.365 +/− 0.321	67.7 +/− 14.4	16.5 +/− 4.36	51.2 +/− 11.4	0.326 +/− 0.064	3.04 +/− 0.375	0.781 +/− 0.255
	Spring	1,410 +/− 715	53.1 +/− 54.7	0.245 +/− 0.187	75.8 +/− 14.0	17.4 +/− 3.02	59.2 +/− 12.8	0.302 +/− 0.061	3.23 +/− 0.502	1.05 +/− 0.219
State	Anesthetized	1,525 +/− 709	53.1 +/− 33.7	0.223 +/− 0.158	74.3 +/− 13.3	18.9 +/− 3.59	55.8 +/− 12.2(a)	0.351 +/− 0.080 (a)	3.37 +/− 0.463	1.06 +/− 0.211
	Conscious	1,940 +/− 1,210	88.7 +/− 72.8	0.301 +/− 0.246	72.0 +/− 13.0	18.9 +/− 4.16	53.1 +/− 10.5	0.360 +/− 0.078	3.06 +/− 0.551	1.16 +/− 0.453
Radiotransmitter	Pre	1,880 +/− 1,120	84.8 +/− 63.8	0.186 +/− 0.061	73.0 +/− 11.7	20.9 +/− 3.03 (a)	52.5 +/− 9.15	0.407 +/− 0.045 (a)	3.43 +/− 0.298 (a)	1.14 +/− 0.316
	Post	1,850 +/− 1,060	77.8 +/− 65.8	0.372 +/− 0.293	70.1 +/− 13.9	17.5 +/− 4.27	52.6 +/− 11.4	0.338 +/− 0.086	2.93 +/− 0.667	1.17 +/− 0.490
	Removal	1,330 +/− 569	38.8 +/− 15.7	0.255 +/− 0.198	76.7 +/− 14.3	17.1 +/− 3.02	60.5 +/− 12.9	0.290 +/− 0.054	3.22 +/− 0.523	1.00 +/− 0.168
Time in captivity	0–30 days	1,680 +/− 904	62.8 +/− 50.5	0.282 +/− 0.223	72.7 +/− 13.0	18.7 +/− 3.88	54.4 +/− 11.1	0.353 +/− 0.079	3.28 +/− 0.452	1.08 +/− 0.384
	30–60 days	1,870 +/− 1,320	76.3 +/− 67.7	0.250 +/− 0.197	74.0 +/− 13.1	18.6 +/− 3.86	55.1 +/− 11.7	0.348 +/− 0.084	3.20 +/− 0.330	1.17 +/− 0.289
	>60 days	1,590 +/− 568	101.0 +/− 74.8	0.153 +/− 0.048	74.7 +/− 16.3	20.7 +/− 3.64	54.0 +/− 13.0	0.391 +/− 0.050	2.90 +/− 1.14	1.13 +/− 0.278

Different letters indicate significant differences ($P < 0.05$) between conditions.

AST, Aspartate aminotransferase; Ca, calcium; CK, creatine kinase; g/L, gram per liter; mmol/L, millimole per liter; P, phosphorus; Unit/L, unit per liter.

From Bryant GL, Fleming PA, Twomey L, et al: Factors affecting hematology and plasma biochemistry in the Southwest carpet python (*Morelia spilota imbricata*). *J Wild Dis* 48(2):282-291, 2012.

TABLE 8-10

Hematologic and Plasma Biochemical Values That Differed Significantly (*p* < 0.05) between Sexes in Massasauga Rattlesnakes (*Sistrurus catenatus catenatus*) from Illinois

Parameter	Sex	Mean +/− SD	Min/Max
PCV	Male	27.4 +/− 4.9	17.0–34.0
	Female	17.6 +/− 6.8	7.0–25.0
Azurophils (/μL)	Male	3264 (a)	806–17013
	Female	919 (a)	522–4065
Glucose (mg/dL)	Male	90.0 +/− 42.0	29.0–189.0
	Female	50.9 +/− 20.5	28.0–89.0
Calcium (mg/dL)	Male	11.9 +/− 1.0	10.5–14.3
	Female	18.2 +/− 9.2	7.2–32.8
Phosphorus (mg/dL)	Male	2.6 +/− 1.4	1.0–6.3
	Female	4.3 +/− 1.7	1.6–6.2

(a) = median–non-normally distributed data.

mg/dL, Milligram per deciliter; *μL*, microliter; *PCV*, packed cell volume.
From Allender MC, Mitchell MA, Phillips CA, et al: Hematology, plasma biochemistry, and antibodies to select viruses in wild-caught Eastern Massasauga rattlesnakes (*Sistrurus catenatus catenatus*) from Illinois. *J Wild Dis* 42(1):107-114, 2006.

microbiology techniques; molecular identification is often needed. Sensitivity profiles are often highly variable within genera, making specific identification important for rational antimicrobial drug choice. Some of the clinically important genera in the Actinobacterium include *Mycobacterium*, *Nocardia*, *Actinomyces*, *Arcanobacterium*, *Trueperella*, *Dermatophilus*, and *Devriesea*. Granulomatous lesions are common, and one study found that 25.6% of granulomatous lesions in reptiles contained *Mycobacterium* sp. Multiple drug therapy for months or longer, ideally based on sensitivity profiles, is indicated.[30] The most clinically important genus in the Chlamydiae is *Chlamydophila*, and *C. pneumoniae* is not uncommon in snakes. Granulomatous lesions are common, and one study found that 64.4% of granulomatous lesions in reptiles contained Chlamydiales. Treatment with azithromycin or doxycycline for 6 weeks is indicated.[30] The most clinically important genus in the phylum Tenericutes is *Mycoplasma*. *Mycoplasma* sp. may be seen in snakes in association with pneumonia; the species found in snakes have yet to be named. Treatment with azithromycin or doxycycline for 6 weeks is indicated, but the possibility of carrier status after treatment should be considered.

Fungal Diseases

Fungal disease has been documented in all orders and suborders of the Reptilia except the Rhynchocephalia (tuataras). Although mycosis in captive reptiles is less commonly encountered than bacterial disease, it does occur with regularity and is likely both underestimated and underdiagnosed. Mycoses in reptiles were historically blamed on poor husbandry. Most of the organisms associated with documented reptile mycoses are heavily sporulating fungi, and if conditions are favorable (large amounts of organic debris, high humidity, unsanitary conditions), spore contamination in an enclosure may quickly reach sufficient levels to challenge the immune system of the reptiles housed within it. Isolating multiple species of fungi from a lesion is not uncommon. It has been documented that reptiles can normally harbor a large number (up to 15) of different saprophytic and pathogenic fungi on their skin.[23] Cytologic examination of the skin lesion or biopsy evaluation is essential to directing the diagnostic plan. Diagnosis of a fungal disease should be made

only when culture and histopathology confirm the specific pathologic condition associated with the organism. Treatment should follow antifungal culture and sensitivity testing.

Ascomycetous fungi in the order Onygenales have emerged as primary causes of fungal disease in squamates worldwide. The order Onygenales also contains most significant fungal pathogens of mammals including *Blastomyces*, *Histoplasma*, *Coccidioides*, and *Microsporum*. While reptile isolates have often been called the *Chrysosporium* anamorph of *Nannizziopsis vriesii* (CANV), molecular genetic evidence shows that very diverse organisms are represented in reptile disease, and *Nannizziopsis vriesii* does not appear to be a common reptile pathogen. The species most commonly identified as pathogenic in snakes is *Ophidiomyces ophiodiicola*. Infection with *O. ophiodiicola* begins with cutaneous lesions, often on the face, but often disseminates with fatal outcomes. *O. ophiodiicola* has probably been underdiagnosed, especially in earlier reports, due to unfamiliarity leading to misidentification. *O. ophiodiicola* is probably contagious among snakes. *O. ophiodiicola* is best diagnosed through biopsy of lesions, submitted for histological evaluation and sequence-based identification. Also in the clade formerly misidentified as CANV is the genus *Paranannizziopsis*; *P. australasiensis*, *P. californiensis*, and *P. crustacea* are also significant snake pathogens, although primarily in highly aquatic snakes (*Erpeton tentaculatum* and *Acrochordus* sp.). Touch preparation cytology of ulcerated or necrotic lesions may yield characteristic rectangular arthroconidia, suggestive of Onygenales. Culture for Onygenales of reptiles is best accomplished at 25°C (77°F). Voriconazole is currently the drug of choice in snakes diagnosed with infection caused by *O. ophiodiicola*; combination therapy with terbinafine is likely to be synergistic. Studies on therapy of *Paranannizziopsis* have not been done.

Viral Diseases

The family Herpesviridae are large enveloped deoxyribonucleic acid (DNA) viruses that replicate in the nucleus and have significant host fidelity. Herpesviruses are divided into three subfamilies; all herpesviruses of reptiles, including the birds, that have been analyzed to date cluster with the subfamily Alphaherpesvirinae.[17,38] These viruses are known for latency; if an animal is infected, it should be considered to be infected for life. Herpesvirus-like particles were detected in the venom gland of cobras and rattlesnakes in association with poor-quality venom, necrosis of glandular epithelial cells, and hepatic necrosis in two boa constrictors. However, none of the snake herpesviruses has been isolated or had any sequence characterization done to date, so little can be said about epidemiology or diversity.

The family Adenoviridae are large DNA viruses that replicate in the nucleus and have host fidelity. They are enveloped viruses, conferring significant environmental stability.[9] Adenoviruses are divided into six genera; all adenoviruses of squamates that have been analyzed to date cluster in the genus *Atadenovirus*. Persistent infections with atadenoviruses in squamates appear to be common. Lesions that are seen in snakes with adenoviruses include hepatitis, enteritis, gastritis, esophagitis, splenitis, and encephalopathy. There are at least three species-level clades of atadenoviruses reported in snakes so far (snake adenoviruses 1, 2, and 3). Snake adenovirus 1 has been seen in boids and colubrids, snake adenovirus 2 has been seen in viperids and colubrids, and snake adenovirus 3 has been seen in colubrids. Although cidofovir is effective against adenoviruses in mammals, safety, efficacy, and pharmacokinetic data in snakes are lacking.

The family Iridoviridae are large DNA viruses that replicate in the cytoplasm and show significantly less host fidelity than viruses that replicate in the nucleus.[17,38] These viruses are enveloped but have the ability to infect even if the envelope is damaged, rendering them more environmentally stable. In snakes, a member of the genus *Ranavirus* and an unnamed member of a probable novel genus have been identified. The *Ranavirus* was associated with nasopharyngeal ulceration and hepatic necrosis. The other iridovirus was characterized from erythrocytes and is associated with anemia. Iridoviral disease manifestation is temperature dependent; the best therapeutic strategy is to provide temperature options for the snake outside of temperatures at which disease manifests.

The family Papillomaviridae are small, nonenveloped, double-stranded circular DNA viruses. A papillomavirus has been characterized from a diamond python (*Morelia spilota*) with papillomatous skin lesions.[13] Although papillomaviruses have traditionally been considered host specific, some recent data do not support host–pathogen codivergence, and the snake papillomavirus does not cluster with the known papillomaviruses of turtles and birds. Although cidofovir and imiquimod are effective against papillomaviruses in mammals, safety, efficacy, and pharmacokinetic data in snakes are lacking.

The family Paramyxoviridae are enveloped, negative-sense single-stranded ribonucleic acid (RNA) viruses. They are associated with neurologic, respiratory, and acute immunosuppressive diseases in snakes. Two clades of paramyxoviruses are seen in snakes: the genus *Ferlavirus* in the subfamily Paramyxovirinae, and the recently discovered "Sunshine virus," which may represent a new subfamily.[11] Although ribavirin is effective against some paramyxoviruses in mammals, safety, efficacy, and pharmacokinetic data in snakes are lacking. Paramyxoviral disease manifestation appears to be temperature dependent; the best therapeutic strategy is to provide temperature options for the snake outside of temperatures at which disease manifests. While hemagglutination inhibition (HI) titers for ferlaviruses are available, only one assay has published validation. There is significant diversity within the genus *Ferlavirus*; cross-reactivity of antibodies to different genotypes is limited. For most purposes, clinical applicability of HI titers is limited, and the authors (JW) recommend use of PCR with sequencing for most clinical applications.

The family Reoviridae are nonenveloped, segmented double-stranded RNA viruses.[17,38] The segmented nature of the genome enables rapid evolution through reassortment, much like influenza. All reoviruses of snakes characterized to date are in the genus *Orthoreovirus*. Clinical disease in snakes is similar to paramyxoviral disease, but the nonenveloped nature of reoviruses makes them much more stable in the environment. Although mycophenolic acid is effective against some paramyxoviruses in mammals and birds, safety, efficacy, and pharmacokinetic data in snakes are lacking. Reoviral disease manifestation may be temperature dependent, and thermal manipulation should be considered when disease outbreaks occur.

The family Arenaviridae are enveloped, negative-sense bipartite RNA viruses. A recently discovered clade of arenaviruses is strongly implicated as the causative agents for inclusion body disease (IBD) of boas and pythons.[32] The number of species-level genotypes in this clade is growing rapidly. Clinical disease primarily consists of immunosuppression, and the animal is typically overwhelmed by secondary disease. Disease may progress slowly and take months or years. Ribavirin, genistein, and favipiravir are effective against some arenaviruses in mammals, but safety, efficacy, and pharmacokinetic data in snakes are lacking. The chronic nature of IBD differs significantly from mammalian arenaviral infections; and antiviral therapy does not appear promising. Consensus adenoviral, iridoviral, papillomaviral, paramyxoviral, reoviral, or arenaviral polymerase chain reaction (PCR) with sequencing are currently the most straightforward ways to diagnose infection with these viruses; this should be combined with histopathology to determine clinical significance.

Parasitic Diseases

Protozoa and nematodes may be commensal or parasitic, depending on the species of parasite, environment, coinfections, and the general condition of the host. Distinguishing when endoparasites are causing problems may be difficult. Chronic parasitism may have an overall negative effect on the host. The best time to treat snakes against parasites is during the quarantine period, before the animals are introduced into a collection.

Entamoeba invadens is one of the most significant protozoal parasites infecting snakes. This organism has a direct life cycle, and

transmission is through the fecal–oral route.[12] Herbivorous tortoises have been known to harbor this parasite without showing clinical signs. However, in snakes, this amoeba may cause damage to the intestinal mucosa, resulting in hemorrhagic enteritis, colitis, and hepatitis.[12,31] Diagnosis may be made on a direct smear with Lugol iodine or a fecal flotation. In situ hybridization has been effective for speciation in snakes and a commercial PCR assay is under development (Jim Wellehan, University of Florida, personal communication, April 2013). The treatment of choice is metronidazole for trophozoites, with or without combination therapy, and paromomycin for cysts. Colubrids and rattlesnakes may be more sensitive to metronidazole, and these species should be treated at the lower dose and frequency. Temperature may also play a significant role in therapy; multiple studies have shown that infected snakes kept at 33–35°C did not develop clinical disease, whereas infected snakes at 25° consistently died. Because of the severe lesions present, secondary bacterial infections, especially with *Salmonella* species, are common, so antimicrobials should be considered in the treatment plan against amoeba (Table 8-11).[31]

The protozoa *Cryptosporidium* spp. are monogenous (entire life cycle in one host) and are a significant cause of parasitic disease in snakes.[36] Transmission is via the fecal–oral route, and fomite transmission may occur, as these parasites have a thick-walled sporozoite that is resistant to desiccation and most disinfectants (only ammonia, 5%, and formal saline are effective against oocysts).[36] All *Cryptosporidium* spp. have direct life cycles. The two most significant species in snakes are *Cryptosporidium serpentis*, which has gastric tropism and *Cryptosporidium varanii* (formerly *C. saurophilum*), which has small intestinal tropism.[12,36] Snakes infected with *C. serpentis* often present with poor growth, weight loss, regurgitation, and gastric hypertrophy leading to a midbody swelling. The common clinical sign is regurgitation that leads to chronic weight loss and muscle wasting. Snakes infected with *C. varanii* usually present with wasting, poor growth, and diarrhea, with no symptoms of regurgitation. Histopathologically, cryptosporidial organisms have been seen on the gallbladder and intra- and extrahepatic bile ducts.[12] Antemortem diagnosis is made by demonstrating the oocysts in mucus-coated, regurgitated food, gastric lavage samples, in impression smears of biopsy samples, or in feces by using acid-fast stains. A nested PCR with sequence analysis is available (at the University of Florida) for all *Cryptosporidum* spp. and should be used for speciation, as morphology alone cannot distinguish pathogenic from nonpathogenic (mouse) species.[36] For antemortem samples, it is suggested to contact the laboratory first. During quarantine, acid-fast screening of fecal samples with PCR sequencing for any positive results should be considered. Shedding of the organism is transient, so multiple fecal samples may be required for diagnosis. Endoscopic biopsies or laparotomy samples may be evaluated for the presence of the organism. Treatment is unrewarding and has not proven effective. Paromomycin may have some efficacy but needs to be evaluated critically. Nitazoxanide (Navigator, IDEXX Lab Inc., Westbrook, ME) may have promise, based on mammalian data.[36] Consideration should be given to culling confirmed cases from the collection, and prevention through quarantine is the best control method.

The most important and frequently encountered coccidian parasites in snakes are *Eimeria* spp. (direct life cycle), *Isospora* spp. (direct life cycle), and *Caryospora* spp. (direct or indirect life cycle).[34,37] With intestinal *Coccidia* spp., young animals tend to have the heaviest infestations and show the most significant clinical signs.[35] Lesions that have been reported in snakes, include necrotizing cholecystitis, fibrosis and epithelial ulcerations, and catarrhal and diptheroid inflammation of the small intestine.[12,35] Diagnosis may be made by evaluation of fecal material on a direct saline smear or fecal flotation. A nested PCR assay with product sequence analysis is available for all *Coccidia* sp. from the University of Florida. This PCR test with sequence analysis is important, as other coccidian (mouse) species that may be identified from fecal flotation analysis in snakes may not be morphologically distinguishable from pathogenic coccidian species.[35]

TABLE 8-11

Antimicrobials Used to Treat Snakes

Drug	Dose	Comments
Amikacin	3 mg/kg every 72 hours	Use caution in dehydrated snakes or those with renal disease
Azithromycin	10 mg/kg PO every 48–72 hours	
Carbenicillin	400 mg/kg IM every 24 hours	
Ceftazidime	20 mgk/g IM every 72 hours	
Chlorhexidine	Topical 0.05% to 0.1%	Use to clean external topical wounds
Ciprofloxicin	10 mg/kg PO every 24–48 hours	
Enrofloxicin	5–10 mg/kg IM once, then PO every 24 hours	Multiple injections may cause necrosis at injection sites
Itraconazole	5–10 mg/kg PO, SID	Pulse therapy: 1 week on 3 weeks off, may have synergistic effect with terbinafine (use each 1 week per month) Monitor blood values for signs of organ insult
Fluconazole	5 mg/kg PO, SID	Yeasts only
Voriconazole	5–10 mg/kg PO, SID-BID	Monitor blood values for signs of organ insult
Silver-sulfadiazine	Topical	Apply topically for dermatitis and wounds
Terbinafine	10 mg/kg PO, SID	Pulse therapy: 1 week on 3 weeks off, may have synergistic effect with Itraconazole (use each 1 week per month) Monitor blood values for signs of organ insult
Trimethoprim-sulfadimethoxine	20 mg/kg PO or IM every 24 hours	Use caution in dehydrated snakes or those with renal disease

BID, Twice daily; *IM*, intramuscularly; *mg/kg*, milligram per kilogram; *PO*, by mouth; *SID*, once a day.
From Mitchell MA: Snakes. In Michell MA, Tully TN, editors: *Manual of exotic pet practice*, 1st ed, St. Louis, MO, 2009, Saunders.

Although flagellates are commonly encountered in the GI tract of snakes, few reports of lesions associated with flagellates in snakes exist. Many of these organisms are commensals and likely serve an important role in the maintenance of the microecology of the GI tract. Flagellates are often found in the intestinal lumen of clinically healthy snakes, and thus it is often difficult to attribute disease of ill snakes to the presence of flagellates in the fecal sample. The most significant genera in snakes are *Trichomonas*, *Tritrichomonas*, and *Monocercomonas*, the genera most commonly associated with lesions being *Monocercomonas*.[12] Confirmed lesions of *Monocercomonas* include cholecystitis, chronic regurgitation, pneumonia, pancreatic duct lesions, and salpingitis.[12] Clinical signs are generally nonspecific and include lethargy and anorexia. Diagnosis can be made on fecal material by a direct saline smear, and treatment is accomplished with metronidazole.

Digenetic trematodes are only rarely associated with disease in captive-bred snakes. These flukes have an indirect life cycle, which generally is a gastropod, and thus infestations are self-limiting. The most significant order of cestodes found in snakes is the Pseudophyllidea. Pseudophyllideans of the genera *Bothridium* and *Bothriocephalus* are mainly parasites of boid snakes, whereas the genus *Spirometra* is widely distributed among snake genera.[12] The life cycle requires an intermediate host and is thus usually self-limiting in captivity. *Bothridium* and *Bothriocephalus* have been associated with severe edema and hemorrhage in the small intestinal tract as well as mild-chronic enteritis.[12]

Spirometra is widely distributed in snakes, which serve as an intermediate or paratenic, host. The plerocercoid life stage is commonly seen in snakes, especially wild-caught animals, and present as subcutaneous, soft swellings of the body, known as *spargana*.[12] Edema and hemorrhage have been associated with this stage in snakes. Treatment is by surgical incision and extraction. Adults of both parasites are found in the small intestine. Diagnosis of pseudophyllidian infections is based on identification of *Spirometra* larvae on direct smear or of the eggs on fecal flotation. Pseudophyllidean eggs are operculated and float in salt solutions.[12] Treatment may be accomplished with praziquantel.

Renifers, or lung flukes, may be encountered in the oral cavity. Adults migrate from the oral cavity into the lungs and attach to the epithelial lining causing focal lesions, which have been associated with secondary bacterial pneumonia. Another member of the Plagiorchiidae known to infect snakes is *Styphlodora*. This species inhabits the urinary system of snakes, where infections of collecting tubules and ureters are seen. Lesions associated with infection include renal tubular dilatation and chronic interstitial nephritis.[12] Treatment is accomplished with praziquantel.

Nematodes are the most frequently diagnosed endoparasite in snakes. Life cycles can be either direct or indirect, and clinical signs vary with parasite density and location within host tissues. Affected snakes may be asymptomatic or present with diarrhea, intestinal obstruction and torsion, pneumonia, renal disease, and muscle wasting. Most lesions and clinical signs are attributable to larval migration through tissues, with subsequent tissue damage and secondary bacterial infections. Diagnosis may be made by examining a direct fecal smear of fecal flotation. A variety of parasiticides may be used to treat nematodes (Table 8-12).

Pentastomids are an assemblage comprising approximately 100 species of vermiform arthropods that are obligate parasites of the lower respiratory tract of vertebrates.[37] Affected animals may be asymptomatic or have generalized respiratory disease. Taxonomy is in flux, and recent evidence, based on sperm morphology and molecular data, strongly suggests that pentastomes are crustaceans highly adapted to an endoparasitic lifestyle and most closely related to branchiurans, which include *Argulus* spp. or fish lice.[37] All require an intermediate host for completion of the life cycle, and zoonotic potential exists for some species to humans (*Armillifer* and *Porocephalus*). Antemortem diagnosis depends on identification of eggs in lung washes or feces, and survey radiography may provide an indication of infection. Larvae possess hooklets that can be seen inside the thin-walled eggs. Treatment in larger snakes is best accomplished via removal endoscopically. Chemotherapeutic agents that have been used or suggested include diethylcarbamazine, praziquantel, levamisole, thiobendazole, and ivermectin. Ivermectin and fenbendazole administered orally in 4 Boelen's pythons at 200

TABLE 8-12

Parasiticides Used to Treat Snakes

Parasiticide	Dose/Frequency	Indication	Comment
Fenbendazole	25–50 mg/kg PO SID 1–3 days; repeat in 14 days	Nematodes	25 mg/kg for ball pythons; monitor heterophil counts for declines
Ivermectin	0.2 mg/kg PO or SQ, every 10 days for 2 to 4 Tx	Ectoparasites and nematodes	Do not use in indigo snakes or debilitated snakes
Levamisole	5–10 mg/kg intracoelomically once; repeat in 2 weeks	Lungworms	Drug has narrow range of safety Do not use in debilitated snakes
Metronidazole	25–50 mg/kg PO once; repeat every 7 days for 2 to 3 Tx 25–50 mg/kg PO every 2 to 3 days for 3–5 Tx	Flagellated protozoa *Entamoeba invadens* (clinical snakes)	Use lower dose for indigo snakes, milk snakes, king snakes, and rattlesnakes
Ponazuril	5–20 mg/kg PO SID ×28 days	Coccidia	Dose and frequency based on mammal data; an empirical dose of 30 mg/kg (two doses 48 hours apart) has been used in bearded dragons
Toltrazuril	5–20 mg/kg PO SID ×28 days	Coccidia	A frequency of SID for 3–5 days has been effective anecdotally
Nitazoxanide	25 mg/kg PO SID for 5 days, then 50 mg/kg PO SID ×23 days	Coccidia/cryptosporidia	Not critically evaluated in reptiles
Amprolium hydrochloride	10 mg/kg PO SID ×7–12 days	Coccidia	Potential thiamine deficiencies; may be less effective than the other drugs
Sulfadimethoxine	90 mg/kg PO once, then 45 mg/kg SID ×7–10 days	Coccidia	Potential folic acid deficiencies; may be less effective than the other drugs
Trimethoprim/Sulfamethoxazole	30 mg/kg PO SID ×2d, then q48h ×26 days	Coccidia	Potential folic acid deficiencies; may be less effective than the other drugs
Praziquantel	5–8 mg/kg PO or IM once; repeat in 14 days	Cestodes/trematodes	
Paromomycin	50–100 mg/kg PO SID ×28 days	*Cryptosporidium* cysts	

IM, Intramuscularly; *mg/kg*, milligram per kilogram; *PO*, by mouth; *SID*, once a day; *SQ*, subcutaneously; *Tx*, treatment(s).

microgams per kilogram (μg/kg), and 100 milligrams per kilogram (mg/kg) respectively, for 3 consecutive days seemingly resolved the infection. However, this dose of fenbendazole may cause significant bone marrow suppression and damaged gut epithelium in many species. Because pentastomes are crustaceans, it has been suggested that therapeutics for fish lice may be more appropriate than anthelmintics, but this has not been investigated in snakes. The drug with the best evidence for anti-pentastomid use is loperamide; it has not been investigated in snakes.

Mites and ticks are in the subclass Acari within the class Arachnida. Aside from being a distinct lineage, ticks are simply a group of large mites. Ticks are a common finding on wild-caught snakes and are commonly found around the eyes and within the gular fold but may be found anywhere on the body. Although good documentation is lacking for snakes, ticks are known vectors of disease and should be manually removed. It is important to grasp the tick near its attachment (mouth parts) to prevent body remnants leading to granuloma or abscess formation.

Ophionyssus natricis is the common snake mite. This ectoparasite can be devastating in snake collections. Both larval and adult forms of the mite are parasitic and may become reproductive within 2 to 2.5 weeks and live for 5 to 6 weeks. *O. natricis* may serve as a vector for disease transmission and has been shown to transmit *Aeromonas hydrophila*. It has been postulated that snake mites may play a role in the transmission of inclusion body disease but this has not been substantiated.

A variety of parasiticides have been used to eliminate mites, including bathing the snake in water or applying mineral oil topically, topical and parenteral ivermectin, organophosphates, topical permethrin, and topical pyrethrins. Treatment must be two-fold, including both the snake and the environment. Provent-a-Mite (Pro Products, Mahopac, New York) has been found to be both effective and safe when the directions on the label are followed.[14]

Noninfectious Diseases

Nutritional Diseases

Primary nutritional disease in snakes is not well documented and seems to be uncommon. Husbandry may play an important role in improper nutrition. Snakes housed under the wrong temperatures may be exposed to hypothermia or hyperthermia, which will negatively affect feeding and digestion. Both temperature extremes will lead to anorexia and regurgitation if food is taken. Obesity is the most common nutritional disorder observed in captive snakes. Obesity may lead to a number of health problems, and reproduction is often very poor in both females and males. Leaner food items should be offered, especially to snakes that feed on mammalian prey. Young rats and mice have less fat than older adult breeders, and rabbits, in general, are leaner than rodent prey. Reducing the weight of an obese snake should be done slowly over a period of 6 to 12 months; rapid reduction of food may lead to hepatic lipidosis in some cases.[28]

Captive snakes should not be fed wild-caught prey items. These wild prey items often harbor parasites, may be exposed to pesticides or insecticides, and may have accumulated biotoxins in their tissues. Rodent suppliers who use pesticides to manage ectoparasites in their operation should be asked to stop the use of pesticides a minimum of 3 weeks before shipment. The few snakes that are fed primary insect prey should have these items treated, as in the case of an insect-eating lizard (dusting with a vitamin or calcium powder, feeding high-quality diet 24 hours prior to feeding), to avoid nutritional secondary hyperparathyroidism (NSHP). Dusting with a calcium or vitamin source has also been suggested for snakes fed neonate rodents to improve the calcium content of the food item.

Piscivorous snakes fed a strictly fish diet may be predisposed to thiamine and vitamin E deficiencies (although this is not well documented). Signs of thiamine and vitamin E deficiencies are neurologic and include loss of righting reflex, abnormal locomotion, muscle tremors, and blindness. Thiamine (25 mg/kg, IM) once a day for 72 hours followed by oral dosing at the same rate seems to be corrective.[22] Vitamin E deficiencies leading to steatitis may occur when snakes are fed fish high in polyunsaturated fats. Feeding a variety of fish species, and not a high percentage of fatty, cold water fish, is an effective preventive strategy.

QUARANTINE

The goal of a quarantine is to allow animals to be monitored for disease for a sufficient period to avoid introducing infectious agents into a collection. Therefore, it is critical to first understand what is already in a collection before deciding what needs to be kept out. Progression of infectious diseases in snakes may be significantly slower; quarantine periods of at least 90 days are recommended. Standard quarantine surveillance protocols used for snakes in zoos have become somewhat dated. Although it is often recommended that titers for ferlaviruses be run, besides the complications of ferlavirus titers mentioned earlier, the focus of pathogen testing in quarantine should not be directed toward pathogens that manifest disease relatively rapidly, since part of the point of extended quarantine is to allow disease to manifest. Testing should be targeted toward agents causing chronic diseases that may take longer than a quarantine period to manifest, especially those that are environmentally stable and have direct life cycles, thus posing a greater collection threat. Some of the snake pathogens that merit most significant consideration for quarantine testing include adenoviruses, arenaviruses, *Chlamydophila pneumoniae*, and *Cryptosporidium* sp.

REFERENCES

1. Acierno MJ, Mitchell MA, Zachariah TT, et al: Effects of ultraviolet radiation on plasma 25-hydroxyvitamin D3 concentrations in corn snakes (*Elaphe guttata*). *Am J Vet Res* 69:294–297, 2008.
2. Allender MC, Mitchell MA, Phillips CA, et al: Hematology, plasma biochemistry, and antibodies to select viruses in wild-caught Eastern Massasauga rattlesnakes (*Sistrurus catenatus catenatus*) from Illinois. *J Wild Dis* 42(1):107–114, 2006.
3. Banzoto T, Russo E, Toma AD, et al: Evaluation of radiographic, computed tomographic, and cadaveric anatomy of the head of boa constrictors. *Am J Vet Res* 72:1592–1599, 2011.
4. Bergmann PJ, Irschick DJ: Vertebral evolution and the diversification of squamate reptiles. *Evolution* 66:1044–1058, 2012.
5. Bertelsen MF, Mosely CA, Crashaw GJ, et al: Inhalation anesthesia in Dumeril's monitor (*Varanus dumerili*) with isoflurane, sevoflurane and nitrous oxide: Effects of inspired gasses in induction and recovery. *J Zoo Wildl Med* 36:62–68, 2005.
6. Bertelsen MF: Squamates (snakes and lizards). In West G, Heard D, Caulkett N, editors: *Zoo animal and wildlife immobilization and anesthesia*, ed 1, Ames, IA, 2007, Blackwell.
7. Bryant GL, Fleming PA, Twomey L, et al: Factors affecting hematology and plasma biochemistry in the Southwest carpet python (*Morelia spilota imbricata*). *J Wild Dis* 48(2):282–291, 2012.
8. Dutton CJ, Taylor P: A comparison between pre- and posthibernation morphometry, hematology, and blood chemistry in viperid snakes. *J Zoo Wildl Med* 34(1):53–58, 2003.
9. Garner MM, Wellehan JFX, Pearson M, et al: Characterization of enteric infections associated with two novel atadenoviruses in colubrid snakes. *J Herp Med Surg* 18:86–94, 2008.
10. Goris RC: Infrared organs of snakes: An integral part of vision. *J Herpetol* 45:2–14, 2011.
11. Hyndman TH, Marschang RE, Wellehan JFX, Nicholls PK: Isolation and molecular characterization of sunshine virus, a novel paramyxovirus found in Australian Snakes. *Infect Genet Evol* 12(7):1436–1446, 2012.
12. Jacobson ER: Parasites and parasitic diseases of reptiles. In Jacobson ER, editor: *Infectious diseases and pathology of reptiles—color atlas and text*, ed 1, Boca Raton, FL, 2007, CRC Press.
13. Lange CE, Favrot C, Ackermann M, et al: Novel snake papillomavirus does not cluster with other non-mammalian papillomaviruses. *Virol J* 8:436, 2011.
14. Lock BA, Stahl SJ: Ectoparasites. In Mayer J, Donnelly TM, editors: *Clinical veterinary advisor—Birds and exotic pets*, ed 1, St. Louis, MO, 2013, Saunders.
15. Machado CC, Silva LF, Ramos PR, et al: Seasonal influence on hematologic values and hemoglobin electrophoresis in Brazilian boa constrictor amarali. *J Zoo Wildl Med* 37(4):487–491, 2006.
16. Mader DR, Bennett RA, Funk RS, et al: Surgery. In Mader DR, editor: *Reptile medicine and surgery*, ed 2, St. Louis, MO, 2006, Saunders.
17. Marschang RE: Viruses infecting reptiles. *Viruses* 3:2087–2126, 2011.
18. McCracken H: Organ location in snakes for diagnostic and surgical evaluation. In Miller RE, editor: *Zoo and wildlife medicine, current therapy*, ed 4, Philadelphia, PA, 1999, Saunders.
19. McFadden MS, Bennett RA, Kinsel MJ, et al: Evaluation of the histologic reactions to commonly used suture materials in the skin and musculature of ball pythons (*Python regius*). *Am J Vet Res* 72:1397–1406, 2011.
20. McFadden MS, Bennett RA, Reavill DR, et al: Clinical and histologic effects of intracardiac administration of propofol for induction of anesthesia in ball pythons (*Python regius*). *JAVMA* 239:803–807, 2011.
21. Mitchell MA: Ophidia (snakes). In Miller ER, Fowler ME, editors: *Zoo and wild animal medicine*, ed 5, St. Louis, MO, 2003, Saunders.
22. Mitchell MA: Snakes. In Michell MA, Tully TN, editors: *Manual of exotic pet practice*, ed 1, St. Louis, MO, 2009, Saunders.
23. Sigler L, Hambleton S, Paré JA: Molecular characterization of reptile pathogens currently known as members of the *Chrysosporium* anamorph of *Nannizziopsis vriesii* complex and relationship with some human-associated isolates. *J Clin Microbiol* 51:3338–3357, 2013.
24. Pees MC, Kiefer I, Ludewig EW, et al: Computed tomography of the lungs of Indian pythons (*Python molurus*). *Am J Vet Res* 68:428–434, 2007.
25. Pyron RA, Burbrink FT, Colli GR, et al: The phylogeny of advanced snakes (Colubroidea), with discovery of a new subfamily and comparison of support methods for likelihood trees. *Mol Phyl Evol* 58:329–342, 2011.
26. Salakij C, Salakij J, Apibal S, et al: Hematology, morphology, cytochemical staining, and ultrastructural characteristics of blood cells in king cobras (*Ophiophagus hannah*). *Vet Clin Pathol* 31(3):116–126, 2002.
27. Scheelings FT, Baker RT, Hammersley G, et al: A preliminary investigation into the chemical restraint with alfaxalone of selected Australian squamate species. *J Herp Med Surg* 21:63–67, 2011.
28. Simpson M: Hepatic lipidosis in a black-headed python (*Aspidites melanocephala*). *Vet Clin North Am Exot Anim Pract* 9:589–598, 2006.
29. Sladky KK, Kinney ME, Johnson SM: Analgesic efficacy of butorphanol and morphine in bearded dragons and corn snakes. *JAVMA* 233:267–273, 2008.
30. Soldati G, Lu ZH, Vaughan L, et al: Detection of mycobacteria and chlamydiae in granulomatous inflammation of reptiles: A retrospective study. *Vet Pathol* 41:388–397, 2004.
31. Stahl SJ: Entamoebiasis. In Mayer J, Donnelly TM, editors: *Clinical veterinary advisor—Birds and exotic pets*, ed 1, St. Louis, 2013, Saunders.
32. Stenglein MD, Sanders C, Kistler AL, et al: Identification, characterization, and in vitro culture of highly divergent arenaviruses from boa constrictors and annulated tree boas: Candidate etiological agents for snake inclusion body disease. *Mol Biol* 3:180–225, 2012.
33. Tsuihijii T, Kearney M, Rieppel O: Finding the neck-trunk boundary in snakes: Anteroposterior dissociation of mycological characteristics in snakes and its implications for their neck and trunk body regionalization. *J Morphol* 273:992–1009, 2012.
34. Wack RF, Hansen E, Small M, et al: Hematology and plasma biochemistry values for the giant garter snake (*Thamnophis gigas*) and valley garter

snake (*Thamnophis sirtalis fitchi*) in the Central valley of California. *J Wildl Dis* 48(2):307–313, 2012.

35. Wellehan JF, Stahl SJ: Coccidiosis. In Mayer J, Donnelly TM, editors: *Clinical veterinary advisor—Birds and exotic pets*, ed 1, St. Louis, MO, 2013, Saunders.

36. Wellehan JF, Stahl SJ: Cryptosporidiosis. In Mayer J, Donnelly TM, editors: *Clinical veterinary advisor—Birds and exotic pets*, ed 1, St. Louis, MO, 2013, Saunders.

37. Wellehan JF, Stahl SJ: Pentastomes. In Mayer J, Donnelly TM, editors: *Clinical veterinary advisor—Birds and exotic pets*, ed 1, St. Louis, MO, 2013, Saunders.

38. Wellehan JFX, Johnson AJ: Reptile virology. *Vet Clin N Am Exot Anim Pract* 8:27–52, 2005.

39. Wiens JJ, Hutter CR, Mulcahy DG, et al: Resolving the phylogeny of lizards and snakes (Squamata) with extensive sampling of genes and species. *Biol Lett* 8(6):1043–1046, 2012. published online 19 September 2012.

40. Young BA, Morain M: The use of ground-borne vibrations for prey localization in the Saharan vipers (*Cerastes*). *J Exp Biol* 205:661–665, 2002.

41. Young BA: Snake bioacoustics: Toward a richer understanding of the behavioral ecology of snakes. *Quart Rev Biol* 78:302–325, 2003.

CHAPTER 9

Ratites or Struthioniformes: Struthiones, Rheae, Cassuarii, Apteryges (Ostriches, Rheas, Emus, Cassowaries, and Kiwis), and Tinamiformes (Tinamous)

Maya S. Kummrow

RATITES

General Biology

Ratite is not a strict taxonomic term; it is used to refer to flightless birds that do not have a keel but have, rather, a flat "raft-like" breast.[2,19] In general, ratites are classified in one order, Struthioniformes, with four suborders with distinct geographic distributions: (1) Struthiones are endemic to the African continent (apart from introduced populations in Australia), (2) Rheae in South America, (3) Casuarii in Australia and New Guinea, and (4) Apteryges in New Zealand.[19]

Struthiones include one family, Struthionidae, and one species with currently four recognized subspecies: (1) the North African ostrich (*Struthio camelus camelus*), (2) the Somali ostrich (*S. c. molybdophanes*), (3) the Massai ostrich (*S. c. massaicus*), and (4) the South African ostrich (*S. c. australis*).[19] Many farm populations (*S. c. domesticus*) are hybrids of various subspecies. Although ostrich farming became well established on the African, American, European, and Australian continents in the second half of the 20th century, wild ostriches have become exceedingly rare in some parts of their range. South Africa and East Africa still hold strong populations, but most of the *S. c. camelus* subspecies populations in West and North Africa are considered endangered.[14,19] The Rheidae, the only family to the suborder Rheae, are endemic to the Neotropical Region and include two species: (1) the Common or Greater Rhea (*Rhea americana*) and (2) the Darwin's or Lesser Rhea (*Pterocnemia pennata*). Although neither species is reckoned to be in immediate danger, both have been listed as near-threatened, and their numbers are declining in most parts.[19] The close genetic relationship between the families Dromaiidae (emus) and Casuariidae (cassowaries) is recognized by the common suborder Casuarii. Emus consist of one single species (*Dromaius novaehollandiae*) and occur in stable populations on mainland Australia, and the cassowaries constitute three clearly distinguishable species (Southern cassowary, *Casuarius casuarius*; Dwarf cassowary, *C. bennetti*; Northern cassowary, *C. unappendiculatus*), with a high number of subspecies.[19] All three species occur in altitudinally separate habitats in New Guinea, and the Southern cassowary also occurs in the northern parts of Australia. Because of defragmentation and reduction of their rain forest habitat, cassowaries are considered endangered.[19,41] The fifth ratite family, the kiwis (Apterygidae), is endemic to New Zealand and consists of three species (Brown Kiwi, *Apteryx australis*; Little Spotted Kiwi, *A. owenii*;

Great Spotted Kiwi, *A. haastii*). Habitat destruction, inadvertent poisoning and trapping for pest control, and introduced predator species have greatly reduced their numbers and rendered some populations endangered, but because of their reclusive way of living, their status is poorly known.[29]

Whereas emus occur in a wide variety of habitats, ostriches prefer open semi-arid areas with short grass and are well adapted to hot and dry environments.[14,18,19] Rheas are characteristic to the semi-arid tall grass steppe and other savannah-type habitats of South America, but they like the vicinity of water or wetlands for breeding.[19] Cassowaries and kiwis are most typically found in rain forest habitats,[19,41] but because of destruction of habitat, kiwis are also to be found in other habitats with relative high humidity, adequate soil texture, and density of vegetation to dig their burrows. All ratites may swim.[19]

Ostriches and rheas are gregarious, diurnal birds, with males being territorial and entertaining polygamous social structures during breeding season.[14,18,19] Emus are usually found alone or in pairs except when they form large groups on the move or in places where water and food are abundant. Cassowaries are shy, solitary, and territorial all year round, with a mostly crepuscular activity pattern. Kiwis are almost entirely nocturnal, take refuge in earth burrows during the day, mate for life, and show strong attachment to their territory.[19]

Unique Anatomy

Except for the kiwi, the ratites are the largest birds in the world (Table 9-1). Ratites lack a keel, and as the need for flight is absent, ratites lack clavicles (except emus) and triosseus canals, the thoracic girdle is modified by fusion of scapula and coracoid, and the only pneumatized bone is the femur in ostriches and emus. The wings are vestigial and carry variable numbers of claws (two in ostriches, one in rheas, none in emus and cassowaries) and are used for balance and display behavior. Ratites have long, heavily muscled legs, which enable them to run at high speeds; they also use their legs for defense and offense, kicking forward, with cassowaries using both feet at once. Ratites lack a patella. Whereas emus, cassowaries, and rheas have tridactyle feet with a nail on all toes, the ostrich only has two toes (didactyl) with a nail on the larger, medial toe only. Cassowaries carry a daggerlike, dangerously sharp claw on the inner toe. Kiwis have a small fourth toe pointing caudally with a spurlike nail.[18,19,52,53]

TABLE 9-1

Morphologic and Reproductive Aspects of Ratites

	Ostrich	Emu	Rhea	Cassowary	Kiwi
Size (m)	2.5–3.0	1.5–1.8	1.5–1.7 (Common> Darwin's)	1.7–2.0	0.3–0.6
Max. weight (kilogram [kgl])	120–160	38–55	25	60–85	1–4
Gender size	M > F	F > M	M > F	F > M	F > M
Breeding strategy	Polygamous	Paired for breeding	Polygamous	Paired for breeding	Paired for life
Eggs No/female/year	<100	7–20	10–15	3–6	1–3
Color	cream	dark green granular	yellow- greenish	light, bright green	white
Weight	1–2 kg	500–700 grams (g)	400–600 g	600–700 g	400–500 g
Incubation (days)	39–44	56–61	39–42	60	71–78 (–92)
Incubating partner	M (night), F (day)	M	M	M	M
Parental care	M (+F), 1 year	M	M, 4–6 months	M	M (+ F)

M, Male, *F,* female.
From Del Hoyo J, Andrew E, Sargatal J: Order Struthioniformes. In Del Hoyo J, Elliott A, Sargatal J (eds): *Handbook of the birds of the world,* Volume 1, Barcelona, Spain, 1992, Lynx Editions.

In ratites, the barbules, although present, do not interlock, giving the ratite feathers the particular fluffy appearance sought after for decoration and fashion.[18,19] Feathers of the emu and cassowaries have a double shaft.[53] Down feathers are rare or absent, and ratites continuously molt. The plumage of kiwis has a shaggy appearance because of the hard, hairlike, waterproof distal ends. Cassowaries have a unique protuberance on the head, called *casquet* or *helmet.* Brightly colored wattles are only present in the Northern and Southern species and likely function as a social signal.[19,41,53]

The respiratory system in ratites is comparable with that of other avian species with 10 air sacs.[6,7] In the emu, the complete cartilaginous tracheal rings in the distal trachea are interrupted by a 6- to 8-cm long ventral cleft, where a thin membrane forms a large, expandable pouch to produce the characteristic booming sound.[19,52,53] Respiration rates of ostriches fall within two ranges, either within a low range of 3 to 5 breaths per minute (breaths/min) or a high range of 40 to 60 breaths/min when panting in response to heat stress.[53] Ratites have a slightly lower core body temperature compared with other birds; kiwis, especially, have a low average basal temperature of 38° C, approximating that of mammals.[47]

All ratites lack a true crop, but considerable differences exist in the musculature and enzyme secretory function of the gastric compartments and characteristics of the intestinal tract, reflecting adaptations to different diets.[18,52,53] Having adapted to a rough, fibrous diet, both ostriches and rheas rely on a small glandular patch in the proventriculus but show a large, thick-walled ventriculus with a distinct koilin layer. Other than in the rhea, in which the proventriculus is significantly smaller than the ventriculus, both compartments are similarly sized and connected by a large, rather indistinct sphincter in the ostrich and small stones for grinding are physiologically found in both compartments. Ostriches show a unique arrangement of the two gastric compartments, with the thin, saclike proventriculus taking a turn and the gizzard being located cranioventrally. Whereas the rhea largely depends on enormous paired ceca for effective hindgut fermentation, the ostrich has a particularly voluminous colon and long rectum and relatively smaller ceca. Spiral folds within the cecal lumen provide an increased surface area for fermentation. Following the adaption to a more nutritive and less fibrous diet, the proventriculus in emus and cassowaries is comparably large and diffusely glandular, whereas the small ventriculus is thin walled and lacks a koilin layer altogether in the cassowaries. The paired ceca in emus and cassowaries are vestigial and of minor functional importance, particularly in the cassowary. The gastrointestinal (GI) passage time is approximately 48 hours and 18 hours in ostriches and rheas, respectively, but only 7 hours in emus.[53] In all ratites, a particularly

strong rectal–coprodeal sphincter results in separate defecation and voiding of urine: feces are stored in the rectum, whereas urine is mainly stored in the proctodeum, which acts as "bladder."[18] Ratites lack a true bursa; instead, the bursa of Fabricius in the ostrich and emu forms an integral part of the dorsolateral wall of the proctodeum. No gallbladder exists in the ostrich, but one is present in the other ratites.[53]

Male ratites have an intromittent reproductive organ. In adult ostrich males, the flaccid phallus is up to 20 cm long and lies folded in a phallic pocket in the ventral wall of the proctodeum; when erect, it may reach a length of 40 cm and physiologically deviates to the left.[18,53] It serves to transport sperm via a dorsal sulcus (in the ostrich and kiwi) or a central cavity (in the rhea, emu, cassowary) but has no urinary function.[53] Manual gender determination may be easily conducted in young birds at 1 to 3 months: the clitoris and the phallus are similarly sized but differ in shape and in the presence of the seminal groove.[18] Female reproductive organs are similar to those of other avian species; usually only the left ovary and oviduct develop.[53] Kiwis, however, are among the very few avian species with paired ovaries.[29]

Although the larger ratites have acute eye sight,[53] the nocturnal kiwi mostly relies on its strong sense of smell with its nostrils at the distal tip of the beak and excellent hearing, as evidenced by large earholes. Kiwis lack a pecten, and their vision is rather poor.[19]

Special Housing Requirements

Ostriches and, to a lesser extent, emus and rheas are reared as farm animals for meat, feathers, and hides in Africa, Europe, Australia, and South and North Americas.[18,19,52] Ostriches and rheas may be kept in large groups; however, during breeding season, males become territorial, so harem groups are advisable.[18] Emus are usually kept in pairs. In zoologic institutions, ostriches, rheas, and emus are commonly included in multispecies exhibits with other herbivores. In the wild, ostrich groups move and feed with herds of hoofstock, but they tend to avoid close contact with other animals. If startled or challenged, ostriches may react with panicky escapes; therefore, exhibits need to provide sufficient space and structures to allow avoidance or flight behavior. Barriers have to be easily visible, as ostriches, emus, and rheas tend to get entangled and caught in piles of branches, wires, and dry moats. Large ratites are usually kept in open paddocks and fenced pastures.[18] Ratites need indoor enclosures or at least dry shelters to be protected against wind and precipitation. They may tolerate cold temperatures and even snow for short periods, but they are sensitive to cold-wet conditions.[45] As waterproofing is impossible because of the lack of interlocking barbules, ratites get sodden in rain, and they lack down feathers for insulation.[19] Indoors areas with heated or at least well-insulated flooring are imperative for hatchlings and juveniles.[18]

Cassowaries may also be kept in pairs and may tolerate each other, but it is advisable to keep them separate for incubation of the eggs and rearing of the chicks.[23,41] Keeping kiwis in captivity is not easy; usually, only the Brown Kiwi is kept in zoologic institutions but is very rarely bred. Kiwis are to be kept in pairs as they take mates for life. Deep earth floors for burrowing, high humidity, and dense vegetation are important factors in their exhibit.[19]

Feeding

Ostriches and rheas are exclusively vegetarian and selective grazers with very efficient fiber utilization in postgastric microbial fermentation. Green annual grasses and forbs are preferred, although leaves, flowers, fruit from succulent and woody plants, and, rarely, insects and small invertebrates are also consumed.[18,19] Because of the economic interest in ratite farming, a large body of information on the nutritional requirements of ostriches is available. Complete diets are commercially available in pelleted form, which should be supplemented with high-quality roughage and vegetation for adequate fiber intake and enrichment.[13,52,53] Having adapted to an arid environment, absence of drinking is possible in adult ostriches, rheas, and emus if succulent food is fed, but reduced weight gain and impaired reproduction are often caused by inadequate water supply.[19,52] Emus are omnivorous but show a highly selective behavior for nutritious food items. In the summer time, a large part of their diet consists of insects.[19] Cassowaries are largely frugivorous but may also consume fungi, insects, and small vertebrates.[41] Wild kiwis consume almost exclusively invertebrates from the forest floor, but their captive diets are generally meat and fruit, with much higher carbohydrate and water content and lower crude fat compared with the diet in the wild.[19,39]

Restraint and Handling

While chicks and kiwis may easily be restrained manually, catch pens or chutes are most appropriate for adult, large ratites. Ratites jump, kick, and slash in a forward direction; therefore, manual restraint of large ratites may be dangerous and requires experienced personnel.[47,52] The risk of injury from the daggerlike claw does not allow for manual restraint of adult cassowaries.[47] Ostriches, emus, and rheas may be approached from behind or the side. At least three people are needed to handle an adult bird, but care needs to be taken not to grab the bird by the neck (neck hooks are not recommended), the legs, or the vestigial wings or to interfere with respiration during straddling.[47,52,53] In ostriches, lowering the head quickly to the ground prevents them from kicking, and they may even assume sternal recumbency. Darkness has a calming effect on ratites, and hooding is one of the best aids to handle manually restrained ostriches.[52] Other ratite species are less tolerant of hooding, and the effect is unpredictable.[53] As ratites are prone to exertional myopathy, chemical restraint is advisable for any longer procedure to reduce stress and risk of injury to birds and handlers.[52]

Whereas most other birds and chicks are not recommended to be fasted for anesthesia, adult large ratites may be fasted for 12 to 24 hours and water withheld for up to 4 hours prior to anesthesia to reduce the risk of regurgitation and aspiration.[42,52,53] Chicks and kiwis are usually just manually restrained for induction via face mask and maintained, ideally intubated, on isoflurane inhalation. For remote injection of anesthetic drugs in larger birds, the ideal dart placement is perpendicular into the proximal thigh muscle.[53] Underdosing may result in overexertion during the excitatory phase and should be avoided. Benzodiazepines (diazepam or midazolam 0.3 to 1 milligram per kilogram [mg/kg]) and α_2-agonists (xylazine 0.2 to 3 mg/kg, medetomidine 0.05 to 0.5 mg/kg) are commonly used alone or in combination with butorphanol (0.1 to 0.2 mg/kg) for sedation and premedication, but times to effect and efficacy are highly variable and depend on the disposition of the bird.[42,52,53]

Ketamine (3 to 20 mg/kg) or telazol (2.3 to 4.9 mg/kg) are commonly used as induction agents but need to be combined with benzodiazepines or α_2-agonists to prevent muscle rigidity and rough induction and recoveries.[47,53] Injectable agents rarely provide anesthesia of sufficient duration for longer procedures, and inhalants (usually isoflurane) are commonly used for maintenance.[42,52,53] Intubation is achieved easily with the tracheal opening readily visible at the base of the tongue.[47] The unique tracheal cleft in emus necessitates wrapping of the lower neck with an elastic bandage to avoid insufflation of the pouch.[47,53] Alternatively, intravenous (IV) maintenances on a triple-drip combination (ketamine, xylazine, and guaifenesin) or propofol infusion are described in the literature.[47] Ratites appear rather refractory to the sedative effects of potentiated opioids but show excessive running or frenzied activity during the excitatory phase and apnea during anesthesia.[47] However, combinations of thiafentanil, α_2-agonists, and telazol have shown promising results in emus and rheas.[6,17,38]

Monitoring via pulsoxymetry is possible on the ulnar vein or intermandibular tissue.[47] Supplementation of vitamin E or selenium, nonsteroidal anti-inflammatory agents, and adequate infusion therapy may be advisable to prophylactically address exertional myopathy.[47] Recovery should occur in a dark, padded room, or the birds need to be supported until they are able to maintain normal head position. Sternal recumbency is not a problem, but lateral recumbency over a long time might result in peroneal nerve paralysis, so careful padding is crucial.[53] A body wrap may help to control the recovery process.[52] Haloperidol administration achieved long-term sedation in adult ostriches for transport and reduction of aggression, lasting for 20 hours.[38] For short transports, azaperone is useful as it provides little muscle relaxation but good tranquilizing effects for up to 24 hours.[47]

Surgery

One of the most commonly described surgical interventions in ratites is proventriculotomy to address gastric impaction and ingestion of foreign bodies.[3,33,52,53] Juvenile ostriches are most commonly affected, but cases in juvenile rheas and an adult kiwi have been reported.[24,25] The proventriculus in ostriches is palpated in the left paramedian quadrant over the xiphoid. A left lateral approach over the proventriculus is preferred. Failure to adequately absorb the yolk sac may necessitate removal of the yolk sac in chicks, which is usually performed with a ventral midline approach, cranial of the umbilicus to beyond the extension of the yolk sac.[52,53] After excising the umbilical cord, the yolk sac is lifted out of the coelomic cavity and the duct ligated. Any spillage of yolk requires vigorous rinsing with warm saline. As in all other birds, egg binding may have to be addressed surgically, and castration of male ratites has been performed successfully.[18,53]

Wound management and orthopedic surgery are commonly necessary, as traumatic injuries are frequent in ratites.[52,53] These procedures follow the same principles as in any other species, considering the requirements to support heavy weights and bipedal locomotion in these large and rather nervous animals.[52]

Other Pharmaceuticals

In most countries, no drugs have been licensed for ratites, and chemical therapeutics need to be used in an off-label manner compatible with the local veterinary authority guidelines. Because of the lack of large pectoral muscles, the preferred injection sites in ratites are the epiaxial or proximal leg muscles.[53] IV access is possible at the right jugular vein and medial metatarsal or ulnar veins. If IV access is not possible, intraosseous catheters in the ulna or tibiotarsus may be placed in juvenile birds.[47] Only few pharmacokinetic studies in ratites exist, and most drug therapies are extrapolated from commonly known avian dosages. However, several studies found differences in the pharmacokinetic profiles not only between ostriches and other avian species but also between emus and ostriches. Therapeutic success should therefore be carefully monitored and evaluated.[11,53]

Physical Examination and Diagnostics

Blood sampling is, as in most avian species, most convenient from the large right jugular vein of the neck or the medial metatarsal vein in young or anesthetized adult birds.[18,52] Because of the highly movable skin along the neck, placement of a permanent catheter into the jugular vein may be very difficult, and the ulnar or medial metatarsal veins are preferred for IV catheters.[53] Lithium-heparin or citrate should be used as anticoagulants, as EDTA (ethylenediaminetetraacetic acid) causes hemolysis.[18,53] Reference ranges for blood values are comparable with those in other avian species but vary considerably in the literature; single samples may, therefore, be difficult to interpret, and trends in multiple, sequential samples are most useful to evaluate the progress of disease in an individual bird.[18,52,53] Physical examination in ratites is similar to that in other avian species.[53] Ratites are very sensitive to stress-associated diseases, so careful risk assessment of the necessary diagnostic steps and treatments is necessary. Full body survey radiographs (e.g., for suspected gastric impaction) are best accomplished with large ratites standing, either sedated or hooded in manual restraint, with a horizontal beam against a radiographic plate attached to the wall.[52]

Disease—General

Increased demand of ostrich products and worldwide ostrich trade in the 1990s raised the question of their disease status regarding poultry diseases (e.g., avian influenza, Newcastle disease) and led to the legal classification of ostriches as "poultry" in most jurisdictions with application of the same restrictions.[2] Most diseases in ratites are, therefore, described for the economically interesting species such as ostrich, emu, and rhea. For cassowaries and kiwis, not many publications are readily available, but both species appear susceptible to the same types of diseases that are described for other ratites and avian species. Exceptions are discussed below.

Infectious Disease

GI infections are very common in chicks and juvenile ratites. Yolk sac retention and infection is a multifactorial disease causing mortalities in chicks up to 2 weeks of age.[21] Source of infection either originates from egg contamination or naval infection. *Escherichia coli* is often involved and responds poorly to antibiotics, necessitating surgical removal or aspiration of the yolk.[18,22,52,53] Enteritis in chicks and juveniles is often caused by failure to establish a balanced gut flora, the use of antibiotics, lack of fibers in the diet, hypothermia, excessive coprophagy, and poor hygiene. A multitude of bacterial pathogens such as pathogenic strains of *E. coli*, *Salmonella* spp., *Klebsiella*, *Aeromonas* sp., *Pseudomonas* sp., and certain strains of *Campylobacter jejuni* (enteritis, hepatitis in chicks) and *Clostridium perfringens* may be involved.[15,18,44,52,53] Spirochete-associated (*Serpulina hyodysenteriae*) necrotizing typhlitis was diagnosed most frequently in young rheas in summer and fall.[28,53] Viral (avian influenza virus, coronavirus, rotavirus) or protozoal pathogens (cryptosporidia, *Histomonas meleagridis*) have also been identified in ratites with GI problems.[15,18,53] Fungal proventriculitis and ventriculitis are common sequelae to gastric impaction, and *Macrorhabdus ornithogaster* has caused severe losses in juvenile ostriches.[15,18,26,53]

Respiratory diseases are commonly caused by infections with *Pasteurella* sp., *Pseudomonas* sp., *Bordetella* sp., *Haemophilus* spp., *Staphylococcus* spp., *Streptococcus* sp., *Corynebacterium* sp., *Mycoplasma* spp., and *Chlamydophila psittaci* in predisposed birds because of hypothermia, stress, and overcrowding, or poor air quality.[18,44,52,53] Respiratory aspergillosis caused by *Aspergillus fumigatus* and other *Aspergillus* spp. is a common problem in juveniles or compromised adults in stressful or suboptimal management conditions.[15,18,52,53] Antifungal prophylaxis should be considered during antibiotic treatment or stressful situations such as transports and translocations.

Acute deaths in juvenile emus from *Erysipelothrix rhusiopathiae* septicemia has been reported several times. The disease could be controlled with antibiotic treatment, improved husbandry management, and annual vaccination of birds.[49,53] The ostrich is the only

avian host susceptible to *Bacillus anthracis*, but cases have become extremely rare.[49,53] Mycobacteriosis, commonly caused by *Mycobacterium avium*, occurs occasionally in zoo ratites but is very rare in farms. It is hardly ever a herd problem but often affects individual birds; however, because of the theoretical zoonotic potential, this pathogen has attracted a lot of attention. Clinical signs either reflect localized lesions (granulomatous lesions at conjunctiva, cloaca, phallus) or generalized infection (GI, liver) in which the animals slowly waste away. Culture and polymerase chain reaction (PCR) assay on tubercles is considered the gold standard diagnosis, but as no effective treatment exists, affected birds should be culled.[15,53]

Cryptococcus neoformans var. *gattii* (serotype B) was identified in a kiwi with disseminated infection in the heart, kidney, liver, oviduct, and pancreas. Eucalyptus mulch was thought to be the source of infection. Because of their lower body temperature compared with other birds, kiwis are thought to be more susceptible to cryptococcosis.[27]

Ostriches, emus, and rheas are among birds that are highly susceptible to avian influenza, and various strains have been identified in ratites, including H7N1, H5N9, H5N2, H9N2, and H10N7. The pathogenicity in ratites depends on the viral strains, with particularly high mortality reported in H7N1 outbreaks among juvenile ostriches. Chicks are more susceptible than adults, and secondary bacterial respiratory and intestinal infections sometimes mask the underlying viral infection.[12,52] Despite the highly contagious nature of avian paramyxovirus serotype 1 (Newcastle disease) during an outbreak, chronic neurologic disease in ostriches tends to spread relatively slowly through the population, is usually limited to a small number of birds (mostly juveniles), and may therefore be controlled with vaccinations. Emus have tested serologically positive, but no cases of clinical disease have been described.[2,12,30,52] In contrast to the pathogenesis in most other avian species, eastern equine encephalitis virus does not cause neurologic disease in emus and rheas but shows a unique visceral tropism, primarily leading to GI symptoms.[52,53,55] Avian poxvirus may manifest as either wet or dry forms. Vaccination with fowl pox vaccines has proven effective in ostriches.[12,52,53] Bornavirus infection has been reported to have resulted in outbreaks of paresis and general malaise, followed by anorexia, depression, and death from dehydration in ostrich chicks in intensive farming conditions.[12,53] Both adenovirus and circovirus were isolated from sick ostrich chicks and were suspected to be implicated in the "chick-fading syndrome."[22,40,53] Miscellaneous viral pathogens reported in ratites include infectious bursal disease virus (only experimental disease, no natural infections reported),[35,53] rotaviruses, orthoreoviruses, and reoviruses (serologically positive samples or viral isolation, but clinical relevance remained unclear),[18,53] and Crimean-Congo hemorrhagic fever (CCHF), a tick-transmitted disease occurring across the African continent, that causes a short, symptomless viremia in sheep, cattle, and ostriches and has fatal zoonotic potential (through handling of tick-infested ostriches or through contact with infected ostrich blood during slaughter).[12]

Two cases of spongiform encephalopathy in adult ostriches in German zoos have been histologically described, but the etiology was never confirmed with electronmicroscopy.[18]

Parasitic Disease

A range of endoparasites were identified in ratites, of which GI nematodes are of most significant clinical importance, as they cause economic losses in ratite farming.[18,36,53] In ostriches, the trichostrongylid nematodes *Libyostrongylus douglassii* (most common), *L. dentatus*, and *L. magnus* are found in the openings of the deep proventricular glands and under the koilin layer of the proventriculus and the gizzard. Heavy parasitic load may lead to proventriculitis with associated weight loss and anemia and to high mortality in chicks and juveniles.[15,18,36,53] The parasite appears to be rather host specific but may infect other ratites such as rheas. Similarly, in rheas, *Sicarius uncinipenis*, a reddish worm, inserts itself between the koilin layer and the ventricular mucosa and leads to destruction of the koilin layer.[53,56] In addition, the large-intestine nematodes

Paradeletrocephalus minor and *Deletrocephalus dimidiatus* are considered to be of some relevance because of their blood-feeding habits, which may, in high infections, be associated with an anemia syndrome in rheas.[36,56] *Trichostrongylus tenuis* has been found in the ceca of emus, and pathogenicity is comparable with that in game birds. A low burden might remain clinically unapparent, but large numbers of parasites may result in bloody diarrhea, progressive anemia, and toxemia.[36,53] *Codiostomum struthionis* is a slightly larger helminth, which inhabits the distal cecum and upper rectum of adult ostriches but is mostly clinically inapparent.[18,36,53] *Houttuynia struthionis* is a large tapeworm, which inhabits the small intestine of ostriches and rheas, causing ill-thrift in young ostriches.[15,18,36,53] *Fasciola hepatica* has been associated with subacute and chronic hepatitis in emus. Antiparasitic treatment with triclabendazole may be necessary in severely affected birds, and separation of hoofstock carriers and pasture management are recommended. Although no reports of clinically apparent fasciolosis exist, chronic fasciolosis was identified in the livers of healthy slaughtered rheas.[36,54] The finding of extraintestinal filarial worms (*Dicheilonema rhea, D. spicularia, Contortospiculum rhea, Paronchocerca struthionis, Struthiofilaria megalocephala*) in the coelomic cavity, musculature, lungs, and air sacs of ratites is, however, mostly incidental. Attempted antifilarial treatment may be detrimental because of the immune response to the dead parasites.[53] *Syngamus trachea* and *Cyathostoma variegatum* have been found in apparently healthy ratites, but high parasitic burden and accompanying stressors may lead to respiratory clinical signs, especially in juvenile birds.[36,52,53] Fatal cerebral nematodiasis caused by *Baylisascaris procyonis* and *Chandlerella quiscalis* larvae migrans are primarily reported in emus and ostriches but also occasionally in other ratites in North America. Songbirds are the reservoir for *C. quiscalis*, and the parasite is transmitted by Culicoides mosquitoes, whereas *B. procyonis* is harbored by raccoons and directly transmitted from raccoon latrines near ratite enclosures. Prophylaxis with oral ivermectin, fenbendazole, or pyrantel tartrate is recommended in endemic areas.[10,15,53]

Cryptosporidium sp. are specific to ostriches and infect the bursa, rectum, and pancreas, causing severe chick losses in farms in South Africa.[36] Although coccidiosis is common in emu chicks, no clinical cases have been reported in ostriches.[36] *Entamoeba struthionis* is highly prevalent but nonpathogenic, and *Balanthidium struthionis* cysts may be confused with coccidial oocysts.[18,36] *Histomonas meleagridis* derived from poultry may cause similar disease (typhlohepatitis) in ostriches.[36,53] *Toxoplasma gondii* serology studies revealed only a rare risk of disease despite potential susceptibility.[20] Coccidiostats in ratite rations are not recommended and possibly also dangerous, as some of the ionophore coccidiostats are toxic for ratites.[18]

Ectoparasites such as feather lice (*Struthiolipeurus struthionis, S. rheae*), thribs (*Limothrips denticornis*), and quill mites (*Gabucinia* spp., *Struthiopterolichus* sp.) may cause pruritus, cellulitis, excessive pruning, and feather and skin destruction.[15,36] Hippoboscid flies (*Struthiobosca struthionis*) may be the cause of considerable irritation and act as disease vector.[18] A number of ixodid ticks are known to infect ostriches, and their potential to transmit diseases needs to be considered.[53]

Antiparasitic treatment in ratites follows the principles of treatment in other avian species. However, toxicologic side effects have been noted with several products, and the reader is referred to the toxicology section.[15]

Noninfectious Disease

"Chick fading syndrome" is a multifactorial disease complex that relates to improper incubation and rearing techniques and possibly viral infections.[18,22,40,53] Affected chicks often hatch with increased generalized edema, are weak, are reluctant or unable to exercise, and show delayed or inappropriate intake of food. Subsequent problems such as yolk sac retention and infection, leg deformities, gastric stasis and impaction, and secondary infections are responsible for major mortalities in 1- to 3-week-old chicks.[18] Cloacal prolapse in less than 3-month-old chicks is often associated with insufficient hydration

and enteritis and may be treated with reposition of the cloaca followed by purse string suture and supportive care.[44]

Deformities of legs are identified as one of the most important constraints to farm ostrich production but also happen in other ratites. Tibiotarsal rotation, rolled toes, slipped tendons, and bowed legs appear at different stages of growth, and the multiple etiologic factors include protein content of feed and other nutritional factors (minerals, trace elements), trauma, flooring (pen design), inadequate exercise, availability of water, and genetic predisposition. Rolled toes happen by medial displacement of the toe pad and happen most frequently in chicks less than 2 weeks of age. Vitamin B deficiency was hypothesized on the basis of "curled toe paralysis" syndrome in poultry, but the pathogenesis differs. Splinting and trimming nails work in most cases, but often spontaneous resolution also occurs by the age of 4 weeks. Tibiotarsal rotation and bowed tarsometatarsal bones occur in 2-week to 6-month-old chicks and may be caused by an inappropriate diet (high protein; excessive vitamin supplementation; deficiencies of calcium, manganese, and niacin), and rapid early growth rates. Slipped tendon corresponds to lateral displacement of the gastocnemius tendon of the tibiotarsometatarsal joint mostly in older chicks or the Achilles tendon medially over the tarsometatarsophalangeal joint in younger birds, often because of abrupt movement ("waltzing"). Similarities to perosis in poultry because of magnesium deficiency have not been proven.[18,41,44,53]

Gastric impaction is another common disease of juvenile ratites less than 6 months old and appears to be stress related. Impaction of the proventriculus with foreign body material because of abnormal compensatory picking (disorientation stress, desertion stress, or frustration with regard to finding food from change of location or diet), with or without stasis of the ventriculus with accumulation of natural substrates, and koilin hypertrophy frequently occur simultaneously, and the clinical signs and treatment are identical. Clinical signs are nonspecific (loss of appetite, lethargy, weight loss, dehydration, scant defecation), and successful treatment depends on early recognition of the syndrome; regular weight checks, serial contrast radiographic examinations, and auscultation and palpation of the left cranial quadrant after withholding food for 12 hours are the helpful measures.[18,44,46,53] If impaction is suspected, medical treatment may be tried with high-energy liquid (vegetable oil), gastric lavage and emulcents and laxatives, metoclopramide, and systemic antibiotics.[3] However, if no improvement is seen in over 24 hours or presence of foreign bodies is confirmed radiologically, surgical intervention (proventriculotomy) is mandatory and has a good prognosis if attempted early. As birds mimic each other's behavior, all birds must be checked if one bird is affected.[33,52]

Nutritional diseases include obesity; metabolic bone disease in chicks; white muscle disease induced by vitamin E or selenium deficiency; vitamin B (pantothenic acid) deficiency caused by high grain rations, resulting in retarded growth and skin crust formation on eyelids and corners of the beak; vitamin A deficiency in rheas, associated with runny eyes, abscesses, on the palate, and stunted growth; and vitamin E–associated encephalomalacia in emus, resulting in neurologic disease and sudden deaths.[4,18]

The excitable disposition of ratites predisposes them to capture myopathy after exertion, heat, recovery from anesthesia, and entrapment. Treatment is rarely successful, but one report describes successful treatment of a rhea with IV fluids, esophagostomy-tube feeding, long-term sedation, treatment with muscle relaxants, dexamethasone, and antibiotics, and sling and physiotherapy, all resulting in resolution after 23 days. Proper management, restraint, transport, and capture techniques are important preventive measures.[47,48,50]

Female reproductive tract infections and egg binding are important causes of poor fertility in captivity.[53] Transcutaneous ultrasonography is a useful noninvasive technique to monitor ovarian (in) activity and to diagnose reproductive pathologies, with the probe placed directly behind the thigh on the ventrolateral, featherless part of the abdomen.[8]

Miscellaneous conditions include trauma to neck and legs,[52,53] subchondral cysts, bone sequestration, and arthritis as a cause of lameness in ostriches and emus,[9,51] phallus prolapse and lesions and testicular cysts in adult males,[1,53] aortic dissection and aneurysm,[5] a hereditary form of neuronal gangliosidosis in emus,[7] behavioral abnormalities (excessive feather pecking, stargazing in close confinement, imprinting on humans),[43] and a most likely genetically related, noncontagious, mechanobullous skin disorder with skin sloughing and coagulative skin transudate in juvenile ostriches.[37]

Toxicities

Drug-related toxicities have been reported from lindane-containing antiparasitic products (benzene hexachloride, morantel), ionophore coccidiostats, lincomycin, dynamulin, streptomycin, and colistin antibiotics.[18] Selenium toxicities from oversupplementation has resulted in high mortality in ostrich and emu chicks.[32] Ingestion of parsley was associated with photosensitivity, avocado with epicardial edema and myocardial degeneration, acorns with enteritis, and oak leaves with fatal nephritis (cassowary).[18,31] Fungal toxins such as sporodesmin and aflatoxin in moldy feed lead to liver damage and immunosuppression. *Clostridium botulinum* toxicities (from occasional intake of bones, carcass in hay) were associated with paralysis in wild ostriches.[18] Their curious nature and long necks predispose ratites to accidental intoxication with pest control agents such as rat poisoning (anticoagulant warfarin).[18]

Reproduction

Differences in reproduction between the five ratite species are listed in Table 9-1.[18,19] Male ostriches sexually mature at 4 to 5 years of age and the hens slightly earlier, and they remain reproductive for up to 40 years. Their sexual activity is seasonal and associated with the photoperiod, rainfall, and availability of food. Males become territorial during the breeding season and display an impressive courtship behavior. Territorial males dig shallow nest scrapes, in which several visiting females contribute eggs to a communal clutch, leading to multiple maternity and paternity in one clutch, but only the "major" female and the resident territorial male provide incubation and parental care. More eggs (40–60) are laid in the nest than may be incubated, and the major female ejects surplus eggs from the incubated central clutch of approximately 20. Incubation is carried out by both genders, with the male bird mostly sitting during the night. Hatching in the nest occurs after average incubation duration of 42 to 43 days and over 4 to 5 days. Parental care is provided by both parents, and chicks are abandoned at the age of 1 year.[18,19,53] Ostrich eggs are unusual for their large size and low shell conductance, which makes them prone to insufficient water loss and results in edematous and malpositioned chicks.[18] The ostrich has been farmed for over 100 years, and the production has gained global importance in the past few decades. The main constraints of the ostrich production are high rate of infertility, low hatchability, and post-hatch problems such as leg deformities and fading chick syndrome.[18,53] As a consequence, a wealth of literature on ostrich production is available, and the reader is referred to it. Briefly, artificial incubation protocols consist of preincubation storage of the eggs at approximately 20°C for 7 to 10 days, incubation at temperatures of 36°C to 36.5°C and comparably low humidity at 20% to 25% to reach 8% to 18% loss of egg weight until pipping. Vertical position of the eggs during incubation appears beneficial, and frequent turning of the eggs is crucial.[16,53] Sperm collection and artificial insemination have been attempted but are not commonly practiced.[42]

Like ostriches, rheas practice polygamous reproduction, with one male competing for several females to lay eggs in a communal nest. Parental care is performed exclusively by males, with females restricting their investment to the production and laying of eggs.[19]

Although kiwis pair for life, emus and cassowaries only pair for the breeding season.[19,23,41] Incubation and rearing of chicks is performed exclusively by the males in all three species; however, kiwi females may be partly involved.[19] Kiwis have the largest egg-to-body ratio, with eggs reaching up to 20% of the female's body weight.[29] The clutches are considerably smaller (2–3 eggs) and

incubation time significantly longer (63–92 days) than in other ratites.[19]

Preventive Medicine

Quarantining new birds for at least 30 days, fecal parasitologic examinations, and serologic testing for avian influenza and Newcastle disease are, if not mandatory per regulations, strongly advised.[18,52,53] Although no vaccinations are licensed for use in ratites, the use of commercial vaccines for domestic hoofstock and poultry against enterotoxemia (clostridial toxins B and D), *Mycoplasma gallisepticum*, anthrax, Newcastle disease, avian pox, and avian influenza have shown promising results and may be advised in endemic areas. Tick and rodent control should be part of the routine prophylactic measures.[52,53]

TINAMOUS (ORDER TINAMIFORMES, FAMILY TINAMIDAE)

Biology and Reproduction

Tinamous are exclusively neotropical, medium-sized, plump, terrestrial but nonetheless flighted birds. As one of the oldest avian families in the New World, they are thought to come from the same stock as the Struthioniformes. The close relationship between ratites and tinamous is reflected in similarities in bone structures (especially the palate), eggshell structure, and thermoregulatory and metabolic physiology. The subfamily Tinaminae (forest tinamous) includes 29 species, which are primarily found in tropical and subtropical forests and are differentiated from the second subfamily Rhynchotinae (steppe tinamous, 18 grassland species) by the presence of nostrils in the distal half of the bill. Tinamous are shy and elusive birds and good runners when startled. Their diet is extremely variable and opportunistic, including plant material (fruit, seeds, leaves, flowers, roots), invertebrates, and small vertebrates. Forest dwelling species generally have a larger part of fruit in their diet, whereas grassland species take a greater proportion of seeds.[19,34]

During breeding season, males attract several females to lay eggs in a communal nest on the ground. The male solely takes care of incubation and rearing of the chicks. Tinamous eggs are elliptical to spherical, shiny, and uniformly but brightly colored in varying colors, depending on the species. Clutches contain up to 16 eggs, and incubation is relatively short (16–20 days). The precocial chicks become independent from the male's care within 10 to 20 days, and sexual maturity is reached at approximately 1 year of age.[19]

Anatomy

The external appearance of tinamous closely resembles that of Old World partridges or pheasants, reaching 15 to 50 centimeters (cm) in height and 50 to 1800 grams (g) in weight, depending on the species. Similarly, the wings are small in relation to the plump body. The tail is rudimentary and useless for steering, so flight cannot be kept up for long distances and does not appear particularly coordinated. Tinamous feathers have a unique structure, with the barbules being joined together in a solid mass and producing a whistling noise during flight. Feathers on the back and rump are easily shed as a defensive measure. Unlike Struthioniformes, tinamous have highly developed powder-downs for waterproofing the feathers. Females of some species are more brightly colored than males and are heavier. Tinamous have three forward facing toes and one absent or rudimentary hind-toe, and some species may be differentiated by the colors of the tarsi.[19]

Diseases

Reports on captive and wild tinamid diseases are scarce, with a limited number published in Portuguese. The few captive populations are mostly in private hands, and veterinary monitoring has been poor. A recent health survey in private collections in Brazil revealed a small percentage of animals serologically positive to infectious bursal disease virus.[34] All animals were serologically negative to avian paramyxovirus serotype 1; however, in an experimental study, experimental and natural seroconversion was shown. Serology results for *Mycoplasma gallisepticum* and *M. synoviae* were variable, depending on the tests, or negative. Despite serologically positive birds for *Salmonella pullorum* and *S. gallinarum*, bacteriologic examinations were negative. Fecal examinations revealed *Capillaria* spp., *Eimeria rhynchoti*, *Strongyloides* spp., *Ascaridia* spp., and unknown sporozoa and several louse species that were externally parasitizing on the animals.[34]

ACKNOWLEDGMENTS

The author thanks Dr. Dale Smith and Dr. Pia Krawinkel for their valuable contributions to this chapter.

REFERENCES

1. Aire TA, Soley JT, Groenewald HB: A morphological study of simple testicular cysts in the ostrich (*Struthio camelus*). Res Vet Sci 74:153–162, 2003.
2. Alexander DJ: Newcastle disease in ostriches (*Struthio camelus*)—a review. Avian Pathol 29:95–100, 2000.
3. Aslan L, Karasu A, Okzan C, et al: Medical and surgical treatment of gastric impaction in juvenile ostriches. J Anim Vet Adv 8:1141–1144, 2009.
4. Aye PP, Morishita TY, Grimes ABS, et al: Encephalomalacia associated with vitamin E deficiency in commercially raised emus. Avian Dis 42:600–605, 1998.
5. Baptiste KE, Pyle RL, Robertson JL, et al: Dissecting aortic aneurysm associated with a right ventricular arteriovenous shunt in a mature ostrich (*Struthio camelus*). J Avian Med Surg 11:194–200, 1997.
6. Beest JT, McClean M, Cushing A, et al: Thiafentanil-dexmedetomidine-telazol anesthesia in greater rheas (*Rhea americana*). J Zoo Wildl Med 43:802–807, 2012.
7. Bermudez AJ, Freischiitz B, Yu RK, et al: Heritability and biochemistry of gangliosidosis in emus (*Dromaius novaehollandiae*). Avian Dis 41:838–849, 1997.
8. Bronneberg RGG, Taverne MAM: Ultrasonography of the female reproductive organs in farmed ostriches (*Struthio camelus* spp.). Theriogenology 60:617–633, 2003.
9. Burba DJ, Tully TN, Jr, Pechman RD, et al: Phalangeal amputation for treatment of osteomyelitis and septic arthritis in an ostrich (*Struthio camelus*). J Avian Med Surg 10:19–23, 1996.
10. Campbell GA, Hoover JP, Russell WC, et al: Naturally occurring cerebral nematodiasis due to *Baylisascaris* larval migration in two black-and-white ruffed lemurs (*Varecia variegata variegata*) and suspected cases in three emus (*Dromaius novaehollandiae*). J Zoo Wildl Med 28:204–207, 1997.
11. Clarke CR, Kocan AA, Webb AI, et al: Intravenous pharmacokinetics of penicillin G and antipyrine in ostriches (*Struthio camelus*) and emus (*Dromaius novaehollandiae*). J Zoo Wildl Med 32:74–77, 2001.
12. Cooper RG, Horbanczuk JO, Fujihara N: Viral diseases of the ostrich (*Struthio camelus* var. *domesticus*). Anim Sci J 75:89–95, 2004.
13. Cooper RG, Jaroslaw O, Horbanczuk JO, et al: Nutrition and feed management in the ostrich (*Struthio camelus* var. *domesticus*). Anim Sci J 75:175–181, 2004.
14. Cooper RG, Mahrose KMA, Horbanczuk JO, et al: The wild ostrich (*Struthio camelus*): A review. Trop Anim Health Prod 41:1669–1678, 2009.
15. Cooper RG: Bacterial, fungal and parasitic infections in the ostrich (*Struthio camelus* var. *domesticus*). Anim Sci J 76:97–106, 2005.
16. Cooper RG: Handling, incubation, and hatchability of ostrich (*Struthio camelus* var. *domesticus*) eggs: A review. J Appl Poult Res 10:262–273, 2001.
17. Cushing A, McClean M: Use of thiafentanil-medetomidine for the induction of anesthesia in emus (*Dromaius novaehollandiae*) within a wild animal park. J Zoo Wildl Med 41:234–241, 2010.
18. Deeming DC: *The ostrich, biology, production and health*, Cambridge, United Kingdom, 1999, CABI Publishing University Press.
19. Del Hoyo J, Andrew E, Sargatal J: Order Struthioniformes. In Del Hoyo J, Elliott A, Sargatal J, editors: *Handbook of the birds of the world*, vol 1, Barcelona, Spain, 1992, Lynx Editions.
20. Dubey JP, Scandrett WB, Kwok OCH, et al: Prevalence of antibodies to *Toxoplasma gondii* in ostriches (*Struthio camelus*). J Parasitol 86:623–624, 2000.
21. Dzoma BM, Dorrestein GM: Yolk sac retention in the ostrich (*Struthio camelus*): Histopathologic, anatomic, and physiologic considerations. J Avian Med Surg 15:81–89, 2001.
22. Eisenberg SWF, van Asten AJAM, van Ederen AM, et al: Detection of circovirus with a polymerase chain reaction in the ostrich (*Struthio camelus*) on a farm in The Netherlands. Vet Microbiol 95:27–38, 2003.
23. Fisher GD: Breeding Australian cassowaries *Casuarius casuarius* at Edinburgh zoo. Int Zoo Yearbook 8:153–156, 1968.
24. Frasca S, Khan MI: Multiple intussusceptions in a juvenile rhea (*Rhea americana*) with proventricular impaction. Avian Dis 41:475–480, 1997.
25. Gasthuys F: Successful vetriculostomy for removal of foreign bodies in a kiwi (*Apteryx australis mantelli bartlett*). J Zoo Anim Med 18:166–167, 1987.
26. Gulbahar MY, Agaoglu Z, Biiyik H, et al: Zygomycotic proventriculitis and ventriculitis in ostriches (*Struthio camelus*) with impaction. Aust Vet J 78:247–249, 2000.
27. Hill FI, Woodgyer AJ, Lintott MA: Cryptococcosis in a North Island brown kiwi (*Apteryx australis mantelli*) in New Zealand. J Med Vet Mycol 33:305–309, 1995.
28. Jensen NS, Stanton TB, Swayne DE: Identification of the swine pathogen *Serpulina hyodysenteriae* in rheas (*Rhea americana*). Vet Microbiol 52:259–269, 1996.
29. Jensen T, Durant B: Assessment of reproductive status and ovulation in female brown kiwi (*Apteryx mantelli*) using fecal steroids and ovarian follicle size. Zoo Biol 25:25–34, 2006.
30. Jorgensen PH, Herczeg J, Lomniczi B, et al: Isolation and characterization of avian paramyxovirus type 1 (Newcastle disease) viruses from a flock of ostriches (*Struthio camelus*) and emus (*Dromaius novaehollandiae*) in Europe with inconsistent serology. Avian Pathol 27:352–358, 1998.
31. Kinde H: A fatal case of oak poisoning in a double-wattled cassowary (*Casuarius casuarius*). Avian Dis 32:849–851, 1988.
32. Kinder LL, Angel CR, Anthony NB: Apparent selenium toxicity in emus (*Dromaius novaehollandiae*). Avian Dis 39:652–657, 1995.
33. Komnenou ATh, Georgiades GK, Savvas I, et al: Surgical treatment of gastric impaction in farmed ostriches. J Vet Med Assoc 50:474–477, 2003.
34. Marques MVR, Ferreira FC, Jr, De Assis Andery D, et al: Health assessment of captive tinamids (Aves, Tinamiformes) in Brazil. J Zoo Wildl Med 43:539–548, 2012.
35. Mendes AR, Luvizotto MCR, Ferrari HF, et al: Experimental infectious bursal disease in the ostrich (*Struthio camelus*). J Comp Pathol 137:256–258, 2007.
36. Nemejc K, Lukesova D: Parasite fauna of ostriches, emus and rheas. Agr Tropica Subtropica 45:455–510, 2012.
37. Perelman B, Cognano E, Katchko L, et al: An unusual mechanobullous skin disorder in ostriches (*Struthio camelus*). J Avian Med Surg 9:122–126, 1995.
38. Pfitzer S, Lambrechts H: The use of haloperidol during the transport of adult ostriches. Tydskr S Afr Vet Ver 72:2–3, 2001.
39. Potter MA, Hendricks WH, Lentle RG, et al: An exploratory analysis of the suitability of diets fed to a flightless insectivore, the North Island brown kiwi (*Apteryx mantelli*), in New Zealand. Zoo Biol 29:537–550, 2010.
40. Raines AM, Kocan A, Schmidt R: Experimental inoculation of adenovirus in ostrich chicks (*Struthio camelus*). J Avian Med Surg 11:255–259, 1997.
41. Romagnano A, Hood RG, Sbedeker S, et al: Cassowary pediatrics. Vet Clin Exot Anim 15:215–231, 2012.
42. Rybnik PK, Horbanczuk JO, Lukaszewicz E, et al: The ostrich (*Struthio camelus*) ejaculate: effects of the method of collection, male age, month of the season, and daily frequency. Br Poultry Sci 53:134–140, 2012.
43. Samson J: Behavioral problems of farmed ostriches in Canada. Can Vet J 37:412–414, 1996.
44. Samson J: Prevalent diseases of ostrich chicks farmed in Canada. Can Vet J 38:425–428, 1997.

45. Schrader L, Fuhrer K, Petow S: Body temperature of ostriches (*Struthio camelus*) kept in an open stable during wintertime in Germany. *J Therm Biol* 34:366–371, 2009.

46. Shwaluk ThW, Finley DA: Proventricular-ventricular impaction in an ostrich chick. *Can Vet J* 36:108–109, 1995.

47. Siegal-Willott J: Ratites. In West G, Heard D, Caulkett N, editors: *Zoo animal and wildlife immobilization and anesthesia*, Ames, IA, 2008, Blackwell Publishing.

48. Smith KM, Murray S, Sanchez C: Successful treatment of suspected exertional myopathy in a rhea (*Rhea americana*). *J Zoo Wildl Med* 36:316–320, 2005.

49. Swan RS, Lindsey MJ: Treatment and control by vaccination of erysipelas in farmed emus (*Dromaius novaehollandiae*). *Aust Vet J* 76:325–327, 1998.

50. Tully TN, Jr, Hodgin C, Morris JM, et al: Exertional myopathy in an emu (*Dromaius novaehollandiae*). *J Avian Med Surg* 10:96–100, 1996.

51. Tully TN, Jr, Martin GS, Haynes PF, et al: Tarsometatarsal sequestration on an emu (*Dromaius novaehollandiae*) and an ostrich (*Struthio camelus*). *J Zoo Wildl Med* 27:550–556, 1996.

52. Tully TN, Jr: Ratites. In Tully TN, Dorrestein GM, Jones AK, editors: *Handbook of avian medicine*, Philadelphia, PA, 2009, Saunders.

53. Tully TN, Shane SM: *Ratite management, medicine, and surgery*, Malabar, Florida, 1996, Krieger Publishing Company.

54. Vaughan JL, Charles JA, Boray JC: *Fasciola hepatica* infection in farmed emus (*Dromaius novaehollandiae*). *Aust Vet J* 75:811–813, 1997.

55. Veazey RS, Vice CC, Cho DY, et al: Pathology of eastern equine encephalitis in emus (*Dromaius novaehollandiae*). *Vet Pathol* 31:109–111, 1994.

56. Zettermann CD, Nascimento AA, Tebaldi JA, et al: Observations on helminth infections of free-living and captive rheas (*Rhea americana*) in Brazil. *Vet Parasitol* 129:169–172, 2005.

CHAPTER 10

Sphenisciformes (Penguins)

Roberta S. Wallace

BIOLOGY

Penguins are flightless pelagic birds that are widely distributed along the coastal areas of the southern hemisphere, from cold tolerant species inhabiting Antarctica and the subantarctic areas, to temperate species found near the equator.[37] Currently, 6 genera and 18 recognized species (Table 10-1) exist, with the rockhopper penguin (*Eudyptes chrysocome*) recently being split into two distinct species on the basis of morphologic, vocal, and genetic distinctions: the northern rockhopper penguin (*Eudyptes moseleyi*) and the southern rockhopper penguin (*Eudyptes chrysocome*).[17] Penguins are long lived, with captive individuals frequently living to be 25 to 30 years of age. Age of sexual maturity varies among species but usually occurs around 3 to 5 years of age. Penguins are generally monogamous. Some species mate with one partner each season but change partners in successive breeding seasons, whereas other species form strong pair bonds that last for the life of the individuals. Occasionally, extra-mate pairing occurs. Males and females share the responsibility for incubation and chick rearing. Most species have a clutch of two eggs and use a variety of nest types: under rocks or bushes, in small cavities, or in shallow scrapes. Some build nests out of stones or dig deep burrows. Incubation generally lasts 37 to 45 days. Aptenodyptes is the exception, laying only one egg per clutch and incubating the egg on its feet for 62 to 67 days.[37]

UNIQUE ANATOMY AND CLINICAL RELEVANCE

Penguin species have a very similar body shape that allows for efficient swimming, diving, and porpoising but vary in height and weight. The little blue penguin is the smallest, standing 40 centimeters (cm) tall and weighing about 1 kilogram (kg), whereas the emperor penguin is the largest and may reach a height of 130 cm and weigh up to 38 kg. Despite the size differences among species, all penguins share several unique anatomic features.

1. The trachea bifurcates at different levels in most penguin species; the area of bifurcation may be seen radiographically. Use of an endotracheal tube may result in unilateral intubation, but with the efficiency of the avian pulmonary–air sac system, this usually does not lead to the problems of hypoventilation or hypo-oxygenation seen in mammals. The medial cartilaginous septum is easily traumatized, and if the tracheal size diminishes distal to the bifurcation, tracheal trauma may occur if an inappropriately sized tube is used.

2. Penguins lack a crop. The large stomach has two distinct chambers: the proventriculus and the ventriculus. The proventriculus stores food to feed chicks. Therefore, before administering oral medications, consideration must be given to penguins feeding small chicks, as toxic doses of medication may be regurgitated to the chick. Foreign objects often settle in the distal aspect of the ventriculus and radiographically appear to be in the distal intestine near the cloaca. This frequently leads clinicians to erroneously believe that the object is about to pass through on its own. Usually, endoscopy or surgery is needed for foreign body retrieval.

3. Feathers are short and dense in number and highly waterproof, providing a watertight and highly insulating layer. In preparation for surgery, it is easier and less traumatic to the underlying skin if the feathers are shaved rather than plucked. The feather shafts will fall out, and normal feathers will grow back during the next molt. Until that time, heat loss will occur in cold ambient temperatures and in water, but in captivity, the penguin may compensate for the loss. In the wild, successful rehabilitation of oiled birds requires complete waterproofing before the birds are released to prevent debilitating heat loss.

TABLE 10-1

Status of Wild Penguin Species Populations

Genus	Common Name	Scientific Name	Population Trend	2012 IUCN Status	Estimated Breeding Pairs in Wild
Aptenodytes	Emperor penguin	A. forsteri	Stable	Near threatened	238,000
Aptenodytes	King penguin	A. patagonicus	Increasing	Least concern	*2,000,000
Eudyptes	Southern rockhopper penguin	E. chrysocome	Decreasing	Vulnerable	1,230,000
Eudyptes	Macaroni penguin	E. chrysolophus	Decreasing	Vulnerable	9,000,000
Eudyptes	Northern rockhopper penguin	E. moseleyi	Decreasing	Endangered	265,000
Eudyptes	Fiordland penguin	E. pachyrhynchus	Decreasing	Vulnerable	5,000–6,000
Eudyptes	Snares penguin	E. robustus	Stable	Vulnerable	31,000
Eudyptes	Royal penguin	E. schlegeli	Stable	Vulnerable	850,000
Eudyptes	Erect-crested penguin	E. sclateri	Decreasing	Endangered	67,000
Eudyptula	Little penguin (Fairy or Blue penguin)	E. minor	Decreasing	Least concern	<1,000,000
Megadyptes	Yellow-eyed penguin	M. antipodes	Decreasing	Endangered	3500
Pygoscelis	Adélie penguin	P. adeliae	Increasing	Near threatened	2,370,000
Pygoscelis	Chinstrap penguin	P. antarcticus	Increasing	Least concern	9,000,000
Pygoscelis	Gentoo penguin	P. papua	Decreasing	Near threatened	387,000
Spheniscus	African penguin	S. demersus	Decreasing	Endangered	26,000
Spheniscus	Humboldt penguin	S. humboldti	Decreasing	Vulnerable	†45,000 (all ages)
Spheniscus	Magellanic penguin	S. magellanicus	Decreasing	Near threatened	1,300,000
Spheniscus	Galápagos penguin	S. mendiculus	Decreasing	Endangered	600

*International Penguin Conservation Working Group (www.penguins.cr).
†Wallace, unpublished data.
From International Union for Conservation of Nature, 2012: *Red List of Threatened Species Version 2012.2*: www.iucnredlist.org. Accessed December 24, 2012.

4. Penguin bones are not pneumatic and are much denser than in other species of birds; therefore, intraosseous catheterization for administration of fluids may be quite difficult.
5. Countercurrent heat exchange mechanisms are well developed in the feet and flippers to aid in thermoregulation. This, along with the insulation provided by feathers, may lead to hyperthermia during anesthetic procedures, especially in the Antarctic and subantarctic species. Ice packs placed on the feet and flippers will help prevent hyperthermia.
6. Daily activities of penguins have both aquatic and terrestrial components. The visual system has anatomic features that allow penguins to have normal sight in either environment. Although the corneal shape is flatter than in mammals, the ultrastructure is similar.[26] The nictitating membrane is transparent to allow normal vision while providing protection to the cornea when the penguin is under water. When performing ocular surgery, the nictitating membrane must be identified and retracted to avoid accidental incision.
7. Salt glands in the orbital region handle the excess salt in a marine environment. The glands will atrophy in captive penguins maintained in a fresh water environment unless supplemental salt is provided. However, studies have shown that atrophied glands will become functional rapidly if exposed to a saline environment.[20]

IDENTIFICATION METHODS

The use of flipper bands in the wild is controversial.[2,15] However, most institutions successfully use flipper bands on captive penguins. Color cable ties and metal or silicone flipper bands may be used. Bands should be tightened to the point where a finger may be slipped between the band and the flipper. As cable ties may continue to tighten after application, the fastener should be glued so that it does not slip and impede blood circulation to the flipper. During molt, flippers swell, potentially restricting circulation. Band tightness must be monitored and bands replaced with looser bands, if needed. Small metal rings may be placed in the interdigital webbing of the foot. Microchips may be placed subcutaneously in the loose skin of the back of the neck, on top of the head, or in the fleshy part of the foot in the front of the tarsus. Chicks weighing as little as 500 grams (g) may be microchipped. For smaller collections, identification of adults may be done on the basis of photographs of spot patterns of the breast feathers after molt into adult plumage.[24]

SEXING

Penguin species are only subtly dimorphic, males generally being slightly larger with bigger and thicker bills, but overlap in size exists between sexes. Although research on morphometrics has been published, it is unreliable for captive Humboldt penguins and thus might be expected to be unreliable for other penguin species. DNA (deoxyribonucleic acid) sexing from feather, blood, or egg membranes is highly reliable and is the recommended method for sexing penguins.[24]

SPECIAL HOUSING REQUIREMENTS

To successfully manage penguins in captivity, exhibits must be designed to meet the physical, behavioral, and psychological needs of the species. As colony birds, penguins should not be housed alone, and the AZA Penguin Taxonomic Advisory Group (TAG) recommends a minimum of 10 birds. Air and water quality, lighting, and type of substrate must be considered for optimal health as well as protection from land and air predators. The various penguin species have widely differing environmental requirements, and it must be ensured that in a mixed species exhibit, penguins with similar requirements are housed together. Indoor exhibits are generally preferred to facilitate control of air and water temperatures for the various species, decrease exposure to disease vectors, and provide protection from predators. *Aptenodytes*, *Pygoscelis*, *Eudyptes*, and *Megadyptes* species are best kept indoors under refrigerated conditions (<9°C). Temperate climate species are often exhibited outdoors and may tolerate temperature ranges from freezing to 30°C. In cold climates, pools should be prevented from freezing, and penguins should have access to shelters with supplemental heat. Misters may be used during warm weather to aid in cooling the birds. An indoor area with climate control capability should be available for protection from extreme heat and humidity and for nesting. Mosquitoes are the vectors for several diseases in penguins (see list below); therefore, mosquito control is paramount for penguins housed outdoors. This includes removing standing water on a weekly basis; applying larvicide to standing water that cannot be removed, including any drains in the penguins' indoor and outdoor enclosures; and minimizing foliage near animal exhibits. Exposure to mosquitoes may be reduced by bringing the penguins indoors during peak mosquito hours (dusk to dawn), ensuring that door sweeps and screens are in good condition, placing screens over intake fans, and providing fans, wherever possible, to keep the air moving to discourage mosquitoes.[24]

The AZA Penguin TAG recommends minimum land and water surface areas for exhibition and holding. Additional space should be provided to allow for a full range of species-appropriate behaviors, including nesting (species other than *Aptenodytes*). For king and emperor penguins, the minimum land and water surface areas for exhibit and holding are 18 square feet for the first six birds and 9 square feet for each additional bird, with a minimum pool depth of 4 feet. For all other species of penguins, the recommendations are 8 square feet for the first six birds, 4 square feet for each additional bird, and a minimum pool depth of 2 feet. Ideally, larger water areas should be provided to encourage swimming to help prevent obesity and pododermatitis. A separate holding area should be provided for birds with behavioral problems or noncontagious health problems that require separation from the flock. Quarantine facilities with separate air and water systems should be available for newly acquired birds or birds with infectious diseases. Water may be either fresh water or salt water, and recent studies show that salt supplementation is not needed for penguins in fresh water exhibits. Water cleanliness and clarity may be maintained with the use of sand and gravel filters, judicious addition of chlorine to keep coliform counts to a minimum, and surface skimmers to remove excess fish oil and debris from the surface of the water. Lighting indoor exhibits should mimic the natural light cycle with gradual increasing and decreasing of daylight hours. Inappropriate lighting may lead to poor molt cycles and decreased reproductive success.[24] Spheniscid species enjoy climbing, so exhibits designed to allow climbing provide enrichment.

FEEDING AND NUTRITION

In the wild, penguins feed on pelagic schooling fish species, squid, and crustaceans (mostly euphasid species). Food consumed varies with availability and season. In captivity, the type of prey items fed by a given institution is often limited and dictated by cost and availability from commercial fisheries. Feeding several different types of whole prey is recommended to provide a complete nutrient profile and so that the birds do not "imprint" on one item to the exclusion of others. In most cases, the prey items are frozen. Fish should be individually quick frozen (IQF) instead of in large blocks, stored at −18° to −30°C, and used within 4 to 6 months to ensure optimal nutritional quality. Institutions should consider whether the food items used are being harvested in an ecologically sustainable fashion.[10] If appropriate species of prey are unavailable or the condition of the fish is less than ideal, three types of a nutritionally complete powder (reconstituted into a gel) are commercially available as substitutes for low-fat fish, high-fat fish, or squid and crustacean diets.

The size of the fish must be appropriate for the species. If an item must be cut because it is too large, all portions should be fed to ensure ingestion of the entire nutrient supply of the item. To prevent bacterial growth, food should be thawed in a refrigerator in clean containers, then kept refrigerated or on ice until the time of feeding. Using running water for thawing may wash away many of the water-soluble nutrients, but in some institutions, the fish is quickly rinsed in cold water just prior to feeding to remove any surface contaminants. Extensive vitamin supplementation is not needed if penguins are fed good-quality whole-food items thawed appropriately. Recommendations are limited to vitamin E at 100 international units per kilogram (IU/kg) and thiamine at 25 to 30 milligrams per kilogram (mg/kg) of diet fed on a wet weight basis. Supplements should be added to the fish immediately before feeding to prevent breakdown by the enzymes and oxidants in the fish. Salt supplementation is not needed.[10]

Most institutions hand-feed individual penguins, especially if they are receiving medication or vitamin supplements. Complete hand-feeding may cause penguins to become lazy and develop poor swimming habits; therefore, some pool feeding is recommended, but feeding must be observed to ensure that all individuals are eating enough. Penguins may consume up to 20% of their body weight daily, with increased consumption during the few weeks prior to molt, and during chick rearing. Consumption usually decreases drastically during molt with frequent skipped feedings. Penguins may gain more than 25% of their body weight prior to molt and then rapidly return to premolt weight or slightly below by the end of molt.[37]

RESTRAINT AND ANESTHESIA

Penguins are sturdy and may tolerate handling for minimally invasive procedures. Several different methods exist for capturing the animal, with initial restraint often done by grabbing the back of the head or very high on the neck and then lifting and supporting the belly with the other hand. Grabbing penguins by the flippers should be avoided, since the flippers may dislocate or fracture. Two people should work together when capturing and restraining king and emperor penguins. People capturing the birds should wear eye protection, especially with king penguins. Once the bird has been secured, a black bag may be placed over its head with the beak and nares exposed. Noninvasive procedures may require only minimal restraint. Stronger restraint is needed for procedures that require the bird to be immobile. One method involves placing the penguin between the handler's legs such that the flippers are held secure. In this way, the handler's hands are free to restrain and position the head and neck to facilitate procedures such as blood collection or banding. With king and emperor penguins, a second person may be needed to avoid injury to the bird or handlers. Other methods of restraint include using large diameter PVC pipes or traffic cones to secure the bird. Air kennel or large tubs may be used for transport.

Animals should be fasted 18 to 24 hours prior to anesthesia to prevent regurgitation and aspiration of gastric contents. Isoflurane or sevoflurane are the most commonly used gas anesthetics. A facial cone is used for induction, with subsequent intubation, if desired. Shallow breathing or breath holding (dive reflex) may occur, resulting in a chronic excitement phase and swimming-like behavior. Assisted ventilation two to three times per minute may achieve a smoother plane of anesthesia. Midazolam given intramuscularly or intranasally may be used for sedation for minor procedures or to reduce the stress of handling. Sedation may then be reversed with flumazenil. Ketamine or diazepam given intramuscularly for induction has been recommended over isoflurane for Little (Fairy or Blue) penguins (*Eudyptula minor*) because of the fragile nature of this species and its tendency to traumatize itself during anesthetic induction with isoflurane. However, recovery is prolonged compared with using isoflurane alone. If cold climate species are anesthetized for extended periods, ice, ice packs, or other ways to prevent hyperthermia should be used during the anesthetic procedure.

BLOOD SAMPLE COLLECTION

Blood may be collected from a variety of sites, including the jugular, medial metatarsal, interdigital, and brachial veins (the brachial vein is also a good site for intravenous [IV] catheterization). Blood may also be collected from a venous sinus located on the dorsal aspect of the vertebral column at the base of the tail. The amount of blood that may be removed follows normal avian standards of no more than 1% of body weight. Each institution should establish its own set of normal blood parameters for every species maintained. If no institutional norms exist, the International Species Information System has norms for most species. Otherwise, zoos that have the penguin species in question may be contacted. As Galápagos penguins are rarely kept in captivity, values for this species are not readily available, but values obtained from the wild population have been published.[33] Postprandial increases in uric acid occur; therefore, penguins should be fasted for accurate uric acid assessment.[9] Both egg-laying and molt may have a temporary effect on specific blood chemistry values.[38] As with other avian species, increases in cholesterol, calcium, phosphorus, and occasionally alkaline phosphatase are often seen in reproductively active females.[21]

SURGERY

Surgery has been successfully performed on a variety of penguin species. It is important to remember to keep Antarctic and subantarctic species cool during surgery. Standard surgical technique is employed. Intubation, standard patient monitoring, and fluid administration are generally easy to perform. Birds should be kept out of the water until the skin incision has healed.

BLOOD TRANSFUSIONS

Blood transfusions may be performed when birds are severely anemic from malaria, blood loss, or clotting disorders. Transfusions may stabilize a bird until a diagnosis is made and treatment initiated, and is indicated when the packed cell volume (PCV) drops rapidly into the teens or lower and does not stabilize. If the PCV stabilizes, penguins generally have a good bone marrow response, if not debilitated by concurrent disease or old age, and generally respond well to supportive care alone (fluids, oral or injectable iron supplementation, oxygen and B-vitamins). In malarial birds with a stable PCV in the teens, transfusion appears to shorten the convalescent time until the treatment with chloroquine or primaquine takes effect. Homologous transfusions are preferred, since the blood cells probably remain in the recipient's circulation longer. Instructions for transfusion may be found in the *Penguin Husbandry Manual*.[24]

BACTERIAL AND FUNGAL DISEASES

Penguins are susceptible to a variety of bacterial diseases, including outbreaks caused by *Erysipelothrix*,[4] mycobacteria,[13,22] *Edwardsiella*,[23] *Plesiomonas*,[23] and *Chlamydophila*.[14] Although few pharmacokinetic studies exist,[35] various antibiotics have been used successfully in penguins (Table 10-2). The diagnosis of *Chlamydophila* in live birds is complicated by confusion with regard to the testing methods of various laboratories and how to interpret test results to determine whether illness is caused by active infection. A thorough understanding of the latest diagnostic techniques, what each test result signifies, and its validity in penguins is needed. Doxycycline is the drug of choice for treatment. *C. psittaci* is a zoonotic disease, and risk of transmission to the public or to the animal care staff is real. Affected birds or flocks should be quarantined to protect other collection birds as well as the staff. Persons working with ill birds should wear protective clothing, including N-95 masks.

The primary fungal disease causing illness in penguins is aspergillosis. The causative agent is *Aspergillus* spp., typically *A. fumigatus*. The organism is ubiquitous in the outdoor environment and is often found in indoor exhibits. It may exist at low levels without causing problems in healthy and well-adapted penguins. Disease frequently occurs in stressed or debilitated animals. Stressors associated with aspergillosis include substandard air quality, poor ventilation, elevated ammonia levels, overcrowding, excessive environmental heat or cold, and social incompatibility. Historically, many severe outbreaks of aspergillosis have occurred after major environmental changes, especially those involved with social factors such as

TABLE 10-2

Antimicrobials and Parasiticides Commonly Used in Penguins

Generic Name	Route of Administration	Dosage	Comments
Itraconazole	PO	5–10 mg BID	Until signs resolve; manufacturer's product (not generic) must be used
Voriconazole	PO	10 mg/kg BID	Until signs resolve
Terbinafine	PO	15 mg/kg q24h	Can combine with itraconazole
Clotrimazole	Nebulize	1% solution 15 minutes BID	Until signs resolve
Amphotericin B	Nebulize	0.3–1 mg/mL of saline 15 minutes BID	Until signs resolve
Amphotericin B	IV	1.5 mg/kg BID–TID	3–5 days
Enrofloxacin	PO, IM	15 mg/kg BID	2–4 weeks
Trimethoprim sulfa	PO	50–100 mg/kg q12h	7–10 days
Cephalexin	PO	50–75 mg/kg BID	10–21 days
Clindamycin	PO	75 mg/kg BID	10–14 days
Ivermectin	PO, SQ	0.2–0.4 mg/kg	Repeat in 7–14 days, if needed
Praziquantel	PO, IM, SQ	15–20 mg/kg	Use the higher doses orally; repeat in 2 weeks
Fenbendazole	PO	20–50 mg/kg ×3 days	Repeat in 2 weeks

bid, Twice daily; *IM*, intramuscular; *IV*, intravenous; *mg/kg*, milligram per kilogram; *PO*, oral; *q12h*, every 12 hours; *q24h*, every 24 hours; *SQ*, subcutaneous; *TID*, three times daily.
Note: For antimalarial drug treatments, see individual disease writeup.

introduction to a new social group, or inappropriate, prolonged, or stressful relocation. Exposure to new *Aspergillus* species may occur via new substrate or change in location. Construction in the area of the exhibit may increase exposure to fungal spores.

Signs are often nonspecific, and early diagnosis is difficult. Signs include open-mouth breathing, coughing, altered vocalization, inappetence, weight loss, lethargy, weakness, and self-isolation. A complete blood cell count (CBC) may show a moderate to marked leukocytosis with monocytosis, and changes in the protein electrophoretic pattern compatible with chronic inflammation may be present. Serologic titers to *Aspergillus* may be useful, but it is difficult to differentiate an acute infection from previous exposure. Fungal cultures of the throat, trachea, or air sacs may grow the causative agent. Radiography, fluoroscopy, or computed tomography (CT) is helpful in identifying pulmonary or air sac granulomas or general cloudiness of air sac or lung fields.

Success of treatment depends on the stage and severity of disease when diagnosed. Antifungal drugs may be given systemically (orally or intravenously), by nebulization, or intratracheally. Treatment is typically long term, frustrating, and often unsuccessful if begun in the later stages of disease. Several drugs have been used (see Table 10-2), but, again, few pharmacokinetic studies in penguins have been done.[3,31] If itraconazole is used, the manufacturer product, not the generic form, must be used.[31] Supportive care may include fluids given by gavage, subcutaneously, or intravenously and fish gruel by gavage. For indoor exhibits, maintaining good air quality is crucial for disease prevention. If the air filtration system in a penguin exhibit is shut down, it is recommended that the system run for at least a week after it is restarted before putting penguins back into the exhibit. Air cultures and disinfection for *Aspergillus* sp. should be taken at this time. Regular fungal air cultures may be taken from the exhibit area to monitor levels of *Aspergillus*. Prophylactic antifungal drugs, typically 10 mg/kg itraconazole given orally once a day should be administered when shipping, relocating, or introducing new birds to an exhibit. It is crucial to avoid shipping or relocating penguins during molt (including the premolt and immediate postmolt periods).[24]

PARASITIC DISEASES

Malaria is the most significant parasitic disease in captive penguins housed outdoors. Malaria is caused by a blood parasite carried by mosquitoes, biting flies, or both. The causative agent is a *Plasmodium* organism, usually *P. relictum* or occasionally *P. elongatum*. Wild birds serve as reservoir hosts. Most cases of penguin malaria occur in animals that are currently or have historically been housed outside. Penguins of all ages may be clinically affected, but susceptibility is highest during first exposure; therefore, chicks and juvenile birds, naïve adults previously housed indoors, or those that have been transported from areas with low mosquito or malaria problems are at higher risk of disease. The mortality rate from novel malaria infection is high, and stressors such as molt, chick rearing, or poor husbandry may increase mortality. Blood samples may be collected every 2 weeks from birds considered at high risk and stained smears of the blood checked for the presence of malarial organisms. Unfortunately, this test is not very sensitive, as malarial organisms are often visible only after the onset of severe clinical signs or during necropsy when organisms may be seen in blood smears or splenic impressions.[8]

A serologic test has been validated for black-footed penguins (*Spheniscus demersus*) and may be useful for other Spheniscid species.[8] Research is underway to try to detect malarial organisms in blood using polymerase chain reaction (PCR) techniques, but accurate tests have yet to be developed.

Clinical signs for malaria may vary and range from acute death with or without dyspnea to lethargy, inappetence, pale mucous membranes (from anemia), and behavioral separation from the group.

Malarial infection has both tissue and blood phases, and treatment targets both phases. Standard treatment is with 5 mg/kg

chloroquine every 12 hours for four doses, or four doses of mefloquine at 0, 12, 24, and 48 hours.[32,36] Concurrent treatment with primaquine for 10 to 14 days is needed to treat exo-erythrocytic forms. Prophylaxis during the mosquito season (potentially year round in some locations) may be attained using 1.25 mg/kg primaquine daily or mefloquine 30 mg/kg once a week if primaquine is not available. A compounded capsule containing 125 mg sulfadiazine, 4 mg pyrimethamine, and 0.4 mg folic acid administered every other day to penguins weighing 3 to 5 kg has also been used for prophylaxis. Pyrimethamine is a folic acid inhibitor and is teratogenic and may cause fetal malformations if given to laying females. Doxycycline is used in humans for both treatment and prevention of malaria, but to date, no studies have been published indicating dose or efficacy in birds. Administration of any prophylactic treatment is risky in adults that are feeding chicks, as the parent may regurgitate the medication to a small chick. Discontinuing treatment for a week or two while the chick is small should be considered. Then treatment may be restarted first in the parent that is less involved in feeding the chick. If using the every-other-day therapy, the parents should be treated on alternate days to minimize the chance that the chick might receive two doses in a day.

Deaths from toxoplasmosis have occurred in black-footed penguin chicks exposed to cat feces.[27] Signs were primarily neurologic, with death occurring within 24 hours. Aside from the direct threat of predation that cats may pose to penguins, *Toxoplasma* oocysts transmitted from infected cat feces pose a risk; therefore, penguin exhibits should be secured to prevent entry by domestic cats.

VIRAL DISEASES

A number of viruses may cause encephalitis in birds. Disease spread is usually through the bite of an infected mosquito, and wild birds may act as reservoirs for the virus. Some evidence suggests that bird-to-bird transmission occurs via semen and other infected bodily fluids. Diseases relevant to penguins include eastern equine encephalitis (EEE) and West Nile virus (WNV). Both EEE and WNV have been reported in Spheniscid penguins, and these penguins may have high rates of morbidity and mortality in response to these diseases.[11,34]

WNV is caused by a flavivirus. Species susceptibility to severe morbidity and mortality varies widely, with penguins being one of the more highly susceptible avian groups (see Chapter 77). Birds that survive infections are assumed to have some latent immunity to reinfection, but it is not known how long this immunity lasts. Acute death may occur with few premonitory signs, or death may occur within 3 to 4 days. Clinical signs, when present, include anorexia, weakness (lying down frequently), and vomiting, with inability to retain even small amounts of water or oral electrolyte solutions. Dyspnea from excessive mucoid tracheal or pulmonary secretion may occur. In Humboldt penguins, neurologic abnormalities are not common. No specific treatment exists for this disease; therapy is limited to supportive care. With supportive care, the course of the disease may be protracted, with death occurring after a couple of weeks. Recovery may be prolonged in those animals that survive, with weakness and decreased appetite lasting for several weeks. Antifungal or antibacterial therapy may be given, as needed, for secondary infections. Oral supplementation of fluids or gruel is not recommended until the penguin's condition has stabilized, as sick birds tend to vomit. Virus may be shed in the respiratory secretions, and horizontal transmission of the virus to humans from avian species has been documented.[7] Therefore, WNV should be considered a zoonotic disease, and appropriate protective clothing should be worn when working around infected birds.

Vaccination is recommended for susceptible species. At this time, no vaccines produced specifically for birds are commercially available. Two vaccines developed for horses have been used. Innovator (Pfizer) is a killed vaccine. Its efficacy, as measured by serologic titers, differs in different avian species. Recommendations are to vaccinate susceptible birds three times at 3- to 4-week intervals and then annually 1 month prior to the mosquito season.[24] Recombitek (Merial) is a live recombinant canarypox vaccine. Anecdotal reports of this being used exist, but efficacy is currently unknown.

EEE is caused by an alphavirus. This disease was reported in a group of African penguins housed outdoors.[34] Common signs included acute anorexia, lethargy, intermittent vomiting, bile-stained diarrhea, and self-isolation. Ataxia developed after 3 to 4 days, progressing to recumbency and seizures in about 25% of affected penguins. Signs in less severely affected penguins began to resolve in 6 to 9 days but only after 14 days in more severely affected penguins. A hemagglutinin inhibition test for titers to the EEE virus may confirm exposure to the disease, and although no reference limits for penguins exist, a rising titer in samples taken 2 to 4 weeks apart suggests true infection. No specific treatment is available, and therapy is limited to supportive care, including anticonvulsants to control seizures. Antifungal or antibacterial therapy should be provided, as needed, for secondary infections. A killed vaccine against EEE is available for horses, and although the required dose and efficacy for penguins has not been determined, some institutions in EEE-endemic areas have opted to use this vaccine.

Avian pox has occurred in both captive and wild penguin populations.[18] Both diphtheritic and cutaneous forms may manifest. Currently no treatment exists, and supportive care must be provided while the disease runs its course, usually lasting 2 to 3 weeks. The virus may survive for prolonged periods in the scabs or other dried secretions, so meticulous disinfection of any areas where ill animals were housed is necessary to prevent transmission.

NONINFECTIOUS DISEASES

Pododermatitis (bumblefoot) continues to cause problems in captive penguins. Factors associated with pododermatitis include decreased swimming (sedentary behaviors) and prolonged standing on hard, abrasive surfaces or on surfaces with excessive moisture or fecal contamination. The original lesion may result from a puncture wound or soft tissue damage caused by pressure necrosis. Once the epithelium is compromised, secondary bacterial invasion may occur, resulting in deep soft tissue infections. If left untreated, severe complications, including mineralized soft tissue and osteomyelitis, may occur. Therapy should be aimed at protecting the foot from further damage, instituting local and systematic treatment of the lesion, and altering the environment to prevent future occurrences, for example, improving hygiene and changing to an appropriate substrate or flooring. Treatments that have been used include systemic antibiotics; local antibiotics with or without dimethyl sulfoxide (DMSO); topical ointment; surgical debridement; cryotherapy; and chronic bandaging in conjunction with various salves and ointments, accompanied by intermittent debridement of devitalized tissue. Often initial improvement is seen, but the condition tends to recur once therapy is discontinued. When bandaging, it is helpful to provide padding to minimize pressure on the wound site. Gauze, waterproof cast padding, and booties made from soft material have all been used. Healing efficiency may be improved with proper debridement and the use of hydroactive dressings. Booties may be made from neoprene dive suits or are commercially available in various sizes. Prevention is key, as treatment is typically long term and frustrating. Penguins should be encouraged to swim, and appropriate substrate free of standing contaminated water should be provided. Anecdotal evidence suggests that allowing birds with bandages to swim in salt water may promote healing.

Preen gland infections have been reported in penguins.[19] The specific etiology is unknown, but predisposing factors include sedentary birds with decreased swimming patterns, nonpreening birds that do not molt regularly, and nutritional deficiencies. Early diagnosis and treatment may prevent impaction. In birds that do not respond to symptomatic or antibiotic therapy, surgical removal may be needed to avoid rupture and secondary septicemia. Encouraging swimming, particularly with nesting birds, may be beneficial. If birds are temporarily housed without a pool, daily showers may stimulate preening.

Gastrointestinal foreign bodies may cause significant morbidity and death.[25] Young penguins and nesting females, in particular, will investigate small and novel items and may ingest them. Ingested items have included nesting material, bristles from cleaning brushes, coins, lead pellets, and molted tail feather shafts. When metal objects are ingested, zinc, lead, and other heavy metal toxicities are possible. Although penguins regurgitate easily, foreign objects usually remain in the stomach and tend not to pass into the intestinal tract. Treatment is usually by endoscopic or, less frequently, surgical removal.

Pathology of the reproductive system is uncommon in penguins, although salpingitis, egg binding, and cloacal prolapse occur. Treatment for egg binding is similar to that in other avian species. Birds may benefit from calcium supplementation. Manual extraction of the egg is preferable, but surgical removal of the egg may be required. Removal of the entire oviduct may be necessary if egg retention leads to oviductal rupture or necrosis. The toxic effects of lead and zinc on the smooth muscle of the uterus and oviduct may predispose to egg retention.

Various neoplasms have been reported in penguins including T-cell lymphoma,[30] melanoma,[28] carcinomas,[12,29] and adenocarcinomas.[39]

Nutritional disorders may occur with poor-quality or improperly handled fish. Thiamine deficiency occurs when fish quality is compromised. Incoordination and "stargazing" are occasionally reported as clinical symptoms. Differential diagnoses for nonspecific signs of central nervous system involvement include viral, parasitic, or bacterial encephalitis; fungal granuloma; sepsis; and tumors. Metabolic bone disease has been reported in several hand-raised penguin chicks.[1] Poisoning by domoic acid was reported to cause the total loss of a rockhopper penguin collection.[6] Exposure came from ingesting fish contaminated by the algal toxin. Consideration should be given to the source of the fish (caught in shallow versus deep water) fed to penguins.

CONSERVATION

The conservation status of the penguin species is given in Table 10-1. Many populations have declined rapidly in the last 70 years, although for a few species the numbers are stable or increasing, with expanding ranges.[16] Reclassification of the rockhopper penguin from one to two distinct species has conservation implications, since the northern population is smaller and more fragmented compared with the southern population. Many penguin species live in rather inaccessible areas without direct daily contact with humans, but nonetheless human activities affect these populations. Threats include climate change or El Niño, overfishing, entanglement in fishing nets, habitat loss and destruction, predation, and human disturbance. Oiling has caused significant deaths in some species.[5] Various conservation measures have been undertaken to protect specific penguin populations, and these include establishment of natural reserves, some of which include no-fishing areas in the water adjacent to these reserves, providing barriers to protect colonies from predators, observation and monitoring of guano harvesting to minimize poaching and disruption of nesting areas, temporary relocation of entire colonies to prevent oiling, and controlled access and viewing by ecotourists.

ACKNOWLEDGMENTS

The author would like to thank Mary Kazmierczak and Jennifer Rohrer for assistance in the preparation of this chapter and for editorial help.

REFERENCES

1. Adkesson MJ, Langan JN: Metabolic bone disease in juvenile Humboldt penguins (*Spheniscus humboldti*): Investigation of ionized calcium, parathyroid hormone, and vitamin D3 as diagnostic parameters. *J Zoo Wildl Med* 38:85–92, 2007.

2. Barham PJ, Underhill LG, Crawford RJM, et al: Impact of flipper-banding on breeding success of African penguins (*Spheniscus demersus*) at Robben Island: Comparisons among silicone rubber bands, stainless-steel bands and no bands. *Afr J Marine Sci* 3:595–602, 2008.

3. Bechert U, Christensen JM, Poppenga R, et al: Pharmacokinetics of orally administered terbinafine in African penguins (*Spheniscus demersus*) for potential treatment of aspergillosis. *J Zoo Wildl Med* 41:263–274, 2010.

4. Boerner L, Nevis KR, Hinckley LS, et al: Erysipelothrix septicemia in a little blue penguin (*Eudyptula minor*). *J Vet Diagn Invest* 16:145–149, 2004.

5. Boersma PD, Stokes DL: Conservation: Threats to penguin populations. In Williams TD, editor: *The penguins*, New York, 1995, Oxford University Press.

6. Broadbent R: Deaths in rockhopper penguins. *Vet Rec* 164:127–128, 2009.

7. Campbell G, Lanciotti R, Bernard B, et al: Laboratory-acquired West Nile virus infections—United States, 2002. *MMWR Morb Mortal Wkly Rep* 51:1133–1135, 2002.

8. Cranfield MR: Sphenisciformes (penguins). In Fowler M, editor: *Zoo and wild animal medicine*, ed 5, Philadelphia, PA, 2000, Saunders, pp 103–110.

9. Cray C, Stremme DW, Arheart KL: Postprandial biochemistry changes in penguins (*Spheniscus demersus*) including hyperuricemia. *J Zoo Wildl Med* 41:325–326, 2010.

10. Crissey SD: *Handling fish fed to fish-aating animals: A manual of standard operating procedures.* Beltsville, MD, 1998, US Dept Agr, Agr Res Serv, Natl Agr Libr.

11. Davis MR, Langan JN, Johnson YJ, et al: West Nile virus seroconversion in penguins after vaccination with a killed virus vaccine or DNA vaccine. *J Zoo Wildl Med* 39:582–589, 2008.

12. Ferrell ST, Marlar AB, Garner M, et al: Intralesional cisplatin chemotherapy and topical cryotherapy for the control of choanal squamous cell carcinoma in an African penguin (*Spheniscus demersus*). *J Zoo Wildl Med* 37:539–541, 2006.

13. Fisher KJ, Reavill DR, Weldy SH, et al: *Mycobacterium genavense* in a black-footed penguin (*Spheniscus demersus*). *Proc Am Assoc Zoo Vet* 211, 2008.

14. Garner MM, Jencek JE, Dunker FH, et al: An outbreak of *Chlamydophila psittaci* in an outdoor colony of Magellanic penguins (*Spheniscus Magellanicus*). *Proc Am Assoc Zoo Vet* 140, 2006.

15. Gauthier-Clerc M, Gendner JP, Riibic CA, et al: Long-term effects of flipper bands on penguins. *Proc R Soc Lond B (Suppl)* 271:S423–S426, 2004.

16. International Union for Conservation of Nature 2012: Red List of Endangered Species Version 2012.2. www.iucnredlist.org. Accessed December 24, 2012.

17. Jouventin P, Cuthbert RJ, Ottvall R: Genetic isolation and divergence in sexual traits: evidence for the northern rockhopper penguin *Eudyptes moseleyi* being a sibling species. *Mol Ecol* 15:3413–3423, 2006.

18. Kane OJ, Uhart MM, Rago V, et al: Avian pox in Magellanic penguins (*Spheniscus Magellanicus*). *J Wildl Dis* 48:790–794, 2012.

19. MacCoy DM, Campbell TW: Excision of impacted and ruptured uropygial glands in three gentoo penguins (*Pygoscelis papua*). *Proc Am Assoc Zoo Vet* 259–260, 1991.

20. Mazzaro LM, Tuttle A, Wyatt J, et al: Plasma electrolyte concentrations in captive and free-ranging African penguins (*Spheniscus demersus*) maintained with and without dietary salt supplements. *Zoo Biol* 23:397–408, 2004.

21. Monroe A: Annual variations in plasma retinol and α-tocopherol levels in gentoo and rockhopper penguins. *Zoo Biol* 12:453–458, 1993.

22. Napier JE, Hinrichs SH, Lampen F: An outbreak of avian mycobacteriosis caused by *Mycobacterium intracellulare* in little blue penguins (*Eudyptula minor*). *J Zoo Wildl Dis* 40:680–686, 2009.

23. Nimmervoll H, Wenker C, Robert N, et al: Septicaemia caused by *Edwardsiella tarda* and *Plesiomonas shigelloides* in captive penguin chicks. *Schweiz Arch Tierheilkd* 153:117–121, 2011.

24. *Penguin husbandry manual*, ed 3, 2005, AZA publication, pp. 101-102.

25. Perpinan D, Curro TG: Gastrointestinal obstruction in penguin chicks. *J Avian Med Surg* 23:290–293, 2009.

26. Pigatto JAT, Laus JL, Santos JM, et al: Corneal endothelium of the Magellanic penguin (*Spheniscus Magellanicus*) by scanning electronic microscopy. *J Zoo Wildl Med* 36:702–705, 2005.

27. Ploeg M, Ultee T, Kik M: Disseminated toxoplasmosis in black-footed penguins (*Spheniscus demersus*). *Avian Dis* 55:701–703, 2011.

28. Rambaud YF, Flach EJ, Freeman KP: Malignant melanoma in a Humboldt penguin (*Spheniscus humboldti*). *Vet Rec* 153:217–218, 2003.

29. Renner MS, Zaias J, Bossart GD: Cholangiocarcinoma with metastasis in a captive Adélie penguin (*Pygoscelis adeliae*). *J Zoo Wildl Med* 32:384–386, 2001.

30. Schmidt V, Philipp HC, Thielebin S, et al: Malignant lymphoma of T-cell origin in a Humboldt penguin (*Spheniscus humboldti*) and a Pink-backed pelican (*Pelecanus rufescens*). *J Avian Med Surg* 26:101–106, 2012.

31. Smith JA, Papich MG, Russell G, et al: Effects of compounding on pharmacokinetics of itraconazole in black-footed penguins (*Spheniscus demersus*). *J Zoo Wildl Med* 41:487–495, 2010.

32. Tavernier P, Sagesse M, Van Wettere A, et al: Malaria in an eastern screech owl (*Otus asio*). *Avian Dis* 49:433–435, 2005.

33. Travis EK, Vargas FH, Merkel J, et al: Hematology, serum chemistry, and serology of Galápagos penguins (*Spheniscus mendiculus*) in the Galápagos Islands, Equador. *J Wildlife Dis* 42:625–632, 2006.

34. Tuttle AD, Andreadis TG, Frasca S Jr, et al: Eastern equine encephalitis in a flock of African penguins maintained at an aquarium. *J Am Vet Med Assoc* 22:2059–2062, 2005.

35. Wack AN, KuKanich B, Bronson E, et al: Pharmacokinetics of enrofloxacin after single dose oral and intravenous administration in the African penguins (*Spheniscus demersus*). *J Zoo Wildl Med* 43:309–316, 2012.

36. Willette M, Ponder J, Cruz-Martinez L, et al: Management of select bacterial and parasitic conditions of raptors. *Vet Clin North Am Exot Anim Pract* 12:491–517, 2009.

37. Williams TD: *The penguins*, New York, 1995, Oxford University Press.

38. Williams G, Ghebremeskel K, Keymer IF, et al: Plasma α-tocopherol, total lipids and total cholesterol in wild rockhopper, Magellanic and gentoo penguins before and after moulting. *Vet Rec* 124:585–586, 1989.

39. Yonemaru K, Sakai H, Asaoka Y, et al: Proventricular adenocarcinoma in a Humboldt penguin (*Spheniscus humboldti*) and a great horned owl (*Bubo virginianus*): Identification of origin by mucin histochemistry. *Avian Pathol* 33:75–79, 2004.

CHAPTER 11

Gaviiformes, Podicipediformes, and Procellariformes (Loons, Grebes, Petrels, and Albatrosses)

Luis R. Padilla

GENERAL BIOLOGY

The three orders included in this chapter comprise a taxonomically diverse group of aquatic birds that are rarely kept in captivity. Despite some similarities in lifestyle and natural history, the three orders are not taxonomically related to each other. The Gaviiformes (loons) share many traits with the Podicipediformes (grebes) and were once believed to be related to each other, but they are considered examples of convergent evolution and not taxonomic relatedness.

Podicipediformes are considered a primitive, distinct lineage of birds with no close relatives, but the Phoenicopteres (flamingoes) may be their nearest taxonomic relatives. The Procellariformes, which includes the albatrosses, petrels, shearwaters, storm petrels, and diving petrels, may be a sister group to the Spheniciformes (penguins). Table 11-1 summarizes the general biologic features of the families in these three orders, and Table 11-2 summarizes select species information.

The Order Podicipediformes is limited to one extant family (Podicipedidae), which includes all the grebes. Approximately 22 species of grebes are recognized worldwide, classified in six genera. Grebes are small- to medium-sized, heavy-bodied birds with long necks and feet set far back on the body. They have an almost exclusive aquatic lifestyle and are limited in mobility when on land. Grebes inhabit freshwater and inland wetland habitats, although some species overwinter in salt water and may be migratory. Some species congregate in flocks of hundreds to thousands of birds and may migrate en masse, but most species are solitary or found in small groups. On average, male grebes are larger than females. Most species exhibit seasonally dichromatic plumage, and molt occurs on nonbreeding grounds. Grebes forage by diving for prey and are highly adapted divers and agile swimmers.

Members of the Order Gaviiformes, commonly known as loons or divers, are limited to one genus (*Gavia*) in one family (Gaviidae). There are five recognized species of loons worldwide. The term "loon" is used in North America and is synonymous with "diver" in the Old World. Loons are geographically limited to the Northern hemisphere (North America and Eurasia). Loons are long and heavy-bodied birds with webbed feet set far back on the body. Like the grebes, their lifestyle is almost exclusively aquatic, and they may have limited mobility on land. Breeding occurs near fresh water, but birds overwinter in marine environments and are migratory.

The Order Procellariformes includes the albatrosses, mollymawks, petrels, storm petrels, shearwaters, and diving petrels. Considerable size diversity exists within this order—from the small storm petrels that weigh 25 grams (g) as adults, to the albatrosses that exceed 10 kg and are among the largest birds capable of flight. The order is composed of four families: (1) Diomedeidea (albatrosses and mollymawks), (2) Procellaridae (petrels and shearwaters), (3) Hydrobatidae (storm petrels), and (4) Pelecanoidea (diving petrels). On the basis of recent molecular data, the Pelecanoidea, which consists of only one genus, should be classified as a subfamily within the Procellaridae.

Procellariformes are oceanic, pelagic species that spend very limited time on land except during nesting or breeding season. They are highly migratory, skilled long-distance fliers who may also be good swimmers. These birds rely on dynamic soaring and slope soaring to cover long distances in flight while conserving energy, and this is particularly true of the larger-bodied albatross species. Long distance migrations, sometimes for hundreds and thousands of miles, are essential for foraging on specialized diets in specific foraging grounds. Procellariformes are present throughout the world, but a distinct predominance of species exists in the Southern Hemisphere.

The Family Diomedeidae, which includes the albatrosses and mollymawks, comprises entirely pelagic oceanic species. Mollymawks are medium-sized albatrosses limited to southern oceans. The taxonomy of this family has undergone frequent revisions and has been the source of ongoing debate. As many as four genera have been proposed, with at least two being widely accepted. The number of distinct species ranges from 13 to 24, depending on taxonomic revisions. The greatest diversity of species occurs in the Southern Hemisphere. It has been hypothesized that the calmer winds found in the doldrums of the equator pose a geographic barrier to the northern dispersal of the albatross species. Many of the albatross species are threatened or at risk of extinction.

The albatrosses have the largest wingspans of any bird and may measure over 11 feet in some species, although the wing profile is only obvious in flight. The majority of flight is energy-efficient gliding, relying on wind speed. During calm wind conditions, albatrosses often choose to sit on the water. The family is extremely colonial, and birds nest in remote, isolated islands, with pairs that remain together for life. Birds feed by floating on the water surface and picking the prey around them.

The Family Procellaridae encompasses the petrels, shearwaters, and fulmars and includes a large number of small pelagic birds with drab plumage, which only come to shore during the breeding season. Most species migrate over long distances. Although found in all oceans, species diversity peaks in the Southern Hemisphere. The taxonomy of the Procellaridae is in a constant state of revision, with differences in opinion on numbers of distinct species (70–80) and genera (12–14). The Procellaridae have stout bodies with short tails, webbed feet, and monochromatic plumage that varies on the amount of black, gray-brown, and white coloration. Most species are colonial and nest in remote oceanic islands, primarily in underground burrows.

The Family Pelecanoidea, the diving petrels, consists of four species in a single genus (*Pelecanoides*) and is likely a subgroup of the Procellaridae and not a distinct family. Diving petrels are auk-like species, with geographic ranges limited to the southern oceans, but are some of the most numerous aquatic bird species. Most diving petrels are small, weighing between 100 and 200 g and have a characteristic black-and-white plumage. Diving petrels feed exclusively by underwater pursuit-diving of fish, squid, crustaceans, and other invertebrate prey. Some species of diving petrels may dive distances exceeding depths of 80 meters (m). Their small, stocky wings are also used for paddling and propulsion in the water.

The Family Hydrobatidae includes roughly 20 species of storm petrels, distributed in seven genera, although the taxonomy is being

TABLE 11-1

Basic Biology and Geographic Distribution

Order	Geographic Distribution	Natural Diet	Lifestyle	Unique Features
Order Podicipediformes				
Family Podicipedidae (Grebes)	Worldwide except Oceania, around freshwater wetlands	Fish, amphibians, insects, aquatic invertebrates	Some species migratory Nest on floating platforms built of aquatic vegetation as isolated pairs, but may be semi-colonial in prime habitat	Weak fliers (some species are flightless), clumsy on land Strong swimmers and divers
Order Gaviiformes				
Family Gaviidae (Loons/ divers)	Northern parts of Northern Hemisphere	Fish, insects, crustaceans	Migratory Breed on fresh water, winter on salt water Nest on ground, close to water	Very adept swimmers and divers, strong fliers
Order Procellariformes	Occur in all seas of the world, majority of species in Southern Hemisphere	Fish, marine invertebrates (cephalopods, crustaceans, insects), plankton, carrion		"Tube" extension of the nares, horny plates on bill
Family Diomedeidae (Albatrosses)	Oceans worldwide except North Atlantic, Arctic, and tropical doldrums		Migratory species Colonial species that nest on oceanic islands	Capable of long distance gliding
Family Procellaridae (Shearwaters, petrels)	Oceans, seas worldwide		Migratory species Colonial species that nest in underground burrows or on ledges of sea cliffs	Pelagic species, rely on primarily gliding
Family Hydrobatidae (Storm-Petrels)	Oceans, seas worldwide except Arctic		Most species migratory Colonial species nest in burrows or rock crevices	Flutter over the water
Family Pelecanoididae* (Diving Petrels)	Southern oceans		Nonmigratory Live in small colonies, nest in burrows or under rocks	Weak fliers, excellent swimmers, strong divers

*Recent data suggest that the Family Pelecanoididae should be a subfamily within the Procellaridae.

TABLE 11-2

Information on Selected Species

Family	Species	Common	Weight (kg)	Distribution	Comments
Gaviidae	*Gavia immer*	Common Loon	2.6–3.0	North America, Iceland, Greenland	
Gaviidae	*Gavia stellata*	Red-throated loon	1.6–2.0	Circumpolar	
Podicipedidae	*Podilymbus podiceps*	Pied-billed grebe	0.25–0.57	Americas	Most widespread American grebe species
Podicipedidae	*Podiceps nigricollis*	Eared grebe	0.20–0.74	North and Central Americas	Most abundant grebe in the world
Diomedeidae	*Phoebastria immutabilis*	Laysan Albatross	2.3–3.5	Northern Pacific Ocean to Hawaiian Islands	
Diomedeidae	*Diomedea exulans*	Wandering albatross	6.5–8.5	Southern Hemisphere	
Procellaridae	*Puffinus puffinus*	Manx Shearwater	0.4–0.5	North Atlantic	
Procellaridae	*Fulmarus glacialis*	Northern Fulmar	0.4–1.0	Northern Hemisphere	
Hydrobatidae	*Oceanites oceanicus*	Wilson's Storm Petrel	0.03–0.04	Worldwide except North Pacific and extreme North Atlantic	May be most abundant seabird worldwide

constantly revised and debated. Storm petrels are small, delicate birds with relatively large heads. In most species, the long legs dangle below the body, and the feet patter on the surface of the water when near the surface, giving the impression of the bird walking on the surface of the water. These pelagic species are found in all oceans. These birds may congregate in very large numbers. Storm-petrels feed primarily on phytoplankton and small invertebrates, with fish being consumed occasionally. Storm petrels are often predated by other birds and by introduced mammalian predators.

The members of the three orders included in this chapter face similar threats to their continued existence: anthropogenic habitat disturbance and modification, pollution, overharvesting, and (4) predation by introduced species. Some families (e.g., Diomedeidae) contain a large number of species at some risk of extinction. For primarily inland aquatic species (loons and grebes), the threats include the draining of wetland areas, human disturbance, pollution (specifically heavy metals and pesticides), and exposure to coastal oil spills during overwintering in marine environments. Marine seabirds are threatened by overharvesting for food, feathers, and oil; accidental bycatch during fishing operations; habitat disturbance of nesting grounds (including guano harvesting); pollution; and predation by introduced species (rats, cats, pigs, mongoose). Introduced predators may destroy or eat the eggs, the chicks, and the adults sitting on nesting sites, causing a significant impact on the populations in a relatively short timespan. Large-scale harvesting of fish by indiscriminate use of explosives, an illegal practice in many countries, may have a significant impact by affecting large groups of birds during feeding congregations. In addition, long-line fishing operations present a specific risk to many Procellariiformes, as the birds get accidentally entangled in lines and die by drowning. Many species are prone to ingesting indigestible pieces of waste and garbage created by humans, specifically plastic, and this has been a threat to albatross species and their chicks. The epidemiology of infectious diseases has not been extensively studied in colonies, but the risk of virulent diseases spreading could be significant to the continued survival of some species, in particular those with limited nesting sites or isolated populations. The introduction and spread of foreign infectious diseases to established, naive colonies could have a significant effect at the population level.

UNIQUE ANATOMY

Members of all three orders have webbed feet. In loons and grebes, the feet are positioned caudally on the body and are the primary form of propulsion when swimming. The caudal positioning of the feet often limits the locomotor capabilities of these birds.

Grebes have specialized, lobated digits, which are specifically used for propulsive locomotion in the water. The tarsi are laterally compressed and the anterior digits (2, 3, and 4) have excess "lobes" of skin capable of contracting or expanding as the bird paddles when swimming. The nails are flat on the foot and do not extend like claws. As the foot is advanced in a cranial direction, the lobes are collapsed to minimize the profile and decrease the friction and drag against the water. The lobes are flared as the foot pushes back to form a paddle effect and propel the bird forward during a stroke. As highly adapted divers with caudally positioned feet, grebes have difficulty launching from the water for flight and often must use the rapid movements of their wings to propel themselves across the surface of the water before becoming airborne. Additional adaptation to swimming and diving in loons and grebes are a predominance of non-pneumatic bones and a decreased air sac system, which allow them better control of buoyancy.

Members of the Procellariiformes have a characteristic tubelike extension of the nares extending on the dorsal aspect of the bill, well-developed salt glands, and a good sense of smell that is used for both prey detection and recognition of nesting sites. Some species use the large webs on their feet for maneuvering in flight as well as in swimming. All members have well-developed salt glands, which are located dorsal to the orbit and are used in salt homeostasis by excreting salt in drops over the bill. It is an adaptation that allows the ingestion of saltwater and saltwater prey without the need to drink fresh water. Salt metabolism is also regulated by renal excretion. The sense of smell is well developed in Procellariiformes, and many species may detect the smell of certain oils in the water for locating food in the open sea. The sense of smell also serves a purpose in locating nesting sites or burrows, and this function may even be more significant than prey detection in some species of diving feeders, which may rely on few olfactory cues for prey location. Many species are well adapted for nocturnal vision, which may be crucial for the underground nesting species and for predator avoidance when returning to nesting sites at night. In some species, nocturnal vision likely is an adaptation for feeding at night.

Most Procellariiform species are highly adapted for long distance flight and gliding, an energy-conserving strategy that allows the larger mass birds to travel long distances. The diving petrels are highly adapted for feeding underwater—including adaptations such as auk-like black-and-white cryptic coloration, a gular pouch, and short wings.

With the exception of the Pelecanoididae, Procellariiformes may accumulate gastric oils in their proventriculus. This is an adaptation to concentrate lower-volume, high-caloric meals and occurs both by physiologic regulation and specialized anatomy. The oils are not secretory products but, rather, derived from dietary lipids and concentrated by regulating the amount of lipid emptying. The location of the pylorus is an adaptation to retain lipids while allowing water-soluble ingesta to pass through. Lipid emulsifiers of intestinal origin may be refluxed in a retrograde fashion and may play a role in gradual lipid metabolism without entering the intestines.[15] When handled, all species may regurgitate gastric oils, but some species (e.g., northern fulmar, *Fulmarus glacialis*) are capable of forcefully expelling the gastric oil as a defense mechanism.

Most species of grebes (Podicipediformes) routinely ingest their own feathers. Feather ingestion varies with season and type of ingested prey. Ingested feathers contribute bulk to bind undigested stomach contents and allow the formation of uniform, bound pellets. These pellets, which are excreted regularly, may play a role in gastric parasite control[14] and slowing gastric transit time to maximize digestive efficiency.

SPECIAL HOUSING REQUIREMENTS

With the exception of wild birds being temporarily housed for rehabilitation purposes, the birds in this chapter are not routinely housed in captivity. The caudal positioning of the feet of these birds renders them almost incapable of ambulating on land, so they need special accommodations. Birds should be given access to large pools of water, if possible. Providing proper padding to avoid ulcers and pressure sores on the keel and the ventrum is essential. In addition, vigilance to detect the development of pododermatitis and provision of clean, padded substrates to avoid it are essential, since a lot of aquatic or pelagic species are not adapted to spend significant amounts of time weight bearing on their feet.

Salt water should be used when housing marine species, but many species adapt well to housing in fresh water. Holding pools should be designed for ease of cleaning and draining. The large amount of oils in the diets of aquatic birds often soil the water quickly. In temporary housing arrangements, draining and refilling pools at regular intervals help keep the water fresh, but more elaborate filtration systems capable of handling the oils and organic matter produced by these species may be necessary for long-term holding. Attention should be given to concrete or flooring substrates surrounding the pools, as the porous surfaces may be difficult to disinfect properly. The use of rubber mats may provide surfaces that facilitate cleaning and also provide additional traction and padding. Excessively smooth surfaces may predispose the birds to tendon or joint injuries.

Monitoring ambient temperature is an important factor in the holding environments. Birds that are highly adapted to life in the oceans may not thermoregulate as well in limited spaces or when housed indoors. Stressed birds may generate endogenous heat from muscle activity or continuous attempts to escape, and their bodies may overheat. Birds with compromised feather function may suffer from hypothermia. Social species may be particularly stressed when the birds are held in isolation. If conspecifics are not available, mirrors may be used judiciously.

The propensity of many aquatic birds to regurgitate or expel gastric oils when handled (as in the Procellariformes) warrants special consideration. A bird that gets soiled by its own regurgitant should be properly washed, as the oils may compromise feather function and thermoregulation.

The translocation of hand-reared chicks has been advocated as a tool for establishing safety populations of endangered *Procellariform* species. Between 1997 and 2008, a large-scale trial of relocating chicks of eight petrel species was done in New Zealand with burrow-nesting birds of four genera.[10] The birds were placed in artificial burrows and hand reared until fledged by feeding a pureed diet of canned sardines and water into the crop. This diet worked well for all species regardless of their natural diet, and a majority of birds fledged near the expected natural fledging weight. Some translocation attempts to historical colony sites have been supplemented by continuously playing recorded vocalizations, which attract conspecifics to the site. Likewise, short-tailed albatross (*Phoebastria albatrus*) chicks have been successfully translocated between islands and hand reared to fledging.[2]

FEEDING AND DIET

The birds in these orders feed primarily on other aquatic animals: fish, invertebrates (squid, krill, crustaceans, shellfish, plankton, insects, etc.), or carrion. In general, most rely on calorically dense diets rich in fat, protein, or both. The diversity of species makes a summary of specific diets beyond the scope of this chapter, and readers are encouraged to consult the natural history of particular species of interest. Emaciation and cachexia from malnourishment is the most common cause of morbidity in aquatic birds in captivity.

Loons feed primarily on live fish but will also eat aquatic invertebrate prey. Grebes have diets that may vary seasonally and include fish, amphibians, and aquatic invertebrates. The taxonomic diversity in Procellariformes groups also includes a large variety of feeding preferences. Albatross species differ in the percentage of squid, fish, or carrion that they normally take as part of their diet, and in some instances, the species of squid and fish prey is important. Giant petrels are opportunistic feeders, taking carrion when available (and often relying on the carcasses of marine mammals) but catching live invertebrate or fish prey. The prions (family Procellaridae) are specialized filter-feeders, relying on highly adapted beaks with lamellae along the mandible to eat small food particles from the water.

Artificial diets should be supplemented with thiamine if frozen fish are being fed. Vitamin E is often added as a supplement to aquatic animal diets, but attention should be given to dosage to avoid antagonism of other vitamins. The addition of 25 to 30 milligrams (mg) of thiamine and 100 mg of vitamin E per kilogram of fish is a recommended amount when feeding most species. The addition of salt supplements has been advocated to prevent atrophy of the salt gland in marine birds fed freshwater fish or maintained in freshwater systems for prolonged periods. Diets containing deboned fish, which may be given to sick individuals or chicks, should be supplemented with calcium to avoid metabolic bone disease.

When hand-rearing or giving supplements to chicks, a general approach has been to duplicate adult diets and puree them into liquid forms that may be fed by tube to most altricial species. As discussed earlier, feeding Procellariform chicks these slurries, with canned whole sardines as the base, suggests that this may be a practical and suitable strategy for some species.[3] Precocial species (grebes) may be fed small-sized prey items, including live fish, that are supplemented with insects (crickets, mealworms) to stimulate self-feeding behaviors. Prey size is an important consideration in the bird's acceptance of offered prey.

RESTRAINT AND HANDLING

Birds in these taxa may be handled using basic precautions appropriate for their size, powerful beaks, and sharp nails. The wings must be protected, as even seemingly minor injuries could affect their ability to forage and migrate. Handlers should take precautions to avoid injury to their eyes, hands, and face caused by the birds' powerful beaks. Light gloves and eye protection are sufficient for handling most species, and towels may be used for safe restraint.

The foul-smelling oily secretions regurgitated or expelled when the birds are handled require special consideration. Besides the unpleasant effects on the handlers, the tenacious nature of these oils may cause damage to feather function and thermoregulation if the substance adheres to a bird's own plumage. Beaks should not be held shut without close monitoring, as it may lead to accidental ingestion of regurgitated oils and may restrict respiration. The excretion of salt in marine birds may be impaired by holding a bird's mouth tightly shut.[19]

No specific anesthetic techniques unique to this group of birds exist, although the same considerations as for handling—attention to body temperature, feather function, regurgitation and possible aspiration—are applicable.

SURGERY (COMMON AND SPECIAL CONSIDERATIONS)

Surgical interventions may be necessary for injured birds in rehabilitation settings, and in these cases, basic avian surgical techniques should be followed. Surgical placement of internal telemetry devices, which has found applications for monitoring bird populations and objectively assessing the success of rehabilitation-and-release efforts, is also applicable to the species in these orders. Species-specific differences in surgery-related morbidity and mortality have been suggested, and caution should be used when extrapolating between species. Surgical technique and surgeon's skill, size of device, anesthesia management, species' physiology, temperament, and underlying health or social conditions may all affect the outcome of the surgical placement of these devices. Descriptions of specific surgical techniques in Procellariformes, Gaviiformes, or Podicipediformes have been limited at the time of writing this chapter. In a short (9 day) study in wild western grebes (*Aechmophorus occidentalis*),[4] postoperative survival improved when the surgical techniques improved waterproofing, decreased communication into the coelom, and improved the seal around a protruding antenna. These general considerations are likely applicable to successful outcomes in all aquatic taxa. The specific measures taken in this study included offsetting the body wall incision from the skin incision, applying tissue adhesive glue to the subcutaneous space between the two incisions, applying a waterproof sealant to the skin incision after closure, and using porcine small intestine submucosa at the site of the antenna egress.

PHYSICAL EXAMINATION AND DIAGNOSTICS

Physical examination of these birds should follow general principles of avian medicine. Expediency is essential to minimize handling time and associated stress. Scoring body condition may be difficult until a veterinarian has reached enough familiarity with the anatomy of the pectoral musculature of some of these species. Many healthy birds will feel lighter than their body size and wing span would

TABLE 11-3

Representative Hematology and Biochemistry Parameters

	Laysan Albatross (*Phoebastria immutabilis*)[21]	Waved Albatross (*Phoebastria irrorata*)[13]	Hawaiian Dark Rump Petrel (*Pterodroma phaeopygia*)[21]	Southern Giant Petrel (*Macronectes giganteus*)[20]	Common Loon (*Gavia immer*)[5]
White blood cells ($\times10^9$/µL)	19.52 +/– 4.49	5.9 +/– 2.4	10.94 +/– 3.46	4.0 +/– 1.2	17 +/– 6.2
Heterophils ($\times10^9$/µL)	10.21 +/– 3.31	3.9 +/– 1.77	3.39 +/– 1.50	2.1 +/– 0.7	See below
Lymphocytes ($\times10^9$/µL)	3.80 +/– 1.19	1.8 +/– 0.89	4.36 +/– 2.59	1.2 +/– 0.5	See below
Monocytes ($\times10^9$/µL)	0.02 +/– 0.04	0.1 +/– 0.1	0.10 +/– 0.11	0.2 +/– 0.1	See below
Eosinophils ($\times10^9$/µL)	4.40 +/– 2.28	0.1 +/– 0.1	1.99 +/– 1.24	0.4 +/– 0.2	See below
Basophils ($\times10^9$/µL)	1.09 +/– 0.46	0.0 +/– 0.0	1.11 +/– 0.53	0.006 +/– 0.023	See below
PCV (%)	39 +/– 3	38.2 +/– 5.1	49 +/– 4	47.4 +/– 4.0	47 +/– 4.7
Total Protein (g/dL)		4.5 +/– 0.6	3.1 +/– 0.5	6.2 +/– 1.1	3.9 +/– 0.5
Calcium (mg/dL)	11.5 +/– 4.0	9.8 +/– 1.1	7.0 +/– 1.6	9.1 +/– 1.2	
Phosphorous (mg/dL)	4.3 +/– 1.7	3.4 +/– 0.8	0.8 +/– 0.3	2.4 +/– 2.0	
Glucose (mg/dL)	162 +/– 34	229.4 +/– 35.4	329 +/– 43	285 +/– 39	189.2 +/– 45
Uric Acid (IU/L)	2.5 +/– 0.7	4.4 +/– 2.7	7.3 +/– 4.4	8.9 +/– 2.3	
AST (IU/L)	139 +/– 18	117.6 +/– 46.9	212 +/– 116	93.1 +/– 29.6	
Sodium (mEq/L)		152.7 +/– 6.2		154.5 +/– 15.5	
Chloride (mEq/L)		118.0 +/– 7.7		121.3 +/– 5.8	
Albumin (g/dL)	1.9 +/– 0.2	1.8 +/– 0.2	1.5 +/– 0.2	1.5 +/– 0.3	
Globulin (g/dL)	3.1 +/– 0.3	2.8 +/– 0.5	1.7 +/– 0.4	2.3 +/– 0.86	

Reported reference parameters: Heterophils: 32 +/– 11%, mononuclear cells: 37 +/– 13.7%, eosinophils: 31+/– 11.5%, and basophils: 0%.
g/dL, Gram per deciliter; *IU/L*, international unit per liter; *mEq/L*, milliequivalent per liter; *mg/dL*, milligram per deciliter; *µL*, microliter

suggest on first impression, and objective monitoring of body weight should be used as a baseline. Special attention should be given to plumage (for parasites, waterproofing, flight feather quality); to the tubular structures of the nares (for patency), and to the feet (for evidence of pododermatitis). The open oral cavity should be visualized, and the coelomic cavity should be palpated carefully for evidence of foreign bodies (specifically, ingested pieces of plastic).

Venipuncture may be accomplished using the same landmarks and anatomic sites as in other bird species. Reference ranges are available for very few species, and even these should be used with caution in interpreting health status, as differences in sampling techniques, sample handling, analytic techniques, and laboratory equipment may not be applicable. Table 11-3[5,13,20,21] summarizes relevant blood work parameters for representative species.

DISEASE

General

Reports of diseases affecting members of the orders in this chapter come from distinctly different sources, introducing a sampling bias not unique to these birds. The bulk of the health-specific literature derives from the study of free-ranging populations, data collected during mass mortality or morbidity events, and from rehabilitation efforts. Many pelagic species are not even available for examination until breeding season, and carcasses may not be retrievable, representing only a portion of these birds' life history. The diseases discussed in the following sections of this chapter represent unique diseases of significance, and this is not a comprehensive list of avian diseases that may affect these birds.

Infectious Disease

The dynamics of infectious diseases in colonial nesting pelagic species have not been well studied and are areas of specific interest for the conservation of species and protecting them against the introduction of novel pathogens.

Viral Diseases

A novel herpesvirus (Gaviid herpesvirus-1) was recently described from two stranded common loons suffering from ulcerative tracheitis and showing lesions similar to those caused by infectious laryngotracheitis virus in chickens.[16] As a newly identified virus, its significance in loon populations is currently unknown.

Avian poxviruses have been reported in different species of Procellariformes. Although mosquitoes are the primary vectors of transmission of poxviruses, transmission by contact may also occur during feeding of chicks by infected parents. Manx shearwaters (*Puffinus puffinus*) are affected by cutaneous, self-limiting pox lesions on the feet, which may be confused with the lesions caused by puffinosis virus. Cutaneous pox lesions are common in Laysan albatross (*Phoebastria immutabilis*) chicks during high rainfall but do not have an effect on fledgling success at the population level.[22] Since 2004, cutaneous and diphtheritic pox lesions have been identified in giant petrels (*Macronectes giganteus*) from Antarctica,[17] although the overall impact at the population level and the reasons for the apparent emergence of this disease are not currently known.

Puffinosis is an epizootic viral disease of Manx shearwaters (*Puffinus puffinus*),[19] presumed to be caused by a coronavirus. Regular epizootics affect general juveniles near fledging, causing high mortality after a period of blisters on the web of the feet and, sometimes, conjunctivitis. It is thought that the virus overwinters in other species such as fulmars and gulls, suggesting that other Procellariformes are susceptible. In one instance, it was suspected that the black-browed albatross served as an intermediate host between shearwaters and penguins.[5]

Serological evidence of adenoviral infections is common during health surveys of aquatic birds,[5] but the significance is often not clear, since links to clinical disease are missing and because most serologic testing has some limitations. Antibodies to avian influenza viruses and evidence of viral presence are common in seabird colonies. Some strains of avian influenza may be present at enzootic levels and circulate in seabird colonies, often being shared between species, but documentation of the dynamics and epidemiology of these viruses is limited. The globalization of trade and travel and related agricultural practices carry the potential to increase contact between domestic animal strains (poultry, swine, human) of influenza and those present in seabird colonies, warranting special vigilance.

Bacterial Diseases

Chlamydophila psittaci is a common zoonotic concern cited in aquatic bird populations and a concern in colonial nesting species. Between 1930 and 1938, 174 cases of human infection with *C. psittaci* were reported in the Faroe Islands.[6] These cases were characterized by high human mortality, prompting an investigation that linked human infections to the preparation of wild-caught juvenile fulmars for cooking and a ban on fulmar consumption until 1954. A recent survey has shown that *C. psittaci* is still endemic in the Faroe Island fulmar population at a relatively high (10%) prevalence, but human infections are not common despite the resumed harvesting of fulmars for human consumption at high numbers (estimated at 50,000 to 100,000 juvenile fulmars per year).[6] *C. psittaci* should be considered a zoonotic concern in working with seabirds of unknown status and of specific concern in Procellariformes.

Avian cholera (*Pasteurella multocida*) has been reported in a southern Giant petrel[9] and has been isolated from grebes,[19] in which it may occur concurrently with other diseases. *Salmonella* bacteria are often isolated from carnivorous and piscivorous birds. *Salmonella* spp. (multiple serotypes) have been documented in overwintering loons in Florida and in eared grebes. Chronic salmonellosis has been documented in an eared grebe (*Podiceps nigricollis*),[3] and morbidity and mortality likely occur with certain strains in all species.

Fibrinous airsacculitis caused by infections with *Nocardia asteroides* has been reported in albatrosses. Air sac lesions are tightly adherent fibrinous plaques or exudates adhering to the wall of the air sacs. Nocardial airsacculitis may be seen as incidental pathologic findings in Laysan albatross chicks.[18]

Fungal Diseases

Respiratory infections with aspergillus have been commonly reported in overwintering loons. In addition, many aquatic birds are susceptible to aspergillus infections during periods of stress and during rehabilitation. Fatal fungal nephritis was documented in a gray headed albatross.[19]

Parasitic Diseases

Most reports of parasites of the aquatic birds in these orders are mentioned as incidental findings or reported in the ecologic or evolutionary science literature. The clinical significance of parasite infestations is not often clear, but special attention should be paid to birds with concurrent disease, as the parasites may impose an additional physiologic burden for recovery. A listing of parasites or an in-depth discussion of parasite diversity are beyond the scope of this chapter. Ectoparasites (lice and mites) are common findings, and specialized parasites of feathers, nares, and respiratory tract exist, often adapted and co-evolved with their host species. Some topical ectoparasite treatments may affect a bird's waterproofing ability, and caution is warranted when selecting products.

In grebes, intestinal, ventricular, and proventricular nematodes are commonly reported. The parasites of notable clinical relevance are *Eustrongylides tubifex* and *Contracaecum* spp., including *C. ovale*,[19] which shows high specificity for Podicipediformes. *E. tubifex* may cause verminous coelomitis in many bird species, including grebes and loons, and has an indirect life cycle that requires two intermediate hosts. Cestodes are very common in grebes. For instance, in the western grebe, 11 species of cestodes have been documented, but no obvious clinical disease.

Intestinal trematodes are a common finding in debilitated wild loons or in birds affected by concurrent disease, including toxicities. *Cryptocotyle* spp. is often seen in common loons in the maritime provinces of Canada.[1] Renal coccidiosis, caused by *Eimeria gaviae*, has been reported in a common loon.[19]

Few clinically significant parasites have been documented in Procellariformes, which is likely a function of their pelagic lifestyle and not of absence of helminthes. A case report of *Anisakis* sp. causing proventricular perforation in a greater shearwater (*Puffinus gravis*) showed that this common parasite of marine mammals may be a lethal aberrant host in this species.[12]

Limey disease is caused by a renal coccidian (*Eimeria* spp.) that affects the flightless chicks of the Tasmanian mutton bird (also known as short-tailed shearwater; *Puffinus tenuirostris*). Affected birds have "limey" staining and pasting of the vent and poor body condition.[19] These clinical signs are neither unique nor specific to coccidian nephritis, and other diseases may be lumped with the common name of this disease if gross signs are the only basis for a diagnosis.

Noninfectious Disease

Large-scale mortality events of eastern grebes have been periodically reported in North America, and the cause is often undetermined, as in a 1992 mass mortality event involving over 150,000 eared grebes (*Podiceps nigricollis*) in the Salton Sea in California.[7] It has been theorized that weather conditions during migration may play a role in these events, but the grebes' tendency to congregate in large numbers prior to migration, limited agility in flight, and flying at night lead to interspecific collisions and crashes of large groups of birds at once.

During their coastal migration, loons and grebes may become victims of oil spill events. Procellariformes are also susceptible to damage by oil, but their choice of offshore feeding sites may protect them. The success of operations that rescue, stabilize, treat, and rehabilitate oiled grebes and loons for return to the wild depends on many factors, and results may be variable. Besides the physical damage caused to the feathers and the integument, oil negates the thermoregulatory and waterproofing capabilities of an aquatic bird's plumage, leading to energy lost through loss of body heat. Accidental ingestion of oil may have toxic systemic effects. A mass stranding of 14 species of birds, including loons and grebes, was attributed to surfactant-like proteins produced on the water surface by organic matter associated with a red-tide event caused by the dinoflagellate *Akashima sanguinea*.[8]

Albatrosses, petrels, and other marine fish-eating animals are susceptible to accidental death by drowning caused by fishing operations. Line fishing is particularly dangerous to birds that follow ships in their search of fish and may get caught and dragged by the fishing line, eventually dying by drowning. The impact at the population level is difficult to quantify.

Accidental ingestion of plastic has long been recognized as a problem in Laysan albatrosses in the Hawaiian Islands but has now been recognized as a worldwide concern that may affect many seabird species. Direct morbidity or mortality from mechanical obstruction may occur, but ingested plastic can also cause chronic physiologic stress as a result of malnourishment.

Nutritional Diseases

Emaciation and cachexia are common signs in many aquatic bird species, specifically loons, presenting for rehabilitation. The underlying cause is often not found.

Metabolic bone disease was documented in two northern royal albatross chicks (*Diomedea sanfordi*) that were being hand reared shortly after hatching and fed an unsupplemented diet of primarily (deboned) fish filets and gastric oil harvested from sooty shearwaters.[11] After these cases, chicks have been successfully hand reared on a diet of whole fish and no gastric oil and have showed no evidence of fibrous osteodystrophy.

Toxicities

Mercury has been identified as a concern for the survival of common loon populations in northern United States and the Great Lakes region. After entering a water source, elemental mercury is converted into a biologically active form by bacteria. This biologically active

TABLE 11-4

Reproductive Parameters of Select Species

	Common Loon	Least Grebe	Wandering Albatross	Wilson's Storm Petrel	Northern Fulmar
Latin name	*Gavia immer*	*Tachybaptus dominicus*	*Diomedea exulans*	*Oceanites oceanicus*	*Fulmarus glacialis*
Family	Gaviidae	Podicipedidae	Diomedidae	Hydrobatidae	Procellaridae
Sexual maturity	1 year	1 year	8–9 years	Unknown	8–10 years
Eggs per clutch	1–3	4–6	1	1	1
Incubation period	28 days	21 days	75–82 days	39–48 days	52–53 days
Fledging age	56 days	Unknown	278 days	70–75 days	46–51 days
Nest	Mound of plant material around lakeshore	Floating nest made of vegetation in shallow water	Mound of mud and vegetation on ridge	Underground burrows	Grass ledge or ground vegetation

form, methylmercury, enters the food chain and accumulates in fish. Inland piscivorous birds such as loons and grebes, are at high risk of mercury exposure. Exposure varies according to local concentrations in the water as well as lake conditions. Although overt signs of mercury toxicity have been difficult to demonstrate, mercury may have reproductive effects at the population level, and some evidence suggests effects on eggs, chicks, and hatchability.

Lead poisoning has been documented in common loons and Pacific loons. Birds ingest toxic levels of lead derived from fishing sink weights or from spent lead shot. Clinical signs are primarily neurologic but may be limited to subtle paresis or partial paralysis.

Birds of all three orders are susceptible to the biotoxins produced by algal blooms and by domoic acid toxicity and have been affected in mass mortality events affecting multiple species. Avian botulism type E has been reported in grebes and in loons. Botulism type C has been seen in grebes.

REPRODUCTION

Most knowledge on the reproductive biology of the birds in these orders comes from observations and studies of free-ranging species. Table 11-4 summarizes biologic data on some common species.[19]

PREVENTIVE MEDICINE

Because many grebes and loons are prone to aspergillosis during periods of stress or during prolonged captivity, the use of antifungals has been advocated as a prophylactic treatment when working with these species. It is reasonable to assume that this practice is also applicable to Procellariiformes. Pharmacokinetic data are extrapolated from other species, and the Sphenisciformes may be the best available model for Procellariiformes.

REFERENCES

1. Daoust P, Conboy G, McBurney S, et al: Interactive mortality factors in common loons from maritime Canada. *J Wildl Dis* 34(3):524–531, 1998.
2. Deguchi T, Jacobs J, Harada T, et al: Translocation and hand-rearing techniques for establishing a colony of threatened albatross. *Bird Cons Int* 22(1):66–81, 2012.
3. Dunmay RM, Stroud RK, Locke LN: *Salmonella enteritidis* isolated from an eared grebe (*Podiceps nigricollis*). *J Wildl Dis* 19(1):63–64, 1983.
4. Gaydos JK, Massey JG, Mulcahy DM, et al: Short-term survival and effects of transmitter implantation into western grebes using a modified surgical procedure. *J Zoo Wildl Med* 42(3):414–425, 2011.
5. Haefele HJ, Sidor I, Evers DC, et al: Hematologic and physiologic reference ranges for free-ranging adult and young common loons (*Gavia immer*). *J Zoo Wildl Med* 36(3):385–390, 2005.
6. Herrmann B, Persson H, Jensen JK, et al: *Chlamydophila psittaci* in fulmars, the Faroe Islands. *Emerg Infect Dis* 12(2):330–332, 2006.
7. Jehl JR: Mortality events of eared grebes in North America (Mortandad en masa de individuas de Podiceps nigricollis en Norte América). *J Field Ornithol* 67(3):471–476, 1996.
8. Jessup DA, Miller MA, Ryan JP, et al: Mass stranding of marine birds caused by a surfactant-producing red tide. *PLoS ONE* 4(2):e4550, 2009.
9. Leotta GA, Rivas M, Chinen I, et al: Avian cholera in a southern giant petrel (*Macronectes giganteus*) from Antarctica. *J Wildl Dis* 39(3):732–735, 2003.
10. Miskelly CM, Taylor GA, Gummer H, et al: Translocations of eight species of burrow-nesting seabirds (genera *Pterodroma*, *Pelecanoides*, *Pachyptila* and *Puffinus*: Family Procellariidae). *Biol Cons* 142(10):1965–1980, 2009.
11. Morgana KJ, Alleya MR, Gartrella BD, et al: Fibrous osteodystrophy in two northern royal albatross chicks (*Diomedea sanfordi*). *New Zealand Vet J* 59(5):248–252, 2011.
12. Nemeth NM, Yabsley M, Keel MK: Anisakiasis with proventricular perforation in a greater shearwater (*Puffinus gravis*) off the coast of Georgia, United States. *J Zoo Wildl Med* 43(2):412–415, 2012.
13. Padilla LR, Huyvaert KP, Merkel J, et al: Hematology, plasma chemistry, serology and *Chlamydophila* status of the waved albatross (*Phoebastria irrorata*) on the Galápagos Islands. *J Zoo Wildl Med* 34(3):278–283, 2003.
14. Piersma T, Van Eerden MR: Feather eating in great crested grebes *Podiceps cristatus*: A unique solution to the problems of debris and gastric parasites in fish-eating birds. *Ibis* 131(4):477–486, 1989.
15. Place AR, Stoyan AC, Ricklefs RE, et al: Physiological basis of stomach oil formation in Leach's storm-petrel (*Oceanodroma leucorhoa*). *The Auk* 106(4):687–699, 1989.
16. Quesada RJ, Heard DJ, Aitken-Palmer C, et al: Detection and phylogenetic characterization of a novel herpesvirus from the trachea of two stranded common loons (*Gavia immer*). *J Wildl Dis* 47(1):233–239, 2011.
17. Shearn-Bochsler V, Green DE, Converse KA, et al: Cutaneous and diphtheritic avian poxvirus infection in a nestling southern giant petrel (*Macronectes giganteus*) from Antarctica. *Polar Biol* 31:569–573, 2008.
18. Sileo L, Sievert PR, Samuel MD: Causes of mortality of albatross chicks at Midway Atoll. *J Wildl Dis* 26(3):329–338, 1990.
19. Stoskopf MK: Gaviiformes (loons), Podicipediformes (grebes), and Procellariiformes (albatrosses, fulmars, petrels, storm petrels, and shearwaters). In Fowler ME, Miller RE, editors: *Zoo and wild animal medicine*, ed 5, St. Louis, MO, 2003, Saunders, pp 110–122.
20. Uhart MM, Quintana F, Karesh WB, et al: Hematology, plasma, biochemistry and serosurvey for selected infectious agents in southern giant petrels from Patagonia, Argentina. *J Wildl Dis* 39(2):359–365, 2003.
21. Work TM: Weights, hematology and serum chemistry of seven species of free-ranging tropical pelagic seabirds. *J Wildl Dis* 32(4):643–657, 1996.
22. Young LC, VanderWerf EA: Prevalence of avian pox virus and effect on the fledging success of Laysan Albatross. *J Field Ornithol* 79(1):93–98, 2008.

CHAPTER 12

Pelecaniformes (Pelicans, Tropicbirds, Cormorants, Frigatebirds, Anhingas, Gannets)

Sharon Redrobe

BIOLOGY

The Order Pelecaniformes was previously defined as comprising birds that have feet with all four toes webbed. Hence, they were formerly also known by such names as *totipalmates* or *steganopodes*. The group included frigatebirds, gannets, cormorants, anhingas, and tropicbirds.[2] The current International Ornithological Committee classification now groups pelicans with the Families Threskiornithidae (ibises and spoonbills), Ardeidae (herons, bitterns, egrets), Scopidae (hamerkop), Balaenicipitidae (shoebill), and Pelicanidae (pelicans). Previously included families are now classified in the Order Suliformes, that is, Fregatidae (frigates), Sulidae (gannets and boobies), and Phalacrococorcidae (cormorants and shags).[3] However, for the purposes of consistency and for this chapter, the previous grouping of Pelecaniformes (pelicans, tropicbirds, cormorants, frigatebirds, anhingas, gannets) will be used with a focus on pelicans (Table 12-1). Most of the birds in this order have large beaks relative to their head size and a distensible pouch formed by the floor of the mouth, between the mandibles. The natural range of the species extends around the world, mainly in the tropical areas. The species most commonly maintained in captivity are the pelicans and cormorants but the others rarely so.

UNIQUE ANATOMY

The most obvious distinguishing feature of the pelican, besides being large birds, is the gular pouch. The floor of the mouth is greatly enlarged to form the pouch used for scooping up water and prey and then draining the water before swallowing the captured prey. The large beak ends in a pronounced downward facing hook. The tongue is significantly reduced in size. The pelicans are among the largest flying birds and yet are relatively light because of the extensive air sac diverticula between the skeletal muscles of the neck and the breast. These air pockets under the skin are readily palpated when the birds is restrained. The subcutaneous air sacs are known to anatomically connect with the respiratory system, and the bird maintains inflation by the closing of the glottis. The subcutaneous air pockets are presumed to act as a shock absorber when the bird hits the water at speed during a dive and also assist in floating. Males are generally larger than females and have longer bills. Several other species, for example boobies and gannets, as mentioned earlier, also have extensive subcutaneous air sacs. The external nares are not patent in some birds in this order, including brown pelicans, cormorants, boobies, and gannets, perhaps as an adaptation to diving. The rest of the Order Pelecaniformes comprises long-legged birds that hunt or scavenge prey near lakes or rivers and are relatively slender in body shape. The gular pouch is used for courtship displays in frigatebirds and absent in the tropicbirds. Birds of this order are typically carnivorous (primarily fish eating). The proventriculus and the ventriculus are both thin and extensible in the pelican and cormorant species and relatively indistinguishable. The pylorus is very well defined and well muscled, and this may be an adaptation to prevent foreign bodies and bones entering the small intestine.

SPECIAL HOUSING REQUIREMENTS

In common with many other marine species, Pelecaniformes typically have supraorbital salt glands that may atrophy in captivity if they are housed on fresh water. When birds are transferred between institutions, the salinity of the water should be noted, and it must be ensured that the birds are transferred between the same systems; in the case of transference from a freshwater environment to a saline environment, supplementation with dietary salt (if a pool of increasing salinity cannot be provided) should be carefully instigated to reactivate the salt glands without risking salt poisoning. The birds should be carefully monitored during this process. This process should also occur prior to release from a freshwater or a low-salt facility. Birds in this order are characteristically semi-aquatic birds that dive from a great height into water to capture prey. It may be challenging to replicate this behavior in captivity, but the birds should certainly be provided with pools that permit swimming and surface diving. Maintenance of adequate water hygiene, using appropriate surface skimmers and other measures, will be required to prevent the accumulation of fish oils damaging the feathers. Sufficient dry land area is required, especially for pelicans, cormorants, and anhingas, which have feathers that tend to get waterlogged. The substrate needs to be supportive and noninjurious, as all birds in this order, particularly the heavier species, are prone to pododermatitis.

FEEDING

The natural diet of pelicans is quite varied and related to their aquatic habitat, including fish (up to 30 centimeters [cm] long), crustaceans, amphibians, turtles, and occasionally other birds. The way different species of pelican feed varies. For example, the brown pelican feeds by diving into water, whereas the white pelican species feed cooperatively by herding fish and dipping their beaks into the water to scoop the fish out. Cormorants and anhingas are surface divers and capture their prey underwater. Tropicbirds, boobies, and gannets are plunge divers. Frigatebirds are renowned scavengers and steal food from other birds. Birds in captivity need to adapt to taking dead fish, and training may be required when presenting the fish in a manner dissimilar to their wild presentation. Throwing fish into the air is the least natural presentation of fish, but the movement may stimulate attack and feeding. If feeding fish that has been frozen, supplementation with vitamins is often required; further information on fish handling as food and supplementation will not be covered in this chapter.

RESTRAINT AND HANDLING

In general, restraint of these species is simple, with the birds being captured in a net or herded into a corner, the beak restrained in one hand initially, and then the body and wings restrained under the other arm. As the nares are not patent in some species (brown pelicans, cormorants, boobies, and gannets), the beaks should be held

TABLE 12-1

Biological Data for Selected Pelecaniformes

Scientific Name	Common Name	Weight (Adults, kg)	Distribution
Phaethon rubricauda	Red-tailed tropicbird	0.64–1.1	Tropical Indian and Pacific Oceans
Fregata magnificens	Magnificent frigatebird	1.2–1.6	Tropical Atlantic and Pacific Oceans
Sula sula	Red-footed booby	0.85–1.0	Tropical Indian, Pacific, and Atlantic Oceans
Morus bassanus	Northern gannet	2.2–3.6	Newfoundland, Iceland, and Great Britain
P. bougainvillii	Guanay cormorant	1.55–3.2	Western South America
Anhinga anhinga	Anhinga	1.23–1.27	Southern North America to Argentina
Pelecanus occidentalis	Brown pelican	2.05–4.1	Coastal southern North America and Central and South America
Pelecanus erythrorhynchos	American white pelican	6.18–8.0 (males); 4.21–8.0 (females)	Coastal and inland North and Central America
Pelecanus rufescens	Pink-backed pelican	3.86–5.55 (males); 3.42–4.57 (females)	Sub-Saharan Africa

Adapted from Weber M: *Zoo and wild animal medicine*, 5th ed, St. Louis, MO, 2003, Elsevier. Chapter 13: Pelecaniformes.

slightly open during restraint to prevent asphyxia. When stressed, some birds (gannets and pelicans) may inflate their subcutaneous air sac diverticulae that may easily be palpated by the handler as crepitus under the skin; this may be an alarming finding to the novice. Staff should consider wearing eye protection when handling birds such as the anhingas, which have long sharp beaks.

SURGERY AND ANESTHESIA

Inhalant anesthesia using isoflurane is a simple and easy way of anesthetizing Pelecaniformes. The long beak makes application of a mask difficult; a useful tip is to use a disposable rectal glove as a makeshift mask for induction. Pelecaniformes are easily intubated with an uncuffed endotracheal tube. Nitrous oxide should be avoided because it has been reported to cause significant expansion of the subcutaneous air sacs of a pelican.[9] Endotracheal intubation of some species may be challenging because of the crista ventralis, a septum or projection across the lumen of the trachea just inside the glottis. Intubation is readily achieved using a smaller tube, with the awareness that the inhalation anesthesia may be less efficient and the bird will also be breathing room air, that the airway is less protected, and that assisted ventilation will be less effective. As with other bird species, the addition of ketamine (3 milligrams per kilogram intramuscularly [mg/kg, IM]) and butorphanol (1 mg/kg, IM) provides more controlled anesthesia suitable for surgery and endoscopy (personal communication, author).

Surgery, particular to this group of birds, is performed for repair of the pouch.[12] Special considerations include establishing that subramal and ventral gular blood supply is intact, as no evidence of anastomoses between these vessels exists, so vascular damage to these areas may result in poor wound healing. Full thickness suture patterns should also be avoided when repairing laceration of the pouch to avoid compressing the vascular layer. The pouch should be repaired by separating the epithelial layers and suturing them separately using a simple interrupted pattern.

Flight is often restricted in the larger species such as pelicans, as their size necessitates very large (and relatively expensive) meshed aviaries to permit free flight; they are therefore often restrained in large, open-topped areas by such methods as feather clipping, feather follicle extirpation, or pinioning. Clinicians should note that in some countries, pinioning (amputation of the wing tips) is legally performed by nonprofessionals in very young birds. In other countries, pinioning is legally restricted; for example, it is considered "an act of veterinary surgery" in the United Kingdom and, as such, may only be performed by a veterinary surgeon (on a bird of any age) and must be performed with the bird under general anesthesia if the bird is over 10 days old.

Currently, few publications on pelican surgery exist in the literature, but a case of successful keratoplasty performed on the left cornea of a young adult female California brown pelican (*Pelecanus occidentalis*) for the treatment of vision-threatening corneal scarring has been reported.[5]

DIAGNOSTICS

Blood collection is similar to that in other birds, with the metatarsal veins being the most accessible. Blood collection via the jugular vein or the wing veins may be challenging in pelicans because the subcutaneous air pockets make visualization and palpation of the vessels difficult. Complete blood cell count and serum biochemistry values are comparable with those performed in other avian species (Table 12-2).

DISEASES

General

Pelecaniformes are susceptible to a wide range of diseases noted to affect other avian species. Diseases particularly noted in captivity include aspergillosis, pododermatitis, endoparasitism, and vitamin deficiencies and other conditions associated with the feeding of frozen fish. In general, diagnosis and treatments are similar to those in other avian species.

Infectious Disease

Bacterial enteritis has been reported in captive pelicans and cormorants. *Escherichia coli*, *Proteus* spp., *Salmonella* spp., and *Campylobacter* spp. have been cultured from affected animals. Fatal *Clostridium perfringens* enteritis has been diagnosed in a captive brown pelican, and contaminated fish was suspected to be the source of the infection.

Viral diseases reported in Pelecaniformes include infections with West Nile virus, Newcastle disease virus, and poxvirus. Avian influenza vaccination has a mixed result in the Pelecaniformes; a study reported that the commercially inactivated H5N2 vaccine (manufactured for domestic poultry) elicited only a partial response in cormorants and no immune response in pelicans.[7]

Parasitic Diseases

Pelecaniformes may harbor parasites typically infesting many bird species in captivity, typically ascarids, which are trematodes that are routinely treated with fenbendazole or albendazole (Table 12-3). External parasitism is common but rarely leads to clinical signs, and treatment is routine. A study of the parasites of the American white pelican found 75 different species of parasites, the majority of which

TABLE 12-2

Reference Ranges for Hematologic and Serum Biochemical Parameters of Selected Pelican Species*

Test	Units	American white pelican, *Pelecanus erythrorhynchos*			Brown pelica, *Pelecanus occidentalis*			Pink-backed pelican, *Pelecanus rufescens*		
		Reference Interval	Mean	Median	Reference Interval	Mean	Median	Reference Interval	Mean	Median
White Blood Cell Count	*10∧9 cells/L	4.56–32.02	14.02	12.93	3.85–25.40	11.25	10.32	0.00–41.07	19.23	16.37
Red Blood Cell Count					1.63–3.89	2.78	2.76	1.67–3.38	2.55	2.52
Hemoglobin	g/L	95–191	140	143	115–198	156	157	56–186	121	121
Hematocrit	L/L	0.314–0.560	0.436	0.434	0.330–0.559	0.457	0.458	0.289–0.564	0.43	0.435
MCV						171.4	167.3	116.7–222.8	168.6	169.8
MCH								25.5–70.4	48.6	47.9
MCHC	g/L	267–409	341	338	245–411	325	328	161–407	287	284
Heterophils	*10∧9 cells/L	2.41–20.02	8.14	6.9	1.71–14.76	6.25	5.54	0.00–25.13	12.23	10.34
Lymphocytes	*10∧9 cells/L	0.90–14.11	4.76	3.98	0.43–9.34	3.3	2.67	0.00–9.18	4.07	3.36
Monocytes	*10∧6 cells/L	68–2227	580	374	50–2049	639	472	0–1658	669	576
Eosinophils	*10∧6 cells/L	63–1310	420	289	50–1419	402	296	0–1637	653	512
Basophils	*10∧6 cells/L	0–789	335	282	47–1117	371	270		387	310
Glucose	mmol/L	7.51–17.35	11.87	11.56	5.46–17.86	12.41	12.39	5.47–16.88	10.79	11.18
Blood Urea Nitrogen	mmol/L	0.0–3.1	1.4	1.1	0.0–2.9	1.4	1.2			
Creatinine	µmol/L	0–66	29	24	0–80	40	35			
Uric Acid	µmol/L	97–870	376	330	162–1238	511	436	0–896	448	391
Calcium	mmol/L	2.01–2.76	2.35	2.36	1.85–3.15	2.41	2.38	1.79–2.92	2.37	2.36
Phosphorus	mmol/L	0.25–1.91	0.89	0.83	0.46–2.73	1.24	1.08	0.26–2.01	1.21	1.13
Ca/Phos ratio		1.7–8.4	3.9	3.6	0.9–6.6	3.2	3	0.8–4.5	2.8	2.7
Sodium	mmol/L	139–159	150	150	138–164	149	150		151	151
Potassium	mmol/L	1.5–6.4	3.1	2.8	1.4–6.2	2.9	2.8		4.2	3.9
Na/K ratio		23.0–101.7	55.1	52.5	23.2–113.3	56.5	51	16.4–60.1	37.8	38.2
Chloride	mmol/L	100–125	113	113	95–122	111	112			
Total Protein	g/L	31–59	43	42	28–63	45	44	20–60	43	40
Albumin	g/L	10–22	15	15	9–25	16	16	6–22	14	14
Globulin	g/L	16–42	27	27	11–47	28	27	9–44	28	26
Alkaline Phosphatase	U/L	362–2317	1281	1339	225–2161	1176	1193	0–1192	536	484
Lactate Dehydrogenase	U/L	0–1035	557	511	0–1750	893	684			
Aspartate Aminotransferase	U/L	60–466	181	155	104–840	301	247	0–770	352	311
Alanine Aminotransferase	U/L	0–71	34	33	0–132	56	40		64	57
Creatine Kinase	U/L	223–1405	609	531	290–3246	1138	920	0–1808	937	744
Gamma-glutamyltransferase	U/L	0–9	4	3	0–15	6	5		5	5
Amylase	U/L	0–3969	1737	1586	466–5728	3178	3097	472–2822	1631	1647
Total Bilirubin	µmol/L	0.0–9.6	4.2	3.8	0.0–12.8	5.1	3.7			
Cholesterol	mmol/L	2.57–6.73	4.7	4.73	2.98–9.89	5.54	5.41	0.32–5.83	3.4	3.07

*Values from ISIS, USA, downloaded at Twycross Zoo, U.K., January 2013.

ALK. PHOS., Alkaline phosphatase; *ALT (SGPT)*, alanine transaminase (serum glutamic pyruvic transaminase); *AST (SGOT)*, aspartate aminotransferase (serum glutamic-oxaloacetic transaminase); *BUN*, blood urea nitrogen; *CPK*, creatine phosphokinase; *fL*, fluid ounce; *g/L*, gram per liter; *GGT*, gamma-glutamyl trans-peptidase; *HCT*, hematocrit; *HGB*, hemoglobin; *LDH*, lactate dehydrogenase; *MCH*, mean corpuscular hemoglobin; *MCHC*, mean corpuscular hemoglobin concentration; *MCV*, mean corpuscular volume; *mmol/L*, millimole per liter; *µmol/L*, micromole per liter; *RBC*, red blood cell; *SD*, standard deviation; *WBC*, white blood cell; *Units/L*, units per liter.

From Teare JA, ed: 2013, American White Pelican; Brown Pelica; Pink Backed Pelican_No_selection_by_gender__All_ages_combined_Standard_International _Units__2013_CD.html *in* ISIS Physiological Reference Intervals for Captive Wildlife: A CD-ROM Resource, International Species Information System, Bloomington, MN.

TABLE 12-3

Common Parasites of Pelecaniformes

Parasite (Type)	Site Typically Found	Clinical/Pathologic Findings
Contracaecum (ascarid)	Ventriculus, distal esophagus, gular pouch	Ulcerative gastritis, if present in large numbers
Phagicola longa, Mesostephanus appendiculatoides (trematodes)	Intestines	Mild histologic changes only
Piagetiella sp. (pouch lice)	Gular pouch	Severe hemorrhagic stomatitis in debilitated pelicans and cormorants

TABLE 12-4

Reproductive Characteristics of Pelecaniformes

Parameter	Pelicans	Cormorants	Gannets	Boobies	Tropicbirds
Maturity (approx.)	3–4 years	2–4 years	5 years	1–6 years	4 years
Eggs/clutch (approx.)	2–4	2–4	1	1–3 (facultative siblicide may occur)	1
Incubation period (approx.)	28–35 days	24–31 days	42–46 days	40–45 days	40–46 days
Incubation method	Under foot webs	On foot webs	Under foot webs	Under foot webs	Insulated in breast feathers

cause little or no clinical signs.[8] Fenbendazole is reported to be effective in brown pelicans at a relatively low dose of 22 mg/kg and effectively treated *Contracaecum multipapillatum, Mesostephanus appendiculatoides*, and *Phagicola longus*.[1] Fatal enteritis and bone marrow damage have been seen in pink-backed pelicans following administration of fenbendazole. Affected birds were found dead or exhibited respiratory distress and died shortly after presentation. In treatment with benzimidazoles, the recommendation is to medicate the birds individually or to hand-toss medicated fish to individuals, rather than treating an entire group with medicated fish placed in a pan.

Toxicities

Poisoning with marine toxins, including domoic acid and brevetoxin, has been reported in brown pelicans, Brandt's cormorants, and double-crested cormorants.[4] Pelicans affected by domoic acid poisoning exhibited slow, side-to-side head motion, fine motor tremors, scratching at the pouch, and vomiting, whereas affected cormorants were unusually docile when approached by humans.[13] Cormorants affected by brevetoxicosis showed ataxia, disorientation, and intention tremors.

Botulism, caused by ingestion of the toxin produced by *Clostridium botulinum*, has been reported in Pelecaniformes birds and has been associated with up to 20% of a population die-off in the western population of the American white pelican.[10]

Noninfectious Disease

Osteodystrophy caused by dietary calcium, vitamin D_3 deficiency, or both has been reported in captive raptors fed all-meat diets and in cormorants (*Phalacrocorax auritus*).[6] Reports of neoplasia are rare but include skin melanoma diagnosed in a pelican throat pouch in addition to a multicentric T-cell lymphoma. The pelican was found dead but a clinical history of T-cell lymphoma did not exist.[11]

REPRODUCTION

Reproduction has been low for most of the Pelecaniformes species maintained in captivity and may be caused, in part, by the small flock sizes that are maintained (Table 12-4). Mature white pelicans have a keratinized growth on the dorsal maxilla during the breeding season; this growth is shed at the end of the season. Both sexes incubate eggs and participate in rearing chicks.

REFERENCES

1. Grimes J, Suto B, Greve JH, et al: Effect of selected anthelmintics on three common helminths in the brown pelican (*Pelecanus occidentalis*). *J Wildl Dis* 25:139–142, 1989.
2. Hedges SB, Sibley CG: Molecules vs. morphology in avian evolution: The case of the "pelecaniform birds." *PNAS* 91(21):9861–9865, 1994.
3. International Ornithological Committee (2 January 2012): *Ibises to Pelicans & Cormorants. 2012 IOC World Bird Names: Version 3.2*: <www.WorldBirdNames.org>. Accessed 22 January 2013.
4. Kreuder C, Bossart GD, Elie MS: Clinicopathologic features of an epizootic in the double-crested cormorant (*Phalacrocorax auritus*) along the Florida gulf coast. In *Proceedings of the annual meeting of the American Association of Zoo Veterinarians*, Omaha, NB, 1998, pp 161.
5. Lynch GL, Scagliotti RH, Hoffman A, Dubielzig R: Penetrating keratoplasty in a California brown pelican. *Vet Ophthalmol* 10:254–261, 2007.
6. Nichols D, Montali RJ, Pickett C, Bush C: Rickets in double-crested cormorants (*Phalacrocorax auritus*). *J Zoo Anim Med* 14:115–124, 1983.
7. Oh S, Martelli P, Hock OS, et al: Field study on the use of inactivated H5N2 vaccine in avian species. *Vet Rec* 157(10):299–300, 2005.
8. Overstreet RM, Curran S: Parasites of the American white pelican. *Gulf Caribbean Res* 17:31–48, 2005.
9. Reynolds WT: Unusual anaesthetic complication in a pelican. *Vet Rec* 113:204, 1983.
10. Rocke T, Converse K, Meteyer C, McLean B: The impact of disease in the American white pelican in North America. *Waterbirds* 28(sp1):87–94, 2005.
11. Schmidt V, Philipp HC, Thielebein J, et al: Malignant lymphoma of T-cell origin in a Humboldt penguin (*Spheniscus humboldti*) and a pink-backed pelican (*Pelecanus rufescens*). *J Avian Med Surg* 26(2):101–106, 2012.
12. Williams TD, Gawlowski PQ, Strickland DM, et al: Surgical repair of the gular sac of the brown pelican (*Pelecanus occidentalis*). *J Zoo Anim Med* 19:122–125, 1988.
13. Work TM, Barr B, Beale A, et al: Epidemiology of domoic acid poisoning in brown pelicans (*Pelecanus occidentalis*) and Brandt's cormorants (*Phalacrocorax penicillatus*) in California. *J Zoo Wildl Med* 24:54–62, 1993.

CHAPTER 13

Ciconiiformes (Herons, Ibises, Spoonbills, Storks)

Terry M. Norton and Douglas P. Whiteside

GENERAL BIOLOGY

The Order Ciconiiformes comprises medium- to large-sized, charismatic wading birds that are popular in zoologic collections. This group has a worldwide distribution in temperate, subtropical, and tropical climates. The five families include Ardeidae (herons, bitterns, and egrets), Balaenicipitidae (shoebills), Ciconiidae (storks), Scopidae (hammerkopfs), and Threskiornithidae (ibises and spoonbills).[11,24] Over 26 species are considered near threatened, vulnerable, or endangered by the International Union for the Conservation of Nature.[30] Many species are long lived, with some of the larger species living for 40 to 50 years.[8]

Most species are sexually monomorphic with similar feathering; however, females are usually smaller than males. Gender determination may be accomplished through DNA (deoxyribonucleic acid) analysis of whole blood or blood feathers. Other techniques, which have proved successful, include measurements of bill length, tibiotarsal length, and body length.[51,68,70]

UNIQUE ANATOMY

Most Ciconiiformes species have long legs and elongated toes with slightly webbed feet. The middle toe may be well developed for feather maintenance. Most have long necks with 15 to 20 vertebrae. Herons have a modified sixth cervical vertebra, which allows the neck to be held in an S-shape during flight. Many species have bare portions to the head and neck. Herons have powder-down feathers; however, adult storks, ibises, and spoonbills lack this feature.

Storks lack syringeal musculature, and most are mute. Bill clattering is an important form of communication, especially in Ciconiidae. Openbill storks have a distinct separation between their rhamphotheca and gnathotheca, whereas the other stork species have variably tapered long beaks.[18]

SPECIAL HOUSING REQUIREMENTS

In a captive environment, meeting the physical, social, and psychological needs of the species through appropriate exhibits, social groupings, and opportunities to express species-appropriate behaviors will maximize their welfare. Large meshed exhibits, which allow uninterrupted flight, are most ideal. Where this is not possible, feather clipping may be performed to keep birds in open exhibits. Pinioning is not recommended, as it potentially interferes with breeding ability and may violate legal regulations in some countries. A water feature such as a pond or small lake should be available. Natural substrate with low, wide stumps is preferred, and trees should be available for perching. Many zoologic facilities successfully display various Ciconiiformes species in mixed-species exhibits; however, care should be taken because interspecific aggression–related trauma has been documented. When these birds are housed with larger species, a safety zone should be established that allows the birds ability to enter while preventing access by the larger species.

FEEDING

Most Ciconiiformes species are aquatic carnivores, and fish, amphibians, aquatic insects, molluscs, small mammals, birds, and reptiles are part of the diet in the wild; however, not all species feed on all of these. Some are generalists, whereas others are specialists. For example, openbill storks feed on freshwater snails (*Pilia* spp.) and bivalve mollusks almost exclusively. Adjutant storks are part-time scavengers at kills of large predators; however, they feed their young only live-caught prey. Some ibises hunt for insects in grasslands. Spoonbills have large, flat, spatulate bills and feed by wading through shallow water, sweeping the partly opened bill from side to side. The moment any small aquatic creature—an insect, crustacean, or tiny fish—touches the inside of the bill, it is snapped shut.[10,18]

In a captive environment, Ciconiiformes species are fed a variety of fish, whole vertebrate prey (e.g., rodents, juvenile rabbits, day-old chicks, and amphibians), nutritionally balanced ground-meat carnivore products, insects, earthworms, and commercially prepared carnivore and avian dry and semi-dry pelleted diets. As in other carnivore species, it is important to avoid excessive amounts of vitamin A in the diet. Chicks are fed regurgitated food, so appropriate food sizes are important. For growing chicks, it is important to supplement the diet with calcium (e.g., bone meal, calcium lactate) and to ensure that they have access to dietary sources of vitamin D (as found in whole prey food items) and exposure to natural or artificial ultraviolet B (UVB) light. Where fish is a predominant portion of the diet, it is essential to supplement with vitamin E and thiamine to offset the peroxidation and thiaminase activity in frozen fish.[18,69] Roseate spoonbill and scarlet ibis require supplementation with special pigments (synthetic canthaxanthin) in their diet so that they can exhibit normal natural brilliant feather and skin coloration similar to flamingos. In the wild, they obtain these pigments from feeding on aquatic invertebrates. Newly hatched chicks of these species will lack pigment.

RESTRAINT AND HANDLING

Appropriate planning should take place prior to capture or immobilization. Capture myopathy is not uncommon in Ciconiiformes. Care should be taken when handling and restraining to prevent injury to the bird and to the handler. Ensuring that an appropriate number of people are present is paramount, particularly with larger birds. Birds may be initially netted, or herded into a smaller space, for hand capture. The long legs and the beak should be controlled to prevent trauma. Personal protective equipment such as safety glasses or face shields is recommended, particularly with aggressive individuals. Some handlers place a large syringe case or a similar apparatus over the beak as an additional safety measure for species with sharp-tipped bills.

Anesthetic techniques are similar to those used for other large avian species. To accommodate the large bill, anesthetic masks often need to be fabricated from plastic syringe cases, bottles, cones, obstetric gloves, or sheets of rubber. Induction and maintenance with gaseous anesthetics (isoflurane or sevoflurane) in oxygen at appropriate flow rates is most commonly used for anesthesia. Intubation is typically straightforward; however, it should be performed with utmost care to minimize trauma and resultant inflammation, as postintubation tracheal granulomatous obstruction has been reported in some species of Ciconiiformes.[48,64] Many of the Ciconiiformes species have a crista ventralis in the center of the glottis, which may make intubation a bit more challenging. Induction with an intravenous (IV) agent such as propofol (5–7 milligrams per kilogram [mg/kg] to effect) is also effective. Where gaseous anesthesia is not possible, a combination of intramuscular (IM) medetomidine (0.1 mg/kg), ketamine (5–10 mg/kg), and midazolam (0.1 mg/kg) has proven successful for immobilization in larger stork species and would likely work well in other Ciconiiformes species. While the bird is under anesthesia, monitoring of end tidal carbon dioxide is strongly recommended, as ventilation may be affected by patient positioning and significant dead space may exist in the long trachea and air sacs. Intermittent positive pressure ventilation during anesthesia is successful in reducing hypercapnea. During recovery from anesthesia, the bird should be held or semi-confined (e.g., in a padded crate) until it is capable of standing to prevent injury. It is best to avoid keeping the legs in one position for the entire procedure or surgery.

SURGERY (COMMON AND SPECIAL CONSIDERATIONS)

Traumatic injury, either self-inflicted or from intraspecies or interspecies aggression, is the most frequent cause for surgery encountered in a captive setting. Techniques used in other avian species are applicable. The novel use of hinged braces as an external support device for soft tissue joint injuries has been described in storks.[36] Beak prosthetics have also been used successfully. In northern climates, ischemic necrosis from frostbite may necessitate amputation when medical management is not successful. Necrosis of the cervical throat sac was documented in a marabou stork that was managed successfully with surgical resection and supportive care (Donna Todd, personal communication, 2011).

Postintubation tracheal obstruction has been reported in storks and often requires surgical management via tracheal resection and anastomosis or laser ablation.[48,64]

Multimodal analgesia is an important component of surgical management. Pharmacokinetic and clinical efficacy studies of analgesics have not been published for any Ciconiiformes species, so extrapolation is made from other avian species. Local anesthetics (lidocaine 1 mg/kg, bupivacaine 1 mg/kg), meloxicam (0.3–0.5 mg/kg, IM, once daily [SID]), and the opioid butorphanol (0.5–1.0 mg/kg, IM, every 4–6 hours [q4-6h]) have been used successfully by the authors of this chapter.

OTHER PHARMACEUTICALS

No published studies of pharmacokinetics or clinical efficacy exist for Ciconiiformes species. Extrapolation for drug dosages is based on published studies and experience with other avian species. Fenbendazole toxicity has been reported in marabou storks at a dosage of 60 mg/kg, so caution is advised when using this anthelmintic in Ciconiiformes.[6]

PHYSICAL EXAMINATION AND DIAGNOSTICS

A systematic approach to the physical examination should always be followed. Ciconiiformes may be safely physically restrained for the examination.

Specimen collection and handling are the same as in other avian species. Venipuncture may be accomplished from the jugular vein, the medial metatarsal vein, or the ulnar vein. As many storks will defecate and urinate on their legs to keep cool, it is important to clean the metatarsus prior to blood collection to avoid false elevations in uric acid.

Erythrocyte morphology and hematologic and serum biochemistry parameters have been studied in juveniles and adults of several Ciconiiformes species.[1,2,9,12,16,28,31,39,55,57,58,65] The hematocrit, the erythrocyte count, and the hemoglobin concentration increase from hatching to adulthood, and this is thought to be related to oxygen demands for flight.[2,55] Gender- and age-related alterations to serum biochemical values have been noted, especially in total protein, albumin, uric acid, cholesterol, and aspartate aminotransferase.[31,39] The interpretation of hematologic and serum biochemical values is similar to that in other avian species. Spoonbills and scarlet ibises have pink plasma, which should not be confused with hemolysis. Reference ranges for species held in captivity are available from the International Species Information System (www.isis.org).

DISEASE

General

Ciconiiformes species are not exquisitely sensitive to infectious disease, and many of the diseases reported are not unique to their taxon.

Infectious Disease

Infectious diseases reported in Ciconiiformes include Ciconiiformes hepadnaviruses in gray herons and white storks, viral hemorrhagic enteritis in storks (inclusion body disease), avian poxvirus, avian paramyxovirus, West Nile virus, eastern equine encephalitis, mycobacteriosis, chlamydiosis, salmonellosis, aspergillosis, and candidiasis.[20,23,32,33,41,44,45,50,53,71] Bumblefoot and several cases of vegetative endocarditis caused by gram-positive cocci were reported in Waldrapp ibises.[22] Salmonellosis has been the cause of clinical disease and mortality in a variety of Ciconiiformes rookeries and is a potential zoonosis, especially as increased development causes closer interactions between humans and wildlife.[41,53] *Campylobacter jejuni* isolated from several wild Ciconiiformes in the family Ardeidae has the potential to cause clinical disease and is a zoonosis (Table 13-1).[35]

Parasitic Diseases

Only a few parasites have been associated with disease in Ciconiiformes. *Eustrongylides ignotus* is most common in great blue herons (*Ardea herodius*), great egrets (*Casmerodius albus*), and snowy egrets (*Egretta thula*) but also occurs in a variety of Ciconiiformes. Two intermediate hosts are required for its transmission. Larvae perforate the ventriculus, with resultant hemorrhage and bacterial peritonitis that may progress to fibrous peritonitis with extensive adhesions.[60]

Heartworm infection with *Paronchocerca ciconarum* has been reported in saddle-billed, marabou, white, and white-necked storks, with pulmonary artery thrombosis and thickening and myocardial degeneration.[15] The trematode, *Chaunocephalus ferox* has been associated with granulomatous enteritis in white, black, black-necked, and Asian openbill storks.[27] *Mesaulus grandis* (trematode of intestine and coelomic cavity), *Phagicoloa longus* (trematode, intestine), *Pergosomum* spp. (trematode, gallbladder and liver), and *Paroncocerca ciconarum* (nematode, myocardial degeneration) have been found in various Ciconiiformes species.[20] Other significant helminth parasites include *Cathaemasia* spp. (esophageal flukes in maribou, white, and black storks), *Clinostomum complanalum* (trematode in oral cavity in several Ciconiiformes species) *Syncuaria* sp. (ventriculus nematode), and *Thelaszia* spp. (conjunctival sac nematode).[20,40,63] Although other nematodes and cestodes have been described, they are considered nonpathogenic.[47] Giardiasis has been reported in a white stork.[21] Hematozoa include *Haemoproteus crumenium, Haemoproteus brodkorbi,* and *Haemoproteus peircei*.[17,19] Numerous species of lice also have been described.[66] *Sarcocystis* sp. cysts have been found in the muscle of several Ciconiiformes species.[62] Visceral and subcutaneous acariasis caused by hypopi of *Hypodectes propus bulbuci* (mite) has been reported in the cattle egret and other Ciconiiformes species.[25]

Noninfectious Disease

Trauma is the most common noninfectious disease of Ciconiiformes in captivity. Musculoskeletal abnormalities in growing chicks, ingestion of foreign objects, and dermatologic issues such as pododermatitis caused by inappropriate substrates may be encountered.[26,69] Atherosclerosis has been reported in herons.[69]

Nutritional diseases include hypovitaminosis E, hypothiaminosis, and metabolic bone disease. Although typically a disease of captivity,

TABLE 13-1

Important Select Diseases

Disease	Etiology	Epizootiology	Clinical Signs	Diagnosis	Management
Viral hemorrhagic enteritis (Inclusion body disease)	Ciconid herpesvirus-1	Contact with infected birds or contaminated environment Fecal–oral route	Peracute to acute mortality; depression, anorexia, drooping wings, vomiting, hemorrhagic diarrhea; moderate leukocytosis, heteropenia, lymphocytosis, monocytosis	Hemorrhagic enteritis, especially ileum and proximal colon; hepatomegaly Intranuclear inclusion bodies in gastrointestinal tract, liver, spleen, reproductive tract, and lung Virus isolation; electron microscopy; PCR	Supportive therapy Isolation of infected individuals
West Nile virus	Flavivirus	Indirect transmission by arthropod vector (mosquito); possible direct fecal–oral transmission	Ataxia, weakness, tremors, abnormal head posture, sternal recumbency, acute mortality	Multifocal acute hemorrhages, nonsuppurative meningoencephalitis, myocarditis, splenitis, hepatitis, enteric lesions Serology, immunohistochemistry, in situ hybridization, electron microscopy	Consider vaccination in susceptible species
Equine encephalitides	Eastern equine encephalitis virus	Susceptible species include snowy egret, great egret, glossy ibis, roseate spoonbill, and cattle egret	None to anorexia, lethargy, drooping wings, ataxia, bloody discharge from mouth, death	Serology, viral isolation, electron microscopy	Insect control
Poxvirus infection	Avipoxvirus	Insect vector likely	Verrucous cutaneous pox lesions on legs, feet, beak, eyelids	Histologic features and electron microscopy	Insect control Treat supportively
Salmonellosis	*Salmonella typhimurium*	Direct contact, fecal oral, zoonotic concern	Emaciation, focal liver necrosis, and a caseonecrotic enteritis	Histology, culture	Supportive therapy
Fungal pneumonia	*Aspergillus fumigatus; Lichthiemia corymbifera; Rhizopus* sp.; opportunistic zygomycetes	Young chicks <3 weeks of age most susceptible	Respiratory signs; anorexia, weakness, acute mortality	Severe granulomatous pneumonia with fungal elements on histology Fungal culture, PCR	Supportive therapy Minimize stresses during growth

naturally occurring secondary nutritional hyperparathyroidism was described in the nestlings of two colonies of cattle egrets (*Bubulcus ibis*). Adults were feeding chicks exclusively insects low in calcium because of the depletions of small mammals in the area.[54] Steatitis is a common problem in Ciconiiformes species maintained in captivity or undergoing rehabilitation and occasionally in free-ranging birds.[52,69] Vitamin E deficiency is often the underlying cause associated with ingestion of rancid fish oils or high dietary levels of polyunsaturated fat. Large amounts of firm subcutaneous and coelomic fat comprising necrotic adipose tissues with infiltrates of heterophils and macrophages are often found.[49] One study has suggested that the cyanobacterial toxin microcystin could cause steatitis.[56]

Degenerative cardiac disease has been documented in saddle-bill, painted, and marabou storks.[7,34] Further investigation into heart disease in storks is ongoing.

Published reports of neoplasia in Ciconiiformes are rare. Successful treatment of a squamous cell carcinoma in a juvenile white stork has been described.[42] Other published cases of neoplasia include seminoma in a sacred ibis, osteosarcoma in boat-billed heron, retrobulbar teratoma in great blue heron, undifferentiated carcinoma attached to viscera in an Australian bittern, and chondrosarcoma on the nictitating membrane in a free-ranging great white heron.[38,61,69]

Toxicities

Owing to their aquatic carnivorous lifestyle, free-ranging Ciconiiformes species are at a higher risk for toxicities from environmental pollutants such as lead, mercury, and other heavy metals, arsenic, and organophosphates and carbamate pesticides. Such exposure may lead to disrupted bone metabolism in chicks or to alterations in adrenocortical stress responses or thyroid hormone status. The pathogenesis and treatment are similar to those in other avian species.[3,37,46,59,69] Sodium toxicity was reported in captive juvenile great blue herons fed a diet of herring in brine; clinical signs consisted of lethargy, dyspnea, regurgitation, anorexia, and postmortem lesions involving the kidneys.[5]

REPRODUCTION

In general, most Ciconiiformes species are socially monogamous, but many species are genetically promiscuous. Pair bonding is important in most species and may span a single season or multiple years. Each species of Ciconiiformes have elaborate behavioral courtship displays; exhibits should allow for these important breeding displays to occur.[13,14,43] Most are communal breeders, with some exceptions (bitterns, night herons, black storks, and hadada, spot-breasted, and oriental crested ibises). Breeding colonies commonly comprise mixed species. Ciconiiformes species range from solitary nesters that maintain large territories to semi-colonial species to highly colonial nesters. It is recommended that colonial species be maintained in species-appropriate groups to stimulate reproductive behaviors and nest building in conspecifics, and semi-colonial or solitary nesting storks should be maintained in pairs.[13,68]

Nest size tends to be large, so provision of appropriate platforms and nesting material (twigs, leaves, grasses, and straw) is important. Nests usually are built in trees (bitterns are the exception). The female constructs the nest from plant material, which is usually brought to the site by the male. Copulation often takes place in the nest itself. Artificial insemination has been used in some stork species. Clutch size for the various species ranges from two to five eggs and are incubated by both sexes. Many Ciconiiformes species will double clutch if the first eggs are removed for artificial incubation. The incubation period is dependent on the species but, in general, ranges from 29 to 35 days. Hatching is often asynchronous.[4,13,29,43,69]

Parental infanticide of smaller chicks, especially in larger clutches, has been reported in white storks, and black-necked storks and saddle-bill storks may become aggressive toward their chicks as they mature.[67]

PREVENTIVE MEDICINE

All birds should receive annual preventive health examinations, which should include complete physical examination, weighing, and assessment of blood parameters. Where indicated, additional diagnostics may include radiography and ultrasonographic evaluation. Fecal examinations are indicated annually or more frequently if parasite issues are identified.

REFERENCES

1. Aengwanich W, Tanomtong A, Pattanarungson R, et al: Blood cell characteristic, hematological and serum biochemistry values of Painted Stork (*Mycteria leucocephala*). J Sci Technol 24(3):473–479, 2002.
2. Alonso JC, Huecas V, Alonso JA, et al: Hematology and blood chemistry of adult white storks (*Ciconia ciconia*). Comp Biochem Physiol 98(3–4): 395–397, 1991.
3. Baos R, Blas J, Bortolitti GR, et al: Adrenocortical responses to stress and thyroid hormone status in free-living nestling white storks (*Ciconia ciconia*) exposed to heavy metal and arsenic contamination. Environ Health Perspect 114(10):1497–1501, 2006.
4. Barnhill RA, Weyer D, Young WF, et al: Breeding biology of jabiru (*Jabiru mycteria*) in Belize. Wilson Bull 117(2):142–153, 2005.
5. Bennet DC, Bowes VA, Hughers MR, et al: Suspected sodium toxicity in hand-reared great blue heron (*Ardea herodias*) chicks. Avian Dis 36:743–748, 1992.
6. Bonar CJ, Lewandowski AH, Schaul J: Suspected fenbendazole toxicity in 2 vulture species (*Gyps africanus*, *Torgus tracheliotus*) and marabou storks (*Leptoptilos crumeniferus*). J Avian Med Surg 17(1):16–19, 2003.
7. Bronson E, Wack A, Rosenthal S, et al: Cardiac disease in a saddle-billed stork (*Ephippiorhynchus senegalensis*). Proc Am Assoc Zoo Vet 52:2008.
8. Brouwer K, Jones ML, King CE, et al: Longevity and breeding records of storks Ciconiidae in captivity. Int Zoo Yearbook 31:131–139, 1992.
9. Chou SJ, Shieh YC, Yu1 CY: Hematologic and biochemistry values for black-faced spoonbills (*Platalea minor*) with and recovering from botulism. J Wildl Dis 44:781–784, 2008.
10. Clancy GP: The feeding behavior and diet of the black-necked stork *Ephippiorhynchus asiaticus australis* in northern New South Wales. Corella 36(1):17–23, 2011.
11. Clements JF, Schulenberg TS, Iliff MJ, et al: The eBird/Clements checklist of birds of the world: Version 6.7. 2012. <http://www.birds.cornell.edu/clementschecklist/downloadable-clements-checklist>: Accessed November 27, 2012.
12. Coke RL, West GD, Hoover JP: Hematology and plasma biochemistry of captive puna ibis (*Plegadis ridgewayi*). J Wildl Dis 40(1):141–144, 2004.
13. Coulter MC, Balzano ST, Johnson RE, et al: *Conservation and captive management of storks*, Athens, Greece, 1989, Proceedings of an international workshop.
14. Datta T, Pal BC: Polygyny in the Asian openbill (*Anastomus oscitans*). Auk 112(1):257–260, 1995.
15. Echols MS, Craig TM, Speer BL: Heartworm (*Paronchocerca ciconarum*) infection in 2 saddle-billed storks (*Ephippiorhynchus senegalensis*). J Avian Med Surg 14(1):42–47, 2000.
16. Dutton CJ, Allchurch AF, Cooper JE: Comparison of hematologic and biochemical reference ranges between captive populations of northern bald ibises (*Geronticus eremite*). J Wildl Dis 38(3):583–588, 2002.
17. Fedynich AM, Bryan AL, Harris MJ: Hematozoa in the endangered wood stork from Georgia. J Wildl Dis 34(1):165–167, 1998.
18. Fidget AL, Dierenfeld ES: Minerals and stork nutrition. In Fowler ME, Miller RE, editors: *Zoo and wild animal medicine, current therapy*, ed 6, St. Louis, MO, 2007, Saunders, pp 206–213.
19. Forrester DJ, Greiner EC, Bennet GF, et al: Avian haemoproteidae.7. A review of the haemoproteids of the family Ciconiidae (storks) and descriptions of *Haemoproteus brodkorbi* sp. nov. and *H. peircei* sp. nov. Can J Zool 55:1268–1274, 1977.
20. Fowler M: Storks and flamingos. In Fowler ME, editor: *Zoo and wild animal medicine*, ed 2, Philadelphia, PA, 1986, Saunders, pp 328–331.
21. Franssen FF, Hooimeijer J, Blankenstein B, et al: Giardiasis in a white stork in the Netherlands. J Wildl Dis 36(4):764–766, 2000.

22. Greenwood AG, Marshall J, Tinsley EGF: Vegetative endocarditis in a Waldrapp ibis. *Avian Pathol* 25:387–391, 1996.

23. Gómex-Villamandos JC, Hervás J, Salguero FJ, et al: Haemorrhagic enteritis associated with herpesvirus in storks. *Avian Pathol* 27:229–236, 1998.

24. Hancock JA, Kushan JA, Kahl MP: *Storks, ibises, and spoonbills of the world*, London, UK, 1992, Academic Press.

25. Hendrix CM, Kwapien RP, Porch JR: Visceral and subcutaneous acariasis caused by hypopi of *Hypodectes propus bulbuci* in the cattle egret. *J Wildl Dis* 23(4):693–697, 1987.

26. Henry PY, Wey G: Balança G: Rubber band ingestion by a rubbish dump dweller, the white stork (*Ciconia ciconia*). *Waterbirds* 34(4):504–508, 2011.

27. Höfle U, Krone O, Blanco JM, et al: *Chauocephalus ferox* in free-living white storks in Central Spain. *Avian Dis* 47(2):506–512, 2003.

28. Hollamby S, Afema-Azikuru J, Sikarskie JG, et al: Clinical pathology of nestling marabou storks in Uganda. *J Wildl Dis* 40(3):594–599, 2004.

29. Imanuddin AM: Breeding success and chick development of milky stork (*Mycteria cinera*) in Palua Rambut Wildlife Sanctuary. *Hayati* 10(2):76–80, 2003.

30. IUCN: *IUCN Red List of Threatened Species*. Version 2012.2. 2012. www.iucnredlist.org. Accessed November 27, 2012.

31. Jerzak L, Sparks TH, Kasprzak M, et al: Blood chemistry in white stork *Ciconia ciconia* chicks varies by sex and age. *Comp Biochem Physiol B* 156:144–147, 2010.

32. Kaleta EF, Kummerfeld N: Herpesvirus and Newcastle disease viruses in white storks (*Ciconia ciconia*). *Avian Pathol* 12(3):347–352, 1983.

33. Kaleta EF, Mikami T, Marschall HJ, et al: A new herpesvirus isolated from black storks (*Ciconia nigra*). *Avian Pathol* 9(3):301–310, 1980.

34. Kapustin N, Weldon AD, Teare JA, et al: Echocardiographic assessment in adult saddle-billed storks (*Ephippiorhynchus senegalensis*): Normal and abnormal findings. *Proc Am Assoc Zoo Vet* 227–228, 2010.

35. Keller JI, Shriver WG, Waldenstro J, et al: Prevalence of *Campylobacter* in wild birds of the mid-Atlantic region, USA. *J Wildl Dis* 47(3):750–754, 2011.

36. Klein PN, Cranfield MR, Wagner RA: The novel use of hinged braces as external support devices for soft tissue joint injuries in long-legged birds. *Proc Am Assoc Zoo Vet* 332–333, 1997.

37. Kwon YK, Wee SH, Kim JH: Pesticide poisoning events in wild birds in Korea from 1998 to 2002. *J Wildl Dis* 40(4):737–740, 2004.

38. Kubo M, Kobayashi K, Masegi T, et al: A case of chondrosarcoma in a free flying great egret. *J Wildl Dis* 43(3):542–544, 2007.

39. Lanzarot MP, Barahona MV, San Andrés MI, et al: Hematologic, protein electrophoresis, biochemistry and cholinesterase values of free-living black stork nestlings (*Ciconia nigra*). *J Wildl Dis* 41(2):379–386, 2005.

40. Liptovszky M, Majoros G, Perge E: *Cathaemasia hians* in a black stork (*Ciconia nigra*) in Hungary. *J Wildl Dis* 48(3):809–811, 2012.

41. Locke LN, Ohlendorf HM, Shillinger RB: Salmonellosis in a captive heron colony. *J Wildl Dis* 2(10):143–145, 1974.

42. Lopez-Beceiro AM, Pereira JL, Barreiro A, et al: Squamous cell carcinoma in an immature common stork (*Ciconia ciconia*). *J Zoo Wildl Med* 29(1):84–86, 1998.

43. Mace M, Ranger W, Lewins E, et al: Breeding and hand-rearing Storm's storks *Ciconia stormi* at the Zoological Society of San Diego. *Int Zoo Yearbook* 40:254–260, 2006.

44. Malkinson M, Banet C, Weisman Y, et al: Introduction of West Nile virus in the Middle East by migrating white storks. *Emerg Infect Dis* 8(4):392–397, 2002.

45. McLean RG, Crans WJ, Caccamise DF, et al: Experimental infection of wading birds with eastern equine encephalitis virus. *J Wildl Dis* 31(4):502–508, 1995.

46. Meharg AA, Pain DJ, Ellam RM, et al: Isotopic identification of the sources of lead contamination for white storks (*Ciconia ciconia*) in a marshland ecosystem (Doñana, S.W. Spain). *Sci Total Environ* 300:81–86, 2002.

47. Mellen JW, Dronen NO: Some digenetic trematodes from a wood ibis *Mycteria Americana*, including a new species of Ascocotyle. *Trans Am Microsc Soc* 106(3):269–272, 1987.

48. Miller M, Weber M, Mangold B, et al: Tracheal resection and anastomosis in storks. *Proc Annu Conf Assoc Avian Vet* 201–205, 2001.

49. Neagari Y, Arii S, Udagawa M, et al: Steatitis in egrets and herons from Japan. *J Wildl Dis* 47(1):49–55, 2011.

50. Olias P, Gruber AD, Winfried B, et al: Fungal pneumonia as a major cause of mortality in white stork (*Ciconia ciconia*) chicks. *Avian Dis* 54(1):94098, 2010.

51. Ong HKA, Chinna K, Khoo SK, et al: Morphometric sex determination of milky and painted storks in captivity. *Zoo Biol* 31:219–228, 2012.

52. Pavlat J, Beach H, Platter-Rieger M, et al: Steatitis in herons and egrets in Southern California. In *Proceedings: International wildlife rehabilitation council 27th annual conference*, Oakland, California, 2004, International Wildlife Rehabilitation Council, pp 1–6.

53. Phalen DN, Drew ML, Simpson B, et al: *Salmonella enterica* subsp. *enterica* in cattle egret (*Bubulcus ibis*) chicks from central Texas: prevalence, serotypes, pathogenicity, and epizootic potential. *J Wildl Dis* 46:379–389, 2010.

54. Phalen DN, Drew ML, Contreras C, et al: Natural occurring nutritional hyperparathyroidism in cattle egrets (*Bubulcus ibis*) from central Texas. *J Wildl Dis* 41(2):401–415, 2005.

55. Puerta ML, Muñoz Pulido R, Huecas V, et al: Hematology and blood chemistry of chicks of white and black storks (*Ciconia ciconia* and *Ciconia nigra*). *Comp Biochem Physiol* 94A(2):201–204, 1989.

56. Rattner AB, McGowan CP: Potential hazards of environmental contaminants to avifauna residing in the Chesapeake Bay estuary. *Waterbirds* 30(Special Publication 1):63–81, 2007.

57. Salakij C, Slakij J, Narkkong NA, et al: Hematology, morphology, cytochemistry and ultrastructure of blood cells in painted storks (*Mycteria leucocephalus*). *Kasetsart J (Nat Sci)* 37:506–513, 2003.

58. Salakij C, Slakij J, Rochanapat N, et al: Hematology, morphology, and cytochemistry of blood cells in lesser adjutant (*Leptoptilos javanicus*) and greater adjutant (*Leptoptilos dubius*). *Kasetsart J (Nat Sci)* 38:400–408, 2004.

59. Smits JE, Bortolitte GR, Baos R, et al: Disrupted bone metabolism in contaminant-exposed white storks (*Ciconia ciconia*) in southwestern Spain. *Environ Pollut* 145:538–544, 2007.

60. Spalding MG, Forrester DJ: Pathogenesis of *Eustrongylides ignotus* (Nematoda: Dioctophymatoidea) in Ciconiiformes. *J Wildl Dis* 29(2):250–260, 1993.

61. Spalding MG, Woodard JC: Chondrosarcoma in a wild great white heron from southern Florida. *J Wildl Dis* 28(1):151–153, 1992.

62. Spalding MG, Atkinson CT, Carleton RE: *Sarcocystis* sp. in wading birds (Ciconiiformes) from Florida. *J Wildl Dis* 30(1):29–35, 1994.

63. Stoskopf MK, Patton S, Bueding E: Treatment of two marabou storks (*Leptoptilos crumeniferus*) infested with the esophageal fluke (*Cathaemasia spectabilis*). *J Zoo Wildl Med* 13(3):51–55, 1982.

64. Sykes JM, Neiffer D, Terrell S, et al: Post-intubation tracheal obstruction in birds—22 cases from two institutions. *Proc Am Assoc Zoo Vet* 95–96, 2011.

65. Szabó Z, Beregi A, Vajdovich P, et al: Hematological and plasma biochemistry values in white storks (*Ciconia ciconia*). *J Zoo Wildl Med* 41(1):17–21, 2010.

66. Thompson GB: A list of the type-hosts of the Mallophaga and the lice described from them: Order Ciconiiformes. *Ann Mag Nat Hist* 11(5):297–308, 1940.

67. Tortosa FS, Redono T: Motives for parental infanticide in white storks *Ciconia ciconia*. *Ornis Scand* 23(2):185–189, 1992.

68. Urfi AJ, Kalam A: Sexual dimorphism and mating pattern in the painted stork (*Mycteria leucocephala*). *Waterbirds* 29(4):489–496, 2006.

69. Waters M: Ciconiiformes (herons, ibises, spoonbills, storks). In Fowler ME, Miller RE, editors: *Zoo and wild animal medicine*, ed 5, St. Louis, MO, 2003, Saunders, pp 122–129.

70. Weckhauf R, Handschuh M: A method for identifying the sex of lesser adjutant storks *Leptoptilos javanicus* using digital photographs. *Cambod J Nat Hist* 1:23–28, 2011.

71. Zangger N, Müller M: Endemic poxvirus infection in white storks (*Ciconia ciconia*) and black storks (*Ciconia nigra*) in Switzerland. *Schweiz Arch Tierheilkd* 132(3):135–138, 1990.

CHAPTER 14

Phoenicopteriformes

Fabia S. Wyss and Christian J. Wenker

BIOLOGY

Flamingos are popular zoo birds because of their elegance and brilliant coloration. They are closely related to grebes (Podicipediformes)[15] and currently divided into six different species, belonging to three genera (*Phoenicopterus, Phoenicoparrus, Phoeniconaias*) within the family Phoenicopteridae (Table 14-1). These birds live in large colonies and are adapted to extreme habitats, for example, lakes with high salinity and alkalinity where no other vertebrates could survive. Flamingos are among the longest-lived bird species, and captive individuals in zoos may reach a lifespan of up to 70 years.[45] All flamingo species are highly nomadic when searching for feeding and nesting sites, but movement patterns vary individually, temporally, and spatially among subpopulations and reflect adaptation to varying water levels and food availability.[5,39]

UNIQUE ANATOMY AND PHYSIOLOGY

The plumage color is caused by carotenoids (canthaxanthin, astaxanthin, and phoenicoxanthin) found in algae, crustaceans, and mollusks. After 4 to 6 years, greater flamingos display their adult plumage and turn from gray-brown to pink, which is a sign of sexual maturity.[20] Preen oils containing carotenoids are excreted by the uropygial gland and are applied as additional cosmetic coloration of the feathers.[3] The flamingo's neck is proportionally the longest in birds and has 17 cervical vertebrae.[11] Flamingos regulate their body temperature by resting on one or both legs,[6] in different water depths, or both.

Sex determination may be performed using polymerase chain reaction (PCR) of feather bulbs by isolating deoxyribonucleic acid (DNA) of the *CHD-W* and *CHD-Z* genes (females) or the *CHD-Z* genes only (males).[7] Tarsometatarsal length rather than simple size is a tool for sex determination in Caribbean, greater, and Chilean flamingos older than 1.5 years, with males having larger tarsometatarsi.[46]

Flamingos are divided into two groups according to their diets: (1) the Phoenicopterus species, which possess a shallow bill and feed primarily on arthropods and mollusks, and (2) the deep-billed Phoenicoparrus and Phoeniconaias species, which feed on algae and diatoms. Flamingos are filter-feeders and hold their bill upside down when feeding (Figure 14-1). Food-rich mud or water is pumped and released by tongue movements into and out of the oral cavity. Internal horn lamellae localized at the upper and lower bills trap the food items. Spines on the tongue act as a comb to clean the lamellae. Flamingos "walk-feed," moving forward with the bill in the substrate, or "stamp-feed," treading on the spot to stir up food.[7] Excessive salt is secreted by nasal salt glands.[1]

Unlike other filter-feeding birds, flamingos are able to see the tip of their bill in their binocular field, probably to be able to accurately place the bill when feeding chicks.[26] At the same time, the chicks orient themselves toward the black bill tip, which is present in all species.

SPECIAL HOUSING REQUIREMENTS

Several water ponds of different depths should be offered to stimulate foraging. A marsh area with reeds (cut short) offers additional enrichment with natural plankton. Flamingos were observed to sleep in full sun during the day; different resting sites and microhabitats in the enclosure, exposed to the sun at different times of day, stimulate the birds to move. Exciting experiences made while moving to different places of the enclosure enhances binding of the flock and breeding pairs and stimulates synchronization of mating.[44] A 3.5 square meters (m²) feeding pool, 10 to 15 centimeters (cm) deep, has been recommended for flamingos.[43] However, if floating pelleted food is used, this may be dispersed on all water surfaces, thus expanding the feeding range and feeding time (see Nutrition). A salt water pond as a disinfectant foot bath[14] is no longer recommended because it was observed that it increased already existing foot lesions.[49] Concrete, vinyl or rubber lining, and grass were all shown to be inadequate flooring substrates for the flamingo feet.[30] Covering the concrete floor with 10-cm fine granular sand led to a significant decrease in foot lesions in indoor and outdoor enclosures.[53] Any temperature below 15°C has been identified as a risk factor for pododermatitis.[30] Although indoor housing also increases the risk for pododermatitis,[30] a heated house with a sand substrate should be available for flamingos in temperate or cold climate zones. The house should be adjacent to the outdoor enclosure so that the birds may be kept inside during cold nights and allowed to go out during the warmer times of the day.[43] The flamingo outside enclosure should be secured (e.g., using electric wire) against predators.

Feather clipping, pinioning and feather follicle extirpation are acceptable methods to prevent the birds from flying.[23] Pinioned male flamingos have shown difficulties in maintaining their balance during mating.[43] Feather follicle extirpation has been successfully performed in many zoo birds, including flamingos.[23] Feather follicle atrophy by laser, successfully used in pelicans and cranes, may provide a less traumatic and faster means for flight restraint in birds.[8] Vegetation planted in and around the enclosure blocks any runways that flamingos could use to rise into the air. Nevertheless, flamingos are still able to take off when a gusty wind occurs.[43] At the Copenhagen Zoo, a 1100 m² aviary (approximately 50 × 40 m area; height 10 m) was opened in 2011 for flamingos, ibises, and spoonbills. However, the flamingos do not fly in there.[10] If locations for resting, feeding, drinking, and breeding are close, flamingos seem to prefer walking between sites.

Banding flamingos with rings that may be read easily from long distances helps gain knowledge about captive and wild flamingo colonies (Figure 14-2).[9,43] Color rings (for small captive colonies) or rings with a binary coding system or letter combinations (bigger captive and wild colonies) may be used (see website http://www.birdband.com).

REPRODUCTION

Group courtship display (raising necks, looking around, calling and simultaneous head flagging, walking close together, ritualized wing salute, etc.) is performed by both sexes and is assumed to stimulate the synchronization of breeding. Warm mild rain fall in spring may stimulate greater flamingos to walk to the nesting site. Nests are dispersed irregularly but may be built closely together (2.8 nests per m² for greater flamingos) in the wild as well as in captivity.[38,47] Flamingos usually lay one egg, incubated by both sexes over 28 to 30 days.[11] Captive flamingos are susceptible to unusual disturbances, and eggs are easily damaged or abandoned.[47] Chicks hatch with their eyes open and with pink or red legs and bills that turn black within the first week. Flamingo chicks are fed by their parents with an initially dark red and later pale red to yellow high energy "crop milk," containing canthaxanthin and white and red blood cells, produced

TABLE 14-1
Biologic Information about Flamingos

Scientific Name	Phoenicopterus Ruber Roseus	Phoenicopterus Ruber Ruber	Phoenicopterus Chilensis	Phoeniconaias Minor	Phoenicoparrus Andinus	Phoenicoparrus Jamesi
Common name	Greater flamingo	American/Caribbean flamingo	Chilean flamingo	Lesser flamingo	Andean flamingo	James's/Puna flamingo
Body weight	2–4 kg	2.2–2.8 kg		Approx. 2 kg		
Distribution[11]	Africa, Mediterranean, southwestern Asia	Caribbean, northern South America, Mexico, Galapagos	Southwestern South America; up to 4500 meters a.s.l.	East, West, and South Africa, South Asia	Peru, Bolivia, Chile, Argentina (high Andean plateaus and lower)	Peru, Bolivia, Chile, Argentina (high Andean plateaus and lower)
Red list cat. / Wild pop. size[19]	Least concern 500–700 x10^3	Least concern	Near threatened 300 * 10^3	Near threatened 2–3 * 10^6	Vulnerable 40 * 10^3	Near threatened 106 * 10^3

A.s.l, Above sea level.
Figure 1 courtesy Zoo Basel; Figure 2 courtesy Dace Vitola; Figures 3, 5, and 6 coursey Omar Rocha; and Figure 4 courtesy Fabia Wyss.

by glands in the upper digestive tract.[25] Fledging occurs within 2 to 3 months of age; at that time, the filter feeding apparatus is developed.[11,47]

Breeding behavior has been successfully stimulated in small flamingo flocks in several institutions by the use of artificial nests, loud speakers and mirrors around the breeding site to "increase" the size of the group, and dummy eggs and application of "mild warm rain" with a sprinkler.[50]

FEEDING

Commercially prepared diets with all essential nutrients, including canthaxanthin, are available, but self-mixed diets are used by some institutions. Floating pellets remain on the water surface for some hours and provide excellent enrichment, and waste is minimized. Floating extrudate products with sprayed-on oil should be avoided because they were found to create an oil film on the water surface, and subsequently, flamingos were reported to have difficulties cleaning their plumage. Duckweed may be offered as a supplement, as it contains a broad spectrum of natural carotenoids. In multispecies exhibits, care should be taken to ensure that flamingos do not feed on other large food items, as this may lead to bill impaction and subsequent improper feeding, anorexia, and emaciation.[16]

Canthaxanthin, besides being responsible for the coloration of the feathers, is primarily a potent antioxidant. It accumulates in egg yolk and is assumed to be beneficial for the protection of the embryonic chick.[48] A breeder formulation with elevated protein content should be used during the breeding and hatching season, that is, for 6 to 8 months per year.

RESTRAINT AND HANDLING

All capture operations should be planned well in advance; enough staff as well as a small round or oval pen should be available prior to capture (Figure 14-3). During the roundup to direct the birds into the pen, it must be ensured that the flamingos stay together and do not run. Flamingos should be grasped one by one. The wings should be kept closed near the flamingo's body, and the legs should not be pulled toward the body. The body is held near the handler's hip. A light blindfold, with the bill and nares exposed, may be used to calm the bird. Release should be as quiet as possible. Placing one hand at the animal's sternum helps it to find its balance. Close inspection of the animals in a release pen is recommended to avoid the stressful recapture of the whole group in the exhibit if one animal is not well.

ANESTHESIA AND SURGERY

Isoflurane administered through an inhalation mask is the anesthesia of choice. Premedication is desirable, and a drug combination with ketamine, medetomidine, and butorphanol is currently being investigated.[21] Animals are handled carefully to avoid capture-related stress and hyperthermia, and legs should not be pulled toward the body to maintain optimal perfusion. Essential monitoring includes respiratory rate, heart rate, and body temperature, as well as pulse oximetry, electrocardiography, and ultrasonic Doppler probes.

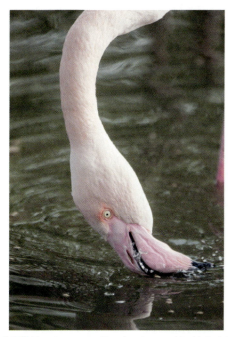

FIGURE 14-1 Flamingos are filter-feeders and hold their bill upside down when feeding. They are able to create a vortex effect.

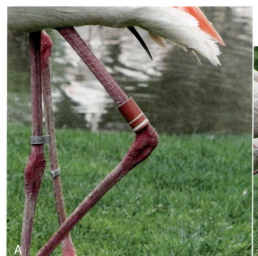
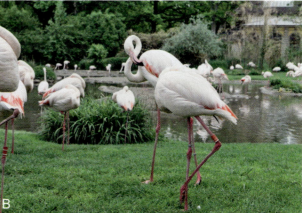

FIGURE 14-2 A, Large colored plastic rings provide better visibility from a distance than rings with numbers. This example shows a binary system with four positions from top to bottom: No line = 0, thin line = 1, thick line = 2. So this flamingo is identified as 0 0 1 2 (*red left*). **B,** Same animal and picture from a larger distance. Lines on ring are still visible.

Recovery is prolonged in anesthetized flamingos that become hypothermic, and fatalities may result. Intubation is difficult because of the limited opening of the bill and because of the back of the tongue blocking the passage of an adequately sized endotracheal tube.

Surgical techniques in flamingos are similar to those in other birds. Pinioning, feather follicle extirpation, laparoscopy, fracture repair, and debridement of pododermatitis are the most common surgical procedures.

PHYSICAL EXAMINATION AND DIAGNOSTICS

In general, the diagnostic workup in flamingos corresponds to that in other birds. During physical examination, the highly specialized bill should be checked for any impacted material that prevents accurate filtration; bill impaction may be visible from a distance because of retrograde displacement of the tongue, which creates gular enlargement.[16] No closed septum exists between the nares; therefore, when looking through one nare during lateral inspection, the other nare can be seen. The plantar feet should be examined thoroughly because of the high prevalence of pododermatitis in captive animals. The type and the extent of foot lesions should be determined (Figure 14-4).[29,51] Blood is preferably collected from the jugular, the medial metatarsal or the ulnar vein. Pressure should be applied on the puncture site long enough to control bleeding and to prevent hematoma formation, especially in juveniles. Blood smears are screened for hemoparasites. Hematologic and biochemical reference values have been published for several flamingo species and ages (Table 14-2, 14-3, and 14-4). Pink-orange plasma and serum coloration is physiologically caused by high xanthoid and carotenoid contents.[12] Packed cell volume (PCV) increases with age and may indicate increased requirements of oxygen during growth. Neither the nutritional status nor the body condition of chicks was related to PCV.[4] Cholesterol plasma levels may be used to predict the body condition of flamingo chicks as they are negatively correlated.[2]

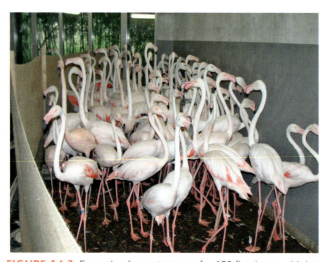

FIGURE 14-3 Example of a capture pen for 120 flamingos with jute curtain.

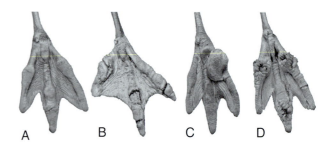

FIGURE 14-4 Classification of foot lesions in captive flamingos. A, Hyperkeratosis. B, Fissures. C, Nodular lesions. D, Papillomatous growths. (Courtesy of American Association of Zoo Veterinarians.)

TABLE 14-2

Reference Range for Hematologic Parameters in Flamingos

Parameter (mean ± SD)	Caribbean[28] Juvenile/ Adult	Chilean[36] Adult	Greater[56] Juvenile Captive/Wild	Lesser[17] Adult
	n = 13–28*	n = 32	n = 16–27*	n = 10
RBC (×10⁶/μL)	1.48 ± 0.19	2.84 ± 0.51	—	2.7 ± 0.1
Hemoglobin (g/dL)	13.4 ± 2.2	16.9 ± 1.9	12.2 ± 1.0	16.8 ± 1.6
PCV (%)	47.9 ± 5.1	46 ± 5	40.6 ± 4.2	50 ± 3
MCV (fL)	326.7 ± 47.1	163.9 ± 26.3	—	188 ± 6
MCH (pg)	91.6 ± 17.2	55.5 ± 7.6	—	62.0 ± 5.4
MCHC (g/dL)	28.1 ± 3.9	34.6 ± 1.9	—	33.0 ± 2.5
WBC (×10³/μL)	8.71 ± 3.67	6.65 ± 3.28	11.7 ± 4.2	6.0 ± 2.0
Heterophils (×10³/μL; %)	3.57 ± 3.17; 39.86 ± 20.98	2.57 ± 1.39; 26.7 ± 7.2	5.26 ±2.39; 46.0 ±13.8	4.63 ± 1.85; 77 ± 8
Lymphocytes (×10³/μL; %)	4.51 ± 2.82; 52.21 ± 22.35	4.91 ± 2.04; 67.4 ± 7.3	4.86 ± 2.34; 41.4 ±12.3	1.21 ± 0.56; 21 ± 7
Monocytes (×10³/μL; %)	0.39 ± 0.28; 5.07 ± 4.15	0.06 ± 0.07; 0.59 ± 0.59	0.40 ± 0.34; 3.3 ± 1.9	0.10 ± 0.15; 1.4 ± 2.1
Eosinophils (×10³/μL; %)	0.08 ± 0.20; 0.86 ± 2.03	0.55 ± 0.50; 5.76 ± 3.20	0.90 ± 0.72; 7.3 ± 4.6	0; 0
Basophils (×10³/μL; %)	0.16 ± 0.22; 2.00 ± 2.65	0.01 ± 0.02; 0.18 ± 0.39	0.26 ± 0.23; 2.1 ± 1.6	0.06 ± 0.08; 1.2 ± 1.6

*n varies between parameters; range indicating minimal and maximal number of animals sampled.

fL, femtoliter; *g/dL*, grams per deciliter; *μL*, microliter; *MCH*, mean corpuscular hemoglobin; *MCHC*, mean corpuscular hemoglobin concentration; *MCV*, mean corpuscular volume; *PCV*, packed cell volume; *pg*, picogram; *RBC*, red blood cell; *WBC*, white blood cell.

TABLE 14-3

Reference Range for Plasma Biochemical Parameters in Flamingos

Parameter (mean ± SD)	Caribbean[28] Juvenile/adult	Chilean[36] Adult	Greater[56] Juvenile Captive/Wild	Andean[32] Juvenile, Wild
	n = 13–28*	n = 32	n = 16–27*	n = 14
Total protein (g/dL)	4.06 ± 0.45	5.3 ± 0.5	3.44 ± 0.33	2.9 ± 0.4
Albumin (g/dL)	—	2.77 ± 0.44	1.43 ± 0.16	1.4 ± 0.3
Globulin (g/dL)	—	1.57 ± 0.46	2.02 ± 0.22	1.5 ± 0.2
Chloride (mEq/L)	116.9 ± 3.3	103.5 ± 10.3	119.5 ± 5.9	—
Sodium (mEq/L)	149.8 ± 5.	161 ± 7	156.4 ± 3.9	—
Calcium (mg/dL)	13.37 ± 4.29	12.4 ±2.0	10.77 ± 0.60	14.8 ± 3.2
Phosphorus (mg/dL)	3.93 ± 1.44	36.22 ± 5.57	6.03 ± 0.62	5.2 ± 1.5
Potassium (mEq/L)	2.84 ± 0.50	3.1 ± 0.6	2.82 ± 0.46	—
Magnesium (mEq/L)	—	2.2 ± 0.6	1.44 ± 0.15	—
Glucose (mg/dL)	197.8 ± 46.2	202.9 ± 40.4	152.7 ± 36.1	—
Uric acid (mg/dL)	12.92 ± 4.69	6.00 ± 2.60	5.26 ± 2.72	—
Urea (mg/dL)	—	1.45 ± 0.70	0.65 ± 0.32	—
Creatinine (mg/dL)	—	0.50 ± 0.10	0.20 ± 0.01	0.11 ± 0.06
Cholesterol (mg/dL)	—	320.0 ± 88.8	286.6 ± 56.7	461 ± 76
Triglycerides (mg/dL)	—	247.0 ± 79.7	116.8 ± 79.6	—
ALP/AP (Units/L)	166.0 ± 128.8	48.1 ± 15.9	796 ± 120.7†	—
AST (Units/L)	273.0 ± 103.4	74.7 ± 29.6	222.2 ± 61.8	269 ± 63
CK (Units/L)	1058 ± 1096	541 ± 345	2254 ± 1013	—
LDH (Units/L)	267.5 ± 452.8	238 ± 126	606.1 ± 164.6	—
ALT (Units/L)	—	18.2 ± 5.7	16.4 ± 5.6	48 ± 26

*n varies between parameters, range indicating minimal and maximal number of animals sampled.
†n = 5 for ALP/AP.
ALP/AP, Alkaline phosphatase; *ALT*, alanine aminotransferase; *AST*, aspartate aminotransferase; *CK*, creatine kinase; *g/dL*, gram per deciliter; *LDH*, lactate dehydrogenase; *mEq/L*, milliequivalents per liter; *mg/dL*, milligram per deciliter; Units/L, units per liter.

TABLE 14-4

Reference Ranges for Plasma Vitamin and Mineral Levels in Flamingos

	Greater[54] Juvenile, Captive	Greater[54] Juvenile, Wild
Vitamin A (mg/dL)	0.06 ± 0.01	0.06 ± 0.01
Vitamin E (mg/dL)	1.00 ± 0.32	0.74 ± 0.22
Copper (μg/dL)	40.9 ± 16.5	32.5 ± 2.4
Zinc (μg/dL)	164.3 ± 55.3	177.9 ± 23.7

mg/dL, Milligram per deciliter; *μg/dL*, microgram per deciliter.

Radiography, ultrasonography, laparoscopy, or endoscopy may be performed as in other birds.

THERAPEUTICS AND INTENSIVE CARE

Pharmacologic studies have not been performed in flamingos, and thus drug dosages have to be extrapolated from other bird species. Recumbent flamingos are placed in a sling for recovery (Figure 14-5).[11] Food, water, and heat should be provided. Tube feeding may be necessary, although flamingos are able to fast for several days. To

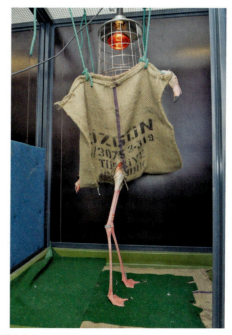

FIGURE 14-5 Recumbent flamingo placed in a sling for recovery. This procedure requires constant monitoring.

reduce stress in hospitalized animals, it is beneficial to provide a partner animal or to use mirrors and loudspeakers to mimic a flamingo colony. Preventive antifungal therapy for aspergillosis should be considered. Regular exercises and physiotherapy on the ground or in the water are used for rehabilitation.

DISEASES

Pododermatitis

Pododermatitis is probably the most important health problem in captive flamingos. It is a multifactorial disease, and colder regions, temperatures below 15°C, and indoor housing were shown to influence the extent of this disease.[30] Hyperkeratosis, fissures, and nodular lesions develop at the plantar surface of the feet of juvenile greater flamingos as early as at 2 to 3 months of age. Papillomatous growths, a fourth type of lesion, were not seen before 5 months of age and appeared significantly less often in flamingos younger than 1 year than in all other age groups.[51] The prevalence of nodular lesions with ulceration was increased in greater flamingos weighing more than 4 kg, but none of the other lesions was affected by body weight. The number of foot lesions was much smaller in birds housed in enclosures with water ponds that had natural substrate (e.g., sand) compared with those in exhibits with pools that had a concrete floor.[51] A 10-cm cover of fine granular sand with a grain size less than 1 mm in diameter improved foot lesions markedly.[53] Nutrition may play a role in the onset of pododermatitis: low zinc levels were suspected to weaken the cornified epidermis and facilitate the onset of the disease.[54] No evidence for the presence of papillomavirus, previously discussed as etiologic agent,[42] was found when histology, PCR, immunohistochemistry, and electron microscopy were performed.[52] A novel bacterium, *Arsenicicoccus dermatophilus*, was found to invade the cornified epidermis of juvenile flamingos' feet that macroscopically appeared unaffected.[14] This organism is suspected to be responsible for a primary inflammation, which causes the different types of foot lesions if the factors described above are suboptimal.[52]

Capture Myopathy

Long-legged waders such as flamingos are prone to capture myopathy.[35] Cases in Chilean, Caribbean, and greater flamingos were mostly fatal despite intensive treatment.[18] Animals usually die because of massive myoglobinuric tubulonephrosis and kidney failure, but a peracute shock syndrome has been reported in other animals[35] and was probably the cause of death in two Caribbean flamingos.[18] One Caribbean flamingo survived and was released back into the group after 12 days of treatment. The following measures are recommended to treat capture myopathy in flamingos: placing affected birds in a sling to prevent further muscle damage; supporting the kidney function by providing fluids; reducing inflammation and pain using nonsteroidal anti-inflammatory drugs (NSAIDs) or opioids; providing benzodiazepines for muscle relaxation and to reduce muscle spasms (midazolam, diazepam), sodium bicarbonate to reduce metabolic acidemia, and vitamin E or selenium as an antioxidant; and providing supportive treatment (force feeding, warmth) and physical therapy. Since capture myopathy is difficult to treat, prevention is very important.

Trauma

Trauma such as fractures, luxations, and soft tissue injury was diagnosed in 28% of all necropsy reports of greater flamingos from the Zoo Basel from 1972 to 2012 (n = 124); among these cases, 35% were killed by predators, mostly red foxes. Other predators may include badgers, coyotes, raccoons, or dogs. Leg fractures are common in startled, captured, or restrained flamingos. Fractures of the tibiotarsal and tarsometatarsal bone occur most often.[11] Interdigital webs and digits are prone to be affected by frostbite. Clinical signs include lameness and darkening and eventual necrosis of the affected tissue.

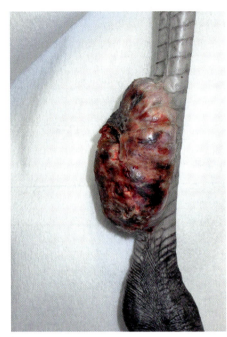

FIGURE 14-6 A slightly bleeding and rapidly growing tumor-like nodule of the skin, proximal to the tibiotarsal–tarsometatarsal joint of a juvenile flamingo, was histologically confirmed as avipox infection after surgical excision.

Infectious Disease

West Nile virus (WNV) has been isolated from a dead Chilean flamingo, following cases of human encephalitis in the United States.[41] The vaccination of adult flamingos and 1-month-old flamingo chicks with a killed WNV vaccine (intended for horses) failed to produce a demonstrable virus-neutralizing activity or antibody response.[33,40] Avipox infections are characterized by slightly bleeding and rapidly growing skin tumors (Figure 14-6). Following surgical removal, virostatic therapy with famciclovir was successfully performed in two cases.[34] Massive die-offs in lesser flamingos were reported from Lake Bogoria and Lake Nakuru, Kenya, and an infection with *Mycobacterium avium* serovar I was suspected.[22] Like other birds, flamingos are susceptible to aspergillosis. In the Zoo Basel, aspergillosis was diagnosed in postmortem examinations in 7 of 124 animals, including three animals that had been intensively treated for capture myopathy; therefore, preventive systemic antifungal drugs (e.g., itraconazole) are recommended for flamingos in stressful disease conditions or in an intensive care situation. Parasites, including *hemoproteus* sp. and *plasmodium* sp.,[13] cestodes,[37] nematodes, flagellates, lice, and mites (all from the Zoo Basel survey) were reported in individual flamingos.

Noninfectious Disease

Atherosclerosis was associated with several unexplained collapses or deaths during stressful situations and was diagnosed in 14% of the necropsy reports from greater flamingos in the Zoo Basel from 1972 to 2012 (n = 124). Affected flamingos were between 14 and 50 years old. Amyloidosis of various organs (6%) and gout (renal or visceral, 4%) were other, noninfectious findings. Limb deformities were reported in various flamingo species;[55] in the greater flamingos of the Zoo Basel, this was a cause for euthanasia or an incidental finding in 9% of the birds. Surgical correction and various banding techniques could be successful treatment options.[55]

Toxicities

Another differential diagnosis of the massive die-offs of lesser flamingos at Lake Bogora and Lake Nakuru, Kenya, as well as at Lake Manyara, Tanzania, was the intoxication with cyanobacterial toxins, as indicated by the presence of cyanobacteria and hepatotoxins (microcystin -LR, -RR, -LF, -YR) and neurotoxins (anatoxin-a) in the stomach contents, and the observation of neurologic signs in the birds after being at the lake.[24,31] Lead poisoning by the ingestion of lead shots was suspected to be the cause of death of wild greater flamingos with severe emaciation, inability to fly, and bile-stained diarrhea.[27]

TRANSPORT

For short transfers or air transports, flamingos may be placed in boxes one by one, just large enough to enable the birds to stand and lift their heads. For longer road transfers, flamingos should be kept in groups in narrow transport pens with padded walls and griped floors, for example, in a horse transporter with flexible compartments. Transport during hot days should be avoided.

ACKNOWLEDGMENTS

We thank the following persons for their valuable contributions to this chapter: Adelheid Studer-Thiersch, Friederike von Houwald, Bruno Gardelli, Arnaud Béchet, Anne-Sophie Deville, Madeleine Leutenegger, Beatrice Steck, Stefan Hoby and Marcus Clauss.

REFERENCES

1. Almansour MI: Anatomy, histology and histochemistry of the salt glands of the greater flamingo *Phoenicopterus ruber roseus* (Aves, Phoenicopteridae). *Saudi J Biol Sci* 14:145–152, 2007.
2. Amat JA, Hortas F, Arroyo GM, et al: Interannual variations in feeding frequencies and food quality of greater flamingo chicks (*Phoenicopterus roseus*): Evidence from plasma chemistry and effects on body condition. *Comp Biochem Physiol* 147:569–576, 2007.
3. Amat JA, Rendón MA, Garrido-Fernández J, et al: Greater flamingos (*Phoenicopterus roseus*) use uropygial secretions as make-up. *Behav Ecol Sociobiol* 65:665–673, 2011.
4. Amat JA, Rendón MA, Ramírez JM, et al: Hematocrit is related to age but not to nutritional condition in greater flamingo chicks. *Eur J Wildl Res* 55:179–182, 2009.
5. Amat JA, Rendón MA, Rendon-Martos M, et al: Ranging behaviour of greater flamingos during the breeding and post-breeding periods: Linking connectivity to biological processes. *Biol Conserv* 125:183–192, 2005.
6. Anderson MJ, Williams SA: Why do flamingos stand on one leg? *Zoo Biol* 29:365–374, 2010.
7. Balkiz Ö, Dano S, Barbraud C, et al: Sexing greater flamingo chicks from feather bulb DNA. *Waterbirds* 30:450–453, 2007.
8. Baumgartner K, Kempf H, Will H, et al: Feather follicle atrophying by laser—an improvement of exstirpation for animal welfare reasons. *Proc Int Conf Dis Zoo Wild Anim* 25–28, 2012.
9. Béchet A, Johnson AR: Anthropogenic and environmental determinants of greater flamingo *Phoenicopterus roseus* breeding numbers and productivity in the Camargue (Rhone delta, southern France). *Ibis* 150:69–79, 2008.
10. Bertelsen MF, personal communication, 2012.
11. Brown C, King CE, Mossbarger S, et al: *Flamingo taxon advisory group husbandry manual*, 2002.
12. Burgdorf-Moisuk A, Wack R, Ziccardi M, et al: Validation of lactate measurement in American flamingo (*Phoenicopterus ruber*) plasma and correlation with duration and difficulty of capture. *J Zoo Wildl Med* 43:450–458, 2012.
13. Ferrell ST, Snowden K, Marlar AB, et al: Fatal hemoprotozoal infections in multiple avian species in a zoological park. *J Zoo Wildl Med* 38:309–316, 2007.
14. Gobeli S, Thomann A, Wyss F, et al: *Arsenicicoccus dermatophilus* sp. nov., a hypha-forming bacterium isolated from the skin of greater flamingos (*Phoenicopterus roseus*) with pododermatitis. *Int J Syst Evol Microbiol* 63:4046–4051, 2013.
15. Hackett SJ, Kimball RT, Reddy S, et al: A phylogenomic study of birds reveals their revolutionary history. *Science* 320:1763–1768, 2008.
16. Hammer S, Jensen S, Borjal R, et al: Bill impaction in a group of captive Caribbean flamingos (*Phoenicopterus ruber ruber*). *J Zoo Wildl Med* 38:465–470, 2007.
17. Hawkey C, Hart MG, Samour HJ: Normal and clinical haematology of greater and lesser flamingos (*Phoenicopterus roseus* and *Phoeniconaias minor*). *Avian Pathol* 14:537–541, 1985.
18. Hebel C, personal communication, 2012.
19. International Union for Conservation of Nature: *Red list of threatened species:* Version 2012.2, Switzerland, 2012, IUCN.
20. Johnson AR, Cezilly F, Boy V: Plumage development and maturation in the greater flamingo (*Phoenicopterus ruber roseus*). *Ardea* 81:25–34, 1993.
21. Kempf H, personal communication, 2012.
22. Kock ND, Kock RA, Wambua J, et al: *Mycobacterium avium*-related epizootic in free ranging lesser flamingos in Kenya. *J Wildl Dis* 35:297–300, 1999.
23. Krawinkel P: Feather follicle extirpation: Operative techniques to prevent zoo birds from flying. In Miller RE, Fowler ME, editors: *Zoo and wild animal medicine*, vol 7, St.Louis, MO, 2012, Saunders, pp 275–280.
24. Krienitz L, Ballot A, Kotut K, et al: Contribution of hot spring cyanobacteria to the mysterious deaths of lesser flamingos at Lake Bogoria, Kenya. *FEMS Microbiol Ecol* 43:141–148, 2003.
25. Lang EM: Flamingos raise their young on a liquid containing blood. *Experientia* 19:532, 1963.
26. Martin GR, Jarett N, Tovey P, et al: Visual fields in flamingos: Chick-feeding versus filter feeding. *Naturwissenschaften* 92:351–354, 2005.
27. Mateo R, Carles Dolz J, Aquilar Serrano JM, et al: An epizootic of lead poisoning in Greater flamingos (Phoenicopterus ruber roseus) in Spain. *J Wildl Dis* 33:131–134, 1997.
28. Merritt EL, Fritz CL, Ramsay EC: Hematologic and serum biochemical values in captive American flamingos (*Phoenicopterus ruber ruber*). *J Avian Med Surg* 10:163–167, 1996.
29. Nielsen AMV, Nielsen SS, King CE, et al: Classification and prevalence of foot lesions in captive flamingos (Phoenicopteridae). *J Zoo Wildl Med* 41:44–49, 2010.
30. Nielsen AMV, Nielsen SS, King CE, et al: Risk factors for foot lesions in captive flamingos (Phoenicopteridae). *J Zoo Wildl Med* 43:744–749, 2012.
31. Nonga HE, Sandvik M, Miles CO, et al: Possible involvement of microcystins in the unexplained mass mortalities of lesser flamingos (*Phoeniconaias minor Geoffroy*) at Lake Manyara in Tanzania. *Hydrobiologia* 678:167–178, 2011.
32. Norambuena MC, Parada M: Serum biochemistry in Andean flamingos (*Phoenicoparrus andinus*): Natural versus artificial diet. *J Zoo Wildl Med* 36:434–439, 2005.
33. Nusbaum KE, Wright JC, Johnston WB, et al: Absence of humoral response in flamingos and red-tailed hawks to experimental vaccination with a killed West Nile virus vaccine. *Avian Dis* 47:750–752, 2003.
34. Ochs A, Aue A, Hentschke J, et al: Successful surgical and virustatic therapy of tumorous avipoxvirus infection in an Andean (*Phoenicoparrus andinus*) and James flamingo (*Phoenicoparrus jamesi*) at Berlin Zoo. *Verhandlungsbericht Erkrankungen bei Zootieren* 42:86–91, 2005.
35. Paterson J: Capture myopathy. In West G, Heard D, Caulkett N, editors: *Zoo animal and wildlife immobilization and anesthesia*, Ames, IA, 2007, Blackwell Publishing, pp 115–121.
36. Peinado VI, Polo FJ, Viscor G, et al: Haematology and blood chemistry values for several flamingo species. *Avian Pathol* 21:55–64, 1992.
37. Poynton SL, Mukherjee G, Strandber JD: Cestodiasis with intestinal diverticulosis in a lesser flamingo (*Phoeniconaias minor*). *J Zoo Wildl Med* 31:96–99, 2000.
38. Samraoui B, Ouldjaoui A, Boulkhssaïm M, et al: The first recorded reproduction of the greater flamingo *Phoenicopterus roseus* in Algeria: Behavioural and ecological aspects. *Ostrich: J Afr Ornithol* 77:153–159, 2006.
39. Sanz-Aguilar A, Béchet A, Germain C, et al: To leave or not to leave: Survival trade-offs between different migratory strategies in the greater flamingo. *J Anim Ecol* 81:1171–1182, 2012.
40. Siegal-Willott JL, Carpenter JW, Glaser AL: Lack of detectable antibody response in greater flamingos (*Phoenicopterus ruber ruber*) after vaccination against West Nile virus with a killed equine vaccine. *J Avian Med Surg* 20:89–93, 2006.

41. Steele KE, Linn MJ, Schoepp RJ, et al: Pathology of fatal West Nile virus infections in native and exotic birds during the 1999 outbreak in New York City, New York. *Vet Pathol* 37:208–224, 2000.

42. Studer-Thiersch A, Von Houwald F, Heldstab A: *Some remarks on foot infections in flamingos*, Heidelberg, 2005, EAZA Bird TAGs Meeting.

43. Studer-Thiersch A: Behavioural considerations in flamingo enclosure design, Heidelberg, 2005, EAZA Bird TAGs Meeting.

44. Studer-Thiersch A: Behavioural demands on a new exhibit for greater flamingos at the Basel Zoo, Switzerland. *Waterbirds* 23(spec. publ. 1):185–192, 2005.

45. Studer-Thiersch A: Longevity and value of veteran flamingos in zoological collections, Flamingo. *Bulletin of the IUCN-SSC/Wetlands International FLAMINGO SPECIALIST GROUP*, 2008.

46. Studer-Thiersch A: Tarsus length as an indication of sex in the flamingo genus Phoenicopterus. *Int Zoo Yearbook* 24:240–243, 1986.

47. Studer-Thiersch A: What 19 years of observation on captive greater flamingos suggest about adaptation to breeding under irregular conditions. *Waterbirds* 23:150–159, 2000.

48. Surai PF: The antioxidant properties of canthaxanthin and its potential effects in the poultry eggs and on embryonic development of the chick. Part 2. *World's Poultry Sci J* 68:717–726, 2012.

49. von Houwald F, personal communication, 2012.

50. White D, Kenward M, Forsyth S, personal communication, 2012.

51. Wyss F, Wenker C, Hoby S, et al: Factors influencing the onset and progression of pododermatitis in captive flamingos (Phoenicopteridae). *Schweizer Archiv für Tierheilkunde* 155:497–503, 2013.

52. Wyss F, Wenker C, Hoby S, et al: Pododermatitis in captive flamingos (Phoenicopteridae)—a comprehensive study with detailed histological investigation. *2011 Proc Ann AAZV Conf* 92, 2011.

53. Wyss F, Wenker C, Hoby S, et al: The effect of finely granular sand on pododermatitis of captive greater flamingos (*Phoenicopterus roseus*). *Anim Welf* 23:57–61, 2014.

54. Wyss F, Wolf P, Wenker C, et al: Comparison of vitamin A and E, copper and zinc plasma levels in free-ranging and captive greater flamingos (*Phoenicopterus roseus*) and their relation to pododermatitis. *J Anim Physiol Anim Nutr*, in review, 2014.

55. Zollinger TJ, Backues KA, Burgos-Rodrigez AG: Correction of angular limb deformity in two subspecies of flamingo (*Phoenicopterus ruber*) utilizing a transphyseal bridging technique. *J Zoo Wildl Med* 36:689–697, 2005.

56. Zoo Basel, unpublished data: Reference ranges from captive greater flamingos from Zoo Basel and from wild greater flamingos from the Camargue, France.

CHAPTER **15**

Charadriiformes

Stephanie McCain

GENERAL BIOLOGY

Charadriiformes are a diverse group of birds with three suborders: Alcae, Charadrii, and Lari.[6] The suborder Alcae includes the auks, with 22 species. The suborder Charadrii includes 203 species in 12 families, including avocets, ibisbills, jacanas, oystercatchers, plovers, sandpipers, snipes, stilts, thick-knees, and others. The suborder Lari contains 105 species and includes gulls, terns, skimmers, and skuas. Charadrii live, breed, and forage along the water's edge, whereas Alcae and Lari are more aquatic. Charadrii are birds of the open, except the woodcock, which inhabits edges of wet, wooded areas, and solitary and spotted sandpipers may be found at heavily forested ponds and lakes, from sea level to high in the mountains. Shorebirds migrate over long distances; the red knot migrates from the Arctic region to Tierra del Fuego. Most shorebirds are gregarious, and mixed flocks of several species are frequently seen.

UNIQUE ANATOMY

A wide variation in appearance exists among the birds in this order. Alcids are generally small- to medium-sized birds with stocky bodies and short wings and tail. Charadrii tend to be long-legged and have a remarkable variety of bill shapes and sizes, from the long, down-curved bill of the curlew to the short, stubby plover's bill. The Lari suborder comprises species ranging in size from small to large and slender- to heavy-bodied, long-winged birds. The skimmers have a unique bill structure, with a very narrow and long lower bill compared with the upper bill. The crop and the gizzard are often simple and reduced.

SPECIAL HOUSING REQUIREMENTS

Consideration must be given to land, water, and air space for these birds, and requirements will vary by species. Various substrates have been used successfully. Pools should be easy to clean and sized appropriately for the species and number of birds. Air quality may be important in preventing respiratory fungal infection,[8,9] and exhibit design should consider open-air exhibits or those with proper ventilation and facility for purification. Quarantine and hospitalization should take place in appropriate-sized enclosures that allow for inclusion of a pool. A pool should be large enough for all birds housed in the room to enter the water all at once and should be located away from the entrance so that the birds feel safe in the pool when a staff member enters the room. A sandy shore or soft soil is recommended, as it allows normal feeding behavior. Adequate privacy and hiding places should be provided.

FEEDING

Marine diets typically consist of fish or invertebrates. Captive diets may consist of these items or may also include commercial diets such as those prepared for birds of prey or flamingos. Following proper fish handling and storage guidelines is essential. Most shorebirds have a carnivorous nutritional feeding strategy referred to as *fauni- vora*. Faunivora is the digestive ability to separate digestible soft tissues from relatively indigestible components in prey items such as insects and invertebrates.[14] The gizzard in these shorebirds is adapt- able, with a large proventriculus for protein breakdown.[14] Depending on the species of shorebird, the diet may consist of marine worms, fly larva, beetles, crustaceans, mollusks, small fish, seeds, and occa- sionally berries.

RESTRAINT AND HANDLING

Manual restraint is appropriate for most Charadriiformes species. If possible, the target individual should be restricted to a small area rather than caught in a large enclosure. The smaller the area and the fewer the birds in the area, the easier it is to catch the targeted bird. A net may be used to catch quick birds. A light towel or gloves may be helpful for restraint, particularly in alcids. If necessary, the pool should be drained or dropped. Alcids should be restrained by using one hand to secure the head and the other to secure the wings and by holding the bird against the body. In larger charadrii, the wings should be secured by holding the body tucked under one arm to help prevent causing any damage to the bird. A finger should be placed between the bird's legs for better control and to ensure that the legs do not rub together. The head should be restrained with the other hand. Care should be taken with the beak, as it may cause injury to the handler; however, covering of the nares should be avoided. In some cases, a second person may be helpful to restrain the head. In the case of small charadrii, the bird may be held upright against the handler's body with one hand to secure the wings and one hand to secure the beak (Figure 15-1). In even smaller species such as plovers, the restrainer may hold the bird in one hand with the back of the bird against the palm of the hand and the head between the index and middle fingers.

The most common anesthetic agents used in Charadriiformes are isoflurane and sevoflurane. These may be administered via a face mask after manual restraint. Face masks may be fabricated from empty syringe cases with part of a disposable glove placed over the end to better fit long-beaked birds. Intubation should be performed when control of the airway is desired, as in prolonged procedures or if the bird is not ventilating well on its own. Breath holding may be seen in diving species.

Anesthetic monitoring is similar to that in other birds. Use of a thermometer, electrocardiography, Doppler, pulse oximetry,

capnography, and blood gas analysis may all be useful. Birds should be restrained during recovery and not allowed to recover in a crate, as they tend to flap as they recover and may injure themselves. The same restraint methods should be used, as described above, making sure that keel movement is not restricted.

SURGERY

The most common surgical procedures include fracture repair, treat- ment of pododermatitis, and pinioning for flight restriction. The long legs of many Charadriiformes species are susceptible to trauma, especially during restraint. Treatment of pododermatitis is similar to that used in other avian species. The main methods of restricting flight include pinioning chicks, regular wing trimming, and the use of covered enclosures. Pinioning is more invasive, but regular clip- ping, which is the alternative, requires frequent restraint, which may result in injury. The pros and cons should be discussed at each institution. (Also see Chapter 65.)

OTHER PHARMACEUTICALS

Pharmacologic data are lacking in Charadriiformes, and dosages for most drugs are extrapolated from other avian species. Because of the susceptibility of alcids to aspergillosis, many institutions prophylacti- cally treat these birds with antifungals (e.g., itraconazole) beginning a few days prior to shipment.

Endoparasites may be treated with pyrantel, fenbendazole, or ivermectin, as appropriate. Capillaria is a relatively common parasitic disease of Charadriiformes and may be difficult to get rid of. Infesta- tion with ectoparasites may be treated with ivermectin.

PHYSICAL EXAMINATION AND DIAGNOSTICS

Physical examination is easily completed during manual restraint. Blood samples may be collected under manual restraint or general anesthesia. The jugular vein, ulnar vein, and metatarsal vein are all commonly used sites. Care must be taken to provide adequate hemo- stasis when using the ulnar or metatarsal vein, as these sites are prone to hemorrhage for a longer period compared with the jugular vein. A wrap may be applied to the leg for a brief period, if necessary. Reference values for hematologic and biochemical parameters of selected species are listed in Tables 15-1 and 15-2.[12]

DISEASES

Infectious Diseases

Bacterial infections may be primary or secondary. *Salmonella* spp., *Erysipelothrix* spp., *Campylobacter* spp., *Chlamydophila* spp., and *Yer- sinia* spp. have been reported in Charadriiformes and have zoonotic potential.[2] *Mycoplasma* spp. are also occasionally encountered. *Myco- plasma* spp. have been isolated from stone curlews, with most birds having no associated pathologic findings.[23] *Mycobacterium avium* infection is uncommon but should be considered with any radio- graphic evidence of bony lesions, particularly when other diagnostics support an infectious cause.[2] Laughing gulls are considered highly susceptible to avian mycobacteriosis.[11] Wounds and pododermatitis lesions may become infected with a variety of bacteria, which may lead to osteomyelitis. *Klebsiella pneumoniae* often is implicated in cases of respiratory tract disease in captive Charadriiformes and was implicated in mortality of black stilt chicks.[21]

Avian influenza is not rare in Charadriiformes. Typically, it causes an inapparent or subclinical infection. A mortality event occurred in wild common terns in South Africa in 1961, but this is not typical.[10] In shorebirds, 10 of the 15 hemagglutination type and 8 of the 9 neuraminidase type have been identified, and many of the combina- tions are unique to Charadriiformes. The H9 and H13 types pre- dominate. The avian influenza type H5N1 has been identified in shorebirds.

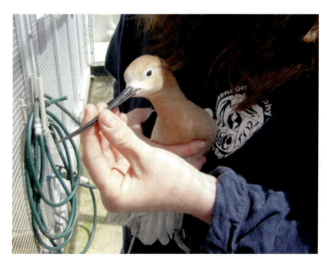

FIGURE 15-1 Proper restraint of smaller Charadriiformes species such as plovers. The restrainer may hold the bird in one hand, with the back of the bird against the palm of the hand and the head between the index and middle fingers.

TABLE 15-1

Reference Intervals for Hematological Parameters of Selected Species.[12]

Parameter	Tufted puffin (*Fratercula cirrhata*) (*N*)	Black-necked stilt (*Himantopus mexicanus*) (*N*)	Cape thick-knee (*Burhinus capensis*) (*N*)	Inca tern (*Larosterna inca*) (*N*)	Masked lapwing (*Vanellus miles*) (*N*)
Leukocytes (×10³/µL)	1.57–18.37 (111)	0.68–11.69 (59)	4.37–27.53 (65)	1.97–21.17 (275)	1.03–14.36 (72)
Hematocrit (%)	34.7–58.8 (118)	37.5–63.6 (68)	39.3–54.4 (66)	40.3–58.6 (285)	31.3–55.5 (70)
MCHC (g/dL)				23.9–40.0 (74)	
Heterophils (×10³/µL)	1.06–10.67 (108)	0.00–6.61 (59)	1.46–19.14 (65)	0.67–8.91 (270)	0.42–8.23 (71)
Lymphocytes (×10³/µL)	0.15–8.05 (110)	0.00–6.12 (59)	0.50–10.52 (65)	0.54–12.10 (275)	0.19–7.51 (70)
Monocytes (×10³/µL)	0–0.79 (71)	0–0.62 (43)	0–1.68 (58)	0.04–1.34 (242)	0–325 (50)
Eosinophils (×10³/µL)		0–0.86 (45)	0–2.93 (55)	0.02–0.47 (183)	0–1027 (52)
Basophils (×10³/µL)	0–0.99 (59)	0–0.43 (44)	0–1.05 (48)	0.06–2.15 (670)	0–531 (48)

MCH, Mean corpuscular hemoglobin; *MCHC,* mean corpuscular hemoglobin concentration; *MCV,* mean corpuscular volume.
From Teare JA, ed: 2013, "Tuffed Puffin; Black-necked Stilt; Cape Thick Knee; Inca Tern; Masked Lapwig;_No_selection_by_gender__All_ages_combined_Conventional American Units and Values__2013_CD.html" in ISIS Physiological Reference Intervals for Captive Wildlife: A CD-ROM Resource., International Species Information System, Bloomington, MN.

TABLE 15-2

Reference Intervals for Serum Biochemistry Parameters of Selected Species.[12]

Parameter	Tufted puffin (*Fratercula cirrhata*) (*N*)	Black-necked stilt (*Himantopus mexicanus*) (*N*)	Cape thick-knee (*Burhinus capensis*) (*N*)	Inca tern (*Larosterna inca*) (*N*)	Masked lapwing (*Vanellus miles*) (*N*)
Glucose (mg/dL)	239–471 (102)	156–367 (54)	147–420 (64)	192–448 (241)	197–415 (69)
Blood Urea Nitrogen (mg/dL)	1–5 (48)			1–10 (103)	
Creatinine (mg/dL)	0.0–0.5 (44)		0.0–0.7 (29)	0.1–1.1 (116)	
Uric Acid (mg/dL)	3.5–27.3 (103)	0.0–13.8 (52)	1.5–19.6 (64)	2.6–25.0 (239)	1.4–20.8 (71)
Calcium (mg/dL)	8.4–11.7 (103)	7.0–10.9 (52)	7.8–10.9 (61)	7.5–11.1 (220)	6.4–11.5 (68)
Phosphorous (mg/dL)	0.0–6.2 (56)	0.0–6.6 (41)	0.0–6.4 (49)	0.4–6.7 (191)	0.0–7.0 (67)
Sodium (mEq/L)	140–176 (53)	137–175 (33)	143–163 (58)	139–166 (194)	143–167 (53)
Potassium (mEq/L)	0.5–3.9 (52)	0.0–8.9 (31)	0.3–3.9 (55)	1.0–6.8 (191)	0.0–6.9 (52)
Chloride (mEq/L)	108–127 (43)		108–126 (43)	98–127 (166)	112–132 (39)
Cholesterol (mg/dL)	144–583 (92)	106–395 (39)	146–429 (39)	204–462 (178)	113–304 (50)
Triglycerides (mg/dL)				19–74 (42)	
Total Protein (g/dL)	2.9–5.7 (114)	2.3–4.7 (52)	2.4–5.0 (61)	2.6–5.2 (235)	2.2–4.6 (70)
Albumin (g/dL)	0.9–2.9 (87)	0.5–2.0 (36)	0.5–2.2 (50)	0.7–2.2 (184)	0.0–2.8 (58)
Globulin (g/dL)	0.3–3.7 (87)	1.1–3.3 (37)	0.8–3.8 (50)	0.5–3.4 (193)	0.2–3.6 (58)
AST (IU/L)	65–331 (102)	51–336 (52)	84–605 (62)	78–412 (219)	131–422 (67)
ALT (IU/L)	6–79 (41)		0–150 (30)	8–66 (135)	
Total bilirubin (mg/dL)	0.0–0.7 (37)		0.0–0.7 (33)	0.0–1.3 (130)	
Amylase (U/L)				209–1417 (64)	
ALP (IU/L)	0–60 (29)	0–413 (37)	4–59 (35)	64–410 (163)	0–118 (38)
LDH (IU/L)	0–1011 (37)		0–4260 (30)	114–782 (121)	0–2209 (27)
CPK (IU/L)	145–1431 (96)	0–1157 (47)	0–796 (50)	72–720 (190)	218–2318 (66)

AST, Aspartate aminotransferase; *ALT,* alanine aminotransferase; *ALP,* alkaline phoshatase; *LDH,* lactate dehydrogenase; *CPK,* creatine phosphokinase.
From Teare JA, ed: 2013, "Tuffed Puffin; Black-necked Stilt; Cape Thick Knee; Inca Tern; Masked Lapwig;_No_selection_by_gender__All_ages_combined_Conventional American Units and Values__2013_CD.html" in ISIS Physiological Reference Intervals for Captive Wildlife: A CD-ROM Resource., International Species Information System, Bloomington, MN.

Paramyxovirus type 1 has been isolated from tufted puffins,[24] and Newcastle disease virus and infectious bursal disease virus have been detected serologically in wild Charadriiformes.[2] The significance of these diseases is unknown. A mortality event has been associated with a reovirus in American woodcock,[7] and avian pox has been diagnosed in a royal tern,[13] sanderlings,[15] and stone curlews.[16] Puffinosis is a serious viral disease of unknown cause.[20] It is associated with annual mortality in Manx shearwaters (*Puffinus puffinus*) and is thought to be spread by the trombiculid mite (*Neotrombicula autumnalis*).[22]

Aspergillosis is not uncommon in captive Charadriiformes, although it is rare in free-ranging populations. *Aspergillus fumigates* is the most common causative agent. Stress and subsequent immunosuppression likely play a role in the pathogenesis of the disease in birds in captivity. The fungus is generally acquired through the respiratory tract, causing lesions in the air sacs, lungs, and even the central nervous system and eyes. Significant changes with animal management (e.g., newly introduced birds and exhibit construction), and inherent social or physiologic stressors such as breeding, molting, and interspecies competition for territory and food, are major factors that enhance the birds' susceptibility to fungal disease. Auks undergo annual molt of flight feathers, and this period may be associated with reduced appetite and increased susceptibility to disease, including aspergillosis.[22] Poor air turnover, excessive humidity, and certain types of substrates may increase fungal growth and sporulation within the exhibit. Diagnosis and treatment of aspergillosis are discussed elsewhere.[4,5,19]

Parasitic Diseases

A variety of endoparasites and ectoparasites have been seen in Charadriiformes.[17,18,24] The most common reports include cestodes and capillaria.[2] Cestodes are more common in wild-caught birds than in the captive born because of the lack of a suitable intermediate host. Capillaria has a direct life cycle and is easily transmitted between birds. Several species of ticks have been identified on wild birds and, although are not considered significant themselves, may carry hemoparasites and viruses.[17,20,24] *Cyclocoelum* sp. trematodes have been seen in shorebirds and may be associated with respiratory infection, airway obstruction, and acute death. Lice do not generally affect feather quality; however, they may cause pruritus.

Noninfectious Diseases

The most common noninfectious diseases in captive Charadriiformes include trauma, pododermatitis, and circumferential foreign body entanglement of the digits.

Trauma, either from accidents or from interspecies aggression, is not uncommon. Treatment of fractures or ligament repair should follow standard avian techniques and must allow the bird to be functional. Some instances may require limiting access to water. In cases of beak trauma, it is important to restore the functionality of the beak. Birds may require nutritional support during treatment or repair.

Pododermatitis may occur in nearly all Charadriiformes species and may be seen at any age. Although a number of predisposing factors such as stress and nutrition may play a role in the occurrence of pododermatitis, other factors such as substrate quality, character, and cleanliness seem to predominate in the development of clinical disease. Prevention is key to management. Sand substrate has been used successfully and should be cleaned of debris and feces at least daily. Sand depth must be adequate to ensure proper drainage. Pine shavings should be used with caution, as they have been associated with pododermatitis in shorebirds. Adequate space for exercise is important in prevention as well.[3] Treatment of pododermatitis depends on the severity of the lesion and may include anti-inflammatories, antibiotics, bandaging, or surgical intervention.

Foreign objects such as thread, hair, and other stringlike material may wrap around the digits and cause avascular necrosis. If identified quickly, damage may be minimized; however, the need for partial amputation is not uncommon. Walk-through exhibits should be monitored closely to prevent problems caused by foreign objects.

Metabolic bone disease has been seen in American avocets and black-winged stilts. Scissor bill and curly toe may result from inappropriate incubation and are seen in avocets and stilts.[2] Corrective trimming may be attempted to realign the bill, although some deviation may persist. It is important to ensure adequate nutritional intake during this time. Curly toe may often be corrected with splints and appropriate substrate.

Neoplasms have not been commonly reported. A report of a suspected teratoma in a black-headed gull has been published.[1]

Chicks are susceptible to such problems as yolk sac infection or retention, sepsis, dehydration, hypothermia, weakness, splayed leg, constipation, trauma, poor feeding reflex or appetite, and poor weight gain. Early recognition and treatment are often necessary to prevent long-term complications or mortality. Thermoregulatory, hydration, and nutritional support of chicks are all critical.

Toxicities

Conditions caused by environmental contaminants such as pesticides, heavy metals, industrial chemicals, and petroleum products are common in free-ranging shorebirds but are not typically seen in captive settings.

REPRODUCTION

Most shorebird species are monogamous, at least for a particular season. Black oystercatchers, long-billed dowitchers, marbled godwits, and long-billed curlews are thought to be strictly monogamous. Most nests are simple scrapes on bare earth or in short vegetation. Egg clutches usually contain two to four mottled, speckled eggs. The eggs are pear shaped so that they pack snugly into the nests and may be easily incubated. The background color ranges from cream or gray to pale green or brown. Development of the embryo is rapid; eggs hatch in 3 to 4 weeks after fertilization. Time to hatching may be as short as 17 days in the smaller species or as long as 30 days in larger species. Most shorebirds incubate the eggs for 22 to 24 days. Hatchlings of most species are precocial, being able to run about and feed themselves soon after birth. Most species leave the nest within 24 hours after hatching

Most alcid species breed in colonies on islands and cliffs, and they are usually monogamous through their entire breeding life. Most reach sexual maturity around 4 to 5 years of age. They have low reproductive rates, usually producing a single egg, although *Cepphus* guillemots and *Synthliboramphus* murrelets usually lay two eggs. The incubation period ranges from 27 to 29 days in *Alle* to 41 to 46 days in puffins.[6] Most alcids are semi-precocial and are fed by both parents.

PREVENTIVE MEDICINE

Routine health inspections by a veterinarian are recommended, at least annually, and should include a complete physical examination, including body weight, blood collection for complete blood cell count, and biochemical panel, protein electrophoresis, and radiography. Fecal parasite screening should be performed twice yearly. It may be appropriate to take a representative group sample when a number of birds are housed together.

No specific vaccinations are recommended at this time, although Charadriiformes species have been shown to be competent reservoirs for West Nile virus, so vaccination may have to be considered.[25]

ACKNOWLEDGMENTS

The author acknowledges Dr. Mike Murray for his assistance with this chapter.

REFERENCES

1. Baker JR, Chandler DJ: Suspected teratoma in a black headed gull (*Larus ridibundus*). *Vet Rec* 18:60, 1981.
2. Ball RL: Charadriiformes (gulls, shorebirds). In Fowler ME, Miller RE, editors: *Zoo and wild animal medicine*, ed 5, Philadelphia, PA, 2003, Saunders.
3. Chang Reissig E, Tompkins DM, Maloney RF, et al: Pododermatitis in captive-reared black stilts (*Himantopus novaezelandiae*). *J Zoo Wildl Med* 42:408–413, 2011.
4. Cray C, Watson T, Rodriguez M, et al: Application of galactomannan analysis and protein electrophoresis in the diagnosis of aspergillosis in avian species. *J Zoo Wildl Med* 40:64–70, 2009.
5. Cray C: Diagnosis of aspergillosis in avian species. In Fowler ME, Miller RE, editors: *Zoo and wild animal medicine*, ed 7, Philadelphia, PA, 2012, Saunders.
6. Del Hoyo J, Elliot A, Sargatal J: *Handbook of the birds of the world, hoatzin to auks*, ed 3, Barcelona, Spain, 1996, Lynx Edicions.
7. Docherty DE, Converse KA, Hansen WR, et al: American woodcock (*Scolopax minor*) mortality associated with a reovirus. *Avian Dis* 38:899–904, 1994.
8. Dykstra M: A comparison of sampling methods for airborne fungal spores during an outbreak of aspergillosis in the forest aviary of the North Carolina Zoological Park. *J Zoo Wildl Med* 28:454–463, 1997.
9. Faucette TG, Loomis M, Reininger K, et al: A three-year study of viable airborne fungi in the North Carolina Zoological Park R.J.R. Nabisco Rocky Coast Alcid Exhibit. *J Zoo Wildl Med* 30:44–53, 1999.
10. Friend M, Franson JC, editors: *Field manual of wildlife diseases: general field procedures and diseases of birds*, Athens, Georgia, 1999, U.S. Geological Survey.
11. Hejlicek K, Treml F: Comparison of the pathogenesis and epizoologic importance of avian mycobacteriosis in various types of domestic and free living syntropic birds. *Vet Med* 40:187–194, 1995.
12. International Species Information System (ISIS): *Physiological data reference values*, Apple Valley, MN, 1999, International Species Information System.
13. Jacobson ER, Raphael BL, Nguyen HT, et al: Avian pox infection, aspergillosis, and renal trematodiasis in a royal tern. *J Wildl Dis* 16:627, 1980.
14. Klasing KC: *Comparative avian nutrition*, Cambridge, U.K., 1998, Cambridge University Press.
15. Kreuder CA, Irizarry-Rovira AR, Janovitz EB, et al: Avian pox in sanderlings from Florida. *J Wildl Dis* 35:582–585, 1999.
16. Lierz M, Bergmann V, Isa G, et al: Avipoxvirus infection in a collection of captive stone curlews (*Burhinus oedicnemus*). *J Avian Med Surg* 21:50–55, 2007.
17. Muzaffar SB, Jones IL: Parasites and diseases of the auks (Alcidae) of the world and their ecology—a review. *Marine Ornithol* 32:121–146, 2004.
18. Muzzafar SB: Helminths of murrelets (Alcidae: *Uria* spp.): Markers of ecological change in the marine environment. *J Wildl Dis* 45:672–683, 2009.
19. Oglesbee BL: Mycotic diseases. In Altman RB, Clubb SL, Dorresein GM, et al, editors: *Avian medicine and surgery*, Philadelphia, PA, 1997, Saunders.
20. Pokras MA: Clinical management and biomedicine of sea birds. In Rosskopf WJ, Woerrpel RW, editors: *Diseases of cage and aviary birds*, ed 3, Baltimore, MD, 1996, Williams and Wilkins.
21. Reed CEM, Sancha SE, Fraser I: Growth and mortality of black stilt or kaki *Himantopus novaezelandiae* chicks at the Department of Conservation, Twizel. *Int Zoo Yearbook* 37:340–345, 2000.
22. Robinson I: Seabirds. In Tully T, Lawtin MPC, Dorrestein GM, editors: *Avian medicine*, Woburn, MA, 2000, Butterworth-Heinemann.
23. Schmidt V, Spergser J, Cramer K: Mycoplasmas isolated from stone curlews (*Burhinus oedicnemus*) used in falconry in the United Arab Emirates. *J Zoo Wildl Med* 40:316–320, 2009.
24. Stoskopf MK, Kennedy-Stoskopf S: Aquatic birds. In Fowler ME, Miller RE, editors: *Zoo and wild animal medicine*, ed 2, Philadelphia, PA, 1986, Saunders.
25. Travis D: West Nile virus in birds and mammals. In Fowler ME, Miller RE, editors: *Zoo and wild animal medicine*, ed 6, Philadelphia, PA, 2008, Saunders.

CHAPTER **16**

Anseriformes

Kay A. Backues

TAXONOMY AND BIOLOGY

Until recently, the order Anseriformes ("waterfowl,") has contained two families: (1) Anatidae, which includes the familiar ducks, geese, and swans and (2) Anhimidae, which includes the three species of very "un-duck-like" screamers native to South America. Recently, the Australian magpie goose, *Anseranas semipalmata* has been elevated to its own unique familial status on the basis of genetic studies, and the family Anseranatidae has increased the number of families under Anseriformes to three[30,31] (Figure 16-1).

UNIQUE ANATOMY

The anatomic features of Anatidae and Anseranatidae are familiar to most veterinary practitioners—webbed feet, soft sensitive bills, relatively long necks with short legs, strong wings, and plumage that often includes heavy down feathers. The family of screamers is a bit more unusual. Aptly named for their loud raucous territorial calls, screamers lack the webbed feet and the soft, skin-covered bill of other Anseriformes. In addition, screamers possess complex systems of subcutaneous air sacs that may be contracted rapidly, an action that reportedly may produce a crackling sound![4] Additionally, they have extensive pneumatization of their bones, and even their phalanges may be pneumatized. They do not have distinct pterylae, or feather tracts; instead, their feathers are evenly distributed all over their bodies. Wild screamers are strong flyers and tend to form monogamous pairs, although large seasonal congregations occur, too. These birds are entirely herbivorous, and their tongues are keratinized and not fleshy as those of other Anseriformes species.[4]

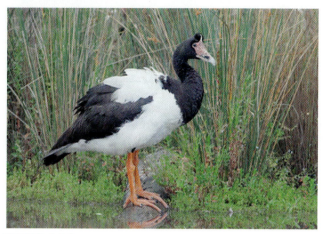

FIGURE 16-1 The Australian magpie goose at Tidbinbilla Nature Reserve, Australia. This species has recently been assigned its own genus, Anseranatidae. (Courtesy of Leo Berzins.)

Screamers are most often encountered in zoologic collections and have bred well in captivity.

The Anatidae family contains the majority of species in this order, comprising approximately 150 species of ducks, geese, and swans.[8] Referred to as waterfowl, they are important agricultural production animals, common zoo and private collection species, as well as frequently encountered wild bird species worldwide. Anatidae species range in size from a mere 275 grams (g) to 12 kilograms (kg) and include the heaviest birds capable of true flapping flight—the swans.[19] Species such as the bar-headed goose (*Anser indicus*), which migrates over the Himalayas, represent some of the most remarkable vertebrate athletes in existence.[19] The extensive seasonal migrations and the social nature of most species, both wild and domestic, expose these birds to many environments as well as to potential toxins and infectious diseases. In urban and suburban settings, the endemic wild species have adapted to human-dominated environments and mingle with domestic species. The opportunity for disease transmission, to the detriment of wild, captive, and domestic populations, has occurred repeatedly and continues to be a major concern for the agricultural industry and with regard to conservation efforts.[10]

HOUSING REQUIREMENTS

Waterfowl, as their name implies, do best with constant access to clean water. Large, outdoor, planted enclosures with ponds, pools, or lakes are preferred. High stocking rates of waterfowl will lead to loss of turf and compaction of soil around lakes and ponds and promote unsanitary conditions associated with infectious diseases.[3] For domestic and captive species, ensuring a place of refuge from predators (e.g., an island) and shelter from adverse weather is recommended. When artificial pools are provided, gently sloped sides to the pool are recommended to reduce abrasions to the plantar surface of the feet. Hospitalized waterfowl should have access to soft matted areas to cushion their feet and prevent abrasions that may lead to pododermatitis.

FEEDING

The National Research Council (NRC) requirements for commercially raised ducks and geese are well established and provide a general reference for waterfowl diets.[26] However, the overall protein and energy levels of commercially available waterfowl feeds are designed for maximum growth rates and should not constitute the sole diet of captive nonproduction animals. Herbivorous and granivorous, Anseriformes species do well when fed commercially available duck and/or poultry diets designed for maintenance as a base diet, with the addition of leafy greens and live insects, access to pasture and grazing, or both. The more carnivorous or piscivorous species require diets based on chopped fish or other specific dietary items. Table 16-1[17] lists selected nutritional deficiencies documented in Anseriformes.

REPRODUCTION AND NEONATAL CARE

In the family Anseriformes, males have an intromittent copulatory organ attached to the ventral wall of the cloaca. This spiral-shaped phallus may be extruded manually from the first day of life by applying pressure to both sides of the cloaca; thus many species may be sexed at an early age.[19] Sex determination by this method in adult nonsexually dimorphic Anseriformes species may be challenging, even with the use of sedation, with or without anesthesia, to relax the cloaca. Swans and geese form a lifetime pair-bond and may not form another bond if one member of the pair dies. Male ducks generally are not involved in egg incubation and may or may not breed with the same female in subsequent breeding seasons. Anseriformes young are precocial and leave the nest within hours of hatching, follow their mother, and are known for their strong imprinting instincts. Care of artificially brooded ducklings is similar to that of poultry chicks, by providing a round basin with central heat source. A round pen or basin of 0.5 to 1.0 square feet (ft^2) per duckling is recommended for raising domestic ducklings, with a brooder temperature maintained at 85°F to 90°F for the first 2 to 3 weeks.[6] An infra-red heat lamp positioned approximately 2 feet from the floor of the center of the pen provides warmth, and the ducklings may move closer to or away from it, as needed. Brooders should provide a soft but nonslip substrate to prevent spraddle or splay-leg in young ducklings, and the depth of substrate will depend on the species raised. Newspaper is not recommended unless it is shredded or pelleted to prevent it from becoming slippery; hay and straw beddings have been associated with aspergillosis.[17] Most exotic species of ducks and geese that are similar to their domestic counterparts may be initially reared on a chick starter crumble that contains approximately 20% protein. The crumble may be wetted into a mash and the mash supplemented with grazing opportunities, whenever possible, to provide exercise as well as a diet of fresh greens. If grazing is initially not available, chopped fresh greens and live insects are both well accepted by neonatal waterfowl of most species. Food and water containers should have low sides to prevent very young ducklings from becoming wet. Neonatal ducklings are susceptible to chilling as their down is not waterproof. Chilled ducklings are poorly responsive and do not feed well.[6] Ducklings may also become exhausted and drown if unable to exit the water container. Once they are no longer reliant on an external heat source, young waterfowl may be transitioned into larger holding facilities with pools or ponds that allow easy exit from the water. Predation from raptors, mammals, and reptilian carnivores, especially aquatic turtles in well-established ponds, are significant risks for young waterfowl that are housed outdoors.

RESTRAINT

Restraint of captive waterfowl includes netting and herding for the catch-up, culminating in manual restraint. Some Anatidae species undergo a postbreeding molt, during which all the remiges, or flight feathers, are lost en masse in a very short period (hours to days) rendering them flightless for several weeks.[19] In both wild and captive environments, this flightless period may be used opportunistically to herd and capture large numbers of waterfowl in some settings. When manually restraining waterfowl, handlers should take special precaution to avoid painful bites and scratches. Larger species may inflict strong and painful blows from their wings.

Once captured, smaller species may be held single-handedly by restraining the animal with the wings folded or with fingers of one

TABLE 16-1

Selected Nutritional Diseases of Anseriformes

Disease	Cause	Clinical Signs	Comments
Perosis	Manganese, choline deficiency may be seen at hatching, or in first few weeks of life May also have genetic component in some domestic breeds	Deformities of tarsometatarsal bone, medial luxation of Achilles tendon, and non–weight-bearing on affected limb	Occurs mainly in captive ducklings and goslings Prevent by supplementing hen's diet with manganese Surgical correction, including stabilization of the tendon is sometimes successful
Angel wing	Excess dietary protein suspected to contribute Manganese deficiency or excess dietary energy also may be factors	Lateral rotation of distal carpometacarpal bone; inability to fly; twisted appearance to distal wing	Occurs mainly in tropical and temperate species; occurs in captivity and in the wild May be corrected with taping the wing in normal position if caught early Prevent by restricting dietary protein
Rickets	Vitamin D deficiency	Poor growth and lameness	Occurs mainly in captive ducklings Correct by feeding balanced diet
Hypovitaminosis A	Vitamin A deficiency	Ducklings show ataxia, poor growth, paresis, paralysis, and death; adults have white nodules in esophageal mucosa, and cachexia	Occurs in captive and free-ranging waterfowl feeding strictly on grains throughout winter Need to balance diet Correct or prevent by feeding fresh leafy greens or allowing access to grazing
Thiamin (B_1) deficiency	—	Stargazing and weight loss in ducklings	Disease of captivity; treat with supplemental thiamin at 100 μg/L in drinking water
Niacin (vitamin B_6) deficiency	Ducklings have a higher requirement for niacin than the young of other avian species	Leg deformities such as bowed legs; weakness and poor growth	Disease of captivity; prevent by supplementation of feed with niacin or 7.5% brewer's yeast. Ducklings have higher requirement for niacin compared with other species

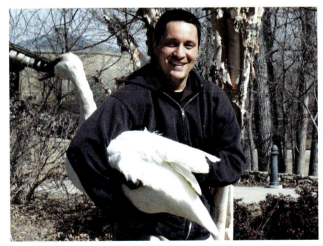

FIGURE 16-2 Restraint of an adult trumpeter swan. the bird should be held facing away from the restrainer to protect the face and eyes, but the bird is still capable of biting.

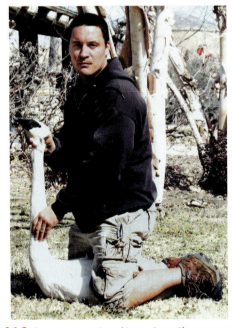

FIGURE 16-3 Straddle restraint of large Anseriformes such as swan may be useful for collection of blood, administration of oral medications, and other procedures.

hand under each wing supporting the proximal humerus and the other hand supporting the bird's abdomen. Supporting even small species only by the wings may lead to musculoskeletal injury, especially if the bird struggles. In one incident, a mallard-sized bird restrained only by the wings fractured a coracoid bone while struggling. Neurologic damage from such restraint has also been reported.[17]

In the case of larger species such as geese and swans, it is typical to hold the bird, wings folded and facing backward, under the arm of the handler (Figure 16-2). Large, relatively calm species may also be straddled on the ground to be restrained for oral administration of medications, gavage feeding, and minor procedures such as blood collection. Handlers must take special care not to put their body weight on the bird, but use their legs to keep the wings restrained and their hands to control the bird's head and neck (Figure 16-3).

SURGERY AND ANESTHESIA

Anesthesia should be administered to waterfowl for all but minor nonpainful procedures. Anesthesia or sedation is also often used as a method of safe restraint for nonpainful diagnostics such as radiography where manual restraint would be unsuccessful or contraindicated. Fasting for several hours is recommended prior to anesthesia. Prior to anesthesia, the crop should be palpated and its size and fullness assessed. If large amounts of food have been stored in the crop, non-emergency anesthetic procedures should be delayed. Inhalation anesthesia with isoflurane or sevoflurane is the most common in-hospital method for anesthetizing waterfowl. Induction is typically via a face mask. Intubation with a noncuffed endotracheal tube is recommended for all anesthetic procedures of more than 10- to 15-minute duration. Dose-dependent respiratory depression is seen in most anesthetized waterfowl, so occasional positive pressure ventilation is recommended. Waterfowl anesthetized with inhalant agents have been noted to present what is described as "rollercoastering" while anesthetized. The birds appear to be deeply anesthetized with slowing heart rate and respiratory rate but then suddenly lighten in their anesthetic depth, arouse, and move. This phenomenon may be associated with partial pressure of carbon dioxide (PCO_2) chemoreceptors in the lung that influence respiratory drive.[17,23] The addition of sedatives such as butorphanol and midazolam to the anesthesia regimen appears to lessen the degree of this fluctuating anesthetic depth in many waterfowl. Another complication in waterfowl is the development of thick mucus in the trachea or glottis during anesthesia. Mucus may completely plug the endotracheal tube or glottis during anesthesia or recovery and, if not removed, will lead to death of the bird. Thus, airway patency should be regularly checked during anesthetic episodes, the endotracheal tubes cleared, and the airway monitored until the bird has completely recovered. The most important piece of anesthetic equipment to ensure successful anesthesia of waterfowl is an attentive and experienced attendant whose sole responsibility should be the monitoring of anesthetic delivery, depth, and the patient's vital signs during the entire anesthesia and recovery periods. An in depth review of anesthesia techniques and respiratory physiology of waterfowl as it pertains to anesthesia is published in detail elsewhere.[23]

Preparation of Anseriformes patients for surgery should take into account the individual species' need for waterproofing and insulation. The feathers of Anseriformes species do not typically epilate easily, and most have small, tightly-packed contour and down feathers to provide waterproofing and insulation, respectively. The minimum amount of feathers should be plucked at the surgical site to provide a sterile field, and special care should be taken to avoid or decrease skin damage from plucking these tightly adherent feathers. Presurgically, only one feather or a few feathers at a time should be plucked and pulled in the direction that the feather lies to prevent tearing or bruising the skin. In addition, most waterfowl species do not have large apteria, and down feathers are evenly distributed over the entire body.[19] Postsurgical care must take into account the loss of waterproofing and insulating properties caused by feather plucking. Following major surgical procedures, the bird may need to be withheld from access to water or swimming, depending on ambient and water temperatures, until significant feather regrowth occurs. The most common surgical procedure performed on captive waterfowl is pinioning. Done at 1 to 6 days of age, it is a relatively minor procedure that typically does not require plucking or general anesthesia, although a small amount of local anesthetic may be injected at the site prior to the procedure. The surgical site should be lightly prepped with a suitable topical disinfectant. The distal wing tip may then be clamped with a small hemostat, and the wing tip may be sharply removed distal to the clamp or directly amputated with a sharp pair of tissue scissors. Several minutes of moderate digital pressure at the amputation site is recommended to ensure hemostasis. It is common to apply a drop of skin glue at the site. The site of amputation is typically at the middle or proximal metaphyseal region of the metacarpal bones. The alula is often used as an external marker

for the appropriate length at which to set the clamp and cut through the soft, cartilaginous major and minor metacarpal bones, but the length of the pinioned wing should be individualized for the species and the collection's preferences. Neonatal pinioning has few adverse effects, whereas pinioning an adult bird is a major surgical procedure that requires careful tissue handling, attention to hemostasis, postoperative bandaging for at least 1 to 3 days, and postoperative pain relief. Adult pinioned birds are highly prone to repeated trauma to the pinioned site and often develop large fibromatous nodules that may be unaesthetic and prone to hemorrhage. The options of surgical feather follicle extirpation or laser ablation have been investigated as an alternative to the surgical pinioning of adult birds.[20,29] In a study of two species of Anseriformes, the primary feathers were cut, a diode laser tip placed into the cut calamus of the treated primary flight feathers, and the follicle ablated with a total dose of 20 Joules of energy.[29] Postoperatively, the treated wings showed swelling, edema, ulceration, and serosanguineous oozing. These side effects were deemed minor and completely resolved in all treated birds within 12 weeks. The laser treatment resulted in successful prevention of feather regrowth in 65% of treated follicles.[29] The options of surgical follicle extirpation or nonsurgical follicle destruction in lieu of surgical pinioning should be considered for limiting flight in adult Anseriformes and warrant further study. For further information, see Chapter 65.

ANALGESIA

The use of analgesics is necessary to provide humane care for painful injuries and procedures. Many publications have shown that different classifications of analgesics such as nonsteroidal anti-inflammatory drugs (NSAIDs) and opiates may have measureable effects in birds.[25] However, the proof of analgesic efficacy, safety, proper dosage, and duration of analgesia for these drugs in many avian species, including Anseriformes, needs further study. Existing data demonstrating that analgesics administered to waterfowl do have some benefit via inhalant-anesthetic sparing effect are corroborated by the author's experience.[23,25] Both NSAIDs and opiates have been tested at various dosages in birds and some waterfowl species with varying results.[2, 25] However, NSAIDs such as flunixin meglumine and ketoprofen have been shown to have side effects in many species of birds, including waterfowl. Flunixin meglumine was shown to reduce the production of cyclooxygenase (COX) enzyme-2, COX-2, but its use was associated with muscle necrosis at the site of injection in mallard ducks.[21] Ketoprofen was associated with mortality in one study of eider ducks but has been used in studies of other waterfowl.[24] Use of analgesics for painful procedures or injuries is considered part of humane care and best practice in modern veterinary medicine but is not without risk because of the lack of data on safety and efficacy in individual species. The extreme sensitivity of some Old World vultures to the NSAID diclofenac is an example of the variability of safety in different species to different drugs.[27] The selection of an analgesic for use in any species should be based on a combination of the practitioner's experience and a review of studies that show, at a minimum, the safe use of the selected drug in a particular species or a closely related species.

DIAGNOSTICS

The majority of diagnostic procedures for Anseriformes do not differ from those performed on other avian species. The long neck of many waterfowl species makes jugular venipuncture the preferred site for blood collection; other sites include the medial metatarsal or brachial veins. As in other birds, the right jugular is larger than the left and is the preferred site for obtaining larger quantities of blood. The venipuncturist holds the bird's head and palpates the vein or at least the jugular groove cranial to the epaxial musculature and lateral to the trachea. This procedure works best if the neck is extended fully and the bird is adequately restrained. The medial metatarsal vein is found on the medial side of the tarsometatarsus; as in other birds, the site is an alternative for obtaining small quantities of blood. The brachial vein courses across the wing near the elbow and is easily found on most waterfowl species, but because of the limited soft tissue around the vein, venipuncture from this site is more likely to result in hematoma formation. Once obtained, blood may be placed in heparinized blood tubes or microtainers for a complete blood cell count or chemistry panel analysis. Some hematologic and plasma biochemistry reference ranges for selected Anseriformes species may be found in reference 5.

INFECTIOUS DISEASE

The classic infectious diseases of waterfowl, for example, avian cholera and duck viral enteritis, have not significantly changed in

their epizootiology, clinical signs, diagnosis, and management. An excellent review of the basic biology of these diseases is still sound.[15] Current outbreaks, locations, and ongoing research about mortality in free-living waterfowl is monitored in the United States by the United States Geological Service (USGS). The National Wildlife Health Center (NWHC) of the USGS produces quarterly mortality reports and actively continuing mortality event surveillance for many infectious as well as noninfectious diseases seen in free-ranging waterfowl and other animal species. These wildlife mortality events are compiled from local, state, and regional authorities and made available for easy reference at the NWHC website (www.nwhc .usgs.gov). A chart of selected infectious diseases of waterfowl are listed in Table 16-2.[12,17,28] A list of selected antibiotics used in waterfowl are listed in Table 16-3.[5,11,14,17]

TABLE 16-2

Selected Infectious Diseases of Waterfowl

Disease, Agent	Epizootiology	Signs	Gross Lesions or Diagnosis	Management
Aspergillosis *Aspergillus fumigatus*	Ubiquitous airborne spores, poor ventilation, moldy feed	Respiratory signs, dramatic weight loss or acute death	Clinical suspicion; radiology and serology	Itraconazole, terbinafine, amphotericin-B, supportive care
Avian cholera *Pasturella multocida*	Aerosolized excrement and respiratory secretions, fecal oral transmission, carrier state in recovered birds	Peracute death with birds in good body condition, neurologic signs	Gross petechiae on heart, serosal membranes, focal hepatic necrosis. Culture of blood, liver, or bone marrow	Individual birds may respond to antibiotics, isolate affected birds. Carcasses should be collected and buried
Avian bornavirus Mononegavirus (See text in this chapter for detailed discussion)	Fecal-oral transmission, vertical through egg suspected. Carrier state common, intermittent shedding	Few signs in carrier. Bird appears "sick," weak, unable to fly. Neurologic signs	Grossly maybe in poor condition, gastrointestinal impaction or dysfunction. RT-PCR of cloaca. Oropharyngeal swabs may underestimate. RT-PCR of brain tissue. Serologic tests, IFA, and serology available. Histologic examination of nonsuppurative encephalomyelitis and ganglioneuritis	No known treatment available. Affected birds should be eliminated from collections
Chlamydiosis *Chlamydophila psittaci*	Respiratory secretions and fecal material; asymptomatic carrier state	Sinusitis, conjunctivitis, diarrhea, ataxia, and neurologic signs	Hepatomegaly, splenomegaly, pneumonia and airsacculitis. Paired antibody titers, culture, or antigen-based tests for PCR from fecal, cloacal, tracheal, or choanal swabs	Zoonotic disease. Caretakers should wear appropriate PPE. Isolate affected birds and use chlamydiocidal disinfectants. Chlortetracycline and doxycycline orally. Reportable disease in some states
Duck plaque Duck viral enteritis Herpesvirus	Fecal–oral transmission, horizontal transmission via contact with infected birds. Carrier state common	Seasonal occurrence. Some bodies of water known for repeated outbreaks. Peracute death, with birds in good body condition or with depression, hematochezia, epiphora, ulcer under tongue in carrier	Grossly characteristic annular bands of necrotic intestinal mucosa with overlying hemorrhagic bands typical in domestic ducks and mallards. Myocardial petechiation. Virus isolation from liver, spleen. Characteristic histologic appearance of lymphoid aggregates	Isolate carrier birds or prevent access of unaffected birds to potentially affected environments, particularly affected bodies of water. Depopulation and attenuated live-virus vaccine. Carcasses should be collected and buried

TABLE 16-2

Selected Infectious Diseases of Waterfowl—cont'd

Disease, Agent	Epizootiology	Signs	Gross Lesions or Diagnosis	Management
HPAI -H5N1-Asian strain type A orthomyxovirus (See text for detailed discussion)	Fecal-oral transmission, and respiratory secretions Carrier state is poorly documented compared with LPAI	Acute death, dullness, paresis, paralysis, tremors, torticollis, nasal discharge, diarrhea May resemble other acute bacterial and viral diseases in a multibird mortality event	Marked congestion of lungs, and brain airsacculitis, congestion of various organs, hemorrhagic intestines, focal necrosis, and friable liver	Cloacal or choanal swabs of living birds If suspected, state and federal regulatory agencies should be contacted
Salmonellosis *S. typhimurium* *S. paratyphi*	Fecal-oral transmission Environmental contamination with feces of numerous other animals Transovarian vertical transmission and fecal contamination of eggs	Primarily seen in ducklings and captive waterfowl Peracute death, lethargy, diarrhea, ataxia, and conjunctivitis	Hepatosplenomegaly, multifocal necrosis of liver, no lesions in acute cases Culture of the organism from parenchymous organs	Removal of carrier adults from breeding flocks
Tuberculosis *Mycobacterium avium*	Fecal-oral transmission, ingestion of high numbers of organisms Environmental persistence of organisms may last years	Progressive weight loss, cachexia, leukocytosis, characteristic osteolytic bone lesions on radiographs Death	Emaciated carcass, multifocal granuloma in liver, GIT and other organs, secondary amyloidosis from chronic inflammation Acid-fast staining of affected organs at necropsy or biopsy	Euthanasia of infected birds, increased surveillance of birds in contaminated environments Disinfection of exhibit with tuberculocidal disinfectants and removal of top 6–7 inches of soil substrate

GIT, Gastrointestinal tract; *HPAI*, highly pathogenic avian influenza; *LPAI*, low pathogenic avian influenza; *RT-PCR*, real-time polymerase chain reaction.

TABLE 16-3

Selected Antibiotics Recommended for Anseriformes

Generic Name	Trade Name	Dosage	Route of Administration	Interval
Ampicillin	Amp-Equine	100 mg/kg	IM	Every 4 hours
Amoxicillin trihydrate	Amoxi-Tabs Amoxi-drops	300 mg/L	In drinking water	Provide every other day for 3 treatments
Ceftiofur	Naxcel	2–4 mg/kg	SQ	Every 24 hours
Ceftiofur crystalline-free acid (CCFA)	Excede	10 mg/kg	IM	Every 72 hours
Cefquinome		5 mg/kg	IM	Every 24 hours
Chlortetracycline	Aureomycin	300–1000 mg/kg of feed	PO	Daily
Doxycycline	Vibramycin	25–50 mg/kg	PO	Every 12 hours
Enrofloxacin	Baytril	10–15 mg/kg	PO or IM	Every 12 hours, Avoid repeated injection
Oxytetracycline	Liquamycin, LA-200	200 mg/kg	IM	Every 24 hours for 5–7 days
Trimethoprim-sulfamethoxazole	Septra	75 mg/kg	PO or IM	Every 12 hours
		0.04% feed	PO	Daily
Tylosin	Tylan	20–30 mg/kg 500 mg/L in water	IM PO in drinking water	Every 8 hours for 3–7 days 3–28 days
Marbofloxacin	Zeniquin	2 mg/kg	PO or IM	Every 24 hours

IM, Intramuscular; *mg/kg*, milligram per kilogram; *mg/L*, milligram per liter; *PO*, oral; *SQ*, subcutaneous.

Two major diseases are relatively new in their appearance and importance in Anseriformes health and are more thoroughly discussed below.

Avian Bornavirus

The discovery of avian bornavirus (ABV) and its recognition as the agent of avian disease has been relatively recent. Bornavirus is a non-enveloped negative strand ribonucleic acid (RNA) virus. It is a member of the Order Mononegavirales. Because it uniquely replicates in the cell nucleus, it has been classified in its own family, Bornaviridae.[28] In 2008, ABV was identified as the causative agent of proventricular dilatation disease (PDD) in psittacines, but the primary reservoir for ABV appears to be waterfowl.[13] The first ABV was isolated from a wild bird species, a Canada goose (*Branta canadensis*), and free-living waterfowl, and subsequent surveys for ABV have been primarily conducted in North America.[28] A number of wild waterfowl species that have been found to be infected with ABV include *B. canadensis*, mute and trumpeter swans (*Cygnus olor, C. buccinator*), pintails (*Anas acuta*), gadwalls (*A. strepera*), mallards (*A. platyrhynchos*), redheads (*Aythya americana*), American widgeon (*A. americana*), and northern shoveler (*A. clypeata*). ABV appears to be of low pathogenicity to most waterfowl, and long-term intermittent shedding in apparently healthy birds has been documented. Viral shedding has been confirmed with real-time polymerase chain reaction (RT-PCR) samples of fecal, cloacal, and oropharnygeal swabs of surveyed wild waterfowl species. Prevalence rates vary for tested waterfowl species tested using fecal swabs, at less than or equal to 10%, but fecal swabs may underestimate ABV infection rates. Survey reports using RT-PCR on brain tissue samples from sacrificed or hunter-killed waterfowl showed much higher prevalence rates, varying from 22% to as high as 50%.[28] The difference in prevalence rates is likely related to intermittent fecal shedding by infected birds. Transmission appears to be the fecal–oral route, and vertical transmission has been suggested in one study of hatching eggs of domestic ducks.[28] The percentage of wild waterfowl infected appears to vary by geographic location sampled and may be associated with habitat factors that promote transmission of the virus. ABV infects the central and enteric neurologic tissues of birds, inducing an inflammatory response, which then leads to neuronal and glial cell loss. The histologic characteristics of a nonsuppurative encephalomyelitis and ganglioneuritis similar to that seen in psittacine PDD is also commonly found in clinically ill waterfowl. An inapparent carrier state is likely the most common form of disease in waterfowl, and carriers should be considered a source of infection to other birds. Clinically affected waterfowl present as sick, weak, unable to fly, and neurologically impaired and potentially have an impacted upper gastrointestinal tract. Antemortem detection of ABV may be performed using RT-PCR on freshly plucked contour feathers that include the calamus, or crop biopsies, and reverse enzyme-linked immunosorbent assay (rELISA) on serum at avian specialty laboratories. Indirect fluorescent antibody (IFA) and Western blot are additional antemortem serologic tests. Unfortunately, currently available antemortem tests cannot differentiate diseased birds from unapparent carriers.[28] Neither cloacal or vent swabs nor fecal samples are recommended for routine screening because of intermittent viral shedding. Postmortem detection of ABV RNA using RT-PCR is best performed on brain tissue samples, proventricular tissue samples, or both. Most commercially available tests for ABV have been developed for the psittacines, so contacting the laboratory for estimates of the test efficacy in a particular waterfowl species is recommended. The identification of new ABVs will likely continue, as their distribution is predicted to be worldwide in waterfowl, although few studies have been conducted outside of North America.

Avian Influenza

The family Orthomyxovirus, genus Influenza A, contains the highly variable enveloped RNA virus of avian influenza virus (AIV). Historically, these viruses were of little consequence causing disease in their normal Anseriformes and Charadriiformes hosts. The recent emergence of new, highly pathogenic strains of avian influenza virus has elevated their importance in agricultural, wildlife disease surveillance and conservation, as well as in human health protection. The influenza virus types are named for their combinations of surface glycoproteins, hemagglutinin (H, 16 subtypes), and neuraminidase (N, 9 subtypes). These combinations also determine their virulence. The hemagglutinin subtypes of H5 and H7 are associated with increased pathogenicity in birds.[18] The virus's designation as either low pathogenic avian influenza (LPAI) or high pathogenic avian influenza (HPAI) is based on the particular virus's pathogenicity to domestic chickens. LPAI in waterfowl is transmitted via the fecal–oral route, and its prevalence has been shown to peak in *A. platyrhynchos* in late summer and early fall associated with premigration staging areas.[32] Other free-living species of waterfowl and shore birds routinely are found positive for LPAI throughout the world. The epidemiology varies with regard to species and with regard to species population differences such as age, environment, and season.[32] Although HPAI-H5N1 infections have been detected in asymptomatic wild waterfowl, the virus is more likely to be detected in clinically affected birds, and early detection strategies have focused heavily on morbidity and mortality events.[18,32] Like LPAI, HPAI's transmission is by the fecal–oral route through contaminated water sources and fomites, but it additionally has a respiratory component and may be spread by direct contact and via respiratory secretions.[10,18] HPAI-H5N1 has caused numerous wild waterfowl deaths, has a mortality rate approaching 100% in domestic chickens, and has caused infection and death in numerous other atypical species, including canids, felids, mustelids, viverids, suids, lagomorphs, and primates.[10] Cases of human HPAI-H5N1 infection have been reported, with an alarmingly high mortality rate of almost 60%. In a report of 499 known infected individuals from 15 countries from 2003 to June 2010, the disease was reported to have been fatal in 295 cases.[34] Since its first appearance in China in a domestic goose in 1996 and the first verified outbreak in wild migratory waterfowl in 2005, HPAI-H5N1 has emerged as an endemic virus in Eurasia and North Africa. It is now believed to have been continuously circulating in Asia, Europe, and Africa since 2003.[9,34] Human activity, agricultural environments, and specific farming practices (e.g., free-grazing of domestic waterfowl) consistently play key roles in the occurrence, maintenance, and spread of HPAI-H5N1.[34] To date, the virulent Asian subtype of HPAIV-H5N1 has not been isolated in the United States, Canada, South America, or Australia. Numerous U.S. agencies have tested thousands of wild and domestic birds, and to date, only LPAI versions of H5N1 have been found (mostly in wild birds) and have been genetically confirmed as North American LPAI strains with no lineage or similarities to the H5N1-HPAI Asian strain. Readers are referred to the World Animal Health Interface Database for the most current information regarding HPAI outbreaks. At this website (www.oie.int), member countries of the World Organization for Animal Health (OIE) report various disease outbreaks by country and year.

Clinical signs of HPAI in poultry range from decreased egg production to peracute death, but clinical signs such as diarrhea and neurologic signs reflect the virus's target organs: the gastrointestinal tract and the nervous system. Neurologic signs include depression, paresis, and paralysis (with or without tremors), and an intermittent head shake or head tilt. Characteristic respiratory rales, sinusitis, epiphora, edema of the head, and cyanosis and hemorrhage of the wattles and comb are also seen in poultry. Anseriformes species may present with clinical signs such as inactivity, dullness, weakness, staggering, and acute death. In some birds, only a clear nasal discharge, lacrimation, or mild diarrhea has been noticed before death.[18] The clinical signs of HPAI in waterfowl are nonspecific and resemble those of other highly pathogenic infectious diseases. Differential diagnoses in waterfowl should include other flock mortality events, including septicemic diseases such as avian cholera, viral diseases such as duck viral enteritis, or exotic Newcastle disease, and acute poisonings such as botulism.[18] Gross pathology of waterfowl dying of HPAI has included congestion and edema of various organs, pericardial effusions, thickened air sacs, red-brown mottling of the pancreas, hemorrhage in the duodenum, and a friable liver with foci of necrosis. Histopathologic lesions consisted of congestion and multifocal necrosis in multiple organs, including the spleen, the liver, and the gastrointestinal tract. Marked congestion and edema in the lungs, cerebral congestion, with or without multiple small foci of necrosis, and mild gliosis or multifocal nonsuppurative meningoencephalitis are also significant.[9]

Diagnostic testing for avian influenza in the United States is generally performed by specialized county, state, regional, or national laboratories such as the U.S. Department of Agriculture (USDA)-approved laboratories in the National Animal Health Laboratory Network (NAHLN). Wild bird samples are tested at the USGS

National Wildlife Health Center (NWHC) laboratory in Madison, Wisconsin. Current NWHC surveillance testing is passive and confined to mortality events that involve 500 or more birds, characteristics of AIV, or ongoing mortality. The samples are screened for influenza A viruses by virus isolation or RT-PCR performed on cloacal or pharyngeal swab specimens. The U.S. Interagency Strategic Plan recommends obtaining both cloacal and pharyngeal swab specimens from wild birds. Currently, any H5 or H7 avian influenza subtypes, regardless of pathotype, are immediately notifiable to authorities in all states, federally notifiable to USDA-APHIS-VS, and internationally notifiable to OIE. In the United States, the USDA has jurisdiction over matters relating to avian influenza. The federal government is the regulatory authority for matters relating to HPAI

TABLE 16-4

Selected Parasitic Diseases of Anseriformes

Disease	Etiology	Location in Host		Diagnosis	Management
		Adult	**Immature**		
Leeches	*Theromyzon* spp.	Nasal cavity, pharynx, and conjunctiva	—	Examination of trachea, nasal cavity, and eyes	Manual removal; drain and disinfect pond
Coccidiosis, renal	*Eimeria truncate* *E. boschadis* *E. somateriae*	Kidney	Kidney	Fecal flotation, intestinal lesions, and oocysts in renal impression smears	Use of amprolium and sulfonamides; segregation of young birds to minimize their exposure
Coccidiosis, intestinal	*Eimeria* spp. *Tyzzeria* spp. *Isospora* spp. *Wenyonella* spp.	Intestinal mucosa	Intestinal mucosa	Fecal flotation and intestinal lesions containing merozoites	Amprolium and sulfonamides
Sarcosporidiosis	*Sarcocystis rileyi*	Intestinal tract of opossums and skunks	Muscle tissue of waterfowl	Characteristic macroscopic appearance of white cysts in striated muscle on muscle biopsy	Not pathogenic
Nematodiasis, tracheal (gape worm)	*Cyathostoma bronchialis*	Tracheal mucosa	—	Fecal flotation; adults in tracheal mucus	Fenbendazole and ivermectin
Nematodiasis, myocardial	*Sacronema eurycerca*	Heart	Microfilaria in biting lice and blood of bird	Microfilaria on blood smear	Louse control with pyrethrins; treatment for *Sacronema* sp. unknown
Nematodiasis, proventricular	*Echinuria uncinata*	Proventricular mucosa and submucosa	Water fleas (*Daphnia* spp.)	Recovery of adults from proventricular nodular lesions	Increase water flow to decrease *Daphnia* spp.; use of ivermectin and fenbendazole
Nematodiasis, ventricular	*Amidostomum* sp. *Epimidiostomum* sp.	Ventriculus and subepithelial	Feces and water (direct life cycle)	Fecal flotation	Ivermectin and fenbendazole
Cestodiasis	Numerous species	Intestinal tract lumen	Aquatic crustacean	Fecal flotation	Praziquantel
Trematodiasis	Numerous species, Non-native genuses: Cyathocotyle, Leyogonimus, and Sphaeridiotrema may cause fatal disease in lesser scaup duck, American coot	Intestinal tract, bile duct, and respiratory tract	Mollusks are intermediate hosts	Fecal flotation	Difficult to control; use of levamisole and praziquantel

viruses and their eradication, whereas the state governments regulate matters relating to LPAI viruses in domestic poultry. The legal authority to conduct an emergency eradication program is shared by the state and federal governments, and the specifics are determined by both on a case-by-case basis. Any suspect cases should be reported immediately to the appropriate state veterinarian and to the USDA. Authorities should be consulted regarding regulations for sending samples to authorized diagnostic laboratories.

The potential for the spread of HPAI-H5N1 from Eurasia to North America is logistically possible via human activities or wild waterfowl migratory flyway overlaps across the Bering Sea. Prevention of cross-contamination is extremely difficult in public parks where wild and domestic waterfowl intermingle but may also be challenging in zoos and private collections with outdoor bird enclosures. In the somewhat more controlled environment of a zoologic or private collection, captive waterfowl and other AIV-susceptible species may be afforded some protection from disease with a good veterinary medical preventive health program and preplanning. Regardless of pathogenicity, prevention of AIV transmission between wild birds and captive waterfowl must focus on the exclusion of wild birds and their feces from collection birds.[18] Effective general sanitation and hygiene measures will help prevent fomite transmission between areas inside and outside the facility. An established veterinary medical preventive health plan that includes quarantining and screening of incoming animals, routine medical care of collection animals, postmortem examinations and appropriate testing on collection animal deaths are all useful strategies in preventing the introduction of any contagious disease into an animal collection and will provide the foundation for surveillance, prevention, and control in a collection should HPAI enter the country or region. The Association of Zoo and Aquariums (AZA), in conjunction with the American Association of Zoo Veterinarians (AAZV), compiled an extensive document to help U.S. facilities plan and prepare for the protection of animal care staff and valuable and endangered animal collections should HPAI occur in the United States and in the region of a facility.[1] Use of this document, in conjunction with a cooperative working relationship with local and federal agencies involved in animal disease outbreaks, is recommended as a foundation for an individualized preparedness policy for waterfowl and zoologic collections.

PARASITIC DISEASE

Selected parasitic diseases are listed in Table 16-4[12,17] and selected antiparasitic medications are listed in Table 16-5.[17]

NONINFECTIOUS DISEASE

Toxicity

The aquatic habitat of waterfowl and their feeding behavior may expose waterfowl to environmental toxins. Lead exposure from the ingestion of lead shotgun pellets and fishing tackle is still a major cause of waterfowl mortality in the United States despite the outlawing of lead shot use in waterways since 1991. Overall, the number of lead toxicity cases verified by the NWHC has continued to decrease. Eagles have become the predominant species affected. However, large quantities of lead are still present in the silt and mud bottoms of ponds, lakes, and waterways where waterfowl hunting has continued through most of the 20th century.[12] Annual variation in rainfall and drought conditions may lead to increased access and ingestion in both free-ranging and captive waterfowl.[7] Lead toxicity and other selected toxicities seen in waterfowl are listed in Table 16-6.[7,12,16]

Pododermatitis

Pododermatitis, also known as bumblefoot, is a chronic infection, with abscess development on the plantar surface of the feet. It is a common condition of waterfowl and other shore and water birds typically associated with captive environments. Husbandry and sanitation are considered crucial to bumblefoot prevention. Treatment of pododermatitis may be frustrating, and resolution is unlikely without improvement of husbandry-related issues. Depending on the severity and duration of lesions, treatment includes thorough debridement and cleaning of lesions, padded bandaging of the feet, and long-term antibiotic therapy. Severe chronic pododermatitis may lead to osteomyelitis of the bones of the affected foot, tenosynovitis of its tendons and ligaments, or both and these sequelae carry a grave prognosis for the affected bird. The chronic inflammation of pododermatitis has been linked to amyloidosis of the organs of affected waterfowl.

Amyloid Deposition

Waterfowl are well documented to form amyloid deposits secondarily to chronic inflammatory conditions. Swans appear to be especially sensitive to the development of amyloid deposits and have been mentioned as possible research candidates for the study of amyloidogenesis in humans.[33] In two separate pathology reviews of waterfowl, both the trumpeter swan and mute swan were noted to have high incidences of amyloid deposition in parenchymous organs at necropsy, particularly in the spleen and liver, and to a lesser degree

TABLE 16-5

Parasiticides Recommended for Anseriformes

Generic Name	Trade Name	Dosage	Route of Administration	Comments
Amprolium	Corid	0.5-1.0 mL/L of 9.6% solution	PO in drinking water for 5 days	Coccidia
Fenbendazole	Panacur	5-15 mg/kg	PO every 24 hours for 5 days	Nematodes
Ivermectin	Ivomec	0.2 mg/kg	PO, SQ, or IM once	Nematodes
Levamisole	Tramisol	20-50 mg/kg once	PO	Nematodes and trematodes (low therapeutic index)
Praziquantel	Droncit	10-20 mg/kg 10 mg/kg	SQ or IM; repeat in 10 days PO, SQ, or IM every 24 hours for 14 days	Cestodes Trematodes
Pyrantel pamoate	Strongid, Nemex	7 mg/kg	PO repeat in 14 days	Nematodes
Sulfadiazine- trimethoprim		60 mg/kg	PO every 12 hours for 3 days, then off 2 days, and then on 3 days	Coccidia

IM, Intramuscular; *mg/kg,* milligram per kilogram; *mL/L,* milliliter per liter; *PO,* oral; *SC,* subcutaneous.

TABLE 16-6

Selected Toxins Reported in Waterfowl

Toxin/Sources	Seasonality	Clinical Signs	Clinical Pathology	Diagnosis	Gross Findings	Treatment
Lead (Pb) Plumbism Shot pellets, fishing weights, smelter pollution	Autumn, winter, early spring	Weakness, emaciation Bile-stained diarrhea at vent, GIT stasis and impaction, wing paralysis, neurologic signs	Hypochromic anemia Low hemoglobin and MCHC, other changes associated with starvation, blood lead levels most helpful >0.5 ppm consistent with lead poisoning, prognosis worse for >1.0 ppm	Blood lead levels Metallic foreign bodies in GIT on radiography Pb levels on postmortem, liver preferred tissue	Emaciated carcass, severe atrophy of pectoral musculature, distention or impaction of esophagus and proventriculus common in geese Distended gallbladder, bile staining of ventriculus, visceral gout, myocardial degeneration	Supportive care, chelation therapy, removal of further lead from GIT via oral medications or mechanical removal with extreme caution
Zinc (Zn) Pennies minted after 1983, galvanized metal, smelter pollution	None More common in captive birds	Weakness, ataxia, paresis, paralysis, and weight loss	Anemia, body condition variable with duration Zn levels variable >3 ppm suspicious >10 ppm diagnostic	Blood Zn levels, Metallic foreign bodies in GIT on radiography Zn levels on postmortem tissues Pancreas is tissue of choice; liver and kidney	Weight loss	Supportive care, chelation therapy similar to Pb poisoning treatment Mechanical removal of Zn may lead to rapid recovery as levels not stored in tissues similar to Pb
Botulism *Clostridium botulinum* toxin type C	Summer into fall; year round in warm climates Spores are persistent so die-offs tend to recur at specific bodies of water	Weakness, paralysis of membrane nictitans, ascending paralysis, flying with head drooped, death by drowning, predation	Birds dying in good body condition, maggots in ventriculus	Season, clinical findings associated with mass mortality events, mouse inoculation of affected birds blood	Carcass in good body condition Absence of gross and histologic lesions	Affected birds may recover with protection from elements and predation supportive care
Petroleum Any petroleum product Oil spills, open pits and tanks	None Coastal near major oil ports or near production facilities	Oiled birds stranded on shoreline, weakness and hypothermia	Anemia from oil ingestion, pneumonia, and secondary aspergillosis	Mass oiling events highly publicized, but small local events common as well	Carcass typically in good body condition because of acute nature of exposure topical oil present Feathers not waterproof, and bodies wet Oil may be found in GIT and airways from ingestion and aspiration	Intensive supportive care and oil removal via repeated washings Bird will need time to "re-waterproof" feathers once cleaned
Algae toxins, two types common Red tide, *Gymnodinium breve*	Red tide Summer in southern coastal area	Weakness, head droop, diarrhea, lacrimation, oral and nasal discharge, dyspnea	Severe dehydration HCT 50% to 70%	Toxins cannot be detected in tissues Collect toxins from environment	Few gross lesions	Supportive care, no specific treatment
Blue-green cyanobacterium, *Anabaena flos-aquae* Avian vacuolar myelopathy New unknown species of cyanobacterium	Summer freshwater Typical blue-green "algae" and new AVM bacteria	*Typical:* Neuroparalytic swallowing, regurgitation, opisthotonus, convulsions and death *New:* Cyanobacteria Ataxia, inability to walk, fly, and swim; blindness	*Typical:* Depolarization at neuromuscular junction *New:* Cyanobacteria neurotoxin	*Similar:* Toxins cannot be detected in tissues Organisms in GIT and toxin collection from environment	Few gross lesions *New:* Cyanobacteria associated with microscopic vacuolization of the white matter in the central nervous system	No known treatment Supportive care

GIT, Gastrointestinal tract; *HCT,* hematocrit; *MCHC,* mean corpuscular hemoglobin concentration.

in other organs.[22,33] In both studies, diseases that caused significant chronic inflammation, such as aspergillosis and pododermatitis, were highly associated with the presence of amyloid deposition.

REFERENCES

1. AZA Animal Health Committee: *Avian influenza: Guidelines for prevention and control in AZA member institutions*, November 18, 2005.
2. Baert K, De Backer P: Comparative pharmacokinetics of three non-steroidal anti-inflammatory drugs in five bird species. *Comp Biochem Physiol C Toxicol Pharacol* 124:25–33, 2003.
3. Cambre RC: Water quality for a waterfowl collection. In Fowler ME, Miller RE, editors: *Zoo and wild animal medicine*, vol 4, Philadelphia, PA, 1999, Saunders, pp 292–299.
4. Carboneres C: Screamers. In Del Hoyo J, Elliott A, Sargatal J, editors: *Handbook of the birds of the world*, vol 1, Barcelona, Spain, 1992, Lynx Edicions, pp 528–535.
5. Carpenter JW, Marion CJ, editors: *Exotic animal formulary*, St. Louis, MO, 2013, Elsevier.
6. Coates WS, Erenest RA: *Raising ducks in small flocks,* Publication #2980, 2000, University of California Cooperative Extension Service.
7. Degernes LA: Waterfowl toxicology: A review. *Vet Clin Exotic Anim* 11:283–300, 2008.
8. Dickinson EC, editor: *The Howard & Moore complete checklist of the birds of the world*, ed 3, Princeton, NJ, 2003, Princeton University Press.
9. Ellis TM, Bousfield RB, Bissett LA, et al: Investigation of outbreaks of highly pathogenic H5N1 avian influenza in waterfowl and wild birds in Hong Kong in late 2002. *Avian Pathol* 33(5):492–505, 2004.
10. Gilbert M, Philippa J: Avian influenza H5N1 virus: Epidemiology in wild birds, zoo outbreaks, and zoo vaccination policy. In Fowler ME, Miller RE, editors: *Zoo and wild animal medicine*, vol 7, St. Louis, MO, 2012, Elsevier, pp 343–348.
11. Goudah A: Hasabelnaby: The disposition of marbofloxacin after single dose intravenous, intramuscular and oral administered to muscovy ducks. *J Vet Pharmacol Ther* 34:97–201, 2010.
12. Green DE, Hines MK, Russell RE, et al: *U.S. Geological Survey, National Wildlife Health Center, report of selected wildlife diseases 2011: U.S. Geological Survey Scientific Investigations Report, 2012–5271*, 32 pages plus 1 appendix, 2012.
13. Honkavuori KS, Shivaprasad HI, Williams BL, et al: Novel bornavirus in psittacine birds with proventricular dilation disease. *Emerg Infect Dis* 14:1883–1886, 2008.
14. Hope KL, Tell LA, Byrne BA, et al: Pharmacokinetics of a single intramuscular injection of ceftiofur crystalline-free acid in American black ducks (*Anas rubripes*). *AJVR* 73(5):620–627, 2012.
15. Humphreys PN: Ducks, geese, swans, and screamers (Anseriformes). In Fowler ME, editor: *Zoo and wild animal medicine*, Philadelphia, PA, 1986, Saunders, pp 333–363.
16. Katavolos P, Staempfli S, Sears W, et al: The effect of lead poisoning on hematologic and biochemical values in trumpeter swans and Canada geese. *Vet Clin Pathol* 36(4):341–345, 2007.

17. Kearns K: Anseriformes (waterfowl, screamers). In Fowler ME, Miller RE, editors: *Zoo and wild animal medicine*, St. Louis, MO, 2003, Saunders, pp 141–149.
18. Kelly TR, Hawkins MG, Sandrock CE, et al: A review of highly pathogenic avian influenza in birds, with an emphasis on Asian H5N1 and recommendations for prevention and control. *J Avian Med Surg* 22(1):1–16, 2008.
19. King AS, McClelland J: *Birds, their structure and function*, ed 2, Sussex, England, 1984, Bailliere Tindall.
20. Krawinkel PH: Feather follicle extirpation: Operative techniques to prevent zoo birds from flying. In Fowler ME, Miller RE, editors: *Zoo and wild animal medicine*, vol 7, St. Louis, MO, 2012, Elsevier, pp 275–280.
21. Machin KL, Tellier LA, Lair S, et al: Pharmacodynamics of flunixin and ketoprofen in mallard ducks (*Anas platyrhynchos*). *J Zoo Wildl Med* 32(2):222–229, 2001.
22. Meyerholz DK, Vanloubbeeck YE, Hostettter SE, et al: Surveillance of amyloidosis and other disease at necropsy in captive trumpeter swans (*Cygnus buccinators*). *J Vet Diag Invest* 17(3):295–298, 2005.
23. Mulcahy DM: Free-living waterfowl and shorebirds. In West G, Heard D, Caulkett N, editors: *Zoo animal and wildlife immobilization and anesthesia*, Ames, IA, 2007, Blackwell Publishing, pp 299–324.
24. Mulcahy DM, Tuomi P, Larsen RS: Differential mortality of male spectacled eiders (*Somateria fischeri*) and king eiders (*Somateria spectabilis*) subsequent to anesthesia with propofol, bupivacaine, and ketoprofen. *J Avian Med Surg* 17(3):117–123, 2003.
25. Murphy JP, Hawkins MG: Avian analgesia. In Fowler ME, Miller RE, editors: *Zoo and wild animal medicine*, vol 7, St. Louis, MO, 2012, Elsevier, pp 312–323.
26. Subcommittee on Poultry Nutrition, National Research Council: *Nutrient requirements of poultry*, 9th rev. ed, Washington, DC, 1994, The National Academic Press.
27. Oaks LJ, Meteyer CU: Nonsteroidal anti-inflammatory drugs in raptors. In Fowler ME, Miller RE, editors: *Zoo and wild animal medicine*, vol 7, St. Louis, MO, 2012, Elsevier, pp 349–355.
28. Payne SL, Delnatte P, Jiahan G, et al: Birds and bornaviruses. *Anim Health Res Rev* 13(2):145–156, 2012.
29. Shaw SN, D'Agostino J, Davis MR, et al: Primary feather follicle ablation in common pintails (Anas acuta acuta) and a white-faced whistling duck (*Dendrocygna viduata*). *J Zoo Wildl Med* 43(2):342–346, 2012.
30. Sibley CG, Ahlquist JE: *Phylogeny and classification of birds: A study in molecular evolution*, New Haven, CT, 1990, Yale University Press.
31. Sibley CG, Monroe BL: *Distribution and taxonomy of birds of the world*, New Haven, CT, 1990, Yale University Press.
32. Stallknecht DE, Brown JD: Wild birds and the epidemiology of avian influenza. *J Wildl Dis* 43(3):S15–S20, 2007.
33. Tanaka S, Dan C, Kawano H, et al: Pathological study on amyloidosis in *Cygnus olor* (mute swan) and other waterfowl. *Med Mol Morphol* 41(2):99–108, 2008.
34. Xin H, Hui LA, Tian AB, et al: Global occurrence and spread of highly pathogenic avian influenza virus of the subtype H5N1. *Avian Dis* 55:21–28, 2011.

CHAPTER 17

Falconiformes (Falcons, Hawks, Eagles, Kites, Harriers, Buzzards, Ospreys, Caracaras, Secretary Birds, Old World and New World Vultures)

Claude Lacasse

The taxonomy of the order Falconiformes has been the subject of debate but the order usually includes five families: (1) Cathartidae (New World vultures), (2) Accipitridae (hawks, eagles, kites, harriers, buzzards, and Old World vultures), (3) Falconidae (falcons, falconets, kestrels, merlins, hobbies, and caracaras), (4) Pandionidae (ospreys), and (5) Sagittariidae (secretary birds).[8,11]

Because of the endangered status of several species, recent decades have seen an increase in environmental awareness and conservation efforts involving raptors. Some examples are the captive breeding and management of the Mauritius kestrel (*Falco punctatus*); the European Bearded Vulture (*Gypaetus barbatus*) Reintroduction Project; and the conservation breeding and release program of the California condor (*Gymnogyps californianus*).[39,55] The Spanish imperial eagle (*Aquila adalberti*) is one of the most endangered species of birds of prey in the world.

UNIQUE ASPECTS OF BIOLOGY AND ANATOMY

The anatomy and biology of raptors is very similar to those of other avian species except for some modifications that give them great hunting capabilities. A table of maximum recorded life spans for selected raptor species has been published.[29]

Special Senses

Falconiformes are generally diurnal and rely heavily on sight to locate food.[71] They may perceive ultraviolet light and have a visual field of about 250 degrees, 50 degrees of which is binocular.[12] Each eye has two foveae, enabling two planes of vision (the temporal fovea for binocular vision and the central fovea for monocular vision). The exceptions are Andean condors (*Vultur gryphus*) and black vultures (*Coragyps atratus*), which have only a nasal fovea.[33] The pecten is plicated in most raptors.[39]

About 10 to 18 ossicles overlap to form a ring encircling the sclera. The sphincter and dilator muscles of the pupil are striated; therefore, unlike mammals, voluntary control may be possible, and atropine has no effect.[71] Raptors lack consensual pupillary light reflexes. A slight degree of anisocoria is normal. The pupils of birds that are stressed, especially *Accipiter* species, become dilated and less responsive to light, and the menace reflex might be absent.[45]

In most raptors, the sense of smell is poorly developed, except in vultures.[71] Most Falconiformes do not have a sense of hearing that is as developed as in Strigiformes; the exception are the harriers, which have a similar facial disk, which directs sounds toward the acoustic meatus.[12] Taste buds are located on the base of the tongue.[61]

Beak

A feature unique to raptors and fundamental to their carnivorous lifestyle is their stout, sharply hooked beak. Falcons have a notch on their maxilla, behind the tip of the upper beak, which forms the tomial tooth that is believed to enable them to easily sever the neck of vertebrate prey. It is important to preserve the tomial tooth when performing any repairs or trimming of the beak.[71] If cracks appear in the beak, these should be filed back above the start of the crack.[8] Overgrowth of the upper beak is seen in raptors on a diet exclusively of day-old chicks.[29]

Feathers, Skin, and Glands

With the exception of the northern harrier (*Circus cyaneus*), American kestrel (*Falco sparverius*), and merlin (*Falco columbarus*), the plumage of North American raptors is not sexually dimorphic.[71]

The integrity of the primary remiges and tail rectrices is of the utmost importance for flight performance in species destined for release.[61] Tail feathers of hospitalized raptors should be protected from breakage and soiling by using a tail guard made from an envelope of heavy paper or file folders placed over the tail feathers and affixed to the covert feathers with adhesive tape (Figure 17-1). The technique of feather repair (or imping), involving total or partial feather replacement or splinting may be very beneficial in hastening the return of flight after feather damage.[61]

Most raptors molt their feathers in symmetrical pairs, one from the right and one from the left, once per year in the early summer, usually after breeding. This graduated symmetrical molt means that only a slight flying handicap exists during the 6 months required for molting.[71] The steppe buzzard (*Buteo buteo vulpinus*) exhibits bizarre chaotic molt pattern.[12] Molting in Old World vultures may extend up to 2 to 3 years.[8] Some species such as goshawks and eagles molt only partially each year, which permits some degree of distinguishing second- and third-year birds. Once adult plumage is obtained, age cannot be determined by plumage characteristics.[52]

Induction of molting has been achieved by manipulating the photoperiod or by oral administration of exogenous thyroid hormone. The photoperiod is advanced to 18 to 20 hours of light per day after a period of 4 to 6 weeks of less than 10 hours of light per day. Molting will start within a few weeks and may be completed over 4 to 5 months. The onset and rate of molt with thyroxine administration tends to be very rapid, some birds losing most of their flight feathers nearly simultaneously. Quality of regrown feathers from a forced molt often is less than natural molts.[71] Increased ambient temperature may speed up molting, and corticosteroids may retard the progression of a molt.[8]

As in other avian species, stress marks appear as lines across one or more feathers because of an interruption in the normal flow of nutrients during its growth. Cystine deficiency may lead to weak and broken feathers.[8,71]

The "pinching off" syndrome is described as follows: normal growth of a feather occurs for one-half to two thirds of its normal

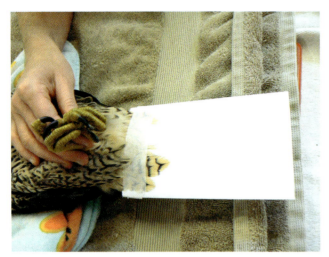

FIGURE 17-1 Tail guard made from an envelope of heavy paper placed over the tail feathers and affixed to the covert feathers with adhesive tape.

growth, after which blood supply withdraws and the feather pinches off in a characteristic hour-glass presentation. The cause of the syndrome has been attributed to quill mites and to viral or genetic etiology.[44,71]

Skin sweat glands are absent. Infection of the uropygial gland is rare in raptors, but adenocarcinoma and blockage may occur.[8] The adrenal glands are paired structures except in a few species such as the bald eagle (*Haliaetus leucocephalus*) that has fused glands.[61]

In the Savanna hawk (*Buteogallus meridionalis*), the supraorbital or salt gland, a paired glandular structure with ducts opening in the nasal cavity, contributes to water and electrolyte homeostasis.[39]

The Harris' hawk (*Parabuteo unicinctus*) is the only species of raptors that shows psychological feather plucking, and a temporary beak modification technique to prevent self-mutilation in this species has been described.[8,64]

Seborrhea sicca (dry skin) is encountered in eagles, especially on the feet of captive birds.[8,12] Large pealike subcutaneous abscesses caused by staphylococci are frequently seen in raptors.[8] Other skin infections are relatively uncommon in birds of prey.[12] Papillomatosis is occasionally seen on the feet and eyelids of raptors.[12]

Feet

Raptors use their feet to capture their prey. They have thick scales to protect their feet from injury and strong toes that terminate in strongly curved triangular talons.[20] Hard papillae on the plantar surface assist in grasping.[12] Vultures do not need to capture live animals, so their talons are blunt.[12]

The digital flexor tendons have unidirectional, interlocking ratcheting mechanisms that resist digital extension when the toes are clenched, a mechanism that makes it difficult to pry open the feet of a restrained raptor.[52]

Ospreys (*Pandion haliaetus*) have enlarged, highly curved talons, with specialized little spines (spicules) on the ventral surface of the foot, which enable them to grab and hold slippery fish. Ospreys also have the ability to swivel their fourth digit to the rear, making them semi-zygodactylous. All the other Falconiformes species are anisodactyl and perch with three digits forward and one backward.[8]

The talon of the third digit has a specialized sharp edge on the medial side, used for feather grooming, which should be preserved during any trimming and reshaping.[71] To trim the talons and beak, guillotine-type nail clippers, utility knife, flat and round metal files, or hand-held Dremel hand drill may be used.[61]

Talons may be accidentally torn off. Treatment is accomplished by quickly controlling bleeding, painting the surface with a protective material (e.g., fingernail polish), and affixing a protective cover such as plastic syringe case, vinyl nail caps, or multiple layers of cyanoacrylate glue, with either antibiotic powder and talcum powder or fine sodium bicarbonate powder.[61,71] Regrowth of a talon will take up to 6 months.[71]

Nares

Nares of falcons, *Buteo* species, and eagles have a bony baffle, or operculum, thought to facilitate air flow in the nostrils during high-speed flight.[71]

Gastrointestinal Tract

All Falconiformes species, except the bearded vulture, have a crop for the storage of food.[31] The stomach of raptors is simple. The pH of the stomach is approximately 1.0 in diurnal raptors prior to eating (1.7 in hawks), and they are capable of digesting bones.[12] The ceca is absent or vestigial.[71] The gall bladder is usually present.[8] The small pancreas is located within the duodenal loop.[12] The cloaca is similar to other avian species.[71]

Escherichia coli, *Proteus* spp., coagulase-negative *Staphylococcus* sp., *Micrococcus* sp., *Corynebacterium* sp., *Bacillus* sp., *Streptococcus* sp., and *Salmonella* sp. have been isolated from the lower intestines, cloaca, and fecal samples of healthy raptors.[12,37]

Respiratory System

The epiglottis is absent, and the trachea contains complete cartilaginous rings.[71] Normal flora of the choana should be predominantly gram positive, including coagulase-negative *Staphylococcus* sp., *Micrococcus* sp., *Corynebacterium* sp., and *Pasteurella* sp.[8,37]

Urogenital System

In contrast to other birds, many Falconiformes of the families Cathartidae, Accipitridae, and Falconidae have two ovaries and two oviducts. It seems unlikely that both ovaries are fully functional.[61] No phallus is present.[8]

Musculoskeletal Anatomy

Many good diagrams of the anatomy of the wing and pelvic limb of raptors are available.[8,39] The femur and humerus are usually pneumatized.[8] In the genus *Falco*, two sesamoid bones are present in the metacarpophalangeal joint and one sesamoid bone in the interphalangeal joint of the major digit. Two intratendinous ossifications are present in the region of the carpometacarpus and the major digit.[39] An *os prominens* is present at the cranial margin of the carpus in *Buteo* and *Accipiter*, articulating with the distal radius.[39] In falcons, the tarsometatarsus has a medullary cavity running the whole length of the bone. In hawks and eagles, the medullary cavity is absent from the proximal third of the tarsometatarsus.[8]

HOUSING

Both indoor facilities (called *mews*) and outdoor facilities should be provided. Minimum dimensions for a typical 1-kilogram (kg) raptor housed singly are 2 × 3 × 2.5 meters (m) high.[71] Shade is important. Some species, including highly migratory species, small-sized *Accipiter* species, and southern temperate zone species (e.g., Harris' hawk), cannot tolerate cold and must have supplemental heat when the ambient temperature drops below 0° C. Eagles, red-tailed hawks, goshawks, and most falcons may tolerate extreme cold, as long as they are protected from wind.[52] Temperature tolerance guidelines and minimum size requirements have been established for many species.[29] Water must be provided at all times for drinking and bathing.

Accipiter cannot be housed with other species, and the sexes of merlins and Northern goshawks (*Accipiter gentilis*) should be housed separately, since the larger female may kill her mate. A table of compatible species has been published.[8,71]

Perches must be considered carefully with regard to size, shape, covering materials, and placement to maintain foot health and comfort. Falcons require broad, flat perches, covered with artificial turf, whereas buteos and goshawks are maintained on perches elliptical in cross-section, sized proportionately to their feet, and wrapped with sisal rope.[71] Multiple perches may be detrimental if the birds hop with hard landing, rather than flying, subjecting their feet to bruising.[52]

FEEDING AND NUTRITIONAL DISORDERS

All raptors are carnivores. Most Falconiformes obtain a lot of their total daily fluid intake with their food, but they should have access to fresh drinking water daily.[8]

The smaller raptors eat approximately 20% of their body weight daily, the medium-sized birds eat approximately 10% to 15% of their body weight, and the large birds eat 6% to 8% of their body weight. Regular weighing of birds is important to ensure adequate dietary intake.[71] When assist-feeding or force-feeding, the stomach capacity of raptors is 40 milliliters per kilogram (mL/kg).[32] Hills A/D (Topeka, KS) or Oxbow Carnivore care (Murdock, NE) may be tube-fed in anorectic birds.

A reduction in food intake is observed in warm weather. A bird that is stressed or has additional energy requirements (e.g., during breeding or molting) will benefit from additional essential amino acids and vitamins. Breeding females should receive calcium and vitamin D_3 supplement. Raptor chicks are born with little or no gut flora, and enteritis with bacterial overgrowth is common. The use of probiotics in the first 14 days will reduce such infections.[8]

Several raptor species egest (regurgitate) castings composed of the undigested remains of the bones and fur of their prey.[71] The casting material is usually regurgitated 12 to 18 hours after ingestion, but hawks may eat more than one meal before casting.[12,32]

Raptors need a diet consisting of the whole bodies of prey species such as domestic quails, chicks, mice, rabbits, and other small birds and rodents. Pigeons are a special risk to raptors because of their high prevalence of trichomoniasis and should be frozen and thawed before feeding.[8]

Buzzards have a nonspecialized diet and may be scavengers.[8] Vultures are obligatory scavengers that may encounter long periods of food deprivation between feedings.[39] Most vultures tend to have a calcium-deficient diet because they usually ingest meat and viscera. They depend on large predators to provide them with bone fragments.[12] Ospreys require fish. If frozen fish are to be used for food, thiamine needs to be supplemented at 1 to 3 mg/kg.[12]

A fatty liver–kidney syndrome of merlins, possibly from excessive feeding of day-old chicks and inbreeding, has been recognized.[12]

Small raptors, particularly *Accipiter*, are prone to neurologic signs and collapse from hypoglycemia if deprived of food or flown too light in weight on a cold or windy day.[8]

Bird presenting with neurologic signs that have been fed an all-meat diet should be given glucose, B vitamins (particularly thiamine), vitamin A, and calcium supplementation.[71]

Young secretary birds (*Sagittarius serpentarius*) fed on standard raptor diets may suffer a calcium-to-phosphorus imbalance because their principal food in the wild is snakes, which are high in calcium phosphate.[12]

Secondary nutritional hyperparathyroidism (metabolic bone disease) occurs in raptors, and clinical signs are similar to those seen in other avian species. Raptors need vitamin D_3, and they cannot utilize vitamin D_2.[12] The calcium-to-phosphorus ratio should be 2:1. This disease, which is problematic in captive raptors, has also been encountered among free-flying vultures in regions where other large predators that would normally crush the bones in carcasses have been eliminated or when parents select pieces of china or plastic instead of bone to supplement the diet of their chicks.[52,61]

Thiamine deficiency is associated with loss of appetite, "star gazing," muscle weakness, tremors, opisthotonus, seizures, and death. Thiamine deficiency is most commonly observed in juveniles consuming all-meat diets or piscivorous birds fed thawed fish.[71]

Treatment includes thiamine by intramuscular injection and diet supplementation. The derangement may become permanent and unresponsive to therapy if not dealt with immediately.[71]

Vitamin A deficiency causes similar signs as in other species, including white pustules along the mouth, esophagus, crop, and nasal passages; caseous nodules blocking salivary glands, syrinx, or the area under the eyelids; xerophthalmia; polyuria or polydipsia; gout; reduced egg and sperm production; hyperkeratosis of plantar surface of feet, which predisposes to bumblefoot; and reduced immune response leading to diseases such as aspergillosis.[71]

Signs of vitamin E deficiency include poor muscle function, muscular dystrophy, spastic leg paralysis, degeneration of pipping muscle in neonates with poor hatchability, spraddle legs, muscle twitching, encephalomalacia, incoordination, torticollis, testicular degeneration, infertility, and steatitis.[71]

RESTRAINT AND HANDLING

Falconry hoods block visual stimuli and have a calming effect, resulting in slower heart rate.[12] Alternatively, the bird's head may be covered with a lightweight towel or cloth.

The feet of raptors must be the first concern for restraint. However, falcons and vultures bite fiercely, as do some eagles.[52] Once restrained, the index finger of the handler should always be placed between the bird's legs to prevent injuries to the legs and provide a good grip.

Methods to restrain hooded raptors from the fist or wild raptors in a box or from a perch have been described.[8,61] Condors, large vultures, and eagles should be captured and restrained by two persons. The use of protective gloves is recommended. One person approaches the bird from behind and above with a large blanket and covers the bird, finding the upper legs through the blanket and quickly restraining one leg in each hand. The bird is then lifted and the wings tucked between each arms into the handler's body. The second person may restrain the head as soon as possible (Figure 17-2). Vultures may regurgitate food from their crop when handled.[61]

Capture myopathy has been reported in secretary birds. Clinical signs include depression, limb paresis or paralysis, hock-sitting, lateral or sternal recumbency, and death.[61]

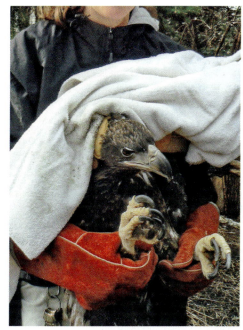

FIGURE 17-2 Two-person manual restraint of an eagle.

Some kites and hawks will lie in sternal recumbency and feign death when approached.

ANESTHESIA

It is difficult—if not impossible—to conduct an adequate physical examination on a struggling raptor. Raptors should be fasted for 6 to 8 hours before anesthesia.[61] Isoflurane is administered as in other avian species, via a facemask, intubation, an air sac cannula, or a chamber. Arrhythmias with the use of isoflurane have been reported in bald eagles.[2] Sevoflurane may also be used.

Injectable anesthetics are unreliable and should only be used if gaseous anesthesia is not available. Ketamine with xylazine has been reported as effective in raptors but has also caused deaths attributed to severe sinus bradycardia.[61] Intravenous (IV) ketamine may cause convulsions, prolonged apnea, or immediate cardiac arrest in a number of raptors.[61] When using xylazine alone, raptors may show a hypersensitivity to external stimuli.[61] Tiletamine zolazepam (Telazol) is suitable to produce anesthesia via parenteral injection.[39] Death with the use of alphaxalone has been reported in red-tailed hawks, with high prevalence of sinus arrest and tachycardia.[12] Use of continuous rate infusion (CRI) propofol has been studied in red-tailed hawks; it had minimal effects on blood pressure, but effective ventilation was reduced. Prolonged recovery periods with moderate-to-severe excitatory central nervous system (CNS) signs may occur in this species with propofol.[28] Ketamine or tiletamine zolazepam have been used orally in bait.[39,61] Buprenorphine does not appear to be effective in birds of prey.[12] The author of this chapter prefers to use butorphanol as an analgesic, but the frequent administration needed sometimes negates the benefits in highly stressed birds.

SURGERY

Surgical conditions in raptors are similar to those in other avian species. Some details of orthopedic surgical techniques are covered later in this chapter. Whole limb amputation usually causes bumblefoot on the remaining foot.[8] A scale has been established to serve as a guide to surgeons for digit amputation. If the bird is missing both second digits, one or both halluxes, or all of these parts, it is considered not releasable.[10] In male raptors, loss of a wing may be problematic, as the male bird uses its wings to maintain its position on the female during mating.[8]

DIAGNOSTICS

The hematologic assessment may be accomplished by drawing blood from the basilic, metatarsal, ulnar, or right jugular veins. Packed cell volume (PCV) and total plasma solids may be determined, and a blood smear is used for differential counts as well as for detecting parasites and cellular abnormalities.[12,71] Many publications have described the reference values for hematology and biochemistry in many species of Falconiformes.[8,61]

Raptors show a predominantly heterophilic leukogram with leukocytes similar to other avian species. Falconiformes species have relatively large erythrocytes (up to 16 ×8 micrometers [μm]). Mild heterophilia without severe toxic changes, lymphopenia, or both might indicate stress in raptors.[12] California condors demonstrate a unique stress leukogram, with white blood cell (WBC) counts ranging between 25 and 30 ×10^3, thus masking leukocytosis associated with infection.[15]

Since elevated plasma uric acid concentrations occur postprandially in healthy raptors, blood for uric acid analysis should not be taken until 24 hours after the last meal.[8] Increased plasma urea concentration is observed in dehydrated individuals. In prerenal function disorders the ratio between urea and uric acid is high (>6.5 in peregrine falcon).[39]

Protein electrophoresis has been shown to play an important role in the diagnosis of chlamydophilosis and aspergillosis in raptors and species-specific reference values are available.[23,36,61] Falcons with confirmed aspergillosis possibly show lower serum prealbumin values compared with healthy falcons.[36]

Radiography is an important diagnostic tool. The caudoplantar view of the foot is particularly useful in assessing chronic bumblefoot.[61] Gastrointestinal (GI) tract contrast study using fluoroscopy may be performed with the bird standing on a perch or in a cardboard box. Barium sulfate is administered orally at 0.025 to 0.05 milliliter per gram (mL/g) bodyweight. Falcons and hawks have an empty tract after 8 hours.[61] In raptors, a recent meal would fill the proventriculus and gizzard and spread the liver shadow, making the liver appear larger, and this must be differentiated from pathologic changes.[8] Cardiac size during radiographic examination has been studied in some Falconiformes.[4] IV iohexol increases the contrast of the kidneys.[8]

Reference values for B-mode (two-dimensional) echocardiography have been reported for some diurnal raptors.[61] Electrocardiographic (ECG) reference values have been published for conscious golden eagles (*Aquila chrysaetos*) and buzzards (*Buteo buteo*) anesthetized with isoflurane.[16,27]

Microbiologic examination may consist of cultures taken from the oral pharynx and trachea and from freshly voided feces.[61] Castings may be used for parasitologic or microbiologic investigations as well as be radiographed to detect metallic objects.[12]

Comprehensive urinalysis data from healthy falcons have been published.[70] Most raptors are positive for blood in urine because of their meat diet. Severe liver disease (e.g., falcon herpes virus) or inanition may increase the secretion of biliverdin, which results in lime-green urine and urates.[12,61] Screening for intestinal parasites is done through fecal examination—both direct smear as well as flotation.

In falcons, the "stress or endurance test" may be performed for the assessment of air sacculitis. After 5 to 10 minutes of rest, the falcon is allowed to fly suspended from a leash for an average of 30 seconds. If the bird requires longer than 2 to 3 minutes to return to normal, radiology or endoscopy is indicated.[61]

Endoscopic examination or biopsy is best performed by a lateral approach through the caudal thoracic air sac into the abdominal air sac.[39]

Mydriasis for ophthalmic examination may be performed with the use of anesthesia with isoflurane.[39] Topical application of the neuromuscular blocking agent rocuronium bromide (0.12 mg per eye) induces mydriasis without adverse effects in European kestrels (*Falco tinnunculus*).[5] Mean intraocular pressure values have been published for some Falconiformes species.[54]

Computed tomography (CT) may be used to demonstrate the lesions of aspergillosis and the structures of the head.[12] Magnetic resonance imaging (MRI) has been shown to be superior to radiography in evaluating spinal cord trauma in bald eagles.[66]

THERAPEUTICS

Only a few pharmacokinetic studies, including those for terbinafine, marbofloxacin, enrofloxacin, itraconazole, piperacillin, and tramadol, have been performed in raptors.[7,22,26,34,56,65] A formulary for Falconiformes, with information collated from personal experiences and many textbooks and journals, is provided in Table 17-1. Drug toxicities are covered later in this chapter. Maintenance fluid requirement is 40 to 60 mL/kg/day. A maximal fluid administration rate of 80 to 90 mL/kg/hr may be used for shock therapy. Boluses of fluids at 10 mL/kg/min are well tolerated and usually yield satisfactory results.[32]

INFECTIOUS DISEASES

The most common bacterial, fungal, and viral infections of Falconiformes are summarized in Table 17-2. Aspergillosis is covered under management-related diseases.

Text continued on p. 136

TABLE 17-1

Formulary of Drugs Used in Falconiformes

Drug (Generic)	Dose (mg/kg)	Frequency	Route	Comments
ANTIBIOTICS				
Amikacin	15	BID	IM	
Amoxicillin	150	BID	IM/PO	
Amoxicillin/clavulanic acid	150	BID	PO	
Amoxicillin-LA	150	SID	IM	
Ampicillin	15	BID	IM	
Carbenicillin	100-200	TID	IM	
Cefazolin	50-100	BID	IM/PO	
Cefotaxime	75-100	BID	IM	
Cephalexin	40-100	TID/QID	IM/PO	
Cephalothin	100	BID	IM	
Chloramphenicol	50	TID	IM	
Ciprofloxacin	50	BID	PO	
Clindamycin	50-100	SID-BID	PO	
Clofazimine	1.5	SID	PO	For tuberculosis
Cloxacillin	250	BID	PO	
Cycloserine	5	BID	PO	For tuberculosis
Doxycycline	50	BID	PO	
Enrofloxacin	15	SID-BID	IM/PO	Can cause emesis/anorexia
Erythromycin	60	BID	PO	
Ethambutol	20	BID	PO	For tuberculosis
Gentamicin	2.5	TID	IM	
Lincomycin	50-75	BID	IM/PO	Intra-articular 0.25-0.5 ml
Marbofloxacin	10	SID	PO	In Eurasian buzzards
Metronidazole	50	SID	PO	
Oxytetracycline	25-50	TID	IM/PO	
Long-acting injection	50-200	Every 3-5 days	IM	
Piperacillin	100	QID	IM	In red-tailed hawks
Ticarcillin	200	BID	IM	
Tobramycin	5-10	BID	IM	
Trimethoprim-sulfadiazine	20-30	BID	SC	
	60	BID	PO	
Tylosin	30	BID	IM	
ANTIPROTOZOALS/ANTIHELMINTICS				
Amprolium	30	SID	PO	Thiamine deficiency (merlins)
Carnidazole	20-25	Once	PO	
Chloroquine	20-25	Once	PO	Use with primaquine
	10-15	At 12, 24, 48 hours		
Chlorsulon	20	Every 2 weeks × 3 doses	PO	
Clazuril	5-10	Every 3 days ×3 doses or SID × 2 days	PO	
Doramectin	1		SC/IM	
Fenbendazole	20-25	SID	PO	
	100,	Once		
Ivermectin	0.2-1.0	Every 14 days × 2-3	SC/IM/PO	
Levamisole	20-40	Once	PO	
	10-20	Once	SC	
Mebendazole	20	SID	PO	
Mefloquine	30	At 0, 12, 24, 48, 72 hours, then weekly	PO	

Continued

TABLE 17-1

Formulary of Drugs Used in Falconiformes—cont'd

Drug (Generic)	Dose (mg/kg)	Frequency	Route	Comments
Metronidazole	50-100	SID	PO	
Moxidectin	0.5	Once	PO	
Praziquantel	5-10 or 50	SID; repeat in 14 days	PO/SC/IM	
Primaquine	0.75-1.0	Once or SID ×2	PO	Use with chloroquine
Pyrantel	20	Once	PO	
Pyrimethamine	0.25-0.5	BID	PO	
Quinacrine	5-10	SID	PO/IM	
Toltrazuril (Baycox)	15-25	SID ×2 days or every other day ×3 doses	PO	Repeat in 2 weeks
LEAD TREATMENT				
Calcium-EDTA	50-100	BID	IV/IM	
Dimercaptosuccinic acid	30	BID	PO	5 days on/2 days off (3–5 weeks)
D-Penicillamine	55	BID	PO	
Vitamin C	250	SID	PO	
Zinc	25	SID	PO	
ANTIFUNGALS				
Amphotericin B	1.5	TID	IV (slow)	With 10–15 mL/kg fluids
Fluconazole	5	SID–BID	PO	
Flucytosine	20-30 40-50	QID TID	PO	
Itraconazole	Prophylaxis: 10 Therapeutic: 10-15	BID for 5 days; then SID for 3 weeks	PO	Gyrfalcons only 8 mg/kg; anorexia or regurgitation
Ketoconazole	60 25	BID BID	PO IM	
Nystatin	300,000 Units/kg	BID-TID	PO	
Terbinafine	22	SID	PO	In red-tailed hawks
Voriconazole	10-15	BID	PO	
SEDATIVES/ANESTHETICS/ANALGESICS				
Alphaxalone	5-10		IV	Deaths in red-tailed hawks
Atropine	0.1	Every 3–4 hours	IV/IM	
Butorphanol	1-4	TID–QID	IM	
Diazepam	0.5-1.5	As needed	IV/IM	
Ketamine	5-30 May be given with medetomidine at low end of dose		IM	May cause cardiac arrest or apnea or convulsions; 100 mg/kg in a piece of meat
Medetomidine	0.15-0.35 (with ketamine)		IM	Atipamezole to reverse
Midazolam	0.5-1.0	TID	IV/IM	
Propofol	1.33		IV	1 mg/kg/min CRI
Tiletamine/Zolazepam	5-30		IM	80 mg/kg in an oral bait
Tramadol	5	BID	PO	In bald eagles
Xylazine	1.0-2.2 (with ketamine)		IV/IM	Yohimbine to reverse
ANTI-INFLAMMATORIES AND STEROIDS				
Carprofen	1-2	SID-BID	PO/IM	
Dexamethasone	0.5-2.0	One dose	IV/IM	
Flunixin meglumine	1-10	SID	IM	
Ketoprofen	1-5	SID	IM	
Meloxicam	0.5	BID	IM/PO	
Methylprednisolone acetate	0.5-1.0	Once	IM	
Prednisolone sodium succinate	10-20	Once	IM/IV	
Triamcinolone	0.1-0.2	Once	IM	

TABLE 17-1

Formulary of Drugs Used in Falconiformes—cont'd

Drug (Generic)	Dose (mg/kg)	Frequency	Route	Comments
NEBULIZATION				
Amphotericin B	100 mg in 15 mL saline			
Clotrimazole	7%-10% solution			With 5% DMSO in polyethylene glycol
Enrofloxacin	100 mg in 10 mL saline			
Enilconazole	1 mL in 9 mL saline			
Gentamicin	50 mg in 10 mL saline			
Terbinafine	1 mg in 1 mL saline			
MISCELLANEOUS				
Acyclovir	333	BID	PO	
	80	TID	PO	
Aminoloid	0.25-0.75	Once, repeat in 14 days	IM	Induction of molt
Biotin	0.05	SID (30–60 days)	PO	Aid in beak or claw regrowth
Calcium glubionate	25-150	BID	PO	
Calcium gluconate/ borogluconate 10%	1-5 mL/kg	Once	IV/SC	
Cisapride	0.25	TID	PO	
Dextrose 50%	1-2 mL/kg	As needed	IV slowly	
Doxapram	10	Once	IV	
Dinoprost	0.02-0.1	Once	Topical	On cloaca; for egg binding
Furosemide	0.5-2.0	As needed - QID	IV/IM	
Imidocarb dipropionate	5	Once, repeat in 1 week	IM	To treat *Babesia shortii*
Iron dextran	10	Weekly	IM (deep)	
Isoxsuprine	5-10	SID	PO	For wing tip edema
Lactulose	0.5 mL	As needed	PO	
Leuprolide acetate	250 µg/kg	Every 14–21 days	IM	
Mannitol	0.25-2.0		IV slowly	
Metoclopramide	2	TID	IV/IM/PO	
Oxytocin	3-5 IU/kg		IM	
Pralidoxime chloride	100	Repeat after 6 hours	IM	
Propentofylline	5	BID	PO	For wing tip edema
Ranitidine	0.2-0.5	BID	IM	
Sucralfate	25	TID	PO	
Thiamine	10-50	SID	PO	
Thyroxine	100-800 µg/kg	Daily	PO	
Vitamin A	<20000 IU/kg	Weekly	IM	
Vitamin B complex	10-30 (of thiamine)	Every other day-weekly	IM	
Vitamin E/selenium	0.05 mg selenium and 3.4 IU vitamin E	Repeat at 72 hours	SC	
Vitamin K$_1$	0.2-2.2	TID, then SID	IM	

From references 7, 8, 12, 14, 22, 26, 28, 29, 32, 34, 39, 52, 56, 61, 65, and 71.

BID, Twice daily; *DMSO,* dimethyl sulfoxide; *EDTA,* ethylenediaminetetraacetic acid; *IM,* intramuscularly; *IU/kg,* international units per kilogram; *IV,* intravenously; *µg/kg,* microgram per kilogram; *mL/kg,* milliliter per kilogram; *PO,* by mouth; *QID,* four times daily; *SC,* subcutaneously; *SID,* once daily.

TABLE 17-2

Infectious Diseases of Falconiformes

Agents	Hosts	Clinical Signs/Pathology	Transmission	Diagnostic	Treatment/Prevention
BACTERIA/FUNGI					
Mycobacterium avium/intracellulare complex and *M. genavense* (avian tuberculosis)	Uncommon in raptors in North America; endemic other parts of the world	Chronic wasting disease affecting liver, intestines, lungs, bone marrow, and subcutis	Direct contact	Leukocytosis (heterophilia/monocytosis); acid-fast staining of feces/bone marrow/biopsy of tubercules; PCR; radiology; histopathology	Euthanasia recommended; combination of enrofloxacin, cycloserine, ethambutol, or clofazimine
Chlamydophila psittacii (chlamydophilosis)	Not common; antibodies detected in healthy free-ranging raptors	Sinusitis, rhinitis, air sacculitis, conjunctivitis, green stained urates, anorexia, weight loss; hepatomegaly, splenomegaly, pancreatic lesions in a red-tailed hawk	Direct contact	PCR ELISA Histopathology	Doxycycline Azithromycin
Clostridium perfringens (enterotoxemia)	All	Acute death or diarrhea, dehydration, shock; severe hemorrhagic enteritis, liver necrosis, acute heart muscle degeneration	Endogenous (GI tract flora) or toxin in food improperly managed (e.g., not properly frozen)	Gram stain on feces	Metronidazole; emptying of stomach; activated charcoal; supportive care; intravenous bovine hyperimmune serum
Bacillus anthracis (anthrax)	Rare	Vultures resistant	Raptors play role in epidemiology	Gram stain on feces (spores)	
Pasteurella multocida (fowl cholera)	All	Acute, septicemic disease; death in 24-36 hours Oral abscesses (*Buteo*)	Direct contact; recovered birds likely carriers		Penicillin G, cefazolin, trimethoprim-sulfa, amikacin; poultry vaccine
Mycoplasma spp.	In respiratory tract of healthy wild raptors	Air sacculitis, pneumonia; poly-arthritis in black vulture due to *M. corogypsi*			Tetracyclines; tylosin; spectinomycin; enrofloxacin
Candida albicans	Isolated from GI tract of healthy raptors	Anorexia, flinging food, regurgitation, diarrhea, weight loss; gray-green amorphous diphtheritic membranes in oral cavity and crop	Associated with malnutrition, prolonged use of antibiotics, and poor husbandry	Cytology (Diff-Quik or Gram stain); culture (Sabouraud agar)	Nystatin; miconazole gel directly to esophagus or crop; ketoconazole; itraconazole; fluconazole
Malassezia sp.	Harris' hawks	Feather loss; greasy skin			
VIRUSES					
Herpesvirus (fatal hepatosplenitis or inclusion body disease)	Falconid HV1 (mainly gyrfalcons and hybrids); Accipitrid-HV1 (*Accipiter*)	Weakness, anorexia, regurgitation, lime green urates, diarrhea, sudden death; necrosis of liver and spleen; eosinophilic intranuclear inclusion bodies; viral stomatitis	Virus has crossed over the adapted host barrier from pigeons to accidental falcon host; some birds may be latent carriers	Profound leukopenia 24-48 hours preceding death Virus isolation Histopathology	No treatment; avoid feeding contaminated pigeons; attenuated herpesvirus vaccine (Central Veterinary Research Laboratory, Dubai)

	Species affected	Clinical signs	Transmission	Diagnosis	Treatment/Prevention
Adenovirus	Nonnative, tropical falcons reared in temperate zones and fed poultry	Sudden death or acute illness (2–4 days) with anorexia and lethargy; basophilic intranuclear inclusions in spleen, liver, intestine, and pancreas	Fecal–oral route and aerosols; peregrine falcons are possible reservoirs	Histopathology PCR	No treatment. Avoid co-housing of nestling falcon species; quarantine and strict hygiene
Poxvirus	All	Dry/cutaneous form; nodular encrustations on cere, eyelids, and feet that progress through papule to vesicles, pustules, then scabs; no clinical signs unless obstructing mouth or eye; common bacterial and *Candida* infections	Biting arthropods (mosquitoes) or direct contact with infected birds or fomites	Histologic examination of biopsies: ballooning of epithelial cells and intracytoplasmic inclusion (Bollinger bodies); electron microscopy	Topical antiseptic compounds, vitamin A, and systemic antibiotics; surgical removal; usually self-limiting; pigeonpox or turkeypox vaccines; attenuated falconpox vaccine in Middle East; insecticide spray to reduce vectors
Newcastle disease	Falcons in Middle East; Vultures resistant except bearded vultures	Fatal; GI signs and later CNS signs; vomiting of semi-digested blood; petechial hemorrhages in GI tract; death in captive bearded vultures	Close contact or consumption of contaminated food (poultry or pigeons) Insects, rodents, and humans are potential mechanical vectors	Virus isolation	Commercial vaccine used for poultry (should not be given to birds intended for release); new falcon vaccine in Middle East
West Nile virus	Prevalence highest in red-tailed hawks, Cooper's hawks, goshawks, and golden eagles	Lethargy, cachexia, ataxia, tremors, seizures, visual impairment; chronic disease/death due to myocarditis (goshawks), lymphoplasmacytic and histiocytic encephalitis, endophthalmitis and pancreatitis	*Culex* mosquitoes Birds are primary vertebrate reservoir hosts	Heterophilia; IgM-capture enzyme-linked immunosorbent assay; plaque reduction neutralization test; virus isolation	Supportive Vaccines (West Nile Innovator—Fort Dodge)
Influenza virus	All	Low pathogenic/fatal highly pathogenic	Direct contact or ingestion of prey		

From references 8, 12, 39, 42, 51, 52, 58, 60, 61, 62, 63, 68, 69, 71.
CNS, Central nervous system; ELISA, enzyme-linked immunosorbent assay; GI, gastrointestinal; IgM, immunoglobulin M; PCR, polymerase chain reaction.

Parasitic Diseases

Ectoparasites

Most ectoparasites are commensal on raptors. With debilitation or stress, their numbers may increase resulting in immunosuppression and anemia. Pyrethrin and fipronil sprays effectively kill most ectoparasites.[71] Multiple lice species have been reported in Falconiformes, including *Crasperdorrhynchus, Laemobothrion, Colpocephalum, Degeeriella,* and *Falcolipeurus.*[12,43,61] Flea infestations are generally rare in raptors, but a number of species are sometimes found in the nests of Falconiformes. The stickfast flea *Echidnophaga gallinacea* actually attaches itself to the skin of the host.[12] Ticks are occasionally found on raptors, on the less feathered parts of the head and under the thighs. Subcutaneous hemorrhage and edema of the head have been reported with *Ixodes ricinus* in captive birds of prey.[19] Blow-fly larvae infestation (myiasis) may be found in the external auditory canals of nestling raptors, especially hawks, but usually they do not cause permanent damage. They should be mechanically removed with forceps by placing a drop of mineral oil or saline in the ear, forcing the worms to get their spiracles out into the open air for breathing. Wounds may also be affected by myasis.[12,71] The mite *Knemidokoptes* may affect the scales of feet and create the typical honey-combed skin. It should be treated with liquid paraffin and ivermectin.[8,12,41] The red mite *Dermanyssus gallinae* may be found on birds housed in wooden mews or in aviaries and may cause feather loss or broken feathers, mainly in juveniles. The preferred treatment is with ivermectin, and the premises should be sprayed with an insecticide.[8] A comprehensive checklist of parasitic mites of Falconiformes has been published.[49] Hippoboscidae (flat flies) such as *Ornithomyia avicularia* are commonly found on birds of prey and may cause significant blood loss in very young birds.[8] They may be removed manually or the raptor dusted with pyrethrin (0.5% to 2%), malathion (5%), or carbaryl (0.5%).[12]

Endoparasites

A review of endoparasites of raptors has been published.[39] The main endoparasites and blood parasites of Falconiformes are reviewed in Tables 17-3 and 17-4.

MANAGEMENT-RELATED DISEASES

Management failure is the main cause of bumblefoot and fungal infections such as aspergillosis.

Aspergillosis

One of the most devastating diseases of captive raptors is fungal infection of the respiratory system caused by *Aspergillus fumigatus.* Among North American raptors, goshawks, gyrfalcons, immature red-tailed hawks, and golden eagles are more likely to develop the disease. Raptors originating from arctic or subarctic climates, as well as ospreys and rough-legged buzzards (*Buteo lagopus*) are also reported as being particularly at risk.[12,61] Aspergillosis is one of the most important mortality causes in captive bearded vultures in the European Bearded Vulture Project.[39] Aspergillosis in gyrfalcons is a serious problem for falconers and becomes apparent when the birds are approximately 10 weeks of age.[61]

Aspergillosis is not transmissible among birds.[8] Infection occurs by inhalation of the ubiquitous spores. Acute aspergillosis is the product of inhalation of overwhelming numbers of spores from the environment, whereas the chronic forms usually develop as a result of low-level exposure coupled with compromised immune function caused by recent capture, change of ownership, poor ventilation, neonatal and geriatric conditions, corticosteroids, respiratory irritants, or lead poisoning.[61,71] Localized forms involve granuloma formation in the syrinx or the sinuses.[61]

The respiratory tract is most often affected, but the spores may migrate to other organs. Ocular and skin infections have been reported. The interclavicular air sac is more often affected in gyrfalcons than in other raptors. When respiratory signs or weight loss

become apparent, the disease usually has developed extensively.[61] An alteration or loss of voice is pathognomonic for the syringeal form of aspergillosis, and complete obstruction of the respiratory tract may occur.[8]

A diagnosis is made by observing elevated total WBC count (heterophilia and monocytosis), radiography, and deep tracheal or air sac cultures. Indirect enzyme-linked immunosorbent assay (ELISA) for *Buteo* species is available, but specific conjugates must be made for use in falcons and *Accipiter* species. A polymerase chain reaction (PCR)–based test is available in the United States. Protein electrophoresis may demonstrate an increase in β- and γ-globulins.[61] Endoscopic examination of the trachea and air sacs is invaluable in confirming the diagnosis and establishing the prognosis.[71]

One recommended treatment consists of oral itraconazole twice a day for 5 days and then once daily for 1 to 3 months; nebulization with clotrimazole, two 1-hour sessions per day for 4 to 8 weeks; and amphotericin B given intratracheally or injected into posterior thoracic air sacs (percutaneous puncture—approximately 1 mg/kg diluted to 1–3 mL in water—or applied directly to air sac lesions via endoscope). Amphotericin B may also be administered intravenously.[71] Voriconazole may be given orally, 1 hour before or after feeding, twice a day for 4 days, followed by once-a-day administration.[14] A liquid form may also be concurrently nebulized.[66] Fluconazole appears to be ineffective.[8] A 1:250 dilution of F10 has been used to nebulize raptors with aspergillosis, alone or in combination with oral itraconazole.[61] Birds with severe respiratory signs have a poor prognosis, and surgical removal of localized lesions is needed.[71]

Prophylaxis using itraconazole for 3 to 4 weeks is recommended for captive-held raptors undergoing a change in management and for injured raptors after admission to a rehabilitation center. For young gyrfalcons 40 to 45 days of age, daily administration of itraconazole or terbinafine is initiated and continued until the onset of cooler weather.[52,71]

Bumblefoot

Bumblefoot is a degenerative, inflammatory foot condition most often found in Falconidae. The condition is initiated by abnormal pressures placed on the bird's feet by improperly shaped perches or inappropriate perching substrate and housing arrangements. In rare instances, the condition may result from trauma. Inactivity, lack of exercise, and hypovitaminosis A may play a role in the occurrence of bumblefoot.[71] Infection is usually secondary. The bacterium most commonly isolated is *Staphylococcus aureus.* Other agents such as *Streptococcus* sp., *E. coli, Proteus* sp., *Pasteurella* spp., *Pseudomonas aeruginosa, Klebsiella* sp., *Clostridium* sp., *Corynebacterium* sp., *Nocardia* sp., *Actinomyces* sp., *Candida* sp. and *Aspergillus* sp. have also been isolated.[39,61] Bumblefoot has been classified by different authors into three stages or five stages.[12,47] Severely swollen feet should always be examined radiographically.[61]

The treatment of bumblefoot involves removal of the underlying causes and management of the wound. In early type 1 cases, application of skin tougheners (camphor spirits and tincture of benzoin) along with alteration of perch size or covering material will suffice.[71] It appears that bumblefoot types 1 and 2 may heal spontaneously if the bird is released or given freedom of a large aviary.[12] When ulceration, swelling, and inflammation have occurred, treatment involves surgical debridement, irrigation with sterile saline or 0.5% chlorhexidine, and protective ball bandaging or application of a custom-made polypropylene foam shoe. Culture and determination of antibiotic sensitivity is essential for systemic antibiotic selection. Cephalosporins, fluoroquinolones, lincomycin, and clindamycin typically yield the best results.[61,71] Swelling may be reduced 1 to 2 days prior to surgical debridement by the application of a cocktail of 0.5 mL dimethylsulfoxide, 0.2 mL dexamethasone, and 0.3 mL of enrofloxacin 100 mg/mL.[71] The use of slow-release antibiotic-impregnated methylmethacrylate beads in conjunction with surgical debridement and a course of systemic antibiotic therapy have improved the outcome of bumblefoot and reduced recurrence. Antibiotics that may be incorporated in the beads include piperacillin, rifampicin,

TABLE 17-3

Endoparasites of Falconiformes

Parasites	Hosts	Clinical Signs	Life Cycle	Treatment
Trichomonas gallinae (flagellate) (Frounce)	Wild pigeons; wild/captive raptors; wild peregrine falcons appear to have innate resistance	Yellow caseous plaques on tongue, pharynx, esophagus, crop (Figure 17-3); may invade sinuses, ear, trachea; liver necrosis; secondary *Pseudomonas aeruginosa*	Direct ingestion of infected pigeons; also direct contact or ingestion of contaminated food/ water	Metronidazole; carnidazole (some resistance reported); Surgery; Freeze pigeons for 24 hours
Caryospora spp.	*C. neofalconis* in juvenile merlins (UK)	Lethargy, weight loss, anorexia, green/bloody diarrhea; acute death	Direct and indirect; rodents are intermediate hosts	Clazuril; toltrazuril Prophylaxis: Clazuril at 17–20 days and 6 weeks of age
Sarcocystis spp. *Sarcocystis calchasi* sp. nova	All raptors; mortality in free-ranging bald and golden eagles (*S. falcatula*) Northern goshawk/ European sparrowhawk	Neurologic signs in Northern goshawk and golden eagle; usually inapparent; tissue cysts in muscles Fatal in pigeons; asymptomatic in raptors	Indirect; raptors are definitive or intermediate hosts; rodents are intermediate hosts Domestic pigeons are intermediate hosts	
Toxoplasma gondii	Usually resistant	Intermediate hosts (no clinical signs)	Feeding on other intermediate hosts	
Syngamus trachea *Cyathostoma* spp.	All	Obstruction of trachea, dyspnea, coughing, head shaking; *C. lari* in conjunctival sac and nasal or orbital cavities	Direct or via paratenic hosts (earthworms, snails, invertebrates)	Fenbendazole; mebendazole; thiabendazole; ivermectin; physical removal
Serratospiculum spp. or *Serrato-spiculoides* spp. (Filarid nematodes)	Falcons (*S. seurati* in tropical countries; *S. amaculata* in North America)	Found in air sacs; usually not pathogenic but can cause air sacculitis, peritonitis and death	Indirect; intermediate hosts: grasshoppers and beetles	Ivermectin; fenbendazole Removal of dead worms endoscopically is controversial
Capillaria spp.	All	White diphtheritic membranes in esophagus, crop, oral cavity, pharynx Mortalities in gyrfalcons	Direct or ingestion of paratenic hosts (mollusks, earthworms)	Mebendazole; fenbendazole; moxidectin; levamisole
Eucoleus aerophilus	Peregrine falcon	Fatal pneumonia		
Trichinella pseudospiralis	All raptors—rare	Adult worms in intestines; decreased reproduction in American kestrels; paralysis in Cooper's hawk	Direct (eating infected prey)	Fenbendazole
Ascarids	Pathogenic only in young raptors	Weight loss, ileus, intestinal impaction and rupture		Ivermectin; fenbendazole
Contracaecum spp. *Porrocaecum* spp.	May affect juvenile raptors	Usually in stomach; weight loss, intestinal obstruction	Insectivores are paratenic hosts	Ivermectin; fenbendazole
Cyrnea spp. *Synhimantus* spp. (spirurid nematodes)	All	Incidental finding in proventriculus; heavy infection with *S. laticeps* caused ulcers in a buzzard	Intermediate hosts are flies and beetles	Fenbendazole
Tapeworms: *Ligula* spp., *Cladotaenia* spp., *Paradilepis* spp.	All	Usually not pathogenic; heavy infestation of *C. globifera* caused ileus in buzzards	Intermediate hosts are rodents and fish	Praziquantel
Acanthocephalids: *Centrorhynchus kuntzi*, *C. spinosus*	Raptors are definitive hosts; may be pathogenic in juveniles	Asymptomatic; adults in small intestine; larvae in esophagus of kestrel and red-shouldered hawk	Intermediate hosts are rodents	
Flukes (Trematodes): *Strigea* spp., *Neodiplostomum* spp., *Nematostrigea* spp.	Mainly fish-eating birds; *N. serpens* is specific to osprey	Cholangitis, hepatitis; adults may be found in bile and pancreatic ducts; intestinal intussusception in kestrel	Indirect: two intermediate hosts (snail and vertebrate)	Praziquantel

From references 8, 12, 18, 38, 42, 43, 48, 53, 58, 66, 74.

amoxicillin, clindamycin, enrofloxacin, pefloxacin, and gentamicin. The beads may be left in place indefinitely and have caused no clinical problems for periods up to 1 year.[39] Meloxicam and carprofen are both useful for analgesia.[61] Some practitioners administer vitamin A routinely for bumblefoot.[12] Five elements are key for the prevention of bumblefoot: (1) providing a nutritious, balanced diet and preventing obesity; (2) providing perches of appropriate size, shape, and appropriate cover (e.g., Astroturf); (3) providing adequate maneuvering space for free-lofted birds so that they can land normally; (4) keeping the talons at appropriate lengths and blunting the talon tips of captive birds not used for hunting; and (5) providing exercise and observing the feet regularly to recognize the condition early.[61,71]

NONINFECTIOUS DISEASES

Toxicities

The use of organochlorines has been greatly restricted since the early 1970s because of their known negative effect on populations of raptors, including the peregrine falcons, European sparrow-hawks, and California condors.[12,15] The main toxicities in Falconiformes are summarized in Table 17-5.

Neoplasms

The reader is directed to a survey that reported 122 neoplasms of 39 types in 44 species of Falconiformes and Strigiformes.[39] Raptors may present with any type of neoplasia.

Trauma

Trauma is usually the most common cause of presentation of raptors in rehabilitation centers. Clinical signs associated with spinal trauma include flaccid paralysis of the pelvic limbs, inability to manipulate tail feathers, and loss of cloacal tone. Radiology is generally not useful initially, but increased areas of density may be seen 2 to 3 weeks after the injury.[71] MRI defines spinal damage more effectively.[66] Treatment consists of supportive care, including manual voiding of the cloaca at least once a day and short-acting steroids, which are

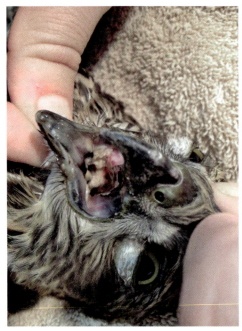

FIGURE 17-3 *Trichomonas gallinae* in the oral cavity of a goshawk.

TABLE 17-4

Blood Parasites of Falconiformes

Parasites	Hosts	Target Cells	Clinical Signs	Vectors	Treatment
Leucocytozoon spp. (*L. toddi* is the most common)	All raptors	Leukocytes and erythrocytes; cell-distorting (nucleus forming a crescent)	Non-pathogenic (adults) central nervous system disease or blindness in wild juvenile nankeen kestrels	Black flies (*Simulium* spp.)	Usually ineffective; quinacrine and trimethoprim or sulfamethoxazole
Hemoproteus spp. (*H. tinnunculus*, *H. brachiatus*, *H. elani*, *H. nisi*, *H. janovyi*)	All raptors; usually non-pathogenic	Erythrocytes; encircles the nuclei producing halter-shaped appearance	Severe anemia in Harris' hawks; prolonged rehabilitation time and higher mortality rate; reduced reproductive rate in kestrels	*Culicoides* spp.	Chloroquine and primaquine, followed by chloroquine every 24 hours for 1 week (to reduce parasitemia)
Plasmodium relictum (avian malaria)	All, but mainly gyrfalcons and hybrids	Erythrocytes; displace the nucleus	Depression and anorexia to severe dyspnea with sudden death; anemia, biliverdinuria, hepatomegaly, splenomegaly	Mosquitoes (Culicidae)	Mefloquine; chloroquine/ primaquine, then chloroquine at 12, 24, and 48 hours; prophylaxis with mefloquine or chloroquine or primaquine weekly
Hemogregarines or Trypanosomes		Nonpathogenic			
Babesia shortii	All prairie falcons		Blindness or mortality in prairie falcon nestlings	Ixodid ticks	Imidocarb dipropionate
Hepatozoon neophrontis	Black or Egyptian vultures, osprey, *Accipiter*	Large monocytes		Ticks	

From references 12, 39, 50, 53, 61, 71.

TABLE 17-5

Toxicities of Falconiformes

Toxicity	Species	Sources	Clinical Signs	Diagnostic	Treatment
Lead	All; common in California condors and eagles	Consumption of shot preys	Similar to other avian species; pathognomonic "holding hands" (rest on hocks with one foot grasping the other); proventricular dilatation, crop stasis	Whole blood lead levels (blood levels >0.4 ppm/40 µg/dL); Radiography	Ca EDTA; dimer-captosuccinic acid, vitamin C, zinc; removal of lead (gastric lavage or endoscopy)
Organophosphates or carbamates	UK: common buzzard, red kites North America: bald eagle; Mississippi kites	Cholinesterase-inhibiting compounds	Bradycardia, ataxia, weakness, salivation, paralysis, head tremors	Plasma B esterases	Atropine, supportive care, diazepam, pralidoxime
Alphachloralose	Eagles, buzzards, harriers	Pigeon bait	Incoordination, lethargy, death		Recover without treatment (24–36 hours)
Ammonium chloride	Falconry birds around Persian Gulf	To improve appetite and hunting ability	Vomit immediately after oral administration; if unable to vomit, death occurs from hyperammonemia		
Fenbendazole	African white-backed and lappet-faced vultures		Fatal; profound leukopenia; secondary septicemia		
Anticoagulants	All	Ingestion		Low packed cell volume	Therapy for blood loss; vitamin K₁
Diclofenac	Long-billed, slender-billed, and Oriental white-backed vultures	Ingestion: tissues of livestock	Decline in populations; severe visceral gout		
Mercury	Bald eagles (Great Lakes)		Levels capable of causing subclinical neurologic signs		

From references 3, 8, 9, 12, 15, 21, 39, 40, 46, 52, 55, 57, 59, 61, 71.
Ca EDTA, Calcium ethylenediaminetetraacetic acid; *µg/dL*, microgram per deciliter; *ppm*, parts per million.

thought to be effective only if given within 12 to 24 hours of the traumatic event. A withdrawal response within the first 3 to 5 days of treatment is an indicator of a favorable outcome.[71]

Some raptors, for example, sparrow hawks, have a tendency to fly into windows in the excitement of the chase. Concussed birds have reduced response to stimuli, slow pupillary reflexes, and depression. They should be kept at a lower temperature to prevent further intracranial vasodilation, and seizing birds may be treated with benzodiazepines.[8,32]

Wounds involving loss of tissue on the head are frequently encountered in *Accipiter* species. A sliding pedicle graft technique (bilateral Z-plasty) to repair these deficits has been described.[8] Useful reviews of wound management and the use of skin flaps and grafts in raptors have been published.[10,24,67]

Brachial plexus avulsion presents with paralysis of the affected wing.[8] Repeated wing tip injuries from crashing into the fences or walls of their enclosures may lead to ulcerative wounds, fibrosis, and ankylosis of the joint. Treatment consists of debriding the fibrous tissue, applying sutures, and placing bandage anchored to the feathers.[61]

"Blain" is a bursitis of the carpus with blister on the joint. It is often diagnosed in tethered birds of prey that incur repeated injury to the ventral aspect of the wing hitting the floor when attempting to escape from an approaching handler. Treatment is with drainage, topical and systemic antibiotics, and suitable bandages.[12,61]

A syndrome of edema, avascular necrosis, and dry gangrene around the base of the distal primary feathers has been commonly diagnosed in birds of prey (wing tip edema). The exact etiology is unknown, but cold weather is probably responsible. Species originating from warmer climates are more commonly affected when kept tethered and less active. Treatment includes attempts to restore adequate blood circulation by massaging, warming the bird, and administration of antibiotics and corticosteroids. Prognosis is reserved, as in many birds the distal wing tip sloughs off and is lost. The bird should be encouraged to continue flying. Laser therapy may be used to assist tissue recovery. Use of oral vascular stimulants such as isoxoprine or propentofylline or topical vascular stimulants such as Preparation-H may be attempted.[8]

Although elbow luxation carries a poor prognosis, moderate success has been reported with the surgical repair of closed caudodorsal elbow luxations, followed by immobilization for a few days with transarticular external skeletal fixator or "figure-of-eight" wing wrap.[1] Luxations of the carpal joint are best treated with the use of external fixation devices.[61] Stifle luxations may be repaired with a transarticular external skeletal fixator. Luxations of the shoulder are typically managed with cage rest and bandaging of the wing to the body, but surgical repair may also be attempted.[61] Metacarpophalangeal joint luxation has been treated successfully with arthrodesis using a type 1 external skeletal fixator to stabilize the joint.[72]

Tendons of the digits may be injured by ring constriction, trauma from anklets, entanglement in jesses, bites from prey, infection, and collisions with cars. The key to successful surgical tendon repair is the use of a vascularized pedicle between the tendon and the tendon sheath. A waiting period of several weeks after the initial trauma is recommended to allow vascularization of the damaged tendon. Tendon autograft has been performed.[39]

Although multiple other techniques have been reported in the literature, the external skeletal fixator–intramedullary pin tie-in fixator (TIF) yields exceptional results in a variety of long bone fractures. It consists of the insertion of an intramedullary pin that fills approximately three quarters of the bone marrow cavity and two to four external skeletal fixator (ESF) positive-profile threaded pins placed at the proximal and distal ends of the affected bone. The intramedullary pin is bent at a 90-degree angle at its exit point and rotated into the same plane as that of the ESF pins. Latex tubing filled with acrylic is placed onto the pins to hold everything together. Wing coaptation by figure-of-eight bandaging is usually not needed. Phased disassembly (dynamization) of the fixation is recommended.[39]

Most forelimb fractures may be repaired with the TIF applied to the ulna and stabilization of the radius with retrograde placement of an intramedullary (IM) pin. The ulna must be pinned in a normograde fashion. If the radius is intact and the ulnar fracture is stable, a figure-of-eight bandage might be sufficient. With proximal radial fractures, the proximal fragment is usually too short for pinning, and coaptation for 3 to 4 weeks is most commonly used. Distal radial fractures are best managed by intramedullary pinning.[61]

When using bandages, passive range of motion physical therapy under anesthesia should be undertaken within the first week to prevent patagial contraction.[61] Radio-ulnar synostosis (the bony bridge between the ulna and the radius) is a common complication of external coaptation. Surgical excision of the bony union with the application of a polypropylene mesh implant between the two bones has restored wing function in a Mississippi kite.[6]

For tarsometatarsus fractures, coaptation with tape splint, combined with taping the hock in flexion so that the tarsometatarsus is splinted by the tibiotarsus, is effective in small birds. Type 2 ESF is applicable for larger birds. Fractures of the metacarpus and carpometacarpus are best corrected by immobilization using an external splint or bandage or type 1 ESF. It is recommended that application of fixation be delayed by 5 to 7 days after the injury to allow soft tissue to recover.[61]

Fractures of the mandible respond well to the intramedullary fixation technique or an external fixation device.[8,12] Coracoid fracture may be treated conservatively with cage rest or with IM pin or plate fixation.[13] Fractures of the pelvis may heal without external support if the bird is kept restricted and no neurologic damage has occurred.[8] A review of fracture prevalence and healing rates has been published.[8] Fractures with devitalized, necrotic or infected bone close to joints, or with extensive soft tissue damage, are not likely to heal.[8]

Low Condition and Sour Crop

Low condition may result from having been maintained at flying weight for too long, the inadequate daily provision of food, or an abrupt decrease in temperature. The affected bird is depressed, weak, profoundly anemic, hypoproteinemic, cachectic, dehydrated, and hypotensive. Once fed, GI stasis occurs, and the food in the crop begins to putrefy, leading to "sour crop," toxemia, and rapid death. Treatment consists of aggressive fluid therapy, with blood transfusion if PCV is below 20%, keeping the bird warm, and antimicrobial therapy. If the crop has soured, the contents should be removed, under anesthesia, after intubation, by retrograde massage and

irrigation of the crop with warmed saline. Injectable ranitidine stimulates crop motility. Liquid food items given by crop or stomach tube are introduced after a minimum of 12 hours of fluid therapy. Solid food, devoid of feathers, fur, or bone and well-moistened in saline, should be reintroduced slowly.[71]

Ocular Disorders

Wild raptors have a high prevalence of traumatic eye disorders. Vitreous hemorrhage, retinal detachment, and tearing may be seen after accidents or gunshot wounds.[61] Many traumatized birds show fundus disorders often without any changes in the anterior segment or other external signs of trauma. Intravitreal hemorrhages may take months for resorption, if they resorb at all.[39] Tears in the iris and uveitis are also seen commonly after trauma. Secondary cataract may occur with extensive damage of the iridial tissue, but small tears usually heal uneventfully following local corticosteroid and antibiotic treatment.[61] Corneal injuries and keratitis may also occur in raptors after accidental collisions.[61] A temporary tarsorrhaphy may be performed to address chronic keratitis, with the use of sterile rubber bands as stents to minimize pressure-induced necrosis of the lid margin.[45]

Ocular conditions may be found with systemic infections with *Salmonella*, mycobacterial infections, paramyxovirus, herpesvirus, and *Toxoplasma*.[39] Causes of cataract formation may be congenital, inherited, senile, or a sequel to trauma or uveitis. Removal by phacoemulsification or extracapsular extraction is effective.[45] Microphthalmos appears to be one of the most common congenital ocular lesions.[45]

Enucleation has been described in birds of prey.[45] The author prefers evisceration of the eye, removing all soft tissue structures and leaving the bony structures intact. The globe is then flushed until the socket is clean and the eyelid margins freshened and sutured together. The release of a one-eye raptor is controversial, and the ability to hunt live preys must be determined.

Other Conditions

Amyloidosis is seen in association with some chronic infections (e.g., aspergillosis, tuberculosis, bumblefoot, trichomoniasis) in Falconiformes. In hunting falcons in the United Arab Emirates, it presents as a fatal syndrome of wasting, weight loss, and green mutes. Amyloid is usually found in most organs, including the liver, spleen, kidney, and adrenal glands. A semi-quantitative serum test for falcon serum amyloid A has been developed.[25]

In Falconiformes, gout has recently been associated with *Clostridium perfringens* infection.[61] Articular gout in raptors is rare. Allopurinol treatment is controversial and has been reported to actually cause hyperuricemia.[39] Successful treatment of a red-tailed hawk with acute obstructive uric acid nephropathy has been documented with IV and subcutaneous (SC) saline and furosemide.[39]

A syndrome of bilateral paralysis of the legs with clenched digits is sometimes seen in raptors, especially goshawks. Some cases respond to B-vitamin complex injections, but postmortem examination of affected goshawks has revealed no specific lesions.[12]

Impaction of the crop may occur with casting material or indigestible, oversized items.[12] Crop rupture or ingluviotomy must be repaired in two layers, the crop being sutured separately from the skin.[10] Impaction of the ventriculus and intestinal tract of falcons with sand has been reported.[61] Motion sickness has been reported in birds of prey, so they should not be transported with food in their upper alimentary tract.[12] Trash ingestion was the most important mortality factor in nestling California condors in the reintroduction program from 1992 to 2009.[55]

Sinusitis is usually caused by mechanical obstruction with dust and sand in captive Falconiformes species.[61] It should be treated with nasal flushing with saline and antibiotics.[8] Rhinoliths are typically related to bacterial, mycoplasmal, fungal, or viral infection.[8]

Atherosclerosis may be a cause of sudden death in overfed aviary birds.[8] Right-sided congestive heart failure with cardiomyopathy has been reported in a captive red-tailed hawk.[35]

A condition resembling "stroke" is recognized in raptors, particularly old birds, when the birds suddenly collapse and show weakness and incoordination. They usually recover within a few hours but may remain partly paralyzed or become comatose and die acutely.[12]

Avian vacuolar myelinopathy, first recognized in 1994, is a neurologic disease affecting bald eagles, American coots (*Fulica americana*), and other birds in the southeastern United States. The disease is seasonal and appears to involve cyanobacteria in the order Stigonematales.[73] Birds of prey acquire the disease via ingestion of tissues from affected coots.[17]

REPRODUCTION

Reproductive biologic data of some common raptors species have been published.[8] Male birds are generally sexually mature 1 to 2 years before female birds.[8]

In most species, female birds are approximately 30% heavier than males, but a considerable overlap exists between the sexes in some species.[8] Vultures are conventionally dimorphic.[52] Endoscopic visualization of the gonads is used to determine the gender of raptors. Determination of gender may also be achieved by using the molecular method.[39] A noninvasive intracloacal ultrasonography protocol has been described for sexing in birds of prey.[30]

Because of the demands for conservation and to provide birds for falconry, many species of raptors have been bred successfully in captivity.[52] Incubators are usually kept between 36.75 to 37.75° C with a relative humidity of 40% to 45%.[8] Incubation requirements for some commonly reared Falconiformes species have been described.[61] Young are altricial.[8]

Artificial insemination is used in some centers. Breeding activity is mainly stimulated, in temperate regions, by a decreasing day length prior to an increasing day length. Semen samples may be obtained by massage techniques. Handlers may train sexually imprinted males to copulate.[8] Sperm concentration of some falcons is low compared with that of domestic birds.[12]

Fatal malposition in the egg, yolk sac infection, and bacterial enteritis caused by *Salmonella* and *Campylobacter* have been observed in California condor chicks in breeding programs.[15]

Splay legs occur when the young bird attempts to stand but its leg muscles are not strong enough. Placing with other chicks to encourage huddling may prevent this condition.[8] Bilateral valgus deformity of the distal wings (angel wings) was reported in a 4-week-old northern goshawk. The condition resolved with bandage and physical therapy.[75] Cannibalism is well recognized among the nestlings of free-living birds, particularly larger species such as eagles, and it may also occur in captivity.[12]

When a young raptor has been reared by hand, it grows up thinking it is human (imprinting). It will scream for food at the human and present itself as a mate to the handler. To avoid this phenomenon, chicks should be reared with others or fed with gloved or puppet hand and prevented from seeing the handler. In species of a nervous disposition such as sparrow hawks, the period of sensitivity to imprinting decreases rapidly at around 18 days of age. In other species, this period of sensitivity declines more gradually up to 16 weeks of age.[8]

As in other avian species, egg binding may be associated with low dietary calcium or vitamin D_3, physical or psychological trauma, or other diseases. Treatment consists of administration of oxytocin, calcium gluconate, or calcium borogluconate. Dinoprost may be applied directly onto the cloacal mucosa.[8] Oviductitis and egg peritonitis are usually associated with gram-negative bacteria.[12]

REFERENCES

1. Ackermann J, Redig P: Surgical repair of elbow luxation in raptors. *J Avian Med Surg* 11(4):247–254, 1997.
2. Aguilar RF, Smith VE, Ogburn P, Redig PT: Arrhythmias associated with isoflurane anesthesia in bald eagles (*Haliaeetus leucocephalus*). *J Zoo Wild Med* 26(4):508–516, 1995.
3. Aguilar RF, Yoshicedo JN, Parish CN: Ingluviotomy tube placement for lead-induced crop stasis in the California condor (*Gymnogyps californianus*). *J Avian Med Surg* 26(3):176–181, 2012.
4. Barbon AR, Smith S, Forbes N: Radiographic evaluation of cardiac size in four falconiform species. *J Avian Med Surg* 24(3):222–226, 2010.
5. Barsotti G, Briganti A, Spratte JR, et al: Safety and efficacy of bilateral topical application of rocuronium bromide for mydriasis in European kestrels (*Falco tinnunculus*). *J Avian Med Surg* 26(1):1–5, 2012.
6. Beaufrere H, Ammersbach M, Nevarez J, et al: Successful treatment of a radioulnar synostosis in a Mississippi kite (*Ictinia mississippiensis*). *J Avian Med Surg* 26(2):94–100, 2012.
7. Bechert U, Christensen JM, Poppenga R, et al: Pharmacokinetics of terbinafine after single oral dose administration in red-tailed hawks (*Buteo jamaicensis*). *J Avian Med Surg* 24(2):122–130, 2010.
8. Beynon PH, Forbes NA, Harcourt-Brown N, editors: *Manual of raptors, pigeons and waterfowl*, Gloustershire, U.K., 1996, British Small Animal Veterinary Association.
9. Bonar CJ, Lewandowski AH, Schaul J: Suspected fenbendazole toxicosis in 2 vulture species (*Gyps africanus, Torgos tracheliotus*) and Marabou storks (*Leptoptilos crumeniferus*). *J Avian Med Surg* 17(1):16–19, 2003.
10. Burke HF, Swaim SF: Amalsadvala T: Review of wound management in raptors. *J Avian Med Surg* 16(3):180–191, 2002.
11. Clements JF: *The Clements checklist of birds of the world*, ed 6, Ithaca, NY, 2007, Cornell University Press, pp 34–53.
12. Cooper JE: *Birds of prey: Health and disease*, ed 3, Oxford, U.K., 2002, Blackwell Science Ltd.
13. Davidson JR, Mitchell MA, Ramirez S: Plate fixation of a coracoid fracture in a bald eagle (*Haliaeetus leucocephalus*). *J Avian Med Surg* 19(4):303–308, 2005.
14. Di Somma A, Bailey T, Silvanose C, Garcia-Martinez C: The use of voriconazole for the treatment of aspergillosis in falcons (*Falco* species). *J Avian Med Surg* 21(4):307–316, 2007.
15. Ensley PK: Medical management of the California condor. In Fowler ME, Miller RE, editors: *Zoo and wild animal medicine, current therapy*, ed 4, Philadelphia, PA, 1999, Saunders, pp 277–292.
16. Espino L, Suarez ML, Lopez-Beceiro A, Santamarina G: Electrocardiogram reference values for the buzzard in Spain. *J Wild Dis* 37(4):680–685, 2001.
17. Fischer JR, Lewis-Weis LA, Tate CM: Experimental vacuolar myelinopathy in red-tailed hawks. *J Wild Dis* 39(2):400–406, 2003.
18. Forbes NA, Simpson GN: *Caryospora neofalconis*: An emerging threat to captive-bred raptors in the United Kingdom. *J Avian Med Surg* 11(2):110–114, 1997.
19. Forbes NA, Simpson GN: Pathogenicity of ticks on aviary birds. *Vet Record* 133(21):532, 1993.
20. Fowler DW, Freedman EA, Scannella JB: Predatory functional morphology in raptors: Interdigital variation in talon size is related to prey restraint and immobilization technique. *PLoS ONE* 4(11):e7999, 2009.
21. Franson JC: Parathion poisoning of Mississippi kites in Oklahoma. *J Raptor Res* 28:108–109, 1994.
22. Garcia-Montijano M, Gonzalez F, Waxman S, et al: Pharmacokinetics of marbofloxacin after oral administration to Eurasian buzzards (*Buteo buteo*). *J Avian Med Surg* 17(4):185–190, 2003.
23. Gelli D, Ferrari V, Franceschini F, et al: Serum biochemistry and electrophoretic patterns in the Eurasian buzzard (*Buteo buteo*): Reference values. *J Wild Dis* 45(3):828–833, 2009.
24. Gentz EJ, Linn KA: Use of a dorsal cervical single pedicle advancement flap in 3 birds with cranial skin defects. *J Avian Med Surg* 14(1):31–36, 2000.
25. Hampel MR, Kinne J, Wernery U, et al: Increasing fatal AA amyloidosis in hunting falcons and how to identify the risk: A report from the United Arab Emirates. *Amyloid* 16(3):122–132, 2009.
26. Harrenstien LA, Tell LA, Vulliet R, et al: Disposition of enrofloxacin in red-tailed hawks (*Buteo jamaicensis*) and great horned owls (*Bubo virginianus*) after a single oral, intramuscular, or intravenous dose. *J Avian Med Surg* 14(4):228–236, 2000.
27. Hassanpour H, Moghaddam AKZ, Bashi MC: The normal electrocardiogram of conscious golden eagles (*Aquila chrysaetos*). *J Zoo Wild Med* 41(3):426–431, 2010.

28. Hawkins MG, Wright BD, Pascoe PJ, et al: Pharmacokinetics and anesthetic and cardiopulmonary effects of propofol in red-tailed hawks (*Buteo jamaicensis*) and great horned owls (*Bubo virginianus*). *Am J Vet Res* 64(6):677–683, 2003.

29. Heidenreich M: *Birds of prey: Medicine and management*, Oxford, U.K., 1997, Blackwell Science Ltd.

30. Hildebrandt T, Pitra C, Sommer P, Pinkowski M: Sex identification in birds of prey by ultrasonography. *J Zoo Wild Med* 26(3):367–376, 1995.

31. Houston DC, Copsey JA: Bone digestion and intestinal morphology of the bearded vulture. *J Raptor Res* 28:73–78, 1994.

32. Huckabee JR: Raptor therapeutics. *Vet Clinic North Am Exot Anim Pract* 3:91–115, 2000.

33. Jones MP, Pierce KE, Ward D: Avian vision: A review of form and function with special consideration to birds of prey. *J Exot Pet Med* 16(2):69–87, 2007.

34. Jones MP, Orosz SE, Cox SK, Frazier DL: Pharmacokinetic disposition of itraconazole in red-tailed hawks (*Buteo jamaicensis*). *J Avian Med Surg* 14(1):15–22, 2000.

35. Knafo SE, Rapoport G, Williams J, et al: Cardiomyopathy and right-sided congestive heart failure in a red-tailed hawk (*Buteo jamaicensis*). *J Avian Med Surg* 25(1):32–39, 2011.

36. Kummrow M, Silvanose C, Di Somma A, et al: Serum protein electrophoresis by using high-resolution agarose gel in clinically healthy and *Aspergillus* species-infected falcons. *J Avian Med Surg* 26(4):213–220, 2012.

37. Lamberski N, Hull AC, Fish AM, et al: A survey of the choanal and cloacal aerobic bacterial flora in free-living and captive red-tailed hawks (*Buteo jamaicensis*) and Cooper's hawks (*Accipiter cooperii*). *J Avian Med Surg* 17:131–135, 2003.

38. Larrat S, Locke S, Dallaire AD, et al: Fatal aerosacculitis and pneumonia associated with *Eucoleus* sp. (Nematoda: Capillaridae) in the lungs of a peregrine falcon (*Falco peregrinus*). *J Wild Dis* 48(3):832–834, 2012.

39. Lumeij SJ, Remple JD, Redig PT, et al, editors: *Raptor biomedicine*, ed 3, Lake Worth, FL, 2000, Zoological Education Network.

40. Meteyer CU, Rideout BA, Gilbert M: Pathology and proposed pathophysiology of diclofenac poisoning in free-living and experimentally exposed Oriental white-backed vultures (*Gyps bengalensis*). *J Wild Dis* 41(4):707–716, 2005.

41. Miller DS, Taton-Allen GF, Campbell TW: *Knemidokoptes* in a Swainson's hawk, *Buteo swainsoni*. *J Zoo Wild Med* 35(3):400–402, 2004.

42. Mirande LA, Howerth EW, Poston RP: Chlamydiosis in a red-tailed hawk (*Buteo jamaicensis*). *J Wild Dis* 28:284–287, 1992.

43. Morishita TY, Mertins JW, Baker DG, et al: Occurrence and species of lice on free-living and captive raptors in California. *J Avian Med Surg* 15(4):288–292, 2001.

44. Muller K, Altenkamp R, Brunnberg L, et al: Pinching off syndrome in free-ranging white-tailed sea eagles (*Haliaeetus albicilla*) in Europe: Frequency and geographic distribution of a generalized feather abnormality. *J Avian Med Surg* 21(2):103–109, 2007.

45. Murphy CJ: Ocular lesions in birds of prey. In Fowler ME, editor: *Zoo and wild animal medicine, current therapy*, ed 3, Denver, CO, 1993, Saunders, pp 211–221.

46. Murray M, Tseng F: Diagnosis and treatment of secondary anticoagulant rodenticide toxicosis in a red-tailed hawk (*Buteo jamaicensis*). *J Avian Med Surg* 22(1):41–46, 2008.

47. Oaks JL: Immune and inflammatory responses in falcon staphylococcal pododermatitis. In Redig PT, Cooper JE, Remple JD, Hunter DB, editors: *Raptor biomedicine*, Minneapolis, MN, 1993, University of Minnesota Press, pp 72–82.

48. Olias P, Olias L, Krucken J, et al: High prevalence of *Sarcocystis calchasi* sporocysts in European Accipiter hawks. *Vet Parasitol* 175(3–4):230–236, 2011.

49. Philips JR: A review and checklist of the parasitic mites (Acarina) of the Falconiformes and Strigiformes. *J Raptor Res* 34(3):210–231, 2000.

50. Raidal S, Jaensch SM: Central nervous disease and blindness in Nankeen kestrels (*Falco cenchroides*) due to a novel Leucocytozoon-like infection. *Avian Pathol* 29:51–56, 2000.

51. Redig PT, Tully TN, Ritchie BW, et al: Effect of West Nile virus DNA-plasmid vaccination on response to live virus challenge in red-tailed hawks (*Buteo jamaicensis*). *Am J Vet Res* 72(8):1065–1070, 2011.

52. Redig PT: Falconiformes (vultures, hawks, falcons, secretary bird). In Fowler ME, Miller RE, editors: *Zoo and wild animal medicine*, ed 5, St. Louis, MO, 2003, Saunders, pp 150–161.

53. Remple JD: Intracellular hematozoa of raptors: A review and update. *J Avian Med Surg* 18(2):75–88, 2004.

54. Reuter A, Muller K, Arndt G, Eule JC: Reference intervals for intraocular pressure measured by rebound tonometry in ten raptor species and factors affecting the intraocular pressure. *J Avian Med Surg* 25(3):165–172, 2011.

55. Rideout BA, Stalis I, Papendick R, et al: Patterns of mortality in free-ranging California condors (*Gymnogyps californianus*). *J Wild Dis* 48(1):95–112, 2012.

56. Robbins PK, Tell LA, Needham BA, Craigmill AL: Pharmacokinetics of piperacillin after intramuscular injection in red-tailed hawks (*Buteo jamaicensis*) and great horned owls (*Bubo virginianus*). *J Zoo Wild Med* 31(1):47–51, 2000.

57. Roy C, Grolleau G, Chamoulaud S, Riviere J: Plasma B-esterase activities in European raptors. *J Wild Dis* 41(1):184–208, 2005.

58. Ruder MG, Feldman SH, Wunschmann A, McRuer DL: Association of *Mycoplasma corogypsi* and polyarthritis in a black vulture (*Coragyps atratus*) in Virginia. *J Wild Dis* 45(3):808–816, 2009.

59. Rutkiewicz J, Nam DH, Cooley T, et al: Mercury exposure and neurochemical impacts in bald eagles across several Great Lakes states. *Ecotoxicology* 20(7):1669–1676, 2011.

60. Saggese MD, Noseda RP, Uhart MM, et al: First detection of *Bacillus anthracis* in feces of free-ranging raptors from Central Argentina. *J Wild Dis* 43(1):136–141, 2007.

61. Samour J, editor: *Avian medicine*, ed 2, Philadelphia, PA, 2008, Mosby, p 525.

62. Shivakoti S, Ito H, Otsuki K, Ito T: Characterization of H5N1 highly pathogenic avian influenza virus isolated from a mountain hawk eagle in Japan. *J Vet Med Sci* 72(4):459–463, 2010.

63. Shrubsole-Cockwill AN, Millins C, Jardine C, et al: Avian pox infection with secondary *Candida albicans* encephalitis in a juvenile golden eagle (*Aquila chrysaetos*). *J Avian Med Surg* 24(1):64–71, 2010.

64. Smith SP, Forbes NA: A novel technique for prevention of self-mutilation in three Harris' hawks (*Parabuteo unicinctus*). *J Avian Med Surg* 23(1):49–52, 2009.

65. Souza MJ, Martin-Jimenez T, Jones MP, Cox SK: Pharmacokinetics of intravenous and oral tramadol in the bald eagle (*Haliaeetus leucocephalus*). *J Avian Med Surg* 23(4):247–252, 2009.

66. Stauber E, Holmes S, DeGhetto DL, Finch N: Magnetic resonance imaging is superior to radiography in evaluating spinal cord trauma in three bald eagles (*Haliaeetus leucocephalus*). *J Avian Med Surg* 21(3):196–200, 2007.

67. Stroud PK, Amalsadvala T, Swaim SF: The use of skin flaps and grafts for wound management in raptors. *J Avian Med Surg* 17(2):78–85, 2003.

68. Tell LA, Ferrell ST, Gibbons PM: Avian mycobacteriosis in free-living raptors in California: 6 cases (1997–2001). *J Avian Med Surg* 18(1):30–40, 2004.

69. Travis D: West Nile virus in birds and mammals. In Fowler ME, Miller RE, editors: *Zoo and wild animal medicine, current therapy*, ed 6, St. Louis, MO, 2008, Saunders, pp 2–9.

70. Tschopp R, Bailey T, Di Somma A: Silvanose C: Urinalysis as a noninvasive health screening procedure in Falconidae. *J Avian Med Surg* 21(1):8–12, 2007.

71. Tully TN, Dorrestein GM, Jones AK, editors: *Handbook of avian medicine*, ed 2, Philadelphia, PA, 2009, Saunders, pp 25–55, 209–242.

72. Van Wettere AJ, Redig PT: Arthrodesis as a treatment for metacarpophalangeal joint luxation in 2 raptors. *J Avian Med Surg* 18(1):23–29, 2004.

73. Wiley FE, Wilde SB, Birrenkott AH, et al: Investigation of the link between avian vacuolar myelinopathy and a novel species of cyanobacteria through laboratory feeding trials. *J Wild Dis* 43(3):337–344, 2007.

74. Wunschmann A, Rejmanek D, Conrad PA, et al: Natural fatal *Sarcocystis falcatula* infections in free-ranging eagles in North America. *J Vet Diagn Invest* 22(2):282–289, 2010.

75. Zsivanovits P, Monks DJ, Forbes NA: Bilateral valgus deformity of the distal wings (angel wing) in a northern goshawk (*Accipiter gentilis*). *J Avian Med Surg* 20(1):21–26, 2006.

CHAPTER 18

Galliformes

Teresa Y. Morishita

Galliformes species are characterized as birds that are medium to large bodied, have rounded wings, have a well-developed keel bone, and have strong legs with four digits that are designed for their terrestrial life.[17] Galliformes are one of the first bird orders to be associated with humans and among the first domesticated.[17] They remain diverse with regard to their domestication, ranging from the common barnyard poultry species to the more exotic species found in zoologic settings and captive breeding programs. In a zoologic setting, aviary collections may include the more exotic members of Galliformes, whereas places such as children's zoos may have the common domesticated chicken and turkeys. The more exotic Galliformes species are usually housed as breeding pairs, and collections of domesticated Galliformes species are housed in small flocks. It is important to consider disease transmission between domesticated species of Galliformes and that of the exotic Galliformes collection. Although diseases and their treatment and control are often extrapolated from those diseases well described in domestic Galliformes species,[5] exotic ones seem to be fairly hardy under captive conditions.

Within Galliformes, relatedness among the various species has been debated. Relatedness has been based on deoxyribonucleic acid (DNA),[63] and more recent phylogenetic trees have been based on mitochondrial DNA.[26] The major divisions of the Galliformes are found in Box 18-1. For a complete listing of genus and species worldwide, including natural histories, comprehensive pictorial atlases are readily available.[11]

The majority of exotic Galliformes species housed in zoologic parks are the guans, chalacas, currasows, pheasants, peafowl, and guinea fowl. In some captive conditions, guinea fowl are considered the "watch dogs" of Galliformes and have been used for rodent control and alerting other species to impending danger with their shrill calls.[19] In some zoologic settings, guinea fowl are usually kept in mixed exhibits. Peafowls are often allowed free roam access in zoologic settings, and this may present problems if they have contact with both the exotic and domestic species of Galliformes kept on site. The same concern applies to free-roaming jungle fowl.

CLINICAL SIGNIFICANCE OF UNIQUE ANATOMY AND PHYSIOLOGY

Some Galliformes species have portions of their integumentary system that are unfeathered, including areas of the head. The most extreme elaborate unfeathered areas are found in turkeys, with their bare heads, ornamental caruncles, and the *snood*, a fleshy skin appendage found near the upper beak between the eyes.[17] For Galliformes, unfeathered areas of the head may be prone to frost bite in environments with extreme winter conditions.[66]

Since the Galliformes species are terrestrial birds, their adaption to ground dwelling has been cryptically colored feathers in brown, black, and gray.[17] Some Phasianidae, especially the males, are brightly colored in red, yellow, and silver feathered patterns.[12,20] The peacock, a member of the Phasianidae family, has elongated uppertail coverts with the characteristic eyespots that are used in mating displays.[17] Most young of the Galliformes species are covered in down when they hatch; however, members of the Megapodiidae family are fully feathered and capable of flight when they emerge from their mound nests.[17] Although many of the male of the Galliformes species are brightly colored compared with the more drab-colored females, both males and females of guinea fowl are similar in appearance, having

the same plumage, markings, and colorations that make visual sexing guinea fowl difficult.[19] Guinea fowl also have a unique characteristic of having tiny white dots over their entire plumage.[19]

The beaks of the Galliformes species are short, stout, and generally conical in shape, with an arched culmen and with the tip of the maxilla slightly overlapping the mandible.[17] The beak is used to pick up grains and small insects and does not have the crushing power as seen in other seed eaters.[17] In a captive setting, beaks will not overgrow and need not be trimmed unless malocclusion exists.[35] The main injury that has been associated with the beak is related to wire gauge size of the housing. If too large a gauge size is used and the bird's beak may fit through the cage wiring, traumatic damage to the beak may occur if the bird becomes spooked and jerks its beak backward.[35] Lacerations of the beak may be prevented with appropriate cage gauge size.[35]

Galliformes species have digits that are arranged in the anisodactyl position with three digits facing forward and one digit, often referred to as the *hind toe*, facing backward.[17] The hind toe is often reduced in size. In some species within Galliformes, differences exist. In Phasianidae and Numidadae, the hind toe is elevated and not in contact with the ground.[17] However, in the Megapodiidae and Cracidae families, the hind toe is on the same level as the ground.[17] Some members of the Phasianidae have spurs on the tarsus; and some members such as the grouse have feathered tarsi and digits.[17] The spurs do not need to be medically managed but may cause injuries for zoo staff when the bird is captured, handled, or both. If spurs are to be removed, caution should be exercised during surgical removal.[9,35]

All members of the order Galliformes are known as granivorous birds and have a well-developed muscular ventriculus (gizzard) because of the striated muscle layers.[8,17] In addition, Galliformes species have well-developed ceca.[8,17] Although domesticated Galliformes species have been provided grit in their diets, it is not required for digestion.[35] Under natural exhibit conditions, exotic species may have small stones in their gizzards and observed as incidental findings during necropsy.[29] In addition, it should be noted that Galliformes species are curious, and if exposed to environmental conditions they are not accustomed to, they may ingest excessive grass, flooring substrates, and even feathers to form an impaction (blockage) in the gizzard that needs to be surgically removed.[29,35,39,40,50,56] This may be prevented by obtaining a history on the previous housing conditions provided to the birds.

Radiographic Anatomy Considerations

The general body-shape of Galliformes is rounded and the visceral organs are compact. Hence, it may be difficult to visualize individual visceral organs such as the heart, liver, and ventriculus.[65] The manus is shorter than or about the same length as the antebrachium or the brachium.[65] Radiographically, a sesamoid bone is seen proximal to the carpus, located within the tendon of the tensor propatagialis muscle.[65] Since the legs of Galliformes were developed for a terrestrial life style, the femur, tibiotarsus, and tarsometatarsus are all relatively long.[65] In some birds, the length of the femur may be two thirds the length of the tibiotarsus.[65]

Behavioral Aspects

Galliformes species have ritualized feeding habits that are incorporated in their courtship behavior and are especially noted in quails,

BOX 18-1 Bird Families within the Galliformes Order

Family	Examples of Species
Phasianidae*	Chickens, grouse, partridge, pheasant, quail, turkey
Odontophoridae	New World quail
Numididae	Guineafowl
Cracidae	Chachalaca, guan, curassow
Megapodiidae	Brush-turkey, mallee fowl

*The family Phasianidae has often been subdivided into the families Meleagrididas and Tetraonidae as its own families.
From del Hoyo J, Elliott A, Sargatal J, eds: *Handbook of birds of the world, Vol 2, New World Vultures to Guineafowl*, Barcelona, Spain, 1994, Lynx Edicions, pp 277–567.

pheasants, and peacocks.[12,17] These ritualized feeding behaviors displayed in courtship behavior is often referred to as *tidbitting* and involves the male bowing in front of the female with wings and tail outstretched to varying degrees, and beak pointing to the ground.[17] Guinea fowl are rather aggressive and may chase other Galliformes and bird species away, so care must be used if they are placed in mixed species avian exhibits.[19]

HUSBANDRY

Husbandry and management requirements for Galliformes depend on the species and numbers. In general, a pair of pheasants would need a minimum of 200 square feet with tragopans needing closer to 400 square feet; for a basic enclosure.[20] For smaller Galliformes, 100 to 150 square feet may be adequate.[20] One of the most important considerations in facility design is to predator-proof the enclosures and to determine the size of the netting's gauge and type.[20,22] If wire netting is used, it is necessary to extend the netting at least 12 inches into the ground to prevent predators from digging through and gaining access into the exhibit areas.[20,22] With regard to the netting gauge, a determination needs to be made if the exhibit is primarily designed to keep the Galliformes species in the enclosure or if the primary purpose is to prevent small birds such as house sparrows from entering the enclosures and having contact with the Galliformes species.[35] With recent concerns of diseases such as avian influenza among free-living birds and Galliformes, prevention of pest avian contact is of utmost importance. However, in geographic regions with heavy snow, the concern with exhibit collapse exists if snow is not removed and allowed to accumulate on small-gauge wiring.[35] In addition, the smaller gauges will also hinder the public's clear view of the birds on exhibit. In terms of design, a long aviary with narrow frontage is preferred, as it would provide enough space for the birds to retreat to the back of the exhibit if they need to feel safe.[20,35] An aviary with shallow depth and long frontage will provide better viewing but would not allow a retreat area for the birds.[20] With multiple adjacent aviaries housing Galliformes, it has been recommended to have a solid partition that is 18 to 24 inches in height to prevent aggression or to have small-gauge netting to prevent contact between adjacent exhibits.[20,35] Exotic Galliformes species such as pheasants may be highly aggressive and, if crowded, may display intraspecies aggression and incur skin wounds that could result in gangrenous dermatis.[48]

Perches should be placed in a sheltered area. Consideration should be given for birds that have long tail feathers. For these birds, perches should not be located close to exhibit walls and caging, as this could damage or break the feathers as the birds turn on their perches.[20]

Housing requirements are simple. Some species are fairly hardy, and all that is required is a simple A-frame structure.[20,23,24,35,40] Those species from neotropical and tropical environments may need supplemental heat during inclement weather. For such species, indoor housing with supplemental heat may be needed, depending on environmental conditions.

Since Galliformes tend to reside in flocks, single bird exhibits should be avoided. A breeding pair for exotic Galliformes is ideal. A single guinea fowl will tend to vocalize more than normally as they prefer to be in flocks, with a minimum of three birds.[19] In the case of domestic species such as chickens in the children's zoo or farm sections, the birds should be kept in all-hen groups. If roosters are to be included in the group, at least two males should be placed in a flock, with six to seven females per male.[35,50] Caution should be used in dealing with single-rooster flocks, as these roosters tend to be more aggressive to both keepers and visitors.[35,50] Having two roosters in the flock will allow the roosters to establish a pecking order.[35,50]

BIOSECURITY AND QUARANTINE

It is of utmost importance to perform the necessary tests to fully evaluate the health and exposure of newly acquired exotic Galliformes during the quarantine period.[14,35] The quarantine period may start from a minimum of 2 weeks for commercial and backyard poultry species[35,46]; this period is insufficient for exotic Galliformes. For exotic Galliformes, or for domestic Galliformes destined for a children's zoo, a minimum of 45 to 60 days would be more appropriate. The reason for this recommended time is the 2-week incubation time of most documented diseases in domestic Galliformes, and the time needed for diagnostic test result reporting also needs to be taken into account.[35] Although domestic poultry have a 2-week to 30-day quarantine period, their prior history is documented, and thus their disease exposure history may already be known.[35] In addition, if disease does occur, domestic Galliformes housing areas are more easily cleaned and disinfected.[35] However, one of the challenges in housing exotic Galliformes in public displays that recreate their natural settings for enrichment is that they are extremely difficult to thoroughly clean and disinfect once a disease has been established.[35,39,40] This is why a complete disease assessment needs to be performed during the quarantine period. Moreover, for collections involving areas of public display, major renovations to the environment may be limited for disease control purposes.[35] For example, roundworms may survive in the soil for at least 7 years, and in heavy nematode infestations in Galliformes, it is recommended to turn over the top 3 to 5 inches of soil to reduce exposure of the birds to infective ova and to top-dress (place new floor substrate) the top of the flooring to reduce exposure of birds to infected ova.[35,39,40] However, this would be impractical for areas of public display. Hence, the quarantine period is very important to determine the presence of diseases in new acquisitions to prevent and minimize the contamination of the aviary environment.

On arrival, shipping containers should be examined and feces present collected so that the first round of fecal examination may be performed to evaluate for the presence of endoparasites. This should be repeated at 2-week intervals for at least three successive collections to ensure the detection of endoparasites. False-negative test results may occur if the birds were in an early stage of infection, so serial testing is necessary. Table 18-1 lists the recommended tests that should be performed in the quarantine period and the rationale.

A physical examination and additional testing, including fecal examination (for internal parasites), serologic monitoring, and hematologic and biochemical monitoring, are highly recommended.[35,43,44] The time needed in the quarantine period is well worth the prevention of seeding the exhibit area with infectious agents and parasites.[46]

Nutrition and Feeding

Although specific diets may be created for each species, it is often difficult to find nutritionists and feed mills, and the feed may be cost prohibitive. The nutritional diets of pheasants most closely align with

TABLE 18-1

Recommended Procedures and Tests for Exotic Galliformes in Quarantine and Duration of Recommended Testing

Procedure/Test	Rationale	Ideal
Physical examination	Examine the birds for external parasites, especially lice and mites. Mites have a wide host range and live also in the environment. If detected while the birds are on exhibit, control may be difficult with restrictions on chemical exposure to species and environment. Early mite infections start near the vent and ventral abdomen region, so scrutinize these areas during physical examination.	Some species may be fractious to handling. Even in the absence of parasite detection, treat with antiparasitic agent, and repeat in 2 weeks because of generalized 2-week life cycles of external parasites. For exotic Galliformes, have at minimum three successive 2-week treatment plan.
Serologic testing	Collect serum to determine exposure to *Mycoplasma*, a bacterium that may be spread via vertical and horizontal transmission and may impact captive breeding programs. If detected, clearing breeders of the infection may be attempted as described for commercial poultry. Although this disease may cause minimal clinical impact as a sole disease, it may impact the severity of other respiratory diseases. Other serologic tests to perform include those for Newcastle disease and avian influenza exposure.	Test all birds on arrival. Allow at least 2 weeks for testing results to be completed. Establish collaborative relationship with state diagnostic laboratories that may perform such tests, as they are commonly used in the commercial poultry industry. Some states monitor for diseases within the state, so costs may be minimal. Collect serum 3 weeks after initial blood collection to detect early infections that may not have been previously detected, as antibody levels did not raise to detectable levels.
Hematologic and biochemical values	When collecting blood, also make blood smears to evaluate for blood parasite presence.	Because of the existence of a variety of exotic Galliformes species for which established values have not been determined, it would be helpful to collect "baseline" levels in birds whenever the opportunity arises. Since exotic Galliformes species are not usually handled once on exhibit, the quarantine period is a good opportunity to get species-specific data.
Parasite fecal examination	Minimal cost necessitates the need to perform such tests. Some infective ova of nematodes may survive in the soil for prolonged periods, so it is best to detect such infections before the exhibition area becomes "seeded" with parasites, which would necessitate lifelong treatment of the collection.	Treat for nematodes, cestodes, and trematodes on arrival of the birds and 2 weeks thereafter to ensure detection of developing stages. For exotic species, have a minimum three successive, 2-week treatment plan. Check feces before releasing the birds into the exhibit area.

those of domesticated turkeys, and feeds produced for turkeys provide almost all the basic requirements of most pheasant species.[20] Starter diets for chicks usually contain 28% to 30% protein.[20] Diets for growing birds contain 20% to 24% protein, whereas protein levels needed for maintenance range from 13% to 15%.[20] If breeding of pheasants is required, a 17% to 20% protein level is recommended. Guinea fowl starter diets should contain 24% protein for the first 4 weeks and 22% between 4 and 8 weeks of age.[19] Guinea fowl may then be maintained at 18% protein.[19]

Besides a balanced diet, fresh greens are also recommended.[19] Fresh grass clippings may be provided, but caution should be used to ensure that the birds do not gorge on grass as crop and gizzard impactions may occur.[35] More digestible green leafy lettuce, along with carrots and fruits such as apples, oranges, bananas, and grapes, is often popular. Mealworms as live insect food also provide enrichment and are recommended for captive birds.[20] Overexposure to new items may lead to curiosity and potential ingestion and impaction of indigestible materials.[35,50]

Since exotic Galliformes species are usually fed balanced rations, the occurrence of nutritional diseases is rare. Nutritional deficiencies may occur if feed storage conditions are inadequate. Food should be stored in a cool, dark, rodent-proof container, away from sun and moisture to avoid degradation of vitamins and mold development,

respectively. Feed mixing errors that directly affect the birds or indirectly affect their offspring may occur.[27]

It is important that newly hatched young Galliformes be directed to water drinkers, and marbles must be placed in water troughs such that the water levels do not cover the marbles, as some young Galliformes, especially guinea fowl, have a tendency to explore the water and will often get their down wet. Having wet down will chill the young chick and may increase chick mortality.[35]

RESTRAINT AND HANDLING

In general, Galliformes species may be handled without chemical restraint. To restrain Galliformes, the bird should be grasped across the back to control its wings, since they may be easily broken if the bird flaps them to escape.[50,66] After gaining control of the bird, one hand should be quickly placed between the bird's legs, with the legs controlled between the handler's fingers. The legs should be grasped firmly but loosely and close to the body. The bird should then be gently flipped so that one side of its body is placed against a hard, nonmovable surface.[50] Once the bird feels secure, it will become calm. In the case of a fractious bird, it may be necessary to place a dark-colored cloth over its head to keep it calm.[50]

Although handler injuries are usually not serious, caution should be used when handling Galliformes species with tarsal spurs.[50] Handler safety measures should include face and head protection during handling of birds that are nervous and unpredictable.[50]

It is difficult to capture guinea fowl as they are fearful unless they have experienced extensive handling as young chicks. Guinea fowl should never be picked up by the wings as the feathers surrounding the wings are loosely attached and will result in their loss.[19] Unlike in other Galliformes, the legs of guinea fowl are extremely fragile and may be easily broken. To restrain a guinea fowl, one hand should be used to close the wings while pushing the bird's body to the ground. At the same time, the other hand should be placed over the closed wing to pick the guinea fowl straight up. The key is to prevent the bird from flapping its wings and constantly kicking its legs.[19]

In a zoologic setting, it may be difficult to monitor the health of Galliformes species that are allowed free-roaming status, including peafowl, jungle fowl, and guinea fowl. Hence, accessing health status of these birds and other birds in the collection is necessary before they are allowed free-roam access.

SURGERY AND ANESTHESIA

Flight Restriction

While exotic species of Galliformes tend to be terrestrial species, they are capable of flight for short distances. Most captive Galliformes are housed in aviary situations where escape opportunities are limited and measures for flight control and restriction are unnecessary. However, flight restriction may be needed for those species that may have free access to the grounds. The most common species allowed free-roam access include jungle fowl, peafowl, and guinea fowl. The least invasive flight control method is wing clipping, but it is only a temporary measure. See Chapter 65 for more information on avian deflighting techniques.

Spur Management

In some Galliformes species such as pheasants, peafowl, and jungle fowl, a pointed spur (calcar) projects caudomedially from the medial surface of the tarsometatarsus. The spur is composed of the bony calcarial process that is ankylosed to the tarsusmetatarsus and covered by a sharp pointed horny covering.[9,65] Removal of the spur, if deemed necessary, should be considered a surgical procedure. Spurs should never be removed with guillotine-type nail clippers.

DIAGNOSTICS

For the diagnosis of diseases in captive exotic Galliformes species, some of the well-developed tests used in the commercial poultry industry may be adapted.

Serologic Monitoring

Serologic monitoring is one of the most important tools for determining disease exposure, chronicity of disease, effectiveness of vaccination programs, and disease epidemiology.[44,50,53] To minimize stress in captive species, every instance that calls for the capture of the birds should be used for collection of blood also if such procedures do not stress the birds too much. This will allow for the monitoring of disease and for the banking of serum for disease monitoring or for future disease investigation.[35,39,44] Blood collection from Galliformes is fairly simple, and three main sites may be used: the right jugular vein along the neck, the wing (brachial) vein, and the leg (tarsal) vein.[21,44] Depending on the size of the bird, each approach has its advantages. In smaller birds such as quails or in young chicks, the jugular vein is the preferred site. The wing vein is most often preferred for adult birds. No more than 1% of a bird's body weight should be collected (i.e., 1 mL/100 gm), and in general, for the total volume blood collected, a yield of 50% serum may be harvested.[21,41]

Hematologic and Biochemical Evaluation

Collection of blood to establish hematologic and biochemical values is important to assess the health of individual birds. It is recommended that a baseline value be established first for each individual species at the time of quarantine because it may be assumed that the bird would be healthy at that point in time. Tables 18-2 and 18-3 provide hematologic and biochemical values for selected exotic Galliformes species as previously reported.[1,4,13,16,18,25,68,69]

Fecal Examination

Fecal flotation and sedimentation examinations are often considered first in fecal diagnostics; however, for Galliformes species, it is also important to evaluate the physical condition of feces. Galliformes have formed feces, composed of the fecal portion, which is dark green to brown in color, and a white uric acid portion, often referred to as the *white cap*, from the urinary system.[32,54] The color and consistency of the feces and the urate portion may provide some clues to the bird's health.[32] In the case of Galliformes with a well-developed cecum, it is important to recognize the two physical forms of feces. As mentioned above, the normal droppings of Galliformes contain the fecal portion as well as a white urate portion. Birds on commercial diets have more well-formed feces.[32] The color of the fecal portion may indicate abnormalities. Normal coloration may range from brown to green and depends on the bird's diet. Red coloration may indicate hemorrhage within the intestines if it is incorporated within the fecal material, and this should be distinguished from red coloration on the surface, which would indicate blood from the cloaca, from the reproductive tract, or both.[32,54] Other colors that may be observed include bright green, indicating lead poisoning, which is, however, rare in exotic Galliformes species unless they have been exposed to lead-based paints under captive conditions.[32,54] Yellowish colored feces, often referred to as *sulfur color droppings*, are characteristic findings in birds with histomoniasis.[32,54] Watery diarrhea may indicate potential viral infections or parasitic infections such as coccidia, and it is often accompanied by blood in more severe infections.[32,54] The presence of tapeworm segments may also be visually apparent in birds that are heavily infested.

The second type of normal feces observed in Galliformes is the cecal dropping. These droppings occur usually at night, are dark brown to black in color, are loose and tenacious in consistency, and represent the contents of the cecum. It is important to recognize that sporadic cecal droppings are normal.[32] However, an increased number of cecal droppings may indicate stress.[32]

Diagnostic tests for parasites are the same as those used to diagnose parasites in other animal species. In exotic Galliformes, it is not sufficient to perform only a simple flotation examination, as exotic species may have parasites such as flukes and tapeworms that will be missed if only flotation exams are performed.

Radiography

Radiography has been frequently used in Galliformes to estimate obesity, organ enlargement, impaction and the presence of foreign bodies within the digestive system, crop distension, respiratory tract infections, and impacted oviducts.[10,65]

DISEASES

Numerous species of exotic Galliformes exist, and many diseases in these species have not been well documented or reported. To identify potential diseases that may occur within a collection, it is always important to remember family relationships. In general, many of the exotic Galliformes species housed in captivity, for example, peafowl, pheasants, and guinea fowl, are more closely related to the domestic turkey, and thus their susceptibility to diseases is more commonly related to the diseases reported in domestic turkeys.[40,50] Knowing these phylogenetic relationships among Galliformes is important, and a classic example is histomoniasis. Chickens may serve as inapparent carriers of the parasite *Histomonas meleagridis* and may

TABLE 18-2

Reference Ranges for Hematology Parameters for Selected Species of Galliformes

	Domestic Chicken	Domestic Turkey	Wild Turkey	Ring-Necked Pheasant	Guinea Fowl	Peafowl	Bobwhite Quail	Chacalaca	Wattled Curassow
Family	Phasiandae	Phasiandae	Phasiandae	Phasiandae	Numididae	Phasiandae	Odontophonidie	Cracidoe	Cracidoe
Parameter									
Red blood cell (cells × 10⁶/mL)	2.2–3.3	2.3–2.8		2.2–3.6	1.7–2.8	2.1	3.4–5.4	2.7	3.23 ± 0.35
Packed cell volume (%)	24–43	36–41	31–42	28–42	39–48	33–41	38	35–45	42 ± 4.4
Hemoglobin (g/dL)	8.9–13.5	10.3–15.2		8.0–18.9	11.4–14.9	12.0	11.6–15.8		15.2 ± 2.0
MCV (fL)	120–137	129		104–150					131.9 ± 13.1
MCH (pg)									47.4 ± 5.3
MCHC (g/dL)									36.0 ± 3.8
White blood cell (cells × 10³/mL)	19.8–32.6	23.5–26.8	10.3–46.5		15.5				20.9 ± 14.3
Heterophils (%)	19.8–32.6	43.4	39.1–59.4	48.0	43.5				25
Lymphocytes (%)	54.0–75.0	50.6	40.7–73.7	34.0	36.2				60
Eosinophils (%)	1.5–2.7	0.9		1.0	7.4				2
Monocytes (%)	8.1–16.5	1.9	0–8.5	8.0	8.4				8
Basophils (%)	1.7–4.3	3.2	0–4.7	10.0	4.5				4.8

From references 1,4,16,18,25,68,69; as summarized by Drew (13) with modifications.

fl, Femtoliter; *g/dL*, gram per deciliter; *MCH*, mean corpuscular hemoglobin; *MCHC*, mean corpuscular hemoglobin concentration; *MCV*, mean corpuscular volume; *mL*, milliliter; *pg*, picogram.

transmit this disease to turkeys and closely related Galliformes species such as peafowl and pheasants. For this reason, collections that allow jungle fowl to roam free may pose a risk to exotic pheasant collections.

Box 18-2 features the Disease Risk Awareness Questionnaire (DRAQ), which allows facilities to assess the high risk of disease for an exotic Galliformes collection, depending on the type of exhibits. If disease does occur, it is important to have an accurate diagnosis so that an effective cleaning and disinfection program may be established on the basis of the causative agent identified. Various disinfectants may then be used as in domestic Galliformes.[52] Although vaccination has been used in domestic Galliformes,[31] its use in exotic Galliformes is limited.

Disease Management

A variety of diseases have been documented in domestic Galliformes species such as chickens and turkeys and game birds such as pheasants and quail,[5,33,37,43,50,64] and data on many of the diseases seen in these species may be extrapolated to exotic Galliformes species.

The prevalence of disease depends on the exposure and potential risk factors of the collection. Infectious diseases tend to be more common under intensive commercial poultry production; however, exotic and free-living species are relatively free of infectious diseases unless exposed. In most Galliformes species housed in zoologic collections, noninfectious diseases and parasitic diseases appear to be of greater importance. The diagnosis of parasitic diseases is fairly simple with the use of standard parasitologic techniques, and treatment of such diseases is fairly simple with drug classes effective against specific parasites. It is highly recommended that veterinarians overseeing such collections of exotic Galliformes and pathologists performing necropsies on such species collect parasites to facilitate the expansion and documentation of parasite species in exotic Galliformes.[55]

A multitude of diseases in domestic Galliformes has been documented. For all practical purposes, the most important diseases that may be of concern in exotic Galliformes, as related to risk factors and captivity purpose, are presented in Tables 18-4, 18-5, and 18-6. The diseases discussed below are in terms of special consideration for exotic Galliformes collections. Further information on diseases may be acquired from more detailed reports on poultry diseases.[5,33,37,43,50,54,55,64]

Viral Diseases

Avian encephalomyelitis is a viral disease that has been reported in coturnix quail and pheasant chicks and is characterized by tremors and incoordination of the head, neck, and limbs.[64] The disease is spread from infected hens to chicks, so knowing the source of the birds is necessary if hatching eggs are obtained for aviary or captive breeding collections. No effective treatment exists, so knowing the disease status of parental sources and ensuring that hatching eggs are from immune parental sources are of utmost importance. This disease is more of concern for captive breeding programs.

TABLE 18-3

Reference Ranges for Serum Biochemical for Selected Galliformes

	Domestic Chicken	Domestic Turkey	Wild Turkey	Ring-Necked Pheasant	Guinea Fowl	Peafowl	Bobwhite Quail	Chacalaca	Wattled Curassow
Family	Phasiandae	Phasiandae	Phasiandae	Phasiandae	Numididae	Phasiandae	Odontophonidie	Cracidoe	Cracidoe
Parameter									
Total protein (g/dL)	3.3–5.5	4.9–7.6	3.6–5.5	6.9	3.5–4.4				4.0 + 0.7
Albumin (g/dL)	1.3–2.8	3.0–5.9	1.1–2.1	5.2					
Globulin (g/dL)	1.5–4.1	1.7–1.9		1.7					
Calcium (mg/dL)	13.2–23.7	11.7–38.7	11.4–14.6	14.1–15.4					11.8 + 1.2
Phosphorus (mg/dL)	6.2–7.9	5.4–7.1							
Sodium (mEq/L)	131–171	149–155		164–172	149–157	154–162		158–164	161 + 5
Potassium (mEq/L)	3.0–7.3	6.0–6.4							4.3 + 1.5
Chloride (mEq/L)									
Creatinine (mg/dL)	0.9–1.8	0.8–0.9							0.3 + 0.1
Uric acid (mg/dL)	2.5–8.1	3.4–5.2	3–17	2.3–3.7	2.9–5.1	1.8–3.7		3.7–7.9	10.0 + 3.6
Glucose (mg/dL)	227–300	275–425	215–500	335–397		273–357		235–345	309 + 47
ALT (IU/L)									34 + 13.6
AST (IU/L)			255–499						14 + 6.
GGT (IU/L)									
LDH (IU/L)			420–1338						
Bilirubin (mg/dL)									0.3 + 0.1

From references 1,4,16,18,25,68,69; as summarized by Drew (13) with modifications.
ALT, Alanine aminotransferase; *AST*, aspartate aminotransferase; *g/dL*, gram per deciliter; *GGT*, gamma-glutamyl transpeptidase; *IU/L*, international unit per liter; *LDH*, lactate dehydrogenase; *mEq/L*, milliequivalent per liter; *mg/dL*, milligram per deciliter.

Galliformes species are susceptible to avian influenza virus. In captive settings, exposure is primarily from infected free-living birds, especially free-living waterfowl that have access to zoologic collections or from new avian acquisition from countries that have a high prevalence of avian influenza. Peafowl are less susceptible than other Galliformes species, but all Galliformes are considered susceptible.[64] Exposure to free-living birds places birds at a higher risk of a disease outbreak.

Quail bronchitis has been reported in bobwhite quails.[64] Affected birds have respiratory distress and catarrhal tracheitis. In addition, some birds may have watery diarrhea. Chickens may be inapparent carriers of the disease, so a higher risk exists in facilities with children's zoo or barnyard exhibits and free-roaming jungle fowl on premises. Birds may be treated for secondary bacterial infection.[64]

Disease caused by avian pox virus has been reported in Galliformes species. It has been well documented in domestic chickens and turkeys, and quail have also been reported to be affected.[7,64] The dry form of the disease involves scabbing on the unfeathered portions of the bird's body, usually involving the head and feet. Lower rate of mortality is associated with the dry form. However, the wet form causes plaques within the oropharynx of birds, and occlusion of the trachea and oropharynx may interfere with eating and breathing. The wet form of avian pox is associated with higher mortality. Prevention of this disease is achieved by vaccination and effective mosquito control programs.[33,44,64]

Pheasants, chukars, and guinea fowl are susceptible to rotaviruses, and clinical signs of affected birds include diarrhea and stunting.[64] Necropsy of affected birds reveal increased fluid and gas within the intestines. Electron microscopy and immunofluorescence staining have been used to diagnose infections.[64] A higher risk of this disease exists in facilities with children's zoo or barnyard exhibits and free-roaming jungle fowl on the premises, as domestic chickens and turkeys may serve as sources of infection.

Equine encephalitis is an acute disease that may affect pheasants and chukars. Affected pheasants have leg paralysis, torticolis, and tremors.[40,64] No gross lesions are seen on necropsy. A commercially available vaccine may be used to protect valuable species, but its efficacy has not been explored in more exotic species.[64] Mosquito control is necessary. It is important to be informed about this disease if it has been reported in the vicinity of the zoologic park or captive breeding facility so that appropriate control strategies may be developed.

BOX 18-2 Disease Risk Awareness Questionnaire (DRAQ) for Captive Exotic Galliformes

1. Do you have a barnyard facility that houses common domestic Galliformes such as chickens and turkeys and an aviary housing exotic Galliformes?
   a. *Yes:* Caution should be used because of the disease transmission potential between domestic Galliformes and exotic Galliformes.
   Recommendation: Have separate caretakers for these sections to prevent cross-transmission. Obtain health history and vaccination history of the domestic Galliformes, as they will be the likely source of infectious diseases to the exotic Galliformes.
   b. *No:* If only one of these types of Galliformes is present, less concern exists with disease transmission between these two groups. Proceed with routine avian health management programs.

2. Do you have free-roaming Galliformes such as jungle fowl, peafowl, and guinea fowl on grounds?
   a. *Yes:* These free-roaming birds may serve to transmit diseases between domestic and exotic Galliformes, depending on the diseases present in the domestic and exotic Galliformes population.
   Recommendation: Depending on the species status (endangered, threatened, etc.) of the captive exotic Galliformes, it may be recommended to remove free-roaming species from the grounds or minimize access between the domestic and exotic Galliformes groups.
   b. *No:* If you have both domestic and exotic Galliformes on site, ensure that no contact exists between groups by minimizing zookeeper duties between these two groups.

3. For the housing of exotic Galliformes, do you have barriers between the separate species?
   a. *Yes:* This will provide some protection of cross-transmission for respiratory diseases, but do not have false sense of security that this will entirely prevent diseases.
   b. *No:* It would be important to determine the presence of respiratory diseases to prevent cross-transmission of disease and to know what species present a risk to others in the collection.
   Recommendation: Perform serologic tests to establish a baseline.

4. Do free-living bird species such as passerines have the ability to contact exhibit birds?
   a. *Yes:* An increased surveillance should be made for diseases such as Newcastle disease, avian influenza, mycoplasmosis, salmonellosis, and chlamydiosis.
   Recommendation: Try to limit wild bird access to food and water to avoid contamination at these sites. For exotic Galliformes, caging diameter may help to prevent contact. For domestic Galliformes, feeding may occur indoors prior to release in an outdoor exhibit or when birds are being cooped in the evening. Also, contact state diagnostic laboratories to determine disease prevalence in the region.
   b. *No:* Less risk potential for diseases exists.

5. Does a history of mosquito-borne infections exist in the environment?
   a. *Yes:* Ensure that mosquito control methods are in place.
   Recommendation: Use of mosquito fish in aquatic exhibits may prevent mosquito larvae development. Avoid having standing pools of water. It may be necessary to vaccinate exotic Galliformes for arthropod-bone diseases. Long-term solutions may require indoor housing for Phasanidae species, which are susceptible to such diseases as those caused by equine encephalitis virus and West Nile virus.
   b. *No:* Less risk potential for these diseases exists.
   Recommendation: Keep abreast of mosquito-borne diseases though periodic contact with state diagnostic laboratories and public health departments; local mosquito control divisions will have information on diseases in the region.

TABLE 18-4

Viral Diseases That Should Be Considered for Captive Exotic Galliformes Depending on Risk Factor and Captivity Purposes

	Risk Factor/Captivity Purpose					
Viral Disease	Captive Breeding Facility	Mosquito Exposure	Free-Living Waterfowl	Free-Living Passerine	High Prevalence in County of Acquisition	Facility Design and Close Contact with Other Galliformes
Avian encephalomyelitis	✓					
Avian influenza			✓	✓	✓	
Newcastle disease			✓	✓	✓	
Quail bronchitis						✓
Avian pox		✓				✓
Rotavirus infection						✓
Equine encephalitis		✓				
Laryngotracheitis						✓
Marble spleen disease						✓

Laryngotracheitis, also known as *infectious laryngotracheitis*, was once only reported in chickens; however, pheasants and peafowl have also been reported to be affected.[64] This upper respiratory disease is transmitted via aerosols from infected birds or by ingestion. Since it is a herpesvirus, affected birds carry this disease for life and may manifest signs when under stress.[33] In its most severe form, it may cause open mouth breathing and emesis of blood in affected birds. It would be difficult to see blood on colored feathers, but it is most noticeable on light-colored plumage. Vaccination is not an option in exotic species, as the vaccine is a live modified virus and vaccinated birds will remain carriers for life. It is unknown how exotic Galliformes will react to the vaccine strains. This disease

TABLE 18-5

Bacterial Disease That Should Be Considered for Captive Exotic Galliformes Depending on Risk Factor and Captivity Purposes

Bacterial Disease	Risk Factor/Captivity Purpose					
	Captive Breeding Facility	Mosquito Exposure	Free-Living Waterfowl	Free-Living Passerine	High Prevalence in County of Acquisition	Facility Design and Close Contact with Other Galliformes
Avian tuberculosis				✓	✓	✓
Bordetellosis						✓
Avian cholera			✓	✓	✓	✓
Infectious coryza						✓
Mycoplasma gallisepticum	✓			✓		✓
Necrotic enteritis						✓
Ulcerative enteritis						✓
Salmonellosis	✓		✓	✓		✓

TABLE 18-6

Parasitic Disease That Should Be Considered for Captive Exotic Galliformes Depending on Risk Factor and Captivity Purpose

Parasitic Disease	Risk Factor/Captivity Purpose					
	Captive Breeding Facility	Mosquito Exposure	Free-Living Waterfowl	Free-Living Passerine	High Prevalence in County of Acquisition	Facility Design and Close Contact with Other Galliformes
Protozoan						
Coccidiosis						✓
Cryptosporidiosis						✓
Histomoniasis						✓
Blood parasites		✓			✓	✓
Nematodes						
Intestinal worms						✓
Crop worms						✓
Proventricular worms						✓
Gizzard worms						✓
Cecal worms						✓
Eye worms					✓	
Tracheal worms					✓	✓
Heart worms		✓			✓	✓
Subcutaneous/Connective					✓	✓
Coelomic cavity tissue worm					✓	✓
Cestodes					✓	✓
Trematodes					✓	✓
External Parasites						
Fleas						✓
Mites				✓		✓
Lice						✓
Scaly-leg mite				✓		✓

should be considered if free-roaming domestic chickens and jungle fowl are kept on site.

Marble spleen disease has been reported in ring-necked pheasants.[64] It is caused by an adenovirus. Affected birds have a swollen, marbled, colored spleen and a swollen liver. Affected pheasants may have pulmonary edema and die suddenly. A commercial vaccine is recommended for pheasants in aviary collections if this disease is prevalent in the area.[64]

Bacterial Diseases

Avian tuberculosis is caused by the bacterium *Mycobacterium avium*. In zoologic settings, avian tuberculosis has been reported in other bird species in aviary collections. Galliformes species are susceptible to infection by *M. avium*. Avian tuberculosis tends to be a chronic condition, and affected birds often do not demonstrate any clinical signs until death.[40] On physical examination, emaciation and a prominent keel bone are seen. Transmission is via ingestion of contaminated feed, water, and exposure to contaminated feces from infected birds. Wild birds such as sparrows, starlings, and pigeons may disseminate the bacteria to exotic Galliformes. Necropsy often reveals granulomatous lesions in the intestines, liver, and spleen. Treatment is not recommended unless endangered species are affected.[64]

Bordetellosis has been reported primarily in turkeys, but quails and partridges have also been reported to be affected.[64] It is caused by the bacterium *Bordetella avium*. Transmission is primarily through inhalation of infectious aerosols. Affected birds have catarrhal rhinitis. Sanitation of water systems may help prevent future outbreaks.[28,33] This should not be a problem in zoologic settings unless domestic turkeys are present; transmission may be from contaminated clothing and footwear, so caretakers of a children's zoo should not be assigned care of exotic Galliformes collections.

Avian cholera affects a wide range of avian species, including many Galliformes species. Sulfadimethoxine is the drug of choice. Sulfaquinoxaline and sulfamethazine have been very effective in treating affected birds. Rodent control is an effective measure to reduce the incidence of avian cholera, as this disease has been associated with rodents for other zoo-housed aviary species.[33,38] This disease should be considered if free-ranging passerine and waterfowl are present and if facilities house children's zoo or barnyard exhibits with domestic chickens. Chickens may serve as reservoirs and not demonstrate any clinical signs. However, turkeys, peafowl, and pheasants are often affected with unilateral or bilateral infraorbital sinusitis.

Infectious coryza is caused by the bacterium *Hemophilus paragallinarium*. This is a disease primarily reported in chickens, but pheasant, guinea fowl, and turkeys have also been reported to have this disease.[64] It should be noted that recovered birds may serve as carriers. Transmission is from infected aerosols from direct contact of infected birds or by ingestion of contaminated water and feed. This bacterium may also be transferred from contaminated clothing and fomites. Affected birds have upper respiratory infection, often with swelling of the infraorbital sinuses.[33,40] This disease should be considered if domestic chickens are housed on site with exotic Galliformes. Sulfa drugs, tetracycline, and erythromycin have been effective.[64]

The general terminology of mycoplasmosis refers to disease caused by species belonging to the *Mycoplasma* genus of bacteria. This disease is transmitted via horizontal as well as vertical transmission. Free-living passerines have been reported with *Mycoplasma*.[2] In exotic Galliformes, vertical transmission may disseminate this disease among aviary and zoologic collections. Birds infected with *Mycoplasma* often do not display any clinical signs of disease. This bacterium does not cause any problems unless a concurrent respiratory infection exists, in which case clinical signs could become more severe. This organism has been reported in pheasants, partridges, pea fowl, guinea fowl, and quail.[64] In some aviary collections of exotic peafowl, up to 100% of the birds may be infected, with initial clinical signs reported as bilateral or unilateral swollen infraorbital sinuses (Morishita, unpublished data). Treatment of affected birds has been effective with tylosin, erythromycin, baytril, lincomycin, and spectinomycin.[64] Tylosin in water has been effective in bringing the infection under control.[64] All incoming exotic Galliformes species entering zoologic facilities and in captive breeding facilities during the quarantine period should be monitored for this disease through serologic examinations.

Necrotic enteritis is caused by the bacterium *Clostridium perfringens* and is often associated with intestinal injury initiated by coccidia. Chukar partridges and pheasants have been known to be infected with this disease.[64] Affected birds have mucoid and often bloody diarrhea. A number of antibiotics may be used to treat the infection and include bacitracin, lincomycin, streptomycin, and tetracycline.[64] This is a soil-borne disease and is usually prevalent in high-density captive breeding conditions. It is usually not a problem in zoologic aviaries, but it may occur when birds are temporarily crowded during maintenance of pens.

Ulcerative enteritis is also known as *quail disease* and is caused by the bacterium *Clostridium colinum*. It has been reported in quails and pheasants.[64] Affected quails have a white watery diarrhea that is characteristic of this disease. Affected birds become depressed and are often found dead. Typical lesions at necropsy include ulcers in the small intestines and cecum. The liver may have tan or yellow focal lesions. Neomycin may be provided in the water.[64]

Paratyphoid *Salmonella* infections have been reported in exotic Galliformes species. Over 2000 species of *Salmonella* exist, and they have a wide host range. Many Galliformes species do not show any signs and yet shed the bacteria. Culture of feces when birds are in quarantine is recommended to determine prevalence, but this needs to occur for several successive collections, as shedding may be sporadic.[35] Maintaining *Salmonella*-free conditions may be impracticable, as the large variety of host species would be difficult to control. Moreover, free-living waterfowl and passerines have been documented to carry *Salmonella* species in their feces.[15,57]

Other Bacterial Diseases

There are other bacterial diseases such as botulism that may affect exotic Galliformes, but this is probably seen in facilities with a known history of botulism on the premise, for example, those with wetland environments[7] or high-density avian exhibits, which are not usually common in zoologic facilities but may be an issue in captive breeding facilities.

Parasitic Infections

Coccidiosis is caused by the parasite *Eimeria* which is highly host specific. Documented cases have been reported in pheasants, quails, chukars, guinea fowl, and peafowl.[64] Sulfadiomethoxine is the preferred drug, as it is safer.[64] Amprolium in water is a safe and effective drug for the treatment of coccidiosis.[64] This disease is of concern in newly acquired birds, which should be evaluated during the quarantine period to prevent future oocyst buildup in exhibits. Although it has been shown that coccidiosis tends to be host specific,[55] this disease in exotic Galliformes needs to be documented for host range species specificity. Since coccidiosis is host specific and exotic Galliformes are not housed in large numbers, disease outbreaks are minimal unless oocyst buildup occurs over time.

Cryptosporidium has been reported in quails, pheasants, and peafowl and affects the respiratory and digestive systems.[64] Effective sanitation measures for prevention are important, as no effective treatment exists. Assessment for this parasite should be performed during the quarantine period to prevent seeding of spores in the facility.

Guinea fowl are susceptible to the parasite *Histomonas meleagridis*.[19] Chukars, grouses, quails, partridges, pheasants, and peafowl have also been reported to be affected.[64] Sudden death may occur, and affected birds may have sulfa colored droppings. Necropsy may reveal depressed, craterlike lesions in the liver and cecal cores. Cecal cores have also been reported in other diseases such as salmonellosis, coccidiosis, and colibacillosis,[29,51,54] so it is necessary to confirm hertomoniasis with parasite identification from intestinal scrapings and other clinical signs. Metronidazole, dimetridazole, and ipronidazole have been used for treatment.[6,64] This disease may be common in zoologic facilities. Domestic chickens may carry this parasite and not demonstrate any clinical signs; however, turkeys, peafowl, and pheasants are highly susceptible, and high mortality may be seen. Facilities with free-roaming peafowl and children's zoo or barnyard areas are at higher risk (Morishita, unpublished data).

Blood Parasites

Hemoproteus has been reported in quails,[64] *Leucocytozoon neavel* in guinea fowl,[64] *Plasmodium* spp. in pheasants and guinea fowl.[55,64]

Guans, curassows, and chachalacas have also been documented to have *Hemproteus*.[3] Assessments for blood parasites should be performed during the quarantine period. Mosquito control is important in areas with mosquitos.

Roundworms

Crop worms that have been found in the crop also invade the esophagus, since the crop is actually an outpocket of the esophagus. *Capillaria* species have also been reported in exotic Galliformes species, with earthworm as the intermediate host.[55] *Capillaria contorta* has been reported in guinea fowl, partridges, pheasants, quails, and turkeys.[55,64] *Capillaria annulata* has been reported in grouses, guinea fowl, partridges, pheasants, quails, and turkeys.[55,64] *Gongylonema* species such as *Gongylonema ingluvicola* affect the crops of partridges, pheasants, quails, and turkeys.[55,64] Beetles and cockroaches serve as intermediate hosts.[55] If these worms are detected on site, control of intermediate hosts is warranted.

Worms in the proventriculus belong to the species *Dispharynx*, including *Dispharynx nasuta*, and have been reported in grouses, guinea fowl, partridges, pheasants, and quails.[55,64] Pill bugs and sow bugs may serve as intermediate hosts for *Dispharynx* species.[55,64] Affected birds may appear emaciated. Thiabendazole has been effective as treatment.[64]

Other genera found in the proventriculus include *Tetrameres*. Cockroaches and grasshoppers serve as intermediate hosts.[55,64] *Tetrameres americana* has been reported in grouses, quails, and turkeys.[55,64] In addition, *T. fissispina* has been reported in guinea fowl, quails, and turkeys; and *T. pattersoni* has been reported in quails.[55,64] Affected birds appear emaciated and may be anemic. Fenbendazole has been effective in the treatment of this parasitic infection.[64]

Cyrnea colini has been reported in grouses, prairie chickens, quails, and turkeys and use the cockroach as the intermediate host.[55,64] *Cyrnea pileata* has been reported in quails.[55,64] *Physaloptera acuticauda* has been reported in prairie chickens and pheasants.[55,64]

The "gizzard worms," *Cheilospirura spinosa*, have been reported in grouses, partridges, pheasants, quails, and turkeys.[55,64] The species *C. hamulosa* has been reported in grouses, guinea fowl, and turkeys.[55,64] Phenothiazine and fenbendazole have been effective.[64] Affected birds may have hemorrhagic and necrotic gizzard linings. Grasshoppers and beetles are intermediate hosts for this genera.[55] Another genus, *Cyrnea eurycerea*, has been reported in pheasants, quails, and turkeys.[55,64] *Epomidiostomum uncinatum* and *Streptocara crassicuada* have been reported in prairie chickens.[55,64]

Ascaridia galli has been reported in turkeys and in quails.[55,64] *A. numidae* has been reported in guinea fowl.[55,64] *A. bonasae* has been reported in grouses; and *A. compare* has been reported in grouses, partridges, pheasants, and quails.[55,64] *Trichostrongylus*, also found in the intestines of quails and guinea fowl, has a direct lifecycle.[55] Fenbendazole is the drug of choice.[64]

Capillaria species are more commonly associated with the crop, and certain other species have also been reported in the small intestines. For example, *C. anatis* has been reported in partridges, quails, and turkeys; *C. bursata* has been reported in pheasants and turkeys; *C. caudinflata* in grouses, guinea fowl, partridges, pheasants, quails, and turkeys; and *C. obsignata* in guinea fowl, quails, and turkeys.[55,64] Most species use earthworms as the intermediate host.[55] *C. phasuanina*, also reported in the cecum, has been reported in the partridge, pheasant, and guinea fowl.[55,64] *C. tridens* has been reported in wild turkeys.[55,64] This disease is best prevented by evaluating its prevalence during the quarantine period.

In the cecum, *Heterakis gallinarum* may be found in many exotic Galliformes species, including grouses, guinea fowl, partridges, pheasants, and quails.[55,64] This worm is unique in that it may also play a role in histomoniasis, an important disease in Galliformes. *H. isolonche* has been reported in the grouse, pheasant, prairie chicken, and quail.[55,64] *H. gallinarum* and *H. isolonche* do not need an intermediate host to perpetuate their lifecycles.[55]

Other genera of nematodes reported in the ceca include *Sublura*, including the species *S. brumpti* in the grouse, guinea fowl, partridge, pheasant, quail, and turkey, and *S. strongylina* in the guinea fowl and quail.[55,64] *Sublura* genera use beetles, grasshoppers, and cockroaches as intermediate hosts.[55] The genera *Aulonocephalus* has also been reported in exotic Galliformes species, including *A. lindaquisti* and *A. quaricensis* in the quail and *A. pennula* in turkeys.[55,64]

Two additional genera in exotic Galliformes species include *Strongyloides avium* in the grouse, quail, and turkey and *Trichostrongylus tenuis* in the guinea fowl, quail, and turkey.[55,64]

The eye parasite *Oxyspirura mansoni*, has been reported in the grouse, guinea fowl, peafowl, and quail.[55,64] The cockroach serves as the intermediate host.[55] Affected birds may have conjunctivitis and protrusion of the third eyelid. Severe infections result in damage to the eye, as the bird tries to remove the irritation. Tramisol and ivermectin have been effective for the treatment of this parasite.[64] *O. petrowi* has been reported in the grouse, pheasant, and prairie chicken.[55,64]

The tracheal parasite, *Syngamus trachea*, has been reported to affect the guinea fowl, partridge, peafowl, pheasant, and quail.[55,64] Affected birds may have open mouth breathing and severe respiratory distress. Increased mortality is seen in young birds. Earthworms may serve as intermediate hosts.[55] *Splendidofilaria californiensis* has been recovered from the heart of quails.[55,64]

In exotic Galliformes species, nematodes in the subcutaneous tissue are often underdiagnosed, as subcutaneous tissues may not be examined as thoroughly during necropsy. Examination of subcutaneous tissues during a necropsy is warranted to establish prevalence. However, subcutaneous parasites cause minimal effects in Galliformes. *Singhfilaria hayesi* has been reported in quails and turkeys; and *Splendidofilaria pectoralis* has been reported in the grouse.[55,64,69] *Chandlerella chitwoodae* has been reported in the connective tissue of the grouse.[55,64]

Nematodes in the body cavity have been more frequently reported in other bird orders such as Piciformes (woodpeckers) and herons, *Aproctella stoddardi* has been reported in quails and turkeys, and *Cardiotilaria niles* has been reported in prairie chickens.[55,64]

Numerous tapeworm genera exist, including *Amoebotaenia*, *Choanotaenia*, *Davainea*, *Drepanidotaenia*, *Hymenolepis*, *Imparmargo*, *Metroliasthes*, and *Raillietina* has been reported in exotic Galliformes species (guinea fowl, peafowl, pheasants, quails, and turkeys).[55,64] Weight loss has been noted in severely affected birds.

Numerous genera of flukes have been reported in exotic Galliformes species.[55] They are often missed if only fecal flotation examinations are performed.[55] Necropsy may detect specimens as incidental findings. For example, a sudden death of two vulturine guinea fowl housed in a zoo was submitted for necropsy. No clinical signs were noted in the birds' histories, but the two birds had numerous intestinal flukes identified as *Morishitium*.[60] Hence, examinations of intestinal contents is warranted for many exotic Galliformes species.

External Parasites

Sticktight fleas (*Echidnophaga gallinacean*) have been reported in pheasants and quails.[55,60,62]

Ornithonyssus sylvarium is the northern fowl mite and has a wide host range, so physical examination of these birds should be performed. Since the host range is extensive, free-living passerine may disseminate this parasite in aviary collections.[55,61] Mites may live for some time away from live birds, so control of mites needs to include disinfection of the housing, which may be difficult under zoologic conditions.

Lice are highly host specific. Lice infestation may be prevented by examining birds during the quarantine period.[55,61] If lice cannot be detected on physical examination, bird feathers must be examined for evidence of nits. Nits may appear along the feathers but often occur at the base of the feather shaft. Examining for eggs is important, as sometimes birds are dusted at preshipping sites but may still carry nits that may hatch within 2 weeks. The entire lifecycle of lice occurs on live birds.

Knemidocoptes mutans is known as the scaly leg mite and has a wide host range. The scales of the bird's feet are upturned because of the burrowing mite. In severe infections, loss of digits has been reported in chickens.[58] Galliformes housed in facilities with exposure to free-living birds have a higher risk.

REPRODUCTION

The main reproductive diseases in Galliformes are impacted oviducts and an associated colibacellosis.[10,34] Galliformes have a functioning left ovary.[67] Frequently, the precursor to an incident of impacted oviducts is a prior respiratory disease. Hence, the bird's health history should be evaluated. If breeding of Galliformes is desired, the enclosure should be set to contain nest boxes that are easily accessed by staff for egg collection for artificial incubation. Nest boxes should measure 18 inches in length and 12 inches in height and 12 inches in width with a 3- to 4-inch lip in the front to retain the nest material within the nest boxes.[19] A layer of straw is placed to line the box. The diet should also be transitioned from a maintenance diet to a breeding diet. Since most exotic Galliformes species such as pheasants are seasonal breeders, the diet should be transitioned in early February.[20]

Mating pairs occur among the guinea fowl.[19] Good fertility may be achieved with a ratio of one male to 4 to 5 females.[19] Unlike in other Galliformes species, guinea fowl eggs are tear-drop shaped.[19] Other exotic Galliformes species should be maintained as breeding pairs.[3]

TABLE 18-7

Reproductive Parameters of Selected Species of Galliformes

Family	Common Name	Clutch Size	Incubation Period (Days)
Megapodidae	Australian brush turkey	5–35	45–90
Cracidae	Curassow	2	28–32
Tetraonidae	American woodcock	4	19–22
	Ruffed grouse	8–14	24–26
Phasianidae	Blood pheasant	5–12	27–29
	Tragopan	2–6	28
	Monal	5	27
	Jungle fowl	5–10	21
	Eared pheasants	5–8	26–27
	Crested pheasants	4–9	22–24
	Ring-necked pheasants	8–12	23
	Argas pheasants	2	25
	Peafowl	2–8	26–28
	Quail	5–12	16–21
	Partridge	3–15	24–26
	Black francolin	8–12	18–19
	Erckel's francolin	5–10	21–23
	Greater prairie chicken	12	23–26
	Roul'roul	4–6	18–22
Numididae	Guinea fowl	6–20	26–28
Meleagrididae	Turkey	8–15	28
Opistocomidae	Hoatzin	2–3	Unknown

As summarized by Drew ML: Galliformes (pheasants, grouse, quail, turkeys, chacalacas, currasows, hoatzins). In Fowler ME, Miller RE (ed): *Zoo and wildlife medicine*, 5th ed. St. Louis, MO, 2003, Saunders.

If a captive breeding program is desired, eggs should be collected once a day. In extremely hot weather, collection should be done twice a day. Eggs should be immediately incubated; if a synchronous hatch is desired, the eggs may be refrigerated until a clutch is obtained.[59] Hatchability decreases the longer eggs are refrigerated; and eggs should not be kept longer than 5–7 days as hatchability will decrease.[59]

A large variation exists in the number of days needed for incubation of the eggs of exotic Galliformes species. Table 18-7 provides common incubation times for exotic Galliformes species.[13] Since artificial incubators are used in most zoologic and private aviary settings, once the eggs are collected, it is important to write the name of the species, the date of collection, and the potential hatch date on the egg so that these dates may be monitored.[59,64] Light colored eggs should be "candled" to observe if a chick is developing. Chick development may be best confirmed about 4 to 5 days after the start of incubation.[59] If no chick development is noted in any of the eggs, it is best to remove those eggs, as they may pose a risk for other incubating eggs. Infertile eggs or eggs in which the embryo has died early in incubation are excellent source of nutrients for bacteria such as *Pseudomonas* and may cause the egg to explode within the incubator.[59] These exploding eggs may spread infection to other eggs in the incubator and may cause egg mortality or early chick infections.

Guinea fowl eggs have a thicker shell and require more humidity and a slightly higher temperature compared with the chicken egg.[19] Hence, they are often incubated with waterfowl eggs.

Eggs incubated under poor sanitation or those with poor shell quality may result in chicks with an increased incidence of omphalitis caused by bacteria such as *Escherichia coli*, *Staphylococcus aureus*, *Klebsiella* spp., *Streptococcus* spp., and *Proteus* spp.[36,42,45,49] Although *Enterococcus* species may be isolated, it is rarely associated with omphalitis.[47]

Artificial heaters have been used for large breeds after hatching, but caution should be exercised when using gas heaters because of the risk of toxic gas buildup.[30]

REFERENCES

1. Amand WB: Clinical pathology. In Fowler ME, editor: *Zoo and wildlife medicine*, Philadelphia, PA, 1978, Saunders.
2. Aye PP, Morishita TY, Bills B: Conjunctivitis in Ohio's free-living passerines. *Wildl Rehab* 15:165–168, 1998.
3. Bennett GE: Gabaldan A, Ullva G: Avian haemoproteidae. The haemoproteids of the avian family Cracidae (Galliformes); The quans, curassows, and chachalacas. *Can J Zool* 60:3105–3112, 1982.
4. Bounous DL, Wyatt RD, Gibbs PS, et al: Normal hematologic and serum biochemical reference intervals for juvenile wild turkeys. *J Wildl Dis* 36:393–396, 2000.
5. Calnek BW, Barnes HJ, Beard CW, et al: *Diseases of poultry*, Ames, IA, 1991, Iowa State University Press.
6. Carpenter N: Anseriform and galliform therapeutics. *Vet Clin North Am Exot Anim Pract* 3:1–17, 2000.
7. Davidson WR, Nettles VF: *Field manual of wildlife diseases in the southeastern United States: Southeastern cooperative wildlife disease study*, Athens, GA, 1988, University of Georgia Press.
8. Davis MF, Morishita TY: *Poultry necropsy basics. Extension Factsheet, Veterinary Preventive Medicine, Factsheet #VME-11-2001*, Columbus, OH, 2001, The Ohio State University Extension.
9. Davis MF, Ebako G, Morishita TY, et al: *Medical management of the rooster spur. Extension Factsheet, Veterinary Preventive Medicine, Factsheet #VME-014-02*, Columbus, OH, 2002, The Ohio State University Extension.
10. Davis MF, Ebako GM, Morishita TY: A golden comet hen (*Gallus gallus forma domestica*) with an impacted oviduct and associated colibacillosis. *J Avian Med Surg* 17:91–95, 2003.
11. del Hoyo J, Elliott A, Sargatal J, editors: *Handbook of birds of the world*, vol 2, New World Vultures to Guineafowl. Barcelona, Spain, 1994, Lynx Edicions, pp 277–567.

12. Delacour J: *Pheasants of the world*, Hindhead, England, 1977, World Pheasant Association and Spur Publications.

13. Drew ML: Galliformes (pheasants, grouse, quail, turkeys, chacalacas, currasows, hoatzins). In Fowler ME, Miller RE, editors: *Zoo and wildlife medicine*, ed 5, St. Louis, MO, 2003, Saunders.

14. Ebako GM, Morishita TY: Preventive medicine for backyard chickens. In *Extension Factsheet, Veterinary Preventive Medicine, Factsheet #VME-12-2001*, Columbus, OH, 2001, The Ohio State University Extension.

15. Fallacara DM, Monahan CM, Morishita TY, et al: Survey of parasites and bacterial pathogens from free-living waterfowl in zoological settings. *Avian Dis* 48:759–767, 2004.

16. Gerlach H: Galliformes. In Altman RB, Clubb SL, Dorrestein GM, Quesenberry K, editors: *Avian medicine and surgery*, Philadelphia, PA, 1997, Saunders.

17. Gill FB: *Ornithology*, New York, 1990, W.H. Freeman and Company, p 529.

18. Gylstorff I, Grimm F: *Vogelkrankheiten (bird diseases)*, Stuttgart, Germany, 1987, Verlag Eugen Ulmer.

19. Hayes C: *Raising turkeys, ducks, geese, pigeons, and guineas*, Blue Ridge Summit, PA, 1987, TAB Books Inc., p 354.

20. Howman K: *Pheasants of the world: Their breeding and management*, Blaine, WA, 1993, Hancock House Publishers, p 184.

21. Ison AJ, Spiegle SJ, Morishita TY: *Poultry blood collection. Extension Factsheet, Veterinary Preventive Medicine. Factsheet #VME-22-04*, Columbus, OH, 2004, The Ohio State University Extension.

22. Ison AJ, Spiegle SJ, Morishita TY: *Predators of poultry. Extension Factsheet, Veterinary Preventive Medicine, Factsheet #VME-22-05*, Columbus, OH, 2005, The Ohio State University Extension.

23. Johnsgard PA: *The grouse of the world*, Lincoln, NE, 1983, University of Nebraska Press.

24. Johnsgard PA: *The quails, partridges, and francolins of the world*, Oxford, U.K., 1988, Oxford University Press.

25. Johnson-Delaney CA: *Exotic companion medicine handbook for veterinarians*, Lake Worth, FL, 1996, Wingers Publishing, Inc.

26. Kan XZ, Yang JK, Li XF, et al: Phylogeny of major lineages of galliform birds (Aves: Galliformes) based on complete mitochondrial genomes. *Genet Mol Res* 9:1625–1633, 2010.

27. Latshaw JD, Kobalka P, Morishita TY, et al: Selenium toxicity in breeding ring-necked pheasants (*Phasinus colchicus*). *Avian Dis* 48:935–939, 2004.

28. Morishita TY: *A word about … disinfectants. California Poultry Letter,* Cooperative Extension, Davis, CA, 1990, University of California-Davis.

29. Morishita TY: Establishing a differential diagnosis for backyard poultry flocks. In *Proceedings of the 1990 Annual Conference of the Association of Avian Veterinarians*, Phoenix, Arizona, 1990, Association of Avian Veterinarians, pp 136–146. September 10–15.

30. Morishita TY: *Ventilation and toxic gases. California Poultry Letter,* Cooperative Extension, Davis, CA, 1991, University of California-Davis.

31. Morishita TY: *Vaccines and their implications to poultry health. California Poultry Letter,* Cooperative Extension, Davis, CA, 1992, University of California-Davis.

32. Morishita TY: May you judge a fecal sample by its color? In *Proceedings of the 43rd Western Poultry Disease Conference*, Sacramento, CA, 1994, p 7.

33. Morishita TY: Respiratory syndromes in backyard poultry. In *Core Seminar Proceedings of the Association of Avian Veterinarians Annual Conference*, Reno, Nevada, 1994, pp 35–44.

34. Morishita TY: Common reproductive problems in the backyard chicken. In *Section 11: Topics in clinical medicine, Main Conference Proceedings, Association of Avian Veterinarians Annual Conference*, Philadelphia, PA, 1995, pp 465–467.

35. Morishita TY: Poultry management 101: Poultry management topics for avian veterinarian. In *Section 7: Practice Management. Main Conference Proceedings, Association of Avian Veterinarians Annual Conference*, Philadelphia, PA, 1995, pp 327–331.

36. Morishita TY: Egg diagnostic techniques. *Ohio State Univ Vet Extension Newslett* 23(3):2–3, 1995.

37. Morishita TY: Common infectious diseases in backyard chickens and turkeys (from a private practice perspective). *J Avian Med Surg* 10(1):2–11, 1996.

38. Morishita TY, Lowenstine LJ, Hirsh DW, et al: *Pasteurella multocida* in psittacines: Prevalence, pathology and characterization of isolates. *Avian Dis* 40:900–907, 1996.

39. Morishita TY: Doctoring the fowl patient. In *113th Annual Convention, Ohio Veterinary Medical Association. Annual Conference Proceedings, February 20–23, 1997*, Columbus, OH, 1997, Hyatt Regency, 4, pp 319–321.

40. Morishita TY: Fowl patients and pheasant experiences. In *113th Annual Convention, Ohio Veterinary Medical Association Annual Conference Proceedings, February 20–23, 1997*, Columbus, OH, 1997, Hyatt Regency, 4, pp 322–323.

41. Morishita TY: Blood collection techniques for backyard chicken flocks. *Ohio State Univ Vet Extension Newslett* 23(4):7, 1997.

42. Morishita TY: Egg diagnostic techniques. In *114th Annual Convention, Ohio Veterinary Medical Association Annual Conference Proceedings*, vol 3, Session (Small Ruminant) 391. Columbus, OH, 1998, p 5.

43. Morishita TY: Clinical assessment of chickens and waterfowl in backyard flocks. *Vet Clin North Am Exot Anim Pract* 2(2):383–404, 1999.

44. Morishita TY: Backyard poultry medicine: Vaccination strategies and serological monitoring. In *115th Annual Convention, Ohio Veterinary Medical Association Annual Conference (Midwest Veterinary Conference) Proceedings*, vol 3, (Session 374). Columbus, OH, 1999, pp 467–469. February 18–21.

45. Morishita TY: Maximizing your poultry necropsy skills. In *116th Annual Convention, Ohio Veterinary Medical Association Annual Conference (Midwest Veterinary Conference) Proceedings*, vol 3, Columbus, OH, 2000, pp 457–463.

46. Morishita TY: *Biosecurity for poultry. Extension Factsheet, Veterinary Preventive Medicine, Factsheet #VME-9-2001*, Columbus, OH, 2001, The Ohio State University Extension.

47. Morishita TY: Enterococcosis. In *The Merck veterinary manual*, ed 10, Whitehouse Station, NJ, 2010, Merck & Company, Inc., pp 2419–2420. (Invited Author).

48. Morishita TY: Gangrenous dermatitis. In *The Merck veterinary manual*, ed 10, Whitehouse Station, NJ, 2010, Merck & Company, Inc., p 2478. (Invited Author).

49. Morishita TY: Streptococcosis. In *The Merck veterinary manual*, ed 10, Whitehouse Station, NJ, 2010, Merck & Company, Inc., p 2468. (Invited Author).

50. Morishita TY: Backyard poultry medicine: Working with fowl patients. In *Proceedings of the 26th Annual Avian and Exotic Medicine Symposium*, Davis, CA, 2011, Avian and Exotic Medicine Club, School of Veterinary Medicine, University of California—Davis, p 3. April 30–May 1.

51. Morishita TY, Bickford AA: Pyogranulomatous typhlitis and hepatitis in market turkeys. *Avian Dis* 36:170–175, 1992.

52. Morishita TY, Gordon JC: *Cleaning and disinfection of poultry facilities. Extension Factsheet, Veterinary Preventive Medicine, Factsheet #VME-013-02*, Columbus, OH, 2002, The Ohio State University Extension.

53. Morishita TY, Greenacre CB: Biosecurity and zoonotic diseases. In Greenacre CB, Morishita TY, editors: *Backyard poultry medicine and surgery: A guide for veterinary practitioners*, Ames, IA, 2014, Elsevier.

54. Morishita TY, Porter RE, Jr: Gastrointestinal and hepatic diseases. In *Backyard poultry medicine and surgery: A guide for veterinary practitioners*, Ames, IA, 2014, Elsevier.

55. Morishita TY, Schaul JC: Parasites of birds. In Baker DG, editor: *Flynn's parasites of laboratory animals*, Ames, IA, 2007, Blackwell Publishing Professional, pp 217–302.

56. Morishita TY, Aye PP, Harr BS: Crop impaction resulting from feather ball formation in caged layers. *Avian Dis* 43:160–163, 1990.

57. Morishita TY, Aye PP, Ley EC, et al: Survey of pathogens and blood parasites in free-living passerines. *Avian Dis* 43:549–552, 1999.

58. Morishita TY, Johnson G, Thilstead J, et al: Scaly-leg mite infestation associated with digit necrosis in bantam chickens. *J Avian Med Surg* 19:230–233, 2005.

59. Morishita TY, Rutllant-Labeaga J, Karcher D: Egg diagnostics. In Greenacre CB, Morishita TY, editors: *Backyard poultry medicine and Surgerysurgery: A guide for veterinary practitioners*, Ames, IA, 2014, Elsevier.

60. Morishita TY, Sawa TR, Nagano CM, et al: Intestinal trematodes: An occasional finding in poultry. In *Proceedings of the 39th Western Poultry*

Disease Conference, Sacramento, CA, 1990, Association of Avian Pathologists, p 119. March 4–6.

61. Pickworth CL, Morishita TY: *Common external parasites in poultry: Lice and mites. Extension Factsheet, Veterinary Preventive Medicine, Factsheet #VME-18-03*, Columbus, OH, 2003, The Ohio State University Extension.

62. Pickworth CL, Morishita TY: *Less common external parasites in poultry. Extension Factsheet, Veterinary Preventive Medicine, Factsheet #VME-19-03*, Columbus, OH, 2003, The Ohio State University Extension.

63. Randi E, Csaikl U, Csaikl F: DNA analysis of Galliformes species: New aspects for phylogenetic relationships. *Biochem Systematics Ecol* 17:77–81, 1989.

64. Schwartz DL: *Grower's reference on gamebird health*, Okemos, MI, 1995, AVION, Inc., p 357.

65. Smith SA, Smith BJ: Bobwhite quail. In *Atlas of avian radiographic anatomy*, Philadelphia, PA, Philadelphia, PA, 1992, Saunders, pp 187–206.

66. Spiegle SJ, Ison AJ, Morishita TY: *Performing a physical exam on a chicken. Extension Factsheet, Veterinary Preventive Medicine, Factsheet #VME-20-04*, Columbus, OH, 2004, The Ohio State University Extension.

67. Spiegle SJ, Ison AJ, Morishita TY: *The making of an egg. Extension Factsheet, Veterinary Preventive Medicine, Factsheet #VME-21-04*, Columbus, OH, 2004, The Ohio State University Extension.

68. Tocidlowski ME, Norton TM, Young LA: Medical management of curassows. In *Proceedings American Association of Zoo Veterinarians*, 1999, AAZV.

69. Vollmerhaus B, Sinowatz F: Atmungsapparat. In Nickel R, et al, editors: *Lehrbuch der anatomie der haustiere, band v. anatomie der vogel*, Berlin, Germany, 1992, Verlag Paul Parey.

CHAPTER 19

Gruiformes (Cranes, Limpkins, Rails, Gallinules, Coots, Bustards)

Robert A. MacLean and Hugues Beaufrère

BIOLOGY

The order Gruiformes has historically been problematic to classify and does not seem to be a monophyletic group as at least four different clades exist in it. It includes the families Gruidae (cranes, 15 species), Psophiidae (trumpeters, 3 species), Rallidae (rails, crakes, soras, gallinules, swamphens, takahes, moorhens, and coots, 138 species), Sarothruridae (flufftails, 7 species), Heliornithidae (sungrebes, and finfoots, 3 species), and Aramidae (limpkins, 1 species). The orders Otididiformes (bustards, 26 species), Eurypygiformes (sunbitterns and Kagus, 2 species), Cariamiformes (seriemas, 2 species), and Mesitornithiformes (mesites, 2 species, and monias, 1 species) are traditionally included in the Gruiformes but are now largely separated because of morphologic and phylogenetic distinctions.[12]

This chapter presents information derived primarily from experience with managing cranes, as more published data are available, with some additional information provided for bustards, coots, and rails. Sustained efforts are ongoing to maintain, breed, and rear many species of Gruiformes for captive management and for reintroduction efforts. Much of our scientific knowledge, captive management techniques, and veterinary experience derive from these programs. According to the International Union for Conservation of Nature (IUCN) and Convention on International Trade in Endangered Species (CITES) (websites accessed November 16, 2012), of the 15 extant species of cranes, 14 species and subspecies are vulnerable or endangered; in bustards, 6 species are vulnerable or endangered; and in rails, 35 species are vulnerable or endangered, and one, the Guam rail (*Gallirallus owstoni*), is extinct in the wild (reintroduction efforts are ongoing).

Cranes are found throughout the world except in the neotropics and the Antarctic. They differ from herons and egrets in that many crane species have bright-red thick skin covering parts of the head and neck and have perforate nares. Cranes are long-lived, with a captive lifespan that may reach 50 years. Crane adults, with the exception of the African crowned cranes (*Balearica* spp.), have a long, convoluted trachea that is enclosed within the bones of the keel, which is thought to be an adaptation for producing their loud bugling call (Figure 19-1). Cranes share this tracheal characteristic only with swans (Cygninae). An extremely long and coiled trachea is also a characteristic of trumpeters (Psophiidae), but the tracheal elongation is subcutaneous.

FEEDING

Cranes are omnivorous and are known to eat a variety of foods, including grains, fish, amphibians, mollusks, rodents, and insects. For practical reasons, most captive cranes are fed commercially produced pelleted diets that have been specifically developed for cranes.[10,51,58]

RESTRAINT AND HANDLING

Cranes may sustain leg and wing injuries during capture, and they are prone to skin lacerations from their sharp toenails when mishandled. The recommended method of capture is to gently herd or push the bird into a corner or other confined space using raised arms, brooms, or both. The folded flight feathers (or bustle) may be grasped by the handler with one hand, maintaining the wings in a closed position, and the free arm may grasp around the body and wings while directing the head and neck behind them. The hand holding the bustle may then be used to restrain the legs at the hock

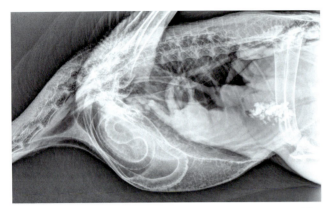

FIGURE 19-1 Lateral radiograph of a wild whooping crane (*Grus canadensis*), subsequently diagnosed with aspergillosis. Note the convoluted trachea that penetrates and is enclosed within the bones of the sternum, a characteristic of most species of cranes.

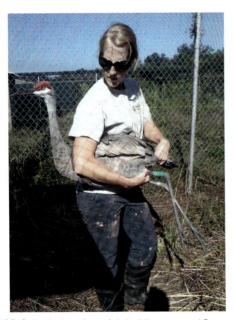

FIGURE 19-2 Technique for safely holding a crane (*Grus canadensis pulla*); one hand supports the body, and the other grasps the legs at the hocks. (Courtesy of Megan Savoie.)

using one or two fingers between the hocks. The bird is picked up, and the legs are extended parallel to the ground (Figure 19-2). For the bird that insists on facing the handler prior to capture, handlers should gently grasp the neck and direct the head behind them to initiate the grab.[10] Safety eyewear is highly recommended. Caution is advised, as aggressive cranes may cause serious injury, including punctures and lacerations. Other recommendations for restraint and handling have been outlined elsewhere.[63]

Kori bustards (*Ardeotis kori*) are powerful birds with very strong legs capable of leaping high into the air and upon restraint may cause substantial injury to themselves and to the handlers. Experienced handlers are strongly recommended for bustards (see the AZA Gruiformes TAG 2009 Kori Bustard [*Ardeotis kori*] Care Manual, Association of Zoos and Aquariums).

Chemical restraint is appropriate for extensive handling or prolonged procedures to reduce stress-related complications, including hyperthermia and capture myopathy. Inhalant anesthesia, using isoflurane or sevoflurane administered via a mask; intubation, using an uncuffed endotracheal tube; and intermittent positive pressure

ventilation (IPPV) are the preferred techniques for chemical restraint in captive Gruiformes. An appropriate facemask to accommodate the long beak of the crane may be made using a 60-milliliter (mL) plastic syringe case. Appropriate assessment of vital signs is recommended and should include monitoring of heart rate via Doppler blood flow monitor, end-tidal carbon dioxide (CO_2) and respiratory rate with the use of a capnograph, and core body temperature (published recommended values for cranes are not available but seem comparable with those for birds of similar size). The minimum alveolar concentration (MAC) in Mississippi sandhill cranes is 1.34% ± 0.14%, and cranes are susceptible to dose-dependent, isoflurane-induced respiratory depression and hypotension, particularly under spontaneous ventilation.[40] Therefore, it is recommended that a multimodal approach to anesthesia and controlled ventilation be used in these species. In addition, cranes have larger tracheal dead space compared with most birds, and inadequate ventilation and hypercapnia are frequently accompanied by bradycardia. Moreover, the interval between respiratory arrest and cardiac arrest may be very short in birds, leaving little time to respond. To reduce the chance for injury during recovery, the bird should be manually restrained in a quiet place, hooded or in low light, until it is likely to stand on its own when released.

Mild to moderate sedation with midazolam (0.5 to 1.5 milligrams per kilogram [mg/kg]) and butorphanol (0.5 to 1.5 mg/kg) intramuscularly (IM) may be adequate for minor procedures and more prolonged handling such as bandaging or diagnostic imaging in cranes. Diazepam (0.5 to 1.0 mg/kg, orally [PO]) lasts 4 to 6 hours and is useful for tranquilization for procedures such as shipping agitated birds. Sedatives may be reversed for a rapid recovery, if necessary or desired. Local anesthetics (lidocaine 0.5 milliliters [mL], xylocaine 0.5 mL, or bupivacaine up to 2 mg/kg) may be infiltrated into areas for minor procedures such as wound suturing or implanting subcutaneous radio transmitters.[51]

For field work, cranes have been successfully anesthetized with ketamine and xylazine (10–15 mg/kg ketamine, 1 mg/kg xylazine, IM), ketamine and diazepam (10–15 mg ketamine, 0.2–0.5 mg/kg diazepam, IM) combinations, or with propofol (PropoFlo Injectable, Abbott Laboratories, North Chicago, IL) as a bolus intravenously (IV) or as a continuous rate infusion (CRI).[51] A mixture of alphaxolone and alphadolone has also been used successfully in cranes for short procedures (6.5–7.0 mg/ kg, IV).[2] Alpha-chloralose (0.39–0.48 gram per cup [g/cup], or 280 mL, of corn) has been used to capture wild cranes and cranes that have escaped from zoos or private collections; however, the ingested dosage is variable, and an increased risk of capture myopathy exists.[29,49]

DIAGNOSTIC PROCEDURES

Blood may be collected from the right jugular vein or from the medial metatarsal vein. Although very rare, jugular lacerations resulting in death have occurred in a struggling crane, so appropriate caution is advised. The basilic or ulnar veins may also be used but are not recommended in alert cranes. Normal blood values of select cranes and bustards are listed in Table 19-1.[10,16,24,28,32,35,54] Hemolysis induced by EDTA (ethylenediaminetetraacetic acid) has been reported in crowned cranes, so heparin is recommended in these species.[9] The looping trachea present in other crane species may lead to the buildup of mucus or fluids at certain points and result in severe dyspnea; because of this unique anatomy, any tracheal flushes should be used with extreme caution.[51]

MEDICAL TREATMENTS

Most medical treatments, procedures, and therapeutic regimens appropriate for use in other avian species should be generally applicable to Gruiformes and Otididae. Drug selection, dosage, route and frequency of administration may vary. Refer to Tables 19-2[4,7,10,15,39,47,48] and 19-3[7,8,10,48] for antimicrobials and anthelmintics commonly used in cranes.

TABLE 19-1

Hematologic and Serum Biochemical Reference (Mean [Range] or Mean +/− SD) Values for Select Captive Gruiformes

Measurement	Sandhill Crane	Whooping Crane	Siberian Crane	Red-Crowned Crane	Wattled Crane	Eurasian Crane[a]	Kori Bustard[a]
HEMATOLOGY							
PCV (%)	43 (37–49)	42 (38–48)	45 (40–50)	39 (33–45)	45 (40–50)	42.9 ± 0.9	47 ± 5
Hb (g/dL)	13.5 (10.5–18.7)	14.4 (13.0–16.7)	—	—	—	14.8 ± 0.4	14.1 ± 0.2
RBC ($\times 10^6$/μL)	2.5 (1.9–3.3)	2.2 (1.8–2.6)	—	—	—	2.47 ± 0.07	2.3 ± 0.1
WBC ($\times 10^3$/μL)	13.0 (6.2–22.6)	18.2 (12.2–25.1)	10.8 (6.5–15.0)	14.9 (6.3–23.5)	12.7 (3.2–22.2)	21.9 ± 1.3	7.3 ± 0.4
Heterophils (%)	37 (21–56)	56 (38–74)	53	41	48	51.8 ± 2.3	55 ± 4*
Lymphocytes (%)	58 (40–74)	41 (21–60)	39	48	39	35.8 ± 2.8	30 ± 3*
Monocytes (%)	2.3 (0–10)	2 (0–6)	3	6	5	3.0 ± 0.3	8 ± 1*
Eosinophils (%)	2 (0–5)	1 (0–5)	5	5	8	3.4 ± 0.4	5 ± 1*
Basophils (%)	2.6 (0–5)	—	—	—	—	1.5 ± 0.2	3*
CHEMISTRY							
Albumin (g/dL)	1.5 (1.0–4.5)	1.5 (1.2–1.7)	1.4 (1.2–1.5)	1.2 (1.1–1.3)	1.1 (1.0–1.3)		1.6 ± 0.08
Albumin or globulin	0.63 (0.38–1.32)	0.65 (0.57–0.76)	0.6 (0.5–0.7)	0.6 (0.5–0.7)	0.6 (0.4–0.6)		1.2 ± 0.06
ALP (Units/L)	164 (34–423)	46 (28–72)	45 (28–68)	226 (128–409)	37 (13–61)		—
ALT (Units/L)	50 (19–162)	53 (42–71)	16 (6–25)	30 (18–67)	11 (10–11)		16 ± 2.2
AST (Units/L)	181 (16–260)	261 (133–612)	182 (117–254)	208 (108–456)	189 (148–230)		227 ± 11
Calcium (mg/dL)	9.7 (8.8–10.9)	9.1 (8.3–9.7)	10.5 (9.5–11.2)	10.8 (10.4–11.2)	10.8 (10.3–11.6)		12.5 ± 0.8
Chloride (mEq/L)	108 (101–115)	107 (102–113)	109 (106–113)	107 (104–110)	108 (105–111)		115 ± 1
Chol (mg/dL)	128 (87–187)	148 (96–200)	212 (148–286)	170 (140–217)	147 (120–188)	200 ± 9	120 ± 7
Creatinine (mg/dL)	0.7 (0.4–1.2)	0.6 (0.4–0.8)	0.3 (0.3–0.4)	0.3 (0.2–0.4)	0.4 (0.3–0.5)		0.57 ± 0.04
Globulin (g/dL)	2.3 (1.8–3.4)	2.3 (1.8–2.8)	2.3 (1.9–2.7)	2.1 (1.9–2.3)	2.0 (1.8–2.1)		1.3 ± 0.1
Glucose (mg/dL)	247 (87–323)	232 (210–267)	266 (209–314)	267 (239–328)	266 (246–293)		241 ± 8.5
LDH (Units/L)	278 (108–488)	440 (178–975)	202 (100–323)	288 (161–372)	137 (55–249)		3863 ± 307
P (mg/dL)	3.6 (1.7–5.4)	2.8 (2.0–4.1)	3.8 (1.9–5.8)	3.5 (2.0–4.4)	2.7 (1.6–5.7)		4.1 ± 0.2
K (mEq/L)	3.4 (2.2–4.8)	3.4 (2.6–4.2)	2.9 (1.6–4.0)	2.8 (1.6–4.0)	3.2 (2.0–3.9)		2.9 ± 0.2
TP (g/dL)	3.9 (2.9–7.9)	3.8 (3.1–4.4)	3.6 (3.1–4.1)	3.3 (2.9–3.6)	3.1 (2.8–3.4)	4.9 ± 0.1	3.0 ± 0.2
Sodium (mEq/L)	148 (142–160)	147 (140–152)	149 (146–151)	148 (143–150)	146 (144–153)		154 ± 1
Uric acid (mg/dL)	9.7 (4.1–24.6)	8.1 (6.5–10.2)	9.0 (5.5–12.6)	7.8 (4.2–11.3)	7.7 (5.4–11.1)	2.9 ± 0.4	7.9 ± 0.5

ALP, Alkaline phosphatase; *ALT*, alanine aminotransferase; *AST*, aspartate aminotransferase; *Chol*, cholesterol; *g/dL*, gram per deciliter; *Hb*, hemoglobin; *K*, potassium; *LDH*, lactate dehydrogenase; *mEq/L*, milliequivalent per liter; *mg/dL*, milligram per deciliter; *μL*, microliter; *P*, phosphorus; *PCV*, packed cell volume; *RBC*, red blood cells; *TP*, total protein; *Units/L*, units per liter; *WBC*, white blood cells.
[a]Reported as mean ± standard error of mean (*Note:* sem = sd/√n).
*Calculated from reported mean absolute values.

TABLE 19-2

Antimicrobial Agents Commonly Used in Cranes

Agent	Dosage
ANTIBIOTICS	
Amikacin	10 mg/kg, IM, every 12 hours
Ampicillin	20 (to 100) mg/kg, IM, every 12 hours
Carbenicillin	100 mg/kg, IM or IV, every 12 hours
Cefazolin sodium	25–30 mg/kg, IM or IV, every 8 hours
Cefotaxime sodium	50–100 mg/kg, IM, every 8 hours
Cephalexin	35–50 mg/kg, PO, every 6 hours (PK)
Cephalothin	100 mg/kg, IM, SQ, every 6 hours (PK)
Chloramphenicol	100 mg/kg, SQ, every 8 hours
Enrofloxacin	8–15 mg/kg, PO or IM,* every 12 hours
Gentamicin	5 mg/kg, IM, every 8 hours (PK)
Piperacillin	100 mg/kg, IM, every 4–6 hours†
Trimethoprim–sulfamethoxazole	16–24 mg/kg (based on trimethoprim) PO every 12 hours
Tylosin	15 mg/kg, SQ, every 8 hours (PK)
ANTIMYCOTICS	
Amphotericin B	5–10 mg/15 mL water; nebulize 20 minutes every 8 hours
Clotrimazole	30 mg (3 mL) in glycerol glycolate; nebulize 20 minutes every 8 hours
Flucytosine	100 mg/kg, PO, every 8–12 hours
Itraconazole	5–10 mg/kg, PO, every 12 hours
Nystatin	300,000 IU/kg, PO, every 12 hours

*Because these drugs have the potential to cause necrosis when administered intramuscularly, oral administration is preferable or it should be diluted in subcutaneous fluids.
†According to pharmacokinetics in parrots, hawks, and owls.
IM, Intramuscularly; IU/kg, international unit per kilogram; IV, intravenously; mg/kg, milligram per kilogram; mL, milliliter; PO, by mouth; PK, pharmacokinetic study; SQ, subcutaneously.

INFECTIOUS DISEASE

Bacterial Diseases

Infectious diseases in cranes appear to be mainly bacterial in origin and sporadic in occurrence, and they are found primarily in birds that may have been predisposed to infection by environmental or population stresses.[10] A wide variety of bacteria have been isolated from cranes, including *Salmonella* spp., *Pasteurella multocida*, *Mycobacterium avium* and *M. tuberculosis*, *Clostridium* spp., *Erysipelothrix*, *Campylobacter* spp., *Streptococcus* spp., and numerous members of the Enterobacteriaceae (e.g., *Escherichia coli*, *Proteus vulgaris*, *Pseudomonas aeruginosa*, and *Bacillus* spp.).[10,21,30,62,65] The significance of most of these organisms in cranes is incompletely understood, and normal flora is reported to vary with crane species.[30,45]

Eye infections involving the cornea in crane chicks caused by *Pseudomonas aeruginosa* may be severe and lead to loss of vision in the affected eye; therefore, antibiotic treatment of corneal trauma is recommended in chicks.[45] Multiple subspecies of *Salmonella* have been cultured from wild and captive cranes, and the findings are frequently incidental, with no apparent clinical signs being present. *Salmonella*, however, has also been associated with enteritis, septicemia, and death.

Mycobacterium avium has been isolated from captive cranes, wild whooping cranes, and wild sandhill cranes. *M. avium* and salmonellosis are frequently associated with crowding, a contaminated environment, or both and should be recognized as potential dangers

where birds congregate.[62] Signs of infection in birds are variable and may be nonexistent, making diagnosis in living birds difficult. One 5-year-old wild whooping crane that was found debilitated by *M. avium* was successfully managed for over 2 years with antibiotic therapy.[49]

Viral Diseases

Viral diseases such as avian pox and Newcastle disease, which occur in most species of birds, also occur in cranes.[51] Three viral diseases have been identified as potential problems in captive cranes maintained in North America: (1) eastern equine encephalitis (EEE), (2) West Nile virus (WNV) disease, and (3) inclusion body disease of cranes (IBDC), also known as gruid herpesvirus type 1 disease. Another viral disease, infectious bursal disease (IBD), has the potential to cause morbidity and mortality in cranes.[51]

IBDC virus has been isolated from cranes in outbreaks in North America, Austria, France, Japan, and the former Union of Soviet Socialist Republics. Clinical signs were mostly nonspecific, and a herpesvirus was characterized. The antibody response noted in some surviving cranes lasts for several years, and these birds should be considered carrier animals of IBDC. A survey of wild sandhill cranes in Wisconsin and Indiana did not find any exposure to IBDC, indicating that positive, potentially subclinically infected captive birds should not come in contact with naïve wild cranes.[10] One study has demonstrated an absence of vertical transmission of the virus in a pair of seropositive black-necked cranes (*Grus nigricollis*).[26] No known treatment or vaccine exists for IBDC at the present time.[52]

EEE virus is an arbovirus (alphavirus, togaviridae) transmitted by the vector mosquito *Culiseta melanura*, which occurs sporadically in a sylvatic cycle. It infects a wide variety of indigenous bird species in the Americas, primarily in the eastern United States, and an epizootic of EEE was reported in captive whooping cranes in 1984.[17] Some birds died without any premonitory signs, and others showed signs of lethargy, ataxia, and paresis before death.[10] When the virus successfully invades the central nervous system, affected birds become depressed, lethargic, uncoordinated, and paralyzed, and they assume abnormal postures, especially of the head and neck.[48] Whooping cranes exhibit mainly the viscerotropic form of the disease with minimal neural involvement but with coelomic gross lesions while Mississippi sandhill cranes have been diagnosed with the neurotropic form.[17,44,68]

WNV is another arbovirus belonging to flaviviruses, flaviviridae, and is transmitted by *Culex* spp. Significant mortality has occurred in Mississippi and Florida sandhill crane chicks.[51] Adult birds, however, seemed to be relatively resistant to the virus, as experimental infection failed to induce death in sandhill cranes despite viremia.[49] Clinical signs include lethargy, weakness, ataxia, weight loss, and inappetence. Several other captive crane species have had WNV antibodies detected in postmortem examinations. Mortalities are rare, even without implementation of routine WNV vaccination in some captive flocks, but still occur occasionally. WNV antigen has also been associated with mortalities in Aramidae and Rallidae in North America (WNV Affected Species List 2005, March 2005, National Wildlife Health Center, Madison, WI).

IBD is a viral disease (avibirnavirus, birnaviridae) with an acute onset that targets the lymphoid tissue of the bursa, resulting in immunosuppression. Among young chickens, IBD is highly contagious. Seropositivity to IBD was associated with the deaths of captive-raised and released whooping cranes in Florida, and the virus was subsequently shown to be endemic in the region.[6] At this time, the course of IBD in cranes is not well documented, but it is thought to have been associated with fatal cases. Housing cranes in an exhibit with or near chickens or turkeys should be avoided to reduce exposure to IBD.

Mycotic Diseases

Oral candidiasis is treated in cranes using oral nystatin.[10] Aspergillosis has been diagnosed in young and adult captive cranes and has caused the deaths of numerous crane chicks, some as young as 9

TABLE 19-3

Antiparasitic Agents Commonly Used in Cranes

Agent	Dosage	Comments
Albendazole	20 mg/kg, PO; repeat in 7 days	Trematodes (some)
Amprolium	0.0125 mg/kg of feed, continuous 0.025 mg/kg of feed for 14 days 0.006% in drinking water, continuous	Coccidiosis: Prophylactic Coccidiosis: Therapeutic Coccidiosis
Carbaryl powder (5%)	Topical, weekly or biweekly, prn	Ectoparasites; use sparingly
Fenbendazole	50–100 mg/kg, PO; repeat in 14 days, prn	Intestinal strongyles, ascarids
	50 mg/kg, PO, for 5 days; repeat in 14 days	Gapeworms and capillarids
Ivermectin	0.2 mg/kg, SQ; repeat in 14 days	Nematodes and mites
Levamisole	40 mg/kg (25 mg/kg in chicks), PO; repeat in 14 days, prn	Intestinal strongyles, ascarids, and capillarids
Monensin	90 g/ton of feed, 99 ppm (continuous or seasonally)	Coccidiosis, recommended for the prevention of visceral coccidiosis
Ormetoprim-sulfadimethoxine	0.015% ormetoprim and 0.026% sulfadimethoxine in food continuously for 3 weeks	Coccidiosis
Praziquantel	6 mg/kg, PO or IM; repeat in 10–14 days	Cestodes and trematodes
Pyrantel pamoate	4.5 mg/kg, PO; repeat in 10–14 days	Intestinal nematodes
Pyrethrin powder (0.10%)	Topical; repeat in 7–14 days, prn	Ectoparasites; apply lightly
Pyrethrin 0.03%, piperonyl butoxide 0.30% spray	Topical; repeat in 3 to 7days, prn	Ectoparasites; apply lightly
Sulfachlorpyridazine	1 tsp/gal (1.3 mL/L) drinking water for 7–14 days	Coccidiosis
Sulfadimethoxine	50 mg/kg, PO, every 24 hours for 14 days	Coccidiosis
Thiabendazole	100 mg/kg, PO; repeat in 7–14 days	Intestinal strongyles and ascarids
Trimethoprim-sulfamethoxazole	16–24 mg/kg (based on trimethoprim), PO, every 12–24 hours	Coccidiosis

g/ton, Gram per ton; *IM*, intramuscularly; *mg/kg*, milligram per kilogram; *mL/L*, milliliter per liter; *PO*, by mouth; *ppm*, parts per million; *prn*, pro re nata (as circumstances require); *SQ*, subcutaneously; *tsp/gal*, teaspoon per gallon.

days. Published treatments are similar to those in other birds.[48] The use of voriconazole in cranes has not been reported.

Parasitic Diseases

Parasites are present in most wild and in many captive cranes, although the burdens are usually light.[10] Parasite prevalence in the environment will frequently increase in captivity or in areas where wild birds congregate. Clinical signs of parasitism are usually absent and, when they occur, are frequently nonspecific. Parasitism generally increases the susceptibility of an animal to disease, predation, malnutrition, and other mortality factors, thus reducing the chances of survival for the bird.[10]

Protozoa

At least three species of blood protozoans, *Haemoproteus antigonis, H. balearicae,* and *Leucocytozoon grusi,* have been found in cranes with at least one reported chick mortality.[10,18,60] Two captive Mississippi sandhill crane chicks in separate seasons became ill with severe anemia and lethargy and were diagnosed with a heavy burden of *Haemoproteus* spp. Both recovered with a single blood transfusion and treatment with atovaquone proguanil (20 mg/kg, PO, q24h 3 doses) (authors' experience). *Spironucleus* (formerly *Hexamita*) and *Spironucleus*-like spp. were associated with necrotizing enteritis and the death of captive demoiselle (*Anthropoides virgo*) in Europe and sandhill cranes in Florida. *Plasmodium* sp., *Nuttalia* sp., and non-*Eimeria* tissue coccidia (*Lankesterella* or *Atoxoplasma* spp.) have been reported in cranes, but their significance to the health of wild and captive cranes is unknown.[10]

Coccidia are considered a potentially important cause of mortality of captive cranes. Coccidia probably infect all species of cranes, and under certain conditions cause morbidity, diarrhea, and death. The coccidia *Eimeria gruis* and *E. reichenowi* are common parasites of sandhill and whooping cranes, and their presence has been reported

in at least three other crane species in captivity. Although coccidiosis generally is recognized as a disease of the intestinal tract, *Eimeria* infections in cranes, and in particular, *E. reichenowi*, is especially pathogenic because infection may become systemic with widespread extraintestinal dissemination of developmental stages.[59] This is known as disseminated visceral coccidiosis. Necropsy of naturally infected adult birds revealed multifocal nodules in many organs, including the alimentary tract and the lung, air sacs, trachea, and nares (Figure 19-3). In experimentally infected sandhill crane chicks, morbidity and death occurred at the peak of merogony (9 to 11 days following infection). Lesions identified in postmortem examination included granulomatous pneumonia and tracheitis, hepatitis, myocarditis, splenitis, and enteritis.

Eimeria represent a significant health problem for captive crane rearing facilities. Concentrations of these parasites in the substrate may increase substantially because of the direct life cycle, thus increasing the risk of overwhelming infection. Appropriate countermeasures include parasite surveillance, pen rotation, and separation of cranes by age class.[51] The anticoccidial monensin has been shown to be effective in cranes as prophylaxis.[8] It may be milled into the feed at 90 grams per ton (g/ton; 99 parts per million [ppm]) and fed continuously or for 2 months prior and 2 months after the chick-rearing season.[48] Additional references and more specific information on this common disease in cranes can be found elsewhere.[59]

Endoparasites

Although endoparasites may cause illness in cranes under certain conditions, their overall impact in wild and captive cranes is probably of low significance.[10] *Capillaria, Eucoleus, Ascaridia,* and *Syngamus* (gapeworms) species, however, are known pathogens, occasionally resulting in debilitation or death. Gapeworms may cause pneumonia and may obstruct the trachea, resulting in asphyxiation; ivermectin and fenbendazole have been effective treatment

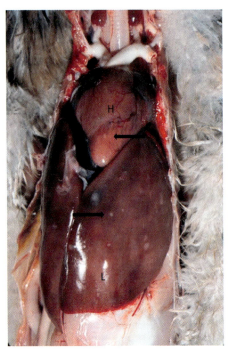

FIGURE 19-3 Granulomas (*arrows*) present in the liver (*L*) and heart (*H*) of a Mississippi sandhill crane (*Grus canadensis pulla*) that died of disseminated visceral coccidiosis caused by *Eimeria* spp. (Courtesy USGS National Wildlife Health Center.)

(see Table 19-3). Acanthocephalans, or spiny-headed worms, may perforate the intestine and lead to a fatal coelomitis. No effective anthelmintic is available, but controlling arthropods may aid in preventing transmission. Water rallidae are affected with a wide range of helminths with complex life cycles; coots, specifically, are susceptible to gastrointestinal (GI) trematodes and the gizzard worm *Amidostomum fulicae*.[22,33]

Ectoparasites
At least five species of mites (order Acarina) and four species of biting lice (order Mallophaga) have been reported in cranes. Severe cases of ectoparasites, especially in chicks, may be debilitating. Control is achieved by dusting cranes with antiparasitic powder (see Table 19-3). Biting and stinging insects, including bees (*Apis* spp.), wasps (*Vepis* spp.), black flies (*Simulium* spp.), and deer flies (*Chrysops* spp.) will attack cranes, causing localized inflammation of the skin, excessive preening, discomfort, and stress. Occasionally, the mucous membranes in the mouth will swell because of an inflammatory response resulting from an insect sting. This is a common occurrence in chicks around fledging age.[51]

NONINFECTIOUS DISEASE
Trauma
The most frequent cause of trauma in captive birds is intraspecific aggression, which often results in soft tissue trauma to the head and neck and occasional skull fractures. Aggression in cranes is often associated with the formation of dominance hierarchies and the mate selection process, including defense of territory, food, or water.[10] Any disruption of the social order also may result in aggression, including moving a new crane into an established pen.[48] In general, forming a new social group in a new and neutral pen is best; alternatively, introducing an individual crane into an adjacent pen for a few weeks before allowing it to join a group may be effective.[10] In another form of aggression, parents may attack and occasionally kill their chicks.

An underlying factor may be a sick or lethargic chick, parental disturbance (redirected aggression), or an abnormal appearance of the chick (wound or deformity).[48]

Aggression, collision with sharp objects, and self-inflicted wounds may cause lacerations. A struggling crane may lacerate itself with a sharp toenail while being captured.[10] Trauma also may rupture air sacs, resulting in subcutaneous emphysema or audible and focal abnormal respiratory sounds in chicks and adults. Minor cases of air sac rupture may resolve without medical intervention, but severe cases may result in extensive subcutaneous emphysema over the entire body.[48] Air may be withdrawn with a syringe, needle, and a three-way valve. If the affected area is limited, a pressure bandage may prove helpful. In the most severe cases, surgical insertion of a Penrose drain through the skin into the air-filled subcutaneous spaces is required to resolve the problem. The crane should be administered antibiotics and the drains cleaned with an appropriate antiseptic solution (e.g., 1% povidone-iodine solution) twice daily. After 1 to 2 weeks, the drains may be removed and cultured.[48]

Trauma to the beak is also relatively common in captive cranes, usually associated with pen fencing. With minor fractures of the tip of the beak (distal 2 to 3 cm), the two ends may be trimmed evenly to facilitate grasping and feeding. More proximal fractures require medical or surgical repair. Dental acrylic and Kirschner wires may be used to create a splint around the fracture (acrylic alone will not adhere to the rhamphotheca for sufficient time) (Figure 19-4). The splint is left in place for 3 to 4 weeks.[48]

Trauma also may result in injuries to toes or in fractures, especially of the long bones (see Orthopedic Conditions and Fractures). Neck fractures resulting in death occur in captive cranes, usually associated with a flight response into caging. Trauma is a leading cause of mortality in wild and reintroduced cranes and bustards, especially from collisions with power lines.[20,21,34,43] Interestingly, one study has shown that these birds are essentially blind in the direction of flight while scanning the terrain below.

Predation is a significant cause of mortality in wild and reintroduced cranes and remains a constant concern and cause for vigilance in captive cranes.[13,21]

Orthopedic Conditions
Disorders in Chicks
Hand-raised cranes are predisposed to leg disorders, which include deformities in the proximal ends of the tibiotarsus and tarsometatarsus, the distal end of the tibiotarsus, and the intertarsal and tibiofemoral joints.[10,51] These conditions are thought to result from an inordinately rapid weight gain during the first 4 weeks combined with insufficient limb strength but may also be related to nutritional deficiencies, hatching difficulties, improper substrate, improper handling or other physical injury, or a combination of these factors.[48] Detection involves monitoring the chick's gait and monitoring weight gain daily.[48] Exercise is known to reduce the incidence of leg deformities in captive crane chicks. In the United States, captive whooping crane and sandhill crane chicks are walked and placed in a pool for swimming several times a day for 10 to 30 minutes. Exercise may also be encouraged by placing food and water on opposite ends of the pen. If weight gain exceeds 10% per day (up to 15% at one facility), feed withholding—that is, food offered for no more than 15 minutes four times during the day and feed provided *ad libitum* overnight—should be considered.

Crooked toes are common in very young captive chicks and may also be associated with the subsequent development of limb deformities. Splinting the toes at the first sign of deviation is recommended; encircling the toe in a mildly adhesive reinforced packing tape for 2 to 3 days may be effective.

Using natural incubation, hatching, and rearing (parent or foster) of chicks also appears to reduce the occurrence of leg and toe abnormalities. Chicks will continually follow their parents in search of insects and other foods, and this provides adequate exercise on an uneven and varied surface. Diets formulated to contain low levels of

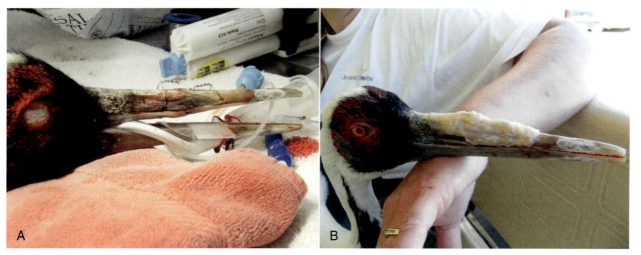

FIGURE 19-4 Beak repair in a white-naped crane (*Grus vipio*). **A,** Orthopedic wire is positioned through the beak on opposite sides of the fracture to aid in securing the splint. **B,** Cold-curing methylmethacrylate acrylic is used to splint the fracture. (Courtesy of Barry Hartup, DVM.)

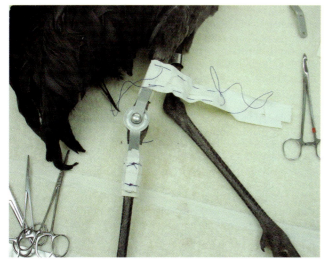

FIGURE 19-5 Application of a Belmont splint to support intertarsal joint trauma or abnormality in a crane. (Courtesy of Barry Hartup, DVM.)

methionine or sulfur-containing amino acids also appear to be effective in reducing chick growth rates.[10]

Other problems known to occur in captive crane chicks include broken blood feathers and deformities of the carpal joint (angel wing) and beak; treatment is similar to those reported for other avian species.

Arthritis

Arthritis involving the joints of the legs is also a common problem in captive cranes. Although trauma is the most common cause, septic arthritis, arthritis secondary to congenital or developmental deformities, and immune-mediated arthritis also have been documented.[14,38,41,47,52] Degenerative osteoarthritis of the hocks is common in captive Siberian cranes (*Grus leucogeranus*).[37] A 4% per year incidence of intertarsal joint trauma was estimated at the International Crane Foundation (Figure 19-5).[38]

Fractures

Fractures of the long bones are a serious problem in cranes because of an inordinately high rate of complications and subsequent death

or euthanasia.[51] Techniques for fracture repair are similar to those used in other avian species. Recombinant human bone morphogenic protein was used successfully in repairing an open comminuted humeral fracture in a whooping crane and may aid in improving outcomes.[57] When a failure occurs in the distal pelvic limb, it is possible to amputate the leg at or just above the fracture site and build a prosthetic leg for the crane. The prosthesis may be made from a thin-walled PVC pipe and held onto the stump of the leg using adhesive tape, which is usually wrapped up around the hock to avoid slippage. The tape and the prosthesis should be changed every 30 to 60 days. One Mississippi sandhill crane lived for 20 years with such a device.[51] A comfortable prosthesis must be attained quickly to avoid life-threatening pododermatitis in the remaining foot. Recently, a titanium prosthesis was implanted in a white-naped crane; appropriate osteointegration was observed on subsequent histopathology after the bird was euthanized because of apparently unrelated complications.[56]

Exteriorized Yolk Sac

A common problem in hatchling chicks is an exteriorized yolk sac. This is thought to occur from inadequate incubation parameters or infection, usually from *E. coli*, and treatment for this condition has been described elsewhere.[61]

Capture Myopathy

Capture myopathy (exertional rhabdomyolysis) has been observed after manipulation or immobilization of cranes[9,25,48,66] and bustards.[1,53] Clinical signs include peracute death from cardiac failure; apparent pain, stiff movement, and swollen, hard muscles that are warm to the touch; trauma to the limbs from struggling; or a combination of all of these signs. As in other species, serum elevations in muscle-associated enzymes are useful in diagnosing a myopathy.[25,51] Treatment consists of supportive care (which may include physical support in a sling apparatus), physical therapy, IV fluids, corticosteroids, vitamin E and selenium, and antibiotics.[5,9,51]

Foreign Bodies

Cranes commonly pick up small objects, including pieces of metal, and may ingest them. These objects may then persist in or even penetrate the ventriculus or other portions of the gastrointestinal tract (GIT). Clinical signs and treatment are similar to those described for other birds. To reduce the chance of foreign body ingestion, it is imperative to remove all such objects in new or recently renovated enclosures with the aid of a rolling magnet and a metal detector. Tracheal foreign body (a kernel of corn) has been reported in a whooping crane and has also occurred in a Mississippi sandhill crane.[31,47]

Neoplasms

Although rare, neoplasms have been reported in cranes and include renal adenocarcinoma, renal carcinoma, lymphocytic and granulocytic leukemias, cholangiocarcinoma, leiomyosarcoma, and hematopoietic stem cell neoplasia.[10,23,48,51] Hepatocellular carcinoma, osteosarcoma, and malignant peripheral nerve sheath tumor have also been observed (authors' experience).

Toxins

Cranes have died from lead intoxication through ingestion of fishing weights, lead shot, and lead-based paint.[36,67] *Clostridium botulinum* toxin has killed cranes in at least one North American zoo, and botulism should be considered whenever cranes present with progressive paralysis.[10] Famphur, an organophosphorus, anticholinesterase insecticide used almost exclusively on livestock, caused the death of wild cranes in Georgia in 1988.[19] This pesticide was intentionally used in corn by local farmers to target birds presumed to be feeding on their crops. An incident in Japan involving another organophosphate, fenthion, killed several red-crowned cranes.[64] Anticholinesterase poisoning should be considered as a possible differential diagnosis when wild birds in otherwise good condition are found dead.[10,21]

In the 1980s, an estimated 9500 sandhill cranes died in Texas and New Mexico because of *Fusarium* species toxicosis from contaminated peanuts.[55] Clinical signs included inability to hold the heads straight while flying or standing. Necropsy lesions included multiple muscle hemorrhages and submandibular edema. Tilling peanut fields in the fall reduced this cause of crane mortality.[10] Mycotoxins were also responsible for numerous deaths and high morbidity in captive cranes in Maryland in 1987, where minute levels of both deoxynivalenol toxin and mycotoxin t-2 were found in the pelleted feed. The birds showed a reduction in pelleted feed consumption, weight loss, and a progressive weakness, sometimes collapsing when stressed. Treatment included supportive care, fluids, and replacement of the contaminated pellets.[47]

The American coot is one of the main species affected by avian vacuolar myelinopathy suspected to be caused by a neurotoxic amino acid BMAA (β-N-methylamino-L-alanine) synthetized by epiphytic cyanobacterial species.[3] Environmental selenosis has been reported in American coots and was characterized by muscle atrophy, ascites, and feather loss from the head.[46] Rallidae are also frequently affected by environmental oil contamination (authors' experience).

Other Conditions

Other conditions that also occur in cranes occasionally include egg retention (egg binding), prolapsed cloaca, pododermatitis, aspiration pneumonia, ophthalmic disorders, frostbite (toes and wattles), hypothermia, hyperthermia, dermatitis, zinc toxicity from coin ingestion, and insect bite hypersensitivity.[27,40,48] Treatment of these conditions in cranes is similar to that for other species. Venomous snakebites have been reported to occur periodically at one crane rearing facility in Louisiana; immediate treatment with antivenin has appeared to be successful in improving outcomes in these cases (authors' experience). Other reported pathologies include cataracts, atherosclerosis, chronic enteritis, postintubation tracheal stenosis, and ventricular and atrial septal defects in chicks.[41,51]

REPRODUCTION

Cranes are territorial during the breeding season and generally build nests of sedges and other emergent vegetation in marshy areas. The female generally lays two eggs, and both parents share in brooding activities during the 30-day incubation period. Hatching takes 12 to 24 hours following pipping. The chicks are precocial and are cared for by both parents. The young are often extremely aggressive toward their siblings, which may result in the death of one or both chicks.[10]

Cranes are often monogamous for life, although new bonds often are established rapidly after a separation or when one member of a pair dies. Sandhill cranes generally form bonds when they are 2 to 3 years old and usually breed for the first time in the third or fourth year. Breeding may be delayed in captive birds if they are not separated from other conspecifics after pairing. In addition, aggression among pairs kept in a community enclosure may result in substantial injury and mortality. For these reasons, as soon as newly formed pairs are identified, they should be moved from community pens to separate breeding enclosures.

Cranes often re-nest if their first clutch is lost before the middle of the incubation period. Removing completed clutches for artificial or foster incubation may increase total egg production. Captive crane production may be enhanced by using semen collection, artificial insemination, and extending the photoperiod by artificial illumination.[35] Moreover, cryopreservation of crane semen has proven successful, with the production of apparently healthy chicks after artificial insemination.[42]

PREVENTIVE MEDICINE

A preventative medicine program should be developed for captive cranes and include an annual health examination (physical examination, complete blood cell count, and serum biochemistries), parasite surveillance, control, and treatment where indicated (to limit or prevent parasite burdens, especially coccidia), and vaccinations as warranted locally to meet the specific needs of the flock.

In North America, captive adult cranes are currently vaccinated for EEE virus and WNV annually after receiving an initial series as chicks. Equine vaccine products are commonly used, with preference given to killed vaccines. A 0.25 mL dose of ENCEVAC (Intervet, Inc., Millsboro, DE) given intramuscularly and repeated 3 to 4 weeks later appears to be effective in immunizing whooping crane chicks against EEE virus. An annual booster is recommended.[50,51] Interestingly, an experiment failed to demonstrate seroconversion using a killed EEE vaccine in sandhill cranes; however, this species appears resistant to clinical disease from the virus.[11,50] West Nile–Innovator (Wyeth/Fort Dodge Laboratories, Madison, NJ), a killed vaccine, is shown to protect young sandhill and whooping cranes at an intramuscular dose of 1 mL given as a three-dose series; however, the sandhill cranes did not appear to seroconvert.[49] Booster vaccinations are given in July or early August, as the mosquito activity and potential spread of EEE is greatest in late summer and fall.[49] The recombinant WNV vaccine (Recombitek) has not been evaluated in cranes.

The preventative program should include testing all resident, incoming, and outgoing cranes for IBDC antibody titers and removing or isolating any positive birds (the disease has not been isolated from wild North American cranes, so it is critical to identify any potential carriers).[51]

ACKNOWLEDGMENT

The authors wish to acknowledge that this chapter is an update to previous versions of this work by Dr. James Carpenter and is meant to supplement the extensive body of work compiled through his efforts and by veterinarians and researchers who have devoted their lives to preserving rare and threatened species of Gruiformes. Please see previous editions of this book for direction to additional literature sources.

REFERENCES

1. Bailey TA, Nicholls PK, Samour JH, et al: Postmortem findings in the United Arab Emirates. *Avian Dis* 40:296–305, 1996.
2. Bailey TA, Toosi A, Samour JH: Anaesthesia of cranes with alphaxolone-alphadolone. *Vet Rec* 145:84–85, 1999.
3. Bridigare RR, Christensen SJ, Wilde SB, Banack SA: Cyanobacteria and BMAA: Possible linkage with avian vacuolar myelinopathy (AVM) in the

south-eastern United States. *Amyotroph Lateral Scler* 10(Suppl 2):71–73, 2009.

4. Bush M, Locke D, Neal LA, Carpenter JW: Pharmacokinetics of cephalothin and cephalexin in selected avian species. *Am J Vet Res* 42:1014–1017, 1981.

5. Businga NK, Langenberg J, Carlson L: Successful treatment of capture myopathy in three wild greater sandhill cranes (*Grus Canadensis tabida*). *JAMS* 21:294–298, 2007.

6. Candelora KL, Spalding MG, Sellers HS: Survey for antibodies to infectious bursal disease virus serotype 2 in wild turkeys and sandhill cranes of Florida, USA. *J Wildl Dis* 46:742–752, 2010.

7. Carpenter JW, editor: *Exotic animal formulary*, 4th ed, Philadelphia, PA, 2012, Saunders.

8. Carpenter JW, Novilla MN, Hatfield JS: Efficacy of selected coccidiostats in sandhill cranes (*Grus canadensis*) following challenge. *J Zoo Wildl Med* 36:391–400, 2005.

9. Carpenter JW, Thomas NJ, Reevees S: Capture myopathy in an endangered sandhill crane (*Grus Canadensis pulla*). *J Zoo Wildl Med* 22:488–493, 1991.

10. Carpenter JW: Gruiformes (cranes, limpkins, rails, gallinules, coots, bustards). In Fowler ME, Miller RE, editors: *Zoo and wild animal medicine*, 5th ed, St. Louis, MO, 2003, Saunders.

11. Clark GG, Dien FJ, Crabbs CL, et al: Antibody response of sandhill and whooping cranes to an eastern equine encephalitis virus vaccine. *J Wildl Dis* 23:539–544, 1987.

12. Clements JF, Schulenberg TS, Iliff MJ, et al: *The eBird/Clements checklist of birds of the world: Version 6.7*, 2012: http://www.birds.cornell.edu/clementschecklist/downloadable-clements-checklist. Accessed February 15, 2013.

13. Cole GA, Thomas NJ, Spalding M, et al: Postmortem evaluation of reintroduced migratory whooping cranes in Eastern North America. *J Wildl Dis* 45:29–40, 2009.

14. Curro TG, Langenberg J, Paul-Murphy J: A review of lameness in long-legged birds. In Jenkins JR (ed): *Proceedings of the annual conference of the Association of Avian Veterinarians*, New Orleans, LA, 1992, pp 265–269.

15. Custer RS, Bush M, Carpenter JW: Pharmacokinetics of gentamicin in blood plasma of quail, pheasants, and cranes. *Am J Vet Res* 40:892–895, 1979.

16. D'Aloia ME, Samour JH, Bailey TA, et al: Normal blood chemistry of the kori bustard (*Ardeotis kori*). *Avian Pathol* 25:161–165, 1996.

17. Dein FJ, Carpenter JW, Clark GG, et al: Mortality of captive whooping cranes caused by eastern equine encephalitis virus. *J Am Vet Med Assoc* 189:1006–1010, 1986.

18. Dusek RJ, Spalding MG, Forrester DJ, Greiner EC: *Haemoproteus balearicae* and other blood parasites of free-ranging Florida sandhill crane chicks. *J Wildl Dis* 40:682–687, 2004.

19. Eisler R: Famphur hazards to fish, wildlife, and invertebrates: A synoptic review. In *U. S. National Biological Survey Biological Report*, 1994, p 20.

20. Fanke J, Wibbelt G, Krone O: Mortality factors and diseases in free-ranging Eurasian cranes (*Grus grus*) in Germany. *J Wildl Dis* 47:627–637, 2011.

21. Deleted in proof.

22. Fedynich AM, Thomas MJ: Amidostomum and epomidiostomum. In Atkinson CT, Thomas NJ, hunter DB, editors: *Parasitic diseases of wild birds*, Ames, IA, 2008, Wiley Blackwell.

23. Frazier KS, Herron AJ, Hines II ME, et al: Metastasis of a myxoid leiomyosarcoma via the renal and hepatic portal circulation in a sarus crane (*Grus antigone*). *J Comp Pathol* 108:57–63, 1993.

24. Gee GF, Carpenter JW, Hensler GL: Species differences in hematological values of captive cranes, geese, raptors, and quail. *J Wildl Manage* 45:463–483, 1981.

25. Hanley CS, Thomas NJ, Paul-Murphy J, Hartup BK: Exertional myopathy in whooping cranes (*Grus Americana*) with prognostic guidelines. *J Zoo Wildl Med* 36:489–497, 2005.

26. Hartup B, Clyde VL: Lack of evidence for vertical transmission of inclusion body disease in black-necked cranes (*Grus nigricollis*) at the International Crane Foundation. In Baer CK (ed): *Proceedings of the AAZV, AAWV, AZA/NAG Joint Conference*, Madison, WI, 2005, Omnipress.

27. Hartup BK, Schroeder CA: Protein electrophoresis in cranes with presumed insect bite hypersensitivity. *Vet Clin Pathol* 35:226–230, 2006.

28. Hawkey C, Samour JH, Ashton DG, et al: Normal and clinical haematology of captive cranes (Gruiformes). *Avian Pathol* 12:73–84, 1983.

29. Hayes MA, Hartup BK, Pittman JM, Barzen JA: Capture of sandhill cranes using alpha-chloralose. *J Wildl Dis* 39:859–868, 2003.

30. Hoar BM, Whiteside DP, Ward L, et al: Evaluation of the enteric microflora of captive whooping cranes (*Grus Americana*) and sandhill cranes (*Grus canadensis*). *Zoo Biol* 26:141–153, 2007.

31. Howard PE, Dien J, Langenberg JA, et al: Surgical removal of a tracheal foreign body from a whooping crane (*Grus americana*). *J Zoo Wildl Med* 22:359–363, 1991.

32. Howlett JC, Samour JH, D'Aloia MA, et al: Normal haematology of captive adult kori bustards (*Ardeotis kori*). *Comparat Haematol Int* 5:102–105, 1995.

33. Huffman JE: Trematodes. In Atkinson CT, Thomas NJ, Hunter DB (eds): *Parasitic diseases of wild birds*, Ames, IA, 2008, Wiley Blackwell.

34. Jenkins AR, Smallie JJ, Diamond M: Avian collisions with power lines: A global review of causes and mitigation with a South African perspective. *Bird Conservat Int* 20:263–278, 2010.

35. Jones KL, Nicolich JM: Artificial insemination in captive whooping cranes: Results from genetic analyses. *Zoo Biol* 20:331–342, 2001.

36. Kennedy S, Crisler JP, Smith E, Bush M: Lead poisoning in sandhill cranes. *J Am Vet Med Assoc* 171:955–958, 1977.

37. Langenberg JA, Businga NK: Epizootic hock osteoarthritis in captive Siberian cranes (*Grus leucogeranus*). In Baer CK (ed): *Proceedings of the annual conference of the American Association of Zoo Veterinarians*, Columbus, OH, 1999, pp 277–278.

38. Linn KA, Templer AS, Paul-Murphy JR, et al: Ultrasonographic imaging of the sandhill crane (*Grus canadensis*) intertarsal joint. *J Zoo Wildl Med* 34:144–152, 2003.

39. Locke D, Bush M, Carpenter JW: Pharmacokinetics and tissue concentrations of tylosin in selected avian species. *Am J Vet Res* 43:1807–1810, 1982.

40. Ludders JW, Rode J, Mitchell GS: Isoflurane anesthesia in sandhill cranes (*Grus canadensis*): Minimal anesthetic concentration and cardiopulmonary dose-response during spontaneous and controlled breathing. *Anesth Analg* 68:511–516, 1989.

41. MacLean R, Beaufrère H, Heggem B, et al: Presumed reactive polyarthritis and granulomatous vasculitis in a Mississippi sandhill crane (*Grus canadensis pulla*). *JAMS* 27:309–314, 2013.

42. Maksudov GY, Panchenko VG: Obtaining an interspecific hybrid of cranes by artificial insemination with frozen-thawed semen. *Biol Bull* 29:311–314, 2002.

43. Martin GR, Shaw JM: Bird collisions with power lines: Failing to see the way ahead? *Biol Conserv* 143:2695–2702, 2010.

44. McLean RG, Ubico SR: Arboviruses in birds. In Thomas NJ, Hunter DB, Atkinson CT (eds): *Infectious diseases of wild birds*, Ames, IA, 2006, Blackwell, pp 17–62.

45. Miller PE, Langenberg JA, Hartmann FA: The normal conjunctival aerobic bacterial flora of three species of captive cranes. *J Zoo Wildl Med* 26:545–549, 1995.

46. Ohlendorf HM: Selenium. In Fairbrother A, Locke LN, Hoff GL, editors: *Noninfectious diseases of wildlife*, 2nd ed, Ames, IA, 1996, Iowa State University Press.

47. Olsen GH, Carpenter JW, Langenberg JA: Medicine and surgery. In Ellis DH, Gee GF, Mirande CM, editors: *Cranes: Their biology, husbandry, and conservation*, Washington, DC, 1996, US Department of the Interior, National Biological Service.

48. Olsen GH, Carpenter JW: Cranes. In Altman RB, Clubb SL, Dorrestein GM, Quesenberry K, editors: *Avian medicine and surgery*, Philadelphia, PA, 1997, Saunders.

49. Olsen GH, Miller KJ, Docherty DE, et al: Pathogenicity of West Nile virus and response to vaccination in sandhill cranes (*Grus Canadensis*) using a killed vaccine. *J Zoo Wildl Med* 40:263–271, 2009.

50. Olsen GH, Turell MJ, Pagac BB: Efficacy of eastern equine encephalitis immunization in whooping cranes. *J Wildl Dis* 33:312–315, 1997.

51. Olsen GH: Cranes. In Tully TN, Dorrestein GN, Jones AK, Cooper JE, editors: *Handbook of avian medicine*, 2nd ed, New York, 2009, Saunders.

52. Olsen GH: Orthopedics in cranes: Pediatrics and adults. *Semin Avian Exotic Pet Med* 3:73–80, 1994.
53. Ponjoan A, Bota G, García de la Morena EL, et al: Adverse effects of capture and handling little bustard. *J Wildl Manage* 72:315–319, 2008.
54. Puerta ML, Alonso JC, Huecas V, et al: Hematology and blood chemistry of wintering common cranes. *Condor* 92:210–214, 1990.
55. Roffe TJ, Stroud RK, Windingstad RM: Suspected Fusariomycotoxicosis in sandhill cranes (*Grus canadensis*): Clinical and pathological findings. *Avian Dis* 33:451–457, 1989.
56. Rush EM, Turner TM, Montgomery R, et al: Implantation of a titanium partial limb prosthesis in a white-naped crane (*Grus vipio*). *J Avian Med Sci* 26:167–175, 2012.
57. Sample S, Cole G, Paul-Murphy J, et al: Clinical use of recombinant human bone morphogenic protein-2 in a whooping crane (*Grus americana*). *Vet Surg* 37:552–557, 2008.
58. Serafin JA: The influence of diet composition upon growth and development of young sandhill cranes. *Condor* 84:427–434, 1982.
59. Spalding MG, Carpenter JW, Novilla MN: Disseminated visceral coccidiosis in cranes. In Atkinson CT, Thomas NJ, hunter DB, editors: *Parasitic diseases of wild birds*, Ames, IA, 2008, Wiley Blackwell.
60. Spalding MG, Erlandsen SL, Nesbitt SA: Hexamita-like species associated with enteritis and death in captive Florida sandhill cranes (*Grus canadensis pratensis*). *J Zoo Wildl Med* 25:281–285, 1994.
61. Stewart J: Ratites. In Ritchie BW, Harrison GJ, Harrison LR, editors: *Avian medicine: Principles and application*, Lake Worth, FL, 1994, Wingers.
62. Stroud RK: Avian tuberculosis and salmonellosis in a whooping crane (*Grus americana*). *J Wildl Dis* 22:106–110, 1986.
63. Swengel SR, Carpenter JW: General husbandry. In Ellis DH, Gee GF, Mirande CM, editors: *Cranes: Their biology, husbandry, and conservation*, Washington, DC, 1996, US Department of the Interior, National Biological Service and Baraboo, Wisconsin, International Crane Foundation.
64. Tahara R, Nagahora S, Watanabe Y, Kurosawa N: Determination of fenthion in dead Japanese cranes. *J Yamashina Inst Ornithol* 38:56–59, 2006.
65. Thoen CO, Himes EM, Barrett RE: *Mycobacterium avium* serotype 1 infection in a sandhill crane (*Grus canadensis*). *J Wildl Dis* 13:40–42, 1977.
66. Windingstad RM, Hurley SS, Sileo L: Capture myopathy in a free-flying greater sandhill crane (*Grus Canadensis tabida*) from Wisconsin. *J Wildl Dis* 19:289–290, 1983.
67. Windingstad RM, Kerr SM, Locke LN: Lead poisoning of sandhill cranes (*Grus canadensis*). *Prairie Naturalist* 16:21–24, 1984.
68. Young LA, Citino SB, Seccareccia V, et al: Eastern equine encephalomyelitis in an exotic avian collection. In LaBonde J, Doolen M, Murray M, Tully TN, Jr (eds): *Proceedings of the annual conference of the Association of Avian Veterinarians*, Madison, WI, 1996, Omnipress, pp 163–165.

CHAPTER 20

Columbiformes

Zoltan S. Gyimesi

GENERAL BIOLOGY

The order Columbiformes comprises a single family (Columbidae), which includes over 40 genera and 300 species of extant pigeons and doves. The term "pigeon" is typically used for larger species, whereas the term "dove" applies to most of the smaller species, although these terms may be interchangeable. Pigeons are believed to be the earliest domesticated avian species and have been used as a source of meat and fertilizer, as a method of long distance communication prior to the telegraph, and as a laboratory animal.[28,34] Domestic columbids, including homing or racing pigeons, and the many varieties kept for exhibition and hobby (Figure 20-1) are descendants of the "urban pigeon" or rock dove (*Columba livia*).

Columbiformes species have a widespread distribution found on every continent except Antarctica. Although many species are quite numerous, some of the populations inhabiting small islands are in danger of extinction. The dodo (*Raphus cucullatus*) and the passenger pigeon (*Ectopistes migratorius*) are two well-known Columbiformes species that have been driven to extinction by human activity.

Pigeons and doves are typically tree-dwelling species, but some cliff-dwelling and ground-dwelling species occur as well. Tropical fruit doves spend most of their time in trees, feeding, roosting, and nesting there, and many other species nest in trees but forage on the ground. Rock doves in cities have adapted to using man-made structures such as buildings and bridges for roosting and nesting.

UNIQUE ANATOMY

Pigeons and doves have plump, stocky bodies, small heads and beaks, and relatively short legs and necks. They stand on anisodactyl feet (three toes forward, one toe backward). They are heavily feathered and lack a lateral cervical apterium (featherless tract), which complicates jugular venipuncture. Some tropical species are brilliantly colored or have ornamental crests or eye rings, but most pigeons and doves have more muted gray or brown coloring, perhaps with some iridescence. Males are generally larger, but gender determination may be challenging without DNA or laparoscopic sexing, as most species lack sexual dimorphism. Pigeons and doves tend to display a simple song and exhibit a wide range of soft calls and coos. They possess a fleshy cere, and the beak is not hard or powerful. The uropygial gland is either rudimentary or absent. Waterproofing and maintenance of plumage relies on powder from specialized feathers distributed via preening.[31,34]

Pigeons and doves have a prominent crop. Under the influence of prolactin, hyperplasia of the crop mucosa, with subsequent crop milk production, occurs in both males and females during brooding and raising of squabs. Crop milk is a cheesy, semi-solid, nutritious substance derived from desquamated crop epithelial cells. A vascular plexus in the cervical skin, from the cranium to the crop, has numerous functions such as sexual and territorial display, thermoregulation, and possibly facilitation of nutrient and enzyme deposition

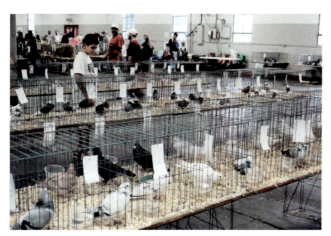

FIGURE 20-1 A variety of domestic pigeons exhibited at a state fair.

during lactation.[31,34] The gizzard, or ventriculus, is muscular and harbors ingested grit in granivorous species but is less muscular, more saccular, and typically devoid of grit in specialized frugivores. Ceca are highly rudimentary in columbids, and a gall bladder is absent in many genera but present in others, including *Ptilinopus*, *Ducula*, and *Gymnophaps*.[14] Columbids possess a long keel that supports a well-developed pectoral muscle mass, allowing for their characteristic explosive flight when taking off.

SPECIAL HOUSING REQUIREMENTS

Although many of the temperate species are cold hardy and may be housed outdoors year round in most climates, tropical columbids require indoor housing, at least during the cold season. Studies suggest that tropical fruit doves have a lower basal metabolic rate compared with other birds, including granivorous columbids, and are more intolerant of temperature extremes.[30] All columbids require shelter and protection from predators, including raptors, terrestrial carnivores, rats, and feral dogs and cats. Hobbyists typically maintain domestic pigeons in protected lofts that vary in design, depending on the particular requirements of the pigeon variety and the number of birds housed. Breeds kept for their flying abilities need ample room to fly freely to maintain physical conditioning and fitness.

Despite being a peace symbol, columbids are not docile and may be intolerant of conspecifics or other species. Aviaries should be well planted to offer cover and visual barriers, and ample roosting sites should be provided. A variety of natural perching is ideal. New groups of columbids should be closely monitored for signs of aggression. Overcrowding may lead to stress and disease. Favored roosting areas should be identified, and attention should be given to the subsequent accumulation of feces below these sites. If breeding is desired, a variety of species-appropriate nesting opportunities should be provided. Enclosures should be well ventilated but not drafty. Flooring may be concrete in off-exhibit holding pens or consist of a variety of natural substrates such as soil, mulch, and gravel in zoo exhibits. Columbids enjoy bathing in shallow water, so enclosures should include a suitable water feature. Particularly sensitive or wary species, newly acquired birds in quarantine, or columbids in off-exhibit breeding programs may benefit from more privacy; sheeting hung outside their aviary functions as an effective visual barrier to foot traffic. Similarly, padded ceilings, when feasible in smaller aviaries, decrease the risk of head trauma when birds startle and fly upward.

FEEDING

In nature, pigeons and doves feed on a wide variety of vegetable matter, with seeds, legumes, fruits and berries, young leaves, buds, and flowers forming most of the diet.[28,31,34] Invertebrates such as insects, snails, and earthworms are occasionally consumed,

particularly by ground-foraging species. Granivorous pigeons will find seeds by flicking extraneous material out of the way with their beak and swallowing seeds whole. Fruit doves are highly arboreal, capable of clinging tightly to branches as they forage and reach to pluck bite-sized morsels of food. Rock doves may be agricultural pests, but other columbid species play important roles in the dispersal of the seeds of fruiting plants.[37] In contrast to most birds that need to take in water and throw their heads back to swallow, pigeons and doves drink actively via suction by placing their beak in water up to their nares.

In captivity, granivores should be provided an appropriate, commercially available avian crumble or pellet. Columbids do not typically eat finely ground feeds. When necessary, birds may be conditioned to eat pellets by soaking them in fruit juice or offering a formulation that is brightly colored. Pelleted feeds are often combined with a variety of seeds and legumes, diced vegetables and fruit, and cultivated insects. Complete formulated diets are readily available for domestic pigeons, and nutritional requirements have been reported elsewhere.[29,31,34] For frugivorous doves, a higher proportion of chopped fruits and berries are offered. The fruit dove diet may also be supplemented with nectar. Species more prone to iron overload may benefit from a ration lower in iron and vitamin C and supplemented with dietary tannins. Husbandry staff should be aware that captive fruit doves have a tendency to accumulate soft foods on the beak and feathers around the mouth. Rations may need to be fortified with vitamin and mineral supplements, particularly calcium, as seed, fruit, and insect diets are typically not complete in themselves.

Multiple feeding stations should be offered at various perch levels, even on the floor if necessary, to allow subordinate animals to feed. Positioning food and water bowls under roosting sites should be avoided. Food bowls may be swarmed by ants in aviaries and may impact feeding. This may be managed with shallow water moats and pest control practices.

RESTRAINT AND HANDLING

Exotic pigeons and doves maintained in large aviaries may be conditioned to feed at food stations within smaller catch pens to facilitate trapping. Birds in small pens or aviaries may be captured for examination by using soft mesh nets. Dimming the lights prior to capture may decrease panic and "fright flights" and facilitate a smoother, safer catch. Exotic pigeons and doves have a tendency to drop contour feathers as an adaptation to avoid capture by a predator. Quick, decisive captures, covering the head, and using a soft towel will decrease struggling, and minimize the risk of injury and feather loss. The wings should be folded and secured close to the body during manual restraint and examination (Figure 20-2). The duration of restraint events should be minimized. Placing columbids in padded, darkened crates is ideal for birds in need of being transferred to other locations. Capture and handling of domestic varieties are typically easier on both the handler and the bird, as they tend to be more accustomed to close observation and manual manipulation. The beak and feet of columbids do not pose a danger to handlers.

ANESTHESIA

As in most avian species, inhalant anesthetic agents such as isoflurane or sevoflurane via a non-rebreathing system are preferred for induction and maintenance of general anesthesia. Prior to certain procedures, a surgical plane of anesthesia should be reached, as painful stimuli may induce powerful wing flapping that risks injury to the bird. As with other birds, respiratory rate and depth must be constantly monitored. For surgical procedures, endotracheal intubation is recommended to better control the airway. With small patients, clinicians should be mindful of kinking or obstruction of the endotracheal tube lumen by secretions or lubricant.

Injectable protocols are rarely indicated but ketamine at 20 to 50 milligrams per kilogram (mg/kg), alone or combined with diazepam

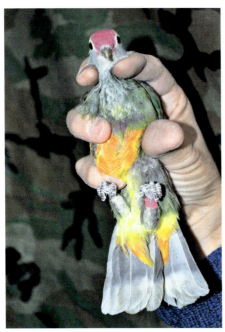

FIGURE 20-2 One-hand restraint of a Mariana fruit dove (*Ptilinopus roseicapilla*).

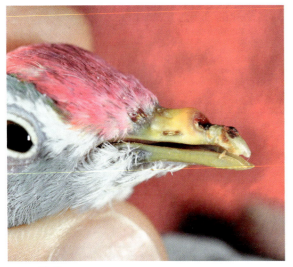

FIGURE 20-3 Beak trauma in a beautiful fruit dove (*Ptilinopus pulchellus*).

(0.5–1.0 mg/kg) or xylazine (2.0 mg/kg), intramuscularly (IM), intravenously (IV), or intraosseously (IO) has been reported.[17,31] Medetomidine, by itself or combined with other drugs, may yield variable results and profound bradycardia and bradypnea.[1,27]

SURGERY

Surgical procedures and approaches are similar to those in other birds of comparable size; however, the relatively long keel in columbids may complicate surgical access to some coelomic organs. Because of their tendency to launch into explosive flight when threatened, beak (Figure 20-3) and head injuries are not uncommon. Despite the presence of a cervical vascular plexus, a pedicle advancement flap from the dorsal cervical skin is still a viable option for cases of head trauma when the skull is exposed (Figure 20-4).[10] Hens with dystocia or salpingitis not responding to medical management may require exploratory laparotomy. As with other captive birds, the

most commonly seen leg fractures tend to involve the tibiotarsus. Stabilization of these fractures may require both internal fixation and external coaptation.

DIAGNOSTICS

General anesthesia is often indicated to facilitate safe and thorough physical examination, radiography, and sample collection. Jugular venipuncture is possible but complicated in columbids because of the pigmentation of the skin, the presence of the vascular plexus, and the lack of a featherless tract. The combination of patience, good lighting, and dampening of the cervical plumage with isopropyl alcohol allows for phlebotomy from the right jugular vein in most species. Other options for blood collection include the basilic (wing) veins, which are visible in the medial elbow region, and the medial metatarsal veins; however, these sites typically yield a lesser volume compared with the jugular vein and post-phlebotomy hemostasis may be prolonged. Blood values for selected species are included in Table 20-1.

Swabbing of the crop with saline-moistened cotton-tipped applicators followed by microscopy is a routine method for screening for *Trichomonas gallinae*. Similarly, cytologic evaluation of crop and cloacal swabs may be performed to evaluate bacterial and fungal flora present. Combined conjunctival–choanal–cloacal swabs for molecular testing are recommended as a component of *Chlamydophila psittaci* screening.

INFECTIOUS DISEASES

Table 20-2 summarizes selected infectious diseases in columbids.

Bacterial Diseases

Free-ranging *Columba livia* are known to be carriers of *Chlamydophila psittaci*; however, fortunately, the genotype most prevalent in pigeons tends to exhibit low virulence and relatively low zoonotic risk potential.[5,6,15,28,31] Morbidity and mortality, as well as shedding of *Chlamydophila*, increase in pigeons when infected concurrently by other pathogens. Flock treatment of infected zoo birds has been described.[25] Columbids are susceptible to fatal *Salmonella* infections, specifically the *Typhimurium* var. Copenhagen strain of *Salmonella enterica* is a major disease issue in *Columba livia*.[12,15,28,31,33,38] Mycobacteriosis is not uncommon in zoo columbids, and infections may be widely disseminated by the time a diagnosis is made. Other bacterial agents reported to cause disease in columbids include *Escherichia coli*, *Pasteurella*, *Haemophilus*, *Pseudomonas*, *Klebsiella*, *Clostridium*, *Yersinia*, *Streptococcus*, *Staphylococcus*, and *Mycoplasma*.[6,15,28,31,38]

Fungal Diseases

Candida albicans is considered a commensal organism in the gastrointestinal (GI) tract of columbids but is an opportunistic pathogen.[18] With stress, disease, immunosuppression, and long-term antimicrobial therapy, yeast overgrowth may occur and lead to morbidity and mortality if left untreated. Aspergillosis occurs in columbids, typically following inhalation and, less commonly, ingestion of the saprophyte. Cryptococcosis has been reported rarely in pigeons and doves and may initiate granuloma formation in invaded tissues.[11,26,36] Given the zoonotic risk and poor prognosis, euthanasia should be considered for confirmed cases. Zoonotic potential also exists following human exposure to fungi that may concentrate in pigeon guano, including *Cryptococcus*, *Histoplasma*, *Blastomyces*, and *Candida*.[26]

Viral Diseases

Columbids are susceptible to strains of both Newcastle disease and a distinctly separate strain of paramyxovirus type 1 (PMV-1), which causes severe neurologic signs in pigeons and doves and yet is only mildly pathogenic to poultry.[21,28] Pigeonpox is transmitted through arthropods and contact with infected birds and may lead to the development of debilitating lesions. Pigeon circovirus infections tend to induce immunosuppression and secondary infections; feather loss

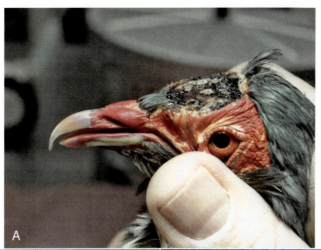

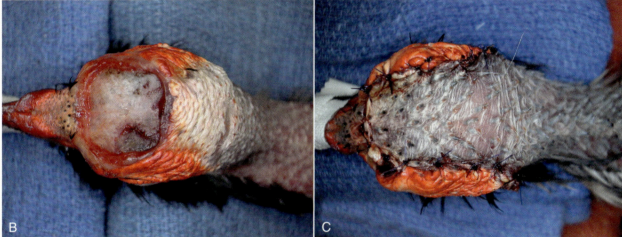

FIGURE 20-4 Head trauma and skull exposure in a Papuan mountain pigeon (*Gymnophaps albertisii*) and treatment via surgical debridement and dorsal cervical single pedicle advancement flap. **A,** The pigeon on presentation. **B,** Appearance after anesthesia, regional plucking, and debridement. The initial repair failed due to graft necrosis. **C,** Second attempt 1 week later resulted in a successful outcome.

or feather dystrophy are rare.[21,28] Herpesvirus infections may cause conjunctivitis, respiratory signs, pharyngitis, and esophagitis in affected birds.[6,15,21,28] Young birds are most susceptible to clinical herpesvirus and adenovirus infections. Pigeons appear to be resistant to West Nile virus encephalitis and to both high and low pathogenic strains of avian influenza virus.[21]

PARASITIC DISEASES

See Table 20-2 for selected parasitic diseases in columbids. Trichomoniasis, caused by the protozoan parasite *Trichomonas gallinae*, is a worldwide disease entity in wild and captive pigeons and doves.[4,31] The severity of the disease depends on the virulence of the strain, the immune status of the bird, and the magnitude of debility from concurrent diseases. Clinical coccidiosis and *Hexamita columbae* infections tend to occur in juvenile pigeons.[15,19,28,31] Sarcocystosis may cause an acute fatal pneumonia in Old World columbids, and morbidity and mortality associated with this parasite make it important to protect collection birds from contact with roaming opossums (*Didelphis virginiana*) and their feces (Figure 20-5).[9,24,32] Other protozoa that may infect columbids include *Toxoplasma gondii*[9,35] and *Cryptosporidium*,[9] as well as several genera of hemoprotozoa, including *Haemoproteus*, *Plasmodium*, and *Leucocytozoon*.[3,12,15,28,31,38] *Leucocytozoon* has been shown to affect survival in endangered juvenile Mauritius pink pigeons (*Columba mayeri*).[3]

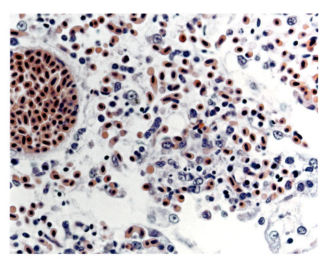

FIGURE 20-5 Pulmonary edema, histiocytic inflammation, and intravascular elongated protozoal meront with zoites (*Sarcocystis* sp.) in the lung of a magnificent fruit dove (*Ptilinopus magnificus*) (H&E stain, ×1000). (Courtesy of Rita McManamon.)

TABLE 20-1

Blood Values for Selected Columbiform Species*

Parameter	Jambu Fruit Dove, Ptilinopus jambu	Mauritius Pink Pigeon, Columba mayeri	Nicobar Pigeon, Caloenas nicobarica	Victoria Crowned Pigeon, Goura victoria
Erythrocytes (x10⁶/µL)	—	3.32; 2.52–4.14 (50)	3.46; 2.07–4.74 (100)	2.44; 1.64–3.22 (64)
Hematocrit (%)	50.3; 37.6–62.1 (190)	48.9; 36.8–61.0 (246)	49.3; 36.8–59.0 (417)	37.7; 27.6–47.7 (222)
Hemoglobin (gm/dL)	14.2 (36)	15.8; 8.9–23.4 (85)	16.4; 11.3–22.4 (108)	13.5; 9.3–17.6 (82)
Leukocytes (x10³/µL)	8.99; 2.04–23.33 (188)	11.21; 2.22–28.42 (227)	10.80; 3.12–25.26 (391)	14.40; 3.61–34.21 (211)
Heterophils (x10³/µL)	3.04; 0.69–8.50 (183)	3.24; 0.44–8.98 (220)	5.29; 0.99–12.82 (388)	6.48; 0.96–15.99 (210)
Lymphocytes (x10³/µL)	4.64; 0.43–13.50 (186)	6.43; 0.98–19.38 (227)	4.40; 0.75–12.25 (389)	6.06; 0.79–18.62 (208)
Eosinophils (cells/µL)	317; 0–808 (111)	399; 0–1046 (104)	196; 42–562 (130)	340; 0–824 (88)
Monocytes (cells/µL)	495; 41–1838 (156)	595; 53–1979 (188)	668; 55–2233 (337)	1109; 87–4125 (179)
Basophils (cells/µL)	328; 0–834 (88)	200; 0–468 (78)	237; 39–639(181)	361; 0–863 (103)
Glucose (mg/dL)	264; 162–370 (128)	300; 185–405 (185)	260; 188–341 (324)	309; 212–412 (164)
Uric acid (mg/dL)	10.9; 2.8–22.8 (133)	6.3; 1.5–15.1 (213)	6.2; 1.9–13.3 (346)	5.0; 1.1–12.3 (173)
Calcium (mg/dL)	8.4; 5.5–10.7 (119)	9.7; 6.8–13.2 (189)	9.3; 7.2–11.9 (312)	10.3; 8.4–13.3 (163)
Phosphorus (mg/dL)	4.7; 0.0–8.7 (102)	4.0; 0.6–9.5 (153)	3.3; 1.1–7.5 (250)	5.3; 2.0–9.9 (149)
Sodium (mEq/L)	156; 135–179 (74)	157; 139–175 (97)	153; 140–176 (181)	155; 138–171 (117)
Potassium (mEq/L)	2.3; 0.5–4.0 (74)	2.7; 0.7–4.5 (93)	2.8; 1.3–4.8 (180)	4.4; 3.0–6.6 (121)
Chloride (mEq/L)	117; 98–137 (46)	115; 98–133 (72)	116; 104–130 (151)	114; 102–126 (88)
Total protein (gm/dL)	3.6; 1.9–5.2 (114)	4.4; 2.5–6.6 (204)	3.5; 2.3–5.3 (305)	3.7; 2.4–5.2 (140)
Albumin (gm/dL)	2.2; 0.0–4.3 (81)	2.0; 0.8–3.9(124)	1.6; 0.8–3.2 (228)	1.7; 0.8–2.6 (130)
Globulin (gm/dL)	1.6; 0.0–3.6 (61)	2.1; 0.0–4.6(124)	1.8; 0.0–3.1 (222)	1.9; 0.6–3.2 (113)
Alk Phos (IU/L)	183; 0–409 (46)	118; 0–277 (75)	95; 19–302 (163)	45; 0–117 (91)
AST (IU/L)	289; 71–594 (136)	170; 41–443 (194)	133; 41–318 (340)	154; 69–311 (168)
CK (IU/L)	1473; 0–3228 (81)	602; 154–1747 (141)	431; 79–1329 (278)	515; 127–1415 (128)
Cholesterol (mg/dL)	308; 116–496 (54)	385; 218–543 (102)	333; 226–476 (209)	179; 100–256 (108)

*Blood values are listed as the mean followed by the reference interval using conventional American units (sample size in parentheses). No reference interval is provided for hemoglobin in Jambu fruit doves due to an insufficient sample size.

Alk Phos, Alkaline phosphatase; *AST,* aspartate aminotransferase; *CK,* creatine kinase; *g/dL,* gram per deciliter; *mEq/L,* milliequivalent per liter; *mg/dL,* milligram per deciliter; *µL,* microliter; *IU/L,* international unit per liter.

From Teare, JA, ed: 2013, ISIS Physiological Reference Intervals for Captive Wildlife: A CD-ROM Resource., International Species Information System, Bloomington, MN. The compiled data include no selection by gender and all ages are combined. Birds included were classified as healthy at the time of sample collection.

Nematodes reported to occur in pigeons include *Ascardia columbae, Capillaria* spp., *Ornithostrongylus* spp., *Syngamus trachea,* as well as two spirurid parasites, *Dispharynx* and *Tetrameres.*[15,22,31,38] With *Dispharynx* and *Tetrameres,* which are proventricular worms, antemortem diagnosis and management may be difficult. Cestode and trematode infections are more seldom observed. Ectoparasites reported in columbids include pigeon flies (hippoboscids), lice, mites, and more rarely, sticktight fleas[13] and ticks.[31]

NONINFECTIOUS DISEASES

Morbidity and mortality from traumatic injuries is very common in captive columbids,[12] likely related to their inclination to fight with aviary-mates during the reproductive cycle and their tendency to launch into sudden flight when frightened. Neoplastic disease is occasionally seen in older birds, and a variety of neoplasms have been observed.[9,12] Dystocia and yolk coelomitis occasionally occur in hens. Fruit doves (*Ptilinopus* spp.) and imperial pigeons (*Ducula* spp.) are more prone to hepatic or multisystemic hemosiderosis; however, hemochromatosis is rare.[9,20]

TOXINS

Benzimidazole anthelmintics such as albendazole and fenbendazole should be used very cautiously with columbids, if used at all. Toxicosis is dose related, and these drugs have been demonstrated to cause damage to developing feathers, weight loss, intestinal mucosal damage, bone marrow hypoplasia, leukopenia, and death.[16] A wide variety of toxins may affect free-ranging pigeons and doves.[31,38] Some wild Columbiformes species have been studied as indicators of environmental pollution, as they are known to bioaccumulate heavy metals such as lead, cadmium, copper, and zinc in their bones, soft tissues, and feathers.[7,8,23]

REPRODUCTION

Columbiformes species form monogamous pairs, at least seasonally. Nests typically consist of a platform or a shallow cup made with twigs and dry stems and tend to be loose and flimsy in construction; however, some species do build stronger and more substantial nests. In nature, most species are solitary nesters, but some such as the Nicobar pigeon (*Caloenas nicobarica*) nest in colonies. One or two eggs are typically laid per clutch. Both sexes incubate the eggs and develop marked mucosal hyperplasia of the crop during brooding in preparation for feeding the young. Incubation times range from 10 to 30 days, depending on species.[31,34] Squabs are altricial, and crop milk is the primary food for the first 7 to 10 days of life.[2] Gradually, it is mixed with the adult diet as it is regurgitated to developing nestlings and fledglings. Crop milk is a holocrine secretion consisting of 50% dry-matter (DM) protein (sloughed epithelial cells), 45% DM fat (lipid droplets), and negligible carbohydrates (no lactose).[2] It is easily digestible and is also an important source of immunoglobulins. This energy-dense food is responsible for the rapid growth and short fledging times (10–40 days) observed in columbids.[31,34] Pigeons and

TABLE 20-2

Selected Bacterial, Fungal, Viral, and Parasitic Diseases of Columbiformes

Disease	Etiologic Agent	Transmission	Signs	Diagnosis	Management and Treatment
Chlamydiosis, ornithosis	*Chlamydophila psittaci*	Contact with droppings and secretions of infected birds	Nonspecific; oculonasal discharge, conjunctivitis, respiratory signs, diarrhea, enteritis	Serologic testing; antigen/DNA detection in blood, swabs, or tissue; culture	Doxycycline (typically 45 day course)
Salmonellosis, paratyphoid	*Salmonella* spp.	Fecal-oral	Nonspecific; diarrhea, enteritis, hepatitis, arthritis, neurologic signs	Isolation of organism via culture	Antimicrobial therapy based on culture and sensitivity results
Mycobacteriosis, "avian TB"	*Mycobacterium avium* subsp. *avium*; also *M. genavense* and *M. intracellulare*	Environmental exposure	Nonspecific; weight loss, diarrhea, "poor doer," rough plumage, hepatosplenomegaly	Antemortem diagnosis is challenging; examination, radiography, hematology; presumptive diagnosis if compatible acid-fast bacilli are observed in biopsy or cytology	Typically euthanasia; consider treatment only in very valuable birds
Candidiasis, thrush	*Candida albicans*	Normal flora; direct contact	Anorexia, weight loss, regurgitation due to pseudomembranous inflammation in the oral cavity, esophagus and crop	Cytology of crop or oropharyngeal swab demonstrating characteristic budding yeast	Nystatin, imidazoles (fluconazole, etc.)
Aspergillosis	*Aspergillus* spp.	Environmental exposure	Anorexia, weight loss, lethargy, respiratory signs	Antemortem diagnosis is challenging; examination, radiography, hematology, *Aspergillus* antibody and antigen testing combined with protein electrophoresis, demonstration of organism via cytology or culture, laparoscopy	Prognosis is guarded to poor in many cases; surgical removal of aspergilloma(s), prolonged antifungal therapy
Paramyxovirus	Paramyxovirus type 1	Contact with carrier feral birds or fomites	Polyuria, diarrhea, CNS signs	Serologic testing, antigen detection	No treatment, supportive care; vaccination of other birds in the loft is recommended to pigeon hobbyists in the face of an outbreak

Continued

TABLE 20-2

Selected Bacterial, Fungal, Viral, and Parasitic Diseases of Columbiformes—cont'd

Disease	Etiologic Agent	Transmission	Signs	Diagnosis	Management and Treatment
Pigeonpox	Poxvirus	Contact with diseased birds or mechanical transmission via biting insects	Cutaneous form—epidermal hyperplasia on non-feathered parts of the body; Diphtheritic form—diphtheritic membranes in the oral cavity, esophagus, trachea, usually accompanied by respiratory signs	Characteristic lesions, biopsy/histopathology	No treatment; supportive care; vaccines are available
Spiruridosis, proventricular worms	*Tetrameres, Dispharynx*	Ingestion of intermediate or paratenic host	Variable but emaciation and regurgitation are possible	Identification of larvae, eggs, or adult nematodes	No proven treatment; high dose ivermectin, levamisole, and benzimidazoles have been attempted; breaking the life cycle is difficult
Sarcocystosis	*Sarcocystis* spp.	Ingestion of sporocysts	Variable and depends on susceptibility of bird infected; may see respiratory, muscular, neurologic signs, or peracute death	Hematology, plasma chemistries, identify organism in tissue biopsy, serologic testing, protein electrophoresis	If bird survives peracute disease, treat with a sulfonamide combined with pyrimethamine; toltrazuril, ponazuril
Coccidiosis	*Eimeria* spp. predominantly	Fecal-oral; ingestion of oocysts	Clinical disease most common in juveniles; anorexia, dehydration, cachexia, and diarrhea	Oocysts in feces	Amprolium, sulfonamides, toltrazuril, ponazuril
Trichomoniasis, canker	*Trichomonas gallinae*	Direct contact with infected birds or contaminated water	Anorexia, lethargy, frequent swallowing movements, dyspnea, associated with ulceration and inflammation of the upper gastrointestinal tract; with or without development of caseous lesions; omphalitis may occur in squabs	Identification of protozoa in wet mounts obtained from crop/oral cavity	Nitroimidazoles (carnidazole, metronidazole, ronidazole, etc.)

doves exhibit high fecundity, and the relatively short time investment in incubating and raising a clutch allows hens to recycle and produce multiple broods each breeding season. Eggs may be artificially incubated at temperatures between 37.2° C and 37.5° C;[31] however, successful hand-rearing of hatchlings remains a challenge.

PREVENTIVE MEDICINE

Effective preventive health programs begin with sound, "all-in, all-out" quarantine practices. A minimum of 45 days quarantine length has been recommended for newly acquired columbids, as in psittacines. Screening for *Chlamydophila* and *Trichomonas*, along with other infectious agents and parasites, is indicated during this period. Newly acquired columbids or birds that have been moved to new aviaries should be closely monitored for signs of social dysfunction or maladaptation and anorexia. Birds should be individually identified with colored leg bands with or without implanted microchips. High-quality and complete nutrition, attention to hygiene, and appropriate housing and husbandry are critical. Birds should be protected from predators and from vectors of disease, and a fecal testing program should be in place to monitor for endoparasitism. Sick birds should be isolated, and complete necropsies with histopathologic examination should be performed on deceased birds. Although seldom applied to exotic columbids in zoological parks, commercial vaccines are available for domestic pigeons against certain infectious agents, including poxvirus, PMV-1, and *Salmonella*.

ACKNOWLEDGMENTS

The author would like to acknowledge the Exotic Animal Pathology Service at the University of Georgia for the production of Figure 20-5 and his father, Sandor Gyimesi, a pigeon enthusiast, for cultivating his interests in the animal kingdom.

REFERENCES

1. Atalan G, Uzun M, Demirkan I, et al: Effect of medetomidine-butorphanol-ketamine anaesthesia and atipamezole on heart and respiratory rate and cloacal temperature of domestic pigeons. *J Vet Med A Physiol Pathol Clin Med* 49:281–285, 2002.
2. Baer CK: Comparative nutrition and feeding considerations of young Columbidae. In Fowler ME, Miller RE, editors: *Zoo and wild animal medicine*, ed 4, Philadelphia, PA, 1999, Saunders, pp 269–277.
3. Bunbury N, Barton E, Jones CG, et al: Avian blood parasites in an endangered columbid: *Leucocytozoon marchouxi* in the Mauritius pink pigeon, *Columba mayeri*. *Parasitology* 134:797–804, 2007.
4. Bunbury N: Trichomonad infection in endemic and introduced columbids in the Seychelles. *J Wildl Dis* 47:730–733, 2011.
5. Dickx V, Beeckman DS, Dossche L, et al: *Chlamydophila psittaci* in homing and feral pigeons and zoonotic transmission. *J Med Microbiol* 59:1348–1353, 2010.
6. Esposito JF: Respiratory medicine in pigeons. *Vet Clin Exot Anim* 3:395–402, 2000.
7. Fedynich AM, Fredricks TB, Benn S: Lead concentrations of white-winged doves, *Zenaida asiatica* L., collected in the Lower Rio Grande Valley of Texas, USA. *Bull Environ Contam Toxicol* 85:344–347, 2010.
8. Frantz A, Pottier MA, Karimi B, et al: Contrasting levels of heavy metals in the feathers of urban pigeons from close habitats suggest limited movements at a restricted scale. *Environ Pollut* 168:23–28, 2012.
9. Garner MM: Personal communication, 2012.
10. Gentz EJ, Linn KA: Use of a dorsal cervical single pedicle advancement flap in 3 birds with cranial skin defects. *J Avian Med Surg* 14:31–36, 2000.
11. Griner LA, Walch HA: Cryptococcosis in Columbiformes at the San Diego Zoo. *J Wildl Dis* 14:389–394, 1978.
12. Griner LA: Order Columbiformes. In *Pathology of zoo animals*, San Diego, CA, 1983, Zoological Society of San Diego, pp 205–214.
13. Gyimesi ZS, Hayden ER, Greiner EC: Sticktight flea (*Echidnophaga gallinacea*) infestation in a Victoria crowned pigeon (*Goura victoria*). *J Zoo Wildl Med* 38:594–596, 2007.
14. Hagey LR, Schteingart CD, Ton-Nu HT, et al: Biliary bile acids of fruit pigeons and doves (Columbiformes): Presence of 1-beta-hydroxychenodeoxycholic acid and conjugation with glycine as well as taurine. *J Lipid Res* 35:2041–2048, 1994.
15. Harlin R, Wade L: Bacterial and parasitic diseases of Columbiformes. *Vet Clin Exot Anim* 12:453–473, 2009.
16. Howard LL, Papendick R, Stalis IH, et al: Fenbendazole and albendazole toxicity in pigeons and doves. *J Avian Med Surg* 16:203–210, 2002.
17. Kamiloglu A, Atalan G, Kamiloglu NN: Comparison of intraosseous and intramuscular drug administration for induction of anaesthesia in domestic pigeons. *Res Vet Sci* 85:171–175, 2008.
18. Koochakzadeh A, Ehsan MR, Jahany S, et al: Ingluvial fungal flora of rock doves (*Columba livia*). In Bergman E, editor: *Proceedings of the Association of Avian Veterinarians Annual Meeting*, 2010, pp 289–290.
19. Krautwald-Junghanns ME, Zebisch R, Schmidt V: Relevance and treatment of coccidiosis in domestic pigeons (*Columba livia* forma *domestica*) with particular emphasis on toltrazuril. *J Avian Med Surg* 23:1–5, 2009.
20. Lowenstine LJ, Munson L: Iron overload in the animal kingdom. In Fowler ME, Miller RE, editors: *Zoo and wild animal medicine*, ed 4, Philadelphia, PA, 1999, Saunders, pp 260–268.
21. Marlier D, Vindevogul H: Viral infections in pigeons. *Vet J* 172:40–51, 2006.
22. Martinez-Carrasco C, Martinez CM, de Ybáñez Mdel R, et al: Tetrameriosis in feral pigeons from Murcia, Southeastern Spain. *Prevent Vet Med* 90:284–286, 2009.
23. Nam DH, Lee DP: Monitoring for Pb and Cd pollution using feral pigeons in rural, urban, and industrial environments of Korea. *Sci Total Environ* 357:288–295, 2006.
24. Olias P, Gruber AD, Heydorn AO, et al: A novel Sarcocystis-associated encephalitis and myositis in racing pigeons. *Avian Pathol* 38:121–128, 2009.
25. Padilla LR, Flammer K, Miller RE: Doxycycline-medicated drinking water for treatment of *Chlamydophila psittaci* in exotic doves. *J Avian Med Surg* 19:88–91, 2005.
26. Pollack C: Fungal diseases of Columbiformes and Anseriformes. *Vet Clin Exot Anim* 6:351–361, 2003.
27. Pollack CG, Schumacher J, Orosz SE, et al: Sedative effects of medetomidine in pigeons (*Columba livia*). *J Avian Med Surg* 15:95–100, 2001.
28. Powers LV: Veterinary care of Columbiformes. In Bergman E, editor: *Proceedings of the Association of Avian Veterinarians Annual Meeting*, 2005, pp 171–183.
29. Rupiper DJ, Ehrenberg M: Diagnostic procedures for pigeon loft management. In Kornelsen MJ, editor: *Proceedings of the Association of Avian Veterinarians Annual Meeting*, 1994, pp 225–230.
30. Schleucher E: Metabolism, body temperature, and thermal conductance of fruit-eating doves (Aves: Columbidae, Treroninae). *Comp Biochem Physiol Mol Integr Physiol* 131:417–428, 2002.
31. Schultz DJ: Columbiformes (pigeons, doves). In Fowler ME, Miller RE, editors: *Zoo and wild animal medicine*, ed 5, St. Louis, MO, 2003, Saunders, pp 180–187.
32. Suedmeyer WK, Bermudez AJ, Barr BC, et al: Acute pulmonary *Sarcocystis falcatula*-like infection in three Victoria crowned pigeons (*Goura victoria*) housed indoors. *J Zoo Wild Med* 32:252–256, 2001.
33. Suedmeyer WK, Bermudez A, Shaiken L: Osteolysis and hepatomegaly caused by *Salmonella typhimurium* in a Temminck's fruit dove (*Ptilinopus porphyrea*). *J Avian Med Surg* 12:184–189, 1998.
34. Vogel C, Gerlach H, Löffler M: Columbiformes. In Ritchie BW, Harrison GJ, Harrison LR, editors: *Avian medicine: Principles and application*, Lake Worth, FL, 1994, Wingers Publishing, pp 1200–1217.
35. Waap H, Cardoso R, Leitão A, et al: In vitro isolation and seroprevalence of *Toxoplasma gondii* in stray cats and pigeons in Lisbon, Portugal. *Vet Parasitol* 187:542–547, 2012.
36. Werther K, de Sousa E, Alves Júnior JRF, et al: *Cryptococcus gattii* and *Cryptococcus albidus* in captive domestic pigeons (*Columba livia*). *Braz J Vet Pathol* 4:247–249, 2011.
37. Wotton DM, Kelly D: Frugivore loss limits recruitment of large-seeded trees. *Proc Biol Sci* 278:3345–3354, 2011.
38. Zwart P: Columbiform medicine. In Fowler ME, editor: *Zoo and wild animal medicine*, ed 3, Philadelphia, PA, 1993, Saunders, pp 240–244.

CHAPTER 21

Psittaciformes

J. Jill Heatley and Juan Cornejo

GENERAL BIOLOGY

Psittaciformes is a homogeneous order of over 350 extant species of parrots grouped in about 84 genera.[12] The three superfamilies consist of Strigopoidea, which includes the kakapo (*Strigops habroptilus*), the kea and the kaka (*Nestor* spp.); Cacatuoidea, which includes the black and white cockatoos (Cacatuoidea, Calyptorhynchinae, and Cacatuinae), and the cockatiel (Nymphicinae, 1 sp.); and Psittacoidea, which comprises the remaining 326 species.[26,59] Parrots are found mainly in the tropical and subtropical regions of the Southern Hemisphere, with the greatest diversity in the New World and Australia. Most parrots are diurnal and arboreal. Common habitats include moist forest, woodland, and savanna; few species prefer open areas. Their bright colors, mimicry ability, and charisma have made parrots popular in captivity for centuries. In part because of this popularity and in part because of loss or degradation of their habitat, parrots are the most endangered birds in the world. At least nine species have become extinct since 1600, over 25% of the extant species are listed as threatened, and an additional 11% are listed as near threatened.[25]

UNIQUE ANATOMY

The most remarkable anatomic characteristic of the parrots is their broad, hooked bill and the complex associated musculature. The upper mandible is prominent and down-curved and fits over the broad shorter up-curved lower mandible. The upper mandible articulates with the skull, allowing extensive movement of both mandibles and an increased biting pressure. Most Psittaciformes species have a thick, muscular tongue, which, when used in combination with the bill, is an effective tool to manipulate and process food. In the subfamily Loriinae (lories and lorikeets) the tongue tip is further modified with erectile dermal papillae for gathering nectar and pollen. Parrots have short tarsi and zygodactyl (yoke-toed) feet, and the first (hallux) and fourth toes orient posteriorly, as an adaptation for climbing trees and manipulation of objects. The head is proportionally large and broad, the neck is short, and the ceca are vestigial or absent. Most species have brightly colored plumage, and only a few species have sexual dimorphism, apparent to the human eye. Juvenile parrots often have slightly dull plumage and a darker iris compared to adults. Parrots vary widely in size, from the Hyacinth Macaw (*Anodorhynchus hyacinthinus*) reaching 100 centimeters (cm) to the flightless Kakapo weighing up to 3 kilograms (kg) to the 8-cm 10-gram (g) pygmy parrots (*Micropsitta* spp.). The superfamily Cacatuoidea is distinguished by the presence of a gall bladder, the superficial position of the left carotid artery, the ossified orbital ring in the skull, the absence of blue and green plumage colors, and the presence of a movable feathered crest.[2,38,53]

SPECIAL HOUSING REQUIREMENTS

Because of their powerful beaks and propensity to chew, parrots are best housed in metal enclosures. Galvanized box wire mesh of 1 × 1 inch is an option for many species; however, some of the larger macaws and cockatoos require more secure welds, and may be able to navigate complex locking systems. New galvanized wire should be washed with a 1:10 vinegar solution and rinsed with water to remove the deposits of zinc that are likely to be toxic. Young or small birds with bills that fit into mesh of this size may be more at risk of toxicity when this type of enclosure is used.

Except in large aviaries, it is difficult to maintain live plants in parrot enclosures. A soft substrate such as bark chips, sand, or soil is best, as it can be easily cleaned and dried to avoid fungal overgrowth. Suspended cages that limit access to feces or discarded food are a popular option for housing breeding pairs. Most parrots are not cold hardy and should not be kept below 50° F (10° C) without supplemental heat. Acclimatization may facilitate the parrot to tolerance of approximately 30° F (0° C) for short periods, with protection from the elements during inclement weather. Daily access to fresh air and sunlight are highly recommended for the health and well-being of these species and to promote good bone density and feather quality. To fulfill their enrichment and chewing needs, parrots should also be provided with a regular supply of fresh branches to minimize damage to the perches and live plants in their enclosures. See Table 21-1 for breeding parameters of common species in North American zoos.

FEEDING

In the wild, most parrots consume a variety of plant-based diets (seeds, fruits, buds, bark, roots, flowers, nectar) that include occasional insects and are generally classified as herbivores.[29] Field conditions make determination of food sources and quantification of food consumption challenging. Thus, little information on the nutritional content of wild adult parrot diets exists[3,14] despite an increasing volume of research on the nutrition of captive Psittaciformes.[8,11,16,22,28,30–33,44,45,50,57,58,61] Because of a lack of complete understanding of nutritional requirements for growth and maintenance in captive parrots, malnutrition is still one of the main concerns in the care and propagation of this group, and providing nutritionally adequate diets remains a serious concern.[21,23,31,43,48]

Parrot diet formulation must account for caloric density, as this determines how much food the bird will eat and, thus, the amount of each nutrient consumed.[29] For this reason, diets of free-ranging parrots will tend to be deficient if extrapolated to captive birds. Most recommended diets for Psittaciformes are based on studies on poultry modified by research for small granivorous species (budgerigars, *Melopsittacus undulatus,* and cockatiels, *Nymphicus hollandicus*); therefore, it is unlikely that they adequately model all the dietary requirements of the diverse members of the order.

Traditional diets of captive parrots have been seed based. Most commercial seeds are high in fat; have a low calcium-to-phosphorus (Ca:P) ratio; and low levels of Ca, P, sodium (Na), zinc (Zn), iron (Fe), lysine, and vitamin A, based on metabolic energy needs.[24,56] Thus, deficiencies of these nutrients are common in captive parrots.[54,56] The addition of fruits and vegetables to a seed mix will not always result in a complete and balanced diet, as parrots will preferentially consume high-energy seeds.[4,10,24,54] Formulated processed diets available from many manufacturers provide the best available option for complete nutrition. To fulfill parrots' environmental enrichment needs, these diets may have up to 25% fresh low-energy-density vegetables and fruits added and still be within recommended dietary ranges.[4,25,55] Lories and lorikeets (Loriini) have unique anatomic adaptations to feed on nectar and pollen, and their diet in captivity should ideally be liquid.[13,60] Several nectar products are commercially available to provide parrots with complete

TABLE 21-1

Characteristics of Common Psittaciforme Species Kept in North American Zoos (as of 31 December, 2011)*

Rank	Number of Individuals	Common Name	Latin Name (number of species)	Clutch Size	Incubation Time (days)	Nesting Period (weeks)	Sexual Maturity (years)	Median Lifespan (years)	Maximum Lifespan (years)	Adult Weight (grams)	Outdoor Breeding Aviary Length x Width x Height (feet)	Nest box Length x Width x Height [Entrance Diameter] (inch)	Ring Inside Diameter (mm)	CITES Appendix
1	5766	Budgerigar	*Melopsittacus undulates*	4–6	18	4	1	5	18	26–35	3 × 3 × 3, suspended	5 × 5 × 7 [2]	4	Non-CITES
6	1346	Rainbow lorikeet	*Trichoglossus haematodus* subsp.	1–3	24–25	7–8	1	7	38	75–157	9 × 9 × 3, suspended	9 × 9 × 20 [3.5]	6.5	CITES II
7	830	Cockatiel	*Nymphicus hollandicus*	4–5	18–19	4–5	1	9	36	80–100	6 × 3 × 3, suspended	6 × 6 × 16 [2.5]	5.5	Non-CITES
27	322	Blue-and-yellow macaw	*Ara ararauna*	1–3	25–27	12–14	3–4	21	48	995–1380	20 × 9 × 6	20 × 20 × 40 [6]	14	CITES I
51	207	Sun conure	*Aratinga solstitialis*	4–5	23	7–8	2–3	19	30	120–130*	9 × 3 × 3, suspended	9 × 9 × 20 [3.5]	6	CITES II
52	204	Scarlet macaw	*Ara macao*	1–4	28	12–13	4–5	21	48	900–1490	20 × 9 × 6	20 × 20 × 40 [7]	14	CITES I
66	166	Green-winged macaw	*Ara chloropterus*	2–3	26–28	12–14	4–5	19	63	1050–1708	20 × 9 × 6	20 × 20 × 40 [7]	14	CITES II
77	144	Hyacinth macaw	*Anodorhynchus hyacinthinus*	2–3	29	14–16	5–6	22	54	1435–1695	30 × 8 × 8	22 × 22 × 40 [8]	15	CITES I
82	129	Military macaw	*Ara militaris*	2–4	28	13	3–4	20	54	972–1134	20 × 9 × 6	20 × 20 × 35 [6]	14	CITES I
84	126	Grey parrot	*Psittacus erithacus*	2–3	26	11	3–4	9	48	402–490	9 × 3 × 3, suspended	11 × 11 × 24 [5]	10	CITES II
86	125	Masked lovebird	*Agapornis personatus*	3–8	20–22	4–5	1	6	24	43–47	6 × 3 × 3, suspended	5 × 5 × 10 [2]	4.5	CITES II
88	122	Fischer's lovebird	*Agapornis fischeri*	3–8	20–22	4–5	1	8	32	42–58	6 × 3 × 3, suspended	5 × 5 × 10 [2]	4.5	CITES II
Other		Cockatoos	*Cacatua* spp. (12)	1–4	20–29	7–14	2–5	10–13	30–93	300–975	9 × 3 × 3, suspended 15 × 6 × 6	10 × 10 × 18 [4] 12 × 12 × 26 [6]	10–14	CITES I and II
Other		Conures	*Pyrrhura* spp. (17) *Aratinga* spp. (20)	2–9	22–30	6–9	1	14–28	19–35	65–196	6 × 3 × 3, suspended 9 × 3 × 3, suspended	8 × 8 × 15 [2.5] 10 × 10 × 20 [3.5]	5.5–6	CITES II
Other		Amazons	*Amazona* spp. (30)	2–6	24–28	8–10	2–3	9–35	22–67	206–610	9 × 3 × 3, suspended	12 × 12 × 24 [5]	9–12	CITES I and II

References from 7,12,15,27, and 63.
*Suggested outdoor aviary, nest box, and leg band are based on author experience (JC).

nutrition, and fruits and vegetables may be added to provide diversity and enrichment.

RESTRAINT AND HANDLING

Capture of parrots in large enclosures may be challenging. Training birds to station, target, load into carriers, or present at the side of the cage is recommended to facilitate examination and preventive medical procedures. Otherwise parrots may be netted or restrained initially with a towel. Nets with mesh size smaller than the bird's head and feet to lessen the risk of entanglement, a net hoop that is wide enough to cover the entire animal, and a net with fabric that is long enough to allow the bird to be secured into the bottom by folding over (locking) of the net should be chosen. Once the birds are captured, two handlers are required to extract large parrots from the net while avoiding the claws and bill.

Physical restraint and handling are acceptable in most parrot species. Even the largest of parrot species may be adequately restrained by two people with appropriate handling skills. Correct methods for handling Psittaciformes include aspects that limit the likelihood of damage to the handler, the examiner, and the patient. For handler protection, the patient should be held in such a way as to not be injured by the bill and the claws. The keel should be allowed to move freely for respiration, the wings held to the side of the body to avoid damage to the appendages, and the feet adequately restrained to allow easy examination. Generally, a complete ring made with the thumb and the forefinger and placed below the mandible allows for neck extension and good restraint while allowing excellent airflow to the bird's respiratory system. No attempt should be made to restrain parrots by gripping the lateral aspects of the mandible, as the delicate bones in this area as well as the tissues of the bare facial patch on some parrots may be seriously damaged. The bill, which has approximately 400 pounds or greater of bite force in some species, cannot be adequately restrained by using this method. Insertion of the thumb or other digit into the gular area beneath the mandible of the beak for extension of the head is also not recommended, as the glottis may be, inadvertently, obstructed in this manner. In small parrots, the entire body may be cupped in the palm of the hand, while the head, held between the index and middle finger, is extended to allow adequate restraint. The bird's body should always be supported. The overlapping signet ring formation of the trachea allows fairly firm restraint in this manner without risk of tracheal collapse.

Although some may prefer lightweight leather gloves for field work with parrots, these provide little protection from the crushing force of the bill. Similarly, a towel only provides a "hide" or foil for the holders' hands, much like the cape of a matador. Ear plugs are also recommended if the parrot is anticipated to be so loud that the staff must raise their voices to communicate during examination to avoid damage to the human auditory system; even parrots that are quite small, for example, the sun conure (*Aratinga solstitialis*), may emanate sound meant to be heard over long distances.

Much work has been accomplished lately in these intelligent species on positive reinforcement training for a variety of medical examinations and procedures. Birds have been trained to target, station, load into carriers, and accept medications from syringes and intramuscular injections. Whenever possible, these techniques should be incorporated into the daily care and enrichment of Psittaciformes to reduce stress and increase veterinary ability to provide medical care without undue stress to the patient.

Sedation of Psittaciformes species with midazolam and butorphanol, which may be given intranasally (IN) or intramuscularly (IM), has become popular for use with companion parrots and has also been used in the zoo setting.[37] Based on the tolerance of different species to these drugs, it is advisable to begin with a low dose and to have reversal drugs available. Additional medications used for pain control in these species include meloxicam, carprofen, and tramadol. For anesthesia, induction with sevoflurane or isoflurane via a face mask is most commonly used; Generally, parrots are not intubated for short-term anesthesia (<20 minutes); an uncuffed endotracheal tube is used if intubation is necessary. Fasting to ensure an empty crop is recommended prior to anesthesia induction. Parrots may also be intubated through other air sacs when access to the oral cavity, bill, or trachea is desired for surgery. Excellent reviews of avian anesthesia, applicable to parrots, may be found elsewhere.[19]

SURGERY (COMMON AND SPECIAL CONSIDERATIONS)

Common surgical procedures include endoscopy for internal examination, gender determination, and biopsy. Tumor removal, bill repair or restructuring, amputation or other orthopedic repair, and reproductive system surgery are also common. Surgical approaches should be tempered by constraints of patient positioning to allow free keel mobility and observation. Additionally, surgical preparation and perioperative care should incorporate techniques to avoid excessive heat loss and to provide heat supplementation, for example, minimal feather removal, use of noncooling or warmed liquids, and transparent draping. Flammable liquids as preparatory agents must be avoided when electrosurgical, radiosurgical, or laser surgical techniques are used.

Foreign body removal is often an indication for veterinary intervention. However, in parrots, alternatives to exploratory coeliotomy should be considered, as proventriculotomy, ventriculotomy, and enterotomy are not without risk of morbidity and mortality. In many cases, flexible or rigid endoscopy, accompanied by ingluviotomy if necessary, is a reasonable alternative approach for foreign body removal; use of neodymium magnets embedded in the end of flexible tubing for removal of metal objects has also been successful as a less invasive, although blind, method if fluoroscopy is not available. Because of the tough ventricular koilin lining and the very muscular ventriculus, foreign objects that are not obstructive may not need removal, as they will be disintegrated slowly by normal GI action and motility. However, this same action often results in continuing toxic insult and blood accumulation if the object contains lead, zinc, or copper.

As neoplasms are not uncommon in these long-lived species, tumor removal should be followed up with histopathologic examination to provide an appropriate standard of care for parrots.

Principles for surgical approach, orthopedic repair, and amputation of pelvic and thoracic limbs to be used in parrots have been published.[41] Many captive parrots do well with coaptive or conservative management of thoracic and pelvic limb injuries as flight and full talon function are not required for eating and perching. Surgery to limit flight is not recommended in these species because of their longevity and predisposition to atherosclerosis and obesity. Surgery or repair of the bill is challenging because of the numerous functional joints and fragile bones in this area. Computed tomography (CT) is recommended prior to bill surgery to determine the best approach for surgical correction. Correction of bill malformation in these species (scissor bill, mandibular prognathism) is best attempted when the birds are young.[2] Many parrots with complete or partial loss or malformation of the upper or lower bill may adapt to feeding and maintain normal body weight and social bonds.

Reproductive surgery is a common concern in female parrots which produce too many eggs. Some parrots may lay eggs until total body calcium stores become depleted, resulting in pathologic fractures, tetany, and paresis. Salpingohysterectomy does not guarantee cessation of ovulation, and ovary removal is challenging because of proximity to the adrenal gland, the cranial pole of the kidney, and local vessel anatomy. Hormonal modulation via synthetic gonadotropin-releasing hormone (GnRH) agonists may decrease reproductive organ activity, facilitating surgical intervention or negating the need for surgical intervention. However, environmental factors, species factors, and individual patient factors all affect reproductive activity, so treatment and environment should be modified accordingly for best patient outcome.

Surgery for cloacal prolapse is common for *Cacatua* spp. Although surgical reduction of vent aperture or tacking of the extruded cloaca may reduce the prolapse in the short term, hormonal and inappropriate physical stimulation of the birds and the inappropriate bonding behavior of keepers or owners may result in breakdown of this repair, which is associated with morbidity and mortality.[46] Surgery alone will not often repair a behavioral, hormonal, and usually longstanding, problem. Because the cloaca is the nexus of three different systems, cloacal prolapse may involve not only the GI tract but also the urinary and reproductive tracts. Care should be taken to discern which aspects of these systems are prolapsed prior to attempting surgical repair and to counsel the primary caretaker to correct any behavioral problems prior to attempting this non-emergency surgery.

OTHER PHARMACEUTICALS

Numerous pharmaceuticals are of use in Psittaciformes. Pharmacologic concerns in parrots include regurgitation (in macaws) after administration of trimethoprim sulfa and upon recovery from isoflurane or sevoflurane anesthesia. Birds should be allowed to regurgitate without restraint to avoid aspiration. Doxycycline, a drug commonly used in Psittaciformes to treat chlamydial infection, is an effective chelator; however, administration of supplemental calcium should be considered in young growing birds or possibly in hypocalcemic hens when using this drug. Administration of long-acting topical steroids such as triamcinolone, commonly available for use in companion mammals, or long term administration of systemic steroids are *not* recommended for use in parrots, as they may cause overwhelming fungal infection and mortality. Although pharmacotherapy is often used in an attempt to control feather-destructive behavior, a full diagnostic workup is necessary to rule out medical causes and to assess baseline health status prior to administration of behavioral modification drugs. In-depth assessment of the enrichment needs of the parrot patient, prior to drug administration, is also highly recommended.

PHYSICAL EXAMINATION AND DIAGNOSTICS

Physical examination of parrots should progress in a manner similar to that in other species. However, observational examination should proceed prior to physical examination to avoid unexpected patient death resulting from physical restraint. Parrots often mask signs of illness until decompensation is near total and mortality is impending. Therefore, when severe clinical signs of illness are apparent on observational examination, full physical examination may be forgone in the critical patient to preserve life via critical supportive therapies such as provision of warmth, oxygen, and fluids; administration of antibiotics; and pain control. After patient stabilization, a more complete physical examination may be performed on the live parrot.

Physical examination should progress in a timely manner, and sometimes a stepwise physical examination with periods of rest for the patient may be indicated. Based on observational examination of the patient, if the neurologic, respiratory, and musculoskeletal systems of the patient appear to be in order, physical examination generally proceeds from head to toe as with companion mammals. Special attention should be given to examination of the choanal papilla; symmetry; body condition; auscultation of the lungs, air sacs, and heart; palpation of the pulse and assessment of venous refill time on the wing; hydration; and the ventrum of the feet. Examine the vent for mucous membrane roughening associated with papillomas. Grip and strength of the bill and feet and the withdrawal response of the limbs, as well as joint mobility, should be assessed. Coelomic palpation in most parrots will reveal a concave conformation, and the ventriculus is often palpable. The jugular apteria and ears should also be assessed, as trauma is often obscured until the feathers are parted to observe the transparent skin and subcutaneous tissues. Feathers should be observed for stress lines, fractures, or color changes, and the bill should be assessed for weakness or overgrowth. The uropygial gland, present in most parrots but absent in *Amazona* and *Anodorhynchus* spp., should be visualized and palpated.

DISEASE

Common infectious diseases of concern are listed in Tables 21-2, 21-3, and 21-4. Few bacterial diseases of parrots are transmissible to man, but infection with *Chlamydia* spp. is the most important exception. Clostridial infection, pasteurellosis, and multiple gram-negative bacterial infections are of most immediate concern for parrot health, as they may lead to rapid sepsis and acute death. Mycobacterial disease is not uncommon in parrot species; zoonotic potential, challenging assessment and diagnosis, and the necessary prolonged multidrug therapy often result in euthanasia of these patients. *Salmonella* spp. as well as methicillin-resistant *Staphylococcus aureus* and other multidrug-resistant bacteria may be carried by parrots, and although morbidity is likely in the avian patient, concern with regard to infection is primarily based on zoonotic potential. Numerous bacteria with possible human pathogenicity have now been cultured from apparently healthy captive and free-living parrots.[62] Similarly, normal flora of humans may pose some risk to the health of parrots.[6] Bacterial diseases of particular significance to both parrot and human health are listed in Table 21-2.

Viral diseases of most concern for parrots are given in Table 21-3. For more complete information, excellent texts are available.[49] Avian influenza virus, Newcastle's disease virus (paramyxoviruses), psittacinepox virus, West Nile virus (WNV), and avian adenovirus rarely cause disease in Psittaciformes.

Most fungal diseases of concern for parrots are associated with poor husbandry or other causes of immune system suppression (see Table 21-4). Free-living parrots in their native habitat are attacked by numerous parasites, which appear unable to complete their lifecycle in North America. Sarcocystosis and toxoplasmosis are diseases of importance, and hemoparasites, *Giardia* or *Hexamita*, ascarids, red mites, *Eimeria*, keds, lice, and *Knemidokoptes* are parasites of most concern in parrots in zoologic collections. Table 21-5 lists parasites of most concern for zoologic collections and those that are population limiting in free-living parrots.

Noninfectious diseases of concern in parrots are mainly related to husbandry and nutritional issues, although endocrine and neoplastic diseases also occur. Feather-destructive behavior is a common problem in captive parrots. With this syndrome, it may be very challenging to elucidate the medical or behavioral cause; and treatment may be equally frustrating. It is important to assess for underlying health issues and provide environmental enrichment to the affected parrots prior to placing them on psychotropic drugs for this disorder.

Nutritional disorders are a common concern in captive parrots, as many vitamin and nutrient needs of these species remain unknown. Vitamin A deficiency, obesity, atherosclerosis, and hemachromatosis are still relatively common in these species. Definitive diagnosis of vitamin deficiency remains challenging, as vitamin levels from healthy free-living parrots are largely unknown. Endocrine diseases such as diabetes mellitus and hypothyroidism are rare but have been reported in these species. Diagnosis of endocrine diseases is often hindered by lack of parrot-appropriate diagnostic reagents.

Trauma is not uncommon as many species are territorial and agonistic, particularly during breeding season in the wild. As an intelligent and active group, parrots often also encounter trauma because of poor decisions or curiosity. Flying toward moving objects such as ceiling fans or into solid objects, becoming caught on an object within their environment and causing further severe damage to the limb while attempting to free itself, and having limbs severed or mauled by predators from outside the enclosure are common presentations.

Text continued on p. 184

TABLE 21-2

Selected Bacterial Diseases of Psittaciformes

Bacterial Disease	Etiology	Epizootiology	Signs	Diagnosis	Management
Chlamydiosis, ornithosis, parrot fever, psittacosis	*Chlamydia psittaci* Obligate intracellular bacteria, gram negative. Life cycle consists of the infectious elementary body, which may survive outside the host and infects the host epithelial cells, becoming the reticulate body, which exists inside the host and reproduces by binary fission. Only the elementary body is immunogenic, as the reticulate body evades the host immune system inside the cell.	All parrots are susceptible and disease is circumglobal. Parrots seem particularly suited to harbor this pathogen. Incubation ranges from 3 days to 2 months. Duration of immunity is negligible after infection and treated birds may become reinfected. Antibodies are not protective.	Parrots may harbor *C. psittaci* without clinical signs. When present, clinical signs are often nonspecific, as the organism affects the gastrointestinal tract, liver, and the respiratory and neurologic systems. Birds often appear depressed and lethargic and may have bright green stools because of liver disease. Disease may be limited to the upper respiratory system or conjunctivitis. Clinical signs may mimic heavy metal intoxication.	Chlamydiosis is often a diagnostic challenge in the live bird. Isolation of the organism for definitive diagnosis requires specialized media and is rarely pursued based on expense. Elementary body agglutination was the preferred test for diagnosis of active infection, especially when combined with an immunoglobulin M (IgM) titer; however, this test is no longer commercially available. Most commonly, a choanal or cloacal swab is submitted for polymerase chain reaction (PCR) testing to determine if the organism is being shed. The presence of the organism, consistent clinical signs, and severe leukocytosis are often combined to make a diagnosis consistent with suspicion of chlamydiosis. PCR and detection of intracytoplasmic chlamydial inclusions often found in the enlarged liver or spleen at necropsy are diagnostic. Special stains or indirect fluorescent antibody (IFA) testing are helpful for detection of these inclusions, which are rare in oral, ocular or respiratory secretions or conjunctival scrapings.	This zoonotic organism may cause mild to severe respiratory disease in humans with flu-like symptoms. However, disease is rare in humans with less than 50 cases confirmed since 1996. Treatment in humans and birds is prolonged (at least 45 days) because of the occult and protracted lifecycle of *C. psittaci*. Tetracyclines, doxycycline, azithromycin, or fluoroquinolones may be used for treatment. This organism and the required repeated testing are the primary reasons for Psittaciformes to be quarantined and carefully screened prior to entry into a zoologic collection for 45 to 60 days. Required treatment and additional testing in cases of positive birds may prolong required isolation. No vaccine is available. Elementary bodies are environmentally stable but may be inactivated with ultraviolet (UV) light, 70% ethanol, quaternary ammonium, or 3% hydrogen peroxide.
Clostridium	*Clostridium perfringens* Gram-positive, rod-shaped, anaerobic, spore-forming bacterium that is ubiquitous in nature and a common component of decaying vegetation.	Ingestion of clostridial organisms generally occurs because of spoiled high-sugar (nectar or fruit) food stuffs. Spoilage may occur within hours in hot weather. Some parrots such as the Kakapo may have clostridial organisms normally within their gastrointestinal (GI) tracts.[55]	Birds often die acutely without clinical signs. Parrots that survive longer may show lethargy, depression, and dehydration; foamy malodourous droppings caused by gas production of some organisms may be observed. Observed clinical signs prior to death are the exception rather than the rule and usually limited to parrots that are not nectivores.	Antemortem diagnostics are often limited in these cases because of the extremely unstable nature of the patient. Radiography and fecal cytology may provide supportive evidence of spore-forming, gas-producing bacterial infection. The bird may be in poor condition or more often very good body condition at necropsy with minimal gross signs. Diagnosis is often made after death histologically. Necrosis of the GI mucosa and colonization of villi by large gram-positive rods consistent with *Clostridium* spp. are found.	*C. perfringens* is a common cause of foodborne illness in humans but has minimal zoonotic potential, as it occurs in aviaries. Supportive care should include hydration, antibiotic treatment with appropriate spectrum, and antiendotoxin treatment. Prognosis in all but the most stable cases, where findings may be incidental, is guarded. Appropriate disinfection of food containers and utensils should occur daily if not more often to maintain cleanliness, and sugar-containing food should be removed

Disease	Etiologic Agent	Hosts / Transmission	Clinical Signs	Diagnosis	Treatment / Prevention
					and replaced as often as every 4 hours in hot weather, which is conducive of growth of these organisms. Facilities which cannot adhere to these standards or have continuing outbreaks should consider limiting nectivores in their collections. *C. perfringens* enterotoxin (CPE), which mediates disease, is inactivated at 74° C (165° F)
Colibacillosis Coligranuloma	*Escherichia coli* Gram-negative, facultative anaerobic, rod-shaped bacterium, common in the lower intestine of many mammals.	All parrots considered susceptible; but reported in the Amazon parrot, Hyacinth macaw, budgerigar, lories, and lorikeets.	Young birds may have navel illness. Signs may be insidious and nonspecific. The bird may fail to thrive or have ill thrift, but no signs are pathognomonic.	Diagnosis in the live bird relies on diagnosis of bacterial infection based on culture of the affected area, blood culture, or fecal culture. Gram stain of the affected system that shows heavy growth of gram-negative rods may be supportive of the diagnosis. Classically, granulomas are found in the intestinal tract and liver at necropsy.	As a normal component of GI flora in most humans, it is of minimal zoonotic risk. Prompt, appropriate antibacterial treatment and aggressive supportive care are important in these cases, as the birds are often found severely compromised, septic on presentation, or both. Affected birds should be isolated until the infection is resolved. Glove use and appropriate sanitation and disinfection are required. Sodium hypochlorite is an effective disinfectant.
Mycobacteriosis	*M. genavense* *M. avium* *M avium intracellulare complex* *M. tuberculosis* Zoonotic potential depends on mycobacterial species identified.	All parrots susceptible; immunocompromised individuals are at most risk. Many mycobacteria are common soil saprophytes or found in water sources. Transmission is generally considered to occur by the fecal–oral route.	Classic clinical signs are that of a bird with ravenous appetite, which continues to lose weight, as mycobacterial disease most often affects the GI tract in birds. However, clinical signs are often insidious and may mimic many other diseases. Signs may occur in any system, including the respiratory system, eyes, skin, muscle, and bone. Common signs include dysfunction and enlargement or nodular swelling in the affected area.	Acid-fast staining of feces or affected organs; histopathology and acid-fast staining, PCR, and culture remain the gold standard but are expensive and slow. Diagnosis may be made on the basis of associated complete blood cell count (CBC) (often, but no guarantee of elevated white blood cell [WBC] count >30,000) but must be confirmed by biopsy or cytological sampling and PCR or culture of the affected organ, usually at necropsy. Affected organs at necropsy (classically the liver and spleen) may be found enlarged, pale, or both and have white-yellow nodules. Diagnosis of mycobacteriosis in the live bird is challenging, and a single negative screening sample (usually obtained from the liver) does not guarantee that the animal is free of mycobacterial disease.	Although the zoonotic potential of parrot-associated mycobacteriosis appears very low, the public should not be exposed to infected parrots. Treatment with multidrug therapy, similar to that of humans, has been attempted in some parrots. Preventive measures include obtaining a full history on any birds donated to the collection and limiting contact with free-living birds. Specific disinfectants available and labeled as mycobactericidal should be used in bird quarantine areas.

Continued

TABLE 21-2

Selected Bacterial Diseases of Psittaciformes—cont'd

Bacterial Disease	Etiology	Epizootiology	Signs	Diagnosis	Management
Pasteurellosis	*P. multocida* Small gram-negative coccobacillus. Nonmotile, penicillin-sensitive, facultative anaerobe.	Parrots appear exquisitely sensitive to a variety of bacterial pathogens, most importantly *P. multocida*, found in the mouths of predators. Parrots are unlikely to survive for more than 24 hours after predator attack because of overwhelming sepsis, likely to occur without antimicrobial support.	Parrots maintained outside are often mauled through the cage as they sleep. The next morning they may be miraculously found to be alive because of the effects of shock, only to perish from overwhelming sepsis a few days later if appropriate and aggressive therapy is not instituted. Drooping or missing appendage(s), blood in the enclosure, and multiple missing feathers are classic presenting signs. Absence of bite marks does not negate the possibility that a predatory attack has occurred. Avian stoic behavior, feathers, and skin are very good at obstructing the health care professional from recognizing serious damage and inflammation.	Because of the extremely unstable nature of many of the cases, extensive diagnostics are often forgone; a presumptive diagnosis and aggressive supportive care, including hydration, warmth, and appropriate antibiotic administration, which should initially be parenteral and include a gram-positive spectrum, are provided. Flouroquinolones alone may not provide adequate gram-positive antibacterial spectrum for these cases. CBC may demonstrate left shift and leukopenia in severely affected cases, as well as anemia from blood loss. Many cases with severe damage to the appendage may require amputation to resolve local infection.	Zoonotic potential is low (humans obtain the organism from bites or scratches from domestic pets) from the parrot, but gloves should be worn when handling any parrot wound or abrasions to minimize colonization by normal human bacterial flora. Provide predator-proof enclosures, especially at night. Prompt attention and aggressive antimicrobial and supportive care to these cases is essential for the best outcome. Amputation of the affected portion of the limb should be considered in refractory cases that have been stabilized. Immediate anaerobic and aerobic cultures are indicated. As a microaerophilic bacterium, this organism is unlikely to survive for long in the environment, However, polymicrobial infections are common in cases of animal attack; therefore, wound cover and glove use, as well as enclosure disinfection with steam, are recommended.
Salmonellosis	*Salmonella* spp. Gram-negative bacterium.	In captivity salmonella carriage and salmonellosis are common in parrots; however, *prevalence* in wild parrots appears low. Transmission is by the fecal–oral route. Food contamination is common.	Clinical signs include those related to sepsis (lethargy, depression) and those related to gastroenteritis (anorexia, weight loss etc.). Birds may die acutely with minimal clinical signs.	Diagnosis may be challenging in the live bird, as culture is the gold standard but requires selective media; and *Salmonella* spp. are intermittently shed. Birds may remain carriers for prolonged periods without clinical signs, although this has not been specifically proven in parrots. A bird with consistent clinical signs, and fecal Gram staining consistent with gram-negative bacterial infection should prompt cloacal bacterial culture collection immediately prior to institution of treatment.	Salmonellosis is a zoonotic pathogen. Affected birds should be isolated until the infection resolves. Treatment should include hydration support and antibacterials if leukocytosis and signs of illness or sepsis are present. Caretakers should wear gloves when handling birds and masks when washing down enclosures. Appropriate sanitation and disinfection, including hand washing, are required. Birds used for educational display and that may come in direct or indirect audience contact should be screened, more than once, for salmonellosis. Parrots should be kept separate and handled separately from raptors and reptiles.

References from 9, 18, 35, 39, 42, 51, 52, and 62.

TABLE 21-3

Select Viral Diseases of Psittaciformes

Viral Disease	Etiology	Epizootiology	Parrot Clinical Signs	Diagnosis	Management
Avian bornavirus (ABV)	Bornaviridae Enveloped single-strand RNA virus Multiple genotypes	This virus is widespread in free-living birds. Transmission and pathogenesis of the disease in companion birds are still under active investigation. Infection rate may be as high as 15%. How long birds shed, maintain, or incubate the virus until disease is apparent is unknown. Latent shedding is likely. However, once infected, birds likely shed the virus for life. It is likely that some infected birds are never affected by disease. Likely transmitted vertically by aerosol, contact, or ingestion. Virus may be shed in urine, feces, tears, and oral secretions.	Neurologic syndrome, in which affected birds may have gastrointestinal and neurologic signs, including blindness, ataxia, weakness, weight loss, inability to perch, or passage of undigested food. The birds may succumb to opportunistic gastrointestinal infection or starvation caused by inability to ingest and digest food.	PCR, VI, IFA of cell culture, IHC, Western blot Crop biopsy and histopathology. Antibody test not commercially available. When present, gross lesions consist of dilated proventriculus and cardiac enlargement. Histopathology of proventricular dilatation disease is characterized by nonsuppurative inflammation in the central, peripheral and autonomic nervous systems.	No proven zoonotic potential. Care limited to supportive with easily digestible high calorie food, NSAIDs, monitor gastrointestinal flora in affected birds. Screen for viral infection and shedding via PCR. Maintenance of an ABV free collection preferred but is rarely currently feasible. Testing and separation is difficult based on intermittent shedding and latency of virus. No recommended commercially available vaccine. Appropriate disinfection uninvestigated. As a cell associated virus, likely easily inactivated.
Avian influenza	Orthomyxoviridae Influenza A virus Enveloped single-stranded RNA virus	Despite worldwide distribution by waterfowl, the serotypes which affect poultry are not of great risk to parrots. Flu isolates from parrots are limited to: H5N2, H5N1 and H9N2 and H7N1. Transmission: Aerosol, contact, ingestion, fomites	Range from subclinical infection to severe lethargy and depression to peracute death. Gastrointestinal, respiratory, and neurologic systems are often affected	VI, PCR, VN, AGID When present gross findings may include airsacculitis, necrotic debris in the sinuses or trachea, and inflammation and congestion of the brain, lungs, and gastrointestinal tract.	Avian and other influenza viruses have zoonotic potential in humans. Influenza A is rare in parrots and rarely affects humans, cats or dogs. No known human illness or fatality has been linked to a parrot influenza virus infection. Isolation and supportive care for 4 weeks post resolve of clinical signs, if present. No vaccine approved for use in parrots. Quarantine screening not prudent unless clinical signs are present, or dictated by recent importation. Virus inactivated by most disinfectants and sunlight.
Avian polyoma virus (APV)	Polyomaviridae Non-enveloped, double-stranded DNA virus	Budgerigars often considered the reservoir species, however APV is worldwide in free-living Passeriformes and has a broad host range. Transmission of APV within breeding populations of parrots appears rare. Transmission: Aerosol, contact, ingestion, vertical, fomites	Acute death, feather abnormalities, SQ hemorrhage, crop stasis, clinical signs are of particular concern and severity in large nestling Psittaciformes which usually do not survive; infection of adult birds is of minimal consequence.	IFA, EM, VN, PCR Gross findings include feather abnormalities, hydropericardium, enlarged heart, swollen liver, congested kidneys, and hemorrhage into body cavities. Large basophilic nuclear inclusion bodies in spleen, liver, kidneys	Polyoma viral infection is limited to birds. Isolation and supportive care for affected birds. APV vaccine available. Keep parrots and free living Passeriformes separated. Consider quarantine screening in actively breeding programs with juvenile birds susceptible to disease. Disinfection: Phenolics, sodium hypochlorite.

Continued

TABLE 21-3

Select Viral Diseases of Psittaciformes—cont'd

Viral Disease	Etiology	Epizootiology	Parrot Clinical Signs	Diagnosis	Management
Newcastle's Disease	Paramyxoviridae Enveloped single-stranded RNA virus, serotypes 1, 2, 3, and 5	Paramyxoviruses are found worldwide and are of concern based on threat of highly virulent strains (VVND, a reportable strain of PMV-1 which has been eradicated from the US) causing shortage of poultry as human food supply. Respiratory and fecal shedding primarily. Transmission via aerosol, ingestion or fomites.	Signs range from subclinical to peracute death. Gastrointestinal respiratory and development of central nervous systems signs which may persist for months are expected.	PCR, VI, HI, AGID, ELISA Few gross lesions reported specifically for parrots. If present, lesions may include, enlarged heart and spleen, pericardial effusion, mucus in urinary tract, brain hyperemia, hemorrhage in the trachea, and ovary hemorrhage and edema of the respiratory and gastrointestinal tracts.	Zoonotic risk of conjunctivitis is low. Based on the risk of devastation this disease can cause in poultry flocks, infected birds are often euthanized. Screen imported or unknown history parrots in quarantine for PMV. Disinfectants: detergents, chloramine 1%, sodium hypochlorite, Lysol, phenol, and 2% formalin.
Psittacine Beak and Feather Disease	Circoviridae Non-enveloped, single-stranded DNA virus	Naturally occurring in Australian parrots, all parrots are considered susceptible. Transmission likely aerosol, ingestion, and possibly horizontal. Virus in feather dander and crop secretions. Surviving birds are considered resistant. Incubation period weeks to years.	Sudden death occurs in peracute and acute forms. In the chronic form, progressive symmetric feather dystrophy and loss and beak deformities from necrosis and hyperplasia of epidermal cells. Beak deformities are found only in select species and depend on additional factors. Immunosuppression and opportunistic infection often lead to morbidity and mortality.	HA, HI, EM, PCR, histopathology of feathers and skin. Gross necropsy lesions are as seen clinically. Basophilic intranuclear and intracytoplasmic inclusion bodies within feather epithelial cells or macrophages	Psittacine Beak and Feather Infection is limited to birds No vaccine commercially available. Clinical patients are given supportive care and isolated. Quarantine testing recommended Virus may persist in feather dander and feces. Disinfectants: Sodium hypochlorite, chlorine dioxide, glutaraldehyde
Psittacid Herpes Virus (PsHV)	Herpesviridae Double-stranded DNA virus Multiple genotypes	PsHV-1 host range includes Amazon, Conure, Cockatiel, Cockatoo, Macaw, and African Grey Parrots and probably many others. PsHV-2 isolated from African Gray parrots, pathogenicity unclear. Latent infection and intermittent shedding common. Transmission: aerosol, contact, ingestion	Acute death, depression, anorexia, diarrhea, tremor, mucosal papillomas. Association with liver carcinomas suggested.	EM, PCR When present, gross findings may include necrosis, congestion and hemorrhage in liver, spleen, kidneys, and intestines. Cowdry type A intranuclear inclusion bodies in liver, kidneys, spleen, pancreas, intestines.	No zoonotic potential. Maintain birds with papillomas separately, monitor for hepatic tumor occurrence. Care for mucosal papillomas, or Pacheco's disease outbreak, is supportive although antiviral administration may be attempted. Unstable virus inactivated by most disinfectants. Screen birds in quarantine carefully for mucosal papillomas and viral shedding. Inactivated vaccine does not stop viral shedding.

From references 2, 6, 19, 37, 41, 46, and 62.
AGID, Agar gel immunodiffusion; *DNA,* deoxyribonucleic acid; *ELISA,* enzyme-linked immunosorbent assay; *EM,* electron microscopy; *HI,* hemagglutination inhibition; *IFA,* indirect fluorescent antibody; *IHC,* immunohistochemistry; *NSAIDs,* nonsteroidal anti-inflammatory drugs; *PCR,* polymerase chain reaction; *RNA,* ribonucleic acid; *SQ,* subcutaneous; *VI,* viral isolation; *VN,* virus neutralization.

TABLE 21-4

Select Fungal Diseases of Psittaciformes

Fungal Disease	Etiology	Epizootiology	Clinical Signs	Diagnosis	Management
Aspergillosis	*Aspergillus* spp. *A. fumigatus* *A. niger* *A. flavus*	Saprophyte ubiquitous in ventilation ducts and soil. Inhalation of spores results in respiratory infection and inflammation, secondary infection with opportunistic bacteria (*Pseudomonas* spp.) common. Host immunosuppression likely required. Shipping, quarantine, malnutrition, surgery, exposure to smoking or prolonged illness +/– antibiotic therapy likely predispose parrots to infection.	Most often clinical signs stem from respiratory tract infection; signs of upper or lower tract respiratory dysfunction may be present. Infection may spread hematogenously to any other organ. Disease progression is often insidious, with the patient failing to respond to treatment for presumed bacterial disease. The classic clinical sign is loss of voice or voice change because of fungal colonization of the syrinx. However, progressive weight loss, dyspnea, and other nonspecific signs of illness are also common. Disease may be limited to rhinitis or sinusitis.	Diagnosis in the live parrot may be challenging. PCR is prone to false positives because of environmental contamination. Serology is not well validated for use in the many parrot species and connotes only exposure and a functioning immune system. False negatives and positives occur. Imaging is poorly sensitive. Cytologic or histopathologic examination and culture of affected tissue may be definitive, but collection of specimens has risk in the patient with respiratory compromise. A presumptive diagnosis is often made in birds with consistent clinical signs, immunocompromise, and hematology suggestive of chronic disease. Diagnosis at necropsy is straightforward: the fungus is often green and found in the caudal air sacs, lungs, and at the syrinx.	Human aspergillosis is rare and comes from the environment, not birds. Treatment should be crafted and monitored carefully based on the patient's tolerance and needs and is often prolonged. Options for antifungal therapy are many but medications may be delivered IT, IV, PO, and via nebulization. Surgical or endoscopic debulking of large granulomas or those obstructing the airways may also be therapeutic. Parrots should be maintained in well-ventilated, clean enclosures without hay. The organism prefers damp fecal soiled litter, which parrots are prone to create. Topical steroids and exposure to cigarette smoke should be avoided. *Aspergillus* spp. may colonize brooders, nest boxes, and incubators; thorough preseason and postseason cleaning or replacement is necessary for these areas.
Avian gastric yeast (Previously called Megabacteria)	*Macrorhabdus ornithogaster* Anamorphic, ascomycetous yeast	Found in the avian stomach, this often benign fungus may cause acute hemorrhagic disease in budgerigars and parrotlets and a chronic wasting disease of cockatiels and budgerigars. The organism is intolerant of the low pH (0.7–2.3) of the avian stomach. *M. ornithogaster* colonizes the isthmus and modifies the environment to pH 3–4 to permit growth. The organism is microaerophilic and uses multiple sugars.	When present, birds may suffer weight loss (going light); diarrhea, or pasted vent. Acute death is caused by separation of ventricular koilin lining, and acute hemorrhage may also occur.	Diagnosis may be accomplished with fecal staining and examination or PCR; however, shedding is intermittent. The organism may be cultured with select culture media and conditions.	Avian gastric yeast affects only select avian species. Treatment options are poorly investigated. Antifungal therapy, cimetidine to change gastric pH, and treatment with sodium benzoate could be attempted in ill parrots. The organism may survive for only a limited time in the environment; normal disinfection should eliminate this organism.

Continued

TABLE 21-4

Select Fungal Diseases of Psittaciformes—cont'd

Fungal Disease	Etiology	Epizootiology	Clinical Signs	Diagnosis	Management
Candidiasis	*Candida* spp. *C. albicans* *C. tropicalis* *C. famata* *C. glabrata* *C. parapsilosis* Part of yeast microbiota in apparently healthy cockatiels	Opportunistic infection commonly encountered in budgerigars, cockatiels, and cockatoos. Immunocompromise is common in parrots affected by candidiasis. Juvenile birds with immature immune systems and adult birds affected by stress, viral infections, malnutrition, or administration of corticosteroids are more susceptible to candidiasis. Prolonged broad-spectrum antibiotic treatment may also predispose parrots to infection. Candidiasis commonly affects the mucosa of the oropharynx, esophagus, and crop. Local infections of the oral cavity, bill, sinuses, and gastrointestinal tract also uncommonly occur; external skin lesions and systemic infections are rare.	Clinical signs vary, depending on the area affected. Most commonly gastrointestinal signs such as crop slowing or stasis are seen. Small pin-point plaques may be seen in the oral cavity; an odor may emanate from the crop; and the crop mucosa may be palpably thickened. Regurgitation, polydipsia, or anorexia may also occur. Gas may sometimes be palpable in the gastrointestinal tract. External infections may result in feather loss, local irritation or erythema, and moistened skin or bill flakiness or other abnormal growth.	Diagnosis is commonly based on cytology, although organisms also grow readily in culture. Biopsy and histopathologic examination may be necessary for confirmation of lesions in the bill or boney tissues. Clinical signs should be combined with the presence of large numbers of yeast and/or pseudohyphae to confirm diagnosis. However, presumptive diagnosis and treatment trial are common, especially in juvenile birds with clinical signs, where tissue invasion and lack of large numbers of yeast for cytologic diagnosis are common.	Candidiasis is often environmentally acquired in immunocompromised humans and has not been linked to birds. Treatment choices are based on the severity of yeast infection. Superficial or nonsystemic infection in parrots without concern of immunosuppression may be treated topically with antifungals, and supportive care such as probiotics may also be instituted. Parrots with severe, invasive, or systemic infection causing organ dysfunction (such as crop stasis) or those with immunocompromise and overwhelming infection, should be treated with systemic antifungals, and topical and systemic treatment may also be combined. Systemic infection or deep-seated infection may require prolonged treatment and carries a poor prognosis. Implement contamination is often implicated in repeat infections; sanitization of feeding implements (such as feeding tubes) should occur on a daily basis.

From references 2, 5, 20, and 47.
IT, Intratracheally; *IV*, intravenously; *PCR*, polymerase chain reaction; *PO*, orally.

TABLE 21-5

Select Parasitic Diseases of Psittaciformes

Parasitic Disease	Etiology	Epizootiology	Clinical Signs	Diagnosis	Management
Miasis, bots fly strike	*Philornis* spp. Calliphoridae Diptera: Muscidae	While population limiting in some free-living South American parrot populations, these parasites are not common in North American zoo collections. In nature, the egg is deposited on the skin of the nestling, pupates subcutaneously, and emerges prior to fledging. Causes nestling morbidity and mortality.	Subcutaneous swellings, local infection, inflammation, nestling debilitation.	Clinical signs and physical extraction of larvae. Speciation requires the fly to pupate to adulthood.	Maggots may be mechanically removed if causing morbidity and the site cleaned and disinfected. Use of chemical pesticides in free-living parrots' nests is not recommended.
Scaly leg mites	*Knemidokoptes* spp. *Cnemidokoptes pilae* in budgerigars	Common in budgerigars, rare in other parrots. Immunocompetent individuals are not often affected. Mite's entire life cycle is on the host. Other birds become infected via prolonged direct contact with infested birds or surroundings.	Brittle flaky, powdery, white, porous, proliferative encrustations near the bill, cere, and occasionally the periorbital area, legs, or vent.	Presumptive diagnosis is based on clinical signs, and resolution with treatment is acceptable; but confirmation with skin scrape and microscopic examination may be necessary.	Administer antiparasitics (ivermectin is most commonly used) orally or parenterally at recommended doses for at least 3 treatments. Topical treatment is not recommended. No known zoonotic potential, but mites are likely class specific rather than host specific. Apparent resistant or recurrent infestation may alert the veterinarian to underlying disease and or immunosuppression.
Sarcocystosis	*Sarcocystis* spp. *S. falcatula* is commonly implicated, but many other species exist	Birds are the intermediate host in the two-host life cycle. Opossums are the definitive host for *S. falcatula*, and shed fecal oocysts. *Sarcocystis* spp. are also carried by other wildlife and domestic predator species. Cockroaches and flies may transport fecal oocysts. Old world Psittaciformes species are susceptible to the acutely fatal form of sarcocystosis; however, New World birds may also be affected by the tissue cyst and neurological forms.	The organism may encyst in or otherwise cause damage to the lungs, muscles, central nervous system, or heart. Death without premonitory signs is the common presentation because of pneumonitis. However, birds may show dyspnea, lethargy, weakness, and ataxia.	Multiple forms of disease occur, making diagnosis challenging. Grossly encysted parasites may resemble "rice breast disease" caused by *S. rileyii* or streaks mimicking white muscle disease. Cardiac enlargement and reddened lungs are also common findings. PCR and histopathologic diagnosis at necropsy is most common. Microscopic examination will reveal banana-shaped merozoites grouped within spherical to spindle-shaped cysts. Increased AST and CPK activity caused by tissue damage may occur.	Humans are affected on rare occasion by sarcocystosis, which occurs via ingestion of poorly cooked meat. Parrots should not be eaten. Parrot areas should be kept clean and free of wildlife intermediate hosts, their feces, or transport hosts. Supportive care, anti-inflammatories, and antiprotozoal drugs should be used. Relapse and nonresponse to treatment are common.

From references 1 and 40.
AST, Aspartate aminotransferase; *CPK*, creatine phosphokinase; *PCR*, polymerase chain reaction.

Diseases associated with advanced age such as cataracts, degenerative arthritis, neoplasia, atherosclerosis, and obesity are common in parrots.[36]

Toxicities of major concern for parrots include lead, zinc, nicotine, PTFE (polytetrafluoroethylene, i.e., teflon, more specifically the fluorocarbon gas it releases when overheated), and plant-based toxicities such as avocado toxicity, chocolate toxicity, and aflatoxicosis. Excellent reviews are available for the diagnosis and treatment of parrot intoxication.[34] The natural grinding ability of the parrot's GI tract, an innate curiosity about and attraction to shiny objects, and the formidable ability to dismantle and ingest very hard objects with the bill make these species particularly prone to heavy metal toxicity. Tests for lead and zinc may be performed from a single sample of approximately 0.5 milliliters (mL) of whole blood placed in a green-top, lithium heparin, microtainer (plastic stoppered) tube. Radiography may or may not be useful in diagnosis, as birds may have high blood burdens of metal without evidence of metallic objects remaining in the GI tract. Supportive care is extremely important in these cases, as toxins often affect GI tract motility, which results in weight loss, anorexia, and extreme dehydration. Specific chelation should be considered for cases of heavy metal toxicity. However, chelation is not without risk and may cause renal insult and lowering of other cations necessary for body function; definitive diagnosis of heavy metal toxicity is advised prior to administration of prolonged chelation.

REPRODUCTION

Most parrot species nest in natural cavities found in palms and other trees and in cliffs. Some species excavate cavities in sand walls, termitaries, or the ground.[12] The monk parakeet, *Myopsita monachus*, is the only species that constructs a nest using plant materials. Eggs are white and usually are laid every second day. Clutch size usually ranges from one to five, with some of the smaller species having as many as eight eggs. In Psittacoidea, incubation usually starts with the first egg, and hatch occurs asynchronously, whereas in Cacatuoidea, incubation is usually delayed until the penultimate egg is laid. Incubation time ranges from 14 days in some *Forpus* spp. to 33 days in the palm cockatoo (*Probosciger aterrimus*). The altricial chicks hatch with no or sparse down, with the eyes closed. Parrots grow slowly in comparison with other altricial species of similar size, and chicks stay in the nest between 1 (budgerigar, *Melopsittacus undulatus*) to 3½ months (kakapo). Chicks are fed by regurgitation for up to several months after fledging by the female or both parents. Large species typically may take 4 or 5 years to attain sexual maturation, whereas small species attain sexual maturity in 1 to 2 years. Most species are monogamous and, at least in the larger species, pair for life. However, parrots are quite social and often flock during the nonbreeding season. Reproductive details of common parrot species held in North American zoos are compiled in Table 21-1.

With most Psittaciformes species, the best results are obtained by keeping them in monogamous pairs year round; however, some breeders find it beneficial to flock the birds in big aviaries after the breeding season to recreate their natural social dynamics. Infertility is a common cause of breeding failure in captive Psittaciformes species. Besides different physiologic reasons, infertility may stem from pair incompatibility, which may be alleviated by providing parrots the opportunity to choose their mates. This may be achieved by holding several birds of both sexes in a large aviary and removing pairs to breeding cages as they show signs of bonding.

In the case of pairs that fail to incubate their eggs or that have the habit of breaking them, artificial incubation and use of a foster pair of the same or similar species are options. Artificial incubation parameters for most parrots are 37.2° C to 37.5° C. Relative humidity (RH) should be adjusted to achieve the desired weight loss by the end of the incubation period of 14% to 18% of the laying weight (usually 45% to 55% RH). Better results are often obtained when the eggs are naturally incubated for the first third of the incubation period. Most parrots will lay a replacement clutch if the first is removed completely. "Double clutching" is often used by breeders to maximize production. Eggs are collected from the nest and pooled for artificial incubation followed by hand rearing of the chicks. Although parrots may produce a replacement clutch several times, double clutching should be used cautiously, as overuse may risk hypocalcemia in the female. When possible, the last clutch should be left to be incubated, hatched, and fed by the parents so that they experience successful reproduction. Artificially incubated eggs may also be returned to the pair for hatching if the pair had been left to incubate dummy eggs.

Hand rearing is a common practice for the propagation of Psittaciformes, both for the pet market and for conservation aviculture. Hand feeding of home-made diets for Psittaciformes has largely been replaced by commercially available products. However, nutritional evaluation of these products for hand rearing has revealed a wide range of physical and nutritional characteristics, including dietary insufficiencies and excesses.[61] Because the most critical part of the hand rearing process is the first week of the chick's life, allowing parental feeding of chicks during this period increases the chances of survival during hand feeding. Birds propagated for breeding programs, particularly if hand reared, will benefit if flocked as subadults to allow proper socialization and acquisition of natural skills. For reproductive parameters, suggested breeding aviary dimensions, and nest box sizes of common species in North American zoos, see Table 21-1.

PREVENTIVE MEDICINE

Pathogens of most concern in parrots undergoing quarantine are *Chlamydia*, psittacid herpesvirus, avian bornavirus, polyoma virus, and psittacine beak and feather disease virus. Additional routine tests recommended in these species include a complete blood cell count (CBC), which is an excellent indicator of often occult inflammation, and a plasma biochemical panel, which should include uric acid and bile acids. Parasitologic testing should include fecal examination via both fecal flotation and wet mount or direct smear. Birds with outdoor access may have significant endoparasitic burdens despite low egg counts or lack of parasitic ova in feces. Therefore, prophylactic anthelmintics, administered at dosages below reported toxicities in other species, is indicated. A yearly recommended health maintenance examination, which may include grooming of beak and nails and full physical examination, should also include a CBC, plasma chemistry panel, and fecal testing for parasites. In parrots without signs of GI or upper respiratory illness, a choanal or cloacal culture or Gram staining of this flora is unlikely to be diagnostically rewarding. However, in parrots that are routinely used in educational venues or are exposed to immunocompromised persons, especially children, assessment for zoonotic bacterial pathogens such as *Salmonella* spp. is highly recommended. Routine vaccination is not recommended for most parrot species. Polyoma vaccination may be considered in birds that are considered for breeding or are exposed to a large collection and to outdoor birds. WNV generally causes little disease in most parrot species, and vaccination may not provide protection.[17]

ACKNOWLEDGMENTS

We thank the Schubot Exotic Bird Health Center for their support of this work and Dr. Tom Tully for his manuscript review.

REFERENCES

1. Allgayer MC, Guedes NMR, Chiminazzo C, et al: Clinical pathology and parasitologic evaluation of free-living nestlings of the hyacinth macaw (*Anodorhynchus hyacinthinus*). *J Wildl Dis* 45:972–981, 2009.
2. Altman R, Clubb S, Dorrestein GM, et al: *Avian medicine and surgery*, St. Louis, MO, 1997, Saunders.
3. Brightsmith DJ, McDonald D, Matsafuji D, et al: Nutritional content of the diets of free-living scarlet macaw chicks in southeastern Peru. *J Avian Med Surg* 24:9–23, 2010.

4. Brightsmith DJ: Nutritional levels of diets fed to captive Amazon parrots: Does mixing seed, produce, and pellets provide a healthy diet? *J Avian Med Surg* 26:149–160, 2012.

5. Brilhante RS, Castelo-Branco DS, Soares GD, et al: Characterization of the gastrointestinal yeast microbiota of cockatiels (*Nymphicus hollandicus*): A potential hazard to human health. *J Med Microbiol* 59:718–723, 2010.

6. Briscoe JA, Morris DO, Rosenthal KL, et al: Evaluation of mucosal and seborrheic sites for staphylococci in two populations of captive psittacines. *J Am Vet Med Assoc* 234:901–905, 2009.

7. Brouwer K, Jones ML, King CE, et al: Longevity records for Psittaciformes in captivity. *Int Zoo Yb* 37:299–316, 2000.

8. Brue RN: Nutrition. In Ritchie B, Harrison GJ, Harrison LR, editors: *Avian medicine: Principles and application*, Lake Worth, FL, 1994, Wingers Publishing, pp 63–95.

9. Bush JM, Speer B, Opitz N: Disease transmission from companion parrots to dogs and cats: What is the real risk? *Vet Clin North Am Small Anim Pract* 41:1261–1272, 2011.

10. Carciofi AC, Saad CEDP: Nutrition and nutritional problems in wild animals. In Fowler M, editor: *Biology, medicine, and surgery of South American wild animals*, Ames, Iowa USA, 2001, Iowa State University Press, pp 425–436.

11. Carciofi AC, Sanfilippo LF, De-Oliveira LD, et al: Protein requirements for blue-fronted Amazon (*Amazona aestiva*) growth. *J Anim Physiol Anim Nutr* 92:363–368, 2008.

12. Collar N: Family Psittacidae. In Hoyo J, Elliott A, Sargatal J, editors: *Handbook of the birds of the world*, Barcelona, Spain, 1997, Lynx Edicions, pp 280–479.

13. Cornejo J, Clubb S: Analysis of the maintenance diet offered to lories and lorikeets (Psittaciformes; Loriinae) at Loro Parque Fundación, Tenerife. *Int Zoo YB* 39:85–98, 2005.

14. Cornejo J, Dierenfeld ES, Bailey CA, et al: Predicted metabolizable energy density and amino acid profile of the crop contents of free-living scarlet macaw chicks (*Ara macao*). *J Anim Physiol Anim Nutr (Berl)* 96:947–954, 2012.

15. Dunning J: *CRC handbook of avian body masses*, Boca Raton, FL, 1993, CRC Press.

16. Earle KE, Clarke NR: The nutrition of the budgerigar (*Melopsittacus undulatus*). *J Nutr* 121:S186–S192, 1991.

17. Glavis J, Larsen RS, Lamberski N, et al: Evaluation of antibody response to vaccination against West Nile virus in thick billed parrots (*Rhynchopsitta pachyrhyncha*). *J Zoo Wildl Med* 42:495–498, 2011.

18. Gomez G, Saggese MD, Weeks BR, et al: Granulomatous encephalomyelitis and intestinal ganglionitis in a spectacled Amazon parrot (*Amazona albifrons*) infected with *Mycobacterium genavense*. *J Comp Pathol* 144:219–222, 2011.

19. Gunkel C, Lafortune M: Current techniques in avian anesthesia. *Semin Avian Exot Pet Med* 14:263–276, 2005.

20. Hannafusa Y, Bradley A, Tomaszewski EE, et al: Growth and metabolic characterization of *Macrorhabdus ornithogaster*. *J Vet Diagn Invest* 19:256–265, 2007.

21. Harper EJ, Skinner ND: Clinical nutrition of small psittacines and passerines. *Semin Avian Exot Pet Med* 7:116–127, 1998.

22. Harper EJ: Estimating the energy needs of pet birds. *J Avian Med Surg* 14:95–102, 2000.

23. Harrison GL, McDonald D: Nutritional considerations. In Harrison GL, Lightfoot TL, editors: *Clinical avian medicine*, vol I, Palm Beach, FL, 2006, Spix Publishing, pp 108–140.

24. Hess L, Mauldin G, Rosenthal K: Estimated nutrient content of diets commonly fed to pet birds. *Vet Rec* 150:399–404, 2002.

25. International Union for Conservation of Nature: *Red list of threatened species*, Cambridge, UK, 2012, IUCN.

26. Joseph L, Toon A, Schirtzinger EE, et al: A revised nomenclature and classification for family-group taxa of parrots (Psittaciformes). *Zootaxa* 3205:26–40, 2012.

27. Juniper T, Parr M: *Parrots: A guide to parrots of the world*, Yale University Press, New Haven CT, 2003, Christopher Helm Publishers, Incorporated.

28. Kamphues J, Otte W, Wolf P: *Effects of increasing protein intake on various parameters of nitrogen metabolism in grey parrots (Psittacus erithacus*

erithacus), First International Symposium Pet Bird Nutrition, Hannover, Germany, 1997, pp 118, Oct 3–4.

29. Klasing KC: *Comparative avian nutrition*, New York, 1998, CAB International.

30. Koutsos EA, Klasing KC: Vitamin A nutrition of growing cockatiel chicks (*Nymphicus hollandicus*). *J Anim Physiol Anim Nutr* 89:379–387, 2005.

31. Koutsos EA, Matson KD, Klasing KC: Nutrition of birds in the order Psittaciformes: A review. *J Avian Med Surg* 15:257–275, 2001.

32. Koutsos EA, Smith J, Woods LW, et al: Adult cockatiels (*Nymphicus hollandicus*) metabolically adapt to high protein diets. *J Nutr* 131:2014–2020, 2001.

33. Koutsos EA, Tell LA, Woods LW, et al: Adult cockatiels (*Nymphicus hollandicus*) at maintenance are more sensitive to diets containing excess vitamin A than to vitamin A–deficient diets. *J Nutr* 133:1898–1902, 2003.

34. LaBonde J: Toxicity in pet avian patients. *Semin Avian Exot Pet Med* 4:23–31, 1995.

35. Ledwon A, Szeleszczuk P, Zwolska Z, et al: Experimental infection of budgerigars (*Melopsittacus undulatus*) with five Mycobacterium species. *Avian Pathol* 37:59–64, 2008.

36. Lightfoot T: Geriatric psittacine medicine. *Vet Clin North Am Exot Anim Pract* 13:27–49, 2010.

37. Mans C, Guzman DS, Lahner LL, et al: Sedation and physiologic response to manual restraint after intranasal administration of midazolam in Hispaniolan Amazon parrots (*Amazona ventralis*). *J Avian Med Surg* 26:130–139, 2012.

38. Mayr G: Parrot interrelationships—morphology and the new molecular phylogenies. *Emu* 110:348–357, 2010.

39. Nouri M, Gharagozlou M, Azarabad H: Lymphoid leucosis and coligranoluma in a budgerigar (*Melopsittacus undulatus*). *Int J Vet Res* 5:5–8, 2011.

40. Olah G, Vigo G, Ortiz L, et al: *Philornis* sp. bot fly larvae in free living scarlet macaw nestlings and a new technique for their extraction. *Vet Parasitol* 196:245–249, 2013.

41. Orosz S, Ensley P, Haynes C: *Avian surgical anatomy: Thoracic and pelvic limbs*, Philadelphia, PA, 1992, Saunders.

42. O'Toole D, Mills K, Ellis R, et al: Clostridial enteritis in red lories (*Eos bornea*). *J Vet Diagn Invest* 5:111–113, 1993.

43. Petzinger C, Heatley JJ, Cornejo J, et al: Dietary modification of omega-3 fatty acids for birds with atherosclerosis. *J Am Vet Med Assoc* 236:523–528, 2010.

44. Pryor GS, Levey DJ, Dierenfeld ES: Protein requirements of a specialized frugivore, Pesquet's parrot (*Psittrichas fulgidus*). *Auk* 118:1080–1088, 2001.

45. Pryor GS: Protein requirements of three species of parrots with distinct dietary specializations. *Zoo Biol* 22:163–177, 2003.

46. Radlinsky MG, Carpenter JW, Mison MB, et al: Colonic entrapment after cloacopexy in two psittacine birds. *J Avian Med Surg* 18:175–182, 2004.

47. Ratzlaff K, Papich MG, Flammer K: Plasma concentrations of fluconazole after a single oral dose and administration in drinking water in cockatiels (*Nymphicus hollandicus*). *J Avian Med Surg* 25:23–31, 2011.

48. Ritchie B, Harrison G, Harrison L: *Avian medicine: Principles and applications*, Lake Worth, FL, 1994, Wingers Publishing Inc.

49. Ritchie B: *Avian viruses: Function and control*, Lake Worth, Florida, 1995, Wingers Publishing Inc.

50. Roudybush TE, Grau CR: Food and water interrelations and the protein requirement for growth of an altricial bird, the cockatiel (*Nymphicus hollandicus*). *J Nutr* 116:552–559, 1986.

51. Schmidt V, Schneider S, Schlomer J, et al: Transmission of tuberculosis between men and pet birds: A case report. *Avian Pathol* 37:589–592, 2008.

52. Shitaye EJ, Grymova V, Grym M, et al: *Mycobacterium avium* subsp. *hominissuis* infection in a pet parrot. *Emerg Infect Dis* 15:617–619, 2009.

53. Smith GA: Systematics of parrots. *Ibis* 117:18–68, 1975.

54. Ullrey DE, Allen ME, Baer DJ: Formulated diets versus seed mixtures for psittacines. *J Nutr* 121:S193–S205, 1991.

55. Waite DW, Deines P, Taylor MW: Gut microbiome of the critically endangered New Zealand parrot, the kakapo (*Strigops habroptilus*). *PLoS ONE* 7:e35803, 2012.

56. Werquin GJ, De Cock KJ, Ghysels PG: Comparison of the nutrient analysis and caloric density of 30 commercial seed mixtures (in toto and dehulled) with 27 commercial diets for parrots. *J Anim Physiol Anim Nutr (Berl)* 89:215–221, 2005.

57. Westfahl C, Wolf P, Kamphues J: Estimation of protein requirement for maintenance in adult parrots (*Amazona* spp.) by determining inevitable N losses in excreta. *J Anim Physiol Anim Nutr (Berl)* 92:384–389, 2008.

58. Westfahl CP, Wolf P, Kamphues J: Estimation of inevitable macro mineral losses in amazons (*Amazona* spp.) as basis for the calculation of maintenance requirement. *Arch Anim Nutr* 63:75–85, 2009.

59. White NE, Phillips MJ, Gilbert MT, et al: The evolutionary history of cockatoos (Aves: Psittaciformes: Cacatuidae). *Mol Phylogenet Evol* 59:615–622, 2011.

60. Wolf P, Habich AC, Burkle M, et al: Basic data on food intake, nutrient digestibility and energy requirements of lorikeets. *J Anim Physiol Anim Nutr (Berl)* 91:282–288, 2007.

61. Wolf P, Kamphues J: Hand rearing of pet birds—feeds, techniques and recommendations. *J Anim Physiol Anim Nutr (Berl)* 87:122–128, 2003.

62. Xenoulis PG, Gray PL, Brightsmith D, et al: Molecular characterization of the cloacal microbiota of wild and captive parrots. *Vet Microbiol* 146:320–325, 2010.

63. Young AM, Hobson EA, Lackey LB, Wright TF: Survival on the ark: Life-history trends in captive parrots. *Anim Conservat* 15:28–43, 2012.

CHAPTER 22

Cuculiformes (Cuckoos, Roadrunners)

Douglas P. Whiteside

GENERAL BIOLOGY

The order Cuculiformes comprises small- to medium-sized birds, with a worldwide distribution in forests and woodlands of temperate, subtropical, and tropical climates. Most are arboreal, although some are ground dwelling. They range in length from 16 to 70 centimeters (cm) and in weight from 17 grams (g) (little bronze cuckoo, *Chrysococcyx minutillus*) to 770 g (buff-headed coucal, *Centropus milo*).[31] Globally, most Cuculiformes populations are stable; however, 18 species are classified as vulnerable, near threatened, or endangered by the International Union on the Conservation of Nature (IUCN).[19]

Historically, this order used to include three families: (1) the Cuculidae, (2) the Musophagidae (turacos, plantain eaters, and go-away birds), and (3) the Opisthocomidae (hoatzin); however, most taxonomists have elevated the last two families to separate orders. The Cuculidae family is currently divided into five subfamilies comprising 32 genera; the brood parasitic cuckoos and malkohas (Cuculinae, 88 species), the couas and Old World ground cuckoos (Couinae, 13 species), the coucals (Centropodinae, 26 species), the anis and Guira cuckoos (Crotophaginae, 4 species), and the New World ground cuckoos (Neomorphinae, 10 species).[13,31]

Although most cuckoos are diurnal, they are often highly secretive, with many species vocalizing only at night. Their vocalizations are species specific and are often used to identify cryptic species. Sexual dimorphism occurs in some species, with females being larger than males in 71% of the species with parenteral care, while males are larger in 84% of the brood parasitic species. Almost all parenteral species (95%) are monomorphic, on the basis of their plumage, whereas 41% of the Old World brood parasitic species and malkohas are dimorphic.[25,31] In monomorphic species, gender determination may be accomplished through deoxyribonucleic acid (DNA) analysis of whole blood or blood feathers or via laparascopy.[34]

UNIQUE ANATOMY

Zygodactyly is one of the most distinctive features of cuckoos. The body forms of the Cuculidae vary, depending on their lifestyle, with arboreal cuckoos having long tails and slender bodies and terrestrial cuckoos being heavy bodied and proportionately longer tarsi. Well-developed eyelash feathers are a characteristic feature of cuckoos. The bill has no cere, is usually slender, and is slightly arched. The tarsi are often unfeathered and scutellate. The uropygial gland is prominent. Depending on the species, the wing has 10 primary and 9 to 13 secondary remiges, and usually 10 retrices exist, with only 8 in the anis and the Guira cuckoo. During molting of the wing feathers, the odd numbered primaries are shed and regrow first followed by the even numbered primaries, a pattern that is unique to cuckoos. The young of several cuckoo species may be distinguished by the unique pattern of white to yellowish-tan papillate patches in the oropharyngeal cavity.[7,31]

SPECIAL HOUSING REQUIREMENTS

The Cuculidae are not commonly found in zoologic collections, although globally several members of the cuckoo family are represented in institutions, including several species of cuckoo (Guira, fan-tailed, hawk, channel-billed, squirrel, and Renault's ground cuckoos), malkohas, yellow bill coul, coua, coucal, and roadrunners.[20]

Appropriate exhibits, coupled with suitable social groupings and opportunities to express species-appropriate behaviors, are important to maximize the physical and mental well-being of these birds. For arboreal species, large meshed exhibits with appropriate perching and plantings that allow for uninterrupted flight are most ideal, and terrestrial species may be housed in planted exhibits with natural substrates. Feather clipping may be performed to keep the birds in open exhibits. In general, cuckoos are not tolerant of cold environmental temperatures (less than 5° C or 40° F), so additional heat sources should be provided when the birds are housed outdoors in temperate climates. Some species of anis may adapt to cooler climates by lowering their body temperature at night (nocturnal torpor) and will demonstrate sunning behaviors to increase their body temperature.[1]

Most species of cuckoos are not housed in mixed species exhibits because of their aggressive nature, as they will prey on smaller birds or their eggs and offspring.[24,31] A few species are amenable to being housed with other birds; for example, roadrunners have been displayed successfully with burrowing owls. Intraspecific aggression may also be an issue, as most cuckoos are solitary in nature. A notable exception is the Guira cuckoo, which is a social species with communal nesting activities and postnatal group affiliations.[1,27,31]

FEEDING

Diets of Free-Ranging Birds

Free-ranging cuckoos are carnivorous, with most being insectivorous, preying on noxious insects such as caterpillars that are often avoided by other birds. They remove the indigestible and toxic leaf products within the intestines of the caterpillars by beating them or wiping them back and forth on branches or by passing them back and forth through their bills before ingesting them. The hairs on the caterpillars are indigestible as well and form a mat within the ventriculus, and the mat is later egested as a pellet. Other prey items, depending on the cuckoo species, include locusts, grasshoppers, millipedes, centipedes, spiders, phalangids, terrestrial snails, tree frogs, lizards, snakes, and mice. Brood parasitic species often take eggs from the nest of their host, whereas coucals and roadrunners consume nestling birds. The diet of a few of the Old World species such as cous, some malkohas and coucals, channel-billed cuckoo, dwarf koel, and common koel consists mainly of fruits (figs, tamarinds, berries, and palm oil fruits) with occasional insects. During the breeding season, roadrunners feed predominately on snakes and lizards, often beating their prey repeatedly against a rock.[1,31,36]

Diets of Captive Birds

Diets in captivity should approximate the feeding ecology of the species. Depending on the species, captive cuckoos may be fed a variety of insects, earthworms, small vertebrate prey items (e.g., juvenile mice, amphibians, anoles) and nutritionally balanced, commercially prepared avian and insectivore semi-moist pelleted diets. For omnivorous species such as Guira cuckoos, chopped mixed fruits and vegetables may be added. Invertebrate prey items should be dusted with calcium powder, and particularly for growing chicks, it is important to ensure they have access to dietary sources of vitamin D and exposure to natural or artificial ultraviolet B (UVB) light to prevent metabolic bone disease. Roadrunners do well on a mixture of vertebrate and invertebrate food items combined with commercial diets. Whole-prey items should be of appropriate size, if chicks are present, to prevent choking hazards. Some species of strictly insectivorous cuckoos such as the Diederik cuckoo (*Chrysococcyx caprius*), the emerald cuckoo (*Chrysococcyx cupreus cupreus*), the shining bronze cuckoo (*Chalcites lucidus lucidus*), and the great spotted cuckoo (*Clamator glandarius*) are difficult to maintain in captivity, as they will only eat live food items.[1,31]

RESTRAINT AND HANDLING

Care should be taken when handling and restraining cuckoos, especially the smaller species, to prevent injury to the bird. Physical restraint and anesthetic techniques are similar to those used for other similar-sized avian species. Induction and maintenance with gaseous anesthetics (isoflurane or sevoflurane) in oxygen at appropriate flow rates is most commonly used for anesthesia. Intubation is

straightforward. During recovery from anesthesia, birds should be confined in a quiet holding cage, until they are capable of standing, to prevent injury.

SURGERY (COMMON AND SPECIAL CONSIDERATIONS)

Surgical management of traumatic injuries, either self-induced or from intraspecies or interspecies aggression, is the most frequent surgical problem encountered in a captive setting. Techniques used in other avian species are applicable.

Multimodal analgesia is an important component of surgical management. Pharmacokinetic and clinical efficacy studies of analgesics have not been published for Cuculiformes, so data are extrapolated from studies on other avian species.

OTHER PHARMACEUTICALS

No published studies of pharmacokinetics or clinical efficacy exist for Cuculiformes species. Extrapolation for drug dosages is based on published studies and experience with other avian species.

PHYSICAL EXAMINATION AND DIAGNOSTICS

A systematic approach to the physical examination should always be followed. Cucidae species may be safely restrained for the examination, although anesthesia may be indicated for prolonged procedures or for stressed individuals.

Specimen collection and handling is analogous to other avian species. Venipuncture may be accomplished from the jugular vein, the medial metatarsal vein, or the ulnar vein. Interpretation of hematologic and serum biochemical values is similar to other avian species. Reference ranges for species held in captivity are available from the International Species Information System (www.isis.org).

DISEASE

General

Cuculiformes species are not exquisitely sensitive to infectious disease, and the few diseases reported are not unique to their taxon.

Infectious Disease

Infectious diseases are not commonly reported in Cuculiformes but include avian poxvirus affecting the feet and legs of Diederik cuckoos (*Chrysococcyx caprius*) and other cuckoos, aspergillosis, and candidiasis. *Chlamydophila* has been detected in the Guira cuckoo and the common cuckoo. Guira cuckoos may shed *Salmonella* spp. and *Yersinia pseudotuberculosis* asymptomatically in feces. Osteomyelitis has been noted in the tibiotarsus of a Renauld's ground cuckoo.[1,21,33,35]

Parasitic

Only a few parasites have been described in Cuculidae. This includes bloodborne parasites (*Haemoproteus* sp., *Plasmodium* sp., *Leucocytozoon centropi*), *Sarcocystis falcatula* and *S. corderoi*, *Isopora* sp., filarid nematodes (*Pelecitus*, *Struthiofilaria*, and *Cardiofilaria*), *Geopetitia*, *Dispharynx nasuta* in the smooth billed ani, ascarids (*Ascaridia cuculina*) in the common cuckoo (*Cuculus canorus*), and *Ascardia circularis* and *A. trilabium* in the greater coucal (*Centropus sinensis*).[2-6,10-12,14,15,23,32,37] A new species of nasal mite (*Sternostoma* sp.) was described in the common cuckoo.[8] A biting lice species (*Cuculicola latirostris*) has been found in the common cuckoo, and a chewing lice species (*Osborniella guiraensis*) has been described in a Guira cuckoo.[29] Myiasis has been associated with *Protocalliphora* sp.[26]

Noninfectious Disease

Trauma, either self-induced or from intraspecies or interspecies aggression, is the most common noninfectious disease of Cuculiformes in captivity. Pododermatitis from inappropriate perching or substrates may be encountered. Metabolic bone disease in growing chicks, egg binding, and poorly calcified eggshells have been documented in Guira cuckoos. Fatal foreign body ingestion has been reported in the greater roadrunner; one case involved ingestion of a cocklebur, and the second case was a juvenile that choked after ingesting a Texas horned lizard.[1,16,18]

Published reports of neoplasia in the cuckoo family are rare. Reported tumors include a cavernous hepatic hemangioma and an invasive squamous cell carcinoma of the rhamphotheca.[1,9]

TOXICITIES

Toxicities have not been described in Cuculiformes. If encountered, the pathogenesis and treatment would be extrapolated from the literature and from experience with other avian species.

REPRODUCTION

Although cuckoos are well recognized for their brood parasitic reproductive behavior, as a group, they have a wide diversity of breeding behaviors and parental care. In fact, approximately two thirds of cuckoo species, including couas, coucals, malkohas, roadrunners, and most of the American cuckoos build their own nest in trees, bushes, low shrubs, or the ground, depending on the ecology of the species. Only 56 Old World species and 3 New World species are obligate brood parasites. The majority of species are monogamous, but polyandry does exist in some species such as the African black coucal (*Centropus grilli*) and possibly in other coucals. Communal nesting occurs in the Guira cuckoo and the anis, although the female may remove other birds' eggs when laying its own.[17,22,30,31]

Nonparasitic cuckoos, like most other nonpasserines, lay white eggs, but many of the brood parasitic species lay colored eggs that closely resemble the eggs of their hosts. Other species lay dark "cryptic" eggs to hide them from host birds that lay their light eggs in dark, domed nests. The female cuckoo will often ingest or push the host's eggs from the nest to make space for its own eggs. In some cases, if the host rejects the cuckoo's egg, the cuckoo will completely destroy the host's clutch.[31]

Clutch size for the various species ranges from two to eight eggs. The incubation period is dependent on the species but, in general, ranges from 9 to 14 days. Young cuckoos are altricial. In the parasitic species, the cuckoo egg hatches earlier than the host's, and the cuckoo chick grows faster; in most cases, the chick evicts the eggs or young of the host species. Although on some occasions nonparasitic cuckoos parasitize other species, the parent still helps feed the chick. Parental infanticide of smaller chicks has been documented in Guira cuckoos.[28, 31]

PREVENTIVE MEDICINE

All birds should receive annual to biennial preventive health examinations that include complete physical examination, weight measurement, and assessment of blood parameters. Where indicated, radiography or other additional diagnostics may be indicated. Fecal examinations are indicated annually or more frequently if parasite issues are identified.

REFERENCES

1. Abou-Madi: Cuculiformes (cuckoos, roadrunners). In Fowler ME, Miller RE, editors: *Zoo and wild animal medicine*, 5th ed, St. Louis, MO, 2003, Saunders, pp 211–213.
2. Ashford RW: Blood parasites of Ethiopian birds. General survey. *J Wildl Dis* 12:409–426, 1976.
3. Atkinson CT: Haemoproteus. In Atkinson CT, Thomas NJ, Hunter DB, editors: *Parasitic diseases of wild birds*, Ames, IA, 2008, Wiley-Blackwell, pp 13–34.
4. Bartlett CM: Filarioid nematodes. In Atkinson CT, Thomas NJ, Hunter DB, editors: *Parasitic diseases of wild birds*, Ames, IA, 2008, Wiley-Blackwell, pp 439–462.
5. Bartmann A, Amato SB: Dispharynx nasuta (Nematoda: Acuariidae) em Güira Güira e Crotophaga ani (Cuculiformes: Cuculidae) no estado do Rio Grande do Sul, Brasil. *Cien Rural* 39:1152–1158, 2009.
6. Carreno RA: Dispharynx, Echinuria, and Streptocara. In Atkinson CT, Thomas NJ, Hunter DB, editors: *Parasitic diseases of wild birds*, Ames, IA, 2008, Wiley-Blackwell, pp 326–342.
7. Cook HL: What is your diagnosis? *J Avian Med Surg* 25(1):57–60, 2011.
8. Dimov I, Knee W: One new species of the genus Sternostoma (Mesostigmata: Rhinonyssidae) from *Cuculus canorus* (Cuculiformes: Cuculidae) from Leningrad Province, Russia. *J Acarol Soc Jpn* 21(2):141–146, 2012.
9. Effron M, Griner L, Benirschke K: Nature and rate of neoplasia found in captive wild mammals, birds, and reptiles at necropsy. *J Natl Cancer Inst* 59(1):185–198, 1977.
10. Fedynich AM: Heterakis and Ascaridia. In Atkinson CT, Thomas NJ, Hunter DB, editors: *Parasitic diseases of wild birds*, Ames, IA, 2008, Wiley-Blackwell, pp 388–412.
11. Forrester DJ, Greiner EC: Leucocytozoonosis. In Atkinson CT, Thomas NJ, Hunter DB, editors: *Parasitic diseases of wild birds*, Ames, IA, 2008, Wiley-Blackwell, pp 54–107.
12. Galindo P, Sousa O: Blood parasites of birds from Almirante, Panama with ecological notes on the hosts. *Rev Biol* 14(1):27–46, 1966.
13. Gill F, Donsker D, editors: *IOC World Bird Names* (v 3.2), 2012. www.worldbirdnames.org. Accessed November 27, 2012.
14. Greiner EC, Bennett GF, White EM, et al: Distribution of the avian hematozoa of North America. *Can J Zool* 53:1762–1787, 1975.
15. Greiner EC: Isospora, Atoxoplasma, and Sarcocytis. In Atkinson CT, Thomas NJ, Hunter DB, editors: *Parasitic diseases of wild birds*, Ames, IA, 2008, Wiley-Blackwell, pp 108–119.
16. Griner LA: Order Cuculiformes. In Griner LA, editor: *Pathology of zoo animals*, San Diego, CA, 1983, Zoological Society of San Diego.
17. Goymann W, Wittenzellner A, Wingfield JC: Competing females and caring males. Polyandry and sex-role reversal in African black coucals, *Centropus grillii*. *Ethology* 110(10):807–823, 2004.
18. Holte AE, Houck MA: Juvenile greater roadrunner (Cuculidae) killed by choking on a Texas horned lizard (Phrynososmatidae). *Southwest Nat* 45:74–76, 2000.
19. International Union for the Conservation of Nature: *IUCN Red List of Threatened Species*. Version 2012.2, 2012. www.iucnredlist.org. Accessed December 21, 2012.
20. International Species Inventory System: *ISIS Species holding*, www.isis.org. Accessed December 21, 2012.
21. Kaleta EF, Taday EMA: Avian host range of *Chamydophila* spp. based on isolation, antigen detection and serology. *Avian Pathol* 32(5):435–462, 2003.
22. Karubian J, Carrasco L, Cabrera D, et al: Nesting biology of the banded ground cuckoo (*Neomorphus radiolosus*). *Wilson J Ornith* 119(2):221–227, 2007.
23. Kinsella JM, Forrester DJ: Tetrameridosis. In Atkinson CT, Thomas NJ, Hunter DB, editors: *Parasitic diseases of wild birds*, Ames, IA, 2008, Wiley-Blackwell, pp 376–383.
24. Komar O, Thurber WA: Predation on birds by a cuckoo (Cuculidae), mockingbird (Mimidae) and saltator (Cardinalidae). *Wilson Bull* 115(2):205–208, 2003.
25. Krüger O, Davies NB, Sorenson MD: The evolution of sexual dimorphism in parasitic cuckoos: Sexual selection or coevolution? *Proc R Soc B* 274:1553–1560, 2007.
26. Little SE: Myiasis in wild birds. In Atkinson CT, Thomas NJ, Hunter DB, editors: *Parasitic diseases of wild birds*, Ames, IA, 2008, Wiley-Blackwell, pp 546–556.
27. Macedo RH: Reproductive patterns and social organization of the communal Guira cuckoo (*Guira guira*) in central Brazil. *Auk* 109(4):786–799, 1992.
28. Macedo RHF, Melo C: Confirmation of infanticide in the communally breeding Guira cuckoo. *Auk* 116(3):847–851, 1999.

29. Marrietto-Gonçalves GA, Martins TF, Filho RLA: Chewing lice (Insecta, Phthiraptera) parasitizing birds in Botucatu, SP, Brazil. *R bras Ci Vet* 19(3):206–212, 2012.
30. Ohmart RD: Observations on the breeding adaptations of the roadrunner. *Condor* 75:140–149, 1973.
31. Payne RB: *The Cuckoos*, Oxford, U.K., 2005, Oxford University Press.
32. Peirce MA, Adlard RD: The haemoproteids of the Cuculidae. *J Nat Hist* 39(25):2281–2287, 2005.
33. Rothschild BM, Panza RK: Epidemiologic assessment of trauma-independent skeletal pathology in non-passerine birds from museum collections. *Avian Pathol* 34(3):212–219, 2005.

34. Santamaria CA, Kelly S, Schulz GG, et al: Polymerase chain reaction-based sex identification in the greater roadrunner. *J Wildl Manag* 74(6):1395–1399, 2010.
35. Van Ruper C, Forrester DJ: Avian pox. In Thomas NJ, Hunter DB, Atkinson CT, editors: *Infectious diseases of wild birds*, Ames, IA, 2007, Blackwell Publishing, pp 131–176.
36. Whelchel AW, Lansford KC: California least tern chick predation by greater roadrunner. *Southwest Nat* 51(4):562–564, 2006.
37. Yabsley MJ: Eimeria. In Atkinson CT, Thomas NJ, Hunter DB, editors: *Parasitic diseases of wild birds*, Ames, IA, 2008, Wiley-Blackwell, pp 162–180.

CHAPTER 23

Strigiformes

Julia B. Ponder and Michelle M. Willette

BIOLOGY

The order Strigiformes comprises 220 to 225 extant species of owls divided into two families: Tytonidae (barn owls) and Strigidae (true owls). The two genera of barn owls, Tyto and Phodilus, represent less than 20 species. Most of the species living today are classified as Strigidae, which includes approximately 25 genera.[26] Although the question has not been completely resolved at this time, recent systematics have aligned owls more closely with nightjars than diurnal birds of prey. Using the Sibley-Ahlquist taxonomy, the most recent addendum to the American Ornithologists' Union combines Caprimulgiformes with Strigiformes (although they are discussed in separate chapters for the purposes of this book).[50]

With lineages extending back 70 to 80 million years, owls are one of the oldest groups of land birds.[26] Modern day extinctions of owls such as the laughing owl (*Sceloglaux albifacies*) of New Zealand and the Mauritius owl (*Mascarenotus sauzieri*) are thought to be the result of habitat alteration and persecution.[54] Habitat destruction is the greatest concern for many at-risk owl populations, including the Blakiston's fish owl (*Bubo blakistoni*), the northern spotted owl (*Strix occidentalis caurina*), and many tropical owl species. A new species, the Rinjani scops owl (*Otus jolandae*) in Indonesia, has recently been discovered.[46]

Owls are found worldwide with the exception of Antarctica and some very remote islands. Most owls are nocturnal, with some species demonstrating crepuscular behavior and a few species hunting during the day.

ANATOMY AND PHYSIOLOGY

Owls possess several unique anatomic and physiologic adaptations relative to other birds or even other raptors. The skull design optimizes two critical senses for owls—hearing and vision. In up to one third of all owl species worldwide, large ear openings are placed asymmetrically on each side of the head to facilitate vertical location of sound. The right opening points upward and the left downward. The asymmetrical placement is critical for species that are nocturnal hunters, those that reside north of 35 degrees latitude where heavy snow cover often prevents visualization of prey, or both.[31] Horizontal location of sound is assisted by a wide skull.

Another cranial adaption in owls is found in the large, forward-facing eyes, which provide 60 to 70 degrees of binocular vision and a high level of stereoscopic vision for judging distances. The eyes are tubular in shape and have relatively large corneas for gathering light. The retina is specialized for dim-light vision, possessing more rods than cones (up to 56,000 per millimeter square [mm^2] in the tawny owl, *Strix alluco*), and the rods contain high levels of rhodopsin, a light-absorbing pigment.[31] In many species, the retina also has a tapetum lucidum, a reflective layer that increases the amount of light each rod receives. Unlike some other bird species, owls cannot detect ultraviolet (UV) light. Owls are far sighted and use the tactile bristle feathers around their beaks to feel objects up close.

Owls have several unique anatomic differences in their gastrointestinal (GI) tracts relative to diurnal raptors. Unlike hawks, they do not possess a *crop* (dilation of the esophagus that stores food). Ingested food passes directly into the proventriculus, or glandular stomach. The pH of the ventriculus in owls averages 2.2 to 2.5 and does not provide sufficient acidity to break down fur, feathers, or bones. Through muscular contractions, the ventriculus forms a *pellet*, a compact bundle of indigestible foodstuffs, which is then cast at a meal-to-pellet interval of 10 to 13 hours.[11] Owls do possess *ceca*, paired secretory organs at the juncture of the ileum and the colon. Fermentation (especially of cellulose), water and calcium resorption, and microbial action of both beneficial and disease-causing organisms occur in the ceca.[33] Because of the blind-ended nature of these organs, food stuffs remain longer than in the rest of the GI tract, resulting in a product that is brown, homogeneous, and odiferous when excreted. Owls may eliminate their cecal contents in response to stress.

The foot of an owl is zygodactylous. When perched, digits 2 and 3 face anteriorly and digits 1 and 4 face posteriorly. Digit 4, however, is opposable and may assist in the restraint of prey by being placed in the forward position. The distal tibiotarsus is more rounded in owls compared with hawks, relating to the zygodactylous positioning of the digits. The tendons associated with the muscles of the tibiotarsus are calcified, providing increased strength to leg muscles, which are exposed to high stress forces.[58]

Determination of the age (aging) of owls on the basis of the molt pattern of flight feathers has been studied in a variety of North American owl species. The identification of multiple generations of feathers may be aided by using UV light to fluoresce porphyrin pigments. Distinct molting patterns may assist in the aging of many owl species up to age 3 or 4.[59]

Reverse dimorphism exists in many owl species. For example, size may often be used to sex snowy owls (*Bubo scandiaca*), northern saw-whet owls (*Aegolius acadicus*), boreal owls (*Aegolius funercus*), and great gray owls (*Strix nebulosa*), since less overlap exists in weight ranges between the sexes. In the northern saw-whet owl, wing chord measurements may also be used.[37] In the snowy owl, distinct plumage differences, such as the number of bars on the tail and the amount of spotting on the back of the head may also be used to determine sex.[47]

MANAGEMENT

Housing

It is critical to have a working knowledge of each owl species' natural history to understand their captive housing and management needs. The choice of caging material and design should ensure that feathering is not damaged as the bird moves around the enclosure. Wood and some plastics may be good choices, whereas metal caging (chain-link, metal mesh, etc.) may be extremely damaging to the feathers, feet, and ceres of raptors. Consideration should be given to the flooring substrate if the owl will spend any amount of time on the ground. Small gravel (average 5 mm diameter) is the preferred choice for substrate that comes in direct contact with the bird. Most enclosures work best with two to three solid sides, multiple, strategically placed perches, access to water for bathing and drinking, and at least one area in which the bird may hide from the elements or from being viewed by the public. Shelter boxes are recommended for cavity nesters.[2]

Multiple owls may be maintained in one enclosure, although it is safest to not mix species in one display. Within a species, multiple-bird housing may work very well, but if the enclosure is not large enough to allow for personal space, aggression may occur. Aggression may also be a problem with new introductions into an established exhibit; adequate monitoring should be ensured. As many owls kept in exhibits have disabilities, their additional needs should also be considered when housing multiple birds together.

Diet

Owl diets[2,3] are diverse and vary by species in relationship to size, habitat, and feeding behavior. Small rodents comprise the bulk of most diets, but owls are opportunistic and feed on insects, invertebrates, fish, amphibians, reptiles, birds, small mammals, and bats. Captive diets include mice, rats, day-old chicks, quail, fish, chicken, guinea pig, and rabbit. Wild or domestically raised pigeons should not be fed to owls because of the risk of trichomoniasis and a host of viral diseases. Feeding hunter-killed prey sources carries the risk of lead poisoning from spent lead ammunition. Dead wild rodents and birds should also not be fed to owls, as these prey items may be a source of poisoning or diseases such as West Nile virus (WNV) infection.

The food should be presented on a raised feeding area, which is easily accessed and protected from the elements and contamination from vermin. Most owl species should be fed once a day; smaller species may require twice-a-day feeding. Feeding is usually done late in the day. Exceptions include freezing temperatures and accommodating species that are more active during the day.

A wide variety of whole-prey items should be offered. Food should be wholesome, freshly killed, or properly frozen and thawed to prevent nutrient loss and to limit microbial load. The intestines of previously frozen mammals and poultry (except day-old chicks) should be removed, as these items are a potential source of

Clostridium. Intake should be monitored, and uneaten food should be promptly removed. Supplementation is not usually required if owls are fed good-quality whole food items. Exceptions are thiamine and vitamin E supplementation needed for diets high in fish content, breeding situations, and growing chicks.

A source of water for drinking and bathing should always be made available, except during freezing temperatures and in medical housing.

Hunting behavior may be used for behavioral enrichment in some species. Live crickets, mealworms, crayfish, frogs, and fish have been introduced into owl enclosures. A diet of live food may carry some risks, including parasites, injuries from the prey, and poor public reception.

Management of Feet, Feathers, Beaks, and Talons

Perches should be placed strategically to help the bird feel comfortable in the enclosure and provide enriching views. Since owls perch in areas where they feel safe and not necessarily on perches that are the best for the health of their feet, it is critical to provide them with several suitable perches. For most owl species, rounded or beveled perches work best. These may consist of dowels, beveled 2 × 4 inch (or 5 × 10 cm) wooden boards cut at species-specific angles or natural branches (oak is recommended) of varying diameter.[2] Generally, a rounded perch should not be so wide that the owl's foot is flattened when the bird perches. Also, if natural branches are used, they must be replaced every few months or sooner when the bark wears off, leaving a smooth surface. If an owl develops bumblefoot, perch locations, sizes, and substrates should be evaluated, focusing on those the owl uses most frequently. The location of the lesions on the feet may further assist in identifying the problem.

Feathers may be damaged by perches, enclosure walls, ceiling, and floors. Bent, tipped, or broken feathers are all signs of management problems and need to be addressed to stop further damage. For example, perches should be placed far enough from the wall so that when a bird turns around, it does not brush or rub its wing or tail feathers against the wall. Broken feathers may be repaired by a process called *imping*, in which a molted feather from the same species, sex, and feather position is used to replace the broken one. A short piece of whittled bamboo (or guitar string in small owls) is glued into the hollow shaft of the broken feather and used to secure the replacement feather.[2] To prevent breakage, bent feathers may be straightened either with a feather straightener or a small moist rag heated for 30 seconds in the microwave oven.

In captivity, the beaks and talons of owls need regular maintenance, as they grow throughout the year. In the wild, natural wearing and reshaping occur with exposure to varying weather conditions, larger bone sizes of prey, and a variety of uneven surfaces that owls rub (feak) their beaks on to clean and maintain the shape. The manual trimming and reshaping of beaks is called *coping* and is most often done with a rotary tool such as a Dremel rotary tool. When using the tool, care must be taken to ensure that the facial bristle feathers do not get caught by the rotating bit. If this happens, serious injury may result.

PREVENTIVE MEDICINE

Recommended preventive medical measures of owls include monitoring weight on a frequent basis; routine physical examinations; obtaining baseline hematology and chemistry values; baseline radiography; periodic fecal examinations; serology, as appropriate; plasma banking, as practical; vaccinations in species susceptible to WNV; and prophylactic medication in species susceptible to plasmodiasis and aspergillosis. Blood smears and the buffy coat should be evaluated for hemoparasites.

DIAGNOSTICS

As in all species, a thorough, systematic examination is the cornerstone diagnostic and should be conducted in a fashion similar to that in other birds. Appropriate restraint is required for handler and patient safety and to minimize patient stress. Traditional diagnostic tests such as hematology and blood chemistry, imaging, parasitology, bacteriology, cytology, and necropsy are all applicable to owls, although it may be difficult to find species' normal values to compare results. Often, only a single case report or the result from a closely related species is available for comparison. Establishing baseline values for hematology, chemistry, and radiology during routine physical examinations may provide important information to offset these challenges. Select hematology and chemistry results are listed in Table 23-1.

A significant portion of the recent diagnostic literature pertaining to owls is focused on the eye. Owl eyes are frequently traumatized because of their size and prominence, and significant numbers of owls are presented for rehabilitation at wildlife hospitals. The use of tonometry, B-mode ultrasonography, and electroretinography to examine owl eyes have all been reported.[29]

INFECTIOUS DISEASE

Owls are susceptible to a wide range of viral, bacterial, fungal, and parasitic diseases. The most commonly seen infectious diseases in owls are summarized in Table 23-2 and have been reviewed in the literature.[27,60] During the recent emergence of WNV in North America, Strigiformes species were found to be susceptible to natural infection.[13] Signs of WNV in owls are primarily neurologic, with owls not demonstrating the retinal lesions seen in hawks. Vaccination is recommended for owls in exhibits or those used for education, which are at risk of exposure. Killed, recombinant, and vectored equine vaccines have all been used safely; their efficacy is not known, but anecdotal evidence suggests some level of protection.

Many of the infectious diseases found in owls may be easily prevented in captivity. Vectorborne diseases such as WNV and malaria may be reduced through control of and protection from vectors. Risk of foodborne illnesses such as clostridiosis, salmonellosis, and trichomoniasis may be reduced through careful handling of food (freezing and thawing practices) as well as avoiding feeding inappropriate food items such as pigeon. Aspergillosis, a common infectious disease of captive birds, may often be prevented in susceptible birds. It is rare in owls overall, but susceptibility is associated with specific species (northern owls, especially snowy owls), immunosuppression, and massive spore exposure. It is also a common sequela to debilitating conditions such as starvation and toxicity. As the prevention of aspergillosis is much easier and more effective than treatment, it is recommended that any susceptible bird be put on prophylactic antifungal therapy.

Raptors are hosts to many intestinal parasites.[30] Although the parasites are not often pathogenic, the risk remains, especially in captivity and during periods of stress. Diagnosis is made on the basis of direct and flotation fecal examinations. Treatment is similar to that in other avian species.

Infectious Pododermatitis (Bumblefoot)

Bumblefoot is a common problem seen in captive raptors and is almost always associated with inadequate management techniques. Diagnosis is based on history, physical examination, culture and sensitivity of open wounds, and radiology to evaluate the extent of bone involvement. Treatment varies, depending on severity.[42] Bacteria may play an important role in the pathogenesis of the disease, but bacterial infection is usually secondary. Heavier-bodied species such as snowy owls are more susceptible to bumblefoot compared with other species.

Effective management is crucial to the prevention of bumblefoot. Providing species-appropriate perches (size, shape, and substrate) in enclosures and routinely monitoring the bird's feet is important, as is managing weight to prevent obesity. Early signs of bumblefoot such as flattening of the papilla on the plantar surface of the foot and reddening or thinning of the epithelium should lead to management changes and treatment of the foot through bandaging or

application of skin tougheners such as Tuf Foot or camphor and benzoin. The fundamental goal of treatment is protection of the foot and removal of weight-bearing from the affected tissue with the use of bandaging techniques such as ball bandages, "shoes," and interdigital bandages.[7]

NONINFECTIOUS DISEASE

Eye Trauma

The large prominent eyes of owls make them susceptible to trauma. A complete ophthalmic examination, including assessment of the fundus, should be performed as part of any physical examination. This is best performed in a darkened room, with the bird under manual restraint; the authors have found it advantageous to use the PanOptic ophthalmoscope in owls because of its increased magnification and field of view. Ultrasonography may aid in the evaluation of the posterior segment in cases of anterior segment opacity or vitreal hemorrhage.[29] In many species of owls, the posterior aspects of the globe may be visualized through the aural aperture (Figure 23-1). Because of this close association, eye trauma is often seen concurrently with aural trauma or blood in the ear opening. This access to the posterior segment also facilitates diagnostics, including vitreal aspiration for cytology and culture; instillation of therapeutic medication; and ocular surgery.

As head trauma may often accompany eye trauma, a thorough neurological examination should also be performed. Stoic or fractious behavior in many owl species or in individual birds may make vision or neurologic assessments challenging.

Anticoagulant Rodenticides

Owls are at significant risk for secondary poisoning from anticoagulant rodenticides. Clinical signs include pallor of mucous membranes and a marked anemia, particularly in the absence of any traumatic injury. In addition, the affected bird may be weak or quiet, blood clotting may be slow after venipuncture, or the bird may show extensive bruising. A normal thrombocyte estimate in the face of prolonged bleeding or clotting times may be indicative of exposure to anticoagulant rodenticides. *Prothrombin time (PT)*, a screening test for the extrinsic coagulation pathway, has been measured in various avian species, and a 25% increase above reference range PT is considered indicative of exposure to anticoagulant rodenticides.[49] As avian PT evaluation is complicated by a lack of standardized avian thromboplastin, *Russell's Viper Venom Time (RVVT)*, which shows less analytic variability, has been used to detect vitamin K deficiency in birds. A modified *whole blood clotting time* may also be performed as a screening test. Blood is collected into several uncoated capillary tubes and the tubes broken in half at 1-minute intervals until a clot forms. The normal clotting time in psittacine birds is less than 5 minutes.[35] Definitive diagnosis of anticoagulant rodenticide exposure requires identification of the compound in blood, tissues, or ingesta.

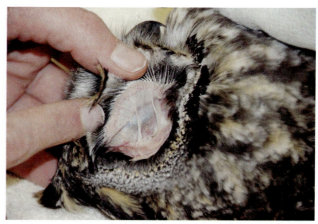

FIGURE 23-1 The right ear opening of a long-eared owl (*Asio otus*).

TABLE 23-1

Select Physiological Reference Intervals for Select Owl Species[25]

Tests	Units	Short-eared Owl (*Asio flammeus*)		Burrowing Owl (*Athene cunicularia*)	
		Mean	Reference Interval	Mean	Reference Interval
White Blood Cell Count	$*10^3$ cells/μL	8.62	0–17.16	7.44	2.20–16.49
Red Blood Cell Count	$*10^6$ cells/μL			2.44	*
Hemoglobin	g/dL				
Hematocrit	%	43.40	33.00–53.1	44.70	29.40–55.00
MCV	fL			179.00	*
MCH	pg				
MCHC	g/dL				
Heterophils	$*10^3$ cells/μL	3.67	0–8.74	4.00	0.97–10.92
Lymphocytes	$*10^3$ cells/μL	3.55	0.00–7.55	2.53	0.50–6.82
Monocytes	cells/μL	378.00	0–1286	278.00	0–1199
Eosinophils	cells/μL	663.00	0–2924	338.00	0–1704
Basophils	cells/μL	131.00	0.00–572	169.00	0.00–915
Glucose	mg/dL	299.00	212–395	321.00	209–450
Blood Urea Nitrogen	mg/dL				
Creatinine	mg/dL				
Uric Acid	mg/dL	9.10	0–16.70	8.60	1.80–25.90
Calcium	mg/dL	9.20	7.30–10.80	9.40	7.30–12.00
Phosphorus	mg/dL	4.70	*	3.90	1.30–9.10
Ca/Phos ratio				3.00	1.00–6.70
Sodium	mEq/L			153.00	135–169
Potassium	mEq/L			2.50	0.30–4.50
Na/K ratio				67.10	7.50–116.80
Chloride	mEq/L			118.00	107–128
Total Protein	g/dL	3.30	1.90–4.40	3.50	2.50–4.80
Albumin	g/dL	1.60	0.50–2.50	1.60	0.80–3.30
Globulin	g/dL	1.80	0.60–2.80	1.90	0.30–3.10
Alkaline Phosphatase	IU/L			55.00	0–106
Lactate Dehydrogenase	IU/L			367.00	0–1071
Aspartate Aminotransferase	IU/L	250.00	0–447	164.00	68–322
Alanine Aminotransferase	IU/L			120.00	12–215
Creatine Kinase	IU/L	446.00	0–1012	428.00	94–1235
Gamma-glutamyltransferase	IU/L				
Amylase	IU/L			731.00	211–1296
Total Bilirubin	mg/dL				
Cholesterol	mg/dL			250.00	99–378

*Sample size is insufficent to produce a valid reference interval.
From Teare, J.A. (ed.): 2013, "Select Owl Species _No_selection_by_gender_All_ages_combined_Conventional_American_Units_2013_CD.html" *in* ISIS Physiological Reference Intervals for Captive Wildlife: A CD-ROM Resource., International Species Information System, Bloomington, MN.

Eurasian Eagle Owl (*Bubo bubo*)		Verreaux's Eagle Owl (*Bubo lacteus*)		Snowy Owl (*Bubo scandiacus*)		Great Horned Owl (*Bubo virginianus*)	
Mean	Reference Interval	Mean	Reference Interval	Mean	Reference Interval	Mean	Reference Interval
12.77	3.76–30.69	14.00	0–26.53	9.78	3.06–26.11	13.08	4.14–27.71
				2.39	1.33–3.46	2.28	1.39–3.16
				11.10	4.5–17.4	13.40	8.02–18.30
39.60	29.10–47.80	36.50	26.10–46.70	43.00	28.10–54.10	41.30	32.60–51.20
				184.50	110.00–256.90	176.50	134.80–221.50
				42.50	10.40–68.40	58.80	37.30–81.30
				25.00	10.80–38.08	32.20	22.90–41.30
6.88	1.76–18.59	7.81	0–16.52	4.78	1.25–12.71	7.37	2.14–17.13
4.68	0.87–14.50	4.72	0–11.84	3.74	0.74–12.05	4.18	0.88–11.01
394.00	0–1952	328.00	0–899	271.00	0–1192	537.00	0–2215
595.00	0–3401	879.00	0–2857	226.00	0–1322	599.00	0–3174
147.00	0.00–770	99.00	0–420	83.00	0–511	196.00	0–1157
350.00	281–426	317.00	222–409	335.00	221–456	336.00	256–417
				7.00	1–12	6.00	0–11
				0.30	0–0.70	0.50	*
9.20	2.50–22.90	8.80	0–17.40	9.00	2.60–20.20	9.00	3.00–19.80
9.80	8.00–13.00	10.00	8.00–11.70	9.50	7.40–11.60	9.40	7.70–11.60
5.60	0.60–9.60	4.70	1.70–8.00	4.80	1.50–10.30	5.30	1.90–11.40
1.90	0.70–3.10	2.20	0.60–3.60	2.40	1.00–5.00	2.20	0.90–4.80
155.00	142–167	155.00	143–165	156.00	140–174	157.00	143–173
3.10	0.90–5.00	3.20	1.80–4.50	3.00	1.50–6.10	3.00	1.20–5.00
55.10	16.40–87.90	50.80	27.30–72.30	58.00	27.50–103.40	57.80	25.10–120.20
119.00	107–129	120.00	*	116.00	107–127	118.00	101–130
3.70	2.50–5.20	4.40	3.10–5.70	4.00	2.40–6.50	3.80	2.60–5.60
1.80	0.10–3.20	1.60	0.80–2.40	1.50	0.90–2.50	1.60	0.80–3.10
1.60	0–3.50	2.80	1.70–3.90	2.30	0.30–4.60	2.30	0.40–4.40
31.00	5–58			39.00	11–111	51.00	16–163
274.00	0–628			662.00	0–1812	490.00	0–1134
164.00	55–331	142.00	36–230	272.00	108–570	188.00	86–347
38.00	*			34.00	0–66	32.00	0–70
485.00	0–1080	298.00	0–596	584.00	140–1592	633.00	128–1688
						5.00	0–16
679.00	*			270.00	97–435	385.00	0–830
				0.20	0–0.40	0.20	0–0.60
191.00	105–280	218.00	89–330	237.00	143–364	184.00	112–298

TABLE 23-2

Select Infectious Diseases of Owls

Disease	Etiology	Clinical Signs	Diagnosis	Treatment[8,55]	Prevention[8,55]	Comments
West Nile virus infection[27,62]	West Nile virus (Flavivirus)	Anorexia, weight loss; depression, ataxia, seizures, sudden death; "bobble head"	Clinical signs; time of the year; splenomegaly (radiography); RT-PCR, HAI, IHC; necropsy findings	Meloxicam (0.5–1.0mg/kg PO q12–24h) or other anti-inflammatories; supportive care	Mosquito netting, eliminate mosquito breeding grounds, bring birds indoors, vaccination	Zoonosis
Hepatosplenitis[16,44]	Columbid herpesvirus 1	Usually acute death, depression	Necropsy findings; PCR	No effective treatment	Do not feed pigeons	
Mycobacteriosis[6,21,39,53]	Mycobacterium avium	Debilitation; weight loss; diarrhea; "punched-out" lesions in the bones (radiography)	CBC; acid-fast cytology; PCR; culture	Generally not undertaken; protocols available		Reported to be zoonotic
Clostridiosis[60]	Clostridium perfringens	Anorexia; diarrhea; enlarged intestinal loops (radiography)	Fecal cytology	Metronidazole (50 mg/kg, PO, q12h); if acute toxicity: empty stomach, activated charcoal	Do not feed food items that were not properly acquired, stored and thawed	
Salmonellosis[22,51,57]	Salmonella spp.	Dehydration; green urates; depression; elevated liver enzymes	Fecal culture	Supportive care	Do not feed food items that were not properly acquired, stored and thawed	Potential zoonosis
Aspergillosis[5]	Aspergillus spp.	Clinical signs referable to the respiratory tract; green mutes	History; clinical signs; CBC (leukocytosis, monocytosis, increased total solids); radiography; endoscopy with culture and cytology; PCR	Voriconazole (12.5 mg/kg, PO, q12h ×10T then q24h ×6T)	Prophylactic itraconazole (7 mg/kg, PO, q12h ×10T then q24h ×16T): susceptible species, changes in management, serious medical conditions	Northern owl species
Candidiasis[27]	Candida spp.	Anorexia, reluctance to swallow, "food flicking"; regurgitation; lesions oral cavity or esophagus	Culture of oropharynx or esophagus; cytology	Nystatin (100,000 Units/kg, TO, q12h ×6–14T)		
Malaria[60]	Plasmodium spp.	Anorexia; depression, lethargy; jade-green mutes; labored respirations; anemia	Visualization of parasite in blood smear	Mefloquine hydrochloride (30 mg/kg, PO, at times 0 hr/12 hr/24 hr/48 hr)	Mosquito netting, eliminate mosquito breeding grounds, bring birds indoors; prophylactic mefloquine for susceptible species (30 mg/kg, PO, q7d)	Northern owl species
Trichomoniasis[9,60]	Trichomonas gallinae	"Food flicking"; oral ulcers (mild), caseous lesions upper GIT (severe), invasion of the parasite into bone or soft tissue (very severe)	Wet mount cytology oral lesion; InPouch TF test	Carnidazole (20 mg/kg, PO, q24h for 2–5 times); metronidazole; surgical debridement of caseous plugs	Do not feed pigeons or wild caught passerine species	

CBC, Complete blood cell count; GIT, gastrointestinal tract; HAI, hemagglutination inhibition; hr, hour; IHC, immunohistochemistry; mg/kg, milligram per kilogram; PO, orally; RT-PCR, real-time polymerase chain reaction; TF, Tritrichomonas foetus

Treatment for rodenticide toxicity begins with the removal of any toxin remaining in the digestive tract and mitigating its effects with an activated charcoal lavage. Successful treatment of rodenticide-poisoned birds has been reported with the use of 2.5 milligrams per kilogram per day (mg/kg/day) of phytonadione (vitamin K_1), a dose extrapolated from small animal medicine.[35] Vitamin K_1 may be given orally or parenterally, and it is recommended that initial doses be given parenterally until the patient is stable. If the patient presents with a packed cell volume (PCV) of less than 20%, or if during treatment the PCV drops below 20%, the blood loss may be treated with a transfusion from a healthy, conspecific individual. To prevent additional blood loss, the intraosseous (ulna or tibiotarsus) mode of administration is recommended.

Hepatic Lipidosis

Hepatic lipidosis, a condition seen with increasing frequency in captive small owl species, has been diagnosed in several species of owls.[25] It results from an excessive accumulation of lipids within the hepatocytes. Etiologies include an improper diet with excessive fat or carbohydrates or lack of lipotrophic factors; fat mobilization caused by anorexia, the increased lipogenesis resulting from diabetes or egg-laying; or decreased fatty acid oxidation or secretion in the liver. Diagnosis is made on the basis of signalment, history, clinical signs, and supportive testing. Patient obesity, increased plasma aspartate aminotransferase (AST), cholesterol, and bile acids, and an enlarged liver on palpation or radiography are indicative of the condition. The diagnosis may be confirmed by liver aspiration or biopsy; however, caution should be exercised, as bleeding may occur if clotting proteins are lacking. It is worth noting that evaluation of the body condition score (BCS) is extremely subjective and should not be used as the sole criterion to determine obesity. The BCS should be evaluated in conjunction with weight, level of flight activity, and diet. The authors are aware of cases of hepatic lipidosis in owls with extremely poor BCS. Hepatic lipidosis carries a poor prognosis, and treatment requires supportive care with easily digestible alimentation. It may take weeks or months to resolve the condition.

Synovial Chondromatosis

As a broad range of neoplasms have been described in owl species, in both captive and free-ranging individuals, neoplastic disease should be considered a differential diagnosis when consistent with clinical signs.[14] In the authors' experience, the most commonly seen neoplasm in free-ranging owls is synovial chondromatosis in the great horned owls (*Bubo virginianus*), primarily affecting the scapulohumeral joints.[52] The condition is characterized by the formation of chondral or osteochondral nodules in the synovial tissue of joints, tendon sheaths, or bursae. The etiology of these lesions in raptors is unknown. Diagnosis is made on the basis of signalment, clinical signs, and radiographic signs. Affected joints are firm and enlarged with limited range of motion. Patients are often severely debilitated because of inability to hunt. Radiography indicates mineralized nodules surrounding single or multiple joints (Figure 23-2). No treatment is available for this disease.

RESTRAINT

Behavioral Restraint

Whether the captive owl is on display or presented on the handler's fist in educational programs, operant conditioning may increase the owl's comfort level and enrichment and also assist in management procedures.[15] Training may be used to facilitate medical procedures and for daily management processes. For example, owls may be trained to allow someone to lift up a foot to check the condition of the pad or to allow instillation of eye drops without physical restraint.

Owls that are imprinted on humans may be highly tractable when immature but may display territorial behaviors, including aggression, as adults. Behavioral training is difficult, but critical, because unintentional reinforcement of some behaviors in young imprinted birds

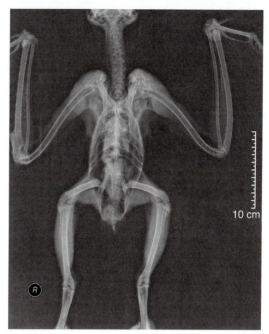

FIGURE 23-2 A radiograph of a great-horned owl (*Bubo virginianus*) with synovial chondromatosis. This owl, admitted in August 1999 with a right ulna fracture, was banded and released back into the wild in October 1999. It was readmitted in 2011 in poor body condition, with poor range of motion of both shoulders, and a fracture of the left radial carpal bone.

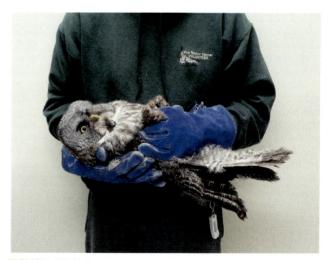

FIGURE 23-3 Proper restraint for safely carrying an owl (*Strix nebulosa*).

often leads to undesirable adult behaviors. Imprinted owls may also display unusual behaviors that may be unhealthy, for example, ingesting foreign materials and self-plucking or mutilation.

Manual Restraint

The main goals of proper handling are to ensure the safety of the owl, the handler, and any other participants in the procedure; to minimize stress; to maintain feather condition; and to provide proper positioning for procedures. Protective eyewear and gloves should always be used. Control of both legs of the owl is critical as its main defense is use of its powerful feet and sharp talons. Controlling the wings at all times is also important to prevent injury to the bird (Figure 23-3).

Common capture techniques used with captive owls include casting off a glove, body grab, leg grab, and use of a net for small species. Each technique is employed under appropriate circumstances and has both advantages and disadvantages. The most important factor is to have a well-thought out plan and have the proper personnel and equipment to implement the plan.

Anesthesia, Chemical Restraint, and Pain Management

Full anesthesia is most appropriately achieved through the use of gas anesthetics such as isoflurane, desflurane, or sevoflurane. Use of rompun, ketamine, or both is discouraged in owls because of species variability in response, especially in *Bubo* spp.[45] Response in *Strix* species is acceptable. Other injectables such as medetomidine or dexmedetomidine and midazolam have anecdotally been used successfully in owls; brief research on the use of propofol has been published.[20,32] Propofol may prove to be the most useful short-term anesthetic agent in situations where gaseous agents are not available. Current analgesic agents of choice include torbugesic (anesthetic-sparing and intraoperative or postoperative analgesia at 1 to 3 mg/kg; typically 0.3 mg/kg) and meloxicam (well tolerated at doses up to 1 mg/kg and four times in 24 hours [q24h]).

Monitoring of body temperature during anesthesia is important, especially in northern species of owls such as great gray owls (*Strix nebulosa*) and snowy owls (*Bubo scandiacus*), as they have a heavy coat of down insulation and tend to overheat quickly. Ice packs may be placed on the extremities to reduce body temperature, when necessary.

Readers are referred to other comprehensive guidelines on avian anesthesia, including intubation, ventilation, and anesthesia by air sac cannulation.[19,41]

SURGERY

Few surgical procedures or approaches are unique to owls. Unique adaptations of two procedures are discussed below.

As previously discussed, owl eyes are extremely large compared with those of other species and are frequently involved in trauma. In addition to trauma, owls may present with intraocular and post-orbital tumors, abscesses, or panophthalmitis. Occasionally, extensive pathology leaves enucleation as the only treatment option. Enucleation is used to decrease the likelihood of secondary complications or to make the owl more comfortable when the conditions mentioned above are present. The extensive aural opening in the owl has been used to modify the approach to enucleation of the eye and presents an option to the globe-collapsing procedure used in other avian species. An advantage of the transaural approach is that it allows for complete histological examination.[34] It is worth noting that enucleation results in significant disfigurement to the face and facial disk, likely impacting the owl's hearing, and may also affect the bird's balance for a short time. An alternative to enucleation is evisceration, a procedure in which the sclera and associated ossicles are left in the orbit. This procedure is contraindicated if infection or neoplasia is present, or if complete histologic examination is required.

Like many other raptors, owls are frequently seen for long-bone fractures. Repair of the tibiotarsus, which has unique anatomy in the owl and is often fractured secondary to tethering in captivity, is presented here as an example of surgical repair of a long bone. The most commonly used technique for repairing tibiotarsal fractures is the external skeletal fixator–intramedullary pin tie-in (ESF–IM tie-in), which has been described in the literature and has been used in avian orthopedics since 1995 (Figure 23-4).[38] The choice of intramedullary pin size in the tibiotarsus must take into consideration that the bone has a triangular shape proximally and flattens ventrodorsally as it nears the tarsometatarsal joint; the narrowest part of the bone may be evaluated most easily on a lateral radiographic view. In addition, placement of external fixator pins in the distal limb is assisted by knowledge of the location of the extensor canal, which

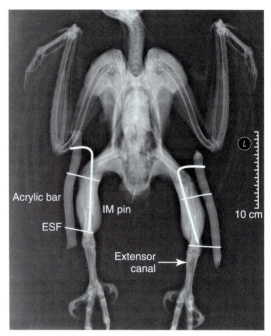

FIGURE 23-4 A radiograph of a great-horned owl (*Bubo virginianus*) with external skeletal fixator–intramedullary tie-in fixation on both tibiotarsi. The arrow is pointing to the extensor canal.

is on the metatarsus in an owl, rather than on the distal tibiotarsus as in diurnal raptors. Alignment of the fracture site is critical, as is reestablishing normal bone length. Failure to do so may result in uneven weight bearing over the long term and the development of bumblefoot in the contralateral foot. As uneven weight bearing is also a concern during the healing phase, it is recommended that a prophylactic bandage be applied to the contralateral foot during recuperation. The mean healing time for a tibiotarsal fracture in raptors is 31 days.[55] Dynamic destabilization of the fixation, with removal of the intramedullary pin after 10 to 14 days, is recommended to prevent the likelihood of damage to the stifle.

Coracoid fractures occur infrequently in owls and may be successfully managed through coaptation.[40] Treatment consists of application of a body wrap,[7] cage rest, and regular physical therapy for approximately 3 weeks. Bandaging of any type may present challenges in owls, as many species are known for their chewing tendencies. Often, close monitoring of some conditions without bandaging is more successful than frequent replacement of bandages. A layer of duct tape over a bandage (not directly on the feathers) may be required in owls.

THERAPEUTICS

Given the ever-increasing number of therapeutic medications available, as well as ongoing research, veterinarians are urged to consult a current formulary and review the current literature prior to initiating treatment with any drug. In general, drugs used in other raptor species are safe to use in owl species. An exception may be intravenous administration of enrofloxacin. Two great horned owls (*Bubo virginianus*) showed acute weakness, bradycardia, and peripheral vasoconstriction during intravenous injection of enrofloxacin. The same response was not seen in red-tailed hawks (*Buteo jamaicensis*).[18]

The authors currently do not use any topical, oral, or parenteral steroids in owls because of the risk of immunosuppression.[23] An exception is the use of methylprednisolone sodium succinate for the treatment of acute spinal cord injuries (30 mg/kg, intramuscularly [IM]; two treatments 12 hours apart).

REPRODUCTION

Most owls in the family Strigidae are monogamous; many pairs having strong pair-bonds that last over multiple seasons. Extra-pair copulations and polygamy are seen in strigids; polygamy is observed particularly during seasons of prey abundance.[43] Breeding in the tropics may occur in any month, whereas in other regions, it may be seasonal, depending on the weather, temperature, or breeding activity of the mammalian prey species. Two main kinds of nest sites are found in the family Tytonidae: (1) those in natural cavities, typically in trees; and (2) those in grassy areas, where nests may be contained safely in dense vegetation. Strigids use stick nests made by other birds, cliff ledges, cavities, and grassy sites, whereas the burrowing owl (*Athene cunicularia*) uniquely nests in burrows in the ground. Manmade structures such as churches, towers, barns, castles, abandoned cottages and warehouses, chimneys, and other structures that provide a cavity may also be used. Nest-type affinity varies among the species.

Clutch size is variable across the family Tytonidae, ranging from 1 to 2 eggs in the greater sooty owl (*Tyto tenebricosa*) to 2 to 14 eggs in the common barn owl (*Tyto alba*). Strigids' largest clutch contains nine eggs, with four to seven eggs on average. Average interval between egg laying in owls is 1 to 2 days and may be up to 4 days. Eggs that are hatched asynchronously result in chicks in the nest having significant differences in age. If food becomes scarce, the oldest remain well fed, whereas the youngest may starve. Most strigids only breed once per season, primarily because of the length of the breeding cycle. Incubation period may range in the family Tytonidae from 29 to 34 days in the common barn owl (*Tyto alba*) to 40 to 42 days in lesser sooty owl (*Tyto multipunctata*). In strigids, it ranges between 22 days (small species) and 32 days (larger species). The female incubates the eggs, as she possesses a brood patch, and the male brings food to the female while she tends the nest. The female is primarily responsible for protecting the chicks from predators. When the chicks hatch, she does not leave the nest unattended until the youngest chick is approximately 2 weeks old. The chicks huddle together to minimize heat loss. Fledge age may range from 42 to 90 days, depending on the species, and chicks are given food by parents long after fledging.[10]

The Association of Zoos and Aquariums (AZA) manages five species of owls in zoos or related institutions in a Species Survival Plan (SSP) or studbook program, which includes the burrowing owl (*Athene cunicularia*, SSP); the Eurasian eagle owl (*Bubo bubo*, SSP); the spectacled owl (*Pulsatrix perspicillata*, SSP); the snowy owl (*Bubo scandiacus*, studbook); and the Verreaux's eagle owl (*Bubo lacteus*).[4] This management attempts to maintain the genetic diversity of each of the species bred in captivity. Managed owls are used for education programs or for ex situ conservation, in an attempt to sustain captive populations. The Raptor Taxon Advisory Group (TAG) meets every 3 years, reviewing the owls that remain in zoos and recommending phase-outs to make space for managed species. Permanently injured owls from wildlife rehabilitation centers are also commonly displayed in zoos. Although these birds may not be bred in captivity, they are useful to increase public awareness of native owl species.

CONSERVATION MEDICINE

Like other birds of prey, owls are excellent biosentinels.[61] Owl species are widely distributed, territorial, and generally nonmigratory. North American migratory species include the short-eared owl (*Asio flammeus*), the long-eared owl (*Asio otus*), and the Northern saw-whet owl (*Aegolius acadicus*). Owls, in general, have a high reproductive rate and trophic status. As such, owls bioaccumulate many substances through their prey and have been shown to be sensitive to a wide variety of environmental contaminants, including pesticides, polychlorinated biphenyl (PCB), and heavy metals.[48]

Owls are at significant risk for poisoning from anticoagulant rodenticides. A recent paper analyzed the livers from 164 owls; 70% of the livers had residues from at least one rodenticide, 41% contained residues of more than one rodenticide.[1] Another paper estimated that "a minimum of 11% of the sampled great horned owl (*Bubo virginianus*) population is at risk of being directly killed by second-generation anticoagulant rodenticides."[56] The Environmental Protection Agency (EPA) recently banned numerous mouse and rat poison products to protect children, pets, and wildlife from accidental exposure.[12]

Owls may also serve as biosentinels for zoonotic diseases such as WNV infection that involve enzootic or sylvatic transmission cycles. Many owl species are susceptible to WNV infection,[17] and detection of WNV in raptor species may be used as an early warning system with regard to threat to human and equine health along with other techniques.[36] WNV infection in some owl species may have public health implications. For example, experimentally infected great horned owls developed a viremia sufficient to infect mosquitos, and thus it was demonstrated that the owls could serve as amplifying hosts.[28] These same owls shed large quantities of virus in oral and cloacal secretions, which could be a source of infection for human handlers.[29]

ACKNOWLEDGMENT

The authors wish to acknowledge Patrick Redig, Lori Arent, Gail Buhl, and Irene Bueno-Padilla, from The Raptor Center, and Jaime Ries, from the Minnesota Zoo, for their contributions to this chapter.

REFERENCES

1. Albert CA, Wilson LK, Mineau P, et al: Anticoagulant rodenticides in three owl species from Western Canada, 1988–2003. *Arch Env Cont Tox* 58(2):451–459, 2010.
2. Arent LA: *Raptors in captivity: Guidelines for care and management*, Blaine, ID, 2007, Hancock House.
3. Association of Zoos and Aquariums: *Raptor TAG: Owl care manual*, Silver Spring, CO, (in prep), AZA.
4. Association of Zoos and Aquariums: *Raptor TAG: Raptor Taxon Advisory Group Regional Collection Plan*, ed 2, Silver Spring, CO, 2008, AZA.
5. Beernaert A, Pasmans F, Van Waeyenberghe L, et al: Aspergillus infections in birds: A review. *Avian Pathol* 39(5):325–331, 2010.
6. Biet F, Boschiroli ML, Thorel MF, Guilloteau LA: Zoonotic aspects of *Mycobacterium bovis* and *Mycobacterium aviam-intracellulare complex* (MAC). *Vet Res* 36(3):411–436, 2005.
7. Bueno-Padilla I, Arent LA, Ponder J: Tips for raptor bandaging. *Exotic DVM* 12(3):25–43, 2010.
8. Carpenter JW, Mashima TY, Rupiper DJ: *Exotic animal formulary*, St. Louis, MO, 2005, Saunders.
9. Cover AJ, Wallace MH, Thomas MT: A new method for the diagnosis of *Trichomonas gallinae* infection by culture. *J Wildl Dis* 30(3):457–459, 1994.
10. del Hoyo J, Elliott A, Sargatal J: *Handbook of the birds of the world*, vol. 5, *Barn-owls to hummingbirds*, Barcelona, Spain, 1999, Lynx Edicions.
11. Duke GE, Evanson OA, Jegers A: Meal to pellet intervals in 14 species of captive raptors. *Comp Biochem Physiol* 53(1):1–6, 1976.
12. Environmental Protection Agency: *Cancellation process for 12 D-Con mouse and rat poison*, <http://www.epa.gov/pesticides/mice-and-rats/cancellation-process.html>. Accessed March 15, 2013.
13. Fitzgerald SD, Patterson JS, Kiupel M, et al: Clinical and pathologic features of West Nile virus infection in native North American owls (Family Strigidae). *Avian Dis* 47(3):602–610, 2003.
14. Forbes NA, Cooper JE, Higgins RJ, et al: Neoplasms in birds of prey. In Lumeij JT, Remple D, Redig P, editors: *Raptor biomedicine*, vol. 3, Lake Worth, FL, 2000, Zoological Education Network.
15. Friedman SG: *The ABC's of behavior*, <http://thegabrielfoundation.org/files/friedman/ABC.pdf>. Accessed March 15, 2013.
16. Gailbreath KL, Oaks JL: Herpesviral inclusion body disease in owls and falcons is caused by the pigeon herpesvirus (*Columbid herpesvirus 1*). *J Wildl Dis* 44(2):427–433, 2008.

17. Gancz AY, Barker IK, Lindsay R, et al: West Nile virus outbreak in North American owls, Ontario, 2002. *Emerg Infect Dis* 10(12):2135–2142, 2004.

18. Harrenstein LA, Tell LA, Vulliet R, et al: Disposition of enrofloxacin in red-tailed hawks (*Buteo jamaincensis*) and great horned owls (*Bubo virginianus*) after a single oral, intramuscular, or intravenous dose. *J Avian Med Surg* 14(4):228–236, 2000.

19. Hawkins MG, Pasco PJ: Cagebirds. In West G, Heard DJ, Caulkett N, editors: *Animal and wildlife immobilization and anesthesia*, Ames, IA, 2007, Wiley Interscience Blackwell (Online service).

20. Hawkins MG, Wright BD, Pascoe PJ, et al: Pharmacokinetics and anesthetic and cardiopulmonary effects of propofol in red-tailed hawks (*Buteo jamaicensis*) and great horned owls (*Bubo virginianus*). *Am J Vet Res* 64(6):677–683, 2003.

21. Heatley JJ, Mitchell MM, Roy A, et al: Disseminated mycobacteriosis in a bald eagle (*Haliaeetus leucocephalus*). *J Avian Med Surg* 21(3):201–209, 2007.

22. Heidenreich M: *Birds of prey: Medicine and management*, Oxford, U.K., 1997, Blackwell Science.

23. Huckabee JR: Raptor therapeutics. *Vet Clin North Am Exot Anim Pract* 3(1):91–116, 2000.

24. International Species Information System: *ISIS Physiological reference intervals for captive wildlife: A CD-ROM resource*, Eagan, MN, 2013, ISIS.

25. James SB, Raphael BL, Clippinger T: Diagnosis and treatment of hepatic lipidosis in a barred owl (*Strix varia*). *J Avian Med Surg* 14(4):268–272, 2000.

26. Johnsgard PA: *North American owls: Biology and natural history*, Washington, DC, 1988, Smithsonian Institution Press.

27. Jones MP: Selected infectious diseases of birds of prey. *J Exot Pet Med* 15(1):5–17, 2006.

28. Komar N: West Nile virus: Epidemiology and ecology in North America. *Adv Virus Res* 61:185–234, 2003.

29. Labelle AL, Whittington JK, Breaux CB, et al: Clinical utility of a complete diagnostic protocol for the ocular evaluation of free-living raptors. *Vet Ophthalmol* 15(1):5–17, 2012.

30. Lacina D, Bird DM: Endoparasites of raptors. In Lumeij JT, Remple D, Redig P, et al, editors: *Raptor biomedicine*, vol. 3, Lake Worth, FL, 2000, Zoological Education Network.

31. Lynch W: *Owls of the U. S. and Canada. A complete guide to their biology and behavior*, Baltimore, MD, 2007, John Hopkins University Press.

32. Mama KR, Philips LG, Pascoe PJ: Use of propofol for induction and maintenance of anesthesia in a barn owl (*Tyto alba*) undergoing tracheal resection. *J Zoo Wildl Med* 27(3):397–401, 1996.

33. Meyer W, Hellman AN, Kummerfeld N: Demonstration of calcium transport markers in the ceca of owls (Aves: Strigiformes), with remarks on basic ceca structure. *Eur J Wildl Res* 55(2):91–96, 2009.

34. Murphy CJ, Brooks DE, Kern TJ, et al: Enucleation in birds of prey. *J Am Vet Med Assoc* 183(11):1234–1237, 1983.

35. Murray M, Tseng F: Diagnosis and treatment of secondary anticoagulant rodenticosis in a red-tailed hawk (*Buteo jamaicensis*). *J Avian Med Surg* 22(1):41–46, 2008.

36. Nemeth N, Kratz G, Edwards E, et al: Surveillance for West Nile virus in clinic-admitted raptors, Colorado. *Emerg Infect Dis* 13(2):305–307, 2007.

37. Pyle P, Howell SNG, DeSante DF, et al: *Identification guide to North American birds, part 1*, 1997, Slate Creek Press.

38. Redig PT, Cruz L: Fractures. In Samour J, editor: *Avian medicine*, New York, 2008, Mosby.

39. Redig PT, Cruz-Martinez L: Raptors. In Tully TN, Dorrestein GM, Jones AK, editors: *Handbook of avian medicine*, ed 2, St. Louis, MO, 2009, Saunders.

40. Redig PT, Francisco ON, Froembling M, et al: Coracoid fractures: An assessment of conservative management. In Martel A, editor: *10th European Association of Avian Veterinarians Conference Proceedings*, Antwerp, Belgium, 2009.

41. Redig PT, Ponder J, Willette ME: Raptor anesthesia. In West G, Heard D, Caulkett N, editors: *Zoo animal and wildlife immobilization and anesthesia*, ed 2, Ames, IA, in press—expected publication 2014, Wiley.

42. Remple JD: A multifaceted approach to the treatment of bumblefoot in raptors. *J Exot Pet Med* 15(1):49–55, 2006.

43. Reynolds RT, Linkhart BD: Extra-pair copulation and extra-range movements in flammulated owls. *Ornis Scandinavica* 21(1):74–77, 1990.

44. Rose N, Warren AL, Whiteside D, et al: Columbid herpesvirus-1 mortality in great horned owls (*Bubo virginianus*) from Calgary, Alberta. *Can Vet J* 53(3):265, 2012.

45. Samour JH, Jones DM, Knight JA: Comparative studies of the use of some injectable anesthestic agents in birds. *Vet Rec* 115(1):6–11, 1984.

46. Sangster G, King BF, Verbelen P, et al: A new owl species of the genus Otus (Aves: Strigidae) from Lombok, Indonesia. *PloS* 8(2):e53712, 2013.

47. Seidensticker MT, Holt DW, Detienne J, et al: Sexing young snowy owls. *J Raptor Res* 45(4):281–289, 2011.

48. Sheffield SR: Owls as biomonitors of environmental contamination. In Duncan JR, Johnson DH, Nicholls TH, editors: *Biology and conservation of owls in the Northern hemisphere*, 2nd International Symposium, St. Paul, MN, 1997, US Department of Agriculture.

49. Shlosberg A, Booth L: *Veterinary and clinical treatment of vertebrate pesticide poisoning—a technical review*, Lincoln, New Zealand, 2006, Landcare Research.

50. Sibley CG, Ahlquist JE: *Phylogeny and classification of bird*, New Haven, CT, 1990, Yale University Press.

51. Smith KE, Anderson F, Medus C, et al: Outbreaks of salmonellosis at elementary schools associated with dissection of owl pellets. *Vector Borne Zoonotic Dis* 5(2):133–136, 2005.

52. Stone EG, Walser MM, Redig PT, et al: Synovial chondromatosis in raptors. *J Wildl Dis* 35(1):137–140, 1999.

53. Tell LA, Ferrell ST, Gibbons PM: Avian mycobacteriosis in free-living raptors in California: 6 Cases (1997-2001). *J Avian Med Surg* 18(1):30–40, 2004.

54. International Union for the Conservation of Nature: *The IUCN Red list of Threatened Species*, <http://www.iucnredlist.org/>. Accessed March 15, 2013.

55. The Raptor Center, University of Minnesota, unpublished data.

56. Thomas PJ, Mineau P, Shore RF, et al: Second generation anticoagulant rodenticides in predatory birds: Probabilistic characterization of toxic liver concentrations and implications for predatory bird populations in Canada. *Environ Int* 37(5):914–920, 2011.

57. Tizard I: Salmonellosis in wild birds. *Semin Avian Exot Pet* 13(2):50–66, 2004.

58. Ward AB, Weigl PD, Conroy RM: Functional morphology of raptor hindlimbs: Implications for resource partitioning. *Auk* 119(4):1052–1063, 2002.

59. Weidensaul CS, Colvin BA, Brinker DF, et al: Use of ultraviolet light as an aid in age classification of owls. *Wilson J Ornithol* 123(2):373–377, 2011.

60. Willette M, Ponder J, Cruz-Martinez L, et al: Management of select bacterial and parasitic conditions of raptors. *Vet Clin North Am Exot Anim Pract* 12(3):491–517, 2009.

61. Willette MW, Ponder JB, McRuer D, Clark EE: Wildlife Health Monitoring in North America: From sentinel species to public policy. In Aguirre AA, Ostefeld RS, Daszak P, editors: *New directions in conservation medicine*, New York, 2012, Oxford University Press.

62. Wünschmann A, Shivers J, Bender J, et al: Pathologic and immunohistochemical findings in goshawks (*Accipiter gentilis*) and great horned owls (*Bubo virginianus*) naturally infected with West Nile virus. *Avian Dis* 49(2):252–259, 2005.

CHAPTER 24

Caprimulgiformes (Nightjars and Allies)

Rosemary J. Booth

BIOLOGY

The order Caprimulgiformes (nightjars and allies) comprises five families and 120 species of large-eyed, wide-mouthed, superbly camouflaged birds. Family Podargidae (frogmouths), Family Aegothelidae (owlet-nightjars), and Family Caprimulgidae (nightjars and nighthawks) are predominantly from Australasia. The European nightjar (*Caprimulgus europaeus*) is migratory between Europe and Africa. Family Steatornithidae (oilbirds) and Family Nyctibiidae (potoos) are from South America. Despite their superficially similar external appearances, taxonomists argue that Caprimulgiformes birds differ distinctly in many anatomic features. Strong evidence suggests sister taxa status between Aegothelidae (owlet nightjars) and the diurnal Apodiformes (swifts and hummingbirds) and that perhaps all six families belong to a clade with a shared common ancestor.[20] Caprimulgiformes species also share morphologic affinities with Strigiformes (owls).[9]

Most birds in this order are nocturnal and insectivorous and live in bonded pairs during the breeding season, but the oilbirds set themselves apart by living in colonies in caves by day and feeding on fruit by night.

The tawny frogmouth (*Podargus strigoides*) will be the main focus of this chapter because among the members of this order, it is the most commonly maintained one in captivity, with 273 specimens in 92 institutions worldwide (International Species Information System [ISIS], 2012).

UNIQUE ANATOMY

Plumage

A distinctive feature of all Caprimulgiformes species is their excellent camouflage. Species that roost and nest in the open by day rely on their cryptic coloring and cryptic postures for protection (Figure 24-1). Nightjars roost and nest on the ground, and their colors match their local substrate. When danger approaches, birds of this order flatten their plumage, extend their neck, close their eyes to mere slits and remain motionless to blend into the background. The plumage of all Caprimulgiformes species is not only intricately shaded but also soft, loose, and fluffy, facilitating both camouflage and silent flight.[5]

Sensory rictal bristles on the face are another feature of the order, although they are absent in potoos. These bristles also assist with camouflage by obscuring the outline of the beak.

A naked vestigial uropygial gland is present in most species but absent in frogmouths and potoos, which maintain their plumage with the assistance of large femoral powder down patches. Powder down is absent in the other families.[5,20]

Special Senses

Because all Caprimulgiformes species are nocturnal or crepuscular, they have large eyes and a reflective tapetum lucidum to assist with low-light hunting. Evidence suggests that they require at least the light of dawn or dusk or bright moonlight to hunt successfully. Oilbirds also have a well-developed olfactory organ to assist with location of aromatic fruits.[5]

Respiratory System

Most Caprimulgiformes species produce their vocalization via a tracheobronchial syrinx. Oilbirds have an asymmetrical bronchial syrinx with which they produce echolocating sonar clicks, which enable them to navigate in the absolute darkness of roosting caves (Figure 24-2).[5,13,25]

Gastrointestinal System

All Caprimulgiformes species have a vestigial, flaplike tongue, which contributes little to the swallowing process (Figure 24-3). Caprimulgiformes species have no crop, and large ceca (5 centimeters [cm] in tawny frogmouths) are present in all species except owlet-nightjars.[5,20]

Musculoskeletal System

All Caprimulgiformes species have anisodactylous feet, with digit 1 pointing backward and digits 2 to 4 pointing forward. Digit 2 is quite mobile.[9,12] The feet are small and weak.

SPECIAL PHYSIOLOGY

Low Basal Metabolic Rate

Caprilmulgiformes species have low basal metabolic rates (BMRs) compared with other birds, with the Podargidae having the lowest avian metabolic rate (40% to 70% of the BMR for an equivalent-sized nonpasserine). This low BMR is reflected in unusually low physiologic values of body temperature in the order of 37°C to 38.5°C, heart rate of 125 to 150, and respiratory rate of 10 to 20.[9,16] Tawny frogmouths and potoos are heat tolerant but will pant when the ambient temperature exceeds 40°C.[16,17]

Facultative Heterothermy

Facultative heterothermy, or *torpor*, is a physiologic state characterized by episodes of reduced BMR and low body temperature in response to low ambient temperature. Tawny frogmouths are one of the avian species that may use torpor to conserve energy in response to low ambient temperature, food shortage, or both. Nightly torpor bouts may last for several hours, and the body temperature may drop to 29°C.[15] Daily torpor has been observed in seven orders of birds, particularly Caprimulgiformes and Trochilidae, and is employed at a variety of ambient temperatures and seasons.[3] The smaller Caprimulgiformes species employ torpor during the day, whereas tawny frogmouths have been observed to regularly use shallow torpor for several hours during the night following a bout of foraging at dusk, then rewarming at dawn for a second bout of foraging.[15]

In the Arizona desert, some common poorwills (*Phalaenoptilis nuttalli*), which weigh 45 gram (g), undergo true hibernation lasting for up to 85 days in winter.[10] Other individuals and close relatives use the alternative strategy of migration. In hibernating poorwills, body temperature falls to as low as 4.8°C, and BMR may drop by 93%.[2]

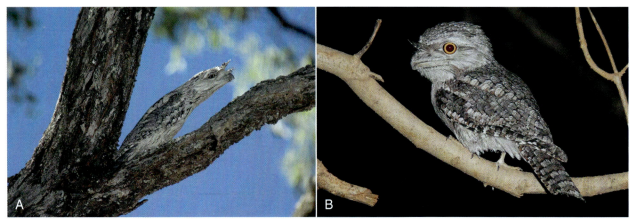

FIGURE 24-1 **A,** Diurnal roosting behaviour of the tawny frogmouth (*Podargus strigoides*) demon-strating camouflaged plumage, cryptic posture, and perch selection. **B,** Nocturnal hunting behavior from an elevated perch. (Courtesy John Young www.johnyoungwildlife.com.)

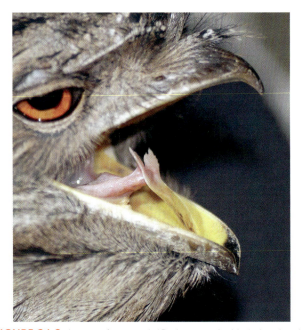

FIGURE 24-2 A tawny frogmouth (*Podargus strigoides*) showing the wide gape, vestigial tongue, and sensory rectal bristles. (Courtesy of Pauline Gaven.)

SPECIAL HOUSING REQUIREMENTS

Aviaries should be large enough to allow flight when the birds are active at night, with a recommended minimum measurement of 3 meters (m) width, 6 m length, and 3 m height. Large-gauge wire mesh may be used to allow nocturnal insects to enter the aviary. Vegetation should simulate a eucalypt woodland, and natural perching should have a range of diameters and heights to allow choice and avoid pododermatitis. An undercover area, approximately one third of the aviary, should contain high perching for day time roost-ing in an area visible to the public. Frogmouths often choose to roost in sites exposed to heavy rain. Hollow logs placed vertically and forked perching with thick textured bark in a colour that blends with the birds' plumage makes an attractive display (see Figure 24-1). A natural aviary substrate provides extra prey and behavioral enrich-ment, and a sand area under roosting perches facilitates cleaning. The diurnal roosting behavior and temperament of tawny

frogmouths allows a unique display opportunity in that they may be placed on a perch outside an aviary or in a classroom, and they will usually sit tight for hours if provided with some browse for cover and minimal supervision.

Owlet-nightjars roost in hollows during the day and so are not suited to outdoor displays unless perspex viewing ports or spy cameras are used. Owlet-nightjars require at least two horizontally placed roosting logs or nest boxes per bird, fixed high on walls in a sheltered area of the aviary.[3] Nocturnal house displays have been tried with varying success.

Tawny frogmouths acquire most water from their food or from rain. Their legs are unsuited to walking to the edge of a pond to drink. An elevated, broad, shallow water supply should be available near the favored roost site, and a range of perching should be avail-able so that the birds may sit in the rain if they choose to. Nightjars have been observed taking water on the wing, much like swallows, and skimming along the surface of a lake.

FEEDING

Diet of Free-Ranging Birds

Most members of this order are adapted to a diet of nocturnal insects and small vertebrates, with the exception of the oilbird, which is a frugivore. The wild tawny frogmouths diet consists of 78% insects, 18% other invertebrates (worms, slugs, and snails), and 4% verte-brates (small mammals, amphibians, reptiles, and birds).[9] The pro-portion of vertebrates in the diet increases in winter when insects are less abundant. The heavily ossified and muscled bills of Caprimul-giformes species form a stong snap trap, enabling them to eat larger prey, which they crush or vigorously beat on branches before swallowing.[9]

Most food is obtained by pouncing to the ground from a tree or other elevated perch. Flying insects are caught on the wing and swallowed whole. Ingested grit and stones help break down prey.[5,9,11]

Oilbirds eat the fruits of a wide range of tree species, predomi-nantly palms, laurels, and incense trees. They feed on the wing and swallow the fruits (up to 6 cm in diameter) whole. The seeds are regurgitated, and mounds of decaying seeds are left on the floor of their roosting caves.[5]

Diet of Captive Birds

Captive Caprimulgiformes species require a high-protein insectivore or carnivore diet. The tawny frogmouth may be maintained on whole mice, chopped day-old chicks, and a variety of insects, including grasshoppers, crickets, mealworms, and cockroaches plus good-quality insectivore or carnivore mix molded into balls. Calcium

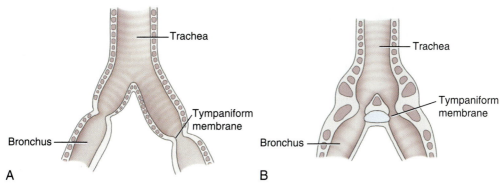

FIGURE 24-3 The asymmetrical bronchial syrinx of the oilbird, which may produce clicks used for echolocation (**A**) compared with the tracheobronchial syrinx of the other Caprimulgiformes (**B**). (Courtesy of Mark Blyde.)

supplementation is required with a diet of juvenile rodents or day-old chicks. Providing inactive food in a dish, either on a perch or on the ground, does not trigger a hunting response in most birds, and hand feeding is usually required. Most tawny frogmouths readily gape for food after a short time in captivity. The gaping begins as a threat response but is eventually conditioned to a useful feeding routine. A range of light sources and moth traps may be used to attract nocturnal insects to the aviary to supplement the diet.

Rescued wild frogmouths, owlet-nightjars, and nightjars rarely self-feed, so initial force-feeding and then hand feeding are usually required until release. Nightjars have a large stomach capacity accounting for 20% to 25% of a bird's body weight when full.[19]

The general rule of feeding 10% to 25% body weight applies, with smaller and younger birds requiring the high end of this range. Sedentary birds maintained in a thermoneutral environment obviously require less food compared with mobile birds with thermoregulatory needs.

RESTRAINT AND HANDLING

Most Caprimulgiformes are docile birds in captivity and are assessed as low risk or innocuous to handlers. Usually, handlers do not need gloves or protective clothing to protect themselves, but a towel is useful to handle aggressive wild frogmouths. Most species adopt their stick posture when approached during the day and are then easy to capture by hand. Net capture may be required at times, and the occasional individual may be aggressive and fly at the face of keepers when approached. Such birds may generally be gradually conditioned with food rewards to remain perched. The beak of a tawny frogmouth may exert significant crushing force, so handlers should avoid bites by grabbing wild or aggressive birds from behind and controlling the head. The feet of Caprimulgiformes are weak and harmless. The smaller species drop their feathers to avoid predation, so they must be handled gently but firmly. Owlet-nightjars are nervous birds but are caught easily during the day from their roost logs or boxes.

ANESTHESIA AND SURGERY

Preanesthetic evaluation is recommended, as well as stabilization of dehydrated or debilitated birds with warmed subcutaneous lactated Ringer solution (up to 40 milliliters per kilogram [mL/kg]). Isoflurane administered via a T-piece and face mask and then via endotracheal tube is the anaesthetic of choice (typically 5% induction, 1% to 2.5 % maintenance to effect). The epiglottis is absent in avians, which increases their susceptibility to aspiration. For birds weighing 200 to 400 g, fasting for 2 to 4 hours, followed by intubation with an uncuffed tube, is advisable. The phalanges make a suitable

attachment point for pulse oximetry. The birds should be placed in lateral or ventral recumbency as soon as possible after surgery to reduce inspiratory effort.

Traumatic injuries requiring surgery are common. Closed midshaft fractures of the radius or ulna where one bone is still intact have an excellent prognosis, with a "figure-of-eight" support bandage immobilizing the elbow and the carpus for 2 to 3 weeks, followed by early ambulation to avoid contracture of the patagium. Open fractures carry a worse prognosis, but surgical repair is certainly possible. Fractures within a centimeter of a joint have an unfavorable prognosis because of the possibility of arthrodesis caused by diffuse calcification common in avian fracture healing. Serious oral injuries, including beak fractures, pharyngeal lacerations, and tongue injuries, may occur from mouth-to-mouth fighting between incompatable individuals. Pharyngeal wounds may be so deep that they progress to osteomyelitis and septicemia.[21] Beak fractures may be repaired successfully by wiring. The tongue also may be injured during force-feeding, as it may be pushed back and creased, later dropping off at the site of trauma.[21] Injured tongues generally heal well. Tawny frogmouths have a high risk of trauma caused by motor vehicles because automobile lights illuminate prey, which attracts the birds to approach the roads for foraging. Owlet-nightjars and nightjars are at greater risk of predation becaue of their small size and ground dwelling habits.

Cataracts are common in captive and rescued tawny frogmouths, generally occurring secondary to trauma and may be removed via phaco-emulsification if preoperative electroretinography indicates retinal health and a likely return of sight.

Nociception in birds is similar to that in mammals.[18] Meloxicam is the analgesic and anti-inflammatory agent of choice at a dose of 0.3 to 0.5 mg/kg intramuscularly (IM), intravenously (IV), or orally (PO), twice daily (BID).[18] Other nonsteroidal anti-inflammatory drugs (NSAIDs; diclofenac, carprofen, flunixin, ibuprofen, and phenylbutazone) have been associated with nephrotoxicity, visceral gout, and mortality in Caprimulgiformes species, but with administration of meloxicam to over 700 birds from 60 species, no mortalities have been reported.[7]

DIAGNOSTICS
Clinical Examination

A full clinical examination involves a systematic examination of the external features, examination of all orifices for discharges, and evaluation of all body systems. Initial examination is best carried out in the aviary to assess locomotion, particularly the ability to fly and wing symmetry, and behavior prior to handling. Respiratory effort should be judged from a distance when the bird is at rest on its perch. Assessment of preening activity requires examination of the

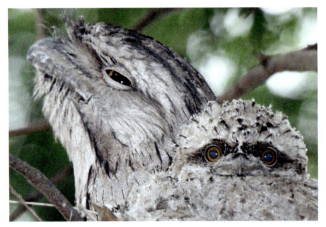

FIGURE 24-4 Normal tawny frogmouth nestlings have cloudy eyes which clear soon after fledging. (Courtesy of Larry Dunis.)

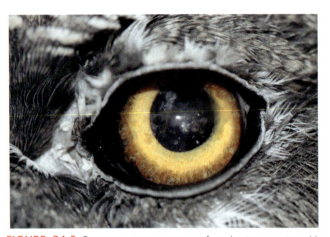

FIGURE 24-5 Common consequences of ocular trauma, torn iris fibrils, and calcification of the anterior lens capsule. Such injuries often accompany hemorrhages of the pectin. (Courtesy of Rosemary Booth.)

powder down patches in species in which the uropygial gland is absent.

Particular attention should be paid to the eyes, especially if the bird is not flying, as flight is dependent on sight in birds. The large eyes of the Caprimulgiformes species are highly prone to traumatic injury (Figure 24-4). Opthalmoscopy is obligatory in traumatized birds, as hemorrhages in the pecten oculi is a common occurrence and carries a poor prognosis for rehabilitation of wild birds.[14] Mydriasis is best achieved under general anesthesia, since the iris of birds contains striated intraocular musculature, which responds poorly to atropine or tropicamide.[14] Bilateral homogeneous ocular cloudiness is normal in tawny frogmouth and owlet-nightjar nestlings, but the eyes clear as the birds mature (Figure 24-5).

Because the Caprimulgiformes species have a low BMR, the expected physiologic values are as follows: heart rate 120 to 150, respiratory rate 10 to 20, and body temperature 37°C to 38.5°C. As body temperature is volatile in birds during handling, cloacal temperature is not always a useful measure.

Body weights of wild and captive tawny frogmouths show seasonal variation, with peaks in autumn and early winter. Gut fill also contributes to body weight, and a full stomach in nightjars may weigh 20% to 25% of total body weight. An attempt to weigh birds should always be made before feeding and at the same time each day.

Hard data on longevity is scarce, partly because many captive birds arrive as unreleasable adults. Tawny frogmouths have a life expectancy of around 15 years.

Blood Collection, Hematology, and Serum Biochemistry

The jugular vein, visible in the featherless tract on the right side of the neck, is the preferred venipuncture site; however, it may be obscured completely by subcutaneous fat in tawny frogmouths in prewinter conditions, and the cutaneous ulnar vein should be used.[21] Reference ranges for hematologic and serum biochemistry values for tawny frogmouths are presented in Table 24-1 (ISIS, 2013). *Haemoproteus* and *Leucocytozoon* organisms may be seen in the erythrocytes of a range of Caprimulgiforme species and are generally nonpathogenic.

DISEASES

Published reports on the viral diseases of wild birds may underrepresent the true extent of viral infections in a particular order of birds. It is necessary to remain constantly vigilant for possible zoonotic or notifiable diseases when handling sick and injured wildlife. Particular care is required when handling wild birds that are in poor body condition, which is evidence of underlying systemic disease.

Infectious Disease

Inclusion body hepatitis from suspected adenovirus infection is a common finding in wild tawny frogmouths in eastern Australia. Affected birds show weakness, depression, or secondary traumatic injury and generally die while in care. At necropsy, the liver is found enlarged and friable. Histopathologic examination demonstrates foci of acute hepatocellular necrosis, with intranuclear eosinophilic to basophilic inclusion bodies in hepatocytes at the margins of these lesions.[23] Cutaneous poxlike lesions have been seen on the face and feet of several wild frogmouths. Histopathologic findings are typical of avianpox, with epithelial proliferation and abundant intracytoplasmic pox inclusions.

Erysipelothrix rhusiopathiae has caused septicemia and sudden death in tawny frogmouths. Necropsy findings have demonstrated pericarditis and hepatomegaly, with clumps of intracellular gram-positive bacteria in the vessels and hepatic sinusoids. Rodents and insects may act as vectors for this disease.[21]

Aspergillosis with pneumonia and airsacculitis may occur in hospitalized wild birds. Prophylactic oral itraconazole at 20 mg/kg, once daily (SID), is recommended for Caprimulgiformes species in situations of long-term stress.

Cryptococcus neoformans has been cultured from the fresh feces of a captive tawny frogmouth but has not been identified as a cause of disease in the species.[24]

Parasitic Diseases

Ectoparasites

The most common and obvious parasites of tawny frogmouths are two species of flat fly in the family Hippoboscidae: *Ornithoica podargi* and *Ornithomya fuscipennis* (Figure 24-6). These are biting flies known to transmit *Haemoproteus* in other avian species. They may be controlled with topical permethrin sprays or carbaryl powder. Heavy burdens may be debilitating.

Other ectoparasites identified in the Caprimulgiformes species include ticks (*Haemaphysalis bremneri*), lice (*Podargoecus tasmaniensis* and *Nyctibicola* spp.), and feather mites (*Ascouracarus vassilevi* and *Nyctibiolichus* spp.).[21]

Endoparasites

Eosinophilic meningoencephalitis caused by *Angiostrongylus cantonensis* is an emerging disease in free-living tawny frogmouths in Australia. Histologic surveys from the Sydney region have suggested a dramatic increase in the incidence of this disease in tawny frogmouths over the last 2 decades.[18] *A. cantonensis* is a nematode, which

TABLE 24-1

Reference Values for Hematologic and Biochemical Analysis for *Podargus strigoides**

Test	Units	Mean	Standard Deviation	Minimum Value	Maximum Value	Sample Size	Animals
White blood cell count	*10^3/μL	12.7	6.3	2.40	43.20	124	77
Red blood cell count	*10^6/μL	2.2	0.5	0.60	3.15	42	28
Hemoglobin	g/dL	13.5	3.3	8.40	23.80	42	25
Hematocrit	%	41.0	4.7	29	53	131	83
Mean corpuscular volume	fL	184.7	34.7	125	272	40	27
Mean corpuscular hemoglobin	pg/cell	63.4	21.9	38	111	25	15
Mean corpuscular hemoglobin concentration	g/dL	32.9	6.7	19	54	41	25
Platelet count	*10^3/μL	7.0	0.0	7.0	7.0	1	1
Heterophils	*10^3/μL	6.1	4.0	1.11	30.20	121	74
Lymphocytes	*10^3/μL	5.0	3.2	0.36	18.10	120	73
Monocytes	*10^3/μL	0.8	0.7	0.05	3.54	95	60
Eosinophils	*10^3/μL	0.7	1.1	0.04	6.72	80	50
Basophils	*10^3/μL	0.7	0.6	0.06	3.04	90	57
Calcium	mg/dL	9.8	2.4	0.0	19.4	89	70
Phosphorus	mg/dL	3.7	2.2	1.1	9.0	54	43
Sodium	mEq/L	154	7	140	166	37	29
Potassium	mEq/L	2.7	0.9	1.3	4.9	38	29
Chloride	mEq/L	113	9	84	135	29	22
Bicarbonate	mEq/L	19.3	2.2	16.0	21.0	4	3
Carbon dioxide	mEq/L	22.8	5.6	17.0	35.0	8	5
Iron	μg/dL	250	0	250	250	1	1
Magnesium	mg/dL	1.70	0.00	1.70	1.70	1	1
Blood urea nitrogen	mg/dL	4.0	2.0	2.0	8.0	33	26
Creatinine	mg/dL	0.4	0.2	0.1	0.9	29	24
Uric acid	mg/dL	6.4	4.0	0.0	20.9	102	74
Total bilirubin	mg/dL	0.2	0.2	0.0	0.6	25	19
Direct bilirubin	mg/dL	0.0	0.1	0.0	0.1	4	3
Indirect bilirubin	mg/dL	0.3	0.2	0.0	0.5	4	3
Glucose	mg/dL	314	84	33	574	85	66
Cholesterol	mg/dL	308	75	158	478	54	40
Triglyceride	mg/dL	283	523	36	2290	19	15
Creatine phosphokinase	IU/L	979	639	186	3421	56	49
Lactate dehydrogenase	IU/L	345	342	52	1800	45	38
Alkaline phosphatase	IU/L	120	121	6	675	58	45
Alanine aminotransferase	IU/L	28	45	1	259	42	31
Aspartate aminotransferase	IU/L	229	99	63	639	102	77
Gamma glutamyltransferase	IU/L	38	91	0	295	10	10
Amylase	U/L	598	294	265	1483	14	12
Total protein	g/dL	4.3	0.9	2.3	7.0	89	71
Globulin	g/dL	2.1	0.6	0.8	3.6	44	36
Albumin	g/dL	2.0	0.4	1.3	3.0	47	38
Fibrinogen	mg/dL	125	50	100	200	4	4

*From up to 124 samples from up to 83 individuals from 30 institutions.

fL, Femtoliters; *g/dL*, gram per deciliter; *IU/L*, international unit per liter; *mEq/dL*, milliequivalent per deciliter; *mg/dL*, milligram per deciliter; *μL*, microliter; *pg*, picogram.

requires an invertebrate intermediate host, mainly slugs and snails, and a definitive terrestrial mammalian host, usually *Rattus* spp. Paratenic hosts, in which the parasites do not develop to the next stage, may be either invertebrates or vertebrates and include species that eats mollusks, including humans and tawny frogmouths. In paratenic hosts, ingested third stage larvae migrate to the brain via the bloodstream. Affected humans report severe headaches, stiff necks, and clouded consciousness and paralysis of the fifth cranial nerve.[26] Eosinophilic meningoencephalitis should be suspected as a differential diagnosis in tawny frogmouths presenting with

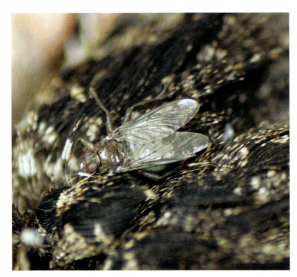

FIGURE 24-6 Hippoboscid flies are a common ectoparasite of tawny frogmouths (*Podargus strigoides*). (Courtesy of Pauline Gaven.)

neurologic signs, including bad temper and reluctance to fly. In humans, peripheral blood and cerebrospinal fluid (CSF) eosinophilia strongly support a diagnosis of *Angiostrongylus* meningoencephalitis but may appear only late in the course of illness or occasionally not at all.[22] Enzyme-linked immunosorbent assay for *A. cantonensis* antigen is available and may be performed on serum or CSF. Paired tests may be required. Immune responses provoked by dead worms may cause severe inflammation, so the use of anthelmintics in treatment is a risk that must be assessed. Treatment with corticosteroids is primarily aimed at reducing inflammation and intrathecal pressure. The disease may be fatal, but humans generally recover over a period of weeks.[22] Tawny frogmouths with a presumptive diagnosis based on the presence of neurologic signs and eosinophilia have been treated with a combination of ivermectin (0.2 mg/kg, subcutaneously [SQ], weekly ×3) and dexamethasone (1 mg/kg, IM, SID, reducing the dose over 3 weeks) and have shown clinical improvement within 3 weeks.

Occasionally, *Capillaria*, ascarid, and cestode ova are detected on routine fecal flotations. *Capillaria* may be treated with albendazole orally at 50 mg/kg, SID, for 3 days, or ivermectin at 0.2 to 0.4 mg/kg, SQ or pour-on topically. Ascarids may also be treated with fenbendazole at 100 mg/kg and cestodes with praziquantel at 10 mg/kg.

Haemoproteus transmitted by ectoparasites has been identified in the erythrocytes of 16% of 106 Caprimulgiformes species examined.[1] Although reports of clinical disease are lacking, heavy burdens may be significant.

Juvenile tawny frogmouths are susceptible to potentially fatal coccidiosis, which may be treated with toltrazuril (25 mg/kg, PO, two doses 7 days apart).

Noninfectious Disease

Toxicity
The presence of pesticides in the tissues of species high in the food chain is not unusual. The clinical significance of these toxins is not always clear, and the potential for chronic low-grade effects also exists. Tawny frogmouths have been assessed for organochlorine and organophosphate toxicity, which they may acquire through ingestion of poisoned insects or through inhalation or percutaneous absorption through aerosols. Rapid use and depletion of fat stores during times of stress such as migration or reduced food supply may mobilize fat-stored organochlorines, which may become concentrated in the brain, resulting in acute toxicity.[6]

Potentially toxic tissue concentrations of the lipophilic organochlorines have been demonstrated in small numbers of birds and have been linked to clinical signs, including abnormal diurnal activity, weakness, inability to fly, seizures, and opisthotonus.[4] The total organochlorine concentrations in eight tawny frogmouths were 13 to 66 mg/kg in the liver and 11 to 29 mg/kg in the brain.[4] The toxic doses of organochlorines are highly variable, but it has been shown that 5 parts per million (ppm) dieldrin or 50 ppm DDT in the brain of mallards is indicative of acute toxicity (NB: ppm = mg/kg).[8] Neurologic signs are not specific to poisoning, and assessment for head trauma, starvation, eosinophilic meningoencephalitis, toxoplasmosis, and other causes should be considered. Treatment of suspected poisoning cases with anticonvulsants, anticholinergics, or both has not been successful.

Postmortem diagnosis of poisoning may be achieved if funding is available, a short list of likely toxins exists, and a local laboratory is willing and able to test the liver, brain, and adipose tissue of the dead birds. To diagnose organophosphate poisoning, a decrease in brain cholinesterase activity of 50% or more from normal is evidence of lethal exposure to a cholinesterase-inhibiting compound (OP, or carbamate pesticide).[6] As a general rule, mortality associated with neurologic signs and the absence of lesions suggesting another cause of death are suggestive of poisoning.[8]

Nephritis and Renal Gout
Nonsuppurative interstitial nephritis with severe nodular fibrosis and secondary renal gout was idenitfied at postmortem examination in a geriatric captive tawny frogmouth, which had developed nonspecific clinical signs of weight loss, inappetence and lethargy, heterophilia (10.2 × 10^3 per microliter [μL]), azotemia (urea 6.2 milligrams per deciliter [mg/dL]), and elevated aspartate aminotransferase (AST; 271 units per liter [Units/L]). Renal gout is a common nonspecific consequence of reduced glomerular filtration rate (GFR) in birds.

REPRODUCTION

Sexual dimorphism exists in tawny frogmouths. All rufous and chestnut forms are female. All males are gray and generally larger and have a broader bill. Females, however, may be gray, and the weight ranges overlap.[9] Males generally weigh 450 to 600 g and females 300 to 500 g, but seasonal and geographic variations exist. Tawny frogmouths are monogamous and pair for life. During the breeding season, pairs perform a low drumming duet. The nest site is usually a horizontal fork in a large eucalyptus tree. The nest is a flimsy twig platform lined with leaves. Both parents build the nest and incubate the eggs, the better camouflaged and larger males incubating by day and the females incubating at night. Mates bring food to each other at the nest. Incubation takes 28 to 30 days, and fledging occurs at 27 to 31 days.[12] The young remain with the parents for several months after fledging and undertake a slow continuous molt ("staffelmauser") to adult plumage by the end of the first year.[9] Sexual maturity occurs by 9 to 12 months.[9,12]

Tawny frogmouths are seasonal breeders, reproducing once per year in the spring, with a clutch size of one to three eggs (usually two). The eggs are laid 1 to 2 days apart, with incubation beginning from the laying of the first egg. The semi-altricial hatchlings weigh 17 to 19 g, are covered in white down, and have their eyes closed until around Day 4. Hatching is asynchronous, but simultaneous fledging occurs; that is, the youngest chick is disadvantaged and may meet with misadventure on the ground.[9,12] The chicks have a slow growth rate because of the low BMR, gaining 6 to 10 g per day when parent reared.[12] Hand raising is straightforward but takes longer than with most other birds, but the delightful temperament of these birds makes it a very rewarding experience.

Nightjars nest on the ground in a shallow depression and rely on camouflage to avoid detection. Owlet-nightjars nest in tree hollows lined with leaves. Oilbirds nest in caves and make a nest from decaying fruit seeds and saliva, as do swifts.

ACKNOWLEDGMENT

The author is grateful to Kim Maciej for providing access to ISIS data; to John Young, Pauline Gaven, and Larry Dunis for granting permission to use their photos; to Mark Blyde for illustrating the syrinx; and to Rebekah McKee for editorial assistance.

REFERENCES

1. Atkinson CT, Thomas NJ, Hunter DB: *Parasitic diseases of wild birds*, Ames, IA, 2008, Wiley-Blackwell.
2. Brigham RM, Kortner G, Maddocks TA, Geiser F: Seasonal use of torpor by free-ranging Australian owlet-nightjars. *Physiol Biochem Zool* 73(5): 613–620, 2000.
3. Brigham RM, Woods CP, Lane JE, et al: Ecological correlates of torpor use among five caprimulgiform birds. *Acta Zoologica Sinica* 52(Suppl): 401–404, 2006.
4. Carney T: *Breeding action plan: Australian owlet-nightjar, Aegotheles cristatus cristatus*, Sydney, Australia, 2000, Australasian Regional Association of Zoological Parks and Aquaria.
5. Charles JA: Organochlorine toxicity in tawny frogmouths. In *Proceedings of the Australian Committee of the Association of Avian Veterinarians*, Dubbo, Australia, 1995, pp 135–141.
6. Cohn-Haft M, Cleere N, Holyoak DT, Thomas BT: Order Caprimulgiformes. In del Hoyo J, Elliott E, Sargatal J, editors: *Handbook of the birds of the world, Vol. 5, Barn owls to hummingbirds*, Barcelona, Spain, 1999, Lynx Edicions, pp 244–386.
7. Cuthbert R, Parry-Jones J, Green RE, Pain DJ: NSAIDS and scavenging birds: Potential impacts beyond Asia's critically endangered vultures. *Biol Lett* 3(1):91–94, 2007.
8. Friend M, Franson JC. Organophosphorus and carbamate pesticides. In Ciganovich EA, editor: *Field manual of wildlife diseases, general field procedures and diseases of birds*, Madison, WI, 1999, USGS, pp 287–294.
9. Higgins PJ, editor: *Handbook of Australian, New Zealand and Antarctic birds, Vol. 4, Parrots to dollarbird*, Melbourne, Australia, 1999, Oxford University Press, pp 963–1048.
10. Jaegar EC: Further observations on the hibernation of the poor-will. *Condor* 51(3):105–109, 1949.
11. Jenkinson MA, Mengel RM: Ingestion of stones by goatsuckers (Caprimulgidae). *Condor* 72:236–237, 1970.
12. Kaplan G: *Tawny frogmouth*, Collingwood, VIC, 2007, CSIRO Publishing.
13. Konishi M, Knudsen EI: The oilbird: hearing and echolocation. *Science* 204(27):425–427, 1979.
14. Korbel R: *Avian ophthalmology—principles and application proceedings of Australasian Committee Association of Avian Veterinarians and Unusual and Exotic Pet Veterinarians*, Melbourne, Australia, 2012, pp 1–8.
15. Kortner G, Brigham RM, Geiser F: Torpor in free-ranging tawny frogmouths (*Podargus strigoides*). *Physiol Biochem Zool* 74(6):789–797, 2001.
16. Lasiewski RC, Bartholomew GA: Evaporative cooling in the poor-will and the tawny frogmouth. *Condor* 68:253–262, 1966.
17. Lasiewski RC, Dawson WR, Bartholomew GA: Temperature regulation in the little Papuan frogmouth, *Podargus ocellatus. Condor* 72:332–338, 1970.
18. Lierz M, Korbel R: Anesthesia and analgesia in birds. *J Exot Pet Med* 21:44–58, 2012.
19. Marshall JT: Hibernation in captive goatsuckers. *Condor* 57(3):129–134, 1955.
20. Mayr G: Phylogenetic relationships of the paraphyletic caprimulgiform birds (nightjars and allies). *J Zool Syst Evol Res* 48(2):126–137, 2010.
21. McCracken H: Caprimulgiformes (goatsuckers). In Fowler M, Miller RE, editors: *Zoo and wild animal medicine*, ed 5, St. Louis, MO, 2003, Saunders, pp 224–231.
22. Mindlin GB, Laje R: *Physics of birdsong*, Berlin/Heidelberg, Germany, 2005, Springer-Verlag.
23. Roberts FHS: *Australian ticks*, Melbourne, Australia, 1970, CSIRO Publishing.
24. Rose AB: Mass of wild birds of the Order Caprimulgiformes. *Aust Bird Bander* 14(2):50–51, 1976.
25. Snow J: *Husbandry guidelines for tawny frogmouth* Podargus strigoides *(Aves: Podargidae)*, Richmond, Australia, 2008, Western Sydney Institute of TAFE.
26. Suthers RA: Variable asymmetry and resonance in the avian vocal tract: A structural basis for individually distinct vocalisations. *J Comp Physiol [A]* 175:457–466, 1994.

SUGGESTED READING

1. Bech C, Nicol SC: Thermoregulation and ventilation in the tawny frogmouth, *Podargus strigoides*: A low metabolic avian species. *Aust J Zool* 47:143–153, 1999.
2. Brigham RM: Daily torpor in a free-ranging goatsucker, the common poorwill (*Phalaenoptilus nuttallii*). *Physiol Zool* 65(2):457–472, 1992.
3. Friend M, Franson JC. Chlorinated hydrocarbon insecticides. In Ciganovich EA, editor: *Field manual of wildlife diseases, general field procedures and diseases of birds*. Madison, WI, 1999, USGS, pp 295–302.
4. Ma G, Dennis M, Rose K, et al: Tawny frogmouths and brushtail possums as sentinels for *Angiostrongylus cantonensis*, the rat lungworm. *Vet Parasitol* 192:158–165, 2013.
5. Maa TC: Genera and species of Hippoboscidae (Diptera): Types, synonymy, habitats and natural groupings. *Pacific Insects Monogr* 6:1–185-186, 1963.
6. Mawson PM, Angel LM, Edmonds SJ: A checklist of helminths from Australian birds. *Rec S Aust Mus* 19(15):219–325, 1986.
7. Palma RL, Barker SC: Phthiraptera. In Wells A, editor: *Zoological catalogue of Australia*, vol 26, Melbourne, Australia, 1996, CSIRO Publishing, pp 81–247, 333–361, 373–396.
8. Prior DS, Konecny P, Senanayake SN, Walker J: First report of human angiostrongylus in Sydney. *Med J Austr* 179(8):430–431, 2003.
9. Puette M, Latimer KS, Norton TM: Epicardial keratinaceous cyst in a tawny frogmouth (*Podargus strigoides plumiferus*). *Avian Dis* 39(1):201–203, 1995.
10. Reece RL, Beddome VD, Barr DA, et al: Common necropsy findings in captive birds in Victoria, Australia (1978–1987). *J Zoo Wildl Med* 23(3):301–312, 1992.
11. Rose KA: Common diseases of urban wildlife. In Bryden DI, editor: *Wildlife in Australia: Healthcare and management. Proceeding 327, Postgraduate committee in Veterinary Science*, Sydney, Australia, 1999, University of Sydney, pp 365–429.
12. Staib F, Schultz-Dieterich J: *Cryptococcus neoformans* in fecal matter of birds kept in cages: Control of *Cr. Neoformans* habitats. *Zbl Bakt Hyg I Abt Orig B* 179:179–186, 1984.
13. Suthers RA, Hector DH: The physiology of vocalization by the echolocating Oilbird, *Steatornis caripensis. J Comp Physiol [A]* 156:243–266, 1985.
14. Syed S: Angiostrongylus cantonensis (on-line), Animal Diversity Web, 2001. http://animaldiversity.ummz.umich.edu/accounts/Angiostrongylus _cantonensis/. Accessed March 15, 2013.
15. Williams NA, Bennett GF, Mahrt JL: Avian Haemoproteidae. 6. Description of *Haemoproteus caprimulgi* sp. nov., and a review of the haemoproteids of the family Caprimulgidae. *Can J Zool* 53(7):916–919, 1975.

CHAPTER 25

Musophagiformes

Maryanne E. Tocidlowski

GENERAL BIOLOGY AND ECOLOGY

The family Musophagidae is made up of the group of birds called *turacos*, including plantain-eaters and go-away birds. They are naturally found in the sub-Saharan region of Africa occupying the forest, woodland, and savanna regions. Previously, turacos had been placed in the order Cuculiformes, but evidence led to placing them in their own order Musophagiformes.[9,15] They were associated with cuckoos because of a particular anatomic feature, that is, zygodactyl toes, in which digits 2 and 3 face forward and digits 1 and 4 face backward, although digit four is flexible and may face toward the back or the front. Other than the toe arrangement, no other commonalities between cuckoos and turacos exist.[21,22]

The family Musophagidae is divided into six genera (*Turaco, Ruwenzorornis, Musophaga, Corythaixoides, Crinifer,* and *Corythaeola*), which contain 23 species and 38 subspecies. Others have divided the turacos under a suborder Musophagae, which is further subdivided into three groups of *Corythaeolinae* (1 species *Corythaeola*), *Criniferinae* (5 species *Corythaixoides* and *Crinifer*), and *Musophaginae* (17 species *Turaco, Ruwenzorornis, Musophaga*).[22]

Turacos are long-lived, medium- to large-sized birds, ranging in body weight from 200 to 400 grams (g) with the great blue turaco weighing up to and over 1 kilogram (kg). They have long tails, conspicuous head crests, stout beaks, and colorful feathering. Most species of turacos have unique pigments in their feathers: *turacoverdin,* a true green pigment found only in these birds, and *turacin,* a true red pigment. These pigments are copper based and not made from carotenoids as in other bird species. This pigmentation specialty in turacos has been well described.[9,22] During handling, the feathers may exfoliate easily as a defense mechanism. Turacos are sexually monomorphic, with the exception of the white-bellied go-away bird, in this species the female's beak is a dull green and the male's is black. Sexing may be done by feather or blood deoxyribonucleic acid (DNA) analysis or laparoscopic examination.[10,14] Turacos are arboreal, gregarious, active birds. They are poor flyers but are able to run in the trees and foliage quite well. Anatomically, turacos are similar to other bird species with the exception that they have little or no ceca, a distensible esophagus with no crop, a thick muscular proventriculus and a thin-walled ventriculus, a relatively larger liver for its body size, and a short intestinal tract.[11] Turacos regurgitate food when stressed or captured. It is important to allow this to occur so that the bird does not aspirate food particles.

HOUSING

Turacos are active birds and require space to move around. Flight cages or aviaries that are heavily planted seem to work best in providing perching, shelter, and hiding places. During the colder months, access to indoor housing, a shelter, or windbreak with a heat source is needed, as turacos are susceptible to hypothermia and frostbite. During the hotter months, these birds cool themselves by gular fluttering and sitting in the shade and enjoy bathing in a sprinkler or water bath. They may be housed with other species but may become territorial and aggressive toward others, especially birds of similar size. Caution must be taken, even with bonded pairs, that birds are not aggressive toward each other. Occasional separation of birds may be needed to inhibit an aggressive bird attacking its cage

mate. Juveniles should be separated from the parents once they are able to feed themselves reliably.[3,20]

DIET

The dietary requirements of turacos have not been well established. The family Musophagidae is generally vegetarian, tending more toward frugivory and folivory, but do occasionally supplement their diet with various small invertebrates, especially around breeding season.[12,18] Contrary to its name Musophagidae, turacos and plantain-eaters (*Crinifer* sp.) do not ingest bananas or plantains (Musa).[21] In captivity, turacos have been fed various diet formulations. A good general diet should consist of a parrot pellet or soft-bill-type pellet with fruit mix and chopped greens, supplemented with a small amount of invertebrates and possibly a meat offering during breeding season. Corythaixoides, Crinifer, and Corythaeola species should be given more greens and leaf browse compared with other turaco species. Mixing the ingredients of the offered diet should help prevent specific item selection by the birds.[14,20]

RESTRAINT AND HANDLING

Turacos are great runners on branches, which makes them hard to catch. They typically do not bite but will rake with sharp claws. They exfoliate feathers easily when held and sometimes will become overly stressed. Regurgitation of recently eaten food is also common. Inhalation anesthesia is more commonly used for advanced restraint and surgical procedures. It has been suggested that turacos be given time to calm down prior to exposure to isoflurane inhalant anesthesia because of issues caused by stress.[12,18,23]

PHYSICAL EXAMINATION, DIAGNOSTICS, AND THERAPY

Examination of turacos may be done under manual or chemical restraint. A thorough examination should include assessment of plumage quality and skin condition, uropygeal gland evaluation, assessment of beak and cere (nares) quality, oral and choanal visualization, feet and nail check, cloaca check, ophthalmic visualization, otic review, auscultation of heart and lungs, coelomic palpation, musculoskeletal review, and assessment of body weight and condition. Blood may be collected from the right jugular vein for larger quantities and the wing vein for smaller samples.[14] Clinical pathology data from three common turaco species are provided in Table 25-1. Fecal examination should be done on a regular basis. Turaco feces are typically moist and soft to loose. Familiarity with normal turaco feces is helpful when determining if the bird has dehydration, diarrhea, or enteritis. Direct wet mount examination should be done to visualize protozoans; centrifugation of a flotation solution for checking for parasitic ova; and culture if an enteric pathogen is suspected. Cytologic staining (with Romanovsky's type, Gram, or acid-fast stain) of fecal smears is helpful if enteritis is suspected. Additional testing (for *Cryptosporidium* and *Giardia*; viral culture; electron microscopy) may be applied, where deemed necessary. Medications used to treat turacos are similar to those reported for other avian species. Turacos may be individually identified by a leg bracelet or a transponder chip placed in the left pectoral muscle mass.

TABLE 25-1

Representative ISIS Mean Blood Values for Three Turaco Species

Parameter	Units	*Musophaga rossae*	n	*Corythaixoides leucogaster*	n	*Tauraco erythrolophus*	n
WBC	x10³/mm³	10.7	95	11.9	33	7.2	32
RBC	x10⁶/mm³	3.13	39				
HGB	gm/dL	16.6	30				
HCT	%	47.8	94	47.6	34	43.4	38
Heterophils	x10³/mm³	3.74	93	4.47	33	3.45	32
Lymphocytes	x10³/mm³	5.02	93	5.46	33	2.55	30
Monocytes	x10³/mm³	0.82	83	0.94	27	0.47	28
Eosinophils	x10³/mm³	0.25	60	0.44	29		
Basophils	x10³/mm³	0.41	67			0.11	19
Glucose	mg/dL	279	91	269	32	278	34
BUN	mg/dL	3.0	41				
Uric acid	mg/dL	14.8	87	9.9	31	7.2	32
Calcium	mg/dL	9.4	90	10.2	31	9.1	35
Phosphorus	mg/dL	4.5	67			4	25
Na	meq/l	154	64			155	19
K	meq/l	2.3	58			3.4	18
Cl	meq/l	113	51			116	13
Cholesterol	mg/dL	158	65			174	23
Triglycerides	mg/dL	119	31				
Total protein	gm/dL	3.5	89	4.1	32	3.7	34
Albumin	gm/dL	1.3	63			1.7	30
Globulin	gm/dL	2.2	63			1.8	30
AST	IU/L	247	90	304	32	208	33
ALT	IU/L	37	46				
Total bilirubin	mg/dL	0.3	41				
Alk phosphatase	IU/L	85	59				
LDH	IU/L	729	39				
CPK	IU/L	289	65			266	25
GGT	IU/L	6	15				

From Teare JA, ed: 2013, *"Jambu Fruit Dove/Mauritius pink pigeon/Nicobar pigeon/Victoria crowned pigeon_No_selection_by_gender__All_ages _combined_Standard_International_Units__2013_CD.html" in* ISIS Physiological Reference Intervals for Captive Wildlife: A CD-ROM Resource., International Species Information System, Bloomington, MN.

SHIPMENT AND QUARANTINE

Prior to shipping, a thorough examination should be performed to make sure that the bird is healthy and will survive the shipping process. Shipping containers should meet or exceed International Air Transport Association (IATA) regulations. The bird should be placed under 30-day quarantine once it arrives at the receiving institution. During this time, it should be introduced to the new diet and observed for behavior, eating, drinking, and eliminations. Testing should include multiple fecal examinations (2–4) and treatment if positive; complete physical examination; blood collection for complete blood cell count (CBC) and biochemistry; body weight; and confirmation of identification. Prophylactic treatment for parasites is sometimes done during the quarantine period.

DISEASES

In general, turacos as a group appear to be fairly hardy birds but may be susceptible to diseases that affect other bird species. The Houston Zoo has housed over 1000 turacos of various species over the past 30 or more years. Review of the Houston Zoo antemortem and postmortem medical records and the literature has identified health problems that have affected this group of birds. Treatment is based on general avian medicine as no pharmacokinetic studies have been done in the Musophagidae. A basic summary of general causes of death in the Musophagidae collection at the Houston Zoo for the past 25 years (n = 193) has been listed in Table 25-2. This list reflects problems that may be found in the live birds of the collection that may be treated and is organized by age groups: perinatal and nestlings (0–30 days of age), fledglings and juvenile birds (1–11 months of age), and adults (1–28 years of age).

General health problems included aggression-induced trauma from cagemates and predators, leading to cuts, laceration, and possible death. Young birds are susceptible to dehydration and hypothermia, whereas older birds may present with issues of sepsis, amyloidosis, and unidentified diseases.

Digestive problems are common, ranging from *Candida* fungal infections, aerobic and anaerobic bacterial enteritis and sepsis[7] leading to possible morbidity, regurgitation, diarrhea, intussusception, and possible rectal or cloacal prolapses.[5] Foreign body ingestion or impaction from ingested materials with resulting intussusception

TABLE 25-2

General Summary of Turaco Deaths at the Houston Zoo 1988–2012 (N = 193)

Age Range	n	Category/Details
0–30 days	26	Digestive-enteritis, perforation, torsion, impaction, starvation
n = 95	25	General: trauma, sepsis, hypothermia, dehydration, neglect
	15	Unknown cause of death
	12	Musculoskeletal: rotational deformity, trauma, rickets, deformity
	8	Respiratory: pneumonia, tracheitis, asphyxiation, drowning
	6	Abnormal hatch, position, drowning
	1	Cardiac: necrosis, unknown
	1	Urogenital: renomegaly
	1	Neurologic: anencephaly
1–11 months	14	Digestive: enteritis, esophagitis, *Cryptosporidium*, perforation
n = 35	6	Respiratory: fungal, impacted trachea (self-feeding)
	5	Musculoskeletal: rotational deformity, rickets
	3	General: *Mycobacterium*, perforation
	2	Gout, visceral
	2	Unknown
	2	Euthanized following contact with *Mycobacterium*-positive birds
	1	Ocular: lens degeneration
1–28 years	28	General: sepsis (suspected), trauma, amyloid, *Mycobacterium*, unknown
n = 62	8	Digestive: enteritis, perforation, impaction, candidiasis, hepatic necrosis, esophagitis
	7	Respiratory: tracheal obstruction, dyspnea, sinusitis, pneumonia, lung hemorrhage, anesthetic
	6	Urogenital: egg binding, yolk peritonitis, kidney disease
	3	Integumentary: mycobacterium, neoplasia, dermatitis
	3	Musculoskeletal: rotational, frostbite
	3	Vascular: leukemia, lymphoma, hematoma
	3	Euthanasia because of issues related to age or quality of life
	1	Ocular: blindness, unknown etiology
	1	Cardiac: myonecrosis

has also been noted.[23] Hemosiderosis and issues related to iron storage in the liver have been previously documented in turacos,[23] although it does not seem to be common in the birds raised in the Houston Zoo. Endoparasites, including various nematodes and coccidia, as well as cryptosporidium protozoal infections, have been found in the Houston collection.*

Respiratory diseases vary widely, from tracheal obstruction, aspiration, and gaping (from parasites) causing dyspnea and distress to infections such as aspergillosis, bacterial sinusitis, and pneumonia.

*Tocidlowski, ME, Personal Communication, Houston Zoo, Inc., 2013.

Musculoskeletal problems may cause limping and lameness, and fractures may be found and repaired. Constriction by improperly fitting leg bands has occurred, and frostbite is possible from low temperatures. Rickets and rotational deformities may occur in young birds with inadequate diets.

Ectoparasites, broken feathers, broken nails, lacerations, bumble foot from inadequate perching, and rare skin masses have affected the integument.

Other miscellaneous diseases and medical issues include viral infections (avian influenza[13]), egg binding, ocular abnormalities (cataracts, corneal mineralization, trauma to the eyes or eye structures), otic issues (external ear infections), neurologic problems of unknown etiology (ataxia, head tilt), visceral gout, and hematologic issues (protozoan infections[2] and leukocytosis). Neoplasia seems to be rare in Musophagidae.

According to reports in the literature, captive turacos appear to be susceptible to mycobacterial infections.[3,17,24] At the Houston Zoo, 6 of 193 (3%) turaco deaths were attributed to *Mycobacterium* organisms. It seems that turacos may be susceptible to mycobacterial infection if exposed, but they do not appear to carry or harbor the bacterium any more than any other bird species.[4]

REPRODUCTION

Turacos become sexually active in their second year. Courtship may include vocalizing, chasing, mutual feeding, flashing, billing, and wing spreads. Both sexes participate in building a large, usually flimsy, twig-and-stick nest in a tree or platform provided. Two to three eggs are laid and incubated by both sexes. If eggs are pulled when the hen is done laying the clutch, she will usually reclutch. Incubation periods vary among the species, ranging from approximately 16 to 31 days. When chicks hatch, they are semi-precocial with downy feathering and open eyes and are well developed. Both sexes feed the chick by regurgitation of food. Chicks will start to fledge at about 2 to 3 weeks of age, but the parents will continue to feed the young for several months thereafter. Occasionally, one adult will become aggressive toward the chick or its mate and needs to be separated from the enclosure. Chicks may be raised successfully by one parent. Turacos in captivity are generally very tolerant of nest monitoring and invasion by staff, which is important to chick survival. At the Houston Zoo, young chicks and eggs have been cross-fostered to other pairs of turacos (not necessarily the same species) that were sitting on eggs or pulled for hand-raising.[20] One pair accepted additional eggs after sitting for only 6 days on its own eggs.[1]

NEONATOLOGY

Hatchling turaco chicks are active, gregarious birds. Attitude is one of the best monitoring tools for chick health. Turaco eggs hatch after an incubation ranging from as little as 16 to 18 days in *Tauraco hartlaubi*, 24 to 26 days in *Musophaga rossae*, and 29 to 31 days in *Corythaeola cristata*.[22] Eggs may be parent incubated and raised, fostered to other turaco pairs of the same or different species, or artificially incubated and hand raised. Turaco pairs are generally tolerant of some nest invasion to check on chicks, remove for weighing, supplementation, or treatment. It is suggested that chicks be closely monitored for the first few weeks to make sure that they do not succumb to illness or parental neglect. Body weight loss is common in the first 1 to 3 days, but chicks should grow at a constant rate after that. Details on turaco rearing have been previously documented.[1,6]

Chicks should be "bright-eyed," aware of human presence, sometimes vocalize, or try to bite. They often gape to take food from anyone offering it. If a turaco chick is subdued or looks "sleepy-eyed," a basic examination, weight evaluation, and diagnostics should be performed. Chicks are susceptible to digestive tract infections, so fecal cytology or swabs of the oral cavity, deep esophagus, and cloaca (if no feces available) should be evaluated for signs of fungal or bacterial overgrowth, particularly *Candida* or spore-forming bacteria. Other conditions that may arise include trauma from parents, parental neglect, poor doing, sepsis, and stunted growth of unknown etiology. Physical problems such as curled toes or rotated feet or legs should prompt evaluation of nest materials and positioning. Treatment for conditions that arise in turaco chicks is the same as that for other bird species.[8,16,25]

REFERENCES

1. Bailey H: How to grow a turaco. In *Proceedings of the Turaco and Cuckoo Workshop*, Tucson, AZ, 2002, Avian Scientific Advisory Group, AZA Regional Workshop, pp 28–42.
2. Bennett GF, Peirce MA: The haemoproteids of the avian orders Musophagiformes (the turacos) and Trogoniformes (the trogons). *Can J Zool* 68:2465–2467, 1990.
3. Brannian RE: Diseases of turacos, go-away birds, and plantain-eaters. In Fowler ME, editor: *Zoo and wild animal medicine*, ed 3, Philadelphia, PA, 1993, Saunders, pp 237–240.
4. Converse KA: Avian tuberculosis. In Thomas NJ, Hunter DB, Atkinson CT, editors: *Infections Diseases of Wild Birds*, Ames, IA, 2007, Blackwell Publishing, pp 289–302.
5. Cornelissen JM: Intussusception of the intestinal tract in the intestinal tract in a white-cheeked turaco. *J Avian Med Surg* 7:218–219, 1993.
6. Davis KJ: Turacos. In Gage LJ, Duerr R, editors: *Hand-rearing birds*, Ames, 2007, Blackwell Publishing, pp 289–295.
7. Dhillon AS, Shafar D: *Yersinia pseudotuberculosis* infection in two toco toucans and a turaco. *Proc Int Conf Zool Avian Med* 1:37–38, 1987.
8. Flammer K, Clubb SL: Neonatology. In *Avian medicine: Principles and applications*, Lake Worth, FL, 1994, Winger publishing Inc., pp 805–838.
9. Gamble KC: Musophagiformes (Turacos). In Fowler ME, editor: *Zoo and wild animal medicine*, ed 5, Philadelphia, PA, 2003, Saunders, pp 232–234.
10. Ingram K: Hummingbirds and miscellaneous orders. In Fowler ME, editor: *Zoo and wild animal medicine*, ed 2, Philadelphia, PA, 1986, Saunders, pp 448–466.
11. Johnston GB: Comparative anatomy of Musophagidae (Turacos). *AFA Watchbird* 43–45, 1999, Austin, Tx.
12. Johnston GB: Turacos, diet and gastrointestinal morphology. *Avicultur Soc Am Avicultur Bull* 27:10–15, 1998.
13. Lernould JM, Louzis C, Andral B: Influenza infection of turacos (Musophagidae). *Proc Int Symp Dis Zoo Anim* 26:363–368, 1984.
14. Phalen DN, Tocidlowski M, Faske JS: Turacos: Husbandry, management, and medical considerations. *Proc Assoc Avian Veterinarians* 187-203: 1999.
15. Sibley CG, Ahlquist JE, Monroe BL: A classification of the living birds of the world based on DNA-DNA hybridization studies. *Auk* 105(3):409–423, 1988.
16. St. Leger J: Nondomestic avian pediatric pathology. In Broome KK, Rupley AE, editors: *Veterinary clinics of North America: Exotic animal practice*, New York, 2012, Elsevier, pp 233–250.
17. Stamper MA, Norton T, Loomis M: Acid fast bacterial infection in four turacos. *J Avian Med Surg* 12(2):108–111, 1998.
18. Sun C, Moermond TC, Givnish TJ: Nutritional determinants of diet in three turacos in a tropical montane forest. *Auk* 114(2):200–211, 1997.
19. Teare JA, Teare Med. A.R.K.S: *International Species Information System*, version 5.54.e, Egan, MN, July 2012, ISIS.
20. Todd W: *Turaco TAG husbandry manual*, Houston, TX, 1998, Houston Zoological Gardens.
21. Turaco. (2013, January 11): In *Wikipedia, The Free Encyclopedia*: http://en.wikipedia.org/w/index.php?title=Turaco&oldid=532515542. Accessed January 16, 2013.
22. Turner DA: Family Musophagidae (turacos). In Del Hoyo J, Elliott A, Sargatal J, editors: *Handbook of the birds of the world*, vol 4, Barcelona, Spain, 1997, Lynx Edicions, pp 480–506.
23. Waine J: *Pathology and diseases of touracos*, 2000, International Touraco Society, pp 29–36.
24. Wilson SC, Carpenter JW, Veatch J: Investigation of suspected mycobacteriosis in a group of tropical birds at the Topeka Zoological Park. In *Proceedings of the American Association of Zoo Veterinarians*, 1994, pp 163–166.
25. Worell AB: Current trends in avian pediatrics. *J Exot Pet Med* 21:115–123, 2012.

CHAPTER 26

Trochiliformes (Hummingbirds)

Cornelia J. Ketz-Riley and Carlos R. Sanchez

BIOLOGY

Traditionally, hummingbirds were classified in the order Apodiformes.[27,28] According to the new SAM (Sibley/Ahlquist/ Monroe) classification using molecular techniques, hummingbirds are placed in their own order: Trochiliformes,[29] with the family Trochilidae, divided into two subfamilies, the Phaethornithinae (hermits) and the Trochilinae (typical hummingbirds). The Trochilidae family contains more than 335 species.[27,35]

In this chapter, we are focusing on the true hummingbirds. Most of them weigh between 6 and 12 grams (g) with the smallest, the bee hummingbird (*Mellisuga helenae*), weighing at 2 g and the giant hummingbird (*Patagona gigas*) at 20 g.[5] Hummingbirds are important pollinators of a number of plants, even being the only pollinators for some plants.[11,28] Free-ranging hummingbirds live between 6 to 12 years, but in captivity, they may live up to 17 years.[27,28,35] Hummingbirds, particularly males, are very colorful, with bright iridescent feathers on the tail, crest, and throat patches, the so-called *gorgets*.[27,29,35] Male hummingbirds are generally highly territorial and show impressive courtship displays.[27,28,35]

Hummingbirds are found only in the Western Hemisphere. Although their range extends far north to Alaska and Labrador in

Canada and to the Strait of Magellan in the south, they are predominately tropical and subtropical, with most of the species found in Brazil and Ecuador.[27,28] The status and population trends for most of the hummingbirds are listed as unknown by the International Union for the Conservation of Nature (IUCN).

ANATOMY AND PHYSIOLOGY

Hummingbirds have the highest metabolic rates relative to body size of any animal. Average temperature ranges from 36.5°C to 43.3°C, with around 39°C at resting. Resting respiratory rate is about 250 breaths per minute, up to 400 breaths per minute at flight. Normal heart rate is 500 to 600 beats per minute (beats/min) with up to 1260 beats/min during flight.[11,27,28] The heart is proportionally the largest among all birds, representing greater than 2% of the total body weight.[11,27,28]

Hummingbirds present a number of unique anatomic and physiologic adaptations. Long wings with long carpal and metacarpal bones and a very short, stout humerus bone, as well as a unique shallow cup-and-ball joint that attaches the coracoid bones to the sternum,[28,33,35] enable the hummingbird to hover in the air and to fly forward and backward.[5,28,29] They may reach speeds up to 15 meters per second (m/sec; 54 kilometers per hour [km/hr]) during flight and flap their wings 12 to 80 times per second while hovering.

Hummingbirds have an extendable tongue that forms two parallel C-shaped grooves of keratinized membranes around a rigid supporting rod with a bifurcated end (Figure 26-1).[13] The grooves function like rods, drawing nectar via capillary action, but also like a fluid trap for the nectar.[12,25,28,29]

Gastrointestinal Tract and Energy Metabolism

The digestive tract of hummingbirds includes a small crop and a short intestinal tract and lacks a cecum and a gallbladder. The crop

emptying time of about 4 minutes is the rate-limiting factor in hummingbird feeding. During an intestinal transit time of about 15 minutes, 99% of ingested glucose is absorbed.[12,16] The flight muscles are composed mostly of fast oxidative-glycolytic fibers, allowing the bird to sustain high aerobic power.[33] Mitochondria in hummingbird muscles are able to oxidize carbohydrates equally well as fat.[34] The carbohydrate oxidation of newly consumed nectar supports the high adenosine triphosphate (ATP) demands during short-term hovering flight.[34] Fat oxidation is selected during long migratory flights.[34] To prepare for long-distance migration, hummingbirds may rapidly gain as much as 72% of their body weight in fat. Their liver is one of the most metabolically active known, with the highest levels of enzymes for lipid synthesis.[22,32]

Most hummingbirds seem to have the ability to use arthropods as an alternative energy source when access to floral nectar is scarce.[23]

Energy Conservation

To conserve energy, hummingbirds spend the majority of their day sitting or perching and only an estimated 10% of their day-time flying and hovering while feeding in short meals.

Another effective way to save energy during cold nights or prior to migration is going into a torpor.[9,16,28,29] The metabolic rate may drop to one fifteenth of its normal rate,[29] body temperature as low as 8°C, the heartbeat reduces to 30 to 50 beats/min and the respiratory rate lowers to 50 breaths per minute with apnea episodes of up to 5 minutes.[11,21,28] The birds are cold to the touch; they perch with fluffed feathers and closed eyes and their bill pointed straight up. When in torpor, the birds barely respond to stimuli or seem uncoordinated.[21,31]

Osmoregulation

Hummingbirds depend almost entirely on a liquid diet of floral nectar. To meet their metabolic demands, they may consume more than three times their body mass in fluid per day.[2] The high

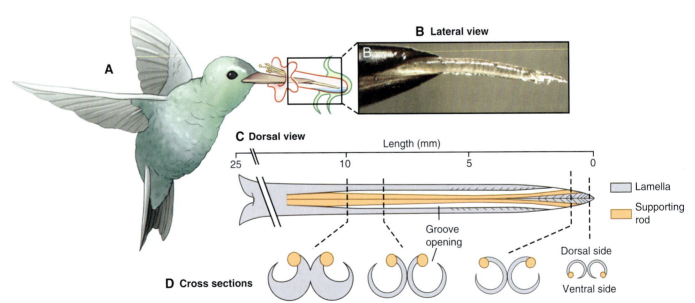

FIGURE 26-1 **Hummingbird tongues. A,** Nectarivores use their tongue (yellow) for food gathering. **B,** Lateral picture of a postmortem ruby-throated hummingbird tongue tip protruding from the bill. **C,** Dorsal view of the morphology of a hummingbird tongue showing open-sided grooves and lamellar region of the tip (approximately 6 millimeters [mm]). Base of the tongue is to the left. **D,** Cross-sectioning of the distal tongue; green arrows identify the placement of the cross-sections. Black lines indicate the same structures in dorsal and cross-sectional views. Note the position of supporting rods from the base of the grooves to the tongue. Unlabeled scale bars, 0.5 mm. (Used with permission from Rico-Guevara A, Rubega M: The hummingbird tongue is a fluid trap, not a capillary tube. *PNAS* 108(23):9356–9360, 2011.)

metabolism depends on an efficient way to extract energy and nutrients from this liquid diet. Processing a large quantity of water for energy coverage requires highly specialized kidneys and gastrointestinal tract.[2,9,18] In hummingbirds, more than 99% of nephrons do not possess a Henle loop and cannot concentrate urine.[4,15] Hummingbird kidneys are structurally similar to those of reptilians and their waterflux rate close to that of amphibians, and these birds are still able to maintain a high metabolic level of an endotherm animal, which makes them very unique animals.[2,9,10,15,16]

Nervous System

Hummingbirds have a large head in relationship to the body, with one of the relatively largest brains of any bird species.[36] Because of an enlarged hippocampus, hummingbirds are able to remember spatial location and distribution of high-nectar flowers.[35]

SPECIAL HOUSING REQUIREMENTS

Since males of many species are highly territorial around their food sources, multiple feeding stations should be available on exhibit. One station for every two birds has been reported to be adequate.[21] Feeding stations should be in open areas to allow free flight and aerial displays. Optimal ambient temperatures depend on the species. Generally, species from temperate zones are more cold tolerant compared with tropical and subtropical species.

Ideally, hummingbird aviaries should be supplied with extensive planting for perching and hiding places. Water should be available in the form of streams, waterfalls, or a pond to provide ample water access. Otherwise, bathing can be encouraged by providing shallow water bowls or daily misting or hosing of the foliage.[21,31] Shelter from extreme weather conditions as well as from aggressive conspecifics needs to be available. If mixed with other bird species, the other birds should be of similar size and not very territorial. Any windows of the enclosure should be positioned on a slight downward angle and preferably covered with branches. Feeding stations, water features or bird-attractive plants or flowers should be placed either more than 30 feet from any window or within 3 feet because of reduced velocity within this short distance. Small enclosures of about 3 to 5 feet long by 1.25 to 1.75 feet deep and 2 feet high are possible for individual housing or introduction.

FEEDING

Hummingbirds are specialized nectarivores that feed mainly on floral nectar containing basically sucrose, glucose, and fructose.[16] The remaining diet consists of arthropods as the main source of protein.[28,29,31] Consumption of sand and ash by female hummingbirds is possibly associated with higher mineral requirements during reproductive activity.[31] Many of the plants pollinated by hummingbirds are bright red, yellow, or orange in color and have long, tubular corollas and little or no scent. The shape of the bill in a hummingbird determines the species of flowers from which it may obtain nectar.[11,29,30] Published lists of adequate flowers for the various hummingbird species should be consulted for proper planting in hummingbird aviaries.[11,31] These flowers should provide low nutrient diets with minimum of 20% sugar and at least 3% protein.[3,19,21] A commercial diet or regular table sugar, at 1 part to 4 parts of water, have been successfully used in zoologic collections but should only be used as a supplement to natural flower nectar. Fruit flies or other small insects should be available as an additional protein source.[3,19,21] Honey should not be used as part of the diet because of its rapid fermentation that allows bacterial and yeast (*Candida*) overgrowth. The addition of any coloring to the nectar seems unnecessary, as hummingbirds are more attracted to visual beacons than to color. The added dye could potentially cause deleterious health effects.

Hummingbird diets provide a rich growth medium for microbes. To avoid fermentation, feeders should be protected from direct sunlight, frequently replaced, and thoroughly cleaned.

PHYSICAL RESTRAINT AND HANDLING

Hummingbirds are not easy to capture because of their speed and maneuverability. In the wild and large areas, mist nets may be used, and in smaller enclosures small hand nets are useful. However, extreme caution should be taken to avoid injuries. Darkening the room may help with capture. A simple method to trap hummingbirds is the use of a pull-string trap with a feeder inside to attract the hummingbird. The bird may then be manually restrained by using cupped hands gently restricting the movement of the wings. Hummingbirds may be transported in wooden boxes after loosely wrapping them in cloth jackets with their heads exposed for frequent feeding.[1,21,31]

SURGERY AND ANESTHESIA

Inhalation anesthesia is the preferred method for anesthesia. Isoflurane remains the most common gas anesthetic used in avian species, but sevoflurane and desflurane also may be used.[8] Induction is achieved by manual restraint and delivery of the gas via a custom-fit face mask.

The most common indication for surgical procedures is the repair of skeletal fractures. Tape splints are often used to repair long-bone fractures.[21] Cloth jackets are useful to immobilize the bird and potentially allow wing fractures to heal. Hummingbirds should be fed frequently during hospitalization.[31]

DIAGNOSTICS

Mammography radiography provides a greater detail and quality compared with digital radiography or standard radiography, so their use is the technique of choice for hummingbirds.[14]

Phlebotomy on hummingbirds is performed as in other bird species, via the jugular vein or the femoral vein or artery.[21,31] Toe-nail clipping should only be considered as the last resort or during field studies.[9,10] Up to 20 microliters (μL) of blood may be safely collected on a 4.5-g hummingbird, which may be used to evaluate cell counts and morphology via blood smears.[21] The erythrocytes of hummingbirds are minuscule and have the highest density for any bird.[11]

Hummingbird fecal matter is normally liquid and should be free from *Enterobacteriacae* bacteria.[26]

DISEASES

Reviews of necropsy reports have revealed no unique cause of death for this group. Of 50 hummingbird deaths, cause of death was noninfectious in 44%, infectious in 52%, and undetermined in 4% (Northwest ZooPath, Smithsonian National Zoological Park, unpublished data).

Infectious Disease

The most commonly reported infectious disease in hummingbirds is oral candidiasis with characteristic oral white plaques. The lesions may cause inability to swallow or regurgitate, leading to inanition. Tongue necrosis and beak deformities may further prevent the animal from feeding.[21,31] Diagnosis and treatment with nystatin or other antifungal agents are similar to those in other avian species.

Other infectious diseases reported on hummingbirds are chlamydiasis, mycobacteriosis, salmonellosis, aspergillosis, and other fungal diseases (Table 26-1).[20,21,27,31]

Avian poxvirus has recently been reported for the first time in hummingbirds. Wartlike lesions, confirmed as pox with polymerase chain reaction (PCR), electron microscopy (EM), and histopathology, were found at the base of the bill, wings, and legs in free-ranging Anna's hummingbird (*Calypte anna*) (Figure 26-2).[7]

Parasitic Diseases

Nectar mites that are transported by hummingbirds in their nasal cavities from flower to flower should not be considered parasites.[28]

TABLE 26-1

Selected Infectious Diseases of Hummingbirds

Disease	Causative Agent	Epizootiology	Clinical Signs	Diagnosis	Management
Candidiasis	*Candida albicans*	Poor sanitation immunosuppression	White raised plaques with catarrhal-mucoid exudates in oral cavity, crop, esophagus; dysphagia, regurgitation; tongue and beak necrosis	Direct smear	Antifungal agents, hygiene, supportive care
Salmonellosis	*Salmonella* sp.	Poor sanitation	Gastroenteritis	Culture	Antibiotics
Tuberculosis	*Mycobacterium avium, M. intracellulare,* possibly other spp.	Poor sanitation	Emaciation, weakness, dyspnea	Histopathology, acid-fast stain; culture, polymerase chain reaction test	Sanitation; depopulation
Aspergillosis	*Aspergillus* sp.	Poor sanitation	Dyspnea, weakness	Direct smear, culture; histopathology	Sanitation; antifungal agents

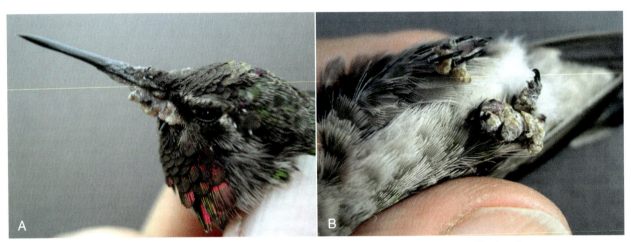

FIGURE 26-2 A, Anna's hummingbird (*Calypte anna*) with pox lesions on skin around beak and eyes. **B,** Anna's hummingbird (*Calypte anna*) with pox lesions on skin of legs and feet. (From Godoy LA, Dalbeck LS, Tell LA, et al: Characterization of avian poxvirus in Anna's Hummingbird [Calypte Anna] in California, USA, Journal of Wildlife Diseases 49:978-985, 2013.)

Other external parasites such as feather mites and enteric parasites have been found in hummingbirds, but parasite-related diseases are not common among these birds.[21,31] Adverse reaction to ivermectin diluted with propylene glycol has been described in emerald hummingbirds (*Amazilia amazilia*).[26,31] The affected birds showed central nervous system depression and seizures that were responsive to steroid and supportive treatment.[31]

Noninfectious Disease

Trauma and inanition were the most common noninfectious causes of death, according to the review of necropsy reports. Injuries to the keel are highly likely to heal, whereas trauma to the head or neck has a rather poor prognosis.

Nutritional Disorders

Inanition is most common in captive hummingbirds with limited access to feeders or lack of protein supplementation.

Migratory species may be prone to hepatic lipidosis because of lack of exercise and high caloric intake. Treatment includes diet change and increase in exercise, as well as administration of choline, methionine, vitamin B$_{12}$, or inositol via a nectar diet.[21]

Lysosomal storage disease has been reported in three captive Costa's Hummingbirds. Two of the birds showed neurologic signs before death. Treatment is symptomatic.[24]

Hummingbirds may be susceptible to iron toxicosis because of exposure to high-iron diets. It is recommended that the diet for hummingbirds contain less than 20 milligram per kilogram (mg/kg) of iron.[6] Nectar diets should be chosen carefully, as many products show levels above 20 mg/kg.[6] White sugar should be used for nectar preparation, as brown sugar contains molasses with iron.

REPRODUCTION

Most hummingbird species are polygynous and only gather for courtship and copulation. They normally hatch two white eggs in cup-shaped nests and have two to three clutches per season.[29,36] Females incubate the eggs for 13 to 19 days. They leave the nest very frequently for food intake. Fluctuating temperatures do not seem to interfere with normal egg development.[17] Chicks are altricial, with eyes closed and almost no feathers. Females feed their young with nectar and small insects twice per hour until the chicks fledge at 20 to 35 days.[11,29]

ACKNOWLEDGMENTS

The authors would like to thank Drs. Michael Garner and Timothy Walsh for their help with this chapter.

REFERENCES

1. Bailey TA: Capture and handling. In Samour J, editor: *Avian medicine*, London, U.K., 2000, Mosby.
2. Beuchat CA, Calder WA, III, Braun EJ: The integration of osmoregulation and energy balance in hummingbirds. *Physiol Zool* 63(6):1059–1081, 1990.
3. Brice AT, Grau CR: Hummingbird nutrition: Development of a purified diet for long term maintenance. *Zoo Biol* 2:233–238, 1989.
4. Casotti G, Beuchat C, Braun EJ: Morphology of the kidney in a nectarivorous bird, the Anna's hummingbird, *Calypte anna*. *J Zool Lond* 244:175–184, 1998.
5. Fernandez JM, Dudley R, Bozinovi F: Comparative energetic of the Giant hummingbird (*Patagonia gigas*). *Physiol Biochem Zool* 84(3):333–340, 2011.
6. Frederick H, Dierenfeld E, Irlbeck N, et al: Analysis of nectar replacement products and a case of iron toxicosis in hummingbirds. *NAG Proc* 38–43, 2003.
7. Godoy LA, Dalbeck LS, Tell LA, et al: Characterization of avian poxvirus in Anna's hummingbird (*Calypte anna*) in California, USA. *J Wildl Dis* 49(4):978–985, 2013.
8. Granone TD, de Francisco ON, Killos MB, et al: Comparison of three different inhalant anesthetic agents (isoflurane, sevoflurane, desflurane) in red-tailed hawks (*Buteo jamaicensis*). *Vet Anaesth Analg* 39(1):29–37, 2012.
9. Hargrove J: Adipose energy stores, physical work, and the metabolic syndrome: Lessons from hummingbirds. *Nutr J* 4:36, 2005.
10. Hartman Bakken H, Sabat P: Gastrointestinal and renal responses to water intake in the green-backed firecrown (*Sephanoides sephanoides*), a South American hummingbird. *Am J Physiol Regul Integr Comp Physiol* 291:830–836, 2006.
11. Johnsgard PL: *The hummingbirds of North America*, ed 2, Washington, D.C., 1997, Smithsonian Institution Press.
12. Karasow WH, Phan D, Sando J, et al: Food passage and intestinal nutrient absorption in hummingbirds. *Auk* 103(3):453–464, 1986.
13. Kim W, Peaudecerf F, Baldwin M, et al: The hummingbird's tongue: a self-assembling capillary syphon. *R Soc B Proc* 279:4990–4996, 2012.
14. Krautwald-Junghans ME: Birds. In Pees M, Reese S, Tully T, editors: *Diagnostic imaging of exotic pets: Birds, small mammals, reptiles*, Hannover, Germany, 2011, Schlütersche.
15. Lotz C, Martinez del Rio C: The ability of rufous hummingbird *Selasphorus rufus* to dilute and concentrate urine. *J Avian Biol* 35:54–62, 2004.
16. Martinez del Rio C, Schondube JE, McWhorter TJ, et al: Intake responses in nectar feeding birds: digestive and metabolic causes, osmoregulatory consequences and coevolutionary effects. *Am Zool* 41:902–915, 2001.
17. Masters Vleck C: Hummingbird incubation: Female attentiveness and egg temperature. *Oecology* 51(2):199–205, 1981.
18. McWhorter TJ, Martinez del Rio C: Does gut function limit hummingbird food intake? *Physiol Biochem Zool* 73(3):313–324, 2000.
19. Meadows MG, Roudybush TE, McGraw KJ: Dietary protein level affects iridescent coloration in Anna's hummingbird, *Calypte anna*. *J Exp Biol* 215:2742–2750, 2012.
20. Meteyer CU, Chin RP, Castro AE, et al: An epizootic of chlamydiosis with high mortality in a captive population of euphonias (*Euphonia violaceas*) and hummingbirds (*Amazilia amazilias*). *J Zoo Wildl Med* 23(2):222–229, 1992.
21. Orr K: Trochiliformes (Hummingbirds). In Fowler ME, Cubas ZS, editors: *Biology, medicine and surgery of South American wild animals*, Ames, IA, 2001, Iowa State University Press.
22. Powers DR, Nagy KA: Field metabolic rate and food consumption by free-living Anna's hummingbirds (*Calypte anna*). *Physiol Zool* 61(6):500–506, 1988.
23. Powers DR, Van Hook A, Sandlin EA, et al: Arthropod foraging by a southeastern Arizona hummingbird guild. *Wilson J Ornithol* 122(3):494, 2010.
24. Proudfoot JS, Garner MG, Prieur D, et al: Lysosomal storage disease in Costa's hummingbirds (*Calypte costae*). *AAZV/IAAAM Proc* 305–306, 2000.
25. Rico-Guevara A, Rubega M: The hummingbird tongue is a fluid trap, not a capillary tube. *PNAS* 108(23):9356–9360, 2011.
26. Ritchie BW, Harrison GJ: Formulary. In Ritchie BW, Harrison GJ, Harrison LR, editors: *Avian medicine: Principles and application*, Lake Worth, FL, 1994, Wingers Publishing.
27. Saldenberg AB, Teixeira RH, Astofli-Ferreira SC, et al: *Serratia marcescens* infection in a Swallow-tailed hummingbird. *J Wildl Dis* 43(1):107–110, 2007.
28. Sargent R, Sargent M: Hummingbirds. In Elphick C, Dunning J, Sibley D, editors: *The Sibley guide to bird life and behavior*, New York, 2001, Alfred A. Knopf.
29. Schuchmann K: Family Trochilidae. In Del Hoyo J, Elliott A, Jordi S, editors: *Handbook of the birds of the world*, vol. 5, Barcelona, Spain, 1999, Lynx Edicions.
30. Sibley CG, Ahlquist JE: *Phylogeny and classification of birds*, New Haven, CT, 1990, Yale University Press.
31. Shima A: Trochiliformes (Hummingbirds). In Fowler ME, Miller RE, editors: *Zoo and wild animal medicine*, ed 5, St. Louis, MO, 2003, Saunders.
32. Suarez RK, Brown GS, Ho-Chachka PW: Metabolic sources of energy for hummingbird flight. *Am J Physiol* 251(20):R537–R542, 1986.
33. Ward BJ, Day LB, Wilkening SR, et al: Hummingbirds have a greatly enlarged hippocampal formation. *Biol Lett* 8(4):657–659, 2012.
34. Warrick D, Hedrick T, Fernandez MJ, et al: Hummingbird flight. *Curr Biol* 22(12):472–477, 2012.
35. Welch KC, Jr, Hartman Bakken B, Martínez del Rio C, et al: Hummingbirds fuel hovering flight with newly ingested sugar. *Physiol Biochem Zool* 79(6):1082–1087, 2006.
36. West GC, Butler C: *Do hummingbirds hum? Fascinating answers to questions about hummingbirds*, Piscataway, NJ, 2010, Rutgers University Press.

CHAPTER 27

Apodiformes and Coliiformes

Carlos R. Sanchez

TAXONOMY AND BIOLOGY

For the past 150 years, the taxonomic classification of the order Apodiformes has included three living families: Apodidae (Swifts), Hemiprocnidae (treeswifts), and Trochilidae (hummingbirds).[6,8,10,11,26] New studies on molecular evolution have revealed that swifts and hummingbirds diverged in recent times from one another; accordingly, hummingbirds were placed in their own order: Trochiliformes.[8,22] This chapter will discuss Apodidae and Hemiprocnidae families only.

The divisions within the Apodidae family remain uncertain, but two subfamilies are generally recognized: (1) the Cypseloidinae with 13 species (primitive American swifts) and (2) the Apodinae with 79 species in three tribes: Collocaliini, Chaeturini, and Apodini (swiftlets, needletails [or spinetails], and typical swifts, respectively).[8,21] An important distinction between these three tribes is that only the swiftlets and the typical swifts use saliva to glue building materials together to make rudimentary nests. None of the Cypseloidinae species uses saliva for this purpose. Apodidae species are found on all continents but Antarctica and inhabit mostly in tropical and temperate areas and close to water with an abundance of insects.[6,8] The species that breed outside the tropics are forced to migrate over long distances because of the extreme seasonal variability of insect abundance in the temperate zones. Swifts present considerable variations in size. The smallest swiftlet (the pygmy swiftlet) weighs only 5.4 grams (g) and measures 9 centimeters (cm) long, whereas the largest one (the purple needletail) weighs 184 g and measures 25 cm.[7] The plumage of swiftlets is a dull light brown color, and these birds are considered one of the most aerial of all birds, eating, bathing, drinking, roosting, and possibly even copulating in midair.[8,17] They possess a small beak but a large gape that facilitates the aerial capture of flying insects. These small birds are long lived, with life-span reported up to 26 years.[8]

The Hemiprocnidae family comprises one genus with four species of treeswifts also referred as crested swifts. They are distributed from India and South East Asia through Indonesia to New Guinea, the Philippines, and the Solomon Islands. Treeswifts exhibit a wide range of habitat preferences, from deciduous savannah to evergreen rainforest. They differ from other swifts in that their plumage is softer and glossy and they possess long wingtips and long forked tails. Some of them have crests or other facial plumes.[7] Slightly larger than most swifts, their total length ranges from 15 to 31 cm, with weights ranging from 21 to 80 g.[21,26]

The order Coliiformes consists of one family (Coliidae) and six species of mousebirds; they are alternatively referred as *coly* and *colies*. They are found in sub-Saharan Africa, and this order is the sole order of birds restricted to the Afro-tropical region.[10] All mousebirds measure 28 to 40 cm from the tip of the beak to the tip of the tail, weighing between 40 and 70 g.[9] Their plumage is soft, and their tails are slender and long (up to two thirds of the total length of the bird); the two central tail feathers are further elongated. In some species, the tail is so elongated and stiff that it resembles the tail of a rodent.[6] This characteristic and their sneaky movements through vegetation, similar to small rodents, give them the name "mousebird." A unique feature of this group is the way they perch or "hang." They suspend their bodies vertically with their tails pointing downward with their feet widely splayed at the level of the upper breast or neck area while keeping their heads right side up.[9,10] It is their sleeping position of choice. Mousebirds are one of the few groups of birds that do not possess feather tracts.

Status and Conservation

The International Union for the Conservation of Nature (IUCN) *Red List of Threatened Species* lists the status for all mousebirds and treeswifts species to be of "Least Concern," with most of their population trends as stable or increasing.

Of the 101 species of swift listed, only 11 are either near threatened or vulnerable. The Guam swiftlet (*Collocalia bartschi*) is classified as endangered because it has undergone a rapid population decline, presumably owing to pesticide use and predation by the introduced brown tree snake to Guam. Because of their dependence on trees for nesting, factors that affect the wild population of certain swift species in the Western Hemisphere include mortality caused by insect outbreaks and disease, tree harvesting, wildfire, climatic shifts, and habitat changes in the winter range.[5]

UNIQUE ANATOMY

Apodiformes possess several unique anatomic features. Like their close relatives from the family Throchilidae (hummingbirds and hermits), they have small feet that are used to perch but are not useful for walking or climbing. Although small, their feet have great strength; this, together with the sharpness of their curved nails, the calluses on their tarsi, and the stiff tail feathers, allows them to grip onto vertical surfaces. The primitive American swifts (Cypseloidinae), the swiftlets (Collocaliini), and the needletails (Chaeturini) have anisodactyl feet, in which the hallux is directed backward, whereas the second, third, and fourth digits are directed forward.[8] In the typical grasping position, all Apodinae have their hallux and second digit spread medially and oppose the third and fourth digits, which are spread laterally as in the grasping positions of chameleons and koalas.[8] Half or more of the long wing is composed of a long carpus, metacarpus, and phalanx bones. In contrast, they have remarkably short humerus, radius, and ulna. Also, as in hummingbirds, their coracoid is strong and is attached to the sternum by a unique shallow cup-and-ball joint.[6,17,21] The long carpometacarpus supports 9 or 10 long primary feathers and a group of 8 to 11 shorter secondary feathers.[8] All of these birds have a claw on the manus. Swifts have no ingluvia (crop) or ceca, but a gall bladder is present.[21,22]

The main difference between treeswifts and the typical apodid swifts is that treeswifts have a nonreversible hallux that allows them to perch on branches and twigs. Treeswifts lack the claw on the manus. Their tails have a deep fork, accounting for 45% to 70% of the tail length; this is considerably larger than that of the typical swift.[26]

Mousebirds are classified in their own group (Coliiformes) because they have some unique anatomic features not found on any other birds. Thanks to a special arrangement of muscles and tendons, including two small inner muscles unique to the group and an extension to the hallux of the extensor digitorum longus, they have an incredibly flexible foot structure, which allows them to oppose one or two toes or to turn all four forward.[6,10,22] The position of the toes may change continually and may be different in either foot at the same time. With all four digits pointing forward, a mousebird may hang from a twig, or with the toes facing in opposite directions, it may grasp and perch; the position of the toes change very rapidly, accounting for some of the sudden movements only mousebirds can make. This is the equivalent of having anisodactyl, zygodactyl, or pamprodactyl feet all at once.[10] Another unique anatomic feature is the presence of an "anatomic device," similar to the ones bats have, which allows them to perch without any additional energy expenditure. The thick flexor tendons of the toes are covered with striated epithelium and pass through a grooved sheath that restrains slippage. These tendons do not insert at the bases of the outer phalanges but do so more distally; so when the leg is flexed, the claws move downward and automatically "engage" in grasping position.[10] This mechanism is so effective that dead birds have been found still perched. Their wings have 10 primaries and 10 ancillary feathers; they do not possess down feathers. Their intestinal tract is short and wide, lacking ceca as might be expected of frugivores birds.

SPECIAL PHYSIOLOGY

Members of the Apodidae family show several physiologic adaptations to high-altitude flying. Their erythrocytes are larger than those of other bird species, facilitating oxygen exchange. Their hemoglobin is sensitized for optimal delivery of oxygen in conditions of low oxygen pressure, and their oxygen affinities are higher than in other small species of birds such as passerines.[8,19] Similarly, the erythrocytes of mousebirds are noticeably larger (in length, width, and volume) than those of other birds. The hemoglobin content per erythrocyte is relatively low in mousebirds.[2]

Torpor has been reported in a number of Apodiformes and Coliiformes species.[9,14,17,20,21] Like hummingbirds, they use torpor as a way to save energy during cold nights, when food is scarce, or prior to migration. It is a hibernation-like state, in which their metabolic rate is reduced down to one fifteenth of its normal rate, thus saving up to 60% of energy expenditure. During torpor, their heart rate is reduced by about 20%, and cardiac output decreases by around 50%; body temperature may decrease down to 18° C.[2,10,21] Apodiformes and Coliiformes are capable of spontaneous arousal from this torpid state.

In addition to torpor, Coliiformes present behavioral traits associated with evolutionary thermal physiology. Clustering and sun bathing, or sunning, along with torpor, ensure the survival of the mousebird in harsh environments, particularly because their food is of very low caloric value and sometimes is scarce. During sun bathing, they fluff their feathers, exposing their heavily pigmented skin to the sun, spread their wings in an arc, and stretch and tilt their backs exposing the ventral surface of their bodies to solar radiation.[9,10] Irrespective of weather conditions, it is common to see mousebirds hanging from branches in clusters of half a dozen to a dozen birds or more. Sometimes, in harsh conditions, several clusters form one ball. Mousebirds sleep, belly to belly against each other, with the head hunched between the shoulders, minimizing the body surface area exposure to climate elements. Clustering behavior allows mousebirds to save up to 50% of energy expenditure.[10,21]

SPECIAL HOUSING REQUIREMENTS

Because of their almost exclusive aerial existence and feeding habitats, swifts are not at all suited for captivity.[17] Swifts need a large open space for flying to be aerobically fit at release time. For rehabilitation of swift fledgling, individuals should be placed in an artificial chimney inside an outdoor flight cage (24 feet long, 12 feet wide, and 8 feet high). Screen netting, textured plywood, or a combination of both is required on the interior for clinging.

Mousebirds use clustering to save energy and share body heat, as they are susceptible to cold temperatures. This must be taken into consideration when housing Coliiformes, particularly if housing a single individual. Supplemental heat is recommended for groups of mousebirds and is mandatory for single birds kept outside in other than mild weather.[9]

FEEDING

In the wild, all species of swifts feed exclusively on insects and spiders, although exact details of what prey are taken has not been studied in detail for most species.[8] Their beaks are small, but these birds have a wide gape that allows them to catch insects while they are on the wing with their mouths open. Many of the swifts pursue their food at great heights, and therefore a proper feeding environment is difficult to reproduce in captivity. When in captivity, swifts should ideally be offered harvested *Diptera* flies. Other insects that may be used for the diet of swifts during rehabilitation include silent crickets, brown crickets (both with the legs removed), greater wax moth larva, and mealworms, along with vitamin and mineral supplements. Treeswifts are aerial feeders, but little is known of specific prey they catch. Treeswifts eat flying insects such as bees, beetles, wasps, small flies, and termites. In addition to these insects, the moustached treeswift (*Hemiprocne mystacea*) is reported to consume ants.[26] It is not understood how treeswifts deal with bee venom.

Mousebirds diets are not highly specialized; they feed mainly on many types of fruits, but they also eat buds, flowers, shoots, leaves, and nectar, as well as insects such as aphids.[10] Native, non-native, and even ornamental plants and plant parts are consumed. Although ingestion of eggs and nestlings of other birds has been reported in the wild, mousebirds in captivity do not appear to show interest in animal products other than ant pupae, which they occasionally feed to their chicks.[6,10] Coprophagy is normal behavior; the adults will consume their offspring's feces, and a mixture of regurgitated food and feces is fed back to the nestlings.[9] In captivity, mousebirds are easy to feed because of their non-specialized diet. They are hardy eaters, and even wild-caught animals are easy to transition to captive diets. Because these birds are mainly frugivorous, chopped fruit should be the basis of their diet. It is recommended that a mixture of at least five types of fruits and vegetable plus pellets be offered daily; ripe pears and grapes are reported to be some of their favorites. Commercial pellets should be medium sized and low in iron. A single brand or a mix of brands may be used, and the food may be served dry or soaked in water or fruit juice.[9,21] Mealworms and waxworms may be added a few times a week to the diet. Hard-boiled egg, mashed and mixed together with other food, as a source of calcium, vitamins, and protein, has been recommended for aviculturists during the breeding season.[9]

RESTRAINT AND HANDLING

Gentle manual restraint is adequate for Apodiformes and Coliiformes. As with other species of birds, darkening the room will be helpful in capturing these species.

SURGERY AND ANESTHESIA

Gas anesthesia (isoflurane or sevoflurane) is the preferred method for induction and maintenance of anesthesia in Apodiformes and Coliiformes. To avoid trauma during induction in a chamber, it is better to manually restrain the bird and deliver the gas via a homemade face mask (e.g., modified syringe-case). It has been speculated that mousebirds may be particularly sensitive to inhalant anesthesia, as evidenced by associated high mortality during anesthetic procedures, but further scientific documentation is needed to support this assumption.[9]

Swifts suffer skeletal fractures frequently when flying onto objects, and the most common surgical procedure in this group is the repair of these fractures. Because of their high-altitude flying, swifts must recover full flying capabilities to be released back into the wild. With the exception of radius or ulna fractures, most other wing bone fractures, as well as coracoid, clavicle, and scapula fractures have a poor prognosis, and euthanasia should be considered. For the repair of radius and ulna fractures a combination of 0.4- to 0.5-millimeter (mm) intramedullary pins and "figure-of-eight" bandages have been successfully used. Once the fracture is healed, physiotherapy must follow. Tape splinting is the most common technique used to repair leg fractures.

Leg and foot injuries are not uncommon in mousebirds because of their tendency to hang and their strong grip. Severe lacerations, non-reparable luxations, and exposed fractures may require amputation of the affected digit, foot, or leg. Surgical amputation techniques are similar to the ones used in any other bird. Mousebirds cope well once the amputation site has healed. Standard avian techniques for bone fracture repair apply for uncomplicated fractures.

DIAGNOSTICS

For most species of Apodiformes and Coliiformes, the most common venipuncture site is the jugular vein. In larger individuals, the ulnar or brachial veins are additional options. The erythrocytes of Coliiformes and Apodiformes are larger in length, width, and volume than in most other bird species.[8,19] Hematologic and biochemical parameters for selected species of mousebirds are available in the previous edition of this book as well as in the International Species Information System (ISIS) reference range database.

Traditional radiography and digital radiography are routinely used in avian practice. For members of the Apodidae and Hemiprocnidae families with a body weight less than 40 g, digital radiography is not adequate.[18] Mammography units or mammography film with standard units provide better film details and better-quality films for the smaller species.

DISEASES

Swifts are rarely kept in captivity, and therefore the scientific literature on swift diseases is limited. Most swifts brought to rehabilitation centers present with trauma, malnutrition, or a combination of both.

One review of captive mousebird necropsies revealed trauma as the most important cause of death. Of the 168 mousebird deaths, 59% had noninfectious causes, 36% had infectious causes, and 5% had undetermined causes (Northwest ZooPath, unpublished data). These results are similar to another review of 21 mousebird deaths, in which 62% of the causes of death were noninfectious, 19% infectious, and 19% undetermined.[15]

Infectious Disease

No infectious diseases are unique to Apodiformes or Coliiformes. During rehabilitation, swifts have a high propensity to aspergillosis and candidiasis, both likely associated to improper husbandry, poor feeding techniques, or inadequate usage of antibiotics. Standard diagnosis and therapeutic approaches used for other avian species are used in these birds as well. Significant mortality in little swifts (*Apus affinis*) was caused by *Erysipelothrix rhusiopathiae*–associated septicemia; the origin of the infection was suspected to be the ingestion of water from contaminated sewage.[25] The common swift (*Apus apus*) has been implicated in the introduction, amplification, and spread of West Nile virus in France.[1]

Salmonellosis has been reported in mousebirds but *Salmonella* ssp. also appears to be commonly isolated from healthy blue-naped mousebirds (*Urocolius macrourus*).[21] Other cloacal isolates from clinically normal mousebirds include *Enterococcus* sp., *Escherichia coli*, and *Enterobacter* sp.[13] The last two organisms were recovered from the pulmonary lesions of a blue-naped mousebird with bacterial cholecystitis with disseminated acute necrotizing pneumonia and myocarditis.[13] Systemic toxoplasmosis was confirmed with immunohistochemistry in a colony of speckled mousebirds.[23] Many aviculturists consider pseudotuberculosis one of the most devastating diseases in their collections.[9] The review of 168 necropsy reports yielded only one case of yersiniosis. As with swifts, aspergillosis may occur in Coliiformes because of improper husbandry practices, particularly in caged birds (as opposed to birds housed in open aviaries).

Parasitic Diseases

A large variety of ectoparasites, including lice, flies of the Hippoboscidae family, ticks, and mites have been reported in swifts.[8,17,21,25] Although these ectoparasites do not cause clinical disease or have effect on reproductive success in most cases, heavy infestation of biting lice could affect birds during stressful or physically demanding times such as migration.[9,21,24] *Microfilaria* sp., *Plasmodium* sp., *Leucocytozoon* sp., *Trypanosoma* sp., *Haemoproteus* sp., *Haemogregarina* sp., and *Atoxoplasma* sp. have all been reported in swifts and swiftlets.[3,4] Because most of the swifts seen in captivity are wild birds in rehabilitation, it is not uncommon to find tapeworms in their feces. Treatment with suitable anthelmintics is indicated.

The *Hyalomma rufipes* tick has been recovered from the red-faced mousebird (*Urocolius indicus*); this tick may transmit *Anaplasma marginale*, *Rickettsia* sp., and *Babesia* sp. in Africa. In South Africa, it is the most important vector of Crimean-Congo hemorrhagic fever virus to humans.[16] Microfilaria, *Haemoproteus* sp., and *Leucocytozoon* sp. have been reported in mousebirds.[4,21] Sarcocystis cysts have also been found in the red-face mousebird in Africa, but like in many other bird species, it is likely of no clinical significance.[12]

Noninfectious Disease

Trauma (from flying into objects, injury caused by dogs or cats, burns, or malicious acts) and inanition are frequent causes of mortality in swifts, but reports of other noninfectious diseases are almost non-existent. During the past 10 years, rehabilitators have gained a wealth of experience and knowledge on the care of malnourished and injured swifts; success is possible if trauma is detected early on and is not severe. Chimney swifts may be poisoned by toxic fumes, and the prognosis in these cases is poor.[21]

In aviculturist circles, cold is considered the number one killer of mousebirds in captivity.[9] The mousebird necropsy review revealed that almost 60% of the 168 deaths were attributed to noninfectious causes. The vast majority of the noninfectious cases were trauma related but also included shock, malnutrition or inanition, and gout. Anesthesia- or surgery-related deaths represented 7% of the noninfectious causes of death. In the same review, hepatic lipidosis was noted on a significant number of birds, but it was determined not to be the cause of death and is considered to be of little clinical importance.[21] Nevertheless, overweight birds may be prone to reproductive problems such as the laying of infertile clutches.[9] Because of their mostly frugivorous nature, mousebirds are fed low-iron pellets in captivity, although no conclusive evidence that this family is prone to iron storage disease (hemochromatosis) exists.

REPRODUCTION

In swifts, the breeding season is timed with the availability of insects. Pairs are together for long periods but will nest in large colonies. Most swifts make rudimentary nests. Because swiftlets and the typical swifts use saliva to build their nests, the sublingual glands in both sexes are markedly enlarged. Treeswifts use saliva not only to build the nest, but in some species, it is thought that they use it to glue their eggs to the nest. Needletails and primitive American swifts do not use saliva for nest building. In the Apodidae family, the eggs are dull white in color and, although small, have high yolk content. Clutch size is variable and ranges from a single egg up to seven eggs, and this seems to be related to weather.[6,8,26]

Laparoscopic surgery or deoxyribonucleic acid (DNA) sex determination in mousebirds is necessary before pairing them, as they are sexually monomorphic. Surgical sexing should be performed when the bird is mature at 8 months of age. Pairs are monogamous and long lasting. Frequently, mousebird pairs receive assistance from helpers for nest building, incubating, and caring for the young. Mousebirds build their nests as an open bowl structure in trees and bushes. Clutches sizes are small, with only two to four eggs. The eggs are remarkably small, oval in shape, noticeably rough-textured, and whitish with or without markings. On hatching, the altricial young weigh 2 g or less and are blind.[10] In the wild, predation (by reptiles and other birds) and nest destruction by rain or wind are the main causes for the low nestling survival rates.[10] In captivity, predation, overfeeding with secondary aspiration, and malnutrition have been considered important causes for neonatal mortality in blue-naped mousebirds.[21]

TABLE 27-1

Reproductive Characteristics of the Most Common Coliidae Found in Captivity

Parameter	Blue-Naped Mousebird (*Urocolius macrourus*)	White-Backed Mousebird (*Colius colius*)	Speckled Mousebird (*Colius striatus*)	White-Headed Mousebird (*Colius leucocephalus*)	Red-Faced Mousebird (*Urocolius indicus*)
Number of eggs	2–3	3 or more	1–4	1–3	2–4
Incubation period (days)	12.5 +/–0.8	13	10–14	14	10–15
Nestling period (days)	10–12	12	10	17–18	14–20
Method of feeding	Regurgitation	Regurgitation	Regurgitation	Regurgitation	Regurgitation
Life span (years)	8–13	7–8	Up to 12.3	8–10	8

From references 9, 10, 14, and 21.

Table 27-1 lists the reproductive characteristics of the most common Coliidae found in captivity.

ACKNOWLEDGMENTS

The author would like to thank the generous contribution of pathology information by Dr. Michael Garner.

REFERENCES

1. Jourdain E, Toussaint Y, Lebond A, et al: Bird species potentially involved in introduction, amplification and spread of West Nile virus in a Mediterranean wetland, the Camargue (Southern France). *Vector Borne Zoonotic Dis* 7(1):15–31, 2007.
2. Prinzinger R, Misovic A, Kleinschmidt T: Analysis of blood component in blue naped mousebirds *Urocolius macrorus*. *Ostrich* 65:311–315, 1994.
3. Bennett GF, Peirce MA, Earlè RA: An annotated checklist of the valid avian species of Haemoproteus, Leucocytozoon (Apicomplexa: Haemosporida) and Hepatozoon (Apicomplexa: Haemogregarinidae). *Systemat Parasitol* 29:61–73, 1994.
4. Bennett GF, Whiteway M, Woodworth-Lynas C: *A host parasite catalogue of the avian haematozoa*, St. John's, Newfoundland, 1982, Department of Biology, Memorial University of Newfoundland, pp 15–16, 28, 73–74.
5. Bull EL: Declines in the breeding population of Vaux's swift in Northeastern Oregon. *W Birds* 34:230–234, 2003.
6. Burnie D: *Smithsonian nature guide to birds*, New York, 2012, DK Publishing, pp 208–211, 218–219.
7. Burton M, Burton R: *International wildlife encyclopedia*, ed 3, Tarrytown, NY, 2002, Marshal Cavendish Corporation, pp 1676–1677.
8. Chantler P: Family Apodidae (swifts). In del Hoyo J, Elliott A, Sargatal J, editors: *Handbook of the birds of the world*, vol 5, Barcelona, Spain, 1999, Lynx Edicions, pp 388–457.
9. Davis KD: *Mousebirds in aviculture (e-book)*, Creswell, OR, 2012, Birdhouse Publications.
10. de Juana E: Family Coliidae (mousebirds). In del Hoyo J, Elliott A, Sargatal J, editors: *Handbook of the birds of the world*, vol 6, Barcelona, Spain, 1999, Lynx Edicions, pp 60–77.
11. Dickinson E: *The Howard and Moore complete checklist of the birds of the world*, ed 3, Princeton, NJ, 2003, Princeton University Press, pp 255–278.
12. Erickson AB: Sarcocystis in birds. *Auk* 57(4):514–519, 1940.
13. Ferrel ST, Phalen D, Weeks BR: Bacterial cholecystitis with cardiac and pulmonary dissemination in a blue-naped mousebird (*Urocolious macrorus*). *Avian Dis* 44:460–464, 2000.
14. Finke C, Misovic A, Prinzinger R: Growth, the development of endothermy and torpidity in blue-naped mousebirds (*Urocolius macrourus*). *Ostrich* 66:1–9, 1995.
15. Griner LA: *Pathology of zoo animals*, San Diego, CA, 1983, Zoological Society of San Diego, p 241.
16. Hasle G, Horak IG, Grieve G, et al: Ticks collected from birds in the northern provinces of South Africa, 2004-2006. *Onderstepoort J Vet* 76:167–175, 2009.
17. Ingram K: Hummingbirds and miscellaneous orders. In Fowler ME, editor: *Zoo and wild animal medicine*, ed 2, Philadelphia, PA, 1986, Saunders, pp 447–456.
18. Krautwald-Junghanns ME, Pees M, Reese S, Tully T: *Birds: Diagnostic imaging of exotic pets. Birds, small mammals, reptiles*, Hannover, Germany, 2011, Schlütersche, pp 1–136.
19. Palomeque J, Planas J: Erythrocyte size in some wild Spanish birds. *Rev Esp Fisiol* 37:17–22, 1981.
20. Prinzinger R, Göppel R, Lorenz A, et al: Body temperature and metabolism in the red-backed mousebird (*Colius castanotus*) during fasting and torpor. *Comp Biochem Physiol A Physiol* 69:689–692, 1981.
21. Pye G: Apodiformes and Coliiformes (Swifts, Swiftlets, Mousebirds). In Fowler ME, Miller RE, editors: *Zoo and wild animal medicine*, ed 5, St. Louis, MO, 2003, Saunders, pp 239–245.
22. Sibley CG, Ahlquist JE: *Phylogeny and classification of birds: A study in molecular evolution*, New Haven, CT, 1990, Yale University Press, pp 357–363, 391–401.
23. Stidworthy M: Toxoplasmosis: A serious exotic disease for ex situ captive wildlife. In *Proceedings of the British Veterinary Zoological Society*, Spring Meeting, Jersey, U.K., 2009, Durrell Wildlife Conservation Trust, p 32.
24. Tompkins DM, Jones T, Clayton TH: Effect of vertically transmitted parasites on the reproductive success of Swifts (*Apus apus*). *Funct Ecol* 10(6):733–740, 1996.
25. van Vuren M, Brown JMM: Septicaemic *Erysipelothrix rhusiopathiae* infection in the little swift (*Apus affinis*). *J S Afr Vet Assoc* 61(4):170–171, 1990.
26. Wells DR: Family Hemiprocnidae (treeswifts). In del Hoyo J, Elliott A, Sargatal J, editors: *Handbook of the birds of the world*, vol 5, Barcelona, Spain, 1999, Lynx Edicions, pp 458–467.

CHAPTER 28

Trogoniformes

Genevieve Dumonceaux and Donald L. Neiffer

BIOLOGY

The order Trogoniformes (trogons and quetzals) consists of a single family (Trogonidae), 6 genera, and 39 species. Most taxonomists recognize two subfamilies: Apalodermatinae (3 African species) and Trogoninae, which is split into tribe Harpactini (11 Asian species) and tribe Trogonini (25 New World species).[12,18,20]

Trogonid distribution is roughly pantropical, with species approximately centered around the tropical forests of Malaysia and Indonesia and the equatorial forests of the Amazon and Congo river basins.[8,14] A variety of trogonids are found in Costa Rica, including the black-headed trogon (*Trogon melanocephalus*), Baird's trogon (*Trogon bairdii*), the violaceous trogon (*Trogon violaceus*), the elegant trogon (*Trogon elegans*), the collared trogon (*Trogon collaris*), the orange-bellied trogon (*Trogon aurantiiventris*), the black-throated trogon (*Trogon rufus*), the slaty-tailed trogon (*Trogon masena*), the lattice-tailed trogon (*Trogon clathratis*), and the resplendent quetzal (*Pharomacrus mocinno*).[1,9]

Trogonids use different sylvan habitats that range in elevation from sea level to more than 3,500 meters (m; 11,500 ft.). Although some species require primary forests, others flourish in secondary forest, forest fragment, logged forest, scrub, and agricultural land.[14] The insectivorous red-headed trogon (*Harpactes erythrocephalus*) of Nepal inhabits middle- and lower-storey forests at elevations from 250 m up to 1830 m.[10]

Deforestation threatens trogonids worldwide. The Javan trogon (*Apalharpactes reinwardtii*) is on the International Union for the Conservation of Nature (IUCN) Red List as endangered. Twelve species are listed as near threatened. The resplendent quetzal (*Pharomachrus mocinno*), a species limited primarily to the remote and mist-draped cloud forests of middle America, is also listed by CITES (Appendix 1). The authors refer the readers to the IUCN website for more details, as the status of each species may change over time. Habitat loss, collection for zoos and aviaries, and the feather trade have raised concerns about this species' status.[8] Human activities that disrupt breeding, habitat, and food sources adversely affect trogonid populations.

UNIQUE ANATOMY

The foot anatomy of trogonids is described as *heterodactylous*, a term used for the toe arrangement in which the first and second toes are oriented posteriorly, with the hallux in the lateral position (heterodactylous toe). The anterior toes of most New World trogons are partially united, presumably an adaptation for nest excavation.[14]

Muscle distribution reflects aerial foraging. The heart is large, and the pectoral muscle complex accounts for approximately 20% of body weight, whereas the muscles of the relatively small feet and short legs represent only about 3%.[8,14,19] The muscles of the feet and legs are underdeveloped to the degree that trogonids are unable to turn around on a perch without the assistance of the wings.[8] Walking and hopping are rare except in the elegant trogon.[8,14]

Trogonid integument is bright and colorful, with soft, dense, and dry-textured feathers. Sexual dichromatism exists in all species except the Cuban trogon (*Priotelus temnurus*) and is most marked in the quetzals, in which, besides being more brightly colored, males also sport elongated and modified upper tail-coverts. These "tail feathers" are longest (48 to 96 centimeters [cm]) in the resplendent quetzal.[14]

Trogon is Greek for "to gnaw or eat" and refers to the structure and function of the beak. The cutting edges of the maxilla, the mandible, or both are variably serrated in most New World species and probably aid in securing live prey or large fruit. These serrations, along with the decurved tip of the bill (present in all species), are also useful in cutting food items into smaller pieces.[8,14] Most species have short, triangular tongues, with backward-pointing projections that probably aid in holding and swallowing prey.[14] The Cuban trogon is an exception, having a relatively long tongue with a bifurcate tip that may be involved in nectar feeding.[7,8] All trogonids have short bills with an unusually wide base, which provides a large gape in relation to bill length and allows for ingestion of large food items.[14] Resplendent quetzals, which regularly consume the large drupes (median diameter of 18 millimeters [mm]) of the laurel family (Lauraceae) that they have collected in flight, have several morphologic adaptations for a highly frugivorous diet.[1,19] In addition to a wide gape, this species has flexible mandibles and clavicles, which enable swallowing of fruits 3 to 4 mm wider than one would predict from gape measurements.[19] The long esophagus (up to 12 cm) is thin walled, elastic, and ringed by circular muscles presumably important in regurgitation of large seeds; no crop is present. The proventriculus is expansible and lined with glandular tissue in a pattern of closely packed hexagons. The ventriculus is large (external diameter of 2.5 cm) and muscular.[19] The paired ceca (each 4.5 cm long) are well developed and make up 15% total intestinal length, which suggests that some fermentative digestion occurs.[14] The Cuban trogon, a primarily fruit-eating species, also lacks a crop and possesses a large ventriculus (1.8 cm diameter) and an even larger ceca (18% to 26% total intestinal length).[7,17] Examination of the gastrointestinal (GI) tracts of six other New World trogons also has revealed proportionally long ceca.[14,17]

SPECIAL PHYSIOLOGY

In a review of avian metabolism, which compared over 350 species from more than 70 families, a low resting metabolic rate for the tropically adapted black-throated trogon (*Trogon rufus*) was reported.[4] If typical of the family, limits on the climatic tolerances of all trogonids, both wild and captive, may exist. The distribution of New World species supports this theory. The relatively large 5 quetzal species and the eared trogon occupy mostly temperate high-altitude forests; the 8 mostly midsized species occupy intermediate altitude or temperature ranges; and the 9 smaller species occupy low-altitude tropical ranges.[14]

HOUSING AND FEEDING REQUIREMENTS

Trogonids tend to be subcanopy or middle-strata hunters. They usually perch upright on horizontal branches between foliage and trunk and sit quietly for extended periods and move only their head through 180 degrees as they search for food and predators. The most common feeding behavior is termed "perch and pounce" or "sally-gleaning." Birds plucks food items during graceful sallies without alighting beside fruit, plant, insect, or vertebrate prey.[1,8] Occasionally, some species such as the resplendent quetzal descend to the ground during pursuit of insects and lizards. Because of their weak feet and legs, trogonids have difficulty reaching for items from their perches, particularly those below them.[14,19] As such, trogonid enclosures should contain multiple horizontal branches, with some positioned over feeding stations, where the birds may perform sallies should they choose. Placement of plants and other structures within these areas should allow for unimpaired flight. Feed bowls should be shallow, with edges textured for perching so that the birds may alight and reach their food with minimal effort. Chronic pododermatitis has been reported in a pavonine (*Pharomachrus pavoninus*) and a golden-headed quetzal (*Pharomachrus auriceps*), and rotation of perches of different sizes and textures is recommended.

Trogonid diets vary from completely insectivorous to mostly frugivorous. In Africa, exclusive insectivory exists, presumably because of exclusion from other foods by other avian families early in trogonid evolution. Although they are predominantly insectivorous, many Asian species consume fruit and vegetation in moderate quantities. The greatest variation among trogonid diets is seen in the New World biogeographic zone, with its relatively large niche width and species divergence.[8] Here, progression from exclusive or primary insectivory to primary frugivory directly correlates with increased body size and altitude and a decrease in insect life.[12] Progression during development also exists. The golden-headed quetzals are known to feed exclusively insects to their chicks for the first 3 days of the chicks' lives. When this feeding strategy was employed in a group of these birds in captivity, digestive issues decreased, and chick survival increased.

Diets offered to captive trogonids consist of a mixture of vegetables (avocado, grape, apple, pear, melon, berries, banana, papaya, cactus, tomato, peas, corn, cooked potato, carrot) and vertebrate animal matter (pinky mice, hard-boiled egg, bird of prey diet), and insects (mealworms, waxworms, crickets, occasionally locusts). Pelleted diets have also been offered in some collections (soft bill diet, soaked dog food). Trogonids are susceptible to hemosiderosis and hemochromatosis, and limiting dietary iron should be considered. Trogonids must consume carotenoids to maintain their bright colorations,[6,13] and addition of a synthetic mixed carotenoid product to the diet is recommended.

The physiologic dependence on surface water is unknown, although drinking from a pool has been observed in wild elegant trogons.[8,15] Bathing has also been observed in wild elegant trogons,[15] a wild Malabar trogon (*Harpactes fasciatus*),[8] a captive golden-headed quetzal,[5] and captive resplendent quetzals. On the basis of this information, provision of pool-type water sources is recommended.

Regular nail and beak trimming has been reported necessary for captive golden-headed quetzals. Providing vertically positioned soft or semi-decayed logs and food items sized such that the birds must cut them may decrease the need for these procedures and serve as enrichment by increasing foraging and digging behaviors.

Institutions in the United States that successfully breed some species of trogons have useful clinical databases on several adults

and chicks. One of the more commonly identified problems with parent-reared chicks is parents feeding substrate materials to chicks within several days of hatching. In one of these institutions, chick losses involving white-tailed trogons (*Trogon viridis*) occurred most frequently within the first 14 days after hatching. Birds living past this age, in general, tended to do well and grew to a size and age that allowed safe transfer to other institutions.

LONGEVITY

Trogonids may be long lived in captivity. Two resplendent quetzals housed at the Bronx Zoo lived for 17 and 21 years, respectively.[14] One wild-caught golden-headed quetzal at the Houston Zoo lived for over 21 years, and a second housed at the Denver Zoo has reached 19 years of age. A breeding pair of white-tailed trogons (*Trogon viridis*) at the National Aquarium in Baltimore is over 16 years of age at the writing of this chapter. Historically, wild-caught animals have not fared as well in the United States. Historical acquisition or disposition information for United States institutions has revealed that 55% of wild-caught trogonids (80% quetzals) died within 1 year and 88% within 4 years.

RESTRAINT AND ANESTHESIA

Care must be taken when manually restraining trogonids because the skeleton is fragile, feathers are easily removed, and the skin tears easily.[8,13,18] Stress-induced death from physical restraint has occurred in healthy trogonids; therefore, the birds' reactions should be closely observed.[13] Use of inhalant anesthesia with isoflurane has been reported in captive trogonids; this agent should be used for invasive procedures or for birds that struggle excessively.[17] Captive-reared and hand-reared individuals appear to handle restraint better overall compared with their wild counterparts.

DIAGNOSTICS

Diagnostic testing on trogonids is similar as in other avian species. Hematologic and plasma biochemical reference ranges for selected species are listed in Table 28-1.

DISEASES

Parasitic Diseases

Table 28-2 lists parasites reported in wild and captive trogonids. Wild and captive species are hosts to multiple parasites. Treatment of parasites for these animals is with the usual anthelmintics and doses used in other avian species.

TABLE 28-1

Reference Ranges for Hematologic and Plasma Biochemical Parameters of Selected Captive Trogonid Species

Parameter	Golden-Headed Quetzal (*Pharomachrus auriceps*) (N)	Crested Quetzal (*P. antisanus*) (N = 1)	White-Tailed Trogon (*Trogon viridis*) (N)	Blue-Tailed Trogon (*Harpactes reinwardti*) (N = 1)
Leukocytes ×10³/µL	5.484 ± 5.384 (11)	8.800 ± 0	J 5.693 ± 1.879 (12) A 6.27 ± 2.055 (7)	12.485 ± 0
Heterophils ×10³/µL	2.059 ± 1.626 (11)	6.160 ± 0	J 1.336 ± 616 (13) A 2.311 ± 689 (7)	7.491 ± 0
Lymphocytes ×10³/µL	3.236 ± 3.032 (11)	2.288 ± 0	J 2.578 ± 1.432 (13) A 1.902 ± 0.974 (7)	2.622 ± 0
Monocytes ×10³/µL	0.534 ± 0.607 (11)	0.352 ± 0	J 0.253 ± 0.163 (11) A 0.535 ± 0.173 (6)	0.749 ± 0
Eosinophils ×10³/µL	0.317 ± 0.426 (11)	0.000 ± 0	J 0.396 ± 0.176 (12) A 1.284 ± 0.395 (5)	0.874 ± 0

Continued

TABLE 28-1

Reference Ranges for Hematologic and Plasma Biochemical Parameters of Selected Captive Trogonid Species—cont'd

Parameter	Golden-Headed Quetzal (*Pharomachrus auriceps*) (N)	Crested Quetzal (*P. antisanus*) (N = 1)	White-Tailed Trogon (*Trogon viridis*) (N)	Blue-Tailed Trogon (*Harpactes reinwardti*) (N = 1)
Basophils ×10³/µL	0.067 ± 0.110 (11)	0.000 ± 0	J 1.018 ± 0.334 (11) A 0.916 ± 0.429 (7)	0.749 ± 0
Erythrocytes ×10⁶/µL	3.53 ± 0.45 (6)	1.41 ± 0	2.49 ± 0.360	—
PCV (%)	52.3 ± 4.4 (7)	40 ± 0	J 52.6 ± 2.55 (13) A 55.4 ± 4.5 (6)	50 ± 0
Hemoglobin (g/dL)	17.1 ± 1.9 (6)	12.9 ± 0	J 19.85 ± 0.7 A 18.2 ± 5	—
MCV (fL)	152.5 ± 12.1 (4)	284.7 ± 0	193 ± 25.5	—
MCH (mg/dL)	48.7 ± 4.9 (6)	91.8 ± 0	—	—
MCHC (µg)	31.5 ± 3.7 (4)	32 ± 0	J 38 ± 1.5 (11) A 32.5 ± 4.5 (2)	—
Total protein (g/dL)	2.9 ± 0.8 (9)	5.2 ± 0	J 3.6 ± 0.38 (13) A 3.73 ± 0.31 (6)	3.9 ± 0
Albumin (g/dL)	1.0 ± 0.2 (3)	—	J 2 ± 0.23 (6) A 0.96 ± 0.15 (3)	0.8 ± 0
Globulin (g/dL)	1.8 ± 0.1 (2)	—	A 1.6 ± 0.2 (3)	—
Calcium (mg/dL)	9.1 ± 0.5 (6)	15.1 ± 0	J 9 ± 0.6 (16) A 8.4 ± 0.5 (3)	11.8 ± 0
Phosphorus (mg/dL)	3.5 ± 1.6 (3)	—	J 4.5 ± 1.2 (16) A 3.8 ± 0.1 (3)	3.7 ± 0
Sodium (mEq/L)	158 ± 4 (6)	—	J 155 ± 3.9 (16) A 157 ± 1 (3)	—
Potassium (mEq/L)	2.4 ± 1.1 (4)	—	J 3 ± 0.86 (14) A 2.4 ± 0 (3)	—
Chloride (mEq/L)	121 ± 2.3 (2)	—	A 123 ± 2.5 (2)	—
Creatinine (mg/dL)	0.1 ± 0 (1)	—	—	—
Urea nitrogen (mg/dL)	2 ± 0 (1)	—	—	—
Cholesterol (mg/dL)	276 ± 17 (3)	—	—	370 ± 0
Triglycerides	293 ± 111 (3)	—	—	—
Glucose (mg/dL)	245 ± 84 (6)	288 ± 0	339 ± 0 J 292 ± 24 (17) A 354 ± 75 (4)	332 ± 0
Total carbon dioxide	18 ± 0 (1)	—	—	—
Manganese (mEq/L)	—	—	—	2.6 ± 0
ALP (Units/L)	231 ± 179 (4)	—	A 69 ± 40 (3)	83 ± 0
AST (Units/L)	93 ± 20 (7)	—	203 ± 69 J 191 ± 48 (17) A 210 ± 67 (4)	263 ± 0
ALT	26 ± 10 (4)	—	A 47 ± 28 (3)	81 ± 0
LDH (Units /L)	215 ± 132 (3)	—	A 99 ± 30 (3)	265 ± 0
CPK (Units /L)	450 ± 472 (3)	—	J 295 ± 95 (13) A 245 ± 201 (4)	703 ± 0
GGT (Units /L)	7 ± 0 (1)	—	A 8.3 ± 3.2 (3)	6 ± 0
Uric acid (mg/dL)	11.0 ± 4.8 (6)	—	J 6 ± 1.9 (11) A 8.5 ± 3.8 (4)	8.6 ± 0
Total bilirubin (mg/dL)	0.4 ± 0.2 (4)	—	—	—
Amylase (Units /L)	324 ± 26 (3)	—	—	—
Reference (Unpublished data)	Houston Zoo, Denver Zoo, Philadelphia Zoo	Philadelphia Zoo	National Aquarium in Baltimore	San Diego Zoo

ALP, Alkaline phosphatase; *AST*, aspartate aminotransferase; *CPK*, creatine phosphokinase; *fL*, femtoliter; *g/dL*, gram per deciliter; *GGT*, gamma-glutamyl transferase; *LDH*, lactate dehydrogenase; *MCH*, mean corpuscular hemoglobin; *MCHC*, mean corpuscular hemoglobin concentration; *MCV*, mean corpuscular volume; *mEq/dL*, milliequivalent per deciliter; *PCR*, polymerase chain reaction; *PCV*, packed cell volume; *mg/dL*, milligram per deciliter; *µL*, microliter; *Unit/L*, unit per liter.

TABLE 28-2

Parasites Reported in Captive and Free-Ranging Trogonids

Parasite	Hosts	Site/diagnosis/comments	Reference
Protozoa			
Flagellates			
Hemoflagellates			
Trypanosoma sp.	*Trogon massena**	Blood smear	3
Enteric flagellates			
Giardia sp.	*Pharomachrus antisanus*	Fecal examination	San Diego Zoo[†]
	Harpactes reinwardtii	Small intestine histopathology	
Trichomonas sp.	*P. auriceps, P. pavoninus*	Fecal examination	San Diego Zoo[†]
Unidentified flagellate	*P. auriceps*	Intestinal tract necropsy	Houston Zoo[†]
	T. viridis	Mortality attributed to overgrowth	National Aquarium,
		Fresh fecal examinations on chicks	Baltimore
Sarcodina			
Unidentified amoeba	*P. pavoninus*	Fecal examination	San Diego Zoo[†]
Sporozoans			
Hemosporozoans			
Haemoproteus	*Harpactes ardens*, H. duvaucelli*,*	Blood smear	2
trogonis	*H. erythrocephalus*, H. oreskios**		
	T. rufus, T. violaceus**		
Haemoproteus sp.	*T. clathratus*, T. comptus* ,*	Blood smear	3
Leucocytozoon sp.	*P. moccino,*H. oreskios**	Blood smear	3,12
Plasmodium sp.	*T. mexicanus*, T. violaceus**	Blood smear	3
Coccidia			
Sarcocystis sp.	*H. reinwardtii*	Sarcocystis-like cysts in brain at necropsy	San Diego Zoo[†]
Unidentified coccidia	*P. auriceps*	Fecal examination	Denver Zoo[†]
Nematodes			
Spirurida			
Acuarioidea			
Acuariidae			
Dispharynx nasuta	*P. auriceps*	Embryonated ova in feces	San Diego Zoo[†]
		Treated with 70 mg/kg fenbendazole once daily (SID) ×7 days	
Filarioidea			
Onchocercidae			
Unidentified species	*P. antisanus, H. reinwardtii,*	Adult filariid in pulmonary artery	San Diego Zoo[†]
	T. personatus	Microfilaria present in tissue (lung) impression or histopathology	
	T. clathratus, T. massena*,*	Microfilaria present on blood smear	3
	*T. violaceus**		
Habronematoidea			
Habronematidae			
Cyrnea semilunairs	*T. collaris*, T. melanurus**	Proventriculus, small and large intestine	16
Enoplida			
Trichinelloidea			
Trichuridae			
Unidentified—	*P. auriceps, P. pavoninus,*	Fecal examination. Treated with 20–50 mg/kg	San Diego Zoo[†]
Capillaria	*H. reinwardtii, T. personatus*	fenbendazole orally (PO) SID ×5 days; repeat in 1 week	
Other Nematodes			
Unidentified	*P. antisanus, P. auriceps*	Fecal examination.	Houston Zoo[†]
strongyle-type egg		Likely *Ornithostrongylus* sp.	Philadelphia Zoo[†]
or larvae		Treated with ivermectin 0.3–0.5 mg/kg ivermectin PO or subcutaneously (SQ), repeat in 3 weeks, or levamisole 25–35 mg/kg PO as single treatment	
Cestodes			
Unidentified cestode	*P. mocinno*	Several tapeworm cysts found in pectoral musculature at necropsy	Philadelphia Zoo[†] 9
		Unidentified cestodes have also been reported in an unidentified *Trogon* sp. and *Pharomachrus* sp. at necropsy	

Continued

TABLE 28-2

Parasites Reported in Captive and Free-Ranging Trogonids—cont'd

Parasite	Hosts	Site/diagnosis/comments	Reference
Trematodes Unidentified trematode	*P. antisanus*	Fluke ova found in fecal examination	San Diego Zoo[†]
		Urinary trematodiasis present with distended left ureter No inflammatory reaction or changes in adjacent kidney Trematode characterized by a thin spinose cuticle, a terminal sucker, and no body cavity	Wildlife Conservation Society[†]
Lice Mallophagan (biting louse) *Trogonirmus elegans*	*T. elegans* *	Integument	15
Mites Unidentified feather mite	*P. moccino*	Infestation resulted in abnormal molts Treated with topical insecticidal powder and normal molts resumed	Miquel Alvarez, Del Toro Zoo[†]

*Samples from free-ranging specimens.
[†]Unpublished data.

Infectious Disease

Fungal Diseases

Aspergillosis has been a significant disease in captive quetzals. Necropsy or mortality information for 76 wild-caught quetzals—including resplendent, golden-headed, and crested (*Pharomachrus antisanus*) quetzals—revealed aspergillosis-associated mortality in 22 birds (29%), with most dying within 1 year and 50% within 6 months of arrival at their institutions.[11] Other recorded fungal infections include peracute GI zygomycosis in an adult golden-headed quetzal and enteric candidiasis in an 8-day-old golden-headed quetzal. Similar to many other avian species, trogon and quetzal chicks appear to be prone to *Candida* infections secondary to other infections, antibiotic use, and other immunosuppressive events. Ventricular candidiasis has been a frequent finding in several white-tailed trogon chicks that have succumbed to enteric bacterial overgrowth at a young age.

Bacterial Diseases

Disseminated mycobacteriosis has been reported in two Cuban trogons, a crested quetzal, and two golden-headed quetzals; all three quetzals had concurrent aspergillosis. Other bacterial infections recorded in captive birds include pseudotuberculosis in an unspecified trogonid, bacterial enteritis in an unspecified trogonid,[13] disseminated granulomatous disease caused by an unidentified gram-positive filamentous bacterium in a golden-headed quetzal, and two cases of bacterial sinusitis in golden-headed quetzals and one white-tailed trogon chick. One of these last two cases had concurrent pneumonitis, and the other previously had been treated for *Aspergillus* sp. sinusitis. In the latter quetzal case, *Pseudomonas aeruginosa*, *Proteus mirabilis*, *Enterococcus* sp., *Escherichia coli*, and α-hemolytic *Streptococcus* sp. were identified on culture. The condition was successfully treated with piperacillin. As with other avian families, bacterial overgrowth of the intestinal tract is a risk in hand-reared trogonidae chicks.

Noninfectious Disease

Neoplastic Diseases

Biliary adenoma has been reported in a resplendent quetzal.[11] A granulosa cell tumor with liver metastasis was noted in a medical report of an 18-year-old, female golden-headed quetzal.

Nutritional Disorders

General malnutrition and wasting have been seen in a number of trogonids. Most of these have been recent captures; many of these birds display varying degrees of hepatic lipidosis.[11] Iron-storage disease (hemochromatosis) was reported in a crested quetzal, with death attributed to the condition. Hemosiderosis was detected in a second crested quetzal and a golden-headed quetzal at necropsy and in two clinically normal golden-headed quetzals via hepatic biopsy. A condition felt to be related to a high-fruit diet has been reported in 14 quetzals and 1 *Trogon* sp., whereby focal to diffuse accumulation of large, refractile, pigment particles—thought to be primarily lipofuscins but with some iron also present—were observed in the liver. Hepatic necrosis and chronic inflammation commonly were associated with larger areas of pigment accumulation.[11] Other presumptive nutrition-related disorders include bilateral cataract development in a hand-reared golden-headed quetzal,[5] and atheroma of the great vessels of the heart in an unspecified trogonid.[13]

GI obstruction and hypomotility in neonatal golden-headed quetzals was seen in the Houston Zoo. Changing the diet of the parents and thereby changing the diets of the chicks to a higher-protein, lower-carbohydrate diet during the first 3 days of the chicks' lives seemed to resolve this issue.

Trauma

Trogonids are monogamous and territorial and are maintained as individuals, pairs, or small family groups. In single-species exhibits, intraspecific aggression has rarely been reported, but in mixed-species exhibits, trauma and death from aggression (presumably interspecific) has been reported more frequently. Exhibit-related trauma, including drowning and running into objects, have also been reported, with a greater prevalence in mixed-species enclosures. Parental trauma to chicks has been noted.

Diseases of Unknown Etiology

Gastrointestinal System

Ulcerative ventriculitis with acute hemorrhage was reported in a resplendent quetzal. Acute enteritis was reported in Cuban trogons, and chronic enteritis characterized by moderate diffuse lymphoplasmacytic infiltrates in the lamina propria of the small intestine was described in a crested quetzal. Small intestinal obstruction was

TABLE 28-3

Reproductive Parameters for Captive Trogonids at Three Institutions

Species	Breeding Season	Housing and Nest Sites	Eggs, Incubation, and Fledging	Comments	References
Golden-headed quetzal (*Pharomachrus auriceps*)	January–September in captivity April–June in wild	*Housing:* Sole species in 3 × 3 × 2.7 m high, planted, indoor exhibit. Adjacent to larger aviary. *Nest site:* 1.8 m tall hollow palm log resting vertically on floor. Before each nesting, log firmly packed with dried leaves to midpoint followed by pine shavings to level of opening located on side. Excavated to depth of 45.7 cm on one occasion. Excavation may take upwards of 2 weeks.	*Eggs:* 1–2, grayish blue. *Incubation:* 16–20 days. *Fledging:* 24–30 days (Parent-raised), hand-raised chicks independent at 7–14 weeks.	Most chicks produced by wild-caught birds. Clutches have been laid <1 month after previous brood has fledged. Most chicks parent-raised, but several pulled at 11–14 days due to parental neglect. See Table 29-1 for dietary information.	Houston Zoological Gardens, Houston, TX, USA (unpublished data)[5,14]
White-tailed trogon (*Trogon viridis*)	July–October in captivity December–July in wild	*Housing:* Mixed avian species indoor aviary measuring 6 × 5 × 2.6 m high. Heavily planted and adjacent to larger aviary. *Nest site:* Birch tree with a natural cavity 20 cm deep with an 8.5 cm diameter opening. Cavity filled with sand and wood shavings. Opening located approximately 1.6 m from the ground. Excavation up to 15 cm noted.	*Eggs:* 2, white. *Incubation:* 18 days; 37.4° C, 55% humidity in incubator. *Fledging:* hand-raised chick flying at 18 days but not independent until day 30.	Wild-caught breeding only. Second clutch laid 2 months after eggs of first clutch pulled at around day 13. Hand rearing at 50% humidity and 33°C. See Table 29-1 for dietary information. Chicks pulled because of adults inadvertently feeding bark and fibers with food with associated mortality.	Vogelpark-Walsrode, Germany (unpublished data)[18]
White-tailed trogon (*Trogon viridis*)	January–August in captivity December–July in wild	*Housing:* Mixed species (mammals, birds, reptiles, amphibians) large walk-through indoor aviary *Nest sites:* Nest box (medium parrot-sized) covered with cork bark, inside and out, with a small hole at opening that requires some excavation by birds. Box angled slightly forward (hole facing down) and attached to a large epiphyte tree. This tree is a manmade structure covered with cork bark and live plants.	*Eggs:* 2, white. *Incubation:* 18 days estimated. *Fledging:* 20–25 days. Hand-raised chick fully dependent until 18 weeks of age.	All chicks have been parent-hatched and most parent-raised. See Table 29-1 for dietary information on hand-reared chick. Birds initially attempted to excavate palm logs but were unsuccessful. Nest box attached to artificial tree after birds observed digging a hole in cork bark covering structure.	National Aquarium, Baltimore, MD, USA (unpublished data).

reported in two resplendent quetzals; a food item (piece of orange) was identified in the duodenum in one case. Hepatitis—usually acute—has been reported in Cuban and elegant trogons and in resplendent quetzals. In some collections, digestive impactions in chicks result from parents feeding inappropriate nondigestible materials such as wood shavings and cork pieces.

Urogenital System

Mortality associated with egg-binding has been reported in a blue-tailed trogon (*Harpactes reinwardtii*). Reported primary renal diseases have included glomerulonephritis, renal amyloidosis, and nephrosclerosis in resplendent quetzals, and peracute nephrosis in a golden-headed quetzal.

Nervous System

Encephalitis was reported in a resplendent quetzal, which developed progressive incoordination, inability to perch, and wasting over a month. Histopathology revealed neuronophagia, satellitosis, and focal gliosis. Brain abscessation has also been reported in a resplendent quetzal.

REPRODUCTION

Little information about the breeding behavior, nest sites, or eggs is available for over 25% of trogonid species.[13] Only the resplendent quetzal, golden-headed quetzal, and white-tailed trogon (*Trogon viridis*) have reproduced in captivity.[5,18] Table 28-3 summarizes reproductive information for the last two species.

In the wild, breeding coincides with food availability and is dependent on geography.[14] Singing males have been observed in 12 species, and occasional dual-species assemblages have been reported in Africa and the New World. During these events, males may chase one another, but physical contact is generally avoided. Although the behavior attracts females and the majority of participating males are bachelors, it is not felt to serve solely a pair-forming function; even paired males may leave their mates temporarily to join the assemblage.[8,14]

Both sexes share in nest site preparation and use elevated cavities. Sites are classified as either open niche, with the incubating or brooding adult largely visible from the front of the opening, or as sites with an upward slanted tube leading to a fully enclosed chamber.[8] Most species use preexisting holes that require minimal excavation in decaying trees or stumps, natural cavities in living trees, dead bamboo (orange-breasted trogon, *Harpactes oreskios*), or old woodpecker holes.[14] However, among the New World genus *Trogon*, full excavation of nest sites is often performed. The trogonid beak is poorly designed for this task; considerable energy and time are expended, with multiple sites often abandoned after the birds strike substrate that is too hard or two soft. Besides decaying wood, several *Trogon* sp. excavate arboreal termitaries. The violaceous trogon (*Trogon violaceus*) also excavates vespiaries (wasp nests) and occasionally arboreal ant nests, the latter behavior being unique to New World birds.[8] Although trogons cohabitate with termites, wasps and ants are removed or eaten or forced to vacate.[8,14] The violaceous trogon is also unique in its excavation of arboreal fern-root masses and other epiphytes.[8,14] Successful nest sites provided for captive trogonids are described in Table 28-3. Provision of nest sites that require some excavation appears to be critical to success in most cases. Patience is required because interest in nest sites may be delayed. For example, at Vogelpark Walsrode (VW), Germany, a pair of white-tailed trogons introduced to an exhibit showed no interest in the provided nest for 3 years.

Usually two to three eggs are laid in the unlined nest, with both parents sharing in the 16- to 21-day incubation. Brood rearing is also performed by both parents, with the chicks fed bill-to-bill or via regurgitation of recently captured prey items. Although most species feed only insects to their nestlings, the violaceous trogon also feeds small fruits. The resplendent quetzal initiates the feeding of fruit,

especially lauraceous varieties, to their young starting at age 11 days.[14,19] During brood rearing at the Houston Zoo, golden-headed quetzals shifted dietary preferences with an increase in avocado, animal protein, and mealworm consumption (see Table 28-3).[5,14] Nest sanitation is not performed, and chick feces, regurgitated seeds, and chitinous insect remains may accumulate considerably.[14,15] Hand rearing has usually been required in golden-headed quetzals because of parental neglect or disinterest in the eggs, the chicks, or both (see Table 28-3). In at least one institution in the United States, chick mortality was highest within the first 14 days after hatching in white-tailed trogons regardless of rearing history. Hand rearing at VW was required because of the mortality associated with the adults inadvertently feeding bark and fibers with food to the chicks. Successful hatching of white-tailed trogons at VW occurred with incubators set at 37.4° C and 55% humidity.

Like other hole-nesting birds, trogonid chicks have papilla-like calluses on the undersides of their tarsi, which seem to function as nonslip cushions or for resting on the hard nest substrate and may also aid in climbing out of the nest cavity. Fledging occurs in 14 to 31 days, although the chick may depend on adults for up to 17 weeks, given the rather specialized food-catching behavior of trogonids.[14] See Table 28-3 for description of captive fledging dates and behavior. First basic plumage is quickly assumed, and, except in some larger species, the young bird resembles the adult of the respective sex.[8] Adult plumage is gained by approximately 1 year of age,[8] and on the basis of the production of viable offspring from captive-hatched golden-headed quetzals, sexual maturity is determined to be attained by 2 years of age.[14]

ACKNOWLEDGMENT

This chapter would not have been possible without the generous contributions of husbandry, medical, and pathology information from the following individuals: Martin Vince, Riverbanks Zoo; Donna Ialeggio and John Trupkiewicz, Philadelphia Zoo; Shirley Lliso and Marianne Tocidlowski, Houston Zoo; Jeff Baier, Denver Zoo; David Rimlinger, Ilse Stalis, and Meg Sutherland-Smith, San Diego Zoo; Christopher Hanley, Toledo Zoo; Dieter Rinke, Vogelpark Walsrode, Germany; Jill Arnold, Carey Rowsom, Brent Whitaker, and Leigh Clayton, National Aquarium in Baltimore; Abenamar Pozo and Jacqueline Sigler, ZOOMAT; Miquel Alvarez, Del Toro Zoo, Chiapas, Mexico; Paul Calle and Barbara Mangold, Wildlife Conservation Society; Mark Bremer, Jessica Hampton and Robert Wagner, National Aviary in Pittsburgh; Josef Lindholm, Caldwell Zoo; and Eric Miller and John Sykes, Saint Louis Zoo. I would also like to thank Tobias Kruhm and Eduardo Valdes, Walt Disney World, for the translation of the German and Mexican literature.

REFERENCES

1. Attenborough D: *The life of birds*, Princeton, NJ, 1998, Princeton University Press, pp 85–87.
2. Bennett GF, Peirce MA: The haemoproteids of the avian orders musophagiformes (the turacos) and Trogoniformes (the trogons). *Can J Zoo* 68: 2465, 1990.
3. Bennett GF, Whiteway M, Woddworth-Lynas C: A host-parasite catalogue of the avian haematozoa. *Mem Univ Nfld Occas Pap Biol* 5, 1982.
4. Bennett PM, Harvey PH: Acting and resting metabolism in birds: Allometry, phylogeny, and ecology. *J Zoo* 213:327–363, 1987.
5. Berry RJ: Breeding the golden headed quetzal. *AFA Watchbird* 13:24–31, 1986/1987.
6. Bruning D: Use of canthaxanthin to maintain the natural colour of captive birds at Bronx Zoo. *Int Zoo YB* 11:215, 1971.
7. Clark HL: Notes on the anatomy of the Cuban trogon. *Auk* 35:286–289, 1918.
8. Espinosa De Los Monteros A: Phylogenetic relationships among the trogons. *Auk* 115:937–954, 1998.

9. Garrigues R, Dean R: *The birds of Costa Rica: A field guide*, Costa Rica and New York, 2007, Comstock Publishing Associates, pp 140–144.
10. Grimmett R, Inskipp C, Inskipp T: *Helm field guides: Birds of Nepal*, New Delhi, India, 2000, Prakash Book Depot, p 72.
11. Griner LA: *Pathology of zoo animals*, San Diego, CA, 1983, Zoological Society of San Diego.
12. Huff CG, Wetmore A: Blood parasites of birds collected in four successive years in Panama. *Bull Wildl Dis Assoc* 3:1978, 1967.
13. Ingram K: Hummingbirds and miscellaneous orders. In Fowler ME, editor: *Zoo and wild animal medicine*, ed 2, Philadelphia, PA, 1986, Saunders, pp 447–456.
14. Johnsgard PA: *Trogons and quetzals of the world*, Washington, DC, 2000, Smithsonian Institution Press.
15. Kunzman MR, Hall LS, Johnson RR: Elegant trogon (*Trogon elegans*). In Poole A, Stettenheim P, Gill F, editors: *The birds of North America*, Philadelphia, PA, 1998.
16. Magalhares-Pinto R, Correa-Gommes D: Nematodes of Amazonian birds. *Mem Inst Oswaldo Cruz Rio de Janeiro* 80:213–217, 1985.
17. Miller WDW: Relative length of the intestinal caeca in trogons. *Auk* 35:480, 1918.
18. Rinke D, Müller M, Magnus W: Erfahrungen mit WeiBschwanz-Trogonen (*Trogon viridis*). *Gefiederte Welt* 120:345–347, 1996.
19. Wheelwright NT: Fruits and the ecology of resplendent quetzals. *Auk* 100:286–301, 1983.
20. Williams JG, Arlott N: *A field guide to the birds of East Africa*, Glasgow, Scotland, 1981, William Collins Sons and Company Ltd., pp 122–123.

CHAPTER 29

Coraciiformes (Kingfishers, Motmots, Bee-Eaters, Hoopoes, Hornbills)

Kathryn C. Gamble

TAXONOMY AND BIOLOGY

The order Coraciiformes includes four suborders (Alcedines, Meropes, Coracii, Bucerotes), with 10 families distributed respectively into the suborders as 3, 1, 3, and 3. It is a highly eclectic grouping of birds composed of kingfishers, todies, motmots, bee-eaters, rollers, cuckoo-rollers, ground-rollers, hoopoes, woodhoopoes, and hornbills. Birds in this order are generally diurnal (except the hook-billed kingfisher, *Melidora macrorrhina*) and found in the Old World (except todies, motmots, and some kingfisher species).[2] They are generally nonmigratory, although some startling exceptions in the *Merops* bee-eaters and rollers have been documented. Each family, and often even genus, is so phenotypically distinct that it is difficult to confuse their identification with any other bird species, but they rarely ever seem to resemble other species within their own order.

Extensive natural history descriptions for this order have been provided in a prior edition,[4] where the topic was reviewed in its entirety, and no additions or changes have been made thereafter.

UNIQUE ANATOMY

Coraciiformes species generally are large headed, with short, hooked beaks and weak, short legs. Although exceptions to each of these characteristics exist, for example, the sharp beaks of the kingfishers or the delicate beaks of the hoopoes and wood hoopoes and the longer legs of the ground-rollers and ground hornbills, which move confidently by striding rather than hopping as typically seen in other species of this order. Coraciiformes species do share varying arrangements of syndactylism,[2] including fusion of pedal digits 3 and 4 in kingfishers, bee-eaters, hoopoes, and woodhoopoes; fusion of pedal digits 2 and 3 in rollers; central fusion of all pedal digits in hornbills; and zygodactylous pedal digits in ground-rollers and cuckoo-rollers. Additionally, all species lack the stylohyoideus muscle, which minimizes tongue mobility and affects feeding style, and ceca,[1] but all have a primitive bony stapes within the middle ear.

In Bucerotes, the molting patterns of the remiges and rectrices are characteristic of the order and are extremely complex. In *Momotus* species, the characteristic streamers of the central pair of rectrices terminate in diamond or oval racquets, and are created as the weakly attached barbs along that plume are lost from a normally erupted feather.[2] Bee-eaters present intercalated covert feathers along their primaries, whereas hornbills have no primary covert feathers. Most members of this order present brightly colored plumage, including the scarlet gorget characteristic of todies, although in hornbills spectacular keratin coloration is concentrated in the bare skin and beak rather than in the plumage. Most unusually, in the Asian hornbills in *Buceros*, the beak and casque coloration is based in orange and yellow carotenoid pigments as cosmetic oil obtained from the uropygial gland.[2]

The beak of the hornbill needs to be discussed in detail, as each of the 52 extant species develops an ornamentation on the dorsal rhinotheca (casque), which is unique to this group.[2] In all but one species, the structure is an air-filled chamber created of a thin bony layer surrounded by keratin, although in some species (*Tockus* and *Ocycerous*), the casque is simply a ridge. The exception of the helmeted hornbill (*Rhinoplax* [*Buceros*] *vigil*) is the casque of the male that is immense and essentially solid; it is made of an "ivory," which weighs nearly 10% of the bird's body

TABLE 29-1

Supplemental Biology for the Order Coraciiformes[2,4]

	Weight	Length	Free-Ranging Diet	Captive Diet
Kingfisher	Micronesian 58–66.5 grams (g)[19]		Never plants	Supplement with calcium, multi-vitamins during hand rearing[10]
Tody	5–9 g		Limited vegetation	
Motmot	Blue-crowned 105–125 g[19]	Blue-crowned 38–43 centimeters (cm)		
Bee-eater	Most spp. 20–90 g Carmine 44–61 g Rainbow 20–30 g	Carmine 24–27 cm, tail 9 cm		Mixed carotenoid supplementation specific for carmine and rainbow[3,10]
Roller	80–214 g		Chicks fed exclusively protein for first 14 days of nesting	
Woodhoopoe	Green 54–99 g	Green 32.5–37 cm		
Hornbill			Omnivores with increased protein and fig consumption associated with reproduction; African *Tockus* primarily insectivorous; African *Bucorvus* essentially carnivorous; Asian *Buceros* omnivorous with marked protein consumption; all other species predominantly frugivorous	Despite differences in diets, *Buceros* and *Aceros* hornbills did not have differing protein metabolism;[6] caution indicated for iron-sensitive *Aceros* sp.[9]

NOTE: As Table 29-1 in the previous edition[4] was well detailed and extensively reviewed, this current table only provided updates or amendments to the previously published data. No changes of any kind were needed for data on ground-rollers, cuckoo-rollers, or hoopoes.

weight as compared with the estimated 3% to 5% in other *Buceros* species.[2,8] The true purpose of the casque is unknown, although it has been proposed to be a resonance chamber or a hammer for nest excavation. It is presumed to be a signaling mechanism, particularly for gender and maturity, as it varies so markedly by species, gender, and age. Systematic imaging and skeletal preparation have identified relationships of this casque space within the paranasal sinus system.[8] Specifically, *Buceros* hornbills were not found to connect the casque space to the maxillary sinus, whereas other species were demonstrated to do so. All species assessed did present a casque sinus located between the casque and the calvarium.

Another unique feature of the bucerotids is the normal presence of subcutaneous emphysema. This air sac system begins to develop in the chick under the skin of the shoulders and then moves to cover the entire body by the time of fledging.[2]

Additional taxonomic description has been provided in a prior edition,[4] and the taxonomy was reviewed in its entirety with no additions or changes for anatomy, measurements, or dietary habitats made thereafter; the exceptions have been discussed above and are listed in Table 29-1.

SPECIAL PHYSIOLOGY

The non-hornbill species of the order overall do not tolerate extreme temperatures well. Generally, the taxon-specific approach to colder ambient temperatures is communal nocturnal roosting, especially documented in bee-eaters and woodhoopoes, and morning sunbathing.[2] The exception to this cold management is found in the todies (see extensive accurate description provided in the prior edition[4]) and includes heterothermy, reduced basal metabolic temperature, and torpor; these adaptive mechanisms are employed most notably in females.[2] These approaches are rare within other avian species, specifically *heterothermy*, which has been documented in two families of Passeriformes (Nectariniidae–sunbirds; Pipridae–manakins) and in Apodiformes (hummingbirds), and *torpor*, which has been

documented in four orders—Apodiformes, Caprimulgiformes (nightjar), Coliiformes (mousebirds), Procellariiformes (petrels)—and in only one family within Passeriformes—Hirundinidae (swallows). Bee-eaters have thin plumage on their medial thighs, which allows dissipation of excess heat when the legs are lowered during flight.[2]

Most other taxon-specific details have not changed from the prior edition[4] and exceptions are discussed later in this chapter.

HOUSING REQUIREMENTS

In the prior edition of this text, details regarding the natural habitats and reproductive parameters of this order were reviewed and have not changed thereafter.[4] In spite of the several highly cooperative breeding techniques used by these species, it is important to note that many of the Coraciiformes species are highly territorial; this can complicate mixed-species displays, particularly those containing kingfishers, motmots, rollers, and wood hoopoes.[2]

FEEDING

In the prior edition of this text, details on the natural and captive diets documented were reviewed and have not changed thereafter.[4] An additional detail that has to be noted is that reduced tongue mobility, as a result of lack of the retractor musculature, affects the ability of the Coraciiformes species to manipulate food. It is the beak that manipulates food items dexterously, and the manipulation ends with a head tossing technique that moves the food to the caudal oral cavity to be swallowed. The green woodhoopoe (*Phoeniculus pupureus*) has gender differences in beak length and size, which affects the type and size of insect prey each gender most successfully obtains.

As food items are swallowed intact, nearly every species of the order has been confirmed to employ mashing or often "whacking" of food items held in the beak to soften fruits, kill prey and break its bones, or remove spines or barbs.[2] This approach is particularly important for birds such as bee-eaters that consume venomous prey or when chicks are fed. Because of their consumption of whole-prey food items, many of the Coraciiformes species—even chicks—regurgitate pellets of indigestible material. This finding is particularly noteworthy in bee-eaters but rarely seen in hoopoes and never in todies.

Hornbills can be categorized by their means of food carriage to the nest to feed chicks as those that carry single or multiple items, those that swallow and regurgitate the food item, and those that carry the food item intact in the beak.[2] The smallest African species (*Tockus*) carry single food items in the bill tip, whereas the largest African species (*Bucorvus*) carry multiple items aligned along the beak path. The arboreal African species found in the genera *Bycanistes* and *Ceratogymna* are mainly frugivorous and similar to the Asian hornbill frugivores of the genera *Anthracoceros*, *Aceros*, and *Rhyticeros*, as they swallow a number of fruits and then regurgitate them singly to feed the chicks at the nest. Interestingly, the Asian species in *Ocyceros* that most phenotypically resemble *Tockus* was differentiated by its carriage of multiple ingested fruit items for regurgitation. The largest Asian hornbills of *Buceros* and *Rhinoplax* feed multiple ingested fruits to chicks by swallowing and then regurgitating the food, whereas individual prey items are carried in the beak and presented to the chicks.

REPRODUCTION AND NEONATAL CARE

In the prior edition of this text, details on breeding behavior, egg appearance and number, and periods of incubation and nesting were reviewed and have not changed since[4] except as follows. To the extent known, rollers are considered monogamous. Bee-eaters produce up to 8, rather than 10, eggs; hoopoes produce 4 to 8 eggs, on average; palearctic hoopoes produce up to 12 eggs; and woodhoopoes produce an average of 2 to 5 eggs.[2,4] A species-specific detail to note is that each one of the 1 to 4 eggs laid by a female tody is 26% of its body mass. Each egg has a large yolk in proportion to its size because of longer incubation duration by 1 week compared with similarly sized bird's eggs, and this imparts a rosy-sheen to the white shell. This prodigious commitment of resources is similar to that measured in only two other avian families, Apterygidae (kiwi) and Hydrobatidae (storm petrel), whereas in most other avian species, a given egg makes up between 1.8% to 11% of the female's body weight.[2]

Coraciiformes neonates are hatched altricial, with prognathism that is maintained for several days. As the order members are cavity-nesters, often with minimal nest material, the chicks have prominent tarsal callosities to cushion this area. They are all gymnopedic, except for the montane blue-throated motmot (*Aspatha gularis*), cuckoo-roller, hoopoe, and green woodhoopoe. However, all Coraciiformes species have quill-like eruptions of their developing feathers, which persist in the waxy sheaths for a protracted time. As the majority of the order is naked of other plumage at this stage, the chick has a startling appearance that has been described as resembling a "hedge-hog," a "pincushion," or a "porcupine." The chicks essentially fledge with a duller version of the adult plumage.

Some species-specific information with regard to the cavity nesting of Coraciiformes is presented in Table 29-2. These factors affect housing, nesting provision, and chick rearing potential. The asynchronous hatching of the laughing kookaburra (*Dacelo novaeguinaea*) is particularly noteworthy, as siblicide of the younger chicks is frequent when resources are limited.[2] This species, by an unknown mechanism, also manipulates the gender of its chicks with the first eggs nearly always being male and second eggs being nearly always female. With the gender disparity of females of larger size than males in the Alcedines, this arrangement provides a catching-up potential for the second chick while permitting the first chick to establish itself. A second species-specific occurrence would be one egg from each green woodhoopoe clutch often failing to hatch, which appears to be a population-adaptive mechanism in wild populations.[2] Finally, as with adults, tody chicks are particularly vulnerable to cold temperatures. They are documented to huddle closely within the nest for warmth in a more taxon-typical manner to thermoregulation as compared with the adults of this species.[2]

TABLE 29-2

Nesting Characteristics of the Order Coraciiformes[2]

	Location	Appearance	Annual Replacement	Hatching Synchronicity
Kingfisher	Mud bank (most); tree; termite mound	Excavated or preformed chambers	Reused	Synchronous, except pied kingfisher (*Ceryle rudis*) and laughing kookaburra (*Dacelo novaeguineae*)
Tody	Earth embankment	Excavated burrows or tunnels	Replaced	Unknown
Motmot	Earth embankment	Excavated burrows	Replaced	Synchronous, except turquoise-browed motmot (*Eumomota superciliosa*)
Bee-eater	Earth embankment	Excavated holes	Replaced	Asynchronous
Roller	Tree (nearly all); earth	Excavated or enlarged holes	Unknown	Asynchronous
Ground-roller	Ground or earth embankment; except tree short-legged roller (*Brachypteracias leptosomus*)	Excavated burrows	Unknown	Unknown
Cuckoo-roller	Tree	Preformed cavity	Unknown	Unknown
Hoopoe	Rock; tree (secondary)	Preformed cavity	Reused but annual change to pair using	Asynchronous
Woodhoopoe	Tree	Preformed cavity	Unknown	Variable synchronicity
Ground hornbill	Flat ground	Minimal excavation	Variable, generally area reused	Synchronous
Hornbill	Tree	Excavated or enlarged cavities	Variable, generally reused	Asynchronous

It is important to note that nesting material is limited in the typical Coraciiformes environment in captive hand-rearing situations. Ventricular impaction with plant material resulting in death has been reported in juvenile Micronesian kingfishers (*Todiramphus* [*Halcyon*] *cinnamominus*).[13]

RESTRAINT AND HANDLING

Smaller Coraciiformes species, as well as small hornbills, can be captured, as described in the prior edition,[4] by using an appropriate-sized net and then restrained manually in a routine manner. However, adult hornbills, especially those other than *Tockus* species, generally should be captured by using direct manual restraint; netting must be followed by secure restraint of the bird's very strong beak and head movements. Hornbills are particularly amenable to operant conditioning, so routine training for weighing or for crating for transport should be considered.

SURGERY AND ANESTHESIA

No particular difference exists in the consideration of manual restraint versus anesthesia for Coraciiformes compared with other avian species. When the ability to restrain is limited or the required procedural intervention is more complex than physical examination and blood collection, anesthesia is recommended. Hornbills have external nares located near the head, and often in birds with larger casques routine facemask application is precluded; as an alternative to chamber induction, an appropriately sized plastic bag can be used to cover the head of the manually restrained bird and infused with inhalant anesthesia; this is an excellent induction approach prior to endotracheal intubation for longer procedures.

Surgical approach for Coraciiformes is not widely different from that for other similarly sized birds; however, the hornbill's casque and paranasal sinuses have to be taken into consideration while determining the surgical approach. Published reports of systematic imaging and skeletal preparation have provided surgical anatomic description of the casque space in relation to the paranasal sinuses.[8]

DIAGNOSTICS

Phlebotomy in Coraciiformes is routine, both in approach and volume limitations, as in other avian species. Subcutaneous emphysema of the Bucertoid may occasionally make it challenging to perform needle insertion along the venous furrows.

In the prior edition of this text, clinical pathology reference values were tabulated for several species of Coraciiformes.[4,19] At that time, it was noted that the data provided were derived from the classification of all individuals in the sample set regardless of age. In review, it was noted that using either all individuals or only adults did not change the data markedly, the exception being the alkaline phosphatase of the Abyssinian ground hornbill (*Bucorvus abyssinicus*), in which case exclusion of the data set to adults (22 international units [IU] ± 8) reduced this value from that for all birds (94 IU ± 129). This change was attributed to the long-lived nature of the species of this order and because 50% of the all-inclusive data set was for sub-adults. Table 29-3 provides both the number of birds sampled for reference ranges from the original table and additional reference values for other commonly displayed hornbill species.

INFECTIOUS DISEASE

No additional infectious disease concerns have been added to this edition of the text, as this taxon of birds does not have a particular disease predisposition, except the Micronesian kingfisher, in which hepatic mycobacteriosis has been repeatedly documented. Although the prior description remains accurate for the species,[4] more recent epidemiology has assessed this as a disease of environment rather than direct contagion.[21] Since the last edition,[4] a novel, somewhat

unexpected, atypical mycobacterial infection with *Mycobacterium simiae* has been documented in this kingfisher species.[20] With this apparent species proclivity, it is recommended that complete mycobacterial species identification be performed in suspected avian mycobacteriosis cases.

PARASITIC DISEASE

The information provided in the previous edition of this text is still current.[4] In the last decade, however, two reports of parasitic diseases of concern to this taxon have been documented. In three wrinkled hornbills (*Aceros* [*Rhyticeros*] *corrugatus*), deaths, disseminated granulomatous disease, and proventricular spirurid infection were identified. These animals presented as typically ill birds with abdominal distension.[5] The parasite—confirmed in only one case as *Microtetrameres*—was not identified with routine fecal parasite evaluations and seemed apparently unresponsive to usual anthelminthic protocols.

Even more recently, increasing reports of air sac trematodiasis have been associated with blue-crowned motmots (*Momotus momota*) in multiple U.S. and European collections.[15] These Cyclocoelidae digenean infections—not all, but many, in the genus *Szidatitrema*—seem to originate in wild-caught birds and have become established in coincident snail populations found within the animal's exhibit. Captive-born birds as well as passerines sharing habitats with motmots have become infected. Death has occurred in juvenile motmots and passerines because of suffocation by adult trematodes or egg-induced respiratory secretions. Diagnosis by using fecal flotation and sedimentation has been challenging because of inconsistent passage of eggs, so motmots in quarantine should be screened specifically and for multiple days. Although direct assessment of air sacs through endoscopy is possible, the procedure is highly invasive in smaller birds, and complete direct removal of adult trematodes is not possible. The diagnostic value of tracheal swabbing and lavage currently is under assessment (K. Delaski, personal communication). Treatment with praziquantel, clorsulon, and ivermectin has been reported to have little success in motmots, although passerines may be cleared of the parasite. This finding provides supporting evidence that the motmot is an adapted host and perhaps should be maintained separately from other bird species unless confirmed clear of trematodes.

NONINFECTIOUS DISEASE
Neoplasia

The most important neoplastic concern for Coraciiformes is squamous cell carcinoma of the casque in the giant hornbill (*Buceros bicornis*). The presentation, diagnostics, and possible treatments for this disease have been reviewed extensively elsewhere.[7] Only one new case has been reported in the United States but three have occurred on two other continents. Antioxidants such as carotenoids, which are present in the uropygial gland secretions of *Buceros* and transferred to the casque, may be contributory to neoplasia risk factors (K.C. Gamble, data in preparation, 2013).[17]

Carcinoma and squamous metaplasia in the uropygial gland have been reported in a single collection in the carmine bee-eater (*Merops nubicus*), which is another Coraciiformes species that is highly reliant on dietary carotenoids.[3,12] In five birds presented from a flock of 10, no etiologic viral agent or hypovitaminosis A was identified as an alternative explanation.

Iron Storage Disease

This issue is covered in more detail in another chapter in this text. Despite minimal data for confirmation (Table 29-4), a generally held concept is that Asian hornbills are uniformly susceptible to iron storage disease.[9,14,18] Many species of these genera are sympatric in areas of southern mainland Asia and associated islands. On the basis of an analysis of feeding strategies and dietary composition,[2,6] it seems unreasonable to assign a taxon-wide susceptibility.

TABLE 29-3

Clinical Pathology Mean and Standard Deviation for Selected Hornbill Species of the Order Coraciiformes[19]

	Von der Decken's (14)	Wreathed (18)	Wrinkled (35)	Rhinoceros (24)
WBC (1000/μL)	6.31 ± 5.90	15.95 ± 13.44	17.64 ± 10.41	17.46 ± 8.15
RBC (10^6/μL)	3.59 ± 0.59	3.00 ± 0.50	2.82 ± 0.61	3.43 ± 1.87
Hemoglobin (g/dL)	8.2 ± 1.3	15.0 ± 3.0	15.8 ± 2.5	13.6 ± 2.3
PCV (%)	45.4 ± 5.2	47.4 ± 6.8	48.9 ± 6.1	45.9 ± 5.9
Heterophil (1000/μL)	3.12 ± 3.31	10.21 ± 11.43	8.10 ± 5.6	8.98 ± 4.05
Lymphocyte (1000/μL)	2.68 ± 2.82	4.50 ± 2.87	7.18 ± 5.84	7.61 ± 5.32
Mon ocyte (1000/μL)	0.34 ± 0.43	0.60 ± 0.53	1.25 ± 1.07	0.82 ± 0.66
Eosinophil (1000/μL)	0.28 ± 0.42	0.83 ± 0.86	1.67 ± 2.49	0.87 ± 2.05
Basophil (1000/μL)	0.19 ± 0.03	0.23 ± 0.19	0.93 ± 1.22	0.22 ± 0.12
Calcium (mg/dL)	8.2 ± 1.0	7.6 ± 1.0	8.5 ± 1.2	9.4 ± 1.6
Phosphate (mg/dL)	3.1 ± 2.1	3.3 ± 1.1	4.0 ± 2.1	5.9 ± 3.7
Sodium (mEq/L)	159 ± 5	149 ± 10.0	161 ± 11	156 ± 9
Potassium (mEq/L)	3.5 ± 0.8	3.3 ± 1.3	3.4 ± 1.1	4.3 ± 1.3
Chloride (mEq/L)	121 ± 7	109 ± 17	116 ± 8	116 ± 6
Uric acid (mg/dL)	10.1 ± 8	8.9 ± 5.1	0.2 ± 0.1	7.9 ± 4.1
Total bilirubin (mg/dL)	1.1 ± 0	0.2 ± 0	0.2 ± 0.1	0.1 ± 0.1
Glucose (mg/dL)	343 ± 50	258 ± 49	250 ± 44	218 ± 46
Cholesterol (mg/dL)	85 ± 31	144 ± 33	109 ± 41	159 ± 49
CPK (IU/L)	560 ± 245	602 ± 212	454 ±223	1618 ± 550
ALP (IU/L)	144 ± 61	32 ± 10	44 ± 19	83 ± 112
ALT (IU/L)	23 ± 13	72 ± 130	26 ± 13	28 ± 10
AST (IU/L)	135 ± 42	291 ± 125	162 ± 62	259 ± 66
Total protein (g/dL)	2.9 ± 0.6	4.2 ± 0.5	3.7 ± 0.8	4.2 ± 0.7
Globulin (g/dL)	1.1 ± 0.3	2.2 ± 0.4	1.8 ± 0.4	2.0 ± 0.7
Albumin (g/dL)	1.6 ± 0.5	1.9 ± 0.4	1.8 ± 0.4	1.9 ± 0.5

ALP, Alkaline phosphatase; *ALT*, alanine aminotransferase; *AST*, aspartate aminotransferase; *CPK*, creatine phosphokinase; *mEq/dL*, milliequivalent per deciliter; *mg/dL*, milligram per deciliter; *μL*, microliter; *PCV*, packed cell volume; *RBC*, red blood cell; *IU/L*, international unit per liter; *WBC*, white blood cell.
NOTE: For this chapter, maximum number of birds contributing samples is provided following the species name. For comparable table (Table 30-2) in the preceding edition,[4] these sample sizes were: Micronesian kingfisher (73), blue-crowned motmot (33), carmine bee-eater (20), lilac-breasted roller (30), common hoopoe (28), green woodhoopoe (21), Abyssinian ground hornbill (45), and great Indian hornbill (41).

TABLE 29-4

Mean and Standard Deviation of Plasma Iron Concentrations (μg/dL) for Selected Hornbill Species of the Order Coraciiformes[19]

Abyssinian Ground (8)	African Ground (3)	Giant Indian (4)	Rhinoceros (1)	Wreathed (2)	Wrinkled (1)*	Silvery-cheeked (2)
102 ± 34	92 ± 18	801 ± 678	139	257 ± 19	135 ± 59	111 ± 53

NOTE: Number of birds contributing samples is provided following the species name. One specimen (*) provided multiple samples to the database.

In 2012, database analysis of 334 complete hornbill necropsies, spanning a 20-year period, confirmed that in 10% (15 of 149) of African hornbills and 23% (43 of 185) of Asian hornbills, iron storage disease was the primary cause of death.[9] Analysis of data on Asian hornbills focused on the four genera with more than 10 individuals in the overall database, including *Buceros* (79), *Aceros* (54), *Rhyticeros* (23), and *Anthracoceros* (19). Only *Aceros* presented increased evidence of iron storage disease, as 32% of the 43 cases were confirmed attributable to iron storage disease, whereas in each of the other genera 21% to 24% were confirmed. The analysis was extended to those species with greater than 20 individuals in the overall database, including giant hornbill (*Buceros bicornis*) (53), rhinoceros hornbill (*Buceros rhinoceros*) (26), wrinkled hornbill (*Aceros (Rhyticeros) corrugatus*) (33), and wreathed hornbill (*Rhyticeros undulatus*) (23). Iron storage disease was present predominantly in two species: wrinkled hornbills (24%) and wreathed hornbills (30%), compared with *Buceros* at 7.5% and 19% in giant and rhinoceros hornbills, respectively.

On the basis of this analysis, it was recommended that the two *Aceros* species be considered iron sensitive because of their primarily frugivorous diet, which seems a predisposing factor for other avian taxa with iron sensitivity.[9] Since the Asian hornbill has been managed historically as iron sensitive, the evaluated data may underestimate the actual prevalence of the problem. Treatment for iron storage disease has been accomplished through routine chelation, with success rates similar to those documented for other iron-sensitive species.[17] For *Aceros* and *Rhyticeros* species, particularly wrinkled hornbills and wreathed hornbills, and perhaps even more for frugivorous African species, dietary iron should be restricted through accurate and complete feed analysis of low-iron products and through limitation of animal protein.[16] Additionally, provision of dietary tannin may help restrict absorption of ingested iron. However, these restrictions must be lifted during breeding activities and nesting.[16] This approach reflects the natural tendency of this taxon to increase dietary protein intake during these times and provides the needed nutritional support for the chicks as well as for the female that is not only caring for the chicks but also undergoing a complete molt of remiges and rectrices. In another iron-sensitive avian species, intermittent dietary iron restriction seemed to minimize its storage concerns while permitting reproductive success.[11]

Atherosclerosis

Interestingly, with their reliance on uropygial gland carotenoids, aortic and primary artery atherosclerosis has been reported increasingly as a primary cause of death in giant hornbills (K.C. Gamble, data in preparation, 2013).[17]

REFERENCES

1. Clench MH: The avian cecum: Update and motility review. *J Exp Zool* 283:441–447, 1999.
2. Del Hoyo J, Elliott A, Sargata J: *Handbook of the birds of the world*, vol 6, Barcelona, Spain, 2001, Lynx Edicions, pp 129–523.
3. Dierenfeld E, Sheppard C: Canthaxanthin pigment does not maintain color in carmine bee-eaters. *Zoo Biol* 15(2):183–185, 1996.
4. Dutton CJ: Coraciiformes (kingfishers, motmots, bee-eaters, hoopoes, hornbills). In Fowler ME, Miller RE, editors: *Fowler's zoo and wild animal medicine*, ed 5, St. Louis, MO, 2003, Saunders, pp 254–260.
5. Ferrell ST, Pope KA, Gardiner C, et al: Proventricular nematodiasis in wrinkled hornbills (*Aceros corrugatus*). *J Zoo Wildl Med* 40(3):543–550, 2009.
6. Foeken SG, de Vries M, Hudson E, et al: Determining nitrogen requirements of *Aceros* and *Buceros* hornbills. *Zoo Biol* 27(4):282–293, 2008.
7. Gamble KC: Squamous cell carcinoma in *Buceros* hornbills. In Miller RE, Fowler ME, editors: *Fowler's zoo and wild animal medicine*, ed 7, St. Louis, MO, 2011, Saunders, pp 281–285.
8. Gamble KC: Internal anatomy of the hornbill casque described by radiography, contrast radiography, and computed tomography. *J Avian Med Surg* 21(1):38–49, 2007.
9. Gamble KC, Garner MM, Wolf C: Iron storage disease susceptibility profiles in Asian hornbills. In *Proceedings of the American Association of Zoo Veterinarians Annual Meeting*, Oakland, CA, 2012, pp 187–189.
10. Graham KT: www.coraciiformestag.com. Accessed 13 January, 2013.
11. Helmick KE, Kendrick EL, Dierenfeld ES: Diet manipulation as treatment for elevated serum iron parameters in captive Raggiana bird of paradise (*Paradisaea raggiana*). *J Zoo Wildl Med* 42(3):460–467, 2011.
12. Howard L, Lamberski N, Newton AL: Uropygial gland inflammation, neoplasia, and surgical resection in six Northern carmine bee-eaters (*Merops nubicus nubicus*). In *Proceedings of the American Association of Zoo Veterinarians Annual Meeting*, Tampa, FL, 2006, p 18.
13. Kinsel MJ, Briggs MB, Crang RJE, et al: Ventricular phytobezoar impaction in three Micronesian kingfishers (*Halcyon cinnamomina cinnamomina*). *J Zoo Wildl Med* 35(4):525–529, 2004.
14. Klasing KC, Dierenfeld ES, Koutsos EA: Avian iron storage disease: Variations on a common theme? *J Zoo Wildl Med* 43(Suppl):S27–S34, 2012.
15. Libert C, Joet D, Ferté H, et al: Air sac fluke *Circumvitellatrema momota* in a captive blue-crowned motmot (*Momotus momota*) in France. *J Zoo Wildl Med* 43(3):689–692, 2012.
16. Olsen GP, Russell KE, Dierenfeld E, et al: A comparison of four regimens for treatment of iron storage disease using the European starling (*Sturnus vulgaris*) as a model. *J Avian Med Surg* 20(2):67–73, 2006.
17. Petzinger C, Heatley JJ, Cornejo J, et al: Dietary modification of omega-3 fatty acids for birds with atherosclerosis. *J Am Vet Med Assoc* 236(5):523–528, 2010.
18. Sandmeier P, Clauss M, Donati OE, et al: Use of deferiprone for the treatment of hepatic iron storage disease in three hornbills. *J Am Vet Med Assoc* 240:75–81, 2012.
19. Teare A: *Reference ranges for physiological values for captive wildlife, 2002 edition*, Apple Valley, Minnesota, 2002, International Species Information System.
20. Travis (Crook) EK, Junge RE, Terrell SP: Infection with *Mycobacterium simiae* complex in four captive Micronesian kingfishers. *J Am Vet Med Assoc* 230(10):1524–1529, 2007.
21. Witte CL, Hungerford LL, Papendick R, et al: Investigation of factors predicting disease among zoo birds exposed to avian mycobacteriosis. *J Am Vet Med Assoc* 236(2):211–218, 2010.

CHAPTER 30

Piciformes (Honeyguides, Barbets, Woodpeckers, Toucans)

John M. Sykes IV

BIOLOGY

The order Piciformes comprises four families: (1) Indicatoridae (honeyguides); (2) Capitonidae (barbets); (3) Picidae (woodpeckers); and (4) Ramphastidae (toucans, toucanets, aracari). The jacamars (Galbulidae) and puff birds (Bucconidae) are now considered part of the order Galbuliformes. Galbuliformes and Piciformes have historically been grouped together, as they are both zygodactylous and have similarities in tendon structure. However, the current thought is that zygodactyly has evolved separately in different taxa (including in Psittaciformes and Cuculiformes), so this trait does not imply a close evolutionary relationship. Galbuliformes species are typically insectivorous, neotropical, perching birds and are not often kept in captivity.[8]

Piciformes species are zygodactylous (digits 2 and 3 point forward, and digits 1 and 4 point backward), have unique and similar flexor tendon pattern in the leg, have a well-developed sehnenhalter of the tarsometatarsal trochlea, have short incubation times, have altricial (naked and blind) young, are cavity nesters, and lack down feathers as adults.[8,16,26] Honeyguides (Indicatoridae; 17 species; 10–20 centimeters [cm] long) are relatively small birds from sub-Saharan Africa and southern Asia. Wax, either in the form of a waxy coating of some insects or from honeybee nests, composes some portion of their diet. Adults have thickened skin, potentially as a protective mechanism against bee-stings, as they are not immune to this venom. They are brood-parasites, and their hatchlings will kill the host hatchlings. Barbets (Capitonidae; 82 species; 9–33 cm long) are pantropical and may be found in Asia, Africa, and Central and South Americas. They typically have a large head, short neck, and strong bills. Barbets are found primarily in forested areas and generally need a habitat with sufficient dead wood for excavation of nesting and roosting sites, although three species of the *Trachyphonus* genus nest in cavities in the ground. Woodpeckers (Picidae; 216 species; 8–50 cm long) have a cosmopolitan distribution (although not found in Australia or Antarctica). They are found typically in arboreal habitats such as tropical and temperate forests, but certain species live in sparsely treed areas, including deserts and rocky hillsides. The Ramphastidae family includes toucans, toucanets, and aracaris (34 species; 34–56 cm long). These birds are neotropical and found only in Central and South Americas. They typically have large brightly colored bills and are often found in the forest, although some species are present in woodlands and savannas. They typically nest in existing cavities, so their habitat may be limited by the presence of preexisting nest cavities.[8] As honeyguides are not often kept in captivity, the rest of this chapter will focus primarily on toucans and provide available information on barbets and woodpeckers.

UNIQUE ANATOMY

Barbets have a short tongue with a brushy tip and bristles around the bill.[8] Woodpeckers have anatomy designed to prevent head injury during hammering into wood, including a straight bill, specialized microstructure of the cranial bones to increase their strength, a modified hinge between the skull and mandible that redirects the force away from the brain, and modifications to the structure of the eye.[8,34,40] These birds also have a long tongue, with sublingual glands that produce a sticky substance. The tongue muscles are supported by an extensive hyoid apparatus that extends around the back of the skull and over the head and may enter the nares in some species (Figure 30-1).[8] Many woodpecker and neotropical barbet species are dimorphic.[7,16]

Toucans have serrated edges to their long and colorful bills. The bill is lightweight and composed of bony struts (Figure 30-2). Many functions have been proposed for this beak, including its use in courtship and foraging. One recent theory proposes that the beak may be used as an effective thermoregulator, similar to elephant ears.[30] The tongue is laminated along the sides and tends to be brush-like toward the tip (Figure 30-3). The tail vertebrae are modified such that these birds may rotate the tail forward until it touches the head, and they often sleep in this position with the tail forward and the head curved back.[8] Ramphastids also have a ventral deviation of the trachea at the thoracic inlet, which should not be interpreted as abnormal (see Figure 30-2). With the exceptions of some toucanets (*Selenidera* spp.), the green aracari (*Pteroglossus viridis*), and the lettered aracari (*P. inscriptus*), toucans are monomorphic. Toucans lack a crop.[8]

The nestlings of Piciformes species generally have some type of hypotarsal heel pad near the hock that they rest on the ground instead of standing on their feet. This feature fades as the nestlings mature.[7,8]

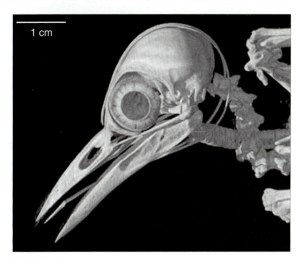

FIGURE 30-1 Composite computed tomography image of the skull of a golden-fronted woodpecker (*Melanerpes aurifrons*). Note how the hyoid apparatus wraps around the back and top of the skull, nearly reaching the nares. (Photo courtesy of Digimorph.org; reprinted with permission.)

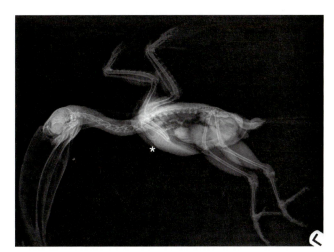

FIGURE 30-2 A lateral whole-body radiograph of a keel-billed toucan (*Ramphastos sulfuratus*). Note the minimal bony component to the bill and the ventral deviation of the trachea at the thoracic inlet (*asterisx*). This deviation is normal in Ramphastids. (Photo courtesy of J. Sykes, Wildlife Conservation Society.)

SPECIAL HOUSING REQUIREMENTS

As both barbets and woodpeckers excavate their own nesting and roosting cavities, these species may be destructive to wooden structures. Some of this behavior may be redirected by including enrichment items such as soft or rotting logs in the enclosure. Care should be taken to keep the enclosure free of blind-ended tight cavities. Barbets have been known to enter cavities such as the ends of hollow bamboo or paper towel rolls and be unable to back out. Barbets are generally kept in pairs or family groups. It may be useful to drill pilot holes in logs to encourage nest excavation and breeding for barbets, although woodpeckers will often use preexcavated nest boxes. Many of the Piciformes species may be territorial during breeding.[32]

Toucans are very active and need an appropriate amount of space. These birds do occasionally prey on smaller birds, particularly nestlings, and so may be difficult to keep with other species, as they may eliminate the breeding potential of other birds in the exhibit. The

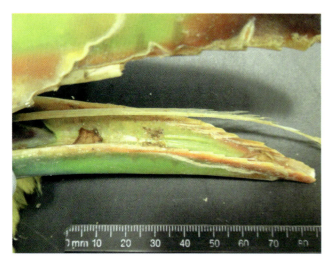

FIGURE 30-3 The tongue of a keel-billed toucan (*Ramphastos sulfuratus*). Note the laminated sides and brushlike tip. (Photo courtesy of D. McAloose, Wildlife Conservation Society.)

most successful housing for breeding activity is a large private outdoor enclosure. Breeding pairs should be visually separated from each other. Some species are somewhat cold tolerant but are susceptible to frostbite and should be kept indoors during the colder months in temperate climates.[16,32] Young birds may be prone to flying into mesh and damaging their bills, which are generally soft early in life. Care should be taken to avoid startling these young birds and to provide a large enough enclosure so that they can move away from people.[32] Adults are active and curious, so they may trap their heads in small holes or forked branches and may ingest foreign objects in the enclosure.[16] Ramphastids are reported to be particularly prone to yersiniosis, likely transmitted from rodents. Thus, food pans should be elevated off the ground, ideally on freestanding structures and preventive rodent control measures routinely employed.[32]

FEEDING

Barbets are primarily frugivorous but will eat arthropods. Woodpeckers are primarily insectivorous but will eat fruits, nuts, seeds, and sap. Toucans are primarily frugivorous. All these groups will feed insects, and often animal protein, to their nestlings. As toucans are particularly prone to hemochromatosis (iron storage disease), the iron in their diet should be limited. A number of low-iron complete pellets are commercially available. The appropriate upper limit of dietary iron is debatable. Pellets should contain less than 150 to 200 parts per million (ppm) iron,[32] and the total iron content of the diet should probably be less than 40 ppm.[7] Canine kibble is generally too high in iron for these birds. As in humans, highly acidic foods increase the absorption of iron from the stomach, so it is often recommended not to feed acidic fruits such as citrus, tomatoes, or strawberries to toucans.[7,16,32] Some institutions attempt to use dietary tannins to help bind the iron and make it less available for absorption. Methods for adding these tannins include soaking the food in brewed tea or sprinkling tea leaves over the diet. It is unclear if these types of measures alter the uptake of iron in birds, but they are not likely to be particularly harmful.[32]

RESTRAINT, ANESTHESIA, SURGERY, AND DIAGNOSTICS

Restraint and medical techniques are similar to those for other birds. Some of the larger specimens may bite, so their heads should be restrained as for psittacines. Anesthesia is most often accomplished

by using inhaled isoflurane. Custom-made masks (such as those made out of plastic soda bottles) are required to fit the long toucan beak into the mask to deliver the isoflurane to the nares. These birds may be easily intubated with an uncuffed endotracheal tube, although in the author's practice, most toucans are maintained by using a laryngeal mask airway to decrease the risk of postintubation tracheal stenosis.[29] Bill fractures are not uncommon in toucans. These wounds may be initially bandaged to control hemorrhage, and repair may be attempted with the use of dental restoratives and prosthetics.[7] Blood may be collected from the right jugular vein or the ulnar vein in larger animals. Selected hematology and biochemical parameters are listed in Tables 30-1 and 30-2.

Reports on the normal cloacal flora for three species of toucans and two species of aracaris have been published. Normal flora include typical gram-negative enteric bacteria (*Escherichia coli*, *Klebsiella* spp., *Enterobacter* spp.) in addition to gram-positive cocci, including *Staphylococcus* spp. and *Streptococcus* spp.[5]

DISEASES

Barbets

Little published information on the causes of morbidity or mortality in Piciformes other than ramphastids is available. A review of 164 necropsy records of barbets from 1939 to 2012 from the author's institution has revealed that 7% (12/164) died of metabolic causes, 15% (25 of 164) of trauma, and 28% (46 of 164) of infectious or inflammatory conditions, and the diagnosis remained open for 45% (75 of 164). Causes for inflammation where an etiology was determined included aspergillosis, pancreatic tremadodiasis, ventricular candidiasis, and disseminated mycobacteriosis. Two cases of neoplasia were identified: a pulmonary fibrosarcoma and a ventricular sarcoma. Although not widely reported in Piciformes other than ramphastids, 7 birds showed evidence of significant iron storage at the time of death: 5 showed hemosiderosis, and 2 showed hemochromatosis. Of these 7 birds, iron storage was thought to be related to the cause of death in 3 birds, whereas the other 4 had died of other causes.[18] In a similar review at a different institution, mycobacteriosis, aspergillosis, and air sac nematodiasis were occasionally seen in barbets.[12]

Incidental renal trematodiasis caused by *Tanaisia zarudnyi* was found in two captive barbets. The life cycle of this parasite involves snails, which may have been present in the enclosure.[23] Lesions similar to proventricular dilatation disease were seen in a bearded barbet (*Lybius dubius*). The bird was found dead with no antemortem signs. Intestinal dilatation was present, and lymphoplasmacytic infiltrates were seen in the ganglia of the gastrointestinal (GI) tract and skeletal muscle fibers.[19]

Woodpeckers

A review of 147 necropsy records of woodpeckers from 1939 to 2012 from the author's institution identified a cause of mortality in 51% (75 of 147), though in many cases, the cause remained undetermined because of postmortem autolysis or other reasons (72 of 147). Captive individuals made up 67% of cases (99 of 147) and free-ranging North American species 8% (12 of 147). Captivity status could not be determined for 24% (36 of 147), and these cases were not included in further analysis. Some etiologies, including arteriosclerosis (1 of 99), foreign body impaction or obstruction (3 of 99), and metabolic causes (9 of 99) such as hepatic lipidosis, were seen only in captive animals. Infection or inflammation caused 30% of deaths in captive animals (30 of 99), primarily of the GI tract (12 of 30) or respiratory tract (13 of 30), including one case of mycobacteriosis. Trauma as a cause of death was seen in 12% of captive animals (12 of 99). In free-ranging birds found on zoo grounds or presented for rehabilitation to the author's facility, trauma was the most common cause of death (7 of 12), followed by infection and inflammation (2 of 12), including one case of West Nile virus.[18]

In the literature, trematodiasis caused by *Tanaisia* spp.[3] and a lethal ventricular *Procyrnea* infection[25] have been reported. Protozoal

TABLE 30-1

Hematology Values in Toucans[1]

Parameter	Toucans[2] Mean	Toucans[2] Range	n	Toucans[3] Range	Toco-Toucan[4] (Ramphastos toco) Mean	Toco-Toucan[4] (Ramphastos toco) Range	n	Red-Breasted Toucan[4] (Ramphastos dicolorus) Mean	Red-Breasted Toucan[4] (Ramphastos dicolorus) Range	n
Erythrocytes (×10⁶/mm³)				2.5–4.5	2.49	2.24–2.74	7	2.04	1.53–2.55	6
PCV (%)	49.8	42–60	86	45–60	46	44–47	7	43.50	33–53	6
Hemoglobin (g/dL)					16.40	14.61–18.19	7	15.46	13.12–17.80	6
MCV (fL)					195.60	176–214	7	193.43	160–226	6
MCH (pg)					65.10	53–76	7	75.82	68–80	6
MCHC (g/dL)					35.30	31–39	7	35.99	30–41	6
Leukocytes (/mL)	13,500	8,000–18,000	86	4,000–10,000	5,500	2,100–8,800	3	8,000	3,500–12,400	5
Heterophils (%)	51.9	41–62	86	35–65	56	36–76	3	61	35–85	5
Heterophils/µL					3,730	536–6,923	3	4,680	1,162–8,197	5
Lymphocytes (%)	50.5	35–70	86	25–50	32	11–52	3	36	10–61	5
Lymphocytes/µL					2,060	992–3,127	3	3,240	423–6,056	5
Eosinophils (%)	0.67	0–3	86	0–1	0	0–1	3	1	0–2	5
Eosinophils/µL					0	0–63	3	50	0–95	5
Monocytes (%)	0	0–2	86	0–4	0	0–1	3	0	0–1	5
Monocytes/µL					0	0–20	3	0	0–60	5
Basophils (%)	0	0–1	86	0–5	0	0–1	3	0	0–1	5
Basophils/µL					0	0–20	3	0	0–11	5
Plasma protein (g/dL)								4.4	3.4–5.3	5

fL, Femtoliter; *g/dL*, gram per deciliter; *MCH*, mean corpuscular hemoglobin; *MCHC*, mean corpuscular hemoglobin concentration; *MCV*, mean corpuscular volume; *mL*, milliliter; *µL*, microliter; *PCV*, packed cell volume; *pg*, picogram.
[1]Reprinted from Cubas ZS: Piciformes (woodpeckers, barbets, puffbirds, jacamars, toucans). In Fowler ME, Miller RE (eds): *Zoo and wild animal medicine*, 5th ed. Philadelphia, PA, 2003, Saunders, pp. 261–266.
[2]Fudge AM: *Laboratory medicine: Avian and exotic pets*. Philadelphia, PA, 1999, Saunders.
[3]Cornelissen H, Ritchie BW: Ramphastidae. In Ritchie BW, Harrison GJ, Harrison LR (eds): *Avian medicine: Principles and application*. Lake Worth, FL, 1994, Wingers Publishing.
[4]Correia LS: *Laboratório ambiental*, Cascavel, PR, Brazil, 1999, Editora Universitária Edunioeste.

TABLE 30-2

Selected Serum Biochemical Values in Toucans[1]

Parameter	Toucans[2] Mean	Toucans[2] Range	n	Toucans[3] Range	Toco-Toucan[4] Mean	Toco-Toucan[4] Range	n
Total protein (g/dL)	3.5	2.8–4.4	86	3–5			
Albumin (g/dL)	2.1	1.4–2.4	86				
Globulin (g/dL)	1.79	1.4–2.2	86				
A:G ratio	1.42	0.92–2.67	86				
Calcium (mg/dL)	10.2	8.8–11.8	86	10–15			
Cholesterol (mg/dL)	175.1	104–254	86				
Glucose (mg/dL)	297.9	222–363	86	220–350			
LDH (IU/L)	257.6	180–319	86	200–400			
AST (IU/L)	243.3	141–340	86	130–330			
ALP (IU/L)	43.3	14–88	86				
Bile acid (µmol/L)	54.4	16–86	86				
Uric acid (IU/L)	7.93	2.4–14	86	4–14			
Plasma iron (µg/dL)				<350	104	88–119	11
TIBC (µg/dL)				<550	389	348–430	11
PST (%)					27	20–33	12

A:G ratio, Albumin:globulin ratio; *ALP*, alkaline phosphatase; *AST*, aspartate aminotransferase; *g/dL*, gram per deciliter; *IU/L*, international unit per liter; *LDH*, lactate dehydrogenase; *µg/dL*, microgram per deciliter; *µmol/L*, micromole per liter; *mg/dL*, milligram per deciliter; *PST*, percentage of saturation of transferring; *TIBC*, total iron binding capacity.
[1]Reprinted from Cubas ZS: Piciformes (woodpeckers, barbets, puffbirds, jacamars, toucans). In Fowler ME, Miller RE (eds): *Zoo and wild animal medicine*, 5th ed. Philadelphia, PA, 2003, Saunders, pp. 261–266.
[2]Fudge AM: *Laboratory medicine: Avian and exotic pets*. Philadelphia, PA, 1999, Saunders.
[3]Cornelissen H, Ritchie BW: Ramphastidae. In Ritchie BW, Harrison GJ, Harrison LR (eds): *Avian medicine: Principles and application*. Lake Worth, FL, 1994, Wingers Publishing.
[4]From Carlos Eduardo Silveira Goulart, TECSA Laboratories; Belo Horizonte, MG, Brazil.

meningitis caused by toxoplasmosis has been seen,[11] and lead intoxication has been found in two species of free-ranging woodpeckers.[17]

Ramphastids

Significant infectious diseases reported in ramphastids include gram-negative sepsis, mycobacteriosis, clostridiosis, herpesviral hepatitis, candidiasis, aspergillosis, and penicilliosis.

Bacterial sepsis caused by *Escherichia coli*, *Salmonella* spp., *Providencia* spp., and *Klebsiella pneumoniae* has been seen,[12,37,38] although many of these bacteria are part of normal cloacal flora.[5] Toucans are reported to be sensitive to sepsis caused by *Yersinia pseudotuberculosis*. This disease is thought to be spread by rodents in the enclosure, so proper hygiene and rodent control are important when housing these species.[7,16,32,38] Sepsis and disseminated bacterial disease caused by *Coxiella*-like bacteria,[24] *Bacteroides* spp.,[16] and mycobacterial species[20] have also been reported.

Ulcerative enteritis caused by *Clostridium colinum* has been reported in a group of toucans. Six individuals died over a 4-month period. The birds were found dead with no premonitory clinical signs. Necrotizing hepatitis and enteritis were identified on postmortem examination. These birds had elevated iron levels in their tissues, which was postulated to have contributed to the death of the birds.[33]

Candidiasis is not uncommon in chicks and young animals.[7,16] Pneumonia and airsacculitis caused by *Aspergillus* spp. and *Penicillium* spp. have been reported.[1,7] Typical antifungal treatments such as nystatin, ketoconazole, and itraconazole, as used in other birds, may be used to treat these infections in Piciformes.

A case of herpesviral hepatitis was reported in a toucan (species unknown). This bird was in contact with five macaws that had died of a herpesviral hepatitis at the same time, but the virus appeared to be distinct from Pacheco's herpesvirus.[4]

Capillariosis is a major cause of mortality in captive toucans. The parasites cause lethargy, diarrhea, dehydration, hypoproteinemia, anemia, and emaciation. They may be treated with fenbendazole at 50 to 100 milligrams per kilogram (mg/kg), once daily (SID), for 5 days.[7] A filarial worm, *Pelecitus* sp., has caused tenosynovitis in the legs of a channel-billed toucan (*Ramphastos vitellinus*) with microfilariae seen in the lungs and legs.[15] *Toxoplasma* organisms have been recovered from the muscle tissue of a keel-billed toucan (*R. sulfuratus*), but the infection was likely not causing disease in this bird.[9]

Ramphastids are particularly prone to hemochromatosis. Unlike hemosiderosis, in which accumulation of iron in tissues does not result in inflammation or pathology, hemochromatosis results in cellular and functional derangements. It is unclear what factors cause some species to be more severely affected by this disease compared with others. It is postulated that species from environments low in iron or that consume diets typically low in iron have evolved to absorb and retain iron more efficiently. Alternatively, the lack of tannins in captive diets, which may be present in free-ranging diets, may contribute to the development of the condition, and stress may play a role as well.[14] Clinical signs in affected birds may include lethargy, dyspnea, anorexia, poor feathering, and neurologic signs (i.e., hepatic encephalopathy).[7,27] Birds may be found dead with no premonitory signs. Ascites or hepatomegaly may be identified on physical examination or via radiology or other imaging modalities. Liver function tests or enzymes may be altered on a standard biochemical panel. Tests that measure or estimate the iron content of the blood (e.g., total iron binding capacity or transferrin levels) are not often helpful in the diagnosis of this disease in birds. Definitive antemortem diagnosis may be made via histologic examination of a liver biopsy. Necropsy findings include hepatic congestion, enlargement, and discoloration, as well as fibrosis, cirrhosis, and ascites. Treatment may include regular phlebotomy or administration of iron-chelators such as deferoxamine (100 mg/kg, SID, subcutaneously [SQ])[6] or deferiprone (50 mg/kg, orally [PO], twice daily [BID] for 30 days).[36] Preliminary use of the drug deferasirox in a group of oropendolas in the author's practice resulted in white discoloration of the feathers.[21] Serial liver biopsies are generally recommended to monitor the efficacy of treatment. The iron content may be measured by using chemical tests or may be estimated by special staining and image analysis.[22] The author has used magnetic resonance imaging (MRI) to measure the iron content of the liver of a uakaris (*Cacajao calvus*), as has been reported in humans and gerbils,[2,35] and this modality may hold promise as a diagnostic tool in avian medicine. Because of the significance of the disease and difficulty in treatment, prevention is critical in these birds. Dietary iron should be strictly limited (20–60 ppm) except when raising chicks which need animal-source protein for growth.[7,38] For more in-depth discussion of this disease, the reader is referred to Chapter 69 of this text.

Nutritional secondary hyperparathyroidism (metabolic bone disease) has been reported in young toucans. The bill may become particularly soft and easily damaged with this condition. A calcium supplement may be added to the diet when raising chicks to help prevent this problem.[38] Diabetes mellitus has been reported in tocos (*R. toco*) and keel-billed toucans. This condition may be treated with insulin,[38] although one case of successful treatment with somatostatin has been reported.[13] Keel-billed toucans may be particularly sensitive to propylene glycol. Significant morbidity and mortality occurred when diets using propylene glycol as a preservative were fed to these birds.[39]

REPRODUCTION

General reproductive parameters are provided in Table 30-3. As discussed above, all Piciformes species are cavity nesters. They tend to have short incubation periods, which results in altricial young that take some time to mature. Barbets and woodpeckers generally excavate their own nests, whereas toucans generally use existing cavities that they occasionally enlarge.[32] Woodpeckers will use nest boxes, if provided, and creating pilot holes into which barbets may excavate may be helpful. Toucan cavities may be made by carving out the center of a log and creating an entry hole on one side. Ends of the log may then be capped with plywood. Some species may want to do some of their own excavation. In these cases, premade cavities may be filled with mud, shavings, and moss creating a relatively soft substrate for the birds to dig into.[32] Recommended sizes for toucan cavities are 70 to 100 cm long and 20 to 30 cm in diameter, with an 8- to 10-cm wide entrance hole; and for toucanets and aracaris, the measurements are 70 to 100 cm length 12 to 15 cm diameter for the cavity and 6 to 7 cm width for the entrance hole.[7] For successful reproduction in toucans, mate compatibility, appropriate housing, appropriate diet, and good general health are important. Finding or creating compatible pairs may be challenging. Incompatible pairs are not generally aggressive but are indifferent to each other. This may improve over time, or other pairings may be tried. Signs of good compatibility include the birds sitting close together, touching bills, and offering food items to each other.[16] Enclosures should be large and visually screened from other toucans. Adults may often be stimulated to take care of the young when live insects are offered.

Artificial incubation parameters for woodpeckers are 37.5° C and 55% humidity to start with. Humidity should be adjusted to achieve a 12% to 15% weight loss from laying to hatching.[32] Nestling woodpeckers may be presented for hand rearing to wildlife rehabilitation centers. These birds should be warmed and rehydrated prior to starting the feeding. They may be fed high animal-protein diets initially, as for passerines. As they age, they should be presented with a variety of food items such as insects, nuts, berries, and sap, using different methods, to encourage foraging behavior. Hatchlings need to be fed every 20 to 30 minutes for 12 to 14 hours per day, and fledglings may be fed every 45 minutes for the same period. Woodpeckers do not tend to gape and are stimulated to open the mouth when the beak is touched. Birds should reach adult weight by age 2 to 3 weeks.[10]

Artificial incubation parameters for toucans are 36.9° C to 37.2° C, with humidity maintained at 65%. Humidity should be adjusted as for woodpeckers (see above).[28] When hatchlings are moved to a brooder, temperature may be decreased slightly to 36.1° C and

TABLE 30-3

Reproductive Characteristics of Piciformes

Family	Number of Eggs/ Clutch	Incubation Period (days)	Time to Fledging (days)	Diet for Nestling	Parent Incubating/ Care
INDICATORIDAE Honeyguides	1*	12–18	38–40	Insects, fruits, beeswax, and larvae	Brood parasites of hole-nesting species Nestlings fed by the hosts
PICIDAE Woodpeckers, piculets, flickers, sapsuckers	2–9	11–17	18–25	Insect larvae, flying insects, fruits, nuts, sap	Both sexes incubate the eggs and feed the young
Wrynecks	5–10	12–13	25–26	Ants, other insects, spiders and fruits	Both parents feed and brood the young
MEGALAIMIDAE Asian barbets	2–5	12–15	31	Fruits and insects Large species may take young birds, lizards and mice	Both sexes care for the young
LYBIIDAE African barbets	3–4†	18–19†	33†	Fruits (figs), insects, and snails	Both sexes care for the young
CAPITONIDAE New World barbets	1–5	13–17	31	Fruits, insects, spiders, and small vertebrates	Both sexes care for the young
RHAMPHASTIDAE Toucan and toucanets	2–4	15–16	43–50	Fruits, seeds, and berries but also insects, spiders, lizards, and eggs and nestlings of other birds	Both parents incubate the eggs and feed the young

*One (rarely two) in each of several host's nest.
†Data for black-collared barbet (*Lybius torquatus*).
Reprinted from Cubas ZS: Piciformes (woodpeckers, barbets, puffbirds, jacamars, toucans). In Fowler ME, Miller RE (eds): *Zoo and wild animal medicine*, 5th ed. Philadelphia, PA, 2003, Saunders, pp. 261–266.

humidity increased to 93% to 95%. Because of the lack of a crop, ramphastids must be fed small amounts at a time, so it takes longer to feed these birds than with a psittacine of comparable size (i.e., food must pass to the proventriculus before more may be given, so a large bolus cannot be given, as may be done in birds with crops).[28] Many institutions treat hatchlings with oral nystatin to help prevent GI candidiasis, which is common in these birds.[28,31] Hand-fed commercial formulas are developed for parrots, with the addition of animal protein such as pinkie mice as well as fruit.[28,31] Hatchlings should be fed a liquid diet every 60 to 90 minutes for 14 hours of the day for the first week. After that time, they may eat small pieces of solid food six to seven times per day. In the wild, toucans do not generally offer their chicks fruit until they are 4 to 7 days old.[31] For parent rearing, crickets, mealworms, boiled eggs, and pinkie mice may be provided as high-protein sources.[7] Chicks fledge in 6 to 7 weeks and may feed independently by 10 to 12 weeks.

ACKNOWLEDGMENT

The author would like to thank Dr. A. Harley Newton, for compiling the mortality data on barbets and woodpeckers, and Dr. M. Clancy, for aid in manuscript preparation.

REFERENCES

1. Aho RB, Westerling B, Ajello L, et al: Avian penicilliosis caused by *Penicillium griseofulvum* in a captive toucanet. *J Med Vet Mycol* 28:349–354, 1990.
2. Bonkovsky HL, Rubin RB, Cable EE, et al: Hepatic iron concentration: Noninvasive estimation by means of MR imaging techniques. *Radiology* 212:227–234, 1999.
3. Byrd EE, Denton JF: The helminth parasites of birds. I. A review of the trematode genus *Tanaisia* skrjabin, 1924. *Am Midl Nat* 43:32–57, 1950.
4. Charlton BR, Barr BC, Castro AE, et al: Herpes viral hepatitis in a toucan. *Avian Dis* 34:787–790, 1990.
5. Cornelissen JMM, van den Brink ME, Bakker MH, Koopman JP: Cloacal microflora of healthy hornbills, toucans, and aracaris. In *Proceedings of the First Conference of the European Committee of the Association of Avian Veterinarians*, Vienna, Austria, 1991, pp 453–460.
6. Cornelissen H, Ducatelle R, Roels S: Successful treatment of a channel-billed toucan (*Ramphastos vitellinus*) with iron storage disease by chelation therapy: Sequential monitoring of the iron content of the liver during the treatment period by quantitative chemical and image analyses. *J Avian Med Surg* 9:131–137, 1995.
7. Cubas ZS: Piciformes (woodpeckers, barbets, puffbirds, jacamars, toucans). In Fowler ME, Miller RE, editors: *Zoo and wild animal medicine*, ed 5, Philadelphia, PA, 2003, Saunders, pp 261–266.
8. Del Hoyo J, Elliott A, Sargatal J, editors: *Handbook of the birds of the world*, vol. 7. Barcelona, Spain, 2002, Lync Edicions.
9. Dubey JP, Velmurugan GV, Morales JA, et al: Isolation of *Toxoplasma gondii* from the keel-billed toucan (*Ramphastos sulfuratus*) from Costa Rica. *J Parastiol* 95:467–468, 2009.
10. Duerr RS: Woodpeckers. In Gage LJ, Duerr RS, editors: *Hand-rearing birds*, Ames, IA, 2007, Blackwell Publishing, pp 347–354.
11. Gerhold RW, Yabsley MJ: Toxoplasmosis in a red-bellied woodpecker (*Melanerpes carolinus*). *Avian Dis* 51:992–994, 2007.

12. Griner LA: Pathology of zoo animals, San Diego, CA, 1983, Zoological Society of San Diego, pp 246–250.

13. Kahler J: Sandostatin® (synthetic somatostatin) treatment for diabetes mellitus in a sulfur breasted toucan (*Ramphastus sulfuratus sulfuratus*). In *Proceedings of the Association of Avian Veterinarians*, Reno, NV, 1994, pp 269–273.

14. Lowenstine LJ, Munson L: Iron overload in the animal kingdom. In Fowler ME, Miller RE, editors: *Zoo and wild animal medicine*, ed 4, Philadelphia, PA, 1999, Saunders, pp 260–268.

15. Madani SA, Dorrestein GM: Filarial tenosynovitis caused by *Pelecitus* species (Spiurida, Filarioidea, Onchocercidae) in the legs of a channel-billed toucan (*Ramphastos vitellinus*). *J Avian Med Surg* 26:36–39, 2012.

16. Mikich SB, Jennings J, Cubas ZS: Order Piciformes (Toucans, Woodpeckers). In Fowler ME, Cubas ZS, editors: *Biology, medicine, and surgery of South American wild animals*, Ames, IA, 2001, Iowa State University Press, pp 180–199.

17. Morner T, Petersson L: Lead poisoning in woodpeckers in Sweden. *J Wildl Dis* 35:763–765, 1999.

18. Newton A: Personal communication, 2013.

19. Perpinan D, Fernandez-Bellon H, Lopez C, Ramis A: Lymphoplasmacytic myenteric, subepicardial, and pulmonary ganglioneruritis in four nonpsittacine birds. *J Avian Med Surg* 21:210–214, 2007.

20. Portaels F, Realini I, Bauwens L, et al: Mycobacteriosis caused by *Mycobacterium genavense* in birds kept in a zoo: 11-year survey. *J Clin Microbiol* 34:319–323, 1996.

21. Raphael B: Personal communication, 2013.

22. Roels D, Ducatelle R, Cornelissen H: Quantitative image analysis as an alternative to chemical analysis for follow-up of liver biopsies from a toucan. *Analyt Quantitative Cylol Histol* 18:221–224, 1996.

23. Rotstein DS, Flowers JR, Wolfe BA, Loomis M: Renal trematodiasis in captive double-toothed barbets (*Lybius bidentatus*). *J Zoo Wildl Med* 36:124–126, 2005.

24. Shivaprasad HL, Cadenas MB, Diab SS, et al: Coxiella-like infection in psittacines and a toucan. *Avian Dis* 52:426–432, 2008.

25. Siegel RB, Bond ML, Wilderson RL, et al: Lethal *Procyrnea* infection in a black-backed woodpecker (*Picoides arcticus*) from California. *J Zoo Wildl Med* 43:421–424, 2012.

26. Simpson SF, Cracraft J: The phylogenetic relationships of the Piciformes (Class Aves). *Auk* 98:481–494, 1981.

27. Spalding MG, Kollias GV, Calderwood Mays MB, et al: Hepatic encephalopathy associated with hemochromatosis in a toco toucan. *J Am Vet Med Assoc* 189:1122–1123, 1986.

28. St. Leger J, Vince M, Jennings J, et al: Toucan hand feeding and nestling growth. *Vet Clin North Am Exotic Anim Prac* 15:183–193, 2012.

29. Sykes JM, Neiffer D, Terrell S: Review of 23 cases of post-intubation tracheal obstructions in birds. *J Zoo Wildl Med* 44:700–713, 2013.

30. Tattersall GJ, Andrade DV, Abe AS: Heat exchange from the toucan bill reveals a controllable vascular thermal radiator. *Science* 325:468–470, 2009.

31. Vince M: Toucans. In Gage LJ, Duerr RS, editors: *Hand-rearing birds*, Ames, IA, 2007, Blackwell Publishing, pp 355–360.

32. Vince M, Holland G, Schroeder D: Piciformes. In Holland G, editor: *Encyclopedia of Aviculture*, Surrey, BC, 2007, Handcock House, pp 207–225.

33. Walker RL, Anderson MA, Loretz KJ: Ulcerative enteritis in toucans. In *Proceedings of the 39th Annual Meeting of American Association Veterinary Laboratory Diagnosticians*, Little Rock, AK, 1996, p 19.

34. Wang LZ, Zhang HQ, Fan YB: Comparative study of the mechanical properties, microstructure, and composition of the cranial and beak bones of the great spotted woodpecker and the lark bird. *Sci China Life Sci* 54:1036–1041, 2011.

35. Wang ZJ, Lian L, Chen Q, et al: 1/T2 and magnetic susceptibility measurements in a gerbil cardiac iron overload model. *Radiology* 234:749–755, 2005.

36. Whiteside DP, Barker IK, Conlon PD, et al: Pharmacokinetic disposition of the oral iron chelator deferiprone in the domestic pigeon (*Columba livia*). *J Avian Med Surg* 21:121–129, 2007.

37. Wilson RB: Hepatic hemosiderosis and *Klebsiella* bacteremia in a green aracari (*Pteroglossus viridis*). *Avian Dis* 38:679–681, 1994.

38. Worell AB: Ramphastids. In Tully TN, Dorrestein GM, Jones AK, editors: *Handbook of avian medicine*, ed 2, Philadelphia, PA, 2000, Saunders, pp 297–311.

39. Worell AB: Suspected propylene glycol sensitivity in keel-billed toucans. In *Proceedings of the Association of Avian Veterinarians*, Portland, OR, 2000, pp 199–203.

40. Wygnanski-Jaffe T, Murphy CJ, Smith C, et al: Protective ocular mechanisms in woodpeckers. *Eye* 21:83–89, 2007.

CHAPTER 31

Passeriformes (Songbirds, Perching Birds)

Joseph A. Smith

GENERAL BIOLOGY

The species in the order Passeriformes are often referred to as "passerines" or "perching birds." This is the most diverse order of birds, comprising more than half the known bird species, more than half the bird genera, and more than half the bird families. Passerines have a worldwide distribution and inhabit all but the circumpolar habitats. Passerines are often the most abundant bird taxa in any given habitat. Passerines are relatively small birds, the largest species being the common raven, which weighs greater than 1.5 kilograms (kg), and the smallest being the short-tailed pygmy-tyrant with an average weight of 4.2 grams (g).

The order Passeriformes is often subdivided into suboscines and oscines, the latter often being referred to as "songbirds." Suboscines include the suborders Eurylaimi (broadbills, asities, pittas), Furnarii (ovenbirds, woodcreepers, antbirds), and Tyranni (cotingas, manakins, tyrant-flycatchers). Suborders Acanthisittae (New Zealand wrens) and Menurae (scrub-birds, lyrebirds) are often considered intermediate groups. All other passerines are in the subdivision of oscines.

UNIQUE ANATOMY

Passeriformes species are thought to be monophyletic, with the following anatomic features consistent across all species: (1) an aegithognathous palate, (2) unique syringeal anatomy, (3) an incumbent hallux (digit 1 is at the same level as the other digits of the foot) creating an anisodactyl foot, (4) unique arrangements of plantar tendons, (5) the tensor propatagialis brevis, which attaches to the forearm as well as the humerus, (6) bundled spermatozoa with a coiled head and large acrosome, and (7) distinctive foot anatomy, which allows independent action of the hallux.[10,34]

Passerines have a crop, but the cecum is vestigial or absent in most species. The right and left nasal sinuses do not communicate as they do in psittacines. The cranial thoracic air sacs and the clavicular air sacs are fused in passerines, resulting in seven total air sacs rather than the usual nine seen in other birds. Most passerines have 10 primary remiges, although in some oscines the tenth primary is reduced or vestigial.[10] Oscines have complex muscle morphology of the syrinx that allows for complex vocalizations, which are often learned. These traits make some passerines excellent mimics (e.g., mockingbird, mynah, etc.). The syrinx of suboscines is more basic and therefore produces less complex vocalizations. Several species of pitohui are known to have batrachotoxins in their skin and feathers, which serve as a toxic chemical defense.[9] Much as in dart frogs, this toxin is believed to originate from insects in the diet.

SPECIAL HOUSING REQUIREMENTS

Although small in size, passerines require ample amounts of enclosure space. In addition to enclosure size, elevated perching opportunities (above any perceived threats) and ample visual barriers (which may be achieved with live or artificial plants) may help to reduce stress in these birds. Chronic stress caused by inadequate enclosures or inappropriate husbandry is a major problem in passerines. Many of the common diseases in passerines (e.g., candidiasis, aspergillosis, mycobacteriosis, atoxoplasmosis) are considered to be caused by opportunistic pathogens that are often associated with immunosuppression resulting from chronic stress. Species-specific temperature requirements, social dynamics, lighting or photoperiod, and diets should also be carefully researched to reduce stress. Nest-building materials given to passerines should be carefully chosen, as some materials (especially fine synthetic fibers) are known to cause leg entanglement and constriction.[23] Small enclosures with wire mesh are known to cause feather damage (particularly rectrices and remiges) when the birds hang on the wire, possibly hindering flight. If a small enclosure is needed for transport or hospitalization, those with smooth, solid walls are preferred over those with wire mesh sides.

FEEDING

Passerines have a metabolic rate that is approximately 60% higher than in other bird taxa. When calculating the basal metabolic rate (BMR) in kilocalories, the formula for passerines is BMR = 129 ($W^{0.75}$), where W is the weight in kilograms. This difference in metabolism may have an effect on drug pharmacokinetics, requiring higher dosages, more frequent dosing intervals, or both in passerines compared with other birds. Daily water requirements for passerines are also higher than for other birds and may be as high as 250 to 300 milliliters per kilogram (mL/kg) daily.

The feeding strategies of passerines are as diverse as the species. The order includes species that exhibit carnivory, frugivory, nectivory, granivory, insectivory, and various combinations of omnivory. Diets for captive birds should replicate the natural history of the species and should be as varied as possible to reduce nutritional deficiencies. Some of the passerine species within the superfamilies Corvoidea, Muscicapoidea, Sylvioidea, and Passeroidea lack the L-gulonolactone oxidase enzyme necessary to synthesize vitamin C and therefore require ascorbic acid in their diet.[7] Some species with red-colored plumage (e.g., some *Carduelis* spp. and some *Euplectes* spp.) require carotenoids in the diet to maintain the normal intensity of the red pigment in the feathers.

Some species of passerines (e.g., tanagers, birds of paradise, starlings, mynahs, and manakins) are sensitive to excess iron in the diet, which leads to iron accumulation (hemosiderosis) and damage (hemochromatosis) in the liver (see Noninfectious Diseases below). Diets containing between 25 and 50 mg/kg iron on a dry-matter basis have been shown to prevent hemochromatosis in iron-sensitive species.[14] However, higher dietary iron content may be needed for breeding birds and growing chicks.[20] Reducing substances that may enhance iron absorption (e.g., citric acid, ascorbic acid), adding substances that may bind to iron in the diet to prevent absorption (e.g., tannins, phytates), or both are additional methods employed to prevent hemochromatosis in iron-sensitive species.[20]

Feeding stations for flocks of passerines should be designed to allow sufficient space for all birds to feed. Multiple feeding stations are recommended to reduce starvation caused by conspecific and interspecific aggression. Perches should be positioned such that feces do not drop below to contaminate the feeding areas. In wild house finches (*Carpodacus mexicanus*), increased risk of mycoplasmal conjunctivitis caused by *Mycoplasma gallisepticum* has been associated with tube-style feeders, and the risk was lowered with platform-style feeding stations.[12]

RESTRAINT AND HANDLING

All passerines may be manually restrained safely for short, nonpainful procedures. Longer or painful procedures should be performed with the birds under anesthesia. Initial capture may be difficult and stressful. In large aviaries, smaller capture cages containing feeding stations to attract the birds as well as doors that may be closed remotely are helpful. Birds may either be lured into these capture cages with food, or they may be trained by using operant conditioning to regularly use the cages. Once in a smaller enclosure, hand nets are most often used for capture of passerines. Dimming the room lights may facilitate a quicker capture.

Passerines may be manually restrained by using one of two primary methods, depending on the species and size. The first technique may be used on most species (Figure 31-1). The bird's neck is extended by using the thumb and the forefinger or by using the index and middle fingers, taking care not to apply excessive pressure to the structures within the neck. The body is then supported using the same hand. Pressure should not be exerted on the body cavity, as it may impede movement of the keel and result in hypoventilation, loss of consciousness, and rapid death. For larger passerines, the other hand may need to be used to restrain and extend the feet and legs. The second method of manual restraint is often employed by bird banders and should only be used on the smaller passerine species (Figure 31-2). The tibiotarsi of both limbs are held between the index and middle fingers. The hocks of both limbs are allowed to partially flex, and the tarsometatarsi of both limbs are then held between the index finger and the thumb. The body and the neck are left unrestrained. To avoid excessive strain on the limbs and to aid in normal respirations, the bird should be held in a normal sitting posture, with the majority of the weight resting on the top of the handler's fingers.

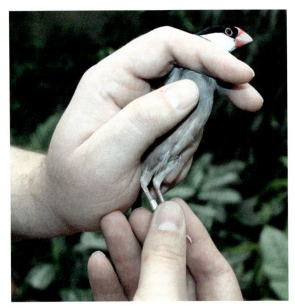

FIGURE 31-1 Restraint of most passerines such as the Java sparrow (*Padda oryzivora*) may be achieved by extending the neck with two fingers and extending the legs with the opposite hand, taking care not to impede normal keel movements and respirations. (Courtesy of the Fort Wayne Children's Zoo.)

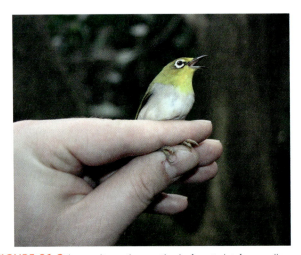

FIGURE 31-2 In an alternative method of restraint for smaller passerines such as the oriental white-eye (*Zosterops palpebrosus*), the tibiotarsi of both limbs are positioned between the index and middle finger, and the tarsometatarsi are held between the index finger and thumb. (Courtesy of the Fort Wayne Children's Zoo.)

ANESTHESIA AND SURGERY

Anesthesia in passerines may be used for proper radiographic positioning, stress reduction during procedures of long duration, and for painful or invasive surgeries or procedures. Gas inhalants, particularly isoflurane, are the most common anesthetic agents used in passerines. The high metabolism and highly efficient air sac system allow for very rapid inductions and recoveries. For the same reasons, passerines may also reach an excessively deep, life-threatening level of anesthesia very rapidly. Therefore, anesthetic monitoring, particularly of heart rate, respiratory rate, and respiratory depth, are critical and should be performed frequently with passerines.

The small size of many passerines poses many challenges during intubation and anesthetic monitoring. Endotracheal intubation with an uncuffed tube should be performed for all but the shortest of anesthetic procedures. Intravenous catheters with the stylet removed may be adapted to serve as an endotracheal tube for smaller species. Heart rate may be monitored with electrocardiography (ECG). Clamping the ECG leads to a small-gauge hypodermic needle that has been placed through the skin may improve the electrical signal and cause less trauma compared with clamping the leads directly to the bird. Heart rate may also be monitored with Doppler heart rate monitor, using a small amount of conductive gel and placing the probe over the mid-antebrachium. Respirations and end-tidal carbon dioxide may be monitored using capnography. Some capnography equipment may not be sensitive enough for the small-sized passerines. Clear surgical drapes allow for visualization of respirations and respiratory depth. Intravenous catheterization, through the jugular, ulnar, or metatarsal veins, may be possible only in the largest of passerines. For smaller species, intraosseous catheterization, with hypodermic needles placed in the distal ulna or proximal tibiotarsus, may be used to provide fluid support or critical care. Size and limitations of current technology make it difficult to obtain blood pressures in passerines. With larger passerines, an indirect systolic blood pressure reading may be obtained by placing a Doppler probe on the mid-antebrachium and placing an appropriately sized cuff around the humerus. Although not validated in passerines, this method may be helpful in monitoring trends and response to fluid therapy in cases of shock.

For surgical procedures, microsurgical instruments, adequate lighting, and magnification using surgical loupes are advantageous. Because of the small size of passerines, orthopedic procedures are often limited to external coaptation and splints. Common surgical indications include trauma, fractures, mass removal, and reproductive abnormalities such as egg binding and yolk coelomitis.

OTHER PHARMACEUTICALS

Most therapeutic drugs used in passerines are the same as those used in other avian species. The higher BMR of passerines should be considered during selection of therapeutic dosages and dosing frequencies, as absorption, time to maximum concentration, and half-life may be altered significantly. Metabolic scaling may be of assistance when estimating dosages or dosing frequencies for some drugs used for the first time in passerines. Commonly used antimicrobial and antiparasitic drugs are presented in Tables 31-1 and 31-2.[13] Because of the wide variations in species and the lack of pharmacokinetic data for most passerines, the use of any therapeutic drug warrants caution and careful monitoring of signs of overdose or lack of efficacy.

PHYSICAL EXAMINATION AND DIAGNOSTICS

The physical examination should be performed in a systematic manner as in other bird species. Some passerine nestlings such as estrildid finches may have very bold and intricate patterns, including tubercles and papillae, within the oral cavity or at the commissures of the beak. These normal, symmetrical patterns, which aid with recognition and feeding of chicks in the nest, should not be confused with lesions. These patterns and structures often disappear as the bird grows older. Other species may have bright red or yellow oral cavity colorations that should not be confused with erythema or jaundice. Auscultation of the heart is easily performed, but identification of murmurs or arrhythmias may be difficult because of the normally rapid heart rate of many passerines. Rates greater than 300 beats per minute (beats/min) are normal in passerines and generally cannot be counted accurately with only a stethoscope. Electronic methods (e.g., pulse oximetry or ECG) may be required to obtain an accurate heart rate.

Venipuncture may be performed with the same technique used in most other avian species. For passerines, the right jugular vein is

TABLE 31-1

Commonly Used Antimicrobial Drugs in Passerines

Drug	Dosage	Comments
ANTIBIOTICS		
Amikacin	15–20 mg/kg SQ, IM, q8-12h	5 days maximum
Amoxicillin trihydrate	150–175 mg/kg, PO, q12h	
Amoxicillin/clavulanate	125 mg/kg, PO, q12h	Dosage based on combined drugs
Azithromycin	43–45 mg/kg, PO, q24h	Intracellular infections
Ceftazidime	50–100 mg/kg, IM or IV, q4-8h	Penetrates the cerebrospinal fluid
Ceftiofur	50–100 mg/kg, q4-8h	
Cephalexin	40–100 mg/kg, PO or IM, q6-8h	
Ciprofloxacin	15–20 mg/kg, PO or IM, q12h	
Doxycycline	7.5–8 mg/kg, PO, q12-24h, 250 mg/L drinking water	Drug of choice for *Chlamydophila* and *Mycoplasma*
Enrofloxacin	10–20 mg/kg, PO, q24h, 200 mg/L drinking water	Broad spectrum
Metronidazole	50 mg/kg, PO, q24h	Anaerobes
Trimethoprim/ sulfamethoxazole	10–50 mg/kg, PO, q24h	Broad spectrum
ANTIFUNGALS		
Acetic acid (vinegar)	16 mL/L drinking water	Gastrointestinal yeast overgrowth
Fluconazole	5–10 mg/kg, PO, q24h	Candidiasis
Itraconazole	5–10 mg/kg, PO, q12h	Aspergillosis prophylaxis
Nystatin	300,000 IU/kg, PO, q12h	Candidiasis; not systemically absorbed
Voriconazole	20 mg/kg PO q24h	Aspergillosis drug of choice

IM, Intramuscularly; *IU/kg,* international unit per kilogram; *IV,* intravenously; *mg/L,* milligram per liter; *mg/kg,* milligram per kilogram; *mL/L,* milliliter per liter; *PO,* orally; *q24h,* once every 24 hours; *SQ,* subcutaneously.

TABLE 31-2

Commonly Used Antiparasitic Drugs in Passerines

Drug	Dosage	Comments
Amprolium	50–100 mg/L drinking water ×5–7days	Coccidiastat
Carnidazole	20–30 mg/kg, PO, q24h ×5 days	*Trichomonas*
Fenbendazole	50 mg/kg, PO, q24h ×3–5 days	
Fipronil	7.5 mg/kg, topically once	Ectoparasites
Ivermectin	0.2–0.4 mg/kg, SQ or IM once	
Metronidazole	30 mg/kg PO once	*Cochlosoma*
Praziquantel	25 mg/kg PO or IM; repeat in 10–14 days	Cestodes
Sulfachlorpyridazine	300 mg/L drinking water ×5 days, off 3 days	*Atoxoplasma*; repeat cycle 4 times
Toltrazuril	12.5 mg/kg, PO, q24h ×14 days	*Atoxoplasma*

IM, Intramuscularly; *IV,* intravenously; *PO,* orally; *q24h,* once every 24 hours; *SQ,* subcutaneously.

(ethylenediaminetetraacetic acid) may be used in some species, but it is known to cause lysis of erythrocytes in some passerines (e.g., corvids). For passerines, the lymphocyte is the predominant WBC, and lymphocytosis may be the primary response to stress. The packed cell volume (PCV) of most passerines falls between 40% and 55%, a PCV of less than 35% indicates anemia. Smears made from the buffy coat of a hematocrit tube increase the likelihood of identifying intracellular parasites such as *Atoxoplasma* spp. within mononuclear cells.[29] The reference intervals for the complete blood count and serum chemistry values for some of the passerines commonly kept in zoos is included in Table 31-3.

Endoscopic sexing of birds has largely been replaced by deoxyribonucleic acid (DNA)-based gender determination. These tests may be performed by using uncontaminated feathers or whole blood. Bone marrow aspirates may be obtained from the proximal tibiotarsus.

DISEASES

General

Because of the high metabolic rate and the bird's inherent instinct to mask clinical signs, the clinical condition of an ill passerine has a high likelihood of deteriorating rapidly once discovered. In the case of a number of diseases in passerines, acute death is the only observed clinical sign. Presentation of an ill passerine warrants rapid and effective treatment of etiologic agents as well as aggressive supportive care. Passerines are particularly susceptible to immunosuppression caused by chronic stress or concurrent disease. Many of the most common diseases associated with captive passerines (e.g., mycobacteriosis, aspergillosis, candidiasis, atoxoplasmosis) have a significant immunosuppressive component to their pathophysiology. During convalescence, quarantine, and transport and following relocation, efforts should be made to minimize stress. Prophylactic treatment with antifungals during periods of stress or during long-term antibiotic use may also be warranted in some species to prevent aspergillosis and candidiasis.

the preferred site. The ulnar or medial metatarsal veins may also be used but may be limiting because of the small size. Clinicians should be very careful about the volume of blood collected. For healthy, hydrated passerines, blood up to 1% of the bird's body weight may be obtained (i.e., 1 mL for every 100 g of body weight). This volume should be reduced in debilitated birds or those with a history of blood loss. Lithium heparin may be used as an anticoagulant for passerines, although it may affect the complete blood cell count (CBC) through clumping of white blood cells (WBCs), artifactual changes during the staining process, or both. EDTA

TABLE 31-3

Reference Intervals for the Complete Blood Count and Serum Chemistry Values for Some of the Passerines Commonly Kept in Zoos*

Common Name	Common Shama Thrush	Raven	Golden-breasted Starling	Azure-winged Magpie	White-headed Buffalo Weaver	Fairy Bluebird	Red-billed Leiothrix	Bali Mynah	Red-capped Cardinal	Taveta Golden Weaver	Superb Starling	Blue-grey Tanager
Scientific Name	Copsychus malabaricus	Corvus corax	Cosmopsarus regius	Cyanopica cyana	Dinemellia dinemelli	Irena puella	Leiothrix lutea	Leucopsar rothschildi	Paroaria gularis	Ploceus castaneiceps	Spreo superbus	Thraupis episcopus
WBC ($\times 10^3$ cells/µL)	0.00–16.63 (7.87)	0.00–16.99 (8.61)	1.84–23.88 (8.83)	0.00–13.34 (6.66)	1.92–29.99 (9.72)	2.21–33.41 (11.94)	0.00–14.02 (6.41)	2.01–27.97 (10.00)	0.00–17.76 (7.56)	0.00–21.16 (9.40)	1.21–24.98 (7.97)	1.82–22.65 (7.68)
Hematocrit (%)	37.1–59.9 (48.5)	28.8–52.3 (42.9)	35.1–63.4 (49.1)	38.1–60.2 (49.1)	37.0–61.4 (51.4)	37.7–61.9 (50.5)	36.9–57.3 (46.4)	35.1–54.3 (44.2)	40.1–68.1 (54.1)	37.2–55.3 (46.3)	34.0–58.8 (47.6)	43.1–59.6 (51.1)
Heterophils ($\times 10^3$ cells/µL)	0.00–7.11 (2.61)	0.00–7.75 (3.92)	0.44–6.73 (2.32)	0.00–5.00 (2.24)	0.22–8.22 (2.80)	0.30–8.37 (2.83)	0.00–2.67 (1.09)	0.69–7.62 (2.92)	0.00–3.24 (1.45)	0.00–4.82 (1.98)	0.15–6.12 (1.82)	0.15–4.96 (1.40)
Lymphocytes ($\times 10^3$ cells/µL)	0.00–9.53 (4.08)	0.00–8.51 (3.61)	0.55–16.78 (5.47)	0.00–8.61 (3.58)	0.82–15.67 (5.11)	0.55–20.84 (6.31)	0.00–9.32 (3.91)	0.54–18.53 (5.54)	0.00–13.32 (5.12)	0.00–12.95 (5.53)	0.36–15.50 (4.47)	0.60–15.76 (4.70)
Monocytes ($\times 10^3$ cells/µL)	0.00–0.600 (0.184)	0.00–0.532 (0.178)	0.00–1.460 (0.298)	0.00–0.578 (0.166)	0.00–1.290 (0.270)	0.00–2.173 (0.506)	0.00–0.681 (0.219)	0.00–1.218 (0.284)	0.00–0.301 (0.087)	0.00–1.189 (0.155)	0.00–1.078 (0.224)	0.00–1.862 (0.363)
Eosinophils ($\times 10^3$ cells/µL)	0.00–0.893 (0.276)	0.00–0.885 (0.264)	0.00–1.053 (0.130)	0.00–0.377 (0.089)	0.00–1.789 (0.355)	0.00–1.697 (0.304)	0.00–1.298 (0.230)	0.00–1.371 (0.269)	0.00–0.245 (0.068)	0.00–1.004 (0.305)	0.00–1.656 (0.274)	0.00–0.567 (0.106)
Basophils ($\times 10^3$ cells/µL)	0.00–1.835 (0.632)	0.00–1.653 (0.363)	0.00–1.366 (0.244)	0.00–0.413 (0.092)	0.00–3.189 (0.521)	0.00–5.616 (1.185)	0.00–1.557 (0.511)	0.00–1.631 (0.328)	0.00–0.814 (0.166)	0.00–1.361 (0.454)	0.00–2.089 (0.352)	0.00–3.093 (0.651)
Glucose (mg/dL)	NA	302–464 (377)	218–474 (333)	205–542 (369)	214–507 (372)	188–412 (298)	NA	203–443 (324)	NA	NA	237–448 (345)	139–464 (297)
Uric acid (mg/dL)	NA	0.8–18.3 (6.1)	3.5–32.8 (13.5)	0.0–26.7 (13.5)	3.0–28.8 (11.5)	3.0–22.5 (10.2)	NA	2.3–20.7 (8.8)	0.0–24.6 (10.6)	0.0–23.4 (11.5)	3.3–27.9 (11.8)	1.4–18.8 (8.1)
Calcium (mg/dL)	NA	6.9–9.8 (8.4)	6.4–10.3 (8.2)	7.2–10.3 (8.9)	5.3–10.3 (8.4)	5.9–11.0 (8.5)	NA	6.7–10.3 (8.6)	NA	NA	6.7–10.3 (8.3)	5.4–11.9 (8.6)
Phosphorus (mg/dL)	NA	0.6–5.8 (2.3)	1.3–10.0 (4.3)	0.0–7.2 (3.4)	0.0–7.0 (3.6)	0.9–14.3 (5.0)	NA	0.8–8.5 (3.4)	NA	NA	0.4–8.4 (3.2)	0.0–7.3 (3.4)

Analyte											
Sodium (mEq/L)	NA	143–170 (156)	132–179 (157)	143–177 (161)	142–176 (159)	142–181 (162)	NA	139–177 (158)	NA	144–169 (157)	NA
Potassium (mEq/L)	NA	1.2–5.0 (3.3)	1.0–5.4 (3.4)	0.2–4.4 (2.5)	0.4–4.1 (2.3)	0.7–4.7 (2.8)	NA	1.5–5.6 (3.0)	NA	1.2–4.9 (3.2)	NA
Chloride (mEq/L)	NA	109–131 (120)	91–142 (117)	NA	106–132 (118)	105–134 (119)	NA	99–130 (119)	NA	106–131 (118)	NA
Total protein (g/dL)	NA	2.6–5.3 (3.8)	2.0–5.9 (3.4)	2.1–4.4 (3.3)	1.6–4.8 (3.3)	2.3–6.2 (3.6)	NA	2.5–5.6 (3.8)	NA	2.0–5.2 (3.4)	NA
Albumin (g/dL)	NA	0.8–3.6 (2.0)	0.5–2.7 (1.4)	0.5–3.0 (1.8)	0.2–2.3 (1.3)	0.3–2.8 (1.7)	NA	0.9–3.3 (1.8)	NA	0.5–3.1 (1.5)	NA
Globulin (g/dL)	NA	0.4–3.5 (1.8)	0.5–3.3 (1.9)	0.2–3.0 (1.6)	0.2–3.7 (1.9)	0.4–3.5 (1.9)	NA	0.4–3.6 (2.0)	NA	0.2–3.7 (1.9)	NA
Alkaline phosphatase (IU/L)	NA	0–120 (64)	0–484 (226)	NA	0–345 (164)	0–170 (78)	NA	68–459 (223)	NA	0–479 (246)	NA
Aspartate aminotransferase (IU/L)	NA	132–478 (275)	148–583 (316)	0–884 (458)	64–362 (229)	185–759 (359)	NA	145–507 (282)	NA	136–737 (324)	NA
Creatine kinase (IU/L)	NA	0–318 (157)	75–1333 (448)	0–1087 (530)	0–907 (490)	340–2253 (893)	NA	154–1407 (535)	NA	78–905 (343)	NA
Cholesterol (mg/dL)	NA	93–271 (183)	101–278 (194)	NA	73–345 (216)	63–253 (164)	NA	103–279 (185)	NA	66–204 (137)	NA

*The mean value is listed in parentheses.

NA, Not available.

From Teare JA, ed: 2013, Common Shama Thrush; Raven; Golden-breasted Starling; Azure-winged Magpie; White-headed Buffalo Weaver; Fairy Bluebird; Red-billed Leiothrix; Bali Mynah; Red-capped Cardinal; Taveta Golden Weaver; Superb Starling; Blue-grey Tanger_No_selection_by_gender_All_age s_combined_Conventional_American_Units_2013_CD.html in ISIS Physiological Reference Intervals for Captive Wildlife: A CD-ROM Resource., International Species Information System, Bloomington, MN.

Infectious Disease

Viral Diseases

Avian pox is a significant disease of wild and captive passerines caused by a virus in the genus *Avipoxvirus*.[43] Infections most commonly present as proliferative skin lesions, particularly around featherless regions. Less common presentations include a diphtheritic form, in which necrotic lesions form in the oral cavity and upper respiratory tract, as well as a very rare systemic form. The virus is spread via direct contact or through mechanical vectors such as flies or mosquitoes. Cytology or histopathology of the lesion often reveals characteristic Bollinger bodies (eosinophilic intracytoplasmic inclusions). The cutaneous form may be self-limiting, although surgical removal of the proliferative masses may be necessary if eating, drinking, or respiration is impaired. Supportive care and antibiotics to control secondary infections may also be warranted in some cases. Diphtheritic and systemic infections are usually more severe.

Passerines are known to be affected by and serve as subclinical reservoirs of a wide variety of arboviruses. In North America, passerines are commonly associated with flaviviruses such as West Nile virus (WNV) and St. Louis encephalitis (SLE), as well as togaviruses such as eastern equine encephalitis (EEE), western equine encephalitis (WEE), and Venezuelan equine encephalitis (VEE). A wide variety of other arboviruses in other regions of the world also affect passerines.[24] The rates of morbidity and mortality from infections with arboviruses in passerines vary widely between species. North American corvids and loggerhead shrikes (*Lanius ludovicianus migrans*) have proven to be very susceptible to WNV, presenting with severe neurologic signs and high rates of mortality.[40] Other passerines are known to harbor the virus but have minimal to no clinical signs.[24] Treatment is strictly supportive. Prevention should focus on mosquito control. Vaccination against WNV with DNA vaccines has been used to reduce mortality and morbidity in corvids.[4,41,44]

Canary circovirus (CaCV) is associated with high rates of neonatal mortality in canaries (*Serinus canaria*). A common clinical feature is abdominal enlargement and congestion of the gallbladder, which may be seen through the translucent skin. This has resulted in the clinical syndrome being called "black spot disease" by aviculturists.[28] Hepatic necrosis, splenic inclusions, and inclusions in the bursa of Fabricius consistent with circovirus infection have been reported in zebra finches (*Poephila guttata*) and Gouldian finches (*Chloebia gouldiae*).[28] Circoviruses have also been demonstrated in other passerine species, although the significance remains unclear.[33]

Papillomavirus infections have been reported in common chaffinches (*Fringilla coelebs*), bramblings (*Fringilla montifringilla*), and Eurasian bullfinches (*Pyrrhula pyrrhula*) in Europe.[31] Clinical signs of infection include hyperplastic, locally extensive, papillomatous lesions on the skin of the toes and distal tarsometatarsus. Similar lesions have been observed in other passerine species, although a viral etiology has not always been established.

A finch polyomavirus (FPyV) has been detected in association with disease outbreaks affecting several passerine species that presented with increased fledgling mortality, feather disorders, and feather loss.[46] FPyV and a crow polyomavirus (CPyV) have been identified during screening of wild passerines.[17] Antibodies to polyomaviruses have been found in zebra finches exposed to polyomavirus outbreaks in psittacines.[31] The exact role of polyomaviruses in clinical disease of passerines warrants further investigation.

Avian influenza, an RNA (ribonucleic acid) virus in the family Orthomyxoviridae, affects many bird species, and passerines are no exception.[38] Like with other bird taxa, low pathogenic avian influenza (LPAI) may circulate in a population subclinically or with mild clinical signs. High pathogenic avian influenza (HPAI), on the other hand, may result in severe clinical signs and high rates of mortality. Clinical signs are usually related to pathology within the respiratory tract, although others may be present. Pathogenicity, species susceptibility, and severity and types of clinical signs are all highly variable, depending on the strain.

Avian paramyxovirus type 1 (APMV-1) is the cause of Newcastle's disease and the targeted pathogen of a federally required 30-day quarantine of all birds imported into the United States. Other avian paramyxoviruses such as APMV-2 and APMV-3 include passerines in their range of common hosts.[21] APMV-1 primarily causes neurologic disease and bloody diarrhea in the host. Other types of avian paramyxoviruses have a variable pathogenicity. Some such as APMV-3 do not seem to cause disease in passerines. Others may cause respiratory disease or reproductive abnormalities.[21]

Bacterial Diseases

Avian mycobacteriosis is a common problem in passerines. It is most commonly caused by *Mycobacterium avium*, *M. intracellulare*, and *M. genavense*, although other opportunistic mycobacterial species may also cause disease.[35] The disease is characterized by granulomatous inflammation in any organ, but the gastrointestinal (GI) tract, liver, spleen, bone marrow, and lung are common sites of infection.[5] A vascular form of the disease characterized by aortitis and cardiopulmonary arteritis has been described and anecdotally seems to be a relatively more common presentation in fairy bluebirds (*Irena puella*) as well as in other passerine species.[16,25] Birds affected by avian mycobacteriosis usually present with a marked leukocytosis and nonspecific signs of illness such as lethargy, weakness, anorexia, and chronic weight loss. Diagnosis is aided through identification of acid-fast positive rods in cytologic or histologic specimens, although culture is required for definitive diagnosis. Polymerase chain reaction (PCR) testing may also aid in identification and speciation of some mycobacterial organisms. The site of infection and intermittent shedding of bacteria may make antemortem diagnosis challenging. Recent epidemiologic studies suggest that avian mycobacteriosis is more likely an opportunistic pathogen acquired from the environment, rather than a pathogen that is directly transmitted from bird to bird.[37,45] As treatment is generally unrewarding and not recommended in zoologic settings because of the zoonotic potential, management of the disease is aimed at prevention and reducing stress and other causes of immunosuppression in passerines.

Mycoplasma gallisepticum is the causative agent of mycoplasmal conjunctivitis in passerines. The disease is primarily associated with wild house finches (*Carpodacus mexicanus*), although many other passerine species are reported to be affected.[22] Some passerines such as American goldfinches (*Spinus tristis*) may be subclinically infected and may serve as potential reservoirs.[8] Clinical signs consist primarily of conjunctivitis that presents as periocular swelling and upper respiratory tract exudate that may form a dried crust on the head and face. Affected birds may lose vision and then starve because of inability to acquire food. Transmission occurs both vertically and horizontally, through direct contact, aerosolization, and fomites.[22] The presence and style of bird feeders have been shown to affect the transmission of the disease in wild bird populations.[12] *Mycoplasma sturni* has been found in association with acute conjunctivitis with focal mucosal ulceration in several species of wild passerines.[22] However, the bacteria may also be found in individuals without clinical disease, so its role in the disease remains uncertain.

Avian chlamydiosis is caused by *Chlamydophila psittaci* and affects a wide range of avian hosts, including passerines. The disease may cause acute mortality or nonspecific signs of illness such as fluffed feathers, lethargy, weakness, anorexia, and abnormal droppings. Signs of upper respiratory involvement such as oculonasal discharge and conjunctivitis may also be present. Marked leukocytosis, hepatomegaly, and splenomegaly are diagnostic features that may suggest chlamydiosis, although other etiologies should also be considered. Diagnosis is often achieved with antigen testing such as PCR or immunofluorescent antibody (IFA) testing on blood samples, conjunctival/choanal/cloacal swabs, or tissues. *C. psittaci* is a zoonotic disease causing influenza-like clinical signs in humans. Therefore, routine *Chlamydophila* sp. screening and quarantine measures are warranted for most bird collections, particularly those that feature walk-through aviaries.

Salmonellosis is a significant disease of wild and captive passerines.[6,19] Many species and serotypes of *Salmonella* have been isolated from birds, with *Salmonella typhimurium* being most often associated with clinical disease. Clinical signs include diarrhea and nonspecific signs of disease. Disease severity may be variable and intermittent, including subclinical infections. Septicemia may occur with bacterial lesions occurring in multiple organ systems. Necropsy findings include weight loss, hepatomegaly, splenomegaly, and necrotic inflamed pale foci in the GI tract and other affected organs. Treatment may be difficult and may result in the creation of subclinical carriers. Outbreaks are frequently associated with bird feeding stations, so efforts should be taken to minimize fecal–oral contamination. Yersiniosis, caused by *Yersinia pseudotuberculosis*, causes similar clinical signs and gross lesions in passerines and may be differentiated through bacterial cultures.

Other bacterial pathogens that are also associated with passerines include *Campylobacter jejuni*, which is reported to cause GI signs and nestling mortality in some passerines, including the Gouldian finch. Many species of passerines may be subclinical carriers, however, and serve as a source of infection for other species. Society finches (*Lonchura domestica*) with subclinical disease have been implicated as sources of infection when used to foster Gouldian finch nestlings.[32] Avian cholera, caused by *Pasteurella multocida*, in passerines is most often associated with cat bites.[36] Without rapid treatment, septicemia may result and be rapidly fatal. Erysipelas, caused by *Erysipelothrix rhusiopathiae*, has been associated with disease in wild passerines, including the endangered Hawaiian crow (*Corvus hawaiiensis*).[48] Few clinical signs and gross lesions are present because of the rapidly fatal septicemia that results from infection.[47] Although they usually do not demonstrate clinical disease, passerines are known to play a significant role in the life cycle of many *Borrelia* spp.[26]

Fungal Diseases

Candidiasis is caused by the yeast *Candida albicans* and rarely by other *Candida* spp. The yeast may be found in subclinical individuals and is likely part of the normal GI flora, but opportunistic overgrowth may cause significant disease, including oral or esophageal plaques, crop stasis, diarrhea, regurgitation, and death.[32] Candidiasis is a particular problem in nestlings, in which it may cause significant mortality. Overgrowth of *Candida* spp. occurs with a disruption of the normal GI flora (dysbiosis) possibly because of chronic stress, antibiotic use, and concurrent diseases. During times of stress, yeast levels may be monitored noninvasively by performing Gram staining of the feces. Should yeast levels become mildly elevated (such as might occur during the stress of quarantine), apple cider vinegar has been added in the drinking water of passerines to acidify the GI tract and inhibit yeast proliferation. If clinical signs are present or more significantly elevated yeast levels are detected in feces, antifungal treatment may be warranted.

Aspergillosis may affect any bird species, including passerines. It is caused primarily by *Aspergillus fumigatus*, a saprophytic mold found commonly in the environment. Clinical disease is usually attributed to either abnormally high environmental exposures or immunosuppression of the host. Granulomatous lesions are usually found in the respiratory tract, and clinical signs include dyspnea, voice changes, lethargy, chronic weight loss, and weakness. A combination of terbinafine and voriconazole is the current treatment of choice for aspergillosis in all species. However, supportive care, treatment of secondary or concurrent disease, reduction of environmental exposure, and eliminating sources of chronic stress are also important tenets of the treatment regimen.

Macrorhabdus ornithogaster, also known as *avian gastric yeast* (formerly megabacteriosis), appears as large cigar-shaped organisms on fecal cytology, and has an affinity for the GI tract, particularly the gastric isthmus (connection between the proventriculus and ventriculus). Clinical signs may include undigested seeds in the droppings, diarrhea, weight loss, and death. However, passerines may also be subclinical carriers of the yeast. Avian gastric yeast is reported

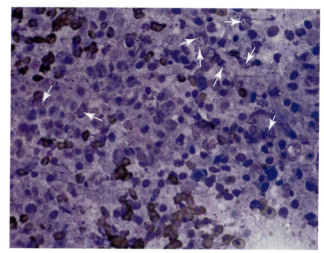

FIGURE 31-3 A splenic impression smear stained with Diff-Quik from a bulbul demonstrates 2 micron intrahistiocytic *Atoxoplasma* organisms (*arrowheads*) characterized by a small colorless halo and occasional indentation of the nucleus. (Courtesy of University of Illinois Zoological Pathology Program.)

to occur commonly in some finch species. Treatment with amphotericin B, nystatin, and fluconazole has been reported.[32]

Parasitic Diseases

Atoxoplasmosis is one of the most important pathogens of captive passerines. The taxonomy of the organism is still being debated, whether to place it in the genus *Isospora* or its own genus *Atoxoplasma*. The organism may be found in virtually every naturalistic or outdoor passerine exhibit. Many passerines may harbor the organism and never exhibit clinical signs. However, for some species, clinical disease may occur and is characterized by significant chick mortality. Adults undergoing stress may also exhibit nonspecific clinical signs such as lethargy, diarrhea, and weight loss. Species known to be particularly susceptible include the Bali mynah (*Leucopsar rothschildi*); *Spreo* spp. starlings; true finches (family Fringillidae), including the canary (*Serinus canaria*); and tanager species (family Thraupidae).[1,11] Diagnosis may be difficult but may be aided by finding oocysts in the feces (which are difficult to differentiate from enteric *Isospora* spp.), finding organisms within mononuclear cells on a buffy coat smear, PCR assay of the liver or other tissues, and cytology or histopathology (Figure 31-3). Prophylactic treatment of susceptible species during breeding with sulfachlorpyridazine or toltrazuril may be successful in reducing chick mortality. A working group was formed to address this disease, and more specific information and recommendations have been made available on the American Association of Zoo Veterinarians website (www.aazv.org).

Cochlosoma spp. are flagellate parasites found in some passerines, particularly finches. Some passerine species such as the society finch may be subclinical carriers and serve as a source of the pathogen for more susceptible species. The disease is a cause of nestling mortality, particularly those foster-reared by society finches.

Avian malaria is caused by a complex of more than 40 species in the genus *Plasmodium*.[2] *Plasmodium relictum* is one of the most widespread species and has played a significant role in the decline of many endangered Hawaiian bird species. In many hosts, infection may not result in any clinical signs. However, susceptible species or individuals may exhibit anemia, lethargy, dyspnea, and signs of generalized illness. The protozoa is spread primarily by *Culex* sp. mosquitoes and may be found as intraerythrocytic inclusions on blood smears (Figure 31-4). Treatment may include antimalarial drugs such as chloroquine or primaquine. Prevention is aimed at controlling the mosquito vector.

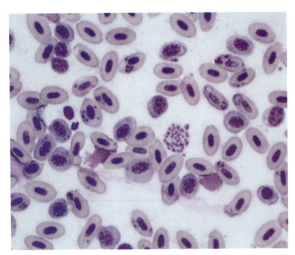

FIGURE 31-4 Avian malaria in a lung impression smear with Giemsa stain from a Hawaiian amakihi (*Hemignathus virens*) demonstrating various life stages of intraerythrocytic *Plasmodium* spp. inclusions. Evidence of polychromasia reflective of a regenerative anemia is also present. (Courtesy of University of Illinois Zoological Pathology Program.)

Other protozoa reported in passerines include *Haemoproteus* spp., *Leucocytozoon* spp., *Isospora* spp., *Eimeria* spp., *Sarcocystis* spp., *Cryptosporidium* spp., *Toxoplasma gondii*, and *Trichomonas* spp. Diseases caused by these organisms are similar to those in other avian taxa.

Passerines may be infected with several significant arthropods. Pediculosis (infection with chewing lice of the order Phthiraptera) may result in pruritus, excessive preening, and poor feather quality. Severe infections may result in weight loss and ill thrift. Treatment with ivermectin or topical fipronil may be successful. The mite *Sternostoma trachaecolum* infects the respiratory tract of passerines and may be fatal. Infections may sometimes by diagnosed by visualizing the mite within the trachea using transcervical illumination. *Knemidokoptes jamaicensis*, a scaly leg mite associated with passerines, causes hyperkeratotic lesions on the legs.[30] Most arthropod infections in passerines may be successfully treated with ivermectin.

Passerines are known to be definitive hosts for avian schistosomes (trematodes of the family Schistosomatidae) and become infected when the intermediate host (snail) is ingested.[15] The infection affects the circulatory system and may result in vasculitis, hemorrhage, respiratory distress, excessive swallowing, and generalized signs of illness. Passerines may also be infected with a wide range of other trematodes, cestodes, and acanthocephalans. All require an intermediate host to complete the life cycle. Cestodes and acanthocephalans usually infect the GI tract and may cause GI obstruction. Trematodes may infect a wide range of tissues. Praziquantel may be used for trematodes and cestodes, but no consistent treatment regimen is known for acanthocephalans.

A wide range of nematodes are known to infect passerines. A few are of particular interest. *Dispharynx nasuta* is a proventricular nematode known to cause ulcerative proventriculitis, anorexia, and death. *D. nasuta* requires terrestrial isopods to complete its indirect life cycle, and preventive measures should aim at breaking that cycle. The gapeworm, *Syngamus trachea*, affects a wide range of avian hosts, including passerines. Paired worms are found in the trachea and syrinx and cause open-mouth breathing, dyspnea, and death. *S. trachea* uses a direct life cycle or may also employ paratenic hosts such as earthworms. Tetrameridosis is caused by nematodes of the family Tetrameridae. Species within the genera *Teterameres*, *Microtetrameres*, and *Geopetitia* are known to infect passerines and are usually found encysted in the wall of the GI tract.[18] The roundworm

Ascaridia galli has been reported in some European passerine species. Larvae of the raccoon roundworm (*Baylisascaris procyonis*) may infect passerines as aberrant hosts, causing neurologic or other clinical signs as the larvae migrate through the brain, spinal cord, and other tissues leaving a path of inflammation. Antemortem diagnosis of *B. procyonis* is nearly impossible. Numerous filarid nematodes have been reported in passerines.[3,39] Capillarid nematodes primarily infect the GI tract, and numerous species are found in a wide variety of passerines, particularly insectivorous and carnivorous taxa.[49]

Noninfectious Disease

Hemochromatosis, also called *iron storage disease*, causes damage of the liver or other organs because of excessive iron deposition within the tissues. Some species are more susceptible and require diet modifications to prevent the occurrence of disease (see Feeding section above). Affected birds often present with nonspecific signs, including lethargy, weight loss, and inactivity. Radiography may reveal hepatomegaly, but a definitive diagnosis may be made with a liver biopsy. Serum iron levels correlate poorly with tissue levels. A low-iron diet combined with either weekly phlebotomy (removing 1% of the bird's body weight in blood once a week) or oral chelation therapy (deferoxamine 100 mg/kg, subcutaneously [SQ], once every 24 hours [q24h]) has been shown to reduce liver iron levels in a European starling model.[27]

Trauma is a common cause of morbidity and mortality in both captive and wild passerines. Collisions with objects that may be difficult to see (e.g., windows, reflective buildings, cellular phone towers, wind turbines, etc.) result in significant mortality each year, particularly with migratory species that may fly at night. Similarly, events that disturb flocks of birds at night (e.g., fireworks) may result in significant mortality as the birds become disoriented and collide with objects in the environment such as power lines. Open-topped posts such as those used for mine claim markers, have recently been identified as a fatal trap for some cavity-nesting species such as cactus wrens (*Campylorhynchus brunneicapillus*) and bluebird species (*Sialia* spp.), which explore the hollow center and cannot climb out. Free-ranging domestic cats, both feral and outdoor pets, have a devastating impact on wild passerines and other wildlife, with estimates of hundreds of millions to billions of wild birds killed annually. If cat attacks are not immediately fatal, secondary infections such as those caused by *Pasteurella multocida* may eventually result in mortality. Entanglement in string, fine filamentous nesting material, or substrates may result in loss of circulation and necrosis of legs or digits.

Chronic stress may result in several fat-related disorders. Obesity may result, as stress mobilizes nutrients that are then stored as fat, particularly in the intracoelomic areas. Stress also affects the way the liver metabolizes nutrients and may result in hepatic lipidosis and hepatic dysfunction. Amyloid deposition in the liver may occur with chronic antigenic stimulation.

Other noninfectious diseases include neoplasia of any tissue, but the prevalence of neoplasia in passerines is relatively lower than in other taxa. Reproductive disorders such as egg binding, yolk coelomitis, hypocalcemia, and chronic egg laying occur commonly in some passerine species and may be treated as in other bird taxa. An emerging epizootic of beak deformities in black-capped chickadees (*Poecile atricapillus*) has recently been described.[42] The syndrome has been named *avian keratin disorder*, but the etiology remains unknown.

Toxicities

Large scale mortality events of wild passerines are occasionally caused by toxins. In most cases, these are intentional poisonings (whether legal or illegal) used to control bird species that are viewed as pests in agricultural areas. Products used for this purpose include strychnine, 4-aminopyridine (Avitrol, Avitrol Corporation, Tulsa, OK 74145), and 3-chloro-p-toluidine (Starlicide, Earth City Resources, Bridgeton, MO 63044). Pesticides such as organophosphates also impact wild passerine populations.

REPRODUCTION

The diverse species of Passeriformes employ almost every reproductive strategy described in birds, including some extreme examples. Monogamy is the most common strategy, although polygyny, polygynandry, and promiscuity are also present in some species. A special type of promiscuity is the phenomenon of a *lek*, which serves as an arena where groups of males congregate to display themselves in an effort to attract a female. Lekking species of passerines (e.g., birds-of-paradise, manakins, cock-of-the-rocks) have evolved to have quite vibrant colors, patterns, modified feather structures, and specialized "dances" to aid in the attraction of a mate. The bowerbirds (family Ptilonorhynchidae) use polygyny, and males use specially designed display areas called *bowers* to attract females. Depending on the species (and individual preferences), the bowers are decorated with "prized" items from the environment. The satin bowerbird (*Ptilonorhynchus violaceus*) has a preference for blue items and will even use scraps of plastic, toys, and other trash in the environment, if the color matches the "decor" of its bower. Some species of passerines are parasitic brooders (e.g., cowbirds, whydahs) and lay their eggs in other bird species' nests to get them to raise their young.

The gonads of both male and female passerines may undergo seasonal enlargement and regression. Passerines may lay from 1 to 12 eggs per clutch, depending on the species. Most eggs are pigmented or patterned in some way. Generally, one egg is laid per day. Incubation varies by species. The pip-to-hatch interval is usually 24 hours or less. Hatchlings are altricial and nidicolous but may grow quite rapidly.

PREVENTIVE MEDICINE

Preventive medicine in passerines should start with ensuring that adequate husbandry practices are in place. Research into the natural biology of the species in question is helpful to ensure that appropriate temperatures, humidity, plant cover, square footage, elevation, lighting, substrate, and diet are used. Proper husbandry will help reduce stress and work toward preventing diseases exacerbated by immunosuppression. Quarantine is an important component of a preventive health plan and usually lasts a minimum of 30 days. During this time, screening for parasites and infectious diseases such as atoxoplasmosis, mycobacteriosis, salmonellosis, and chlamydiosis may be warranted. Regular weight checks and examinations are helpful in assessing the health of passerines on an ongoing basis. Modified scales may be fitted with a perch, and passerines may be conditioned to perch on the scale regularly so that weights are obtained in a minimally stressful manner. The clinician should prepare properly for the physical examination and perform it and any diagnostic procedure as efficiently as possible to minimize stress during handling. Lastly, necropsy and histopathology should be performed on all dead passerines to determine the cause of death and identify potential health risks to other individuals in the collection.

ACKNOWLEDGMENT

The author would like to thank Cheryl Piropato and the Fort Wayne Children's Zoo, for assistance with passerine restraint images, and Mike Kinsel, for assistance with cytologic images.

REFERENCES

1. Adkesson MJ, Zdziarski JM, Little SE: Atoxoplasmosis in tanagers. *J Zoo Wildl Med* 36(2):265–272, 2005.
2. Atkinson CT: Avian malaria. In Atkinson CT, Thomas NJ, Hunter DB, editors: *Parasitic diseases of wild birds*, Ames, IA., 2008, Wiley-Blackwell.
3. Bartlett CM: Filarioid nematodes. In Atkinson CT, Thomas NJ, Hunter DB, editors: *Parasitic diseases of wild birds*, Ames, IA, 2008, Wiley-Blackwell.
4. Bunning ML, Fox PE, Bowen RA, et al: DNA vaccination of the American crow (*Corvus brachyrhynchos*) provides partial protection against lethal challenge with west Nile virus. *Avian Dis* 51(2):573–577, 2007.
5. Converse KA: Avian tuberculosis. In Thomas NJ, Hunter DB, Atkinson CT, editors: *Infectious diseases of wild birds*, Ames, IA, 2007, Blackwell Publishing.
6. Daoust PY, Prescott JF: Salmonellosis. In Thomas NJ, Hunter DB, Atkinson CT, editors: *Infectious diseases of wild birds*, Ames, IA, 2007, Blackwell Publishing.
7. Del Rio CM: Can passerines synthesize vitamin C? *Auk* 114(3):513–516, 1997.
8. Dhondt AA, Dhondt KV, Hochachka WM, Schat KA: Can American goldfinches function as reservoirs for *Mycoplasma gallisepticum*? *J Wildl Dis* 49(1):49–54, 2013.
9. Dumbacher JP, Beehler BM, Spande TM, et al: Homobatrachotoxin in the genus Pitohui: Chemical defense in birds? *Science* 258:799–801, 1992.
10. Feduccia A: The origin and evolution of birds, ed 2, New Haven, CT, 1999, Yale University Press.
11. Greiner EC: Isospora, atoxplasma, and sarcocystis. In Atkinson CT, Thomas NJ, Hunter DB, editors: *Parasitic diseases of wild birds*, Ames, IA, 2008, Wiley-Blackwell.
12. Hartup BK, Mohammed HO, Kollias GV, Dhondt AA: Risk factors associated with mycoplasmal conjunctivitis in house finches. *J Wildl Dis* 34:281–288, 1998.
13. Hawkins MG, Barron HW, Speer BL, et al: Birds. In Carpenter JW, Marion CJ, editors: *Exotic animal formulary*, ed 4, St. Louis, MO, 2013, Elsevier.
14. Helmick KE, Kendrick EL, Dierenfeld ES: Diet manipulation as treatment for elevated serum iron parameters in captive raggiana birds of paradise (*Paradisaea raggiana*). *J Zoo Wildl Med* 42:460–467, 2011.
15. Huffman JE, Fried B: Schistosomes. In Atkinson CT, Thomas NJ, Hunter DB, editors: *Parasitic diseases of wild birds*, Ames, IA, 2008, Wiley-Blackwell.
16. Jimenez-Martinez A, Colegrove K, Terio K, Kinsel M: Granulomatous arteritis in birds with mycobacteriosis. In *Proceedings of the AAZV ARAV Joint Conference*, Los Angeles, CA, 2008, pp 33–34.
17. Johne R, Wittig W, Fernández-de-Luco D, et al: Characterization of two novel polyomaviruses of birds by using multiply primed rolling-circle amplification of their genomes. *J Virol* 80(7):3523–3531, 2006.
18. Kinsella JM, Forrester DJ: Tetrameridosis. In Atkinson CT, Thomas NJ, Hunter DB, editors: *Parasitic diseases of wild birds*, Ames, IA, 2008, Wiley-Blackwell.
19. Kirkwood JK: Salmonellosis in songbirds (Order Passeriformes). In Fowler ME, Miller RE, editors: *Zoo and wild animal medicine: Current therapy*, ed 6, St. Louis, MO, 2008, Saunders.
20. Klasing KC, Dierenfeld ES, Koutsos EA: Avian iron storage disease: Variations on a common theme? *J Zoo Wildl Med* 43:S27–S34, 2012.
21. Leighton FA, Heckert RA: Newcastle disease and related avian paramyxoviruses. In Thomas NJ, Hunter DB, Atkinson CT, editors: *Infectious diseases of wild birds*, Ames, IA, 2007, Blackwell Publishing.
22. Luttrell P, Fischer JR: Mycoplasmosis. In Thomas NJ, Hunter DB, Atkinson CT, editors: *Infectious diseases of wild birds*, Ames, IA, 2007, Blackwell Publishing.
23. Macwhirter P: Passeriformes. In Ritchie BW, Harrison GJ, Harrison LR, editors: *Avian medicine: Principles and application*, Lake Worth, FL, 1994, Wingers Publishing.
24. McLean RG: Ubico SR: Arboviruses in birds. In Thomas NJ, Hunter DB, Atkinson CT, editors: *Infectious diseases of wild birds*, Ames, IA, 2007, Blackwell Publishing.
25. Morton LD, Ehrhart EJ, Briggs MB, et al: Granulomatous aortitis and cardiopulmonary arteritis in fairy bluebirds (*Irena puella*) with mycobacteriosis. In *Proceedings of the American Association of Zoo Veterinarians*, Houston, TX, 1997, pp 272–273.
26. Olsen B: Borrelia. In Thomas NJ, Hunter DB, Atkinson CT, editors: *Infectious diseases of wild birds*, Ames, 2007, Blackwell Publishing.
27. Olsen GP, Russell KE, Dierenfeld E, Phalen DN: A comparison of four regimens for treatment of iron storage disease using the European

starling (*Sturnus vulgaris*) as a model. *J Avian Med and Surg* 20(2):74–79, 2006.

28. Pare JA, Robert N: Circovirus. In Thomas NJ, Hunter DB, Atkinson CT, editors: *Infectious diseases of wild birds*, Ames, IA, 2007, Blackwell Publishing.

29. Partington CJ, Gardiner CH, Fritz D, et al: Atoxoplasmosis in Bali mynahs (*Leucopsar rothschildi*). *J Zoo Wildl Med* 20(3):328–335, 1989.

30. Pence DB: Acariasis. In Atkinson CT, Thomas NJ, Hunter DB, editors: *Parasitic diseases of wild birds*, Ames, IA, 2008, Wiley-Blackwell.

31. Phalen DN: Papillomaviruses and polyomaviruses. In Thomas NJ, Hunter DB, Atkinson CT, editors: *Infectious diseases of wild birds*, Ames, IA, 2007, Blackwell Publishing.

32. Powers LV: Veterinary care of passerines (songbirds). In *Proceedings of the Association of Avian Veterinarians*, Seattle, WA, 2011, pp 135–148.

33. Raidal SR: Avian circovirus and polyomavirus diseases. In Miller RE, Fowler M, editors: *Fowler's zoo and wild animal medicine: Current therapy*, ed 7, St. Louis, 2012, Elsevier.

34. Raikow RJ: Monophyly of the Passeriformes: Test of a phylogenetic hypothesis. *Auk* 99:431–445, 1982.

35. Riggs G: Avian mycobacterial disease. In Miller RE, Fowler M, editors: *Fowler's zoo and wild animal medicine: Current therapy*, ed 7, St. Louis, 2012, Elsevier.

36. Samuel MD, Botzler RG, Wobeser GA: Avian cholera. In Thomas NJ, Hunter DB, Atkinson CT, editors: *Infectious diseases of wild birds*, Ames, IA, 2007, Blackwell Publishing.

37. Schrenzel M, Nicolas M, Witte C, et al: Molecular epidemiology of *Mycobacterium avium* subsp. *avium* and *Mycobacterium intracellulare* in captive birds. *Vet Microbiol* 126:122–131, 2008.

38. Stallknecht DE, Nagy E, Hunter DB, Slemons RD: Avian influenza. In Thomas NJ, Hunter DB, Atkinson CT, editors: *Infectious diseases of wild birds*, Ames, IA, 2007, Blackwell Publishing.

39. Sterner MC III, Cole RA: Diplotriaena, serratospiculum, and serratospiculoides. In Atkinson CT, Thomas NJ, Hunter DB, editors: *Parasitic diseases of wild birds*, Ames, IA, 2008, Wiley-Blackwell.

40. Travis D: West Nile virus in birds and mammals. In Fowler ME, Miller RE, editors: *Zoo and wild animal medicine: Current therapy*, ed 6, St Louis, 2008, Saunders.

41. Turrell MJ, Bunning M, Ludwig GV, et al: DNA vaccine for west Nile virus infection in fish crows (*Corvus ossifragus*). *Emerg Infect Dis* 9(9):1077–1081, 2003.

42. Van Hemert C, Handel CM, O'Hara TM: Evidence of accelerated beak growth associated with avian keratin disorder in black-capped chickadees (*Poecile atricapillus*). *J Wildl Dis* 48(3):686–694, 2012.

43. Van Riper C, III, Forrester DJ: Avian Pox. In Thomas NJ, Hunter DB, Atkinson CT, editors: *Infectious diseases of wild birds*, Ames, IA, 2007, Blackwell Publishing.

44. Wheeler SS, Langevin S, Woods L, et al: Efficacy of three vaccines in protecting western scrub-jays (*Aphelocoma californica*) from experimental infection with west Nile virus: Implications for vaccination of island scrub-jays (*Aphelocoma insularis*). *Vector Borne Zoonotic Dis* 11(8):1069–1080, 2011.

45. Witte CL, Hungerford LL, Papendick R, et al: Investigation of factors predicting disease among zoo birds exposed to avian mycobacteriosis. *J Am Vet Med Assoc* 236(2):211–218, 2010.

46. Wittig W, Hoffmann K, Müller H, Johne R: Detection of DNA of the finch polyomavirus in diseases of various types of birds in the order Passeriformes. *Berl Munch Tierarztl Wochenschr* 120:113–119, 2007.

47. Wolcott MJ: Erysipelas. In Thomas NJ, Hunter DB, Atkinson CT, editors: *Infectious diseases of wild birds*, Ames, IA, 2007, Blackwell Publishing.

48. Work TM, Ball D, Wolcott M: Erysipelas in a free-ranging Hawaiian crow (*Corvus hawaiiensis*). *Avian Dis* 43(2):338–341, 1999.

49. Yabsley MJ: Capillarid nematodes. In Atkinson CT, Thomas NJ, Hunter DB, editors: *Parasitic diseases of wild birds*, Ames, IA, 2008, Wiley-Blackwell.

CHAPTER **32**

Monotremata (Echidna, Platypus)

Peter Holz

BIOLOGY

Taxonomy

The order Monotremata is unique among mammals, as its members lay shell-covered eggs but nurse their young. The two families in this order are Tachyglossidae, which includes the echidnas, and Ornithorhynchidae, which includes the single species of platypus (*Ornithorhynchus anatinus*).

Echidnas are terrestrial mammals with a long, tubular snout, powerful claws, and spines that cover the tail and dorsal surface of the body. The spines are firmly attached to the skin and cannot be pulled out as in the case of porcupine spines. Fur is present between the spines and over the belly. Three species of echidna exist. The short-beaked echidna (*Tachyglossus aculeatus*) is divided into five subspecies: (1) *T. a. acanthion* from the Northern Territory, northern Queensland, inland Australia, and Western Australia, (2) *T. a. aculeatus* from eastern New South Wales, Victoria, and southern Queensland, (3) *T. a. lawesii* from New Guinea, (4) *T. a. multiaculeatus* from South Australia, and (5) *T. a. setosus* from Tasmania. The two species of long-beaked echidna are larger and have fewer, shorter spines and thicker fur compared with short-beaked echidnas. *Zaglossus bartoni* has five claws on the front foot, and *Zaglossus bruijnii* generally has only three. Both are found in New Guinea only.[1]

The platypus is a streamlined, fur-covered aquatic mammal, with a distinctive bill, webbed feet, and a broad flat tail. It is found only in Tasmania and along the east coast of mainland Australia.[4]

The short-beaked echidna and platypus are both listed as common, whereas both species of long-beaked echidna are classified as endangered because of land clearance and hunting.

UNIQUE ANATOMY AND SPECIAL PHYSIOLOGY[1,2,4,12]

See Tables 32-1 and 32-2. Short-beaked echidnas and platypuses are pentadactylous, with echidnas having strong front feet and large pectoral muscles adapted for digging. When approached, the echidna will attempt to bury itself into the ground, rolling into a partial ball with its head tucked under its body and leaving only its spine covered dorsum exposed. This is facilitated by contraction of the panniculus carnosus, which also exists in the platypus, a large muscle under the skin of the back and sides.

Platypus fur is waterproof and has a hair fiber density of 600 to 900 hairs per square millimeter (hairs/mm²) and traps air for insulation. The platypus has no subcutaneous fat (unlike the echidna) but does store fat in its tail, which makes up 40% of its total body fat.

Platypus males possess a sharp spur on each hindlimb, and the spur is connected to a venom gland located in the upper thigh region. The spur is covered by a blunt sheath that erodes away by 9 to 12 months of age. A fleshy collar is present at the base of the spur until about 18 months of age. Spurring and envenomation, although not fatal to humans, is extremely painful and has been known to kill mice, dogs, and other platypuses. Platypuses are more aggressive and their venom more potent during the breeding season (August to October). The venom gland also increases in weight from less than

5 grams (g) to almost 10 g. Therefore, extra care is required when handling these animals during this period. Venom is only produced by sexually mature males from about 4 years of age. Females have a rudimentary spur sheath that is lost around 8 months of age. The spurs are likely used to settle territorial disputes during the breeding season.

Generally, only male echidnas have spurs, which range in length from 4.3 to 15 mm, on their hindlimbs (although some females may have small spurs <2 mm long).[9] Until recently, these were believed to not contain venom. However, new research has found that these spurs connect to a crural gland that contains proteins similar to those found in platypus venom.[10] At this stage, it is unknown if the echidna "venom" is toxic to humans, but echidnas do not strike out with their spurs the way platypuses do.

The echidna's beak and the platypus's bill are equipped with a number of sensitive electroreceptors and mechanoreceptors, which may be used to locate invertebrate prey. The short-beaked echidna has around 400 mucous glands around the snout tip and nostrils. A quarter of these contain sensory nerve terminals. Each sensory gland is surrounded by several noninnervated glands. Approximately seven sensory glands exist per square millimeter. In the long-beaked echidna, all mucous glands are innervated and are found at a density of 12 per square millimeter. Platypuses have around 40,000 receptors, at a density of 30 per square millimeter, arranged in parallel rows from the tip of the bill to the frontal shield, possibly to aid in assessing prey direction. They may detect weak electric fields down to 1.8 (mVcm⁻¹).

Monotreme snouts contain *push rods*, which are believed to be mechanoreceptors (up to 60,000 in the platypus bill, most densely congregated along the border of the upper bill). Each push rod is around 300 micrometers (μm) long and 50 μm wide, with a dome-shaped tip around 25 μm across. As many as 30 to 40 push rods may be present per square millimeter of skin.

The olfactory bulb represents 3.1% of brain volume in the echidna compared with 0.8% in the platypus, and the echidna has 13 times more olfactory nerve fibers. The echidna's prefrontal cortex occupies 50% of the cerebral cortex, which is likely related to the processing of olfactory information.

At the back of the tongue of the platypus are two grooves lined with sensory cells, which are probably involved in taste sensation, and a Jacobson's organ, which consists of two pouches in the roof of the front part of the mouth.

Echidna metabolic rate is one third (in platypuses, half) and oxygen requirements are less than half that of an equivalent-sized dog or cat. Echidnas may hibernate for 6 to 28 weeks, with brief spontaneous arousal every 9 to 12 days, when ambient temperature drops below 12°C. Their body temperature may drop to 4°C, heart rate may decline to 4 to 7 beats per minute (beats/min) and respiratory rate decreases to 0.3 breaths per minute. The echidna thermoneutral range is 20°C to 30°C. Long-beaked echidnas do not appear to hibernate. Monotremes are more susceptible to hyperthermia than to hypothermia. Short-beaked echidnas are unable to sweat or pant, but long-beaked echidnas and platypuses have abundant sweat glands. Platypuses also have two scent glands in the cervical region.

TABLE 32-1

Selected Physiologic Parameters for Echidnas and Platypuses

Parameter	Short-Beaked Echidna	Long-Beaked Echidna	Platypus
Body weight	2–7 kg	Male 5.9–8.0 kg Female 7.4–9.8 kg	Male 1.0–3.0 kg Female 0.7–1.8 kg
Longevity	Up to 50 years	Up to 31 years	Up to 21 years
Heart rate (beats per minute)	50–68 (Rest) 135–145 (Active)		140–230
Blood pressure (mm Hg)	123/96		
Respiratory rate (breaths per minute)	5–6		20–50
Body temperature (°C)	28–33	27–32	29–34
Adrenal weight/Body weight	40 mg/kg		257 mg/kg
Glucocorticoids	0.1 µg/dL		15 µg/dL
Cortisol	0.07 µg/dL		5.4 µg/dL
Corticosterone	0.14 µg/dL		1.8 µg/dL
Cortisone	—		8.2 µg/dL
Aldosterone	0.54 ng/dL		Low

mg/kg, Milligram per kilogram; *µg/dL*, microgram per deciliter.

SPECIAL HOUSING REQUIREMENTS[7]

Echidnas should be provided with a natural soil substrate over a layer of mesh to prevent their attempts to dig out. They must never be kept on concrete surfaces. Alternatively, the walls may be dug down to a depth of 50 centimeters (cm). Peripheral walls should be smooth, solid, and vertical to a height of at least 50 cm. Overhanging structures should be removed, as echidnas may use them to climb out. In the wild, echidnas are solitary. They have home ranges rather than territories, which vary from 45 to 65 hectares (ha). In captivity, they may be housed together as long as a minimum of 5 square meters (m²) of floor space is provided for each animal. In the hospital environment, echidnas may be kept in smooth plastic tubs containing straw or shredded paper to provide shelter and security. Care must be taken to eliminate sharp edges or cavities, as the echidna could damage its beak on these. Wire cages are unsuitable, but plastic garbage bins may be used for short-term confinement. As echidnas are prone to hyperthermia, it is important to provide shelter from heat.

Platypuses require fresh water, for feeding and exercise, and a tunnel system connected to one or more nest boxes. The water needs to be filtered to keep it clean and is commonly replaced at weekly intervals. Pool walls should be 1 to 1.2 m high and at least 0.5 m above the water level to prevent escapes and should contain partially submerged branches and overhanging ledges. Tunnels may be made of marine ply or plastic pipes and should have hatches every meter or so to allow access to the animal. Nesting material such as grass and leaves should be placed in the water during breeding season. Nest boxes may be made of wood, or the platypus may be provided with an area of soil for tunneling and for excavating its own nest. When an area of soil is used, clay soil containing fibrous vegetable matter should be used to prevent possible cave-ins. Platypuses, like echidnas, are cold tolerant but not heat tolerant. Air and water temperatures must be maintained below 27°C.

Platypuses are solitary in the wild. Their home ranges vary from 0.2 to 7.3 km, with some overlap of females and subadults but less of males. In captivity, female–female pairs have been housed together. Male–female pairs should be housed in separate quarters. Adult males should never be housed together.

FEEDING

Free-Ranging Diet[1,4]

Short-beaked echidnas consume predominantly ants and termites (generally preferring termites, as they are more digestible, have higher water content, and live in larger colonies) but will eat other invertebrates such as earthworms and the larvae of beetles and moths. Long-beaked echidnas consume mainly earthworms but will also eat small centipedes, scarab beetle larvae, lepidopteran larvae, and subterranean cicadas.

Platypuses consume aquatic invertebrates such as freshwater crayfish, beetles, midges, snails, crustaceans, and caddisfly and mayfly larvae (*Trichoptera* spp. generally making up over half the diet). Foraging is mainly nocturnal and lasts, on average, 10 to 12 hours per day. Food consumption is 13% to 28% of body weight but may increase to 100% during lactation. They prefer cobbled substrates and avoid mud. Dives usually last between 30 and 140 seconds, but platypuses may remain submerged for up to 10 minutes. Heart rate drops during dives from a range of 140 to 230 to a range of 10 to 120 beats/min. Platypuses usually forage in pools less than 5 m deep, with few dives going deeper than 3 m.

Captive Diet[2,12]

Because of the difficulty in obtaining a regular supply of ants and termites, short-beaked echidnas are generally maintained on an alternative diet based on minced meat. Wild echidnas usually take to this diet within a few days. If not, they may be encouraged to accept it by adding formic acid or "paw paw" to the diet. Echidnas are fed food that is 2% to 5% of their body weight daily. Although they have been successfully maintained on this diet, obesity is common, breeding success is low, and fecal consistency is quite variable compared with wild echidnas. Some institutions provide a breeding (high-fat) diet and a maintenance (low-fat) diet, although evidence that this is better than feeding a constant diet all year round does not exist. Recent research has found that vitamin D levels in the blood of echidnas held at three captive facilities were much higher than in wild ones (335.5 nanomoles per liter [nmol/L], 104.0 nmol/L and 187.2 nmol/L in captive echidnas compared with 24.7 nmol/L in wild echidnas). The health effects are not known, but altering the diet reduced serum vitamin D to wild levels.[13] A suggested echidna diet is given in Table 32-3.

Captive platypuses are fed freshwater crayfish, mealworms, earthworms, fly pupae, and tubifex worms. They consume food that is 15% to 30% of their body weight daily. Feces are unformed, are black, and have a tarry consistency. A suggested diet for platypuses is given in Table 32-4.

Hand Rearing

Monotreme milk composition is presented in Table 32-5,[5] along with two artificial milks for comparison. It is very high in iron but contains very little lactose. The principal carbohydrates are fucosyl lactose and sialyl lactose in echidna milk and difucosyl lactose in platypus milk.

In hand rearing, echidnas and platypuses should be maintained at 20°C to 25°C. They will feed directly from the palm of the hand or out of a small bowl. For echidnas feed 10% to 12% of body weight every 3 to 5 days. Platypuses should be fed food that is 10% to 20% of body weight daily spread over three to six feeds. Between feeds, the animals may be kept in a wooden nest box. High-carbohydrate milks should be avoided, as they will predispose the animals to

TABLE 32-2

Selected Anatomic Parameters for Short-Beaked Echidnas and Platypuses

Spine	Echidna: 7C (bearing ribs), 16T, 3L, 3S, 12Co Platypus: 7C (bearing ribs), 17T, 2L, 2S, 21Co Both vertebral and sternal ribs present, joined by strips of cartilage	Digestive	Teeth absent The echidna tongue is long and slender and may be extended 2–3 cm in the long-beaked echidna and up to 18 cm in the short-beaked echidna The anterior third of the long-beaked echidna tongue has a groove containing three rows of keratinous spines on the upper surface The groove, which allows the echidna to consume its main prey of earthworms, opens when the tongue is protruded, and closes when it is retracted Echidna saliva, which is rich in glycoproteins, is produced by paired sublingual salivary glands Paired submandibular salivary glands are palpable as two firm flattened oval subcutaneous masses on the ventral side of the neck Once consumed prey items are crushed between the keratinous plates at the back of the tongue and the hard palate Juvenile platypuses have one premolar and two molars in each maxilla and two to three molars in each mandible These are lost as the animal matures and are replaced by keratinous pads Food is stored in cheek pouches The monotreme stomach is lined with keratinized stratified epithelium Brunner's glands present Gastric glands absent Gastric pH 6.2–7.4 (echidna) Intestine: 3.5 m long in echidna; 1.5 m long in platypus The echidna small intestinal mucosa has high trehalase activity corresponding to the high trehalose content of termites and ants Lactase and sucrase activity is virtually undetectable Combined pancreatic and bile ducts A small cecum, which is primarily a lymphoid organ, is present in both monotremes Gut transit time: 2 days (echidna), 5 hours (platypus)
Skull	Ectopterygoid bones present Thin zygomatic arches Jugal bone present (platypus only)		
Pectoral girdle	Scapula ×2 Coracoid ×2 Epicoracoid ×2 Clavicle ×2 Interclavicle ×1		
Pelvic girdle	Epipubic bone ×2 Acetabular foramen ×2 In the echidna the head of the femur is inserted horizontally into the acetabulum, projecting at right angles to the body The tibia and fibula are twisted backward so that the feet and claws are directed posteriorly		
Central nervous system	Gyrencephalic (echidna); lissencephalic (platypus) Corpus callosum absent Motor nerve tract crosses in the pons in the echidna (compared with the medulla in most other mammals) Spinal cord terminates at T7 in the echidna compared with L1-L2 in humans		
Auditory	No tympanic bulla Incus and malleus fused and attached to petrous bone (echidna) Cochlea partially coiled and most sensitive to frequencies around 4 kilohertz (kHz) (platypus) and 5 kHz (echidnas) Saccular, utricular, and lagenar macula all present		
Visual	Scleral cartilage present Keratinized cornea (echidna) 10%–15% of photoreceptors are cones (which contain oil droplets) in the echidna, compared with 5% in humans Echidnas have a very flat lens and lack ciliary muscles Accommodation is achieved by protruding the eyes and elongating the eyeballs to vary the distance between the lens and the object Avascular retina Nictitating membrane present (platypus only) 99% decussation of optic fibers at optic chiasma	Miscellaneous	Adrenal glands not divided into a cortex and medulla Medullary tissue located caudally, cortical tissue found cranially Lymph nodes absent Diffuse lymphoid system composed of 0.2–2.0 mm nodules dispersed through lymphatic vessels
Cardiovascular	Chordae tendinae absent; heart valves insert directly onto papillary muscles (echidna) Coronary vein present (empties into right atrium) Right lung lobe ×2 Left lung lobe ×1.		

C, Cervical; *Co,* coccygeal; *L,* lumbar; *S,* sacral; *T,* thoracic.

secondary infection by *Candida* sp. and other infections. Weaning should occur by slowly introducing solid food.

RESTRAINT AND HANDLING[6]

Physical Restraint

When approached, the echidna will quickly dig into the substrate. To bring the echidna out, a spade is required to carefully dig under the animal's body and lift it up. Alternatively, a hindlimb may sometimes be grasped. The entire echidna may then be lifted by the foot and placed in a suitable receptacle such as a plastic garbage can. If the echidna is on a solid surface, it will attempt to curl into a tight ball. In that case, a hand should be slid under the rear of the body and a foot grasped. Alternatively, the entire echidna may be picked up with a towel or while wearing sturdy leather gloves to protect the hands. If picking the echidna up by its leg, it is important to be wary of the cloaca, as stressed echidnas frequently spray urine and feces.

Platypuses are restrained by being held by the tail base. This keeps the spurs away. Docile or hand-raised platypuses may be cradled in the hands. Platypuses are easily transported in bags such as pillow cases.

Chemical Restraint

Intubation of monotremes is not possible because of the narrow oral cavity, small gape, difficulty visualizing the larynx, and presence of a keratinous pad on the dorsal surface of the base of the tongue in echidnas and a bulbous structure (torus linguae) at the base of the tongue in platypuses.

Disturbed echidnas generally roll into a ball, tucking the beak in tightly against the body, making mask induction impossible. Therefore, the echidna may be placed in an induction chamber that is flooded with a mixture of isoflurane and oxygen. Once sedated, the echidna may be maintained on a mask. If an injectable induction is required, several suitable combinations are available: 2 milligrams per kilogram (mg/kg) xylazine and 10 mg/kg ketamine, intramuscularly

TABLE 32-3

Echidna Diet: Amount per Animal

Ingredient	Short-Beaked Echidna Maintenance Diet	Short-Beaked Echidna Breeding Diet
Water	70 mL	70 mL
Minced meat	100 g	110 g
Raw egg (no shell)	24 g	26 g
Glucose monohydrate	45 g	18 g
Bran	17 g	18 g
Olive oil	9 g	14 g
Calcium carbonate	1 g	1 g
Fly pupae	7 g	7 g

g, Gram; *mL*, milliliter.

TABLE 32-4

Platypus Diet: Amount per Animal

Ingredient	Platypus Maintenance Diet	Platypus Breeding Diet	Platypus Lactating Female Diet
Earthworms	60 grams (g)	80 g	120 g
Mealworms	50 g	60 g	100 g
Freshwater crayfish	20–30	20–30	50–70
Fly pupae	40 g	60 g	800 g
Tubifex worms	60 g	80 g	120 g

TABLE 32-5

Monotreme Milk Composition[5,12]

Parameter	Short-Beaked Echidna (Early)	Short-Beaked Echidna (Late)	Platypus	Wombaroo Echidna Milk <30 Days (<210 g)	Wombaroo Echidna Milk >30 Days (>360 g)	Di-Vetalact
Total solids (% wt/wt)		48.9	39.1	21	36	—
Crude lipid (% wt/wt)	1.25	31	22.2	8	16	4
Crude protein (% wt/wt)	7.85	12.4	8.2	7	11.5	3
Carbohydrate (% wt/wt)	2.85	2.3	3.7	5.5	4	5
Calcium milligram per deciliter (mg/dL)		117	191	260	460	100
Phosphorus (mg/dL)		285	133	200	360	70
Magnesium (mg/dL)		16	16	19	34	10
Iron (mg/dL)		3.33	2.11	1.5	2	0.9
Copper (mg/dL)		0.38	0.1	0.24	0.44	0.06
Zinc (mg/dL)		1.51	1.92	0.34	0.6	0.7
Oleic acid %		61.2	25.2			
Palmitic acid %		15.9	17.6			
Palmitoleic acid %		6.2	11.6			
Linoleic acid %		5.1	6.1			
Linolenic acid %		0.8	9.5			
Stearic acid %		3.9	4.0			
Arachidonic acid %	11	0.5	3.1			

(IM) (reversed with 0.1 mg/kg yohimbine intravenously [IV]); 0.5 mg/kg medetomidine and 5 mg/kg ketamine, IM (reversed with 2.5 mg/kg atipamezole IM); or 3 to 10 mg/kg tiletamine and zolazepam, IM. Analgesics that have been used in echidnas include 0.1 mg/kg butorphanol, IM or IV, twice daily (BID); 1 mg/kg buprenorphine IM or IV, once daily (SID); 0.5 mg/kg flunixin, subcutaneously (SC), IM, or IV, SID; 1 mg/kg ketoprofen, SC, IM, or IV, SID; and 0.5 mg/kg meloxicam, SC or IV, SID or 0.2 milliliter (mL), orally (PO; mixed in food), SID.

Platypuses are anesthetized with isoflurane and oxygen via a mask placed over the bill. Injectable agents have rarely been used.

DIAGNOSTICS

Blood Collection[6]

A soft swelling on the dorsal surface of the echidna beak, just caudal to the nostrils, represents a venous sinus (Figure 32-1). This sinus is suitable for blood collection with a 25-gauge needle and 2- to 3-mL syringe. A heparinized winged infusion set (butterfly catheter) reduces the likelihood of the needle coming out of the sinus if the echidna moves. Care must be taken not to exert too much pressure on the syringe, as this will collapse the sinus.[8] The jugular vein may also be used but is more difficult to access because of the echidna's short neck.

In platypuses, a vascular sinus running transversely along the rostral border of the bill is suitable for blood collection (Figure 32-2).

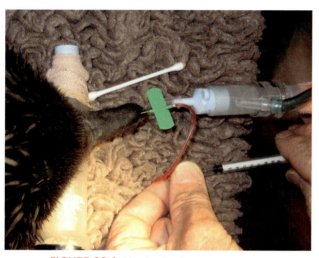

FIGURE 32-1 Blood collection in the echidna.

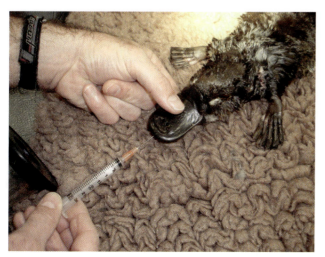

FIGURE 32-2 Blood collection in the platypus.

A 25-gauge needle, attached to a 2- to 3-mL syringe, is inserted either side of the midline. Alternatively, a heparinized winged infusion set may be used, as the needle is less likely to come out of the sinus if the platypus moves. Gentle pressure on the syringe is required to avoid collapsing the sinus. Blood may also be collected from the ventral coccygeal vessels, but it is considerably more difficult.

Monotreme hematology and biochemistry values are provided in Table 32-6. Erythrocytes have very low levels of adenosine triphosphate (ATP; platypus 0.06 and echidna 0.03 millimoles per liter [μmol/L]). Platypus blood contains large numbers of small erythrocytes (10 million/mL[3] of blood), high hemoglobin levels (19 g/100 mL blood), no reticulocytes and neutrophils that commonly contain Dohle bodies.[3] Blood in both echidnas and platypuses has a high oxygen affinity, enabling echidnas to tolerate high levels of carbon dioxide (up to 10%).

DISEASES[2,11,12]

Summaries of echidna and platypus diseases are listed in Tables 32-7 and 32-8.

Internal parasites found in short-beaked echidnas include the cestodes *Echidnotaenia tachyglossi* and *Linstowia echidnae* and nematodes *Parastrongyloides*, *Nicollina*, *Tachynema*, *Tasmanema*, *Dipetalonema*, and *Ophidascaris robertsi*, the python ascarid. Although disease has occasionally been attributed to heavy burdens of *Nicollina* and *Tasmanema*, such findings are usually regarded as incidental. Long-beaked echidnas may be parasitized by trematodes (*Echinostoma* sp.), and nematodes (*Zaglonema ewersi*, *Zaglonema zaglossi*, and *Tridentakis* sp.). Platypuses may also be hosts to trematodes (*Mehlisia ornithorhynchi*, *Maritrema ornithorhynchi*, and *Moreauia mirabilis*) and nematodes (*Tasmanema mundayi* and *Cercophithifilaria johnstoni*). No pathology is usually associated with any of these infections.

No pharmacokinetic studies have been performed on monotremes. Medications used in small animals have been used in monotremes at similar dose rates. No adverse reactions have been reported.

REPRODUCTION[1,4]

Selected reproductive parameters are provided in Table 32-9. Monotremes have a common reproductive and excretory opening called *cloaca*. Testes are internal, and seminal vesicles are absent. Echidnas lack a prostate gland, and platypuses have a disseminated prostate. The vas deferens conveys sperm from the epididymis to the urogenital sinus and then into the penile urethra, which transports only sperm. Urine travels via the ureters to the urogenital sinus. From there, urine enters the cloaca via the urinary papilla, which is situated on the cloacal wall at the ventral base of the penis (Figure 32-3).

The female echidna has two functional ovaries, but in the platypus only the left ovary is functional. The oviducts enter the urogenital sinus. The bladder also attaches to the urogenital sinus, opposite and dorsal to the entry of the ureters (Figure 32-4).

Normally, echidnas are solitary, but during the mating period, they come together to form "trains," in which up to 11 males will follow one female. The time from "train" formation to mating is 7 to 37 days. No trains have been seen in Snowy Mountain echidnas, which form pairs and mate after arousal from hibernation. The most dominant male in the group mates with the female. Copulation lasts 30 to 180 minutes, and females usually only mate once in a season. Within 48 hours of mating, females return to their solitary life, and males wander off to either find another "train" or resume their solitary existence.

Platypuses are also solitary and generally do not breed until at least their fourth year, when they will mate a number of times over several days.

Monotreme egg shells are not mineralized but are leathery. Female echidnas enter a burrow shortly before egg laying. Only the female platypus builds the nest.

TABLE 32-6

Hematologic and Biochemical Values for Monotremes[2,12]

Species	Short-Beaked Echidna		Platypus	
	Mean	SD	Mean	Range
PCV (%)	40.45	5.63	51.00	35.00–62.00
RBC (×10^{12}/L)	6.25	0.85	10.30	7.26–12.10
Hb (g/dL)	14.49	2.58	18.32	13.40–22.30
MCV (fL)	64.91	5.05	50.04	42.00–56.30
MCH (pg)	23.75	4.04	17.84	15.00–34.40
MCHC (g/dL)	35.98	5.01	36.30	32.70–39.90
WBC (×10^9/L)	11.95	5.52	26.03	9.60–40.60
Bands (×10^9/L)	0.08	0.15	0.21	0.00–1.62
Neutrophils (×10^9/L)	6.6	3.86	10.11	1.15–25.17
Lymphocytes (×10^9/L)	5.11	2.51	18.35	3.07–34.51
Monocytes (×10^9/L)	0.3	0.27	0.91	0.00–2.74
Eosinophils (×10^9/L)	0.08	0.17	0.35	0.00–1.22
Basophils (×10^9/L)	0.00	0.00	0.00	0.00
Platelets (×10^9/L)	414.28	125.15	817	262–2144
Total protein (g/L)	76.19	11.51	66.00	57.00–75.00
Albumin (g/L)	37.94	8.37	28.00	22.00–33.00
Globulin (g/L)	38.23	5.22	39.00	25.00–46.00
Glucose (mmol/L)	4.83	1.48	4.47	1.00–8.30
Cholesterol (mmol/L)	4.54	Na	6.60	3.10–9.41
Bilirubin (μmol/L)	5.88	2.85	10.54	3.00–18.00
ALP (Unit/L)	161.17	53.21	238.00	43.00–387.00
ALT (Unit/L)	100.00	32.93		
AST (Unit/L)	321.21	135.71	876.00	535.00–1146.00
LDH (Unit/L)	239.75	136.28	877.00	88.00–1741.00
CK (Unit/L)	79.19	37.76	436.00	107.00–806.00
BUN (mmol/L)	10.55	2.97	30.90	25.90–34.20
Creatinine (mmol/L)	0.07	0.04	0.03	0.01–0.04
Calcium (mmol/L)	2.54	0.35	2.22	1.91–2.55
Phosphorus (mmol/L)	1.76	0.44	2.15	1.19–3.03
Sodium (mmol/L)	138.7	6.06	147	139–156
Potassium (mmol/L)	3.11	0.58	2.61	1.40–4.00
Chloride (mmol/L)	94.66	4.8	112	106–117

ALP, Alkaline phosphatase; *ALT*, alanine aminotransferase; *AST*, aspartate aminotransferase; *BUN*, blood urea nitrogen; *CK*, creatine kinase; *fL*, femtoliter; *g/dL*, gram per deciliter; *g/L*, gram per liter; *Hb*, hemoglobin; *LDH*, lactate dehydrogenase; *MCH*, mean corpuscular hemoglobin; *MCHC*, mean corpuscular hemoglobin concentration; *MCV*, mean corpuscular volume; *μmol/L*, micromole per liter; *mmol/L*, millimole per liter; *PCV*, packed cell volume; *pg*, picogram; *RBC*, red blood cell; *Unit/L*, unit per liter; *WBC*, white blood cell.

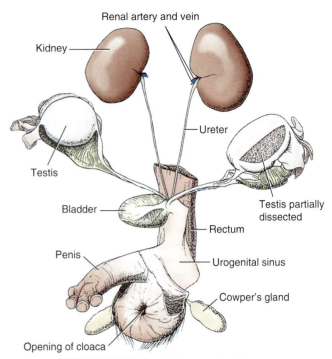

FIGURE 32-3 Male echidna reproductive tract.

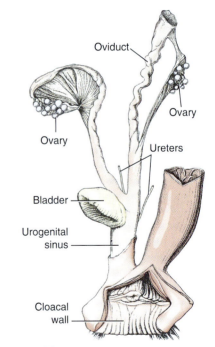

FIGURE 32-4 Female echidna reproductive tract.

Monotremes nurse their young, but they lack nipples, and milk is expressed directly onto the skin of the abdomen in two areas called the *milk patch*, or *areola*, which contains 100 to 150 separate pores. During feeding, the juvenile sucks the milk from the mother's skin and hair. In pregnant echidnas, the enlarged mammary glands form thick "lips" on either side of the midline to create a pouch. This regresses once the young become independent. This does not occur in the platypus.

TABLE 32-7

Selected Echidna Diseases

Disease	Etiology	Clinical Signs and Pathology	Diagnosis	Treatment
Salmonellosis	*S. typhimurium, S. bovis-morbificans, S. dublin, S. saint-paul*	Hemorrhagic diarrhea, weakness, sudden death Enteritis, granulomatous hepatitis, and intestinal intussusception	Fecal culture, necropsy	Antibiotics, fluids
Dermatitis	Bacteria such as *Staphylococcus*, dermatophytes, possible pox	Orthokeratotic hyperkeratosis, suppurative dermatitis	Biopsy, culture, skin scrape, tape prep	Systemic and topical antibiotics, antifungals, antiseptic washes
Coccidiosis	*Eimeria tachyglossi, E. echidnae, Octosporella hystrix*	Depression, lethargy, anorexia, diarrhoea, sudden death Hemorrhagic and necrotizing enteritis or disseminated coccidiosis with foci of necrosis and asexual and sexual life stages scattered through the lung, liver, heart, spleen, kidney and gut	Fecal examination; healthy echidnas also shed oocysts	20 milligrams per kilogram (mg/kg) toltrazuril orally (PO) once daily (SID) 2 days, fluids
Toxoplasmosis	*Toxoplasma gondii*	Nonsuppurative encephalitis, interstitial pneumonia and focal hepatitis, splenitis and nephritis	Necropsy	None
Sparganosis	*Spirometra erinacei* plerocercoids	Large, pale, firm subcutaneous masses	Biopsy, necropsy	Surgical removal
Gastric dilation and gastritis	Feeding high-carbohydrate milk, leading to secondary *Candida, Corynebacterium,* or *Fusobacterium* infection	Sudden death +/− diarrhea in hand raised juveniles Gastritis +/− ulceration and caseous plaques in the stomach and esophagus	Necropsy May observe gastric distention	Prevent by feeding low carbohydrate milk
Piroplasmosis	*Theileria tachyglossi, Babesia tachyglossi* *Hepatozoan tachyglossi*	Probably incidental if <2.5% of erythrocytes infected None	Giemsa-stained blood smear Blood smear–gamonts (8–12 µm, oval with an eccentric nucleus) found in 0%–50% of monocytes	None None
Ticks	*Aponomma concolor, Ixodes* spp., *Amblyomma* spp., *Haemaphysalis* sp.	Anemia, dermatitis	Observation–commonly in ear canals	Ivermectin, fipronil, selamectin, physical removal
Trauma	Cars, dogs, etc.	Beak fractures: difficulty breathing	Radiography	Symptomatic treatment Internal or external fixation is not possible If animals cannot eat or breathe, euthanasia is necessary

TABLE 32-8

Selected Platypus Diseases

Disease	Etiology	Epizootiology	Clinical Signs	Diagnosis	Treatment
Ulcerative mycosis	*Mucor amphibiorum*	Disease only found in Tasmania One study found it in 8% of necropsies Disease likely develops secondary to skin wounds	Granulomatous and ulcerative dermatitis that may spread internally, especially to the lungs Lesions contain 18 micrometers (µm) diameter *Mucor* spherules	Fungal culture, biopsy	Surgery, 0.5 milligram per kilogram (mg/kg) amphotericin B injected into lesion twice weekly Resistant to itraconazole and fluconazole

Continued

TABLE 32-8

Selected Platypus Diseases—cont'd

Disease	Etiology	Epizootiology	Clinical Signs	Diagnosis	Treatment
Cytomegalic inclusion disease	Adenovirus-like: non-enveloped, 80 nanometer (nm) in diameter	Infected renal epithelial cells dramatically enlarged (up to 35 micrometer (µm), instead of 6–10 µm) with eosinophilic intranuclear inclusion bodies	Subclinical with no inflammation	Histology, electron microscopy	None
Leptospirosis	*L. hardjo*	In one study, 50% of platypuses from New South Wales were seropositive and 25% of necropsied Victorian platypuses had mild chronic interstitial nephritis. Zoonosis	Subclinical infection: chronic interstitial nephritis	Serology, histology: silver stain	Not warranted
Ticks	*Ixodes ornithorhynchi*	Vector of *Theileria ornithorhynchi* and *Trypanosoma binneyi*	None	Observation	Ivermectin, physical removal
	Theileria ornithorhynchi	Found in about 1% of erythrocytes	Usually subclinical May cause hemolytic anemia in compromised individuals	Blood smear Infected erythrocytes contain 1–4, 0.5–2.0 µm comma- or crescent-shaped parasites	None
	Trypanosoma binneyi	Found in the blood, lung, liver, and heart in 35% of platypuses in one study	None recorded	Blood smear, polymerase chain reaction	None

TABLE 32-9

Selected Reproductive Parameters for Short-Beaked Echidnas and Platypus

	Short-Beaked Echidna	Platypus
Karyotype	63 males (M), 64 females (F)	52 (M), 52 (F)
Testicular weight	1–3 gram per kilogram (g/kg) (October to March) 8 g/kg (April to September)	1 g (June) 22 g (August to October)
Spermatogenesis	April/May to September	
Mating	June to early September	July to October on the mainland but as late as February in Tasmania.
Gestation	22–24 days	21 days
Number of eggs	1	1–3 (1 or 2 young emerge from the burrow in captivity)
Egg size	13–17 millimeter (mm) 1.5–2.0 g	15–17 mm 1.5–2.0 g
Incubation	10 days	10 days
Hatchling size	13–15 mm 0.3–0.4 g	
Lactation	July/August to January/February	Late September to early March.
Pouch life	45–55 days	No pouch. In the nest for 3 months.
Burrow emergence	January/February	Late January to April on the mainland but as late as May in Tasmania (123–136 days)
Weaning	180–205 days 800–1300 g	120–150 days
Sexual maturity	5–12 years	Can breed at 2 years, but usually not until after 4 years of age
Estrogen (nongravid)		0.01–0.09 nanogram per milliliter (ng/mL)
Estrogen (gravid)		0.16 ng/mL
Progesterone (nongravid)		2.1 ng/mL
Progesterone (gravid)		10.4 ng/mL

Growth is rapid in the echidna, with body weight increasing from 0.5 g to 400 g in 60 days. At one suckling, the young may increase its body weight by 20% in 1 to 2 hours. Suckling intervals may be as long as 5 to 10 days. When weighing around 180 to 260 g, the neonate is left in the plugged nursery burrow with the mother returning at 4- to 6-day intervals to feed it. Age at sexual maturity is unknown.

Platypuses also grow quickly and increase hatching size by 20 times in 14 weeks. By 12 to 18 months, juveniles are close to adult size.

REFERENCES

1. Augee M, Gooden B, Musser A: *Echidna: Extraordinary egg-laying mammal*, Collingwood, Australia, 2006, CSIRO.
2. Booth R, Connolly J: Platypuses. In Vogelnest L, Woods R, editors: *Medicine of Australian mammals*, Collingwood, Australia, 2008, CSIRO.
3. Clark P: *Haematology of Australian mammals*, Collingwood, Australia, 2004, CSIRO.
4. Grant T: *Platypus*, ed 4, Collingwood, Australia, 2007, CSIRO.
5. Griffiths M, Green B, Leckie RMC, et al: Constituents of platypus and echidna milk, with particular reference to the fatty acid complement of the triglycerides. *Aust J Biol Sci* 37:323–330, 1984.
6. Holz P: Monotremes (echidnas and platypuses). In West G, Heard D, Caulkett N, editors: *Zoo animal and wildlife immobilization and anesthesia*, Ames, IA, 2007, Blackwell.
7. Jackson S: *Australian mammals: Biology and captive management*, Collingwood, Australia, 2003, CSIRO.
8. Johnston SD, Madden C, Nicolson V, et al: Venipuncture in the short-beaked echidna. *Aust Vet J* 84:66–67, 2006.
9. Johnston SD, Madden C, Nicolson V, Pyne M: Identifying the sex of short-beaked echidnas. *Aust Vet J* 84:63–65, 2006.
10. Koh JM, Haynes L, Belov K, Kuchel PW: L-to-D-peptide isomerase in male echidna venom. *Aust J Zool* 58:284–288, 2010.
11. Ladds P: *Pathology of Australian native wildlife*, Collingwood, Australia, 2009, CSIRO.
12. Middleton D: Echidnas. In Vogelnest L, Woods R, editors: *Medicine of Australian mammals*, Collingwood, Australia, 2008, CSIRO.
13. Scheelings TF, Haynes L: Effect of diet on serum 25-hydroxyvitamin D concentration in the short-beaked echidna (*Tachyglossus aculeatus*). *Aust Vet J* 90:325–328, 2012.

CHAPTER 33

Marsupialia (Marsupials)

Larry Vogelnest

GENERAL BIOLOGY

Marsupials are an ancient and diverse mammal group, inhabiting a wide range of environments, from high alpine regions to coastal forests and deserts. Many species are arboreal, others are both arboreal and terrestrial, some completely terrestrial, and a few fossorial, and one species, the water opossum (*Chironectes minimus*), is aquatic. Many are nocturnal and some are diurnal or crepuscular. They range in body size from as small as 4 grams (g) up to 85 kilograms (kg). Many species do not live much beyond 10 years. Males of some dasyurids all die in the wild after their first year. A few such as wombats may live up to 30 years.

Numerous defining features of marsupials distinguish them from other mammals: the anatomy of the female reproductive tract; the very short gestation period, with young born in an embryonic state; and a lengthy lactation period, during which the young remain in the pouch. The derivation of the term *marsupial* from "marsupium" and the implication that all female marsupials have a pouch is not correct. The distinction of marsupials from eutherian mammals as not having a placenta is also not correct.

The extant marsupial species are restricted to Australasia and the Americas, with the majority of the 333 species occurring in Australia, New Guinea, and nearby islands. The subclass Marsupialia is divided into seven orders: Didelphimorphia (opossums, 92 spp.), Paucituberculata (shrew opossums, 6 spp.), Microbiotheria (Monito del Monte [*Dromiciops gliroides*]), Dasyuromorphia (dasyurids, 71 spp.), Peramelemorphia (bandicoots and bilby [*Macrotis lagotis*], 21 spp.), Notoryctemorphia (marsupial moles, 2 spp.) and Diprotodontia (koala [*Phascolarctos cinereus*], wombats, possums, gliders, macropods, 140 spp.).[73]

UNIQUE ANATOMY AND PHYSIOLOGY[67,71,73]

Musculoskeletal System

An ossified patella does not exist except in bandicoots and the bilby. Epipubic bones extend from the cranial aspect of the pubis. Paired clavicles are present in all species except in bandicoots and the bilby. Other than in opossums, dasyurids and the numbat (*Myrmecobius fasciatus*), the second and third digits of the hindfoot are syndactylus.

In macropods, the atlanto-occipital articulation is highly flexible, allowing the muzzle to remain horizontal, whether the neck is horizontal or vertical. This may be associated with some weakness at this articulation, possibly accounting for the high incidence of traumatic fractures at this site. The mandibular symphysis of kangaroos and wallabies is unfused and flexible, whereas in the banded hare-wallaby (*Lagostrophus fasciatus*), bettongs, and potoroos, it is fused.

Dentition

Deciduous teeth, apart from the third premolars, degenerate before eruption. Broadly, marsupials may be divided into two groups on the basis of dentition: (1) the *polyprotodonts* (many incisors), including the dasyurids, numbat, opossums, marsupial moles, bandicoots, and bilby, the majority of which are carnivorous or omnivorous; and (2) the *diprotodonts* (two lower incisors), including the macropods, koala, wombats, possums, and gliders, the majority of which are herbivorous. The diprotodonts have a variably sized diastema between the incisors and molars. Wombats are the only diprotodont marsupials with one pair of upper incisors and the only marsupials with hypsodont teeth (rootles and ever growing).[67]

Some species of macropods, particularly those in the genus *Macropus*, exhibit molar progression. Molars erupt caudally and migrate forward throughout life. Cheek teeth are shed from the front as they wear out, replaced functionally by the next tooth. Molar progression is unique to macropods, elephants, and manatees. In the koala, the occlusal surfaces of the molar teeth wear continuously throughout life, and the degree of tooth wear has implications for plane of nutrition.

Gastrointestinal System

Macropods are foregut fermenters. In a process known as *merycism*, macropods, particularly the browsers and grazers, occasionally regurgitate food into their mouths, which involves a rather violent heaving motion with vigorous movements of the forelimbs and the thorax. The bolus is not generally rechewed as in ruminants and is quickly reswallowed.[14] Koalas, wombats, and most possums and gliders are monogastric, hindgut fermenters. Koalas possess the largest cecum relative to body size among all known mammals. The wombat small intestine is short; the colon is large and sacculated; and the cecum is vestigial. In possums and gliders, an expanded cecum is the main site for fermentation in most species. The intestines of the striped possum (*Dactylopsila trivirgata*) and honey possum (*Tarsipes rostratus*) are simple because of the lack of plant material in their diet. Coprophagy of cecal contents occurs in some species of ringtail possums. Dasyurids, bandicoots, and the bilby have simple gastrointestinal tracts.

In females, the urogenital sinus (into which the urethra discharges), together with the rectum, opens into the common vestibule (or cloaca). In males, the penis lies within the common vestibule. The urogenital openings are ventral to the rectum.

Skin

Many species of dasyurids, opossums, and the numbat lack a pouch. Some species develop a temporary pouch from folds of skin on either side of the abdominal teats during lactation. Male marsupials lack teats. Numbers of teats in females varies: 2 in koala, wombats, 4 in macropods, numbat, 4 to 12 in dasyurids, 2 to 6 in possums and gliders, 6 to 8 in bandicoots, bilby, and 4 to 13 in opossums. Marsupials are well endowed with cutaneous glands, which have various functions. Macropods generally have thin skin, particularly in the inner surfaces of the limbs, and is particularly pronounced in the forelimbs, where the vascularity of the subcutis is significantly increased. Wombat skin is considerably thicker than that in other marsupials and quite inelastic, and all three species have a characteristic "sacral plate" on the rump, almost as rigid as bone. Gliders are distinguished from possums by the presence of a gliding membrane extending from the hindlimb to the forelimb.

Sensory Systems

Macropods have a wide field of peripheral vision enabling them to see movement in almost every direction, and binocular vision enables them to have more precise close vision. They have good day and night vision. Despite this, they appear to have difficulty navigating obstacles and barriers that are not solid, especially when alarmed and fleeing. The iris is thick and uniformly brown, and the pupil is circular and may be dilated easily with tropicamide. The fundus is heavily pigmented (usually dark brown) ventrally, whereas dorsally it is usually lighter in color, and in some animals, the choroidal blood vessels may be seen through the pigment. The optic disk sits at the junction between these two zones and is

well vascularized. Retinal vessels are not prominent. All macropods have persistent hyaloid vessels (seen as a tuft of vessels arising from the center of the optic disk and extending anteriorly toward the posterior lens capsule). In most macropods, they are fixed anteriorly and are not easily visualized. If not fixed, they may be seen moving within the vitreous. In many kangaroos, myelination of the nerve fiber layer may be seen extending from around the optic disk. This myelination is generally most obvious in the lateral and medial aspects.[62]

The koala has relatively small, spherical, frontally placed eyes. The cornea occupies a relatively large segment of the globe. A tapetum extends across the retina above the optic disk, and, as in many other marsupials, the retina is essentially avascular except for a small area on the optic disc itself.[56] Mean intraocular pressure is 24.2 ± 6 mm Hg.[26] The iris is usually brown. The pupil is a vertically orientated slit. The lacrimal puncta are slitlike openings just inside the lid edges, 2 to 3 millimeters (mm) from the medial canthus. Dasyurids have a vascular retina. The arteries do not branch but form discrete capillary loops.

Immune System

Significant differences exist in the development of the immune systems of marsupials and eutherian mammals. No lymphoid tissue is present at birth, and the neonate is not immunocompetent. Most species reach immune system maturation at the time of first release from the maternal teat, approximately half way through pouch life. Passive transfer of maternal antibodies occurs throughout lactation, and antibodies are absorbed unchanged across the gut epithelium of the pouch young (PY). This passively acquired immunity is short lived, and most maternal antibody will be lost by about 4 weeks after separation from the mother, with the young only protected by an underdeveloped active immune system. Secretions from the pouch epithelium and macrophages found in marsupial milk may play roles in immunologic protection of the PY.[52]

In healthy macropod PY, the thymi are firm, bulging structures on the ventral side of the neck and may be visualized in unfurred or early furred PY. The thymi regress fully by sexual maturity.[59] Superficial lymph nodes are not palpable in healthy macropods. The superficial inguinal, superficial axillary, rostral mandibular, mandibular, and facial lymph nodes are palpable in healthy koalas. Popliteal and subiliac lymph nodes are absent.[25]

Reproductive System

Marsupials have a diffuse, epitheliochorial choriovitelline placenta. Bandicoots have a diffuse placenta, with both choriovitelline and chorioallantoic contributions.[66] Female reproductive anatomy is similar in all marsupials. Each of the paired lateral uteri opens into a vaginal cul-de-sac through its own cervix. The paired lateral vaginae both open separately into the urogenital sinus at the level of the urethral opening and are separated along their length by a soft tissue median septum (Figure 33-1). During parturition, the fetus tunnels through this septal tissue to form a median vagina. In most marsupials, the median vagina closes rapidly after passage of the fetus and then re-forms with each subsequent parturition. In most macropods, opossums, and the honey possum the median vagina becomes epithelialized after the first parturition and remains patent as a permanent median vagina.[66]

The anatomy of the male reproductive tract is similar in all marsupials. The scrotum is prominent, pendulous, pedunculated (other than wombats), and pre-penile. A strong cremaster muscle retracts the scrotal contents tightly against the body. Seminal vesicles and ampullae are lacking. Accessory sex glands consist of an often large disseminate prostate and one or more pairs of bulbourethral glands. In some species such as bandicoots, the prostate is easily palpated in the abdomen of breeding males.

The Macropodidae are the only marsupials to produce semen, which coagulates to form a seminal plug in the female's urogenital sinus and vaginae after ejaculation[14] and may be seen protruding from the female's common vestibule.

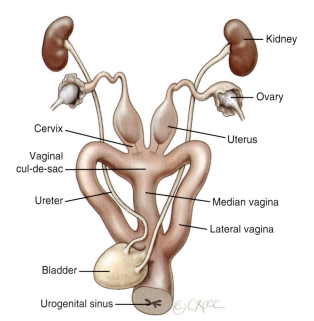

FIGURE 33-1 The female macropod urogenital tract. (Adapted from Vogelnest L and Woods R: Medicine of Australian Mammals, CSIRO 2008, Reprinted with corrections 2010, Illustrator: Beth Croce, Published by CSIRO PUBLISHING, Collingwood, Victoria, Australia, Reproduced with permissions.)

Labels in figure: Kidney, Ovary, Uterus, Median vagina, Lateral vagina, Cervix, Vaginal cul-de-sac, Ureter, Bladder, Urogenital sinus

Urinary System

The urinary system is similar in all marsupials. Unique to marsupials is the path of the ureters from the kidney to the bladder. The ureters pass between the median and lateral vaginae on each side. This anatomy has consequences for surgical procedures of the female reproductive tract. In macropods, the koala, and the wombats, the bladder is intrapelvic when not distended.

The urethra of male macropods has paired valvelike cusps approximately 2 to 3 centimeters (cm) proximal to the external orifice. Each cusp is approximately 5 mm long, with its free margin directed toward the external urethral orifice. A similar but larger pair of cusps lies immediately distal to the urinary bladder sphincter. These cusps may make urethral catheterization difficult. In koalas, two regions of the male urethra may potentially impede catheterization. The first is a narrowing of the lumen and some mucosal irregularity in the vicinity of the openings of the bulbourethral glands. The second is the prostatic sinus, a groove on either side of the urethral crest just distal to the neck of the bladder.

Metabolism and Thermoregulation

Brown adipose tissue, which is used by eutherians to generate heat, has not been found in marsupials.[22] Some marsupials will enter one of two types of torpor. Shallow daily torpor in which the body temperature drops to 11°C to 28°C and lasts 2 to 20 hours occurs in opossums, dasyurids, small possums, and possibly in the numbat and marsupial moles. Deep, prolonged torpor (hibernation), in which body temperature drops to 1°C to 6°C and lasts 1 to 3 weeks occurs in pygmy possums (Burramyidae), the feathertail glider (*Acrobates pygmaeus*), and the Monito del Monte.[21]

Marsupials cannot thermoregulate until about half way through pouch life. Marsupial metabolism is lower than that of eutherians, with macropods at 25% and the koala and hairy-nosed wombats (*Lasiorhinus* spp.) very low at 44%. Basal metabolic rates are highest in the small insectivorous dasyurids (similar to eutherians), whereas rates for other dasyurids are less than half those in eutherian carnivores of similar size.[30] All wombats, in particular the hairy-nosed species, have extremely low requirements of energy, protein, and water. Plasma concentrations of thyroid hormones in wombats are the lowest recorded for any mammal.[4] Koalas and hairy-nosed wombats rarely drink fluids.

Thermoregulation is by evaporative mechanisms (panting, sweating, and licking). A unique feature of kangaroos is that sweating stops as soon as exercise stops, even if body temperature is still elevated and the animal is still panting rapidly.[14,67] A method of evaporative heat loss by spreading saliva on the forearms is common in macropods that have undergone a period of exertion or anxiety. Panting is the major means of evaporative cooling in the koala. Wombats are more tolerant of cold than heat and cannot sweat, using postural thermoregulation or salivating on their forelegs and chest to aid cooling. Dasyurids do not sweat and cope with excessive heat by licking and panting to increase evaporative cooling.

Miscellaneous

Macropods have hearts one-third larger than those of comparably sized eutherian mammals and may move more air through their lungs with each breath.[14] Hand-reared, adult macropods that have a nervous temperament may display a wide-eyed expression and trembling of the head, neck, and upper body when approached. This is termed *tintibulation* and is an apparent expression of anxiety or excitement. In the koala, the linea alba is broad and almost translucent, and no curtainlike omentum exists. Even in healthy, well-nourished captive koalas, fat depots are meager in comparison with those in most eutherian mammals.

SPECIAL HOUSING REQUIREMENTS

Housing requirements for marsupials are diverse.[32,70] Housing for hospitalization of ill or injured marsupials is described in Box 33-1.

FEEDING

Compared with eutherians, most marsupials have a lower basal metabolic rate and therefore lower maintenance requirements for energy, protein, water and other nutrients. Requirements may generally be met with lower food intake and often fairly poor-quality, high-fiber diets. In captivity, marsupials are often fed in excess and fed concentrated diets of low fiber content, which results in obesity and dental and gastrointestinal (GI) disease.[29] Energy intake should be monitored and controlled and activity encouraged through behavioral enrichment. Wild and captive diets have been described.[2,4,17,32,70,71] Hospital and convalescent diets for marsupials are described in Box 33-2.

It is recommended that diets of small macropods be supplemented with vitamin E. Some small macropod species are prone to developing a syndrome of weakness and wasting of the hindlimbs, ultimately progressing to paralysis and death from myopathy. The development of this syndrome is not related to diet alone. Stress caused by overcrowding may increase vitamin E requirement.[30]

Hand Rearing

Successful hand rearing of marsupial PY requires a detailed understanding of neonatal development and physiology, the unique pouch environment, maternal care, passive immunity, development of the immune system, and milk composition.[43] The major challenges in hand rearing marsupials are concerned with simulating the functions of the pouch, which provides a stable thermal environment until the PY becomes endothermic, and providing an appropriate milk substitute that may meet the changing needs of the developing PY until weaning and minimize exposure to pathogens.[9]

The milk of marsupials must support the PY from its embryonic state at birth until independence. The composition, therefore, changes profoundly during the course of lactation. The net effect of these changes is a gradual increase in energy content throughout lactation, meeting the increasing energetic demands of the growing PY as it becomes more active and develops endothermy. Calcium, phosphorus, sodium, and potassium concentrations also change during lactation.[32,43,67]

Marsupial milk has very low levels of lactose, oligosaccharides being the predominant carbohydrates for most of lactation. The

BOX 33-1 Housing Requirements for Hospitalization of Sick or Injured Marsupials

MACROPODS[68]

Enclosure	Simple, solid-walled (no objects protruding from the walls) standard hospital cages to stalls for larger species
Substrate	Rubber matting, wood shavings, straw
Furniture	Rock wallabies and tree-kangaroos should be provided with structures they may sit on top of or climb
Shelter	Structures in which the animal may seek refuge, branches with leaves placed upside down in corners
Other	Consideration should be given to the use of long-acting neuroleptic drugs

KOALAS[8]

Enclosure	Large enclosures allowing climbing both vertically and horizontally
	Intensive care (IC) patients: standard hospital cages
Substrate	IC patients: thick, soft padding covered with towel or blanket
	Plastic floor matting allows urine to drain away
Furniture	At least two resting forks, on the same or separate poles with a horizontal pole connecting the two
	Rough-barked poles are easier to climb
	A gently-inclined pole from the ground to a raised fork may enable a weaker koala to reach an elevated position
	If very weak or unable to climb, a stable fork or other structure for support at ground level will be required
Other	Drinking water should be made available in a stable shallow bowl on the floor

WOMBATS[11]

Enclosure	Robust and escape-proof
	A solid walled den or stall, avoid mesh or chain-link fences, standard hospital cages for IC and juveniles
Substrate	Soil, sand, straw, leaf litter, wood mulch
	If hospitalized for short periods do not need opportunity to dig and should be discouraged for debilitated or ill wombats as they may expend a large amount of energy

Shelter	Burrow substitute to provide shelter and privacy: sturdy wooden box, large diameter concrete pipe, large hollow log
Other	Common wombats <25° C, hairy-nosed wombats <30° C, supplemental heat for debilitated animals

DASYURIDS[28] **AND OPOSSUMS**[35]

Enclosure	10 millimeters (mm) solid wood, glass fronted for small species, standard hospital cages for large species, sturdier accommodation with solid walls for quolls and Tasmanian devils
Substrate	News, shredded or pelleted paper
Furniture	Climbing structures for arboreal species, pool for water opossums
Shelter	Wooden or cardboard nest boxes filled with shredded paper or wood shavings
	Elevated for arboreal species
Other	Supplemental heat may be required
	For opossums 10–30° C (22° C most appropriate), humidity >58%

POSSUMS AND GLIDERS[33]

Enclosure	Standard hospital cages covered with cloth or towel
Substrate	Paper
Furniture	Branches with leaves for cover and climbing
Shelter	Elevated wooden nest box relevant to the size of the animal
Other	Food and water bowls on the floor or elevated

BANDICOOTS AND BILBIES[41]

Enclosure	Standard hospital cages covered with cloth or towel
	Walls should be solid or wire vertical bars, rather than mesh, to prevent nail damage
Substrate	Nonabrasive (epoxy flooring, paper, clean towels)
Shelter	Wooden or cardboard nest box relevant to the size of the animal
Other	Can be kept in such enclosures for lengthy periods while under treatment, avoid frequent handling

BOX 33-2 Hospital and Convalescent Diets for Marsupials[70]

MACROPODS

Offer normal diet

Inappetent animals may be stimulated to eat with fresh grasses, browse, good-quality hay

Offer finely chopped, grated, or cooked food for animals with dental disease or extractions

Intensive care (IC) patients: offer or hand feed specialized herbivore intensive care supplements

KOALAS

Encourage sick koalas to eat leaves

Offer fresh, high-quality leaves of various stages of growth and a variety of species, including known preferred species (sick koalas may change their leaf species preference)

Most do not hand feed and will not generally eat individual leaves removed from branches

May take leaves from small branchlets if not distracted by human presence

Supplementary feeding: low-lactose, high-energy milk powders mixed to a paste with water ± blended leaves

WOMBATS

Better able to tolerate extended periods of inappetence or anorexia because of low metabolic requirements

Offer a higher-energy diet, with greater quantities of foods such as sweet potato, sweet corn, carrot, apple, and higher-protein herbivore pellets

Grate items to tempt reluctant feeders

Tube feed (under general anesthesia) or "assist-feed" with a syringe, energy-rich mixes or specialized herbivore IC supplements for IC patients. Diazepam (0.1 milligram per kilogram [mg/kg], subcutaneously [SC], daily, 30 minutes before offering food) ± vitamin B complex (1 milliliter per kilogram [mL/kg], SC, once daily [SID], for 3 days) may stimulate appetite

DASYURIDS, BANDICOOTS, BILBIES, OPOSSUMS, POSSUMS, AND GLIDERS

Add to standard diet: favorite food items, live insects, cat or dog food, cooked chicken, other meats, semi-solid or liquid convalescent carnivore diets (can be tube fed to IC patients) for carnivores or omnivores; and nectar mixes for possums and gliders

transport of sugars into the intestinal mucosal cells is a relatively slow process. Mother-reared PY drink small volumes frequently. Hand-reared PY are fed larger volumes less frequently. When hand-reared PY are fed milk containing lactose, the capacity of the mechanism for transporting sugars into the cells is exceeded; hence unabsorbed lactose accumulates within the intestinal lumen, increasing the osmolality of the gut contents, resulting in watery diarrhea, dehydration, malabsorption of other nutrients, malnutrition, and retarded growth. Oligosaccharides are significantly larger than lactose and thus exert a lower osmotic effect.[43,49]

Numerous milk formulas have been used. Critical factors in the choice of a formula are low lactose content, and the formula should mirror the changing composition of natural milk from early to late lactation. A number of formulae that satisfy these requirements are available.[43] Nevertheless, hand-reared PY of a wide range of species have thrived on a wide range of formulae, and the formula chosen is not the only key to success. Hygiene, husbandry, stress management, consistency, carer experience, and a maternalistic, nurturing instinct are equally as important.

The weaning process needs to be carefully managed for many species. Herbivorous species require inoculation of the gut with appropriate bacteria at this time. Hand-reared koalas that have not consumed pap must be fed natural pap or a substitute. Macropod and wombat young should be given access to fresh feces from healthy adults or mixed with water or formula and fed as a slurry.

RESTRAINT AND HANDLING

Capture and Physical Restraint

The principles of capture and physical restraint of marsupials is not different from those of other taxa, and appropriate methods have been described.[27,32,70] The unique factor in marsupials is that females may eject the PY during pursuit and restraint. Excessive fear, exertion, or both may result in capture myopathy in macropods (see Box 33-9). Smaller species may spin violently when held by the tail, which results in fractures or dislocations.

Macropods may be caught in large, wide-mouthed hoop nets or by hand by grasping the base of the tail. Koalas may be encouraged to back into a bag. Docile koalas may be picked up from behind, by grasping around the wrists; alternatively, first the wrists and then the ankles may be grasped so that the koala is restrained in a sitting position, facing away from the handler. Wombats may be approached from behind and quickly grasped just behind the front legs with both arms. Small marsupials may be caught in a nest box or small enclosure by hand (protected by small towel or cloth bag) or small net. Larger dasyurids and opossums may be caught in a net or by grasping the tail between midway and the base.

Once captured, the animal should be physically restrained for only minor and quick procedures or anesthetic induction. All but the most tractable animals should be transferred into a bag for examination, drug administration, or transport. The head should remain covered at all times. Macropods held for longer periods should be suspended in bags off the ground. The animals should be kept cool.

Chemical Restraint[27,70]

Injectable chemical restraint agents may be administered by hand, intravenously (IV) or intramuscularly (IM), or remotely by using darts in larger species. In wombats, the sacral plate over the rump makes it impossible to give injections or dart in this area. Inhalational agents may be administered via a face mask or induction chamber (small species) or via an endotracheal tube after induction. Intubation of macropods, koalas, and wombats may be difficult. They have a narrow gape and dental arcade, and the distance from the oral opening to the larynx is substantial. Koalas have a long soft palate. In macropods and wombats, lateral recumbency, with the head extended, is preferable, whereas in koalas, intubation is possible in lateral, sternal, or dorsal recumbency. A long, narrow-bladed laryngoscope, a small rigid endoscope, or a long, curved transilluminator

may be used to visualize the glottis. Long endotracheal tubes are required. A guide stylet may be inserted into the trachea and the endotracheal tube passed over it. Blind intubation may also be achieved by grasping the larynx between the thumb and forefinger of one hand and passing the endotracheal tube over the tongue with the other until the tube touches the glottis. As the animal takes a breath and air is heard rushing through the tube, the tube is inserted into the trachea. Larger dasyurids, possums, gliders, bandicoots, bilbies, and opossums are easily intubated with the aid of a small, narrow-bladed laryngoscope. A stylet may be required. For some possums and gliders, ventral recumbency, with the neck extended and head held vertically (similar to intubating a rabbit), may be used.

Preanesthetic fasting is not generally necessary for macropods, koalas, wombats, bandicoots, and bilbies; however, regurgitation may occasionally occur (particularly in macropods), and intubation is recommended for longer procedures. Preanesthetic fasting for 6 to 8 hours is recommended for dasyurids and 1 to 2 hours for larger possums, gliders, and opossums. In koalas, periods of apnea and, in unintubated animals, respiratory stridor caused by the long soft palate is relatively common. Profound and prolonged tranquillization has been seen in wombats with the use of long-acting neuroleptic agents. Ptyalism, poor relaxation, constant limb and jaw movements, and prolonged recoveries may be seen with tiletamine/zolazepam in some species. In addition tachycardia, respiratory depression, apnea, muscle rigidity and deaths have been seen in possums and gliders.

Box 33-3 provides a list of chemical restraint agents, regimens, and doses used in marsupials.

SURGERY[4]

Common indications for surgery are repair of traumatic injuries (soft tissue and bone), repair of tissues damaged by infectious processes, tumor excision, GI accidents, exploratory laparotomy, and reproductive procedures. Most of the procedures below are described for macropods but are equally applicable to other marsupial species.

Laparotomy

Consideration must be given to the voluminous GI tract in some species, the presence of a pouch (with or without PY) in females, and the epipubic bones. With the animal in dorsal recumbency, a ventral midline approach is used. If access to the caudal abdomen is required, tilt the body head down to about 30 degrees. In both sexes, when access to the cranial abdomen is required, the approach is straight forward. In females with a pouch, the approach will depend on the size of the pouch and the presence of PY. If the pouch is empty or the PY may be temporarily removed, a midline incision may be made inside the pouch, midway between the teats and the cranial border of the pouch. A useful technique is to use stay sutures to hold the pouch open. If a PY is present and cannot be removed, an incision may be made lateral to the pouch opening at the cranial end of the epipubic bone. The skin is then reflected toward the midline to expose the *linea alba*.

In the koala, extreme care is required when opening the abdominal cavity through a ventral midline incision. Subcutaneous fat is absent; the *linea alba* is thin; the abdominal muscles are 2 to 3 mm thick over the ventrolateral abdominal wall; and the cecum and proximal colon lie immediately below the incision site.[8]

Surgical Sterilization

Ovariectomy and Ovariohysterectomy

The animal is prepared as for laparotomy, and the head is tilted down to 30 degrees. An incision is made midway between the tip of the epipubic bones and the pubis. The reproductive tract is visualized, and one side exteriorized with the use of a spay hook. For ovariectomy, one uterus is located, and the corresponding ovary is exteriorized. The fimbria and ampulla of the oviduct are teased off the ovary

BOX 33-3 Chemical Restraint Agents, Regimens, and Doses Used in Marsupials.[27,70]

MACROPODS

Sedation or Tranquillization

- Diazepam 0.1–2 milligrams per kilogram (mg/kg), intramuscularly (IM), 0.1–1.0 mg/kg, intravenously (IV) (individual and species response variable, duration 1–2 hours)
- Midazolam 0.3 mg/kg, IM, 0.2 mg/kg, IV[a]
- Azaperone 2 mg/kg, IM (3–8 hours duration)
- Perphenazine enathate 5 mg/kg, IM (7 days duration)
- Fluphenazine decanoate 2.5 mg/kg, IM (10 days duration)
- Haloperidol decanoate 4–6 mg/kg, IM (duration unknown; possibly up to 30 days)
- Zuclopenthixol acetate 5–10 mg/kg, IM (duration 48–72 hours)

Anesthesia

- Tiletamine/Zolazepam (T/Z) 4–10 mg/kg, IM, 1–3 mg/kg, IV; lower doses for tractable animals, higher for excited animals and western gray kangaroos
- T/Z 2–3 mg/kg, IM + medetomidine (Med) 40 microgram per kilogram (μg/kg), IM, reversal atipamezole (4 × Med dose IM)
- T/Z 3–4 mg/kg, IM + acepromazine 0.3 mg/kg, IM[b]
- Ket 3–5 mg/kg, IM + Med 40–125μg/kg, IM, reversal atipamezole (4–5 x Med dose IM). Use higher doses in nervous or excited animals
- Ket 3–4 mg/kg, IM + Med 50 μg/kg, IM + midazolam 0.02–0.1 mg/kg, IM, reversal atipamezole 0.25 mg/kg, IM[a]
- Alfaxalone 5–8 mg/kg, IM, 1.5–3 mg/kg, IV; very short duration of action
- Isoflurane in oxygen (induction, maintenance, or both)

KOALAS

Sedation or Tranquillization

- Diazepam 0.5–1 mg/kg, IM; 0.5 mg/kg, IV

Anesthesia

- Propofol 2.5–3.0 mg/kg, IV bolus, 4–5 mg boluses for maintenance; short duration of action
- Alfaxalone 3.0 mg/kg, IM, 1.5 mg/kg, IV
- T/Z 5–10 mg/kg, IM, 2.5 mg/kg, IV
- T/Z 3.5 mg/kg, IM + Med 55 μg/kg, IM, reversal atipamezole 2 mg IV
- Isoflurane in oxygen (induction, maintenance, or both)

DASYURIDS

Sedation or Tranquillization

- Diazepam 1–2 mg/kg, IM

Anesthesia

- Isoflurane in oxygen (induction and/or maintenance)
- T/Z 7–10 mg/kg, IM

POSSUMS AND GLIDERS

Sedation Tranquillization

- Diazepam 0.5–1 mg/kg, IM
- Butorphanol tartrate 0.4–1 mg/kg, subcutaneously (SC) or IM

Anesthesia

- Isoflurane in oxygen (induction, maintenance, or both)
- Ket 1–3 mg/kg, IM + Med 20–100 μg/kg, IM, reversal atipamezole 0.05–0.4 mg/kg, IV
- Alfaxalone 5–8 mg/kg IM, 5 mg/kg, IV; rapid short-acting anesthesia in common brushtail and common ringtail possums

WOMBATS

Sedation or Tranquillization

- Diazepam 0.5–1 mg/kg, IM
- Midazolam at 0.5 mg/kg, IM

Anesthesia

- T/Z at 2–9 mg/kg. Effect and duration are dose dependent
- Ket 2 mg/kg, IM + Med 125 μg/kg, IM, reversal atipamezole (4 × Med dose IM)
- T/Z 3 mg/kg, IM + Med 40 μg/kg, IM, reversal atipamazole (5 × Med dose IM)
- Alfaxalone 3–5 mg/kg, IM (effect is dose dependent)
- Isoflurane in oxygen (induction, maintenance, or both)

BANDICOOTS AND BILBIES

Sedation or Tranquillization

- Diazepam 0.5–1 mg/kg, IM
- Midazolam 0.1– 0.2 mg/kg, IM

Anesthesia

- Isoflurane in oxygen (induction, maintenance, or both)

OPOSSUMS

Sedation Tranquillization

- Diazepam 0.5–2 mg/kg, IM, orally (PO), IV[d]

Anesthesia

- Isoflurane in oxygen (induction, maintenance, or both)
- T/Z 15 mg/kg, IM[c]
- Ket 10 mg/kg, IM + Med 100 μg/kg, IM + butorphanol 0.2 mg/kg IM[c]
- Ket 30–50 mg/mg, IM[d]
- Ket 2–3 mg/kg, IM + Med 50–100 μg/kg, IM, reversal atipamezole 0.05–0.4 mg/kg, IV[d]

[a]Joe Smith, personal communication.
[b]Simone Vitali, personal communication.
[c]Doses for Virginia opossum – a euthanasia study so no vital signs and recovery data available.[63]
[d]Doses for Virginia opossum.[35]

to enable clear visualization of the ovarian vessels. The vessels are clamped and ligated, and the ovary is removed. Complications such as pyometra have not been reported.

Ovariohysterectomy is technically more difficult and risky because of limited access and the unique anatomy of the reproductive tract. The only indication for the surgery may be therapeutic reasons. The approach is as for ovariectomy. A hole is made in the broad ligament just lateral but close to the ovaries to avoid catching the ureters (which should be visualized). The ovaries are exteriorized with gentle traction on the suspensory ligament. The vessels are clamped and ligated. Once both ovaries are ligated and detached, the broad ligament is torn off, staying as close to the lateral margins of the blood vessels as possible to avoid damaging the ureters. The uteri are ligated at the immediate proximal end of the cervices (see

Figure 33-1). They are first ligated separately, and then a single ligature may be placed around both uteri. Transfixation ligatures may be required. Once the uteri are removed, a continuous suture to close the stump may be necessary.

Sterilization of koalas and macropods may also be performed via laparoscopic tubal ligation or ovariectomy. The animal is positioned as above. Following routine surgical preparation, the abdomen is insufflated with carbon dioxide (CO_2). Three small incisions are made to allow insertion of the grasping forceps, laparoscope, and cautery scissors into the caudal abdomen. For tubal ligation, each oviduct is visualized and manipulated with the forceps so that transection and cautery may be achieved. For ovariectomy, the ovary is manipulated and elevated with the grasping forceps and removed from the ovarian bursa. Electrocautery (with or without endoclips for large animals) is used to ligate the ovarian vessels. Laparoscopic long-blade scissors are then used to free the ovary from its abdominal attachments. Once free, the cannula is retracted through the skin incision to allow direct removal of the ovary from the abdominal cavity through the incision.

Orchiectomy and Scrotal Ablation

The animal is placed in dorsal recumbency. The scrotal septum is prominent, and the testicles are removed through separate incisions in the scrotum on each side at the most ventral point. A standard open castration technique is used. The incisions are left open. For scrotal ablation, castration is performed, as described above; however, the spermatic cords are severed at as high a point as possible. The scrotal pedicle is cut flush with the abdominal wall. The ligated spermatic cords are pushed through the incision toward the inguinal canal. The wound is closed. Orchiectomy and scrotal ablation in sugar gliders with the use of a CO_2 laser to sever the scrotal stalk has been described.[50]

Vasectomy

With the animal in dorsal recumbency, an incision is made, midway between the testicle and the abdominal wall, in the skin and *tunica vaginalis* over each spermatic cord on the cranial side of the scrotal pedicle. A small portion of the spermatic cord is exteriorized and the vas deferens identified, bluntly dissected out, and exposed. A segment is removed after ligating proximally and distally to the piece being removed. Vas deferens clips may be used. The wounds are sutured.

Orthopedics

All standard orthopedic principles and techniques may be readily applied to fracture repair in marsupials. In macropods, the unique anatomy of the hindlimbs and the massive mechanical stresses that are placed on the bones of the hindlimbs and pelvic girdle during locomotion make adequate stabilization of fractures of these bones difficult. The prognosis for successful repair in adult macropods is generally poor. Hand-reared PY that may be confined to a pouch during convalescence are better candidates for fracture repair. External fixateurs have been used with success to repair fractured tibias in older hand-reared macropods. In small species and perhaps the tamest of larger species, fractures of the metatarsi may be repairable with either internal or external fixation.

Miscellaneous Procedures

Tail amputation has successfully been performed in macropods, with the animals adapting well to the loss of the tail, despite the obvious reliance on the tail for a pentapedal gait.[65,68] Standing up from lateral recumbency may occasionally be a problem. A standard technique for tail amputation is used.

Cataract surgery in macropods is technically easy; however, many cases develop postoperative glaucoma, probably secondary to chronic uveitis. The prognosis even with treatment is poor, and many cases require globe evisceration or enucleation or euthanasia. In PY with galactose-induced cataracts, surgical removal of the lens often reveals extensive opacification of the vitreous, making the prognosis

for return to normal vision poor. Because of these complications it is difficult to justify cataract surgery in macropods.[62]

Conjunctival ablation in koalas may be indicated (as an adjunct to topical treatment, systemic treatment, or both) in chronic cases of chlamydial disease, where proliferative conjunctivae obscure vision.[8]

THERAPEUTICS

Few pharmacokinetic studies have been conducted in marsupials, and drug doses are usually extrapolated from those for domestic animals. As a general rule, drugs seem to be well tolerated and appear to contribute to improvement in clinical condition. It has been proposed that the lower metabolic rate of marsupials should be accounted for by reducing dose and frequency of administration when extrapolating data from eutherian mammals. Recent studies indicate that this is not valid, and some evidence suggests that hindgut-fermenting marsupials may have specific mechanisms for dealing with plant toxins and xenobiotics.[18,44,64]

Several pharmacokinetic and efficacy studies on marsupials have been published.[7,15,16,23,24,37,38,46,48] The koala studies are consistent with what is known about their efficient metabolic pathways and also suggest barriers to oral and subcutaneous absorption.

Very few reports of precautions and adverse drug reactions in marsupials are available. Subadult common ringtail possums (*Pseudocheirus peregrinus*) appear to be particularly sensitive to antibiotics. A dysbiotic syndrome leading to wasting and death (similar to that seen in other hindgut fermenters) has been reported. In macropods there have been anecdotal reports of dysbiosis in macropods, particularly after oral administration of antibiotics (particularly penicillins). Hand-reared PY are prone to developing candidiasis when on antibiotics (see Box 33-6). Mebendazole toxicity has been described in macropods.[58] Wasting and death within 2 to 6 weeks of administration of parenteral oxytetracycline and oral erythromycin has been reported in koalas.[8] Nystatin may induce diarrhea when used at higher doses.

PHYSICAL EXAMINATION AND DIAGNOSTICS[70]

Physical Examination

Wherever possible, physical examination should begin with a distant observation of the undisturbed animal. Many marsupials are nocturnal, and observation in daylight hours may be unrewarding. Body temperature may be obtained by inserting a thermometer into the rectum, which opens into the common vestibule dorsal to the urogenital opening. Body temperatures may range from as low as 31°C to as high as 38°C (some dasyurids); however, in most marsupials, the average is between 35.5°C and 36.5°C. Changes in body condition, hydration status, gut fill, and presence of PY in females should all be considered when interpreting changes in body weight. A numerical body condition scoring system for koalas is available.[8] Hydration is difficult to assess in wombats, as their skin is very thick and inelastic and the oral and conjunctival mucosa may appear dry, even in a well-hydrated animal.

The enormous capacity and prolonged retention time of digesta in the cecum and colon of koalas and wombats are the reasons that healthy koalas have a well-rounded, ovoid body shape and the abdomen of wombats feels full and doughy. After a few days of inappetence, the abdominal girth reduces, and the animal becomes straight-sided or noticeably concave behind the costal arch.

Examination of teeth, particularly in diprotodont marsupials, is important to assess tooth loss, wear, malocclusion, and disease. Advanced tooth loss or wear may be a limiting factor in the recovery from illness or be the primary reason for debility in an older animal (particularly koalas and macropods). In macropods, molar eruption and molar progression may be used to estimate age.[32] The degree of wear of the occlusal surfaces of the upper premolars in koalas is used to estimate age.[8] Uneven tooth wear and malocclusion are often seen in wombats because of their continually growing teeth. The sequence of eruption of premolars and molars and their subsequent wear have been used to determine age in several species of Didelphidae.[67]

It is important to assess for fecal output and consistency. In koalas, fecal pellet counts in the order of 90 to 200 pellets (or more) per 24 hours are expected in normal koalas, whereas counts less than 90 per 24 hours may reflect inappetence or compromised GI function.[8]

The pouch of female marsupials should be examined. Numerous superficial lymph nodes are palpable in healthy koalas. These lymph nodes should be systematically palpated to detect enlargement and asymmetry.

Clinical Pathology

Hematology and Biochemistry

The jugular and cephalic veins are suitable venipuncture sites in most marsupials. The femoral vein is suitable in most except macropods. The lateral caudal (tail) vein is suitable in macropods, possums, some gliders, bandicoots, bilbies, and opossums. Other suitable veins include the recurrent tarsal vein (lateral distal tibia) in macropods and dasyurids; small saphenous vein (runs vertically down the caudal aspect of the lower hindlimb) in koalas; radial, medial metatarsal, and caudal tibial veins in wombats; brachial vein in wombats and opossums; lateral saphenous vein in possums, gliders, bandicoots, bilbies, and opossums; ventral coccygeal vein in possums, gliders, small dasyurids, and opossums; medial metatarsal vein in dasyurids; and brachiocephalic vein in dasyurids, and numbats.[20,27,35,70]

The cytologic characteristics of the blood cells of Australian marsupials have been described.[12] Hematologic and biochemical reference ranges for selected marsupial species are presented in Tables 33-1 to 33-4. Values presented should be regarded as indicative only.

The hematologic and biochemical responses of marsupials to various physiologic and pathologic states have been poorly studied. Changes in marsupials frequently belie the severity of the underlying pathology.[70] Early PY have fetal hematologic characteristics, with up to 100% nucleated erythrocytes at 1 day of age in some species, decreasing over time. Age may also influence leukocyte concentrations. PY have leukocyte characteristics different from those of adults. This varies among species, some having immature and mature myeloid cells with occasional large lymphocytes predominating and immature and mature neutrophils predominating in others. Differential leukocyte concentrations approach that of the adult by mid-to-late pouch life.[12]

Parasitology

Examinations for endoparasites, ectoparasites, and hemoparasites are the same as in other taxa.

Urinalysis

Urine collection may be difficult in marsupials. With patience, free-flowing midstream samples may be collected from tractable animals. Urine may also be collected off the floor or by stimulating the common vestibule in PY. The bladder may be difficult to palpate in macropods, wombats, and koalas, as it often lies within the pelvis and between the epipubic bones. Urine may be collected by expressing the bladder if it is palpable or by ultrasound-guided cystocentesis. The urethral opening in female marsupials is inaccessible for catheterization. Catheterization in male marsupials should only be attempted with the animals under anesthesia. Male macropods and koalas are difficult to catheterize (see Unique Anatomy and Physiology, Urinary System). In the koala, gentle traction to straighten the penis during insertion of the catheter usually facilitates passage of the catheter. The urethral sinus is typically the more problematic area, and cautious exploratory movements of the catheter tip may be required to gain entry to the bladder. The appearance of urine varies with species; however, occasionally red urine may be produced by healthy individuals but is negative for blood. This is most likely caused by the presence of plant pigments. Urine specific gravity is also highly variable among species and may range from 1.010 to 1.045 (macropods), 1.020 to 1.035 (wombats), 1.011 to

TABLE 33-1

Hematology Reference Ranges for Selected Macropod Species and the Virginia Opossum (range or mean ± SD [n])

Parameter	Eastern Gray Kangaroo (n)[31]	Red Kangaroo (n)[31]	Matschie's Tree Kangaroo (n)[31]	Red-Necked Wallaby (n = 47)[12]	Virginia Opossum (n = 17–120)[31]
Packed cell volume, liter per liter (L/L)	0.45 ± 0.06 (52)	0.48 ± 0.07 (216)	0.45 ± 0.07 (198)	0.40–0.56	0.418 ± 0.068
Red blood cells (× 10^{12}/L)	5.8 ± 0.8 (49)	5.2 ± 0.8 (183)	5.8 ± 0.8 (150)	4.4–6.6	5.19 ± 1.73
Hemoglobin, gram per liter (g/L)	154 ± 21 (49)	171 ± 26 (195)	158 ± 23 (164)	140–197	137 ± 22
Mean corpuscular volume, femtoliters (fL)	78 ± 7 (49)	93 ± 7 (182)	79 ± 6 (148)	77–93	84.1 ± 16.9
Mean corpuscular hemoglobin, picogram (pg)	27 ± 3 (49)	33 ± 3 (176)	27 ± 3 (150)	27–33	27.4 ± 4
Mean corpuscular hemoglobin concentration (g/L)	345 ± 13 (49)	354 ± 23 (195)	349 ± 20 (162)	345–376	329 ± 24
Nucleated RBC / 100 WBC	1.0 ± 1.0 (9)	1.0 ± 2.0 (63)	5 ± 8 (52)	0.0–0.1	3 ± 3
White blood cells (× 10^9/L)	6.28 ± 3.04 (53)	4.87 ± 1.82 (208)	5.16 ± 2.74 (197)	3.50–10.50	12.30 ± 6.711
Neutrophils (× 10^9/L)	3.57 ± 2.18 (52)	2.71 ± 1.61 (187)	2.34 ± 1.62 (194)	1.10–5.00	4.142 ± 3.466
Lymphocytes (× 10^9/L)	2.49 ± 1.43 (53)	1.95 ± 1.19 (195)	2.35 ± 1.6 (195)	1.60–5.30	6.529 ± 4.349
Monocytes (×10^9/L)	0.17 ± 0.12 (50)	0.12 ± 0.11 (154)	0.21 ± 0.23 174)	0.00–0.60	0.356 ± 0.305
Eosinophils (×10^9/L)	0.13 ± 0.09 (45)	0.10 ± 0.11 (132)	0.22 ± 0.19 (169)	0.00–0.50	1.392 ± 1.279
Basophils (×10^9/L)	0.06 ± 0.01 (6)	0.03 ± 0.04 (42)	0.06 ± 0.06 (60)	0.00–0.20	0.203 ± 0.176
Platelets (×10^9/L)	186 ± 93 (28)	221 ± 108 (56)	179 ± 114 (17)	136–485	0.30 ± 0.14

For other species of macropod, see Vogelnest and Portas (2008)[68]; for other species of opossums, see Rothstein and Hunsaker (1972)[55] and Evans et al. (2010).[19]

TABLE 33-2

Hematology Reference Ranges for Selected Marsupial Species (range or mean ± SD [n])

Parameter	Koala[a] (n = 14–120)[31]	Southern Hairy-Nosed Wombat (n = 14)[31]	Tasmanian Devil (n = 1-16)[31]	Spot-Tailed Quoll (n = 1–10)[31]	Sugar Glider (n = 18)[31]
Packed cell volume (L/L)	0.359 ± 0.047	0.40 ± 0.04	0.37 ± 0.07	0.49 ± 0.05	0.34–0.50
Red blood cells (× 10^{12}/L)	3.46 ± 0.44	5.1 ± 0.6	6.25 ± 2.19	8.05 ± 0.74	6.3–9.8 (n = 17)
Hemoglobin (g/L)	114 ± 14	142 ± 14	137 ± 22	175 ± 10	122–185
Mean corpuscular volume (fL)	104.3 ± 7.4	79 ± 4	64.5 ± 15.3	61.0 ± 4.1	48–70 (n = 17)
Mean corpuscular hemoglobin (pg)	33.7 ± 2.5	27.8 ± 1.4	23.7 ± 7.0	21.8 ± 2.3	17.8–22.3 (n = 17)
Mean corpuscular hemoglobin concentration (g/L)	318 ± 23	350 ± 15	366 ± 38	358 ± 40	315–394
Nucleated RBC / 100 WBC	9 ± 10		0	1 ± 0	
White blood cells (× 10^9/L)	6.18 ± 2.483	11.4 ± 3.3	6.019 ± 2.481	4.463 ± 2.979	1.3–19.8
Neutrophils (×10^9/L)	2.869 ± 1.766	6.5 ± 2.7	3.749 ± 2.170	1.526 ± 0.577	0.18–4.4
Lymphocytes (×10^9/L)	2.890 ± 1.728	4.3 ± 2.0	2.187 ± 1.107	1.634 ± 0.946	1.12–17.8
Monocytes (×10^9/L)	0.203 ± 0.138	0.4 ± 0.4 (n = 11)	0.102 ± 0.067	0.199 ± 0.150	0.06–0.69 (n = 14)
Eosinophils (×10^9/L)	0.165 ± 0.166	0.3 ± 0.2 (n = 11)	0.163 ± 0.28	0.151 ± 0.158	0.3–0.99 (n = 13)
Basophils (×10^9/L)	0.072 ± 0.037	0.1 ± 0.02 (n = 6)	0.100 ± 0.000	0.014 ± 0.024	0–0.04 (n = 13)
Platelets (×10^9/L)	160 ± 70		226 ± 26	342 ± 69	530–860 (n = 3)

For other species see Vogelnest and Woods (2008).[70]
[a]Blanshard and Bodley (2008)[8] provide additional reference ranges for male, female, wild and captive koalas.

TABLE 33-3

Serum Biochemistry Reference Ranges for Selected Macropod Species and the Virginia Opossum (mean ± SD [n])

Parameters	Eastern Gray Kangaroo[31]	Red Kangaroo[31]	Matschie's Tree Kangaroo[31]	Red-Necked Wallaby[31]	Virginia Opossum[31]
Glucose millimole per liter (mmol/L)	5.9 ± 1.7 (52)	7.0 ± 2.1 (181)	4.9 ± 1.6 (190)	5.9 ± 2.2 (158)	5.439 ± 1.610 (94)
Urea (mmol/L)	8.6 ± 2.9 (52)	8.6 ± 2.9 (188)	8.6 ± 1.8 (191)	8.9 ± 2.5 (156)	12.14 ± 2.856 (100)
Creatinine micromole per liter (µmol/L)	133 ± 53 (52)	133 ± 44 (185)	106 ± 27 (184)	106 ± 35 (155)	53 ± 27 (92)
Uric acid (mmol/L)	0.04 ± 0.03 (8)	0.04 ± 0.04 (78)	0.03 ± 0.02 (63)	0.04 ± 0.03 (57)	0.024 ± 0.018 (23)
Calcium (mmol/L)	2.48 ± 0.23 (49)	2.65 ± 0.30 (184)	2.23 ± 0.18 (183)	2.58 ± 0.23 (155)	2.58 ± 0.25 (95)
Phosphorus (mmol/L)	2.45 ± 0.65 (44)	2.36 ± 0.71 (169)	1.97 ± 0.65 (175)	2.39 ± 0.78 (132)	2.52 ± 0.81 (84)
Sodium (mmol/L)	141 ± 4 (44)	144 ± 5 (170)	140 ± 4 (167)	141 ± 5 (136)	141 ± 5 (73)
Potassium (mmol/L)	4.2 ± 0.8 (46)	4.8 ± 1.0 (170)	4.5 ± 0.8 (166)	4.8 ± 1.2 (136)	4.2 ± 0.7 (73)
Chloride (mmol/L)	102 ± 5 (44)	98 ± 4 (137)	103 ± 4 (144)	97 ± 5 (129)	103 ± 6 (68)
Bicarbonate (mmol/L)	28.3 ± 4.5 (7)	25.5 ± 3.5 (22)	16.7 ± 3.6 (9)	22.1 ± 6.5 (26)	25.1 ± 4.7 (11)
Cholesterol (mmol/L)	2.25 ± 0.67 (35)	2.31 ± 0.67 (144)	4.17 ± 1.19 (159)	2.20 ± 0.67 (141)	3.367 ± 1.166 (85)
Triglycerides (mmol/L)	0.57 ± 0.53 (16)	0.69 ± 0.74 (94)	0.66 ± 0.42 (74)	0.75 ± 0.50 (96)	1.582 ± 1.367 (40)
Total protein gram per liter (g/L) C	60 ± 8 (45)	64 ± 10 (172)	68 ± 8 (171)	62 ± 12 (137)	60 ± 9 (95)
Albumin (g/L) C	38 ± 5 (39)	42 ± 9 (167)	47 ± 6 (161)	41 ± 8 (114)	27 ± 6 (81)
Globulin (g/L) C	23 ± 6 (39)	23 ± 11 (162)	23 ± 10 (159)	25 ± 11 (112)	33 ± 8 (80)
T. bilirubin (µmol/L)	3.0 ± 2.0 (42)	3 ± 3 (172)	3 ± 2 (164)	3 ± 5 (136)	7 ± 3 (78)
D. bilirubin (µmol/L)	3 ± 2 (21)	0 ± 2 (40)	2 ± 2 (38)	2 ± 3 (43)	2 ± 2 (21)
I. bilirubin (µmol/L)	2 ± 2 (21)	2 ± 2 (40)	2 ± 2 (37)	2 ± 2 (42)	5 ± 3 (21)
ALP unit per liter (Unit/L)	1037 ± 775 (46)	824 ± 648 (171)	897 ± 765 (175)	1186 ± 1071 (131)	513 ± 526 (81)
ALT (Unit /L)	56 ± 32 (39)	49 ± 28 (176)	7 ± 7 (157)	45 ± 26 (128)	43 ± 33 (95)
LDH (Unit /L)	95 ± 52 (17)	155 ± 127 (88)	419 ± 227 (81)	578 ± 531 (79)	181 ± 158 (35)
GGT (Unit /L)	18 ± 9 (35)	6 ± 6 (83)	68 ± 42 (104)	46 ± 30 (73)	11 ± 8 (45)
AST (Unit /L)	60 ± 25 (49)	104 ± 65 (179)	45 ± 25 (173)	88 ± 71 (136)	153 ± 90 (92)
CK (Unit /L)	747 ± 762 (28)	638 ± 569 (89)	200 ± 299 (83)	1371 ± 1819 (48)	1803 ± 1206 (46)
Amylase (Unit /L)	87 ± 51 (14)	74 ± 34 (78)	43 ± 26 (68)	68 ± 31 (75)	36.63 ± 12.58 (32)

Continued

TABLE 33-3

Serum Biochemistry Reference Ranges for Selected Macropod Species and the Virginia Opossum (mean ± SD [n])—cont'd

Parameters	Eastern Gray Kangaroo[31]	Red Kangaroo[31]	Matschie's Tree Kangaroo[31]	Red-Necked Wallaby[31]	Virginia Opossum[31]
Lipase (Unit/L)	64.0 ± 130.0 (9)	7.8 ± 11.7 (17)	25 ± 25 (14)	12.5 ± 10.8 (18)	17.51 ± 34.75 (10)
Fibrinogen (g/L)	1.3 ± 0.5 (17)	1.8 ± 1.0 (33)	1.4 ± 1.2 (23)	1.1 ± 0.8 (10)	
Thyroxine nanomole per liter (nmol/L)			12 ± 6 (6)		21 ± 10 (7)

For other species of macropod, see Vogelnest and Portas (2008);[68] for other species of opossums, see Rothstein and Hunsaker (1972)[bb] and Evans et al (2010).[19]

TABLE 33-4

Serum Biochemistry Reference Ranges for Selected Marsupial Species (range or mean ± SD [n])

Parameters	Koala (n = 12–101)[31]	Southern Hairy-Nosed Wombat (n = 14)[31]	Tasmanian Devil (n = 1–16)[31]	Spot-Tailed Quoll (n = 1–10)[31]	Kowari (n = 1–11)[31]	Sugar Glider (n = 18)[31]
Glucose millimole per liter (mmol/L)	5.72 ± 1.61	5.5 ± 1.7	6.27 ± 1.33	5.88 ± 0.94	7.99 ± 3.55	
Urea (mmol/L)	4.64 ± 1.79	10.0 ± 3.9	11.78 ± 3.57	15.35 ± 1.428	26.42 ± 8.21	1.3–6.5 (13)
Creatinine micromole per liter (μmol/L)	115 ± 27	230 ± 40 (11)	62 ± 18	88 ± 18	27 ± 18	27–106 (7)
Calcium (mmol/L)	2.63 ± 0.2	2.3 ± 0.13 (11)	2.28 ± 0.18	2.33 ± 0.28	2.05 ± 0.23	0.3–2.4 (6)
Phosphorus (mmol/L)	1.32 ± 0.39	1.36 ± 0.36 (10)	1.74 ± 0.48	2.26 ± 0.36	1.81 ± 0.42	1.62–3.29 (6)
Sodium (mmol/L)	138 ± 3	142 ± 2 (11)	148 ± 5	147 ± 2	150 ± 0	137–147 (5)
Potassium (mmol/L)	4.5 ± 0.7	4.1 ± 0.5 (11)	5.2 ± 2.1	4.4 ± 0.6	4.4 ± 0	2.7–4.4 (5)
Chloride (mmol/L)	100 ± 4	101 ± 4 (11)	116 ± 4	115 ± 3	112 ± 0	100–107 (5)
Bicarbonate (mmol/L)	20.0 ± 4.4					
Cholesterol (mmol/L)	1.943 ± 0.648	2.5 ± 0.6 (11)	3.42 ± 0.78	3.81 ± 0.8	2.02 ± 0.23	2.6–6.4 (6)
Triglycerides (mmol/L)	1.797 ± 0.588					
Total protein (g/L) C	66 ± 5		60 ± 6	64 ± 14	48 ± 7	
Total protein (g/L) R		62.0 ± 5 (13)				48–71 (12)
Albumin (g/L) C	41 ± 6	34.0 ± 3.0 (10)	33 ± 3	40 ± 2	28 ± 5	32–48 (7)
Globulin (g/L) C	25 ± 6	30.0 ± 6.0 (9)	27 ± 7	21 ± 5	18 ± 2	15–34 (6)
T. bilirubin micromole per liter (μmol/L)	3 ± 3	5.1 ± 3.4	14 ± 14	3 ± 2	10 ± 3	2–10 (12)
D. bilirubin (μmol/L)	0 ± 0		5 ± 5	7 ± 0		
I. bilirubin (μmol/L)	2 ± 2		19 ± 21	0		
Alkaline phosphatase unit per liter (U/L)	203 ± 141	266 ± 125 (10)	104 ± 66	46 ± 11	53 ± 24	148–432 (6)
Alanine aminotransferase (U/L)	11 ± 7	69 ± 32 (13)	26 ± 9	24 ± 14	123 ± 66	28–187 (13)
Lactate dehydrogenase (U/L)	271 ± 140				493 ± 207	210–274 (3)
Gamma glutamyl transpeptidase (U/L)	10 ± 5					7–15 (4)
Aspartate aminotransferase (U/L)	21 ± 10	39 ± 23	87 ± 50	150 ± 85	152 ± 96	19–275 (15)
Creatine kinase (U/L)	271 ± 246	641 ± 587 (9)	1152 ± 1210	288 ± 0	895 ± 1883	224–1463 (5)
Amylase (U/L)	7.96 ± 2.96					
Lipase (U/L)	3.89 ± 2.50					
Fibrinogen g/L	1.08 ± 0.57		0.03 ± 0.00	1.5 ± 1.0	1.0 ± 1.1	
Thyroid hormone (T4) microgram per deciliter (μg/dL)		0.49 ± 0.15 (n=4)[16]				

For other species, see Vogelnest and Woods (2008).

1.030 (brushtail possum), 1.034 to 1.040 (ringtail possum), and greater than 1.060 in koalas. Crystals may be seen in the urine of healthy animals in some species. Koala urine usually gives a false-positive reaction to ketones on reagent strips.

Cerebrospinal Fluid Tap

Cerebrospinal fluid (CSF) may be collected from the lumbar epidural space between the midlumbar to cranial lumbar vertebrae in wallabies. Cisternal CSF tap in the koala is relatively straightforward.[8]

Abdominal Paracentesis and Bone Marrow Aspiration in the Koala

Abdominal fluid is useful in the diagnosis of neoplastic and other disorders. Bone marrow aspiration is used to confirm myelodysplastic disorders and assists with disease staging and assessment of prognosis in cases of lymphoid neoplasia. The wing of the ilium is the most useful site; however, the greater tubercle of the humerus is a reasonable alternative.[8]

Imaging

Digital radiography, ultrasonography, computed tomography (CT), and magnetic resonance imaging (MRI) are all applicable in marsupial medicine. Radiographically, the entire abdomen of healthy koalas has a "ground glass" appearance and contains only scant amounts of gas, in reasonably evenly distributed small bubbles. Individual organs cannot usually be identified. This lack of contrast is caused by the absence of intraabdominal fat, and the cecum and proximal colon occupy the ventral and ventrolateral portions of the entire abdomen. Small quantities of oral barium sulfate given a few hours before abdominal radiography may be a useful marker to help assess gastric emptying and may also enhance interpretation by providing some contrast between loops of bowel.[8]

Organs of marsupials are ultrasonographically comparable with those of domestic species; however, the epipubic bones may interfere with examination of the lower genital tract. In some species, lower abdominal examination is facilitated by inserting the transducer into the pouch.

CT and MRI are particularly useful for diagnosis of craniofacial tumors and cryptococcal granulomas in koalas.[5]

DISEASES

This section will focus on important diseases of marsupials. For a more comprehensive list and further detail, readers are referred to Vogelnest and Woods (2008), Ladds (2009), and the resources of the Australian Wildlife Health Network (www.wildlifehealthaustralia.com.au) and the Australian Registry of Wildlife Health (www.arwh.org).

Infectious Diseases

Important viral, bacterial, and fungal diseases of marsupials are described in Boxes 33-4 through 33-6.

Parasitic Diseases

Free-ranging marsupials are hosts to a spectacular array of parasites, found in almost all organ systems. The majority have little or no impact on the health of the animal. Any pathology is usually an incidental finding at necropsy. In some cases, even heavy burdens of parasites appear to be well tolerated. Important diseases caused by protozoa and ectoparasites are described in Boxes 33-7 and 33-8. Many species of hematozoa and louse and some species of hippoboscid fly are found on marsupials. The helminth parasites of marsupials have been listed, described, and discussed elsewhere.[40,61,70]

Many species of nematodes may be found in the stomach of macropods. Some such as *Strongyloides* spp. may cause severe inflammation and erosive gastritis. Deaths associated with this parasite have occurred in captive macropods. *Globocephaloides* spp. occurs in the duodenum of macropods and feeds on blood, causing anemia and hypoproteinemia. Large numbers may kill captive juvenile kangaroos in situations of high population density. *Hypodontus macropi* has been associated with enteritis and death in macropods. *Marsupiostrongylus* spp. are common parasites of possums and gliders and have been associated with severe verminous pneumonia in common brushtail possums. The filarioid nematode *Pelecitus roemeri* occurs in the subcutaneous and intermuscular connective tissues of the hindlimbs, especially around the stifle joint of macropods.

Neurologic disease associated with the rat lungworm *Angiostrongylus cantonensis* has been reported in macropods, possums, a Tasmanian devil, and a bilby.[42,70] Infection follows the ingestion of third-stage larvae in several species of land mollusks (intermediate hosts), paratenic hosts, or possibly larvae in snail mucous trails. Larval stages of an ascarid nematode of pythons, *Ophidascaris robertsi*, occur commonly in the tissues and organs of dasyurids and bandicoots. Their large size (7–8 cm long) and activity may be highly debilitating, with the worms sometimes protruding through the skin.

Numerous species of capillariid nematodes belonging to the genus *Eucoleus* occur in practically all epithelial tissues of bandicoots. In some cases, these and other endoparasites may be implicated as the cause of enteritis and diarrhea. Attempts at eliminating capillariid nematodes in bandicoots using various anthelmintics are generally unrewarding. Three nematodes, *Physaloptera* (*Turgida*) *turgida*, *Cruzia americana*, and *Didelphostrongylus hayesi*, have been reported to cause significant morbidity and mortality in Virginia opossums (*Didelphis virginiana*) when present in large numbers.[51]

Common wombats infected with *Fasciola hepatica* tend to exhibit extreme (more than in most other marsupials) fibrosis of the bile ducts and liver parenchyma. Similar, but less severe, pathology is seen in small macropods and common brushtail possums. Cysts of *Echinococcus granulosus* are common in the lungs of a variety of free-ranging macropod species. Australian marsupials may serve as intermediate hosts for the cestode *Spirometra erinacei*.

Noninfectious Diseases

Possibly the most important noninfectious cause of morbidity and mortality in free-ranging marsupials is trauma. The incidence in captive animals is lower; however, macropods, because of their often flighty nature, are an exception. Obesity and associated health effects are common in captive marsupials. Other nutrition-related disorders such as metabolic bone disease are also reported. A wide range of neoplastic diseases have been reported in all marsupial orders;[34,40,70] however, the dasyurids are disproportionately overrepresented. Of special note is the Tasmanian devil facial tumor disease, which is having a significant impact on species survival. Gliders, particularly feathertail gliders, have a propensity to develop tumors in association with transponder implants. It is recommended that alternative forms of identification be used in gliders.[33] Important noninfectious diseases of significance are described in Box 33-9.

Toxicities

Important toxicities reported in marsupials include sodium monofluoroacetate (active ingredient of 1080 vertebrate poisons), bufotoxins (toxin of the cane toad, *Bufo marinus*), pindone (anticoagulant lagomorphicide), mebendazole toxicity, and tick paralysis (*I. holocyclus*).[70]

Syndromes of Uncertain Etiology

A few syndromes of uncertain etiology are described in Box 33-10.

REPRODUCTION

The typical marsupial pattern of reproduction is a brief gestation, birth of altricial young, and an extended and sophisticated lactational phase, a significant proportion of which is spent in the pouch. In all marsupials, and unlike in eutherian mammals, conception does not

Text continued on p. 272

BOX 33-4 Infectious Diseases: Viruses[40,70]

POX[3,69]/UNCHARACTERIZED GENERA, ORTHOPOXVIRUS IN COMMON RINGTAIL POSSUMS

Species	Macropods, common ringtail and common brushtail possums
Transmission	Inhalation, penetration of the skin or oral mucosa through microabrasion or arthropod vectors
Clinical signs	Solitary or multiple, variably sized, nodular exophytic lesions, typically on extremities (tail, head, and feet)
	Juveniles or subadults most commonly affected
Pathology	Epidermal hyperplasia, eosinophilic intracytoplasmic inclusions displacing the nucleus of keratinocytes
Management	Typically self-limiting, resolution in uncomplicated cases in 2–3 months, surgically debriding larger lesions may hasten resolution
	Topical or systemic antibiotic, antiseptic and anti-inflammatory therapy

MACROPODID HERPESVIRUS[3,57,72]/ALPHAHERPESVIRUS (MAHV1, 2), GAMMAHERPESVIRUS (MAHV3)

Species	Macropods
Transmission	Direct contact and possibly aerosol over short distances
Clinical signs	MaHV1,2: sudden death, depression, pyrexia, dyspnea, stridor, incoordination, cutaneous and mucosal erythema, conjunctivitis, oral, common vestibule and penile vesicles and ulceration
	MaHV3: mild disease with anogenital ulcerations only to respiratory disease, lethargy, inappetence, ataxia, death in some cases
Pathology	Pulmonary congestion and edema, conjunctivitis, mesenteric lymph node enlargement, hepatic and splenic congestion, multiple pale hepatic foci, diphtheritic plaques on mucosa of esophagus and stomach, focal ulceration and necrosis of genitalia
	Low-grade interstitial pneumonia, generalized multifocal necrosis, severe hepatitis characterized by multifocal necrosis and the presence of intranuclear acidophilic or basophilic inclusion bodies within hepatocytes
Management	Supportive care
	Isolation of positive animals

ENCEPHALOMYOCARDITIS VIRUS[47]/CARDIOVIRUS OF THE FAMILY PICORNAVIRIDAE

Species	Macropods, wombats
Transmission	Rodent reservoir
	Oral, intranasal, intratracheal, aerosol, contamination of wounds
Clinical signs	Sudden death, ataxia, depression, dyspnea, and other signs referable to cardiomyopathy
Pathology	Hepatic and pulmonary congestion, petechial pulmonary hemorrhage, pallor of cardiac muscle
	Myocardial necrosis with mononuclear cell inflammation, pulmonary and splenic congestion, depleted follicular lymphocytes in lymph nodes
Management	Rodent control, vaccination

TAMMAR SUDDEN DEATH SYNDROME[54]/EUBENANGEE SEROGROUP OF THE *ORBIVIRUS* GENUS

Species	Tammar wallabies
Transmission	Insect vectors
Clinical signs	Sudden death, lethargy, depression, ataxia, weakness, lateral recumbency, muscular fasciculations, tachypnea
Pathology	Pulmonary congestion, mottled hepatic parenchyma, hindlimb and inguinal subcutaneous edema, extensive hemorrhage in fascial planes and skeletal muscle of hind limb adductors, inguinal region, ventral thorax, dorsal cervical region, perirenal retroperitoneal area
	Marked diffuse pulmonary and hepatic congestion and lympholysis within lymphoid germinal centers
Management	Control and repel insect vectors

KOALA RETROVIRUS (KORV)[39]/TYPE C ENDOGENOUS GAMMA-RETROVIRUS (SEVERAL VARIANTS NOW IDENTIFIED)

Species	Koalas
Transmission	Vertical, possibly horizontal
Clinical signs	Asymptomatic
	Neoplasia. Signs depend on site and nature of tumor (multicentric lymphosarcoma, alimentary lymphosarcoma, primary lymphoid leukemia, miscellaneous forms)
Pathology	Neoplastic disease (aplastic anemia, myelodysplastic disorders, leukemia, lymphoma), diseases suggestive of immunodeficiency such as stomatitis, glossitis and pharyngitis, fungal dermatopathies, and some gastrointestinal disorders
Management	Supportive care, euthanasia

CHRONIC MENINGOENCEPHALITIS/WOBBLY POSSUM SYNDROME/POSSIBLE NIDOVIRUS FAMILY *ARTERIVIRIDAE*[17]

Species	Common brushtail possums
Transmission	Unknown
Clinical signs	Slowly progressive disease
	Depression, ataxia, blindness, dilated pupils (Australian form)
	Wasting, progressive neurologic signs (ataxia, docility, incoordination), death (NZ form)
Pathology	Nonsuppurative meningoencephalitis, with uvea, optic nerve, optic tract, retina, and cerebellum often involved (Australian form)
	Meningoencephalitis, mononuclear inflammation of other organs, including the liver, kidneys, spleen, lungs, bladder, heart, lymph nodes and muscle (NZ form)

BOX 33-5 Infectious Diseases: Bacteria[40,70]

MYCOBACTERIOSIS/*MYCOBACTERIUM AVIUM, M. AVIUM SUBSP. PARATUBERCULOSIS, M. INTRACELLULARE, M. ULCERANS, M. CHITAE, M. FORTUITUM, M. SMEGMATIS, M. ABSCESSUS*, VARIOUS OTHER ATYPICAL MYCOBACTERIA

Species	Macropods, koalas, dasyurids, numbats, bandicoots, possums
Transmission	Inhalation, puncture (bite) wounds, abrasions
Clinical signs	Depends on location of lesions and often only evident late in disease: weight loss, dyspnea, lameness, abscesses, neurologic signs, blindness, ulcerative to granulomatous skin lesions
Pathology	Lesions evident in a range of organs with lungs, long bones, spinal column, liver, spleen, lymph nodes, and skin most frequently involved
	Pyogranulomatous inflammation, necrosis, mineralization, acid-fast bacilli (AFB)
Management	Surgical resection of localized subcutaneous abscesses, ulcerative or granulomatous skin lesions, antituberculous drugs
	Prognosis generally poor; euthanasia is recommended

ORAL NECROBACILLOSIS (LUMPY JAW)/*FUSOBACTERIUM NECROPHORUM*, OTHER MIXED BACTERIA (MULTIFACTORIAL ETIOLOGY: ENVIRONMENTAL CONTAMINATION, ANAEROBIC CONDITIONS, IMPAIRED HOST RESISTANCE, MUCOSAL DISRUPTION, DIET, REDUCED DENTAL EXERCISE, ORAL/DENTAL TRAUMA, MOLAR PROGRESSION PREDISPOSES)

Species	Macropods (red kangaroos, red-necked wallabies, eastern gray kangaroos overrepresented)
Transmission	Affected animals may contaminate environment, food, water
Clinical signs	Mandibular or facial swelling, draining sinuses, inappetence, dysphagia, halitosis, ptyalism, ocular discharge, blepharospasm, conjunctival hyperemia, unilateral nasal discharge
	Signs of systemic illness may be apparent following hematogenous spread and will reflect location of secondary abscesses
Pathology	Periodontitis, alveolitis, osteomyelitis
	Early lesions: soft tissue cellulitis, surrounding a necrotic core
	Chronic lesions: extensive and expansive subperiosteal bone necrosis and proliferation
	A common sequela is the presence of abscesses in visceral organs
Management	Tooth extraction, surgical debridement of necrotic bone, establish drainage, copious lavage with saline and topical chlorhexidine (solution, gel or varnish)
	Initial, frequent and aggressive therapy under anesthesia improves success
	Antimicrobial therapy (clindamycin, metronidazole, oxytetracycline, penicillin) continued until after complete resolution of lesions
	Analgesia, neuroleptics
	Euthanasia of advanced cases
	Control of predisposing factors; vaccination

BORDETELLA BRONCHISEPTICA RHINITIS/PNEUMONIA

Species	Macropods, koalas, opossums
Transmission	Inhalation of aerosols, direct contact, contact with nasal secretions
Clinical signs	Serous to mucopurulent nasal discharge, intermittent sneezing, coughing, increased respiratory effort, reduced exercise tolerance, weight loss, with or without diffuse, audible crackles on thoracic auscultation
Pathology	Suppurative inflammation, marked mucosal congestion, ulceration and necrosis of the soft, cartilaginous, and bony tissues of the nasal passages and sinuses
	Peritracheal inflammation and marked pulmonary congestion and consolidation
Management	Long-term antibiotic treatment as indicated by culture and susceptibility, symptomatic therapy (nebulization with acetyl cystine ± antibiotics in saline, bromhexine hydrochloride, thermal support)
	Vaccination using commercial canine vaccines
	Isolate affected animals for treatment during outbreaks

TETANUS/*CLOSTRIDIUM TETANI*

Species	Macropods
Transmission	Spores enter body following penetrating injuries or contamination of wounds
Clinical signs	Recumbency, marked opisthotonos, muscular rigidity with clonic spasms, tetanic spasms precipitated by sensory stimulation, protrusion of nictitating membranes, ptyalism caused by inability to swallow, sudden death
Pathology	Pulmonary congestion, rupture of hindlimb musculature
Management	Treatment rarely successful
	Supportive care, tetanus antitoxin, penicillin, benzodiazepines
	Vaccination

SALMONELLOSIS/*SALMONELLA* SPP.

Species	Macropods, dasyurids, numbats, possums, bandicoots, opossums
Transmission	Asymptomatic carriers, fecal–oral route
Clinical signs	Semi-formed feces through to hemorrhagic diarrhea, colic, anorexia, dehydration, lethargy, sudden death
Pathology	Gastroenteritis, septicemia
	Hemorrhagic enteritis, extensive mucosal and submucosal necrosis
Management	Antibiotics, opioid analgesia, fluids
	Isolate affected animals during treatment

POUCH INFECTION/*PSEUDOMONAS AERUGINOSA, KLEBSIELLA* SPP., *PROTEUS* SPP., VARIOUS OTHER BACTERIA, *CANDIDA ALBICANS*

Species	Macropods, koalas
Clinical signs	Death of pouch young (PY) (in or out of the pouch), moist dirty fur around pouch opening, greasy pouch, pouch discharge, odor
Pathology	Mild dermatitis to pyoderma with pustules, ulceration, and exudate
Management	Lavage pouch with antimicrobial solution, topical antimicrobial cream or ointment, systemic antibiotics in severe cases

CHLAMYDIOSIS[39]/*CHLAMYDIA PNEUMONIA, C. PECORUM*

Species	Koalas
Transmission	Contact, aerosol, venereal

Continued

BOX 33-5 Infectious Diseases: Bacteria—cont'd

Clinical signs	Asymptomatic
	Unilateral or bilateral acute to chronic keratoconjunctivitis
	Brown stained wet fur around common vestibule and rump, dysuria, tenesmus, hematuria, urine scalding
	Debilitation, infertility
Pathology	Keratoconjuctivitis
	Urethritis, cystitis, ureteritis, hydroureter, hydronephrosis, pyogranulomatous chronic interstitial nephritis, chronic urogenital sinusitis
	Unilateral or bilateral inflammation and fibrosis of various parts of the reproductive tract, cystic enlargement of the ovarian bursa
Management	Systemic antichlamydial antimicrobials (enrofloxacin, chloramphenicol), with or without topical for ocular disease (with or without corticosteroids)
	Conjunctival ablation (in severe chronic keratoconjunctivitis)
	Analgesic and anti-inflammatory drugs, supportive care (fluids, supplement feeding), cleaning eyes and perineal soiling

YERSINIOSIS/*YERSINIA PSEUDOTUBERCULOSIS*

Species	Macropods, possums, gliders
Transmission	Wild birds and rodents are likely sources
	Ingestion of contaminated food or water
Clinical signs	Acute: diarrhea (melena), dehydration, depression, septicemia, death
	Chronic: wasting, multisystemic abscessation

Pathology	Enteritis and septicemia, or subacute to chronic multisystemic abscessation
	Necrotic foci in the intestine, liver, spleen, kidneys, lungs, and mesenteric lymph nodes
Management	Poor prognosis
	Pest prevention; improved hygiene and husbandry

PASTEURELLOSIS[6]/*PASTEURELLA MULTOCIDA*

Species	Macropods, possums, gliders, opossums
Transmission	Normal upper respiratory and oral bacterial fauna
	Bites or scratches from animals carrying the bacteria
Clinical signs	Purulent to necrotizing gingivitis, mandibular osteomyelitis, and conjunctivitis (macropods), purulent otitis, abscesses, lethargy, lameness, neurologic signs (head tilt, ataxia)
Pathology	Otitis media or interna, meningitis, meningoencephalitis, abscessation, lymphadenomegaly, pulmonary edema, bronchopneumonia, fibrinous pleuropneumonia, hepatic and splenic congestion, ascites, gastrointestinal hemorrhage
Management	Treatment is generally unrewarding
	Early and aggressive antibiotic therapy may be successful in preventing abscessation and septicemia in bitten possums

Other important bacterial diseases reported in marsupials: tuberculosis (*M. bovis*) in common brushtail possums in New Zealand, erysipelas, mellioidosis, leptospirosis, Tyzzer's disease (*Clostridium piliforme*), botulism, enterotoxaemia (*Clostridium perfringens*), nocardiosis, infectious dermatitis in Virginia opossums (cause of "Crispy ear").

BOX 33-6 Infectious Diseases: Fungi[40,70]

CANDIDIASIS/*CANDIDA ALBICANS*, OTHER *CANDIDA* SPP.

Species	Macropods, koalas, possums, gliders; common in hand-reared pouch young (PY) and animals on antibiotics
Transmission	Normal flora
Clinical signs	Cutaneous: erythema, crusting, fissures, plaques, characteristic sweet odor
	Gastrointestinal: oral plaques ± shallow ulceration, ptyalism, crusting lesions around lips, yellow diarrhea with characteristic sweet odor, oral discomfort resulting in rejection of teat, inappetence, anorexia, weight loss, failure to thrive
Pathology	Affects the superficial layers of squamous epithelium (oral mucosa, esophagus, nonglandular stomach, common vestibule)
	White plaques throughout the tract and ulceration of the gastric mucosa
	Blastospores and mycelia evident, invading stratified squamous epithelium; inflammation associated with mycelial invasion of the deeper epithelial layers

Management	Cutaneous: topical nystatin, miconazole, or terbinafine
	Gastrointestinal: nystatin, itraconazole systemically
	Improve husbandry and hygiene; prophylactic antifungal agent when on antibiotics; probiotics after antibiotics to re-establish microbial flora

DERMATOPHYTOSES/*TRICHOPHYTON MENTAGROPHYTES, T. VERRUCOSUM, MICROSPORUM GYPSEUM, M. CANIS*

Species	Macropods,[10] koalas, possums, bilbies, Virginia opossum
Transmission	Direct or indirect contact, environmental contamination
Clinical signs	Focal, multifocal or extensive nonpruritic alopecia; crusting and scaling; lichenification; erythematous margins to lesions; broken hair shafts; paronychia and nail deformity
	Lesions usually on head, pinnae, tail, extremities but may occur anywhere on the body
Pathology	Folliculitis and hyperkeratosis; hyphae and spores
Management	Itraconazole, griseofulvin or terbinafine ± topical miconazole, enilconazole or terbinafine until 2 weeks after resolution of lesions
	Lesions may be self-limiting

BOX 33-6 Infectious Diseases: Fungi—cont'd

CRYPTOCOCCOSIS/*CRYPTOCOCCUS GATTI, C. NEOFORMANS VAR. GRUBII*

Species	Macropods, koalas, dasyurids, numbats, possums, gliders, bandicoots, bilbies
Transmission	Inhalation of airborne cryptococcal organisms from environmental sources (for *C. gatti*, various *Eucalyptus* species)
Clinical signs	Subclinical
	Signs depend on site of lesions
	Respiratory: sneezing, coughing, nasal discharge, epistaxis, dyspnea, facial distortion, stertor or stridor, weight loss, inappetence, occasionally sudden death
	Neurologic: blindness, nystagmus, whole-body tilt, seizures
	Cutaneous: subcutaneous cervical nodules, dry, scab-covered skin on lateral aspects of hindlimbs (koalas)

Pathology	Localized nasal cavity or sinus granulomas; localized skin nodules containing tenacious yellow-green exudate; granulomatous meningitis and encephalitis, optic neuritis; pneumonia with small, multifocal, gray-to-yellow, nodular lesions throughout pulmonary parenchyma, diffuse alveolar distension with large numbers of spherical basophilic yeasts, focal pulmonary hemorrhage, congestion, atelectasis, fibrinous exudation; pleuritis; pericarditis; peritonitis; disseminated form involving multiple organs and lymph nodes
	Granulomas are pale with firm nodules, or pale with gelatinous foci
Management	Antifungal therapy (itraconazole, fluconazole, amphotericin B) until latex cryptococcal antigen test (LCAT) is negative
	Surgical debulking of lesions[5,74]

BOX 33-7 Parasitic Diseases: Protozoa[40,70]

COCCIDIOSIS/VARIOUS *EIMERIA* SPP. AND *ISOSPORA* SPP.

Species	Macropods (juvenile, hand-reared eastern gray kangaroos particularly susceptible), wombats (disease uncommon), bandicoots, opossums
Transmission	Ingestion, heavy environmental load
Clinical signs	Clinical disease usually limited to juvenile animals less than 12 months of age
	Inappetence, abdominal discomfort, lethargy, diarrhea (often hemorrhagic), dehydration, dependent edema, bruxism, common vestibule prolapse
	Sudden death
Pathology	Hemorrhagic enteritis, villous atrophy, mucosal ulceration, epithelial sloughing, congestion, edema and presence of giant schizonts in the upper small intestine
	Biliary duct hyperplasia and fibrosis and granulomatous lesions in the hepatic portal triads seen with hepatic coccidiosis
Management	Treatment should be initiated on early suspicion of disease
	Toltrazuril, antibiotics for secondary bacterial infection, fluids (orally [PO] or subcutaneously [SC] preferred), homologous plasma transfusions, analgesia

TOXOPLASMOSIS/*TOXOPLASMA GONDII*

Species	Macropods, koalas, wombats, dasyurids, possums, gliders, bandicoots, bilbies, opossums
Transmission	Ingestion of sporulated oocysts in feed contaminated with felid feces or in paratenic hosts
	Disease may result from primary infection following the ingestion of oocysts or recrudescence of latent disease following a period of immune compromise

Clinical signs	Variable and consistent multisystemic disease
	Dyspnea, tachypnea, coughing, malaise, uncharacteristic docility, weight loss, anorexia, lymphadenopathy, diarrhea, blindness, ataxia, circling, incoordination, dysphagia, pyrexia, keratitis, uveitis, chorioretinitis, endophthalmitis, unilateral or bilateral cataracts
	Acute to peracute illness and death
Pathology	An extensive range of lesions affecting various and multiple organs
	Gross lesions may not be evident but may include pulmonary congestion, edema and consolidation, pleural effusion, myocardial hemorrhage and pale streaks, lymph node and adrenal gland enlargement and inflammation, adrenal hemorrhage, splenomegaly, hemorrhagic and ulcerative foci within the stomach and small intestine, brain malacia
	Focal to extensive necrosis, inflammation, hemorrhage, edema in multiple tissues
	Free and intracellular tachyzoites in multiple tissues
Management	Treatment often unrewarding
	Atovaquone, clindamycin, sulfadiazine and pyrimethamine (with folinic acid), trimethoprim-sulfonamide for up to 30 days
	Supportive care
	Exclude cats from feed sheds and enclosures

BABESIOSIS/*BABESIA* SPP.[13,53]

Species	Macropods (eastern gray kangaroos, red-necked wallabies, swamp wallabies), dasyurids (recrudescence thought to contribute to post-mating male mortality in male agile antechinus),[12] bandicoots
Transmission	Arthropod vectors, mainly ticks

Continued

BOX 33-7 Parasitic Diseases: Protozoa—cont'd

Clinical signs	Typically hand-reared eastern gray kangaroo pouch young (PY) between 6 and 13 months of age, failure to thrive, poor body condition, dehydration, pale mucous membranes, polydipsia, polyuria, inappetence, bruxism, lethargy, obtundation, vision deficits (mydriasis, reduced pupillary light reflex [PLR], variable menace response, blindness), conjunctival and scleral hemorrhage, ataxia, seizures, recumbency Regenerative anemia (packed cell volume [PCV] <30%), hypoproteinemia (total plasma protein [TPP] <30 grams per liter [g/L])	Pathology	Parasitized erythrocytes sequestered in a range of organs, schizont-like forms in blood vessels (particularly brain and kidney), increased pigment in Kupfer cells, bone marrow and lymphoid hyperplasia, pulmonary edema and congestion, myocardial degeneration and necrosis, nonsuppurative perivascular myocarditis, nonsuppurative panuveitis or iridocyclitis, lymphocytolysis
		Management	Supportive care, blood transfusions, imidocarb intravenously (IV), phytomenadione may be beneficial. Tick and other vector control

Other important protozoa reported in marsupials: *Besnoitia* spp. in macropods and opossums,[3] *Trypanosoma* spp. in macropods, koalas, wombats, bandicoots, dasyurids, opossums,[45,61] amoebiasis (*Entamoeba histolytica*, other *Entamoeba* spp. in macropods, *Leishmania braziliensis* in didelphid opossums.[20]

BOX 33-8 Parasitic Diseases: Ectoparasites[40,70]

SARCOPTIC MANGE/*SARCOPTES SCABEI* VAR. *CANIS*, *S. SCABEI* VAR. *WOMBATI*

Species	Macropods, koalas, wombats (significant debilitating disease of wild common wombats), possums
Clinical signs	Mild, localized, crusting lesions to a generalized, severe crusting hyperkeratotic dermatosis with alopecia, excoriations, deep fissures, secondary pyoderma, pruritus Mild to severe debility In wombats, severe skin lesions impair vision and movement; affected animals often emaciated
Management	Ivermectin, moxidectin, selamectin Euthanasia in severe cases

FLEAS/*ECHIDNOPHAGA* SPP. ("STICK FAST" FLEAS), *LYCOPSYLLA* SPP. (WOMBAT FLEAS), 32 SPECIES IN DASYURIDS, MANY OTHER SPECIES

Species	Koalas, wombats, dasyurids, numbats, possums, bandicoots, opossums
Clinical signs	Asymptomatic Pruritus, pustules, alopecia, presence of fleas and flea feces in the coat Anemia with heavy infestations In Tasmanian devils and quolls *Uropsylla tasmanica* larvae burrow into the skin

Management	Fipronil, permethrin, ivermectin, selamectin, imidacloprid, lufenuron

TICKS/PARALYSIS TICK (*IXODES HOLOCYCLUS*), MANY OTHER SPECIES

Species	Macropods, koalas, wombats, dasyurids, numbats, possums, bandicoots (principal host for *I. holocyclus*)
Clinical signs	Asymptomatic Heavy burdens may result in anemia Naïve animals infested with *I. holocyclus* may develop ascending flaccid paralysis progressing to recumbency, eventual respiratory failure Localized paralysis near the site of tick attachment
Management	Removal of ticks Supportive care and administration of hyperimmune canine serum for tick paralysis Acaricidal preparations (fipronil, selamectin) Iron supplementation for anemia

Other important ectoparasites reported in marsupials: demodectic mange in koalas and dasyurids, *Thadeua serrata* in wallabies, fur mites (*Koalachirus perkinsi*) in koalas, *Trichosurolaelaps crassipes* in common brushtail possums.

BOX 33-9 Noninfectious Diseases[40,70]

TASMANIAN DEVIL FACIAL TUMOR DISEASE

Species	Tasmanian Devil
Transmission	Biting Transmitted by allograft Lack of genetic diversity at the major histocompatibility complex (MHC) allows tumor cells to grow in genetically similar hosts without evoking an immune response to alloantigens

Clinical signs	Ulcerating solid soft tissue masses, first appearing on head and neck regions and mouth Affected Devils die of starvation, secondary infection in the tumor and metastases within 6–12 months Mortality is 100% Tumors rarely seen in Devils less than 2 years of age

BOX 33-9 Noninfectious Diseases—cont'd

Pathology	Cut surface firm, pale, slightly translucent, fibrous septa, often with necrotic core
	Subepithelial expansile masses of round cells, abundant eosinophilic cytoplasm, high nuclear to cytoplasmic ratio encased in a pseudocapsule
	Mitotic figures 0–12, average 4 per high-power field (hpf)
	Tumor cells Schwann cell origin
	Locally aggressive, metastasize to lymph nodes, other organs
Management	No surgical or medical cure has been effective
	Tumor-free insurance populations have been established

CAPTURE MYOPATHY

Species	Macropods
Pathogenesis	Exertion, fear, anxiety with or without high ambient temperatures result in prolonged sympathetic nervous system stimulation causing ischemia caused by reduced tissue perfusion, lactic acidosis, and muscular adenosine triphosphate reserve depletion
	Cardiovascular and circulatory collapse, muscular compartment syndrome, acute renal failure from ischemia, and myoglobinuric nephrosis
Clinical signs	Dyspnea, tachypnea, tachycardia, hyperthermia, muscular tremors and fasciculations, myoglobinuria, inability to hold head in normal elevated position, stiff gait, weakness, recumbency
	Death within days to weeks after an event
	Creatine kinase (CK) ≥25,000 international units per liter (IU/L)
Pathology	Acute: muscular hemorrhage, congestion and edema, pale and friable musculature, myofiber degeneration, hemorrhage and edema of the interstitium
	Chronic: pale, fibrosed muscle, foci of mineralization, interstitial fibrosis

	Hindlimb adductors, psoas, cervical, dorsal musculature most commonly affected
	Also diaphragm and cardiac musculature
	Swollen kidneys, pulmonary congestion, and edema
	Renal tubular necrosis, pulmonary edema, hepatic and adrenal cortex necrosis
Management	Carefully planned and executed capture and restraint, minimize anxiety, judicious use of anxiolytic and neuroleptic drugs
	Intravenous fluids, sodium bicarbonate, dandrolene sodium, corticosteroids or nonsteroidal anti-inflammatory drugs, lower body temperature

NEPHROPATHY/OXALATE NEPHROSIS[8,60]

Species	Koalas
Pathogenesis	Dehydration, oxalate and calcium, aluminum
	Pathogenesis not fully understood
Clinical signs	Anorexia, rapid weight loss, lethargy, obtundation, dehydration, polydipsia, polyuria, small, dry fecal pellets, emaciation, collapse (prostrate, comatose, hypothermic, bradycardic)
	Azotemia
Pathology	Depends on cause and chronicity of disease
	Oxalate nephrosis: normal to reddened cortical areas with pale corticomedullary streaks, tubule loss, segmental cortical fibrosis, tubule dilation, glomerular atrophy, crystal-associated inflammation
	Typical birefringent calcium oxalate crystal morphology
	Aluminum associated nephropathy: positive staining for aluminum
Management	Poor prognosis
	Aggressive fluid therapy, nutritional supplementation, anabolic steroids

Other important noninfectious diseases of marsupials: hip and shoulder dysplasia in koalas, thermal burns, dental disease and malocclusion in wombats, periodontal disease in possums, gliders, bilbies, and opossums.

BOX 33-10 Syndromes of Uncertain Etiology[40,70]

EXUDATIVE DERMATITIS

Species	Brushtail possums
Pathogenesis	Multifactorial: hypersensitivity to ectoparasites (mites, fleas), bacterial and fungal infection, stress, trauma
Clinical signs	Alopecia, exudation, crusting, ulceration in the lumbosacral region, tail, face, trunk or limbs
	Debility
Pathology	Ulcerative dermatitis, dermal edema, mixed inflammatory infiltrate (eosinophils, mast cells, lymphocytes, neutrophils), epidermal hyperplasia, hyperkeratosis, adnexal gland hyperplasia, bacteria
Management	Acaricides, topical and systemic antibacterials, analgesia
	In severe cases, aggressive initial treatment under anesthesia may be required
	Euthanasia is indicated in severe cases where confounding social factors cannot be addressed

SWOLLEN PAW SYNDROME

Species	Common ringtail possums
Pathogenesis	Unknown; photosensitization, bacterial or viral infection, thermal injury, electrocution, mycotoxicosis, plant toxins
Clinical signs	Edema, ulceration, swelling, gangrene of feet, tenosynovitis, moist ulcerative dermatitis of dorsal nose, moist dermatitis or alopecia, thickening, contraction and necrosis of ear tips, crusting or ulceration of tail tip
	One or more feet missing
Pathology	Avascular necrosis resulting in severe, acute necrosis of extremities, coagulation necrosis, epidermal ulceration, dermal edema
Management	Treatment is usually unsuccessful and prognosis for release is poor
	Euthanasia is usually indicated

Continued

BOX 33-10   **Syndromes of Uncertain Etiology—cont'd**

CECAL STASIS

Species	Common ringtail possums (smallest arboreal folivore with strong preference for eucalypt foliage, will also eat foliage, flowers and fruit from other species of trees and shrubs; unique adaptations to dealing with a primarily folivorous diet, the most important being cecotrophy)		Dysbiosis, altered cecal and colonic development and function, hygiene, husbandry, stress, carer expertise may play a role
Pathogenesis	Unknown	Clinical signs	Distended abdomen, spongy rather than gas filled
	More commonly seen in young hand-reared animals at time of weaning onto solid diet		Muscle wastage; normal, increased, or reduced appetite; acute abdominal pain; restlessness; reduced fecal output; death
	Weaning onto inappropriate diet (high-carbohydrate, fruit-based diets) may play a role	Pathology	Cecum distended with fluid, loss of normal sacculated structure
		Management	Correct diet (native browse, flowers, some vegetable, minimal fruit), metoclopramide, supportive care

TABLE 33-5

Contraceptive Methods including Effects on Behavior in Marsupials[70]

Contraceptive method	Marsupial group	Comments
Gonadectomy, tubal ligation, vasectomy	Most	Castration not usually successful in controlling aggression particularly in hand-reared macropods In macropods, tubal ligation and vasectomy may result in increased aggression between males, as females cycle continually
Progestin implants	Macropods, koalas	Norplant II/Jadelle (levonorgestrel, Bayer Health Care): safe, effective, long term, reversible (reversibility not demonstrated in koalas)
Gonadotropin-releasing hormone (GnRH) agonists Suprelorin (deslorelin, Peptech Animal Health)	Macropods, koalas, possums	Safe, effective, long term, reversible in female macropods with minimal effect on behavior Stage of reproductive cycle, presence or absence of blastocyst, presence or absence of pouch young (PY), removal of PY at time of implanting, occurrence of a postpartum estrus, seasonality of species, and dose of deslorelin influence effectiveness and duration Best results achieved if treatment timed to coincide with anestrus No effect on fertility or behavior in male macropods Effective contraception in female koalas and common brushtail possums, no effect on fertility in males
Immunocontraceptives	Macropods	GnRH vaccines: ineffective in female macropods, effective modification of male sexual behavior and aggression PZP immunization: effective in wallabies
Management techniques	Most	Separation of sexes; removal and euthanasia of early PY (not suitable for long-term population management in macropods as removal of PY will result in recrudescence of a blastocyst in diapause, subsequent birth and postpartum estrus in most species)

interrupt the estrous cycle, but lactation does. Marsupials display five basic reproductive strategies:[66]

1. Possums, the mountain pygmy possum (*Burramys parvus*), gliders, dasyurids, and opossums are polyovular and polyestrous, with a gestation period shorter than the estrous cycle. Postpartum estrus and ovulation are suppressed during lactation.
2. Bandicoots and bilbies are polyestrous and polyovular, with an ultra-short gestation period.
3. Macropods are monovular and polyestrous, with a gestation period of similar length to the estrous cycle. Postpartum estrus and ovulation occur. During lactation, if fertilization has occurred, the embryo remains as a blastocyst in embryonic diapause—except in the western gray kangaroo (*M. fuliginosus*), Lumholtz's tree-kangaroo (*Dendrolagus lumholtzi*), and musky rat-kangaroo (*Hypsiprymnodon moschatus*). This is maintained by the sucking stimulus of the PY. In the eastern gray kangaroo (*M. giganteus*), parma (*M. parma*), and whiptail wallaby (*M. parryi*), postpartum

estrus does not occur, but the females may come into estrus and mate when the PY is older.
4. The honey possum and pygmy possums (except the mountain pygmy possum) are polyestrous and polyovular, with a prolonged gestation and embryonic diapause.
5. The koala and wombat are polyestrous and monovular, with a gestation period shorter than the estrous cycle. In the koala, ovulation is induced by copulation.

Reproductive Management

Reproductive Control (Contraception)
Some marsupial species breed well in captivity and in the wild, and populations may quickly reach high densities. It is, therefore, important that these populations are managed carefully to prevent overcrowding, stress, disease, production of surplus animals, inbreeding, degradation of habitat, and starvation.[1] Contraceptive methods including effects on behavior are described in Table 33-5.

Enhancing Reproduction

Semen collection and cryopreservation, induced superovulation, artificial insemination, oocyte and embryo harvesting, and in vitro fertilization have been carried out in various marsupial species, with variable success.[36,70] Perhaps the greatest success has been in koalas.[2] Cross-fostering has been successful in macropods. The benefit of this procedure in marsupials is that it has the potential to dramatically increase the reproductive rate.[68]

PREVENTIVE MEDICINE

A range of vaccines have been used in macropods and include a multi-serotype vaccine against *Dichelobacter nodosus* for oral necrobacillosis (lumpy jaw), a canine vaccine against *B. bronchiseptica*, an inactivated encephalomyocarditis virus vaccine, and either human or equine tetanus toxoid or a multivalent clostridial vaccine for tetanus prophylaxis.[68] Responses are variable, and sterile abscesses and swellings frequently develop at injection sites with some vaccines. Vaccination of koalas against *B. bronchiseptica* using a canine vaccine appears to reduce the incidence of mortality from infection with *Bordetella* spp.[8] In rabies-endemic countries where the incidence of rabies is high, marsupials in zoos may be at high risk of exposure. In such cases, vaccination is recommended; however, the efficacy of rabies vaccination in marsupials has not been established.

Routine screening for endoparasites is recommended for individuals or groups at least annually or biannually. If parasite burdens are high, particularly if animals are clinically affected, routine anthelmintic treatment is recommended. This should be coupled with improved husbandry, sanitation, substrate changes, and reduction in stocking densities. If ectoparasitism is a problem, routine treatment is recommended. A regular program of weighing and body condition scoring is recommended for some species (e.g., koalas) or individuals. Annual or biennial health checks may be warranted in some species.

ACKNOWLEDGMENT

The author would like to thank Joe Smith, Simone Vitali, Karrie Rose, and Sally Colgan, for information provided, and Kimberly Vinette Herrin, for reviewing the manuscript.

REFERENCES

1. Adderton Herbert C: Long-acting contraceptives: A new tool to manage overabundant kangaroo populations in nature reserves and urban areas. *Aust Mammal* 26:67–74, 2004.
2. Allen CD, Burridge M, Mulhall S, et al: Successful artificial insemination in the koala (*Phascolarctos cinereus*) using extended and extended-chilled semen collected by electroejaculation. *Biol Reprod* 78:661–666, 2008.
3. Australian Wildlife Health Network (AWHN) fact sheets: www.wildlifehealthaustralia.com.au. Accessed 21 December 2013.
4. Barboza PS, Hume ID, Nolan JV: Nitrogen metabolism and requirements of nitrogen and energy in the wombats. *Physiol Zool* 66:807–828, 1993.
5. Bercier M, Wynne J, Klause S, et al: Nasal mass removal in the koala (*Phascolarctos cinereus*). *J Zoo Wildl Med* 43:898–908, 2012.
6. Bertelsen MF, Bojesen AM, Bisgaard M, et al: *Pasteurella multocida* carriage in red-necked wallabies (*Macropus rufogriseus*). *J Zoo Wildl Med* 43:726–729, 2012.
7. Black LA, McLachlan AJ, Griffith JE, et al: Pharmacokinetics of chloramphenicol following administration of intravenous and subcutaneous chloramphenicol sodium succinate, and subcutaneous chloramphenicol, to koalas (*Phascolarctos cinereus*). *J Vet Pharmacol Ther* 36:478–485, 2013.
8. Blanshard WH, Bodley KB: Koalas. In Vogelnest L, Woods W, editors: *Medicine of Australian mammals*, Melbourne, Australia, 2008, CSIRO Publishing.
9. Booth R: Macropods. In Gage LJ, editor: *Hand-rearing wild and domestic mammals*, Ames, IA, 2002, Iowa State Press.
10. Boulton KA, Vogelnest LJ, Vogelnest L: Dermatophytosis in zoo macropods: A questionnaire study. *J Zoo Wildl Med* 44:555–563, 2013.
11. Bryant BR, Reiss A: Wombats. In Vogelnest L, Woods W, editors: *Medicine of Australian mammals*, Melbourne, Australia, 2008, CSIRO Publishing.
12. Clark P: *Haematology of Australian mammals*, Melbourne, Australia, 2004, CSIRO Publishing.
13. Dawood KE, Morgan JAT, Busfield F, et al: Observation of a novel *Babesia* spp. in eastern grey kangaroos (*Macropus giganteus*) in Australia. *Int J Parasitol* 2:54–61, 2013.
14. Dawson TJ: *Kangaroos: The biology of the largest marsupials*, Sydney, Australia, 1995, University of New South Wales Press.
15. de Kauwe T, Black LA, Kimble B, et al: Analgesic drug regimens used for captive koalas in Australia and their perceived efficacy. *Aust Vet J* 2013. in press.
16. Death CE, Taggart DA, Williams DB, et al: Pharmacokinetics of moxidectin in the southern hairy-nosed wombat (*Lasiorhinus latifrons*). *J Wildl Dis* 47:643–649, 2011.
17. Dunowska M, Biggs PJ, Zheng T, et al: Identification of a novel nidovirus associated with a neurological disease of the Australian brushtail possum (*Trichosurus vulpecula*). *Vet Microbiol* 156:418–424, 2012.
18. Eason CT, Wright GRG, Gooneratne R: Pharmacokinetics of antipyrine, warfarin and paracetamol in the brushtail possum. *J Appl Toxicol* 19:157–161, 1999.
19. Evans KD, Hewett TA, Clayton CJ, et al: Normal organ weights, serum chemistry, hematology, and cecal and nasopharyngeal bacterial cultures in the Gray Short-Tailed Opossum (*Monodelphis domestica*). *J Am Assoc Lab Anim Sci* 49:401–406, 2010.
20. Fowler ME: Order Marsupialia (Opossums). In Fowler ME, Cubas ZS, editors: *Biology, medicine and surgery of South American Wild Animals*, Ames, IA, 2001, Iowa State University Press.
21. Geiser F: Hibernation and daily torpor in marsupials: A review. *Aust J Zool* 42:1–16, 1994.
22. Geiser F: Thermal biology and energetics of carnivorous marsupials. In Jones M, Dickman C, Archer M, editors: *Predators with pouches: The biology of carnivorous marsupials*, Melbourne, Australia, 2003, CSIRO Publishing.
23. Govendir M, Hanger J, Loader JJ, et al: Plasma concentrations of chloramphenicol after subcutaneous administration to koalas (*Phascolarctos cinereus*) with chlamydiosis. *J Vet Pharmacol Ther* 35:147–154, 2012.
24. Griffith JE, Higgins DP, Li KM, et al: Absorption of enrofloxacin and marbofloxacin after oral and subcutaneous administration in diseased koalas (*Phascolarctos cinereus*). *J Vet Pharmacol Ther* 33:595–604, 2010.
25. Hanger JJ, Heath TJ: Topography of the major superficial lymph nodes and their efferent lymph pathways in the koala (*Phascolarctos cinereus*). *J Anat* 177:67–73, 1991.
26. Hirst LW, Brown AS, Kempster R, et al: Ophthalmologic examination of the normal eye of the koala. *J Wildl Dis* 28:419–423, 1992.
27. Holz P: Marsupials. In West G, Heard D, Caulkett N, editors: *Zoo animal and wildlife immobilization and anesthesia*, Ames, IA, 2007, Blackwell Publishing.
28. Holz PH: Dasyurids. In Vogelnest L, Woods W, editors: *Medicine of Australian mammals*, Melbourne, 2008, CSIRO Publishing.
29. Hume ID, Barboza PS: Designing artificial diets for captive marsupials. In Fowler ME, editor: *Zoo and wild animal medicine*, Philadelphia, PA, 1993, Saunders.
30. Hume ID: *Marsupial nutrition*, Cambridge, U.K., 1999, Cambridge University Press.
31. *ISIS Reference ranges for physiological values in captive wildlife*, Eagan, Minnesota, USA, 2002, International Species Information System.
32. Jackson S: *Australian mammals: Biology and captive management*, Melbourne, Australia, 2003, CSIRO Publishing.
33. Johnson R, Hemsley S: Possums and gliders. In Vogelnest L, Woods W, editors: *Medicine of Australian mammals*, Melbourne, Australia, 2008, CSIRO Publishing.
34. Johnson-Delaney CA: Practical marsupial medicine. In *Proceedings of the Association of Avian Veterinarians*, 2006, pp 51–60.
35. Johnson-Delaney CA: What every veterinarian needs to know about Virginia opossums. *Exotic DVM* 6(6):38–43, 2005.

36. Keeley T, McGreevy PD, O'Brien JK: Characterization and short-term storage of Tasmanian devil sperm collected post-mortem. *Theriogenology* 76:705–714, 2011.

37. Kimble B, Black LA, Li MK, et al: Pharmacokinetics of meloxicam in koalas (*Phascolarctos cinereus*) after intravenous, subcutaneous and oral administration. *J Vet Pharmac Ther* 36:486–493, 2013.

38. Kirkwood JK, Gulland FMD, Needham JR, et al: Pharmacokinetics of oxytetracycline in clinical cases in the red-necked wallaby (*Macropus rufogriseus*). *Res Vet Sci* 44:335–337, 1988.

39. Krockenberger MB, Higgins DP: Koala Disease. In *Proceedings of the Wildlife Pathology Short Course*, 2012, Australian Registry of Wildlife Health. <www.arwh.org>.

40. Ladds P: *Pathology of Australian native wildlife*, Melbourne, Australia, 2009, CSIRO Publishing.

41. Lynch MJ: Bandicoots and bilbies. In Vogelnest L, Woods W, editors: *Medicine of Australian mammals*, Melbourne, Australia, 2008, CSIRO Publishing.

42. Ma G, Dennis M, Rose K, et al: Tawny frogmouths and brushtail possums as sentinels for *Angiostrongylus cantonensis,* the rat lungworm. *Vet Parasitol* 192:158–165, 2013.

43. McCracken H: Veterinary aspects of hand-rearing orphaned marsupials. In Vogelnest L, Woods W, editors: *Medicine of Australian mammals*, Melbourne, Australia, 2008, CSIRO Publishing.

44. McDowell A, McLeod BJ: Physiology and pharmacology of the brushtail possum gastrointestinal tract: Relationship to the human gastrointestinal tract. *Adv Drug Deliv* 59:1121–1132, 2007.

45. McInnes LM, Gillet A, Ryan UM, et al: *Trypanosoma irwini* n. sp. (Sarcomastigophora: Trypanosomatidae) from the koala (*Phascolarctos cinereus*). *Parasitology* 136:875–885, 2009.

46. McLelland DJ, Barker IK, Crawshaw G, et al: Single-dose pharmacokinetics of oxytetracycline and penicillin G in tammar wallabies (*Macropus eugenii*). *J Vet Pharmacol Ther* 34:160–167, 2011.

47. McLelland DJ, Kirkland PD, Rose KA, et al: Serologic responses of Barbary sheep (*Ammotragus lervia*), Indian antelope (*Antilope cervicapra*), wallaroos (*Macropus robustus*) and chimpanzees (*Pan troglodytes*) to an inactivated encephalomyocarditis virus vaccine. *J Zoo Wildl Med* 36:69–73, 2005.

48. McLelland DJ, Rich BG, Holz PH: The pharmacokinetics of single dose intramuscular amoxicillin trihydrate in tammar wallabies (*Macropus eugenii).* *J Zoo Wildl Med* 40:113–116, 2009.

49. Messer M, Crisp EA, Czolij R: Lactose digestion in suckling macropodids. In Grigg G, Jarman P, Hume I, editors: *Kangaroos, wallabies and rat-kangaroos*, Sydney, Australia, 1989, Surrey Beatty & Sons.

50. Morges MA, Grant KR, MacPhail CM, et al: A novel technique for orchiectomy and scrotal ablation in the Sugar glider (*Petaurus breviceps*). *J Zoo Wildl Med* 40:204–206, 2009.

51. Nichelason AE, Rejmanek D, Dabritz HA, et al: Evaluation of *Cruzia americana, Turgida turgida,* and *Didelphostrongylus hayesi* infection in the Virginia opossum (*Didelphis virginiana*) and risk factors along the California coast. *J Parasitol* 94:1166–1168, 2008.

52. Old JM, Deane EM: Development of the immune system and immunological protection in marsupial pouch young. *Dev Comp Immunol* 24:445–454, 2000.

53. Paparini A, Ryan UM, Warren K, et al: Identification of novel Babesia and Theileria genotypes in the endangered marsupials, the woylie (*Bettongia penicillata ogilbyi*) and boodie (*Bettongia lesueur*). *Exp Parasitol* 131:25–30, 2012.

54. Rose KA, Kirkland PD, Davis RJ, et al: Epizootics of sudden death in tammar wallabies (*Macropus eugenii*) associated with an orbivirus infection. *Aust Vet J* 90:505–509, 2012.

55. Rothstein R, Hunsaker D: Baseline hematology and blood chemistry of the south American Woolly opossum, *Caluromys derbianus. Lab Anim Sci* 22:227–232, 1972.

56. Schmid KL, Schmid LM, Wildsoet CF, et al: Retinal topography in the koala (*Phascolarctos cinereus*). *Brain Behav Evol* 39:8–16, 1992.

57. Smith JA, Wellehan JFX, Pogranichniy RM, et al: Identification and isolation of a novel herpesvirus in a captive mob of eastern grey kangaroos (*Macropus giganteus*). *Vet Microbiol* 129:236–245, 2008.

58. Speare R, Skerratt LF, Berger L, et al: Toxic effects of mebendazole at high dose on the haematology of red-legged pademelons (*Thylogale stigmatica*). *Aust Vet J* 82:300–303, 2004.

59. Speare R: Clinical assessment, diseases and management of the orphaned macropod joey. In *Proceedings 104, Australian Wildlife, Post-Graduate Committee of Veterinary Science*, 1988, pp 211–290.

60. Speight KN, Boardman W, Breed WG, et al: Pathological features of oxalate nephrosis in a population of Koalas (*Phascolarctos cinereus*) in South Australia. *Vet Pathol* 50:299–307, 2013.

61. Spratt DM, Beveridge I, Skerratt L, et al: Guide to the identification of parasites of Australian mammals. In Vogelnest L, Woods W, editors: *Medicine of Australian mammals*, Melbourne, Australia, 2008, CSIRO Publishing.

62. Stanley RG: Marsupial ophthalmology. *Vet Clin North Am Exotic Anim Pract* 5:371–390, 2002.

63. Stoskopf MK, Meyer RE, Jones M, et al: Field immobilization and euthanasia of American opossum. *J Wildl Dis* 35:145–149, 1999.

64. Stupans I, Jones B, McKinnon RA: Xenobiotic metabolism in Australian marsupials. *Comp Biochem Physiol C Pharmacol Toxicol Endocrinol* 128: 367–376, 2001.

65. Suedmeyer K: Tail amputation in a red kangaroo (*Macropus rufus*). In *Proceedings of the Annual Meeting of the American Association of Zoo Veterinarians*, 1998, pp 310–312.

66. Tyndale-Biscoe CH, Renfree M: *Reproductive physiology of marsupials*, Cambridge, U.K., 1987, Cambridge University Press.

67. Tyndale-Biscoe CH: *Life of marsupials*, Melbourne, Australia, 2005, CSIRO Publishing.

68. Vogelnest L, Portas T: Macropods. In Vogelnest L, Woods W, editors: *Medicine of Australian mammals*, Melbourne, Australia, 2008, CSIRO Publishing.

69. Vogelnest L, Stewart S, Sangster C: Poxvirus infection outbreak in common ringtails (*Pseudocheirus peregrines*). *Aust Vet J* 90:143–145, 2012.

70. Vogelnest L, Woods R: *Medicine of Australian mammals*, Melbourne, Australia, 2008, CSIRO Publishing.

71. Walton DW, Richardson BJ: *Fauna of Australia*, Vol. B, Canberra, Australia, 1989, Australian Government Publishing Service.

72. Wilcox RS, Vaz P, Ficorilli NP, et al: Gammaherpesvirus infection in a free-ranging eastern grey kangaroo (*Macropus giganteus*). *Aust Vet J* 89:55–57, 2011.

73. Wilson DE, Reeder DM: *Mammal species of the world: A taxonomic and geographic reference*, ed 3, Baltimore, MD, 2005, Johns Hopkins University Press.

74. Wynne J, Klause S, Stadler CK, et al: Preshipment testing success: Resolution of a nasal sinus granuloma in a captive koala (*Phascolarctos cinereus*) caused by *Cryptococcus gattii*. *J Zoo Wildl Med* 43:939–942, 2012.

CHAPTER 34

Insectivores (Insectivora, Macroscelidea, Scandentia)

Jennifer D'Agostino

BIOLOGY

Insectivora

Insectivores are considered the most primitive of all placental mammals and are believed to be the ones from which present day mammals have evolved. The order consists of six extant families: Erinaceidae (hedgehogs and gymnures), Chrysochloridae (golden moles), Tenrecidae (tenrecs), Solenodontidae (solenodons), Soricidae (shrews), and Talpidae (moles, shrew moles, and desmans). A seventh family, Nesophontidae (West Indian shrews), is considered extinct. The order Insectivora comprises the third largest group of mammals, with over 400 species identified. Some controversy exists in classification within this order, and some have proposed the formation of a new order, Afrosoricida, based on molecular studies. This new order would include the families Chrysochloridae and Tenrecidae. However, most current literature maintains all six families in Insectivora.[18,32]

Insectivores are terrestrial, fossorial, or semiaquatic and are almost completely nocturnal. They are found worldwide except in Australia, Antarctica, and most of South America. Over one third of all species in the order Insectivora are listed on the International Union for the Conservation of Nature (IUCN) Red List, with 21% of those listed as critically endangered and 26.5% as endangered. The major causes of population decline are human-induced habitat loss, fragmentation, and degradation. Overall insectivores are poorly understood, and further study is needed to determine practices that will aid in their conservation. As a group, insectivores make important contributions to the environment by controlling insects that damage crops and controlling vermin. Fossorial species also effectively aerate the soil.[18]

Macroscelidea

This order contains a single family, Macroscelididae, with 15 species of elephant shrews or "sengis." Historically, this group was included in the order Insectivora but has been reclassified into its own order based on genetic and morphologic comparison studies. These species inhabit Africa, including the island of Zanzibar, and occupy a wide variety of habitats. Seven species of elephant shrews are listed on the IUCN Red List. Causes for population decline include habitat fragmentation and land clearing for agriculture. Elephant shrews help control insect populations that might negatively affect human health or agriculture. The golden-rumped elephant shrew (*Rhynchocyon chrysopygus*) has become a symbol for conservation in Kenya.[18,33]

Scandentia

This order contains a single family, Tupaiidae, with 16 species of tree shrews. They are native to Southern and Southeast Asia and inhabit primarily tropical rainforests. This family has historically been very difficult to classify, and some have associated it with the orders Insectivora and Macroscelidea and the infraorder Lemuriformes. On the basis of anatomic and morphologic evidence, they were reclassified into their own order, Scandentia. Most tree shrew species are common; however, there are two species that are considered endangered (*Tupaia longipes* and *Tupaia nicobarica*).[18,34]

UNIQUE ANATOMY

Insectivora

Insectivores are small mammals that typically have long, narrow snouts and five clawed, nonopposable digits on each limb. The pelage consists of short, dense fur; short nonbarbed spines; or a combination of both. External ears are very small or non-existent (Talpidae). Insectivores have very small eyes and poor eyesight, with some species (desmans and moles) being completely blind and lacking a palpebral opening. They have a very keen sense of smell, and the nasal chamber consists of scrolls of coiled bone covered in olfactory epithelium for enhanced olfaction.[18,32] Most talpids have an elongated, mobile snout featuring arrays of small bumps called *Eimer's organs*. Eimer's organs contain a dense array of mechanoreceptors that allow detection of very small surface textures and features.[27] The star-nosed mole (*Condylura cristata*) has a specialized snout that contains 22 fleshy appendages with 25,000 mechanosensory receptors to help it locate food. Solenodons have a small bone called the *os proboscis* at the tip of the nose to support snout cartilage. Vibrissae, located on the snout, ears, tails, and sometimes feet, are large in diameter and relatively rigid, and they aid in the location of prey items.[18,32]

The dental formula in many insectivores is 3/3, 1/1, 4/4, 3–4/3–4, with a total of 44 to 48 teeth, although significant variation does exist within the order. All teeth are rooted but are primitive. Deciduous teeth serve no purpose and are shed very early in life. The upper molar pattern in shrews and moles is dilambdodont (W shaped), whereas tenrecs, solenodons, and golden moles have a zalambdodont pattern (V shaped). The upper molars of hedgehogs and gymnures have four main cusps. Solenodons (*Solenodon* sp.) and some shrews (*Neomys fodiens* and *Blarina* sp.) produce toxic saliva from the submaxillary gland, and the saliva is delivered through deep grooves in the lower incisors.[18,32]

The majority of insectivores have a plantigrade stance, and fossorial species have short, powerful forearms specialized for digging. Talpids have a falciform bone, sometimes called a "sixth digit," which expands the palm and supports the digits. In talpids, the radius articulates with the humerus in an S-shaped cavity, causing the forearm to be permanently rotated outward from the body. This allows the forelimb to act as a spade for digging. Aquatic species have webbed feet with hairy fringes, which allows them to run on water surfaces for several seconds. The tails of moles are able to detect ground vibrations, and *Microgale* has a modified tail that is prehensile.[18,32]

Insectivores have a low, flat skull, with reduced or absent zygomatic arches. The brain is small, and the cerebral hemispheres lack fissures and do not extend over the cerebellum. All species except *Potamogale* spp. have a clavicle. All insectivores lack a cecum, and many species have a cloaca.[32]

In males, the testes are abdominal, inguinal, or in a sac in front of the penis. Some species have a baculum. Females of some species in the Talpidae family have ovotestes with a functional ovarian segment and a larger testicular segment that lacks germ cells. These animals are considered true fertile hermaphrodites.[4]

Armored shrews (*Scutisorex somereni*) have unique interlocking lateral, dorsal, and ventral vertebral spines, which create an exceptionally sturdy vertebral column. Despite this feature, these shrews still have considerable flexibility and may bend dorsoventrally and laterally.[32]

Macroscelidea

Elephant shrews are small mammals with a compact body and a large head. The long, narrow snout moves in a circular motion and is extremely sensitive. Nostrils are located at the tip of the nose, and long vibrissae are present at the base of the snout. Eyes and ears are well developed, and auditory bullae are large. Elephant shrews have well-developed senses of smell, sight, and hearing. They exhibit a digitigrade stance; the hindlimbs are longer than the forelimbs and are useful for running and hopping. The dental formula is 1–3/3, 1/1, 4/4, 2/2–3, for a total of 36 to 44 teeth with dilambdodont dentition. Elephant shrews possess numerous scent glands to mark territory. The braincase is relatively large and much more complex than in the Insectivora species. All species in Macroscelidea possess a cecum, although it may not be functional in all species. In males, the penis is divided into three forks.[18,33]

Scandentia

Externally, tree shrews resemble squirrels but have long snouts. All species except the pen-tailed tree shrew (*Ptilocercus lowii*) have a bushy tail. Tree shrews are quadrupedal and range from arboreal to terrestrial. Tupaiids are adept climbers and swift runners. Their senses of smell and hearing are well developed, and their vision is good. The braincase is relatively large, and the orbits are completely encircled in bone. The dental formula is 2/3, 1/1, 3/3, 3/3, with a total of 38 teeth. The lower incisors are angled forward to form a dental comb that is used in feeding and grooming. Similar to the Macroscelidea and some of the Insectivora species, Scandentia species have dilambdodont dentition.[18,34]

SPECIAL PHYSIOLOGY

Most insectivores have a very high metabolic rate. Compared with most mammals, insectivore body temperatures are usually lower (33° C to 35° C), the exception being *Sorex* spp. (37° C to 38°C). Some species such as the hedgehog exhibit true hibernation for part of the year. They spend the months preceding hibernation building up fat stores. Some species in the families Macroscelididae, Chrysochloridae, and Tenrecidae exhibit torpor (heterothermy) on a daily or seasonal basis when ambient temperatures decrease or food sources become scarce. During hibernation and torpor, heart rate, body temperature, and metabolic rate drop significantly. The body temperature of the Southern African hedgehog (*Atelerix frontalis*) may decrease to 1° C during hibernation.[29] Solenodons and some species of moles and shrews emit high-frequency vocalizations that may have an echolocation function for navigation.

Hedgehogs exhibit a unique self-anointing behavior, also called *anting*. When a new or irritating substance is encountered, the hedgehog will lick the substance until saliva is produced and then vigorously groom its quills. The reason for this behavior is unknown, but theories suggest the method may serve as protection from predators or to apply a unique scent to itself or its home range. This normal behavior and the resultant saliva production are often confused for a disease such as rabies or a dental condition.[18,20,32]

SPECIAL HOUSING REQUIREMENTS

Insectivores are rarely used as exhibit animals because of their secretive nature. Most are nocturnal, and the fossorial species spend most or all of their time underground. For the most part, insectivores are solitary and socialize only during mating and during rearing offspring. In a captive situation, some species may be exhibited in groups without problems; however, significant aggression may be

seen. The most successfully exhibited species include elephant shrews, tree shrews, African hedgehogs, and tenrecs.

Insectivore species have a well-developed sense of hearing; therefore, the area around the exhibit should be kept quiet. Double-glass barriers have been used for this purpose. Walls should be smooth, nonclimbable, and easily cleaned. Absorbent bedding may be used to decrease the exposure of the animals to urine and feces, which may lead to dermatitis. Shrews may become entangled in shredded wood bedding and may be averse to the noise of shredded paper. Litter should be deep enough for the animal to plough through.

A nest box is essential. Insectivores are sensitive to disturbances, so cleaning should be done only as needed. The use of a second enclosure to shift animals may minimize disturbance. Shrews and some other insectivores establish latrines and tend to defecate near water, even if provided in a bottle.

Environmental temperatures depend on the natural history of the species but usually are between 23° C and 28° C. All insectivores should be kept free from drafts and abrupt (greater than 5° C) temperature changes. Cages should be well ventilated. Exhibits should be kept dry to prevent the animals from losing body heat through damp pelage.[2,32]

FEEDING

As would be expected, insects are the bases of the natural diet of most insectivore species. However, most species have varied diets, including small vertebrates, carrion, berries, nuts, and vegetation. Aquatic species prey on worms, crustaceans, fishes, and frogs. Many insectivores have a voracious appetite and consume large quantities of food.[18,20,32–34] Hedgehogs possess chitinase in the gastric mucosa and pancreas, which presumably aids in digestion of the exoskeletons of insects.[6]

In captivity, diets should contain high protein (30%–50%) and moderate fat (10%–20%) content on a dry-matter basis.[6] Commonly exhibited insectivores may be maintained on a commercial cat diet or insectivore diet and on insects. Small amounts of fruit, vegetables, and leafy greens may also be added. Raw meat and eggs should be avoided, as they may harbor *Salmonella* sp. Milk should not be fed, as it may cause diarrhea.[20] Periodontal disease has been reported frequently; therefore, dry food may be beneficial to dental health.[6]

Feed consumption varies widely by species. Some shrew species may eat up to several times their body weight daily. Some species may undergo wide fluctuations in appetite and body weight because of seasonal changes and so may be a challenge to manage. Transient weight gain may be physiologically normal in species that exhibit heterothermy; however, in captive situations, diets may need to be rationed to prevent obesity. Nutritional problems may be the cause of the high rates of early mortality and poor rates of survival frequently seen in insectivores in captivity.[2,18,32]

RESTRAINT AND HANDLING

Many insectivore species are sensitive and prone to stress when handled. Plastic tubes and clear containers may be useful for visual examinations. Hedgehogs and tenrecs tend to roll up when touched, making physical examination difficult without sedation or anesthesia. Species that are habituated to handling may be more easily examined under manual restraint. Light gloves may facilitate handling of species that have spines or those that are venomous.[9]

ANESTHESIA AND SURGERY

Parenteral anesthesia has been described in the literature but is reserved mainly for use in the field or for research purposes (Table 34-1). Parenteral anesthetics may be given by subcutaneous (SQ), intramuscular (IM), or intraperitoneal (IP) injection. IV injection is very difficult in most insectivores, but injections may be given via the cephalic vein or by the intraosseous (IO) route into the femur, humerus, or tibia. Inhalant anesthesia is more commonly

TABLE 34-1

Injectable Restraint Agents Used for Insectivores[5,16]

Generic Name	Dosage (mg/kg)	Route of Administration	Reversal (mg/kg)	Comments
Diazepam	0.5–2.0	Intramuscular	—	Mild sedation
Midazolam	0.25–0.5	Intramuscular	—	Preanesthetic
Ketamine	5.0–20.0	Intramuscular	—	May be used in combination with a benzodiazepine or an α_2-agonist
Medetomidine	0.05–0.1 0.2	Intramuscular Subcutaneous, Intramuscular	Atipamezole 0.3–0.5	Mild sedation Heavy sedation
Xylazine	0.5–1.0	Intramuscular	Yohimbine 0.5–1.0	May be given with ketamine
Tiletamine/Zolazepam	1.0–5.0	Intramuscular	—	Recovery may be prolonged and rough
Ketamine/Medetomidine	5.0/0.1	Intramuscular	Atipamizole 0.3–0.5	Anesthesia
Ketamine/Medetomidine/ Midazolam	20.0/0.2/3.0	Subcutaneous	Atipamezole 1.0 Flumazenil 0.2	

TABLE 34-2

Reference Ranges for Hematologic Parameters of Selected Species[19]

Parameters	African Pygmy Hedgehog (*Atelerix albiventris*)	European Hedgehog (*Erinaceus europaeus*)	Lesser Madagascar Hedgehog Tenrec (*echinops Telfairi*)	Large Tree Shrew (*Tupaia tana*)
Erythrocytes (×10⁶/μL)	5.51 ± 1.82*	6.8 ± 2.69	4.21 ± 0.97	7.82 ± 1.17
Hematocrit (%)	35.5 ± 7.4	34.2 ± 6.5	36.3 ± 10.6	40.7 ± 7.0
Hemoglobin (g/dL)	12.0 ± 2.8	10.5 ± 2.0	12.5 ± 2.5	13.6 ± 2.4
MCV (fL)	66.9 ± 8.9	53.6 ± 19.9	95.9 ± 15.0	52.3 ± 6.1
MCH (mg/dL)	22.4 ± 3.9	17.5 ± 7.5	29.9 ± 1.2	18.4 ± 1.0
MCHC (g/dL)	33.8 ± 4.7	32.3 ± 3.6	31.8 ± 4.6	34.0 ± 3.9
Leukocytes (×10³/μL)	10.94 ± 6.2	15.1 ± 10.17	10.11 ± 3.28	3.44 ± 2.05
Neutrophils (×10³/μL)	5.14 ± 5.24	7.98 ± 6.83	3.43 ± 1.0	2.01 ± 1.96
Band neutrophils (×10³/μL)	0.39 ± 0.34	—	0.26 ± 0.0	0.016 ± 0.026
Lymphocytes (×10³/μL)	4.04 ± 2.25	5.29 ± 3.35	6.18 ± 2.65	1.02 ± 0.48
Monocytes (×10³/μL)	0.34 ± 0.31	0.41 ± 0.21	0.22 ± 0.14	0.28 ± 0.24
Eosinophils (×10³/μL)	1.21 ± 0.93	1.14 ± 0.79	0.51 ± 0.25	0.26 ± 0.36
Basophils (×10³/μL)	0.35 ± 0.29	0.36 ± 0.23	—	0.016 ± 0.032
Platelets (×10³/μL)	226 ± 108	196 ± 120	511 ± 0	811 ± 0

*All values are given as mean ± standard deviation.

fL, Femtoliters; *g/dL,* gram per deciliter; *MCV,* mean corpuscular volume; *MCH,* mean corpuscular hemoglobin; *MCHC,* mean corpuscular hemoglobin concentration; *mg/dL,* milligram per deciliter; *μL,* microliter.

used and is the preferred method in insectivores. Anesthesia may be induced using an induction chamber or a face mask. Because of the small body size of insectivores, intubation may be considerably difficult. Fasting is generally not recommended because of the high metabolic rate and small glucose reserves. High metabolic rate and oxygen requirement make insectivores prone to hypothermia, hypoglycemia, and hypoxemia, so the animals should be monitored closely. Anesthetic events should be kept as short as possible to minimize complications. Isoflurane may increase blood flow to the skin in the smaller species, so a heating pad is recommended to avoid rapid temperature decrease. Insectivores may be monitored by using pulse oximetry, electrocardiography (ECG), or Doppler ultrasonography.[9,14,20]

Some surgical procedures reported in insectivores include enucleation, dental extractions, limb amputations, spay or neuter, biopsy and resection of various neoplasms, and treatment for traumatic injuries and abscesses.

DIAGNOSTICS

Collecting samples from insectivores may be challenging because of their small size, unique anatomy, and tendency for some species to roll into a ball when handled. Blood may be collected from the jugular vein, the cranial vena cava, and the cephalic, femoral, or saphenous veins. Reference ranges for complete blood cell count and serum biochemistry for select species are presented in Tables 34-2 and 34-3. SQ injections may be given in the spiny or furred areas. The dermal layer under the spines is poorly vascularized in hedgehogs, and absorption of drugs or fluids may be delayed in this area. IM injections may be given in the muscles of the hindlimb. The spines of hedgehogs and tenrecs may diminish radiographic details, and often anesthesia is required for proper positioning. With the use of plastic clips or tape, the dorsal skin may gently be pulled away from the chest and abdomen to achieve improved detail.[20]

TABLE 34-3

Reference Ranges for Serum Parameters of Selected Species[19]

Parameter	African Pygmy Hedgehog (*Atelerix albiventris*)	European Hedgehog (*Erinaceus europaeus*)	Lesser Madagascar Hedgehog Tenrec (*Echinops telfairi*)	Large Tree Shrew (*Tupaia tana*)
Total protein (g/dL)	5.8 ± 0.7*	6.0 ± 0.9	7.4 ± 2.2	6.8 ± 1.1
Albumin (g/dL)	2.9 ± 0.4	3.6 ± 0.5	5.0 ± 1.1	3.4 ± 0.4
Globulin (g/dL)	2.7 ± 0.5	2.5 ± 0.7	3.8 ± 0.7	3.8 ± 1.0
Calcium (mg/dL)	8.8 ± 1.4	10.4 ± 2.9	11.1 ± 0.9	9.2 ± 1.3
Magnesium (mg/dL)	2.24 ± 0.12	2.41 ± 0.0	—	—
Phosphorus (mg/dL)	5.3 + 1.9	4.2 ± 0.3	3.9 ± 0.9	6.5 ± 1.7
Sodium (mEq/L)	141 ± 9	—	157 ± 13	162 ± 5
Potassium (mEq/L)	4.9 ± 1.0	—	4.3 ± 1.3	4.8 ± 0.9
Chloride (mEq/L)	109 ± 10	—	120 ± 8	125 ± 13
Creatinine (mg/dL)	0.4 ± 0.2	0.3 ± 0.1	0.5 ± 0.5	0.6 ± 0.4
Urea nitrogen (mg/dL)	27 ± 9	20 ± 6	53 ± 14	27 ± 12
Cholesterol (mg/dL)	131 ± 25	—	108 ± 50	92 ± 33
Glucose (mg/dL)	89 ± 30	105 ± 10	60 ± 33	137 ± 34
Iron (µg/dL)	239 ± 61	—	—	—
Serum enzymes	—			
AST (IU/L)	34 ± 22	65 ± 44	62 ± 17	162 ± 117
ALT (IU/L)	53 ± 24	69 ± 34	133 ± 96	59 ± 33
LDH (IU/L)	441 ± 258	—	—	—
CPK (IU/L)	863 ± 413	—	146 ± 0	607 ± 566
Amylase (Unit/L)	510 ± 170	—	—	2587 ± 845
Alkaline phosphatase (IU/L)	51 ± 21	51 ± 0	23 ± 6	101 ± 58
GGT (IU/L)	4 ± 4	—	124 ± 81	12 ± 4
Lipase (Unit/L)	14 ± 4	—	—	24 ± 0
Total bilirubin (mg/dl)	0.3 ± 0.3	0.2 ± 0.1	0.5 ± 0.3	0.7 ± 0.4
Direct bilirubin (mg/dL)	0.1 ± 0.2	—	—	0.3 ± 0.1
Indirect bilirubin (mg/dL)	0.2 ± 0.2	—	—	0.5 ± 0.1
Trigylcerides (mg/dL)	38 ± 22	—	51 ± 26	130 ± 50
Bicarbonate (mmol/L)	19.6 ± 1.6	—	—	—
Carbon dioxide (mmol/L)	23.3 ± 12.7	—	—	16.5 ± 9.2
Uric acid (mg/dL)	1.0 ± 0.9	—	—	0.2 ± 0.0

*All values are given as mean ± standard deviation.
AST, Aspartate aminotransferase; *ALT*, alanine aminotransferase; *LDH*, lactic acid dehydrogenase; *CPK*, creatine phosphokinase; *GGT*, gamma-glutamyl transferase; *g/dL*, gram per deciliter; *µg/dL*, microgram per deciliter; *IU/L*, international unit per liter; *mEq/L*, milliequivalent per liter; *mg/dL*, milligram per deciliter; *mmol/L*, millimole per liter; *Unit/L*, unit per liter.

DISEASES

Infectious Diseases

Infectious disease has been reported relatively uncommonly in insectivores. Bacterial diseases reported include enteritis caused by *Salmonella* sp., pneumonia caused by *Corynebacterium* sp., and respiratory disease caused by *Pasteurella* sp. and *Bordetella bronchiseptium*.[20] Insectivores may be reservoirs for several bloodborne diseases, including *Rickettsia* spp., *Borrelia burgdorferi*, *Babesia microti*, and *Anaplasma phagocytophilum*, which are transmitted by parasite vectors; however, clinical disease associated with these organisms has not been noted in insectivores.[17,23,28] Several fungal diseases, including adiaspiromycosis, cryptococcosis, paecilomycosis, histoplasmosis, and dermatophytosis, have been reported.[2,12,20,37,39] Viral disease is rare in insectivore species; however, foot and mouth disease and paramyxovirus have been reported.[21] Several species of shrews have been shown to harbor novel hantaviruses.[22] Herpesviral infection has been reported in European hedgehogs (*Erinaceus europaeus*), and one case of an African hedgehog (*Atelerix albiventris*) that succumbed to infection with herpes simplex virus 1 (HSV-1) has been published.[1] The bicolored white-toothed shrew (*Crocidura leucodon*) has been shown to carry bornavirus, suggesting that it may be a reservoir species.[35] Table 34-4 lists commonly used antibiotics and dosages.

Parasitic Diseases

Ectoparasites reported in insectivores include mites (*Caparinia* spp. and *Notoedres* sp.), fleas (many species depending on host), ticks (most notably ixodid species), and myiasis. Internal parasites include coccidia (*Eimeria* and *Isospora* spp.), *Cryptosporidium* spp., lungworms (*Crenosoma striatum*, *Capillaria* spp., and *Eucoleus aerophilus*), nematodes (*Capillaria erinacei*, *Physoloptera clausa*, *Ganglyonema mucronatum*, and *G. neoplasticum*), trematodes (*Brachylaemus erinacei*), and acanthocephalans (*Prosthorhynchus* spp., *Plagiorhynchus cylindraceus*, and *Oliganthorhynchus erinacei*).[7,10,30,31,38] Xenoma-like formation, primarily in the liver, associated with a myxosporean infection (*Soricimyxum fegati*) has been noted in several species of shrews.[8] Table 34-5 lists various anthelmintics and dosages.

TABLE 34-4

Selected Antimicrobials Used in Insectivores[5]

Medication	Dosage (mg/kg)	Route of Administration	Interval
Amikacin	2.5–5	IM	Every 8–12 hours
Amoxicillin	15	PO, SQ, or IM	Every 12 hours
Amoxicillin/Clavulanic acid	12.5	PO	Every 12 hours
Cephalexin	25	PO	Every 8 hours
Chloramphenicol	30–50	PO, SQ, IM, or IV	Every 12 hours
Ciprofloxacin	5–20	PO	Every 12 hours
Clarithromycin	5.5	PO	Every 12 hours
Clindamycin	5.5–10	PO	Every 12 hours
Doxycycline	2.5–10	PO, SQ, IM	Every 12 hours
Enrofloxacin	2.5–10	PO, SQ, or IM	Every 12 hours
Erythromycin	10	PO or IM	Every 12 hours
Gentamicin	2	SQ or IM	Every 8 hours
Metronidazole	20	PO	Every 12 hours
Oxytetracycline	25–50	PO	Every 24 hours
Penicillin G	40,000 IU/kg	SQ or IM	Every 24 hours
Piperacillin	10	SQ	Every 8–12 hours
Sulfadiazine/trimethoprim	30	PO, SQ, or IM	Every 12 hours
Tylosin	10	PO or SQ	Every 12 hours

IM, Intramuscularly; *IU/kg*, international unit per kilogram; *PO*, by mouth; *SQ*, subcutaneously; *IV*, intravenously.

TABLE 34-5

Selected Parasiticides Used in Insectivores[5,24]

Medication	Dosage (mg/kg)	Route of Administration	Interval	Parasite
Amitraz	0.3%	Topical	Every 7 days	Mites
Fenbendazole	10–15 10–30 25	PO PO PO	Every 14 days Every 24 hours Every 10 days	Nematodes
Imidacloprid 10% + Moxidectin 1% (Advocate®)	0.1 mL/kg	Topical	Once	Mites (*Caparinia tripilis*)
Ivermectin	0.2–0.5	PO or SQ	May repeat every 14 days for 3 treatments	Ectoparasites and nematodes
Levamisole 1%	10	SQ	Repeat in 48 hours and as needed every 14 days	Nematodes, including lungworms
Mebendazole	15	PO	Repeat in 14 days	Nematodes
Metronidazole	25	PO	Every 12 for 5 days	Intestinal protozoa
Permethrin	1%	Topical	—	Mites
Praziquantel	7	PO or SQ	Repeat in 14 days	Cestodes, trematodes
Selamectin	6	Topical	—	Ectoparasites
Sulfadimethoxine	2–20 10	PO, SQ, or IM PO	Every 24 hours for 2–5 days Every 24 hours for 5–7 days	Coccidia

PO, By mouth; *SQ*, subcutaneously; *IM*, intramuscularly.

Noninfectious Diseases

Neoplasia in hedgehogs and tenrecs is the most commonly reported noninfectious disease. The organ systems most commonly involved are the integumentary, hemolymphatic, digestive, endocrine and reproductive systems. Most reported neoplasms are malignant, with mammary adenocarcinoma, lymphoma, and oral squamous cell carcinoma being the most common tumor types diagnosed.[15] Other types of neoplasia that have been reported include plasmacytoma, pancreatic carcinoma, papilloma, sebaceous gland carcinoma, myelogenous leukemia, fibrosarcoma, mast cell tumor, amelenotic melanoma, pituitary adenoma, adrenocortical carcinoma, renal transitional cell carcinoma, hepatocellular carcinoma, gastrointestinal adenocarcinoma, thyroid adenoma or adenocarcinoma, multicentric skeletal sarcoma, cutaneous hemangiosarcoma, uterine leiomyosarcoma, astrocytoma, peripheral neurofibrosarcoma and subcutaneous schwannoma.[13,15] Treatment may consist of surgical removal,

TABLE 34-6

Reproductive Characteristics of Selected Insectivores[18,20,25,32–34]

Parameter	Insectivore Species							
	Atelerix albiventris	*Cryptotis parva*	*Echinops telfairi*	*Erinaceus europaeus*	*Macroscelides proboscideus*	*Sorex* spp.	*Tenrec ecaudatus*	*Tupaia* spp.
Breeding	Year round	Seasonal to year round	Seasonal	Seasonal	Seasonal	Seasonal	Seasonal	Seasonal to year round
Gestation (days)	30–40	21–22	57–79	31–35	56–61	18–28	56–64	40–52
Litter size	1–10 (usually 4–5)	1–9	1–10	2–7	1–2	2–12	1–32 (average 15)	1–3
Average birth weight in grams (g)	10	—	15	15	—	0.5	10–18	10–12
Age at weaning (days)	28–42	18–19	30–35	38–45	18–36	21–35	20–35	36

chemotherapy, or radiation therapy. However, most cases are diagnosed late in the disease course, and prognosis is often poor.

A high incidence of cardiomyopathy is seen in African hedgehogs. The disease most commonly affects males over the age of 1 year. Diagnosis is usually late in the disease course, and prognosis is poor. Normal cardiac measurements have been reported in this species and may aid in early diagnosis and monitoring of heart disease.[3]

Wobbly hedgehog syndrome is a progressive neurologic disease commonly reported in African hedgehogs, and a similar disease is seen in European hedgehogs as well. The disease is characterized by the animal's inability to roll into a ball and incoordination progressing to tetraplegia, seizures, and paralysis. In most affected individuals, onset of clinical signs occurs at less than 2 years of age. Histologically, vacuolation of the white matter of the central nervous system with neuronal degeneration is seen. Numerous therapies have been attempted with little success. Some evidence suggests that this disease is hereditary.[11]

Nutritional diseases reported in insectivores include hepatic lipidosis, obesity, and periodontal disease.[6] Ocular diseases include proptosis, corneal ulceration, panophthalmitis, and orbital cellulitis.[26] Intervertebral disk disease has been reported in hedgehogs and is an important differential diagnosis for neurologic disease.[36]

REPRODUCTION

Insectivora

There is little information on the reproductive biology of many insectivores. Most appear to breed seasonally, but some of the smallest, short-lived species breed year round. Insectivores have a chorioallantoic placenta, which allows the young to fully develop in the uterus.[18] Gestation length and litter size vary considerably across the order. A commonly kept insectivore, the lesser hedgehog tenrec (*Echinops telfairi*), has a mean gestation length of 67.5 days (range 57–79 days) with an average litter size of three to five.[25] The tenrec (*Tenrec ecaudatus*) appears to be one of the most prolific mammals, with litter sizes up to 32 reported.[18] Selected reproductive parameters are listed in Table 34-6.

Some species of shrews exhibit *caravanning behavior*: The young follow each other in a single file while gripping the rump of the one in front. The first of the offspring in the line grips the dam's rump.[32]

Macroscelidea

Elephant shrews are generally monogamous. Females exhibit polyovulation, in which up to 100 eggs are ovulated with most becoming fertilized. Only one to three eggs will implant in the uterus and develop. Elephant shrews give birth to precocial young and may

produce several litters per year. The females leave the young alone in the nest most of the time and return to nurse them once daily.[18,33]

Scandentia

Tree shrews are monogamous and form strong pair bonds. In captivity, most species develop a linear hierarchy based on aggression. The dominant male is the only one to mate with the females. Postpartum estrus occurs, and evidence of delayed implantation exists. Tree shrews have endotheliochorial placentation, with two placental disks that attach to specialized pads in the uterine wall. Females give birth to altricial young in a "juvenile nest," which is separate from the "parental nest." Young are suckled once every 48 hours.[18,34]

REFERENCES

1. Allison N, Chang TC, Steele KE, et al: Fatal herpes simplex infection in a pygmy African hedgehog (*Atelerix albiventris*). *J Comp Pathol* 126:76–78, 2002.
2. Barbiers R: Insectivora (Hedgehogs, Tenrecs, Shrews, Moles) and Dermoptera (Flying Lemurs). In Fowler ME, Miller RE, editors: *Zoo and wild animal medicine*, ed 5, St. Louis, MO, 2003, Saunders, pp 304–315.
3. Black PA, Marshall C, Seyfried AW, et al: Cardiac assessment of African hedgehogs (*Atelerix albiventris*). *J Zoo Wildl Med* 42:49–53, 2011.
4. Carmona FD, Motokawa M, Tokita M, et al: The evolution of female mole ovotestes evidences high plasticity of mammalian gonad development. *J Exp Zool* 310B:259–266, 2008.
5. Carpenter JW, Marion CJ: Hedgehogs. In Carpenter JW, editor: *Exotic animal formulary*, ed 4, St. Louis, MO, 2013, Elsevier, pp 455–475.
6. Dierenfeld ES: Feeding behavior and nutrition of the African pygmy hedgehog (*Atelerix albiventris*). *Vet Clin North Am Exotic Anim Pract* 12:335–337, 2009.
7. Dyachenko V, Kuhnert Y, Schmaeschke R, et al: Occurrence and molecular characterization of *Cryptosporidium* spp. Genotypes in European hedgehogs (*Erinaceus europaeus*) in Germany. *Parasitology* 137:205–216, 2010.
8. Dyková I, Tyml T, Kostka M: Xenoma-like formations induced by *Soricimyxum fegati* (Myxosporea) in three species of shrews (Soricomorpha: Soricidae), including records of new hosts. *Folia Parasitol* 58:249–256, 2011.
9. Fowler M: Small mammals. In *Restraint and handling of wild and domestic animals*, ed 3, Ames, IA, 2008, Wiley-Blackwell, pp 257–273.
10. Gaglio G, Allen S, Bowden L, et al: Parasites of European hedgehogs (*Erinaceus europaeus*) in Britain: Epidemiological study and coprological test evaluation. *Eur J Wildl Res* 56:839–844, 2010.
11. Graesser D, Spraker TR, Dressen P, et al: Wobbly hedgehog syndrome in African pygmy hedgehogs (*Atelerix* spp.). *J Exotic Pet Med* 15:59–65, 2009.

12. Han JI, Na KJ: Cutaneous paecilomycosis caused by *Paecilomyces variotii* in an African pygmy hedgehog (*Atelerix albiventris*). *J Exotic Pet Med* 19:309–312, 2010.

13. Harrison TM, Dominguez P, Hanzlik K, et al: Treatment of an amelanotic melanoma using radiation therapy in a lesser Madagascar hedgehog tenrec (*Echinops telfairi*). *J Zoo Wildl Med* 42:151–157, 2010.

14. Heard DJ: Insectivores (Hedgehogs, Moles and Tenrecs). In West G, Heard D, Caulkett N, editors: *Zoo animal and wildlife immobilization and anesthesia*, Ames, IA, 2007, Blackwell Publishing, pp 347–348.

15. Heatley JJ, Mauldin GE, Cho DY: A review of neoplasia in the captive African hedgehog (*Atelerix albiventris*). *Semin Avian Exotic Pet Med* 14:182–192, 2005.

16. Henke J, Reinert J, Preissel AK, et al: Partially antagonisable anesthesia of the small hedgehog tenrec (*Echinops telfairi*) with medetomidine, midazolam and ketamine. *J Exp Anim Sci* 43:255–264, 2007.

17. Hersh MH, Tibbetts M, Strauss M, et al: Reservoir competence of wildlife host species for *Babesia microti*. *Emerg Infect Dis* 18:1951–1957, 2012.

18. Hutchins M, Kleiman DG, Geist V, et al: In *Grzimek's animal life encyclopedia*, vol 12–16, ed 2, Farmington Hills, MI, 2003, Gale Group.

19. International Species Inventory System: *Reference ranges for physiological values in captive wildlife*, Apple Valley, MN, 2002, ISIS.

20. Ivey E, Carpenter JW: African Hedgehogs. In Quesenberry KE, Carpenter JW, editors: *Ferrets, rabbits and rodents clinical medicine and surgery*, ed 2, St. Louis, MO, 2004, Saunders, pp 339–353.

21. Johnson D: Hedgehogs and sugar gliders: Respiratory anatomy, physiology, and disease. *Vet Clin North Am Exotic Anim Pract* 14:267–285, 2001.

22. Kang HJ, Arai S, Hope AG, et al: Novel hantavirus in the flat-skulled shrew (*Sorex roboratus*). *Vector Borne Zoonotic Dis* 10:593–597, 2010.

23. Keesing F, Hersh MH, Tibbetts M, et al: Reservoir competence of vertebrate hosts for *Anaplasma phagocytophilum*. *Emerg Infect Dis* 18:2013–2016, 2012.

24. Kim KR, Ahn KS, Oh DS, et al: Efficacy of a combination of 10% imidacloprid and 1% moxidectin against *Caparinia tripilis* in African pygmy hedgehog (*Atelerix albiventris*). *Parasitol Vectors* 5:158–165, 2012.

25. Künzle H, Poulson Nautrup C, Schwartzenberger F: High inter-individual variation in the gestation length of the hedgehog tenrec, *Echinops telfairi* (Afrotheria). *Anim Reprod Sci* 97:364–374, 2007.

26. Lennox AM: Emergency and critical care procedures in sugar gliders (*Petaurus breviceps*), African hedgehogs (*Atelerix albiventris*), and prairie dogs (*Cynomys* spp.). *Vet Clin North Am Exotic Anim Pract* 10:533–555, 2007.

27. Marasco PD, Catania KC: Response properties of primary afferents supplying Eimer's organ. *J Exp Biol* 210:765–780, 2007.

28. Marié JL, Davoust B, Socolovschi C, et al: Molecular detection of rickettsial agents in ticks and fleas collected from a European hedgehog (*Erinaceous europaeus*) in Marseilles, France. *Comp Immunol Microbiol Infect Dis* 35:77–79, 2012.

29. McKechnie AE, Mzilikazi N: Heterothermy in Afrotropical mammals and birds: A review. *Integr Comp Biol* 51:349–363, 2011.

30. Meredith AL, Milne EM: Cryptosporidial infection in a captive European hedgehog (*Erinaceus europaeus*). *J Zoo Wildl Med* 40:809–811, 2009.

31. Milek JA, Seville S: Species of *Eimeria* and *Isospora* (Apicomplexa: Eimeriidae) from shrews (Insectivora: Soricidae) in Northwestern Wyoming, USA. *Comp Parasitol* 70:72–77, 2003.

32. Nowak RN: Order Insectivora. In *Walker's mammals of the world*, ed 6, Baltimore, MD, 1999, Johns Hopkins University Press, pp 169–243.

33. Nowak RN: Order Macroscelidea. In *Walker's mammals of the world*, ed 6, Baltimore, MD, 1999, Johns Hopkins University Press, pp 1739–1745.

34. Nowak RN: Order Scandentia. In *Walker's mammals of the world*, ed 6, Baltimore, MD, 1999, Johns Hopkins University Press, pp 245–249.

35. Puorger ME, Hilbe M, Müller JP, et al: Distribution of borna disease virus antigen and RNA in tissues of naturally infected bicolored white-toothed shrews, *Crocidur aleucodon*, supporting their role as reservoir host species. *Vet Pathol* 47:236–244, 2010.

36. Raymond JT, Aguilar R, Dunker F, et al: Intervertebral disc disease in African hedgehogs (*Atelerix albiventris*): Four cases. *J Exotic Pet Med* 18:220–223, 2009.

37. Seixas F, Travassos P, Pinto ML, et al: Pulmonary adiaspiromycosis in a European hedgehog (*Erinaceus europaeus*) in Portugal. *Vet Rec* 158:274–275, 2006.

38. Skuballa J, Taraschewski H, Petney TN, et al: The avian acanthocephalan *Plagiorhynchus cylindraceus* (Palaeacanthocephala) parasitizing the European hedgehog (*Erinaceus europaeus*) in Europe and New Zealand. *Parasitol Res* 106:431–437, 2010.

39. Snider TA, Joyner P, Clinkenbeard KD: Disseminated histoplasmosis in an African pygmy hedgehog. *J Am Vet Med Assoc* 232:74–76, 2008.

CHAPTER 35

Chiroptera (Bats)

Elizabeth L. Buckles

OVERVIEW AND NATURAL HISTORY

Bats have always fascinated people. Unfortunately, much of the connotations around them have been negative. Their odd appearances, nocturnal life styles, and the fact they harbor a variety of zoonotic diseases, particularly rabies, have lead them to be feared rather than respected. However, beneath the surface of the legend, they are members of a diverse group of animals, many of which are essential for the maintenance of ecosystems. In fact, because of disease and habitat destruction, humans are a greater threat to bats than they are to humans.[68] Recent events such as the emergence of white nose syndrome (WNS) and the continued recognition of metabolic diseases in captive bats have shown that much more research is needed into the medical and environmental needs of these animals. Improving veterinary care, conservation efforts, and captive husbandry relies on a deeper understanding of bat biology and how these unique animals fit into larger ecosystems.

What *is* known about bats is that they belong to the order Chiroptera, literally meaning "hand wing." Some mammals such as lemurs and squirrels may parachute, but only bats have powered flight. It is this unique anatomic feature and the ability to fly that distinguish bats from all other mammals. Their wings are actually modifications of the standard mammalian hand consisting of elongate, slender phalanges spanned by a thin, tough wing membrane that serves as a flexible airfoil.[38] This anatomy lends a high degree of adaptability and maneuverability to the flight of bats and allows fine adjustments to navigation.

Ancestors of modern bats first appeared, as evidenced by fossil records, approximately 53 million years ago. As is the case today, ancestral bats were distributed worldwide and appear to have been capable of flight. Today, at least 1240 known species of bats exist, accounting for 20% of all known mammals. They are found on all continents except Antarctica and inhabit a variety of environmental and dietary niches.[38]

Traditional subdivisions of Chiroptera are the two suborders Megachiroptera and Microchiroptera.[38] Current theory suggests that both groups evolved from a common flighted ancestor, and this is generally supported by molecular evidence. Fossil evidence shows that these ancestral bats displayed many modern characteristics, including the ability to echolocate and specializations for fruit and nectar feeding.[38] Despite the terminology, it is ecology and anatomy, not size, that distinguishes the groups. Megachiroptera include "fruit bats," which eat fruit, nectar, and pollen. They are efficient climbers, as they have a claw on each wing, and have excellent eyesight. Microchiroptera species may feed on a variety of mammals, reptiles, fish, fruit nectar, and, in some cases, blood. Their eyesight is poor, and they have relatively small eyes. Hence they rely on echolocation for navigation and hunting.[38]

Bats are found in a variety of habitats, ranging from arid to tropical. Some have limited home ranges, and some range widely. Most species of bat are found in tropical or subtropical regions, where they may remain year round. Those inhabiting less temperate areas must adapt to survive inhospitable climates. Some species migrate, whereas others hibernate. Both survival strategies require specializations. Migratory bats have narrow, more pointed wings that provide more efficient wing strokes for sustained flight. Both hibernating and migratory bats have developed life histories, which allow them to increase fat store prior to hibernation, and thus rely on abundant steady food supplies during certain times of the year.[38] Hibernating bats undergo profound physiologic alterations during hibernation, which result in decreased metabolism, body temperature, and modulation of the immune system. Having an abundant food supply available after hibernation is essential for the survival of these bats.[38]

The diets and sizes of modern bats are as diverse as their habitats. At one end of the size spectrum is the Kitti's hog-nosed bat (*Craseonycteris thonglongyai*). This bat may be the world's smallest mammal, with a length of 29 to 33 millimeters (mm) and weighing a mere 2 to 2.6 grams (g).[52,67] Also known as the *bumblebee bat*, it is native to the limestone caves in a small riparian area of Thailand and Burma. At the other end of the spectrum is the giant golden-crowned flying fox (*Acerodon jubatus*), which weighs 1.1 to 1.2 kilograms (kg). Unlike the insectivorous bumblebee bat, this bat is widely prevalent through the Filipino rainforests, where it feeds primarily on figs. Both the flying fox and the bumblebee bat rely heavily on their unique environments, and both are threatened by deforestation and other anthropogenic alterations to their habitats.[52,67]

Approximately 70% of known Chiroptera are insectivorous, and most of the other species are fruit eaters. Insectivorous bats may either hunt their prey on the wing or glean insects from plants.[38,52,67] This distinction becomes important during attempts to get an insectivorous species to adapt to a captive diet. More species with specialized diets include picivorous bats such as the fish-eating myotis (*Myotis vivesi*) and the greater bulldog (*Noctilio leporinus*) bat. The highly specialized vampire bats, including the hairy-legged vampire bat (*Diphylla ecaudata*), white-winged vampire bat (*Diamus youngi*), and the common vampire bat (*Desmodus rotundus*), are hematophagous and are the only known mammals that are obligate parasites.[38] Fruit-eating bats may limit their diets to a small number of fruits, whereas others are more generalized feeders.[38] When designing plans for conservation or for sustaining bats in captivity, it is essential that the normal wild feeding habits of each species be understood so as to provide the proper diet and feeding opportunities.

HANDLING, CAPTIVE MANAGEMENT, AND DIET

Handling of Bats

Regardless of size, bats have the potential to cause injury to handlers. All species of bats have sharp teeth, and many have sharp claws. The degree of physical damage that can be inflicted does depend on the size of the animal, so the extent of personal protective gear depends on the species. At the very least, sturdy, bite-resistant gloves should be worn while handling these animals. Moreover, bats have the potential to spread a variety of zoonotic diseases. The classic bat-associated disease is rabies, but other diseases can also be transmitted. Lysaviruses, filoviruses, and various fungi and bacteria can be potentially spread to humans from bats. Individuals working with bats should know the risks posed by the species in question and should be vaccinated for rabies virus and have their antibody titers checked regularly.

Besides wearing gloves, other precautions include proper training to prevent bites and scratches and wearing personal protective equipment to prevent exposure to aerosols, urine, and feces. These might include goggles, face shields, or both, moisture resistant clothing, and boots that can be washed and disinfected. Individuals performing medical procedures or postmortem examinations on bats should take precautions to avoid needlesticks and ensure that all medical waste, sharps, and equipment are properly disposed of.

Care should also be taken to avoid injuring the bat during handling. Respiratory function of small bats can be compromised by excessive pressure on the chest or neck. The wings of all bats should be cared for during handling. This includes ensuring that the wings are properly immobilized to prevent fractures and that the wing membranes are protected, as these can be torn and may expose the animal to infection and possibly prevent proper mobility.

Proper biosecurity should also be observed when handling both free-ranging and captive bats. In captivity, care must be taken to avoid exposing bats to potentially infectious material from other captive species or having them come in contact with free-ranging bats or other wildlife. In the wild, equipment should be disinfected between visits to different habitats and even between individual bats if infectious diseases are a concern. Biosecurity during fieldwork has become an important part of the management strategy during outbreaks of WNS in North America and is one way officials are trying to prevent the spread of the associated fungus.

Management of Megachiroptera

Megachiroptera are a familiar part of many zoologic collections as popular inhabitants of nocturnal displays. Species such as Egyptian fruit bats are often housed in groups, and their unique appearance and active behaviors make them attractive to the public. Even the larger, more solitary flying foxes may be found in some of the more complete rainforest displays. Despite the fact that these animals are frequently housed in captivity, much needs to be learned about proper husbandry of these animals. What is known is that the husbandry and dietary needs of Megachiroptera are as diverse as the species involved. Thus, a full description of the needs of each species is beyond the scope of this chapter. Moreover, the regulations for housing these animals are also diverse and dependent on government regulations and the type of facility in which the bats are kept. Prior to housing any animals, local regulations governing the maintenance of animals in the facility should be consulted.

In general, as with many nondomestic animals, captive management should be guided by knowledge of the natural history of the species in the wild as well as modifications to account for the captive environment. Factors to consider include the optimal stocking density for a given enclosure, natural photoperiod of the animal, diet and feeding schedule, natural temperature ranges, size of the animal, and cleaning needs of the exhibit.

Providing adequate room for the animals to fly is a major consideration. Not only do bats need facilities that allow flight, they must also be housed in facilities from where they cannot easily escape when personnel need access to feed or clean the exhibit. Safety features such as double doors are highly recommended. Although the ability to provide enough room for sustained flight might be limited by the size of the animal, they should be able to spread their wings and move about the enclosure. Care should be taken to ensure that the animals have enough room to avoid damaging their wing membranes or bones. Species that are known climbers should be provided with branches and other materials on which to climb or suspend themselves. The animals often rest in an inverted position, so they should have enough room to do so without their heads, ears, or edges of the wings contacting substrates, as this might cause trauma that could result in open wounds susceptible to infection.[27,28]

With regard to temperature and humidity, no hard and fast rules exist for the temperature at which an enclosure should be maintained. Many bats may withstand a wide range of temperatures and humidities, but efforts should be made to ensure a constant range, as many of these species are tropical and may not be able to tolerate low temperatures or low humidity for sustained periods. Temperatures between 18° C and 27° C are reported as being adequate, but this may vary with species.[27,28]

Dietary requirements are also diverse. Flying foxes prefer sweet, soft fruits and may be maintained on such foods supplemented with vitamins, bone meal, and milk replacer. However, the actual dietary requirements of many captive species are unclear. The American Zoo and Aquarium Association Chiropteran Taxon Advisory Group provides guidelines for the nutrient and mineral content of fruit bat diet, and many captive colonies of fruit bats thrive on diets based on these guidelines.[19] Nonetheless, more data on nutrient intake and utilization are required to further refine the nutritional recommendations for captive fruit bats and establish the suitability of these recommendations for different species.

Several studies have examined captive diets and have focused on determining if what the bats consume provides the recommended amount of nutrients. Importantly, predicted dietary values and actual dietary values may differ. Specifically, vitamins A and E and cascium (Ca) concentrations have been found to be lower in the actual diet than would be predicted on the basis of the ingredients. Similarly, trace mineral concentrations of phosphorus (P), magnesium (Mg), and zinc (Zn) tend to be higher in left-over food than in the original diet and tend to be high in feces. This discrepancy suggests some dietary selection by the animals or that the animals are obtaining these elements from alternative sources such as from the galvanized materials in enclosures.[23] Maintaining an overall healthy balance of the levels of vitamins in the diet is important, as complex interaction between compounds may affect the absorption and excretion of other nutrients. Deficiencies or excesses have been associated with the development of disease. Vitamin E deficiency has been associated with cardiomyopathy and excess flouride with a syndrome of hyperostosis.[23,25]

As with many frugivores, excess iron in the diet of fruit-eating bats may result in hepatic disease. When tissues levels of iron become high enough, hepatocytes are damaged, leading to hepatic necrosis and scarring of the liver in more chronic situations.[23] This propensity to develop both hepatic hemosiderosis and hemochromatosis likely relates to the relative paucity of available iron in the diets of free-ranging animals. Frugivorous bats may particularly absorb iron efficiently, which leads to excessive absorption when iron levels are high. The regulation of iron levels is complex and is mediated not only by dietary levels but by interactions with other nutrients. High concentrations of vitamin C enhance the absorption of iron

and may potentiate free radical damage to tissues.[25] Furthermore, other dietary constituents found in the wild and not in captivity may serve to mediate iron availability. Tannins, calcium phosphate, egg yolk, and bran may inhibit iron absorption. Ferrous iron itself is transported across enterocyte membranes to the cytoplasm by divalent metal transporter 1 (DMT1). DMT1 may also transport other metal ions such as cobalt, lead, zinc, cadmium, and copper. The presence of these ions in some cases may upregulate DMT1 and thus secondarily lead to increased iron transport. Alternatively, the presence of these metals may competitively inhibit ferrous ion transport.[23,25,40]

Monitoring and treatment of iron storage disease is an important aspect of captive management of frugivorous bats. Although histopathology is the gold standard for the diagnosis of hemochromatosis, less invasive methods such as use of blood parameters may also be used to monitor the development of iron storage disease. Surprisingly, despite the hepatic damage caused by iron accumulation, aspartate aminotransferase (AST) and alanine aminotransferase (ALT) are not useful in detecting iron-induced liver damage. Farina (2005) studied the correlation of various blood parameters to histologic grade of iron deposition and damage in two species of fruit bat, the Egyptian fruit bat (*Rousettus aegyptiacus*), and the island flying fox (*Pteropus hypomelanus*).[25] Serum iron, transferrin saturation, and plasma ferritin showed positive correlation with morphologic hepatic iron concentration.[25] If the product of the serum iron level and the transferrin saturation exceeded 51, the bats had a high probability of iron overload. Products greater than 90 indicated a high probability of hemochromatosis. It has yet to be fully determined if these techniques may be used to monitor efficacy of treatment for iron overload.[25]

Management of iron overload begins with feeding low-iron diets and managing the levels of other vitamins and factors such as vitamin C that may enhance iron absorption. Unfortunately, maintaining low levels of vitamin C in a diet based on fresh fruit is difficult. Treatment for iron overload may also include addition of dietary chelators, phlebotomy, and in some cases an injectable chelator such as deferoxamine mesylate. Addition of even a small amount of tannic acid to the diet has been shown to reduce the absorption of iron up to 40% in captive straw-colored fruit bats (*Eidolon helvum*).[40] However, as noted by Farina, tannins may be bitter and unpalatable and may not be accepted by all individuals.[25]

Management of Microchiroptera

Like Megachiroptera, Microchiroptera species have widely variable habitats, natural histories, and nutritional needs. Compared with fruit bats, these animals are more rarely kept in captivity. Thus, knowledge of proper environmental and dietary management is scant. Depending on the natural habitat of the animal, needs for temperature, photoperiod, and humidity may vary widely.[38] Many species may actively alter their body temperature and lower their metabolic rate, even to their own detriment, if ambient conditions are suboptimal.[2,11] Thus, when housing these animals, it is advisable to provide them with a range of conditions to allow them to choose their own optimal microenvironment.[27,28] As with Megachiroptera, Microchiroptera species rest by hanging by their feet. Thus, areas rough enough for them to grasp must be provided, but care must be taken that the caging material is not so rough that it causes injury to the animals. In some research settings, bats are provided with strips of cloth, and cloth bags are hung along the edges of the habitat to provide rest areas. Whatever is provided, it must be possible to clean it adequately (Buckles, personal observation).

In some situations, inducing hibernation or torpor may be required. This may be a difficult endeavor. Some facilities have successfully housed hibernating bats in refrigerated enclosures. It is important to maintain proper humidity in these enclosures, as cold dry air may cause the bats to rapidly dehydrate. Improper humidity may also allow the bats' wings to be infected by *Pseudomonas* and other bacterial species, causing death from sepsis or toxemia (Buckles, personal observation). Before attempting to have these animals hibernate in captivity, it is best to contact someone with previous experience for advice on the particular situation to maximize the survivability of the bats.

Diet also presents a challenge in these species. Many of the Microchiroptera species are insectivorous, and in the wild, they catch food while in flight. Other insectivorous bats may pick food off a substrate. Adapting any insectivorous bat to a captive diet may require individual attention to each animal to ensure proper food intake.[27,28] Some failures to adapt could be related to the fact that the movements of mealworms do not stimulate the natural prey recognition response. In one study, bats were more prone to accept food if artificial wings, mimicking the flapping frequency of the natural prey items were added to mealworms.[17]

Both obesity and starvation have been reported in captive insectivorous bats. In most cases, animals are fed diets consisting of artificially raised mealworm larvae. Since insectivorous bats will not accept supplementation with commercially available, nutritionally balanced diets, they are limited to this single source of food. The diets of free-ranging bats are composed of a much wider array of insects than is available in captivity and thus provide a more balanced and complete food source.[17] The captive diets may be low in calcium and high in phosphorous. Nutrition may be improved if the insects being raised as a food source are placed on a mineral premix at least 24 hours before feeding them to the bats. In one dietary study, bone densities of captive mustached bats (*Pteronotus parnelli rubiginosis*), an insectivorous species from South America, maintained on unsupplemented insects were examined. The skulls of the captive animals were soft on palpation, and bone density was significantly lower than in free-ranging individuals.[17] Once the mealworms were supplemented with calcium, the bone density of the animals increased, and no statistical difference between the bone density of captive animals fed calcium-supplemented mealworms and their free-ranging counterparts was observed.[17]

Even when on a calcium-supplemented diet, the captive animals tended to have less body mass compared with free-ranging bats. However, within the study group, some animals had significantly higher body weights than did other individuals. It is possible that some individuals adapt better to the captive lifestyle and monopolize the food supply. This in itself may present a problem, since mealworms are innately higher in fat than most insects, placing well-adapted animals at risk for obesity.[17]

Maintaining proper fat metabolism is particularly important in hibernating bats, as the fat depots laid down prior to entering hibernacula are their sole source of energy during this period. Alterations in fat metabolism during hibernation may lead to bats having insufficient energy to survive.[10] Alternatively, altered fat mobilization caused by hibernation may also cause abnormal metabolism and deposition of lipid within hepatocytes, renal tubular epithelial cells, and myocardial cells. Such systemic lipidosis has been documented in greater horseshoe bats (*Rhinolophus ferrumequinum*) dying after transport during hibernation.[31] Additionally, the female's reproductive cycles are suppressed during hibernation by interactions of circulating leptin, insulin-like receptor, and insulin levels. This affects the amount of stored body fat, and changes in the normal lipid or hormonal environment may have adverse effects on the reproductive capability of bats after emergence from hibernation.[61]

DISEASES OF CHIROPTERA

Little is known about pathologic conditions in either Megachiroptera or Microchiroptera. Reports of disease are sporadic, and a great deal of the literature comprises surveys of wild animals that focus on pathogens of significance to human health rather than on disease states of the bats themselves. Sporadic, often anecdotal, reports of unexplained die-offs in fruit bats have been published. These include mortality events in Pacific flying foxes (*Pteropus mariannus*) in Micronesia, a mass mortality of insular flying foxes (*P. tonganus*) in Fiji, and die-offs of unspecified species of fruit bats on the Admiralty and

Solomon Islands. No investigations were conducted as to the cause of these events, but in some cases, these die-offs coincided with outbreaks of infectious diseases such as measles in the local human population. In other cases, introduction of disease by domestic animals was suspected.[38]

Until the emergence of WNS in North America, reports of mass mortalities in Microchiroptera were rare and often attributed to rabies. In the mid-1980s, a thousand dead bats of various species, including *Myotis* spp. and *Lassarius* spp. were found dead in a Canadian lake along with dozens of dead mallards. The animals were in generally good health, and after laboratory tests confirmed the presence of toxic alkaloids, the deaths were attributed to blue-green algae toxicosis, as the algae was found covering the carcasses and in the water.[55] Other causes of significant mortality have been related to barotrauma around wind farms because of bats being unable to navigate successfully past windmills.[51]

A particularly complete evaluation of causes of mortality of German bats has been published.[48] Various bacterial infections, traumatic injuries, and parasitic infections, as well as physiologic diseases such as hypertension, were documented in this study. Additional studies correlated disease development with the physiology and ecology of the various bat species.[48]

Parasitic Infections

Reports of fatal parasitic diseases are rare. However, anyone who has handled free-ranging bats knows that they often are infested with a variety of ectoparasites. In North America, ectoparasites include *Myodopsylla insignnis*, *Spinturnix americanus*, *Cimex adjunctus*, *Macronyssu scrosbyi*, and *Adndrolaelab scasalis*. The number of parasites on a bat may vary with roost size, energy status, and grooming efficacy.[20] Ectoparasites have been reported on captive fruit bats, particularly those that have been recently captured. *Demodex* sp. have been documented in captive Egyptian fruit bats (*R. aegyptiacus*) as an incidental finding. A single wild-caught Egyptian fruit bat (*Rousettus aegyptiacus leachi*) was reported to be infected with a single *Eucampsipoda africana*, a nycteribiid ectoparasite.[53]

Although some ectoparasites do feed on blood, bats appear to be unaffected, and most infestations are self-limiting. This self-limiting nature is likely the immune response. Experimental studies of Serotine bats (*Eptesicus serotinus*) demonstrate that the bats develop a significant inflammatory response after the attachment of bat tick (*Argas vespertilionis*). The initial response consists of neutrophils followed by eosinophils and basophils and centers around the tick's mouth parts. Adenosine triphosphatase (ATPase)–positive cells, presumed to be Langerhans cells, are frequently present in the lesions, and epithelial cell proliferation occurs into the tick mouthparts. It is presumed that this cellular and enzymatic environment is not suitable for the ticks and results in resistance to infection.[21]

A few surveys of wild populations have documented various blood parasites and flagellates. Schizotrypanum has been found in Kuhl's pipistrelles (*Pipistrellus kuhli*). A trypanosome in the subgenus Megatrypanum and a parasite consistent with *Herpetosoma* has been found in naked-rumped tomb bats (*Taphozous nudiventris*).[42] In one study, 16 bats incidentally caught in mist nets meant for birds in Zambia were examined, and 37.5% of these Gambian epauled fruit bats (*Epomophorus gambianus*) were infected with *Hepatocystis epomophori*, a hematozoan parasite.[53]

Endoparasites are found incidentally in Microchiroptera. Digenean flukes, ascarids, cestodes, and coccidia are common intestinal inhabitants (Figure 35-1).[24,41] Renal coccidia are sometimes encountered incidentally on histology.

Some reports of parasite related mortality have been published. Two captive juvenile flying foxes appear to have died because of aberrant migration of the nematode *Toxocara pteropodis*. This nematode is a frequent intestinal parasite of flying foxes (genus Pteropus) inhabiting Oceania and southeastern Asia.[54] Nematodes mature in the intestines of suckling bats, but the animals clear the infection by the time of weaning. Adult bats ingest the eggs and third-stage larvae hatch and migrate to the liver and, in females, to the mammary gland

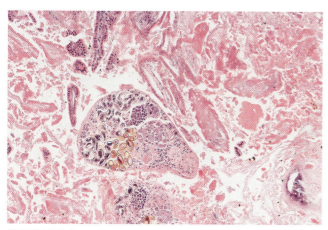

FIGURE 35-1 Photomicrograph showing a Digean fluke in the intestine of a little brown bat (*Myotis lucifugus*). Note the brown, operculated eggs and the lack of inflammatory response to the parasite.

where they are passed to the neonates. Infection is common with approximately 50% of juvenile gray-headed flying foxes (*P. poliocephalus*) in eastern Australia having patent infections. Infected bats do not usually appear ill. Both the reported fatal cases occurred in spectacled flying foxes (*P. conspicillatus*) that had recently been brought into captivity.[54] Both died acutely between 3 and 8 days of capture. In the first, an adult male parasite was found in the gallbladder; in the second, a parasite was found extending from the laryngopharynx into the esophagus.[54]

Another parasite-related mortality occurred in a captive Egyptian fruit bat infected with *Ecephalitozoon hellum*.[15] This was the first report of this disease in a bat. Gross lesions were minimal and consisted of poor body condition, renomegaly, and a mottled liver. Histologically, inflammation was associated with intracytoplasmic microsporidian spores. Lesions were particularly prominent in the urogenital tract and the liver. It is unknown how this bat acquired the infection, but exposure may have occurred because of the proximity of the bat exhibit to an aviary, as microsporidians are known to be passed via bird feces.[15]

Evidence suggests that bats can develop *Angiostrongylus* neuroinfection as the parasite has been detected in black- and gray-headed fruit bats (*Pteropus* spp.) with neurologic disease. Bats developed paresis and eosinophilic and granulomatous reactions to fifth-stage larvae. The clinical syndrome caused by the parasite is indistinguishable from clinical lyssaviral infection.[5]

Bacterial Infections

Numerous scattered cases of bacteria being isolated from a wide variety of bat species have been reported. As with the parasites, many of these published accounts have been the results of population surveys with little or no attempt to identify clinical disease in the bats. Moreover, in some early studies, the species of bat from which the bacteria were isolated was not recorded. Nonetheless, bats do harbor a wide variety of potentially pathogenic bacteria, including *Leptospira, Borrelia, Salmonella, Shigella, Escherichia, Enterobacter, Citrobacter, Proteus, Alcaligenes, Pseudomonas, Pasteurella, Clostridium* bacteroides, *Mycobacterium, Staphylococcus,* and *Yersinia*.[43] In a survey of multiple bat species in Kenya, *Bartonella* spp. were cultured from straw-colored fruit bats (*E. helvum*), Egyptian fruit bats (*R. aegyptiacus*), and long-fingered fruit bats (*Minopterus* sp.).[4] Similarly, a diverse array of *Bartonella* spp. was detected in blood from a variety of Chiroptera species in Guatemala. Isolates were obtained from both Megachiroptera and Microchiroptera, including the common vampire bat (*Desmodus rotundus*).[4]

In one of the more comprehensive pathologic evaluations of mortality of bats in Germany, 500 vespertilionid bats were examined.

Inflammatory lesions associated with bacteria were present in over half the bats. Pneumonia was common, and 22 bacterial species were associated with various lesions.[50] These included *Pasteurella, Enterococcus,* and *Clostridium* species.[50] High genetic diversity in the strains of *P. multocida* found in these bats suggests that some infections did not originate from bats and may have been acquired through cat bites.[49]

A *Pasturella*-like organism has been found in various fruit bats, including two captive epauletted fruit bats (*Epomophorus wahlbergi*). Disease developed just after their release from 30-day quarantine.[35] One bat exhibited no clinical signs, and the other was noted to be anorexic and lethargic just prior to death. Hematology revealed multiple hemogram abnormalities, including a degenerative left shift, in one animal. Postmortem examination demonstrated bite wounds on the wings and ears of one animal and severe necrotizing unilateral pneumonia in both individuals. In one animal, an additional suppurative esophagitis, epicarditis, and an intermandibular abscess were seen. A third bat in the collection developed weight loss, lethargy, anorexia, and pleural effusion. Pulmonary lesions were noted on radiography. *Pasturella*-like organisms and toxic neutrophils were detected on tracheal wash. The animal died, and necropsy revealed multiple inflammatory nodules in the lungs and pleuritis.[35]

The same *Pasturella*-type organism was isolated from subcutaneous abscesses in two little golden-mantled flying foxes (*Pteropus pumilus*) that had been housed with a Wahlberg's epauletted fruit bat (*E. wahlbergi*), in another bat with wing fractures and subcutaneous abscesses, and in a large flying fox (*Pteropus vampyrus*) with radiographic signs of pneumonia. This last animal was treated initially with enrofloxacin but subsequently developed *Staphylococcus aureus* bronchopneumonia and died despite treatment with trimethoprim sulfa. The collection was screened, and the organism was isolated from the pharyngeal swabs of Wahlberg's epauletted fruit bats (*E. wahlbergi*), large flying foxes (*P. vampyris*), island flying foxes (*Pteropus hypomelanus*), and Rodrigues fruit bats (*P. rodricensis*).[35]

One of the more significant reports of bacterial disease in bats involves infection with *Yersinia pseudotuberculosis*. This bacterial disease presented as respiratory and skin infections in a closed colony of Egyptian fruit bats (*R. aegyptiacus*).[16] Initially, 6 of 125 animals died over a 6-week period, and 4 additional bats were euthanized because of poor clinical condition. *Y. pseudotuberculosis* was cultured from 7 of these animals. Of these bats, 2 had acute disease, with sepsis, multi-organ failure, rapid progression, and death. The other 8 exhibited a more chronic disease course, with necrotizing abscesses in multiple organs, especially the liver, spleen, and mesenteric lymph nodes. Subsequently, 12 animals were euthanized to survey the colony. At postmortem, 41.7% of the animals had abscesses in multiple organs. These data, indicating widespread asymptomatic disease, led to the depopulation of the colony.[16] Necropsies revealed that 70% of the bats had gross lesions of lymphadenopathy, hepatic abscesses, and splenomegaly consistent with *Y. pseudotuberculosis*. Histologic lesions ranged from mild, suggestive of sepsis, to severe necrotizing inflammation associated with gram-negative bacteria. The cause of this outbreak was not clear; however, necropsies did reveal some previously undetected diseases in the colony, including an unspecified species of *Demodex Mycobacterium avium* and *Microsporidium hellum*.[40] The disease outbreak began when the population density approached 0.1 bats per cubic foot, and thus population density may have been a factor in the outbreak.[16]

The significance of other bacteria is less clear. A survey of over 2000 bats in Columbia revealed *Salmonella* in asymptomatic Pallas's mastiff bats (*Molossus molossus*), greater fruit-eating bats (*Artibeus lituratus*), and little yellow-shouldered bats (*Sturnira lilium*). *Shigella boydii* has been found in a Bonda mastiff bat (*Molossus bondae*). No associated disease was noted.[3]

Neoplasia

Reports of neoplasia in bats are rare. However, as necropsies are performed on older captive individuals, this may change, as additional cases are documented. In Microchiroptera, neoplasms, including lymphoma in a pallid bat (*Antrozeious pallidus*), subcutaneous leiomyosarcoma in a Townsend's big-eared bat (*Corynorhinus townsendii*), and biliary carcinoma in a pallid bat (*Antrozeious pallidus*), have been reported.[6,12] The lymphoma involved multiple organs and did not seem to be related to retroviral infection.[2] The bat with the biliary carcinoma exhibited nonspecific clinical signs the day before death, and at necropsy, the infiltrative mass primarily affected the left lobe of the liver. Histologically, the mass was composed of irregular ducts lined by cuboidal epithelial cells along with abundant mucin. Multiple metastases were present in the lung. In addition, dilatation of the gastric and esophageal lymphatics and veins with hemorrhage suggested portal hypertension with formation of esophageal varices, common sequelae to this neoplasm in humans.[6]

Several cases of leiomyosarcoma have been reported in Megachiroptera. One was found in the duodenum and extended throughout the abdominal cavity to involve the kidney, stomach, and pancreas of an Egyptian fruit bat (*R. aegyptiacus*). Another was found in the uterus of a Seba's short-tailed bat (*Carollia perspiculatta*), and still another was found in association with a subcutaneous microchip in an Egyptian fruit bat. In the latter case, the neoplasm invaded the dorsal musculature, extended through the diaphragm and liver, and formed small nodules scattered throughout the peritoneal cavity.[60] The widespread metastasis was unusual for a leiomyosarcoma but has been reported in domestic animals.

A more obscure neoplasm has also been reported in an Egyptian fruit bat (*R. aegyptiacus*). The animal was found hypothermic and dyspneic, with tight abdominal musculature. Imaging revealed abdominal fluid, and despite supportive care and abdominocentesis, the animal died. Gross necropsy findings included poor body condition, dehydration, muscular atrophy, and a solid, light-colored mass adherent to the heart and adjacent lung. Histologically, the neoplastic cells were variably immunoreactive for both vimentin and cytokeratin, leading to a diagnosis of sarcomatoid carcinoma.[44] These are rare neoplasms in humans, and very few are diagnosed in veterinary species.[44]

Fungal Diseases—White Nose Syndrome

It is the emergence of a newly described fungal disease that has transformed our understanding of pathogenesis of diseases in Microchiroptera. Until the first cases of WNS were detected in upstate New York, reports of mortality in Microchiroptera were rare. However, WNS has been responsible for the death of over 80% of the bats in some locations, and estimates indicate that the little brown bat, once the most populous bat in North America, could become extinct from the lower 48 states if the mortality trend continues.[29] Researchers during the early stages of the outbreak reported hibernacula floors being covered in dead bats and the carcasses of some animals still clinging to the walls. Sick bats often left hibernation early, only to die in the cold and snow of the winter climate (Buckles, personal communication).

The causative agent of WNS, *Pseudogymnoascus destructans*, is a newly described cold-loving fungus, which thrives at temperatures between 4° C and 10° C, which explains why the disease targets hibernating bats.[8] The fungus forms distinctive white colonies in culture and on the live bats. The conidia of *G. destructans* are sickle shaped and are pathognomonic for infection with *G. destructans*.[45] Despite the emphasis on fungal infections of the nasal planum, wings are often the most involved areas of skin (Buckles, personal observation). Even if the bats survive infection during hibernation, often scars or defects persist in the wings. In some cases, these wounds are incidental, and in others, they may decrease survivability.[57]

Experimentally, *G. destructans* has been shown to be transmissible to healthy bats, and the distinctive lesions of WNS have been reproduced experimentally.[65] These lesions include surface infection, with the fungus progressing to cuplike invaginations of fungal colonies into the dermis and ultimately to invasion of the tissue by fungal hyphae (Figure 35-2). Little or no inflammation is associated with

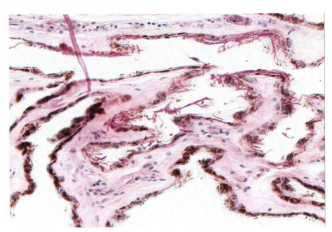

FIGURE 35-2 Photomicrograph of a periodic acid-Schiff stain of *Pseudogymnoascus destructans* infecting the wing of a little brown bat (*Myotis lucifugus*). Hyphae are present on the surface, form small cuplike invaginations, and invade the dermis. Characteristic conidia are present along the surface of the tissue.

the fungal infection.[45] This may be the result of fungal factors or immune downregulation that occurs during hibernation.[13] Bats with WNS arouse frequently from hibernation, which depletes the fat depots essential for winter survival, and affected bats are often depleted of fat stores by late winter[65] (Buckles, personal observation).

The reason for this sudden emergence of a new disease in North American Microchiroptera is unknown. Recent evidence has shown that European bats are infected with *G. destructans* but exhibit little or no mortality.[65] It appears that the North American outbreak is caused by the introduction of the European strains of the fungus into hibernacula and into naive bat populations.[65]

It is hard to overstate the decimation this disease has caused to North American bats, and the enzootic shows no signs of abating. Since detection in New York, WNS has been reported increasingly in a number of states and in Canada (http://whitenosesyndrome.org/). Each time, the appearance of the disease results in the same high mortality rate. The effect that the disease has on the reproductive capacity of those few bats that survive is a focus of current investigation. Current evidence indicates extreme depletions of bat pup numbers in once-healthy maternity colonies (Buckles, personal observation).

Techniques to manage the spread of WNS have been hard to determine. Proposals include providing bats with warm areas in hibernacula, in which they may feed and groom to remove the fungus, and culling of affected bats.[11,32] It appears that if bats are aroused and removed from hibernacula, they may recover from the disease. In one study, bats were removed from the wild, made to emerge from hibernation, and provided with food. In these animals, the *G. destructans* infection was cleared.[46] Although captive treatment of endangered bats may be possible, removal of large numbers of bats from the environment is not feasible. Moreover, *G. destructans* produces large numbers of conidia that contaminate any environment into which bats would be released. To date, no evidence indicates that bats surviving *G. destructans* infection develop sustained immunity to the fungus.

Toxic and Metabolic Diseases

Because many species of Megachiroptera tend to come into human areas, exposure to anthropogenic toxins is always a risk. Two gray-headed fruit bats (*Pteropus poliocephalus*) have been reported to die of lead poisoning.[62] They were found moribund in a suburban back yard. One was in poor body condition and exhibited muscle fasciculation, excess salivation, diarrhea, and ataxia. The second bat was found unable to fly but otherwise normal. It died prior to full veterinary examination. At necropsy, one bat had scattered areas of suppurative bronchopneumonia, and both bats had perivascular hemorrhages in the brain. Intranuclear, eosinophilc, acid-fast inclusion bodies were detected in the kidneys of both bats, and ultrastructural studies showed them to be consistent with lead. In the first bat, lead levels were 20.5 milligrams per kilogram (mg/kg) in the kidney and 59.5 mg/kg in the liver. In the second bat, the levels were 44.6 and 18.7 mg/kg, respectively. The source of lead was unclear, as no metallic lead was found in the bodies. Lead arsenate used by some fruit growers in the area was considered a possible lead source, but this was never proven.[62]

An alopecia syndrome has been reported in four species of fruit bats in Tabasco, Mexico. Affected species include the Jamaican fruit bat (*Artibeus jamaicensis*), the great fruit-eating bat (*A. lituratus*), the little yellow-shouldered bat (*Sturnira lilium*), and the highland yellow-shouldered bat (*S. ludovici*). The hair loss affects areas of the chest, with the highest prevalence of the syndrome being during the dry season in urban areas.[7] Histologically, the affected skin has decreased numbers of hair follicles but no inflammation and no evidence of an infectious etiology. The cause of the syndrome is unclear. Prevalence in urban areas suggests anthropogenic factors. Since more females than males are affected, it may also relate to seasonal feeding and reproductive cycles. Alopecia has been reported sporadically in captive bats and has been attributed to endocrinopathies.[7]

In one of the few reports on drug toxicity, several dog-faced fruit bats (*Cynopterus bachyotis*) developed generalized paralysis after administration of topical ivermectin. The dose of ivermectin given was 1.4 to 1.8 mg/kg. Typical absorption rates in other animals result in a dose of 9 to 12 micrograms per kilogram (μg/kg); so the dose in bats was well within the safe dosage range.[22] The animals that developed clinical signs all died, and postmortem examinations revealed mild to moderate acute renal tubular necrosis, with evidence of regeneration. One bat had a proliferative glomerulonephritis and tubular proteinosis, as well hemorrhagic gastroenteritis. Another had suppurative bronchopneumonia. Not all of the treated bats developed disease, and it is is unclear why some were spared while others were not. Toxicity may be related to the area on which the drug was applied. If the doses were applied in areas of frequent grooming, some drug may have been ingested. Variations in the ability of individuals to metabolize the ivermectin may also be a factor. The reason for the renal lesion is unclear. Similar lesions are seen in humans with ivermectin toxicity, but in humans, they have been linked to factors induced by the death of the parasites.[22]

PUBLIC HEALTH SIGNIFICANCE

With the exception of rabies, no largescale or consistent disease spillover is proven for bats. However, changes in land use patterns, encroachment of humans into previously uninhabited areas, and alterations in climate are increasing the probability of human–bat interactions. Such changes may be at least partly to blame for an increased incidence of vampire bat bites in humans living in areas along the Amazon. In light of changing environmental conditions, bats could serve to maintain pathogens in the environment at low levels, and increased interactions with humans may lead to new opportunities for zoonotic spread.

Rabies and Lyssaviruses

No disease is more associated with bats than rabies is. This invariably fatal neurologic disease is caused by members of the family Rhabdoviridae. Both classic rabies virus and the related lyssaviruses cause fatal disease that is clinically identical to encephalitic disease. Rabies virus is primarily found in New World bats, whereas lyssavirus species are found in Old World bats.[69] Infection occurs primarily through bite wounds, but any wound that results in exposure to infected saliva, tissue, or cerebrospinal fluid may transmit the viruses.

Despite their negative reputation, bats are responsible for only one or two direct bat-to-human rabies transmissions each year in the United States. However, bats may also transmit rabies to wild animals, domestic pets, and livestock. In fact, although most human cases of rabies virus exposure in North America involve bat variants of the rabies virus, actual exposure occurs indirectly through other animals such as livestock or wild carnivores.[37,59] In other areas of the world, particularly where vampire bats come into contact with humans, exposure to bat rabies is more likely to be caused by direct bat-to-human contact.[1]

The actual prevalence of rabies virus infection in bats is unclear. Many studies base prevalence estimates on the numbers of bats testing positive at diagnostic laboratories. Often these animals are tested because of abnormal behavior, which has led to a biased study sample. Under these circumstances, rabies prevalence in some studies is as high as 20.1%.[37] Estimates of rabies prevalence decrease substantially when the sample population is more random. A survey of 1114 silver-haired bats (*Lasionycteris noctivagans*) and hoary bats (*Lasiurus cineresus*) randomly killed at wind farms, resulted in an estimated rabies virus prevalence of only 0% to 1%.[37]

In North America, several of insectivorous bats act as rabies virus reservoirs. The virus is most prevalent in bats that live in large groups, and this increases the probability of bat-to-bat transmission. Serosurveys support the theory that some animals become immune to infection as rabies exposure in bat populations is more prevalent than active rabies. One study conducted in big brown bats (*Eptesicus fuscus*) and little brown bats (*Myotis lucifugus*) showed that active rabies infection in each population was 3% and 0.3%, respectively, whereas seroprevalence was 10% and 20%, respectively.[59] Some individuals in a population appear to develop resistance to the virus, some seroconvert after exposure but do not develop disease, and others may die. In studies on big brown bats, healthy bats were found to have been bitten by known rabid bats and did not develop disease. Other bats in the study were seropositive for rabies virus but did not develop disease. It is theorized that bats may develop a protective antibody response to rabies virus as a result of repeated exposure.[63]

Less is known about the natural history of lyssaviruses. As with rabies virus, exposure to lyssaviruses is common in bats, estimated by some to be 60% to 70%, but the actual risk this poses to humans is not fully understood. Old World bats are reservoirs for 10 of the 11 known lyssaviruses; these include Australian bat lyssavirus, Lagos bat virus, West Caucasian bat virus, and Khujand virus. Countries designated as "rabies free" may have endemic lyssaviruses and have in place control measures similar to those for rabies.[47]

Lyssaviruses appear to be transmitted through bite wounds, and cases of fatal bat-to-human transmission have been documented. The resultant disease in humans is indistinguishable from that produced by the rabies virus, and accurate diagnosis is difficult. The incubation period for development of disease in humans is unknown, and a case of a woman dying of Australian bat lyssavirus encephalitis 2 years after a reported exposure has been reported.[14]

Current control of rabies virus is accomplished by preventive vaccination and post-exposure treatments of humans and animals. In Latin America, where vampire bat (*Desmodus rontundus*) exposure is of particular concern, bat control measures are being explored. Anticoagulants placed on the backs of bats are spread in colonies through allogrooming, which results in hemorrhage and the death of the bat.[1] Although promising, this is a controversial practice, and less lethal measures such as topical administration of vaccines are being researched. Similar to the principle of anticoagulant use, the vaccine is disseminated within the colony through grooming, and vaccine-related mortality is low. Further research is needed to determine if this method will work as a long-term strategy for controlling rabies in wild populations.[1]

Other Potential Zoonoses

Documenting a pathogen in a bat and proving that it may be passed to humans are two different things. Bats are known to harbor a variety of zoonotic bacteria, viruses, and parasites. At least 66 have been detected in bat tissues, and bats probably have a role in the propagation of these organisms.[40] These include rabies, Nipah, Hendra, and severe acute respiratory syndrome (SARS) viruses, which are threats to human health.[14] However, despite this, ungulates, carnivores, birds, and primates are more important sources of zoonoses than are bats.[68] This does not mean that the threat is not serious. Characteristics in the life history of bats certainly favor disease transmission. Some species of bat may live up to 30 years, allowing infectious agents to persist in a population for many years. Flight allows them to spread disease over long distances. Some bats have been shown to wander as much as 393 km in a year.[38]

Flying foxes are of particular interest as vectors because of their propensity to disperse over a large territory and to live in urban areas. Tioman virus, a paramyxovirus isolated from fruit bats (*Pteropus* spp) in Malaysia, is of unknown public health importance, but a correlation may exist between human seroconversion and a history of consuming fruits that have been partially eaten by bats.[70] In the case of the flavivirus Japanese encephalitis virus (JEV), experimental evidence shows that bats may act to pass the virus to mosquitos. JEV causes approximately 40,000 human cases of encephalitis per year, and 25% of cases are fatal.[64]

It is also possible that bats may indirectly pass viruses to humans through domestic animals. Hendra virus, a paramyxovirus, has caused serious outbreaks of human and equine respiratory diseases in Australia. During one outbreak, 21 horses and 2 humans were reportedly affected. Further research pointed to fruit bats and flying foxes as reservoirs for this virus, but little is known about how the virus circulates in the wild population. It appears that humans became infected through exposure to horses, not bats. It is possible that the horses became infected from bat contact.[68]

Similarly, Nipah virus, a paramyxovirus related to Hendra virus, has been isolated from pigs and humans with encephalitis and respiratory illness. This virus appears most prevalent in areas in and around Malaysia and Singapore. Sporadic outbreaks of Nipah virus infection have been documented in these areas, and it appears that humans are most often infected by pigs, but serosurveys indicate that antibodies are prevalent in bats, including Indian flying foxes (*Pteropus giganteus*), the large flying fox (*P. vamprus*), and variable flying fox (*P. hypomelanus*).[68]

Several of the other viruses that bats harbor pose a serious threat to human health. Bats are the only nonprimates known to harbor Marburg virus and Ebola virus.[33,39] Both viruses have been found in multiple species of African insectivorous and fruit-eating bats, including Egyptian fruit bats (*R. aegyptiacus*) and straw-colored fruit bats (*Eidolon helvum*). Prevalence rates of these viruses in the bat populations vary among different surveys. Estimates range from 1.4% to 3.1% prevalence in Egyptian fruit bats from Gabon and the Democratic Republic of Congo to 2.4% to 12% prevalence in other studies. It is known that clinically healthy bats can harbor the viruses and that they can remain seropositive for several months. Histopathology performed on a filovirus-infected bat, captured in Kenya, showed no lesions. Filovirus has been found in a clinically healthy pregnant Egyptian fruit bat (*Rousettus aegyptiacus*), and radio-transmitter studies have shown that at least one bat lived 13 months after being determined to be seropositive for Ebola virus.[17] Neither the exact risk of transmission of filoviruses from bats to humans nor the mode of potential transmission is clear. Scattered cases of human Marburg virus infection have been associated with a history of visits to caves in Africa with large bat populations.[33,39]

Bats have also been implicated as reservoirs for SARS virus, SARS-CoV, which emerged in China and resulted in over 900 human deaths worldwide. SARS-CoV–seropositive species of horse-shoe bats (*Rhinolophus* spp.), and the Leschenault's rousette (*Rousettus leschenaultia*) have been found in China. No illness has been detected in bats, but it is possible that a SARS-CoV–like virus of bats was transmitted to humans through exposure to bats sold as bush meat in local markets.[26]

Nonviral pathogens are also present in bats or have been isolated from guano. As with viruses, the role of bats in disseminating these agents to humans or domestic animals is not always clear, but the potential for transmission does exist. Among diseases caused by fungi, histoplasmosis is the human disease most associated with bats. Guano enriches the soil and results in optimal growth conditions for this fungus.[36] Under proper environmental conditions, the fungus produces spores and may cause an acute respiratory disease when inhaled by humans or other animals. Individuals visiting caves with large bat populations are at particular risk, and the disease has commonly been called "cave sickness."[36] Other at-risk populations include people working around bat feces, and sporadic cases may be associated with colonies of bats living in houses. The role of bats in causing human histoplasmosis is probably limited given that the infection rate among bats seems to be larger than the rates of human infection.[36]

Bats themselves do not frequently succumb to histoplasmosis. In cases of naturally occurring bat infections, infection occurs via inhalation.[36] Histoplasmosis appears to infect and multiply in the intestinal tracts of some bats, and the bats disseminate the fungus both by shedding it in their feces and by producing guano.[36]

Other species of fungi, bacteria, and parasites of bats with the potential to cause human disease have been found in bats, but no clear association exists between any of these agents and outbreaks of human disease. *Wangiella dermatitidis*, a pheohyphomycotic organism that causes skin disease in humans, has been isolated from the internal organs of multiple healthy individuals of bat species, including the pale spear-nosed bat (*Phyllostomus discolor*), the Pallas's mastiff bat (*Molossus molossus*), the little yellow-shouldered bat (*Sturnia lillium*), and the silver-tipped myotis (*Myotis albescens*).[58] *Blastomyces dermatitis* has been isolated from the livers of the lesser mouse-tailed bat (*Rhinopoma hardwickei hardwikei* gray) and *Paracoccidioides brasiliensis*, *Sporothrix schenckii*, *Trichophyton mentagrophytes*, *Microsporum gypseum*, and *M. canis* have all sporadically been found in various species of bats.[56,58] Bacteria such as *Salmonella*, *Shigella*, *Streptococcus*, *Staphylococcus*, *Listeria*, *Leptosporosis*, and *Yersinia* have been isolated from both sick and healthy bats.[3,34] *Streptococcus* and *Staphylococcus* may act as opportunistic pathogens under the right circumstances.[43]

Because of outbreaks of leptospirosis in humans, more organized efforts have been made to determine if bats may transmit the bacteria to people. Surveys of Australian flying foxes (*Pteropus* sp.) detected antibodies to leptospirosis, and bacteria were found in the renal tissue from 11% of individuals and urine from 39% of individuals, indicating the potential for spread.[18] Additionally, some evidence suggests positive leptospirosis titers in humans after exposure to bats.[18]

Zoonotic parasites, including nematodes, cestodes, and protozoa, have been documented in bats. Specifically two species of Schizotrypanum, *T. dionisii* and *T. vespertilonis*, have been found in multiple species of bats, including the common pipistrella (*Pipistrellus pipstrellus*), Leisler's bat (*Nyctalus leisleri*), common noctule (*N. noctula*), the Serotine bat (*Eptesicus serotinus*), and Brandt's bat (*Myotis brandtii*).[30] *T. d. dionisii* has been found in the bat bug *Cimex pipistrella*, a parasite found in many bat roosts, and parasitic pseudocysts containing amastigotes have been found in the thoracic skeletal muscle of *P. pipistrelllus*.[30]

Bats are unique in that regardless of the type of pathogen that they harbor, bats seem to tolerate the infections without developing noticeable disease. This ability for them to act as asymptomatic carriers is one of the most important aspects of bat-associated zoonoses.[14] How bats remain healthy while harboring pathogens that would kill other mammals is unknown. Some evidence suggests that hibernation may alter the immune system of bats.[13] Other evidence suggests that bats co-evolved with these pathogens. Lyssaviruses and rabies viruses seem to have evolved with bats, and Hendra and Nipah viruses are old viruses that may have circulated in flying fox populations throughout evolution.[26] Even if this phenomenon is the result of highly evolved host–pathogen interactions, it is unclear what causes these diseases to emerge and enter human populations. Given the precarious conservation situation of many bat species, further study is needed to determine how pathogens interact with the Chiropteran immune system and what environmental pressure may lead to the spillage of disease from bats to other animals.

CONCLUSION

Chiropterans are a remarkable group of mammals that exhibit a degree of habitat and biologic diversity that is almost unparalleled in the animal kingdom. They have a unique ability to harbor pathogens without succumbing to them, are long lived, and may fly long distances, all of which makes them potential vectors and reservoirs for a variety of diseases. Although much is known about what pathogens are harbored by bats, little is known about the diseases that they succumb to or why they seem to be resistant to numerous pathogens. A more nuanced appreciation of these animals has led to a better understanding of captive bat management, dietary requirements, and habitat needs, but much needs to be learned. Proper captive or wild population management requires an understanding of not only the physiology of the individual species but also their natural history.

Unfortunately, regardless of the diversity of bats in the world, they all have one thing in common—various threats to their survival. These include the emergence of new diseases threatening populations, habitat loss, and anthropogenic threats. No easy answers to these problems exist, with increasing human populations encroaching on bat habitats and the development of even environmentally friendly energy sources such as wind power, which may have a detrimental effect on migratory species. Evidence suggests that climate change may decrease reproductive success in bats. Moreover, the emergence of disease in these very resilient animals is suggestive of more serious environmental problems.[66]

The loss of bats, by whatever means, is not just of academic importance. Some species of bats are essential to pollination of certain plants and in seed dispersal of some trees.[38] Insectivorous bats may play a role in regulating the population of agricultural pests. The loss of bats has the potential to disrupt many ecosystems and negatively impact human food supplies.[9]

Despite all the bad news, efforts are underway to help preserve bat populations. New technologies for wind turbines are being developed to help limit bat mortalities, and studies of bat migration routes are helping to determine where wind farms may be placed and do the least harm.[51] More research is being done on the bat immune system, diseases, and nutritional needs. However, these efforts will not be enough to save many species, and much more comprehensive efforts to understand the biology, ecology, and health of these unique animals are needed to secure their future.

REFERENCES

1. Almeida MF, Martorelli LF, Aires CC, et al: Vaccinating the vampire bat *Desmodus rotundus* against rabies. *Vir Res* 137(2):275–277, 2008.
2. Andreasen CB, Dulmstra JR: Multicentric malignant lymphoma in a pallid bat. *J Wildl Dis* 32(3):545–547, 1996.
3. Arata AA, Vaughn JB, Newell KW, et al: *Salmonella* and *Shigella* infections in bats in selected areas of Colombia. *Am J Trop Med Hyg* 17(1):92–95, 1968.
4. Bai Y, Kosoy M, Recuenco S, et al: *Bartonella* spp. in Bats, Guatemala. *Emerg Infec Dis* 17(7):1269–1272, 2012.
5. Barrett JL, Carlisle MS, Prociv P: Neuro-angiostrongylosis in wild black and grey-headed flying foxes (*Pteropus* spp.). *Aust Vet J* 80(9):554–558, 2002.
6. Beck M, Beck J, Howard EB: Bile duct adenocarcinoma in a pallid bat (*Antrozeous pallidus*). *J Wildl Dis* 18(3):365–367, 1982.
7. Bello-Gutierrez J, Suzan G, Hidalgo-Mihart MG, et al: Alopecia in bats from Tabasco, Mexico. *J Wildl Dis* 46(3):1000–1004, 2010.
8. Blehert DS, Hicks AC, Behr M, et al: Bat white-nose syndrome: An emerging fungal pathogen? *Science (New York, NY)* 323(5911):227, 2009.
9. Boyles JG, Cryan PM, McCracken GF, et al: Conservation. Economic importance of bats in agriculture. *Science* 332(6025):41–42, 2011.
10. Boyles JG, Dunbar MB, Storm JJ, et al: Energy availability influences microclimate selection of hibernating bats. *J Exp Bio* 210(Pt 24):4345–4350, 2007.
11. Boyles JG, Willis CK: Could localized warm areas inside cold caves reduce mortality in hibernating bats affected by white-nose syndrome? *Front Ecol Environ* 2009.
12. Bradford C, Jennings R, Ramos-Vara J: Gastrointestinal leiomyosarcoma in an Egyptian fruit bat (*Rousettus aegyptiacus*). *J Vet Diag Invest* 22(3):462–465, 2010.
13. Buckles EL, Moore MS, Reichard JD, et al: *Histology of the Temporal Progression of WNS and Comparison of the PHA Response of Bats with and without WNS*. Abstracts of Presented Papers and Posters for 2010 White-nose Syndrome Symposium: US Fish and Wildlife Service. A summary of research on the inflammatory response in bats with WNS.
14. Calisher CH, Childs JE, Field HE, et al: Bats: Important reservoir hosts of emerging viruses. *Clin Microbiol Rev* 19(3):531–545, 2006.
15. Childs-Sanford SE, Garner MM, Raymond JT, et al: Disseminated microsporidiosis due to *Encephalitozoon hellem* in an Egyptian fruit bat (*Rousettus aegyptiacus*). *J Comp Pathol* 134(4):370–373, 2006.
16. Childs-Sanford SE, Kollias GV, Abou-Madi N, et al: Yersinia pseudotuberculosis in a closed colony of Egyptian fruit bats (*Rousettus aegyptiacus*). *J Zoo Wildl Med* 40(1):8–14, 2009.
17. Clauss M, Firzlaff U, Castell JC, et al: Effect of captivity and mineral supplementation on body composition and mineral status of mustached bats (*Pteronotus parnellii rubiginosus*). *J Anim Physiol Anim Nutr* 91(5–6):187–192, 2007.
18. Cox TE, Smythe LD, Leung LK: Flying foxes as carriers of pathogenic Leptospira species. *J Wildl Dis* 41(4):753–757, 2005.
19. Crissey SD: Nutrition. In Fascione N, editor: *Fruit bat husbandry manual*, 1995, The Lubee Foundation Inc, AZA Taxon Advisory Group.
20. Czenze ZJ, Broders HG: Ectoparasite community structure of two bats (*Myotis lucifugus* and *M. septentrionalis*) from the Maritimes of Canada. *J Parasitol Res* 34:15–35, 2011.
21. Del Cacho E, Estrada-Pena A, Sanchez A, et al: Histological response of *Eptesicus serotinus* (Mammalia: Chiroptera) to *Argas vespertilionis* (Acari: argasidae). *J Wildl Dis* 30(3):340–345, 1994.
22. DeMarco JH, Heard DJ, Fleming GJ, Lock BA: Ivermectin toxicosis after topical administration in dog-faced fruit bats (*Cynopterus brachyotis*). *J Zoo Wildl Med* 33(2):147–150, 2002.
23. Dierenfeld ES, Seyjagat J: Plasma fat-soluble vitamin and mineral concentrations in relation to diet in captive pteropodid bats. *J Zoo Wildl Med* 31(3):315–321, 2000.
24. Esteban JG, Amengual B, Cobo JS: Composition and structure of helminth communities in two populations of *Pipistrellus pipistrellus* (Chiroptera: Vespertilionidae) from Spain. *Folia Parasitol* 48(2):143–148, 2001.
25. Farina LL, Heard DJ, LeBlanc DM, et al: Iron storage disease in captive Egyptian fruit bats (*Rousettus aegyptiacus*): Relationship of blood iron parameters to hepatic iron concentrations and hepatic histopathology. *J Zoo Wildl Med* 36(2):212–221, 2005.
26. Field HE: Bats and emerging zoonoses: Henipaviruses and SARS. *Zoonoses and Public Health* 56(6–7):278–284, 2009.
27. Fowler ME, Miller RE: *Zoo and wildlife medicine: Current therapy*, ed 4, Philidelphia, PA, 1999, Saunders.
28. Fowler ME: *Zoo and wildlife medicine*, ed 2, Philadelphia, PA, 1984, Saunders.
29. Frick WF, Pollock JF, Hicks AC, et al: An emerging disease causes regional population collapse of a common North American bat species. *Science (New York, NY)* 329(5992):679–682, 2010.
30. Gardner RA, Molyneux DH: Schizotrypanum in British bats. *Parasitology* 97(Pt 1):43–50, 1988.
31. Gozalo AS, Schwiebert RS, Metzner W, et al: Spontaneous, generalized lipidosis in captive greater horseshoe bats (*Rhinolophus ferrumequinum*). *Contem Topics Lab Anim Sci* 44(6):49–52, 2005.

32. Hallam TG, McCracken GF: Management of the panzootic white-nose syndrome through culling of bats. *Conserv Biol* 25(1):189–194, 2011.

33. Hayman DT, Emmerich P, Yu M, et al: Long-term survival of an urban fruit bat seropositive for Ebola and Lagos bat viruses. *PLoS ONE* 5(8):e11978, 2010.

34. Heard DJ, De Young JL, Goodyear B, et al: Comparative rectal bacterial flora of four species of flying fox (*Pteropus* sp.). *J Zoo Wildl Med* 28(4):471–475, 1997.

35. Helmick KE, Heard DJ, Richey L, et al: A *Pasteurella*-like bacterium associated with pneumonia in captive megachiropterans. *J Zoo Wildl Med* 35(1):88–93, 2004.

36. Hoff GL, Bigler WJ: The role of bats in the propagation and spread of histoplasmosis: A review. *J Wildl Dis* 17(2):191–196, 1981.

37. Klug BJ, Turmelle AS, Ellison JA, et al: Rabies prevalence in migratory tree-bats in Alberta and the influence of roosting ecology and sampling method on reported prevalence of rabies in bats. *J Wildl Dis* 47(1):64–77, 2011.

38. Kunz TH, Fenton MB: *Bat ecology*, Chicago, IL, 2003, University of Chicago Press.

39. Kuzmin IV, Niezgoda M, Franka R, et al: Marburg virus in fruit bat, Kenya. *Emerg Infect Dis* 16(2):352–354, 2010.

40. Lavin SR, Chen Z, Abrams SA: Effect of tannic acid on iron absorption in straw-colored fruit bats (*Eidolon helvum*). *Zoo Biol* 29(3):335–343, 2010.

41. Ma JY, Yu Y, Peng WF: A new trematode (Digenea: Mesotretidae) from the horseshoe bat *Rhinolophus ferrumequinum* (Chiroptera: Rhinolophidae) in China. *J Parasitol* 95(3):718–721, 2009.

42. Marinkelle CJ: *Trypanosoma* (*Herpetosoma*) *longiflagellum* sp. N. from the tomb bat, *Taphozous nudiventris*, from Iraq. *J Wildl Dis* 13(3):262–264, 1977.

43. McCoy RH: Bacterial diseases of bats: A review. *Lab Anim Sci* 24(3):530–534, 1974.

44. McLelland DJ, Dutton CJ, Barker IK: Sarcomatoid carcinoma in the lung of an Egyptian fruit bat (*Rousettus aegyptiacus*). *J Vet Diag Invest* 21(1):160–163, 2009.

45. Meteyer CU, Buckles EL, Blehert DS, et al: Histopathologic criteria to confirm white-nose syndrome in bats. *J Vet Diag Invest* 21(4):411–414, 2009.

46. Meteyer CU, Valent M, Kashmer J, et al: Recovery of little brown bats (*Myotis lucifugus*) from natural infection with *Geomyces destructans*, white-nose syndrome. *J Wildl Dis* 47(3):618–626, 2011.

47. Moore PR, Jansen CC, Graham GC, et al: Emerging tropical diseases in Australia. Part 3. Australian bat lyssavirus. *Ann Trop Med Parasitol* 104(8):613–621, 2010.

48. Muhldorfer K, Schwarz S, Fickel J, et al: Genetic diversity of *Pasteurella* species isolated from European vespertilionid bats. *Vet Microbiol* 2010.

49. Muhldorfer K, Speck S, Kurth A, et al: Diseases and causes of death in European bats: Dynamics in disease susceptibility and infection rates. *PLoS ONE* 6(12):e29773, 2011.

50. Muhldorfer K, Speck S, Wibbelt G: Diseases in free-ranging bats from Germany. *BMC Vet Res* 7:61, 2011.

51. Nicholls B, Racey PA: The aversive effect of electromagnetic radiation on foraging bats: a possible means of discouraging bats from approaching wind turbines. *PLoS ONE* 4(7):e6246, 2009.

52. Nowak RM, Walker E: *Walker's bats of the world*, Baltimore, MD, 1994, Johns Hopkins University Press.

53. Peirce MA: Parasites of Chiroptera in Zambia. *J Wildl Dis* 20(2):153–154, 1994.

54. Prociv P: Aberrant migration by *Toxocara pteropodis* in flying-foxes—two case reports. *J Wildl Dis* 26(4):532–534, 1990.

55. Pybus MJ, Hobson DP, Onderka DK: Mass mortality of bats due to probable blue-green algal toxicity. *J Wildl Dis* 22(3):449–450, 1986.

56. Randhawa HS, Chaturvedi VP, Kini S, et al: Blastomyces dermatitidis in bats. First report of its isolation from the liver of *Rhinopoma hardwickei hardwickei* gray. *Sabouraudia* 23(1):69–76, 1985.

57. Reichard JD, Kunz TH: White-nose syndrome inflicts lasting injuries to the wings of little brown myotis (*Myotis lucifugus*). *Acta Chiropterologica* 11(2):457–464, 2009.

58. Reiss NR, Mok WY: Wangiella dermatitidis isolated from bats in Manaus Brazil. *Sabouraudia* 17(3):213–218, 1979.

59. Shankar V, Bowen RA, Davis AD, et al: Rabies in a captive colony of big brown bats (*Eptesicus fuscus*). *J Wildl Dis* 40(3):403–413, 2004.

60. Siegal-Willott J, Heard D, Sliess N, et al: Microchip-associated leiomyosarcoma in an Egyptian fruit bat (*Rousettus aegyptiacus*). *J Zoo Wildl Med* 38(2):352–356, 2007.

61. Srivastava RK, Krishna A: Adiposity associated rise in leptin impairs ovarian activity during winter dormancy in Vespertilionid bat, *Scotophilus heathi*. *Reproduction* 133(1):165–176, 2007.

62. Sutton RH, Wilson PD: Lead poisoning in grey-headed fruit bats (*Pteropus poliocephalus*). *J Wildl Dis* 19(3):294–296, 1983.

63. Turmelle AS, Jackson FR, Green D, et al: Host immunity to repeated rabies virus infection in big brown bats. *J Gen Virol* 91(Pt 9):2360–2366, 2010.

64. van den Hurk AF, Smith CS, Field HE, et al: Transmission of Japanese encephalitis virus from the black flying fox, *Pteropus alecto*, to *Culex annulirostris* mosquitoes, despite the absence of detectable viremia. *Am J Trop Med Hyg* 81(3):457–462, 2009.

65. Warnecke L, Turner JM, Bollinger TK, et al: Inoculation of bats with European *Geomyces destructans* supports the novel pathogen hypothesis for the origin of white-nose syndrome. *Proc Natl Acad Sci U S A* 109(18):6999–7003, 2012.

66. Wibbelt G, Moore MS, Schountz T, Voigt CC: Emerging diseases in Chiroptera: Why bats? *Biol Lett* 6(4):438–440, 2010.

67. Wilson DE, Reeder DM: *Mammal species of the world: A taxonomic and geographic reference*, vol 3, Baltimore, MD, 2005, Johns Hopkins University Press.

68. Wong S, Lau S, Woo P, et al: Bats as a continuing source of emerging infections in humans. *Rev Med Virol* 17(2):67–91, 2007.

69. Wright E, Hayman DT, Vaughan A, et al: Virus neutralising activity of African fruit bat (*Eidolon helvum*) sera against emerging lyssaviruses. *Virology* 408(2):183–189, 2010.

70. Yaiw KC, Crameri G, Wang L, et al: Serological evidence of possible human infection with Tioman virus, a newly described paramyxovirus of bat origin. *J Infect Dis* 196(6):884–886, 2007.

CHAPTER 36

Prosimians

Cathy V. Williams

BIOLOGY

Prosimian primates are composed of lemurs, lorises, pottos, and galagos. The classification of primates remains somewhat controversial, and taxonomic structure continues to be revised as the increasing amount of genetic information is reconciled with earlier methods of classifications based on morphology and fossil records. Most authorities now follow a systematic arrangement in which the primates are divided into two suborders: (1) Strepsirhini (i.e., the tooth combed primates), and (2) Haplorhini, which includes the tarsiers, monkeys, apes, and humans. The Strepsirhine group is further divided into two infraorders: Lorisiformes and Lemuriformes. The infraorder Lorisiformes includes all the extant African and Asian species of lorises, pottos, and galagos, which are represented by nine genera and 18 species of small-bodied, nocturnal primates.[28] The infraorder Lemuriformes is composed of five families endemic to Madagascar: (1) Lemuridae (bamboo lemurs, ring-tailed lemurs, true lemurs, and ruffed lemurs), (2) Indriidae (indri, sifakas, and woolly lemurs), (3) Cheirogaleidae (mouse lemurs, dwarf lemurs, and fork-marked lemurs), (4) Lepilemuridae (sportive lemurs), and (5) Daubentoniidae (aye-aye).

Lemurs are found in a wide range of ecologic niches in Madagascar, including the low to high altitude tropical rain forests on the east coast, the dry deciduous forests of the west, and the spiny deserts of the south. Lorises are native to Southeast Asia and the tropical forests of India and Sri Lanka, and galagos (bush babies) and pottos are distributed throughout Africa south of the Sahara.[28]

Over the last 2000 years, at least 17 species of lemurs have become extinct, and the ranges of most extant species have decreased dramatically, largely because of human activity. All prosimian species are threatened to various degrees in the wild. All members of the family Lemuridae as well as *Nycticebus* sp. (slow lorises) are listed in CITES Appendix I by the International Union for the Conservation of Nature (IUCN). Galagos, pottos, and the slender loris (*Loris tardigradis*) are listed in CITES Appendix II.[18] Habitat destruction is the largest threat; however, hunting for bush meat and capture for sale in the pet trade also contribute to their declining numbers.

Many species are not represented in captivity or are present in only very small numbers. Of the lemur species displayed in zoos, *Lemur catta* (ring-tailed lemur) are most numerous followed by *Varecia* (ruffed lemurs) and *Eulemur* (true lemurs or black and brown lemurs). Increasingly, *Propithecus* (sifaka) and *Daubentoina* (aye-aye) are found on display in North American and European zoos as better husbandry and feeding programs for these species are developed. Galagos, although not present in zoos in large numbers, are often used in research settings.

UNIQUE ANATOMY

Considerable anatomic variations exist among prosimian primates. Adult weights range from 30 grams (g) for the smallest mouse lemur (*Microcebus myoxinus*) to more than 8 kilograms (kg) for the largest lemur species.[24] Table 36-1 contains biologic information on prosimian species commonly kept in captivity.

All prosimians, with the exception of aye-aye (*Daubentonia*), have tooth combs, an adaptation in which the lower incisors together with the lower canine teeth project forward almost horizontally. The tooth comb is used for mutual grooming and self-grooming. The typical dental formula for prosimians is 2/2, 1/1, 3/3, 3/3, although

exceptions exist. In the aye-aye, the dental formula is 1/1, 0/0, 1/0, 3/3. The aye-aye incisors are long, laterally compressed, and continuously growing as in rodents. The roots of the lower incisors are extensive and form a half circle within the mandible, extending caudally into the coronoid process. Sifakas (*Propithecus*) have one less lower incisor (dental formula 2/1, 1/1, 2/2, 3/3), and sportive lemurs (*Lepilemur*) lack upper incisors entirely (dental formula 0/2, 1/1, 3/3, 3/3).[17]

Lorisiform prosimians are small bodied and nocturnal. All have large eyes and superior night vision. Galagos are very active animals and move quickly through forests by leaping from branch to branch. Their body structure is lighter compared with those of lorises and pottos. Hindlimbs are noticeably longer than their forelimbs, and tails are long. In contrast, all limbs of lorises and pottos are of approximately equal length, and tails are short. Locomotion in these species is slow and deliberate. The first digits of both the forelimbs and the hindlimbs of prosimians are opposable to the remaining digits. The second digit of the hindlimb has a claw, which is used for grooming, and all other digits have nails as in other primates.

Among Malagasy prosimians, members of the Cheirogaleidae, Lepilemuridae, and Daubentoniidae are nocturnal as is the genus *Avahi* in the Indriidae family. The remaining species exhibit either diurnal or cathemeral activity patterns. All species have long tails, with the exception of *Indri*, which has a short rudimentary tail. With extremely well-developed hindlimbs, sifaka, *Indri, Avahi*, and *Lepilemur* are vertical clingers and leapers. The remaining lemur species move quadrapedally along tree limbs or leap from branch to branch.[28]

Although all prosimians are monogastric, the length of the intestinal tract as well as the size and conformation of the cecum and large bowel vary, depending on the species. In general, the more folivorous a species, the larger is the cecum and the more pronounced is the ability to use microbial fermentation to derive energy from fibrous diet items. In members of the Indriidae family, the proximal colon forms a spiral and is located in the right anterior quadrant of the abdomen adjacent to the body wall.[17]

SPECIAL HOUSING REQUIREMENTS

Prosimians originate from tropical environments and may be maintained in outdoor enclosures year-round in mild climates. In temperate climates, enclosed environments with supplemental heat should be provided for diurnal lemurs when temperatures drop below 4.5°C to 7°C (40°F–45°F). Nocturnal prosimians are typically housed in indoor environments with temperatures controlled between 21°C to 27°C (70°F–80°F). Adequate shade should be provided in outdoor enclosures.

The size and design of enclosures for prosimians depends on the species, group size and social dynamics, and the reproductive status of individuals. Nocturnal prosimians are generally solitary in nature, although some may tolerate living with related individuals or a member of the opposite sex in captivity. Diurnal lemurs are social and should be housed with a compatible cage mate or social group. Flexible enclosure designs that allow physical separation of group members while maintaining visual contact are preferable, as individuals may require temporary separation for medical or behavioral management. Choosing flooring substrates and cage furniture materials that are sanitized or replaced easily is important for minimizing environmental pathogen loads. Branches and perches are added to

TABLE 36-1

Biological Information for Selected Prosimians

Scientific Name	Common Name	Behavior	Adult Weight (kg)	Geographic Distribution
Cheirogaleus medius	Fat-tailed dwarf lemur	Nocturnal	0.15–0.25	Western Madagascar
Microcebus murinus	Gray mouse lemur	Nocturnal	0.06–0.1	Western Madagascar
Daubentonia madagascariensis	Aye-aye	Nocturnal	2.3–3.0	Eastern and western Madagascar
Eulemur mongoz	Mongoose lemur	Cathemeral	1.1–1.6	Northwestern Madagascar
Eulemur macaco	Black lemur	Cathemeral	2.0–2.4	Northwestern Madagascar
Lemur catta	Ring-tailed lemur	Diurnal	2.0–3.0	Southern Madagascar
Varecia sp.	Ruffed lemurs	Diurnal	3.1–3.7	Eastern Madagascar
Propithecus coquereli	Coquerel's sifaka	Diurnal	3.0–4.5	Western Madagascar
Nycticebus pygmaeus	Pygmy slow loris	Nocturnal	0.35–0.5	Southeast Asia
Galago moholi	Lesser bushbaby	Nocturnal	0.15–0.25	Equatorial Africa
Otolemur crassicaudatus	Thick-tailed bushbaby	Nocturnal	1.1–1.5	Equatorial Africa

maximize the use of vertical and horizontal space. For sifakas, adequate vertical structures are required to accommodate their vertical leaping form of locomotion. Enclosures for multimember groups should contain multiple feeding stations to prevent dominate animals from monopolizing food. The addition of visual barriers allows subordinate animals the option of moving out of sight of dominate individuals and decreases tension and fighting.

Nocturnal species are usually maintained under reversed light cycles for display and to allow husbandry staff to readily monitor behavior and activity. It is important to provide nest boxes or chambers for seclusion when desired. Aye-ayes should be provided with appropriate material to weave nests.

SPECIAL PHYSIOLOGY

Prosimians have a low basal metabolic rate compared with other mammals of similar body size.[34] Behaviors such as basking and huddling are related to energy conservation and thermal regulation. Rectal temperatures of lemurs and bush babies range between 36°C to 37°C (97°F–99°F), with that of lorises somewhat lower between 35°C to 36°C (95°F–97°F).[25,47] Dwarf lemurs (*Cheirogaleus*) and, to a lesser degree, mouse lemurs (*Microcebus*) undergo periods of torpor or hibernation during seasons of the year when food and water are scarce in their native environment. While in torpor, core body temperatures decrease and often match ambient temperatures for prolonged periods of time and metabolic rates slow dramatically. Body temperatures well below 27°C (80°F) are not uncommon in dwarf lemurs during torpor.[9]

Prosimians have no active mechanism for cooling, and temperature regulation is accomplished by limiting activity, seeking cool locations during hot weather, and licking hands to generate evaporative cooling. Capture and handling during warm weather should be done early when outdoor temperatures are cool or in temperature controlled environments.

FEEDING

Feeding strategies in prosimians range from primarily insectivorous for some species of galagos to highly folivorous for members of the Indriidae family. Bamboo lemurs are highly specialized, and bamboo composes 90% to 95% of food consumed in the wild. The ability to successfully maintain many prosimian species in good health in captivity depends, in large part, on providing diets that closely resemble the gross composition of wild diets. The National Resource Council's Nutrient Requirements of Nonhuman Primates contains a summary of differing prosimian feeding strategies.[26] A notable

exception between prosimian and anthropoid primates is the former's ability to synthesize vitamin C endogenously.[27]

Many prosimians do well with diets composed of commercially prepared primate biscuits as a base. Folivorous lemurs such as sifakas and bamboo lemurs require high-fiber biscuits designed for leaf-eating primates, whereas the frugivorous ruffed lemurs are better adapted to biscuits designed for old-world monkeys with intermediate fiber levels. Ring-tailed, black, and brown lemurs do well on biscuits with either moderate or high levels of fiber.

Although useful for providing enrichment and variety in the diet, provision of commercially available fruits and vegetables should be limited as overconsumption contributes to dental disease, diarrhea, obesity, and diabetes. Cultivated fruits and vegetables contain high levels of sugar and starch and low levels of fiber compared with foods consumed in the wild. Domesticated fruits and starchy vegetables such as potatoes, corn, and grains, are high in simple sugars, and alter microbial populations in the hind gut and should be strictly limited or avoided altogether in the diet of folivorous lemurs. The addition of locally available fresh leaves and browse is essential for folivorous species, whereas including live insects or gums is important for species that have evolved to selectively feed on these items. A simple method to calculate the amount to feed a single animal is 25 grams per day (g/day) per animal of primate biscuit and 35 g/day per animal of fruit-and-vegetable mix per kilogram of ideal body weight.

RESTRAINT AND HANDLING

Because prosimians are relatively small, it is feasible to use manual restraint when performing brief examinations or minor treatments. Handlers should wear arm guards to protect themselves against scratches should an animal grasp the handler's forearm. Physical restraint of prosimians weighing less than 1 kg involves initially grasping the animal over the back of the neck and around the mandible with a gloved hand to control the head while using a second hand to control the abdomen and back legs.

An animal weighing between 1 and 4 kg is first netted in its enclosure or out of a transport kennel. The head is controlled by placing one hand around the back of the neck with fingers extending around the jaw to secure the head. The second hand is then placed under the mandible to gain full control of the head and neck. The animal is then brought out of the net and allowed to grasp the handler's arm with front and back limbs (Figure 36-1). If more control is needed, a second handler restrains the hindlimbs above the stifles to prevent injury to the knee joints and extends the legs, while the animal is positioned on either its back or abdomen (Figure 36-2).

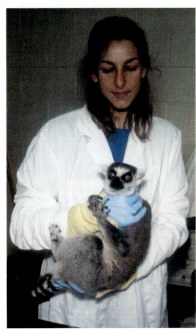

FIGURE 36-1 Single-handler manual restraint of a ring-tailed lemur (*Lemur catta*).

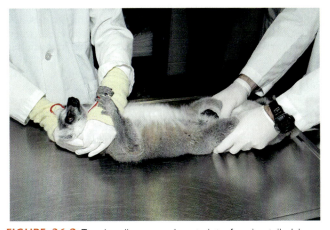

FIGURE 36-2 Two-handler manual restraint of a ring-tailed lemur (*Lemur catta*).

Squeeze cages may be used to restrain medium to large lemurs for the administration of intramuscular injections.

Chemical Restraint

Dosages of sedatives and immobilization agents are given in Table 36-2 and useful combination regimes in Table 36-3. When chemical restraint is needed to facilitate handling or performance of minor procedures, a range of options, spanning mild sedation to full immobilization, is available. Combining agents takes advantage of the synergistic effects of compounds having differing mechanisms of action.

Although ketamine is frequently used in a wide range of primates, it has a number of undesirable side effects in diurnal lemurs. When used alone, the degree and quality of immobilization is inconsistent, vomiting on induction or recovery is common, and seizures may occur even within normal dose ranges. The disadvantages are mitigated somewhat by combining ketamine with other agents; however, full recovery still requires several hours, which is a distinct disadvantage over other options.[45]

Anesthesia and Surgery

When general anesthesia is required, it is desirable to give preanesthetic medications whenever possible, as this provides a

---

TABLE 36-2

Drugs Used for Sedation, Immobilization, and Anesthesia in Prosimians

Agent	Dosage (mg/kg)	Route of Administration	Reversal*
Diazepam	0.25–0.5	PO, IV	Flumazenil
Midazolam	0.1–0.3	IM, IV	Flumazenil
Ketamine†	5–15†	IM	None
Tiletamine/ Zolazepam	5–10	SC, IM	None/ Flumazenil
Dexmedetomidine	0.02	IM	Atipamezole
Butorphanol	0.1–0.4	IM	Naloxone
Fentanyl	0.001–0.03/ hour	IV CRI	Naloxone
Propofol	3–6	IV	None

*Doses for reversal agents: atipamezole (0.2 mg/kg, IM); naloxone (0.02 mg/kg, IM); flumazenil (0.02 mg/kg, IV).
†Ketamine is not recommended for use alone in prosimians.
CRI, Constant rate infusion; *IM*, intramuscularly; *IV*, intravenously; *PO*, orally; *SC*, subcutaneously.

TABLE 36-3

Useful Combination Regimes for Prosimians

Drug Combination	Dosage* (mg/kg)	Duration of Effect (min)	Level of Sedation
Dexmedetomidine/Midazolam	0.02 / 0.2	30	Light to moderate sedation
Midazolam/Ketamine	0.2 / 5–10	20–30	Heavy sedation to complete immobilization
Dexmedetomidine/Ketamine	0.02 / 3–5	10–20	Heavy sedation to complete immobilization
Butorphanol/Dexmedetomidine/Ketamine	0.3–0.4 / 0.02 / 3–5	15–20	Complete immobilization
Butorphanol/Dexmedetomidine/Midazolam	0.3–0.4 / 0.02 / 0.2–0.3	30–50	Complete immobilization
Tiletamine/Zolazepam	5–10	60	Complete immobilization

*All drugs are given intramuscularly.

smoother induction and more stable plane of anesthesia while decreasing the amount of other agents needed to maintain a surgical plane of anesthesia. Isoflurane and sevoflurane are suitable inhalation agents for inducing and maintaining general anesthesia in prosimians. When inducing animals in a chamber or via a mask, sevoflurane is the preferred agent, as it is less irritating to airways, making induction smoother and less objectionable to the patient.

Intubation may be challenging in aye-ayes (*Daubentonia*), sifakas (*Propithecus*), and ring-tailed lemurs (*Lemur catta*) because of the limited visibility of the larynx or the narrow openings between the vocal folds. Intubation is most easily performed in these species by inserting a guide cannula into the trachea and then passing the endotracheal tube over the cannula into proper position. Five-French (5-Fr) polypropylene suction catheters make good guide catheters (Figure 36-3). Once the endotracheal tube is in place the cannula is removed.

Lemurs are highly sensitive to the hypotensive effects of both isoflurane and sevoflurane, so it is important to monitor blood pressure and be prepared to administer intravenous fluids or other supportive measures as necessary when using these agents. Because of their high ratios of surface area to body mass, lemurs develop hypothermia quickly when anesthetized. Heat loss may be minimized by insulating the animals from cold surfaces, providing supplemental sources of warmth, and warming the surgical skin preparation solutions and fluids used for lavage and intravenous administration.

DIAGNOSTICS

Performing a complete physical examination and laboratory evaluation are critical for determining the health status of prosimians as in other taxa. Several sites are accessible for collecting blood samples. The femoral vein or artery in the region of the femoral triangle is the easiest site from where samples can be obtained in most prosimians. The main disadvantage with the site is an increased risk of serious bleeding following collection if the phlebotomist inadvertently hits the artery instead of the vein and adequate attention is not paid to hemostasis. This is particularly true for animals that are manually restrained, as blood pressure may be increased secondary to stress associated with handling. The posterior tibial vein, or small saphenous vein, running up the posterior aspect of the hindlimb, is an ideal site for intravenous injections and indwelling catheter placement (Figure 36-4); however, like the cephalic vein, it tends to collapse easily, making it suitable for collecting only small amounts of blood (typically < 1 milliliter [mL]). Jugular veins may be used for blood collection and catheter placement in anesthetized prosimians; however, the short neck length makes this site less desirable.

Hematology and common serum biochemistry reference values for various species of captive prosimians are provided in Tables 36-4 and 36-5, respectively. Urine is collected by using standard techniques. Cystocentesis and manual bladder compression are easily performed under manual or chemical restraint. Urethral catheterization is straightforward in males but is somewhat more complicated in females, as the position of the urethral orifice varies, depending on the species. In all members of the Lorisidae, the orifice is at the tip of the clitoris, whereas in lemurs, it is located in different positions between the vagina and the base of the clitoris. Urine specific

gravity in healthy lemurs is frequently isosthenuric and not cause for alarm unless other abnormalities are identified on laboratory workup.

Abdominal radiography is frequently unrewarding in lemurs, as their relatively low level of body fat translates into poor resolution of abdominal organs. In sifakas, the location of the spiral colon in the right cranial quadrant lies adjacent to the diaphragm, and the liver lobes are shifted to the left.

INFECTIOUS DISEASES

Infectious and parasitic diseases are summarized in Table 36-6.

Viral Infections

Little is known about the sensitivity of the various prosimian species to viral pathogens. Herpesvirus has been associated with meningoencephalitis in ruffed and ring-tailed lemurs.[20,22] In one report, the virus was identified as *Herpesvirus hominis*, and the route of infection was presumed to be from human exposure. Clinical signs associated with the disease included intermittent hindlimb lameness progressing to seizures, coma, and death. In another report, a herpesvirus was identified in lymphocytes of a slow loris with lymphoma.[41]

A serological survey for viral diseases in wild lemurs tested for adenovirus group–specific antibody, influenza A antibody, influenza B antibody, parainfluenza 1 antibody, rotavirus group–specific antibody, hepatitis A antibody, and hepatitis B surface antigen and found no serum antibody titers. Arbovirus infections of lemurs have been investigated in an effort to determine if lemurs serve as natural reservoirs for pathogens causing human diseases. A small percent of free-ranging lemurs in Madagascar have shown titers to West Nile virus (WNV) and other alphaviruses and flaviviruses, although attempts to isolate viruses from the animals were not successful. Experimental inoculations with WNV and yellow fever virus in lemurs resulted in transient viremia without clinical signs of illness. Antibody titers remained detectable, but viruses could not be isolated after the initial viremia.[33] On the African continent, where yellow fever exists, galagos and pottos may become infected, and clinical disease and death may ensue.[16]

Bacterial Infections

Reports of tuberculosis (TB) in prosimians are rare, which suggests that the disease is uncommon in captivity in developed countries. The intradermal tuberculin test using mammalian old tuberculin (MOT) and thoracic radiography appear to be unreliable methods for diagnosing the disease[21,35] but may provide evidence in support of further diagnostics. In cases of suspected TB, gastric or tracheal lavage and culture is warranted.

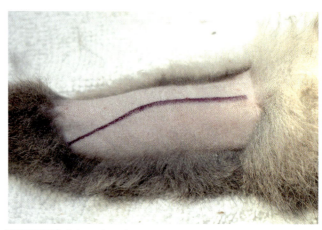

FIGURE 36-4 Location of the posterior tibial (small saphenous) vein in a brown lemur (*Eulemur*).

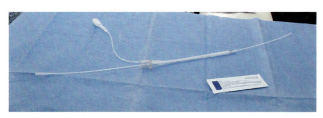

FIGURE 36-3 Endotracheal tube with guide cannula in place.

TABLE 36-4

Reference Values for Hematologic Parameters for Selected Prosimians Species*

Parameter	Pygmy Slow Loris	Greater Bush Baby	Ring-Tailed Lemur†	Black Lemur	Ruffed Lemur†	Aye-Aye‡	Coquerel's Sifaka‡
WBC (×10³/µL)	13.1 ± 7.5	10.9 ± 5.5	8.63 ± 3.84	8.97 ± 3.58	7.75 ± 3.28	11.91 ± 4.18	7.3 ± 3.0
RBC (×10⁶/µL)	5.7 ± 1.3	8.38 ± 1.26	7.63 ± 0.92	8.42 ± 1.29	9.29 ± 1.12	7.2 ± 0.65	8.26 ± 1.34
HCT (%)	42.4 ± 6.3	46.8 ± 5.4	50.4 ± 6.3	47.3 ± 7.0	49.6 ± 5.9	47 ± 5	41.6 ± 7.2
Hemoglobin (g/dL)	14.5 ± 3.0	15.8 ± 2.0	15.5 ± 1.7	15.1 ± 2.2	15.8 ± 1.9	16.0 ± 1.3	13.8 ± 2.3
MCV (fL)	75.1 ± 13.8	55.1 ± 4.8	65.8 ± 6.4	56.8 ± 6.0	53.5 ± 4.6	66.3 ± 3.7	50.6 ± 3.3
MCH (pg/cell)	26.1 ± 3.0	18.6 ± 1.6	20.3 ± 1.6	17.9 ± 1.4	17.1 ± 1.0	22.2 ± 1.1	16.8 ± 1.1
MCHC (g/dL)	35.0 ± 5.3	34.0 ± 1.5	31.1 ± 2.3	32.1 ± 2.6	32.2 ± 2.6	33.6 ± 1.7	33.2 ± 1.8
Platelets (×10³/µL)	341 ± 100	300 ± 153	270 ± 109	205 ± 132	351 ± 149	346 ± 78	377 ± 100
Neutrophils (×10³/µL)	3.12 ± 2.20	4.02 ± 4.31	4.34 ± 3.13	4.60 ± 2.33	3.96 ± 1.97	4.36 ± 2.29	4.51 ± 2.44
Bands (×10³/µL)	0.3 ± 0.4	0.53 ± 0	0.18 ± 0.18	0.33 ± 0.57	0.27 ± 0.73	0 ± 0	0 ± 0
Lymphocytes (×10³/µL)	8.51 ± 4.63	5.31 ± 3.12	3.73 ± 1.99	3.76 ± 2.36	3.18 ± 1.93	6.75 ± 3.45	2.42 ± 1.21
Eosinophils (×10³/µL)	0.42 ± 0.39	0.53 ± 0.48	0.35 ± 0.36	0.48 ± 0.5	0.33 ± 0.36	0.14 ± 0.21	0.05 ± 0.07
Monocytes (×10³/µL)	0.66 ± 0.80	0.44 ± 0.37	0.37 ± 0.41	0.3 ± 0.21	0.28 ± 0.24	0.56 ± 0.43	0.28 ± 0.22
Basophils (×10³/µL)	0.21 ± 0.17	0.08 ± 0.02	0.05 ± 0.06	0.1 ± 0.09	0.05 ± 0.05	0.02 ± 0.05	0.02 ± 0.04

*Values are provided as mean plus or minus (±) standard deviation from composite MedARKs records.
†Values provided for animals greater than 2 years of age.
‡From Duke Lemur Center in-house MedARKs normal values.

fL, Femtoliter; *g/dL*, gram per deciliter; *HCT*, hematocrit; *MCH*, mean corpuscular hemoglobin; *MCHC*, mean corpuscular hemoglobin concentration; *MCV*, mean corpuscular volume; *µL*, microliter; *pg*, picogram; *RBC*, red blood cell; *WBC*, white blood cell.

TABLE 36-5

Reference Values for Serum Biochemical Parameters for Selected Prosimian Species*

Parameter	Pygmy Slow Loris	Greater Bush Baby	Ring -Tailed Lemur†	Black Lemur	Ruffed Lemur†	Aye-Aye‡	Coquerel's Sifaka‡
Calcium (mg/dL)	10.4 ± 1.0	9.7 ± 0.7	9.6 ± 0.8	10.5 ± 1.1	9.7 ± 1.0	9.7 ± 0.9	10.6 ± 1.4
Phosphorus (mg/dL)	4.0 ± 1.7	4.1 ± 0.9	5.0 ± 1.7	6.2 ± 1.6	5.7 ± 1.6	5.2 ± 1.6	4.3 ± 2.1
Sodium (mEq/L)	149 ± 10	147 ± 5	148 ± 5	146 ± 5	142 ± 9	143 ± 3.4	148 ± 4
Potassium (mEq/L)	4.1 ± 1.0	4.0 ± 0.7	4.4 ± 0.6	5.5 ± 0.8	4.5 ± 0.7	5.6 ±1.4	4.5 ± 1.5
Chloride (mEq/L)	109 ± 5	111 ± 5	108 ± 6	102 ± 4	103 ± 8	112 ± 3	109 ± 4.2
Magnesium (mg/dL)	2.86 ± 0.36	—	2.03 ± 0.48	1.93 ± 0.43	2.17 ± 0.63	2.13 ± 0.23	1.66 ± 0.3
BUN (mg/dL)	25 ± 11	20 ± 8	21 ± 8	20 ± 8	19 ± 8	15 ± 5	23 ± 6
Creatinine (mg/dL)	0.4 ± 0.2	0.8 ± 0.3	1.0 ± 0.3	0.9 ± 0.2	0.8 ± 0.5	0.7 ± 0.2	0.7 ± 0.2
Total bilirubin (mg/dL)	0.4 ± 0.3	0.1 ± 0.1	0.6 ± 0.4	0.5 ± 0.3	0.3 ± 0.2	0.3 ± 0.1	0.2 ± 0.1
Glucose (mg/dL)	161 ± 62	140 ± 53	144 ± 78	89 ± 34	100 ± 34	156 ± 40	133 ± 32
Creatinine phosphokinase (IU/L)	342 ± 456	142 ± 157	1032 ± 1209	1399 ± 1247	749 ± 692	197 ± 206	306 ± 275
Alkaline phosphatase (IU/L)	76 ± 46	229 ± 211	209 ± 101	221 ± 147	380 ± 196	524 ± 451	214 ± 165
ALT (IU/L)	89 ± 42	50 ± 50	95 ± 59	117 ± 90	109 ± 85	12 ± 8	53 ± 21
AST (IU/L)	117 ± 49	30 ± 13	46 ± 34	39 ± 39	52 ± 35	17 ± 15	26 ± 13
GGT (IU/L)	47 ± 49	14 ± 6	28 ± 18	23 ± 39	15 ± 17	21 ± 11	13 ± 6
Total protein (g/dL)	7.1 ± 1.0	6.9 ± 0.9	7.3 ± 0.8	7.9 ± 0.8	7.6 ± 0.7	6.0 ± 0.6	7.3 ± 1.1
Globulin (g/dL)	3.5 ± 0.8	3.1 ± 0.7	1.6 ± 0.9	2.3 ± 0.6	1.9 ± 0.7	2.2 ± 0.4	2.5 ± 0.9
Albumin	4.1 ± 0.7	3.7 ± 0.8	5.7 ±.09	5.7 ± 0.7	5.7 ± 0.8	3.9 ± 0.4	4.8 ± 0.7
Total thyroxine (T4) (µg/dL)	—	—	4.59 ± 1.73‡	3.01 ± 1.29‡	3.5 ± 1.9	2.1 ± 0.89‡	0.88 ± 0.52‡

*Values are provided as mean plus or minus (±) standard deviation from composite MedARKs records.
†Values provided for animals greater than 2 years of age.
‡Values are provided as mean plus or minus (±) standard deviation from Duke Lemur Center in-house MedArks normal values.

ALT, Alanine aminotransferase; *AST*, aspartate aminotransferase; *BUN*, blood urea nitrogen; *g/dL*, gram per deciliter; *GGT*, gamma glutamyl transferase; *mEq/L*, milliequivalent per liter; *µg/dL*, microgram per deciliter; *mg/dL*, milligram per deciliter; *IU/L*, international unit per liter.

TABLE 36-6

Selected Infectious Diseases of Prosimians*

Disease	Causative Agent	Comments	Signs	Diagnosis	Treatment/ Management
VIRAL					
Meningoencephalitis[22]	Herpesvirus	Likely acquired from humans	Seizures, ataxia, coma	Virus isolation	Supportive care Not prevalent
West Nile fever[33]	West Nile virus	Small percentage of wild lemurs have titers	None detected Transient viremia	Serology	Supportive care Avoid livestock exposure
Borna disease[36]	Bornavirus	Domestic livestock reservoir	Seizures, ataxia, coma	Serology	Supportive care Avoid livestock exposure
Encephalomyocarditis[31]	Encephalomyocarditis virus	Rodent reservoir	Acute death, necrotizing myocarditis	Virus isolation	Rodent control
Epstein Barr disease*	Epstein Barr virus	Documented in captivity, likely acquired from humans	Possible unilateral facial paralysis	Serology	Minimize human contact, wear personal protective equipment (PPE)
Bovine spongiform encephalopathy[3]	Bovine spongiform encephalopathy prion	Processed primate foods containing animal protein	Neurologic symptoms	Postmortem immunocytochemistry of brain tissue	Avoid feed containing beef byproducts
BACTERIAL					
Enterocolitis	Salmonella, Campylobacter, E. coli, Yersinia, Clostridium difficile	Fecal–oral spread Zoonotic potential	Diarrhea, sepsis, abscesses, ulceration	Fecal culture, demonstrate toxins in feces for C. difficile	Antibiotics and fluid support
Listeriosis*	Listeria monocytogenes	Presumed food contamination	Anorexia, lethargy, hepatic abscesses, +/– CNS symptoms	Blood culture	Amoxicillin, supportive care
Septicemia*	Various agents	Fecal–oral, food contamination, breech of intestinal mucosal barrier	Depression, lethargy, anorexia, +/– diarrhea, and death	Blood culture	Aggressive intravenous antibiotic therapy, supportive care
Tularemia[6,16]	Francisella tularensis	Rodent reservoir	Peracute death, pneumonia, hepatitis, and splenitis	Culture	Aggressive antibiotic therapy, supportive care
Tuberculosis[21,35]	Mycobacteria tuberculosis	Infected humans or mammals	None, acute death, granulomatous abscesses	Intradermal skin test unreliable Gastric or tracheal lavage and culture	No information available for prosimians

PARASITIC

Disease	Organism	Host / Zoonotic potential	Clinical signs	Diagnosis	Treatment / Prevention
Cryptosporidiosis*	*Cryptosporidium parvum*	Zoonotic potential	Diarrhea, lethargy, anorexia	Acid fast stain, enzyme-linked immunosorbent assay (ELISA), immunofluorescent antibody (IFA) test of stool	Supportive care; Nitazoxanide decreases shedding and symptoms
Giardiasis*	*Giardia lamblia*	Asymptomatic carriers common; Zoonotic potential	None to varying degrees of diarrhea, lethargy, anorexia	Direct smear of feces, ELISA	Metronidazole, tinidazole
Toxoplasmosis[7,10]	*Toxoplasma gondii*	Feline definitive host	Acute death, lethargy, weakness, +/– neurologic symptoms	Serology, demonstration of tachyzoites in affected organs	Pyrimethamine and sulfadiazine, atovaquone; Prevent exposure to felid feces and contaminated soil
Cerebral larval migrans[8]	*Baylisascaris*	Raccoon (*Procyon lotor*) definitive host.	Central nervous system signs	Postmortem magnetic resonance imaging (MRI)	Prevent exposure to raccoon feces
Ehrlichiosis[43]	*Ehrlichia chaffeensis*	Lone star tick (*Amblyomma americanum*) intermediate host	Anorexia, lethargy, pyrexia, lymphadenopathy	Polymerase chain reaction (PCR), culture, demonstration of morula in lymph node aspirates	Doxycycline; Control ticks and carrier wildlife species
Stomach worm infestation*	*Physaloptera*	Cockroach intermediate host	Vomiting, anorexia, abdominal pain	Fecal examination, endoscopy	Mebendazole, pyrantel pamoate; Vermin control
Bot flies infestation	*Cuterebra* sp.	Obligate parasites of rodents and lagamorphs	Subcutaneous swelling with breathing hole	Visual	Manual larva removal; Topical fipronil is preventive
Hydatid disease[30,37]	*Echinococcus* and *Taenia*	Carnivore definitive host; herbivore or rodent intermediate host	Dependent on location of cysts	Radiography, ultrasonography, aspiration of cysts	Prevent exposure to host feces
Aortic aneurysm[2]	*Spirocerca lupi*	Dung beetle intermediate host	Acute death	Postmortem, ultrasonography	Vermin control
Malaria[14,29]	*Plasmodium* sp.	Mosquito intermediate host	None identified	Blood smear	Mosquito control

Adapted from Junge R: *Zoo and wild animal medicine,* 5th ed. Published by Saunders, St. Louis, MO, 2003, p340.

*Duke Lemur Center, unpublished data.

TABLE 36-7

Antimicrobials Recommended for Prosimians

Generic Name	Dosage (mg/kg)	Route of Administration	Frequency
Amoxicillin	10–20	PO	BID
Ampicillin	10–30	SC, IM, IV	q6-8h
Azithromycin	5–10	PO	q24h
Cefadroxil	20	PO	BID
Cefazolin	10–30	IM, IV	q8h
Ceftazidime	30–50	IM, IV	q8h
Ceftiofur	1.1–2.2	IM	q24h
Doxycycline	5–10	PO	BID
Metronidazole	25	PO	q24h
Trimethoprim/ Sulfamethoxazole	25	PO, IM	BID
Enrofloxacin	5	PO, SC, IM	q24h

BID, Twice daily; *IM*, intramuscularly; *IV*, intravenously; *mg/kg*, milligram per kilogram; *PO*, orally; *q8h*, every 8 hours; *q6-8h*, every 6 to 8 hours; *q24h*, four times every 24 hours; *SC*, subcutaneously.

TABLE 36-8

Parasiticides Used in Prosimians

Generic name	Dosage (mg/kg)	Route of Administration	Organism
Thiabendazole	50	PO for 3–5 days	Nematodes
Pyrantel pamoate	5–10	PO, repeat in 2 weeks	Nematodes
Metronidazole	25	PO q24h	Protozoa
Nitazoxanide	25	PO q24h for 5–7 days	Protozoa
Tinidazole	40–45	PO q24h for 6 days	Protozoa
Fipronil	0.2 mL of 9.8% solution/kg body weight	Topically q6wk	*Cuterebra* sp., ticks

kg, Kilogram; *mg/kg*, milligram per kilogram; *mL*, milliliter; *PO*, orally; *q6wk*, every 6 weeks; *q24h*, every 24 hours.

Sepsis is the most common cause of mortality in Coquerel's sifakas (*Propithecus coquereli*) in captivity; hence, running blood cultures in all animals prior to implementing antibiotic therapy is important. Signs are nonspecific and include lethargy and anorexia with or without diarrhea. Ill sifakas invariably develop intestinal ileus, which often leads to intestinal bloating that may be confused with obstruction. As in other species, sepsis is associated with high mortality rates. Intensive therapy with intravenous antibiotics and fluids, supplemental warmth and oxygen, and correcting pH and electrolyte imbalances may improve outcomes if instituted early.

Lemurs are susceptible to developing *Clostridium difficile* toxemia secondary to antibiotic therapy.[44] Antibiotics alter gastrointestinal microbe populations, creating an environment conducive to *C. difficile* overgrowth. Clinical signs include bloody or severe watery diarrhea, lethargy, and anorexia. Diagnosis is by demonstrating *C. difficile* toxins in feces. The condition is fatal if not promptly treated. Oral metronidazole is usually effective; however, resistant infections may occur. In such cases, vancomycin is the secondary drug of choice. Performing transfaunation or fecal transplants by using the stool of a healthy individual may be beneficial for restoring healthy populations of intestinal microflora. Recommended dosages for antibacterial mediations are listed in Table 36-7.

Fungal Infections

Fungal infections occur rarely in lemurs in captivity. A case of disseminated coccidiomycosis has been reported in a ring-tailed lemur,[5] and an elderly mongoose lemur with uncontrolled diabetes died of disseminated cryptococcosis at the Duke Lemur Center (DLC) (unpublished data). Oral infections with *Candida albicans* may occur in lemurs treated with long-term antibiotics.

Parasitic Infections

Protozoal organisms infecting prosimians include *Entamoeba, Trichomonas, Giardia, Cryptosporidium,* and *Balantidium*. Lemurs are frequently asymptomatic carriers of *Giardia*. Infections resistant to metronidazole may respond to treatment with tinidazole. Sifakas (*Propithecus*) are highly susceptible to developing severe diarrhea associated with *Cryptosporidium* infection. These animals are most susceptible at weaning. Supportive care to prevent dehydration and to correct electrolyte imbalances is critical. Nitazoxanide decreases

the rate of shedding of cysts and the severity of clinical signs but does not cure the infection.

Common nematode parasites include oxyurids, ascarids, and organisms in the genera *Strongylus, Strongyloides, Gongylonema, Physaloptera, Enterobius,* and *Trichuris*. The preferred method for identification depends on the species of nematode and the specific gravity of the ova. The eggs of *Physaloptera* are shed intermittently and are heavier than the specific gravity of most standard fecal flotation solutions. Using Sheather's sugar solution or sodium nitrate solution at a specific gravity greater than 1.24 (e.g., 1.25 to 1.27) for flotation improves the chance of recovery of ova.[11] Parasiticides used in prosimians are provided in Table 36-8. Preliminary evidence suggests that lemurs, particularly sifakas (*Propithcus*), are susceptible to developing transient leukopenia and neutropenia 10 to 14 days following treatment with fenbendazole (unpublished data). Until further information is available, it is advisable to avoid using this drug in lemurs or to monitor white blood cell (WBC) counts if other suitable options are not available.

Infection with *Toxoplasma gondii* is common in captive prosimians and the disease is frequently fatal.[7,10] The disease is transmitted via ingestion of oocysts from infected cat feces, contaminated soil, bedding, or food items. Animals often die acutely. Clinicopathologic changes reflect the multisystemic nature of the infection, with elevated liver and renal function indexes. Diagnosis is often made by histologic examination of tissues in animals that die; however, tachyzoites may be detected antemortem in liver aspirates from infected animals. Determination of toxoplasmosis titers in paired serum samples confirms the diagnosis.

Malaria parasites have been identified in blood samples from a variety of different lemur species in Madagascar.[23,29] Several species of *Plasmodium* have been described; however, there is no evidence that these organisms are pathogenic in the lemur hosts or infect humans.[14] Evaluations of galagos, pottos, lorises, and tarsiers have not led to identification of any *Plasmodium* organisms.[16]

NONINFECTIOUS DISEASES

Selected noninfectious diseases are listed in Table 36-9. A large variety of neoplasms have been reported in lemurs, the most common being those affecting the gastrointestinal system (specifically the liver), the reproductive system, and the hematopoietic system. Readers interested in more detail are referred to a comprehensive retrospective review of spontaneous neoplasia in prosimians by

TABLE 36-9

Selected Noninfectious Diseases of Prosimians

Disease	Cause	Species	Signs	Management
Diabetes mellitus[38,42]	High-carbohydrate diet, obesity, and decreased exercise are factors	Ring-tailed, black and brown lemurs	None to varying degrees of weight loss, polyuria, polydipsia, polyphagia	High-fiber, low-glycemic index diet Oral hypoglycemics, insulin, if needed
Hemosiderosis[15,40, 46]	Increased iron stores in the liver	Ruffed, black and brown, and ring-tailed lemurs	None documented in lemurs ante mortem	Avoid iron-containing supplements Feed diets high in fiber
Trichobezoars[4]	Accumulation of hair in stomach from grooming	Ruffed lemurs	Abdominal discomfort, vomiting	Add laxative to diet Endoscopic or surgical removal
Periarticular hyperostosis[19]	Genetic proliferative bone disease	Black lemurs	Marked swelling of tarsal and stifle joints; renal failure	Nonsteroidal anti-inflammatory drugs may slow progression and alleviate discomfort

Adapted from Junge R: Zoo and *wild animal medicine*, 5th ed. Published by Saunders, St. Louis, 2003, p 343.

Remick.[32] Hepatocellular carcinoma was the most common neoplasm identified in prosimians. Despite attempts to determine factors predisposing prosimians to developing hepatic tumors, no cause has yet been identified.[48]

Renal disease is a common cause of mortality in older prosimians. Species commonly affected include *Eulemur, Varecia, Hapalemur,* and *Loris tardigradis.* Histopathologic changes at postmortem examination include glomerulonephritis, glomerulosclerosis, and chronic interstitial nephritis.[1,13,16] Urethral and ureteral obstructions occur but are not common. Calcium oxalates stones were identified as the cause of ureteral obstructions in two sifakas at the DLC (unpublished data).

Diabetes is common in middle-aged or older lemurs in captivity. Walzer[42] hypothesized that obesity with subsequent hyperinsulinemia is an obligatory stage in the progression to type II, or non–insulin-dependent, diabetes mellitus in lemurs, although four black lemurs at the DLC with no history of obesity developed diabetes, which suggests that obesity is not a requirement. As in other primates, a high-carbohydrate, low-fiber diet, combined with minimal activity, are likely predisposing factors. Because lemurs are prone to developing stress hyperglycemia secondary to handling, the workup for diabetes should always include measuring serum fructosamine or glycated hemoglobin (HbA$_{1c}$) levels to evaluate blood glucose levels over an extended period. Treatment consists initially of modifying the diets to eliminate simple sugars and starches, increase fiber, and feed frequent small meals to minimize spikes in blood glucose. The oral hypoglycemic agents glipizide, metformin, and acarbose have been used successfully in black lemurs and ring-tailed lemurs at the DLC to manage lemurs in the early stages of diabetes (unpublished data). If diet modification and oral hypoglycemics do not sufficiently regulate blood glucose, then insulin therapy is warranted. Glargine insulin (Lantus), a recombinant human product, given once daily subcutaneously, has been used to achieve glycemic control in a ring-tailed lemur.

Hemosiderosis, excess iron accumulation in tissues, was first reported in captive lemurs in the 1980s, prompting concerns that iron accumulation poses a serious health threat to captive lemurs.[1,39] However, more recent studies comparing liver iron levels in multiple species in captivity have failed to substantiate concerns that levels are sufficiently high to cause clinical disease or adversely affect animal health.[15,46] In a study comparing liver iron content in three species of lemurs, iron levels were highest in ruffed lemurs, lowest in ring-tailed lemurs, and intermediate in collared lemurs, which suggests that the physiologic regulation of iron absorption may vary by species.[46]

REPRODUCTION

A summary of reproductive parameters for selected prosimian species is provided in Table 36-10.

Unlike anthropoid primates, prosimians have estrus cycles as opposed to menstrual cycles. With the exception of aye-ayes (*Daubentonia*), lemurs exhibit seasonal estrus cycles and restricted births seasons. Members of the Lorisidae exhibit both patterns, depending on the species. Reproductive morphology of prosimians includes a bicornuate uterus and epitheliochorial placenta in females and an os penis and seminal vesicles in males, aye-ayes being the exception with vestigial seminal vesicles.[17] Mammary glands are pectoral, abdominal, or both in all species except in aye-ayes, which have a pair of inguinal glands. Levels of testosterone and, therefore, testes size and levels of aggression increase during the breeding season in males of seasonally reproductive species.

Contraception

Contraception may be achieved in prosimians either by permanent means such as surgical sterilization or via reversible methods involving hormonal manipulation. In females, injections of repository progesterone (Depo-Provera), 5 milligram per kilogram (mg/kg), intramuscularly (IM), every 40 days in ring-tailed lemurs and every 60 days in other species, render females infertile as do subcutaneous implants of medroxyprogesterone acetate (MGA).

Gonadotropin-releasing hormone agonists (GnRH agonists) Suprelorin (deslorelin) and Lupron are considered safe, reversible contraceptives for both sexes of a variety of mammals, but dosages and efficacy are not yet established for prosimians. Deslorelin has been used with some success to limit intermale aggression in bachelor groups of Coquerel's sifakas (*Propithecus coquereli*) and black lemurs (*Eulemur macaco macaco*) (DLC unpublished data). In contrast, Lupron used in a bachelor group of collared lemurs (*Eulemur collaris*) did not appear to decrease aggression in this species.[12]

MEDICINE

Subcutaneous transponder chips are the recommended method of permanent identification of prosimians in zoologic collections. Transponders are placed subcutaneously between the scapulae. Tattoos may be used as an additional means of identification, if desired. The preferable location is the nonhaired skin of the medial thigh. For animals not on display, applying colored nylon collars with varying shapes of dog tags or shaving a ring of fur from the tail at different

TABLE 36-10

Reproductive Parameters in Selected Prosimian Primates

	Peak Breeding Season *	Days between Cycles	Sperm Plugs?	Gestation (Days)	Peak Birth Season*	Number of Infants	Infant Weight Ranges (grams)	Average Weaning Age
Aye-aye	Year round	35–40	N	157–172	Year round	1	100–120	1–2 years
Collared lemur	Nov–Jan	30	Y	120–128	Mar–May	1–2	60–90	3–4 months
Black lemur	Oct–Jan	33	Y	120–129	Mar–May	1–3	60–90	3–4 months
Mongoose lemur	Nov–Feb	30–38	Y	120–128	Mar–Jun	1–2	55–60	3–4 months
Ring-tailed lemur	Oct–Dec	39	Y	130–136	Mar–May	1–2	60–90	3–4 months
Mouse lemur	Apr–Jun	40–60	Y	57–63	Jun–Aug	1–6	8–9	60 days
Coquerel's sifaka	Jul–Oct		Y†	155–168	Dec–Mar	1	90–115	4–6 months
Ruffed lemur	Jan–Feb	35–44	Y	98–102	Apr–May	1–5	100–125	3–4 months
Pygmy slow loris	Jul–Sept†		Y	183–198	Jan–Apr†	1–4	25–30	4–6 months
Thick-tailed bushbaby	Year round	51		126–136	Year round	1–3	45–50	5 months

*Peak seasons are given for North America.
†Sperm plugs inconsistently produced.

distances from the base provide easy visual aids for differentiating animals, but permanent identification is still required.

Vaccination

Despite lack of information regarding titer responses of prosimians to rabies vaccines, precaution warrants vaccinating individuals with a killed vaccine if a risk of exposure to rabies vectors exists. Vaccination against tetanus is elective, as no information exists regarding the tendency of prosimians to develop the condition. Routine periodic physical examinations, dental prophylaxis, and laboratory testing under anesthesia are recommended for captive prosimians to detect problems early when treatment is most effective.

Transport

Preshipment testing should be performed prior to moving prosimians between facilities. Common preshipment testing includes a physical examination under anesthesia, complete blood cell count (CBC) and chemistry screening, fecal examination for ova and parasites, fecal culture for *Salmonella*, *Shigella*, *Campylobacter*, and *Yersinia*, and TB testing using MOT. Lemurs may be asymptomatic carriers of both *Giardia* and *Cryptosporidium*, so specific testing aimed at detecting these protozoa is recommended to avoid unknowingly introducing these pathogens into a receiving institution. Additional testing is at the discretion of the receiving institution. Animals should be quarantined on arrival before exposure to other animals in the new collection. Governmental regulations need to be considered; however, agencies are often not prepared with appropriate regulations for this taxon.

REFERENCES

1. Benirschke K, Miller C, Ippen R, et al: The pathology of prosimians, especially lemurs. *Adv Vet Sci Comp Med* 30:167–208, 1985.
2. Blancou J, Albignac R: Note sur l'infestation des lemuriens malagaches par *Spirocerca lupi*. *Rev Elev Med Vet Pays Trop* 29(2):127–130, 1976.
3. Bons N, Mestre-Frances N, Belli P, et al: Natural and experimental oral infection of nonhuman primates by bovine spongiform encephalopathy agents. *Proc Natl Acad Sci* 96:4046–4051, 1999.
4. Brockman KD, Willis MS, Karesh WB: Management and husbandry of ruffed lemurs, *Varecia variegata*, at the San Diego Zoo. 3. Medical considerations and population management. *Zoo Biol* 7:253–262, 1988.
5. Burton M, Morton RJ, Ramsay E, et al: Coccidioidomycosis in a ring-tailed lemur. *J Am Vet Med Assoc* 189(9):1209–1211, 1986.
6. Calle P, Bowerman D, Pape W: Nonhuman primate tularemia (*Francisella tularensis*) epizootic in a zoological park. *J Zoo Wildl Med* 24(4):459–468, 1993.
7. Chang J, Kornegay RW, Wagner JL, et al: Toxoplasmosis in a sifaka. In Montali RJ, Migaki G, editors: *The comparative pathology of zoo animals*, Washington, DC, 1980, Smithsonian Institution Press, pp 347–352.
8. Campbell GA, Hoover JP, Russell WC, et al: Naturally occurring cerebral nematodiasis due to *Baylisascaris* larval migration in two black-and-white ruffed lemurs (*Varecia variegata variegata*) and suspected cases in three emus (*Dromaius novaehollandiae*). *J Zoo Wildl Med* 28(2):204–207, 1997.
9. Dausmann KH, Glos J, Ganzhorn JU, et al: Hibernation in the tropics: Lessons learned from a primate. *J Comp Physiol [B]* 175:147–155, 2005.
10. Dubey JP, Kramer LW, Weisbrode SE: Acute death associated with *Toxoplasma gondii* in ring-tailed lemurs. *J Am Vet Med Assoc* 187(11):1272–1273, 1985.
11. Dryden MW, Payne PA, Ridley R, et al: Comparison of common fecal flotation techniques for the recovery of parasite eggs and oocysts. *Vet Ther* 6(1):15–28, 2005.
12. Ferrie GM, Becker KK, Wheaton CJ, et al: Chemical and surgical interventions to alleviate intraspecific aggression in male collared lemurs (*Eulemur collaris*). *J Zoo Wildl Med* 42(2):214–221, 2011.
13. Fitch-Snyder H, Schulze H: *Management of lorises in captivity: A husbandry manual for Asian lorisines (Nycticebus and Loris spp.)*, San Diego, CA, 2001, Zoological Society of San Diego.
14. Garnham P, Uilenberg G: Malaria parasites of lemurs. *Ann Parasit (Paris)* 50(4):409–418, 1975.
15. Glenn KM, Campbell JL, Rotstein D, et al: A retrospective evaluation of the incidence and severity of hemosiderosis in a large captive lemur population. *Am J Primatol* 68:369–381, 2006.
16. Haines DE, editor: *The lesser bushbaby (galago) as an animal model: Selected topics*, Boca Raton, FL, 1982, CRC Press.
17. Hill WC: *Primates: Comparative anatomy and taxonomy, I-Strepsirhini*, New York, 1953, Interscience Publishers, Inc.
18. International Union for the Conservation of Nature: *The IUCN Red List of Threatened Species*: http://www.iucnredlist.org, 2012. Accessed 2/16/2013.
19. Junge R, Mehren K, Meehan T, et al: Periarticular hyperostosis and renal disease in six black lemurs of two family groups. *J Am Vet Med Assoc* 205(7):1024–1029, 1994.
20. Kemp G, Losos G, Causey O, et al: Isolation of *Herpesvirus hominis* from lemurs: A naturally occurring epizootic at a zoological park in Nigeria. *Afr J Med Sci* 3:177–185, 1972.

21. Knezevic AL, McNulty WP: Tuberculosis in Lemur mongoz. *Folia Primatol* 6:153–159, 1967.

22. Kornegay R, Baldwin T, Pirie G: Herpesvirus encephalitis in a ruffed lemur (*Varecia variegata*). *J Zoo Wildl Med* 24(2):196–203, 1993.

23. Landau I, Lepers JP, Rabetafika L, et al: Plasmodies de Lémuriens Malgaches. *Ann Parasitol Hum Comp* 3:171–184, 1989.

24. Mittermeier RA, Louis EE, Richardson M, et al: *Lemurs of Madagascar*, ed 3, Washington, DC, 2010, Conservation International.

25. Müller EF, Nieschalk U, Meier B: Thermoregulation in the slender loris (*Loris tardigradus*). *Folia Primatol* 44:216–226, 1985.

26. National Research Council: Feeding ecology, digestive strategies, and implications for feeding programs in captivity. In *Nutrient requirements of nonhuman primates*, ed 2, Washington, DC, 2003, The National Academies Press, pp 5–40.

27. Nakajima Y, Shantha TR, Bourne GH: Histochemical detection of L-gulonolactone: Phenazine methosulfate oxidoreductase activity in several mammals with special reference to synthesis of vitamin C in primates. *Histochemie* 18:293–301, 1969.

28. Nowak RM: *Walker's mammals of the world*, vol 1, ed 6, Baltimore, MD, 1999, Johns Hopkins University Press.

29. Pacheco AM, Battistuzzi FU, Junge RE, et al: Timing the origin of human malarias: The lemur puzzle. *BMC Evol Biol* 11:299, 2011.

30. Palotay JL, Uno H: Hydatid disease in four nonhuman primates. *J Am Vet Med Assoc* 167(7):615–618, 1975.

31. Reddacliff L, Kirkland P, Hartley W, et al: Encephalomyocarditis virus infections in an Australian zoo. *J Zoo Wildl Med* 28(2):153–157, 1997.

32. Remick AK, Van Wettere AJ, Williams CV: Neoplasia in prosimians: Case series from a captive prosimian population and literature review. *Vet Pathol* 46(4):746–772, 2009.

33. Rodhain F, Petter J, Albignac R, et al: Arboviruses and lemurs in Madagascar: Experimental infection of Lemur fulvus with yellow fever and West Nile viruses. *Am J Trop Med Hyg* 34(4):816–822, 1985.

34. Ross C: Basal metabolic rate, body weight and diet in primates: An evolution of the evidence. *Folia Primatol* 58:7–23, 1992.

35. Schmidt RE: Tuberculosis in a ring-tailed lemur (*Lemur catta*). *J Zoo Wildl Med* 6(3):11–12, 1975.

36. Schuppel von K, Reinacher M, Lebelt J, et al: Bornasche krankheit bei primaten. *Verh ber Erkrg Zootiere* 36:37–42, 1995.

37. Sharar R, Horowitz IH, Aizenberg I: Disseminated hydatidosis in a ring-tailed lemur (*Lemur catta*): A case report. *J Zoo Wildl Med* 26(1):119–122, 1995.

38. Singleton C, Wack RF, Larsen RS: Use of oral hypoglycemic drugs for the management of diabetes mellitus in prosimians. In *Proceedings of the American Association of Zoo Veterinarians*, Tampa, FL, 2006, p 379.

39. Spelman L, Osborn K, Anderson M: Pathogenesis of hemosiderosis in lemurs: Role of dietary iron, tannin, and ascorbic acid. *Zoo Biol* 8:239–251, 1989.

40. Spencer JA, Joiner KS, Hilton CD, et al: Disseminated toxoplasmosis in a captive ring-tailed lemur (*Lemur catta*). *J Parasitol* 90(4):904–906, 2004.

41. Stetter M, Worley M, Ruiz B: Herpesvirus associated malignant lymphoma in a slow loris (*Nycticebus coucang*). *J Zoo Wildl Med* 26(1):155–160, 1995.

42. Walzer C, Jubber-Heiss A: Obesity in the development of diabetes mellitus in ring-tailed lemurs (*Lemur catta*): An obligatory component? *Verh ber Erkrg Zootiere* 37:143–148, 1995.

43. Williams CV, Van Steenhouse JL, Bradley JM, et al: Naturally occurring *Ehrlichia chaffeensis* infection in two prosimian primate species: Ring-tailed lemurs (*Lemur catta*) and ruffed lemurs (*Varecia variegata*). *Emerg Infec Dis* 8(12):1497–1499, 2002.

44. Williams CV: Spontaneous *Clostridium difficile*-associated diarrhea in lemurs. In *Proceedings of the American Association of Zoo Veterinarians*, Milwaukee, WI, 2002, pp 359–364.

45. Williams CV, Glenn KM, Levine JF, et al: Comparison of the efficacy and cardiorespiratory effects of medetomidine-based anesthetic protocols in ring-tailed lemurs (*Lemur catta*). *J Zoo Wildl Med* 34(2):163–170, 2003.

46. Williams CV, Campbell JL, Glenn KM: A comparison of serum iron, total iron binding capacity, ferritin, and percent transferrin saturation in nine species of apparently healthy captive lemurs. *Am J Primatol* 68:1–13, 2006.

47. Whittow GC, Scammell CA, Manuel JK, et al: Temperature regulation in a hypometabolic primate, the slow loris (*Nycticebus coucang*). *Arch Int Physiol Biochim Biophys* 85:139–151, 1977.

48. Zadrozny LM, Williams CV, Remick AK, et al: Spontaneous hepatocellular carcinoma in captive prosimians. *Vet Pathol* 47(2):306–311, 2010.

CHAPTER 37

New World and Old World Monkeys

Paul P. Calle and Janis Ott Joslin

The primate order may be broadly divided into prosimians, New World (NW) and Old World (OW) monkeys, and great apes.[13,15,17,24,47,48] The NW and OW monkeys, which are the subject of this chapter, represent over 270 species, with several new species described in the last decade. NW monkeys are in the Platyrrhini parvorder, which includes the Cebidae, Aotidae, Pitheciidae, and Atelidae families. The Callitrichinae subfamily of the Cebidae family consists of marmosets and tamarins, which are the smallest monkey species. The rest of the NW monkeys are small- to medium-sized monkeys such as squirrel monkeys (*Saimiri* sp.), capuchin monkeys (*Cebus* sp.), spider monkeys (*Ateles* sp.). OW monkeys are all in the Catarrhini parvorder and the Cercopithecidae family. They are medium- to large-sized monkeys such as macaques (*Macaca* sp.) and baboons (*Papio* sp.) (Table 37-1).[17,24,47,48]

NW and OW monkeys exhibit a range of biology, behavior, and environmental niches with adaptations for those specializations and range across Asia, Africa, South America, and Central America. NW monkeys are generally arboreal and live in tropical forests. OW monkeys may be arboreal and inhabit forests or largely terrestrial and live in more open grasslands (i.e., baboon species); the range of

TABLE 37-1

Biologic Information for New World and Old World Monkeys[17,47,48]

Scientific Name[48]	Common Name	Adult Weight (kg)	Geographic Distribution	Identification
FAMILY: CERCOPITHECIDAE				
Subfamily: Cercopithecinae				
Genus: *Allenopithecus*	Allen's swamp monkey	♂‡, 6 ♀+, 3.5	Northwestern Zaire; northeastern Angola	Stocky, pelage olive green dorsally, white ventrally, face pink, longer hair on cheeks; red scrotum, webbing between fingers and toes
Genus: *Cercocebus*	White-eyed mangabey	3–20	Sub-Saharan Africa	Large, slender bodies; under parts fawn or cream; ♂s ischial callosities fused in the midline; moderate ♀ sexual skin swelling
Genus: *Cercopithecus*	Guenon	1.8–12	Sub-Saharan Africa	Medium to large; fur is thick, short, green, yellow, and black; nose spots, moustaches, and beards; slender; long tail; small ischial callosities; blue scrotum
Genus: *Chlorocebus*	Vervet; grivet; African green	5–9	Sub-Saharan Africa (introduced on St. Kitts, Nevus, Caribbean)	Abdominal skin blue; scrotum and ♂ perianal area blue; red penis; long, sharp canines
Genus: *Erythrocebus*	Patas monkey	♂, 7–13 ♀, 4–7	Sub-Saharan Africa; Senegal to Tanzania	Large, slender; long limbs, slender tail; red brown coarse hair; nose dark when young and gray or white in adults; small ischial callosities; blue scrotum
Genus: *Lophocebus*	Crested mangabey	♂, 9–10 ♀, 6.4–7	Across Central Africa	Long limbs and tail; long molars and large incisors; estrous anogenital swelling or reddening
Genus: *Macaca*	Macaque	♀, 2.5–16 ♂, 3.5–18	North Africa; Asia	Medium to large, heavy bodied; brown; narrow nose; sexually dimorphic in size; prominent ischial callosities; cheek pouches
Genus: *Mandrillus*	Drill; mandrill	♂, 25.5–54 ♀, 11.5	West Africa	*M. sphinx*: large, brightly colored muzzle; perianal skin red; scrotum pale purple and pink; long tail. *M. leucophaeus* also has olive green coat; face black with white checks
Genus: *Miopithecus*	Talapoin	♂, 1.2–1.3 ♀, 0.74–0.82	West Central Africa	Small; fur green, speckled with black; pale yellow arms and legs; tail equal in length to body length; sexual skin swelling in ♀s
Genus: *Papio*	Baboon	14–41 ♂s 50% larger	Sub-Saharan Africa	Large dense coat; prominent muzzle; tail moderately long; prominent ischial callosities, continuous in ♂/separate in ♀; ♂ prominent canines
Genus: *Theropithecus*	Gelada baboon; gelada	♂, 20.5 ♀, 13.6	Ethiopian Highlands	Large, rounded muzzle; upper lip long and bulbous; ♂ long dark heavy mane; chest bare patch with color change in ♀ during estrus; ischial callosities; ♂ canines larger
Subfamily: Colobinae				
Genus: *Colobus*	Black-and-white colobus monkey	5.4–14.5	Africa; Senegal to Kenya and Angola	Large, slender body; long tail; coat glossy black, long, with white mantling; prominent nose; ischial callosities; small thumb

TABLE 37-1

Biologic Information for New World and Old World Monkeys—cont'd

Scientific Name[48]	Common Name	Adult Weight (kg)	Geographic Distribution	Identification
Genus: *Nasalis*	Proboscis monkey; long-nosed monkey	♂, 16–22.5 ♀, 7–12	Borneo; Malaysia; Indonesia	Large; hair dark red to brown; bare face; ♂ nose long, wide, hangs over mouth, smaller and upturned in ♀s; large ischial callosity; pot-bellied; 2nd and 3rd toes webbed; small thumb; ♂ 50% larger than ♀
Genus: *Piliocolobus*	Red colobus	♂ 5.8–12.5 ♀ 5.5–9.1	Western; central; eastern Africa	Dark coat and bright red ventrally; bright red cheeks and forearms; long tail; small thumb
Genus: *Presbytis*	Leaf-monkey; surilis; bearded langur; crested langur	5.0–8.1	Sumatra; Java; Borneo; Indonesia	Medium to large; long tail; fur long; face black; newborns often lighter in color and darken with age; opposable thumb; ♂ canines larger
Genus: *Procolobus*	Olive colobus	2.9–11.3	Africa; Senegal to Zanzibar	Juveniles of both sexes have perianal organs that mimic adult ♀ sexual swelling; coat olive-brown or orange-red
Genus: *Pygathrix*	Douc monkey, Douc langur	♂, 11–17 ♀, 6.5–12	China; Indonesia	Large; short fur; thighs, hands, and feet black; legs red; head brown and bright chestnut below ears; face black or yellow; ♂ canines larger
Genus: *Rhinopithecus*	Snub-nosed monkey, golden monkey	♂, 15–19.8 ♀, 6.5–10	Southern China; Northern Vietnam; Myanmar.	Large; robust body and limbs; muzzle white, hairless; coat long, multi-colored (yellowish, brown, or black); upturned small nose, forward pointing nostrils; rounded face; ♂ larger
Genus: *Semnopithecus*	Hanuman langur; sacred langur	♂, 9–20 ♀, 7.5–18	Southern Asia	Grey to brown coat
Genus: *Simias*	Simakobu; pig-tailed snub-nose langur	♂, 7.6–8.7 ♀, 5.2–6.9	Mebtawai Islands	Large; heavy body; long arms; short slightly furred tail; black-brown coat; black hairless face
Genus: *Trachypithecus*	Dusty langur, leaf-monkey; lutung	4.2–14.0	India; China; Indonesia	Dark grey to black; pale markings on body and head; newborn orange or reddish brown (changes to adult color at 3 months)
FAMILY: CEBIDAE **Subfamily: Callitrichinae** Genus: *Callimico*	Goeldi's marmoset, callimico	0.393–0.860	Western Brazil; northern Bolivia; eastern Peru; Columbia	All black; short fur; claws instead of nails except for hallux, which has a nail
Genus: *Callithrix*	True marmoset	0.100–0.453	Upper and middle Amazon; Brazilian coast south of the Amazon	Non-opposable thumbs; claws on fingers except 1st digit of toes; large chisel-like incisors and canines; ♀ external genitalia resembles ♂'s
Genus: *Leontopithecus*	Lion tamarin; lion marmoset	0.6–0.8	Southeast Brazil	Non-opposable thumbs; claws on fingers except 1st digit of toes; fur golden with black markings
Genus: *Saguinus*	Tamarin	0.225–0.900	Rainforests Central and South America	Non-opposable thumbs; claws on fingers except 1st digit of toes; canines larger than incisors

Continued

TABLE 37-1

Biologic Information for New World and Old World Monkeys—cont'd

Scientific Name[48]	Common Name	Adult Weight (kg)	Geographic Distribution	Identification
Subfamily: Cebinae Genus: *Cebus*	Capuchin monkey	1.1–3.3	Honduras to northern Argentina	Short semi prehensile tail; coats black or brown; thumb well differentiated; large big toe; clitoris is prominent; ♂ larger than ♀; ♂ canines larger
Subfamily: Saimiriinae Genus: *Saimiri*	Squirrel monkey	0.75–1.10	South and Central America	Small; fur is short, dense, gray-green to olive; pale on belly; ♂ larger than ♀
FAMILY: AOTIDAE Genus: *Aotus*	Owl monkey, night monkey, douroucouli	0.6–1.0	South and Central America	Only nocturnal New World monkey; grooming claw on 4th digit of both feet; eyes lack tapetum
FAMILY: PITHECIIDAE **Subfamily: Callicebinae** Genus: *Callicebus*	Titi monkey	0.51–0.73	Columbia to Paraguay; south-eastern Brazil	Long, bushy fur; tail long, non-prehensile; form strong pair bonds, often seen sitting side by side with tails entwined
Subfamily: Pitheciinae Genus: *Cacajao*	Uakari	♂, 4 ♀, 2.4–3.5	Northwestern Brazil; eastern Peru; south-western Venezuela	Short tail; hairless bright red face; lower incisors compressed similar to a dental comb; large canines
Genus: *Chiropotes*	Bearded saki monkey	2–4	North central Brazil; Guyana; French Guiana; Surinam; southern Venezuela	Medium size; long thick dark coat; full, bushy beard; long thick tail
Genus: *Pithecia*	Saki monkey	0.7–1.7	Guyana southwest to Peruvian Amazon	Thick, coarse coat: grey or black long hair on head; lower incisors resemble dental combs
FAMILY: ATELIDAE **Subfamily: Alouattinae** Genus: *Alouatta*	Howler monkey	4–10	Southern Mexico to northern Argentina	Large; robust; long fur; prehensile tail hairless on bottom; bare face; large modified hyoid specialized for producing a loud call (larger in ♂); opposable big toe
Subfamily: Atelinae Genus: *Ateles*	Spider monkey	♂, 6–10 ♀, 6–8	Mexico to Brazil	Long, slender arms and legs; pot-bellied; ♀ larger than ♂; small big toe; prehensile hand; thumb small or absent
Genus: *Brachyteles*	Woolly spider monkey, Muriqui	12–15	South-eastern Brazil	Large; thick coat; absent thumb; prehensile tail; naked dark face; no sexual dimorphism; small canines in both sexes
Genus: *Lagothrix*	Woolly monkey	♂, 3.6–10 ♀, 5–6.5	Middle and upper Amazon basin; Eastern Andes; Amazonas in Brazil	Large; long, muscular prehensile tail; dense woolly dark coat; long thumb; widely divergent big toe; ♂ 30% longer than ♀
Genus: *Oreonax*	Yellow-tailed woolly monkey	♂, 5.7 ♀, 8.3	Peruvian Andes	Large; long, muscular, prehensile tail; long, thick, mahogany coat; yellow genital hair tuff under tail; long thumb; widely divergent big toe; ♂ 30% longer than ♀

kg, Kilogram; ‡♂, male; ⁺ ♀, female.

some macaques extends to high elevations (i.e., Japanese snow monkey *M. fuscata*). Most are diurnal, but some are largely nocturnal. In general, monkeys live in medium- to large-sized troops, with a structured dominance hierarchy consisting of a dominant male, multiple females of various ages, and young males. However, some species are more solitary and live in smaller family groups, multi-male troops, or groups in which females are less submissive. They are intelligent and exhibit tool use, prolonged maturation periods, long gestations, extended life spans, complex social relationships that include grooming of troop members, formation of alliances, long-term relationships, use of tactical deceptive behaviors, and infanticide following the ascension of a new male to dominance. They have many valuable environmental roles, including a significant role in seed dispersal.[13,17,24]

Overall, more than half of all nonhuman primate species face the threat of extinction. The greatest threats are posed by habitat destruction, modification, and fragmentation, as well as both the local and the international bushmeat trade.[16,24,41] Because of the threatened and endangered status of many nonhuman primates, obtaining and possessing these species are governed by national and international regulations such as the Convention on International Trade in Endangered Species (CITES), in the United States by the U.S. Fish and Wildlife Service and various state regulations, and similar agencies in other countries.

Monkeys are popular species for exhibition and biomedical research; however, they do not make good pets, and private ownership is illegal in many parts of the world. Because of a shared evolutionary history, human primates are excellent models for nonhuman primate anatomy, biology, physiology, diseases, therapeutics, and pharmacology. Much more is written about human primates in these disciplines, which provides a ready source of comparative medical information that may be applied to the care of nonhuman primates.

UNIQUE ANATOMY

Nonhuman primates have anatomic features very similar to those of humans, including raised papillary ridges (fingerprints); ocular adaptations, including convergent eye sockets resulting in binocular vision, an overlap of visual fields which enables stereoscopic vision, rods and cones for color vision, and a retinal fovea centralis for sharp imaging; grasping hands; large brains; clavicles; two pectoral mammae; and heterodont dentition. The dental formula for all OW monkeys is 2 : 1 : 2 : 3 and 2 : 1 : 2 : 3 and for all NW monkeys 2 : 1 : 3 : 3 and 2 : 1 : 3 : 3 except for the *Callithrix*, *Leontopithecus*, *Saguinus*, and *Cebus*, which have the same dental formula as OW monkeys.

Biologic data for representative species are listed in Table 37-1. Prehensile tails are only found in some NW monkeys such as howler monkeys (*Alouatta* sp.) and spider monkeys, and ischial callosities occur in OW monkeys.[13,17,24] Opposable thumbs are found in most OW monkeys, although some such as colobus monkeys (*Colobus* sp.) have vestigial thumbs. NW and OW monkeys range in size from the smallest monkey species the approximately 120-gram (g) pygmy marmoset (*Callithrix* [*Cebuella*] *pygmaea*), although some prosimians are smaller, to the largest monkey species the approximately 30-kilogram (kg) mandrill (*Mandrillus sphinx*), which has colorful facial ridges and a bare face.

In some species such as baboons, a dramatic sexual size dimorphism in size exists, the males being significantly larger than the females and possessing large canine teeth, which may inflict serious wounds. Howler monkeys have elaborately enlarged hyoid bones that help create the unique vocalization for which they are named; male lion-tailed macaques (*M. silenus*) have a flamboyant gray mane; douc langurs (*Pygathrix sp.*) are strikingly beautiful; and the male proboscis monkeys (*Nasalis larvatus*) have a significantly enlarged nose.

Laryngeal diverticula (air sacs) are present in most NW and OW monkeys, and many OW monkey species also have cheek pouches in which food is stored during foraging. The OW Colobinae subfamily (colobus, langurs, proboscis, etc.) are folivorous, with diets consisting largely of leaves and other vegetation. They possess complex sacculated stomachs in which foregut microbial fermentation takes place, and this deactivates some plant toxins and generates volatile fatty acids that are absorbed as an energy source. Similarly, NW howler monkeys have hindgut fermentation in the cecum and colon.[13,17,24] The complex foreguts of the OW Colobinae and the hindgut of NW howler monkeys are susceptible to protozoal (*Amoeba* sp.) infection. Antibiotic treatment in these species may disrupt normal microbial digestion, resulting in dysbiosis and diarrhea. If this does not resolve with discontinuation of antibiotic treatment, transfaunation of stomach contents from a healthy OW monkey from the same or a closely related species or, in the case of the NW howler monkeys, feces from another howler, may be performed.

SPECIAL HOUSING REQUIREMENTS

Housing for NW and OW monkeys must meet their social, environmental, physical, and behavioral needs, in addition to addressing disease transmission concerns. Because of advances in exhibit design and construction, in medical treatments, and in the art and science of captive care, naturalistic exhibits are much more common than was previously possible.

Effective parasite treatment regimens, in particular, have enhanced the ability to maintain nonhuman primates in naturalistic exhibits. Design of exhibit and off-exhibit holding areas should prevent disease transmission between human and nonhuman primates through the use of glass or physical separation that is adequate to prevent airborne disease transmission between the public or workers and the nonhuman primates. This should be enhanced through management and husbandry protocols to ensure the health and safety of both human and nonhuman primates.

With medium- and large-sized nonhuman primates, it is recommended that the animals be shifted out of the exhibit for servicing. In the United States, nonhuman primate behavioral enrichment is mandated by the United States Department of Agriculture Animal Welfare Act, and all licensed holders are required to have an active behavioral enrichment program. A complex physical environment that usually incorporates arboreal elements, distribution of food and non-food enrichment items throughout the substrate and exhibit, and housing animals in species-specific normal social groups are all critical components in the maintenance of healthy nonhuman primates.[34]

NUTRITION AND DIET

NW and OW monkeys may be either generalized or specialized feeders, with the majority consuming plants, fruits, nuts, insects, and other foods such as small invertebrates.[13,17] Some dietary specializations are a gummivorous diet or a largely frugivorous, herbivorous, omnivorous, faunivorous, or folivorous diet, with the digestive tract adaptations reflecting the species diet. In all cases, replication of the natural diet is recommended. Because the wild diet is varied, the common practice is to offer a variety of food items, in the belief that nonhuman primates will self-select proper food items for a balanced diet. Unfortunately, this is often not the case, and nutritional problems such as obesity, nutritional secondary hyperparathyroidism, gastrointestinal (GI) problems, and hypoproteinemia may result from this feeding strategy. Nonhuman primates will ingest 2% to 4% of their body weight daily. In contrast to wild fruits and vegetables, many commercially available varieties cultivated for human consumption are lower in protein (2% to 6% of dry matter [DM]), calcium (0.03% to 0.3% of DM), and fiber, and higher in sugar, than their wild counterparts. To prevent overconsumption, nonhuman primates should generally be fed no more than 30% of DM as produce. Because produce contains 10% to 20% of DM, canned foods are 40% DM, and biscuits are 90% DM, the diet fed may be 70% produce and 30% biscuits by weight. If a canned diet is fed, 50% produce and 50% canned diet should be fed by weight, which will equal 30% of the DM in produce.[17]

In general, nonhuman primates have a minimal 7% to 10% protein requirement (DM basis), and pregnant or lactating animals require 12.5% protein. The National Research Council (NRC) recommends 16% protein on a DM basis for most nonhuman primates and 25% for New World monkeys.[17] Commercially prepared diets vary from 16% to 26.1% protein (lower protein diets are used for most nonhuman primates and higher protein ones for New World monkeys). Because most nonhuman primates are fed commercial diets along with low-protein items such as fruit, the total diet offered more closely approximates the requirements.

All nonhuman primates require appropriate ratios and amounts of dietary calcium and phosphorus. Calcium deficiency, or imbalance in calcium and phosphorus ratios, will result in metabolic bone disease ("simian bone disease" or rickets). NW monkeys require preformed dietary vitamin D_3 (cholecalciferol). Sunlight or appropriate ultraviolet (UV) wavelength exposure is also important for calcium metabolism. Marmosets have a vitamin D_3 requirement higher than that for other NW monkeys. Additionally, most marmosets and tamarins are fed insects, which are low in calcium. To balance the calcium and phosphorus levels, the insects must be fed a calcium-rich diet (8%) for at least 48 hours before being consumed. Nursing infants also have higher vitamin D requirements for normal skeletal growth, and if this is not met, the infant may develop nutritional deficiency. Both NW and OW monkeys require a dietary source of vitamin C. Signs of deficiency may include gingival hemorrhage, loose teeth, epiphyseal fractures, subperiosteal hemorrhage, decreased polymorphonuclear leukocyte activity, normocytic normochromic anemia, and exophthalmos. In young squirrel monkeys, cephalhematoma is the most common sign of vitamin C deficiency. The requirements for primates have been estimated to be 1 to 25 milligrams per kilogram per day (mg/kg/day), and stress effects on required vitamin C may account for the wide range in the daily requirements.[17]

Folivorous species (Colobinae subfamily) present special feeding challenges and require diets high in fiber. These species typically have either a large complex stomach or enlarged ceca and colon. *Trachypithecus*, *Semnopithecus*, *Presbytis*, and *Colobus* species have sacculated stomachs with two bands of longitudinal teniae. *Presbytis* species have a well-developed intestinal tract.[17] Commercially available diets high in fiber, with a 25% neutral detergent fiber and 12% to 16% acid detergent fiber, may be supplemented with leafy vegetables and browse, more closely approximating natural diets. Feeding frequently (three or more times daily) is important to promote continuous fermentation. Some *Colobus* species develop gluten sensitivity enteropathy when fed diets containing wheat, barley, rye, or oats. Gluten-free high-fiber monkey biscuits (25% neutral detergent fiber) are available and should be fed to *Colobus* species or any monkey with gluten intolerance. Commercial biscuits are formulated to comprise no less than 50% of the diet on an as-fed basis. Any diet changes for folivorous species should be done gradually to allow time for adjustment of gastric microflora. Diets should be supplemented with browse; however, both exhibit plants and browse that are high in lignin or indigestible fibers (e.g., acacia or browse with fibrous bark or foliage) cannot be digested by gastric microflora and may therefore result in phytobezoar obstruction.[5,17] Cebidae species are mostly omnivores and many feed on fruit and leaves. *Aotus* species mainly consume insects and bats, and both have simple stomachs with a variable length small intestine. The faunivores have a simple stomach and hindgut and a long small intestine. Gummivorous species (i.e., pygmy marmosets) have longer retention times for fermentation.[17]

A range of nutritionally complete canned or biscuit primate diets are commercially available, and the NW monkey diets include vitamin D_3. A combination of these commercially prepared diets and a mix of fresh fruits, vegetables, produce, and browse, as indicated by the dietary specialization, are most commonly fed. In addition, a variety of enrichment items should be planned as components of the calculated daily dietary requirements. A good general guide is that enrichment "treats" should constitute less than 10% of the daily dietary requirements to avoid dilution of the nutritional quality of the diet by overconsumption of enrichment "treats." Often these supplemental environmental or behavioral enrichment items are not nutritionally significant but are very important for the psychological and social stimulation they provide.[17,21,22,32] Dietary indiscretion from inappropriate diets, feeding by visitors, or gorging, may lead to GI upset; good exhibit design along with management and husbandry protocols minimize this risk.

RESTRAINT AND HANDLING

Physical restraint is only recommended for smaller nonhuman primate species and should only be performed by experienced handlers. Improperly performed physical restraint may be dangerous and stressful for the nonhuman primate and dangerous for the handler. Nonhuman primates weighing less than about 10 kg (depending on the level of the handler's experience, type of housing, and the monkey's disposition) may be manually restrained using appropriate gloves and nets; however, this is not recommended for macaque species because of the risk of herpes B virus exposure. However, larger or more aggressive monkeys should not be restrained in this way; instead, specialized restraint devices ("squeeze cages") or chemical immobilization should be employed. In addition, behavioral training may be used to enlist the voluntary participation of nonhuman primates in medical and management procedures.

ANESTHESIA AND SURGERY

A number of anesthetic protocols may be used for immobilization and anesthesia of monkeys (http://www.primatevets.org/education).[17,18,29,43] The most commonly employed for medium- to large-sized species are either ketamine alone (6–10 mg/kg, intramuscularly [IM]), or ketamine (2–4 mg/kg, IM) in combination with either medetomidine (0.04–0.06 mg/kg, IM) or dexmedetomidine (0.02–0.03 mg/kg, IM), typically combined in one syringe. When used in combination, the effects of the medetomidine or dexmedetomidine may be antagonized by the administration of atipamezole (IM at 5× the dose of medetomidine or 10× the dose of dexmedetomidine) to significantly shorten recovery time.

Reversal is best accomplished by administering the antagonist about 20 minutes or longer after initial dosing to allow for ketamine metabolism and therefore avoid residual ketamine sedation, which could result in ataxia or disorientation during recovery. If ketamine is not available, a combination of tiletamine and zolazepam may be used 2–5 mg/kg, IM); however, this drug combination results in considerably longer recovery times, which should be considered while planning how and where the monkey will recover from anesthesia. Atropine is not generally administered unless a specific reason for its use exists. All of these protocols are effective in inducing excellent muscle relaxation. Other injectable anesthetic protocols may be used in particular circumstances, to achieve specific purposes, or based on drug availability.

Doses are typically delivered by hand injection to monkeys that are conditioned to voluntarily receive injections or are manually restrained by hand, in a net, or in a restraint device; or the injection is delivered by pole syringe or by dart for other situations. Smaller species such as callitrichids may be anesthetized with an inhalant anesthetic such as isoflurane, administered either via a face mask to a monkey that may be safely manually restrained or by placing the monkey into an induction chamber. Once anesthetized by any method, anesthesia may be prolonged or the anesthetic plane deepened through the administration of inhalant anesthesia via a face mask.

Comfortable positioning, maintaining appropriate body temperature (i.e., provision of a recirculating hot water pad, heating pads, hot water bottles, heat lamps, etc.), and lubrication of the eyes with ophthalmic ointment are all important considerations, especially for prolonged anesthesia. For longer or more complicated procedures, or when a monkey has significant illness, endotracheal intubation is recommended because it allows for better respiratory support, greater control of the anesthetic plane, and a more effective emergency response, as needed. Similarly, in those situations, placement of an indwelling venous catheter is recommended for administration of fluids and immediate access for administration of emergency drugs.

Anesthesia is typically monitored by thoracic auscultation of heart and respiratory rates, observation of mucous membrane color, assessment of peripheral pulse (typically the femoral artery), electrocardiography (ECG) recording, and pulse oximetry. End tidal carbon dioxide (CO_2) measurement, direct and indirect blood pressure monitoring, and assessment of venous or arterial blood gases may also be performed as would be done in humans or domestic animals, as indicated by the animal's condition or duration of anesthesia. Documentation of the anesthetic drugs, doses, intervals, and physiologic parameters in an anesthesia report is valuable for reference during the anesthesia event and for future consultation.

Common surgical procedures of monkeys include repair of lacerations resulting from conspecific aggression; abscess debridement and treatment; dental extractions (especially carnasial tooth root infections resulting in facial abscesses); root canal procedures; and fracture fixation. All are performed by standard veterinary or human pediatric techniques. GI linear foreign bodies from consumption of inappropriate plant material,[5] and similar complications resulting from consumption of other foreign bodies have been observed. Lion-tailed macaques have a predisposition to develop inguinal hernias, and golden lion tamarins (*Leontopithecus rosalia*) more often have congenital diaphragmatic hernias compared with other species; these problems may be surgically corrected.[4,23,28]

Elective surgeries include vasectomy, castration, tubal ligation, and ovariohysterectomy for contraception. Emergency and therapeutic reproductive procedures include cesarean section, treatment of placental abruption or placenta previa, and treatment of endometriosis.[17,26] A postoperative concern is that the monkey with its nimble fingers, may remove the sutures, so suture lines should be buried by using subcuticular patterns, whenever possible. However, in the majority of cases, the monkeys leave the sutures alone.

DIAGNOSTICS

Most diagnostic techniques and options employed for small animals or in human pediatrics are applicable to NW and OW monkeys. Radiography, with routine lateral and ventrodorsal positioning, is standard; for larger species, obese individuals, or folivorous primates that have a large fluid-filled complex stomach, an upright sitting position and horizontal beam radiography will enhance thoracic detail.[17] Mammography machines provide exquisitely detailed radiographic visualization and may be used for whole body radiography in smaller species or to image the extremities of larger species. Ultrasonography is routinely employed using standard techniques and ultrasound probes. For ultrasonographic visualization of the female reproductive tract, if animal and probe sizes permit, intrarectal ultrasonography will provide the best visualization of the ovaries and the uterus. Flexible and rigid endoscopy allow minimally invasive diagnostic and therapeutic procedures to be performed.

The femoral, cephalic, or saphenous veins are usually used for venipuncture, and the femoral artery is readily accessed for arterial sampling.[17] Routine hematologic and biochemical screening and species-specific viral serology are commonly performed. Normal physiologic ranges for representative species are provided in Tables 37-2 and 37-3 (see http://www.primatevets.org/education).[26,35,37,42]

Because of the frequency of enteric and diarrheal diseases in monkeys, fecal examination is one of the most commonly employed diagnostic tests. This should include direct examination of fresh thin fecal smears, as this is especially useful for the detection of protozoa such as ameba; a routine flotation examination for helminth larvae or ova; and a fecal sedimentation examination, which will detect the heavy ova of parasites such as *Prosthenorchis* sp. that are not detected by routine fecal floatation.[26] Flagellates are frequently observed on direct fecal smear examinations of diarrheic feces. Although they rarely may be the cause of enteric disease, in most cases, they are nonpathogenic and are secondary to the change in composition of the feces. They proliferate in the liquid composition of diarrheic feces and are shed because of the increase in fecal frequency. NW monkeys frequently have *Gongylonema* sp. infection of the oral mucous membranes. In addition to fecal screening, a cotton-tipped applicator or similar material may be used to swab along the oral gingival membranes to manually remove the parasites for diagnosis.

Microbial cultures are frequently conducted, and when fecal aerobic culture is performed on feces, a microbiologic enrichment media should be used. This will aid in the culture of enteropathogens such as *Salmonella* sp., *Shigella* sp., and *Campylobacter* sp., all of which are common causes of diarrheal disease in monkeys. Feces may also be submitted for viral screening with electron microscopy (EM) or viral cultures performed. Urine can be collected by urinary catheterization in both male and female NW and OW monkeys if an appropriately sized catheter is available, or by ultrasound guided cystocentesis, manual expression of the urinary bladder, or collected from the substrate for analysis. Other diagnostic tests (cerebrospinal fluid [CSF] collection, thoracocentesis, abdominocentesis, etc.) may also be performed using the same principles and procedures as in other species.

THERAPEUTICS

For most therapeutic agents, dosages for NW and OW monkeys are based on guidelines for human pediatric or domestic small animal patients, although some specific recommendations for nonhuman primates are also available (http://www.primatevets.org/education).[30,35,40,43] Frequently used antibiotics for enteric, respiratory, or systemic bacterial infections are trimethoprim-sulfa combinations; quinolones; and combinations of aminoglycosides and penicillin and its derivatives. Metronidazole, especially benzoyl metronidazole, which improves palatability, is commonly used for enteric protozoal infections. Various anthelmintics are used for helminth infections. Motility modifiers (e.g., loperamide) and symptomatic treatments (e.g., bismuth subsalicylate) may also be used for treatment of diarrheal diseases.

Enteroparasites may be significant causes of morbidity and mortality, especially in newly imported monkeys. A range of parasiticides are recommended (Table 37-4; http://www.primatevets.org/education) for the treatment of commonly encountered parasites (Table 37-5).

Oral dosing may be challenging because of the ability of many NW and OW monkeys to detect medicated food or drink items, and animal care staff has to be resourceful and creative in concealing medications in food or drink vehicles to administer treatments. Intramuscular treatments may be administered during physical and chemical restraint, using behavioral training or a restraint device, or through remote delivery with a dart or pole syringe. Blood transfusions may be conducted after performing major and minor crossmatches to minimize risk of transfusion reactions.[26] Intravenous catheters are usually placed in the cephalic or saphenous veins, and when intravenous therapy is indicated, animals are usually maintained in a restraint device. Despite the monkeys' great intelligence and manual dexterity, they usually tolerate an intravenous catheter, provided the limb is well bandaged. Similarly, casts, other bandages, and sutures may usually be maintained, although this may be challenging in some individuals.

DISEASES

Enteric and respiratory diseases are particularly common in NW and OW monkeys and are caused by a range of pathogens, including parasites, bacteria, and viruses (Tables 37-5 and 37-6).[1,17,49] Zoonotic and anthropozoonotic diseases are also common, and this necessitates the use of personal protective equipment (PPE) and procedures

Text continued on p. 330

TABLE 37-2

Hematological Reference Intervals from Captive Representative Species of New World and Old World Monkeys from Composite MedARKS Records*

Test (Units)[†]	Species						
	Erythrocebus patas[a]	Lophocebus aterrimus[b]	Mandrillus sphinx[c]	Colobus guereza[d]	Saguinus geoffroyi[e]	Ateles fusciceps[f]	Alouatta caraya[g]
White Blood Cell Count (10³ cells/µL)	2.44-14.79 (462)	2.62-13.70 (142)	3.93-20.25 (931)	3.08-12.17 (1455)	4.18-22.31 (247)	3.92-35.10 (201)	5.82-28.56 (687)
Red Blood Cell Count (10⁶ cells/µL)	4.00-7.36 (406)	3.25-7.54 (111)	3.70-5.78 (863)	3.34-5.89 (1358)	4.45-7.02 (191)	4.13-6.83 (266)	3.17-5.85 (642)
Hemoglobin (g/dL)	10.2-18.0 (402)	10.4-19.2 (136)	9.3-13.7 (841)	9.5-15.7 (1416)	9.6-17.6 (204)	10.5-16.7 (275)	10.0-17.0 (646)
Hematocrit (%)	30.6-54.6 (484)	33.3-58.2 (158)	28.9-45.7 (977)	27.5-48.4 (1579)	29.0-55.0 (274)	32.6-53.2 (307)	30.6-55.5 (792)
MCV (fL)	58.5-90.1 (393)	65.5-90.8 (111)	68.0-88.5 (840)	69.8-93.2 (1325)	66.3-90.1 (175)	67.7-90.0 (266)	77.8-108.9 (625)
MCH (pg)	19.8-27.9 (370)	21.7-30.6 (111)	21.5-27.7 (834)	23.4-31.3 (1303)	19.1-30.1 (179)	21.3-28.6 (258)	25.3-34.2 (586)
MCHC (g/dL)	28.6-36.2 (384)	29.0-37.6 (133)	28.3-35.0 (825)	30.5-37.1 (1367)	26.4-36.5 (201)	28.7-35.4 (271)	28.4-36.4 (629)
Segmented Neutrophils (10³ cells/µL)	0.61-10.64 (459)	0.62-7.80 (142)	0.87-15.07 (928)	1.02-7.89 (1449)	2.02-15.72 (246)	0.65-24.68 (198)	1.76-21.28 (685)
Neutrophilic Band Cells (10³ cells/µL)	0.01-0.08 (429)	0.01-0.08 (133)	0.02-0.13 (851)	0.01-0.10 (1356)	0.02-0.11 (243)	0.02-0.22 (176)	0.02-0.16 (631)
Lymphocytes (10³ cells/µL)	0.61-5.91 (456)	1.06-6.70 (140)	1.02-7.89 (918)	0.57-5.84 (1442)	0.69-8.08 (246)	0.60-5.49 (197)	1.37-10.48 (687)
Monocytes (cells/µL)	43-797 (387)	39-656 (132)	61-1153 (836)	51-846 (1318)	67-1186 (223)	51-1350 (178)	93-1469 (607)
Eosinophils (cells/µL)	11-339 (161)	0-446 (118)	47-557 (584)	7-557 (677)	0-374 (82)	49-923 (159)	70-1379 (536)
Basophils (cells/µL)	0-129 (89)		12-236 (190)	4-173 (274)		36-475 (173)	
Platelet Count (10³ cells/µL)	85-590 (195)	82-457 (82)	122-440 (521)	82-542 (725)	81-702 (67)	121-626 (190)	118-565 (343)
Nucleated Red Blood Cells (/100 WBC)			0-136 (50)	0-2 (95)	0-3 (70)	0-1 (42)	0-2 (66)

*Sample Selection Criteria: No selection by gender, all ages combined, animal was classified as healthy at the time of sample collection, sample was not deteriorated.

[†]Values are given as a reference interval (number of samples used to calculate reference interval).

[a]Teare JA, ed: 2013, "Erythrocebus_patas_No_selection_by_gender_All_ages_combined_Conventional_American_units_2013_CD.html" in ISIS Physiological Reference Intervals for Captive Wildlife: A CD-ROM., International Species Information System, Bloomington, MN.

[b]Teare JA, ed: 2013, "Lophocebus_aterrimus_No_selection_by_gender_All_ages_combined_Conventional_American_units_2013_CD.html" in ISIS Physiological Reference Intervals for Captive Wildlife: A CD-ROM., International Species Information System, Bloomington, MN.

[c]Teare JA, ed: 2013, "Mandrillus_sphinx_No_selection_by_gender_All_ages_combined_Conventional_American_units_2013_CD.html" in ISIS Physiological Reference Intervals for Captive Wildlife: A CD-ROM., International Species Information System, Bloomington, MN.

[d]Teare JA, ed: 2013, "Colobus_guereza_No_selection_by_gender_All_ages_combined_Conventional_American_units_2013_CD.html" in ISIS Physiological Reference Intervals for Captive Wildlife: A CD-ROM., International Species Information System, Bloomington, MN.

[e]Teare JA, ed: 2013, "Saguinus_geoffroyi_No_selection_by_gender_All_ages_combined_Conventional_American_units_2013_CD.html" in ISIS Physiological Reference Intervals for Captive Wildlife: A CD-ROM., International Species Information System, Bloomington, MN.

[f]Teare JA, ed: 2013, "Ateles_fusciceps_No_selection_by_gender_All_ages_combined_Conventional_American_units_2013_CD.html" in ISIS Physiological Reference Intervals for Captive Wildlife: A CD-ROM., International Species Information System, Bloomington, MN.

[g]Teare JA, ed: 2013, "Alouatta_caraya_No_selection_by_gender_All_ages_combined_Conventional_American_units_2013_CD.html" in ISIS Physiological Reference Intervals for Captive Wildlife: A CD-ROM., International Species Information System, Bloomington, MN.

MCV, Mean corpuscular volume; MCH, mean corpuscular hemoglobin; MCHC, mean corpuscular hemoglobin concentration; RBC, red blood cell; WBC, white blood cell.

TABLE 37-3

Serum Biochemical Reference Intervals from Captive Representative Species of New World and Old World Monkeys from Composite MedARKS Records*

Test (Units)[†]	Erythrocebus patas[a]	Lophocebus aterrimus[b]	Mandrillus sphinx[c]	Colobus guereza	Saguinus geoffroyi[e]	Ateles fusciceps[f]	Alouatta caraya[g]
				Species			
Glucose (mg/dL)	56–204 (441)	46–169 (148)	45–179 (924)	60–205 (1555)	41–356 (226)	34–206 (275)	62–218 (738)
Blood Urea Nitrogen (mg/dL)	10–36 (448)	6–24 (149)	6–26 (908)	27–72 (1525)	8–36 (215)	5–31 (276)	13–43 (733)
Creatinine (mg/dL)	0.6–1.7 (439)	0.2–1.2 (148)	0.6–2.1 (890)	0.5–1.6 (1498)	0.2–1.2 (200)	0.4–1.5 (270)	0.4–1.8 (737)
BUN/Cr ratio	8.8–39.7 (437)	8.9–53.7 (147)	5.0–27.3 (870)	23.7–96.8 (1469)	11.9–101.1 (195)	5.9–45.1 (259)	10.8–45.7 (721)
Uric Acid (mg/dL)	0.0–0.3 (64)		0.0–1.0 (202)	0.0–0.6 (317)		0.9–8.6 (95)	0.0–0.6 (125)
Calcium (mg/dL)	7.4–10.3 (437)	8.5–11.1 (144)	7.8–11.0 (897)	7.9–10.9 (1492)	6.9–12.2 (203)	7.9–10.9 (266)	7.9–10.8 (726)
Phosphorus (mg/dL)	1.9–7.9 (388)	1.5–6.8 (139)	1.8–9.3 (817)	1.9–9.0 (1395)	1.8–12.7 (181)	2.1–8.5 (223)	2.0–8.7 (665)
Ca/Phos ratio	1.1–4.1 (381)	1.2–5.8 (132)	1.0–4.7 (801)	1.0–4.2 (1368)	0.7–3.9 (173)	1.1–5.0 (223)	0.8–4.6 (664)
Sodium (mEq/L)	138–159 (375)	138–153 (122)	138–157 (820)	137–155 (1316)	132–163 (185)	135–150 (225)	131–146 (676)
Potassium (mEq/L)	2.7–4.7 (373)	2.8–5.4 (120)	2.9–5.1 (799)	3.1–6.0 (1297)	2.2–6.4 (182)	3.2–6.0 (220)	3.2–5.7 (683)
Na/K ratio	30.2–55.4 (373)	26.8–48.2 (121)	24.7–51.6 (819)	22.0–47.0 (1319)	20.2–65.7 (184)	19.1–43.1 (222)	24.6–43.2 (677)
Chloride (mEq/L)	97–118 (350)	101–118 (109)	100–116 (782)	96–112 (1272)	97–118 (167)	95–113 (207)	94–109 (641)
Total Protein (g/dL)	5.1–7.4 (387)	5.6–8.0 (143)	5.4–8.2 (849)	4.9–7.4 (1419)	4.6–7.6 (208)	5.5–8.6 (246)	5.4–8.2 (728)
Albumin (g/dL)	2.1–4.8 (345)	3.5–5.9 (124)	2.8–5.8 (801)	3.2–5.8 (1346)	2.3–4.9 (189)	2.5–6.7 (230)	2.3–5.7 (684)
Globulin (g/dL)	1.4–4.3 (347)	0.7–3.2 (125)	1.0–3.9 (802)	0.5–3.2 (1331)	1.4–5.8 (179)	0.9–4.3 (230)	1.3–4.6 (673)
Alkaline Phosphatase (IU/L)	58–529 (395)	15–277 (118)	51–904 (871)	65–966 (1282)	25–448 (195)	45–449 (244)	51–459 (585)
Lactate Dehydrogenase (IU/L)	0–1110 (95)		137–1344 (292)	187–1405 (463)		0–1578 (64)	180–845 (252)
Aspartate Aminotransferase (IU/L)	26–119 (306)	4–61 (108)	13–71 (803)	14–91 (1162)	81–323 (182)	42–210 (231)	57–221 (685)
Alanine Aminotransferase (IU/L)	16–138 (424)	14–107 (146)	14–116 (848)	6–50 (1404)	9–88 (196)	8–78 (218)	6–49 (687)

Continued

TABLE 37-3

Serum Biochemical Reference Intervals from Captive Representative Species of New World and Old World Monkeys from Composite MedARKS Records—cont'd

Test (Units)[†]	Species						
	Erythrocebus patas[a]	Lophocebus aterrimus[b]	Mandrillus sphinx[c]	Colobus guereza	Saguinus geoffroyi[e]	Ateles fusciceps[f]	Alouatta caraya[g]
Creatine Kinase (IU/L)	75–1280 (156)	0–955 (96)	105–1532 (514)	52–1063 (670)		0–939 (112)	216–1555 (440)
Gamma-glutamyltransferase (IU/L)	19–127 (226)	0–66 (49)	35–156 (477)	39–162 (798)	0–14 (98)	0–20 (87)	13–98 (517)
Amylase (IU/L)	222–989 (267)	55–328 (43)	99–375 (411)	100–396 (670)	0–2146 (75)	87–1270 (147)	48–472 (330)
Lipase (IU/L)	0–161 (89)		6–133 (223)	1–58 (224)		0–155 (52)	2–50 (141)
Total Bilirubin (mg/dL)	0.1–0.8 (394)	0.1–1.0 (141)	0.1–0.7 (880)	0.1–0.8 (1414)	0.1–0.9 (195)	0.1–1.0 (255)	0.1–0.6 (699)
Direct Bilirubin (mg/dL)			0.0–0.3 (256)	0.0–0.4 (340)			0.0–0.4 (225)
Indirect Bilirubin (mg/dL)			0.0–0.5 (252)	0.0–0.5 (339)			0.0–0.6 (224)
Cholesterol (mg/dL)	52–159 (394)	77–182 (119)	65–221 (849)	90–241 (1336)	51–162 (188)	76–278 (219)	85–239 (681)
Triglyceride (mg/dL)	21–142 (186)		28–149 (446)	25–171 (591)		34–204 (119)	36–173 (323)
Bicarbonate (mEq/L)			13.3–34.6 (136)	17.5–35.7 (142)			12.2–32.4 (66)
Magnesium (mg/dL)	0.87–2.05 (88)		0.72–2.43 (135)	1.09–2.50 (95)			0.69–2.61 (102)
Iron (µg/dL)			45–195 (90)	69–218 (92)			34–208 (45)
Carbon Dioxide (mEq/L)	13.3–38.8 (47)		8.8–34.8 (246)	9.5–35.0 (455)		7.1–31.0 (65)	13.2–28.7 (314)

*Sample Selection Criteria: No selection by gender, all ages combined, animal was classified as healthy at the time of sample collection, sample was not deteriorated.

†Values are given as a reference interval (number of samples used to calculate the reference interval).

[a]Teare JA, ed: 2013, "Erythrocebus_patas_No_selection_by_gender__All_ages_combined_Conventional_American_units__2013_CD.html" in ISIS Physiological Reference Intervals for Captive Wildlife: A CD-ROM, International Species Information System, Bloomington, MN.

[b]Teare JA, ed: 2013, "Lophocebus_aterrimus_No_selection_by_gender__All_ages_combined_Conventional_American_units__2013_CD.html" in ISIS Physiological Reference Intervals for Captive Wildlife: A CD-ROM, International Species Information System, Bloomington, MN.

[c]Teare JA, ed: 2013, "Mandrillus_sphinx_No_selection_by_gender__All_ages_combined_Conventional_American_units__2013_CD.html" in ISIS Physiological Reference Intervals for Captive Wildlife: A CD-ROM, International Species Information System, Bloomington, MN.

[d]Teare JA, ed: 2013, "Colobus_guereza_No_selection_by_gender__All_ages_combined_Conventional_American_units__2013_CD.html" in ISIS Physiological Reference Intervals for Captive Wildlife: A CD-ROM, International Species Information System, Bloomington, MN.

[e]Teare JA, ed: 2013, "Saguinus_geoffroyi_No_selection_by_gender__All_ages_combined_Conventional_American_units__2013_CD.html" in ISIS Physiological Reference Intervals for Captive Wildlife: A CD-ROM, International Species Information System, Bloomington, MN.

[f]Teare JA, ed: 2013, "Ateles_fusciceps_No_selection_by_gender__All_ages_combined_Conventional_American_units__2013_CD.html" in ISIS Physiological Reference Intervals for Captive Wildlife: A CD-ROM, International Species Information System, Bloomington, MN.

[g]Teare JA, ed: 2013, "Alouatta_caraya_No_selection_by_gender__All_ages_combined_Conventional_American_units__2013_CD.html" in ISIS Physiological Reference Intervals for Captive Wildlife: A CD-ROM, International Species Information System, Bloomington, MN.

TABLE 37-4

Parasiticides Recommended for New World and Old World Monkeys[2,9, 17,19, 33, 40,43]

Generic Name (Trade Name)	Species	Dosage	Route	Comments
Albendazole (VALBAZEN)	NW and OW	25 mg/kg	PO	For *Filaroides* and *Giardia*: BID for 5 days
Amitraz (Mitaban)	Tamarins	250 ppm solution	TP	For demodectic mange: place in solution for 2–5 minutes Repeat q14d† for 4 treatments or until lesions resolve
Azithromycin (Zithromax)	Macaques	25–50 mg/kg	SQ	For malaria: SID for 3–10 days In humans, combined with chloroquine
	NW and OW	40 mg/kg	IM	Give SID for one day, then 20 mg/kg SID for 2–5 days
Bunamidine (Scolaban)	NW and OW	25–100 mg/kg	PO	For cestodes: give once
Chloroquine phosphate (Arelan)	NW and OW	2.5–5 mg/kg	IM	For *Plasmodium* sp.: SID for 4–7 days, then 0.75 mg/kg primaquine PO SID for 14 days Give chloroquine and primaquine separately to prevent toxicity
	NW and OW	5 mg/kg	PO; IM	For *Entamoeba histolytica*: SID for 14 days
	NW and OW	10 mg/kg	PO; IM	For *Plasmodium*: give once; 6 hours later give 5 mg/kg, and 24 hours later give 5 mg/kg SID for 2 days and then start primaquine PO 0.3 mg/kg SID for 14 days
Clindamycin (Antirobe)	NW and OW	12.5 mg/kg	PO; IM	For toxoplasmosis: BID for 28 days
Dichlorvos (Atgard-V)	NW and OW	10 mg/kg	PO	For *Trichuris* sp.: SID for 1–2 days
	NW and OW	10–15 mg/kg	PO	For gastrointestinal nematodes: SID for 2–3 days
Diethylcarbamazine Citrate (Filaribits)	Owl Monkey	6–20 mg/kg	PO	For *Filariasis* (*dipetalonema*): SID for 6–15 days
		20–40 mg.kg	PO	For *Filariasis* (*dipetalonema*): SID for 7–21 days
	Squirrel Monkey	50 mg/kg	PO	For *Filariasis* (adults and microfilaria): SID for 10 days
Diiodohydroxyquin [iodoquinol] (Yodoxin)	NW and OW	10–13.3 mg/kg	PO	For *Entamoeba histolytica*: TID for 10–20 days Use with metronidazole in severe cases
	NW and OW	13.3 mg/kg	PO	For *Balantidium coli*: TID for 14–21 days
	NW and OW	20 mg/kg	PO	BID for 21 days
	NW and OW	30 mg/kg	PO	SID for 10 days
Dithiazanine sodium (Dizan)	NW and OW	10–20 mg/kg	PO	For *Strongyloides*: SID for 3–10 days
Doxycycline (Vibramycin)	NW and OW	2.5 mg/kg	PO	For *Balantidium*: BID for 1 day, then SID for 10 days
Fenbendazole (Panacur)	NW and OW	10–25 mg/kg	PO	For *Anatrichosoma cynomolgi*: SID for 3–10 days May result in remission
	NW and OW	20 mg/kg	PO	For *Strongyloides* sp. and *Filaroides*: SID for 14 days
	Marmosets	20 mg/kg	PO	For *Prosthenorchis* sp.: SID for 7 days
	NW and OW	25 mg/kg	PO	For *Ancylostoma*: q7d for 2 times
	NW and OW	50 mg/kg	PO	SID for 3–14 days For *Filaroides*: SID for 14 days
Flubendazole 5% (Flubenol)	Baboons	27–50 mg/kg	PO	For *Trichuris* sp.: BID for 5 days
Ivermectin (Ivomec)	NW and OW	0.2 mg/kg	PO; IM; SQ	For *Strongyloides* sp., *Gongylonema* sp., *Pneumonyssus* sp., Anoplura: give once and repeat in 10–14 days
			IM	For *Ancyclostoma duodenale*: give once and repeat in 21 days if needed
		0.4 µg/kg	IM	For: *Strongyloides* sp. in macaques: Dilute with propylene glycol
		0.5 µg/kg	SQ	For *Pterygodermatites* sp.: SID for 3 days. Dilute in sterile water for smaller species (marmosets)
Levamisole (Levasole)	Saki Monkeys	4–5 mg/kg	PO	For oral *Spiruridiasis*: SID for 6 days
	NW and OW	5 mg/kg	PO	Give once and repeat in 3 weeks
	NW and OW	7.5 mg/kg	SQ	For *Trichuris* sp. and *Ancyclostoma* sp.: give once; repeat in 2 weeks
	NW and OW	10 mg/kg	PO	For *Strongyloides* sp., *Filaroides*, *Oesophagostormum* sp. and *Trichuris*
			PO or SQ	For *Strongyloides* sp.: give 2–3 days
	Spider monkeys	10 mg/kg	—	For *Physaloptera* sp.: give for 3 days.
	Tamarins	11 mg/kg	—	For Filariasis: give for 10 days along with thiacetarsamide sodium at 0.22 mL/kg BID for 2 days

Continued

TABLE 37-4

Parasiticides Recommended for New World and Old World Monkeys—cont'd

Generic Name (Trade Name)	Species	Dosage	Route	Comments
Mebendazole (Telminic)	NW and OW	3 mg/kg	PO	For *Ancyclostoma* sp.: SID for 10 days
	NW and OW	15 mg/kg	PO	For *Strongyloides* sp., *Necator*, *Pterygodermatitis*, and *Trichuris*: SID for 3 days For *Ancyclostoma* sp.: SID for 2 days
	NW and OW	22 mg/kg	PO	SID for 3 days and then repeat in 2 weeks
	NW and OW	40 mg/kg	PO	For *Pterygodermatites* sp.: SID for 3 days repeated 3 to 4 times yearly as prevention
	NW	70 mg/kg	PO	For oral spiruridiasis: SID for 3 days Repeat treatment periodically
	Callitrichids	100 mg/kg	PO	For acanthocephalans: treat once every 2 weeks Use as a preventive along with surgical removal of parasite
Mefloquine (Lariam)	NW and OW	25 mg/kg	PO	For malarial: give one dose
Metronidazole (Flagyl) [Metronidazole benzoate (Flagyl-S) may be compounded with flavored syrup, improving palatability]	NW and OW	10–16.7 mg/kg	PO	For *Giardia intestinalis*: TID for 5–10 days
	NW and OW	11.7–16.7 mg/kg	PO	For *Balantidium coli*: TID for 10 days
	NW and OW	17.5–25 mg/kg	PO	For enteric amoebas and flagellates: BID for 10 days
	NW and OW	25 mg/kg	PO	For *Tritrichomonas mobilensis*, *Giardia lamblia*: BID for 5 days
	NW and OW	30–50 mg/kg	PO	For *Balantidium coli*: BID for 5–10 days
Moxidectin (Pro Heart)	NW and OW	0.5 mg/kg	PO; IM	For *Strongyloides* sp.: give one dose
Niclosamide (Yomensan)	NW and OW	100 mg/kg	PO	For intestinal cestodiasis: give one dose
	Owl monkey	150 mg/kg	PO	For intestinal cestodiasis: give one dose
	NW	166 mg/kg	PO	For cestodes, anoplocephalids
Paromomycin (Humatin)	NW and OW	10–20 mg/kg	PO	For *Balantidium coli*: BID for 5–10 days
	NW and OW	12.5–15 mg/kg	PO	For amoebae: BID for 5–10 days; drug has minimal absorption—need to use additional drugs for invasive disease For *Entamoeba histolytica*: BID for 5–10 days
	Owl monkeys	25–30 mg/kg	PO	For enteric amoebiasis: BID for 5–10 days
	Cercopithecids	100 mg/kg	PO	SID for 10 days
Praziquantel (Droncit)	NW and OW	15–20 mg/kg	PO; IM	Treatment for trematodes
	NW and OW	40 mg/kg	PO; IM	For *Schistosoma* sp., other cestodes and trematodes: give once
Primaquine (Primaquine phosphate)	NW and OW	0.3 mg/kg	PO	For *Plasmodium* sp.: SID for 14 days; use with chloroquine
Pyrantel pamoate (Strongid-T)	NW and OW	11 mg/kg	PO	For oxyurids: give once and repeat in 10 days Better than thiabendazole for *Trypanoxyuris micron* in owl monkeys
Pyrimethamine (Daraprim)	NW and OW	10 mg/kg	PO	For *Plasmodium* sp.: give once daily Monitor for signs of folate acid deficiency and treat if needed
Pyrvinium pamoate (Povan)	NW and OW	5 mg/kg	PO	Give once; repeat every 6 months.
Quinacrine (Atabrine)	NW and OW	2 mg/kg	PO	For *Giardia*: TID for 5–7 days May cause GI upset in squirrel monkeys
	NW and OW	10 mg/kg	PO	For *Giardia*: TID for 5 days. Is 70%–95% effective
Ronnel (Ectoral)	NW and OW	55 mg/kg	PO; TP	For lung mites and ectoparasitic mites: give q72h for 4 times and then every 7 days for 3 months topically
Sulfadiazine (Sulfadiazine)	NW and OW	100 mg/kg	PO	For *Toxoplasma*: treat along with pyrimethamine
Sulfadimethoxine (Albon)	NW and OW	50 mg/kg	PO	For coccidiosis: give one dose; then 25 mg/kg/day
Thiabendazole (Thibenzole)	NW and OW	50 mg/kg	PO	For *Strongyloides* sp. and hookworms (*Necator*): SID for 2 days
	NW and OW	75–100 mg/kg	PO	Give once and repeat in 21 days
Tinidazole (Tindamax)	Marmosets	150 mg/kg	PO	For *Giardia*: SID for one day; then give 77 mg/kg SID for 4 days

BID, Twice daily; *IM*, intramuscular; *IP*, intraperitoneal; *NW*, New World monkey; *OW*, Old World monkey; *PO*, per os (orally); *q7d*, every 7 days; *q7h*, every 7 hours; *q72h*, every 72 hours; *SID*, once daily; *SQ*, subcutaneously; *TID*, three times daily, *TP*, topically.

TABLE 37-5

Selected Parasitic Diseases of New World and Old World Monkeys[2,9,17,33,40]

Disease/Zoonotic Risk	Causative Agent	Species Affected	Location in Host	Clinical Signs*	Diagnosis*
PROTOZOAN PARASITES					
PHYLUM SARCOMASTIGOPHORA					
Flagellates (Class Mastigophora)					
Hemoflagellates					
Trypanosomiasis, Chagas disease, sleeping sickness / Zoonotic risk (accidental inoculation/contamination)	*Trypansoma cruzi, T. brucei,* etc.	NW[†] and OW[†]: (pigtail macaques, baboons) housed outside in Texas, Louisiana, Georgia	Trypomastigote in blood of host; amastigote in reticuloendothelial (RE) system	Generalized edema, anemia, hepatosplenomegaly, lymphadenitis, lethargy, weight loss, ECG* changes, dehydration, fetal death	Parasites in blood or body fluids; blood culture; ELISA*; histopathology
Enteric flagellates					
Giardia / Zoonotic	*Giardia lamblia, G. intestinalis*	OW and NW	Duodenum, jejunum, upper ileum	Asymptomatic carriers, usually self-limiting Vomiting and diarrhea	Trophozoites / cysts in feces DFA; fecal EIA
Trichomonas	*Trichomonas* sp.	Titi monkey	Colon	Weakness, diarrhea, dehydration, death	Fecal O and P, necropsy, histopathology
Ameba (Class Sarcodina)					
Amebiasis / Zoonotic	*Entamoeba histolytica*	OW and NW; lesions in NW more severe than in OW	Pathogenic *E. histolytica*: ameba and cysts in cecum, colon. Invasive trophozoites cause abscesses in lung, liver, brain In langurs, proboscis, colobus monkeys causes gastric lesions	Asymptomatic to severe disease (weight loss, lethargy, hemorrhagic diarrhea, rectal prolapse) pulmonary, neurological signs Gastritis (langurs, proboscis, colobus). Virulence depends on strains, host species, nutritional status, gastrointestinal (GI) microflora, environmental factors	Fresh fecal examination for O and P; histopathology. Fecal ELISA Fecal trophozoites may be nonpathogenic
Balamuthiasis	*Balamuthia mandrillus*	Mandrill, colobus monkey	Parasite in brain and other organs Free living in soil	Rapidly developing central nervous system (CNS) signs (limb paresis or paralysis, weakness, lethargy)	IFS, EM to distinguish organism from *Acanthamoeba*
PHYLUM APICOMPLEXA					
Coccidia and coccidian-like parasites (Class Coccidia)					
Cryptosporidiosis / Zoonotic	*Cryptosporidium* sp.	Macaques, a cotton-top tamarin	GI tract	Severe intestinal signs in infants and immune compromised NHPs[†]	Fecal oocysts, DFA, IFA, EIA; histopathology
Toxoplasmosis / Zoonotic	*Toxoplasma gondii*	All primate species; NW more susceptible than OW	Found in any organ but especially in the liver, lymph nodes, and brain	Retinal lesions; respiratory distress and central nervous system signs	Histopathology (IHC) Sabin-Feldman dye test Serology: CF, IFA, HA

Continued

TABLE 37-5

Selected Parasitic Diseases of New World and Old World Monkeys—cont'd

Disease/Zoonotic Risk	Causative Agent	Species Affected	Location in Host	Clinical Signs*	Diagnosis*
Malaria / Zoonotic	Plasmodium sp. (P. knowlesi, P. fragile, P. brazilianum)	All NHPs except tamarins, and marmosets	Asexual phase in NHPs: schizogonic phase in erythrocyte (erthrocytic; blood phase) or in liver (exoerythrocytic; liver phase)	May be fatal even in adults because of destruction of erythrocytes	Identification of organisms in red blood cells PCR, fluorescent antibody, serology
Ciliates (Phylum Ciliophora)					
Balantidiasis / Zoonotic	Balantidium coli	NW: howler monkeys, capuchin monkey, and spider monkey. OW: baboons, rhesus and cynomolgus macaques	Colon and cecum	Usually asymptomatic but can cause ulcerative colitis with diarrhea	Cysts or trophozoites in fresh feces, in colonic ulcers Presence of B. coli in feces may be secondary to a bacterial or viral infection
Metazoan Parasites **Nematodes** **Rhabditoids**					
Strongyloidiasis / Zoonotic	Strongyloides füelleborni, S. cebus	S. cebus: NW (capuchins, squirrel, spider and woolly monkeys). S. fülleborni: OW (guenons, baboons, macaques) Fatalities in patas and woolly monkeys	Infective larvae penetrate skin or oral mucosa; adults in mucosa of duodenum and jejunum Intestinal larvae may re-infect the host (hyperinfection) or penetrate the perineal or perianal skin (autoinfection) S. fülleborni also infects via colostrum and placenta	Signs: asymptomatic; mild dermal erythema, pruritus; sporadic cough, bronchopneumonia, pulmonary hemorrhage, pericarditis; bloody diarrhea, lethargic, anorexia, weight loss, stunted growth, weakness, death	Clinical signs, fecal examination for ova or larvae (rule out free living larvae) Histopathology or gross necropsy
Oxyurids					
Oxyuriasis (Pinworms) / Zoonotic	OW: Enterobius sp. (E. vermicularis) NW: Trypanoxyuris sp., Oxyuronema sp.	OW and NW (marmosets). Infection rare in wild NHPs, occurs in captivity	Adults reside in colon Adult $♀$ deposit eggs in perianal and perineal area; hatch into larvae	Perianal pruritus, restlessness, self-mutilation, increased aggressiveness GI pathology is rare. Overwhelming infection fatal in a spider monkey	Fecal O and P; examine sample of anal area with cellophane tape and perianal or perineal swabs; adult worms coming out of anus
Strongylids					
Oesophagostomiasis / Zoonotic	Oesophagostomum sp. (nodular worm)	OW monkeys: macaques, baboons, guenons, mangabeys NW monkeys: rare	Adults in colon Larvae penetrate colonic mucosa cause large firm encapsulated nodules that rupture releasing larvae to the intestine	Usually asymptomatic Severe infections cause debilitation, unthriftiness, weight loss, abdominal adhesions, ascites, diarrhea, high mortality rate	Larval identification in stool, stool culture; adult identification on necropsy, histopathology

Disease / Zoonotic	Parasite(s)	Hosts	Location / Pathology	Clinical signs	Diagnosis
Ternideniasis / Zoonotic	*Ternidens diminutus*	Asian and African NHPs (baboons, African green monkeys, guenons, macaques, especially *M. arctoides*)	Adults in cecum, colon cause extensive mucosal damage and cystic nodules in the colon wall. Parasites suck blood causing anemia	Asymptomatic in light infections. Signs may include anemia, cystic nodules in colon	Larval identification in stool, stool culture; adult identification on necropsy, histopathology
Ancyclostomatids					
Ancylostomiasis and Necatoriasis / Zoonotic	*Ancylostoma duodenale*, *Necator americanus*	Mandrills, baboons, rare in NW monkeys	Parasites attach to mucosa of small intestine	With heavy infections: debilitation, abdominal distension, dyspnea with exertion, anemia, eosinophilia	Fecal O and P; diagnosis based on larval identification in stool culture. Gross and histopathology
Trichostrongylids					
Molineiasis	*Molineus torulosus*, *M. torulosus*, *M. elegans*, *M. vexillarius*	Owl, capuchins and squirrel monkeys, and tamarins	Adults lay in mucosa of duodenum and pylorus of stomach. In capuchins: parasites, eggs are in serosal nodules in small intestine and in pancreatic ducts	*M. torulosus*: hemorrhagic or ulcerative enteritis and chronic pancreatitis (in capuchins)	Fecal ova or finding worms in association with lesions in GI tract
Spirurids					
Pterygodermitites nycticebi	*Pterygodermatites nycticebi*, *P. alpha*	Callitrichids (marmosets, tamarins)	Natural host: prosimians (slow loris, genus *Nycticebus*). In marmoset and tamarins: (adults in lumen of small intestine (anterior ends imbedded in the submucosa, tunica mucosa, pancreatic duct). Intermediate host: cockroaches (eaten by marmoset)	High morbidity, mortality in golden lion tamarins. Heavy infestations: watery diarrhea containing adult parasites, anemia, leukopenia and hypoproteinemia, generalized weakness	Fecal O and P, finding masses of adult parasites throughout GI tract; histopathology: identification of parasite in tissue tunnels
Gongylonemiasis	*Gongylonema pulchrum*, *G. macrogubernaculum*	OW and NW: Goeldi's marmoset and pygmy marmoset	Adults tunnel into the stratum malpighii of the squamous epithelium in lip, tongue, esophagus and buccal cavity, bronchi and stomach	Usually asymptomatic. Callitrichids show pruritus and ptyalism	Scraping of tongue and oral mucosa to look for eggs
Physalopteriasis	*Physaloptera* sp.: *P. tumefaciens*, *P. dilatata*, *P. caucasica*, *Abbreviata* sp. *A. poicilometra*	OW: macaques, baboons, mangabeys, guenons; NW monkeys: titi monkeys, bearded sakis, marmosets	Worms attached to wall of stomach, esophagus, and small intestine	Gastritis, esophagitis, enteritis	Finding ova in feces. On necropsy, finding adults attached to mucosa of upper GI tract

Continued

TABLE 37-5

Selected Parasitic Diseases of New World and Old World Monkeys—cont'd

Disease/Zoonotic Risk	Causative Agent	Species Affected	Location in Host	Clinical Signs*	Diagnosis*
Filarioidea Filariasis	*Dipetalonema* sp., *Mansonella* sp., *Tetrapetalonema* sp., *Dirofilaria* sp., *Macacanema* sp., *Edesonfilaria* sp., *Loa* sp., *Brugia* sp., *Meningonema* sp.	NW (owl, spider, squirrel, woolly and pale-headed saki monkeys, capuchins and marmosets) OW (macaques, drills, baboons, vervets, mangabeys, colobus, talapoin and patas monkeys)	Adult worms in subcutaneous tissues, thoracic and peritoneal cavity; subserosal connective tissue of abdominal and thoracic cavities Microfilariae in blood Biting and blood-sucking insects (mosquitoes) transfer microfilariae to primate host with blood meal	Asymptomatic, in heavy infestations with *D. graciliformis, D. gracile, D. robini, D. caudispina* or *D. freitas* may cause pleuritis or peritonitis; anemic, eosinophilia, hyperproteinemia, decreased A/G ratio Lesions: hemorrhage, thickening of connective tissues, adhesions in sites where worms are located	Microfilariae in blood, adult worms found in peritoneal cavity
Trichurids Anatrichosomiasis / Zoonotic	*Anatrichosoma cutaneum*	Macaques, langurs, patas monkeys, vervets, baboons, talapoin monkeys, marmosets, and mangabeys	Reside in nasal mucosa and stratum malpighii near basal layer of the skin; ♀ worms migrate through squamous epithelium, forming tunnels depositing embryonated eggs	Asymptomatic or show mild inflammation due to parakeratosis and hyperplasia of nasal mucosa and a subcutaneous foreign body reaction and pruritus Lesions: white tracks on skin on palms of hands and soles of feet with associated lymphadenopathy Tunnels slough releasing eggs; eggs in nasal discharge or passed in feces	Eggs found in nasal swabs, skin scrapings Histopathology of nasal mucosa or epidermis
Trichuris (whipworms) / Zoonotic	*Trichuris trichiura*	OW: (macaques, baboons, African green monkeys) NW: (howler, squirrel, woolly monkeys)	Larvae embedded in mucosa of cecum	Asymptomatic with light infection, heavy infections: severe enteritis, gray mucoid diarrhea, anorexia and death	Fecal O and P
Acanthocephalus (thorny-headed worms) Prosthenorchis	*Prosthenorchis elegans, P. spirula* (both species native to South America, now found where NW monkeys are housed in captivity.)	Marmosets, tamarins, capuchins, squirrel and spider monkeys, and macaques	Adults attach to intestinal mucosa in terminal ileum, cecum, colon with spiny proboscis, causing granulomatous inflammation and peritonitis Parasite may be free in the abdomen Intermediate host: cockroaches (eaten by marmoset)	Asymptomatic with light infections With heavy infections: diarrhea, anorexia, abdominal enlargement, cachexia, dehydration, intussusception, rectal prolapse, pain, debilitation and death	Fecal smears O and P, clinical signs, necropsy, histopathology Proctoscopy to identify adult worm in intestine

	Organism	Hosts	Life cycle	Clinical signs	Diagnosis
Cestodes					
Cestodiasis, Hymenolepiasis (tapeworm) / Zoonotic	*Hymenolepis nana*	Rhesus macaques and squirrel monkeys	Adults in intestine: may autoinfect as eggs hatch in intestine and develop into adults	Usually asymptomatic, may cause catarrhal enteritis, diarrhea, abdominal pain, mesentery lymph node abscessation	Ova, proglottids and/or adult worms seen in feces and gross necropsy
Larval Cestodiasis					
Hydatidosis, Echinococcosis	*Echinococcus* sp.	Hydatid cysts of *E. granulosis* (guenons, colobus monkeys, mangabeys, mandrills, macaques, baboons, marmosets). Cysts of *E. multilocularis* (macaques)	NHPs eat food contaminated with eggs from carnivore or rodent feces. Embryos in GI tract, spread via portal circulation to abdomen, thorax, lungs, liver, retrobulbar, subcutaneous tissues and develop into hydatid cysts which develop brood capsules	Clinical signs (depend on location, size, age of cyst): exophthalmia, abdominal distension, subcutaneous swellings. If hydatid cyst rupture in lungs may cause anaphylactic shock and death	Clinical signs, visualization of cyst by ultrasonography, radiography (for lung cysts and calcified liver cysts) Serological tests: ELISA, WB, IHC, and PCR on affected tissues
Trematodes					
Schistosomiasis	*Schistosoma mansoni, S. haematobium, S. japonicum, S. incognitum*	Baboons, mangabeys, guenons, macaques, squirrel and patas monkeys	Intermediate host: snails release cercariae that penetrates NHP's skin or are ingested and migrate into vascular system; matures to adults in inferior mesenteric veins or portal vein. Adults pass eggs that penetrate vessel wall and accumulate in perivascular tissues (intestines and bladder)	Lesions from eggs deposited in the venules of the urinary bladder and intestines. Some spread to other organs (brain, spleen, liver, etc.) causing a foreign body response with microgranulomas around schistosome eggs. Clinical signs: hematuria, pyrexia, hemorrhagic diarrhea, ascites	Ova in feces or urine. Histopathology, necropsy: adult parasites found in blood vessels. PCR may be used

Continued

TABLE 37-5

Selected Parasitic Diseases of New World and Old World Monkeys—cont'd

Disease/Zoonotic Risk	Causative Agent	Species Affected	Location in Host	Clinical Signs*	Diagnosis*
Annelida					
Trematode dinobdelliasis	*Dinobdella ferox*	Macaques	Leech lays eggs on the water surface, which hatch; immature leech enters NHPs' nose or mouth when the primate drinks. Leech attaches to upper respiratory mucosa, sucks blood, matures, then drops out as a hermaphroditic adult	Asymptomatic with light infection or mild nasal discharge; with heavy infections: restlessness, epistaxis, anemia, weakness, asphyxiation, and death	Nasal examination
ECTOPARASITE INFECTION—MITES (CLASS ARACHNIDA)					
Sarcoptes / Zoonotic	*Sarcoptes scabiei*	Macaques, drills	Adults in skin	Alopecia, hyperkeratosis, flaking skin, suppurative dermatitis pruritis, anorexia, weakness, weight loss, tremors	Clinical signs, O and P in deep skin scrapings, biopsies, feces
Dunnalge, Rosalialges	*D. lambrechti, R. cruciformis*	NW monkeys (marmoset, owl monkeys)	Adults in skin	Dermatitis	Skin scrapings for O and P
Psorergates	*Psorergates pitheci*	Guenons, African greens, baboons, capuchins	Adults in skin	Dermatitis	Skin scrapings for O and P
Respiratory mites					
Pulmonary Acariasis	*Pneumonyssus* sp., *Pneumonyssoides* sp.	*Pneumonyssus simicola*: asymptomatic carriers (macaques, mangabeys, guenons, baboons, langurs, vervet, colobus, proboscis and patas monkeys) *Pneumonyssoides* sp. (woolly and howler monkeys)	*P. simicola* located in lower respiratory tract Mites, eggs, and larvae in lung lesions, pale white, jelly-like masses usually on surface of lungs *Pneumonyssoides* sp. in lungs, larynx, nasal cavities, sinuses	Usually asymptomatic or nasal discharge, sneezing, coughing In douc langurs, proboscus monkeys, lion-tailed, pig-tailed and rhesus macaques may cause massive infestation and death	Lung mites in feces, lung mite larvae in tracheobronchial washing Histopathology necropsy
Nasal Acariasis	*Rhinophaga* sp.: *R. papinois, R. elongate; R. cercopitheci*	Rhesus macaque, baboons, guenons, vervets; chacma baboon	Mites in olfactory mucosa and upper skull: maxillary sinus; nasal cavity; lungs and frontal sinuses	Usually asymptomatic or show excessive mucus	Mites in nasal swabs Necropsy, histopathology

+ ♀, female.

*CF, complement fixation; DFA, direct fluorescent antibody assay; ECG, electrocardiography; EIA, enzyme immunoassay; ELISA, enzyme-linked immunosorbent assay; EM, electron microscopy; HA, hemagglutination assay; IFA, indirect fluorescent antibody assay; IFS, immunofluorescence staining; IHC, immunohistochemistry; PCR, polymerase chain reaction; WB, Western blot O and P, ova and parasite.

†NW, New World monkey; NHP, nonhuman primates; OW, Old World monkey.

TABLE 37-6

Selected Infectious Diseases of New World and Old World Monkeys[2,17,20, 39,43,44,45]

Disease/Zoonotic Risk	Species*	Causative Agents	Epizootiology	Signs	Diagnosis[†]
ENVELOPED DNA VIRUSES **Poxvirus: Orthopoxvirus** Monkeypox / Zoonotic	Tamarin, marmoset, macaque, langur, African green, squirrel and owl-faced monkey	Monkeypox: two clades: Western African and the more virulent Congo Basin (from Central Africa)	Reservoir: western and central Africa—rodents (Africa squirrels) Asymptomatic African green monkeys have high seroprevalence Transmission from African green monkeys to macaques by direct contact, aerosols, biting insects Animals recover with immunity Latent infection possible	Fever, facial edema, lesions on hands/feet, limbs, tongue, oropharynx, trachea, and lung progress from papules to vesicles to umbilicated centers Signs vary between species. Mortality rates: rhesus 0.5%; crab eating macaques 50%; mortality high in langurs with pulmonary lesions	Clinical signs, ELISA,[†] PCR, antigen detection tests, virus isolation, histopathology
Cowpox / Zoonotic	NW* (marmosets, tamarins) and OW (macaques)	Cowpox	Virus may be acquired from wild rodents (*Rattus norvegicus*)	Macaques: oral erythematous papules, vesicles, umbilication Marmosets and tamarins show: papules change to vesicles, umbilication over 4–6 weeks, erosive ulcerative oral lesions; skin hemorrhage on face, palms, soles of feet, scrotum; may be fatal	Clinical signs; histopathology, EM, serology, PCR tests
Yaba Monkey Tumor virus (YMTV) / Zoonotic	Macaques, baboons, sooty mangabeys, African green and patas monkeys. NW resistant to infection	Yatapoxvirus genus	Captive-born African NHPs susceptible; wild caught African NHPs resistant Transmission: inoculation (tattoo), trauma, biting insects NHPs develop high antibody titers No immunological relationship between yaba, vaccinia, and monkeypox Yaba provides immunity against tanapox infection but not vice-versa	Multiple subcutaneous masses (small papules to nodules up to several centimeters wide) on face, hands, and limbs Large masses ulcerate; regress in 6 weeks New lesions may occur while old ones diminish	Clinical signs; histopathology, EM
Yaba-Like Disease Virus (YLDV) [prior names: Benign Epidermal Monkeypox (BEMP); Or-te-ca; Oregon "1211"; Yaba-Related Disease] / Zoonotic	Macaques (rhesus and pig-tailed, bonnet, stump tailed, crab eating, Sulawesi black macaques), Hanuman langurs	Yatapoxvirus genus: related to the human tanapox virus (TPV)	Asian NHPs infected from African NHPs by insect bites, scratches, and tattoo needles	Small red papules, progress to firm, raised, circular lesions (~1 cm diameter) with umbilicated centers often surrounded by hyperemia, than regress in 2 weeks	History of direct or indirect contact between Asian and African NHPs; clinical signs; histopathology

Continued

TABLE 37-6

Selected Infectious Diseases of New World and Old World Monkeys—cont'd

Disease/Zoonotic Risk	Species*	Causative Agents	Epizootiology	Signs	Diagnosis†
Herpesviridae **Alphaherpesvirinae** Genus Simplexvirus					
Macacine herpesvirus 1: Herpes B virus: [Prior names: *Herpesvirus simiae*, Cercopithecine herpesvirus 1] / Zoonotic	Macaques: natural host Fatal infections in capuchins, marmosets, patas, colobus and DeBrazza's monkeys	Macacine herpesvirus 1	Fatal infections rare in macaques, incidence of infection low in stable colonies In wild macaques incidence increases with age Primary infection in infants and juveniles by oral transmission Virus ascends nerve roots to sensory ganglia (trigeminal or dorsal root) establishes latency Recrudescence believed due to stress or immunosuppression Virus may shed without visible lesions; virus recovered from saliva, blood, feces, urine, sera, brain, eye, and kidney	Macaques usually asymptomatic with occasional oral (at mucocutaneous junction) or genital mucosal vesicular lesions, conjunctivitis, nasal discharge Disseminated infection in macaques are rare and usually fatal (e.g., in bonnet macaques: lobar pneumonia, rhinorrhea, hepatic necrosis and conjunctivitis, high mortality) Systemic infections common in crab eating macaques In De Brazza's monkeys: ulcerated eyelids, depression, anorexia, diarrhea, vomiting, high mortality, source was adjacently caged lion-tailed macaques (one De Brazza's had 12+ years persistent infection) Capuchins had persistent infection, source: macaques housed nearby	In macaques: detection of anti-B virus IgG indicates infection but does not predict the potential risk for viral shed nor does a negative result exclude the presence of B virus in the animal Gold standards: virus isolation, serum neutralization tests, PCR for viral DNA and histopathology
Papiine Herpesvirus 2 (Herpesvirus Papio 2) [prior name: Cercopithecine herpesvirus 16]	Natural host: baboon Lethal in one colobus	Papiine herpesvirus 2 (PaHV-2)	Endemic in baboons; oral and venereal transmission; colobus developed severe neurological lesions and died Exposure may be due to enrichment items shared between baboons and colobus housed nearby	Baboons: otic, genital, cutaneous vesicular eruptions, lymphadenopathy, vesicles or pustules coalesced; spread to surrounding tissues Perineal, vulvar, penile lesions may be severe	Baboons: histopathology, molecular techniques Colobus monkey: CNS and adrenal histopathologic lesions Virus identified by molecular techniques
Saimirine Herpesvirus 1 (SaHV1) [prior name: Herpesvirus tamarinus, Herpes T, Marmoset Herpesvirus]	Natural host: squirrel monkeys, capuchins, spider and woolly monkeys may be antibody positive Lethal in marmosets, owl, cebus, and spider monkeys	Saimirine herpesvirus 1	In host species, usually asymptomatic; intermittent asymptomatic viral shed in oral secretions, feces Owl monkeys, marmosets infected from squirrel monkeys experience high mortality; survivors may become virus carriers and shed	Squirrel monkeys: oral lesions or asymptomatic Owl monkeys, marmosets: anorexia, oral lesions, pruritus, sneezing, nasal discharge, diarrhea, swollen eyelids, depression If encephalitis is present: signs and lesions are minimal 76%–100% mortality; death in 2–3 days.	Virus isolation, serological examination, history, histopathology

Agent	Natural host	Transmission/Epidemiology	Clinical signs	Diagnosis
Human Herpesvirus 1 and 2 (HHV1 and HHV2) [prior name: Herpes simplex virus 1 and 2 Herpesvirus hominis]	Lethal in owl monkeys, tamarins, marmosets, and white faced sakis	Direct contact with people with active lesions via animal's conjunctiva or nasopharynx	Conjunctivitis, nasal discharge, ulcerative dermatitis, lingual ulcers, necrotic plaques. In owl monkeys virus has a predilection for cerebral cortex causing encephalitis. Pathogenesis is similar to infections in marmosets and owl monkeys with Saimirine herpesvirus 1	Serology and histopathology. Need to rule out if infection is caused by Saimirine herpesvirus 1
Genus Varicellovirus				
Cercopithecine Herpesvirus 9, (SVV, Simian Varicella Virus, Patas herpesvirus, Varicella-like disease, Liverpool vervet virus (LVV), Medical Lake macaque virus, Delta herpesvirus)	Host species unknown. High morbidity and mortality in OW monkeys: macaques (less severe in Asian macaques), African green, mangabey and patas monkeys. Baboons found to have a 40% seroprevalence with no clinical disease	Several outbreaks in recently imported NHPs spread probably by aerosolization of respiratory secretions caused exanthematous lesions. All but Delta herpes are antigenically related to human herpesvirus 3 (varicella zoster virus, VZV). Reactivation of latent infections may occur	Clinical signs similar between species except in macaques where disease less severe than in African green and patas monkeys: fever, lethargy, generalized hemorrhagic vesicular exanthema starting inguinal area and spreading elsewhere (except palms and soles), lymphadenopathy, abortions and DIC; can progress to hepatitis and pneumonia. High mortality; spontaneous resolution possible. Marked neutrophilic leukocytosis, decreased platelets, increased BUN, AST, ALT. The infection may be asymptomatic	Serology, virus isolation, clinical signs, histopathology
Gammaherpesvirinae				
Callitrichine Herpesvirus 3 (CalHV-3, Marmoset lymphocryptovirus, Marmoset LCV, LCV$_{Cja}$)	Common marmosets	Virus closely related to human Epstein-Barr Virus (EBV). Seroprevalence in wild and captive marmosets is high (up to 65%) but incidence of clinical disease varies between captive populations	Infected common marmosets are usually symptomatic: but may cause weight loss, anorexia, diarrhea, and enlarged mesenteric lymph nodes, palpable abdominal mass. Lymphoproliferative disease and B cell lymphomas	Serology, histopathology. CalHV-3 was in tumor and circulating mononuclear cells
Saimirine Herpesvirus 2 (SaHV-2) [prior name: Herpesvirus samiri]	Asymptomatic in host species: squirrel monkeys. Lethal in naturally infected owl monkeys and in experimentally infected marmosets, tamarins, howler and spider monkeys	Virus transmitted horizontally; squirrel monkeys under 6 months of age are virus free; by 2 years of age, 70%–100% have titers. Owl monkeys contracted the virus from squirrel monkeys; developed lymphoproliferative disease; virus has never been isolated from tumor cells	Squirrel monkeys asymptomatic. Lesions in owl monkeys: lymphoma, lymphoproliferative disease in 50% of infected animals, lymphadenopathy, splenomegaly, and thymic enlargement	Virus is cell-associated; may be recovered from leukocytes, trigeminal ganglia and throat swabs. In owl monkey, histopathology

Continued

TABLE 37-6

Selected Infectious Diseases of New World and Old World Monkeys—cont'd

Disease/Zoonotic Risk	Species*	Causative Agents	Epizootiology	Signs	Diagnosis†
Ateline Herpesvirus 2 and 3 (AtHV-2 and AtHV-3) [prior names: Herpesvirus ateles 2 {HVA-2} and Herpesvirus ateles 2 {HVA-2}]	Asymptomatic in host species, spider monkeys Lethal in experimental infection in tamarins, marmosets and owl monkeys	Ateline herpesvirus 2 and 3	Host species: 60% of spider monkeys have titers. Experimental infection; horizontal transmission occurred between an inoculated marmoset and another marmoset	Asymptomatic in spider monkeys Leukemia and lymphoproliferative disease in 14–40 days after inoculation in marmosets	Serology and histopathology in marmosets
NONENVELOPED DNA-CONTAINING VIRUSES					
Adenoviridae					
Adenovirus infection	Baboons, tamarins, macaques, patas, vervet, squirrel and owl monkeys	Simian Adenovirus, (human adenovirus, SAdV-2, SAdV-3, SAdV-4, SAdV-5, SAdV-9, SAdV-10 and SAdV-20)	Frequently isolated from healthy animals' respiratory and intestinal tract Usually species specific with aerosol and fecal oral transmission Virus may persist in tonsillar tissue and intestinal epithelium Neonates more susceptible than adults Severity varies with species, immune status, age, serotype	Respiratory (nasal discharge, cough, hyperpnea, dyspnea, cyanosis, conjunctivitis); enteric (diarrhea, anorexia, and pancreatitis) Most animals (except neonates which are often more severely affected) recover within 2 weeks Virus shed for weeks	Serology, viral isolation from oral or rectal swabs, histopathology
Papillomas	Colobus, spider and howler monkeys, rhesus and cynomolgus macaques	Alphapapillomavirus genus and Betapapillomavirus genus (in cynomolgus macaques)	Most papillomaviruses are species specific but some strains (RhPV-d) occur in baboons and macaques Rhesus papillomavirus (RhPV) DNA was detected in rhesus macaque penile squamous cell carcinoma ♀s that had sexual contact with this ♂‡ had a >70% incidence of papillomavirus infection and two had cervical neoplasia	Typical lesions of papillomavirus with fibropapilloma lesions (cauliflower-like growth on palms and soles of hands and feet) Cynomologus macaques had a 19% incidence of cervical intraepithelial dysplasia with some developing cervical carcinomas associated with papillomavirus lesions	Gross lesions and histopathology: intranuclear viral particles resemble papillomavirus EM: Immunostaining
RNA VIRUSES					
Rhabdoviridae					
Rabies / Zoonotic: NHPs to human transmission has occurred	Tamarins, marmosets, squirrel monkeys, capuchins, rhesus, crab eating and cynomologus macaques	Rabies virus	Bite wound from rabid animal or modified live vaccination; incubation similar to man; signs in two NHPs 100 and 183 days after exposure Experimental infection in rhesus with furious rabies virus developed signs in 15–35 days; the dumb or paralytic form took up to 105 days	Paralytic form, neurological lesions; animals may be aggressive and bite if provoked; self-mutilation, irritability leading to paralysis of pelvic and pharyngeal muscles, then death	History, clinical signs Fluorescent antibody testing on frozen neural tissues, histopathology

Virus	Agent	Species	Epidemiology/Transmission	Clinical Signs	Diagnosis
Filoviridae—Filovirus **Orthomyxoviridae** Influenza Viruses Type A strains / Zoonotic	Influenza type A strains	Macaques, cebus, African green monkeys, tamarins, baboons, marmoset, squirrel and owl monkeys	Associated with human pandemics. Transmission by aerosolization, contact with humans, or wildlife. Viral strains replicate in the respiratory tract. Bacterial secondary infection common in natural infections	Rhinorrhea, conjunctivitis, coughing, depression, anorexia, GI signs, death from secondary bacterial infections. Gross lesions depend on the strain	History of concurrent infections in caretakers, clinical signs, necropsy, and histopathology, seroconversion by HIA indicates recent infection. Viral culture. IFS
Paramyxovirus Parainfluenza Virus	Parainfluenza virus *Respirovirus* sp. and *Rubulavirus* sp.	Patas, marmoset, crab eating macaque, vervet, and baboon	Transmission: direct contact with infected secretions, aerosols. Spread between species. Respiratory tract viral infection with secondary bacterial infections: 75% mortality in patas monkeys caused by parainfluenza type 3	Many infections mild or asymptomatic. Clinical signs depend on the location within the respiratory tract. Upper and lower respiratory disease, pneumonia, bronchopneumonia mainly in cardiac lobes, fibrinous pleurisy, pericarditis, and peritonitis	Serology demonstrating increased convalescent titers. Viral detection with PCR or IHC. Clinical signs, necropsy, and histopathology
Morbillivirus Measles (rubeola)	Rubeola	Marmosets, tamarins, hairy sakis, macaques, baboon, African green, squirrel, colobus, silver leaf and owl monkeys	Virus acquired from humans by aerosolization; antibodies rare in wild NHPs; up to 100% of animals in captivity have antibodies; mortality rate in OW: 10%; in colobus and silvered leaf monkeys: 100%; in NW: 50%. Rash develops at the end of the viremia. Measles associated with viral induced immunosuppression, which may suppress response to tuberculin skin test; predispose to opportunistic infections	Asymptomatic or mild illness in macaques unless stressed or immunosuppressed. Signs vary depending on the viral strain, species infected: fever, facial edema and erythema, maculopapular rash (rarely on the palmer and planter surfaces) changing to a dry, scaly dermatitis, cough, conjunctivitis, leukopenia, interstitial pneumonia, abortions, acute neurological signs, ataxia, muscle incoordination, and seizures. Colobus, marmosets, owl monkeys show: GI signs and periorbital edema; and a rash may not be present. Animals are infectious prior to showing signs	Clinical signs; necropsy, histopathology, serology, viral isolation

Continued

TABLE 37-6

Selected Infectious Diseases of New World and Old World Monkeys—cont'd

Disease/Zoonotic Risk	Species*	Causative Agents	Epizootiology	Signs	Diagnosis[†]
Paramyxovirus saguinus	Cotton-top tamarins, red chested mustached tamarins, black chested mustached tamarins, and common marmosets	P. saguinus	The origin of the virus is unknown. It is antigenically distinct from measles, but thought to be a variant of measles. Virus shed in feces; transmission is likely fecal–oral. Virus from the original outbreak was inoculated into marmosets and caused the same fatal disease	Enterocolitis, anorexia, diarrhea, dehydration; death within 24 hours with 10% mortality in cotton-top tamarins; almost 100% mortality in red chested mustached tamarins and black chested mustached tamarins without exanthema	Clinical signs, histopathology, viral isolation
Simian hemorrhagic fever virus (SHFV)	Rhesus, stump tailed, crab eating, and pig-tailed macaques Natural host: Patas monkeys (the greatest risk to macaques), rare in baboons and African green monkeys	Simian hemorrhagic fever virus	Highly contagious, fatal infection of macaques. Patas, baboon, and vervet are asymptomatic carriers (may be seronegative and viremic); 50% of wild patas had antibodies. In carriers, virus transmitted horizontally. Macaques acquire virus from carrier NHPs by inoculation, (tattoo machines, biting insects). Virus spreads between macaques by aerosolization, contact, and inoculation. Mortality may reach 100%. Several strains of SHFV have been isolated from Patas monkeys which vary in virulence	Clinical signs: fever, facial erythema and edema, depression, petechial rash, cyanosis, adipsia, epistaxis, vomiting, dehydration, melena, anorexia, retrobulbar hemorrhage, hemorrhagic diathesis and acute diffuse encephalomyelitis. Laboratory results: increased activated partial thromboplastin time and prothrombin time (PT), anemia, and thrombocytopenia. Usually asymptomatic in patas monkeys but may be fatal if a patas monkey is infected with one of the most virulent strains of SHFV while sick from some other cause	Macaques: necropsy and histopathology: thymic cortical necrosis sparing the medulla (unique lesion to SHFV). No hepatic or adrenal necrosis is suggestive of SHFV. Patas monkeys: lysis of peritoneal macrophages. Serological testing (ELISA, immunofluorescence assay), viral isolation
Flaviviral Hemorrhagic Fevers					
Yellow fever / Zoonotic	Guenon, patas, baboon, colobus, marmoset, spider, howler, squirrel, titi, cebus, owl monkey	Yellow fever virus	Virus transmitted by mosquitos (Aedes, Haemagogus, and Sabethes); in Africa and Central and South America. NHPs in Africa and South America support this sylvatic cycle; mangabeys, African green monkeys, guenon, patas, baboon, and colobus asymptomatic. Nocturnal species are susceptible but rarely infected because mosquito vectors are day feeders. Neurotropic and viscerotropic strains are recognized. Disease in NW is more severe. Epizootics occur in howler, squirrel, and spider monkeys. Capuchin and wooly monkeys are resistant	Icterus, hemorrhages, fatty degeneration of the liver, fever, lethargy, jaundice, emesis, and albuminuria	Clinical signs, histopathology. Virus isolation from blood, liver, and spleen

Disease	Species	Agent	Comments	Clinical Signs	Diagnosis
Kyasanur forest disease	Bonnet macaque and Hanuman langur	Kyasanur forest disease virus	Spread by ixodid ticks (*Haemaphysalis*, *Ixodes*, and *Dermacentor*) Virus isolated from bats and rodents Human infection occurred concurrently	High mortality in bonnet macaques and langurs Fever, encephalitis, epistaxis, and bleeding from the GI, leukopenia, anemia, thrombocytopenia	Necropsy histopathology, serology
Flaviviral Encephalitis West Nile Virus	OW and NW	West Nile virus	In outdoor enclosures in Louisiana, baboons, rhesus and pig-tailed macaques had a 36% seroprevalence A natural infection in a Barbary macaque housed outdoors developed neurological signs and died	Most infections are asymptomatic Signs in Barbary Ape were ataxia, nystagmus, cranial nerve deficits, and tremors	Serology, viral isolation, histopathology, IHC, and molecular techniques
Alphaviral Encephalitis Eastern equine encephalitis	Crab eating macaque	Eastern equine encephalitis virus	Mosquito vector	Lethargy, anorexia, and paralysis of rear legs	Clinical signs, histopathology, serology
Picornaviridae Viral hepatitis, hepatitis A / Zoonotic	Woolly monkey, tamarins, macaques, African green monkey, and owl monkey	Hepatitis A virus (HAV)	Spontaneous self-limiting viral infection Acquired from people, NHPs. Virus in liver; shed in feces for 10–30 days after inoculation Transmission by fecal–oral route, incubation 20–50 day; abnormal liver enzymes values Serological evidence of infection documented in captive and wild-caught NHPs	Usually asymptomatic Anorexia, vomiting, fever, diarrhea, lethargy, jaundice, clay-colored stool, elevated liver function tests (ALT and AST increases 2–10 times normal), total serum bilirubin (mild increase) coincide with the development of humeral and cellular immunity	Clinical signs, histopathology, anti-HAV IgM and anti-HAV IgG increase and confirm viral infection
Encephalomyocarditis virus (EMCV)	Rhesus, De Brazza's, owl and squirrel monkeys; mandrill; baboon; vervet; marmosets	Encephalomyocarditis virus	Natural reservoir: feral mice and rats Also carried by raccoons, opossums, and cockroaches Animals infected by feed contaminated with rodent urine or feces Younger animals are more susceptible	Sudden death, myocarditis, encephalitis, vomiting, dyspnea, tachypnea, frothing at nostrils, placental infection and fetal loss; 100% mortality may occur	Viral isolation from organs; necropsy; histopathology; PCR and IHC
Simian Enteroviruses	Rhesus macaques, African green monkeys	SEV-3 (former SV16)	Outbreak with high morbidity and mortality Animals died due to myocarditis and encephalitis	Death without clinical signs, diarrhea, seizures when handled CSF: increased monocytes. Four of 10 brains cultured SEV-3 African green monkeys died with myocarditis and nonsuppurative encephalitis	Viral isolation in significant numbers in body fluids from NHPs with clinical signs; seroconversion during illness

Continued

TABLE 37-6

Selected Infectious Diseases of New World and Old World Monkeys—cont'd

Disease/Zoonotic Risk	Species*	Causative Agents	Epizootiology	Signs	Diagnosis†
BACTERIAL DISEASES					
Gram-Positive Cocci					
Streptococcus pneumoniae [Prior name *Diplococcus pneumoniae, Pneumococcus pneumoniae*]	All NHPs	*S. pneumoniae* Serotypes 2, 3, 6, 14, 18, and 19 (α-hemolytic *Streptococcus*)	Respiratory, aerosol transmission; carriers harbor bacteria in nasal passages, throat. Animals may be predisposed to infection by stress, viral infections, immunosuppression	Asymptomatic carriers; pneumonia, septicemia, bacterial meningitis, purulent conjunctivitis, panophthalmitis, peritonitis, and arthritis	Culture, CSF tap, clinical signs, histopathology
β-Hemolytic Streptococci	Baboons, macaques	*Streptococcus* sp.	Ascending uterine infections	Metritis, fetal sepsis, abortion, neonatal meningoencephalitis, neonatal septic polyarthritis, pneumonia, skin abscesses	Culture and history
Gram-Positive Rods					
Corynebacterium	Macaques, capuchins, languars, tamarin	*C. ulcerans, C. equi, C. renale*	Organism commensal on skin and mucous membranes. Cultured from nasal and conjunctiva swabs, widely found in nature	Bite wounds: abscesses, pulmonary lesions, dyspnea, weight loss, unthriftiness, urinary tract infections, bloody perineal discharge, depression, mastitis	Clinical signs, culture, histopathology, and gross lesions
Listeria	Celebes black apes, wild colobus	*Listeria monocytogenes*	Acquired by eating contaminated food or water	Abortion, stillbirth, neonatal sepsis and meningoencephalitis, fibrinopurulent placentitis	History of reproductive failure; culture, necropsy, and histopathology
Mycobacteriosis / Zoonotic (For Tuberculosis—see text)	All NHPs species are susceptible	Mycobacteriosis is caused by atypical mycobacterium: *M. avium-intracellulare, M. kansasii, M. leprae, M. paratuberculosis, M. gordanae and M. scrofulaceum*	Mycobacteriosis: saprophytic, opportunistic organisms acquired by contacting contaminated water or soil via respiratory, oral or skin contact. NHP species vary in susceptibility to disease	Mycobacteriosis: diarrhea, weight loss, lymphadenopathy, splenomegaly, segmental to diffuse thickening of intestinal mucosa mainly terminal ileum and proximal colon; draining fistula or ulcerated cutaneous lesion	Intradermal tuberculin skin test with Mammalian Old Tuberculin read at 24, 48, and 72 hours; radiographs; antibody based testing (see text); fecal and gastric samples for acid-fast stain, culture and PCR, acid-fast stain; necropsy, histopathology; biopsies may aid in diagnosis and culture is definitive, but only if positive
Nocardia	Macaques, baboon, squirrel monkey	*Nocardia asteroides*	Exists as a saprophyte in decaying vegetation or in richly fertilized soil. Direct contact with wounds, ingestion or inhalation; dissemination in blood or lymphatics to brain or liver	Diarrhea, abdominal distension, dyspnea, epistaxis, weight loss, pain, diarrhea, coma; pulmonary consolidation with hemorrhages, pleural adhesions, abscesses with cavitation, multifocal abscesses in omentum, mesentery, stomach, liver, kidney, brain	Cultures, clinical signs, histopathology

Disease / Type	Host	Agent	Transmission	Clinical signs	Diagnosis
Yersinia / Zoonotic	OW and NW	*Y. pseudotuberculosis* and *Y. enterocolitica*	Food contamination by rodents and birds carry; Fecal–oral transmission	Diarrhea, anorexia, dehydration, suppurative enteric and hepatic lesions, abortions, stillbirths, septicemia, and enlarged cervical lymph nodes in squirrel monkeys	Culture and histopathology, impression smear from necrotic foci
Shigellosis / Zoonotic	OW and NW	*Shigella flexneri* and *S. sonnei*	Fecal–oral transmission; initial infection from humans. Colony infection is probably due to asymptomatic carriers and rodent reservoirs. Stress may be a factor in causing overt disease	Bloody, mucoid, dysentery, weakness, dehydration; facial edema. Macaques: gingivitis, air sac infections and abortion. Leukocytosis with left shift; hyponatremia, hypochloremia. Asymptomatic carriers common	Rectal culture (may require several cultures); necropsy, histopathology; tissue PCR
Salmonellosis / Zoonotic	All NHPs	*Salmonella enterica*, *S. bongori*	Fecal–oral transmission; aerosol transmission is rare. Insects and rodents may be source of infection	Can be asymptomatic carriers, watery to bloody mucoid diarrhea, and dehydration	Culture, gross and histopathology
Escherichia coli / Zoonotic	All NHPs	*E. coli*: enteropathogenic *E. coli* (EPEC); Shiga toxin-producing *E. coli* (STEC), (*E. coli* O157); enterotoxigenic *E. coli* (ETEC); enteroinvasive *E. coli* (EIEC)	Fecal–oral transmission	Diarrhea, pneumonia, enteritis, meningitis, hepatomegaly, splenomegaly	Culture; necropsy, histopathology. Identification of specific serotypes of *E. coli* (reference laboratory to type and isolate), HEp-2 adherence assay, detection of *E. coli* toxin genes by PCR
Tetanus	All NHPs	*Clostridium tetani*	Soil contamination of wounds, post-partum infection, frostbite	Progressive over 1–10 days: lethargic, excessive thirst, unable to prehend food, difficulty swallowing, progressive stiff gait and adduction of forelimbs, biped walking or hopping, piloerection, tenesmus, extensor rigidity exacerbated by noise, seizures, opisthotonos	History and signs; bioassay for tetanospasmin. PCR test for human diagnosis, tetanus IgG (antitoxin) ELISA

Continued

TABLE 37-6

Selected Infectious Diseases of New World and Old World Monkeys—cont'd

Disease/Zoonotic Risk	Species*	Causative Agents	Epizootiology	Signs	Diagnosis†
Bloody-nose syndrome	Cynomologus macaque	*Moraxella catarrhalis*	Aerosol, associated with low humidity (<45%)	Epistaxis, nasal discharge, sneezing, periorbital edema	Signs and culture
Campylobacteriosis / Zoonotic	All NHPs	*Campylobacter fetus, C. jejuni, C. coli, C. laridis, C. sputorum,* and *C. hyointestinalis*	Fecal–oral transmission Recovered NHPs shed bacteria for up to 21 days after diarrhea resolves	Asymptomatic carriers, watery to mucohemorrhagic diarrhea, colitis, electrolyte imbalances, weight loss. *C. fetus* caused fetal death	Culture; histopathology, serology; fluorescent antibody or avidin-biotin antibody staining of intestinal biopsies
Helicobacteriosis	All NHPs	Gastric helicobacters: *Helicobacter pylori, H. heilmannii, H. suis* Enteric helicobactors: *H. cinaedi, Helicobacter sp., H. macacae*	Transmission occurs in young in social groups, likely oral to oral from dam to offspring Some enterohepatic helicobacters are identified with no definitive link of causality	Usually asymptomatic Gastric: gastritis, occasional vomiting, gastric ulcers Enteric: chronic wasting, diarrhea *H. macacae* found in rhesus macaques with endemic diarrhea A novel *Helicobacter* sp. found in cotton-top tamarins with high incidence of IBD, colon cancer, and 8 out of 12 colonic biopsies were PCR positive for *Helicobacter* genus specific primer set, however, causality could not be shown	Gastric helicobacters: gastric endoscopy and gastric biopsy, culture, rapid urease test, *H. pylori* plasma IgG Enteric helicobacters: culture, colonoscopy, colonic biopsies with PCR
FUNGAL DISEASES					
Pneumocystis	Macaques, Goeldi marmosets, owl, white faced saki, Allen's swamp monkey, Hamlyn's monkey, marmosets, and tamarins	*Pneumocystis carinii, P. c. aotus, P.c. callimico, P.c. pithecia, P.c. nigroviridis, P.c. hamlyn*	Pneumocystis species infecting different hosts are genetically distinct taxa Life cycle includes a trophic and cyst (generative) phase	Clinical disease is secondary to immunodeficiency, stress, neoplasia, etc. May be endemic in tamarin colonies Clinical signs in owl monkey with no other concomitant disease: anorexia, progressive weight loss, failure to thrive, death	History (pulmonary disease with immunodeficiency); necropsy; histopathology; bronchoalveolar lavage (BAL)
Microsporidia / Potential zoonotic	*Encephalitozoon cuniculi* NW: squirrel monkey, tamarins, and Goeldi's marmoset *Encephalitozoon* sp. (likely of arthropod origin) in dusty titi monkey. *E. bieneusi* infections in immunocompetent and immunodeficient macaques and a clinically normal marmoset	*Encephalitozoon cuniculi, E. bieneusi*	Life cycle is monoexenous. Transmission: ingestion of spores from food or environment Organism infects intestinal epithelium, spreads hematogenously to organs (vasculature, brain, adrenal gland, heart, lung, kidney, liver, skeletal muscle) *E. bieneusi* infections in immunocompetent and immunodeficient macaques have a predilection for intestinal epithelium, serosa, bile duct, and gall bladder	Usually asymptomatic, seizures, weight loss, respiratory distress No diarrhea or weight loss seen in macaques	Serology: IFA, dot ELISA, and agglutination assays PCR and sequencing Identification of organisms in urine or diluted fecal smears for *E. bieneusi*; in situ hybridization, monoclonal antibodies, EM, histopathology

SYSTEMIC YEAST INFECTIONS

Disease	Species	Organism	Transmission/Epidemiology	Clinical signs/Lesions	Diagnosis
Coccidioidomycosis	All NHPs, baboons and macaques are highly susceptible	*Coccidioides immitis*	Soil saprophyte in semiarid areas in South and Central America, Mexico, and southwestern United States. Transmission: inhalation of arthrospores. Exposure usually in NHPs housed outdoors exposed to dust storms or dust from recent construction with disturbance of virgin (undisturbed) desert	Disseminated disease: lesions in lung, vertebrae, liver, kidneys, spleen, esophagus, and lymph nodes. Nasal discharge, cough, dyspnea, pneumonia, weight loss, lameness, altered gait, paralysis, ascites, failure to thrive	Culture; identification of organism in cytology or histopathology; clinical signs, history, serology (complement fixation or tube precipitin test) or skin testing with coccidioidin, radiography
Histoplasmosis	Baboons	*Histoplasma capsulatum* var. *diboissi* (large-form or African histoplasmosis)	Fungus resides in the soil in Africa, Texas. Transmission: ingestion, inhalation, and direct dermal contact with soil or with infected cage mate by licking or grooming skin lesions	Skin lesions (discrete, elevated, ulcerated granulomas, pustules or papules) on areas that contact ground, scrotum, ears, face, rarely on torso. Radiographic osteolytic lesions under skin lesions on digits, vertebrae, skull. Superficial (associated with skin lesions) and retroperitoneal lymphadenopathy. Discrete nodular liver and testicular lesions	Histopathology, culture, Compliment fixation, immunodiffusion. Differentiation for human infection uses a panfungal PCR with DNA sequencing of polymorphic genome region
Owl monkey fungus	Feral owl monkeys	EM showed the yeast most closely resembled *Loboa loboi*	Disseminated yeast infection	Often asymptomatic; or anorexia, weight loss, lethargy, weakness, and dehydration. The yeast, engulfed by macrophage; may stay dormant for years. Visceral dissemination and multiplication possible. Bone marrow infection may displace blood precursors	Gross and histopathologic lesions; EM, Bone marrow aspirates, cytology. Nonculturable (similar to *Loboa loboi*)

BLASTOMYCETES

Disease	Species	Organism	Transmission/Epidemiology	Clinical signs/Lesions	Diagnosis
Cryptococcus	Tamarins, squirrel monkey, purple faced langur, sooty mangabey, macaques, patas monkey, De Brazza's monkey, guenon	*Cryptococcus neoformans*	Saprophytic soil organism found in pigeon droppings and old nests. Acquired by inhalation and contact	Clinical signs depend on infection location resulting from fungal dissemination. CNS signs: depression, blindness, and seizures	Gross lesions, histopathology, impression smears of skin masses, spinal fluid. Latex agglutination test in serum, urine or CSF. Molecular diagnostics using PCR, culture

‡♂, male; + ♀, female

*NW, New World monkey; OW, Old World monkey; NHP, nonhuman primates.

†CSP, Cerebrospinal fluid; *ELISA*, enzyme-linked immunosorbent assay; *EM*, electron microscopy; *HIA*, hemagglutination inhibition assay; *IFA*, indirect fluorescent antibody assay; *IFS*, immunofluorescence staining; *IHC*, immunohistochemistry; *PCR*, polymerase chain reaction.

to minimize disease transmission between human and nonhuman primates. The most significant zoonotic diseases are caused by viruses and by *Mycobacterium tuberculosis* complex bacteria, especially *M. tuberculosis*. Other commonly encountered medical problems are traumatic injuries from conspecific aggression and geriatric conditions, including osteoarthritis, diabetes, and neoplasia, which are becoming more common as monkeys live longer in zoo collections and research colonies. Common neoplasms include cancer of the GI, integumentary, reproductive, and hematopoietic systems.[21,27] Mycotic infections are not frequently observed in NW and OW monkeys. Although once common, diseases such as lead toxicity, vitamin C deficiency (scurvy), and metabolic bone disease are now rarely observed in well-cared-for primate colonies and zoo collections.[11,32]

Enteric disease is most commonly caused by bacteria, viruses, parasites, or dietary indiscretion, although metabolic or degenerative disorders may also have diarrhea as a component of the clinical presentation. Common bacterial enteropathogens causing enteric disease include enterotoxigenic *Escherichia coli*, *Yersinia enterocolitica* and *Y. pseudotuberculosis*, *Salmonella* sp., *Shigella* sp., and *Campylobacter* sp.; *Campylobacter* sp. is more common in NW monkeys, especially callitrichids.[3,17,39] Although a number of viral diseases may cause enteric disease, they are often not definitively diagnosed because the appropriate diagnostic tests (fecal viral EM or culture) are less commonly performed compared with fecal direct and indirect examination and bacterial culture.

Both helminth and protozoal parasites are common causes of GI disease.[40] Helminth parasites such as *Gongylonema* sp., *Pterygodermatites nycticebi*, and *Prosthenorchis* sp. are particularly hard to control because a range of invertebrates, including cockroaches, may serve as intermediate hosts. *Prosthenorchis* species are significant pathogens because they may penetrate the intestinal wall and cause peritonitis. *Strongyloides* species are also responsible for significant morbidity because of larval migrations, and *S. stercoralis* is particularly pathogenic because of the propensity for autoinfection and resulting hyperinfection. *Entamoeba histolytica* and *Giardia intestinalis* are common protozoal pathogens that cause acute enteritis and may precipitate secondary bacterial septicemic disease. *E. histolytica* causes necroulcerative colitis, and in folivorous species, fatal gastritis is reported. Parasitic diseases can be transmitted from nonhuman primates to humans, but this risk may be minimized by effective hygiene and personal protective procedures.[22,26,40]

Respiratory diseases may be caused by viral infections, but similar to viral causes of enteric diseases, they are less frequently diagnosed, although infections with paramyxoviruses and influenza A and B viruses are common.[23] These viruses often precipitate bacterial infections, of which *Bordetella bronchiseptica*, *Klebsiella pneumoniae*, and *Pasteurella* sp. are common.[17,23,39] In recently imported monkeys, nasal and pulmonary acariasis caused by *Pneumonyssus* sp. or *Pneumonyssoides* sp. may contribute to secondary bacterial infections.[23]

Disease in NW and OW monkeys caused by *M. tuberculosis* complex bacterial infection is less common than it once was. However, it still occurs, especially in nonhuman primates imported from areas of the world where human *M. tuberculosis* infection is prevalent. The infection is originally transmitted to monkeys through contact with infected humans, then monkeys transmit the infection within the group. *M. bovis* is observed even less often but may occur. *M. tuberculosis* complex bacterial infection is less commonly observed in NW monkeys, but they are also susceptible to infection and may develop classic disease (personal communication, Enrique Yarto, DVM, President of Instituto Mexicano de Fauna Silvestre y Animales de Compania, Mexican Institute for Wild and Companion Animals).[36] Although *M. tuberculosis* complex bacterial infection of nonhuman primates is usually a respiratory infection, systemic spread is common. Clinical signs are generally nonspecific, and monkeys may die of disseminated disease without premonitory signs. Tuberculous lesions in NW and OW monkeys do not calcify as often as they do in humans.[12,14,23,26,39] Since the development of

the eyelid intradermal tuberculin test for diagnosis of tuberculosis in monkeys by Dr. Charles Schroeder at the Bronx Zoo in 1938,[38] it has become the standard for nonhuman primate tuberculosis testing. Intradermal testing is performed with 0.1 milliliters (mL) of tuberculin (Tuberculin Mammalian, Human Isolates Intradermic, manufactured by Colorado Serum Company, 4950 York Street, Denver, CO 80216 and distributed by Synbiotics Corp., Animal Health Division, 16420 Via Esprillo, San Diego, CA 92127), except in smaller species in which 0.05 mL is used.[14] The eyelid tuberculin test is commonly referred to as an *intradermal* test but in this test site it is more properly described as an *interdermal* test; true intradermal testing may be performed at other tests sites (chest, abdomen, etc.). The tuberculin test site should be observed at 24, 48, and 72 hours for erythema and induration and described using standard criteria.[14] Test interpretation may be complicated by false-positive, false-negative, and nonspecific responses.[23,26,39] Nonspecific responses are well described in orangutans[7] but also occur in monkey species, especially folivorous species such as langurs and proboscis monkeys. They will also occur if nonhuman primates are vaccinated with Freund's complete adjuvant. Antibody based diagnostic testing (Prima TB STAT-Pak, Chembio Diagnostic Systems, Inc. Medford, NY; http://www.chembio.com/pdfs/PrimaTB-Sell-Sheet-Final.pdf) and γ-interferon assays (PRIMAGAM, Prionics USA, Inc., http://www.prionics.com/diseases-solutions/tuberculosis/PRIMAGAM/; T-SPOT.TB, Oxford Immunotec, Oxford, U.K.) have been developed.[14,39] These tests may also be limited by nonspecificity, have been validated for a limited number of species, and are not always commercially available. Diagnosis should be based not only on the results of the individual's intradermal tuberculin test but also on the history of the individual and the colony or zoo collection with regard to possible exposure to infected humans or nonhuman primates; a complete diagnostic workup should include physical examination, hematologic and biochemical testing, thoracic and abdominal radiography, gastric and tracheal lavage cytology and culture, repeat tuberculin testing (alternating test sites), and comparative tuberculin testing with biologically balanced purified protein derivative (PPD) of *M. bovis* and *M. avium* (PPD Bovis BAL and PPD Avian BAL, NVSL, Ames, IA), and ancillary antibody or antigen testing (Prima TB STAT-Pak, PRIMAGEN, PCR, etc.).[7,14,17,23,26,39] Limited attempts have been made to treat confirmed infections in nonhuman primates. If undertaken, treatment should be based on the antibiotic sensitivity profile of the infecting *M. tuberculosis* strain and be modeled after human combination drug treatment protocols.[14,26,39] *M. avium-intracellulare* complex and *M. paratuberculosis* infections primarily cause chronic GI disease, may be difficult to diagnose, and generally do not respond to treatment.[39]

The most well recognized serious zoonotic disease of monkeys is infection with herpes B virus (*Macacine herpesvirus* 1, previously known as *Cercopithecine herpesvirus-1* or *Herpesvirus simiae*) in macaques.[17,20,45] Although it is harbored asymptomatically or causes mild conjunctivitis or oral vesicular lesions in macaques, human infection is generally fatal. It is less well recognized that this infection has been documented in a range of other OW and NW monkey species such as Patas monkeys (*Erythrocebus patas*), black and white colobus monkeys (*Colobus guereza*), DeBrazza's monkeys (*Cercopithecus neglectus*), capuchin monkeys (*Cebus* sp.), and common marmosets (*Callithrix* [*Callithrix*] *jacchus*).[45] In addition, a very closely related herpesvirus has been described in the silvery langur *Trachypithecus* (*Trachypithecus*) *cristatus*.[6] It should be assumed that this virus may also cause serious human disease, and the same personal protective precautions as one would employ when working with macaques should also be performed when working with all OW monkeys. Taking similar precautions when working with NW monkeys is also advisable.

Because of the close taxonomic relationship between humans and nonhuman primates, a very real risk of anthropozoonotic and zoonotic infections, resulting from trans-species disease transmission, exists. Depending on the infectious agent and infected species, fatalities may result in either nonhuman primates (i.e., *human herpesvirus*

1 or 2 infection of callitrichids and other NW monkeys) or humans (i.e., *Macacine herpesvirus* 1 infection of humans).[11,45] In addition, mixed species exhibits of nonhuman primates potentially pose a risk of interspecific disease transmission between monkey species that may result in fatalities. Some examples include transmission of *Saimiriine herpesvirus 1* (previously named *Herpesvirus tamarinus*) from asymptomatically infected squirrel monkeys to marmosets, tamarins, or owl monkeys, resulting in fatal infections in these species and simian hemorrhagic fever virus transmission from the asymptomatically infected African monkeys species such as Patas monkeys, African green monkeys (*Chlorocebus aethiops*), or baboons (*P. anubis* and *P. cynocephalus*), resulting in fatal infection of Asian macaque species.[17,45] Because of these infectious disease risks, proper personal protective precautions should be incorporated into all management, husbandry, and medical procedures and taken into consideration in exhibit design. Commonly employed precautions include use of PPE: mask and gloves when caring for NW monkeys and prosimians; and mask, face shield, and gloves when caring for OW monkeys and great apes.[26]

Not all diseases of monkeys can be covered in this chapter, but a few are worth mentioning. *Streptococcus zooepidemicus* has caused septicemia and mortality in a number of nonhuman primate species. In many cases, the infection originated from horsemeat-based diets fed to other species in a mixed species exhibit or was transmitted from infected humans.[23] *Francisella tularensis* has caused septicemic disease and mortality in a range of NW and OW monkey species. *Klebsiella pneumoniae* commonly causes peritonitis and mesenteric lymphadenopathy and respiratory disease in NW and OW monkeys.[39] Marmoset wasting syndrome, a multi-factorial disease of callitrichids, causes chronic weight loss and diarrhea. Contributing factors are suboptimal temperatures that place metabolic demands on the animal; chronic or recurrent GI disease caused by bacterial, viral, or parasitic enteropathogens; *Trichospirura leptostoma* infection of the pancreatic ducts resulting in pancreatic dysfunction; inappropriate diets; and gluten intolerance. The outcome of any or a combination of these disease processes is chronic lymphoplasmacytic enterotyphlocolitis, a final common pathway that results in a malabsorption syndrome with chronic diarrhea and weight loss. In advanced stages, it does not respond to any specific or symptomatic therapy because of the structural changes that have occurred in the GI tract. Similar clinical signs in cotton-topped tamarins (*Saguinus oedipus*) may be caused by chronic colitis or colonic adenocarcinoma, which are very well described and commonly observed in this species.[3,21,27] Infection with lymphocytic choriomeningitis virus causes an acute hepatitis with a high mortality rate in marmosets and tamarins. Callitrichids contract the infection through consumption of, or exposure to, feral rodents or through ingestion of neonatal mice ("pinkies") offered as a dietary or enrichment item. The viral agent was originally termed *callitrichid hepatitis virus* until the causal agent was characterized.[3,22,45] Acute, often fatal, gastric dilation is more often observed in monkeys in biomedical research facilities than those in zoo collections.[3,21,26,39] A number of immunosuppressive retroviral infections such as simian immunodeficiency virus (SIV), simian retrovirus (SRV), simian T-cell leukemia virus (STLV), and gibbon ape leukemia virus (GALV) have been described in nonhuman primates in biomedical research settings and in wild populations, but these are rarely observed in zoo collections. Simian foamy virus (SFV) is extremely common across many NW and OW primate species, and humans have become infected from exposure to nonhuman primates; however, to date, no disease in any species has been associated with SFV infection.[20,45]

REPRODUCTION

Most monkeys live in medium- to large-sized social groups. Typically, a dominant male has his harem of reproductive and younger females of various ages, and young males until they disperse from the group, generally when they near sexual maturity. In this social system, the male typically provides little paternal care to his offspring.

However, variation exists across monkey taxa and some species, especially the callitrichids, which live in smaller family groups, where the male plays a significant role in rearing the babies. Callitrichids also have suppression of female reproduction in the family group, with only the dominant female being reproductively active; this is the only nonhuman primate group that typically gives birth to multiple offspring. Monkeys have a long period of parental dependency, during which the juvenile becomes socialized and integrated into the social group.[10,13,24,25,35] Most NW and OW monkey mothers exhibit good maternal care, but in the case of maternal or neonatal illness or maternal death or inexperience, it may be necessary to hand-rear the neonates. In these cases, raising them with conspecifics and/or encouraging early socialization are critically important; otherwise, hand-reared babies will typically be socially incompatible with their conspecifics, hard to introduce to the group, unable to lead a normal social life, and incapable of integrating into a social group.

Both OW and NW monkeys have an estrous cycle, but OW monkeys have a menstrual cycle with menstruation. Some species such as the Japanese snow macaque have a more seasonal pattern of reproduction, whereas others are reproductively active year round. Many OW monkey species have cyclic perineal hyperemia and tumescence ("sex skin"), which reach maximal color and size in the periovulatory period, reflecting elevated estrogen levels; other species such as gelada (*Theropithecus gelada*) also have similar color changes on bare chest patches.[15,24] Most species exhibit a lactational anestrus interval. Males of most species have an os penis. Reproductive physiology is well described for many monkey species and may be monitored by blood, urinary, or fecal sampling.[10,35,46] All NW and OW monkeys have a simplex uterus and hemochorial placentation and may develop reproductive tract problems similar to those of humans (endometriosis, adenomyosis, leiomyomas, placental abruption, placenta previa, ectopic pregnancy, retained placenta, etc.).[8,13,21,26,27] Callitrichids exhibit chorionic placental fusion of fraternal twins, with blood chimerism.[13] Reproductive details for a range of species are listed in Table 37-7.

Because many nonhuman primate species breed very well in captivity, contraception is frequently elected for population management (http://www.stlzoo.org/animals/scienceresearch/contraception center/).[31] Contraception may be reversible or permanent and involve either management actions (single-sex groups or for seasonally breeding species separation of the sexes during the mating season) or medical and surgical methods. For permanent contraception, castration or vasectomy of the male and tubal ligation of the female are most common. Frequently used reversible techniques include subcutaneous implants of long-acting gonadotropin-releasing hormone (GnRH) agonist such as deslorelin (Suprelorin: Peptech Animal Health, North Ryde, NSW Australia) or progestogen such as melengestrol acetate (MGA) (Wildlife Pharmaceuticals, Inc., Windsor, CO); long-acting medroxyprogesterone acetate injections; or immunocontraception with zona pellucida vaccines. NW monkeys have higher endogenous sex steroid levels compared with other primates, and therefore require higher MGA doses to achieve effective contraception. Implants may fail if they are lost through wound dehiscence from grooming of the surgical site or other reasons. Because specific doses, durations of action, and timing of reversibility are not well established for all contraceptive techniques, selection of the most appropriate technique should include a discussion of the advantages and disadvantages of the technique with knowledgeable sources.

PREVENTIVE MEDICINE

A preventive medical program for NW and OW monkeys typically includes either scheduled or opportunistic tetanus and rabies vaccination, routine fecal parasite screening (annually at a minimum, and typically several times a year), and prophylactic parasite treatment protocols based on the parasite history of the colony or zoo collection and fecal parasite results. In many cases, prophylactic

TABLE 37-7

Reproductive Characteristics of Representative Species of New World and Old World Monkeys[17,46]

Parameter	Species							
	Cercopithecus	*Erythrocebus*	*Macaca*	*Papio*	*Callithrix*	*Cebus*	*Saimiri*	*Aotus*
Age of puberty (months)	40–60	M: 28–60 F: 24–42	18–96	M: 48–84 F: 42–60	12–24	M: 84–96 F: 48	M: 48 F: 30	19–30
Estrous cycle (days)	30–36	30–34	24–40	32–36	16–30	18–23	7–16	15–16
Estrous detection	*C. mitis* occasionally shows blood in vaginal swabs	Menses	Menses, perianal swelling or changes in color in *M. nigra, M. mulatta, M. cyclopis, M. nemestrina*; urinary esterone or luteinizing hormone; vaginal cytologic examination; ultrasonography; body temperature; fecal estrogens and progesterone	Perianal sex skin changes; swelling becomes maximum 3–4 days after urinary estrogen levels peak; menses detected with vaginal lavage; fecal estrogens and progestins	Plasma progesterone ≤5 ng/mL before ovulation; urinary and fecal esterone; 17β-estradiol; and progesterone	Serum 17β-estradiol 50–150 ng/mL rises day 0–5 and peaks day 7–10; urinary esterone and luteinizing hormone; plasma progesterone; and vaginal cytologic examination	Vaginal cytologic examination, estrous behavior, blood hormone levels, urinary and fecal esterone, 17β-estradiol, and progesterone	Serum estrogen levels rise from day 0 to peak day 5 and drop to baseline by day 13; urinary and fecal esterone; 17β-estradiol; and progesterone
Gestation (days)	157–213	160–170 (births Dec–Feb)	144–210	154–193	140–150	180	140–180	133–153

Pregnancy determination	Abdominal palpation, ultrasound	Nose of female becomes white during pregnancy	Rectal and abdominal palpation, ultrasound, fecal progestins, urinary esterone conjugates, progesterone metabolites, and urinary and blood chorionic gonadotropin	Rectal palpation, ultrasound, blood and urinary chorionic gonadotropin, blood estradiol and progesterone, and fecal progestins	Urinary chorionic gonadotropin and hydroxypregnenolone; abdominal palpation, ultrasound	Abdominal palpation, ultrasound, urinary esterone, luteinizing hormone, and chorionic gonadotropin	Abdominal palpation at sixth week of gestation, ultrasonography, blood progestins, and urinary chorionic gonadotropin	Abdominal palpation, ultrasound, urinary chorionic gonadotropin and hydroxypregnenolone
Placentation	Chorioallantoic, villous hemochorial placenta, bidiscoid	Chorioallantoic, villous hemochorial placenta, bidiscoid	Chorioallantoic, villous hemochorial placenta, and mono- or bidiscoid	Chorioallantoic, villous hemochorial placenta, and monodiscoid	Chorioallantoic placenta, discoid (often bidiscoid), and hemochorial	Chorioallantoic, trabecular placenta, discoid (often bidiscoid), and hemochorial	Chorioallantoic, trabecular placenta, discoid (often bidiscoid), and hemochorial	Chorioallantoic, trabecular placenta, discoid (often bidiscoid), and hemochorial
Hormone levels **Estrogens** **Nongravid**	—	—	Estradiol 50–450 pg/mL (serum levels)	Estradiol 50–350 pg/mL (plasma levels)	Estradiol 200–1000 pg/mL (plasma levels)	Estradiol 70–540 pg/mL (plasma levels)	Estradiol 190–500+ pg/mL (plasma levels)	Esterone 700–4000 ng/mL (plasma levels); urinary esterone peaks at 49.2 µg/mg creatinine
Nongravid	—	—	<0.5–20 ng/mL (serum levels)	1–8 ng/mL (plasma levels)	5–10 ng/mL (follicular), 10–100 ng/mL (luteal) (plasma levels)	5–100 ng/mL (plasma levels)	70–400 ng/mL (plasma levels)	2–277.8 ng/mL (plasma levels), urinary pregnanediol 19.8 µg/mg

parasite treatments will be administered for both protozoal and helminth parasites.

Other preventive medical procedures are usually based on the medical histories of individual animals or the colony or zoo collection. Annual examinations are recommended by some, but there is not a consensus as to their necessity. The decision to perform annual examinations should be based on a risk-benefit analysis, weighing not only the risks involved in anesthesia but also the difficulty of restraining the monkey, the social repercussions on the individual or group, and the likely benefit from the medical procedure. If performed, annual examinations typically include physical examination, as well as dental evaluation, venipuncture for routine hematologic and biochemical screening, species-specific viral serology, serum banking, vaccinations, tuberculin testing, radiography, and ultrasonography.[26]

Both quarantine and necropsy examinations are components of a preventive medical plan for monkeys. A 31-day quarantine period is typically conducted for new acquisitions. The derivation of a 31-day quarantine interval as a quarantine standard was based on monkeys receiving three tuberculin tests at 14-day intervals, with the final reading of the last tuberculin test result at 72 hours, all of which requires 31 days. During the quarantine period, depending on previous medical history and preshipment testing, physical examination, permanent identification (tattoo, transponder placement, etc.), venipuncture for hematologic and biochemical testing, species-specific viral serology, vaccinations, and radiography are typically performed. In the United States, imported nonhuman primates have to undergo specific quarantine procedures and protocols mandated by the Centers for Disease Control and Prevention (CDC), and facilities must be approved by the CDC for this purpose before they may import nonhuman primates. Necropsies should be conducted on all monkeys that die in quarantine or in the colony or zoo collection. This should include gross necropsy, histologic evaluation of tissue, and appropriate ancillary testing (culture, molecular diagnostics, etc.). Thorough necropsy will not only determine the cause of death but also serves as a way to evaluate the group, species, and colony or zoo collection for the presence of infectious, parasitic, nutritional, toxic, or metabolic diseases that are relevant to the care of the living nonhuman primates.

VACCINATION

All monkeys are susceptible to tetanus. Infection, through wounds or penetrating injuries, and subsequent neurotoxin production usually result in fatal disease, so all the animals should be routinely vaccinated with tetanus toxoid,[26,39] according to human vaccination recommendations. In rabies-endemic areas, NW and OW monkeys in outdoor exhibits should be vaccinated for rabies.[26] Only an inactivated (killed) vaccine should be used to avoid the risk of vaccine-induced disease that may occur when attenuated (modified live) vaccines are used. For both tetanus and rabies vaccination, the vaccine dose is generally adjusted for the smaller size of NW and OW monkeys (typically 0.05–0.1 mL for callitrichids, 0.25 mL for medium-sized primates, and 0.5 mL for larger primates). Although monkeys are susceptible to measles infection, because of the decline in the incidence of human disease achieved through human vaccinations, effective preventive health protocols for monkeys, and adherence to personal protective procedures by staff, monkeys are not routinely vaccinated for this disease. If measles vaccination is elected, care should be exercised in selecting the specific vaccine to minimize the risk of vaccine-induced disease, since most measles vaccines are attenuated (modified live) vaccine viral strains. Other vaccinations such as those against pneumococcosis or leptospirosis may be administered on a case-by-case basis or as a result of local conditions or facility-specific considerations. In these situations, all attenuated vaccines should be employed cautiously because of the risk of vaccine-induced disease, and it is advisable to contact other veterinary practitioners to determine what attenuated vaccines have been safely used in the species of concern.

BEHAVIORAL TRAINING

NW and OW monkeys are highly intelligent and, through positive reinforcement, may learn to perform a range of behaviors that are useful for both medical and management purposes. These include entering and leaving exhibits on cue, shifting between enclosures, entering a crate, entering a restraint device, allowing hand injection of immobilizing agents or medications (such as insulin) by stationing themselves at the bars or cage mesh, voluntary submission for blood sampling, and shifting onto a scale on command to be weighed.[34]

TRANSPORT

Monkeys are generally transported in plastic or wooden crates designed for dogs and cats or specially built for monkeys. In all cases, the crates should be sturdy and in good repair, substantial enough to safely contain the monkey during transport, and prevent people from accessing the monkey in transit. For air transportation, compliance with shipping regulations of the International Air Transport Association (IATA), local and national regulatory agencies, and those of the airline are required. Food and water should be provided in transit in the event the shipment is delayed, and crate construction should ensure that spillage of food, water, or waste material cannot occur. Any necessary preshipment medical testing should be completed, and the health certificate, the medical record, and copies of test results should be included with the shipment.

REFERENCES

1. Abee CR, Mansfield K, Tardif S, et al: *Nonhuman primates in biomedical research*, vol 2, ed 2, London, U.K., 2012, Elsevier.
2. Abramowicz M, Zuccotti G, Pflomm J, editors: *Drugs for parasitic infections*, ed 2, New Rochelle, NY, 2010, The Medical Letter.
3. Brady AG, Carville AAL: Digestive system diseases of nonhuman primates. In Abee CR, Mansfield K, Tardif S, et al, editors: *Nonhuman primates in biomedical research*, vol 2, ed 2, London, U.K., 2012, Elsevier.
4. Bush M, Montali RJ, Kleiman DG, et al: Diagnosis and repair of familial diaphragmatic defects in golden lion tamarins. *J Am Vet Med Assoc* 177(9):858–862, 1980.
5. Calle PP, Raphael BL, Stetter MD, et al: Gastrointestinal linear foreign bodies in silver leaf langurs *Trachypithecus cristatus ultimus*. *J Zoo Wildl Med* 26:87, 1995.
6. Calle PP, Raphael BL, Stetter MD, et al: Novel herpes-B like infection of silver leaf langurs (*Presbytis cristata*). *Proc Am Assoc Zoo Vet P* 457, 1996.
7. Calle PP: Tuberculin responses in orangutans. In Fowler ME, Miller RE, editors: *Zoo and wild animal medicine*, ed 4, Philadelphia, PA, 1999, Saunders.
8. Cline JM, Brignolo L, Ford EW: Urogenital system. In Abee CR, Mansfield K, Tardif S, et al, editors: *Nonhuman primates in biomedical research*, vol 2, ed 2, London, U.K., 2012, Elsevier.
9. Cogswell F: Parasites of non-human primates. In Baker DG, editor: *Flynn's parasites of laboratory animals*, ed 2, Ames, IA, 2007, Wiley-Blackwell.
10. Einspanier A, Gore MA: Reproduction: definition of a primate model of female fertility. In Wolfe-Coote S, editor: *The laboratory primate*, London, U.K., 2005, Elsevier.
11. Fahey MA, Westmoreland SV: Nervous system disorders of nonhuman primates and research models. In Abee CR, Mansfield K, Tardif S, et al, editors: *Nonhuman primates in biomedical research*, vol 2, ed 2, London, U.K., 2012, Elsevier.
12. Frost PA, Calle PP, Klein H, Thoen CO: Zoonotic tuberculosis in nonhuman primates. In Thoen CO, Steele JH, Kaneene JB, editors: *Zoonotic tuberculosis: Mycobacterium bovis and other pathogenic mycobacteria*, Ames, IA, Wiley-Blackwell Publishing. (In Press 2014).
13. Godfrey LR: General anatomy. In Wolfe-Coote S, editor: *The laboratory primate*, London, U.K., 2005, Elsevier.

14. National Institutes of Health Animal Research Advisory Committee Guidelines: *Guidelines for the prevention and control of tuberculosis in nonhuman primates* (May, 12, 2010): <http://oacu.od.nih.gov/ARAC/documents/NHP_TB_Prevention.pdf>. Accessed February 25, 2013.

15. Hartwig W: Primate evolution. In Campbell CJ, Fuentes A, MacKinnon KC, et al, editors: *Primates in perspective*, ed 2, New York, 2011, Oxford University Press.

16. International Union for the Conservation of Nature: *IUCN Red List of Threatened Species.* Version 2012.2: <www.iucnredlist.org>. Accessed January 28, 2013.

17. Joslin JO: Other primates excluding great apes. In Fowler ME, Miller RE, editors: *Zoo and wild animal medicine*, ed 5, St. Louis, MO, 2003, Saunders.

18. Kreeger TJ, Arnemo JM: *Handbook of wildlife chemical immobilization*, ed 4, Sybille, WY, 2012, Terry J. Kreeger.

19. Lang C, Lewis SD: Appendix. In Baker DG, editor: *Flynn's parasites of laboratory animals*, ed 2, Ames, IA, 2007, Wiley-Blackwell.

20. Lerche NW: Common viral infections of laboratory primates. In Wolfe-Coote S, editor: *The laboratory primate*, London, U.K., 2005, Elsevier.

21. Lewis AD, Colgin LMA: Pathology of noninfectious diseases of the laboratory primate. In Wolfe-Coote S, editor: *The laboratory primate*, London, U.K., 2005, Elsevier.

22. Lewis SM, Hotchkiss CE, Ullrey DE: Nutrition and nutritional diseases. In Wolfe-Coote S, editor: *The laboratory primate*, London, U.K., 2005, Elsevier.

23. Lowenstine LJ, Osborn KG: Respiratory system diseases of nonhuman primates. In Abee CR, Mansfield K, Tardif S, et al, editors: *Nonhuman primates in biomedical research*, vol 2, ed 2, London, U.K., 2012, Elsevier.

24. Macdonald DW: *The Princeton encyclopedia of mammals*, Princeton, NJ, 2006, Princeton University Press.

25. MacKinnon KC: Social beginnings the tapestry of infant and adult interactions. In Campbell CJ, Fuentes A, MacKinnon KC, et al, editors: *Primates in perspective*, ed 2, New York, 2011, Oxford University Press.

26. Mahoney J: Medical care. In Wolfe-Coote S, editor: *The laboratory primate*, London, U.K., 2005, Elsevier.

27. Miller AD: Neoplasia and proliferative disorders of nonhuman primates. In Abee CR, Mansfield K, Tardif S, et al, editors: *Nonhuman primates in biomedical research*, vol 2, ed 2, London, U.K., 2012, Elsevier.

28. Montali RJ: Congenital retrosternal diaphragmatic defects, golden lion tamarins. In Hunt RD, Jones TC, Mohr U, editors: *Nonhuman primates II*, Berlin, Germany, 1993, Springer-Verlag, pp 132–133.

29. Olberg R-A: Monkeys and gibbons. In West G, Heard D, Caulkett N, editors: *Zoo animals andand wildlife immobilization and anesthesia*, Ames, IA, 2007, Blackwell.

30. Physicians' Desk Reference Staff: *Physicians' desk reference,*, ed 67. Montvale, NJ, 2013, PDR Network.

31. Porton IJ, Dematteo KE: Contraception in nonhuman primates. In Asa CS, Porton IJ, editors: *Wildlife contraception issues, methods, and applications*, Baltimore, MD, 2005, Johns Hopkins.

32. Pritzker KPH, Kessler MJ: Arthritis, muscle, adipose tissue, and bone diseases of nonhuman primates. In Abee CR, Mansfield K, Tardif S, et al, editors: *Nonhuman primates in biomedical research*, vol 2, ed 2, London, U.K., 2012, Elsevier.

33. Purcell JE, Philipp TP: Parasitic diseases of nonhuman primates. In Wolfe-Coote S, editor: *The laboratory primate*, London, U.K., 2005, Elsevier.

34. Reinhardt V: Environmental enrichment and refinement of handling procedures. In Wolfe-Coote S, editor: *The laboratory primate*, London, U.K., 2005, Elsevier.

35. Rensing S, Oerke A-K: Husbandry and management of new world species: Marmosets and tamarins. In Wolfe-Coote S, editor: *The laboratory primate*, London, U.K., 2005, Elsevier.

36. Rocha VCM, Ikuta CY, Gomes MS, et al: Isolation of *Mycobacterium tuberculosis* from captive *Ateles paniscus*. *Vector Borne Zoonotic Dis* 11:593, 2011.

37. Sasseville VG, Hotchkiss CE, Levesque PC, et al: Hematopoietic, cardiovascular, lymphoid and mononuclear phagocyte systems of nonhuman primates. In Abee CR, Mansfield K, Tardif S, et al, editors: *Nonhuman primates in biomedical research*, vol 2, ed 2, London, U.K., 2012, Elsevier.

38. Schroeder CR: A diagnostic test for the recognition of tuberculosis in primates: A preliminary report. *Zoologica NYZS* XXIII:397, 1938.

39. Simmons J, Gibson S: Bacterial and mycotic diseases of nonhuman primates. In Abee CR, Mansfield K, Tardif S, et al, editors: *Nonhuman primates in biomedical research*, vol 2, ed 2, London, U.K., 2012, Elsevier.

40. Strait K, Else JG, Eberhard ML: Parasitic diseases of nonhuman primates. In Abee CR, Mansfield K, Tardif S, et al, editors: *Nonhuman primates in biomedical research*, vol 2, ed 2, London, U.K., 2012, Elsevier.

41. Strier KB: Conservation. In Campbell CJ, Fuentes A, MacKinnon KC, et al, editors: *Primates in perspective*, ed 2, New York, 2011, Oxford University Press.

42. Terao K: Management of old world primates. In Wolfe-Coote S, editor: *The laboratory primate*, London, U.K., 2005, Elsevier.

43. Valverde CR: Lemoy M: Primates. In Carpenter JW, editor: *Exotic animal formulary*, ed 4, St. Louis, MO, 2012, Elsevier.

44. Voevodin AF, Marx PA, Jr: *Simian virology*, Ames, IA, 2009, Wiley-Blackwell.

45. Wachtman L, Mansfield K: Viral diseases of nonhuman primates. In Abee CR, Mansfield K, Tardif S, et al, editors: *Nonhuman primates in biomedical research*, vol 2, ed 2, London, U.K., 2012, Elsevier.

46. Wheaton CJ, Savage A, Lasley BL: Advances in the understanding of primate reproductive endocrinology. In Campbell CJ, Fuentes A, MacKinnon KC, et al, editors: *Primates in perspective*, ed 2, New York, 2011, Oxford University Press.

47. Wilson DE, Reeder DM: *Mammal species of the world*, ed 3, 2005, Smithsonian Institution. <http://www.vertebrates.si.edu/msw/mswcfapp/msw/index.cfm>. Accessed February 6, 2014.

48. Wilson DE, Reeder DM: *Mammal species of the world: A taxonomic and geographic reference*, ed 3, Baltimore, MD, 2005, Johns Hopkins University Press.

49. Wolfe-Coote S: *The laboratory primate*. London, U.K., 2005, Elsevier.

CHAPTER 38

Great Apes

Hayley Weston Murphy

BIOLOGY

Great apes are a taxonomic family of primates classified as Hominidae and include seven living species in four genera: chimpanzees and bonobos (*Pan*), gorillas (*Gorilla*), orangutans (*Pongo*), and humans (*Homo*).[13] The dental formula for the great apes is: (incisor 2/2, canine 1/1, premolar 2/2, molar 3/3) × 2 = 32. The great apes originate from equatorial Africa (gorillas, chimpanzees, and bonobos) and Southeast Asia (orangutans) and are characterized by the absence of tails and their intelligence, strength, and large size. Table 38-1 gives an overview of their status in the wild. Significant threats to wild great ape populations include the hunting of apes for sale as commercial meat products, widespread habitat loss, and infectious disease threats. Outbreaks of Ebola virus, respiratory disease epidemics, and bacterial and parasitic illnesses have resulted in high morbidity and mortality events, often in association with close contact with humans.[15-17,31,34,36,41,46,48,49,51]

UNIQUE ANATOMY

The great apes are intelligent animals and have great strength and varied facial and vocal expressions. They all have laryngeal sacs, which are thought to be used for vocal resonations; these sacs vary in size and complexity, expanding with age into the pectoral, clavicular, and axillary regions. Mature male orangutans have extensive laryngeal sacs that extend around the mandible toward the ears and cheeks and along the thoracic wall.[21] Orangutan males are the only great apes that develop cheek pads (flanges), which are composed of fat and fibrous tissue.[2] See Figures 38-1, 38-2, 38-3 for examples of adult male Bornean, Sumatran, and hybrid orangutans.

CAPTIVE MANAGEMENT

Standardized Animal Care Guidelines have been published or are in development for all of the great apes kept in captivity and may be accessed at http://www.aza.org/animal-care-manuals.[2] These Animal Care Manuals (ACMs) provide a compilation of animal care and management knowledge that has been gained from recognized species experts, including Association of Zoos and Aquariums (AZA) Taxon Advisory Groups (TAGs), Species Survival Plan® Programs (SSPs), biologists, veterinarians, nutritionists, reproductive physiologists, behaviorists, and researchers.

Special Housing Requirements

Captive great ape enclosures must be designed with the animals' psychological, social, and physical requirements in mind. Husbandry recommendations for great apes are outlined in Table 38-2. Particular attention should be paid to containment requirements for all ages and both sexes and provision of adequate horizontal and vertical spaces to accommodate the complex social interactions of the great apes. A protective barrier between the ape and the human caregiver should enable safe and voluntary interactions between humans and apes. The United States Department of Agriculture (USDA) has regulations to mandate that any facility that is licensed to sell, exhibit, or do research on primates have a plan in place for environmental enhancement adequate to promote the psychological well-being of nonhuman primates.[18] These codes may be found at www.nal.usda.gov/awic/pubs/Legislat/awabrief.shtml.

Feeding

Institutions that house great apes should have sound nutritional programs, and formulation of ape diets should be made in consultation with nutritionists and veterinarians. Diets need to meet the nutritional and psychological needs of the animals throughout their life stages and should be reviewed on a scheduled basis. All of the great apes are primarily herbivorous and require an exogenous source of vitamin C. Diets may vary considerably among institutions and may consist of commercially available pellets, fruits, vegetables, and browse. The caloric needs of the great apes may be estimated by using the equation: ME (kcal) = 100 × body weight (BW)$^{0.75}$ in kilograms.[28] The nutritional requirements for nonhuman primates are available, but it must be recognized that over 250 primate species exist, so defining species-specific requirements is difficult.[28] Nutritional imbalances resulting in health concerns have been seen in captive situations. Vitamin D deficiency has resulted in metabolic bone disease in mother-reared infants that do not have outdoor access and adequate sun exposure. Obesity, diabetes, cardiovascular diseases, behavioral issues, and osteoarthritis are also a concern in captive apes fed inappropriate diets.[4,5,32,50] Diets made up of primarily high-fiber, low-sugar foods may more closely resemble "wild type" diets and may aid in reducing associated dietary health concerns.

PREVENTIVE MEDICINE

The basic components of a medical program for great apes are provided in Table 38-3; these are preshipment health screening and evaluation; quarantine; physical examination, including a comprehensive dental examination; immunoprophylaxis; parasite control; proper nutrition; and monitoring for new medical problems.[2,21] A well-rounded preventive medicine plan for great apes must take into consideration the close taxonomic relationship between these animals and humans to have maximum effectiveness.[17,27,29,31,48,49,51,52]

Anthropozoonoses are of particular concern and should prompt evaluation of potential ape exposures to human caregivers as well as to the public. Potentially immune-compromised individuals, infants and juveniles, naive populations, and geriatric or chronically ill animals and people are at particular risk. Although the zoonotic disease risks are too many to detail in this chapter, a few are worthy of mention because of their documented effects on great apes. Viruses that cause upper respiratory infections such as colds and influenza may be easily transmitted between humans and apes, and close contact with humans, especially young children (or parents of young children), may increase the likelihood of upper respiratory infections in apes.[15,34] Humans with any active upper respiratory infections should not work in close contact with apes or prepare food or enrichment items. Bacterial diseases, especially gastrointestinal (GI) illnesses such as those caused by *Salmonella* sp., *Campylobacter*, *Yersinia*, and *Shigella* sp. may also be of zoonotic concern and result in clinical illnesses.[32,39,40] Devastating losses in wild populations of African great apes from Ebola viruses have also been documented.[36]

Effective preventive medicine protocols need to take into consideration the use of personal protective equipment (PPE; e.g., N-95 masks, protective clothing, gloves, etc.), and cleaning and hygiene regimes, as well as the health of the humans in close contact with the apes.

Health Screening and Evaluation

Preshipment Evaluations

Prior to transfer from one institution to another, it is important to determine the health status of individual animals. This ensures that the animals are healthy enough to withstand the transfer and will not be carrying novel infectious or parasitic diseases into naïve collections. A thorough health history of the individual animal, as well as a review of disease concerns within the originating collection, is warranted before requesting specific preshipment testing. At a minimum, all great apes should have a complete blood cell count (CBC), blood chemistry, endoparasite testing, fecal bacterial cultures, and testing for tuberculosis (TB) exposure. Additional testing options

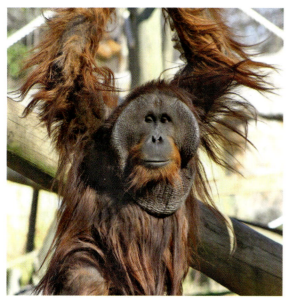

FIGURE 38-1 Adult male Bornean orangutan. (Courtesy Bridget Wright, Zoo Volunteer, Zoo Atlanta, Atlanta, GA.)

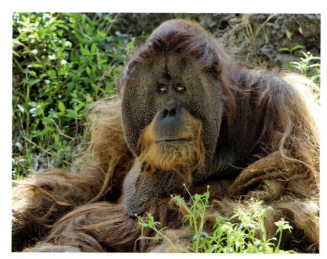

FIGURE 38-2 Adult male Sumatran orangutan. (Photo courtesy Adam K. Thompson-Zoo Atlanta, Atlanta, GA.)

TABLE 38-1

Genus, Species, and Status in the Wild[13]

Genus	Species	Subspecies	Common Name	Weight (adult in kg)	IUCN Status
Pongo	*pygmaeus*	ssp. *morio* ssp. *pygmaeus* ssp. *wurmbii*	Northeast Bornean Orangutan Northwest Bornean Orangutan Central Bornean orangutan	50–100 kg (M) 30–50 kg (F)	Endangered
Pongo	*abelii*		Sumatran orangutan	80–90 kg (M) 33–45 kg (F)	Critically endangered
Gorilla	*beringei*	ssp. *beringei*	Mountain gorillas	180–220 kg (M) 70–90 kg (F)	Endangered
		ssp. *grauri*	Eastern Lowland or Grauer's gorilla	160–250 kg (M) 70–120 kg (F)	
Gorilla	*gorilla*	ssp. *gorilla*	Western lowland gorillas	140–270 kg (M) 70–90 kg (F)	Critically endangered
		ssp. *diehli*	Cross River gorilla	180 kg (M)	
Pan	*troglodytes*	ssp. *ellioti*	Nigerian-Cameroon chimpanzee	40–70 kg (M) 32–47 kg (F)	Endangered
		ssp. *schweinfurthii*	Eastern chimpanzee	45–90 kg (M) 40–80 kg (F)	
		ssp. *troglodytes*	Central chimpanzee	45–90 kg (M) 40–80 kg (F)	
		ssp. *verus*	West African chimpanzee	45–90 kg (M) 40–80 kg (F)	
Pan	*paniscus*		Bonobo	25–45 kg (M) 25–40 kg (F)	Endangered

F, Female; *M*, male;.

will depend on the situation but may include total cholesterol levels, thyroid hormone testing, and screening for more infectious viral and bacterial agents. In adult animals, it is recommended that a complete examination of the cardiovascular health of the animal be performed before shipment occurs. Additionally, because of the high incidence of respiratory disease in orangutans, it is strongly recommended that a thorough evaluation of orangutan respiratory health be done prior to transfer.[2]

Quarantine

Newly acquired animals should go through a quarantine period before being introduced into existing collections. Quarantine periods and examinations may vary greatly among institutions and are dependent on the origin of the animal, evaluation of health and infectious disease status, amount of prearrival screening done, and husbandry adjustments needed. A quarantine period of 30 to 90 days should include one to two physical examinations, consisting of CBC, blood chemistry panels, TB testing, and appropriate infectious disease screening. Parasitic disease risks should be assessed with a minimum of three fecal examinations (floats, centrifugation, sedimentation, or all; direct fecal smears) and bacterial fecal cultures should be done to detect potential pathogens such as *Salmonella*, *Shigella*, *Campylobacter* sp., enterotoxogenic *Escherichia coli* and *Yersinia* spp. If the receiving institution cannot sufficiently quarantine new animals, quarantine may occur at the originating institution as long as the animal is isolated during this time frame and shipped in isolation. The Association of Zoos and Aquariums (AZA) considers this to be an adequate quarantine in these circumstances. If an appropriately designed and physically isolated quarantine facility is not present at either institution, then minimizing infectious disease

risks from newly acquired animals may be attempted by preventing physical, aerosol, and fomite transmission of pathogens and establishing strict cleaning and PPE guidelines. All applicable regulations must be followed and zoonotic disease prevention procedures and staff training protocols established to minimize the risk of transferable diseases. Increased attention to enrichment is necessary when apes are housed in isolation during quarantine periods of any length.

Physical Examinations

Decisions regarding frequency of hands on examinations performed under general anesthesia varies between institutions and should be determined by an institutional and individual animal risk review. Great apes are generally too strong and agile to be handled without the use of chemical immobilizing agents; therefore, for any diagnostic or treatment procedure that requires more than minimal interactions done through operant conditioning, general anesthesia is usually required. Consideration of the collections' historic disease risk analysis, taxonomic recommendations made by species experts, life stage risks (i.e., evaluation of health risks based on age), as well as evaluations of the risks versus the benefits of anesthesia may all factor into the frequency of recommended immobilizations done during an individual animal's life span. Some limited diagnostic procedures including blood collection, auscultation, cursory dental examinations, cardiac echosonographic evaluations, neonatal examinations, blood pressure measurements, and radiography may be done on nonanesthetized animals through training. Figure 38-4 shows an example of a blood pressure monitoring apparatus, and Figure 38-5 shows it in use with an adult male gorilla. Commercial squeeze cages are available for apes but may have limited usefulness in these large and strong animals.

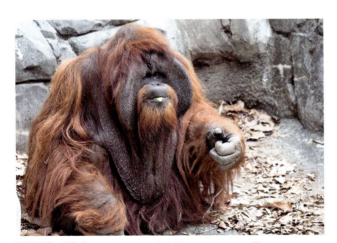

FIGURE 38-3 Adult male hybrid orangutan. (Photo courtesy Adam K. Thompson-Zoo Atlanta, Atlanta, GA.)

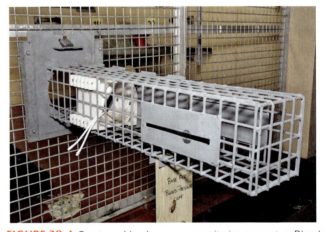

FIGURE 38-4 Great ape blood pressure monitoring apparatus. Blood pressure sleeve is mounted inside of the hard plastic casing. (Photo courtesy Adam K. Thompson-Zoo Atlanta, Atlanta, GA.)

TABLE 38-2

Husbandry Recommendations for Great Apes[2]

Recommendations	Orangutans	Gorillas	Chimpanzees	Bonobos
Temperature	64°F (18°C) to 84°F (28°C)	65°F–85°F	60°F–85°F	64°F (18°C) to 72°F (22°C)
Humidity	30%–70%	30%–70%	30%–70%	50%–60%
Ventilation	10–15 air changes per hour (hr)	10–15 air changes/hr	10–15 air changes/hr	10–15 air changes/hr

Auxiliary ventilation must be provided when ambient temperature is 85°F (29.5°C) or higher.

TABLE 38-3

Recommended Procedures for Scheduled Physical Examinations of Great Apes

Procedure	Frequency	Notes
Physical examination	1–2 times in quarantine, every 1–3 years*	Partial visual examinations may be done through the use of operant conditioning but general anesthesia is needed for a complete physical examination
Dental examination	Every 1–3 years	Complete examination requires general anesthesia
Accurate weights	Monthly	Scales should be designed into holding or exhibit areas
Blood collection	Every 1–3 years, some animals may be trained for voluntary blood draws more frequently	Routine on all: CBC, chemistry panel, viral serology†, serum banking (all ages) Additional tests: thyroid panel, cholesterol, lipid panel, cardiac disease markers
Rectal culture	Every 1–3 years	For *Salmonella*, *Shigella*, *Campylobacter*, *Yersinia*, pathogenic *E. coli* strains
Fecal examination	Every 3–6 months	Includes direct and concentrating techniques (flotation, centrifugation, sedimentation) Additional diagnostics targeting parasites of concern may include *Giardia* and *Cryptosporidium* screening (e.g., IFA, ELISA, PCR), and Baermann technique for identification of select nematode larvae
Mycobacterial testing	Every 1–3 years	Intradermal skin test, lavage (gastric, tracheal, bronchial) ELISA (e.g., ChemBio) PCR testing, γ-interferon testing (e.g., Primagam). Mycobacterial testing results from orangutans are challenging to interpret and many tests have not been validated
Imaging	Every 1–3 years	Radiography (thoracic, abdominal, dental) recommended for all ages +/– Abdominal ultrasound for adults -Echocardiography, blood pressure measurements, ECG; once as juveniles, then every 1–3 years once adults CT imaging of sinuses, air sacs, and thorax recommended to screen for respiratory infections in orangutans when feasible
Vaccinations	Varied frequency	See table 38-4
Identification	Once	Permanent identification for individuals may include natural markings, photographs of facial characteristics, tattoo, transponder chips

*Up to institutional clinical risk assessments for use of general anesthesia.

†Full panel recommended once, then done as needed based on risk assessment. Full panel includes: simian immunodeficiency virus (SIV); simian foamy virus (SFV); simian T-cell lymphotropic virus (STLV); cytomegalovirus (CMV); herpes simplex virus 1 and 2 (HSV-1, HSV-2); influenza A and B (flu A and flu B); parainfluenza 1, 2, and 3; respiratory syncytial virus (RSV); simian adenovirus (SA-8); measles virus; human varicella zoster (HVZ); Epstein-Barr virus (EBV) +/– hepatitis A and hepatitis B; encephalomyocarditis (EMC).

CBC, Complete blood cell count; *CT*, computed tomography; *ECG*, electrocardiography; *ELISA*, enzyme-linked immunosorbent assay; *IFA*, indirect fluorescent antibody; *PCR*, polymerase chain reaction.

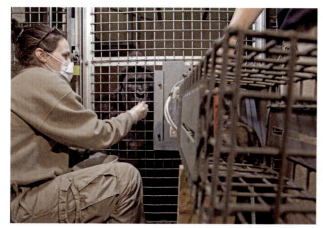

FIGURE 38-5 Gorilla having his blood pressure taken. (Photo courtesy Adam K. Thompson-Zoo Atlanta, Atlanta, GA.)

Immunoprophylaxis

Preventive medicine programs for captive great apes may or may not include a variety of vaccination protocols. Decisions on immunoprophylaxis of great apes are often based on a situational risk analysis taking into consideration geographic disease risks, human interactions, operant conditioning to allow for nonanesthetized access, individual animal disease risk, access to mother-reared infants, and examination frequency. Vaccination of free-living great apes has been proposed as a possible means to mitigate the potentially devastating effects of reverse zoonosis to these vulnerable populations of animals.[41,48,51] Factors such as cost, practicality, and wildlife welfare and management must be considered when evaluating the use of commercially available vaccines in wild populations. Recommendations for human vaccination (with the addition of rabies prophylaxis if the apes may potentially interact with wild mammals) may be used as general guidelines when devising vaccination protocols for great apes and, whenever possible, killed vaccines should be used. In addition, consultations with local public health officials, infectious

TABLE 38-4

Recommended Human Immunization Schedule*

Immunization	Abbreviation	Dosing Schedule
Hepatitis B	Hepatitis B	birth; 1 mo; 6–18 mo
Rotavirus	RV	2 mo; 4 mo
Diphtheria, tetanus, pertussis	DTaP	2 mo; 4 mo; 6 mo; 15–18 mo; 11–12 yr; q10yr
Haemophilus influenzae type b	Hib	2 mo; 4 mo; 12–15 mo
Pneumococcal	PCV	2 mo; 4 mo; 6 mo; 12–15 mo
Inactivated poliovirus	IPV	2 mo; 4 mo; 6-18 mo; 4–6 yr
Influenza	—	Annually
Measles, mumps, rubella	MMR	12–15 mo; 4–6 yr
Varicella	Varicella	12–15 mo; 4–6 yr
Hepatitis A	HepA	12–24 mo; 2nd dose 6–18 mo later
Meningococcal	—	11–12 yr; 16 yr
Human papillomavirus	HPV	3-dose series, beginning at age 9

*From the American Academy of Pediatrics, 2012 Immunization schedule: http://aapredbook.aappublications.org/site/resources/IZSchedule.pdf.
mo, Month; *q10yr,* every 10 years; *yr,* year.

disease experts, and on-line resources for human vaccination schedules, as well as species experts and other zoo and wildlife veterinarians may offer the veterinarian an overview of recommended vaccination protocols being used. The use of vaccinations in great apes is considered "off-label," and therefore specific brand names cannot be given. The American Academy of Pediatrics recommended immunization schedule is outlined in Table 38-4 and may be used as a reference point from which vaccination protocol discussions may be started.

REPRODUCTION

Sexual behaviors and hormonal parameters in great apes have been studied and documented for all great ape genera.[2,3,7,11,35,43] Reproductive parameters are given in Table 38-5. Assisted reproductive techniques have been tried in apes and have met with variable success. Information on contraception of apes may be found at the AZA Wildlife Contraceptive Center (www.stlzoo.org/contraception). Methods for male contraception include vasectomy, vas ligation (potentially reversible), open-ended vasectomy (potentially reversible), and gonadotropin-releasing hormone (GnRH) agonists. Methods of female contraception include intrauterine devices (IUDs), GnRH agonists, progestin contraceptives such as melengestrol acetate (MGA) implants, medroxyprogesterone acetate injections, and levonorgestrel implants, as well as progestin and combination estrogen–progestin oral birth control pills (noncompliance issues have been linked to failures). Hormonal intervention may result in weight gain as in humans; progestins may exacerbate subclinical diabetes, although further studies in apes are needed to clarify whether this also occurs in great apes.[24,25,37]

TABLE 38-5

Reproductive Parameters in Great Apes

Parameter	Gorillas	Chimpanzees	Bonobos	Orangutans
Puberty, age (years)	6–7.5 female (F) 10–15 male (M)	6–10 (F) 7–13 (M)	6–11 (F) 13 (M)	7–10 (F) 7–9 (5–17) (M)
Youngest age to breed (years)	8–10 (M) 6–9 (F)	5–10 (F) 6–13 (M)	10.1 (8.3–14.9 y) (F) 7y (M)	5–7 (F)
Estrous cycle Length (days)	33 (21–49)	36 (28–53)	31–51	28 (23–33)
Menses (days)	1	2–7	3–4	1–4
Receptivity detection (days)	2 (1–4)	6 (may be receptive throughout cycle)	May be receptive throughout cycle	2(1–4)
Uterus	Simplex	Simplex	Simplex	Simplex
Gestation (days)*	255 (237–285)	227 + 12	233–247	245 ± 12
Pregnancy determination	Commercially available urinary human chorionic gonadotropin (hCG) tests	Commercially available urinary hCG tests	10–20× increase in urinary E1C †(10–30 days postestrogen peak); commercially available urinary hCG tests	Commercially available urinary hCG tests (mixed results)
Placentation	Hemochorial, villous, discoid	Hemochorial, villous, discoid	Hemochorial, villous, discoid	Hemochorial, villous, discoid
Luteal phase (days)	11.2 ± 0.8	15 (13–18)	11–15	13.5
Follicular phase (days)	18.14 ± 1.7	20 (15–25)	17–40	12 (11–15)

*Gestation calculations based on three different methods of calculation: days from last menses; days from last tumescence (if present), days from urinary hormonal changes.
†*E1C,* Urinary estrogen conjugates.

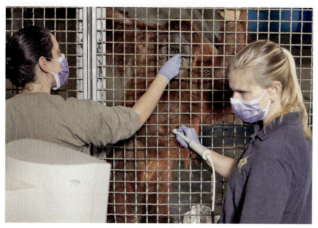

FIGURE 38-6 Gestational ultrasonographic examination on nonanesthetized orangutan. (Photo courtesy Adam K. Thompson-Zoo Atlanta, Atlanta, GA.)

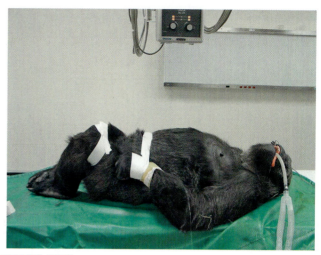

FIGURE 38-7 Positioning a geriatric gorilla for limb support during anesthesia. (Photo courtesy Stephanie Earhart-Zoo Atlanta, Atlanta, GA.)

Reproductive Disorders

Medical problems associated with pregnancy have occurred and may include abortion, placenta previa, endometriosis, pregnancy toxemia, fetal septicemia, retained placenta, dystocia, and congenital defects. Extensive abdominal adhesions are common in great apes and in cases of severe endometriosis and uterine neoplasia, consultation with human oncologic reproductive surgeons may be warranted before attempting surgical removal. Prenatal ultrasonography has been used in nonanesthetized apes to monitor fetal development, and, as in humans, gestational issues may be linked to concurrent health issues such as diabetes, obesity, and hypothyroidism. Figure 38-6 shows gestational ultrasonography performed on a nonanesthetized orangutan for fetal monitoring. Uterine, ovarian, and testicular neoplasia may also affect the great apes, especially older animals.

NEONATAL CARE

Ideally, all healthy ape infants should be left with their natural dam or placed with a comparable ape surrogate for social rearing if maternal rejection or neglect occurs. Newborn apes may not suckle for the first 12 hours, but they should appear bright eyed, strong, and responsive with a strong grip on their mothers. If neonates show signs of weakness, lethargy, diarrhea, or dull eyes, they may deteriorate rapidly. If neonates show signs of illness, they should be assessed quickly, and usually sedation of the dam is necessary to obtain access to the infant. Neonatal physical examinations should include screening for congenital defects, trauma, neonatal disease, malnutrition, or maternal neglect. The timing of these examinations varies widely among institutions, and decisions need to be based on infant's current health, maternal–infant bonding, and risk to the infant if darting the mother is needed to separate the pair. The most common illnesses associated with great ape neonates are hypothermia, hypoglycemia, dehydration, electrolyte imbalance, enterocolitis, respiratory disease, urologic disturbances, and sepsis.[2] Neonates requiring nursery care or treatment are highly susceptible to hypothermia and need to be kept warm, either in incubators or by being held close to the body, until they may maintain their own body temperature. It is recommended that medically stable infants be returned to their dam or surrogate as soon as possible. If this cannot occur, keeping them within auditory, visual, olfactory, and supervised tactile reach of their dam or group is beneficial. Serious, even fatal, respiratory illness may occur in hand-reared infants with prolonged close human contact, so the use of proper PPE (face masks, gloves, etc.) and health of the human caregivers cannot be overemphasized. Most commercially available human infant formulas may be used for feeding great ape neonates. Lactose intolerance and iron sensitivity may occur, so selection of formulas that are soy based and low in iron may be prudent.

GERIATRIC CARE

With the increasing life expectancies seen in captive great apes, challenges in geriatric care and management should be discussed as part of the preventive medicine program. Maintaining a schedule of routine physical examinations and possibly even increasing the frequency of these examinations, balanced with potentially increased anesthetic risks, may be challenging. Common age-related health issues in geriatric apes include renal disease, reproductive disorders, abdominal abscesses, cardiovascular disease, dental issues, vision degeneration, and osteoarthritis.[2,30,32,39,40,50] Specific medical, nutritional, exhibit design, and enrichment protocols may need to be modified for these geriatric challenges. Particular attention should be paid to the prevalence of osteoarthritis when positioning anesthetized geriatric animals, and limb and joint support should be of paramount concern to reduce painful and sometimes long-lasting side effects in recovery. Figure 38-7 shows one method for supporting the limbs of a geriatric, anesthetized gorilla during a procedure.

ANESTHESIA

Thorough physical examinations on great apes require the use of general anesthesia induced via chemical immobilizing agents. No immobilization is completely risk free, so institutional and individual veterinarians must weigh the risk of anesthesia with the benefit of improved diagnostic abilities and thorough physical examinations. A number of commercially available anesthetics may be used alone or in combination to induce and maintain general anesthesia in great apes, and these may be viewed in Table 38-6.[1,44] All apes should be fasted for a minimum of 12 to 24 hours before anesthesia is induced, and water should be withheld for at least 12 hours. If an oral preanesthetic needs to be used, care must be taken to avoid delivering the drug in large volumes of food or liquids, as complications from regurgitation and aspiration may occur during induction. Drug delivery is usually by the intramuscular route, and training the apes for hand injections is preferred. Hand injections of anesthetics via operant conditioning may avoid the stress of darting animals with

TABLE 38-6

Chemical Restraint and Anesthetic Induction Agents Used for Great Apes[21,44]

Generic Name	Orangutan	Chimpanzee	Gorilla	Reversal Agent/ Dose (mg/kg)	Comments
INDUCTION AGENTS					
Ketamine hydrochloride	6–10	5–20	6–10	None	Rapid induction; minimal cardiovascular (CV) and respiratory changes; not reversible; short duration of action
Ketamine/Xylazine	5–7 (K) / 1–1.4 (X)	5–10 (K) / 1 (X)		Yohimbine 0.125–0.25 for X	Rapid induction; CV stable; longer anesthetic times
Ketamine/ Medetomidine	2–7 (K) / 0.03–0.04 (M)	2–5 (K) / 0.02–0.05 (M)	2–5 (K) / 0.02–0.05 (M)	Atipamazole 0.1–0.5 (M)	Spontaneous arousal; potential for CV side effects, reversible
Ketamine/midazolam	1–2 (K) / 0.03 (M)		9 (K) / 0.05 (M)	Flumazenil 0.02–0.1, IV for midazolam only	Shorter duration of effect than telazol; drug volume may be an issue
Tiletamine/Zolazepam (Telazol)	2–6.9	2–6	2–6	Flumazenil 0.02–0.1, IV, for zolazepam only	Smooth inductions; may have prolonged recoveries
Telazol/ Medetomidine	0.8–2.3 (T) / 0.02–0.06 (M)	1.25 (T) / 0.03–0.04 (M)		Atipamazole 0.1–0.25 for medetomidine	Monitor blood pressure and respirations Provide oxygen support
TRANQUILIZERS AND ANALGESICS					
Diazepam	0.5–1.0 PO/IM/IV		0.2, PO	Flumazenil 0.02–0.1, IV	May reduce anxiety; may be used in combination with other drugs for inductions
Midazolam	0.05–0.15 IM/IV/PO			Flumazenil 0.02–0.1, IV	May reduce anxiety; may be used in combination with other drugs for inductions
Butorphenol	0.1–0.2 IM/IV			Naloxone 0.02, IM/IV	May be used in combination with other drugs for inductions
Buprenorphine	0.01–0.02 IM/IV			Naloxone 0.02, IM/IV	May be used in combination with other drugs for inductions May produce respiratory depression
ANESTHETIC MAINTENANCE					
Isoflurane or sevoflurane	0.5–2.5% + or to effect via endotracheal tube	same	same	same	May see dose-dependent hypotension
Propofol	To effect: 25–100 µg/kg/min, IV, OR 50 mg/kg TOTAL DOSE				Monitor blood pressure and respirations May be used for unexpected arousals

IM, Intramuscular; *IV*, Intravenous; *PO*, oral.
All doses given in milligram per kilogram (mg/kg) and given intramuscularly unless stated otherwise.

remote drug delivery systems and will often lead to smoother induction, better planes of anesthesia, lower anesthetic doses, and safer drug deliveries. If this is not an option, remote darting may be used. The use of pole syringes in completely awake apes is not usually successful because of their agility and strength.

Intubation may occur once the ape is sedated enough to have slack jaw tone. Face masks and supplemental gas anesthetic delivery to attain this level of relaxation is sometimes required, and it is important to monitor the animal closely for signs of regurgitation and aspiration during this phase of induction. When using injectable drugs alone, without intubation, supplemental oxygen supplied via a face mask or intranasally via an oxygen line will improve oxygenation. Intubation of great apes may occur in dorsal or lateral recumbency, with the head extended to straighten the airway. A long, curved laryngoscope and an airway exchange catheter may make intubation easier, especially in cases where the animal is regurgitating or when the animal has excessive laryngeal tissue, as is sometimes the case in large male orangutans and gorillas. Laryngeal spasms may occur in apes, so the use of topical local anesthetic sprays may aid intubation.

Great apes have shorter tracheas than would be expected, and it is easy to intubate a main-stem bronchus if care is not taken. Auscultation of all lung fields, using positive pressure ventilation, thoracic radiography, or both, should be performed to confirm tube placement. If pulse oximetry readings are low during gas anesthesia in an intubated animal, withdrawal of the endotracheal tube by a few centimeters may be enough to return the blood oxygen saturation to normal. Cuffed endotracheal tubes should be used; reinforced endotracheal tubes with extended lengths work well in larger animals. Because of the propensity of orangutans to have extensive air sac infections, securing the airway with a cuffed endotracheal tube is essential in these animals when trying to prevent aspiration of infected materials. If the laryngeal air sac contains "fluid" secretions, these animals are at increased risk for aspiration of the fluid via the ostia that connect the air sacs to the trachea, and the anesthesiologist should be prepared to suction, drain the air sac, and maintain upright positioning until intubation.

Maintenance of airways, especially in animals without endotracheal intubation and during the recovery phase of anesthesia, may be difficult, particularly in mature male gorillas and orangutans because of their large size, heavy neck musculature, and the sagittal crest. Hypoventilation may be caused by excessive ventroflexion of the head and subsequent airway occlusion or secondary to large, gas-filled intestines and abdominal pressure on the lungs. Positioning the apes on their sides or propping their upper bodies up at a slight angle, if in dorsal recumbency, with head and neck extended, may help alleviate these issues. During recovery these animals tend to collapse their chins toward their chests which may predispose them to a blocked airway. To avoid this, extubation should occur as far into the recovery period as possible, and the animals should be placed in lateral recumbency with their down arm extended cranially and the head extended.

Hypothermia, hyperthermia, pressure necrosis and potential nerve damage to peripheral limbs, and thermal burns from heating sources are all risks in anesthetized great apes and should be avoided. Recovery on padded or heavily bedded surfaces is preferable. Care should be taken to lubricate the eyes well with sterile lubricating ointments before recovery on bedding to try to avoid corneal abrasions.

SURGERY

Surgical procedures on great apes may occur after trauma (fracture repair, extensive soft tissue injury repair), dental extraction, laparotomy (abscess drainage and removal, hernia repair, reproductive tract surgeries, GI issues, neoplasia), eye, ear, nose, and throat surgeries (cataract removals, otitis interna, sinusitis, etc.), and air sac surgeries.[2,6,20] Orangutans are particularly prone to chronic and

sometimes severe air sac infections, and surgeries such as marsupialization of the air sacs to enhance drainage, tracheal ostea closures, and air sac removal have all been attempted to resolve these issues. Traumatic wounds should be managed using the same principles of wound management that apply to all species. Apes have excellent healing abilities, and except for cases of immediately life-threatening wounds (hemorrhage, vital organ involvement), surgical closure is usually only necessary where serious mechanical damage may occur, serious infection is a risk, and significant defects may result from healing by second or tertiary intention. If skin sutures are used, great apes may pick at them and cause wound dehiscence.

DIAGNOSTICS

Urine Collection

Urine may be collected with the apes under general anesthesia and via cytocentesis or urethral catheterization. Apes may also be taught to urinate on command into specified containers or urine collecting areas.

Cerebrospinal Fluid

Collection of cerebrospinal fluid (CSF) may be necessary to test for encephalopathy and other infectious, inflammatory, or neoplastic processes. The preferred site is the L3-4 lumbar space.

Imaging

Radiography, magnetic resonance imaging (MRI), and computed tomography (CT) have all been performed successfully on great apes. Body size may be a limiting factor, especially with MRI and CT machines. CT has been used in orangutans to assess the extent of respiratory disease and sinus or air sac involvement and infection.[45] Ultrasonography may be used on both anesthetized apes and nonanesthetized apes through the use of operant conditioning. Figure 38-8 shows a nonanesthetized gorilla positioned for echocardiography. Pregnancy monitoring, fetal development, and echosonography have all been performed successfully and may be very useful monitoring aids in situations where anesthesia poses a high risk to the animal.

Blood Collection

Blood may be collected from numerous superficial venous access points, including the femoral vein, the brachial vein, and the

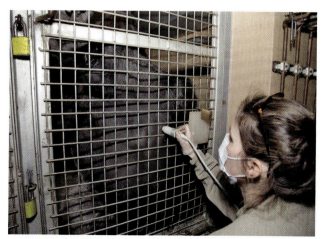

FIGURE 38-8 Position of ultrasound probe for echocardiography on a nonanesthetized gorilla. (Photo courtesy Jodi Carrigan-Zoo Atlanta, Atlanta, GA.)

posterior tibial vein. Arterial samples may be taken from the femoral artery, the dorsal pedal artery, or the radial artery on the medial side of the carpus. If the femoral artery is used, pressure must be applied to that site for at least 10 minutes to prevent hematoma and hemorrhage. Some apes may be trained for voluntary blood draw done through a protective sleeve device.

Hematology

Reference ranges for hematologic parameters of great apes may be found in Tables 38-7 and 38-8.

Therapeutics

Human formularies, in addition to standard veterinary references, may be used for many medication recommendations because of the similarities between great apes and humans.

DISEASES

Infectious Diseases

Viral Diseases

A review of some more frequently isolated viral pathogens associated with great ape respiratory diseases is provided in Table 38-9. Viral respiratory illnesses may cause mild to severe illness, with some resulting in mortalities. Secondary complications from bacterial infections such as *Streptococcus* pneumonia and *Pasteurella multocida* may occur and complicate recovery.[17] Individuals particularly at risk are infants and juvenile animals and geriatric or immunocompromised individuals. Respiratory illnesses have been identified as particularly problematic in captive orangutans, sometimes persisting for years without any visible clinical signs.[20,52] Outbreaks of viral respiratory illnesses in association with human contact have been documented in both captive and wild populations of great apes and may cause significant conservation and zoonotic disease concerns.[15,17,21,34,41,46,48,49,51] Apes with preexisting cardiovascular compromise may also be at increased risk of morbidity and mortality from respiratory tract illnesses and should be monitored closely and given supportive care if affected during outbreaks. Diagnostics for respiratory illness in great apes may be challenging and causative agents are hard to identify. The high frequency of respiratory infections in orangutans makes diagnostic imaging of the sinuses, upper airways, air sacs, and lungs important. Viral isolation and rising paired serum titers may be used to try to isolate viral etiologies, but it is often hard to isolate the cause of the initial illness. Because carriers of human respiratory pathogens are often asymptomatic, wearing of masks (e.g., N95 masks are recommended) should be mandatory for humans in close contact with great apes.

Viral hemorrhagic diseases caused by organisms such as Ebola virus strains should be mentioned because of the toll they have taken on wild populations of African apes. Ebola virus strains have been responsible for catastrophic deaths in wild populations of gorillas and chimpanzees and have happened in close association with human outbreaks.[17,36,41,51]

Research into retroviral infections in apes, their potential to impact ape health and captive ape management, as well as their zoonoses implications, have garnered increasing attention in recent years. Great apes may be naturally infected with a variety of retroviruses, including simian immunodeficiency virus (SIV), simian T-lymphotropic virus (STLV), and simian foamy virus (SFV). Although these viruses have evolved over many generations in the great apes, they have been documented to cause clinical disease in some apes.[27,41] In contrast, simian foamy virus, a retrovirus that is highly prevalent in most nonhuman primates, has not been associated with clinical disease in naturally infected primates. Although it has been shown that human retrovirus infections with human T-lymphotropic virus and human immunodeficiency virus (HIV) originated through multiple independent introductions of simian retroviruses into human populations that then spread globally, little is known about the frequency of such zoonotic events. Recommendations for the prevention of human exposures to simian retroviruses include the use of "universal precautions" and personal protective equipment (e.g., gloves, gowns, face shields or masks, and barrier clothing) when handling primates and primate bodily fluids; aerosol control; proper decontamination techniques; personnel training; and institution-specific medical surveillance programs. Testing to detect these viruses should be done through initial serial serologic screening of all animals for antibodies, which should be followed by additional testing 1 year later to help identify recently exposed animals that may have seroconverted. Serologic testing alone may be sufficient for detection of SIV, STLV, and SFV infection in adult apes. Once an individual nonhuman primate (NHP) has been confirmed to be positive for any retrovirus, it should be considered infected for life, and retesting for that virus is not necessary.

Unique, species-specific hepatitis A and hepatitis B viruses have been documented in chimpanzees, gorillas, and orangutans and may cause clinical disease.[21,22,29] Human herpes virus 1 has also been reported to cause clinical, usually mild, disease in great apes. Many other viruses may be present and may be asymptomatic or cause clinical diseases in apes and include pox viruses, cytomegalovirus, Epstein-Barr virus, and lymphocryptovirus among others.[21]

Bacterial Diseases

Bacterial diseases that have been identified as causing significant morbidity and mortality in great apes may be found in Table 38-10. Therapeutic dosages of antibiotics may generally be inferred from the literature on human dosing. TB cases are rare in great apes because of stringent testing and quarantine procedures put into place in the 1970s and 1980s.[21] TB in great apes is a slowly progressive disease with subclinical signs until the disease is in advanced stages. It is transmitted primarily through aerosolized, infected droplets from diseased individuals, but contaminated food, cages, needles, and bite wounds are all additional modes of potential transmission. Great apes are susceptible to *Mycobacterium bovis*, *M. tuberculosis*, and *M. avium*, but individuals may have reactions after prior exposure to atypical mycobacteria also.[21] Testing for mycobacteriosis is important and may be somewhat problematic, especially in orangutans that may have false-positive reactions to the mammalian old tuberculin (MOT) commonly used for TB testing in primates. No one test is adequate to confirm or rule out TB, and therefore a combination of tests should be performed. Testing may include thorough physical examination, thoracic radiography, CBC, intradermal testing (tuberculin skin test using 0.1 milliliter [mL] of mammalian tuberculin, human isolates, Colorado Serum Co., Synbiotics Corp.), culture of lavaged fluids (gastric, tracheal, or bronchoalveolar), and additional diagnostics. Additional diagnostics include serologic tests, a lateral flow enzyme-linked immunosorbent assay (ELISA) for TB antibodies that may be performed on serum (PrimaTB STATPAK), polymerase chain reaction (PCR)-amplified deoxyribonucleic acid (DNA) probes, and γ-interferon (Primagam) tests and may be valuable to detect subclinical infections. γ-interferon immunoassay is probably a useful screening test in orangutans and is more reliable than multiple antigen ELISA or antigen 85 immunoassay in this species.[2]

Great apes may also suffer from chronic, subclinical, or clinical laryngeal airsacculitis, which may result in significant morbidity and mortality, especially in orangutans.[2,12,20,21,50,52] This disease is characterized by recurrent infections of the upper and lower respiratory tract, including the sinuses, the laryngeal (submandibular) air sac, and the lungs. Bronchoalveolar lavage (BAL), with cytology and aerobic culture, typically reveals neutrophilic inflammation associated with numerous bacteria, including *Pseudomonas aeruginosa*, miscellaneous gram-negative enteric rods (e.g., *Klebsiella* spp.), and gram-positive cocci (e.g., *Staphylococcus* spp., β-hemolytic *Streptococcus* spp.).[2,20] Clinical signs include acute forms, which may

Text continued on p. 351

TABLE 38-7

Reference Intervals for Great Apes

Parameter	Gorilla	Orangutan	Chimpanzee	Bonobo
Erythrocytes × 10⁶cells/μL				
M	4.61	4.79	5.41	5.52
Mdn	*4.59 (3.52–5.87)*	*4.77 (3.72–5.93)*	*5.37 (4.18–6.78)*	*5.51 (3.95–6.76)*
PCV (%)				
M	38.9	38.2	43.5	41.8
Mdn	*38.6 (30.0–49.6)*	*38.0 (29.4–48.3)*	*43.2 (32.2–54.6)*	*41.4 (31.8–52.2)*
Hemoglobin (g/dL)				
M	12.4	11.8	14.0	13.4
Mdn	*12.3 (9.5–15.5)*	*11.8 (9.0–14.7)*	*13.9 (10.3–17.4)*	*13.3 (10.1–17.0)*
MCV (fL)				
M	83.5	79.2	79.6	74.5
Mdn	*83.3 (70.5–96.3)*	*79.5 (65.0–91.3)*	*79.9 (64.8–93.1)*	*74.5 (62.5–87.4)*
MCH (pg)				
M	26.9	24.8	26.0	24.4
Mdn	*27.0 (22.8–30.8)*	*24.8 (20.7–29.0)*	*26.0 (21.4–30.1)*	*24.4 (20.7–30.5)*
MCHC (g/dL)				
M	32.3	31.3	32.5	32.5
Mdn	*32.4 (28.2–35.6)*	*31.3 (27.4–35.3)*	*32.7 (27.9–35.6)*	*32.6 (30.1–34.9)*
Leukocytes × 10³/μL				
M	7.86	9.70	10.43	11.61
Mdn	*7.15 (3.44–16.49)*	*8.90 (4.28–19.52)*	*9.72 (4.24–20.78)*	*10.45 (3.26–27.33)*
Neutrophils × 10³/μL				
M	5.03	5.26	6.77	7.95
Mdn	*4.45 (1.13–12.37)*	*4.46 (1.31–13.17)*	*5.99 (1.15–16.48)*	*6.72 (1.20–21.60)*
Band Neutrophils × 10³/μL				
M	0.04	0.05	0.05	0.06
Mdn	*0.03 (0.01–0.12)*	*0.04 (0.02–0.13)*	*0.05 (0.02–0.12)*	*0.05 (0.01–0.21)*
Lymphocytes × 10³/μL				
M	2.07	3.61	2.90	2.51
Mdn	*1.83 (0.59–4.84)*	*3.22 (1.18–8.40)*	*2.52 (0.76–7.27)*	*2.11 (0.45–7.08)*
Eosinophils cells/μL				
M	191	289	224	259
Mdn	*153 (38–571)*	*223 (48–931)*	*179 (56–671)*	*200 (50–790)*
Monocytes cells/μL				\
M	401	367	341	518
Mdn	*354 (60–1048)*	*302 (64–1083)*	*284 (62–944)*	*428 (84–1618)*
Basophils cells/μL				
M	75	85	93	126
Mdn	*65 (12–191)*	*80 (0–179)*	*85 (10–232)*	*106**
Platelets × 10³/μL				
M	190	205	233	287
Mdn	*189 (2–389)*	*203 (2–371)*	*222 (89–430)*	*263 (132–567)*
Reticulocytes (%)				
M	0.2	*	0.2	*
Mdn	*0.1 (0.0–0.8)*	* (*)	*0.1 (0.0–0.8)*	*
Nucleated RBC/100 WBC				
M	0	1	3	*
Mdn	*0 (0–1)*	*0 (0–3)*	*0 (*)*	*
Body Temp (C)				
M	37.27	36.72	36.94	36.94
Mdn	*37.27 (35.66–38.66)*	*36.77 (34.55–38.66)*	*37.05 (34.66–38.61)*	*37.05 (35.38–38.66)*

All values are given as M = mean; *Mdn = Median*; () = reference interval; *, no value available; (*), no reference value available.

fL, Femtoliter; *MCH*, mean corpuscular hemoglobin; *MCHC*, mean corpuscular hemoglobin concentration; *MCV*, mean corpuscular volume; mg/dL, milligram per deciliter; *μL*, microliter; *PCV*, packed cell volume; *pg*, picogram; *RBC*, red blood cell; *WBC*, white blood cell.

From Teare JA, ed: 2013, Western Gorilla *(gorilla gorilla)*, Orangutan *(pongo pygmaeus)*, Chimpanzee *(Pan troglodytes)*, Bonobo *(Pan paniscus)*—No selection by gender. All ages combined. Standard International Units 2013 CD.html in ISIS Physiological Reference Intervals for Captive Wildlife: A CD-ROM Resource, International Species Information System, Bloomington, MN.

TABLE 38-8

Reference Intervals for Great Apes

Parameter	Gorilla	Orangutan	Chimpanzee	Bonobo
Total Protein (g/dL)				
M	7.2	7.2	7.2	7.2
Mdn	*7.2* (5.7–8.7)	*7.2* (506–8.6)	*7.2* (5.8–8.7)	*7.2* (5.6–8.4)
Albumin (g/dL)				
M	3.8	4.1	3.6	3.6
Mdn	*3.8* (2.8–4.8)	*4.1* (2.9–5.2)	*3.6* (2.5–4.5)	*6.3* (2.3–4.5)
Globulin (g/dL)				
M	3.4	3.0	3.6	3.3
Mdn	*3.4* (1.3–4.9)	*3.0* (1.6–4.3)	*3.6* (2.3–5.1)	*3.5* (0.9–4.7)
Calcium (mg/dL)				
M	9.4	9.5	9.2	9.0
Mdn	*9.4* (8.3–10.6)	*9.5* (8.0–11.0)	*9.2* (7.9–10.7)	*9.0* (8.1–10.2)
Magnesium (mg/dL)				
M	1.70	1.69	1.82	*
Mdn	*1.68* (1.10–2.53)	*1.69* (0.71–2.46)	*1.81* (1.17–2.41)	*
Phosphorus (mg/dL)				
M	4.2	4.1	4.0	3.5
Mdn	*4.1* (2.5–6.1)	*4.1* (2.0–6.6)	*3.8* (1.7–7.2)	*3.4* (1.4–6.5)
Ca/Phos ratio				
M	2.4	2.4	2.6	2.7
Mdn	*2.3* (1.5–3.6)	*2.3* (1.4–4.3)	*2.4* (1.2–5.0)	*2.6* (1.4–5.0)
Sodium (mEq/L)				
M	137	140	141	140
Mdn	*137* (130–145)	*140* (133–148)	*141* (133–151)	*140* (134–147)
Potassium (mEq/L)				
M	4.3	4.1	3.9	3.6
Mdn	*4.3* (3.3–5.7)	*4.1* (3.2–5.7)	*3.9* (2.8–5.3)	*3.6* (2.7–4.8)
Na/K Ratio				
M	32.0	34.4	36.3	39.2
Mdn	*32.0* (23.2–41.3)	*34.5* (22.9–44.7)	*36.0* (25.3–50.1)	*38.5* (28.1–52.9)
Chloride (mEq/L)				
M	101	102	103	102
Mdn	*101* (94–108)	*102* (94–110)	*103* (94–111)	*102* (94–109)
Creatinine (mg/dL)				
M	1.1	1.0	1.0	0.8
Mdn	*1.1* (0.5–1.9)	*0.9* (0.4–1.9)	*1.0* (0.5–1.5)	*0.8* (0.3–1.5)
Urea nitrogen (mg/dL)				
M	10	12	10	9
Mdn	*10* (4–19)	*11* (4–24)	*10* (3–18)	*9* (3–17)
BUN/Cr ratio				
M	10.4	13.1	10.8	12.5
Mdn	*9.4* (3.6–23.3)	*11.5* (4.4–30.3)	*10.0* (3.3–23.1)	*11.4* (3.4–28.9)
Uric acid (mg/dL)				
M	1.2	1.7	2.6	2.3
Mdn	*1.2* (0.2–2.5)	*1.6* (0.3–3.5)	*2.5* (0.9–4.7)	*2.3* (0.9–3.6)
Total bilirubin (mg/dL)				
M	0.5	0.5	0.3	0.3
Mdn	*0.5* (0.2–1.2)	*0.5* (0.2–1.3)	*0.2* (0.1–0.7)	*0.3* (0.1–0.6)
Direct bilirubin (mg/dL)				
M	0.1	0.2	0.1	0.0
Mdn	*0.1* (0.0–0.4)	*0.1* (0.0–0.6)	*0.1* (0.0–0.3)	*0.0* (*)
Indirect bilirubin (mg/dL)				
M	0.3	0.4	0.2	0.3
Mdn	*0.3* (0.1–0.8)	*0.3* (0.1–1.1)	*0.1* (0.0–0.5)	*0.3* (*)
Cholesterol (mg/dL)				
M	256	185	195	224
Mdn	*246* (140–455)	*183* (94–297)	*190* (107–307)	*220* (153–348)
Triglycerides (mg/dL)				
M	116	103	99	80
Mdn	*100* (43–288)	*87* (30–268)	*90* (33–221)	*73* (34–186)

TABLE 38-8

Reference Intervals for Great Apes—cont'd

Parameter	Gorilla	Orangutan	Chimpanzee	Bonobo
Low-density lipoprotein (mg/dL)				
M	106	96	105	106
Mdn	106 (1–249)	101 (6–196)	103 (31–176)	105 (40–170)
High density lipoprotein (mg/dL)				
M	91	54	56	94
Mdn	89 (31–192)	52 (2–103)	52 (3–101)	94 (50–138)
Glucose (mg/dL)				
M	79	95	88	78
Mdn	76 (44–129)	92 (35–166)	84 (44–156)	75 (46–126)
Bicarbonate (mEq/L)				
M	26.5	25.4	27.2	*
Mdn	26.3 (17.3–34.4)	25.1 (16.5–35.8)	27.2 (17.0–36.3)	*
Carbon dioxide (mEq/L)				
M	25.6	25.1	26.1	29.1
Mdn	25.0 (16.4–40.8)	25.0 (15.3–37.8)	25.7 (14.6–37.8)	28.9 (20.3–37.6)
Iron (µg/dL)				
M	92	121	90	113
Mdn	90 (37–177)	121 (28–221)	88 (23–152)	108 (*)
LDH (IU/L)				
M	586	352	485	316
Mdn	434 (210–1644)	256 (129–933)	356 (162–1318)	292 (45–539)
Alk phos (IU/L)				
M	389	234	128	151
Mdn	258 (103–1147)	152 (55–709)	95 (39–443)	93 (51–489)
GGT (IU/L)				
M	25	13	28	10
Mdn	20 (4–76)	11 (3–30)	26 (10–58)	10 (4–21)
CK (IU/L)				
M	269	145	232	157
Mdn	212 (59–791)	120 (32–379)	179 (56–689)	130 (0–340)
AST (IU/L)				
M	31	14	23	20
Mdn	27 (11–75)	12 (4–33)	21 (9–52)	19 (8–38)
ALT (IU/L)				
M	31	20	31	31
Mdn	27 (7–72)	18 (5–47)	28 (11–62)	28 (12–60)
Amylase (IU/L)				
M	28	79	38	17
Mdn	25 (6–68)	70 (27–186)	33 (9–93)	17 (1–32)
Lipase (IU/L)				
M	13	24	32	17
Mdn	6 (0–58)	26 (3–63)	30 (1–70)	16 (0–36)
Thyroxine (µg/dL)				
M	6.3	4.2	8.1	7.7
Mdn	5.8 (3.2–12.4)	3.7 (0.2–10.1)	8.0 (2.9–13.1)	7.2 (1.0–13.4)
Triiodothyronine uptake (%)				
M	39	35	*	*
Mdn	40 (28–53)	38 (10–66)	*	*
Free thyroxine (ng/dL)				
M	1.8	1.9	*	1.6
Mdn	1.7 (0.3–3.0)	1.2 (0.0–4.6)	*	1.5 (0.4–2.6)

All values are given as M = mean; *Mdn = Median*; (reference interval).

g/dL, Gram per deciliter; *IU/L*, international unit per liter; *mEq/L*, milliequivalent per liter; *mg/dL*, milligram per deciliter; *µg/dL*, microgram per deciliter; *mmol/L*, millimole per liter; *mOsmol/L*, milliosmole per liter; *ng/dL*, nanogram per deciliter; *Unit/L*, unit per liter; *, no value available; (*), no reference value available.

From Teare JA, ed: 2013, Western Gorilla *(gorilla gorilla)*, Orangutan *(pongo pygmaeus)*, Chimpanzee *(Pan troglodytes)*, Bonobo *(Pan paniscus)*—No selection by gender. All ages combined. Standard International Units 2013 CD.html in ISIS Physiological Reference Intervals for Captive Wildlife: A CD-ROM Resource, International Species Information System, Bloomington, MN.

TABLE 38-9

Selected Viral Diseases in Great Apes

Disease	Etiology	Epizootiology	Signs	Diagnosis	Management
Adenovirus	Adenovirus / Adenoviridae	Sporadic to epidemic outbreaks Aerosol and fecal-oral route	Cough, tachypnea, dyspnea +/- cyanosis Keratoconjunctivitis +/- Gastrointestinal (GI): diarrhea/hepatitis Asymptomatic infections may occur	Serology; viral isolation	Supportive care, isolation
Influenza	Influenza virus (orthomyxovirus)	Epidemic outbreaks, aerosol transmission	Fever, oculonasal discharge GI: anorexia, lethargy	Viral isolation, seroconversion on hemagglutination-inhibition test	Supportive care +/- Vaccination with human vaccine
Metapneumovirus	Human metapneumovirus	Outbreaks, aerosol transmission	Mild to severe respiratory signs, depression	Viral isolation, PCR	Supportive care
Parainfluenza	Parainfluenza III (paramyxovirus)	Outbreaks via aerosol or direct contact	Upper +/- lower respiratory disease: coughing, sneezing, dyspnea, tachypnea	Virus isolation, paired serum titers	Supportive care
Respiratory syncytial virus	Pneumovirus	Outbreaks may occur, aerosol transmission	Upper respiratory: sneezing, coughing, ocular discharge	Viral isolation, paired serum titers	Supportive care
Varicella virus	Chimpanzee varicella virus; gorilla varicella virus; orangutan varicella virus (alpha herpes virus)	Contact +/- respiratory transmission	Dermatitis: vesicles, usually self-limiting	Virus isolation	Isolation +/- vaccination with human varicella-zoster vaccine
Polio	Poliovirus (enterovirus)	Fecal-oral Outbreaks in wild populations associated with humans	Disseminated spinal cord involvement: paresis, paraplegia, death May also be asymptomatic	Clinical signs	Vaccination
Rabies	Rabies virus	All ages, contact with saliva of infectious animal through bites or dermal compromise	Progressive neurologic disorder, fatal	Clinical signs, immunohistochemistry stains	Vaccination
West Nile virus	West Nile Virus	Mosquito-born	None to encephalitis	Serology, virus isolation, rising titers	Supportive care

		Transmission	Clinical signs	Diagnosis	Treatment/Control
Simian immunodeficiency virus	Retrovirus	Bloodborne, +/– found in feces Vertical and horizontal transmission	None to immune suppression and secondary infections or disorders	Combination of serologic or molecular assays, PCR, Western blot	Supportive care, +/– treat secondary infections and immune stimulation
Simian foamy virus	Spumavirus	Horizontal transmission (biting, sexual contact, blood exposure) through blood and saliva Virus has been found in feces Vertical transmission	No direct association between infection and disease has been proven.	Western blot, serology (ELISA, IFA, RIPA), PCR	None indicated
Simian T-lymphotropic virus (STLV)	Complex retroviruses: three major groups— types 1, 2, 3	Transmission via sexual routes, prevalence increases with age Vertical transmission may occur, possibly via infected cells in milk	STLV-1: persistent lymphocytosis and abnormal T cells, T-cell lymphomas and leukemia, lymphadenopathy, wasting. STLV-2 and STLV-3 have not been documented as being pathogenic in NHPs	Serologic assays (ELISA or particlea agglutination) Western blot	Supportive care, +/– treatment for secondary infections, and immune stimulation
Papilloma virus	Papilloma virus	Young animals through dermal compromise Fomites, direct contact, sexually transmitted	Mucous membranes of the oral cavity and the lower genital tract Dermal or mucosal masses	Biopsy	Usually self-limiting
Measles	Rubeola or morbilivirus	Sporadic outbreaks, epidemics Aerosol transmission	Maculopapular exanthema	Viral isolation, seroconversion, clinical signs	Isolation, vaccination
Filovirus	Marburg virus and Ebola virus Four species of Ebola virus (Ivory Coast, Sudan, Zaire, and Reston)	Sporadic outbreaks, high morbidity and mortality Close contact with infected body fluids, mucous-membrane exposure, +/– aerosols	Severe hemorrhagic fever	Viral isolation, ELISA, PCR	None, usually rapidly fatal and highly zoonotic Barrier isolation
Encephalomyocarditis virus (EMCV)	Picornavirus	Fecal–oral or carried by rodents	Myocarditis, sudden death	Rising serological titers, immunohistochemistry, virus isolation, histopathology	Supportive care, heart failure treatments, rodent control, and good hygiene +/– vaccination

ELISA, Enzyme-linked immunosorbent assay; *IFA*, indirect fluorescent antibody; *PCR*, polymerase chain reaction; *RIPA*, ristocetin-induced platelet aggregation.

TABLE 38-10

Select Bacterial Diseases of Great Apes

Disease	Etiology	Epizootiology	Signs	Diagnosis	Management
Bacterial meningitis	*Streptococcus pneumoniae*	Aerosol	Respiratory signs, head holding, vestibular signs, seizures, dysphagia, blindness, death	Culture, marked leukocytosis, neutrophilia with left sh ft, cerebrospinal fluid (CSF); increased white blood cell (WBC) or protein	Antibiotics, prophylactic antibiotics to exposed animals
Campylobacteriosis	*Campylobacter* sp.	Fecal–oral	Asymptomatic to severe gastrointestinal (GI) signs, usually worse in infants	Culture	Antibiotics and supportive care
Colibacilosis	*E. coli* serotypes: 0119:B14, 055:B5, 026:B6.	Fecal–oral	Lethargy, diarrhea, dehydration Systemic illness; can be rapidly fatal	Culture	Antibiotics, supportive care
Salmonellosis	*Salmonella* sp.	Fecal–oral, more prevalent in young animals	Asymptomatic to severe GI diarrhea, dehydration, anorexia	Culture, leukocytosis with left shift	Antibiotics, supportive care
Shigellosis	*Shigella* sp., *S. flexneri*	Fecal–oral	Asymptomatic to severe GI diarrhea, dehydration, anorexia, arthritis after infection	Fecal culture, degenerative left shift	Antibiotics, supportive care
Yersiniosis	*Yersinia peudotuberculosis, Y. enterocolitica*	Contaminated food or water Direct contact	Death, weakness, depression, watery or hemorrhagic diarrhea, increased abortion and stillbirth rates	Culture, PCR, Pulse-field gel electrophoresis Serotyping by tube agglutination	Rodent control, good hygiene, +/– vaccination
Meloidosis	*Pseudomonas pseudomallei*	Saprophytic, bites or dermal wounds Inhalation and ingestion also possible Long incubation period of months to years possible	Lung, liver, and bone commonly affected but may affect any organ system; so variable signs	Culture	Usually unsuccessful because of resistance
Tuberculosis	*Mycobacterium tuberculosis; M. bovis,* atypical mycobacteriosis	Respiratory route +/– ingestion	Nonspecific and general until advanced disease present. +/– chronic cough and weight loss	Intradermal screening test; culture of gastric, bronchial lavages, enzyme-linked immunosorbent assay (ELISA)	Isolation and treatment Testing keepers and animals regularly

include lethargy, anorexia, moist cough, laryngeal air sac swelling, and pyrexia, and chronic airsacculitis with intermittent nasal discharge, rhinitis, halitosis, and cough. Consultation with a pulmonologist, infectious disease specialist, or both for treatment of affected animals is advantageous. Treatment consists of supportive care, antibiotics, surgical closure of the ostia to prevent future aspiration of air sac contents, air sac removal in extreme cases, or all of these. Air sacs may also be marsupialized to allow drainage of air sac exudate. Topical antibiotic administration via nebulization is recommended in acute cases.

Mycotic Diseases

Mycotic diseases that have been implicated as causing morbidity and mortality in great apes are given in Table 38-11.

Parasitic Diseases

Parasitic diseases may cause significant morbidity and mortality in great apes and are provided in Table 38-12. Management of parasitic disease in captive collections may be performed by a schedule of routine fecal examinations, combined with effective treatment regimes using antiparasitic drugs and environmental management to reduce parasite exposure. Complete fecal evaluations should consist of techniques to maximize results such as fecal flotation, centrifugation and sedimentation, and direct fecal smears. Fecal monitoring should be performed at least twice yearly. Daily cleaning and disinfection protocols, scheduled substrate maintenance, and rotations, as well as vector control, all contribute to the management of parasitism in apes. Ape parasites and the effective therapeutics for parasitic infections may be found in both human and veterinary literature. Collections that house juvenile great apes should pay particular attention to *Strongyloides* spp., *Ancyclostoma duodenale*, and *Necator americanus*, which have all been implicated as a cause of mortality in juvenile orangutans and gorillas.[2,33,38] Elimination of these enteric

infections in adults will help prevent disease in younger animals, and regular repetitive fecal examinations and anthelmintic treatments are recommended especially for pregnant, lactating, and infant animals. The Baermann technique is found to be the most sensitive diagnostic for detecting *Strongyloides* spp. in fecal samples and is recommended as a routine screening diagnostic. Prophylactic antiparasitic treatments targeting *Strongyloides* spp. should be strongly considered, particularly in breeding groups. The most common prophylactic treatment regimen reported is monthly ivermectin. However, other drugs and other dosing intervals have been used for this purpose, and the relative efficacies of the various strategies have not been investigated. Using a rotation of different classes of antiparasitic drugs may be considered in cases where parasite drug resistance is suspected or is a concern.

Although coccidia and oxyurids have been reported in great apes, their clinical significance is not fully known.[2] *Balantidium coli* and *Entamoeba* sp. may be enzootic in some collections, and many animals will be asymptomatic carriers, with no clinical issues until stressors occur (infants, new animals). The most common clinical disease seen will be a diarrheal syndrome (mucosal inflammation or irritation with frequent, mucous, semi-liquid stools) or dysentery (erosive mucositis with rectal urgency, blood, and mucus). Invasive enterocolitis may occur and may lead to ulceration, abscess formation, and perforation.

Cardiovascular Disease

Cardiovascular disease (CVD) is a significant cause of mortality in all four great ape species, but the causes are not clear. Systematic reviews of necropsy reports from zoo gorillas, orangutans, chimpanzees, and bonobos and of wild mountain gorillas have reported a pattern of significant myocardial fibrosis in gorillas, orangutans, chimpanzees, and bonobos.[8] The most common pathology associated with captive ape CVD is structural remodeling, and myocardial fibrosis in the absence of coronary artery disease and

TABLE 38-11

Selected Mycotic Diseases of Great Apes

Disease	Etiology	Epizootiology	Signs	Diagnosis	Management
Candidiasis	*Candida albicans*	Normal saprophyte of mucous membranes and gastrointestinal (GI) and genital tracts Infections secondary to antibiotic therapy and immunosuppression	Dysphagia, excessive salivation, diarrhea	Cytology, culture	Nystatin treatment May treat prophylactically if suspect susceptibility (infants being nursery reared)
Coccidiomycosis	*Coccidiodes immitis*	Saprophytic. Infection via inhalation Lesions most common in bone and lung, but may be disseminated	Initial respiratory, then systemic disease	Radiography, serology, complement fixation test, tube precipitation test Histopathology, culture	Antifungals, largely unsuccessful
Dermatophytosis	*Microsporum canis, Trichophyton rubrum*	Direct contact or fomites contact	Circular lesions, generalize hair loss, scaly, patchy hair loss	Clinical signs, microscopic examination of hair, culture	Systemic or topical antifungal
Pneumocystosis	*Pneumocystis carinii*	Seen in stress or immunocompromise	Respiratory signs, anorexia, pneumonia	Histology	None
Sporotrichosis	*Sporothrix schnekii*	Saprophyte Dermal compromise	Skin nodules, lymph node enlargement	Cytology, culture	None

TABLE 38-12

Selected Parasitic Diseases of Great Apes

Parasite	Location in Host	Clinical Signs	Diagnosis	Treatment
Entamoeba histolytica	Colon and cecum; may go to liver, lung, central nervous system (CNS)	Vomiting, bloody diarrhea, lethargy, dehydration, anorexia	Fecal trophozoites or cysts; examine feces at body temperature Add dilute eosin or Lugol solution to visualize protozoa	Metronidazole, chloroquin, tetracycline, doxycycline, diiodohydroxyquine
Balamutharis mandrillaris	Brain, lung, liver, kidney, mammary gland	Paresis, lethargy	Isolation of organism	No known effective treatment
Balantidium coli	Cecum, colon	May be asymptomatic Ulcerative colitis: watery diarrhea, weight loss, anorexia	Fecal trophozoites or cysts on fresh direct smears or sedimentation	Metronidazole, paramomycin, diiodohydroxyquine, tetracyclines May form cysts that are resistant to temperature extremes and disinfection
Cyclospora spp.	Intestines	Diarrhea	Oocytes in feces	Trimethoprim-sulfamethoxazole
Giardia spp. (*intestinalis, lamblia*)	Small Intestine	Prolonged watery diarrhea, vomiting, dehydration	Iodine-stained wet mount or trichome-stained smear: trophozoites or cysts in feces Biopsy Enzyme-linked immunosorbent assay (ELISA): fecal antigen detection	Metronidazole, furazolidone
Plasmodium sp.	Erythrocytes	None to anemia, collapse, weakness	Blood smear, +/– ELISA	Chloroquin, primaquin
Ancylostoma duodenale	Small intestine	Anemia, dyspnea, debilitation, ascites	Fecal ova, necropsy, larval examination from cultured eggs	Benzimidazole, ivermectin, pyrantel pamoate, levamizole
Ascaris lumbricoides	Intestines	Diarrhea, respiratory signs from larval migrans	Fecal ova	Mebendazole, piperazine
Enterobius vermicularis	Large intestines	Anal irritation and pruritus	Fecal ova, visualization of adults around anal opening, tape impression smears	Hygiene, benzimidazole, ivermectin, pyrantel pamoate, levamizole
Nector americanus	Small intestines	None to potentially severe anemia	Eggs difficult to distinguish from other strongyles	Benzimidazoles, ivermectin, pyrantel pamoate, levamizole, thiabendazole
Strongyloides fulleborni, Strongyloides stercoralis	Intestines, larval migrans: lungs and other organs	Diarrhea, obstipation, urticaria, emaciation, peritonitis, and death	Fecal identification of larvae, Baerman techniques, necropsy identification of adults	Benzimidazoles, ivermectin, pyrantel pamoate, levamizole, thiabendazole
Hymenolepsis nana	Small intestines	Diarrhea, abdominal pain	Fecal ova or proglottids in feces	Praziquantel
Echinococcus sp.	Larvae in abdominal viscera (especially liver), lung, peritoneal cavity, eye	Abdominal distension with fluid wave, exophthalmia, swelling	Ultrasonography (cysts within a cyst), aspiration, surgery	Prevent access to canid feces, surgical removal
Pneumonyssus sp.	Trachea, bronchi, lungs	Coughing, sneezing	Bronchial wash: eggs and larvae seen; fecal examination, necropsy	Ivermectin
Oesophagostomum sp.	Colonic wall, mesentery	Weight loss, debilitation	Fecal oocyte identification	Hygiene, benzimidazole, ivermectin, pyrantel pamoate, levamizole
Sarcoptes scabiei	Skin	Pruritus, alopecia, anorexia	Oocyte, mite in deep skin scrapings	Hygiene, ivermectin
Trichuris trichura	Cecum, colon	Diarrhea, anorexia	Fecal oocyte identification	Hygiene, benzimidazole, ivermectin, pyrantel pamoate, levamizole

cardiomyopathy (including left ventricular hypertrophy and dilated cardiomyopathy), aortic dissections, valvular disease, and electrocardiographic abnormalities have all been observed.[14,19,23,26,42,47] Cardiovascular disease occurs predominately, but not exclusively, in males in the middle to older age groups. Clinical signs of CVD, when present, are rare in apes but have been reported to be lethargy, social withdrawal, peripheral edema, ascites, unilateral paresis, arrhythmias, anorexia, and reluctance to lie down. Sudden cardiac death is often the only sign seen.

A complete cardiac evaluation under anesthesia should include electrocardiography, echosonography, blood pressure measurements, thoracic radiography, blood work (lipid panels, cardiac biomarkers), and retinal examinations.[9,10] α-2 agonists have gained popularity as great ape induction agents because of their reversibility and lowered dose of concomitant drugs needed. The disadvantages include potentials for spontaneous arousals and the cardiovascular effects of α-2 agonists such as peripheral vasoconstriction, increased vascular resistance and bradycardia. Accurate cardiovascular assessment may be challenging when α-2 agonists are used and not reversed prior to the assessment, and caution should be used in individuals with unknown cardiac status. Once an animal has been diagnosed with cardiac disease, α-2 agonists should be avoided.

Institutions may consider training their apes via operant conditioning to participate in nonanesthetized cardiac evaluations by echosonography. Apes have also been conditioned to accept nonanesthetized blood pressure monitoring, and several institutions have successfully used implanted loop recorders to remotely assess heart rate variability and electrocardiography. Interestingly, although ape blood cholesterol levels tend to be higher than in humans, apes rarely develop major coronary artery occlusion, and myocardial infarction is rare.[4,23]

Management of diagnosed CVD in apes has consisted of graduating levels of β-1 or α-1 adrenergic blockers, ace inhibitors, or both, depending on review of cardiac thickening and systolic or diastolic function. The use of diuretics has been limited to individuals with obvious respiratory compromise or fluid accumulation. Potential etiologies for great ape CVD are under investigation and include, but are not limited to, genetic predisposition, hypertension, and nutritional imbalances (dietary sodium levels, lack of fiber, high-carbohydrate diets, and lack of dietary antioxidants). The Great Ape Heart Project (GAHP at www.greatapeheartproject.org) based at Zoo Atlanta, in Atlanta, Georgia, is an international, collaborative effort to investigate great ape CVD and establish uniform diagnostic, treatment, and prevention strategies.

Musculoskeletal Disorders
Musculoskeletal disorders in great apes may result from traumatic injuries, infectious diseases, infections, nutritional imbalances, and congenital defects.[21,32,39,40] Management of these disorders depends on their etiology. Great apes are highly adaptable, and even with permanent musculoskeletal impairments, changes in management and husbandry of these animals, along with effective analgesics, may be very effective for long-term management.

Neoplastic Diseases
Neoplasia has been documented to affect the brain, central nervous system, bone marrow, skin, and reproductive organs of great apes. A link between immunosuppression associated with SIV and STLV-1 may be seen in some lymphomas and leukemias. Consultation with human and veterinary oncologic and surgical oncology specialists is highly recommended in cases of great ape neoplasia.

Dental Diseases
Traumatic tooth injuries may occur frequently and may result in exposure of dentin and tooth roots. Periodontal disease, gingival infections and hyperplasia and retained deciduous teeth may also cause dental issues in apes.

Endocrine Diseases
Thyroid disorders such as hypothyroidism and hyperthyroidism have been reported in great apes. Diabetes (both insulin-dependent and non-insulin-dependent) has also been reported.

Congenital Disorders
Congenital disorders seen in great apes include chromosomal abnormalities, cleft palates, aortic coarctation, atrial septal defects, and conjoined twins.

REFERENCES

1. Adami C, Wenker C, Hoby S, et al: Evaluation of effectiveness, safety and reliability of intramuscular medetomidine-ketamine for captive great apes. *Vet Rec* 171:196, 2012.
2. Association of Zoos and Aquariums: *Animal care manuals* (finalized for chimpanzees, in draft for bonobos, orangutans, and gorillas): www.aza.org/animal-care-manuals.
3. Atsalis S, Margulis SW: Sexual and hormonal cycles in geriatric *Gorilla gorilla gorilla*. *Int J Primatol* 27:1663–1687, 2006.
4. Baitchman EJ, Calle PP, Clippinger TL, et al: Preliminary evaluation of blood lipid profiles in captive western lowland gorillas (*Gorilla gorilla gorilla*). *J Zoo Wildl Med* 37:126–129, 2006.
5. Clyde V: *Bonobo SSP/TAG veterinary advisor annual report*. Prepared for AAZV, 2011: www.aazv.org.
6. de Faber JT, Pameijer JH, Schaftenaar W: Cataract surgery with foldable intraocular lens implants in captive lowland gorillas (*Gorilla gorilla gorilla*). *J Zoo Wildl Med* 35:520–524, 2004.
7. De Lathouwers M, Van Elsacker L: Reproductive parameters of female *Pan paniscus* and *P. troglodytes*: Quality versus quantity. *Int J Primatol* 26:55–71, 2005.
8. Doane CJ, Lee DR, Sleeper MM: Electrocardiogram abnormalities in captive chimpanzees (*Pan troglodytes*). *Comp Med* 56:512–518, 2006.
9. Ely JJ, Bishop MA, Lammey ML, et al: Use of biomarkers of collagen types I and III fibrosis metabolism to detect cardiovascular and renal disease in chimpanzees (*Pan troglodytes*). *Comp Med* 60:154–158, 2010.
10. Ely JJ, Zavaskis T, Lammey ML, et al: Association of brain-type natriuretic protein and cardiac troponin I with incipient cardiovascular disease in chimpanzees (*Pan troglodytes*). *Comp Med* 61:163–169, 2011.
11. Heistermann M, Mohle U, Vervaecke H, et al: Application of urinary and fecal steroid measurements for monitoring ovarian function and pregnancy in the bonobo (*Pan paniscus*) and evaluation of perineal swelling patterns in relation to endocrine events. *Biol Reprod* 55:844–853, 1996.
12. Hill LR, Lee DR, Keeling ME: Surgical technique for ambulatory management of airsacculitis in a Chimpanzee (*Pan troglodytes*). *Comp Med* 51:80–84, 2001.
13. International Union for Conservation of Nature (IUCN): http://www.iucn.org/about/work/programmes/species/our_work/the_iucn_red_list/.
14. Jones P, Cordonnier N, Mahamba C, et al: Encephalomyocarditis virus mortality in semi-wild bonobos (*Pan panicus*). *J Med Primatol* 40:157–163, 2011.
15. Kaur T, Singh J, Tong S, et al: Descriptive epidemiology of fatal respiratory outbreaks and detection of a human-related metapneumovirus in wild chimpanzees (*Pan troglodytes*) at Mahale Mountains National Park, Western Tanzania. *Am J Primatol* 70:755–765, 2008.
16. Kilbourn AM, Karesh WB, Wolfe ND, et al: Health evaluation of free-ranging and semi-captive orangutans (*Pongo pygmaeus pygmaeus*) in Sabah, Malaysia. *J Wildl Dis* 39:73–83, 2003.
17. Köndgen S, Kühl H, N'Goran PK, et al: Pandemic human viruses cause decline of endangered great apes. *Curr Biol* 18:260–264, 2008.

18. Kreger MD: *Environmental enrichment for nonhuman primates resource guide*, AWIC Res Ser 32, 2006: http://www.nal.usda.gov/awic/contact.php.

19. Lammey ML, Baskin GB, Gigliotti AP, et al: Interstitial myocardial fibrosis in a captive chimpanzee (*Pan troglodytes*) population. *Comp Med* 58:389–394, 2008.

20. Lawson B, Garriga R, Galdikas BM: Airsacculitis in fourteen juvenile southern Bornean orangutans (*Pongo pygmaeus wurmbii*). *J Med Primatol* 35:149–154, 2006.

21. Loomis MR: Great apes. In Miller ER, Fowler ME, editors: *Fowler's zoo and wild animal medicine current therapy*, ed 5, Philadelphia, PA, 2003, Saunders.

22. Makuwa M, Souquière S, Telfer P, et al: Hepatitis viruses in non-human primates. *J Med Primatol* 35:384–387, 2006.

23. McManamon R, Lowenstine LJ: Cardiovascular disease in great apes. In Miller ER, Fowler ME, editors: *Fowler's zoo and wild animal medicine current therapy*, ed 7, Philadelphia, PA, 2012, Saunders.

24. Möhle U, Heistermann M, Einspanier A, et al: Efficacy and effects of short- and medium-term contraception in the common marmoset (*Callithrix jacchus*) using melengestrol acetate implants. *J Med Primatol* 28:36–47, 1999.

25. Munson L, Moresco A, Calle PP: Adverse effects of contraceptives. In Asa CS, Porton IJ, editors: *Wildlife contraception: Issues, methods and applications*, Baltimore, MD, 2005, Johns Hopkins University Press.

26. Murphy HM, Dennis P, Devlin W, et al: Echocardiographic parameters of captive western lowland gorillas (*Gorilla gorilla gorilla*). *J Zoo Wildl Med* 42:572–579, 2011.

27. Murphy HW, Miller M, Ramer J, et al: Implications of simian retroviruses for captive primate population management and the occupational safety of primate handlers. *J Zoo Wildl Med* 37:219–233, 2006.

28. National Research Council of the National Academies: *Nutrient requirements of nonhuman primates*, ed 2, Washington, DC, 2003, The National Academies Press.

29. Njouom R, Mba SA, Nerrienet E, et al: Detection and characterization of hepatitis B virus strains from wild-caught gorillas and chimpanzees in Cameroon, Central Africa. *Infect Genet Evol* 10:790–796, 2010.

30. Nunamaker EA, Lee DR, Lammey ML: Chronic diseases in captive geriatric female Chimpanzees (*Pan troglodytes*). *Comp Med* 62:131–136, 2012.

31. Nunn CL, Hare B: Commentary-pathogen flow: What we need to know. *Am J Primatol* 12:1084–1087, 2012.

32. Nunn CL, Rothschild B, Gittleman JL: Why are some species more commonly afflicted by arthritis than others? A comparative study of spondyloarthropathy in primates and carnivores. *J Evol Biol* 20:460–470, 2007.

33. Orihel TC: *Nector Americanus* infection in primates. *J Parasitol* 57:117–121, 1971.

34. Palacios G, Lowenstine LJ, Cranfield MR, et al: Human metapneumovirus infection in wild mountain gorillas, Rwanda. *Emerg Infect Dis* 17:711–713, 2011.

35. Paoli T, Palagi E, Tacconi G, et al: Perineal swelling, intermenstrual cycle, and female sexual behavior in bonobos (*Pan paniscus*). *Am J Primatol* 68:333–347, 2006.

36. Peters CJ, Peters JW: An introduction to ebola: The virus and the disease. *J Infect Dis* 179:ix–xvi, 1999.

37. Portugal MM, Asa CS: Effects of chronic melengestrol acetate contraceptive treatment on perineal tumescence, body weight, and sociosexual behavior of hamadryas baboons (*Papio hamadryas*). *Zoo Biol* 14:251–259, 1995.

38. Rideout BA, Gardiner CH, Stalis IH, et al: Fatal infections with *Balamuthia mandrillaris* (a free-living amoeba) in gorillas and other old world primates. *Vet Pathol* 34:15–22, 1997.

39. Rothschild BM: Primate spondyloarthropathy. *Curr Rheum Rep* 7:173–181, 2005.

40. Rothschild BM, Woods RJ: Spondyloarthropathy as an old world phenomenon. *Semin Arthri Rheum* 21:306–316, 1992.

41. Ryan SJ, Walsh PD: Consequences of non-intervention for infectious disease in African great apes. *PLoS ONE* 6(12):e29030, 2011. doi: 10.1371/journal.pone.0029030.

42. Seiler BM, Dick EJ, Jr, Guardado-Mendoza R, et al: Spontaneous heart disease in the adult chimpanzee (*Pan troglodytes*). *J Med Primatol* 38:51–58, 2009.

43. Shimizu K, Udono T, Tanaka C, et al: Comparative study of urinary reproductive hormones in great apes. *Primates* 44:183–190, 2003.

44. Sleeman JM: Great apes. In West G, Heard D, Caulkett N, editors: *Zoo animal and wildlife immobilization and anesthesia*, Oxford, U.K., 2009, Blackwell Publishing.

45. Steinmetz HW, Zimmermann NE: Computed tomography for the diagnosis of sinusitis and airsacculitis in orangutans. In Miller ER, Fowler ME, editors: *Fowler's zoo and wild animal medicine current therapy*, ed 7, Philadelphia, PA, 2012, Saunders.

46. Terio KA, Kinsel MJ, Raphael J, et al: Pathologic lesions in chimpanzees (*Pan Trogylodytes Schweinfurthii*) from Gombe National Park, Tanzania 2004–2010. *J Zoo Wildl Med* 42:597–607, 2011.

47. Varki N, Anderson D, Herndon JG, et al: Heart disease is common in humans and chimpanzees, but is caused by different pathological processes. *Evol Appl* 2:101–112, 2009.

48. Wallis J, Lee DR: Primate conservation: The prevention of disease transmission. *Int J Primatol* 20:803–826, 1999.

49. Wevers D, Metzger S, Babweteera F, et al: Novel adenoviruses in wild primates: A high level of genetic diversity and evidence of zoonotic transmissions. *J Virol* 85:10774–10784, 2011.

50. Wich SA, Shumaker RW, Perkins L, et al: Captive and wild orangutan (*Pongo* sp.) survivorship: A comparison and the influence of management. *Am J Primatol* 71:680–686, 2009.

51. Woodford MH, Butynski TM, Karesh WB: Habituating the great apes: The disease risks. *Oryx* 36:153–160, 2002.

52. Zimmermann N, Pirovino M, Zingg R, et al: Upper respiratory tract disease in captive orangutans (*Pongo* sp.): Prevalence in 20 European zoos and predisposing factors. *J Med Primatol* 40:365–375, 2011.

CHAPTER 39

Xenarthra

Roberto F. Aguilar and Mariella Superina

BIOLOGY

The superorder Xenarthra consists of 31 extant species of armadillos (Cingulata—Dasypodidae), sloths (Pilosa—Folivora: Bradypodidae and Megalonychidae), and anteaters (Pilosa—Vermilingua: Myrmecophagidae and Cyclopedidae), which are restricted to the New World. This monophyletic group has a fossil history of at least 65 million years and is considered one of the basal clades of placental mammals.[14] Most xenarthrans remain inadequately studied, and taxonomic uncertainties still exist.

The 21 living armadillo species show different degrees of fossoriality and considerable differences in habitat preferences, diet, and behavior. Table 39-1 provides information on selected armadillo species. Some species such as *Dasypus novemcinctus*, *Chaetophractus villosus*, and *Tolypeutes matacus* are commonly kept in zoologic institutions.[53]

The two genera and six species of arboreal sloths are restricted to New World tropical rainforests (Table 39-2). The two species of two-toed sloths (*Choloepus*), which have predominantly nocturnal habits, are relatively common in zoologic collections. The four predominantly diurnal species of three-toed sloths (*Bradypus*) are only rarely kept.[19,33,53]

All four anteater species are myrmecophagous but differ in their habits. Giant anteaters (*Myrmecophaga tridactyla*) are ground dwellers and have a limited ability to climb. Lesser anteaters (*Tamandua* spp.) are predominantly arboreal but also move, feed, and rest on the ground; and silky anteaters (*Cyclopes didactylus*) are strictly arboreal and nocturnal (see Table 39-2).[36]

UNIQUE ANATOMY AND PHYSIOLOGY

The Xenarthra bear several unique anatomic traits such as additional (xenarthrous) joints of lumbar vertebrae; fusion of the ischium to the anterior caudal vertebrae; a secondary scapular spine; extensive retia mirabile in the limbs; paired postrenal venae cavae; and ossified sternal ribs. Their well-developed claws are used for digging, clinging to tree branches, and defense. Except for the toothless Vermilingua, xenarthrans have significantly reduced, homodont, continuously growing teeth that lack enamel. Caniniform teeth are present in sloths. The most conspicuous morphologic feature of armadillos is the presence of a carapace consisting of ossified dermal tissue covered by epidermal scales.[22] Sloths have specialized, large stomachs consisting of several chambers, in which bacterial flora breaks down and ferments rough plant material. They descend to the ground about once a week to defecate.

All Xenarthra have low basal rates of metabolism that are around 40% to 60% of those expected for their body mass.[31] This should be taken into account when medicating them, as drug metabolism may be reduced. Body temperatures of Xenarthra are low and variable. In some cases, they vary according to ambient temperature.[31] At least one species (*Zaedyus pichiy*) may enter torpor and hibernation.[50]

SPECIAL HOUSING REQUIREMENTS

Because of their particular susceptibility to low ambient temperatures, xenarthrans should have access to a heated shelter if ambient temperature drops below 15°C. Access to both sunlight and shaded places will help them thermoregulate. Two-toed sloths tolerate temperatures from approximately 17°C to 35°C and require high humidity levels (60%–80%).

Armadillos should be kept on a soft substrate such as soil, stringbark mulch, or wood shavings, which allow them to dig. Hard flooring such as concrete bears a higher risk of injury because of the armadillos' constant digging attempts. Outdoor facilities require wall footers extending underground for at least 1 meter (m) to keep them from escaping. If kept in pairs or groups, sufficient hiding places must be provided to prevent aggression between conspecifics. Injured armadillos should be separated to prevent cannibalism.

Captive sloths require large spaces with multiple areas to climb, platforms for feeding or resting, and hides. The use of ropes should be avoided as the claws may become entangled. Floors should consist of soil and be devoid of hard or sharp objects to prevent injuries in case of accidental falls.[33,53] *Bradypus* sloths are extremely difficult to maintain in captivity because of their specialized diet, as well as their susceptibility to infectious diseases and management-related diseases. Male sloths may show aggressive behavior when defending territory.[33,53]

Anteaters should be kept on natural flooring. *Tamandua* and *Cyclopes* require numerous branches to climb. *Myrmecophaga* like to bathe and defecate in water and should thus have access to a pool. Rotting logs should be offered to allow anteaters to forage and wear down their claws.

FEEDING

Armadillo species may be classified as carnivores–omnivores, generalist fossorial insectivores, generalist terrestrial insectivores, or specialist insectivores (anteaters and termite eaters) according to their trophic specialization.[43] Captive diets consist of a mixture of beef or dog food, fruit, vegetables, eggs, and vitamin and mineral supplements. Interspecific and seasonal differences are usually not considered in captive diet composition. Pathologies related to inadequate diets are common and include obesity, renal failure, digestive imbalances, hypovitaminoses, and dental disease.[53,54]

The diet of wild sloths is rich in fiber and contains low levels of energy and soluble carbohydrates. Three-toed sloths (*Bradypus*) have a highly selective diet composed of 99% leaves, mainly of *Cecropia*. Individuals of this genus seem to become strongly attached to a specific tree species, and large individual differences seem to exist in the digestive efficiency. Transferring them to a captive diet is difficult.[6,53] The natural diet of two-toed sloths (*Choloepus*) is more varied. In addition to plants, they sometimes eat insects, birds, and small reptiles.[6,53] Captive individuals may eat a wide variety of food items, including fruit and vegetables, commercial small animal preparations, boiled eggs, and cheese. Leaves, flowers, and wild fruit must be offered, and the food must be placed on elevated platforms. Food items should be cut lengthwise to facilitate handling. Sources of animal protein or commercial diets for dogs or primates should not exceed 10% of the diet. Some authors believe that sloths do not drink water but, rather, obtain water from the breakdown of fresh leaves.[30] Clinically, inadequate or imbalanced diets have been implicated in digestive stasis, rectal prolapse, severe diarrheas, dysbiosis, stunted growth, and urolithiasis. Anecdotal reports suggest that some sloths respond well to transfaunation during episodes of suspected dysbiosis.

TABLE 39-1

Biologic Information on Selected Species of Armadillos

Scientific Name	Cabassous spp.	Chaetophractus vellerosus	Chaetophractus villosus	Chlamyphorus truncatus	Dasypus hybridus	Dasypus novemcinctus	Euphractus sexcinctus	Priodontes maximus	Tolypeutes matacus	Zaedyus pichiy
Common name	Naked-tailed armadillo	Screaming hairy armadillo	Larger hairy armadillo	Pink fairy armadillo	Southern lesser long-nosed armadillo	Nine-banded or common long-nosed armadillo	Yellow or six-banded armadillo	Giant armadillo	Southern three-banded armadillo	Pichi
Body weight (kg)	3–6.2	0.85	2.5–3	0.12	2	3–8	3.5–5	30–50	1.5	1
Head-body length (cm)	30–50	23	33	13	30	36–57	45	90	30 (including tail)	27
Conservation status (IUCN)[a]	C. centralis: DD; C. chacoensis: NT; C. tatouay, C. unicinctus: LC	LC	LC	DD	NT	LC	LC	VU	NT	NT
Gestation (days)			68			ca. 140	60–65		104–116	60
Litter size	1	2	Mostly 2	2	8–12[b]	4[b]	1–3	1–2	1	1–2, exceptionally 3
Birth weight (grams)	100–115	50–60	86–115	3–4 cm length	40–45	85	95–115		70–100	45–55
Lactation (months)			2		2	3	1		2.5	1.5
Sexual maturity (months)	9–12	9–12	9			15	9		9–12	9–12

[a]DD, Data Deficient; LC, Least Concern; NT, Near Threatened; VU, Vulnerable. Main threats: hunting, habitat fragmentation, and degradation.
[b]Polyembryony.
References 32, 54, and 59.

TABLE 39-2

Biologic Information on Sloths and Anteaters

Scientific Name	Bradypus pygmaeus	Bradypus variegatus	Bradypus tridactylus	Bradypus torquatus	Choloepus hoffmanni	Choloepus didactylus	Myrmecophaga tridactyla	Tamandua tetradactyla	Tamandua mexicana	Cyclopes didactylus
Common name	Pygmy sloth	Brown-throated three-toed sloth	Pale-throated three-toed sloth	Maned three-toed sloth	Hoffmann's two-toed sloth	Southern two-toed sloth	Giant anteater	Southern tamandua, lesser anteater	Northern tamandua, banded anteater	Pygmy anteater
Body weight (kg)	2.5–3.5	3.9–5.5	3.8–4.5	3.6–4.2	4.5–6.7	4.1–8.5	22–39	3.42–7	3.2–5.4	<0.4
Body length (cm)	48–53	48–80	50–60	50–54	54–72	63–88	174–280	95–130	102–130	3–50
Conservation status (IUCN)[a]	CR	LC	LC	VU	LC	LC	VU	LC	LC	LC / DD[b]
Reproductive period	—	Climate-dependent, breed before rains	Seasonal	Aseasonal, most births between February and April	Slightly seasonal	Aseasonal	Aseasonal	Aseasonal	Aseasonal	December-January
Gestation length	—	6 months	—	—	10 months	10 months	184–190 days	130–160 days	130–150 days	120–150 days
Litter size	—	1	1	1	1	1	1	1	1	1
Birth weight (grams)	—	200–250	300–400	300–400	350–450	—	1200–1500	240–590	—	45–60
First solid food ingestion	—	4 days	3 weeks	2 weeks	2–4 weeks	1–5 weeks	—	—	—	—
Lactation (months)	—	1	>2 months	2–4	—	3–6	6	—	—	—
Independence of offspring (months)	—	6	5	8–11	9	12	9	—	—	—
Sexual maturity Female/Male (years)	—	—	3–6 / 3	—	2 / 3	min. 3 / 4	2 / 2	1 / ?	1 / 1	—

[a]CR, Critically Endangered; DD, Data Deficient; LC, Least Concern; VU, Vulnerable. Main threats: Hunting for food or pet trade, habitat degradation and fragmentation (sloths and anteaters); wildfires, persecution as pest species, road traffic (anteaters).

[b]LC, Main population; DD, Northeastern Brazil subpopulation.

References 1, 19, 25, 28, 34, 55, 60.

Anteaters forage almost exclusively on ants and termites, but the proportion of these insects varies among species, regionally, individually, and seasonally.[44] Giant anteaters (*M. tridactyla*) may also ingest seeds, beetle larvae, and bees, and lesser anteaters (*T. tetradactyla*) consume beetles and seeds. *Tamandua mexicana* has been observed foraging on fruit of the palm *Attalea butyracea*.[3,8,44] Several diets have been formulated for feeding *Myrmecophaga* and *Tamandua* in captivity. Diets are usually based on a semi-liquid mix that contains dog or cat food, lactose-free milk, egg, red meat, and fruit. *Cyclopes didactylus* only ingests arboreal ants, making the formulation of an artificial diet extremely difficult.[2] All anteater species' diets should be supplemented with vitamin K (*Myrmecophaga*: 5 milligrams per day [mg/day]; *Tamandua*: 3 mg/day) and taurine (2.2 grams per day [g/day] for *Myrmecophaga* and *Tamandua*) (Miranda, personal communication). Vitamin K deficiency may lead to hematuria and prolonged bleeding. Taurine deficiency has been associated with dilatory cardiomyopathy. Giant anteaters will develop gastrointestinal (GI) impaction and constipation or chronic soft stool and diarrhea if fiber and chitin levels in the diet are low. The diet of *Cyclopes* should be supplemented with selenium (0.2 g), taurine (0.18 mg), probiotics, vitamins, and minerals (Rojas Moreno, personal communication).

RESTRAINT AND HANDLING

Physical Restraint

Armadillos may defend themselves with their limbs and sharp claws when being caught. Heavy gloves should be used while holding them to avoid scratches. *Euphractus sexcinctus* is the only species that may try to bite. Armadillos are agile and will try to wriggle out of the handler's grip. Applying light lateral pressure on the carapace often calms them down. *Tolypeutes* species roll up into a ball when feeling threatened. They will unroll themselves once they are placed on a hard surface. Large armadillos may be picked up by the lateral edges of the carapace and smaller species grasped by the carapace with one hand. They should only be held by the base of the tail, and their carapace supported with the other hand for short periods.

Two-toed sloths (*Choloepus*) are more aggressive than three-toed sloths (*Bradypus*) and need to be handled more carefully. Adult two-toed sloths may grip the arms or body of the restrainer and inflict severe injuries with their sharp claws or caniniform premolar teeth. Physical restraint must be gentle but firm and performed by at least two persons using leather gloves to hold the feet and the head of the animal. Attempts to force physical restraint on a sloth are likely to be unsuccessful or even dangerous. Infants may feel more comfortable if allowed to grip the arm of a restrainer.

Tamandua and *Cyclopes* may be held using leather gloves by grasping the forearms and head or simply placing them in a cloth bag.[58] In the case of *Cyclopes*, using a cloth bag, to which they may cling, may facilitate manipulation and weighing. *Myrmecophaga* may be restrained using forked wooden sticks or nets, making sure the mouth or lips are not harmed during the capture.[34,58] Special care must be taken to avoid their claws, and gauze and elastic bandages may be placed over them during procedures to avoid potential injury.

Chemical Restraint

Xenarthra have low metabolic rates and low and varying body temperatures. Their chemical restraint must therefore be performed at a stable room temperature. In cool environments, a heat source should be used to avoid significant drops in body temperature. Vital signs should be monitored during the entire procedure. Intubation of anteaters and armadillos may be challenging to impossible, given their peculiar anatomy and prolonged diastemas in a very narrow mouth. Intubation of *Dasypus novemcinctus* may be possible with a polyethylene tube of 0.6 to 1.3 cm diameter and a flexible endoscope.[18] Anesthesia may be maintained with tight-fitting masks, provided secretions are not overabundant. Sloths may usually be intubated by using conventional small animal techniques and materials.

Most inhalation and injectable anesthetics may be used for armadillos (Table 39-3).[12,21,37,54] Considerable interspecific and individual differences have been observed in the duration and depth of anesthesia, and doses may need to be adjusted accordingly.[54] Animals of

TABLE 39-3

Chemical Restraint Agents Used for Selected Xenarthra

	Captive (C), Free-ranging (F)	Generic Name	Dose (mg/kg, IM)	Reversal Agent/Dose (mg/kg)	Comments
Dasypus novemcinctus	F	Ketamine	25	Atipamezole 0.38	
		Acepromazine	0.3		
	F	Ketamine	4–7.5		
		Medetomidine	0.075		
	F	Ketamine	40		Prolonged recovery
		Xylazine	1		
	F	Tiletamine / Zolazepam	8.5		Prolonged recovery
	C	Fentanyl citrate / Droperidol	0.11–0.25 mL/kg		
Tolypeutes matacus	F	Ketamine	20–37	Yohimbine 0.12–0.14	Risk of hypothermia
		Xylazine	0.6–1.25		
	F	Tiletamine / Zolazepam	3.85–11.9		Considerable interindividual variation in degree of muscle relaxation. Severe respiratory depression possible
Zaedyus pichiy	C	Tiletamine / Zolazepam	15		Prolonged recovery
	C	Ketamine	7	Atipamezole 0.4	
		Midazolam	0.05		
		Dexmedetomidine	0.05		

TABLE 39-3

Chemical Restraint Agents Used for Selected Xenarthra—cont'd

	Captive (C), Free-ranging (F)	Generic Name	Dose (mg/kg, IM)	Reversal Agent/Dose (mg/kg)	Comments
Choloepus didactylus	F	Ketamine	10		
		Acepromazine	0.1		
	F	Ketamine	10		
		Xylazine	1		
	F	Ketamine	3	Atipamezole 0.2	
		Medetomidine	0.04		
	C	Ketamine	8–13		Associated with isoflurane anesthesia
		Midazolam	0.22–0.42		
	C	Medetomidine	0.01	Atipamezole 0.05	
		Midazolam	0.21–0.25		
		Butorphanol	0.21–0.25		
	F / C	Tiletamine / Zolazepam	10 / 1.9–6		
Choloepus hoffmanni	C	Ketamine	2.42–2.92	Atipamezole 0.17–0.27	
		Dexmedetomidine Midazolam	0.008–0.016 0.1		
	C	Tiletamine / Zolazepam	4.4		
Bradypus variegatus	F	Ketamine	2.5		
		Medetomidine	0.02		
Bradypus torquatus		Ketamine	1.3		
		Acepromazine	0.1		
Myrmecophaga tridactyla		Ketamine	5–10	Yohimbine 0.12–0.2	No regurgitation
		Xylazine	0.5–1.5		
		Ketamine	2–4	Atipamezole, 5x Medetomidine dose	Good muscle relaxation
		Medetomidine	0.02–0.04		
		Ketamine	5–10	Flumazenile 0.01–0.02	Short procedures
		Midazolam	0.2		
		Ketamine	8.8		Associated with isoflurane anesthesia
		Acepromazine	0.06		
		Diazepam	0.3		
		Buprenorphine	0.006		
		Ketamine	4	Atipamezole 0.15	Rapid induction and recovery after reversion
		Dexmedetomidine	0.015		
		Midazolam	0.1		
Tamandua tetradactyla		Ketamine	20		Good muscle relaxation
		Xylazine	1		
		Ketamine	4–5	Atipamezole 0.15	Rapid induction and recovery after reversion
		Dexmedetomidine	0.02		
		Midazolam	0.1		
		Tiletamine/Zolazepam	15		Rapid induction, prolonged recovery
Cyclopes didactylus		Ketamine	8–12		Short procedures
		Midazolam	0.4		
		Ketamine	4	Atipamezole 0.15	Rapid induction and recovery after reversion
		Dexmedetomidine	0.015–0.03		
		Midazolam	0.1		

IM, Intramuscularly; *mg/kg*, milligram per kilogram; *mL/kg*, milliliter per kilogram.

the genus *Dasypus* seem to be less sensitive to ketamine compared with other Xenarthra and require a higher dose.[21] Premedication with 0.02 to 0.04 mg/kg atropine prevents intensified salivation during anesthesia with ketamine. Inhalation anesthesia with isoflurane is recommended for longer surgical interventions. Induction with masks or in chambers may be problematic because of the armadillos' ability to hold their breath for several minutes.[54]

Chemical restraint of sloths may be risky and even life threatening for the patient. Several authors recommend the use of injectable chemical restraint agents (see Table 39-3).[12,24,27,45,56] Isoflurane

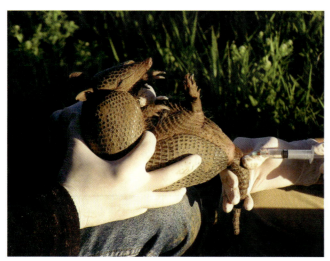

FIGURE 39-1 Blood collection from the ventral coccygeal vein in a southern lesser long-nosed armadillo (*Dasypus hybridus*). (Photograph by M. Superina.)

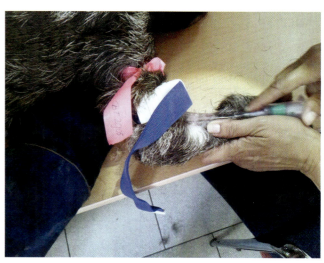

FIGURE 39-2 Blood collection from the brachial vein in a pale-throated three-toed sloth (*Bradypus tridactylus*). (Photograph by M.S. Pool, Green Heritage Fund Suriname.)

anesthesia by means of a facemask, followed by intubation, is recommended rather than fixed anesthesia protocols.

A variety of fixed anesthesia protocols has proven effective in anteaters, both in field and in captive conditions (see Table 39-3).[20,34,46,58] The anesthetic may be injected by hand after physical restraint or darted into the forelimb muscles.

DIAGNOSTICS

In armadillos, the presence of the carapace precludes easy palpation or auscultation. Rectal temperature is difficult to interpret because of the highly variable body temperature of armadillos, which may range from 32°C to 38°C in healthy individuals. Blood is best collected from the ventral tail vein (Figure 39-1). The medial saphenous vein may be used as an alternative, especially for larger volumes or for catheterization.[54] Normal heart rate is around 116 per minute in *Chaetophractus villosus* and 126 per minute in male *Dasypus novemcinctus* or 84 per minute in female *D. novemcinctus*. The respiratory rate in relaxed *C. villosus* and *D. novemcinctus* is 30 to 40 per minute; in the former species, it may rise up to 160 per minute in stress conditions, whereas rates of up to 180 per minute have been measured in the latter at high ambient temperatures.[4,54]

Some diagnostic techniques used for small- and medium-sized mammals may be adapted to sloths. Blood samples may be obtained from the brachial vein (Figure 39-2). The maximum blood volume drawn should not exceed 0.5% of body weight. Urine may be obtained by cystocentesis, using ultrasonography to guide the needle. Body temperature of sloths varies between 32.7°C and 35.5°C and is slightly higher in two-toed sloths than in three-toed sloths.[25] Normal respiratory rates are 10 to 18 per minute in *Choloepus* and 5 to 21 per minute in *Bradypus*. Resting heart rates are 70 to 130 per minute in *Choloepus* and 60 to 110 per minute in *Bradypus*.[24]

In anteaters, blood may be collected from the central coccygeal vein (in *Cyclopes* and *Tamandua*) or the cephalic and medial or lateral saphenous veins (in *Myrmecophaga*).[34] Normal body temperature (Tb), respiratory (RR), and resting heart rates (HR) for anteaters are as follows: *Myrmecophaga tridactyla*: Tb 30°C to 35°C, RR 18 to 26 per minute, HR 60 per minute; *Tamandua tetradactyla*: Tb 30 to 35°C, RR 20 to 25 per minute, HR 80 per minute (Rojas Moreno, personal communication); *Cyclopes didactylus*: Tb 31 to 34.2°C, RR 70 to 90 per minute, HR 60 per minute.[34]

Hematology and serum biochemistry values for selected Xenarthra species are given in Tables 39-4 and 39-5, respectively.

DISEASES

Common diseases of armadillos, sloths, and anteaters are summarized in Tables 39-6, 39-7, and 39-8.

The majority of health problems of captive armadillos are related to poor husbandry and inadequate or imbalanced nutrition. Injuries, especially to the tail and feet, are, by far, the most common health problems of captive armadillos. They accounted for 107 out of 438 pathologies recorded in 44 zoologic institutions.[54] Armadillos' low metabolic rates and body temperatures may predispose them to infections by uncommon or even saprophytic organisms. Prolonged antibiotic treatment may reduce the intestinal microflora that synthesize menaquinones, leading to hypovitaminosis K and spontaneous bleeding. It should therefore be accompanied by vitamin K supplementation. Diseases of the digestive tract (especially enteritis) and nutritional deficiencies are frequent.[53,54] Obesity is a common problem in captive armadillos. The high prevalence of subclinical nephritis in wild *D. novemcinctus* should be taken into account during quarantine and in the formulation of diets. Wild-caught animals may be more susceptible to nephrotoxic drugs and to renal diseases caused by excessive protein in the diet.[49,54] Infectious agents that have been identified in wild armadillos include *Mycobacterium leprae* (only *Dasypus* is susceptible to this pathogen), *Nocardia brasiliensis*, *Paracoccidioides brasiliensis*, *Leptospira interrogans*, *Histoplasma capsulatum*, *Sporothrix schenckii*, and *Salmonella* sp.[33,54]

North American specimens of *D. novemcinctus* seem to carry few parasites, but new imports of other species may be heavily infested with endoparasites or ectoparasites, many of which are specific for xenarthrans or armadillos. GI parasites include cestodes (*Mathevotaenia*), nematodes (*Bairdascaris, Aspidodera, Mazzia, Ancylostoma, Cyclobulura*), Acanthocephala, and protozoans (*Eimeria*). *Dirofilaria immitis* has been identified as the cause of death of a captive three-banded armadillo (*Tolypeutes matacus*), and several wild armadillos were antigen positive for this parasite.[12] Systemic protozoan parasites include *Sarcocystis, Leishmania naiffi, Trypanosoma cruzi, Toxoplasma gondii*, and *Entamoeba histolytica*. The most common ectoparasites include fleas (*Tunga, Malacopsylla, Phthiropsylla*), ticks (*Amblyomma*), and mites (*Dasyponyssus, Ornithonyssus, Sarcoptes*).[33,54] Antibodies against Eastern equine encephalitis virus and Saint Louis encephalitis virus have been found in wild *T. matacus* and *D. novemcinctus*, but their clinical relevance is unknown.[11,13]

Traumatic injuries are common in captive sloths. Branches and posts in their exhibits should be properly affixed. Fractures are

Text continued on p. 365

TABLE 39-4

Reference Ranges for Hematologic Parameters of Selected Xenarthra Species

	Dasypus novemcinctus X ± SD	Dasypus hybridus X ± SD	Chaetophractus villosus X ± SD	Tolypeutes matacus X ± SD	Zaedyus pichiy X ± SD	Choloepus didactylus	Choloepus hoffmanni	Bradypus variegatus	Myrmecophaga tridactyla X ± SD	Tamandua tetradactyla X ± SD
Red blood cells (10^6/µL)	6.6 ± 1.4	5.96 ± 0.68	4.06 ± 0.55	3.37 ± 0.75	4.30 ± 1.05	2.5–2.7	3.85–5.04	3.8–4.4	2.36 ± 0.14	3.15 ± 0.23
Packed cell volume (%)	43.5 ± 5.8	39.67 ± 5.60	36.3 ± 3.9	34 ± 4	49.3 ± 6.0	34.5–36.9	35	32.8–35.6	37.7 ± 1.06	34.8 ± 1.50
Hemoglobin (g/dL)	14.6 ± 1.9	16.84 ± 2.08	11.4 ± 1.5	—	16.0	11.1–11.9	11.7–13.6	10.6–11.5	11.8 ± 0.52	10.73 ± 0.58
Mean corpuscular volume (fL)	66.0 ± 1.8	68.04 ± 14.60	91.6 ± 7.1	—	120.2 ± 30.0	133.4–138.4	—	83–83.07	165.12 ± 8.71	116.06 ± 7.46
Mean corpuscular hemoglobin (pg)	20.1 ± 1.5	28.66 ± 4.60	28.9 ± 2.9	—	—	42.6–44.6	—	25.2–29	51.07 ± 2.27	35.45 ± 2.05
Mean corpuscular hemoglobin concentration (g/dL)	30.6 ± 2.2	42.74 ± 6.56	31.6 ± 2.2	—	—	31.6–32.4	—	31.7–33.1	31.26 ± 0.96	31.14 ± 1.65
White blood cells (10^3/µL)	12.2 ± 6.1	10.08 ± 4.00	9.72 ± 5.30	9.2 ± 4.3	4.7 ± 2.9	17.1–20.1	13.4–21	11.4–12.5	11.87 ± 2.88	8.07 ± 1.04
Neutrophils (10^3/µL)	7.0 ± 4.6	5.72 ± 3.00	51% ± 13	2.40 ± 1.71	2.74 ± 1.93	11.6–14.2	40%–49%	31%–38.6%	72.62% ± 3.67	48.15% ± 4.09
Lymphocytes (10^3/µL)	3.1 ± 2.2	3.46 ± 1.68	36% ± 13	5.58 ± 3.11	1.31 ± 1.08	4.2–5.8	40%–49%	53%–59.8%	18.77% ± 3.17	44.15% ± 4.18
Monocytes (10^3/µL)	0.9 ± 1.1	0.53 ± 0.32	6% ± 3	0.34 ± 0.21	0.19 ± 0.17	0.2–0.4	0%–3%	0%–3%	1.69% ± 0.04	2.00% ± 0.35
Eosinophils (10^3/µL)	0.4 ± 0.8	0.14 ± 0.08	3.9% ± 2.8	0.91 ± 1.01	0.38 ± 0.45	0.2–0.6	0%–5%	—	6.92% ± 1.67	5.69% ± 0.88
Basophils (10^3/µL)	0.1 ± 0.1	0.05 ± 0.08	1% ± 2	0.17 ± 0.09	0.07 ± 0.11	0	1%–3%	0%	0%	0%
Platelets (10^3/µL)	—	—	399 ± 152	—	—	261–319	—	300–348	—	—
References	10, 40	9	5, 39	13	52	57	24	24	34	34

fL, Femtoliter; g/dL, gram per deciliter; µL, microliter.
A conversion table is available in the appendix.

TABLE 39-5

Reference Ranges for Biochemical Parameters of Selected Xenarthra Species

	Dasypus novemcinctus	Dasypus septemcinctus	Chaetophractus villosus	Tolypeutes matacus	Zaedyus pichiy	Choloepus didactylus	Choloepus hoffmanni	Myrmecophaga tridactyla	Tamandua tetradactyla
Total protein (g/L)	62 ± 11.66	60.3 ± 10.50	66.1 ± 6.0	62 ± 8	65 ± 15	82.1–87.9	75	51–71	48–122
Glucose (mmol/L)	0.92 ± 0.41 g/L	0.77 ± 0.25 g/L	1.04 ± 0.24 g/L	4.00 ± 1.11	—	1–1.4	3–38	37–87 mg/dL	48–122 mg/dL
Blood urea nitrogen (mmol/L)	1.39 ± 0.35 g/L	0.23 ± 0.08 g/L	—	13.57 ± 4.28	31.4 ± 10.9	8.5–10.1	6.09	6–40 mg/dL	20–34 mg/dL
Uric acid (µmol/L)	18 ± 11.66 mg/L	2.97 ± 0.59 mg/L	—	—	—	152–176	172.4	0.8–1.2 mg/dL	0.5–1.1 mg/dL
Creatinine (µmol/L)	—	7.88 ± 2.64 mg/L	—	35 ± 18	—	79–89	79.56	—	—
Bilirubin (µmol/L)	—	2.78 ± 0.57 mg/L	—	2 ± 2	—	19.9–29.1	4.78	0.0–0.4 mg/dL	0.0–0.2 mg/dL
Triglycerides (mmol/L)	—	0.46 ± 0.15	0.37 ± 0.16	—	—	0.2–0.4	1.308	17–19 mg/dL	1–15.1 mg/dL
Cholesterol (mmol/L)	—	4.17 ± 1.29	—	3.06 ± 0.67	—	2.6–3	5.04	57–108 mg/dL	97–353 mg/dL
Amylase (Unit /L)	—	80 ± 39	—	2.59 ± 2.04	—	261–351	—	—	—
ALP (Unit/L)	—	80 ± 39	—	—	144 ± 93.5	337–423	—	5–41	7–121
ALT (Unit/L)	—	11 ± 22	—	27 ± 24	8.8 ± 4.3	18–22	—	21–111	48–98
AST (Unit/L)	—	36 ± 34	—	29 ± 21	13.0 ± 7.2	103–121	—	14–50	13–65
CPK (Unit/L)	—	—	—	—	212 ± 237	85–149	—	43–508	0–757
Lactate dehydrogenase (Unit/L)	1587 ± 1422.75	—	—	—	—	1112–1276	—	71–387	0–329
GGT (Unit/L)	—	—	—	41 ± 33	—	2.3–3.7	—	1–85	18–225
Albumin (g/L)	32 ± 5.83	22.3 ± 8.20	37.2 ± 4.0	28 ± 4	3.3 ± 0.4	—	39	24–35	24–34
Globulin (g/L)	—	—	—	36 ± 10	—	—	36	22–44	43–55
Phosphorus (mmol/L)	62 ± 17.49 mg/L	45.3 ± 14.2 mg/L	—	1.42 ± 0.23	—	1.7–2.1	1.48	3.9–5.9	3.0–6.4
Calcium (mmol/L)	98 ± 17.49 mg/L	87.7 ± 15.4 mg/L	—	2.73 ± 0.18	9.8 ± 1.8	2.1–2.3	2.32	7.8–10.0	9.7–13.5
Sodium (mmol/L)	—	—	—	143 ± 6	—	130–136	54.81	133–148	136–144
Potassium (mmol/L)	—	—	—	4.7 ± 1.5	—	5.3–5.9	1.48	4.1–5.9	4.3–5.9
Chloride (mmol/L)	—	—	—	112 ± 5	—	93–97	25.3	101–115	98–108
References	41	7	29, 38, 39	13	52	57	24	34	34

ALP, Alkaline phosphatase; *ALT*, alanine aminotransferase; *AST*, aspartate aminotransferase; *CPK*, creatine phosphokinase; *GGT*, gamma glutamyl transferase; *g/L*, gram per liter; *µmol/L*, micromole per liter; *mmol/L*, millimole per liter; *Unit/L*, unit per liter.
A conversion table is available in the appendix.

TABLE 39-6

Selected Diseases of Armadillos

Disease	Etiology	Clinical Signs	Diagnosis	Management	Comments
Infections, abscesses below carapace and bands	Intraspecific aggression, inappropriate husbandry conditions (rough walls etc.)	(Suppurative) lesions, asymmetric or warmer areas of carapace	Regular, careful examination of carapace, especially of skinfolds between bands	Debridement, antibiotics, vitamin K, intramuscularly (IM), once daily (SID)	Infections or abscesses may extend below carapace and lead to septicemia and death; treatment must be accompanied by improved husbandry conditions
Perionychitis	Animals kept on hard flooring	Prominent lameness	Inspection, radiography to exclude osteomyelitis	Debridement, footbath with 3% tetracycline or 2% nitrofurazone; topical application of antibiotics; amputation in case of osteomyelitis	Treatment must be accompanied by improved husbandry conditions (soft substrate)
Hypovitaminosis K	Oral antibiotic therapy, nutritional deficiency	Spontaneous bleeding, prolonged clotting time	Clinical signs	Vitamin K (e.g., 0.5 milliliters [mL] konakione, IM, SID, or 9–10 milligrams (mg) menadione with food	Animals often die unexpectedly; necropsy reveals multiple hemorrhages (e.g., hemoperitoneum)
Impaction, intestinal obstruction	Ingestion of bedding material	Anorexia, abdominal distension, reduced amount or absence of feces	Radiography	Vegetable oil in food or 20–50 mL mineral oil through stomach tube Gastrotomy in severe cases	Avoid sawdust and shredded paper as bedding materials
Inadaptation to captive diet	Wild-caught individuals often fail to accept artificial diet	Anorexia, cachexia	Anorexia, flattening of convex carapace, isolation from conspecifics, decrease in activity levels	Diet change, offer variety of food items to allow animal to choose Infusions intravenously (IV), intraperitoneally (IP), subcutaneously (SC) In extreme cases, force-feeding with gastric tube (e.g., 2 mm diameter for *Tolypeutes matacus*)	Wild-caught animals often refuse to eat in the presence of humans; leaving the animal alone during feeding time may help
Excessive tooth growth	Inadequate consistency of diet (too soft, too finely chopped)	Anorexia, cachexia	Oral cavity examination	Grinding or extraction of teeth; diet change to incorporate hard items that require animals to chew	
Pneumonia	Stress, suboptimal ambient temperature, elevated dust levels, bacterial infection	Dyspnea, apathy, tremor, somnolence, inappetence, incoordination	Clinical signs	Antibiotics (tetracycline, amoxicillin, enrofloxacin, trimethoprim sulfa), parenteral vitamin supplementation	Often remains undiagnosed and leads to death

From references 33 and 54.

TABLE 39-7

Selected Diseases of Sloths

Disease	Etiology	Clinical Signs	Diagnosis	Management	Comments
Respiratory infections[33]	Bacterial	Weight loss, dehydration (sunken eyes), wet skin, nasal discharge, dyspnea	Clinical signs, radiography, hematology, tracheal wash for culture and antibiography	Trimethoprim–Sulfamethoxazole 20 milligram per kilogram (mg/kg), intramuscularly (IM), once daily (SID), bromhexin, improve environmental conditions	High mortality (>95%) in three-toed sloths
Urolithiasis[42]	Nutritional supplements—excessive minerals	Dysuria	Radiography, ultrasonography	Surgical removal	—
Tympanism[33]	Stress, highly fermentable vegetables	Swollen abdomen, abdominal turgor, dyspnea, tympany on percussion	Clinical signs, radiography, ultrasonography	Abdominocentesis, dimethyl-polysiloxane orally (PO), correction of diet	Death caused by compression of thoracic cavity
Constipation[33]	Stress, dry diets	Absence of defecation for periods >10 days, swollen abdomen	Clinical signs, radiography, ultrasonography	Mild laxatives (mineral oil, psyllium)	Normal gastrointestinal function recovered after 3 weeks or more
Rectal prolapse[33]	Complication following diarrhea or urolithiasis	Prolapse	Clinical signs, ultrasonography	Surgery	—
Gastrointestinal parasites[16,33,48]	*Eimeria choloepi*, Spirurides, Cestodes	Subclinical; uncommon signs: diarrhea, weight loss, hyporexia	Fecal examination	—	Frequent in free-ranging animals, subclinical
Toxoplasmosis[33]	*Toxoplasma gondii*	Acute and lethal: sudden death	Histopathology, polymerase chain reaction (PCR), immunohistochemistry, serology	—	Uncertain transmission (contact with feline feces?)
Ticks[33]	*Amblyomma geayi*, *A. varium*, *Boophylus*	Subclinical; uncommon signs: pruritus, skin irritation	Parasite identification	—	—
Trauma[33]	Incorrectly affixed branches and posts in enclosure	Fractures, muscular paralysis, head trauma, rupture of internal organs	Radiography, computed tomography, ultrasonography	Fractures: surgical orthopedic fixation	Low success of surgical fixation of fractures
Claw injuries	Attacks from humans or domestic animals	Wounds, fracture of claws	Clinical signs, radiography	Wound management; onychectomy[33]	—

TABLE 39-8

Selected Diseases of Anteaters

Disease	Etiology	Clinical Signs	Management	Comments
Bacterial pneumonia	Inappropriate environmental temperature and humidity in enclosures; associated with *Pneumococcus*, *Staphylococcus*, *Streptococcus*	Nasal discharge, excessive ocular secretion, dyspnea, anorexia, and depression; weight loss in chronic cases	Antibiotic therapy, correct temperature and humidity	All species

TABLE 39-8

Selected Diseases of Anteaters—cont'd

Disease	Etiology	Clinical Signs	Management	Comments
Bacterial enteritis	Food or water contaminated with bacterial agents: *Salmonella*, *Shigella*, *Campylobacter*, *Escherichia coli*, *Enterobacter*	Diarrhea—white or yellow feces with mucus and blood; may be accompanied by colic and gas	Fluid therapy, antibiotic therapy—sulfamethoxazole or chloramphenicol	All species in poor captive conditions
Bacterial dermatitis	Skin lesions caused by intraspecific aggression or inadequate enclosures; frequently associated with *Staphylococcus*, *Streptococcus*	Alopecia; pustules, abscesses or purulent skin lesions	Wound cleansing with chlorhexidine or povidone iodine, topical antibiotics, systemic antibiotics (e.g., cephalosporins)	All species in poor captive conditions
Trauma	Intraspecific aggression, inadequate enclosures or hard substrates	Full or partial thickness lacerations to toes or rostrum	Cleansing and wound management	Common in adults, more frequent in males
Hypovitaminosis K	Low levels of vitamin K in diet; malabsorption	Spontaneous hemorrhage—commissure of the mouth, eyelids, and extremities; hematuria	Supplemental vitamin K_1 and probiotics in diet, vitamin K_1 intramuscularly (IM)	Commonly observed in all species of captive anteaters
Hypervitaminosis A and D	Excess of vitamins in diet	Mineralization of soft tissues, difficult locomotion and abnormal posture—vertebral hyperostosis	No treatment described	Captive lesser anteaters, associated with over-supplementation or inappropriate diet
Taurine deficiency	Inadequate or low levels of taurine in diet	Exercise intolerance, dyspnea, ascites, cardiomegaly, cardiac insufficiency, congestive heart failure	Supplemental taurine in diet	Reported in *M. tridactyla* and *T. tetradactyla*
Tongue injuries and constriction	Meat fibers become entangled around tongue	Anorexia, pain, edema, excessive salivation	Correction of diet, removal of tendons and other fibers	Clinical reports and necropsy findings
Chronic diarrhea	Associated with inadequate or very liquid diets	Liquid feces with gas or containing undigested food	Correction of diet	Mainly observed during adaptation to captivity
Gastric or intestinal bloating	Intestinal atony caused by low environmental temperatures	Abdominal distention	Flunixin–meglumine, simethicone, temperature control	May occur in all anteater species, mainly in offspring or juveniles
Epiphora	Stress of captivity or ocular diseases	Excessive tearing, whitish or yellowish discharge	Stress management—eyewash	Mainly observed during adaptation to captivity
Rectal or vaginal prolapse	High stress or aggressive interaction	Exposed vaginal or rectal tissue, edema and congestion	Surgical correction	Few reports, mainly from *T. tetradactyla*

From reference 35.

difficult to repair through conventional orthopedic techniques.[33] Some surgical conditions include correction of rectal prolapse and amputation of injured claws (onychectomy).[33] Nutritional diseases are important in sloths because of their specialized diet.[16,33] *Bradypus* sloths are highly susceptible to stress and prone to suffer dehydration and malnutrition, which, in turn, causes immune suppression. They are prone to respiratory infections, leading to pulmonary edema and death in more than 95% of the cases.[33] Pneumonia caused by *Bordetella bronchiseptica* has been treated successfully with 30 mg/kg trimethoprim-sulfamethoxazole, intramuscularly (IM), once daily (SID) for 7 to 10 days.[26] A comfortable, quiet environment with adequate temperature (24°C–32°C) and humidity (>70%) and a proper diet are key to prevent respiratory diseases. Commensal arthropods are commonly found on the skin of wild sloths. They are of no clinical significance but may become pathogenic under captive conditions. Endoparasites are rare, and treatment is not recommended unless the patient is showing evident clinical signs such as diarrhea, weight loss, or hyporexia. Bacteria such as *Salmonella enteritidis*, *Escherichia coli*, and *Citrobacter freundii* have been isolated from fecal material and many organs.[16] Toxoplasmosis in sloths may be acute and lethal.[33]

Trauma, spontaneous abortion, and dilatory cardiomyopathy caused by taurine deficiency are seen frequently in captive anteaters (Figure 39-3). Chronic diarrhea and soft or pasty stools are common in some giant and lesser anteaters with inappropriate diets or insufficient chitin or fiber. The most common intestinal parasites of anteaters are protozoa, especially *Coccidia*, *Giardia*, and *Amoeba*. The latter may cause severe diarrhea. Metronidazole (10–20 mg/kg) and azythromicin (10–12 mg/kg) are indicated for their treatment, whereas sulfadimethoxine (55 mg/kg first dose, followed by

27.5 mg/kg) is indicated to treat coccidiosis. Infestation with metazoans, especially acanthocephalans, cestodes, trematodes, and nematodes may occur.

THERAPY

Commonly used antibiotics and miscellaneous drugs are summarized in Tables 39-9 and 39-10.

In armadillos, intramuscular injections may be done in the hind limbs. In rolled up *Tolypeutes*, the only access to muscle tissue is at the base of the tail.[37]

The low metabolic rate and the complex GI system of sloths may lead to prolonged elimination time of drugs. Doses should be 25% lower than those for domestic dogs, and the interval of administration should be increased (double than recommended for domestics).[33]

In anteaters, surgery is mostly performed to treat trauma. The most common surgery is onychectomy for trauma caused by improper restraint, inadequate floors, poor substrates, or intraspecific aggression. Trauma may also result in tail-tip fractures or rectal or vaginal prolapse.

High parasite loads leading to weight loss require treatment with fenbendazole (25–50 mg/kg), ivermectin (0.2 mg/kg, subcutaneously [SC], one dose), pyrantel pamoate (10–20 mg/kg) or praziquantel (5 mg/kg).[35]

REPRODUCTION

Reproductive parameters for selected armadillo species are given in Table 39-1. Successful captive breeding of armadillos is uncommon and limited to a few species. Preovulatory genital hemorrhages occur in some species such as *Chaetophractus villosus* and *Tolypeutes matacus* but not in others such as *Dasypus novemcinctus*. At least one species, *Zaedyus pichiy*, is suspected to have induced ovulation.[51] Gestation often remains unnoticed. Radiography, regular weight checks, ultrasonography, and observation of behavioral changes are unreliable methods for pregnancy diagnosis. Fecal hormone analysis is a viable alternative, but fecal progestogen levels remain basal during the first half of pregnancy at least in some species.[51] Wild armadillos give birth inside their burrows, and the offspring do not leave the den until weaned. Captive females should be given the opportunity to dig their burrow or offered a nest box. Females are highly susceptible to external disturbances; stress may suppress ovulation, lead to abortions or induce females to neglect, injure or kill their newborn.

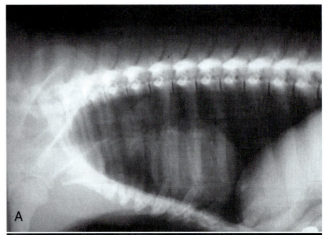
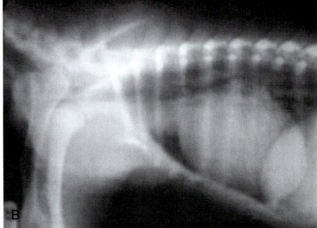

FIGURE 39-3 A, Lateral right recumbent radiograph of a clinically healthy giant anteater (*Myrmecophaga tridactyla*) with mild cardiomegaly secondary to dilatory cardiomyopathy associated with taurine deficiency. **B,** Lateral right recumbent radiograph of a giant anteater (*Myrmecophaga tridactyla*) with severe cardiomegaly secondary to dilatory cardiomyopathy associated with taurine deficiency. The cardiac ejection fraction of the first animal (**A**) was above 50% while the second animal's (**B**) was of 30%. Animal B was in severe failure and died 2 days after this image was taken. (Photograph by R. Aguilar.)

TABLE 39-9

Antibiotic Agents Used in Xenarthra

Generic Name	Taxon	Dose (mg/kg)	Route of Administration	Frequency, Duration	Comments
Amoxicillin	Sloths	10–11	IM, PO	SID, 5 days	
	Anteaters	10	IM, PO	SID–TID, 5 days	Respiratory infections—first choice
Ampicillin	Armadillos	10–20	IM	TID, 5–10 days	
	Sloths	10–20	IM, IV	BID, 5–8 days	IV; effective in septicemia
	Anteaters	10–20	IM	BID, 7–10 days	Dermatitis and pneumonia
Ceftiofur sodium	Anteaters	2.2–4.4	IM	SID–BID, 5 days	Dermatitis and pneumonia
Chloramphenicol	Armadillos	25–75 50–100	IM	BID, 10 days	Bacterial enteritis Pneumonia
	Anteaters	20–100	IM	BID, 7 days	Dermatitis and pneumonia
Doxycycline	Anteaters	5	PO	BID, 5–10 days	Broad spectrum
Enrofloxacin	Armadillos	1.25	IM, PO	BID, 5 days	Hypersensitivity reaction reported in *Z. pichiy*
		2.5–5	IM	SID, 5 days	Generalized or systemic infections

TABLE 39-9

Antibiotic Agents Used in Xenarthra—cont'd

Generic Name	Taxon	Dose (mg/kg)	Route of Administration	Frequency, Duration	Comments
		10	IM	SID, 12 days	*Salmonella* sp. infections
	Sloths	2.5–3.5	IM	SID	Respiratory and urogenital problems
	Anteaters	2.5	IM, PO	SID, 5 days	Broad spectrum
Penicillin G benzatinic and penicillin G procaine	Armadillos	40,000 IU	IM	SID, 5–10 days	
	Anteaters	50,000 IU followed by 10,000 IU	IM, SC	SID, 5–10 days	Can be used as preventive treatment during bacterial culture and while awaiting sensitivity results
Trimethoprim-sulfamethoxazole	Armadillos	15	IM	SID, 5 days	
	Sloths	15–40	IM	SID, 7–10 days	Pneumonia
	Anteaters	15	PO	BID, 3–5 days	Gastrointestinal infections—first choice
		15	IM	SID, 3–5 days	Bone marrow hypoplasia reported in juvenile *T. tetradactyla*

BID, Twice daily; *IM*, intramuscularly; *IU*, international unit; *IV*, intravenously; *mg/kg*, milligram per kilogram; *PO*, orally; *SC*, subcutaneously; *SID*, once daily; *TID*, three times daily.
From references: 15, 17, 23, 26, 34, and 54; Rojas Moreno, personal communication; Brieva, personal communication.

TABLE 39-10

Miscellaneous Drugs Used in Xenarthra

Generic Name	Taxon	Dose (mg/kg)	Route of Administration	Frequency, Duration	Comments
Albuterol sulfate	Sloths	0.042% inhalation solution	Nebulization by facemask	3 mL over 30 minutes	Decongestant or expectorant
Bromhexine	Sloths	0.6	PO	SID, 5–7 days	Decongestant or expectorant
Dexamethasone	Armadillos	0.4	IM	Once	Shock therapy
	Sloths	0.3–0.6	IM	SID, 4 days	Respiratory problems
	Anteaters	2	IM	Once	Shock therapy
Doxapram	Sloths	2–4	IM	Once	Apnea, complications to gas anesthesia
	Anteaters	1–4	IM	SID, 5–10 days	Apnea; anesthetic complications
Flunixin meglumine	Armadillos	2.5	SC	SID, 3 days	Analgesia
	Sloths	1	SC	SID, 3 days	Analgesia, gastrointestinal tract disorders (colic)
	Anteaters	1	SC	SID, 3–5 days	Analgesia, gastrointestinal tract disorders (colic)
Ivermectin	Sloths	0.14	SC	Once or twice a week during 3–4 weeks	Sarcoptic mange
Ketoprofen	Anteaters	1–2	IM	SID, 3–5 days	Anti-inflammatory therapy
Meloxicam	Sloths	0.05–0.1	IM	Q48h, 3–4 doses	Analgesia, anti-inflammatory therapy
Simethicone suspension or tablets	Sloths	50–100 total dose	PO with food	BID to TID	Bloat and overfermentation
Tramadol	Armadillos	0.5	IM	SID–BID	Analgesia May cause anorexia, gastrointestinal tract problems
Vitamin K	Anteaters	5–10 mg	IM	SID, repeat for 1 week	Hypovitaminosis K, coagulation disorders

BID, Twice daily; *IM*, intramuscularly; *IV*, intravenously; *mg/kg*, milligram per kilogram; *mL*, milliliter; *PO*, orally; *Q48h*, four times in 48 hours; *SC*, subcutaneously; *SID*, once daily; *TID*, three times daily.
From references: 17, 23, 26, 34; Superina, unpublished; Aguilar, unpublished; Rojas Moreno, personal communication; Brieva, personal communication.

Offspring mortality may be up to 100% in the presence of males. Therefore, the latter must be separated from the dam prior to birth.[53]

In sloths and anteaters, captive breeding is complicated because of incorrect sexing and the absence of visible behavioral or morphologic signs of estrus. Testes are intraabdominal. Male sloths have a small penis with a small, round opening. The external genitalia of female sloths are smaller than the penis, bear a slit along their length, and are closer to the rectal opening.[25] No changes occur in genital appearance or secretions at the onset of estrus.[24] Reproductive parameters for sloths are given in Table 39-2. Captive breeding has been successful in *Choloepus* but not in *Bradypus*. Infant mortality is extremely high during lactation because of dam rejection or falls.[53] Pregnancy detection, although difficult, has been possible through ultrasonography and radiography. Fecal hormone analyses may be an alternative but require validation.

External genitalia in giant and lesser anteaters are similar to those of sloths. Preovulatory genital bleeding has been reported in *Tamandua* and *Myrmecophaga*, but it is not always recognized. Vaginal cytology may be used for estrous cycle determination in trained giant anteaters.[34] Pregnancy may be detected through fecal hormone analyses or transabdominal ultrasonography. In *Myrmecophaga*, mounting may occur even a few days prior to parturition. The first postpartum estrus occurs during the second half of the lactation period. Spontaneous abortions of unknown etiology or related to hormonal imbalance are common. Stillbirths, incorrect maternal behavior, and male aggression reduce juvenile survival rates to 50%.[34,47] Reproductive parameters for anteaters are given in Table 39-2.

ACKNOWLEDGMENT

The authors thank Claudia Brieva, MV, MSc.; Lizette Bermúdez Larrazábal, Blg., MSc.; Gianmarco Rojas Moreno, MV Esp. MSc.(c); Tiffany Wolf, DVM; and Flávia Miranda, MV, MSc. for their substantial contributions to this manuscript.

REFERENCES

1. Benirschke K: Reproductive parameters and placentation in anteaters and sloths. In Vizcaíno SF, Loughry WJ, editors: *The biology of the Xenarthra*, Gainesville, FL, 2008, University Press of Florida.
2. Bermúdez Larrazábal L: Adaptación al cautiverio del serafín del platanar (*Cyclopes didactylus*). Edentata 12:45, 2011.
3. Brown D: Fruit-eating by an obligate insectivore: Palm fruit consumption in wild northern tamanduas (*Tamandua mexicana*) in Panama. Edentata 12:63, 2011.
4. Burns TA, Waldrip EB: Body temperature and electrocardiographic data for the nine-banded armadillo (*Dasypus novemcinctus*). J Mammal 52:472, 1971.
5. Casanave EB, Polini NN: Comparative study of some haematological parameters of two wild *Chaetophractus villosus* (Mammalia, Dasypodidae) populations. Comp Haematol Int 9:13, 1999.
6. Chiarello AG: Sloth ecology: an overview of field studies. In Vizcaíno SF, Loughry WJ, editors: *The biology of the Xenarthra*, Gainesville, FL, 2008, University Press of Florida.
7. Coppo JA, Quiroz L, Millan S, et al: Valores hemáticos del armadillo *Dasypus* spp. Gaceta Veterinaria (Buenos Aires) 41:493, 1979.
8. Corrêa Vaz V, Santori RT, Jansen AM, et al: Notes on food habits of armadillos (Cingulata: Dasypodidae) and anteaters (Pilosa: Myrmecophagidae) at Serra da Capivara National Park (Piauí State, Brazil). Edentata 13:84, 2012.
9. Cuba-Caparó A: Some hematologic and temperature determinations in the 7-banded armadillo (*Dasypus hybridus*). Lab Anim Sci 26:450, 1976.
10. D'Addamio GH, Walsh GP, Harris L, et al: Hematologic parameters for wild and captive nine-banded armadillos (*Dasypus novemcinctus*). Lab Anim Sci 28:607, 1978.
11. Day JF, Storrs EE, Stark LM, et al: Antibodies to St. Louis encephalitis virus in armadillos from southern Florida. J Wildl Dis 31:10, 1995.
12. Deem SL, Fiorello CV: Capture and immobilization of free-ranging edentates. In Heard D, editor: *Zoological restraint and anesthesia*, Ithaca, NY, 2002, International Veterinary Information Service.
13. Deem SL, Noss AJ, Fiorello CV, et al: Health assessment of free-ranging three-banded (*Tolypeutes matacus*) and nine-banded (*Dasypus novemcinctus*) armadillos in the Gran Chaco, Bolivia. J Zoo Wildl Med 40:245, 2009.
14. Delsuc F, Douzery EJP: Recent advances and future prospects in xenarthran molecular phylogenetics. In Vizcaíno SF, Loughry WJ, editors: *The biology of the Xenarthra*, Gainesville, FL, 2008, University Press of Florida.
15. Diniz LS, Costa EO, Oliveira PM: Clinical disorders in armadillos (Dasypodidae, Edentata) in captivity. Zbl Vet Med B 44:577, 1997.
16. Diniz LS, Oliveira PM: Clinical problems of sloths (*Bradypus* sp. and *Choloepus* sp.) in captivity. J Zoo Wildl Med 30:76, 1999.
17. Diniz LSM, Costa EO, Oliveira PMA: Clinical disorders observed in anteaters (Myrmecophagidae, Edentata) in captivity. Vet Res Commun 19:409, 1995.
18. Divers BJ: Edentates. In Fowler ME, editor: *Zoo and wild animal medicine*, ed 2, Philadelphia, PA, 1978, W.B. Saunders.
19. Emmons LH: *Neotropical rainforest mammals. A field guide*, ed 2, Chicago, IL, 1997, The University of Chicago Press.
20. Fournier-Chambrillon C, Fournier P, Vié JC: Immobilization of wild collared anteaters with ketamine and xylazine hydrochloride. J Wildl Dis 33:795, 1997.
21. Fournier-Chambrillon C, Vogel I, Fournier P, et al: Immobilization of free-ranging nine-banded armadillos and great long-nosed armadillos with three anesthetic combinations. J Wildl Dis 36:131, 2000.
22. Gaudin TJ, McDonald HG: Morphology-based investigations of the phylogenetic relationships among extant and fossil xenarthrans. In Vizcaíno SF, Loughry WJ, editors: *The biology of the Xenarthra*, Gainesville, FL, 2008, University Press of Florida.
23. Gillespie DS: Edentata: Diseases. In Fowler ME, editor: *Zoo and wild animal medicine*, ed 3, Philadelphia, PA, 1993, Saunders.
24. Gilmore DP, Da Costa CP, Duarte DPF: An update on the physiology of two and three toed sloths. Braz J Med Biol Res 33:129, 2000.
25. Gilmore DP, Duarte DF, Da Costa CP: The physiology of two- and three-toed sloths. In Vizcaíno SF, Loughry WJ, editors: *The biology of the Xenarthra*, Gainesville, FL, 2008, University Press of Florida.
26. Hammond EE, Sosa R, Beckerman R, et al: Respiratory disease associated with *Bordetella bronchiseptica* in a two-toed Hoffman's sloth (*Choloepus hoffmanni*). J Wildl Dis 40:369, 2009.
27. Hanley C, Siudak-Campfield J, Paul-Murphy J, et al: Immobilization of free-ranging Hoffmann's two-toed and brown-throated three-toed sloths using ketamine and medetomodine: a comparison of physiologic parameters. J Wildl Dis 44:938, 2008.
28. Hayssen V: *Bradypus torquatus* (Pilosa: Bradypodidae). Mammalian Species 829:1, 2009.
29. Maldonado EN, Casanave EB: Proteínas séricas y proteinograma electroforético de *Chaetophractus villosus* (Mammalia, Dasypodidae). Proceedings, VIII Jornadas Argentinas de Mastozoología, Bariloche, 1993.
30. McKenzie A, Ernst G, Taranu Z: *Behavioural studies and rehabilitation of sloths in Parque Natural Metropolitano*, Washington, DC, 2005, Smithsonian Tropical Research Institute.
31. McNab BK: Energetics, population biology, and distribution of Xenarthrans, living and extinct. In Montgomery GG, editor: *The evolution and ecology of armadillos, sloths, and vermilinguas*, Washington, DC, and London, U.K., 1985, Smithsonian Institution Press.
32. Merrett PK: *Edentates: Project for city and guilds animal management course*, Guernsey Channel Islands, 1983, The Zoological Trust of Guernsey.
33. Messias-Costa A, Beresca AM, Cassaro K, et al: Chapter 24: Order Xenarthra (Edentata) (Sloths, armadillos, anteaters). In Fowler ME, Cubas ZS, editors: *Biology, medicine, and surgery of South American wild animals*, Ames, IA, 2001, Iowa State University Press.
34. Miranda F: *Manutenção de tamanduás em cativeiro*, São Carlos, Brazil, 2012, Editora Cubo.
35. Miranda FR, Costa AM: Xenarthras (tamanduás, tatu e preguiça). In Cubas ZS, Silva JCR, Dias JL, editors: *Tratado de animais selvagens: medicina veterinária*, São Paulo, Brazil, 2007, Roca.
36. Montgomery GG: Movements, foraging and food habits of the four extant species of neotropical vermilinguas (Mammalia; Myrmecophagidae). In

Montgomery GG, editor: *The evolution and ecology of armadillos, sloths, and vermilinguas*, Washington, DC, and London, U.K., 1985, Smithsonian Institution Press.

37. Orozco MM: Inmovilización química de armadillos de tres bandas (*Tolypeutes matacus*) mediante el uso de dos protocolos anestésicos en el Norte Argentino. *Edentata* 12:1, 2011.

38. Polini NN, Casanave EB: Estudio de algunos parámetros bioquímicos de una población salvaje de *Chaetophractus villosus* (Mammalia, Dasypodidae). Proceedings, XIV Jornadas Argentinas de Mastozoología, Salta, 1999.

39. Polini NN, Casanave EB: Estudio poblacional de algunos parámetros de la hemostasia primaria en *Chaetophractus villosus* (Mammalia, Dasypodidae). Proceedings, XIV Jornadas Argentinas de Mastozoología, Salta, 1999.

40. Purtilo DT, Walsh GP, Storrs EE, et al: The immune system of the nine-banded armadillo (*Dasypus novemcinctus*, Linn). *Anat Rec* 181:725, 1975.

41. Ramsey PR, Tyler DFJ, Waddill JR, et al: Blood chemistry and nutritional balance of wild and captive armadillos (*Dasypus novemcinctus* L.). *Comp Biochem Physiol A Comp Physiol* 69A:517, 1981.

42. Rappaport AB, Hochman H: Cystic calculi as a cause of recurrent rectal prolapse in a sloth, *Choloepus* sp. *J Zoo Anim Med* 19:235, 1988.

43. Redford KH: Food habits of armadillos (Xenarthra: Dasypodidae). In Montgomery GG, editor: *The evolution and ecology of armadillos, sloths, and vermilinguas*, Washington, DC, and London, U.K., 1985, Smithsonian Institution Press.

44. Rodrigues FH, Medri IM, de Miranda GHB, et al: Anteater behavior and ecology. In Vizcaíno SF, Loughry WJ, editors: *The biology of the Xenarthra*, Gainesville, FL, 2008, University Press of Florida.

45. Rojas G: Contención farmacológica de perezosos de dos dedos *Choloepus hoffmanni* (Peters, 1858) mediante el uso de ketamina, dexmedetomidina y midazolam, y reversión con atipamezol. *Edentata* 12:20, 2011.

46. Rojas Moreno G: Use of dexmedetomidine, midazolam, ketamine and reversal with atipamezole for chemical immobilization of giant anteaters (*Myrmecophaga tridactyla*), lesser anteaters (*Tamandua tetradactyla*) and silky anteaters (*Cyclopes didactylus*) kept in captivity. In *Proceedings of the American Association of Zoo Veterinarians*, Oakland, CA, 2012, American Association of Zoo Veterinarians.

47. Schauerte N: Untersuchungen zur Zyklus- und Graviditätsdiagnostik beim Grossen Ameisenbären (*Myrmecophaga tridactyla*), doctoral thesis, Giessen, Germany, 2005, Justus-Liebig-Universität.

48. Sibaja-Morales K, de Oliveira J, Jimenez Rocha A, et al: Gastrointestinal parasites and ectoparasites of *Bradypus variegatus* and *Choloepus hoffmanni* sloths from Costa Rica. *J Zoo Wildl Med* 40:86, 2009.

49. Stuart BP, Crowell WA, Adams WV, et al: Spontaneous renal disease in Louisiana armadillos (*Dasypus novemcinctus*). *J Wildl Dis* 13:240, 1977.

50. Superina M, Boily P: Hibernation and daily torpor in an armadillo, the pichi (*Zaedyus pichiy*). *Comp Biochem Physiol A Comp Physiol* 148:893, 2007.

51. Superina M, Carreño N, Jahn G: Characterization of seasonal reproduction patterns in female pichis, *Zaedyus pichiy* (Xenarthra: Dasypodidae) estimated by fecal sex steroid metabolites and ovarian histology. *Anim Reprod Sci* 116:358, 2009.

52. Superina M, Mera y Sierra R: Hematology and serum chemistry values in captive and wild pichis, *Zaedyus pichiy* (Mammalia, Dasypodidae). *J Wildl Dis* 44:902, 2008.

53. Superina M, Miranda F, Plese T: Maintenance of Xenarthra in captivity. In Vizcaíno SF, Loughry WJ, editors: *The biology of the Xenarthra*, Gainesville, FL, 2008, University Press of Florida.

54. Superina M: Biologie und Haltung von Gürteltieren (*Dasypodidae*), doctoral thesis, Zurich, Switzerland, 2000, Universität Zürich.

55. Taube E, Keravec J, Vié JC, et al: Reproductive biology and postnatal development in sloths, *Bradypus* and *Choloepus*: Review with original data from the field (French Guiana) and from captivity. *Mammal Rev* 31:173, 2001.

56. Vogel I, de Thoisy B, Vié JC: Comparison of injectable anesthetic combinations in free-ranging two-toed sloths in French Guiana. *J Wildl Dis* 34:556, 1998.

57. Vogel I, Vié JC, de Thoisy B, et al: Hematological and serum chemistry profiles of free-ranging southern two-toed sloths in French Guiana. *J Wildl Dis* 35:531, 1999.

58. West G, Carter TS, Shaw J: Edentates (Xenarthra). In West G, Heard DJ, Caulkett N, editors: *Zoo animal and wildlife immobilization and anesthesia*, Ames, IA, 2007, Blackwell Publishing.

59. Wetzel RM: Taxonomy and distribution of armadillos, *Dasypodidae*. In Montgomery GG, editor: *The evolution and ecology of armadillos, sloths, and vermilinguas*, Washington, DC, and London, U.K., 1985, Smithsonian Institution Press.

60. Wetzel RM: The identification and distribution of recent *Xenarthra* (=*Edentata*). In Montgomery GG, editor: *The evolution and ecology of armadillos, sloths, and vermilinguas*, Washington, DC, and London, U.K., 1985, Smithsonian Institution Press.

Pholidota

Jason Shih-Chien Chin and Eric Hsienshao Tsao

INTRODUCTION AND IDENTIFICATION

This small order has one extant family (Manidae) and eight species (Table 40-1). The Chinese pangolin (*Manis pentadactyla*), the Sunda or Malayan pangolin (*M. javanica*), the Philippine pangolin (*M. culioensis*), and the Indian or thick-tailed pangolin (*M. crassicaudata*) are prevalent in Asia, whereas Africa is inhabited by the Cape or Temminck's ground pangolin (*M. temminckii*), the giant ground pangolin or giant pangolin (*M. gigantea*), the tree pangolin or African white-bellied pangolin (*M. tricuspis*), and the long-tailed or black-bellied pangolin (*M. tetradactyla*).[5] The Asian species are distinguished from the African species by the presence of hair between the scales.

BIOLOGIC DATA

Anatomy

Pangolins attain a weight of 2 to 35 kilograms (kg) (Table 40-1). Head-and-body length is 300 to 880 millimeters (mm) and tail length 350 to 880 mm.[16] Males are somewhat larger than females. The dorsal surface of the elongate, tapering body is covered with scales composed of cornified epidermis, and the scales overlap in adults but not in the newborns (Figure 40-1). When in danger, pangolins are able to roll into a tight, almost impregnable ball, with only the hard, scaly parts of the body exposed. The scales are attached at the base to the thick skin from which they grow. Scales grow constantly from the base to compensate for wear. Scale pattern, size, shape and number are species characteristic and remain constant through life. The skin is sparsely haired between scales and on the abdomen.

The pangolin's tubular head has a small, toothless mouth, which contains an astoundingly long, sticky tongue. The tongue is 16 to 40 centimeters (cm) in length. In a resting state, the tongue is drawn into its sheath in the chest cavity and connecting with the inner part of xiphisternum. A pair of salivary glands extends from the ventral side of the neck almost to the shoulder. Teeth are lacking, and the lower jawbones are represented by flimsy shafts of bones (Figure 40-2). The small eyes are surrounded by thick lids that provide protection against the bites of ants and termites.

All pangolins have short powerful legs with strong, curved claws. The hindlimbs are long and stouter compared with the forelimbs, and all the limbs have five digits. The central three claws of the forelimbs are much enlarged and are used for digging and breaking open ant and termite nests; they are not used as weapons.

The large stomach is similar in function to the avian gizzard; it is muscular and provided with horny, laminated epithelium. The stomach of the pangolin contains a number of unique anatomic and

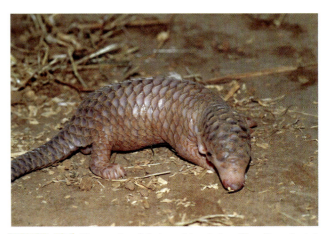

FIGURE 40-1 **The scale of 3-day-old cub is still soft and pink.** (From Chin SC, Lien CY, Chan YT, et al: Monitoring the gestation period of rescued formosan pangolin [*Manis pentadactyla pentadactyla*] with progesterone radioimmunoassay. *Zoo Biol* 31 : 479–489, 2012a.)

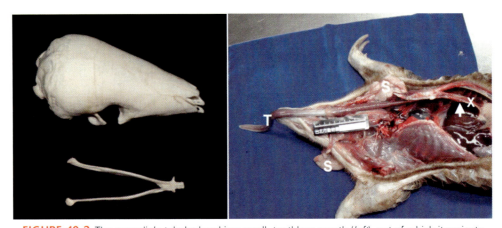

FIGURE 40-2 The pangolin's tubular head is a small, toothless mouth (*left*), out of which it projects an astoundingly long, sticky tongue. The tongue is 16 to 40 cm in length. A pair of salivary glands (*S*) is present at the ventral side of the neck. In the resting state, the tongue is drawn into its sheath in the chest cavity, and the base connects with the medial side (*white arrow*) of the xiphisternum (*X*).

TABLE 40-1

Basic Data for Eight Species of Pangolin

Distribution	Species	Body Weight	Head and Body Length	Tail Length	Common Name
African	*Manis tetradactyla*	2–3 kilograms (kg)	30–40 centimeters (cm)	60–70 cm	Long-tailed pangolin, black-bellied pangolin
	Manis temminckii	2–4 kg	40–70 cm	40–70 cm	Cape pangolin
	Manis gigantea	Up to 33 kg	Up to 180 cm	?	Giant pangolin
	Manis tricuspis	1–2 kg	46 cm	?	Tree pangolin
Asian	*Manis pentadactyla*	Male: up to 9 kg Female: up to 6–7 kg	42–92 cm	28–35 cm	Chinese pangolin
	Manis javanica	Up to 10 kg	Up to 65 cm	Up to 56 cm	Malayan pangolin
	Manis crassicaudata	5–35 kg	45–75 cm	33–45 cm	Indian pangolin, thick-tailed pangolin
	Manis culioensis	Up to 2.7 kg	32–54 cm	29–50cm	Palawan pangolin

histologic characteristics. Previous studies of the stomach of *M. pentadactyla* have reported the structure of the gastric gland and "pyloric teeth."[7]

The stomach of pangolins is C-shaped, with short lesser curvature. At the esophageal junction, the inner smooth muscle is thickened on the greater curvature side. Instead of a mucus-secreting cellular layer, the entire luminal surface of the pangolin stomach is lined with a thick cornified, stratified squamous epithelium, except at the orifices of glands and in the pyloric gland region. The wall of the fundus is thin and devoid of glands. The gastric glands consist of mucus, oxyntic, and pyloric glands. The mucous glands are observed in the lesser curvature, in the greater curvature, and in the pyloric canal, respectively. No sphincter exists at the pyloric–duodenal junction. In the lumen of the pyloric canal region, numerous spines and small pebbles may be observed. The muscle layers in the wall of this region are considerably thickened.[10]

Normal droppings are black or brown in color, dry, and sausage shaped. The white-bellied tree pangolin defecates anywhere; and the Cape and Chinese pangolins bury their dung in scrapes in the ground. The pangolin anus is surrounded by a cluster of large, bean-shaped glands that secrete a noxious fluid used for defense purposes.

BEHAVIOR

Pangolins are largely nocturnal. Although a given species is primarily arboreal or terrestrial, none is restricted to a single plan of locomotion. Pangolins are powerful burrowers and swim adequately. They spend the day in forks or hollows in trees. Arboreal species have prehensile tails to better hold their body positions in trees. Terrestrial species dig a burrow with a terminal den, in which they pass the daylight hours and give birth. The occupant may plug the burrow entrance with dirt.

When walking on all fours, the long front digging claws are curled under, and the animal walks on its knuckles. Pangolins occasionally walk on their hindlimbs, using the tail as a brace. Normally slow and deliberate, an alarmed pangolin will either make for its burrow or curl into an armor-plated ball, twitching its sharp-edged scales to ward off predators. Such a ball is almost impossible for a human to unroll. A predator successful in uncoiling a pangolin may be greeted by a pungent spray of urine or rancid fluid from the glands surrounding the anus.

With their strict nocturnal activity pattern, pangolins never leave the nest box before 4 P.M. in zoologic exhibitions. Over a 10- to 11-hour period, the animals emerge and return to the nest box intermittently, and their active period ends by 02:00 A.M. The length of time when a pangolin remains outside the nest box varies from 30 seconds to 1.5 hours. individual differences exist in the total amount of time spent out of the nest box on any given night. The percentage of the 24-hour day spent outside the nest box averages 5.6% with a range of 2.9% to 7.6%. While in the nest box, pangolins are either coiled as individuals or curled up around each other to sleep. This may provide an important thermoregulatory function to reduce the area of exposed surface per unit body mass and thereby conserve heat. No aggressive behavior has ever been observed in pangolins.[6]

HUSBANDRY

The oldest specimen recorded in captivity is a confiscated male Chinese pangolin, which lived up to 20 years in the Ueno Zoo. Over 70% rescued sick pangolins did not survive their first year in captivity, but the average has been increasing from less than 90 days to more than 1 year.[18] From 2005 to date, 10 pangolins have survived over 5 years and still live well in the Taipei Zoo. One of the Chinese pangolins born in captivity at the Taipei Zoo in 1998 has survived for over 14 years now.

Housing

According to the long-term case studies on maintaining Chinese pangolins, indoor pens measured $120 \times 120 \times 80$ square centimeters (cm^3) and filled to a depth of 10 cm, with a mixture of sterilized dirt and wood shavings as substrate, have been recommended for each pangolin in captivity. A wooden nest box ($40 \times 60 \times 50$ cm^3) divided into two compartments, with similar mixture of dirt and wood shavings substrate for bedding, is placed in each indoor pen.[3] Room temperature is controlled so as to not exceed 28°C (82°F) in the summer and to range between 24°C and 26°C (75 °F–79°F) in the winter. Humidity is maintained at 80% to 100% and photoperiod at 10 hours per day with artificial light year round.[4] The enclosure with regulated temperature (26°C) and photoperiod (10–12 hours light) is important in spatial and thermal environment. When defecating and urinating, pangolins prefer to stand in corners on their hindlimbs, with their forelimbs against the wall. The nest box is used solely for sleeping and therefore must be a relatively clean, easily maintainable enclosure.[6]

FEEDING AND NUTRITION

In the wild, pangolins live on a diet of ants, termites, and various other invertebrates, including bee larvae, flies, worms, earthworms, and crickets, which may be quite difficult for zoos to provide in sufficient quantities. Pangolins in South Africa were reported to feed on 15 species of ants and 5 termite species, with no apparent preferences. All species of pangolins are thought to feed almost entirely on ants and termites. Different species of pangolins have different preferences for various prey species of ants and termites, which are located by scent. A giant pangolin was reported to have 2 liters (L) of 11 species of ants in its stomach. Other pangolins are said to be less catholic. A white-bellied tree pangolin may eat 150 to 200 grams (g) of termites nightly.[14] Quantities of sand and pebbles are ingested along with the insects. This material probably serves a function in the gizzardlike stomach, assisting in the crushing of the tough ant and termite exoskeletons.

A Chinese pangolin was kept at Ueno Zoo, Tokyo, for over 20 years, on a mixture composed of 150 g of ground horse meat, 180 milliliters (mL) of milk, 1 raw egg yolk, 5 g of precooked cereals, 5 g of Esbilac, 1 g of calcium, and 0.2 mL of multivitamins.[11] One Malayan pangolin had been kept at the San Diego Zoo on a blended mixture of 2 tablespoons of ground meat, 1 tablespoon of precooked cereal, 1 ounce (oz) of evaporated cow's milk, 2 oz of water, 1/4 of a raw egg yolk, 1/8 if a teaspoon of brewer's yeast, and 4 meal worms. Four tablespoons were fed twice daily, with the addition of 2 drops of liquid multivitamins in the morning feed.[18]

Increasing the volume of high-protein insects as well as multivitamin and mineral supplements may improve the pangolin's appetite as well as diet palatability, and the animals may become adapted to captive feeding more rapidly (Table 40-2). Since the development of a new diet in 1995, the Taipei Zoo has collected and maintained many pangolins that have lived longer and experienced fewer digestive problems.[18] The addition of a small amount of soil was identified to stabilize fecal flora and helped in the formation of solid feces. Diet passage time could be prolonged from 24 to 48 hours to over 142 hours. Food digestibility was increased from 68% to 82%. The prevalence of hemorrhagic gastric ulcer and enteritis declined significantly.[3] These diets may be fed by placing the mixture in a heavy, flat bowl. The animals lick the food off the bowl. This feeding technique prevents the animal from consuming bedding material or turning the bowl over. Drinking water should be constantly available. Some pangolins appear to enjoy a mud wallow or a spray from a hose.

RESTRAINT

Most pangolins may be handled by grasping the tail or by supporting the curled up animal with outspread hands. The use of leather gloves

TABLE 40-2

Daily Formula for Formosan Pangolin at the Taipei Zoo

Feed	Unit	Amount
Bee larvae	Gram (g)	100
Apple	g	65
Mealworms	g	22.5
Mazuri Insectivore Diet*	g	7.5
Egg yolk	g	10
Mix powder†	g	5–10
Vitamin and mineral supplement‡	g	1.5
Chitin	g	10
Water	Milliliter (mL)	60
Vitamin K	g	1/15
Soil	g	5

*Mazuri 5MK8 Catalog #0050819, from PMI Nutrition International, LLC (Land O'Lakes Purina Feed, LLC), USA.
†Mix powder = coconut powder 300 g + yeast powder 600 g + calcium carbonate 100 g.
‡Vitamin and Mineral Supplement for Pig, China Chemical & Pharmaceutical Co., LD, Taiwan.

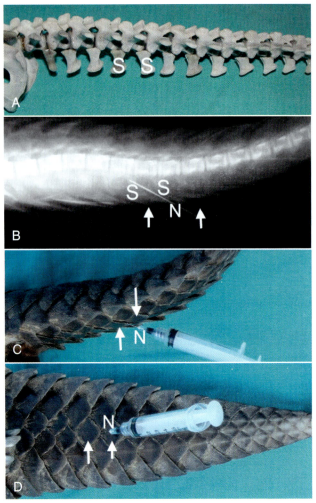

FIGURE 40-3 A, Anatomy of ventral spine (*S*) of coccyx of pangolin. **B,** Lateral view radiograph image of a pangolin's tail. The needle (*N*) has penetrated between the scales (*white arrow*) and has entered the space between the ventral spines (*S*) of the coccyx, where the tail vein existed. **C,** Lateral view of the needle (*N*) inserted. **D,** Ventral site of the needle (*N*) inserted.

may be advisable. If a pangolin is intent on rolling into a ball, it may be difficult to uncoil the animal adequately for examination. The technique for proper physical restraint is to grasp the tail and lift the pangolin in midair. Then it is shaken gently to encourage it to stretch its body. This technique may be used for blood sampling and for administering drugs by injection. After capture, administration of ketamine (10–20 milligram per kilogram [mg/kg]), zoletil (3–5 mg/kg), intramuscularly (IM), allows for short examinations; 5% isoflurane has been used for inducing anesthesia in an induction box and can be followed by administration of 1% to 2% isoflurane via a face mask to maintain for surgical or medical procedures (e.g., amputation of leg or tail, endoscopic and ultrasonographic examinations). Meanwhile, atropine (0.04 mg/kg), subcutaneously (SC), is recommended for salivation control. Trachea intubation has been impossible in pangolins so far.

PHYSIOLOGIC DATA

The body temperature of the pangolins is 32.2 to 35.20° C.[6] Blood samples may be collected when the animal is physically restrained stably, and a 23-gauge 1¼-inch needle may be inserted into the tail vein (not visible) to a depth of more than 2 cm from the ventral side of the tail (Figure 40-3).[3] Some hematology (Table 40-3) and serum biochemistry (Table 40-4) parameters have been identified in Chinese pangolins only (Chin, unpublished).

DISEASES

Survival rates are generally low among captive pangolins. Necropsy reports of 62 Formosan pangolins, mainly from rescue programs based at the Taipei Zoo, were reviewed retrospectively. The male-to-female ratio of cases was 2 : 1. The most commonly observed lesions were found in the lungs (72.5%), followed by the alimentary tracts (67.7%) and the liver (54.8%). Gross lesions of the heart (40.3%), kidneys (30.6%), and genitalia (1.6%) were found less frequently. Also, foreign body obstructions were observed in 3.2% of the cases. In 51.6% of the cases, lesions were found in both the lungs and the alimentary tracts. Significant differences in causes of death between males and females are found only with heart lesions.[4]

Hemorrhagic gastric ulcers with *enteritis* has been considered the major cause of death in rescued pangolins in captivity. Ranitidine (2 to 3 mg/kg) or cimetidine (5 to 10 mg/kg), twice daily (BID), orally (PO), may control early-stage gastric ulcers for 2 weeks. Sucralfate (5 to 10 mg/kg), PO, is administered with hydrogen antagonism on an empty stomach, at least 1 hour prior to meals, for best results in severe cases. Antibiotic therapy for secondary infection prevention is also recommended. Stress and malnutrition had been suspected to be major factors in the past. However, according to a report, an improper diet formula, combined with stress, may have induced nonspecific changes in the microflora in the digestive tract and caused hemorrhagic enteritis in captive pangolins.[1] Routine addition of soil in the daily diet may decrease the prevalence of hemorrhagic gastric ulcer and enteritis.

Infectious respiratory diseases are serious because of its high mortality and morbidity. Clinical syndromes include a runny nose, panting, and dysphagia; in one case, trembling and ataxia were seen at the end stage.[2] Positive results of canine distemper virus (CDV) antibody immunohistochemical stain of tissue blocks in pangolins are considered primary evidences of CDV infection, but no gene has been identified successfully yet. However, positive lesions of CDV have been found in the lungs, digestive tracts, and brains of

TABLE 40-3

Hematologic Parameters for Healthy Formosa Pangolin (*Manis pentadactyla pentadactyla*)

Parameter (unit)	n	Mean ± Standard Deviation	Range (H)*	Range (L)†
White blood cells (10^9/liter [L])	50	7.53 ± 2.08	13.20	3.30
Hemoglobin, gram per deciliter (g/dL)	50	14.24 ± 2.34	18.60	8.30
Hematocrit (%)	50	39.09 ± 6.63	55.30	23.50
Red blood cells (10^{12}/L)	50	5.67 ± 1.03	8.62	3.50
Mean corpuscular volume (%)	50	69.3 ± 5.06	82.30	58.60
Mean corpuscular hemoglobin, picogram per cell (pg/cell)	50	25.24 ± 1.97	28.90	20.10
Mean corpuscular hemoglobin concentration, gram per liter (g/L)	50	36.46 ± 1.17	38.60	31.30
Platelets (10^{12}/L)	50	228.06 ± 136.54	563.00	58.00

*The highest range of data was collected.
†The lowest range of data was collected.
(Chin, unpublished data).

TABLE 40-4

Serum Biochemistry Values for Healthy Formosa Pangolin (*Manis pentadactyla pentadactyla*)

Parameter (unit)	n	Mean ± Standard Deviation	Range (H)*	Range (L)†
Total protein, gram per deciliter (g/dL)	51	7.46 ± 0.84	9.60	5.20
Albumin (g/dL)	50	3.66 ± 0.52	4.50	2.70
Serum glutamic-oxaloacetic transaminase (SGO-T), unit per liter (Unit/L)	32	23.91 ± 11.31	49.00	4.00
Serum glutamic pyruvic transaminase (SGP-T) (Unit/L)	51	156.43 ± 99.81	528.00	46.00
Bilirubin-T, milligram per deciliter (mg/dL)	42	0.42 ± 0.42	1.80	0.10
Blood urea nitrogen (mg/dL)	51	31.95 ± 11.68	87.00	16.50
Creatinine (mg/dL)	51	0.38 ± 0.21	1.30	0.10
Uric acid (mg/dL)	19	0.52 ± 0.38	1.80	0.20
Glucose (mg/dL)	48	85.50 ± 38.55	180.00	34.00
Alkaline phosphatase (Unit/L)	48	209.06 ± 142.71	623.00	42.00
Cholesterol (mg/dL)	50	216.46 ± 88.97	426.00	104.00
Triglycerides (mg/dL)	17	127.53 ± 77.42	315.00	21.00
Amylase (Unit/L)	22	280.00 ± 105.14	538.00	148.00
Calcium (mg/dL)	41	10.64 ± 0.98	12.40	8.20
Phosphorus (mg/dL)	32	5.54 ± 1.06	7.30	4.10
Sodium, millimole per liter (mmol/L)	21	148.86 ± 3.24	156.00	144.00
Potassium (mmol/L)	21	4.94 ± 0.62	5.90	4.00
Chloride (mmol/L)	21	101.90 ± 2.81	107.00	95.00

*The highest range of data was collected.
†The lowest range of data was collected.
(Chin, unpublished data).

pangolins with clinical syndromes. Lesions were also identified in the spleens, testes, and kidneys of different animals.[2] Phylogenetic studies have identified that the pangolin is more closely related to felines than to other animals.[17] CDV infection is a contagious disease found in felids and canids. Stray dogs might be a major source of CDV, and infection may be caused by the population of stray dogs, which has been increasing intensively in exploited housing and farming areas near pangolin habitats in Taiwan.

Parasites may be found generally at the first fecal examination of wild pangolins. Parasitic diseases that have been reported include the tapeworms *Metadavainea aellini*, *Raillietina rahmi*, and *R. anoplocephaloides*. Niclosamide (Yomesan, 157 mg/kg, PO) may be effective against the most common platyhelminths. Large numbers of ova of round worms (*Strongyloides* sp.) and hookworms have been found in pangolin fecal samples. However, the species have not been positively identified. In a field surveillance study, *Ancylostoma* sp.,

Capillaria sp., *Strongyloides* sp. and *Eimeria* sp. were detected in a fecal sample from a Chinese pangolin. Necropsy findings from this animal revealed numerous unattached nematodes in the stomach and esophagus, measuring approximately 5 mm in length. Smaller, U-shaped, thin nematodes were encysted within the mesenteric fat and were also found free in large numbers within the peritoneum. All nematodes were identified as belonging to the genus *Cylicospirura*, but the species was not determined.[7] Thiabendazole (55 to 110 mg/kg active ingredient) or piperazine (88 to 110 mg/kg base).[12,13] No side effects to treatment with thiabendazole (approximately 59 mg/kg) were observed. Ivermectin or doramectin (0.2 mg/kg, SC) is currently recommended.

Biopsy of nodules from the face, ear pinna, groin, and penis of pangolins may reveal parasitic (filarial) dermatitis. Microscopic examinations of the tissue samples submitted have demonstrated extensive eosinophilic infiltration into the dermis, with a heavy

TABLE 40-5

Reproductive Characteristics of Pangolins

Species	Gestation Period	Sexual Maturity	Offspring	Maternal Care
Manis tetradactyla	140 days	Second year	1	?
Manis temminckii	139 days	?	1	?
Manis gigantea	?	?	1	?
Manis tricuspis	150 days.	?	1	?
Manis pentadactyla	318–372 days.	First year	1	5–6 months
Manis javanica	178 days	First year	1	3–4 months
Manis crassicaudata	65–70 days,	?	1 or 2	3 months
Manis culioensis	?	?	?	?

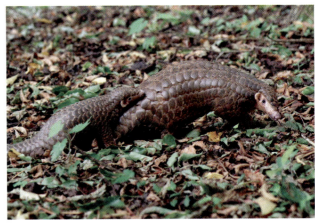

FIGURE 40-4 The young is carried on the back of the mother's tail. (From Chin SC, Lien CY, Chan YT, et al: Monitoring the gestation period of rescued formosan pangolin [*Manis pentadactyla pentadactyla*] with progesterone radioimmunoassay. *Zoo Biol* 31 : 479–489, 2012a.)

perivascular accumulation of eosinophils and lymphocytes. Occasional filarial nematodes, measuring approximately 5 mm in diameter, were seen within the inflammatory nodules. The perivascular inflammatory response suggested that the microfilaria were bloodborne. But species identification was not possible.[6]

When newly imported pangolins are received, they should be examined carefully for ticks (*Amblyomma testudinarium*) under the scales, as these animals are frequently infested. Some of these ticks may have artiodactyls co-hosts. Pangolins have responded to 10% lindane; however, lindane dust at 0.5% concentration should give satisfactory results.[6]

REPRODUCTION

Pangolins are normally solitary, but occasionally a male and a female may live together in the same burrow with their offspring. During copulation, the male mounts the female sideways and forces his genital area under hers. Most African and Asian pangolins give birth to a single young.

The existence of a specific breeding season of the Formosan pangolin (subspecies of the Chinese pangolin) is from September to February; births may occur in captivity from August to January. The gestation period of the Formosan pangolin is estimated to be from 318 to 372 days. The Formosan pangolin can reproduce only once a year.[3]

The gestation period, sexual maturity, and mother's care vary among the species of pangolins (Table 40-5).[15] Regardless of species, the pangolin newborn usually measures 12 to 30 cm in total length and weighs at least 100 to 336 g.[14] The newborn of the African tree pangolin weighs between 90 and 159 g. The newborns are active and well developed, their eyes are open at birth or within a few days, and they urinate and defecate unassisted. Their scales, soft at birth, gradually harden over the next few days. In arboreal species, the young are carried clinging near the base of the female's tail. In terrestrial species, the base of the tail is too wide, and the female stays in the burrow with the young for a time. The Indian pangolin newborn remains in the mother's burrow for 2 to 4 weeks.[9] The young is then carried out on the mother's back or tail outside, where it remains until it is weaned after 3 months.

When the female pangolin sleeps or is alarmed, it curls tightly around the young and defends it vigorously. The mother lies on its back or side to nurse from the single pair of pectoral mammary glands.[14] The newborn is nursed by the mother for 5 to 6 months and accompanies the mother on foraging bouts riding on the base of the tail (Figure 40-4).

The mammary glands of a female Chinese pangolin at the Ueno Zoo dried up 86 days after the birth of a single young. The placenta weighed 13 g and measured $24 \times 3 \times 6.5$ cm. The ear holes were open at 20 days. The young was force-fed 8% Esbilac with a syringe. The young pangolin took adult diet from a pan at 91 days and separated from the mother at 113 days. At 6 months, it was in excellent condition, weighing 2.7 kg.[8]

REFERENCES

1. Chin SC, Yang CW, Chung YH, et al: The effect of diet modification on Formosan pangolin (*Manis pentadactyla pentadactyla*) fecal flora. *Taipei Zoo Bull* 19:51–59, 2007.
2. Chin SC, Guo JC, Chen SY, et al: Contagious viral infection of captive rescued Formosan pangolin (*Manis pentadactyla pentadactyla*). *ASZWM Poster* 2008.
3. Chin SC, Lien CY, Chan YT, et al: Monitoring the gestation period of rescued Formosan pangolin (*Manis pentadactyla pentadactyla*) with progesterone radioimmunoassay. *Zoo Biol* 31:479–489, 2012a.
4. Chin SC, Yu PH, Chan YT, et al: Retrospective investigation of the death of rescued Formosan pangolin (*Manis pentadactyla pentadactyla*) during 1995 and 2004. *Taiwan Vet J* 38(4):243–250, 2012b.
5. Gaubert P, Antunes A: Assessing the taxonomic status of the Palawan pangolin *Manis culionensis* (Pholidota) using discrete morphological characters. *Mammalogy* 86(6):1068–1074, 2005.
6. Heath ME, Vanderlip SL: Biology, husbandry and veterinary care of captive Chinese pangolins (*Manis pentadactyla*). *Zoo Biol* 7:293–312, 1988.
7. Krause WJ, Leeson CR: The stomach of the pangolin (*Manis pentadactyla*) with emphasis on the pyloric teeth. *Acta Anat* 88:1–10, 1974.
8. Masui M: Birth of a Chinese pangolin at Ueno Zoo, Tokyo. *Int Zoo YB* 7:114, 1967.
9. Menzies JA: Feeding pangolins in captivity. *Int Zoo YB* 4:126, 1962.
10. Nisa' C, Agungpriyono S, Kitamura N, et al: Morphological features of the stomach of Malayan pangolin (*Manis javanica*). *Anat Histol Embryol* 39:432–439, 2010.
11. Ogilvie PW, Bridgewater DD: Notes on the breeding of an Indian pangolin at Oklahoma Zoo. *Int Zoo YB* 7:116, 1967.

12. Soifer F: Report of Physiological Normals Committee. In Alderman B, editor: *Proceedings of the American Association of Zoo Veterinarians*, East Lansing, MI, 1970, Michigan State University.
13. Soifer F: Anthelmintics for exotic and zoo animals. In Alderman B, editor: *Proceedings of the American Association of Zoo Veterinarians*, East Lansing, MI, 1970, Michigan State University.
14. Thenius E: Pangolins. In Grzimek B, editor: *Grzimek's Animal Life Encyclopedia*, vol 11, New York, 1975, Van Nostrand Reinhold Company.
15. van Ee CA: A note on breeding the Cape pangolin at Bloemfontein Zoo. *Int Zoo YB* 6:163, 1966.
16. Walker EP: *Mammals of the world*, ed 3, Baltimore, MD, 1975, Johns Hopkins University Press.
17. Murphy WJ, Eizirik E, Johnson WE, et al: Molecular phylogenetics and the origins of placental mammals. *Nature* 409:614–618, 2001.
18. Yang CW, Chen S, Chang C-Y, et al: History and dietary husbandry of pangolins in captivity. *Zoo Biol* 26:223–230, 2007.

CHAPTER 41

Lagomorpha (Pikas, Rabbits, and Hares)

Jennifer E. Graham

BIOLOGY

Leporidae (rabbits and hares) and Ochotonidae (pikas) are the two families in the order Lagomorpha.[27] With a worldwide distribution, this order contains 12 genera and 81 species (Box 41-1). Unlike rodents, lagomorphs have a second set of upper incisors known as "peg teeth." Lagomorphs are born with three pairs of upper incisors, but the most lateral on each side is lost soon after birth. Jaw movements of rabbits, hares, and pikas are vertical or transverse. Lagomorphs are hindgut fermenters, herbivorous, and practice cecotrophy. Although lagomorphs were once classified as rodents, they only illustrate convergent evolution on the basis of their gnawing teeth.[17]

Although rabbits and hares have a short tail, pikas lack a tail.[27] Most lagomorph males have testes located in a scrotum in front of the penis, similar to marsupials, and lack an os penis. Two to five pairs of mammary glands are found in females. Hearing, smell, and touch are well developed, and vocalizations in most species are minimal. Eyes are laterally positioned, providing a circular field of vision. Sensory hairs are positioned around the nose and above the eyes.[17]

The Leporidae family contains 54 species found within 11 genera.[27] Although the term "hare" should probably be reserved for those animals in the Lepus genera, the terms *rabbit* and *hare* are often used interchangeably and applied incorrectly. Hares are born fully furred and precocial, are generally larger, and have ears larger than those of rabbits, with dark ear tips. Rabbits are born naked and blind and usually associate in groups compared with the more solitary hare. Hares and jackrabbits comprise 29 species in the genus Lepus, and rabbits have 25 species, 14 of which are Sylvilagus, or cottontails, in the remaining 10 genera. Unlike many other mammals, female leporids are usually larger than males. The long hindlimbs are well adapted for running, with thick hair, instead of footpads, on the soles of all the feet. The dental formula of leporids is usually (incisor [I] 2/1, canine [C] 0/0, premolar [P] 3/2, molar [M] 3/3) ×2 = 28.

The European wild rabbit *Oryctolagus cuniculus*, which likely originated from the Iberian Peninsula and southern France following the end of the Pleistocene, is the origin of the domestic rabbit.[27]

Domestic rabbits range in size from 1 kilogram (kg) to over 7 kg and are divided into over 60 fancy and fur breeds and over 500 varieties.[33] Box 41-2 lists biologic and physical data of domestic rabbits. Table 41-1 lists hematologic and serum biochemical values of the domestic rabbit and hare.

The family Ochotonidae (pikas, mouse hares, or conies), found in Eurasia and western North America (Figure 41-1), contains one living genus and one recently extinct genus and up to 37 subspecies.[18,27] Pikas have long, fine, dense fur and short legs with five digits on each front foot and four digits on each rear foot. Weight ranges from 125 to 400 grams (g), and both genders are of the same size. The dental formula of pikas is (I 1/1, C 0/0, P 3/2, M 2/3) ×2 = 26. Females have four to six mammae. Males have abdominal testes that descend into the skinfolds at the base of the penis during breeding season.

Pikas are generally social, but the social structure varies. Steppe-dwelling (burrowing) pikas may live in large colonies organized into family units, whereas the species found in talus and boulder-fields defend individual territories (Chris Ray, personal communication, 2012). Pikas gather food in late summer and stack it in heaps called "hay piles"; the weight of food in each pile can be up to 20 kg, and they can survive suboptimal conditions by feeding on these stores. They are primarily diurnal, most active in the early morning and evening, and do not hibernate.[27] The steppe-dwelling pikas may be threatened by human encroachment, but all pikas may be most threatened by climate change.[32]

FEEDING

Domestic rabbits have specific recommended dietary requirements including 13% to 18% dry matter (DM) dietary crude protein; 12% to 16% dietary crude fiber; 7,000 international units (IU) vitamin A per kilogram of food; 40 milligrams (mg) vitamin E per kilogram of food; 2 mg vitamin K per kilogram of food; and 0.5% to 1% DM calcium.[5] Of these requirements, fiber is especially important. Because fiber is essential for the production of short-chain fatty acids and gastrointestinal (GI) motility, diets containing less than 10% crude fiber often result in enteritis.

BOX 41-1 Scientific and Common Names for Commonly Cited Lagomorphs[7]

Scientific Name	Common Name
LEPORIDAE: RABBITS AND HARES	
Sylvilagus aquaticus	Swamp rabbit
S. audubonii	Desert cottontail
S. bachmani	Brush rabbit
S. brasiliensis	Forest rabbit
S. floridanus	Eastern cottontail
S. palustris	Marsh rabbit
Lepus americanus	Snowshoe hare
L. arcticus	Arctic hare
L. californicus	Black-tailed jackrabbit
L. capensis	Cape hare
L. europaeus	Brown hare
L. townsendii	White-tailed jackrabbit
Oryctolagus cuniculus	European rabbit, Old World rabbit, and domestic rabbit
OCHOTONIDAE: PIKAS	
Ochotona princeps	Colorado pika
O. rufescens	Afghan pika

BOX 41-2 Biologic and Physiologic Data of Domestic Rabbits[7,33]

Parameter	Normal Values
Adult body mass of male (buck)	2–5 kilograms (kg)
Adult body mass of female (doe)	2–6 kg
Birth mass	30–80 grams (g)
Respiratory rate	30–60 breaths per minute
Tidal volume	4–6 milliliters per kilogram (mL/kg)
Heart rate	130–325 beats per minute
Rectal temperature	38.5° C–40.0° C (101.3° F–104.0° F)
Life span	5–6 years (up to 15 years)
Food consumption	50 g/kg/day
Water consumption	50–150 mL/kg/day
Gastrointestinal transit time	4–5 hours
Daily urine excretion	10–35 mL/kg/day
Breeding onset of male	6–10 months
Breeding onset of female	4–9 months
Breeding life of female	4 months to 3 years
Reproductive cycle	Induced ovulation
Gestation period	29–35 days
Litter size	4–10
Weaning age	4–6 weeks

TABLE 41-1

Hematologic and Serum Biochemical Values of the Domestic Rabbit[6,7,20] and Hare[12]

Measurement	Normal Values	
	Rabbit	Hare*
HEMATOLOGIC PARAMETERS		
Packed cell volume (%)	30–50	48 (42–55)
Hemoglobin (g/dL)	8.0–17.5	15.8 (13.5–18.4)
Red blood cells (3×10^6/µL)	4–8	7.8 (6.5–9.0)
MCV (µm³)	58.0–75.0	—
MCH (pg)	17.5–23.5	—
MCHC (%)	29–37	—
Platelets (3×10^3/µL)	290–650	—
White blood cells (3×10^3/µL)	5–12	7 (2–16)
Neutrophils (%)	35–55	42 (13–82)
Lymphocytes (%)	25–60	49 (16–80)
Monocytes (%)	2–10	5 (1–16)
Eosinophils (%)	0–5	3 (0–11)
Basophils (%)	2–8	0.5 (0–1.5)
CHEMISTRY PARAMETERS		
Alkaline phosphatase (IU/L)	4–70	—
Alanine aminotransferase (IU/L)	14–80	—
Aspartate aminotransferase (IU/L)	14–113	—
Bicarbonate (mEq/L)	16.2–31.8	—
Total bilirubin (mg/dL)	0–0.75	—
Calcium (mg/dL)	8–14.8	—
Chloride (mEq/L)	92–112	—
Cholesterol (mg/dL)	12–116	—
Creatinine (mg/dL)	0.5–2.6	—
Glucose (mg/dL)	75–150	—
Lactic acid dehydrogenase (IU/L)	34–129	—
Total lipids (mg/dL)	280–350	—
Phosphorus (mg/dL)	2.3–6.9	—
Potassium (mEq/L)	3.5–7	—
Total protein (g/dL)	5.4–7.5	5.6 (2–5)
Albumin (g/dL)	2.5–5.0	—
Globulin (g/dL)	1.5–3.5	—
Sodium (mEq/L)	138–155	—
Triglycerides (mg/dL)	124–156	—
Urea nitrogen (mg/dL)	15–50	—

*Black-tailed jackrabbit (*Lepus californicus*).

g/dL, Gram per deciliter; *IU/L*, international unit per liter; *MCH*, mean corpuscular hemoglobin; *MCHC*, mean corpuscular hemoglobin concentration; *MCV*, mean corpuscular volume; *mEq/L*, milliequivalent per liter; *µg*, microgram; *µL*, microliter; *pg*, picogram.

The preferred diet for the pet rabbit is a high-quality, high-fiber (15% to 16% crude fiber) pelleted diet containing 13% to 18% (ideally 16%) crude protein, at a rate of ¼ cup pellets per 2.3 kg body mass divided into two meals per day.[7] A fiber content below 15% may increase the potential for anorexia and diarrhea, and one greater than 16% reduces feed palatability. However, a fiber content of 18% to 22% helps prevent obesity in pet rabbits and often is used in mature laboratory animals. Some rabbits do well when pellets are offered ad libitum (freely), unless overeating and obesity become problems or an inadequate amount of loose hay is consumed. The pellets are supplemented with loose hay (mixed grass hay, timothy hay, or high-quality dried grass clippings) ad libitum. Alfalfa hay may be offered throughout the growth stages and then discontinued because of its high protein and calcium content. The diet can be supplemented with a small amount of dark fibrous, leafy greens and fresh vegetables (1 cup per 2.3 kg body mass) and small amounts (up to 1 tablespoon per 2.3 kg body mass) of fresh fruit, daily or several times per week. It should be noted that growing rabbits and females in late gestation may require twice as much food, and lactating females may consume three times as much food as an adult in maintenance.

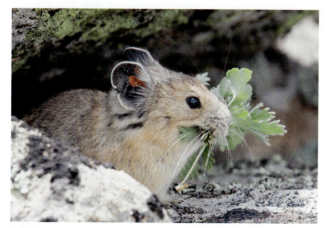

FIGURE 41-1 A Colorado pika (*Ochotona princeps*) gathering food. (Courtesy of N. Zaun, Rocky Mountain National Park, Colorado, 2012).

SELECTED TECHNIQUES

Physical Restraint

The skeleton in rabbits represents only 7% to 8% of the body weight (as opposed to 12% to 13% in cats).[16] Rabbits are prone to fractures of the back and hindlimbs because of hindlimb musculature and the delicate nature of the skeleton. Support of the hindquarters is essential when transporting rabbits to avoid causing injury; rabbits may be carried with one hand under the thorax or holding the scruff, with the second hand supporting the hindquarters. The rabbit should be placed in a cage with its rear facing the back of the cage and the hindquarters supported to reduce chances of injury from the rabbit kicking. A nonslip mat should be used when examining the rabbit or placing the animal in the cage. Alternatively, the rabbit can be wrapped in a towel with the head covered to prevent struggling. A hand may be placed over the eyes to calm the rabbit while using care not to obstruct the nostrils, since rabbits are obligate nasal breathers. Hyperthermia should be avoided when using a towel during handling or examination. Noises or smells from predator animals may stress the sensitive rabbit.

Venipuncture and Injection sites

Multiple sites, including the marginal ear veins, central ear artery, jugular vein, cephalic vein, and the lateral saphenous vein, may be used for venipuncture in rabbits.[16] Use of the ear veins and artery is not ideal because hematoma formation, bruising, or vessel thrombosis and skin sloughing can result. Alcohol may be used to part the fur and visualize the vessel. In some cases, clipping or plucking of the fur may be useful. If clippers are used, care should be taken to avoid damaging the delicate skin of the rabbit. An ideal site for venipuncture is the lateral saphenous vein. The rabbit is restrained in a towel, with the head covered and a rear limb gently extended. The restrainer holds off the vein with pressure across the proximal thigh. The vessel lies across the lateral surface of the tibia just proximal to the hock. Following sample acquisition, gentle digital pressure over the venipuncture site or application of a brief pressure wrap helps prevent hematoma formation.

The cephalic or lateral saphenous veins are the preferred sites for intravenous catheter placement. Intraosseous access is with a spinal needle placed within the trochanteric fossa of the femur. Intramuscular injections may be given into the large lumbar muscles on either side of the spine.[16] Care should be taken to avoid damaging the sciatic nerve if injecting into the hindlimb musculature. If hindlimbs are used for injection, the cranial aspect of the rear leg, the quadriceps, should be used.

Anesthesia

Anesthetic agents can be administered to rabbits in a variety of ways, including topical, injectable, inhalant, and combination protocols.

TABLE 41-2

Chemical Restraint, Anesthetic, and Analgesic Agents Commonly Used in the Domestic Rabbit[7,23]

Agent	Dosage	Comments
Buprenorphine	0.01–0.05 mg/kg, SC, IP, or IV, every 6–12 hours	Analgesia
Butorphanol	0.1–0.5 mg/kg, SC, IM, or IV, every 4 hours	Analgesia
Carprofen	2.2 mg/kg, PO, every 12 hours	Nonsteroidal anti-inflammatory; chronic joint pain
Diazepam	1–3 mg/kg IM	Preanesthetic; tranquilizer
Flunixin meglumine	0.3–2.0 mg/kg, SC, IM, every 12–24 hours	Analgesia; nonsteroidal anti-inflammatory Use for no more than 3 days
Isoflurane	3%–5% induction; 1.5%–3% maintenance	Inhalant anesthetic of choice
Ketamine/ diazepam	15 mg/kg and 0.3 mg/kg, IM, or 20–30 mg/kg and 1–3 mg/kg, IM	Anesthesia Follow with isoflurane
Ketamine/ midazolam	15–25 mg/kg 0.5–1 mg/kg, IM	Anesthesia Follow with isoflurane
Ketoprofen	1 mg/kg, IM, every 12–24 hours	Musculoskeletal pain; nonsteroidal anti-inflammatory
Meloxicam	0.3–1.0 mg/kg, PO, q12-24 hours	Musculoskeletal pain; nonsteroidal anti-inflammatory
Midazolam	1–2 mg/kg, IM	Preanesthetic; tranquilizer
Oxymorphone	0.05–0.2 mg/kg, SC or IM, q8-12 hours	Analgesia
Propofol	2–3 mg/kg (or to effect), IV	Induction after premedication Maintain with approximately 1 mg/kg every 15 minutes
Sevoflurane	To effect	Inhalant anesthesia

IM, Intramuscularly; *IP*, intraperitoneally; *IV*, intravenously; *PO*, orally; *SC*, subcutaneously.

Anesthesia involves many considerations such as stability of the patient, monitoring, anesthetic agents used, and others. The reader should consult additional texts for complete information on anesthesia in rabbits.[14,15,19,21,29]

A variety of injectable anesthetic–analgesic combinations have been used in rabbits. Injectable anesthetic protocols may include parasympatholytics, phenothiazines, benzodiazepines, α_2-adrenergic agonists, ketamine, propofol, tiletamine–zolazepam, and others.[21] Parenteral anesthetics are typically administered via the following routes: subcutaneous, intramuscular, intraperitoneal, intravenous, and intraosseous. In addition, the veterinarian should be aware of the specifics of different anesthetic drugs used in rabbits; for example, the use of tiletamine–zolazepam has been associated with nephrotoxicity in rabbits.[11] Table 41-2 lists agents commonly used in the chemical restraint, anesthesia, and analgesia of domestic rabbits.

Inhalant anesthesia is the primary component of most anesthetic regimens in small mammals.[21] Isoflurane and sevoflurane are commonly used inhalant anesthetic agents. Induction with an inhalant anesthetic is typically administered via a face mask. Premedication and supplemental injectable anesthesia, along with careful restraint to prevent injury, is recommended for rabbits during induction. For maintenance of anesthesia, endotracheal intubation is ideal to protect the upper airway and assist ventilation. Blind and direct techniques may be used to facilitate intubation in rabbits. In either case, it is helpful if the head and neck of the rabbit is hyperextended, as this will allow for the alignment of the larynx and the trachea with the oropharynx.[21] Care should be taken to ensure that the rabbit is adequately premedicated and relaxed to allow for atraumatic intubation. In addition, it is important to avoid overextension of the neck, which could result in damage to the spine. Laryngeal mask airway (LMA) is a new method being used for delivering a gas anesthetic. The LMA is an airway device used as an alternative to a face mask or an endotracheal tube.[3] LMA precludes the need for intubation in rabbits and may minimize laryngeal trauma.

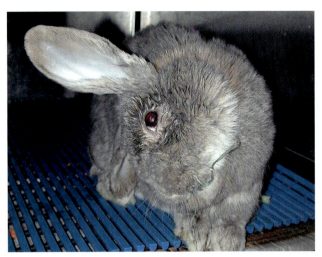

FIGURE 41-2 Torticollis in a rabbit.

INFECTIOUS DISEASES

Bacterial Diseases

Pasteurella multocida is a non–spore-forming, bipolar, gram-negative rod. Although *P. multocida* is a common cause of mortality in brown hares *(Lepus europaeus)* in Europe, the bacterium is associated most commonly with disease in domestic rabbits.[7] *P. multocida* is transmitted from acutely infected rabbits, through direct contact, via fomites, or via inhalation or wounds.[7,25] The incubation period of *P. multocida* is about 2 weeks. In a survey of rabbits with signs of upper respiratory disease, *P. multocida* was the most common isolated bacterium in greater than 50% of rabbits.[30] The bacteria colonize the nares or cause production of nasal exudate if the host is unable to resist infection. Snuffles, a common upper respiratory tract disease in domestic rabbits, is caused by a local overgrowth of *P. multocida* in the nasal epithelium. However, cultures of the nasal epithelium are frequently positive for *P. multocida* in clinically normal adult rabbits housed in institutional colonies (40% to 72%)[10] and in conventional rabbitries (28% to 31%).[9] *P. multocida* may proliferate and spread via the trachea (to the lungs), the nasolacrimal ducts (to the conjunctiva), the eustachian tube (to the middle ear, inner ear, and then the brain), or the bloodstream (septicemia) to the lungs, heart (endocarditis), reproductive organs (orchitis and pyometra-endometritis), skin, and subcutis (subcutaneous abscesses).[7,25] Pasteurellosis infection in the lungs may result in fibrinopurulent pneumonia, pleuritis, and cranioventral pulmonary abscesses. Ophthalmic involvement (conjunctivitis, hypopyon, or retrobulbar abscesses) also may be seen with pasteurellosis. Serologic tests such as enzyme-linked immunosorbent assay (ELISA), and polymerase chain reaction (PCR) tests are available to detect pasteurellosis in rabbits. Culture and sensitivity testing are recommended because organisms other than *Pasteurella* species may be isolated.

Torticollis (head tilt or wry neck) in domestic rabbits usually is caused by the extension of *P. multocida* infection from the nasal cavity to the inner ear via the eustachian tube and middle ear or may arise centrally in the medulla or cerebellum (Figure 41-2).[7] Other causes to consider, although less common, are otitis externa, cranial trauma, listeriosis, encephalitozoonosis, ascarid migration, or extension of ear mite infection. If infection is unilateral, the head of the rabbit tilts down on the affected side. Occasionally, nystagmus may be present. Affected middle ears are characterized by tympanic bullae filled with thick, yellow exudate, which may be seen on radiographic or computed tomography (CT) examination of the skull. The head tilt may or may not respond to antibiotic therapy. Additional supportive care measures, including syringe feeding and protection of the down eye, which may be prone to ulceration from rolling, may be warranted. Prognosis is favorable if a positive response is exhibited within the first week after therapy, and therapy is continued for 1 week after the resolution of clinical signs.

Pasteurella also may cause subcutaneous abscessation. The usual presenting sign is the presence of one or more firm nodules full of thick pus. Aspiration of the nodule is usually unsuccessful. Treatment includes surgical excision and administration of antibiotics for 10 to 14 days. If the abscess cannot be excised, lancing and flushing twice daily with dilute povidone-iodine solution along with antibiotic therapy for 10 to 14 days may be curative. Aerobic and anaerobic cultures and sensitivity testing are appropriate because *Staphylococcus aureus* (sore hocks), *Pseudomonas aeruginosa*, and *Fusobacterium necrophorum* also may cause abscessation.

Enrofloxacin (5–10 mg/kg, orally [PO], every 12 hours for 14 days) is generally effective in treating pasteurellosis in rabbits. Other antibiotics such as chloramphenicol (50 mg/kg, PO, every 12 hours), and ciprofloxacin (20 mg/kg, PO, every 12 hours) have also been used to manage pasteurellosis.[7,25] In addition, nasolacrimal duct flushing and administration of antibiotics into the duct—1 drop of ciprofloxacin in each eye every 8 to 12 hours—is also useful in cases of nasal pasteurellosis. Although more invasive, rhinotomy with surgical debridement has been suggested as an option to manage granulomatous disease of the nasal cavity that is refractory to antibiotic therapy.[30]

Rabbit syphilis, caused by the spirochete *Treponema paraluiscuniculi*, is a contagious but nonzoonotic venereal disease of rabbits.[7,22] Transmission occurs through contact with infected skin or between kits and an infected dam. Crusty ulcers or edematous papules are seen around the lips, eyelids, nose, and perineal region. Diagnosis is based on history, clinical signs, identification of the spirochetes in darkfield microscopic examination of scrapings or smears of the skin lesions. Histologic examination with silver stains of skin biopsy sections may also be used for diagnosis but is considered a low-sensitive test. Serologic testing is available, but false-negatives are possible. Treatment of rabbit syphilis consists of penicillin G benzathine (42,000 to 84,000 international units per kilogram [IU/kg], subcutaneously [SC], every 7 days, three treatments) or parenteral penicillin (40,000 to 60,000 IU/kg, SC, every 24 hours for 5 days). Response is rapid; lesions usually regress dramatically after one injection.

Tularemia, caused by *Francisella tularensis*, has a broad host range but is primarily a disease of lagomorphs and rodents. Among lagomorphs, hares *(Lepus* spp.) and New World rabbits *(Sylvilagus* spp.) are the most important hosts for *F. tularensis*, whereas the European rabbit is relatively resistant to infection. Tularemia is highly infectious, entering the body via arthropod vectors, by direct contact with the blood or tissues or infected animals, by inhalation of infected particles, or by ingestion. In the United States, human cases usually occur during summer from tick bites or from handling rabbits during the fall and winter rabbit hunting season.[7,26]

Clinical signs of tularemia in wild animals have been documented poorly, mainly because of the acute nature of the disease. In more sensitive animals, clinical signs of brief, severe apathy are followed by fatal septicemia. In less sensitive species, nonspecific signs such as depression and elevated body temperature are noted. The organism causes inflammation and necrosis in the lymph nodes, liver, spleen, bone marrow, and lungs, resulting in characteristic multifocal coagulation necrosis of these organs.[7,26] Diagnosis is confirmed by direct or indirect (fluorescent antibody staining, immunofluorescent, or immunohistochemical) methods or culture.

Other bacterial diseases include *Staphylococcus* spp. (most commonly *S. aureus*), a common pyogenic bacteria that causes local abscesses and, less commonly, generalized infections in rabbits and hares. Infected lagomorphs may be listless, emaciated, and lame if tendons or joints are involved. Subcutaneous abscesses may be present. *Sylvilagus* spp. in North America and *Lepus* spp. in Europe and North America have been reported to be naturally infected with *Borrelia burgdorferi* and may serve as reservoirs for the disease. Bacteria most commonly cultured from domestic rabbit abscesses include *S. aureus*, *P. multocida*, *Pseudomonas aeruginosa*, *Proteus* sp., *Fusobacteria* sp., *Bacteriodes* sp., and *Actinomyces* sp.[7] Other bacteria reported less commonly in lagomorphs include *Salmonella* spp., *Campylobacter* sp., *Dermatophilus congolensis*, *Erysipelothrix rhusiopathiae*, *Listeria monocytogenes*, and *Mycobacterium bovis* (in rabbits and hares in New Zealand).[34]

Box 41-3 presents a list of antimicrobial agents commonly used in the domestic rabbit.

Viral Diseases

Rabbit oral papillomatosis virus infection appears restricted to laboratory rabbits, especially New Zealand white rabbits, causing benign oral papillomas on the ventral surface of the tongue. Papillomas start as small millimeter (mm)–sized immobile lesions and may grow into larger (3–5 mm) clusters of pedunculated papules. The lesions are benign and can persist for over 4 months. This virus is different than rabbit (Shope) papillomavirus.

Rabbit (Shope) papillomavirus, also known as *cottontail rabbit papillomavirus*, in the Papovaviridae family, is transmitted by biting arthropods. The virus causes wartlike, keratinized lesions on the skin, with lesions generally around the neck and shoulders in wild cottontail rabbits and around the ears and eyelids in domestic

rabbits.[22] In naturally infected animals, infection may be seen as a cutaneous tumor, most commonly on the legs, especially the dorsal surface of the hindfeet.[7] The tumors are firm, white, and moist on the surface and generally persist for up to 150 days and then disappear. Very young cottontails, however, die about 4 weeks after inoculation. Diagnosis is based on the host, clinical signs, and characteristic microscopic appearance, virus isolation, or both. Surgical removal of lesions and arthropod control is recommended to prevent disease spread.

Rotavirus is highly infectious with a high morbidity and variable (generally low) mortality. Weanling rabbits (2–4 months) are most susceptible, and disease severity is increased with co-infection with another enteric pathogen. Antibodies to rotavirus are found in laboratory, commercial, and pet rabbits, indicating that it can infect most strains. Rotavirus infections are marked by anorexia, dehydration, and green-yellow watery diarrhea. The intestines become distended and congested, with petechial hemorrhages, chronic inflammation, and villous atrophy. Diagnosis requires virus identification, and treatment is with supportive care.

Rabbit hemorrhagic disease virus (RHDV) is a calicivirus of the genus *Lagovirus*, which affects only European rabbits.[1] It was first described in China in 1984 and rapidly spread throughout Asia, Australia, and New Zealand and into Europe, with rare outbreaks in the United States and elsewhere.[8] In 1996, planned dissemination of rabbit hemorrhagic disease was legalized in Australia as a biologic control of rabbit populations. Transmission is via direct contact (with urine, feces, respiratory secretions) and fomite contamination and even by intermediate insect vectors. The disease occurs in rabbits over 2 months of age, as neonatal rabbits are resistant to infection. The virus replicates in the liver, causing severe hepatic necrosis and eventual death from disseminated intravascular coagulation. The clinical presentation and course varies from a peracute disease that lasts only 12 to 36 hours and is followed by sudden death; to an acute or subacute febrile illness, with anorexia, diarrhea (or constipation), neurologic, and other systemic symptoms, lasting a few days to weeks; to a persistent or latent disease with continued virus shedding. Active immunity in recovered rabbits is apparently life-long. Laboratory studies demonstrate a worsening lymphopenia and thrombocytopenia, with eventual prolonged prothrombin and thrombin times. At necropsy, extensive hepatic necrosis, splenomegaly, pulmonary hemorrhage, and evidence of disseminated intravascular coagulation are evident. RHDV is a reportable disease. Vaccination programs using attenuated vaccines have had mixed results. A recombinant vaccine has recently been developed and should be effective in prevention in endemic areas. The virus can be inactivated with 0.5% sodium hypochlorite or 1% formalin. Diagnosis is confirmed by using specific immunohistochemical stains, electron microscopy, or ELISA.

Myxomatosis is a significant disease of European rabbits caused by myxoma virus and is transmitted passively by blood-feeding arthropods or is shed via discharges.[7] Clinical signs vary with the strain of the virus and the nature of the host, with wild rabbits (*Sylvilagus* sp.) developing benign skin tumors and domestic rabbits (*Orytolagus* sp.) developing systemic signs, including swollen eyelids and mucopurulent ocular and nasal discharge. Domestic rabbits may have lethargy, seizures, and a high mortality rate, with surviving rabbits developing edematous nodules on the ears, face, eyelids, and perineum.[22] Diagnosis of myxomatosis is based on clinical signs and pathologic findings (greatly swollen spleen; enlarged, edematous, and often hemorrhagic lymph nodes; hemorrhages; and swollen conjunctiva and nasal mucosa) as well as a history of myxomatosis in the area. Confirmation may be made with electron microscopy, fluorescent antibody, PCR, virus isolation, and antibody levels (ELISA, virus neutralization assays, or complement fixation assays). This disease has been used as a biologic measure for the control of European rabbit populations in Australia since 1950.

European brown hare syndrome is a highly contagious caliciviral infection of free-living and farmed hares characterized by acute necrotic hepatitis.[7] The distribution of European brown hare

---

BOX 41-3 Antimicrobial Agents Commonly Used in the Domestic Rabbit[7,23]

Agent	Dosage
Chloramphenicol	25 milligrams per kilogram (mg/kg), orally (PO), every 8–12 hours
	50 mg/kg, PO, every 8–24 hours
Chlortetracycline	50 mg/kg, PO, every 12–24 hours
	1 gram per liter (g/L) drinking water
Ciprofloxacin	10–20 mg/kg, PO, every 12–24 hours
	1 drop topical in each eye every 8–12 hours*
Enrofloxacin	5–10 mg/kg, PO or subcutaneously (SC), every 12 hours for 14 days
Metronidazole	20 mg/kg, PO, every 12 hours for 3–5 days
Sulfamethazine	1 milligram per milliliter (mg/mL) drinking water
Sulfadimethoxine	10–15 mg/kg, PO, every 12 hours
Trimethoprim/ sulfamethoxazole	15–30 mg/kg, PO, every 12 hours

*For nasal pasteurellosis; maintains therapeutic levels in tear film for at least 6 hours after application (tears drain into nasal sinus).

syndrome corresponds with the distribution of the European brown hare.

In addition, snowshoe hare virus, a member of the California encephalitis complex in *Bunyaviridae,* occurs across the northern part of North America.[34]

Mycotic Diseases

The most commonly reported mycotic infection in rabbits is ringworm (caused by *Trichophyton* and less frequently *Microsporidium*).[7,22] Lesions are seen around the head, legs, feet, and nail beds. Initially, the infected areas may be pruritic and inflamed, later becoming scabby, dry, crusty, and alopecic. Diagnosis is made by growing the fungal organism on a dermatophyte culture medium, direct examination of hair shafts mounted with potassium hydroxide, or fungal-stained skin biopsy samples. Treatment involves antimycotic medications considered safe for kittens, and owners should be advised of the zoonotic risk.

Aflatoxins produced by the fungi *Aspergillus flavus* and *Aspergillus parasiticus* cause liver and biliary damage in rabbits.[28] Rabbits are the species most sensitive to these toxins and serve as an animal model for aflatoxicosis. Outbreaks occur from contaminated feed and are accompanied by anorexia, depression, and weight loss, progressing to icterus and death within 3 to 4 days. On necropsy, livers are congested with periportal and ductal fibrosis, sinusoidal dilation, and hepatocyte degenerative changes. Treatment involves removal of contaminated feed and supportive care.

PARASITIC DISEASES

Coccidia are the most common parasites of the rabbit GI tract, and although they cause significant disease in young (<6 months old) rabbits, they may be incidentally found in fecal studies in adult rabbits.[28] Of the 12 species of the genus *Eimeria*, *E. stiedae* is exclusive to the liver, with the rest causing intestinal disease. Hepatic coccidiosis is ubiquitous in commercial rabbitries and may be fatal in young rabbits by obstructing liver function. Severe disease is marked by anorexia, diarrhea, abdominal bloating, and icterus. Biochemical tests confirm hepatic disease, with elevations in aspartate aminotransferase (AST), alanine aminotransferase (ALT), bile acids, and total bilirubin. On necropsy, the liver is seen studded with nodular, encapsulated abscesses. Oocysts may be identified in bile or feces.

Intestinal coccidiosis is common in rabbits of all ages and most often associated with *E. perforans* infection. Subclinical infection is common, and disease severity varies with age (worse under 6 months), species of *Eimeria*, parasite burden, and condition of the rabbit (stress, poor husbandry, poor diet). Significant disease is marked by diarrhea, with possible mucus or blood, dehydration, and weight loss. Intussusception is a complication of severe disease. Diagnosis depends on histopathology, fecal identification, or both. Molecular assays have been developed to identify intestinal *Eimeria* species. In addition to supportive care, sulfa drugs are most effective at limiting viral multiplication. Sulfadimethoxine (15 mg/kg, PO, four times in 12 hours [q12h]) or trimethoprim-sulfamethoxazole (30 mg/kg, PO, q12h) may be used for 10 days of therapy. Recovering rabbits develop lifelong immunity.

Cryptosporidium parvum infects the small intestine and causes a self-limiting diarrheal illness (4–5 day duration) in young rabbits (peak, 30–40 days old).[28] Illness is accompanied by anorexia, depression, and dehydration. The organism is identified on histopathology. Other than supportive care, no effective treatment is available. Recently, reports of rabbit *Cryptosporidium* species causing zoonotic disease in humans have been reported in several countries.[8]

Passalurus ambiguous, the rabbit pinworm, is found in most rabbits, and even large parasite burdens are not pathogenic. Adult worms reside in the cecum and colon, and transmission is direct through ingestion of eggs during cecotrophy. Diagnosis is often routine, with identification of worms or eggs in feces, although identification should not prompt treatment in most cases. When

treatment is necessary, benzimidazoles such as fenbendazole (10–20 mg/kg, PO, repeated in 10–14 days) are effective.[28]

Vestibular dysfunction (head tilt) in dwarf breeds of domestic rabbits is caused most frequently by *Encephalitozoon cuniculi* (whereas in standard breeds the cause more likely is *Pasteurella multocida*).[7] *E. cuniculi* is an obligate, intracellular, protozoan parasite. Transmission is generally by ingestion or by oral inoculation of infective spores shed in urine, although transplacental transmission also may occur. A positive encephalitozoon titer with compatible clinical signs suggests, but is not conclusive for, encephalitozoonosis. Serologic testing, including complement fixation, ELISA, India ink immunoreaction, indirect fluorescent antibody, or indirect microagglutination, commonly is used. Definitive diagnosis of encephalitozoonosis requires histopathologic identification of the organism. Although many domestic rabbits infected with *E. cuniculi* are asymptomatic, other neurologic signs may include urinary incontinence, stiff rear gait, and posterior paresis. No treatment is effective for encephalitozoonosis, although benzimidazoles have been shown to help decrease neurologic signs.

Cerebrospinal nematodiasis (neural larval migrans), caused by *Baylisascaris* spp., has been reported in rabbits and may produce fatal or severe neurologic disease.

Pelecitus, a filarid, is a common parasite of the legs and joints of various species of rabbits and hares.[2] Microfilaria may be present in blood; no clinical signs have been reported.

Ear mites (*Psoroptes cuniculi*) are common in the domestic rabbit, in which they may cause severe inflammation (Figure 41-3).[22] Treatment of otoacariasis generally involves administering 1% ivermectin (0.2–0.4 mg/kg, SC) and repeating the dose in 10 to 14 days), topical treatment with a combination product containing thiabendazole, dexamethasone, and neomycin (Tresaderm, MSD-AgVet), or a combination of both.[7]

Bots (*Cuterebra* spp.) occur in New World lagomorphs, in which they may produce a granulomatous furuncle within which the larvae complete their development.[31] Warbles (*Oestromyia* sp.) have been reported in pikas.

Endoparasites occur commonly in wild lagomorphs and also occur occasionally in captive species. Lancet flukes (*Dicrocoelium* sp.) are primarily parasites of captive species but have been reported in wild lagomorphs as well.[31] Lagomorphs are also intermediate hosts for cestodes (i.e., *Taenia* spp.), and the larvae are usually in the subcutis and skeletal muscle.

Ectoparasites occur commonly in lagomorphs, and some of the more significant types reported include *Sarcoptes scabiei* (sarcoptic mange, scabies), sucking lice, and a wide range of ticks.

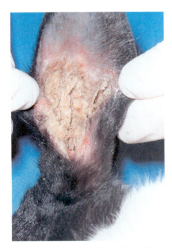

FIGURE 41-3 Otitis externa caused by mites. (From Harcourt-Brown F: Textbook of rabbit medicine, Oxford, United Kingdom, 2002, Butterworth-Heinemann.)

TABLE 41-3

Antiparasitic Agents Commonly Used in the Domestic Rabbit[7,23]

Agent	Dosage	Comments
Albendazole	7.5–20 milligram per kilogram (mg/kg), PO, every 24 hours	Potential treatment for encephalitozoonosis; deaths have been reported
Amprolium (9.6%)	0.4 milliliter per 473 mL(mL/mL) drinking water for 10 days	Coccidiosis
Carbaryl powder (5%)	Topical every 7 days	Ectoparasites. Use sparingly.
Fenbendazole	5–10 mg/kg, PO; repeat in 2 weeks as needed	Intestinal strongyles and ascarids; deaths have been reported
Ivermectin	0.2–0.4 mg/kg, SC, every 10–14 days	Ear mites
Lufenuron (Program, Novartis)	30 mg/kg, PO, monthly	Flea larvicide
Praziquantel	5–10 mg/kg, PO, SC, or IM; repeat in 10 days	Cestodes and trematodes
Pyrantel pamoate	5–10 mg/kg, PO; repeat in 2–3 weeks	Intestinal strongyles and ascarids
Pyrethrins	Use as directed for puppies and kittens	Flea control
Selamectin (Revolution, Pfizer)*	20 mg/kg, topically, q7d	Ectoparasites (ear mites, fleas, and ticks)
Sulfadimethoxine	50 mg/kg, PO, once, then 25 mg/kg, every 24 hours for 10–20 days	Coccidiosis
Sulfamerazine	100 mg/kg, PO, or 0.05%–0.15% in drinking water	Coccidiosis
Sulfamethazine	100 mg/kg, PO, every 24 hours, 0.5%–1.0% in feed, or 0.77 grams per liter (g/L) drinking water	Coccidiosis
Thiabendazole	50–100 mg/kg, PO	Intestinal strongyles and ascarids
Thiabendazole/ dexamethasone/ neomycin (Tresaderm, MSD-AgVet)	3 drops in each ear every 12 hours for 7–14 days	Ear mites; generally concurrent to ivermectin therapy

IM, intramuscularly; *PO*, orally; *SC*, subcutaneously.
*J.W. Carpenter, personal observation.

Table 41-3 lists antiparasitic agents commonly used in the domestic rabbit.

NONINFECTIOUS DISEASES

Gastric Stasis or Ileus and Trichobezoars

The rabbit's GI tract is highly specialized for its high-fiber herbivorous diet; and even minor changes in the diet or digestive process may lead to significant GI disease. GI stasis is the most common disorder, affecting all ages and breeds.

The etiology of GI stasis is often multifactorial. Lack of adequate fiber, either from poor diet or reduced intake, is a primary cause of GI stasis. Diets low in quality grass hay and high in cereal grains and fruits predispose rabbits to GI stasis. In animals receiving an adequate diet, GI stasis may result from reduced intake secondary to any number or combination of factors causing anorexia, including dental disease, dysphagia, pain, anxiety, environmental changes, infection, dysbiosis, neoplasia, chronic disease, drug effects (anesthetics, anticholinergics, opioids, antibiotics), obstruction or foreign bodies, and accidental or forced restriction (preoperative fasting). Restricted water intake and activity will also impair adequate processing of dietary fiber and will promote stasis. In addition to reducing intake, chronic stress causes increased catecholamine signaling acting on the enteric nervous system to impair intestinal motility. Once initiated, dysmotility leads to reduced colonic transit with decreased fecal output, increased dehydration of intestinal contents, dehydration of gastric contents with trichobezoar formation, impaired cecal fermentation, and disruption of the enteric microflora, creating a cycle of further anorexia and worsening stasis.[28]

Physical examination findings correlate with the extent of disease and may be minimal, but most will demonstrate evidence of dehydration, abdominal distension, and gastric tympany. Some animals may be hunched over, grind their teeth, and have abdominal tenderness. Severely ill rabbits progress to hypovolemic shock with reduced blood pressure and altered mentation. Laboratory studies (complete blood cell count [CBC], biochemistry, urinalysis) may be helpful for determination of an underlying cause of anorexia, but most have only nonspecific findings of dehydration or possibly elevated hepatic enzymes from developing hepatic lipidosis. Radiographic studies of the abdomen in two views are essential for examining gastric contents, colonic fecal contents, and, most importantly, severe gas or fluid accumulation suggestive of obstruction, which constitutes a surgical emergency.

Routine GI stasis is treated with comprehensive supportive care, best performed in a hospital setting for close monitoring. Animals should be kept warm in a dark, quiet place to minimize stress. Fluid replacement is achieved with warmed saline (25-35 mL/kg, q8h) and may be given orally or subcutaneously, although animals with severe dehydration will require more aggressive intravenous fluids. Anxiety can be minimized with injectable midazolam (0.25-0.5 mg/kg, intravenously or intramuscularly [IV or IM]), and pain controlled with analgesics such as buprenorphine (0.01-0.05 mg/kg, IM or subcutaneously [SC], every 6-8 hours), which may later be transitioned to meloxicam after adequate hydration (0.2-0.5 mg/kg, IM, SC, or PO, q24h). Once obstruction has been ruled out, prokinetic agents, including metoclopramide (0.5 mg/kg, SC or PO, q8-12h) and/or cisapride (0.5 mg/kg, PO, q8-12h) may be used. Simethicone (20 mg/kg, PO, q8-12h) may be used to reduce gas distension, and ranitidine (2 mg/kg, IV, q24h; 2-5 mg/kg, PO, q12h) used in cases with prolonged anorexia, where gastric ulceration is likely. Nutritional support is essential and may be performed by syringe-feeding an herbivore critical care formulation (15 mL/kg, q8h). Prolonged nutritional support may be provided via a nasogastric tube. Antibiotics should only be used in cases complicated by enterotoxemia and

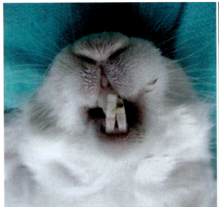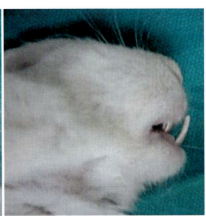

FIGURE 41-4 Malocclusion of incisors in a rabbit. (From Miloro M, Miller JJ, Stoner JA: Low level laser effect on mandibular distraction osteogenesis. *J Oral Maxillofac Surg.* 65(2):168–176, 2007.)

bacterial enteritis. Brushing the hair may be useful in preventing exacerbation of the problem, and supplemental heat may be required in cases of hypothermia.

Antibiotic-Related Toxicities

Diarrheal disease is common in rabbits and frequently results from alterations in the balance of intestinal microflora, or *dysbiosis*, ranging from mild changes causing soft stools, to pathogenic bacterial overgrowth with more significant enteritis, to life-threatening enterotoxemia.[28] Gut flora is sensitive to any type of environmental change. Frequent causes of dysbiosis include poor diet, hypomotility, stress, toxins, and antibiotic use. Indiscriminate antibiotic use, particularly with narrow-spectrum agents that selectively target beneficial gram-positive organisms (penicillins, amoxicillin ± clavulanic acid, cephalosporins, ampicillin, clindamycin, lincomycin), creates optimal conditions for overgrowth of pathogenic species.

Overgrowth of *Clostridium spiroforme* in rabbits causes an often-fatal enterotoxemia from elaboration of bacterial toxin. Adults with dysbiosis may develop enterotoxemia, but weanlings are most susceptible because of their poorly established flora and high gastric pH. Newborns may also develop toxemia from toxin secreted into the milk of infected mothers. In acute infections, rabbits develop watery diarrhea, possibly with blood, that soils the perineum and the legs. The animals become anorexic and decline over 2 to 4 days into a moribund state, with hypovolemic shock leading to death. On necropsy, the cecum, the primary reservoir for bacterial growth, is often seen covered with petechial and ecchymotic hemorrhage that may spread into the appendix and proximal colon. The mucosa may also contain hemorrhage, thick mucus, gas, or pseudomembranes.

Treatment of dysbiosis, enteritis, or enterotoxemia involves aggressive supportive care and correction of hypomotility, as was discussed above. Correction of dehydration and nutritional deficiencies is critical as is providing a warm, safe environment and adequate analgesia. For cases of enteritis caused by bacterial overgrowth, fecal bacterial culture and sensitivity may be helpful to guide antiobiotic therapy with broad-spectrum agents, including trimethoprim-sulfamethoxazole (30 mg/kg, PO, q12h) or enrofloxacin (15 mg/kg, PO, q24h). For enterotoxemia, a dual approach of metronidazole (20 mg/kg, q12h) and cholestyramine (2 g or 20 mL water, q24h, by gavage) may be used to treat *Clostridium* infection and bind its toxin, although *C. spiroforme* has widespread intrinsic and acquired antimicrobial resistance. Preventing dysbiosis with a high-fiber diet and reducing stress are key to prevention.

Malocclusion

Dental malocclusion is a common presenting problem in pet rabbits. Rabbit teeth are elodont (continuously growing or erupting), aradicular (open rooted), and hypsodont (long crowned), and contain incisors and cheek teeth (premolars and molars).[4] Without the regular wear provided by a coarse, abrasive, high-fiber diet, molar crowns elongate and develop sharp points and edges. Buccal ulcerations generally form along the upper arcades and lingual ulcerations along the lower arcades. Eventually, continued growth inhibits normal mouth closure. Congenital deformities may also result in malocclusion and produce dental disease at several months of age. In rabbits with mandibular prognathism, most commonly seen in dwarf rabbits, misalignment causes overgrowth of unopposed incisors, with upper incisors curving inward and upward toward the roof of the mouth and lower incisors curving outward and upward, sometimes into the upper lip or nose (Figure 41-4).

Clinical signs of primary dental disease include anorexia, dysphagia, excessive salivation and drooling, weight loss, emaciation, and changes in fecal appearance and quantity. The presence of facial masses, excessive swelling, exophthalmos, and purulent nasal discharge suggest secondary infection or abscess formation. Rabbits with anorexia or dysphagia from a systemic disease or those with ocular disease restricting feeding may develop secondary dental disease. Diagnosis requires a routine physical examination, including a thorough oral examination of the incisors, cheek teeth, periapical structures, bone, tongue, and oral mucosa. Complete dental examinations require extraoral radiographic studies from multiple projections (lateral, oblique, ventrodorsal, rostrocaudal) using high-definition (mammography) film, as well as a thorough examination with the rabbit under anesthesia, assisted by oral endoscopy, when available. Diagnosis of periapical disease and abscess may be aided by CT, when available. Dental correction involves shortening of overgrown teeth, restoring the occlusal plane, extracting any diseased teeth, and treating abscessation.

Periapical infection, abscessation, osteomyelitis of the surrounding bones, or all of these issues are common sequela in rabbits with dental disease. Treatment typically requires extraction, opening and excising an entire abscess capsule, careful debridement of bone, marsupialization with secondary closure, and packing the surgical site. Antibiotic therapy should be based on culture and sensitivity results and may include combinations of oral and injectable agents, as well as impregnated beads. Surgical treatment must be combined with medical therapy to manage pain, restore health (hydration, diet correction), minimize infection, and minimize the risk of postoperative GI stasis.

Neurologic Conditions

The most common cause of posterior paralysis of acute onset in domestic rabbits is vertebral fracture (generally at the seventh lumbar vertebra) or luxation.[7] The injury often results from improper handling but also may occur in caged rabbits that are startled or frightened. The clinical diagnosis of posterior paresis or paralysis is confirmed radiographically. If treatment is delayed, rabbits with broken backs may become azotemic because of urine retention, so supportive therapy should include manual expression of urine from the bladder. Occasionally, mildly affected rabbits respond to conservative medical management if the spinal cord is not transected. Euthanasia often is indicated.

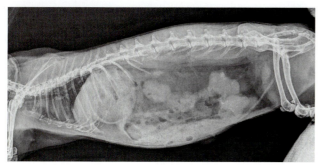

FIGURE 41-5 Uterine adenocarcinoma causing a mineralized caudal abdominal mass in an 8-year-old rabbit.

In addition to trauma and infectious and parasitic agents, other health problems in rabbits include neurologic signs associated with lead poisoning, rabies, herpes simplex virus, fipronil toxicosis, pregnancy toxemia, and heat stroke.[13]

Urogenital Diseases

Rabbit urine is turbid and may vary in color from yellow-orange to red-brown.[7] The color is caused by porphyrin pigment or a food-related metabolite. Pathologic conditions can be ruled out by use of a urine dipstick to determine if blood is present. Thick, white urine in domestic rabbits is not uncommon, however, and indicates the presence of mineral precipitates. Unlike other mammals, calcium absorption and blood calcium concentration are related directly to dietary calcium in rabbits.

Dysuria and hematuria may occur in domestic rabbits and generally are associated with cystitis, cystic calculi, or uterine adenocarcinomata. Cystic calculi (usually composed of calcium carbonate) occur in male and female rabbits. Diagnostics include urine dipstick, urinalysis, CBC, chemistries, culture, radiography, and ultrasonography. Measuring blood calcium concentrations (often as high as 19 milligrams per deciliter [mg/dL]) in rabbits excreting large amounts of urinary calcium is significant. Treatment may include antibiotics (trimethoprim-sulfamethoxazole, chloramphenicol, etc.), manual expression of urine from the bladder (possibly catheterization), fluid therapy, surgery, and modification of the diet. Cystic calculi may be removed surgically. To help prevent calcium sediment or calculi in the bladder, feeding rabbits an appropriate diet (i.e., a diet that does not contain an excess amount of calcium) is important.

Uterine Adenocarcinoma

Decreased litter size in domestic does 3 years of age or older may indicate developing uterine adenocarcinoma (Figure 41-5), the most common neoplasm of female domestic rabbits.[7,24] Adenocarcinomas rarely occur in does younger than 3 years of age; however, the incidence in rabbits older than 3 years ranges from 50% to 80% in certain breeds. Endometriosis, endometritis, and papillary, cystic, or adenomatous hyperplasia may precede the neoplasm. In rabbits, uterine adenocarcinoma is a slow-growing tumor with a 5- to 24-month clinical course. Metastasis occurs late in the clinical course of the disease. Clinical signs are usually inapparent during the hyperplastic stages, although decreased reproductive performance, hematuria or a bloody discharge from the vaginal area, cystic mastitis, or an increase in aggressiveness may be noted in some does. Ovariohysterectomy is the recommended treatment and is successful if done before metastasis has occurred. The prognosis is poor if metastasis has occurred.

REFERENCES

1. Abrantes J, Van Der Loo W, Le Pendu J, et al: Rabbit hemorrhagic disease (RHD) and rabbit haemorrhagic disease virus (RHDV): A review. *Vet Res* 43(12):1–19, 2012.

2. Anderson RC: Filaroid nematodes. In Samuel WM, Pybus MJ, Kocan AA, editors: *Parasitic diseases of wild mammals*, ed 2, Ames, IA, 2001, Iowa State University, pp 342–356.

3. Brain A, Denman W, Goudsouzian N: *LMA instruction manual*, San Diego, CA, 2000, LMA North America.

4. Capello V, Lennox A: Small mammal dentistry. In Quesenberry KE, Carpenter JW, editors: *Ferrets, rabbits, and rodents: Clinical medicine and surgery*, ed 3, Philadelphia, PA, 2012, WB Saunders, pp 452–471.

5. Carpenter J, Kolmstetter C: Feeding small exotic mammals. In Hand M, Thatcher C, Remillard R, Roudebush P, editors: *Small animal clinical nutrition*, Topeka, KS, 2000, Walsworth Publishing Company, pp 947–952.

6. Carpenter JW, Marion CJ: *Exotic animal formulary*, ed 4, St. Louis, MO, 2013, Saunders.

7. Carpenter JW: Lagomorpha (Pikas, rabbits, and hares). In Fowler ME, Miller RE, editors: *Zoo and wild animal medicine*, ed 5, Philadelphia, PA, 2003, Saunders, pp 410–419.

8. Chalmers RM, Robinson G, Elwin K, et al: *Cryptosporidium* sp. rabbit genotype, a newly identified human pathogen. *Emerg Infect Dis* 15(5): 829–830, 2009.

9. Deeb BJ: Respiratory disease and the *Pasteurella* complex. In Hillyer EV, Quesenberry KE, editors: *Ferrets, rabbits, and rodents: Clinical medicine and surgery*, Philadelphia, PA, 1997, Saunders, pp 189–201.

10. DiGiacomo RF, Garlinghouse LE, Jr, Van Hoosier GL, Jr: Natural history of infection with *Pasteurella multocida* in rabbits. *J Am Vet Med Assoc* 183:1172–1175, 1983.

11. Doerning B, Brammer D, Chrisp C, Rush H: Nephrotoxicity of tiletamine in New Zealand white rabbits. *Lab Anim* 42(3):267–269, 1992.

12. Fetters MD: *The domestication, husbandry and some biochemical polymorphisms of the black-tailed jack rabbit*, PhD thesis, Davis, CA, 1970, University of California.

13. Fisher PG, Carpenter JW: Neurologic and musculoskeletal diseases. In Quesenberry KE, Carpenter JW, editors: *Ferrets, rabbits, and rodents: Clinical medicine and surgery*, ed 3, Philadelphia, PA, 2012, Saunders, pp 245–256.

14. Flecknell P, editor: *Anesthesia. Manual of rabbit medicine and surgery*, Quedgeley, U.K., 2000, British Small Animal Veterinary Association, pp 103–116.

15. Flecknell P: *Anesthesia of common laboratory species. Laboratory animal anesthesia*, San Diego, CA, 1996, Academic Press, pp 159–223.

16. Graham J, Mader D: Basic approach to veterinary care. In Quesenberry KE, Carpenter JW, editors: *Ferrets, rabbits, and rodents: Clinical medicine and surgery*, ed 3, Philadelphia, PA, 2012, Saunders, pp 174–182.

17. Grzimek B, editor: *Grzimek's encyclopedia of mammals*, vol 4, New York, 1990, McGraw-Hill, pp 243–324.

18. Hafner D, Smith A: Revision of the subspecies of the American pika. *J Mammal* 91(2):401–417, 2010.

19. Harcourt-Brown F: Anesthesia and analgesia. In Harcourt-Brown F, editor: *Textbook of Rabbit Medicine*, Oxford, U.K., 2002, Alden Press, pp 121–164.

20. Harcourt-Brown F: *Textbook of rabbit medicine*, Oxford, U.K., 2002, Alden Press.

21. Hawkins M, Pascoe P: Anesthesia, analgesia, and sedation of small mammals. In Quesenberry KE, Carpenter JW, editors: *Ferrets, rabbits, and rodents: Clinical medicine and surgery*, ed 3, Philadelphia, PA, 2012, Saunders, pp 429–451.

22. Hess L, Tater K: Dermatologic disease. In Quesenberry KE, Carpenter JW, editors: *Ferrets, rabbits, and rodents: Clinical medicine and surgery*, ed 3, Philadelphia, PA, 2012, Saunders, pp 232–244.

23. Ivey ES, Morrisey JK: Therapeutics for rabbits. *Vet Clin North Am Exotic Anim Pract* 3:183–220, 2000.

24. Klaphake E, Paul-Murphy J: Disorders of the reproductive and urinary system. In Quesenberry KE, Carpenter JW, editors: *Ferrets, rabbits, and rodents: Clinical medicine and surgery*, ed 3, Philadelphia, 2012, Saunders, pp 217–231.

25. Lennox A: Respiratory disease and pasteurellosis. In Quesenberry KE, Carpenter JW, editors: *Ferrets, rabbits, and rodents: Clinical medicine and surgery*, ed 3, Philadelphia, PA, 2012, Saunders, pp 205–216.

26. Mörner T, Addison E: Bacterial and mycotic diseases. In Williams ES, Barker IK, editors: *Infectious diseases of wild mammals*, ed 3, Ames, IA, 2000, Iowa State University Press, pp 303–312.
27. Nowak RM: *Walker's mammals of the world*, vol 2, ed 6, Baltimore, MD, 1999, Johns Hopkins University Press.
28. Oglesbee BL, Jenkins JR: Gastrointestinal diseases. In Quesenberry KE, Carpenter JW, editors: *Ferrets, rabbits, and rodents: Clinical medicine and surgery*, ed 3, Philadelphia, PA, 2012, Saunders, pp 193–204.
29. Paul-Murphy J, Ramer J: Urgent care of the pet rabbit. *Vet Clin North Am Exotic Anim Practice* 1(1):127–152, 1998.
30. Rougier S, Galland D, Boucher S, et al: Epidemiology and susceptibility of pathogenic bacteria responsible for upper respiratory tract infections in pet rabbits. *Vet Microbiol* 115:192–198, 2006.
31. Samuel WM, Pybus MJ, Kocan AA, editors: *Parasitic diseases of wild mammals*, ed 2, Ames, IA, 2001, Iowa State University Press.
32. Smith A, Wetdong L, Hik D: Pikas as harbingers of global warming. *Species* 42(Jan–Jun):4–5, 2004.
33. Vella D, Donnelly TM: Basic anatomy, physiology, and husbandry. In Quesenberry KE, Carpenter JW, editors: *Ferrets, rabbits, and rodents: Clinical medicine and surgery*, ed 3, Philadelphia, PA, 2012, Saunders, pp 157–173.
34. Williams ES, Barker IK, editors: *Infectious diseases of wild mammals*, ed 3, Ames, IA, 2001, Iowa State University.

CHAPTER 42

Rodentia

Enrique Yarto-Jaramillo

BIOLOGY

Rodentia, being represented by nearly half of all placental mammals, is therefore the most diverse animal order comprising 2277 species divided into 33 families. Phylogeny at the family level is still being debated, and more molecular and morphologic studies are needed.[52] Rodent classification is based on morphologic features according to two different systems. Brandt has divided rodents on the basis of the position of masticatory muscles (masseters) into three suborders: Myomorpha, Sciuromorpha, and Hystricomorpha,[26] whereas Tullberg has divided rodents into two suborders known as Sciurognathi and Hystricognathi, according to the position of incisors and the angle of the jaw.[60] Box 42-1 describes the current classification of the order Rodentia.

Classification

Nonetheless, molecular analyses have placed rodents into seven clades: (1) Anomaluromorpha (scaly-tailed flying squirrels, springhares); (2) Ctenohystrica (gundi, porcupines, guinea pigs); (3) Castoridae (beavers); (4) Geomyoidea (pocket gophers, pocket mice); (5) Myodonta (rats, mice, jerbos); (6) Gliridae (dormice); and (7) Sciuroidea (mountain beavers, squirrels, woodchucks).

More recent studies have performed phylogenetic reconstructions that allow the division of those seven clades into three lineages: (1) a "squirrel-related" clade (Sciuriodea and Gliridae); (2) a "mouse-related" clade (Anomaluromorpha, Castoridae, Geomyoidea and Myodonta); and (3) Ctenohystrica.[52]

GEOGRAPHIC DISTRIBUTION

Rodents are naturally found in all continents except Antarctica, inhabiting diverse environments with different living adaptations such as semi-aquatic, terrestrial, arboreal, fossorial, jumping, and gliding.[5]

Rodents may be found from the high arctic tundra to equatorial rain forests, temperate bogs and swamps to hot arid deserts, mountain tops to sandy canyon bottoms.[64] In South America, rodents are the most numerous in species and in abundance compared with other continents, corresponding to approximately 44% of the total amount of native mammals.[48]

In Australia, all of the more than 60 species of rodents belong to the family Muridae, which is the most widespread of all mammalian families in this continent. In recent literature, five groups of rodents (*Pseudomys*, *Uromys*, *Hydromys*, *Xeromys*, and *Pogomomys*) are frequently called the "Old Endemics," referring to the groups that entered Australia at the very end of the Miocene period, approximately five million years ago. True rats are often referred to as the "New Endemics," since they arrived in Australia around one million years ago.[6] Sixteen of the extant Australian rodents are currently threatened (International Union for the Conservation of Nature [IUCN], 2006), all belonging to the Old Endemics.[6]

UNIQUE ANATOMY

In general terms, rodents are characterized by small and compact bodies that are cylindrical to spherical in shape, and short legs; they weigh from less than 10 grams (g) to more than 66 kilograms (kg).[6,64] Hamsters and other rodents have extensive distensible cheek pouches (evaginations of the oral mucosa) that are used to carry food, bedding material, and occasionally the young. Gerbils possess strong claws for burrowing and muscular legs for jumping and standing.[51] Chinchillas have soft fur with 60 hairs per follicle; on either side of the upper lip, they have long vibrissae that are used as sensory organs. Duprasi (*Pachyuromys duprasi*) have developed claws on the front feet and a fleshy tail. Degus are similar anatomically to both guinea pigs and chinchillas. Guinea pigs have large tympanic bullae and four digits on the forelimbs and three digits on the hindlimbs.[27] Hamsters, rats, and mice possess four front toes and five hind toes.

Porcupines have a distinct integument feature as modified hairs that are stiff spines known as *barbed quills* among guard hairs on the back and tail. Porcupines also have thin skin that will tear with the

BOX 42-1 Order Rodentia*

Suborder	Family
Anomaluromorpha	Anomaluridae: scaly-tailed squirrels
	Pedetidae: springhares
Castorimorpha	**Superfamily Castoroidea**
	Castoridae: beavers
	Superfamily Geomyoidea
	Geomyidae: pocket gophers (true gophers)
	Heteromyidae: kangaroo rats and kangaroo mice
Hystricomorpha	**Family incertae sedis Diatomyidae: Laotian rock rat**
	Infraorder Ctenodactylomorphi
	Ctenodactylidae: gundis
	Infraorder Hystricognathi
	Bathyergidae: African mole rats
	Hystricidae: Old World porcupines
	Petromuridae: dassie rat
	Thryonomyidae: cane rats–Parvorder Caviomorpha
	Heptaxodontidae: giant hutias
	Abrocomidae: chinchilla rats
	Capromyidae: hutias
	Caviidae: cavies, including guinea pigs and the capybara
	Chinchillidae: chinchillas and viscachas
	Ctenomyidae: tuco-tucos
	Dasyproctidae: agoutis
	Cuniculidae: pacas
	Dinomyidae: pacaranas
	Echimyidae: spiny rats
	Erethizontidae: New World porcupines
	Myocastoridae: nutria, coypu
	Octodontidae: octodonts
Myomorpha	**Superfamily Dipodoidea**
	Dipodidae: jerboas and jumping mice
	Superfamily Muroidea
	Calomyscidae: mouse-like hamsters
	Cricetidae: hamsters, New World rats and mice, muskrats, voles
	Muridae: true mice and rats, gerbils, spiny mice, crested rat
	Nesomyidae: climbing mice, rock mice, white-tailed rat, Malagasy rats and mice
	Platacanthomyidae: spiny dormice
	Spalacidae: mole rats, bamboo rats, and zokors
Sciuromorpha	Aplodontiidae: mountain beaver
	Gliridae (also Myoxidae, Muscardinidae): dormice
	Sciuridae: squirrels, including chipmunks, prairie dogs, & marmots

*From Latin, *rodere*, to gnaw.
Classification according to Carleton M.D. and Musser G.G. (2005).

slightest pressure.[42] Some rodents such as hamsters have flank glands in the form of dark brown patches, which are used to mark their territory and as sexual stimulation.

Several tail adaptations are present in rodents for a wide variety of functions: fat storage in rock rats (*Zyzomis* spp.), a long tail providing balance when hopping in some mice (*Notomys* spp.), and the ability to shed tail skin when seized by a predator in hopping mice, or a prehensile tail to aid in climbing in the prehensile-tailed rat (*Pogonomys* spp.).[6]

All rodents possess two pairs of continuously growing incisors that confer the ability to gnaw, as well as a monophyodont dentition (no primary teeth are present).[32] They also have a diastema space with no teeth between incisors and molars on each dental arcade. Rodents are divided in two groups on the basis of dentition. Dentition in Muridae (mice, rats, hamsters, and gerbils), Sciuridae, Castoridae, Erethizontidae, and Myocastoridae is classified as *elondont* (grow continually) only for the incisor and as *brachydont* (closed-rooted) for the molars.[51] The brachydont group of rodents consumes diets that are high in caloric energy and not sufficiently abrasive, so their teeth are low crowned with well-rooted premolars and molars. The second group, hystricomorph rodents ("porcupine-like"), including guinea pigs, chinchillas, degus, New World porcupines, agoutis, and others have all teeth open-rooted which grow continually.[27] This group comprises herbivorous rodents whose teeth have evolved to grind abrasive more voluminous diets, as their teeth have large chewing surfaces.[32]

The dental formulas of rodents vary according to different taxonomic families, although in general terms they possess four incisors (I), no canines (C), few premolars (P), and 8 to 12 molars (M). Old world rats and mice (Muridae) have 16 teeth (2 I 1/1, C 0/0, P 0/0, M 3/3), whereas squirrels (Sciuridae) have 20 to 22 teeth (2 I 1/1, C 0/0, P 1-2/1, M 3/3). Other rodent families (Caviidae [guinea pigs]; Chinchillidae [chinchillas]; Hydrochoeridae [capybaras] and Castoridae [beavers]) possess 20 teeth (2 I 1/1, C 0/0, P 1/1, M 3/3).[32]

Rodents do not possess canine teeth, and the Australian species also lack premolars, so the dental formula for these later rodent species is: I 1/1, C 0/0, P 0/0, M 2-3/2-3.[6] Voles are an intermediate group with variation in crown length between species. Incisors in rodents differ from other teeth. Enamel is primarily present on the labial surface and is deposited unevenly. The enamel of most common rodents is white, but some species (chinchillas, hamsters, and others) may have enamel that is orange to yellow in color.

Rodents have a simple stomach with glandular portions, whereas hamsters and other rodent species possess a nonglandular portion (pars cardiaca) or forestomach and a glandular stomach (pars pilorica). Rats have no gallbladders.

In agoutis (*Agouti paca*), guinea pigs (*Cavia porcellus*), coypus (*Myocastor coypus*), and capybaras (*Hydrochoerus hydrochahaeris*) lung anatomy is well described, which might be useful for clinicians to diagnose the location of pulmonary disease and when performing necropsies.[13]

The urinary and reproductive tracts terminate in separate urethral and vaginal orifices in the female. Small rodents are spontaneous ovulators and are polyestrous. Chinchillas have two cervixes and two uterine horns. In most female rodents of both suborders, the genital opening is opened only during the heat season, after parturition, and when an infection occurs.[48]

Most male rodents have open inguinal canals, an os penis, and a complex urogenital system that contains prominent accessory glands.[33] Males of the Dasyproctidae family possess a pair of keratinized lateral accessory structures on the glans in the form of "wings."[48]

The testes usually lie in the scrotum in the breeding season; however, in porcupines, agoutis, chinchillas, cavies, and capybaras, testes lie in the inguinal canal, so no true scrotum is present in these species. A distinct scrotal sac is absent in prairie dogs. One of the most important features to consider in rodent breeding is the precocial nature of the youngsters in the suborder Stricognatha, whereas they are altricial in the suborder Scuirognatha.[48]

Prairie dogs possess a unique anatomic feature: trigonal anal sacs, which are ducts that appear as white papillae beside the anus.[28]

Female house mice have five or more pairs of teats, whereas female Australian native mice have only two pairs of teats, located in the inguinal region.[6]

PHYSIOLOGY

Tables 42-1 through 42-3 provide biologic information on New World and Old World rodents.

TABLE 42-1

Biologic Information of Domesticated Rodents

Common Name	Hamster	Guinea Pig	Rat	Mouse	Chinchilla	Prairie Dog
Scientific name	Mesocricetus auratus	Cavia porcellus	Rattus norvegicus	Mus musculus	Chinchilla lanigera	Cynomys spp.
Family	Cricetidae	Cavidae	Muridae	Muridae	Chinchillidae	Sciuridae
Longevity (years)	1.5–2.0	4.0–5.0	2.5–3.5	1.5–3.0	10–20	6–10
Weight (adults): Male	85–130 grams (g)	900–1200 g	450–530 g	20–40 g	400–500 g	0.5–2.2 g
Female	95–150 g	700–900 g	250–300 g	25–40 g	400–600 g	Males larger than females
Geographic distribution	Middle East	Brazil, Argentina, Peru, and Uruguay	Worldwide	Worldwide	Peru, Bolivia, Chile, Argentina	North America
Dental formula	Incisor (I) 1/1, molar (M) 3/3	I 1/1, premolar (P) 1/1, M 3/3	I 1/1, M 3/3	I 1/1, M 3/3	I 1/1, P 1/1, M 3/3	I 1/1, P 1/1, M 3/3
Water consumption milliliter per 100 gram body weight per day (mL/100 g BW/day)	20	10	10–12	15		Varies, depending on captive diets
Food consumption (g/100 g BW/day)	15	6	10	15	3–6	Calorie consumption varies throughout the year
Rectal temperature ° C	37–38	37.2–39.5	35.9–37.5	36.5–38.0	37–38	35.3–39.0
Heart rate (beats per minute)	250–500	230–380	250–450	325–780	100–150	83–318
Respiratory rate (per minute)	35–135	40–100	70–115	60–220	40–100	40–60
Blood volume milliliter per kilogram (mL/kg)	78	69–75	57–70	76–80	—	60–90

Adapted from References 27, 28, 33, and 48.

Rodents do not pant and have no sweat glands, so their ability to withstand high temperature is very limited. Hamsters, chipmunks, and prairie dogs are permissive hibernators. Other rodents such as woodchucks (*Marmota monax*) do hibernate, presenting an annual cycle of changes in metabolic function during the winter. When ambient temperatures reach 5°C (41°F), they curl up and enter a deep sleep.[33] Prairie dogs may enter a dormant period in inclement weather and tend to gain weight in the autumn as the light cycle and temperature decrease.[28]

Rodents are monogastric, and most practice some degree of coprophagy or cecotrophy, a behavior that involves ingestion of pellets of digestive origin taken directly from the anus, for two reasons: (1) to repopulate the intestinal tract with bacterial flora and (2) to absorb amino acids and vitamins B and K synthetized by those microbes.

Cavies, chinchillas, porcupines, voles, beavers, capybaras, lemmings, and muskrats and other rodents all have complete glandular stomachs, are strict herbivores, and are cecotrophic. They have a prominent cecum and an elongated colon and are hindgut fermenters; bacterial and protozoal fermentation aids in the digestion of cellulose.[6,50]

Carnivorous species such as the water rat (*Hydromys chrysogaster*) have a relatively small stomach, with most (74%) of this organ being composed of glandular tissue.[6] In rats and hamsters, a muscular sphincter limiting the esophagus and stomach prevents these species from vomiting. Insectivorous rodents (grasshopper mice, *Onychomys* sp.; burrowing mice, *Oxymycterus* sp.) have unpocketing and special glandular areas in the stomach.[50]

Rodents in the family Muridae and Cricetidae are omnivorous and coprophagic and have a simple stomach, small intestine, and modest development of the colon and cecum, all of which permits some degree of retention of ingesta for fiber fermentation.

Smell is probably the most important sense in most rodents, since the reproductive cycle, sexual attraction, and parental care are influenced by the acrid odors from glandular secretions. In dasyproctids, a pair of glandular structures in the perianal area secrete acrid odors to mark territory and as a means of sexual communication.[48]

SPECIAL HOUSING REQUIREMENTS

Being such a diverse animal group, rodents have different housing requirements, and most are nocturnal. Among nocturnal rodents, we find the following families: Pedetoidae, Hystricidae, Castoridae, Agoutidae, Chinchillidae, and Dinomyidae.[50]

Australian rodents may be arboreal, terrestrial, aquatic, and burrowing. Rodents are agile and fast, jump high, burrow, and gnaw, and it is of utmost importance to consider these adaptations when designing an enclosure for this animal group, particularly with regard to cleaning.[6] Rodents have been housed singly, in pairs, or in harem groups, although some of them do well in groups, as they are social animals living in large communities in the wild (prairie dogs and capybaras).[28,48]

Diurnal species of rodents include Sciuridae, Caviidae, Myocastoridae, Dasyproctidae, and Octodontidae. Capybaras are crepuscular rodents that live in groups of more than 20 animals, with a dominant male and several females.[48] Agoutis and acouchis (*Myoprocta achouchy*) are examples of South American terrestrial rodents, and coypus (*Myocastor coypus*) capybaras and beavers are aquatic species.[48] Australian rodents are mainly nocturnal or crepuscular, so for display purposes, reversed light cycles are used. It is worthy to

TABLE 42-2

Biologic Information of New World and Old World Rodents

Common Name	Scientific Name	Family	Longevity (years)	Weight (adults) (both sexes)	Geographic Distribution
Capybara	*Hydrochoerus hydrochaeris*	Caviidae	12	30–100 kg	Central and South America
Agouti	*Dasyprocta* spp.	Dasyproctidae	18	3–6 kg	Central and South America
Acouchi	*Myoprocta achouchy*	Dasyproctidae	10	0.6–1.3 kg	South America
Patagonian hare	*Dolichotis patagonum*	Caviidae	10	9–16 kg	Argentina, Paraguay, Bolivia
Rock cavy	*Kerodon rupestris*	Caviidae	11	1 kg	Endemic to eastern Brazil
New World porcupine	*Sphiggurus* spp.	Erethizontidae	12	1.1–1.3 kg	South America
Coendou	*Coendou* spp.	Erethizontidae	12	1.5–2 kg	Central and South America
Lowland paca	*Cuniculus paca*	Cuniculidae	16	6–13 kg	Tropical America, Mexico to Argentina
Pacarana	*Dinomys branickii*	Dinomyidae	10	10–15 kg	Brazil, Bolivia, Colombia, Venezuela
Coypu	*Myocastor coypus*	Myocastoridae	15	7–10 kg	South America
Viscacha	*Lagostomus maximus*	Chinchillidae	9	5–8 kg	Argentina, Bolivia, and Paraguay
Ingram's squirrel	*Sciurus ingrami*	Sciuridae	15	0.25 kg	South America
Crested porcupine	*Hsytrix* spp.	Hystricidae	>20	17–30 kg	Southern Europe, Asia, and Africa
Woodchuck	*Marmot monax*	Sciuridae	15	3–7 kg	North America
Beaver	*Castor* spp.	Castoridae	>20	9–30 kg	North America, Eurasia
Springhaas	*Pedetes capensis*	Pedetoidae	15	4.0 kg	Southern and Eastern Africa
Muskrat	*Ondatra zibethicus*	Cricetidae	6	0.5–1.8 kg	Native to North America, Introduced worldwide
Gray squirrel	*Sciurus carolinensis*	Sciuridae	20	0.4–0.7 kg	North America, U.K. (introduced)
Giant squirrel	*Ratufa* spp.	Sciuridae	19	1.5–2.0 kg	Southeast Asia, India

Adapted from references 27, 28, and 48.

TABLE 42-3

Biologic Data of the Most Common Australian Rodents Kept in Captivity*

Common Name	Spinifex Hopping Mouse	Water Rat	Plains Rat
Scientific name	*Notomys* spp.	*Hydromys chrysogaster*	*Pseudomys australis*
Family	Muridae	Muridae	Muridae
Longevity (years)	3–5.5	2–6	2–3
Weight (adults)	27–45	340–1275	50–80
Geographic distribution	Australia	Australia	Australia

*The physiological parameters of Australian native rodents are likely to be similar to those of domestic rodents.[6]

mention, however, that some rodent species in captivity show a partial shift from nocturnal activity to diurnal activity.[6]

Species of terrestrial (prairie dogs) or arboreal (common dormouse, *Muscardinus avellanarius*) rodents that hibernate or estivate (Sciuridae, Castoridae, Hystricidae, and Chinchillidae) require burrows, nest boxes, and even hollow logs or other types of materials.[50]

Shelter and nest boxes should include rock shelters, tussock grasses, and plastic boxes.[6] For some smaller species of rodents (hamsters, degus, duprasi, chipmunks, prairie dogs), it is advisable to provide deep bedding made of materials such as newspaper, shredded recycled paper pellets, or hardwood shavings for digging and tunneling. Sawdust or sand makes a good substrate for energetic burrowers. Coarse sand may be abrasive, so fine-grained sand is recommended.[6] The printing ink in newspapers is toxic to hamsters.[28,51]

The design of enclosures for rodents depends on the species. Enclosure size must reflect the natural behaviors of the species (arboreal or terrestrial).[6] For domesticated rodents, a minimum space of 0.9 square meters (m^2) per adult (guinea pigs, chinchillas) is recommended. Cages must be made of strong metal, not wood, and should not be larger than 2.5 centimeters (cm), and have fine wire meshing to prevent foot and limb injury. The cage should have a metal support structure, with part of the floor being solid. For smaller terrestrial species, a floor space of 50 × 40 cm is recommended, and for larger terrestrial species such as Australian greater stick-nest rat (*Leporillus conditor*), the minimum recommendation is 200 × 200 cm.[6,28] The cage must be spacious enough for exercise and grazing, according to each species' needs, requiring both horizontal and vertical space with multi-levels and shelves (for chinchillas, New World porcupines, and many zoo rodents).[27,28] Vertical space of up to 2 m is recommended for some arboreal species, and Australian water rats (*Hydromys chrysogaster*) require a minimum space of 300 × 300 cm and a pond of 100 × 100 × 50 cm depth.[6] Many species of zoo rodents burrow, so to prevent escapes from outdoor facilities, it is recommended that the fence be strong, made of concrete or chain-link, and have foundation at least 1 m below ground.[50]

Some rodent species (chinchillas, guinea pigs) are prone to heat stroke at temperatures higher than 25°C and high humidity (>60%). The preferred housing parameters for these species are environmental temperature between 10°C and 24°C and 30% to 60% humidity.[27] Enclosure location must be based on environmental temperatures and ventilation, so enclosures should not be placed in direct sunlight coming in through a window to prevent overheating.[6]

To avoid buildup of ammonia, enclosures must be well ventilated and easy to clean. Frequency of cage cleaning varies according to the density of animals, substrate type, and levels of stress that the animals inside the enclosure experience with this activity.

Porcupines are very sensitive to high environmental temperatures. Shade should be provided in extreme weathers (hot and humid days). Cold and damp conditions are also detrimental for this and other tropical rodent species. Maintaining appropriate conditions in the enclosure is advised. For most small rodent species a normal light cycle (14-hour light, 10-hour dark) is advised.[59]

It is important to note that *Dasyprocta* species prefer eating on elevated surfaces or under and within vegetation, so food items must be placed accordingly for captive agoutis.[40] Furniture for rodent cages or enclosures also depends on the species housed indoors or outdoors and includes exercise wheels, apple or maple branches, PVC pipes and fittings, materials for gnawing, ponds and pools (muskrats, capybaras, beavers, coypus). In captivity, beavers (*Castoridae*) need a pool with tree branches to build a lodge. Coendus, squirrels, chinchillas, and New World porcupines are arboreal and require enclosure furniture that allows them to climb.

Some rodents (Patagonian cavies, agoutis, acouchis) may jump up to 2 m, so enclosure walls must be tall enough to prevent escape. Double doors with secure locking mechanisms are recommended for zoo rodents.[48,50] Species of Australian rodents from arid habitats tend to nest communally, whereas most species of southern Australia and tropical forest live in smaller groups or are solitary, and this must be considered when designing enclosures for these types of rodents.[6]

FEEDING

Diets of Free-Ranging Rodents

Diets for free-living rodents are as diverse as this animal order. Many rodents consume digestible foods such as nuts and seeds, but other rodents may depart from the omnivorous pattern.[31] The rodent gastrointestinal (GI) tract shows great diversity, indicating specialization for a variety of diets.

Rodents have herbivorous and carnivorous feeding adaptations, although the majority of rodents are omnivorous. Capybaras, rock cavies, and chinchillas in the wild feed preferentially on plants, grasses, and barks of small shrubs and bushes. Their natural diet is high in fiber and low in energy content. Capybaras, coypus, and beavers feed preferentially on aquatic plants, which are eaten in the water.[48] Agoutis and acouchis in the wild eat shoots, flowers, fruits, fungi, and roots, whereas coendus, New World porcupines, and squirrels, which are arboreal, feed on leaves, flowers, shoots, and palm tree fruits at tree canopies.[48]

However, evidence supports the classification of the *Dasyprocta* species as a frugivore. *Dasyprocta leporine* is reported to have a wild diet of 87% fruit, 6% animal matter, 4% fibrous foods, and 2% leaves. Currently, any evidence of cecotrophy in agoutis is lacking.[40]

Wild prairie dogs eat grasses, prairie herbs, and weeds. Under natural conditions, prairie dogs have shown three deviations from herbivory: (1) They consume fresh and old scats of American bison; (2) these rodents sometimes also eat insects such as cutworms (Noctuidae) and ground beetles (Carabidae), and short-horned grasshoppers (Acrididae); and, (3) prairie dogs sometimes cannibalize other prairie dogs that have died of natural causes or other unweaned prairie dogs.[25]

In the wild, Patagonian cavies consume vegetation and fruits. They consume leaves of monocot species (70%) and dicot species

(30%). Monocot species include *Chloris*, *Pappophorum*, and *Trichloris*, and the perennial dicots include *Atriplex lampa*, *Lycium*, and *Propsis*.[30]

Desert-living rodents eat succulent plants in the wild to obtain their water supply. Duprasi are omnivorous and eat a considerable amount of insects. Degus in the wild consume herbaceous foliage (60% by volume), with young plants and new leaves preferred over mature plants. Grasses and some seeds seasonally make up the remainder of their diet.[27] The diet of tree squirrels (two genera, *Sciurus* spp. and *Tamiasciurus* spp.) is predominantly seeds (including nuts), fruits, buds, leaves, bark, and fungi. These rodents sometimes eat invertebrates such as beetles, caterpillars, and the larvae of various insects.[20]

Flying squirrels preferentially consume hypogeous mycorrhizal fungi (truffles) over other food items. They also feed on mast-crop nuts, tree sap, insects, carrion, bird eggs and nestlings, buds, and flowers.[20]

Australian water rats are carnivorous, and their natural diet consists of fish, yabbies, prawns, and mollusks, whereas central rock rats are granivorous, and bush rats (*Rattus fuscipes*) eat a great variety of food items such as fungi, leaves, insects, and seeds in nature.[48]

Diets of Captive Rodents

To meet the nutritional and behavioral requirements of a particular rodent species in captivity, it is best to provide a varied diet that reflects the natural diet.[48]

For domesticated rodents, many different commercial diets are available, although pelleted complete feeds are preferred over products that contain a mix of seeds and grains. Fiber digestibility in Patagonian cavies is apparently similar to that of guinea pigs, although the digestibility of crude protein and ash is reported to be lower in Patagonian cavies. Even though Patagonian cavies are closely related to coprophagous guinea pigs, it is not clear whether the cavies are coprophagous as well.[30]

Adapted diets for herbivorous zoo rodents contain a mixture of rodent pellets; high-fiber herbivore pellets (acid detergent fiber higher than 30%), which are low in starches and soluble carbohydrates, low in protein, and high in indigestible fiber; and grasses, vegetables, hays, and small amounts of fruits (Eduardo Valdés, personal communication). Bermuda-grass, brome, fescue, and timothy hay are examples of nutritious foods that may be offered to captive rodents.[25] Clover and alfalfa hays are not recommended for some rodents (guinea pigs) because of their high calcium content, which may lead to calcification within the renal system in adult rodents.[15]

Diets of Patagonian cavies in zoo settings have been reported to consist of commercially produced rodent or primate chow diets, with the addition of leafy greens as the largest proportion, and some fruits.[30] (It should be noted that primate chows, when used, should consist of higher-fiber and low-soluble carbohydrates.)

Excessive levels of some fruits and vegetables (e.g., citrus fruits) may lead to GI disturbances in some rodent species, and excessive levels of high-energy foods (sunflower seeds, dog and cat food) may lead to obesity and nutritional imbalances.[48] The high proportion of seeds and nuts in the diets of wild *Dasyprocta* indicate the need for the selection of foods higher in energy and lower in water content for captive animals to ensure sufficient protein and fats in the diet.[40] Dietary fiber levels for wild *Dasyprocta* are apparently consistent year-round. In captive agoutis, the suggested level of dietary crude fiber for a 2.7-kg animal is 157 g crude fiber per kilogram dry matter (DM) feed.[40] It must be remembered that high-fiber hays and grasses are crucial for captive rodents to ensure normal GI tract function, teeth wearing, and overall health, so they must be provided ad libitum on a daily basis.[15,59] Rodents should be provided with suitable objects to gnaw to allow normal behavior and reduce the incidence of dental disease.[48]

Vitamin and mineral supplements are not required if a balanced (varied) diet is supplied to captive rodents. Unlimited access to clean, fresh water should be ensured for all rodents in captivity, even for desert-living species.

Unique Nutritional Requirements

Guinea pigs and other members of the family Caviidae (capybaras) are incapable of endogenous synthesis of vitamin C (ascorbic acid), since they have a mutated gene for L-gulono-g-lactone oxidase. This enzyme prevents the conversion of L-gulonolactone to L-ascorbic acid.[22,65] Thus, the provision of supplemental vitamin C is an important component of the dietary management of guinea pigs in captivity.

Classification of *Dasyprocta* species as omnivores supports endogenous ascorbic acid synthesis. A study on the biosynthesis of ascorbic acid in the acouchi and agouti further supports endogenous ascorbic acid synthesis in *Dasyprocta*.[40]

RESTRAINT AND HANDLING

Interesting and useful information, including respiratory rate and effort, overall behavior, and gait, may be obtained by examining the rodent as it moves around on the examination table.[33] Some rodent species may also become stressed and collapse during prolonged handling, so minimal handling is advised.[6]

All rodents, including some kept as pets, tend to bite, and improper handling may result in injury to the animal, the handler, or both. Also, handling of small rodents may be challenging, and the key is to maximize diagnostic information while maintaining the safety of both the clinician and the patient.[23,33]

Pet rodents may often be picked up in the palm of the hand or grasped by the tail for transferring or examination.[23] Unlike domesticated rodents, grasping the tail of many Australian rodents may result in the tail skin slipping off or degloving of the tail.[6]

Small rodents such as mice, rats, hamsters, gerbils, duprasi, and chipmunks may be held around the shoulders and pelvic girdle, with the head between the first and second fingers. Firm but gentle pressure, as needed, may prevent the animal from turning the head back to bite, help with performing the examination with the other hand, and, above all, avoid inadvertent ocular prolapse.[51]

Guinea pigs are docile animals and may be carried by supporting its weight in one hand and cupping its dorsum with the other. Chinchillas may be generally handled in the same fashion as guinea pigs, but frequently may be removed from a cage by grasping and lifting the base of the tail, using the opposite hand to support the body.[46]

Prairie dogs may have a strong bond with humans or the social group. However, if untamed, they may roll quickly and bite, squirt musk from the anal sacs, or inflict significant scratches with their long, sharp nails.[28] Gloves may be worn when handling prairie dogs and other aggressive rodents, but gloves limit feel and do not protect the handler against a direct bite.[23,28] Gloves that protect from the bite of a laboratory rodent species may be completely ineffective with a wild rodent such as a marmot or a squirrel.[19] To handle a prairie dog, a small towel may be placed over its head, to prevent biting, and then be lifted, as with guinea pigs and chinchillas.

Degus should be handled in a similar manner to chinchillas, but they seem more inclined to bite. It is advised that degus be restrained with a towel or placed on a nonslip surface for examination.[27] Small laboratory rodents may be transferred from cage to cage by using soft forceps; this same technique is sometimes used for small free-living rodents caught in traps.[23] Plastic tubes are sometimes used for transporting smaller rodents, conducting examinations, taking radiographs, or administering anesthesia.[19] Clear plastic bags may also be successfully used to restrain, measure, and sex rodents, with minimal direct handling.[6]

Agoutis and acouchis may be safely restrained by using a sack with a metal ring attached to one of the bag ends. This method allows the handler to take biomedical parameters while keeping the animal relatively calm.[48] Most rodent species may be netted with a fine mesh, which avoids the entanglement of the claws, and larger species such as capybaras, marmots, and woodchucks may be handled by using specialized squeeze cages.[19] Another option for these and other large rodents is the use of extended nets on the floor on a corridor that may be suspended to bag up the animal once it crosses through.[48]

Porcupines offer a unique challenge, since they have sharp quills and may move back quickly and with great force when they feel threatened. This species also has pathogenic bacteria covering the quills. Some authors recommend purpose-built restraint boxes for handling porcupines.[23]

Special care is required during handling of some species of rodents such as coendus (*Coendu mexicana*) because of their passive defensive abilities. They have modified hair (histriciformes) covered by interwoven scales acting as small tabs, and this warrants specific mechanics during handling to avoid handler injury. Two techniques have proven efficient for handling coendus, depending on the purpose for restraining. One technique requires grasping the animal by the end portion of the tail (where no quills are present), supporting the hindlimbs on a branch or stick, and exposing the hip musculature for injection. Another handling alternative is to force the coendu to enter a PVC tube, where it is immobilized to allow some procedures, including sexing, hand injections, and temperature checking.[48]

Wild rodents in the families Muridae and Sciuridae may be trapped by using wire cage traps and metal box traps (Sherman traps).[53] Aquatic rodents such as beavers, muskrats, and nutrias may be captured in specialized hinged cage traps, called *Hancock* or *Bailey traps*, or wire cage traps set on land.[53] Potential zoonotic threats (Hantavirus infection, tularemia, lymphocytic choriomeningitis virus (LCMV) infection, yersiniosis) should be considered when handling wild or feral rodents, and use of special protective gear is advised.[53]

In handling all rodents, care must be taken to prevent inhibition of respiration or exacerbation of stress during restraint.[27,33] Nervous, distressed, sick, or debilitated rodents benefit from mild sedation for examination, diagnostics, and treatment procedures.[33] Some rodents are prone to "breath holding" when physically restrained, which may cause the rodent to develop hypercapnia and bradycardia. In these species, it is best to use other methods such as an anesthetic chamber for induction.[50]

Chemical Restraint

Basic principles of domestic mammal anesthesiology apply to exotic mammals, although the latter have specific features that must be taken into account when planning an anesthetic procedure. When performed with appropriate equipment and by experienced personnel, chemical restraint reduces stress and the risk of injury.[6] According to a recent report, a higher risk of anesthesia-induced mortality exists in small exotic mammal species compared with that in dogs and cats.[61]

Rodents are often catecholamine-driven prey species that are more easily stressed, are commonly presented in advanced stages of disease (respiratory and nutritional-related issues) with little respiratory and cardiovascular reserve, and have anatomic challenges with regard to procedures such as endotracheal intubation and intravenous access.[14] As rodents are primarily obligate nasal breathers, rodent anesthesia is sometimes complicated by upper respiratory disease such as *Streptococcus* infection in mice and other rodents, hypovitaminosis C and bordetellosis in guinea pigs, chlamydophilosis and adenovirus infection in several rodent species, pasteurellosis and pseudo-odontoma in prairie dogs, and mycoplamosis in rats and other rodents of the family Muridae.[23,28,50] These issues may occur in association with incisor overgrowth, chronic suppurative periodontal disease, and dusty or poorly ventilated environments, all of which are frequent problems in captive rodents.[28]

ANESTHESIA AND SURGERY

Chemical restraint is preferable for wild-caught or rarely handled individuals if a thorough examination or prolonged procedure is necessary.[6] Careful planning and preparation of the sedation or anesthesia procedure greatly contributes to success. This includes stabilizing the patient prior to the procedure (normothermic, rehydrated, good nutrition state and no metabolic derangements), calculating emergency drugs using an emergency drug chart, and preparing equipment and supplies (anesthetic drugs, catheters, fluids, anesthetic circuits according to the size of the rodent, with appropriately sized bags and masks, surgical equipment, preheated disinfectant solutions).[14]

Fasting is not routinely done in small rodents prior to anesthesia, since this exhausts glycogen stores and contributes to ileus in guinea pigs, chinchillas, and other herbivorous rodents.[23] Also, it is important to keep in mind that many rodent species cannot vomit, so withholding food or water for prolonged periods of time before anesthesia is not required. For some rodents, food may be removed approximately 1 hour before anesthesia induction to reduce the presence of food within the oral cavity.[61]

All rodents should be accurately weighed to ensure correct drug and fluid calculations.[61] For all rodents, anesthetic agents that provide a rapid recovery, have specific antagonists, and are easily adjusted with regard to anesthetic depth are preferred.[50]

In rodent species, it is not usually feasible to administer intravenous anesthetics for induction of anesthesia. However, in zoo and pet rodents, intramuscular injections of sedatives, tranquilizers, and anesthetics are possible either by hand injection or remote delivery. Premedicating the rodent with a sedative is often recommended, since this allows for a smooth anesthetic induction. Anticholinergic drugs such as atropine and glycopyrrolate are not routinely administered to rodents as a premedication but are administered to patients that present bradycardia during the anesthetic procedure.[61]

Neither glycopyrrolate nor atropine influence respiration rate, core body temperature, or systolic blood pressure, alone or combined with injectable anesthetics.[23,61] However, glycopyrrolate is more effective in maintaining heart rate within the normal range in rats.[23]

Large doses of parasympatholytics may alter GI motility in hind gut fermenters, including rodents, so the lowest doses are suggested if the use of a parasympatholytic is required.[21]

A balanced approach to anesthesia and analgesia must be taken for each animal, including preanesthetic analgesics, anxiolytics, local or incisional anesthetics, general anesthetics, and post-anesthesia analgesics.[27] Sedatives and tranquilizers may be administered 30 to 60 minutes before induction via a face mask.[50] Benzodiazepines (diazepam 0.1–5 milligrams per kilogram [mg/kg], intramuscularly, intraperitoneally, or orally [IM, IP, or PO]; midazolam 0.1–2 mg/kg, IM, IP, or subcutaneously [SC], depending on the rodent species) provide good sedation and relaxation in rodents and are useful for induction of debilitated patients (midazolam) because of the minimal cardiopulmonary effects of these agents.[23] Diazepam should only be administered IV or PO, although when used IV, the patient must be monitored for hypotension caused by the propylene glycol found in most diazepam formulations.[21]

Because of their intractable natures and the difficulty of handling of many exotics and zoologic species, diazepam has been used IM and even SC. Erratic responses might occur when using intramuscular and subcutaneous delivery of this benzodiazepine.

Midazolam, a short-acting benzodiazepine that is water-soluble, when injected subcutaneously will decrease the excitability of the rodent patient during gas induction. This drug provides adequate effective sedation for approximately 1 hour when used in rodents, and when administered IM or IV in guinea pigs and other rodents, midazolam provides proper sedation for diagnostic procedures (e.g., radiography, ultrasonography).[61] It is worth mentioning that cardiorespiratory side effects associated with midazolam are minimal, so its use is not limited to healthy animals.[27,61] The combination of fentanyl–fluanisone, another sedative used in guinea pigs and other small mammals, produces profound sedation and analgesia.[17]

Injectable anesthesia alone is a practical option for rodents when access to the head and neck is required for any procedure. In small rodents, injectable anesthesia (IP, IM, or SC) is usually administered. Ketamine is one of the anesthetic drugs most commonly used in many small and zoo rodents species, usually combined with sedatives and tranquilizers, although intramuscular injection of the former and of ketamine plus xylazine has been associated with self-mutilation in some species.[23,61,43] Some rodents such as guinea pigs have limb movement at ketamine or tiletamine–zolazepam dosages expected to produce surgical anesthesia.[23] Xylazine, medetomidine, and dexmedetomidine, which are α_2-agonist drugs, combined with ketamine produce muscle relaxation, analgesia, and long duration of effect, and these combinations have been used for short-term immobilization and surgical anesthesia.[23] Recent publications indicate that midazolam enhances the analgesic properties of dexmedetomidine in rats, so it is assumed that this benzodiazepine may be combined with other α_2-agonists to provide adequate sedation and analgesia in rodents and other small mammals. α_2-agonist drugs are reversed with yohimbine, tolazoline, or atipamezole.[23] Nonetheless, many rodents presented to veterinarians are clinically ill, geriatric, and therefore potent α_2-agonists such as dexmedetomidine are only used in young healthy individuals.[4,14] Ketamine–benzodiazepine combinations produce less cardiopulmonary depression and analgesia but good muscle relaxation.[23] Opioids (butorphanol, buprenorphine) and other analgesic drugs may be added to this combination to promote adequate analgesia in rodents.

The tiletamine–zolazepam combination has been used in many laboratory, pet, and zoo rodent species, with variable results, for minor surgery, diagnostic procedures, and routine preventive medicine programs.[23,43] The author of this chapter has used the tiletamine–zolazepam combination at published doses (4–6 mg/kg, IM) in beavers, porcupines, and capybaras for routine health checks and has combined it with opioids (butorphanol 0.1 mg/kg, IM) for wound cleaning and teeth checking or trimming. It has been also used as induction for longer procedures in zoo settings, where inhalant anesthesia has been used subsequently for maintenance.

The combination of medetomidine–midazolam–fentanyl has been used successfully in chinchillas, guinea pigs, rats, mice, and hamsters, and the main advantage of this combination is that it is completely reversible with flumazenil, atipamezole, and naloxone.[35] Midazolam combined with fentanyl–fluanisone produces neuroleptoanalgesia with adequate skeletal muscle relaxation in mice, rats, gerbils, hamsters, and guinea pigs.[4,61]

Parenteral anesthesia is used in rodents when inhalant anesthesia is not available, when handling is stressful or difficult for some zoo rodents, for immobilization of rodents in the wild, to reduce inhalant anesthetic pollution, to enhance analgesia (preemptive analgesia) and for other purposes convenient to the handler or the facility.[23] Propofol, a hypnotic agent, is used in rodents and other species for induction and maintenance of anesthesia when administered as a continuous rate infusion (CRI), manually controlled infusion (MCI), and total intravenous infusion (TIVA) by intermittent bolus. This drug may be diluted with saline for injection in small rodent species. It has a higher elimination clearance and a shorter elimination half-life compared with other injectable agents, and its clearance rate is faster than the liver blood flow.[18,23] Propofol-induced apnea is related to dose, rate of injection, and the concurrent administration of other drugs. Propofol is a poor analgesic.[23] Etomidate is a nonbarbiturate that is an injectable, potent, short-acting, hypnotic, and anesthetic agent. It has been used at a rate of 1 mg/kg in rodents (prairie dogs, chinchillas, guinea pigs) by intravenous delivery for teeth inspection or trimming,[28] so potentially it might be used in other zoo rodent species for the same purposes.

Epidural anesthesia was performed in seven agoutis (*Dasyprocta azarae*) with the use of lidocaine (5 mg/kg) in the lumbosacral space 5 minutes after induction with azaperone, meperidine, xilazine, and ketamine. Duration of analgesia was 80.86 ± 16.1 minutes, and no complications from the epidural technique were observed.[55] Using reversible injectable agents and combinations provides better control of anesthetic depth, less hypothermia, less cardiopulmonary depression, and shorter recovery times.[21]

Inhalant anesthesia is the primary component of most clinical anesthetic regimes, and so is the preferred method for chemical restraint of rodents, since it has the advantage of providing oxygen, resulting in a relatively rapid and smooth induction and recovery, and allows safe and fast titration of the anesthetic dose to the required effect.[6,23]

Preoxygenation (either with an oxygen chamber or an induction chamber) of rodent patients, especially in those undergoing respiratory or cardiac diseases, improves circulatory and tissue oxygen reserves and saturation.[35] Non-rebreathing anesthetic circuits (e.g., Bain circuit or Ayre's T-piece) have low dead space and low resistance and so are recommended for use in small rodents.[61]

Intubation is not easily possible in many species of rodents, so the anesthetic is often administered into a chamber (for small- to medium-sized rodents) or through a tight-fitting mask connected to the breathing system.[23,35] Small- and medium-sized rodents are preferably induced and maintained with an inhalant anesthetic. Rodents such as prairie dogs, chinchillas, squirrels, African pouched rats, maras, and other similar-sized species have been intubated with a 2- or 2.5-mm uncuffed endotracheal tube, with the use of a "blind" technique or with the aid of an otoscope, laryngoscope, or endoscope.[23,28] Endoscopy provides the best visualization of the epiglottis and minimizes trauma during tube placement.[21] Endotracheal tubes are commercially available from the smallest 1-mm internal diameter (uncuffed) to 3-mm (cuffed) and bigger. Actually, for the smallest rodent patients, endotracheal tubes are made from over-the-needle catheters (14 g and bigger) or urinary catheters.[23] In capybaras, endotracheal tubes of 6-mm internal diameter have been used.

The rodent soft palate is fused to the base of the tongue, and entry to the glottis is through the small opening of the palatal ostium, a structure present in chinchillas, guinea pigs, and capybaras.[23] This structure is highly vascular and easily traumatized.[21] Laryngeal masks have been used successfully in rabbits weighing more than 3 kg and so could potentially be useful in similar-sized rodents. This type of mask must be easily inserted and provide a good fit for an adequate seal.[61]

The recommended inhalation agents for rodents are isoflurane and sevoflurane, in a suggested concentration of 3% to 5% for induction and 1.5% to 3% for maintenance of anesthesia for isoflurane, and concentrations of 5% to 6% are recommended for induction when sevoflurane is used. Those levels of gas anesthesia vary, depending on other drugs used prior to the inhaled agent or if any other was used at all.

Isoflurane produces a dose-dependent cardiopulmonary depression, is a poor analgesic, and has the advantage of not sensitizing the myocardium to catecholamine-induced arrhythmias.[23] Sevoflurane is similar to isoflurane, but it produces more rapid induction and recovery, and it is less irritating to inhalation. Guinea pigs are particularly prone to apnea with the use of inhalant anesthetics and require careful monitoring and sometimes the use of a respiratory stimulant (e.g., doxapram at a rate of 5–10 mg/kg, IV or IM) to keep respirations regular.[27]

The small size of rodents makes venous and intraosseous catheterization difficult. Some potential catheterization sites include the cephalic, saphenous, and auricular veins.[23] Intraosseous cannulation may be useful in smaller patients or during cardiovascular collapse. Common sites for intraosseous cannula placement are the trochanteric fossa of the femur, the tibial crest, and the humerus. Depending on the rodent size, products that may be used as intraosseous cannulas include 18-to-24-gauge 1-to-1½ -in. spinal needles or 18- to 25-gauge 1-inch hypodermic needles.[21]

For all rodent species, preemptive analgesia and sedation are critically important. High levels of circulating catecholamines, combined with the stress of handling or restraint, hypoxemia, hypercarbia, and unpredictable responses to anesthetic agents may lead to respiratory and cardiac arrest.[14] The two main groups of analgesic premedication—opioids and nonsteroidal anti-inflammatory drugs (NSAIDs)—are combined or used alone in rodents and other species.[23]

An effective pain management plan should include drugs of different classes and a multimodal approach. Midazolam may also be combined with opioid compounds such as butorphanol to provide additional analgesia.[61] Analgesic medications administered IV as a CRI may be titrated to effect, potentially reducing other drug doses within the anesthetic protocol. Microdose ketamine via intravenous CRI may be an effective analgesic.[21,23] Opioid drugs are effective analgesic agents for the control of acute or chronic visceral pain. In small exotic mammals, including rodents, butorphanol, buprenorphine, and fentanyl are regularly used and well tolerated. The main adverse side effects of opioids in small mammals are drowsiness and respiratory depression, which is dose dependent.[35,61]

Pica and gastric distension have been observed in rats receiving high doses of buprenorphine (0.5 mg/kg, SC).[12] Opioids may also be used for CRI. When used as a low-dose intravenous CRI, opioids do not induce GI stasis in small hind gut fermenters and so may be a part of balanced anesthesia and analgesia protocols. Remifentanil is an ultra-short-acting μ-agonist opioid that is very suitable for CRI in small mammals. Butorphanol has also been used as a CRI, although no published data on small exotic mammals are available.[21]

Tramadol, a synthetic opioid drug, is a centrally acting drug, being both a weak opioid agonist with selectivity for the μ-receptor, and a weak inhibitor of the reuptake of norepinephrine and serotonin. A few studies have been performed in rodents, mainly in laboratory animals. A study in rats showed that tramadol administered intraperitoneally (1–25 mg/kg) showed delayed responses after thermal or ischemic noxious stimuli, and subcutaneously at the site that received noxious stimuli provided local analgesia. The same study found that tramadol and gabapentin worked synergistically to provide analgesia in rats.[56]

The most common NSAIDs drugs used in rodents include meloxicam, carprofen, and ketoprofen. Clinical experience indicates that doses <1 to 2 mg/kg of meloxicam in rats do not adequately alleviate pain after surgery.[61]

Local anesthesia and regional (epidural) anesthesia have proven efficacious in providing good analgesia in rodents for minor procedures such as cesarian section in guinea pigs. Lidocaine and bupivacaine are commonly used local anesthetics that may be applied topically, via tissue infiltration, intra-articularly, as regional nerve block, or by epidural injection.[23,61]

Important nerve blocks for dental surgery in rodents include infraorbital, mental, mandibular, and maxillary nerve blocks. Other sites for nerve blocking in rodents and small mammals are the brachial plexus, the sciatic nerve, and the intratesticular nerve.[21] Volumes of local anesthetic agents used for epidural injection vary between 0.1 and 0.2 milliliters per kilogram (mL/kg).[61]

It is essential to record supportive care and monitoring minute-by-minute in rodents. Eyes should be well lubricated to prevent corneal desiccation and ulceration. The order of loss of reflexes in rodents is as follows: palpebral, pedal, jaw tone, ear pinch reflex (surgical plane).[62] A fixed, dilated pupil that is unresponsive to light is a cross-species indicator of excessive depth.[23]

Monitoring of anesthesia requires recording heart rate, respiratory rate, body temperature, and analgesia. Heart rate varies widely among rodent species and is determined by temperature, size, metabolism, respiratory rate, and the presence or absence of painful stimuli.[21] Quality pediatric stethoscopes, instead of esophageal stethoscopes, are recommended for small species of rodents. Because of the rapid heart rate of many small rodents, electrocardiography (ECG) complexes are assessed with sweep speeds of 100 millimeters per second (mm/s) and 200 mm/s.[21]

The Doppler flow detector is used where major arteries are close to the skin, for example, the ventral aspect of the tail base; the carotid, femoral, and auricular arteries; or directly over the heart. Normal systolic blood pressure measurements obtained with the Doppler range from 90 to 120 millimeters of mercury (mm Hg).[21] Some authors have successfully measured blood pressure in the hindlimbs of guinea pigs, chinchillas, degus, prairie dogs, and other rodents by using a size 1 cuff with sphygmomanometer and audio Doppler ultrasonography just above the medial tarsus.[27]

As in other species, the respiratory rate and character should be monitored closely. In addition to direct monitoring of respiration, respiratory monitors are indicated in monitoring rodent anesthesia protocols, but those that are triggered by a thermistor in the airway function well only in patients weighing more than 500 g. To assess ventilation, end-tidal carbon dioxide ($PET\text{-}CO_2$) monitoring, using a side-stream capnograph, is useful.

Pulse oximetry (SpO_2) is used in many species to evaluate arterial hemoglobin oxygen saturation. It has been evaluated in rats but appears accurate at hemoglobin saturation levels greater than 70%.[23,35] Pulse oximeters may be used on the ears or tongue of guinea pigs, chinchillas, prairie dogs, and other medium-sized rodents, on the feet of most rodent species, and also on the tail, or vaginal or rectal mucous membranes.[21,35]

Some sick or debilitated animals require intermittent positive-pressure ventilation (IPPV) during anesthesia, which, in the case of rodents, is recommended at initial inspiratory pressures of 5 to 10 centimeters of water (cm H_2O) and rates of 6 to 10 breaths per minute.[21]

To reduce the morbidity and mortality associated with anesthetic procedures in rodents, it is of utmost importance to monitor core body temperature. Because of the ratio of large surface area to volume, hypothermia is one of the most frequent complications in anesthetized rodents. An electronic thermometer probe may be fastened to the perineal area to continuously monitor the body temperature.[23,27] Small rodents (less than 500 g) require an ambient temperature of 35°C to 37°C during recovery and larger ones between 25°C and 35°C.[50]

It is recommended that rodents be wrapped in aluminum foil or bubble wrap immediately after induction. Supplemental heating (electric heat pads, heated operating tables, forced warm air blankets, heat lamps, hot water bottles, and towels) should be provided during and after anesthesia. It is of utmost importance to stress that heating devices should not be in direct contact with the animal's skin or body surface to avoid iatrogenic burns.[35,50]

Once the anesthetic procedure has been completed, the animal is placed in a warm, quiet environment and monitored. Monitoring of body functions must continue until the patient is fully alert, since general anesthesia may have adverse effects on gut motility and flora, especially in herbivorous rodents.[27] It is recommended that GI function be assessed, and if necessary, administration of gut motility enhancers (cisapride, metoclopramide, or ranitidine) is advised.

Prolonged recovery is usually caused by hypothermia, hypoglycemia, and anesthetic overdose, altered drug elimination, or all of these factors.

Assisted feeding with the appropriate nutritional products (herbivores, omnivores, and carnivores) is of great importance during recovery in rodents. Ongoing fluid therapy may also be necessary until the animal is able to maintain hydration. Table 42-4 details chemical agents commonly used as sedatives, anesthetics, and analgesics in rodents.

Special Conditions That Require Surgical Intervention

Once chemically immobilized, some common procedures such as incisor trimming (extractions, occlusion adjustments), orchidectomy and vasectomy procedures (frequently reported in domesticated rodents and as a population-control tool in wild agoutis in Brazil), ovariohysterectomy, cesarean section, wound healing (superficial abscesses, trauma, cage-mate bites), orthopedic procedures, mass removals, and ophthalmic disease diagnosis and treatment, among others, are routinely performed in pet and zoo rodents. Anatomic and physiologic rodent features such as an open inguinal canal, the functional cremaster muscle that allows the testicles to migrate into and out of the abdominal cavity, and the considerable amount of fat

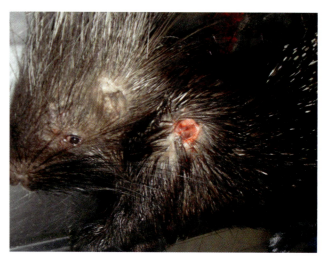

FIGURE 42-1 Crested porcupine (*Hystrix cristata*) with a traumatic skin lesion caused by a dart applied with a blow pipe.

in that area warrant specific care and a precise surgical orchidectomy technique described elsewhere.[3,48]

Computed tomography (CT) was recently used to determine the relevant reproductive anatomy of a male African crested porcupine (*Hystrix africaeaustralis*) and develop a surgical approach for castration. CT imaging confirmed that the testes were located immediately lateral to the prepuce beneath subcutaneous adipose tissue.[49]

Self-mutilation has been reported in rodents and other small mammals after surgical procedures, so gentle handling of tissues and proper analgesia are advised to avoid causing this type of trauma.[50]

Porcupines (*Hystrix africaeaustralis*) have a very thin skin that tears even with slight pressure.[23,42] In the experience of the author of this chapter, traumatic lesions to the skin in this species may even be caused when remote anesthesia is applied by blow pipe (Figure 42-1).

Small-diameter sutures with atraumatic needles such as the ones used for bird skin repair may be useful in porcupines. Figure 42-1 shows a crested porcupine (*Hystrix cristata*) with a traumatic skin lesion caused by a dart applied with a blow pipe.

DIAGNOSTICS

Blood Collection

Even when some blood collection sites have been developed by laboratory animal veterinarians and technicians, some of these locations (orbital venous plexus, cardiocentesis) might seem objectionable when handling pet or zoo rodents. Many rodents do not tolerate the level of restraint required to safely collect an adequate volume for analysis, so they must be sedated or anesthetized.[33,44] It is important to recognize that the blood volume of most small rodents is approximately 6% to 7% of total body weight, and removing a maximum of 10% (a general rule of thumb for most patients) of the blood volume is generally safe.[33] A fresh blood smear should be made at the time of sampling to enable manual hematologic examination if blood volumes are very small.[51] It is also possible to consider drawing 1% of the total body weight in kilograms of blood in healthy rodents (Table 42-5).[44]

The most frequent sites for collecting blood are the femoral, cephalic, lateral tail, saphenous, and jugular veins. A site that has very few reports of complications in some small rodents (hamsters, chinchillas, prairie dogs, rats, chipmunks, squirrels) is the cranial vena cava. Sedation or general anesthesia for successful collection is often required.[41] In members of the Dasyproctidae family, the lateral saphenous vein is a viable option.[48] Prairie dogs are more

TABLE 42-4

Sedatives, Anesthetics, and Analgesics Commonly Used in Rodents (doses are given in mg/kg)

Drug Name	Mouse/Gerbil, Hamster	Rat	Guinea Pig, Prairie Dog, and Chinchilla	Degu	Duprasi	Beaver, Capybara, and Porcupine	Native Australian Rodents	Comments
OPIOIDS								
Buprenorphine	0.05–0.1, SC, q6-12h	0.05–0.1, SC, IM, q6-12h	0.01–0.05, SC, IM, IV, q6-12h	0.05–0.1, SC, q8-12h	0.05–0.1, SC, q1 h	0.01–0.03, IM, SC, q8-12h	—	Can be associated with pica in rats
Butorphanol	1-2, SC, IP, q2-4h	1-2, SC, IM, IV, q2-4h	0.5–1.0, IM, IV, q4h (GP) 0.2–2.0, IM, IV, q2-4h (Ch)	0.4–2.0, IM, q8h	1–5, SC, q4h	0.5, IM, SC, q4h	—	Weaker analgesic than buprenorphine
Hydromorphone	0.2–0.4, SC, q6h	0.2–0.5, SC, q6-8h	0.2–0.5, SC, IM, q6-8h	—	—	—	—	—
Meperidine	10–20, SC, q2-4h	10–20, IM, SC, q2-4h	10–20, IM, SC, q2-4h	10–20, SC, IM	20, SC, IM, q2-3h	—	—	—
Morphine	2–5, SC, IM, q4h	0.5–5, SC, IM, q4h	2–5, SC, IM, q4h	2–5, IM, q4h	2–5, SC, q2-4h	1–3, IM, SC, q4-6h	—	Most commonly used as a single dose preoperatively
Nalbuphine hydrochloride	2–4, SC, IM, q2-4h	1–2, SC, IM, q2-4h	1–2, IM, q2-4h	—	—	—	—	—
Oxymorphone	0.2–0.4, SC, q6-12h	0.2–1.5, SC, q6-12h	0.2–0.5, SC, IM, q6-8h	0.2–0.5, SC, IM, q8-12h	0.2–0.5, SC, IM, q8-12h	—	—	—
NONSTEROIDAL ANTI-INFLAMMATORY DRUGS								
Carprofen	5–10, SC, PO, q12-24h	1–5, SC, PO, q12-24h	1–5, PO, q24h	4, PO, q24h	5, PO, q24h	—	—	—
Flunixin	2.5, SC, q12h	2.5, IM, SC, q12h	1–2, SC, q24	1–2, SC, q24	2–5, SC, q12-24h	0.5, IM, SC, q12-24h	—	Not recommended at least in smaller rodents due to potential renal damage
Ketoprofeno	2–5, SC, IM, q12-24h	2–5, SC, IM, q12-24h	1–2, SC, IM, q12-24h	—	—	1–3, IM, SC, q24h	—	—
Meloxicam	1–5, PO, SC, q24h	0.5–2.0, PO, SC, q24h	0.1–0.3, PO, SC, q24h	0.2–0.4, SC, PO, q24h	0.2–0.4, SC, PO, q24h	0.1–0.3, SC, PO, q12-24h	—	—
Paracetamol	—	—	1–2 mg/mL in drinking water	1–2 mg/mL in drinking water	1–2 mg/mL in drinking water	1–2 mg/mL in drinking water	—	—
OTHER ANALGESICS								
Tramadol	5–40, IP, q12-24h (M) 5–10, PO, q12-24h (H, G)	5–20, PO, SC, IP q12-24h 5–40, SC	5–10, PO, q12-24h	—	—	—	—	—
Gabapentin	50, PO, q24h (H)	—	3–5, PO, q12-24h	—	—	—	—	—
ANESTHETICS								
Ketamine/Acepromazine	50–150/2.5-5.0, IP	50–150/2.5-5.0, IP	20–50/0.5-1.0, IP, IV	—	—	—	—	—
Ketamine/Diazepam	50–100/2-5, IP	40–100/3-5, IP	20–40/1-5, IM	20–30/1-2, IM	Not published	—	—	Poor analgesia
Ketamine/Dexmedetomidine	—	—	40/0.5, IM, IP	—	50/0.5, IP	—	—	—
Ketamine/Medetomidine	50–100/0.1-0.5, IP, IV	45–75/0.3-0.5, IM, IP	5–40/ 0.05-0.5	—	—	3–4/0.03-0.04, IM, IV	—	Lowest doses of ketamine for chinchillas

Continued

TABLE 42-4
Sedatives, Anesthetics, and Analgesics Commonly Used in Rodents (doses are given in mg/kg)—cont'd

Drug Name	Mouse/Gerbil, Hamster	Rat	Guinea Pig, Prairie Dog, and Chinchilla	Degu	Duprasi	Beaver, Capybara, and Porcupine	Native Australian Rodents	Comments
Ketamine/Midazolam	—	5–10/0.25–0.5, IP	5–10/0.5–1.0, IM	—	—	3–4/0.03–0.04, IM, IV	—	—
Ketamine/Xylazine	35–200/2–10, IP	40–100/5–10, IM, IP	20–40/1–2, IM	40/2–4, IM	50/5, IP	5–10/1–2, IM	—	—
Tiletamine/Zolazepam	50–80, IP	5–10, IP, IM	20–40, IM, for chinchillas	—	—	4–6, IM	20–40, IM	Australian brown rat
Propofol	—	7.5–26, IV	2–5, IV	—	—	6–8, IV	—	—
REVERSAL AGENTS								
Atipamezole	≥1, SC, IM, IV	0.1–1, SC, IM, IV, IP	≥1, SC, IM, IV	1, SC, IM, IV, IP	1, SC, IM, IV, IP	—	—	1:1 volume reversal of medetomidine or dexmedetomidine
Flumazenil	—	0.1–1.0, IM, IV, IP	0.05–0.1, SC, IM, IV	0.1, SC	—	—	—	Reversal of benzodiazepines
Naloxone	0.01–0.1, SC, IP	0.01–0.1, SC, IP	0.01–0.1, SC, IP	0.01–0.1, SC, IP	0.01–0.1, SC, IP	—	—	Narcotic reversal
Yohimbine	0.5–1.0, IM, IV	0.2, IV; 0.5 IM	0.5–1.0, IV; 2, IM	2, IM	2, IM	—	—	Reversal for xylazine
LOCAL ANESTHETICS								
Bupivacaine (local and regional blocks)	<2	<2	<2	—	—	—	—	Dosages for local blocks may extend to 2 mg/kg as the maximum dose
Lidocaine (local and regional blocks)	<4	<4	<4	—	—	—	—	Short duration of 20–30 minutes in rats
PREANESTHETICS								
Atropine	0.04 mg/kg, SC, IM	0.05 mg/kg, SC, IP IM, IV	0.05 mg/kg, SC, IM, IV	0.05–0.1 mg/kg, SC, IM	0.1–0.4 mg/kg, SC, IM	0.03 mg/kg, SC, IM	—	Lower doses for herbivores
Glycopyrrolate	0.02–0.5 mg/kg, SC, IM	0.02–0.5 mg/kg, SC, IM, IV	0.01–0.02 mg/kg, SC, IM, IV	0.01–0.02 mg/kg, SC, IM, IV	0.01–0.02 mg/kg, SC, IM, IV	0.01 mg/kg, SC, IM	—	Lower doses for herbivores
SEDATIVES AND TRANQUILIZERS								
Acepromazine	0.5–1.0 mg/kg, IM, IP	0.5–1.0 mg/kg, IM, SC	0.5–2.5 mg/kg, IM, SC	0.5–1.0 mg/kg, IM, SC	0.5–1.0 mg/kg, IM, SC	0.1 mg/kg IM	—	May induce seizures in gerbils
Diazepam	3–5 mg/kg, IP, PO	3–5 mg/kg, IP, PO	1.0–2.5 mg/kg, IM, IP, PO	0.5–3.0 mg/kg, IM	3–5 mg/kg IM	0.1–1.0 mg/kg, IM, IP, PO	—	Erratic results and irritation if given IM
Midazolam	2–3 mg/kg, IM, SC	2.5 mg/kg, SC, IM	0.4–2.0 mg/kg, IM	0.4–2.0 mg/kg, IM	1–2 mg/kg, IM	0.1–0.5 mg/kg, IM	—	Lower doses for premedication
Fentanyl/Fluanisone *Hypnorm	0.2–1 mL/kg, IM	0.2–3.0 mL/kg, IM	0.5–1.0 mL/kg, IM	—	—	—	—	—
Medetomidine	0.03–0.2 mg/kg, SC	0.08–0.2 mg/kg, IM	0.1–0.5 mg/kg, IM, SC	—	—	—	—	Variable effects in guinea pigs
Dexmedetomidine	0.015–0.5 mg/kg, SC, IP	0.015–0.5 mg/kg, SC	0.05 mg/kg, SC, variable effects	—	0.1–0.2, mg/kg, SC	—	—	Half the dose of medetomidine
Xylazine	10–15 mg/kg, IP	10–15 mg/kg, IP	2–10 mg/kg, IM, IP	Not used by itself	Not used by itself	1–5 mg/kg, IM, SC	—	Used more for zoo rodent protocols

*Not readily commercially available in most parts of the world.
IM, Intramuscularly; IP, intraperitoneally; IV, intravenously; SC, subcutaneously.

TABLE 42-5

Hematologic Parameters of Selected Species of Rodents

Common Name	Mouse	Gerbil	Hamster	Degu	Rat	Guinea Pig	Chinchilla	Viscacha	Prairie Marmot	American Beaver
Scientific Name	*Mus musculus*	*Meriones unguiculatus*	*Mesocricetus auratus*	*Octodon degus*	*Rattus norvegicus*	*Cavia porcellus*	*Chinchilla lanigera*	*Lagostomus maximus*	*Cynomys ludovicianus*	*Castor canadensis*
PARAMETERS										
Erythrocytes ×10^6/microliter (μL)	7.5–9.7	7.0 10.0	6.5–7.5	8.69 ± 0.19 male (M)/ 8.94 ± 0.16 female (F)	6.4–8.2*	4–7*	5.6–8.4*	3.78–7.48	5.48–8.08	3.36–3.91
Packed cell volume (PCV) (%)	34–50	41 52	45–52	42–1 ± 0.59 (M)/ 40.0 ± 0.61 (F)	33.0–47.0	35–45		36.22–44.78	32.36–46.41	32.22–40.21
Hemoglobin, gram per deciliter (g/dL)	12.8–16.1	12.1–16.9	15.2–17.4	12.0 ± 0.15 (M)/ 11.7 ± 0.17 (F)	11.2–15.9	10.0–17.2		11.03–15.38	10.26–15.76	11.93–13.52
Mean corpuscular volume (MCV) femtoliter (fL)	73–79		68–74					55.60–90.69	49.38–67.16	91.96–107.51
Mean corpuscular hemoglobin concentration (MCHC) (g/dL)	34 (31–37)		30–34					29.70–35.49	30.30–35.73	33.14–37.24
Leucocytes × 10^3/μL	4.5–9.1	4.3–21.6	6.3–8.9	8.50 ± 0.39 (M)/ 8.20 ± 0.36 (F) +	4.7–9.4	5.5–17.5 (average 11.2) +	5.4–15.6 +	1780–17,450	30–9520	8550–16,500
Neutrophils (%) (Segmented)	21–57	5–34 (total)	16–26 (total)	**	7.0–32.0	22–48	39–54	920–9200	190–4350	4710–11,570
Lymphocytes (%)	49–82	60–95	65–80		57.0–91.0	29–72	45–60	0.0–8190	0.0–4980	1940–6530
Eosinophils (%)	0.3	0–4	0–2		0–4.0	0–7	0–5	100–610	0.0–580	0.0–200**
Monocytes (%)	2 to 8	0–3	0–4		2.0–5.0	1 to 10	0–6	70–500	0.0–190	0.0–150**
Basophils (%)	0–3	0–1	0–2		0–3.0	0.0–2.7	0–1	0.0–0.0	0.0–0.0	0.0–0.0**
Platelets/10^3/μL	421–733	400–600	300–570		411–626	260–740++	200–482++		117,000–735,000	
Reticulocytes/μL						2 to 3	0–2.8	0.0–200	200–3200	0.0–2600**
Fibrinogen (g/dL)									1.94–4.02	3.15–4.31**

*RBC (10^{12}/L); + WBC (10^9/L); ++ Platelets (10^9/L).
**Neutrophil-to-lymphocyte ratio is 40:60 in both males and females.
Adapted from references 27, 28, and 33.

TABLE 42-6

Neutrophil Parameters of Selected Species of Rodents

Common Name	New World Porcupine	Coypu	Agouti	Agouti	Agouti
Scientific Name	*Sphiggurus villosus*	*Myocastor coypus*	*Dasyprocta leporina*	*Dasyprocta primnolopha*	*Dasyprocta primnolopha*
	(free-ranging; *n* = 5)	(free-ranging individuals)	(two different restraint protocols)	(captive animals, males)	(captive animals, females)
PARAMETER					
Neutrophils (bands) (%)	3.4 ± 2.41	0.73 ± 1.14	0.45 ± 0.6	0–5	0–3

Values reported as mean ± standard deviation.
Adapted from reference 48.

challenging, with deeply located jugular veins surrounded by muscle and fat, and the entire cervical region is very short.[44]

To maximize diagnostic value of the blood sample, blood should be collected into a microtainer tube with the appropriate anticoagulant, preferably lithium heparin. Some investigators have found that the quality of blood smear and complete blood cell (CBC) count results from the lithium heparin were comparable with those from an EDTA (ethylenediaminetetraacetic acid) tube. It is also critical to remove the needle and transfer the blood directly into the tube after blood collection to minimize the chances of hemolysis when using small-gauge needles.[44]

For small-sized or critically ill rodents, CBC count using a hemocytometer may be obtained on-site at veterinary and zoo hospitals, along with the hematocrit, total solids, differential white blood cell (WBC) count, and morphologic examination of red blood cells (RBCs) and WBCs (Table 42-6).[41]

Some laboratories require serum or plasma samples for biochemical analyses, although those using plasma samples maximize sample volume. Plasma is preferable to serum because the volume yield of plasma is greater than that of serum for a given amount of blood when whole blood cannot be used.[44]

Point-of-care machines such as the Abaxis VetScan (Abaxis, Union City, CA) perform a diagnostic biochemical panel on 0.13 mL of whole blood.[33] This method is nowadays more commonly used in pet and zoo rodents in clinical practice.

Hematology and Biochemistry

Table 42-7 describes hematology and biochemistry values of selected species of rodents.

The neutrophils of guinea pigs contain eosinophilic-staining granules that are sometimes called *heterophils* and have the same function as in other mammals.[44] A unique leucocyte of the guinea pig is the Kurloff cell, which resembles a lymphocyte but contains round or ovoid inclusions termed *Kurloff bodies*.[46]

In chinchillas, hematologic parameters of note include a higher hemoglobin–oxygen affinity compared with that in other rodents. Also, a seasonal effect is noted, with the RBC count, WBC count, and hemoglobin level being at the highest in winter. The higher WBC count continues into early spring as the reproductive season begins.[27]

The most common disorders of hematology in rodents include different types of anemia, lymphosarcoma (Cavian leukemia or type C retrovirus).[44] In guinea pigs and other rodents, alanine aminotransferase (ALT) activity is low in hepatocytes and therefore is not sensitive or specific as a marker of hepatocellular injury.[46] Gamma glutamyl transferase (GGT) is present in the liver of rodents.[50] Rodents with chronic renal failure may show evidence of increased serum blood urea nitrogen (BUN) levels. Guinea pigs have a longer prothrombin time (PT) compared with many other exotic mammals, so their blood does not clot as quickly as that in the rest of pet mammals studied so far.[41]

Bone Marrow Collection

It is possible to collect a bone marrow sample even in small rodents. The same technique used for domestic animals or for intraosseous catheterization of the femur or tibia may be used.[33]

Indications for collecting bone marrow in rodents are nonregenerative anemia, thrombocytopenias, gammopathy, lymphoproliferative disorders (leukemia), or suspicion of neoplasia and malignancies (lymphoma, mast cell tumors), unexplained fever, or hypercalcemia.[44]

The cellular distribution of bone marrow in guinea pigs is 26.7% erythroblasts, 63.3% myeloid cells, 4.6% lymphocytes, and 5.4% reticulum cells.[46]

Urine Collection

The collection of urine is difficult. Samples for urinalysis, urine culture, and sensitivities should be obtained via cystocentesis under general anesthesia and, if possible, with ultrasonographic guidance.[27] Urethral catheterization and conscious cystocentesis are usually employed with medium-sized and zoo rodents.

Most rodents urinate during handling and when excited. These free-catch samples may be contaminated with fecal and bedding material but could be useful for testing with a urinalysis test strip and to determine specific gravity.[27,33]

In agoutis, urine may be collected in the same fashion as it is collected in domestic cats. In the urinary sediment of agoutis and acouchis, triple-phosphate, calcium-carbonate and amorphous phosphate and urate crystals, spermatozoids, epithelial cells, leucocytes, and thyrosine crystals have been found.[48]

DISEASES

Infectious Diseases

Table 42-8 discusses the most common infectious diseases in this animal group, including those caused by bacterial, fungal, parasitic, and viral pathogens.

Common infectious diseases in free-ranging rodent species include pseudotuberculosis (yersiniosis), dermatomycosis, tularemia (*Francisella tularensis*), and *Pasteurella multocida* infection.[50,51]

In wild capybaras in South America, brucellosis was studied by Bello et al. (1974), who reported a high incidence of this disease diagnosed with serum agglutination tests. A strain of *Brucella abortus* was isolated.[16]

In 1976, Jelambi et al. analyzed 178 serum samples of euthanized capybaras and found 111 (63.3%) positive to different leptospiral serotypes but mainly to *L. canicola*, *L. ballum*, *L. hardjo*, *L. hendomadis*, and *L.wolffi*.[16] Common infectious diseases in captive rodents include Sendai virus infection, salmonellosis, Tyzzer disease, and murine respiratory mycoplasmosis.[50,51]

Text continued on p. 414

TABLE 42-7

Reference Ranges for Biochemical Parameters of Selected Species of Rodents

Common Name	Mouse	Gerbil	Hamster	Degu	Duprasi	Rats	Guinea Pig	Chinchilla	Agouti*
Scientific Name	Mus musculus	Meriones unguiculatus	Mesocricetus auratus	Octodon degus	Pachyuromys duprasi	Rattus norvegicus	Cavia porcellus	Chinchilla lanigera	Dasyprocta primnolopha
	(Mixed sex, n = 50)	(n = 30)	(n = 50)	—	(Obtained under sedation)	(Mixed sex; n = 50)	—	—	—
PARAMETER									
Albumin, gram per deciliter (g/dL)	2.5–4.8	2.5 (2.1–2.9)	3.5–4.9	—	1.7–2.4	2.8–5.3	2.1–3.9	38–56	—
Alkaline phosphatase, international unit per liter (IU/L)	51–285	118 (70–182)	99–186	—	47250	87–381	55–108	6.0–72	38 ± 10
Alanine aminotransferase (IU/L)	29–191	91 (56–165)	—	—	70.0631.0	3680	25–59	10.0–35	20 ± 4.6
Aspartate aminotransferase (IU/L)	—	—	22–128	—	—	—	27–68	96	39 ± 13
Bilirubin, total, milligram per deciliter (mg/dL)	0.1–0.9	—	0.1–0.7	—	1.71–15.39 micromole per liter (µmol/L)	0.20–0.70	0–1.59 µmol/L	5.13–15.4 µmol/L	0.62 ± 0.14
Blood urea nitrogen (mg/dL)	18–29	18 (11–32)	12.0–23.0	—	4.64–13.2 millimole per liter (mmol/L)	11–23.0	3.34–10.33 mmol/L	6.06–16.06 mmol/L	42.6 ± 7.41
Calcium (mg/dL)	8.7–10.1	—	5.3–12.0	—	2.25–2.63 mmol/L	5.7–12.4	2.3–3.1 mmol/L	1.4–3.02 mmol/L	—
Chloride, milliequivalent per liter (mEq/L)	—	—	—	—	—	—	—	—	—
Cholesterol (mg/dL)	—	—	—	—	—	—	0.31–1.67 mmol/L	1.3–7.85 mmol/L	—
Creatinine (mg/dL)	0–1–0.4	0.3 (0.2–0.7)	0.4–1.0	—	17.68–53.04 µmol/L	0.3–0.6	0–77 µmol/L	35.4–114.9 µmol/L	1.4 ± 0.27
Glucose (mg/dL)	90–193	91 (24–117) U/L	37–198	—	6.23–25.14 mmol/L	50–135	3.3–6.9 mmol/L	3.3–6.1 mmol/L	—
Phosphorus (mg/dL)	5.4–9.3	—	3.0–9.9	—	0–78–2.23 mmol/L	6.5–12.2	1.03–6.98 mmol/L	1.29–2.58 mmol/L	—
Potassium (mEq/L)	—	—	—	—	3.0–5.2 mmol/L	—	4.5–8.8 mmol/L	3.3–5.7 mmol/L	—
Sodium (mEq/L)	—	—	—	—	140–160 mmol/L	—	130–150 mmol/L	130–150 mmol/L	—
Total protein (g/dL)	4.6–6.9	5.6 (4.6–6.3)	5.2–7.0	5.70 ± 0.20 (Males) 5.62 ± 0.18 (Females)	—	5.6–7.4	4.7–6.4	4.7–6.4	—

Adapted from references 27, 28, and 33.

TABLE 42-8

Selected Infectious and Zoonotic Diseases of Rodents

Disease	Etiology	Epizootiology	Signs	Diagnosis	Comments
BACTERIAL					
Bartonellosis	Bartonella spp.	Mainly transmitted by vectors An increasing number of animal reservoir hosts, including rodents, have been identified for various Bartonella spp. Bartonella elizabethae, B. grahamii, B. visonii subsp. arupensis, and B. washoensis are all rodent-associated genera which have been implicated in human infections The mechanisms by which humans acquire Bartonella infections from rodents are unknown Likely models of transmission would include direct contact with bacteria shed from rodents and vector transmission by rodent ectoparasites	In humans affected by the rodent-associated Bartonella species, endocarditis, neuro-retinitis, pyrexia, and myocarditis have been diagnosed	Causing a long-lasting intra-erythrocytic anemia; blood smears are suggested for diagnosis Blood culture, biphasic culture, biopsy samples from affected organs Samples from humans suspected of having bartonellosis must be handled as potentially pathogenic with the same standards as if it was a sample for hepatitis B virus, human immunodeficiency virus (HIV), or both	Control of rodents and their ectoparasites
Zoonosis					
Cervical lymphadenitis	Streptococcus zooepidemicus	Associated with feeding of coarse foods in some rodents such as guinea pigs Lesions of lymph nodes may cause an abscess infected with Streptococcus zooepidemicus, Yersinia pseudotuberculosis and other pathogenic bacteria Infected lymph nodes may rupture	Swelling of cervical lymph nodes is the most common clinical sign	History of coarse feed ingestion, bite wounds or other events resulting in oral puncture Culture and CBC and serum biochemistry for septicemia	Surgically excise, flush and drain infected lymph nodes. Important to note that may recur Supportive therapy includes parenteral fluids, nonsteroidal anti-inflammatory drugs, aggressive antibiotic therapy, and surgery if recurrence Separate infected animals from healthy individuals If it recurs and quality of life is low, euthanasia is suggested
Erysipelosis	Erysipelothrix rhusiopatiae	Many rodents have subclinical infection or a carrier state of E. rhusiopatiae. Mice are frequently referred to as carriers of this disease The bacterium persists in soil or dung for 6 months or more as well as in water and animal remains	Rodents may show depression before death since this is an acute disease Chronic disease can cause arthritis, heart failure, or both Clinical signs are often presented in other animal species affected by this bacterium and not commonly in rodents	Culture as it is easily isolated using standard methods	Vaccines for species like pigs and other domestic animals are available Improve management and reduce stressors The key in preventing Erysipelothrix infections in susceptible species rests in limiting exposure to the organism, which can come from several sources, including mice, birds, and other pigs

| Leptospirosis | *Leptospira* spp. | Worldwide public health problem
Rodents are maintenance hosts of serovars *icterohaemorrhagiae* and *ballum*
Other serovars can cause clinical disease in rodents
Over 250 *Leptospira* serovars are known, and each serovar has a preferred animal host
Leptospires are excreted into the environment through the urine of infected animals
Human infections are generally acquired through direct or environmental contact with infected urine
A single report describes a case of human *L. icterohemorragiae* infection acquired from pet rats
Wild rodents are often identified as the source of human infections
Zoonosis | Leptospira infections in rats are subclinical and animals present with minimal or no lesions
In other rodents it may cause fever, inappetence, hemorrhages of mucous membranes, jaundice, red urine, depression, vomiting, and abdominal pain
In humans, the majority of leptospiral infections are subclinical or mild, although a small proportion of patients develop severe icteric illness with renal failure or hemorrhagic pneumonitis | Clinical signs, antibody titers, and culture of urine
Diagnosis is difficult because culture frequently produces negative results | Individuals handling pet rodents must be aware of the risks of contracting leptospirosis and should thoroughly wash their hands with soap and water after handling pet rodents, their cages or other cage implements, and their bedding
Separate maintenance hosts from host in which disease can occur
To reduce the risk of acquiring leptospirosis, individuals should avoid drinking or swimming in water potentially contaminated with animal urine
Individuals with occupational or recreational exposure to contaminated water or soil should wear protective clothing, including gloves, masks, and footwear |
| Listeriosis | *Listeria monocytogenes* | *L. monocytogenes* has been isolated from soil, sewage sludge effluents, and stream water mud and dust
It can usually be acquired from the environment, including the diet, infection occurring by transepithelial invasion of the diet, infection occurring by transepithelial invasion of the intestine or damaged mucosa to the trigeminal nerve and brainstem
It is a serious infection in humans frequently caused by eating food contaminated with *L. monocytogenes*
Listeriosis affects immunocompromised individuals, older adults, pregnant women, and newborns
Zoonosis | Animals affected by the septicemic form of the disease are found dead with no other signs
If the encephalitic form is present, signs vary from depression, ataxia, paralysis, and conjunctivitis
Humans developing fever and chills while pregnant, or individuals sick with fever and muscle aches or stiff neck should seek medical attention immediately | For symptomatic human patients diagnosis is confirmed by isolation of *Listeria monocytogenes* from a normally sterile site such as CSF, blood, or amniotic fluid, placenta, or both | Improve hygiene and locate source of contamination and discard
The risk may be reduced by recommendations for safe food preparation, consumption, and storage
According to the Centers for Disease Control and Prevention (CDC), the general guidelines recommended for the prevention of listeriosis are similar to those used to help prevent other foodborne illnesses such as salmonellosis |

Continued

TABLE 42-8

Selected Infectious and Zoonotic Diseases of Rodents—cont'd

Disease	Etiology	Epizootiology	Signs	Diagnosis	Comments
Murine respiratory mycoplasmosis	*Mycoplasma pulmonis*	Respiratory disease is one of the most frequent problems in rats and mice and may be a complex multifactorial syndrome involving *Mycoplasma pulmonis*, *Streptococcus pneumoniae*, cilia-associated respiratory (CAR) bacillus and Sendai virus Transmission in rodents may be intrauterine or via aerosol This organism survives poorly in the environment and is susceptible to drying It is believed to be commensal and only causes disease in rodents when there is concurrent Sendai virus infection or rising ammonia levels	Clinical disease has only been recorded in rats and mice Clinical signs vary from mild dyspnea to severe pneumonia and death Open-mouth breathing is a poor sign in rodents with this one and other respiratory diseases Other clinical signs might include nasal discharge, weight loss, dyspnea, porphyrin-staining around the eyes, head tilt, and a hunched stance	Clinical signs, radiography showing areas of abscessation or consolidation in lungs Culture on special media	Initial aggressive treatment is rarely curative Several cases require lifelong therapy and many others will never resolve or be well controlled Antibiotics are useful mainly when there is not a mixed viral infection. Fluoroquinolones, tetracyclines, and macrolides are often effective to reduce clinical signs; nonsteroidal anti-inflammatory drugs (NSAIDs), bronchodilators, and mucolytics may be of help as support therapy Environmental adjustments are of utmost importance these include ensuring a dust-free substrate, provision of good ventilation, and regular cleaning of cages to prevent the buildup of ammonia
Mycobacteriosis	*Mycobacterium tuberculosis complex* (*Mycobacterium microti*)	Overt mycobacteriosis is rarely reported in rodents, although some cases are documented Even when rodents are rarely clinically affected by mycobacteriosis, they may serve as a potential reservoir between wildlife, domestic animals, and humans Cases of spontaneous mycobacteriosis in pet rodents have included hairy-footed hamsters (*Phodopus sungorus*) housed in a colony In 2007, disseminated mycobacteriosis was reported in a pet Korean squirrel (*Sciurus vulgaris coreae*) in Spain Another case in a pet squirrel was reported in the Iberian Peninsula This case was diagnosed in a Richardson's ground squirrel (*Spermophilus richardsonii*) **Zoonosis**	Clinical signs reported in rodents affected by mycobacteriosis include cutaneous lesions in the form of ulcerative granulomatous dermatitis, and pulmonary lymph node, intestinal, and renal involvement	Histopathology of affected organs with acid-fast staining and PCR	Other cases of spontaneous mycobacteriosis reported in exotic rodents include capybaras (*Hydrochoerus hydrochaeris*) where *M. bovis*, was confirmed *Mycobacterium tuberculosis* was confirmed in an agouti A porcupine was known to die of tuberculosis in 1944 Vole tuberculosis is the only spontaneous mycobacteriosis of clinical significance to rodents, affecting wild populations of field voles (*Microtus agrestis*), bank voles (*Clethrionomys glareolus*), wood mice (*Apodemus sylvaticus*), and shrews (*Sorex araneus*) in northern England The causative agent of vole tuberculosis is *Mycobacterium microti*

Disease	Organism	Epidemiology	Clinical signs	Diagnosis	Treatment
Pasteurellosis	*Pasteurella multocida* or *Mannheimia haemolytica*	Direct transmission is most important—young infected with commensal strains from dam *Pasteurella* is a significant pathogen in laboratory animals, leading to the development of "Pasteurella-free" animals for research use Strains of *Pasteurella* vary in pathogenicity, with some being more likely to spread via the hematogenous route and causing acute septicemia, generalized disease, and death *Pasteurella multocida* gains entry to the host primarily through the nares or wounds via aerosolization or direct contact with infected animals or fomites Endemic opportunistic pathogens and disease is precipitated by trauma or stress	In prairie dogs, *P. multocida* infection has been associated with pneumonia, rhinitis, and sinusitis In rats and mice, the most common causes of conjunctivitis are not associated with intraocular signs Agents, including *Pasteurella* spp. and *Corynebaterium* spp., may be involved in outbreaks where up to 50% of animals may be affected Respiratory disease is rarely reported in gerbils, although they are susceptible to various pathogens such as *Pasteurella pneumotropica*, *Streptococcuspneumoniae*, and *Bordetella bronchiseptica*, among others	Bacterial culture and antibacterial sensitivity testing can be performed on nasal samples Nasal cavity material can be obtained for culturing, cytology, and staining	Treatment of bacterial respiratory disease should be based on antibiotic sensitivity testing and follow guidelines for antibiotic choice used for treatment in guinea pigs and rabbits Nebulization, bronchodilators, and NSAIDs may decrease the clinical signs of rhinitis, sinusitis, and pneumonia Use of ophthalmic NSAIDs as drops placed in the eyes to reach nasal tissue have been used to reduce local inflammation Reduce stressors and trauma by improving management and veterinary care
Proliferative ileitis ("wet tail") or Proliferative bowel disease (PBD)	*Lawsonia intracellularis*	It is a proliferative enteropathy affecting young hamsters 3–10 weeks of age Underlying stress factors such as weaning and overcrowding can trigger the disease PBD is caused by the same agent in hamsters, ferrets, and pigs and has been implicated in proliferative enteropathies of other species, including rabbits, white-tailed deer, ratite birds, and domestic foals	Clinical signs include anorexia, lethargy, and poor coat appearance, usually followed by diarrhea	History and age ranges in hamsters exhibiting clinical signs of GI tract disease can be of help *Lawsonia intracellularis* is an obligate intracellular organism that cannot be propagated on artificial media, but can be grown in embryonated chicken eggs Polymerase chain reaction (PCR) and indirect fluorescent antibody (IFA) test, which identify the omega antigen common to organisms found in PBD lesions of hamsters, swine, and ferrets Gross histopathologic lesions and observing clinical signs are the diagnostics of choice for clinical cases	Aggressive supportive treatment with fluids and nutritional support is required, along with broad-spectrum antibiotics such as tetracyclines, doxycycline, enrofloxacin, chloramphenicol, neomycin, or trimethoprim Care should be taken when selecting antibiotics for affected rodents Prognosis is poor, since many rodents that survive the infection may develop subsequent obstruction, intussusception, and rectal prolapse

Continued

TABLE 42-8

Selected Infectious and Zoonotic Diseases of Rodents—cont'd

Disease	Etiology	Epizootiology	Signs	Diagnosis	Comments
Rat bite fever	*Streptobacillus moniliformis*	*Streptobacillus moniliforrnis* is the primary cause of human rat bite fever (RBF) in the United States, and *Spirilum minus* causes RBF in Africa *S. moniliformis* inhabits the nasopharynx, middle ear, and respiratory tract of wild rats (*Rattus norvegicus*) and is also present in the blood and urine of infected animals *S. moniliformis* may be transmitted to humans from a bite or scratch from an infected rat, when infected rats are handled, and commonly through the ingestion of water and food with infected rat excreta Mice and gerbils, and apparently squirrels may also be reservoirs of *S. moniliformis* RBF has been reported in Africa, Australia, Europe, Japan, and North and South Americas	*S. moniliformis* infection does not cause clinical signs in rats In humans, clinical signs of RBF infection are nonspecific and include fever, chills, myalgia, headache, and vomiting These signs commonly occur within 7 days of exposure Human patients may also develop a maculopapular rash on the extremities or septic arthritis followed by arthralgia	This disease is diagnosed by detecting the bacteria in skin, blood, joint, fluid, or lymph nodes Serology and PCR may also be used	RBF in untreated patients is responsible for a mortality rate of 7%–10% Individuals at risk for RBF include those with recreational or occupational exposure to rats and children living in rat-infested urban dwellings or rural areas To reduce exposure to *S. moniliformis*, individuals should wear gloves, practice regular hand washing, and avoid hand-to-mouth contact when handling rats or cleaning rat enclosures If a person is bitten by a rat, prompt cleaning and disinfection of the wound is advised, as well as seeking medical attention and reporting their exposure history
		Zoonosis			
Salmonellosis	*Salmonella* spp.	Infection is usually by ingestion of contaminated food or water *Salmonella* can survive for long periods in soil Many human *Salmonella* infections are acquired by contact with animals A multistate human outbreak of multidrug-resistant *Salmonella enterica* serotype *typhimurium* infection was associated with exposure to pet hamsters, mice, and rats A second multistate human outbreak of *S. typhimurium* was associated with feeding frozen vacuum-packed rodents to pet snakes The snakes acquired *S. typhimurium* from frozen feed mice, and human transmission likely occurred through contact	In guinea pigs, salmonellosis results in septicemia and sudden death, rather than enteritis and diarrhea In other rodents, anorexia, lethargy, dehydration, and enteric clinical signs such as diarrhea and abdominal pain Chronic infections may occur, characterized by progressive weight loss, poor general condition, and abortion Pet rodents should be euthanized if diagnosed with salmonellosis because of the zoonotic risk In humans, clinical signs of salmonellosis include gastroenteritis, bacteremia, and subsequent focal infection In hamsters, salmonellosis may cause severe disease with morbidity and mortality	Culture of organism when signs are consistent with salmonellosis It is of utmost importance to consider that hamsters affected by *Salmonella* show clinical signs similar to "wet-tail," a disease caused by *Lawsonia intracellularis*, so *Salmonella* may be underdiagnosed This might put children and adults owning hamsters at greater risk of acquiring salmonellosis When hamsters and any other rodents have diarrhea, fecal cultures should be performed to determine if *Salmonella* species are present	Owners should be aware of the fact that rodents may shed *Salmonella* and expect rodent feces to be potentially infectious Individuals feeding rodents to reptiles should be aware that feeder animals may be infectious and may transmit *Salmonella* infections to the reptiles Detect the source of contaminated food or water and discard it Antibiotic therapy is based on sensitivity testing where antibiotics are effective Reduce stressors on affected animals To reduce zoonotic transmission of *Salmonella*, individuals should thoroughly wash their hands with soap and water after

Disease	Agent	Reservoirs/Transmission	Clinical Signs	Diagnosis	Prevention/Public Health
		with the snakes, their feed, or contaminated environmental surfaces *S. typhimurium* or *S. enteritidis* may cause acute or chronic diarrhea in rodents, though in some cases the feces may be normal **Zoonosis**			handling rodents and rodent-fed reptiles, their cages, or other cage implements, and their bedding It is of utmost importance to consider that clinical signs of *Salmonella*-affected hamsters are similar
Sylvatic plague or Yersiniosis	*Yersinia pestis*	Rodent reservoirs include prairie dogs (*Cynomys* spp.), ground squirrels (*Spermophilus* spp.), antelope ground squirrels (*Ammospermophilus* spp.), chipmunks (*Tamias* spp.), wood rats (*Neotoma* spp.), and mice (*Peromyscus* spp.) Water and food contaminated with feces is major source of infection Ingestion of infected rodents **Zoonosis**	Lymphadenomegaly and subcutaneous hemorrhages in prairie dogs Usually peracute Forms in humans include septicemic, pneumonic, and bubonic plague Gastroenteritis, respiratory distress, mesenteric lymphadenitis, and nonspecific clinical signs such as lethargy and anorexia	Bipolar staining gram-negative coccobacilli on lymph node aspirates Culture on blood agar and immunohistochemistry Mortality and mortality in rodents are substantial and approach 100%	Fleas are a vector for plague Control of rodents and fleas prevents zoonosis Use of gloves, surgical masks, and eye protection is important for handlers processing rodent and rabbit carcasses In cases intended to protect endangered species treatment of the environment to kill fleas may be appropriate
Tularemia	*Francisella tularensis*	Highly infectious organism Ticks and other blood sucking arthropods serve as the most important biological vectors Disease occurs in beavers, muskrats, European brown hares, and ranging hares A single case has been associated with a pet hamster bite Wild rodents with tularemia appear lethargic in the terminal phase and are often preyed upon by other animals continuing the transmission Voles may be reservoirs **Zoonosis**	In humans, tularemia presents as a flulike illness, followed by 1 of 6 clinical syndromes: ulceroglandular, glandular, oropharyngeal, oculoglandular, pneumonic, and typhoidal	Veterinarians should consider tularemia as a differential diagnosis in febrile animals with or without lymphadenopathy in areas were disease is endemic	Tularemia is a notifiable disease in the United States, and cases have been recorded in all states but Hawaii Avoid handling sick or dead animals Tick control and measures to eliminate exposure to ticks The public and veterinarians should be aware that pet hamsters might be a potential source of tularemia

Continued

TABLE 42-8

Selected Infectious and Zoonotic Diseases of Rodents—cont'd

Disease	Etiology	Epizootiology	Signs	Diagnosis	Comments
Tyzzer disease	*Clostridium piliforme* Formerly known as *Bacillus piliformis*	The disease is commonly triggered by underlying stressors such as rehoming, overcrowding, poor husbandry, high environmental temperatures and humidity, prior antibiotic use, heavy parasite burdens, and other diseases Affects all rodents causing infection of the gastrointestinal tract Gerbils and hamsters are more frequently affected, and these rodents suffer higher mortality compared with rats and mice	In gerbils and hamsters, clinical signs are often nonspecific, so may include watery diarrhea, scruffy coat, dehydration, lethargy, and death	Diagnosis is based on postmortem findings such as necrotic foci on liver, and sometimes intestinal lesions Stains such as silver, Giemsa, or PAS are used on affected tissue biopsies	Generalized supportive treatment is rarely successful Oral tetracyclines for 30 days might decrease morbidity in groups as well as treatment of concurrent infections
Yersiniosis	*Yersinia pseudotuberculosis*	Rodents may act as reservoirs of infection The infection may spread to pet rodents via contaminated feed or bedding from wild rodents or birds Euthanasia is advised in pet rodents affected with yersiniosis Water and food contaminated with feces of infected rodents is a major source of infection It has been also considered that ingestion of infected preys might be a major source for predators	Affected rodents may have weight loss, diarrhea, and gradual loss of condition in cases of chronic illness Some animals die acutely with septicemia, whereas others develop a nonfatal infection restricted to the cervical lymph nodes	Lymph node aspirate cultures and blood samples if septicemic At necropsy, some rodents such as guinea pigs present enlarged mesenteric lymph nodes, with necrotic foci in the liver and spleen	Treatment with antibiotics seems effective Care must be taken when administering some classes of antibiotics to herbivorous rodents Avoiding contamination of food and water with feces is a key in prevention
RICKETTSIAE					
Rickettsialpox	*Rickettsia akari*	Member of the spotted fever group Rickettsia is the cause of the mite-borne zoonosis, rickettsialpox This disease was first described in New York in 1946, and most U.S. cases continue to originate in this area It also has been seen in South Africa, Korea, and Russia Rickettsialpox is most likely to occur in crowded urban areas with mouse infested housing	In humans, rickettsialpox causes an ulcerated primary lesion or eschar at the site of inoculation, followed by systemic illness which includes fever, headache, and a generalized papulovesicular rash Sweating, myalgia, and photophobia may also be signs in some human cases	CBC and serology	Rickettsialpox should be considered in any patient with fever and a papulovesicular eruption Other mite rodent species may also be involved in the cycle Control of house mice and their mites is the preventive measure of choice The basic treatment is with doxycycline, but chloramphenicol and azithromycin may work as well

Disease	Organism	Epidemiology / Description	Diagnosis	Treatment / Prevention
		The natural host of *R. akari* is the house mouse (*Mus musculus*), whereas the house mouse mite (*Liponysoides sanguineus*) is the primary vector. Humans are incidental hosts of *L. sanguineus* and become infected when bitten by mites infected with *R. akari* **Zoonosis**		
Murine typhus or Endemic typhus	*Rickettsia typhi*	Rats (*Rattus rattus* and *Rattus norvegicus*) are the primary reservoirs of *R. typhi*, which is an obligate intracellular gram-negative organism. Nonetheless, other mammals such as house mice (*Mus musculus*), opossums, skunks, cats, and dogs may maintain the infection. Vectors include the rat flea (*Xenopsylla cheopis*) and the cat flea (*Ctenocephalides felis*). Humans get infected when infected fleas bite, and feces are inoculated into the bite site. Less than 100 cases have been reported annually in the United States, with cases limited to Texas and Southern California **Zoonosis**	Clinical signs in humans infected with *R. typhi* include fever, headache, and myalgias, followed by a discrete maculopapular rash. The mortality rate for murine typhus is low (1%) with appropriate antibiotics	Serology testing with the indirect immunofluorescence assay is the preferred diagnostic method	Doxycycline is the antibiotic of choice which has been shown to shorten the course of illness. Prevention of murine typhus includes use of flea preventive on dogs and cats, exterminating household rodents, eliminating rodent habitats in or near homes, using pesticides to limit flea infestations, avoiding wild animals, including feral cats and opossums, and using insect repellents
Chlamydophilosis	*Chlamydophila caviae* *Chlamydophila psittaci*	This disease is most commonly caused by *C. caviae*, although *C. psittaci* cases have been reported as well. It is fairly common in guinea pigs, in which it must be differentiated from hypovitaminosis C. *C. caviae* causes guinea pig inclusion conjunctivitis (GPIC). Juveniles are more commonly affected than adults **Zoonosis**	Conjunctivitis is the primary sign in guinea pigs, but it can progress to bronchitis and pneumonia, anorexia, weight loss, and death. Some animals remain asymptomatic, but clinical signs range from mild to severe keratoconjunctivitis with serous to purulent ocular discharge, conjunctival chemosis, follicular hypertrophy, and uveitis	Diagnosis is through cytology and/or PCR of conjunctival scrapings, or histopathology and immunochemistry of respiratory or conjunctival tissues	Tetracyclines works for mild cases or fluoroquinolone ophthalmic ointments or drops. Severe cases may need enrofloxacin orally (PO) or doxycycline parenterally. Stressed or breeding guinea pigs, or those in suboptimal husbandry conditions require prolonged treatment and supportive care. *C. psittaci* is a reportable disease in some public health jurisdictions. Route of transmission of *C. caviae* is still unclear, but it may have zoonotic potential

Continued

TABLE 42-8

Selected Infectious and Zoonotic Diseases of Rodents—cont'd

Disease	Etiology	Epizootiology	Signs	Diagnosis	Comments
FUNGAL DISEASES					
Dermatophytosis	*Trichophyton mentagrophytes*, *Microsporum canis*, *M. gypseum*, and *Epidermophyton*	Direct or indirect contact with carrier animals, with young ones being more susceptible
Guinea pigs, chinchillas, mouse, prairie dogs, and rats are more commonly affected
Dermatophytes infect the epidermis and adnexa, including the hair follicles and hair shaft
Rodents are frequent asymptomatic carriers of ringworm
Ringworm is common in pediatric and geriatric animals because of the decreased host immunity	It is not uncommon in rodents, but can be asymptomatic
Common lesions include irregular patches of alopecia, broken hairs, and variable amounts of redness, crust, and scale
Pruritus is generally absent or minimal	Toothbrushing of the entire animal is suggested for sampling for culture
Microscopy of hair samples is a useful diagnosis
Tricophyton spp. and 50% of *Microsporum* spp. do not fluoresce, so examination with a Wood's lamp is normally unrewarding	Topical or systemic antifungal therapy
Topical therapy to remove spores and systemic therapy to act at the hair follicles
Topical drugs include eniconazole or a miconazole–chlorhexidine shampoo are recommended
Systemic treatment might be given with ketoconazole, itraconazole, or terbinafine
Decontamination of the environment with sodium hypochlorite
The incidence of fungal diseases may also increase with stressors such as overcrowding, heat, humidity, ectoparasitism, old age, youth, or pregnancy
Care should be taken when handling rodents suffering skin diseases because of the zoonotic potential of dermatophytes
Subcutaneous mycoses	*Sporothrix schenckii*	Although many rodent species appear susceptible to infection with this ubiquitous saprophytic fungus, clinical reports are scarce
Reports of sporotrichosis in rats in Brazil have been found in the literature
Rodent bites can transmit the infection to humans as well as contact with domestic cats' skin ulcers	In experimentally infected mice, generalized disease was produced and spread to the liver, lungs, pleura, tail, and extremities
The lesions were suppurative, necrotizing, and fibrosing, as well as macrophagic	Techniques for diagnosis or dermatophytosis used in rodents are the same ones as for other animals, and include cytology, culture, and histopathology
For cytologic evaluation, samples should be mounted in 10% potassium hydroxide (KOH) under a petrolated ringed cover slip	Experimental infection has been created in rats, mice, and hamsters after intraperitoneal or intratesticular injection of the organism
Zoonotic potential
SYSTEMIC MYCOSES					
Adiaspiromycosis	*Chrysosporium parum* and *C. crescens*	Infection is caused by the inhalation of conidia from soil organisms like *Chrysosporium parum* and *C. crescens*
Respiratory infection may be created in many rodents, including free-ranging species
Primary pulmonary mycosis that affects human being as well	Necropsy findings may include gray nodules on the lung surface	Demonstration of spherules and conidia in tissue sections and isolation of the organism
Immunodiffusion test and complement fixation test	**Zoonotic disease**
Care should be taken when handling wild rodents and collecting fecal samples

Disease	Organism	Description	Clinical signs	Diagnosis	Comments
Blastomycosis	*Blastomyces* spp.	Juvenile mice are uniquely susceptible to blastomycosis Susceptibility of mice to this fungal disease persists beyond the development of resistance to other pathogens and the maturation of the immune system			Many experimental studies have been performed on Sendai virus-free mice to get to know more about the extreme susceptibility to this fungal disease
Histoplasmosis	*Histoplasma capsulatum*	Few reports of histoplasmosis in chinchillas, and some others in wild brown rats (*Rattus norvegicus*) in the United States	Respiratory disease was reported in 17 of 130 commercial ranch chinchillas	Histologic confirmation of histoplasmosis was made in only one of the 17 individuals of this report involving commercial ranch chinchillas	*H. capsulatum* was cultured from timothy hay used for food in the case of chinchillas

PARASITIC DISEASES
Parasitic Zoonoses

Disease	Organism	Description	Clinical signs	Diagnosis	Comments
Giardiasis	*Giardia intestinalis* (also known as *G. lamblia* or *G. duodenalis*)	This infection is commonly associated with disease in humans and has been reported in rodents and ferrets The potential zoonotic potential of some species, including *Giardia psittaci* is unknown Cysts are passed in feces and must be ingested to cause the disease	In humans and animals, clinical signs are similar, including severe diarrhea, cramps, gas, and fatigue	Light microscopy, PCR, and indirect immunofluorescense SNAP *Giardia* test (IDEXX Laboratories, Inc.) is available for dogs and cats, although not validated for exotic pets	The only approved treatment of human giardiasis is furazolidone Metronidazole is frequently used, as well as fenbendazole, and albendazole in animals **Zoonosis**
Cryptosporidiosis	*Cryptosporidium parvum*	*C. parvum* is commonly associated with disease in humans Human cases are linked to use of recreational water or after exposure to infected animals Infective oocysts are passed in feces, and infection occurs through ingestion of oocysts contaminating water, food, or the environment Other species of *Cryptosporidium* have been identified such as *C. muris* (rodents), *C. wrairi* (guinea pigs), although these have not been reported to be zoonotic	Some humans and animals can be asymptomatic while others present watery diarrhea, decreased appetite, weight loss, and vomiting	Light microscopy, enzyme-linked immunosorbent assay (ELISA), immunoflourescence, and PCR	No reliable, definitive treatment for animals infected with *Cryptosporidium* In humans, nitazoxanide is approved for treatment **Potential zoonosis**

Continued

TABLE 42-8

Selected Infectious and Zoonotic Diseases of Rodents—cont'd

Disease	Etiology	Epizootiology	Signs	Diagnosis	Comments
Toxoplasmosis	*Toxoplasma gondii*	Felids are the definitive host for *T. gondii* and only felids shed oocysts in feces, but non-felid species, including rodents, may become infected by ingesting bradyzoites	In humans or animals infected during pregnancy, the organism may cross the placenta, infect the fetus, causing abortion or significant disease in the fetus	Fecal examinations on felids to detect oocysts Serology and histopathology in non-felid species	Treatment of asymptomatic animals diagnosed with toxoplasmosis includes clindamycin, pyrimethamine, and sulfonamides Prevent access to cats or to feces of cats, either feral or captive Do not feed uncooked meat **Zoonosis**
Baylisascariasis Larval migrans	*Baylisascaris procyonis* and other *Baylisascaris* sp., apart from *B. laevis*	Definitive hosts are raccoons, skunks, badgers, and bears Humans and other animals, including rodents, may be infected, since large numbers of eggs are environmentally resistant	In animals, including rodents, parasites in the form of larva migrans may infect the liver, lungs, and the central nervous system (CNS) In humans, CNS, visceral organs, and eyes are commonly affected	Clinical signs, history of exposure, serology, brain biopsies, and neuro-imaging	Treatment of humans with clinical signs include anthelmintics such as albendazole, and corticosteroids Patients with neural larva migrans have a grave prognosis In captivity, prevent contact between rodents and the definitive hosts Reduce environmental contamination by treatment of captive procyonids, mustelids, and ursids with anthelmintics **Zoonosis**
Hydatidosis	*Echinococcus multilocularis* *Echinococcus oligarthrus* *Echinococcus vogeli*	Definitive hosts are foxes, South American felids, Central and South American canids Rodents are intermediate hosts for the three species mentioned here *E. multilocularis* is present in the intermediate hosts in the stage of metacestode	Cysts formation in various tissues, including liver *E. multilocularis*-induced disease in rodent is often fatal	In domestic animals and wildlife, diagnosis is accomplished at necropsy	Anthelmintic treatment of definitive host to prevent transmission to rodents, and use of cestocides in infected rodents **Zoonosis**
Cysticercosis, or coenuriasis	*Taenia crassiceps,* *T. twitchelli,* *T. taeniformis,* *T. rileyi, T. parva,* *T. mustelae,* and *T. martis*	Rodents are intermediate hosts from several cestode species *T. twitchelli* is found in the lungs of porcupines	Various tissues affected, including subcutaneous, muscle, mesentery, liver, viscera, and lungs	Morphology of gravid segments from feces and examination of adults recovered after purging the host at necropsy	Anthelmintic treatment is effective **Zoonosis**

Disease	Organism	Description	Pathology	Diagnosis	Treatment/Notes
Hepatic capillariasis	*Calodium hepaticum* (Synonym-*Capillaria hepatica*)	The helminth *Capillaria hepatica* affects the liver of rats and many rodent species	It is located in the liver parenchyma and rats infected with *C. hepatica* regularly develop septal hepatic fibrosis that may progress to cirrhosis in short time. Clinical signs include poor coat condition, lethargy, hepatomegaly, and splenomegaly	Clinical signs, adult worms in the liver at necropsy	Experimental treatment in rodent models has included pentoxifylline, gadolinium chloride, and vitamin A which was considered adequate, since few animals died of infection. Control feral rodent populations. **Zoonosis**
Sarcocystosis	*Sarcocystis* spp.	This intracellular protozoan has a life cycle that includes intermediate hosts (rodents and many other species like humans) and definitive hosts (carnivores)	Protozoans affecting hosts muscles or neural tissues in intermediate hosts	Serology and histopathology	Humans may be intermediate hosts for a variety of *Sarcocystis* species. **Potential zoonosis**
Hepatozoonosis	*Hepatozoon* spp.	*Hepatozoon* is a protozoan that affects different animal species. *H. balfouri* has been found to parasitize rodents in the form of extracellular development of sexual and sporulating species. Found in leucocytes in hosts and in arthropods	Lesions found in various tissues in hosts, including the lungs, heart, skeletal muscles, liver, spleen, and lymph nodes	Gamonts detected in Giemsa-stained preparations of whole blood	Chemotherapeutics not consistently effective and rarely required
Coccidiosis	*Cyclospora* spp., *Eimeria* spp., and *Isospora* spp.	Free-ranging rodents worldwide have been found to have different Coccidia. Samples have been taken from Dipodidae (jumping mice), Erethizontidae (New World porcupines), Muridae (mice and rats), and Cricetidae (voles, lemmings). Located in the intestinal epithelium, causing disease in intensive conditions or immune-suppressed individuals. Frequently cause of illness in young animals	Diarrhea, enlarged abdomen, weight loss, dehydration. Asymptomatic in many cases	Fecal direct cytology. Detection of oocyst in feces	Antiparasitic agents such as metronidazole
Pinworm infections	*Syphacia obvelata* and *S. muris* *Aspicularis* spp. *Dentosmelia translucida*	Located in intestines of rodents. Affect myomorph rodents more frequently	Mild enteritis in young animals. Large worm burdens can cause straining and rectal prolapse	Fecal flotation or adhesive tape strips around anal areas for *Syphacia* eggs	Ivermectin, three doses at 2-week intervals. Good sanitation and treatment for all rodents in building because eggs can be airborne

Continued

TABLE 42-8

Selected Infectious and Zoonotic Diseases of Rodents—cont'd

Disease	Etiology	Epizootiology	Signs	Diagnosis	Comments
Tapeworm infections	*Rodentolepis* (formerly *Hymenolepis*) *nana* Known as dwarf tapeworm Direct life cycle (15 days) and indirect life cycle (via fleas and beetles)	Found in small intestine	Infection is often asymptomatic, but heavy burdens may cause severe gastroenteritis, weight loss, and death	Identification of segments in fecal flotation	Praziquantel or niclosamide Frequent bedding changes and good hygiene **Zoonosis**
	Rodentolepis diminuta (formerly *Hymenolepis diminuta*)	Affects upper small intestine	Infection is often asymptomatic	Identification of segments in fecal flotation	Praziquantel or niclosamide Frequent bedding changes and good hygiene **Low zoonotic risk**
Monanemosis	*Monanema martini* (filaroid nematode) *Monanema joopi*	Lymphatics of the wall of the colon of African murid rodents such as *Acomys spinosissimus* Cutaneous lymphatic vessels of ears and ixodid ticks More susceptible rodent species serve as hosts of this parasite	Low intensity of infection	Soak skin from the ears in saline, and examine saline microscopically	Anthelmintics may be used
Cercopithifilariasis	*Cercopithifilaria johnstoni*	Dermal microfilariae found in many vertebrates in Australia, including rodents Found in subcutaneous connective tissues Lymphatic vessels of the skin, mainly ears, and ixodid ticks (intermediate hosts) Microfilariae are always in the dermis instead of in the blood circulation	Low intensity of infection and examine saline microscopically	Soak skin from the ears in saline Anthelmintics, if needed **May cause zoonosis in tropical and subtropical regions**	Filaroid parasitize wild and domestic animals
Besnoitiasis	*Besnoitia jellisoni*	Definitive host unknown Cysts are found in all internal organs It has been reported in captive maras (*Dolichotis patagorum*)	Fatal interstitial pneumonia in any species	Histopathology to detect cysts	Significance of *B. jellisoni* largely unknown
Frenkeliaosis	*Frenkelia microti* and *Frenkelia glareoli*	Located in the CNS of rodents		Identification of cysts in the CNS	Prevent contact between rodents and the feces of raptors

External Parasites

Ticks (may spread tularemia)	Ticks of the Order Acarina *Ixodes banks* parasitizes beavers, and *Amblyomma americum* parasiticizes squirrels	Located in skin of hosts	Bites of *Ixodes* rarely generate disease	Collection and identification of ticks taken from the host	Control with use of insecticides and habitat modifications
Mites	*Trixacaurus caviae, Myobia musculi, Notoedres muris, Demodex* spp., *Sarcoptes scabiei, Acarus farris, Liponyssus bacoti, Notoedres cati,* and many more	Affect the skin of several species of rodents Many of these genus are species-specific for some rodents	Alopecia, ulceration, dry scaly skin, intense pruritus, thickening of the skin, erythematous and vesicular or papular lesions on tail, limbs, and genitalia	Skin scraping, cytology	Avermectins, NSAIDs, antibiotics, and antifungal medications **Many mites have the potential for zoonoses**
Lice	*Gliricola porcelli, Gyropus ovalis, Polyplax serrata,* suckling lice (Anoplura), biting lice (Mallophaga)	Transmission is by direct contact Stress, inadequate diet, and husbandry, overcrowding, and concurrent disease may trigger a population explosion of lice		Collection from skin and microscopic examination Application of clear cellophane tape to hair coats	Reduce stocking densities Use of pediculicides and disinfection of bedding or caging Important to treat all exposed animals and clean all cages Treatment with ivermectin is usually effective
Fascioliasis	*Fasciola hepatica* (Trematode)	Affects the bile ducts of the liver It has been reported in the beaver and coypu (*Myocastor coypus*) and rats (*R. norvegicus*) Fresh water snails are intermediate host	Fever, jaundice, gastrointestinal disturbances, abdominal pain	Identification of eggs in feces Postmortem identification of adults in the liver	Anthelmintics Role of other natural hosts is considered **Zoonosis**
Myasis	Cuterebrinae (Rodent bots)	Pathogenesis could be similar to that in other mammals such as rabbits, in which larvae of *Cuterebra* species commonly pupate in the subcutis but may migrate aberrantly to other tissues and organs	Subdermal granulomas	Recovery of third instar larvae from furuncle may allow identification	Seen in New World rodents Can be controlled using macrocyclic lactone parasiticides *Cuterebra* infestation can have a negative impact on poorly nourished animals

Continued

TABLE 42-8

Selected Infectious and Zoonotic Diseases of Rodents—cont'd

Disease	Etiology	Epizootiology	Signs	Diagnosis	Comments
VIRAL					
Lymphocytic choriomeningitis	Lymphocytic choriomeningitis (LCMV–Family Arenaviridae)	Wild rodents act as reservoirs. It causes a chronic fatal wasting disease of young hamsters. Virus is shed in urine and saliva. Hamsters and guinea pigs can be a reservoir too. Worldwide distribution.	Individuals are often asymptomatic. Clinical signs depend on age and immune status of infected individuals, and the virulence of the viral strain. Subclinical infection is possible. Reported clinical signs include weight loss, photophobia, tremors, and seizures.	PCR, serological detection of anti-LCMV antibodies or virus isolation from tissue	ZOONOSIS. TREATMENT SHOULD NOT BE ATTEMPTED DUE TO THE ZOONOTIC RISK FROM LCMV.
Omsk hemorrhagic fever	Omsk hemorrhagic fever virus (OHFV–Family Flaviviridae)	OHFV occurs in Northern Siberia regions of Omsk, Novosibirsk, Kurgan, and Tyumen. Vector-borne virus—principally ticks, but direct transmission from urine is possible. The main host of OHFV is rodents. Water vole (*Arvicola terrestris*), and non-native muskrat (*Ondatra zibethica*). *Dermacentor* and *Ixodes* are tick genus involved with transmission. Maintenance hosts are small rodents and shrews.	Weakness, depression, and lethargy in muskrats. In humans, fever, headache, severe muscle pain, cough, dehydration, gastrointestinal symptoms, and bleeding problems.	Virus isolation from blood, or by serologic testing using ELISA	**Zoonosis.** Avoid contact with naturally infected rodent populations.
Hantavirus infections	Hantaviruses (Family Bunyaviridae)	Rodents are a reservoir of hantaviruses. Rodents identified in transmission are Deer mouse (*Peromyscus maniculatus*), Cotton rat (*Sigmodon hispidus*), Rice rat (*Oryzomys palustris*), Whitefooted mouse (*Peromyscus leucopus*). Transmissible through aerosol, breathing dust contaminated with rodent urine or droppings.	Clinical signs are rare in rodents. In humans, Hantavirus pulmonary syndrome (HPS) provokes a severe, and many times fatal respiratory disease.	Serology	**Zoonosis.** There is no specific treatment, cure or vaccine for HPS. Prevent exposure to feral rodents. Due to zoonotic potential preferable to euthanize infected rodents.
Sendai virus infection	Sendai virus (Family Paramyxoviridae) Synonym–Parainfluenzavirus 1	Sendai virus may induce acute respiratory tract disease in laboratory mice, rats, and gerbils. Young infected from dams. Enzootic infection is possible. Sendai virus alone is of little significance in rats, but it causes serious disease in mice. Gerbils can also be carriers.	Respiratory distress, poor coat quality, weight loss, anorexia, neonatal death, dyspnea, sneezing, and more severe signs with concurrent mycoplasma infection.	Serology, histopathology of the lung, fluorogenic nuclease reverse transcriptase polymerase chain reaction.	Supportive treatment, antibiotics, NSAIDs, mucolytics, bronchodilators, diuretics, and oxygen therapy. Eradicate by euthanizing susceptible pups and cease breeding for up to 2 months.

Sialodacryoadenitis	Sialodacryoadenitis virus (Family Coronaviridae)	In ocular infections in mice and rats sialocryoadenitis virus is an important disease of adnexal tissues. It is self-limiting but highly infectious in rats. Enzootic infection in breeding colonies with low morbidity and mortality.	Sneezing, oculonasal discharge, cervical edema, enlarged cervical lymph nodes, necrotic inflamed salivary glands, swelling or infection of the eyes, corneal ulcers and hyphema	Classic swollen neck. Serology and histopathology	No treatment but supportive care and antibiotics for secondary infections. Stop breeding until adults develop immunity.
Papovavirosis in hamsters	Hamster polyomavirus (HaPV) (papovavirus)	Hamster polyomavirus causes cutaneous epitheliomas in Syrian hamsters. High (50%) morbidity in breeding colonies. Virus transmitted via urine and is highly contagious.	The host-specific virus is also thought to cause transmissible lymphoma (abdominal, thoracic, or epitheliotropic) and other skin tumors. Wart-like lesions are seen in young (3-12 months) hamsters around the eyes, mouth, and perianal area.	Classic clinical signs in hamsters	There is no spontaneous resolution. Individual tumors can be removed surgically.
Parapoxvirus disease of red squirrels (Sciurus vulgaris)	Red squirrel parapoxvirus (tentative member of the genus Parapoxvirus)	Gray squirrels (Sciurus carolinensis) are a probable reservoir in United Kingdom and so the source of the virus.	High (60% and more) or gray squirrels apparently healthy were positive in a research study in UK. Erythematous exudative dermatitis with scab formation in red squirrels.	ELISA, virus isolation, and electronmicroscopy	Avoid contact between red and gray squirrels
Fibromas of gray squirrels (Sciurus carolinensis)	Squirrel fibroma virus (genus Leporipoxvirus)	Transmission is probably by biting arthropods. Reported in gray squirrels in the United States	Fibromatosis as multifocal to coalescing, tan, firm cutaneous nodules that may become plaques of pedunculated masses on most parts of the body	Histopathology and isolation. PCR t	Separate affected from non-affected animals. Affected animals may require euthanasia.
Cowpox (Synonyms are carnivorepox, cat pox, elephant pox, ratpox)	Cowpox virus (genus Orthopoxvirus) (CPXV)	Several species or rodents are a probable reservoir of cowpox virus. Infection in humans resulted from direct contact with infected rats. Experimental infection has caused disease in gerbils. Natural reservoir hosts of CPXV are bank voles and wood mice.	Cowpox virus cutaneous infection in humans	Electronmicroscopy of infected tissue, PCR, and virus isolation	**Zoonosis**
Mouse hepatitis	Mouse hepatitis virus (Family Coronaviridae)	Significant variability in the pathogenicity of various strains. Can be enzootic in colonies Epidemic murine illness with high mortality. Can cause a fatal infection. MHV is probably the most important pathogen of laboratory mice.	Some strains of MHV cause a progressive demyelinating encephalitis in mice. Mild signs in enzootic colonies/hunched posture, ruffled coat	Serology via ELISA and/or WA	Eradicate by euthanizing susceptible pups. Obtain replacement stocks from sources known to be free of disease.

Modified from References 1, 11, 29, 39, and 57.

Parasitic Diseases

In captivity, common parasitic diseases include zoonotic threats such as larva migrans (*Baylisascaris* sp. infection), sarcoptic mange, rodentolepis (formerly hymenolepis) infections, and pinworm infections.[50] In the Mexican tropics, captive agoutis (*Agouti paca*) are infested by *Strongyloides* sp., *Eimeria* spp., *Balantidium* spp., *Capillaria* spp., Ascaroidea, *Taenia* spp., and *Trichuris* spp. Reports also indicate the presence of the genus *Nematorpiroides*.[2]

Wild capybaras in South America are known to act as reservoirs of some species of *Trypanosoma* (*T. venezuelense* and *T. evansi*), and acute cases of trypanosomiasis have also been detected in capybaras in Brazil, Argentina, and Paraguay. Several internal parasites have been identified in capybaras in South America, both in captivity and in free-ranging individuals. Among those parasites are trematodes (*Hippocrepis hippocrepis*, *Taxorchis schistocotyle*), Cestodes (*Monoecocestus decresceus*), and nematodes (*Viannella hydrochoeri*, *Protozoophaga obese*, *Dirofilaria acutiuscula*, and *Capillaria hydrochoeri*).[16] Table 42-9 describes antimicrobial, antiparasitic, and antifungal drugs commonly used in rodents.

Bacterial Diseases

Among diseases that involve bacteria and the production of toxins in rodents, it is of utmost importance to consider and recognize antibiotic-associated diarrhea or enterotoxemia, which is caused by *Clostridium* species, which reside in healthy animals. Rodents possess predominantly gram-positive GI flora, susceptible to alteration by the administration of inappropriate antibiotics. GI flora disturbance promotes the proliferation of clostridial species, leading to a modification in the lumen pH and an increased production of volatile fatty acids (VFAs). Those VFAs inhibit normal bacteria (*Lactobacillus* spp. and *Bacteroides* spp.), and this causes production of iota toxins by the resident *Clostridium* species.

Destruction of mucosal epithelium by toxins causes diarrhea and enterotoxemia, sometimes leading to severe disease and death. It is crucial to select appropriate antibiotics for rodents, particularly herbivorous rodents.[51]

Antibiotic Therapy

It is known that herbivorous rodents are susceptible to some antibiotic classes, since they are hind gut fermenters that depend almost entirely on the microbial production of VFAs for energy. Every antibiotic has the potential to disrupt the enteric microbial flora, thus producing enteric dysbiosis and antibiotic-associated enterotoxemia, although drugs such as tetracyclines, chloramphenicol, fluoroquinolones, metronidazole, and aminoglycosides seem to have less impact than others such as penicillins, cephalosporins, lincosamides, and old-generation macrolides. The last are not recommended for treating rodents.[46]

Important notes extracted from other specialized rodent medicine texts suggest that gentamicin may cause renal problems in some rodents (so care must be taken when administering this drug to any species of rodents), and efforts must be made to prevent ingestion through grooming if a topical application was used.[51] Streptomycin may cause ascending paralysis and death in gerbils, hamsters, and mice according to current reports on rodent species.[51] Nitrofurantoin causes neuropathologic lesions in rats.[51]

Zoonoses and Emerging Diseases of Rodents

In recent years, outbreaks of diseases among humans have been caused by rodents, which have been reservoirs of diseases such as monkeypox (orthopoxvirus). Many zoonoses are carried by exotic pets and zoo and wildlife species. In 2006, 2.1 million households owned rodents (including, but not limited to, hamsters, guinea pigs, and gerbils) in the United States.[24,58] Several human activities are

TABLE 42-9

Antimicrobials, Antiparasitic, and Antifungal Drugs Commonly Used in Rodents

Drug	Dose (mg/kg)	Routes (Frequency)	Comments
ANTIMICROBIAL			
Amikacin	10–15.0	SC, IM, IV (BID)	
Azytromycin	15–30	PO (SID)	Doses for most species IP route for mice (75 mg/kg ×5 days)
Cephalexin	50	PO, IM (BID)	For parenteral use only May cause disbacteriosis
Ceftiofur	1	IM (BID)	For pneumonia cases Parenteral use only
Chloramphenicol	20–50	PO, IM (BID)	Ophthalmic ointments also safe for rodents
Ciprofloxacin	10	PO (BID)	Could have less bacterial resistance than enrofloxacin
Doxycycline	2.5	PO (BID)	All species Do not use in young animals May cause disbacteriosis in herbivores
Enrofloxacin	5.0–10.0	PO, SC, IM (SID, BID)	Frequency depends on dose Parenteral injection may cause necrosis if not diluted with saline
Gentamicin	2.0–24.0	IM, SC (SID, BID)	All species May give in combination with enrofloxacin for respiratory infections
Metronidazole	10–40 all species 20–60 in prairie dogs	PO (BID)	Anaerobes and antiprotozoal Use with caution in rodents since taste may reduce food consumption
Oxytetracycline	5.0–50	IM, PO, SC (BID)	Toxicity reported in guinea pigs Use with caution in chinchillas

TABLE 42-9

Antimicrobials, Antiparasitic, and Antifungal Drugs Commonly Used in Rodents—cont'd

Drug	Dose (mg/kg)	Routes (Frequency)	Comments
Tetracycline	10.0–20.0	PO (BID, TID)	Dose indicated for hamsters, gerbils, mice, rats, prairie dogs Toxicity has been reported in guinea pigs
Trimethoprim/sulfa	15–30 all species 48–96 in rats		Tissue necrosis can occur if given subcutaneously
ANTIPARASITIC			
Albendazole	5 (guinea pigs) 25 (chinchillas)	PO (BID)	Use in giardiasis cases
Amitraz	0.3% solution 1.4 milliliters per liter (mL/L)	Topically Topical q7-14d (3–6 treatments)	Use with caution; not recommended in young For demodecosis
Carbaryl powder	5%	Topical q7d ×3 treatments	Ectoparasites
Fenbendazole	20–50	PO (SID ×5 days)	Giardiasis, endoparasites
Imidacloprid	½ kitten dose topically		Prairie dogs
(Advantage, Bayer)	20	Topically q30d	Most species; flea control
Ivermectin	0.2–0.4	SC q7-14d	Ectoparasites and endoparasites Preferred dosage appears to be 0.4 mg/kg, q7d
Pemethrin	0.25% dust in cage		All species; ectoparasites
Piperazine	200–600 3–7 milligrams per milliliter (mg/mL)	PO (SID × 7 days), off 7 days, on 7 days Drinking water × 3–10 days	Nematodiasis Guinea pigs, mice, and rats
Praziquantel	6.0–10 30	PO, SC (repeat in 10 days) PO q14d ×3 treatments	All species of cestodes Gerbils, mice, rats
Pyrantel pamoate	50	PO (SID)	Most species; nematodiasis
Pyrethrin powder		Topical q7d ×3 treatments	All species; ectoparasites
Selamectin	6	Topically q30d	Chinchillas, degus, chipmunks
(Revolution, Bayer)	20–30 15–30	Topically Topically q21-28d × 2 treatments q14d if Demodex	Guinea pigs Most species Use 30 mg/kg with *Sarcoptes*
Sulfadimethoxine	25–50 10–15.0	PO (SID × 10 days) PO (BID)	Chinchillas, guinea pigs, and hamsters to treat coccidiosis To treat coccidiosis in all species
Sulfamerazine	1 mg/mL	Drinking water	To treat coccidiosis in chinchillas, guinea pigs, mice, hamster, rats
Sulfamethazine	1 mg/mL	Drinking water	To treat coccidiosis in chinchillas, guinea pigs, mice, hamster, rats
Thiabendazole	100	PO (SID × 5 days)	Chinchillas, guinea pigs, gerbils, mice, rats, hamsters For the treatment of ascaridiasis
Toltrazuril	10	PO (SID) × 3 days, 3 days off, 3 days on	Drug of choice to treat coccidiosis in all species
(Baycox, Bayer)	25 parts per million per liter (ppm/L)	Drinking water	Most species Use 30 mg/kg with *Sarcoptes*
ANTIFUNGAL			
Captan powder	1 teaspoon per 2 cups of dust		To prevent dermatophytosis between cagemates NOT USED in guinea pigs and duprasi
Griseofulvin	15–50 250	PO (SID × 14–28 days) On feed q10d × 4 treatments	Antifungal for dermatophytosis Prairie dogs
Itraconazole	5.0–10 25	PO (SID × 6 weeks) PO (SID)	Systemic candidiasis Dermatophytosis in chinchillas
Ketoconazole	10.0–40	PO (SID × 14 d)	All species/systemic mycoses; candidiasis
Terbinafine	10.0–30	PO (SID × 4–6 weeks)	Most species/antifungal

BID, Twice daily; *IM*, intramuscularly; *IP*, intraperitoneally; *IV*, intravenously; *SC*, subcutaneously; *SID*, once daily.
Adapted from references 27, 28, and 38.

known as drivers of these and other emerging zoonotic threats, including expansion of human populations worldwide, increased wildlife trade, and encroachment of natural habitats, all of which may increase exposure to zoonotic agents.

In many environments, however, feral rodents live in proximity to humans, domesticated animals, and other wildlife.[24,58] Other activities such as hunting and camping expose humans to wild rodents and to the risk of infectious diseases.[24] Conservation Medicine and One Health concepts propose treating the health of humans, animals, and the environment as a whole to prevent the transmission of zoonotic agents.[36,53,58]

Some of these diverse infectious agents may cause diseases in animals, and these animals may be indicators of the threats to human health. In 2003, an outbreak of monkeypox (orthopoxvirus) was linked to exposure to pet prairie dogs (*Cynomys* sp.), affecting 81 humans in six different states in the United States. It is worth mentioning here that many species of African rodents imported for the pet trade had tested positive for the monkeypox associated with the outbreak, and they had been in contact with prairie dogs. It has been demonstrated that prairie dogs also develop disease and die when infected with monkeypox.[24,58]

Rodent-borne hemorrhagic fevers are zoonotic diseases caused by an ever-increasing collection of Hantaviruses and Arenaviruses carried by rodents. Sin Nombre, Puumala, and Lassa are some of the most representative rodent-borne hemorrhagic fevers. These Hantaviruses cause chronic asymptomatic infection in the rodent host, with long-term shedding of virus in secretions and excretions.[63] Rodents of the genus *Mastomys* spp. carry Lassa arenavirus, which causes Lassa fever in West Africa. Many arenaviruses (Argentinian, Bolivian, and Venezuelan hemorrhagic fevers) have their own rodent hosts. Arenaviruses include other viruses such as LCMV, which poses significant health threats for humans and other animal species.[47,63]

It is important to stress that in many South American countries, some rodent species are a frequent alternative source of meat. For example, in the case of capybaras (*Hydrochoerus hydrochaeris*) in a slaughterhouse in Rio Grande do Sul, Brazil, researchers reported detection of agglutinating antibodies against leptospires in 27% (6 of 22) of all animals. The data presented in this report indicate that a considerable fraction of capybaras in captivity may act as reservoirs for pathogenic leptospires, underlining the occupational risk faced by those working in animal farming and slaughter.[54]

Fungal diseases in nondomestic rodents include "mouse favus," a severe form of ringworm infestation caused by *T. mentagrophytes* var. *quinckeanum*. Although rare, this organism has zoonotic potential, and human infections have been documented.

Organisms causing mycotic diseases in free-ranging or nondomestic rodents are *Candida albicans* in squirrels and European beaver (*Castor fiber*), *Cryptococcus* in beavers, *Emmonsia crescens* in ground and gray squirrels, *Phaeoannellomyces werneckii* in different species of squirrels, *Microsporum cookie* in gray squirrels, and *Trichophyton mentagrophytes* in squirrels and Canadian rodents.[37,45]

Noninfectious Diseases

Corneum Callus

A frequent lesion observed mainly in agoutis (*Dasyprocta* spp.) and acouchis (*Myocprocta acouchy*) is the formation of corneum callus on the metacarpal and calcaneus region. These are keratinized tissue calluses that are extremely resistant, are dark in color, and tend to bend laterally and form tissue expansions that are vulnerable to the tensions caused during restraint. These calluses may potentially peel off when the rodents are handled, leading to lacerations and exposure of bone tissues. This condition is linked to husbandry (substrate types, e.g., concrete and other hard surfaces) and behavior, since agoutis and acouchis have a characteristic behavioral trend of maintaining themselves supported on the tarsi for long periods to manipulate objects with the forelimbs. The pressure on the tarsi seems to increase keratin production, with subsequent local hyperkeratosis and the production of bulky calluses.

Potential complications of these lesions include lacerations, granulation tissue formation, abscesses, bleeding, grave lameness, chronic weight loss, and death.[48]

Dental Diseases: Teeth Overgrowth, Malocclusion, and Odontomas

Diagnosis of dental disease in rodents includes thorough history, clinical signs, extensive physical examination, radiography (including five standard projections: lateral, left-to-right oblique, right-to-left oblique, ventrodorsal or dorsoventral, and rostrocaudal), oral endoscopy with the appropriate instruments (as an integral part of the examination in rodent species, CT, and ancillary diagnostics such as CBC count, biochemical panel, bacterial culture and sensitivity testing (important when dealing with periapical infection and abscesses cases), and histopathology when bone neoplasia is suspected.[9] The goals of dental procedures are to reduce abnormal tooth length, to restore the occlusal plane to as near normal as possible, and to extract diseased teeth.[7,9]

Both pet and zoo rodents frequently have several dental issues because of the anatomy and physiology of their oro-gastrointestinal tract. The teeth of rodents grow continuously (incisors in all species and also molars in some species), any disease or disorder affecting the positioning of teeth within the oral cavity and disrupting normal attritional movements will lead to overgrowth and malocclusion. Maxillary molars and premolars (cheek teeth) are angled outward, whereas mandibular cheek teeth are angled slightly inward.[27,50] Maxillary molars overgrow and laterally injure the buccal mucosa, whereas mandibular molars overgrow medially, potentially injuring or trapping the tongue.[50]

Cheek teeth of guinea pigs have a 30-degree sloped occlusal plane, which slopes from buccal to lingual and dorsal to ventral. The normal oblique angle of the occlusal plane must be carefully assessed, and evaluation should not be affected by improper positioning of the endoscope.[8] Because of the peculiar orientation of cheek teeth and the anatomy of the tongue, abnormal crown elongation always deviates lingually. Unlike in rabbits, the tongue is never traumatized by sharp edges or spurs. Discomfort is a result of entrapment of the tongue by elongated cheek teeth.[8]

Overgrowth and malocclusion in rodents (guinea pigs, chinchillas, prairie dogs, and potentially every single species of rodents), are caused by congenital defects (including conformation), diet (inadequate fiber in all rodent diets), hypovitaminosis C in guinea pigs, trauma, oral abscessation, systemic illness causing anorexia (with subsequent tooth overgrowth), osteoarthritis of the temporomandibular joint and cervical vertebra), and stress (changes in diet, environment), among others.[27,28] Figures 42-2, 42-3, and 42-4 show incisor overgrowth in different species of zoo rodents: agoutis (*Dasyprocta mexicana*), American beavers (*Castor canadensis*), and crested porcupines (*Hystrix cristata*).

In species in which the molars grow continually, molar overgrowth may follow incisor malocclusion. Incisor malocclusion may lead to molar malocclusion, and vice versa, since malocclusion in one area prevents proper attrition of all teeth.[50] The most common early stage of malocclusion of cheek teeth in guinea pigs is elongation of one or both mandibular premolars. Impaction of food and hair is also frequent in guinea pigs with maloccluded cheek teeth. Intermediate stages include malocclusion of the entire mandibular cheek teeth arcade. Coronal elongation and the abnormal occlusal plane must be carefully assessed with endoscopy.

Bridgelike malocclusion of the mandibular premolars is a common finding and represents a more advanced form of cheek teeth malocclusion in guinea pigs. It is caused by coronal elongation and bending over the tongue of both mandibular CT1. Severe coronal elongation, malocclusion, and sharp buccal margins develop at maxillary cheek teeth.[8] Overgrowth of molars in the chinchilla may occur apically and coronally, so the upper pseudo-roots may invade the orbit or the nasal cavity, giving rise to ocular discharge.[50] In chinchillas, no angulation of the cheek teeth occlusal plane (the occlusal surface is flat and rough) is seen, the clinical crowns of

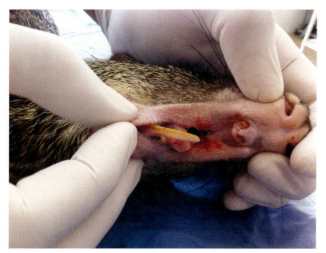

FIGURE 42-2 Incisor overgrowth in an agouti (*Dasyprocta mexicana*).

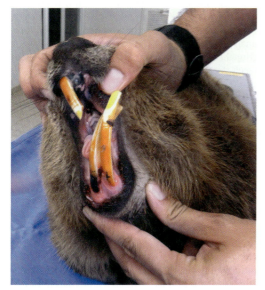

FIGURE 42-3 Incisor overgrowth in an American beaver (*Castor canadensis*).

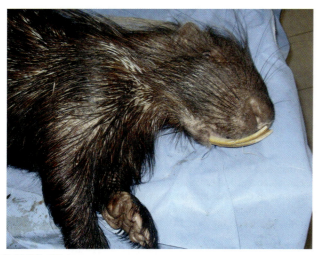

FIGURE 42-4 Incisor overgrowth in a crested porcupine (*Hystrix cristata*).

mandibular arcades are very short, and the mandibular first premolar is triangle shaped.[8] Coronal elongation and malocclusion of cheek teeth occurs in chinchillas and is similar, in some ways, to the disease process in guinea pigs and in rabbits. However, presenting signs and symptoms are usually much less severe compared with those in guinea pigs and vary slightly from the typical presentation in rabbits. Like guinea pigs, chinchillas seldom develop sharp spurs. When present, spurs usually do not traumatize the tongue but, rather, impair its movement and entrap it under the elongated crowns.

Advanced malocclusion shows elongated crowns and widened interproximal spaces. Coronal elongation of maxillary cheek teeth and abnormal sharp edges are frequently accompanied by an increase in the height of both the alveolar crest and the gingival margin. Food impaction between teeth is a common consequence, leading to gingivitis. Cavities are a frequent finding in chinchillas affected by dental disease. Proliferation of the gingiva seems to be associated with increased discomfort and poorer prognosis in chinchillas and makes reduction of crown length more difficult. In case of end-stage dental disease, clinical crowns may be worn out and fractured, and reserve crowns may no longer replace clinical crowns.[8]

Clinical signs described above are indicative of dental disease in rodents, but obtaining a complete clinical history, reviewing diet and feeding habits with the owner and at the zoo facilities, and performing a physical examination are of utmost importance. To detect abnormal teeth overgrowth and malocclusion, a full oral examination must be performed under general anesthesia.[9]

Clinical signs of dental disease in prairie dogs (which, like porcupine-like rodents, are obligate nasal breathers) are mainly respiratory; reduced activity, food intake, and stool production, weight loss or emaciation are other signs.[9,28,65] Geriatric prairie dogs (>6 years of age) may present with molars worn down to the gum line, often with just the necrotic roots visible.[28]

Overgrowth and malocclusion may be treated, and if any underlying cause is identified, it must be also corrected. Mandibular cheek teeth may be corrected by burring. A diamond bur or disk is used to trim the crown of the tooth. Nail clippers should not be used to trim the crown because they may cause teeth to fracture.[27,50] In hystricomorph rodents, reduction of the crowns of incisors is usually performed in conjunction with treatment of cheek teeth. Extraction of incisors is rarely indicated in guinea pigs and chinchillas.[9]

An alternative to trimming teeth is extraction, accessing the molars through buccotomy, which, however, has the attendant risk of food impaction at the buccotomy site resulting in poor healing. Migration of adjacent teeth and super-eruption of opposing teeth may occur in species with brachyodont molars, and in species with elodont molars, the continually opposing teeth pose a problem.[50]

Odontoma is a peculiar form of dental disease and has been reported in many rodent species (rats, mice, guinea pig, prairie dogs, degus, and tree squirrels). The term "odontoma" generally includes both odontogenic tumors (invasive and locally destructive), and tumorlike lesions such as odontogenic dysplasia of incisor teeth, which occurs frequently in prairie dogs and other squirrels (mostly locally compressive in the cranial portion of nasal cavities). Some authors have encountered radiographic abnormalities consistent with this type of lesion in other species such as the pet rabbit, chinchilla, chipmunk, and citellus (*Spermophilus citellus*). In all cases, incisor teeth were affected.[10] Odontoma (dental neoplasia) has been associated with chronic dental disease or mouth trauma from chewing on inappropriate objects such as cage bars. Affected teeth must be removed, and if possible, a permanent opening into the nasal bones caudal to the tumor mass should be left in to facilitate respiration. It is often practically impossible to remove the tumor. Supportive treatment is warranted, since this condition is progressive.[10,28]

Stress Dermatosis

This condition has been seen in agoutis, acouchis, and capybaras, but most cases occur in agoutis (*Dasyprocta* sp.) in zoologic collections, breeding places, and urban areas in Brazil. Its main feature is

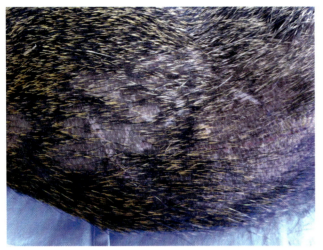

FIGURE 42-5 Stress dermatosis in an agouti (*Dasyprocta mexicana*),with mild signs of skin lesions.

skin lesions on the lumbodorsal region with alopecia and cutaneous lacerations (Figure 42-5). In chronic cases, atriquia, fibrosis, hyperkeratosis, and extensive cutaneous hyperpigmentation are seen. It is important to note that these lesions are secondary to intraspecific aggression when overcrowding is an issue within the enclosure and are frequently misdiagnosed as parasitic dermatitis.[48] Nonetheless, skin scraping and biopsy should be performed to rule out infectious causes.

The long hairs on the dorsum of some rodent species may undergo a form of autotomia (spontaneous casting of a body part) when they get bristled in ritualistic behaviors. Some rodents present tissue fragility, possibly mediated by stress, particularly on the dorsum and tail areas, which leads to lacerations and hair portions peeling off during restraint and immobilization procedures. Direct sunlight over the exposed skin without hair protection causes intense pruritus, which triggers a cycle of self-mutilation with the incisors. This could predispose to abscess and fistula formation, which also causes weight loss, emaciation, myiasis, and death. With extensive lesions, the prognosis is guarded and the recovery is slow, if at all possible. Treatment is symptomatic, and it is suggested to keep the affected individual in a separate, shaded enclosure until complete healing has occurred.[48] Figure 42-5 depicts stress dermatosis in an agouti (*Dasyprocta mexicana*) with mild signs of skin lesions.

Nutritional Diseases

Scurvy in guinea pigs is prevented by the use of proper species-specific commercial diets in which a stable form of vitamin C (as L-ascorbyl 1–2-polyphosphate) has been added to the formulation.[65] Some investigators recommend that supplemental ascorbic acid be provided (10 mg/kg daily to nonbreeding animals, 30 mg/kg daily to pregnant sows).[59]

Obesity is also common in rodents fed high-energy diets (e.g., grain) combined with little exercise. A study reported that captive beavers and woodchucks developed hypervitaminosis D when fed on a commercial primate feed that contained vitamin D_3 or when housed with arboreal species of primates.[50] Herbivorous rodents require a high-fiber diet, and captive management of these species must warrant the provision of feeds containing nondigestible fiber. Consumption of too little fiber causes fur chewing and gut stasis. The resultant change in fermentation rate may disrupt pH and motility and precipitate gastroenteritis.[50]

If fibrous food is lacking in the daily diet of zoo and pet rodents, fur chewing is highly possible and becomes an aberrant behavior that leads to different clinical issues.

Miscellaneous Diseases

Urinary signs such as stranguria and hematuria may be related to cystitis, urolithiasis, and secondary urinary tract bacterial infections. Dysuria and hunched posture are also clinical signs of urinary diseases in rodents.[27,50]

Urinary obstruction may be seen in any rodent and in other small mammals but is common in male guinea pigs. In all cases, relief of obstruction is imperative and must be accomplished rapidly, since hyperkalemia is a common consequence of prolonged urinary tract obstruction. Urinary catheterization is extremely difficult in small rodent species, and cystocentesis is used to relieve bladder overextension temporarily and is performed only once on the same patient. Cystocentesis may be followed by surgical cystotomy, if required.[34]

Vulvar enlargement, discharge, and hemorrhage are clinical signs that may be seen in female rodents suffering cystic ovaries (in guinea pigs, more than 75% of sows between 3 months and 5 years of age; gerbils), pyometra, pregnancy toxemia, endometritis, dystocia, and uterine neoplasia.[22] Affected animals may present with abdominal distention, anorexia, weakness, depression, and hunching in pain. If the cysts are functional, bilateral symmetric hair loss may be seen in the flank region.[22] Ultrasonography and, in cases of larger cysts, radiography may support the diagnosis when the treatment of choice is ovariohysterectomy. Tissues should be sent to histopathology to get an accurate diagnosis. Some authors have reported that therapy with human chorionic gonadotropin (hCG) has been used, but with nonfunctional serous cysts, only temporary or no response to treatment is seen.[22,50]

Amyloidosis in myomorph rodents (mice, rats, hamsters, and gerbils) is caused by deposition of the almost insoluble proteinaceous matrix amyloid in the kidneys, spleen, adrenal glands, or liver, with a higher prevalence in females. Clinical signs depend on the affected organ (failure of the organ) and nephrotic syndrome if the kidneys are involved. Proteinuria, decreased serum albumin, edema, and ascites are common clinical signs. The prognosis is poor, and only supportive care is suggested.[50,51]

In some Australian rodent species, particularly the greater stick-nest rat, genetic predisposition to developing chronic tubular nephropathy, possibly secondary to disorders in oxalate metabolism, leads to a syndrome known as *chronic progressive nephropathy*. Clinical signs include polydipsia or polyuria, wetness around the perineal region, and weight loss.[6]

Reproductive diseases such as uterine prolapse in guinea pigs are commonly associated with parturition. Standard techniques for reinsertion are the same as in other mammalian species, and if the tissue is in poor condition, ovariohysterectomy is recommended after stabilization of the sow.[22,34]

Pyometra is observed clinically in hamsters, gerbils, rats, guinea pigs, chinchillas, chipmunks, and prairie dogs, but it is not common. Diagnosis is made with ultrasonography, radiology, and cytology of the vaginal discharge. Ovariohysterectomy is the treatment of choice.[51]

Ejaculatory plugs are formed in rats and mice from epithelial cells and spermatozoa and are frequently seen in the bladder of males on postmortem examination. Occasionally, these plugs may cause urethral obstruction and must be differentiated from uroliths.[51]

Neoplasia

Numerous tumor types have been seen in rodents and include adenocarcinoma and fibroadenoma of the mammary glands, leiomyomas and leiomyosarcomas of the uterus, ovarian adenocarcinoma, adrenocortical adenoma, pituitary adenomas (chromophobe adenomas of the pars distalis), lymphosarcoma and gastric or cecal adenocarcinomas, skin tumors (trichofolliculomas, liposarcomas, fibropapillomas of the ear canal, melanomas, melanocytomas, epitheliotropic lymphoma), lymphosarcoma or cavian leukemia (type-C retrovirus), insulinomas, alveologenic carcinomas, alveologenic papillary adenomas, hepatic carcinomas, and testicular interstitial cell tumors, among others.[22,46,50,51,65]

Endocrine Diseases

Diabetes mellitus is a spontaneous disease usually seen in 90-day-old Chinese hamsters (associated with autosomal-recessive genes), in guinea pigs, mice, and aged gerbils (as a sequela of obesity and high-calorie diets). Strains of rats used as biomodels for juvenile human diabetes also develop spontaneous diabetes.[50,51] Other reported endocrine diseases in rodents include hyperadrenocorticism (in the hamster in association with adrenocortical adenoma), insulinoma, thyroid adenoma, hypothyroidism, blood vessel mineralization, parathyroid neoplasia, and pituitary adenomas.[50,51] Many of the reported endocrine disease lesions have been diagnosed after death, so the clinical significance in rodents is unknown.

REPRODUCTION

Important aspects of communication in relation to reproduction that have been extensively studied in rodents include chemical factors in urine that accelerate and suppress reproduction, express dominance and territoriality, and serve as cues of genetic compatibility in mate choice.[64] Interesting published data highlight the importance of genetic relatedness in modulating the social behavior of rodents. Social groups of kin most often result from philopatry of daughters, which, in turn, creates advantages for males that disperse to seek unrelated females for mating and to avoid inbreeding or reproduction competition in the natal site. Coloniality and sociality, especially eusociality, depend on kinship and occur in blind mole-rats, North American ground squirrels, desert rodents, some groups of South American rodents, and African mole-rats.[64] Rodents being such a diverse animal group, their reproductive physiology is extremely varied. Larger species (capybaras, acouchis, coendus, New World porcupines) reproduce once a year, and smaller rodents, in general, breed several times in a season.[48,50] Tables 42-10, 42-11, 42-12, and 42-13 present general reproductive parameters of selected species of rodents.

Muridae rodents show estrus shortly after parturition and are extremely prolific.[33,51] It is important to consider breeding female guinea pigs before 6 to 7 months of age to prevent permanent fusion of the pelvic symphisis.[27,46,64] Female degus have no regular estrus cycle, although in wild animals, a pattern of seasonal reproduction characterized by two peaks of parturition (early and late spring) with a non-reproductive period between summer and winter has been

TABLE 42-10

Reproductive Parameters of Selected Rodent Species

	Mouse	Rat	Gerbil	Hamster
Sexual maturity (weeks)	6 both sexes	4–5 both sexes	9–18 male (M) 9–12 female (F)	8 M / 6 F
Estrus cycle (days)	4–5	4–5	4–7	4–5
Estrus length (hours)	9–20	9–20	12–18	8–26
Gestation (days)	19–21	21–23	23–26	15–18
Weight at birth (grams)	1–1.5	4–6	2.5–3.5	1.5–3
Litter size	7–11	6–13	3–8	5–10
Number of pair of teats	5	6	4	6–7
Eyes open (days)	12–14	12–15	16–21	12–14
Altricial or Precocial	Altricial	Altricial	Altricial	Altricial
Weaning (days)	18–21	21	21–28	19–21

Adapted from references 33 and 51.

TABLE 42-11

Reproductive Parameters of Selected Rodent Species

	Guinea Pig	Chinchilla	Degu	Duprasi	Chipmunk	Prairie Dog
Sexual maturity (months)	Male (M): 3–4 Female (F): 2–3	6–8	6 (45 days–20 months)	2.5–3.5	12	2–3
Estrus cycle (days) (average)	15–17	40	Irregular	Breed all year	13–14 (11–21)	Monoestrus
Estrus length (hours)	1 –16	3 –5	Several hours	Similar to gerbils	3	5–6
Gestation (days) (average)	59–72	111	90–93	20–22	31–32 (28–35)	30–37
Weight at birth (grams)	60–100	30–50	14.1–14.6	2.4–2.6	—	—
Litter size (average)	1–6 (3–4)	1–6 (2)	5–6 (1–10)	1–7 (3)	3–5 (1–10)	2–10 (5)
Litters per year	3 t–o 4	2	>1	Several	1	1
Postpartum estrus	Yes	Yes	No	Unknown	No	No
Eyes open (days)	At birth	At birth	At birth	16	—	—
Weaning (days)	14–21	42	28–42	28	42	6 weeks
Comments	Precocial	Precocial	Precocial	Altricial	—	—

TABLE 42-12

Reproductive Parameters of Selected Rodent Species

	Capybara	Agouti	Acouchi	Patagonian Hare	Rock Cavy	New World Porcupine	Coendu	Lowland Paca	Pacarana	Coypu	Viscacha	Ingram's Squirrel
Sexual maturity (months)	15–24	6	8–12	8	5–6	19	19	7		3–7	15	18
Gestation (days) (average)	145–160	103	99	93	65	203	203	115	222–283	128–132	154	44–48
Weight at birth (grams)	1500	140	100		76	40	40	700	900	225	200	>10
Litter size (average)	1–8 (4)	1–3 (2)	1–3 (2)	2–5	1–2 (1)	1–2 (1)	1–2 (1)	1–2 (1)	1–2 (2)	1–10 (5.5)		1–9 (3)
Litters (per year)	1	>2	1	2	5	1	1	1 to 2	1 to 2	2–3	8	2
Lactation (weeks)	16	4	2–3	11	6	10	10	12		6–10	3–8	8

TABLE 42-13

Reproductive Parameters of Selected Australian Rodent Species

	Canadian Beaver (*Castor canadensis*)	Gray Squirrel (*Sciurus carolinensis*)	Woodchuck (*Marmota monax*)	Muskrat (*Ondatra zibethicus*)
Sexual maturity (months)	24	12–18	± 12	12
Estrus cycle (days)	20–21			
Gestation (days) (average)	105–107	44	30–45	28–35

Adapted from: Sainsbury, 2005.

identified.[27] The breeding season of chipmunks in the northern hemisphere is from March to September in response to the lengthening light cycle and increasing temperatures. Ovulation in female chipmunks is spontaneous.[28]

In prairie dogs, spring in the northern hemisphere is the breeding season, and to adapt natural reproductive behaviors in captivity, it is important to consider a colony social situation necessary for successful breeding and rearing.[28] Among Sciuridae and Muridae, many species show anatomic and physiologic changes in males; for example, the gonads are withdrawn into the abdominal cavity after the breeding season and may atrophy.[50] In chipmunks male testicular enlargement starts in January prior to the onset of the female estrus cycle in March.[28]

Many rodents are seasonal breeders and are seasonally polyestrous (e.g., chinchillas in November to May in the northern hemisphere); most beavers in January and February whose copulation occurs in water (here I am indicating that only the beavers copulation occurs in water). A pair of large anal scent glands are present in both sexes in beavers and may be confused with testes. To identify male beavers, the os penis should be palpated by inserting a finger into the cloacal opening.[50]

Various factors, including food availability, temperature, and photoperiod, may affect reproduction in Australian rodents in the wild. Reproduction in captive Australian rodents, including the spinifex hopping mouse, plains rat, and western chestnut mouse, has been successfully accomplished for many generations. Captive breeding of Australian rodents for conservation purposes, reintroduction to the wild, or both has been promoted for Shark Bay mice (*Pseudomys fieldi*), greater stick-nest rats, and central rock rats.[6]

Most rodent species are born naked and helpless and receive care in nests. Species in Hystricognati have long gestation periods in comparison with other rodents, and at birth, they are usually well developed and are usually fully furred, and their eyes are open. They also may survive away from their dam within 2 weeks of birth but usually are suckled longer.[50]

Determining the sex of most rodent species is easy in mature animals, but significantly more challenging in very young ones. Generally, a reliable method to determine sex is to measure the distance between the anus and the genital papilla, as the anogenital distance is greater in males than in females, and the genital papilla is usually more prominent and has a round opening in the male.[33,50,64]

ACKNOWLEDGMENT

The author would like to thank Eduardo Valdés, for his invaluable help and comments on the nutrition and feeding section of this chapter, and to Brandi Graham for assistance with creating the tables in this chapter.

REFERENCES

1. Bangari DS, Miller MA, Stevenson GW, et al: Cutaneous and systemic poxviral disease in red (*Tamiasciurus hudsonicus*) and gray (*Sciurus carolinensis*) squirrels. *Vet Pathol* 46:667–672, 2009.

2. Bautista OMA: *Identificación de nematodos en una población de tepezcuintles (Agouti paca) en cautiverio en la selva de Pipiapán, Veracruz*, Tesis de Licenciatura, 1995, Facultad de Medicina Veterinaria y Zootecnia, Universidad Nacional Autónoma de México, México, D.F.
3. Bennett RA: Soft tissue surgery. In Quesenberry KE, Carpenter JW, editors: *Ferrets, rabbits and rodents: Clinical medicine and surgery*, ed 3, St. Louis, MO, 2012, Elsevier.
4. Boehm CA, Carney EL, Tallarida RJ, et al: Midazolam enhances the analgesic properties of dexmedetomidine in the rat. *Vet Anaesth Anal* 37:550–556, 2010.
5. Brandão J, Mayer J: Behavior of rodents with an emphasis on enrichment. *J Exot Pet Med* 20(4):256–269, 2011.
6. Breed A, Eden P: Rodents. In Vogelnest L, Woods R, editors: *Medicine of Australian mammals*, 2010, CSIRO Publishing.
7. Capello V, Cauduro AM: Clinical technique: Application of computed tomography for diagnosis of dental disease in the rabbit, guinea pig, and chinchilla. *J Exot Pet Med* 17(2):93–101, 2008.
8. Capello V, Lennox A: Advanced diagnostic imaging for dental disease and related complications in rabbits and rodents. In *Proceedings of the 11th Annual Conference, Association of Exotic Mammal Veterinarians*, Oakland, CA, 2012, AAZV.
9. Capello V, Lennox AM: Small mammal dentistry. In Quesenberry KE, Carpenter JW, editors: *Ferrets, rabbits and rodents: Clinical medicine and surgery*, ed 3, St. Louis, MO, 2012, Elsevier.
10. Capello V: Odontomas in rodents: Surgical treatment of pseudo-odontomas in prairie dogs. In *Proceedings of the 11th Annual Conference, Association of Exotic Mammal Veterinarians*, Oakland, Ca, 2012, AAZV.
11. Cardoso R de CA: *Rastreio Virológico em Espécies Selvagens de Roedores Pertenecentes á Fauna Portuguesa*, Lisbon, Portugal, 2011, Maestrado em Microbiologia Aplicada, Faculdade de Ciencias, Departamento de Biologia Vegetal, Universidad de Lisboa.
12. Clark JA, Myers PH, Goelz JE, et al: Pica behavior associated with buprenorphine administration in the rat. *Lab Anim* 47:300–303, 1997.
13. De Andrade AM, Marcel LC, Singaretti F, Fernandes MR: Lobaçao, Árvore Brónquica e Vascularizaçao Arterial do Pulmáo de Paca (*Agouti paca*, LINNAEUS, 1766). *Ciência Animal Brasileira* v9(2):442–448, 2008.
14. Divers SJ: Rabbit and rodent anesthesia. In *Proceedings of the 5th Exotic Animal Medicine for the Clinical Practitioner Conference, sponsored by AAZV*, Oakland, CA, 2012, ACZM.
15. Donnelly TM, Brown CJ: Guinea pig and chinchilla care and husbandry. *Vet Clin North Am Exot Anim Pract* 7(2):351–373, 2004.
16. Estudio de la FAO Producción y Sanidad Animal 122. El capibara (*Hydrochoerus hydrochaerus*). Estado actual de su producción. Por Dr. Eduardo González Jiménez, Universidad Central de Venezuela, 1995.
17. Flecknell PA, Mitchell M: Midazolam and fentanyl-fluanisone: Assessment of anaesthetic effects in laboratory rodents and rabbits. *Lab Anim* 18:143–146, 1984.
18. Fontenot DK, Mylniczenko ND, Fleming GJ: Utilization of continuous rate infusion, manually controlled infusion, and total intravenous infusion for anesthesia and analgesia in zoological collections. In *Proceedings of the American Association of Zoo Veterinarians annual conference*, Oakland, Ca, 2012, AAZV.
19. Fowler ME: *Restraint and handling of wild and domestic animals*, Ames, IA, 2008, Blackwell Publishing.
20. Grant K: Nutrition of tree-dwelling squirrels. *Vet Clin Exot Anim* 12:287–297, 2009.
21. Hawkins MG, Pascoe PJ: Anesthesia, analgesia, and sedation of small mammals. In Quesenberry KE, Carpenter JW, editors: *Ferrets, rabbits and rodents: Clinical medicine and surgery*, ed 3, St. Louis, MO, 2012, Elsevier.
22. Hawkins MG, Bishop CR: Disease problems of guinea pigs. In Quesenberry KE, Carpenter JW, editors: *Ferrets, rabbits and rodents: Clinical medicine and surgery*, ed 3, St. Louis, MO, 2012, Elsevier.
23. Heard DJ: Rodents. In West G, Heard D, Caulkett N, editors: *Zoo animal and wildlife immobilization and anesthesia*, Ames, IA, 2007, Blackwell Publishing.
24. Hill WA, Brown JP: Zoonoses of rabbits and rodents. *Vet Clin Exot Anim* 14:519–532, 2011.
25. Hoogland JL, James DA: Nutrition, care and behavior of captive prairie dogs. *Vet Clin Exot Anim* 12:255–266, 2009.
26. Jaeger J-J: Rodent phylogeny: New data and old problems. In Benton MJ, editor: *The phylogeny and classification of the Tetrapods*, vol 2, Oxford, U.K., 1988, Clarendon Press.
27. Johnson-Delaney C: Guinea pigs, chinchillas, degus and duprasi. In Meredith A, Johnson-Delaney C, editors: *Manual of exotic pets*, ed 5, Gloucester, U.K., 2010, BSAVA.
28. Johnson-Delaney C: Chipmunks and prairie dogs. In Meredith A, Johnson-Delaney C, editors: *Manual of Exotic Pets*, ed 5, Gloucester, U.K., 2010, BSAVA.
29. Juan-Sallés C, Rico-Hernández G, Garner M, Barr BC: Pulmonary besnoitiosis in captive maras (*Dolichotis patagonum*) associated with interstitial pneumonia. *Vet Pathol* 41:408–411, 2004.
30. Kessler DS, Hope K, Maslanka M: Behavior, nutrition, and veterinary care of patagonian cavies (*Dolichotis patagonum*). *Vet Clin Exot Anim* 12:267–278, 2009.
31. Landry SO: The rodentia as omnivores. *Q Rev Biol* 45:351–372, 1970.
32. Legendre LFJ: Oral disorders of exotic rodents. *Vet Clin Exot Anim* 6:601–628, 2003.
33. Lennox AM, Bauck L: Small rodents: Basic anatomy, physiology, husbandry and clinical techniques. In Quesenberry KE, Carpenter JW, editors: *Ferrets, rabbits and rodents: Clinical medicine and surgery*, ed 3, St. Louis, MO, 2012, Elsevier.
34. Lichtenberger M, Lennox AM: Emergency and critical care in small mammals. In Quesenberry KE, Carpenter JW, editors: *Ferrets, rabbits and rodents: Clinical medicine and surgery*, ed 3, St. Louis, MO, 2012, Elsevier.
35. Longley LA: *Anaesthesia of exotic pets*, Philadelphia, PA, 2008, Saunders.
36. Maggi RG, Harms CA, Breitschwerdt EB: Bartonellosis. In Aguirre AA, Ostfeld RS, Daszak P, editors: *New directions in conservation medicine-applied cases of ecological health*, Oxford, U.K., 2012, Oxford University Press.
37. Marshall KL: Fungal diseases in small mammals: Therapeutic trends and zoonotic considerations. *Vet Clin Exot Anim* 6:415–427, 2003.
38. Mayer J: Rodents. In Carpenter JW, Marion CJ, editors: *Exotic animal formulary*, ed 4, St. Louis, MO, 2013, Elsevier.
39. McClure DE: Mycobacteriosis in the rabbit and rodent. *Vet Clin Exot Anim* 15:85–99, 2012.
40. McWilliams DA: Determinants for the diet of captive agoutis (*Dasyprocta* spp.). *Vet Clin Exot Anim* 12:279–286, 2009.
41. Mitchell S: Venipuncture techniques in pet rodent species. *J Exot Pet Med* 20(4):284–293, 2011.
42. Mylniczenko ND: Small mammal potpourri. In *Proceedings of the 5th Exotic Animal Medicine for the Clinical Practitioner Conference*, 2012. sponsored by AAZV and endorsed by the ACZM.
43. Nishiyama SM, Pompermayer LG, Lima de Lavor MS, Silva CLB: Associacao cetamina-xilazina, tiletamina-zolazepam, e tiletamina-zolazepam-levopromazina na anestesia de capivara (*Hydrochoerus hydrochaeris*). *Revista CERES* 53(307):406–412, 2006.
44. Pilny AA: Clinical hematology of rodent species. *Vet Clin Exot Anim* 11:523–533, 2008.
45. Pollock C: Fungal diseases of laboratory rodents. *Vet Clin Exot Anim* 6:401–413, 2003.
46. Quesenberry KE, Donnelly TM, Mans C: Guinea pigs and chinchillas: Biology, husbandry and clinical techniques. In Quesenberry KE, Carpenter JW, editors: *Ferrets, rabbits and rodents: Clinical medicine and surgery*, ed 3, St. Louis, MO, 2012, Elsevier.
47. Rabinowitz PM, Conti LA: *Human-animal medicine: Clinical approaches to zoonoses, toxicants and other shared health risks*, St. Louis, MO, 2010, Elsevier.
48. Ribas LE, Moreira dos Santos SE: Rodentia-Roedores Silvestres (Capivara, Cutia, Paca, Ouriço). In Cubas Z, Ramos JC, Catâo-Dias JL, editors: *Tratado de Animais Selvagens, Medicina Veterinária.*, Sao Paulo, Brasil, 2007, Editora Roca Ltda.
49. Rizzo B, Adkesson M: Use of computed tomography as an imaging guide for castration in the crested porcupine (*Hystrix africaeasutralis*). In

Proceedings of the American Association of Zoo Veterinarians annual conference, Oakland, Ca, 2012, AAZV.

50. Sainsbury AW: Rodentia (Rodents). In Fowler ME, Miller ER, editors: *Zoo and wild animal medicine*, ed 5, St. Louis, MO, 2003, Saunders.

51. Sayers I, Smith S: Mice, rats, hamsters and gerbils. In Meredith A, Johnson-Delaney C, editors: *Manual of exotic pets*, ed 5, Gloucester, U.K., 2010, BSAVA.

52. Shani B-K, Hector M, Osnat P, et al: Rodent phylogeny revised: Analysis of six nuclear genes from all major rodent clades. *BMC Evol Biol* 9:71, 2009.

53. Shury T: Capture and physical restraint of zoo and wild animals. In West G, Heard D, Caulkett N, editors: *Zoo animal and wildlife immobilization and anesthesia*, Ames, IA, 2007, Blackwell Publishing.

54. Silva EF, Seyffert N, Jouglard SDD, et al: Seroprevalência da infeccao leptospiral em capivaras (*Hydrochoerus hydrochaeris*) abatidas em um frigorífico do Rio Grande do Sul. *Pesq Vet Bras* 29(2):174–176, 2009.

55. Singaretti De Olivieira F, Martins LL, Duque JC, et al: Anestesia epidural em cutias (*Dasyprocta azarae*). *Acta Sci Vet* 34(1):89–91, 2006.

56. Souza MJ, Cox SK: Tramadol use in zoologic medicine. *Vet Clin Exot Anim* 14:117–130, 2011.

57. Souza MJ: Bacterial and parasitic zoonoses of exotic pets. *Vet Clin Exot Anim* 12:401–416, 2009.

58. Souza MJ: One health: Zoonoses in the exotic animal practice. *Vet Clin Exot Anim* 14:421–426, 2011.

59. Tamura Y: Current approach to rodents as patients. *J Exot Pet Med* 19(1):36–55, 2010.

60. Tullberg T: Ueber das System der Nagetiere: Eine phylogenetische Studie. *Nova Acta Reg Soc Sci Upsala Ser* 3(18):1–514, 1899.

61. Wenger S: Anesthesia and analgesia in rabbits and rodents. *J Exot Pet Med* 21:71–76, 2012.

62. West G: Rodent medicine. In *Proceedings of the 3rd Exotic Animal Medicine for the Clinical Practitioner Conference*, 2010. sponsored by AAZV and endorsed by the ACZM.

63. Wobeser GA: *Disease shared with humans and domestic animals. Essentials of disease in wild animals*, Ames, IA, 2006, Blackwell Publishing.

64. Wolff JO, Sherman PW: Rodent societies and model systems. In Wolff JO, Sherman PW, editors: *Rodent societies: An ecological and evolutionary perspective*, Chicago, IL, 2007, The University of Chicago Press.

65. Yarto JE: Respiratory system anatomy, physiology and disease: Guinea pigs and chinchillas. *Vet Clin Exot Anim* 14:339–355, 2011.

CHAPTER 43

Cetacea (Whales, Dolphins, Porpoises)

Christopher Dold

BIOLOGY

Cetacea is the order of mammals that includes whales, dolphins, and porpoises. Cetaceans are found throughout the world's oceans but most species types have specific or common ranges (Table 43-1). Fossil evidence indicates that cetaceans are marine mammal descendants, a group of land mammals that were characterized by being even toed and having an oblong skull and slim limbs with significant similarities to that of early whales.[60] The two suborders within the extant order Cetacea are Mysticete and Odontocete. Within the suborder Mysticete, baleen whales, 13 species exist in four families. Baleen whales such as blue and humpback whales are so named for the large plates of keratinized baleen they have instead of teeth. They feed on krill and fish by swallowing large volumes of prey and water and then forcing the water out past the baleen, capturing and then swallowing the prey. At least 70 species exist within the suborder Odontocete, toothed whales, in 40 genera and 10 families. This suborder varies greatly in size—from the largest sperm whale (*Physeter macrocephalus*) to the smallest Hector's dolphin (*Cephalorhynchus hectori*). Toothed whales are known to be social animals that exist in both small and large groups; large groupings of over 100 dolphins are known as *superpods*. Family groups have been documented in several species, and socialized feeding strategies are known to be part of the natural history of these animals. Both aquatic and marine cetacean species exist, and both have evolved anatomically and behaviorally for life in an aquatic environment. Nearly all cetacean species are fish eating, or picivorous, and every species has evolved to specialize in its niche.

The cetaceans found in zoologic parks, oceanaria, and stranding rehabilitation centers are almost exclusively odontocetes (of the families Delphinidae and Monodontidae). Most reported clinical experience has been developed through work with the bottlenose dolphin (*Tursiops truncatus, T. t. gilli*, and *T.t. aduncus*), given its relative ubiquity in zoologic parks and oceanaria, as well as in research and rehabilitation facilities. Other odontocete species, including the killer whale (*Orcinus orca*), the beluga whale (*Delphinapterus leucas*), the Pacific white-sided dolphin (*Lagenorhynchus obliquidens*), the harbor porpoise (*Phocoena phocoena*), the short finned pilot whale (*Globicephala macrorhyncus*), the Commerson's dolphin (*Cephalorhynchus commersonii*), and the spotted dolphin (*Stenella frontalis*), and some freshwater species such as the Amazon river dolphin (*Inia geoffrensis*) are successfully housed in zoos and oceanaria. Husbandry and veterinary care developed for *Tursiops* may generally be extrapolated directly to the other species, with some exceptions, including drug dosing and safety, as well as logistical application of diagnostic and therapeutic techniques.

Since the preponderance of species found in zoologic parks, oceanaria, and rehabilitation settings are odontocetes, this chapter will focus only on their regular as well as medical care, particularly that of members of the families Delphinidae and Monodontidae.

TABLE 43-1

Biological Information of Selected Cetaceans Commonly Housed in Zoological Parks and Oceanaria

Scientific Name	English Common Names	Weight (Adults, kg)	Geographical Distribution	Identification
Tursiops truncatus	Atlantic bottlenose dolphin	150–300	Atlantic Ocean most commonly found along the US east coast and Gulf of Mexico	Prominent rostrum, grey dorsum with white or pink ventrum.
Delphinapterus leucas	Beluga whale	1200–1600	North Pacific, Arctic ocean, Cook Inlet, Alaska, Hudson Bay CAN	Grey as juveniles, all white as adults. Absent rostrum, absent dorsal fin.
Lagenorhynchus obliquidens	Pacific white-sided dolphin	120–160	Widely distributed around the temperate pacific basin	Black dorsum, white side, and white ventrum separated by a black line. Minimal rostrum.
Orcinus orca	Killer whale	2300–5600	Widely distributed	All black with white ventrum and characteristic white false eye patch immediately caudal and dorsal to eyes.

UNIQUE ANATOMY AND PHYSIOLOGY

Whales and dolphins are obligate marine and aquatic swimmers and have distinctive anatomy. They lack hair and hindlimbs, have forelimbs evolved into flippers, tail flukes used for propulsion, and a streamlined body. Further, they have evolved to have a relatively large body size and thick blubber layers to maintain homeothermia in the generally exothermic aquatic and marine environments. Anatomic adaptations of the cardiovascular system to support diving, breath-holds, and temperature conservation include large, distensible veins, venous sinuses, venous valves in the lungs, portal triads of the liver, and a venous sphincter in the common hepatic vein at the junction of the inferior vena cava below the diaphragm. A meshwork of arteries and veins between the thoracic vertebral bodies, called the *rete mirabile*, and periarterial vascular rete represent temperature countercurrent exchange systems. These systems allow cetaceans to peripherally vasoconstrict and still perfuse the brain and other organs with warm, oxygenated blood under the pressure and temperature extremes experienced at depth.

The respiratory system is also adapted for life in the water. The blowhole is the external nasal opening positioned on top of the head of cetaceans. Immediately ventral and lateral to the blowhole are right and left lateral vestibular sacs. Paired internal nares separated by the nasal septum lead to paired nasal cavities that extend ventrally along the cranial aspect of the calvarium to the nasopharynx. The elongated epiglottal and cricoarytenoid cartilages of the larynx are supported laterally by arytenoepiglottal muscles. This structure is frequently referred to as a "goosebeak" because of its shape. It is held in its dorsally oriented position by the nasopharyngeal sphincter muscle along the dorsal oropharynx. The larynx leads to a short trachea. Anterior to the carina is a right-sided accessory bronchus, which leads to the anterior portion of the right lung lobe. Cetaceans also have extensive pulmonary support structures, including complete tracheal and bronchial cartilaginous rings that extend beyond the mainstem bronchi into deep bronchioles, as well as plates and rings of cartilage that extend all the way to the junctions of alveoli. Smooth muscle sphincterlike narrowings occur at the terminal bronchioles. The lungs contain a great amount of elastic tissue. A thick, dense, elastic visceral pleura covers the nonseptate, nonsegmented lungs.

The upper gastrointestinal (GI) tract of odontocetes is dominated by a modified three-chambered stomach. The first chamber (forestomach) is a large, muscular chamber that collects the meal and initiates mechanical digestion. The second chamber (fundic) is the glandular stomach that lies ventrolaterally to the first chamber on the left side of the animal. Digesta leaves the second chamber through a narrow connecting channel on the right side into the elongated pyloric chamber. The terminus of the stomach is referred to as the *duodenal ampula*, which is followed by the small and large intestines that are essentially uniform in diameter all the way to the rectum.

Cetacean kidneys are reniculated as in other marine mammals, including cattle, with whom dolphins share a common ancestor. The evolution of reniculated kidneys in cetaceans is not well understood, but reniculated kidneys have a greater surface area than equally sized nonreniculated kidneys, which may facilitate filtration of larger blood volumes of cetaceans as compared with terrestrial species.

SPECIAL HOUSING REQUIREMENTS

As with other species housed in zoologic parks in the United States, minimal housing requirements for all marine mammals, including cetaceans, are established by the Animal Welfare Act (the Act) written and curated by the United States Department of Agriculture. Routine inspection of zoos, oceanaria, and research facilities and enforcement of the Act are conducted by the Animal Plant Health Inspection Service (APHIS) Animal Care program to ensure that appropriate standards are applied to animal facilities and that proper care is carried out. This includes housing standards and water quality. Minimum space requirements required for housing marine mammals are described by the Act. The size of cetacean habitats is assessed on the basis of depth, volume, surface area, and by a "minimum horizontal distance," which is the usable space across the pool. Cetaceans are divided into special groups, and space requirements include the number of animals allowed per facility. For specifics of housing requirements, the reader is referred to the Act.

As cetaceans are housed exclusively in an aquatic environment, the quality of water is a critical component of the animals' overall health and well being. Water management of cetacean housing habitats exists in two primary forms: open and closed. *Open systems* are lagoon or sea based, and the quality of the water varies, depending on the general environment. *Closed systems* are designed pools that are usually filled with synthetic salt water. A hybrid semi-closed (or semi-open) system relies on access to natural seawater that is pumped into the land-based facility, usually undergoing mechanical filtration prior to use in the animal habitat and again prior to effluence. Closed systems are the most intensively managed, as the water is continuously recycled and only periodically replaced. Further, closed systems may experience shifts in concentration (salinity, acid–base status) because of incidental fresh water additions in the form of rain, and run-off. Marine cetacean water systems should be maintained with a salinity of 27 to 32 parts per thousand (ppt), but short-term variations above or below this range (hours to days) do not pose a significant risk to health.

APHIS regulates the amount of coliform bacteria in marine mammal systems by requiring that samples be collected regularly (weekly) and that the most probable number of coliform bacteria not exceed 1000 per 100 milliliters (mL) of water. This number may be the result of the average of three samples over a 48-hour period. Although coliform bacteria may not ultimately be harmful themselves, they are considered "indicator bacteria" in that their numbers reflect the efficacy of water disinfection. Chlorine-based oxidants and ozone are the principal sterilizing agents applied to marine mammal housing systems. Chlorine reacts with the salts in water to form potent oxidizers that ultimately act as chemical disinfectants.[61] Thus, measures of total chlorine in a system, ideally kept below 1 part per million (ppm), are indirect indicators of oxidation potential.

Chlorine-based oxidants and ozone are highly effective water disinfectants. In fact, they may maintain water in a more sterile condition compared with natural seawater. Future attempts to balance the preservation of beneficial microorganisms against the removal of potentially pathogenic organisms may enhance the overall homeostasis of intensively managed closed water systems. Previous efforts to develop efficacious closed systems—purely biologic filtration systems without chemical or ozone disinfectants (more similar to aquarium systems) while reducing potential risks associated with chlorine oxidant exposure—have shown promise.[68]

Besides water quality and habitat size, the grouping of animals housed together is important. Social groupings and behavioral compatibility of whales and dolphins should be considered in habitat design, as the social compatibility of species may be a significant factor in their health and wellness. Efforts to house conspecifics together are important in their management and are generally recognized as the ideal method of housing, if at all possible.

FEEDING

All cetacean species housed in zoologic parks are piscivorous. Fish species most commonly fed to managed cetaceans include herring (*Clupea herengus*), capelin (*Mallotus villosus*), and squid (*Loligo* spp.). Other species fed less commonly include Atlantic and Spanish mackeral (*Scomber scombrus* and *Scomberomorus maculatus*) and smelt (*Osmerus mordax*). Relative quatities of these fish fed vary, depending on the species of cetacean, but all of the commonly managed whales and dolphins may thrive on these species of fish. A general rule of thumb for adult delphinids and mondontids is to feed 2% to 5% of body weight per day (although it varies with species). Fish quality is paramount to cetacean health. Individually quick frozen (IQF) fish tend to be of higher quality and integrity when thawed for feeding; however, not all species are available as IQF. Fish should remain frozen below −2° C until immediately prior to being fed to cetaceans. Air thawing of frozen fish beginning 24 hours prior to feeding is recommended and is best accomplished in dedicated refrigerators that maintain a constant temperature of not more than 5° C. Thawing in water has been shown to promote bacterial growth and may reduce the nutritional value of the fish. Feeding the whole fish, as opposed to fish cut into small pieces, is recommended to avoid the potentially negative nutritional consequences of loss of organ meats and fats that may accompany the cutting of fish. Spoilage of fish may be subtle and may lead to loss of nutritional value and, in mackeral and tuna species (suborder *Scombroidei*), increases the possibility of scombroid poisoning.

The nutritional composition of the fish species, specifically the fat content, changes seasonally. Therefore, close attention should be paid to the time of year when the lots were harvested and the location where the lots were harvested. Proximate analysis of fish lots is highly recommended to determine the caloric value of fish species, and assessments of peroxidase and histamine levels should be performed to determine the quality and freshness of the fish. In managed cetaceans, body weight should be monitored frequently (twice weekly) to assess any potential errors in feeding plans.

Any potential nutritional disorders are easily avoided with a good quality, well-tended fish diet and proper daily supplementation with multi-vitamins. There are appropriate multi-vitamin supplements developed specifically for piscivorous marine mammals that include vitamins A, E, C, and B complex. Thiamine is a critical component of any cetacean vitamin supplement. Thiamine deficiency, which manifests as depression, body tremors, and central nervous system (CNS) signs (e.g., seizures), is a possible nutritional complication of a frozen fish–based diet. The freeze–thaw cycle of food fish may promote the activity of thiaminases within the fish. Thiamine deficiency is easily avoided with thiamine supplementation at no less than 200 milligrams per kilogram (mg/kg) of fish fed as part of a routine multi-vitamin supplementation program.[40] Thiamine supplements should be added to the fish immediately prior to feeding to assure that thiaminase activity does not reduce the supplement's efficacy.

Although the overall impact of the zoologic community on fisheries is low, current efforts are underway to identify other sustainable fish species to provide a nutritionally balanced diet for whales and dolphins. Several zoologic parks and oceanaria are investigating "novel" fisheries, such as menhaden and mullet, which are smaller in scale, sustainable, and may provide for a more diverse nutritional profile for managed cetaceans. In addition, fish "analogs" made of high-grade sustainable fish meal and supplemented with vitamins, prepared in a gel-based form, offer the potential for "ready to make" diets that may have improved storage capacity and provide inherent nutritional flexibility.

RESTRAINT AND HANDLING

Given the large body size of most cetaceans and their unique anatomy, restraint and handling present unique challenges. Fortunately, whales and dolphins are readily trained with operant conditioning behavioral techniques. These techniques have been comprehensively described by Ramirez.[39] Behavioral training greatly enhances care of cetaceans housed in zoologic parks and significantly reduces the need for physical or chemical restraint. A majority of clinical procedures may be accomplished through operant conditioning techniques: routine care-related behaviors such as presenting for physical examination or sliding onto a scale for body weight measurement, and allowing routine diagnostics such as blood collection, gastric fluid collection, samples of urine, feces, and forced exhaled breath, and even endoscopy may be taught with the use of behavioral training techniques.[4]

Animals may be safely removed from the water for most diagnostic and therapeutic techniques. When necessary, physical restraint of smaller cetaceans (bottlenose dolphin, Pacific white-sided dolphin) may be accomplished. Animals are placed in thick, lined slings or stretchers with holes for the pectoral flippers to pass through (Figure 43-1). Animals may also be handled on the floors of specially designed pools where the water may be rapidly drained or in "false-bottom" pools with rising floors that allow the animals to be lifted mechanically. Most species of dolphins and small whales do well out of the water for extended periods as long as they are protected from contact injuries, overheating, and drying out. This is easily accomplished by keeping the animal on closed-cell foam padding, out of direct sunlight, and by keeping the skin moist or wet. Behavioral desensitization to coming out of the water may be beneficial for some animals. Occasionally, naive dolphins may exhibit dyspnea and tachycardia when removed from the water. These animals will generally calm down and stabilize immediately upon being returned to the water. Distressed dolphins or whales should be immediately placed back into the water and an alternative approach to the medical procedure considered.

Chemical Restraint

Chemical restraint (sedation and, rarely, general anesthesia) may be used for clinical procedures in whales and dolphins. Commonly used sedative medications are discussed below (Table 43-2).

ANESTHESIA AND SURGERY

The practice of general anesthesia in cetaceans is still limited, given their size, and the anatomic and physiologic challenges. Bottlenose dolphins may safely and effectively be placed under general anesthesia, but a cautious, conservative approach is always warranted. Preanesthetic sedation with a benzodiazepine (diazepam or midazolam) facilitates catheter placement. Indwelling peripherally inserted central intravenous catheters (PICC) may be placed in the common brachiocephalic vein and the hepatic vein. Both veins are best catheterized under ultrasonographic guidance. The brachiocephalic vein is deep, is transverse to the ventral midline cervical region and anterior to the manubrium, and is accessed with the animal in right lateral recumbence. The hepatic vein catheter placement may be achieved from both the right and left sides of the animal. In addition to offering the same advantages of the brachiocephalic vein

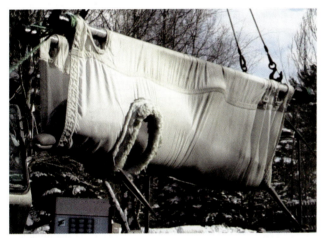

FIGURE 43-1 An Atlantic bottlenose dolphin positioned in a stretcher preparing for a clinical procedure. Note the fleece lining around the holes for the pectoral flippers (Photo Credit: B. Hughes).

(medication and fluid administration), this site carries the added advantage of a lateral approach reducing risk of displacement. Hepatic vein catheterization carries the added risk of hepatic bleeding, so the placement of embolized Gelfoam during removal of the catheter is recommended.[20,22] Indwelling catheter placement when the animals are in the water is not recommended; however, concerted work is ongoing to try to solve the challenge of maintaining a clean catheter and vascular access site and preventing saltwater intrusion.[10]

Propofol achieves smooth and reliable anesthesia when placed into a central vein. Intubation is then performed orally (not generally through the blowhole), with the elongated larynx redirected rostrally by manual manipulation. The trachea is short in cetaceans, and care must be taken not to advance the endotracheal tube past the separate right accessory bronchus. General anesthesia may be maintained with isoflurane, although sevoflurane may improve induction and recovery time. A comprehensive approach to anesthesia monitoring and support is critical, particularly in the presence of general lack of experience and heavy caseload. Applying anesthesia monitoring equipment to patients out of the water and without sedation is as important as applying it to the fully anesthetized patient, if only to help preassess the individual animal's normal heart and respiratory rates, core temperatures, and reflexes.[12]

Respiratory support is generally not necessary in sedated animals that are still spontaneously ventilating. For general anesthesia in dolphins, successful mechanical ventilation is necessary and may be performed with ventilators that allow for an apneustic plateau (prolonged inspiratory hold) in the ventilation cycle. This is particularly true for procedures of longer duration. However, the apneustic plateau ventilatory cycle may not be necessary for shorter procedures.[40] Monitoring end-tidal carbon dioxide ($EtCO_2$) as an indicator of adequate ventilation and perfusion is recommended for dolphins under general anesthesia, and it may be helpful even with dolphins under sedation (not intubated). $EtCO_2$ measurements should always be checked against the patient's partial pressure of CO_2 (pCO_2) before determining just how representative the measured $EtCO_2$ is of true alveolar CO_2. Blood gas levels may be measured as in other animals, and normal ranges appear to be similar to those in other mammals. Because of the vascular anatomy of cetaceans, collecting

TABLE 43-2

Selected Chemical Restraint Agents Used for Cetaceans

Category	Drug Name	Dosage	Route	Comments
Sedatives	Diazepam	0.1–0.2 mg/kg	IM	Intramuscular diazepam is not absorbed as readily as midazolam; longer time to drug effect should be expected.
		0.25–1.0 mg/kg	PO	Larger doses reserved for research or for animals that may have become refractory to smaller oral doses of diazepam.
	Midazolam	0.05–0.15 mg/kg	IM	Provides good plane of sedation lasting about 45–60 minutes. **Flumazenil responsive atrial fibrillation noted in select cases; caution when using in species other than *Tursiops truncatus* **
	Flumazenil	0.005 mg/kg	IM, PO, IV, sublingual	Can be given at equal volume of midazolam when midazolam is 5 mg/ml and flumazenil is 0.5 mg/ml. Usually titrate dose to effect.
	Butorphanol	0.05–0.15 mg/kg	IM	Provides sedation adequate for bronchoscopy and other minor procedures. Possible drug reactions seen when combined with bronchodilators.
	Meperidine	0.1–2.0 mg/kg	IM	Given in combination with midazolam may produce deep level of sedation that is reversible.
	Tramadol	0.15–0.2 mg/kg	PO	Given in combination with diazepam (0.15 mg/kg) provides sedation adequate for tooth extraction.
	[Naloxone]	5–10 mg/kg	IM/IV	Butorphanol and meperidine reversal
	[Naltrexone]	0.005 mg/kg	IM/IV	Opioid reversal

a purely arterial sample or a purely venous sample is possible but difficult. A truly venous sample may be collected from the brachiocephalic and hepatic veins as described above.

Heart rate may be monitored with electrocardiography as in other species. Normal, stable animals should have a profound resting sinus arrhythmia. The sinus arrhythmia will subside under anesthesia and may be overridden if the animal is at all anxious. Perfusion is difficult to measure with standard pulse oximetry; however, use of an impedance probe on the tongue may produce results. Central venous pressure (CVP) may be measured in bottlenose dolphins through an indwelling intravenous catheter placed in the common brachiocephalic vein, as previously described, or by PICC line placed via the hepatic vein into the caudal vena cava under ultrasonographic guidance.[20]

Body temperature may be monitored with a flexible thermometer probe placed rectally to a depth of 15 to 25 centimeters (cm) depending on the animal's size; however, vascular heat exchange systems for internal gonads may interfere with thermometer readings if the probe is placed too deep or too shallow and lead to misinterpretations of core body temperature readings. Depth of anesthesia may be determined through assessment of reflexes as in other mammals. Palpebral and corneal responses, response to manipulation of the blowhole, jaw tone, and swallow reflexes are all appropriate.

DIAGNOSTICS

For the smaller cetaceans, the majority of diagnostic procedures may be performed as they would in terrestrial mammals. As mentioned previously, many procedures may be accomplished without chemical or physical restraint. With large body size (belugas and killer whales) come limitations in the application of diagnostic techniques (imaging and visceral biopsy). Previous editions of this book[40] have stated that cetaceans may mask signs of clinical illness, and the point bears repeating. Factors intrinsic to the animal or present in the environment indicate that serious disease may exist within a dolphin or whale that appears completely normal externally. Bodily functions such as urination and defecation are difficult to appreciate under the best of circumstances and changes in breathing, body posture or other illness cues may be subtle. Therefore, a robust and routine preventive health program is critical. Any small indicators of disease such as partial or complete inappetence should be immediately and thoroughly examined.

Routine preventive care is a mainstay of wellness programming for cetaceans housed in zoos and oceanaria, as regular health assessments may increase the likelihood of early disease detection. A robust preventive care program includes hematology and serum chemistry surveillance at regular intervals, routine physical examinations, and additional routine biologic specimen assessment, including, but not limited to, assessment of urine, feces, gastric fluid, and swabs or forced exhaled breath samples from the blowhole. Multiple health assessments per year are recommended for all managed cetaceans. Body weight should be regularly assessed. A comprehensive visual examination of the animal should be performed, and a hands-on physical examination is valuable despite the limitations with regard to palpation and auscultation in many terrestrial mammals.

Heart rate and body temperature (rectal) should be noted. Respiratory rate and character are important to assess, since changes in breathing, which may be subtle, may still be appreciated. Complete blood cell (CBC) count and serum chemistry analysis should be performed. Multiple phlebotomy sites are available,[12] but the most commonly accessed site for routine blood analysis is a superficial periarterial vascular rete (PAVR) located on both the dorsal and ventral midlines of the fluke blades (Figure 43-2). Blood collected from this and other PAVR sites is nearly always a mixture of arterial and venous blood. Hematology (Table 43-3) and serum biochemistry (Table 43-4) reference values for bottlenose dolphins, killer whales, and beluga whales are included for reference, and excellent discussions of cetacean hematology and clinical chemistry have been reported by Reidarson.[40,41] Reference intervals from both in situ

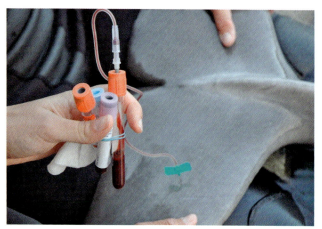

FIGURE 43-2   Routine phlebotomy from the tail periarterial vascular rete (PAVR) in an Atlantic bottlenose dolphin (*Tursiops truncatus*) (Photo Credit: C. Dold).

(free-ranging) and ex situ (housed in zoologic parks or oceanaria) populations of cetaceans are available, and considerable parity exists between the two. Age may affect the reference ranges. Recent work by Venn-Watson et al.[73] suggests that older, managed bottlenose dolphins demonstrate statistically, if not clinically, significant age-related hematologic (red blood cell [RBC] distribution width) and serum chemistry (albumin, globulins, creatinine) changes in animals older than 30 years. Pregnancy-associated alterations are also seen and should be considered when evaluating blood values in pregnant females.[50]

Free-catch urine may be collected from trained animals and through direct catheterization. Male cetaceans have a sigmoid penis and elongated urethra necessitating a longer catheter than might be expected. Gastric samples, fecal samples, and swabs or forced exhaled breath ("chuff") samples from the blowhole are readily collected. Cytologic assessment of these samples may be informative. However, microbiologic assessment is often confusing and may be poorly representative of disease, particularly under the context of a health assessment.

Additional Diagnostics

Ultrasonography is easily performed in cetaceans making it a very good alternative diagnostic tool for the manual palpation and auscultation performed in terrestrial animals. Routine screening scans of the abdomen and thorax may identify abnormalities that may warrant further follow-up.

Ultrasonography is also a valuable imaging tool in the presence of disease. Thoracic[59] and abdominal ultrasonography and examination of peripheral lymph nodes and the thyroid gland may be performed with this diagnostic modality. Several machines work well for ultrasonography in cetaceans, but given their large body size, depth and image quality at 20 to 30 cm is critical. Given that ultrasonography can be performed poolside, with the animals willingly participating in the examination, a portable ultrasound machine works best. Ultrasound-guided needle aspirates and biopsies are readily collected from liver, lymph nodes, and even superficial pulmonary and pleural lesions. The "Bio-Pince" full-core biopsy instrument (Angio-Tech, Denmark) works well for collecting quick, complete organ biopsy samples. Regional anesthesia with 2% lidocaine is recommended prior to biopsy.

Radiography is easily performed in adult bottlenose dolphins and smaller cetaceans.[67] Digital radiography of bottlenose dolphins allows for thorough and detailed examination of the skull, spine, thorax, and abdomen, although the lack of visceral fat limits abdominal radiographic assessments. Larger animals (belugas, pilot whales, and killer whales) are too big for commercially available diagnostic

TABLE 43-3

Reference Ranges for Hematologic Parameters of Selected Cetaceans

Parameter	Unit	Orcinus Orca (Ex Situ)[1]	Tursiops Truncatus (Ex Situ)[1]	Tursiops Truncatus (In Situ)[2]	Delphinapterus Leucas (Ex Situ)[1]	Delphinapterus Leucas (In Situ)[3]
Hemoglobin	g/dL	13.5–15.5	13.5–15.5	12.6–15.7a; 12.0–15.5b	19–22	16.5–22.8
Hematocrit	%	40–46	38–44	37–47a; 35–46b	50–60	43.0–60.0
RBC	M/uL	3.5–4.3	3–3.7	3.3–4.2a; 3.1–3.9b	3–3.4	3.4–4.4
MCV	fL	105–115	115–135	103–124a; 106–131b	163–185	100.0–204.2
MCH	pg	35–40	38–48	35–42a; 36–43b	59–66	44.3–71.4
MCHC	g/dL	34–36	34–46	32–37	36–38	34.5–46.2
Platelets	K/uL	120–230	80–150	104–253	60–130	
MPV	fL	13–17	12–15		11.6–13.4	
N RBC/100WBC		0	0		0–1	
Reticulocyte	%	0.7–2.5	1–2.3		0.3–0.8	
WBC	1000/uL	4–8	5–9	7.1–17.5	5–9.5	12.0–27.8
Bands	%	0–3	1–5		n.d.	
Neutrophils (rel)	%	60–80	56–75		50–70	
Neutrophils (abs)	1000/uL			2.5–9.9		4.4–9.9
Lymphocytes (rel)	%	15–35	13–35		18–34	
Lymphocytes (abs)	1000/uL			0.6–4.2		4.4–7.7
Monocytes (rel)	%	2–8	4–6		4–10	
Monocytes (abs)	1000/uL			0–1.0		0.2–1.6
Eosinophils (rel)	%	1–3	4–18		2–9	
Eosinophils (abs)	1000/uL			1.8–8.1		2.2–4.7
ESR	mm/60min	0–2	4–17		0–9	10.0–40.0
Fibrinogen	mg/dL	170–330	170–400		70–130	76.0–240.0

[1]Reidarson, 2003.
[2]Schwacke, et al. 2008; (a) adult male, (b) adult female
[3]Norman et al. 2012.

radiology equipment to penetrate or image their thorax or abdomen. Skull, teeth, and flippers, however, may be radiographed in these big animals. Computed tomography (CT) is an immensely valuable and powerful diagnostic tool and may be performed in *Tursiops* and smaller cetaceans under appropriate conditions.

Flexible endoscopic examination may be performed in cetacean patients and is useful under behavioral control or under chemical restraint.[13] All modalities of flexible endoscopy may be accomplished, but gastroscopy and bronchoscopy are most commonly performed. Scope sizes and types are best recommended on the basis of use and the size of the animal. However, in the Atlantic bottlenose dolphin, bronchoscopy may be performed with a standard human bronchoscope (60 cm ×5 mm) with an instrument channel that allows for the passage of protected balloon catheter, for bronchoalveolar lavage (BAL), or a protected cytology brush. Topical lidocaine anesthesia improves patient tolerance of bronchoscopy and reduces coughing and bronchospasm. Gastroscopy and colonoscopy may be performed with a standard human colonoscope (200–300 cm ×1 cm). The colonoscope is useful for examination, biopsy, and retrieval of foreign bodies from the upper GI tract.

DISEASES

Selected infectious diseases, parasitic diseases, and noninfectious diseases of odontocete species are summarized in Tables 43-5, 43-6, and 43-7, respectively. The most common infectious agents have been well defined and described by Dunn et al.[15] and Reidarson.[40]

Emerging pathogens and diseases that are getting increasing attention and significance are discussed in more detail below. Overall, bacterial and parasitic lung infections are the diseases most commonly identified in stranded cetaceans,[1] and infectious respiratory disease is the most common general disease category in cetaceans,[71] as it is in many terrestrial species.

Viral Diseases

Viruses are an emerging category of pathogens in cetaceans. The number of known cetacean viruses is relatively low, but new viruses are being revealed by the latest laboratory and diagnostic techniques with increasing regularity and efficiency. Dolphin morbillivirus (also cetacean morbillivirus, pilot whale morbillivirus) is the most well-studied and well-understood cetacean virus, and it is known to cause debilitation, severe pneumonia, and encephalitis. This single-stranded ribonucleic acid (RNA) paramyxovirus is responsible for mortality in in situ populations of cetaceans around the world but appears to be most prevalent in the Atlantic ocean. However, cases have been identified in Australia[64] and in western United States.[42] Polymerase chain reaction (PCR)–based testing is available. Besides mass strandings and mortality events, cetaceans with single-stranded RNA may be infected with morbillivirus, and it should be a primary disease and biosecurity consideration for any rehabilitation facility with resident cetaceans housed in proximity or within the same water system. Further, personnel working with stranded cetaceans undergoing rehabilitation should not work with naive cetaceans without prior decontamination.

TABLE 43-4

Reference Ranges for Serum Biochemical Parameters for Selected Cetaceans

Parameter	Unit	Orcinus Orca[1] (Ex Situ)	Tursiops Truncatus[1] (Ex Situ)	Tursiops Truncatus[2] (In Situ)	Delphinapterus Leucas[1] (Ex Situ)	Delphinapterus Leucas[3] (In Situ)
Glucose	mg/dL	110–135	90–170	60–121	84–124	99.0–159.0
BUN	mg/dL	30–50	42–58	42–76a; 43–75b	47–59	52.0–94.0
Creatinine	mg/dL	0.8–2.0	1.0–2.0	1.0–1.9a; 0.9–1.6b	1.2–1.6	0.1–3.8
Total Bilirubin	mg/dL	0.1–0.2	0.1–0.2	0.0–0.2	0.1–0.2	0.0–0.3
Cholesterol	mg/dL	140–280	150–260	88–236	170–260	126.0–254.0
Triglycerides	mg/dL	80–180	45–170	35–134	81–201	
Total Protein	gm/dL	5.5–7.5	6–7.8	6.7–8.8	5.7–8.7	
Albumin	gm/dL	3–3.7	4.3–5.3	3.8–5.1	4.1–4.7	3.7–5.3
Globulin	gm/dL	2–3.4	1.3–2.5	2.1–2.2	1.6–2.8	2.9–6.0
ALP	U/L	100–700	300–1300	55–342	100–220	330–610
ALT	U/L	10–40	28–60	15–66	3–10	14–38
AST	U/L	35–60	190–300	160–586	45–80	58.0–188.0
GGT	U/L	8–25	30–50	15–33	16–36	19–43
CK II	U/L	60–230	100–250	91–213	80–180	70.0–664.0
LD	U/L	280–400	350–500	329–530	100–220	
Calcium	mg/dL	8–9.5	8.5–10	8.5–10	9.1–10.6	10.7–14.6
Phosphorus	mg/dL	5–7	4–6	3.3–6.8	4.5–5.8	6.4–10.8
Sodium	mEq/L	154–158	153–158	152–160	153–159	157.0–171.0
Potassium	mEq/L	3.5–4.5	3.2–4.2	3.2–4.5	3.5–4.1	2.9–8.5
Chloride	mEq/L	115–125	113–125	107–124	111–120	101.0–118.0
CO2	mEq/L	25–30	23–30		17–38	
Iron	mcg/dL	50–130	120–340	42–144a; 44–156b	195–380	117.0–442.0

[1]Reidarson, 2003.
[2]Schwacke, et al. 2008; a) adult male, b) adult female
[3]Norman et al. 2012.

TABLE 43-5

Selected Infectious Diseases of Cetaceans

Category	Agent	Disease	Treatment/Management/Prevention	Comment
Viral	Herpesvirus	Dermatitis, proliferative genital lesions	Cryotherapy	Sexual transmission likely, lesions are generally self-limiting, significance to reproductive health unknown.
	Morbillivirus	Pneumonia, Encephalitis	Supportive care, euthanasia may be indicated for welfare or biosecurity reasons	Serial PCR testing of whole blood and blow hole swabs or exhaled breath samples are recommended
	Papillomavirus	Proliferative lesions on mucous membranes (frenulum, tongue, penis, vagina)	Cryotherapy, local resection	Oral lesions may undergo neoplastic transformation; metastatic spread possible
	Parainfluenza virus (TtPIV1)	Pneumonia, tracheitis	Supportive care	
	Pox virus	Cutaneous "tattoo" lesions	Not generally required	Commonly found in all delphinidae and monodontidae species
	West Nile Virus	Encephalitis	Supportive care, steroids are contraindicated	Antibodies present in free-ranging bottlenose dolphins
Bacterial	*Bartonella*	Anemia	Appropriate antimicrobial therapy	PCR on whole blood or buffy coat. Consider as differential diagnosis for anemia.

TABLE 43-5

Selected Infectious Diseases of Cetaceans—cont'd

Category	Agent	Disease	Treatment/Management/Prevention	Comment
	Brucella ceti	Abortion, osteomyelitis, discospondylitis	Appropriate antibiotic therapy based on culture and sensitivity	ELISA tests available.
	Erysipelothrix rhusiopathie	Peracute septicemia, "diamond skin disease"	Aggressive antibiotic treatment based on high index of suspicion in non-vaccinated animals.	Vaccination recommended in managed cetaceans
	Mycobacteria spp. (*M. chelonea, M. abscessus, M. marinum*)	Pneumonia, granulomatous dematitis	Appropriate antibiotic therapy based on culture and sensitivity, long-term treatment may be necessary	
	Nocardia spp.	Pneumonia, cutaneous abscessation	Trimethoprim:Sulfadiazine (1:2) formulation plus folic acid supplementation	
	Pseudomonas aeruginosa	Pneumonia	Appropriate antibiotic therapy based on culture and sensitivity	Antibiotic resistance common; reported in free-ranging cetaceans without any clinical exposure.
	Staphylococcus spp.	Pneumonia, septicemia	Appropriate antibiotic therapy based on culture and sensitivity	Antibiotic resistance common; reported in free-ranging cetaceans without any clinical exposure.
Fungal	*Aspergillus* spp.	Invasive pneumonia, obstructive tracheitis	Systemic and aerosol antifungal therapy	Antifungal resistance common
	Candida spp.	Oral form most common, systemic spread possible	Systemic antifungal therapy. Empirical antiyeast treatment during aggressive or long-term antibiotic treatment.	Antifungal resistance common, in vitro sensitivity does not always equate to in vivo efficacy.
	Coccidiomycosis	Pneumonia, systemic spread	Long-term systemic antifungals.	Lifelong antifungal therapy recommended in some cases.
	Cryptococcosis	Bronchopneumonia, systemic spread	Systemic antifungal therapy	
	Lacaziosis	Cutaneous granulomatous disease	Few options. Surgical resection if lesions are interfering with vital functions.	Potentially zoonotic
	Zygomycosis	Pulmonary, cutaneous, abdominal abscessation	Resection and aggressive antifungal treatment recommended.	Fungus is locally aggressive and invasive. High mortality rate associated with class of fungal infection.

TABLE 43-6

Selected Parasitic Disease of Cetaceans

Disease	Etiology	Location in Adult Host	Clinical Signs	Diagnosis	Management/Prevention
Encephalitis	Apicomplexans: *Toxoplasma gondii, Sarcocytis neurona, Neospora caninum*	CNS, cardiac muscle, skeletal, disseminated	CNS signs	Serology, CSF	Unknown, consider clindamycin as safe option. In zoos and oceanaria consider new exposure risks (feral cats, etc.)
	Trematodes: *Nasitrema, Hunterotrema*	Nasal sinuses, large airways	Aberrant migration into the brain causes CNS signs	None; index of suspicion in rehabilitation cases based on signs, and presence in exhaled breath samples.	Praziquantal
Enteritis	Nematodes: *Anisakis, Contraceacum, Pseudoterranova*	Stomach, proximal intestines	Gastric ulceration, enteritis	Fecal float, endoscopy	Ivermectin

Continued

TABLE 43-6

Selected Parasitic Disease of Cetaceans—cont'd

Disease	Etiology	Location in Adult Host	Clinical Signs	Diagnosis	Management/Prevention
	Cestodes: *Strobilocephalus triangularis, Diphylobothrium.*	Intestines, colon		Fecal float, direct examination	Praziquantal
Pneumonia	Nematodes: *Halocercus, Stenurus, Pseudalius*	Lungs and pulmonary arteries	Dyspnea, coughing ("chuffing")	Fecal float, direct exam, worms may be passed from blowhole, visible on bronchoscopic exam	Ivermectin, Fenbendazole
Hepatitis	Trematodes: *Campula, Oschmarinella, Zalophatrema*	Liver and bile ducts	Abdominal signs, elevated hepatic transaminases	Fecal direct, abdominal ultrasound may show distended bile ducts	Praziquantal
Nephritis, mastitis	Nematode: *Crassicauda*	Mammary gland ducts, renal collecting duct	Mastitis, hematuria	Ultrasound	Ivermectin

TABLE 43-7

Selected Noninfectious Diseases of Cetaceans

Disease or Syndrome	Etiology	Prevalence	Signs	Management
Dystocia	May be more commonly associated with death of full-term fetus	Uncommon	Prolonged second stage labor, failure to deliver fetus	Fetotomy and extraction. Weekly ultrasound exams during prenatal period recommended to confirm fetal viability and anticipate problems.
Gastric ulceration	Systemic illness, chronic antimicrobial therapy, *Helicobacter* spp.	Occasional problem	Abdominal discomfort, anorexia, hemorrhagic gastric fluid, regenerative anemia	GI protectants, remove inciting cause. Antibiotic therapy for *Helicobacter* infection.
Hepatitis/hepatopathy syndrome	Unknown (potentially unidentified viral etiology)	Only identified in *T. truncatus*	Partial to complete anorexia, elevated serum hepatic transaminases, +/- increased serum iron and transferrin levels	Corticosteroids, hepatoprotective medications. Therapeutic phlebotomy to treat iron overload may result in improved liver condition.
Intestinal volvulous	Enteritis, hypermotility, may be predisposing diseases	All species	Transient, recurrent, and/ acute abdominal pain/ discomfort	Treatment extremely difficult. Maintain high index of suspicion and use abdominal ultrasonography to early changes.
Oral mass	Oral squamous cell carcinoma	*T. truncatus* most common species	Proliferative or ulcerative lingual and/or frenular lesions. Spread to regional lymphnodes and lungs is possible.	Surgical ressection early in disease recommended. In females, preventing pregnancy may slow development of advanced tumors.
Urolithiasis	Unknown, metabolic vs. dietary	*Tursiops truncatus,* prevalence greater in some managed populations	Hematuria, abdominal pain, azotemia	Oral fluids. Urethroscopy and lithotripsy may be needed for obstructive disease.

Several new viruses have been reported in recent years as diagnostic laboratories specializing in marine mammal disease have become available. These viruses are not always directly associated with disease, but their presence suggests and reinforces the idea that viral diseases may remain undiagnosed in cetaceans. A novel parainfluenza virus (TtPIV-1) was identified in an adult Atlantic bottlenose dolphin and was associated with pneumonia and mortality in this animal.[31] While the virus was not the sole infectious agent found in this case (*Candida glabrata* and a mixed bacterial population were also found), the virus had been isolated before the animal's death and was considered a possibile contributing factor. Other dolphins with evidence of inflammatory respiratory disease within this population developed antibodies to the virus.[72]

An enterovirus was cultured from a tongue lesion of an ex situ bottlenose dolphin with hematologic signs of inflammation.[30] This virus may have been responsible for a small epizootic in this population of managed dolphins as several other animals in this group, also experiencing varying degrees of illness (inflammatory blood changes and reduced appetite), showed elevated antibodies to the same virus. Direct evidence of disease was not confirmed.

Astroviruses have been isolated from marine mammals, including a bottlenose dolphin.[45] Although GI disease was not identified in this animal, astroviruses are known to cause secretory diarrheas in other mammal species.

West Nile virus (WNV) has been reported in a killer whale,[62] and serologic screening of in situ bottlenose dolphins (*Tursiops truncatus*) from the Indian River Lagoon has demonstrated that these free-ranging animals have antibodies to WNV, indicating that free-ranging cetaceans are susceptible to mosquito-borne viral infections.[54] Arbo-viral infection should be included as a differential diagnosis for any cetacean with clinical signs of CNS disease and are not limited to cetaceans with a unique exposure profile.

Bacterial Diseases

Erysipelothrix rhusiopathie is a gram-positive rod bacterium that affects cetaceans, causing either a peracute septicemia and potential mortality, just as in pigs, or a dermatologic, diamond skin disease. It has been reported in both in situ and ex situ delphinids.[26] The bacteria are commonly found in the mucous layer of feed fish, and growth may be promoted in association with poor food handling practices. Diagnosis of the disease may be performed with blood culture; however, given the peracute and often consuming nature of the systemic form, treatment is, and commonly should be, initiated prior to the results of any culture-based testing. Fortunately, *Erysipelothrix* is usually sensitive to a wide variety of antibiotics, including fluoroquinolones and potentiated β-lactams. Additionally, vaccination programs may control the disease in cetaceans.

Nocardia, a gram-positive rod bacterium, has been reported in odontocetes and may cause high mortality with multi-organ disease in some species, including Atlantic bottlenose dolphin (*Tursiops truncatus*), beluga whale (*Delphinapterus leucas*), and killer whales (*Orcinus orca*). The most common presentation of nocardiosis in marine mammals is the systemic form, involving two or more organs. Organs most frequently affected have been reported to be the lungs and thoracic lymph nodes in 8 of 10 cases in cetaceans.[63] However, cutaneous nocardia abscess presentations have been seen in ex situ beluga whales and may be identified prior to systemic spread. These cases may respond well to early, aggressive antimicrobial treatment. Trimethoprim sulfadiazine (1:2 formulation) may be efficacious in reducing, but not eliminating, the risk of bone marrow suppression (Schmitt, personal communication).

Mycobacterial species, including *M. abscessus*, *M. chelonea*, and *M. marinum*, have been reported in ex situ and in situ odontocetes and, being another acid-fast, rod-shaped intracellular bacterium, is a primary differential for *Nocardia*. Respiratory[7] and cutaneous[75] forms have been reported in managed bottlenose dolphins, and serum antibodies have been found in free-ranging Atlantic bottlenose dolphins along the mid-U.S. Atlantic coast.[2] Protracted treatment with appropriate antibiotics may be necessary. Tuberculosis-causing mycobacteria have not been reported in cetaceans.

Brucella infections are another emergent disease in cetacean species. *B. ceti* is the species most commonly identified in cetaceans. This bacterium has caused vertebral osteomyelitis[17] and has been responsible for abortions in bottlenose dolphins.[28] It has been isolated from both managed and in situ cetaceans.[29]

Salmonella newport was isolated from, and was the causative agent for, oomphaloarteritis in a stranded neonatal killer whale (*Orcinus orca*).[8]

Bartonella spp. have been identified with PCR-based testing in both in situ and ex situ odontocetes, including bottlenose dolphins,[19] harbor porpoise, and beluga whales.[24] Transmission of this agent is still poorly understood in cetaceans. It may cause disease and was associated with profound anemia and considered a contributing factor in the death of an ex situ beluga whale. Testing for *Bartonella* infection should be considered in anemic cetaceans.

Antibiotic resistance is important to consider in cetaceans, as in other animals. Antibiotic-resistant bacteria have been isolated from in situ bottlenose dolphins from routine fecal, gastric fluid, and blowhole swab samples collected during health assessments on in situ bottlenose dolphins. *Escherichia coli*, *Pseudomonas* sp., and methicillin-resistant *Staphylococcus aureus* (MRSA) were among bacteria cultured from samples.[53] Therefore, antibiotic resistance is an important consideration even in stranded cetaceans that might otherwise be considered "naïve" to antibiotic treatment.

Fungal Diseases

Invasive fungal infections are found in cetaceans. Coccidiomycosis, cryptococcosis, blastomycosis, histoplasmosis, zygomycotic disease, and invasive aspergillosis have all been reported.[43] Serum-based testing (antigen and antibody) are available for most of these agents; however, sensitivity and specificity for cetaceans have not been evaluated. Diagnostics focused on identifying the organism in vivo are recommended, and in most cases, the affected organs are the lungs and lymph nodes, and cutaneous abscesses also occur. As such, radiography, CT, bronchoscopy with BAL, and ultrasound-guided biopsy or needle aspiration are the diagnostic modalities of choice. Infection with *Aspergillus* spp. is not uncommon in cetaceans. The respiratory system is most commonly affected causing pneumonia and bronchopneumonia. Severe, obstructive trachetitis, with intra-chondral *Aspergillus* invasion has been reported.[11] Mortality is high in these cases. Early identification of changes in respiratory quality and character is important, as these signs may be indicative of large airway disease that may not show expected hematologic changes. Treatment options for obstructive trachetitis are limited. A combination of aerosol therapy and sytemic antfungal therapy may offer the best treatment option. Aerosol therapy allows for aggressive local therapy with potentially toxic antifungals such as amphoteracin B while minimizing negative systemic effects of this medication.

Overgrowth of otherwise normal flora, including *Candida* spp., progressing to oral, urinary, esophageal and regional candidiaisis is possible. The disease syndrome and severity may vary. Overgrowth of *Candida* may be a result of long-term antibiotic therapy, aggressive antibiotic treatment, or both; however, spontaneous disease is possible. Prevention measures include prophylactic oral nystatin (7000–14000 international units per kilogram [IU/kg], two or three times daily [BID/TID]) during antibitotic treatment. Therapy for candidiasis and other fungal infections should generally be based on culture and antimycotic susceptibility testing; however, in vitro antimycotic susceptibility profiles may not always acurately reflect in vivo efficacy. *Candida* spp. show high resistance to itraconazole and fluconazole, but voriconazole has shown efficacy in some cases. For all other fungal infections, long-term and, in some cases, life-long antifungal treatment is necessary.

Lacaziosis (formerly lobomycosis) is a chronic granulomatous skin disease caused by the yeast-like organism *Lacazia loboi* (formerly *Loboa loboi*), which has been shown to affect bottlenose dolphins, particularly from the Indian River Lagoon on the east coast of Florida.[16] This disease is considered potentially zoonotic, as humans are the only other species known to be infected by this organism. One case of presumed transmission from dolphin to human (an aquarium employee) has been reported.[66] The disease is not responsive to medical treatment in dolphins, and repeated surgical excision with wide margins may be necessary.

Parasitic Diseases

Selected parasites found in cetaceans are listed in Table 43-6 and have been extensively reviewed by Dailey.[9] Given that managed whales and dolphins are fed frozen fish with no active or infectious parasite burden, nematode, cestode, and trematode infections are almost exclusively a concern for in situ cetaceans and most relevant in the rehabilitation of stranded whales and dolphins. With the risks of drug resistance developing in these parasites, intervention with appropriate antiparasitic medication is generally reserved for the most severely debilitated animals, and consideration should be given to the prospect of that animal's return to the wild.

Protozoal organisms identified in cetaceans include *Toxoplasma gondii* and *Sarcocystis neurona*. *T. gondii* is a newly emerged pathogen in several marine mammal orders, including cetaceans. This protozoa has also affected in situ species, including Atlantic bottlenose dolphins, Indopacific bottlenose dolphins, spinner dolphins, stripped dolphins, Risso's dolphins (*Grampus griseus*), and beluga whales. It has been reported in ex situ Atlantic bottlenose dolphins and belugas.[14] When disease manifests, it is commonly neurologic as in other animals, although cardiac muscle and systemic manifestations are also possible. A serological survey of 22 St. Lawrence estuary beluga whales indicated an overall seroprevalence of 27%,[27] indicating that *T. gondii* is widespread in this population. Evidence of vertical transmission has also been reported in a stranded Risso's dolphin, with the protozoans identified in fetal tissues and placenta.[44] As cases may be identified before death on the basis of serology, treatment should be directed accordingly. No published treatment regimens are available, but use of clindamycin should be considered safe in most cetacean species.

Noninfectious Diseases

Selected noninfectious diseases have been discussed in Table 43-7. Two diseases of importance have received increased attention recently and are discussed here.

Hepatitis of unknown etiopathogenesis has been reported in Atlantic bottlenose dolphins. The primary behavioral presentation is partial to complete anorexia and may be characterized clinically by an inflammatory blood profile and a progressive rise in hepatic transaminase values (serum alkaline phosphatase [SAP], lactate dehydrogenase [LDH], alanine aminotransferase [ALT], aspartate aminotransferase [AST], gamma glutamyl transferase [GGT]) and dramatic increases in serum iron. The disease syndrome typically waxes and wanes and is recurrent in appearance; it is usually not responsive to antimicrobial therapy and may have variable response to corticosteroid and hepatoprotective treatment. Percutaneous hepatic biopsy should be performed as early in the disease process as is reasonably possible. Given the unknown etiology, it is difficult to rule out the possibility of a viral infection as the initiating cause for disease. The rise in serum iron and shifts in other iron indices, commonly associated with recurrent hepatopathy syndrome in dolphins, are consistent with iron overload disease.[25,69] This iron overload disease has been treated and managed effectively with therapeutic plebotomy. Serial phlebotomies—removing 1 to 3 liters (L) of whole blood (7%–17% of estimated total blood volume) from the distal ventral peduncle PAVR weekly for 20 to 30 weeks—was shown to effectively reduce the serum iron and transferrin levels, along with other hepatic transaminase levels, to within reference range in three adult *Tursiops truncatus*.[21] The relationship between iron metabolism and hepatic disease syndrome is still unknown and requires further investigation. Phlebotomy is a treatment that may be accomplished under behavioral control of the animal and offers an effective option for managing the elevated iron, and, in some cases, the hepatic disease.

Urolithiasis, always associated with ammonium urate stones, is a prevalent disease in some ex situ bottlenose dolphins. The etiopathogenesis of these stones is poorly understood; however, several theories exist. Most prominent and currently investigated theories focus on the fact that uroliths are more commonly identified in managed dolphins than in in situ animals. Accordingly, management practices, particularly focused on nutrition (the kinds of fish fed) and feeding patterns (the timing, amounts, and methods of fish fed) are currently being studied.[6]

Hypocitraturia, documented in some groups of ex situ dolphins,[70] may be a predisposing factor for the development of stones, as is found in some humans with ammonium urate uroliths. The exact mechanism for hypocitraturia in dolphins in unknown. Nephroliths form in the collecting ducts and renal calyx, and disease presents as a chronic, gross hematuria. Changes in serum blood urea nitrogen (BUN) and creatinine and other indicators of kidney disease may not manifest for many years. It is possible for stones to exist without hematuria; however, hematuria identified in a managed bottlenose dolphin should be considered nephrolithiasis until proven otherwise. Ammonium urate stones are radiolucent, so diagnosis is not possible with conventional radiography. CT, nuclear scintigraphy, and renal ultrasonography may identify stones in some dolphins. However, ultrasonography-based diagnosis is variable in efficacy; in some cases, the stones are either too small to be identified by ultrasonography, or the dolphin anatomy itself (blubber thickness, intestinal gas) poses a limitation to clear imaging of the kidneys. Two reports of obstructive urolithiasis, in which stones had migrated to the ureters, urinary bladder, and urethra, have been published.[55,74] Stones may pass spontaneously, but obstruction, particularly of a ureter, should be considered an emergency and should be a differential diagnosis for any dolphin with acute abdominal pain. Dramatic and acute azotemia is usually a confirming sign. The resulting hydroureter may be identified via ultrasonography. To date, only one successful reduction of ureteral obstruction has been reported, and this was accomplished through the use of laser lithotripsy.[55]

REPRODUCTION

An excellent summary of female reproductive parameters was published by O'Brien and Robeck,[35] and selected data from this report are included in Table 43-8. The breadth of understanding of reproductive physiology in bottlenose dolphins, beluga whales, killer whales, and Pacific white-sided dolphins has increased significantly over the past several years, thanks to progressive ex situ research programs.

Anatomy

Cetacean testes are located in the abdomen. Male odontocetes have a fibroelastic sigmoid-shaped penis, similar to that of cattle. In females, the ovaries are located in the abdomen immediately caudal to the kidneys. The ovaries may be readily identified in most Delphinidae and Monodontidae species with ultrasonography; however, they are bordered by the epaxial muscles dorsally and by the abdominal muscles ventrally, leaving a narrow (longitudinally) window in which they may be viewed. Female cetaceans have a bicornate uterus, with relatively long horns and a short body.[47] The cervical complex of most odontocete species consists of a species-specific series of vaginal and cervical folds or rings, which may make endoscopic examination of the uterus challenging.[49,51] The placenta of Delphinidae and Monodontidae species is diffuse epitheliochorial, and as such, the cetacean neonate is dependent on colostrum for immediate postnatal immunity.

Breeding Behavior and Conception

Copulation usually occurs at or near the surface and is exceptionally brief, making observation and confirmation difficult. Females will demonstrate receptivity by lying lethargically at the surface in lateral presentation, swimming in proximity to males (bottlenose dolphins), or exhibiting a "shaking" or rapid side-to-side head movement (Pacific white-sided dolphins).[54] Killer whales have also been observed exhibiting a shaking behavior as well as arching and increased vocalizations (Robeck, personal communication). Often, however, the only observed behavioral change with this matriarchal species may simply be that the female allows the male to approach it or the rest of the group. Generally, copulation is brief but repeated. Reproduction may be monitored with urinary hormone measurements, ovarian ultrasonography, and observation in the preovulatory period to predict and detect ovulation; this may be followed by either

TABLE 43-8

Reproductive Characteristics of Selected Cetacean Species[35]

Species	Reproductive Cycle Length (Days)	Preovulatory Follicle Size (Maximum Diameter, mm)	Gestation Length (Days Post Breeding or AI) Unless Indicated	Reproductive Maturity (Based on Age at First Presumptive Ovulation And/Or Conception) (Years)	Reproductive Seasonality (Based on Cycling and/or Parturition)
Bottlenose dolphin (*Tursiops truncatus*)	33 (31–36)	21 (17–31)	377 (357–399)	4	Seasonal trends
Indo-Pacific bottlenose dolphin (*Tursiops aduncus*)	30 (27–33)	21 (16–23)	370 (352–384)		Seasonal trends
Pacific white-sided dolphin (*Lagenorhynchus obliquidens*)	31 (29–34)	15 (13–18)	356 (348–367)	3	Highly seasonal
Killer whale (*Orcinus orca*)	42 (36–47)	39 (3.1–5.2)	530 (466–561)	6–8	Seasonal trends
Beluga (*Dephinapterus leucas*)	40 (30–49)	29 (2.4–4.2)	471 (450–491)	6	Highly seasonal

introduction of males or artificial insemination. Such planned breeding may enable accurate determination of the conception date, which then may improve prediction of parturition at the end of pregnancy.

Assisted Reproductive Technologies

The development and implementation of management practices that incorporate assisted reproductive technologies (ARTs), including semen cryopreservation, estrus synchronization, and artificial insemination (AI) have increased dramatically in the last 10 years.[35] Although tailored for the reproductive nuances (minor or major) of each species, AI generally consists of estrus synchronization with a progestin (usually altrenogest), with ovulation occuring 20 to 30 days after withdrawal of treatment. Single-dose AI, typically used with sex-selected or genetically valuable semen, requires accurate timing in relationship to ovulation. For this to be accomplished, detection of the luteinizing hormone (LH) surge via urinary hormone monitoring (a minimum of three times daily) and inseminating 28 to 35 hours (species dependent) after LH surge initiation must be accomplished. Semen is deposited in the uterus by using a sterile catheter inserted through the working channel of a flexible endoscope.[37,51,52] In addition to genetic management of ex situ populations, the ability to manage the sex ratio of at least one Delphinidae species, the bottlenose dolphin, has been developed because of the successful application of sperm sorting technology combined with AI techniques with this species.[34,36,49]

Pregnancy Diagnosis

Pregnancy duration is long in cetacean species. From animals with known conception dates and live calves, the mean duration of pregnancy in bottlenose dolphins is 376 days (range 355 to 399 days) and 536 days in killer whales (range 473 to 561 days).[33,50] Pregnancy is best diagnosed with ultrasonography. The developing fetus may be seen easily by the end of the first trimester. Earlier detection of uterine fluid and fetal membranes is possible in bottlenose dolphins as early as day 30 after conception but usually requires 50 to 60 days for confirmation. Serum progesterone levels reach peak values around weeks 9 to 12 following conception, with a mean value of 24 nanogram per milliliter (ng/mL; ± 10.2 standard deviation [SD]) and remaining elevated for the duration of gestation.[33] Weekly blood samples after suspected copulation and conception is recommended to confirm the rise in progesterone levels. Pregnancy is confirmed on the basis of the degree of progesterone persistence, not its increase. Ultrasonography should be performed to support hormonal evidence, as persistant progesterone elevations without pregnancy have been observed.[33] Conversely, in some cases, corpus luteum (CL) failed to maintain confirmed pregnancy, and synthetic

progestins were administered to maintain the pregnancy, although none of these pregnancies were carried to term without parturition complications.[48]

Hematologic and serum chemistry changes do occur in pregnant killer whales, and it is likely that they develop in other cetaceans as well. Changes appear to reflect a progressive, although mild inflammatory state, and include a reduced RBC mass (hematocrit [HCT], hemoglobin [Hb], RBC), decreased serum transaminases, increased fibrinogen and 60-minute erythrocyte sedimentation rate, and an increased serum iron.[50] It is important to distinguish between normal changes associated with pregnancy and possible illness in cetaceans.

Monitoring of pregnancy and the health of the developing fetus with monthly ultrasonographic examinations is recommended. Fetal growth algorithms to predict the parturition date have been determined for bottlenose dolphins.[23] Thorough fetal echocardiography is possible,[57] particularly around months 8 to 9 of gestation. Developmental problems may be diagnosed with ultrasonography, and fetal omphalocele[58] has been reported and was detected at gestational week 16 with the use of ultrasonography. Fetal anencephaly[5] was similarly identified before parturition.

Calving

Vigilant, perinatal observation is important in cetaceans. Regular ultrasonographic examination of the dam to monitor fetal viability and overall health is critical. Dystocias have occurred, and cases are associated with death of the full-term fetus.

The first stage of labor begins with the amniotic sac rupture; however, this stage is typically difficult to appreciate, given that delivery occurs in an aquatic environment. The second stage is indicated by the presentation of tail fluke tips or the fetus being visible within the vulvar opening. The second stage of labor ends with the successful delivery of the calf. It should last 2 hours or less. Oxytocin may be given to delivering females if fetal progression stops. Fluke-first presentation is the most common in all cetaceans; however, successful head-first deliveries have been reported.[46] Twins are exceptionally rare but have been reported in several species, including a common dolphin (*Delphinus delphinus*)[18] and belugas.[38]

Neonatal care continues to improve within zoologic parks and oceanaria. Over the past two decades, the survivability of neonatal *Tursiops* has seen a dramatic increase,[65] above expected natural outcomes, largely because of improvements in neonatal handling and care practices, which include routine health assessments on calves at age 7 days or earlier to monitor weight, collect baseline blood samples, and improve the chances of early disease detection. Handling of calves requires facility design that enables brief separation and safe handling of both dam and calf in shallow water.

Contraception

Options for effective contraception of cetaceans housed within zoos and oceanaria are limited. Given the current population growth and sustainability goals for cetaceans within the global zoologic community, any plans for contraception should be carefully considered before they are put into practice. Separating males and females is a common practice in most zoologic parks and oceanaria. Planned separations specifically to avoid contraception may be accomplished through vigilant monitoring of the estrus cycles of females with ultrasonography and urinary hormone assessment. Regu-mate (altrenogest) (Merck Animal Health, Summit, NJ), 0.05 mg/kg, orally (PO), once daily (SID), may effectively prevent ovulation in bottlenose dolphins, killer whales, belugas, and Pacific white-sided dolphins. However, pregnancy may occur in dolphins and killer whales in spite of contraception with altrenogest. It is not known if this is a result of true "breakthroughs" or if errors in drug adminstration occurred. Deslorelin implants (Suprelorin, Peptech Animal Health, Virbac, Australia) have been used with success for the long term (about 1 year) in the prevention of estrus and ovulation in older female bottlenose dolphins with 9.4-mg implants delivered subcutaneously twice daily (BID). Estrus does appear to return roughly 1 year after dosing.

Luprolide acetate (0.075 mg/kg, intramuscularly [IM], every 28 days) has been successfully used to reduce serum testosterone and produce azoospermia in male bottlenose dolphins.[40] The drug is currently available as a depot formulation from Abbot Laboratories (Chicago, IL). Given the feedback loop mechanism of the synthetic gonadotropin-releasing hormone (GnRH) analog, an increase in cirulating serum testosterone occurs for the first 14 days after treatment begins. Caution is recommended in the use of luprolide acetate, given the limited clinical experience in its use. Megestrol acetate (Meg-Ace, Bristol-Myers Squibb, Plainsboro, NJ) is not a reliable contraceptive in male dolphins, as pregnancies have occurred in females housed with male dolphins that were receiving the synthetic hormone. Further, the drug's glucocorticoid activity may affect adrenal function.

VACCINATION

To date, only one vaccination has been regularly used in cetaceans housed in zoologic parks. *E. rhusiopathie* is a well-established bacterial pathogen of dolphins and the use of the ER BAC PLUS vaccine (Zoetis Animal Health, New York), a liquid, serum-free, clarified bacterin vaccine, has presented a welcome solution to the problem. Experience is limited, although increasing, and the surest indicator that the product provides protection is the apparent decline in new cases since the introduction of vaccine programs in several oceanaria. The product is licensed for use in swine, and any use in dolphins or whales is accordingly considered off-label. Still the most common practice is to follow the manufacturer's handling instructions in detail, to exercise caution with the delivery of every vaccine to every animal, and to be prepared for a hypersensitivity reaction. The vaccine (2 mL) should be delivered intramuscularly. The animal should remain in a shallow pool for 20 minutes to 1 hour after vaccination so that immediate intervention is possible in the event of a hypersensitivity reaction. Some clinicians recommend premedication with diphenhydramine. Appropriate vaccination scheduling is still under investigation, but annual vaccinations after an initial vaccine and a 3-week booster are prudent, particularly in younger cetaceans.

ACKNOWLEDGMENT

The author would like to thank Dr. Judy St. Leger and Dr. Todd Robeck especially, for their critical reviews and recommendations on this chapter. An immense debt of gratitude is owed to the incredible team and community of marine animal veterinarians and health professionals, whose work and knowledge have made this chapter possible. It is because of their great work that we have the collective ability to provide excellent care for the health and well-being of marine mammals every day.

REFERENCES

1. Arbelo M, Los Monteros AE, Herráez P, et al: Pathology and causes of death of stranded cetaceans in the Canary Islands (1999–2005). *Dis Aquat Organ* 103:87–99, 2013.
2. Beck BM, Rice CD: Serum antibody levels against select bacterial pathogens in Atlantic bottlenose dolphins, *Tursiops truncatus*, from Beaufort NC USA and Charleston Harbor, Charleston, SC, USA. *Marine Environ Res* 55(2):161–179, 2003.
3. Begeman L, St Leger JA, Blyde DJ: Intestinal volvulus in cetaceans. *Vet Pathol Online* 2012.
4. Brando SICA: Advances in husbandry training in marine mammal care programs. *Int J Comparat Psychol* 23:791, 2010.
5. Brook F: Ultrasound diagnosis of anencephaly in the fetus of a bottlenose dolphin (*Tursiops aduncas*). *J Zoo Wildl Med* 569–574, 1994.
6. Carlin KP: *Effects of meal size and feeding frequency on selected postprandial blood and urine variable in bottlenose dolphins* (Tursiops truncatus). *Dissertation*, San Diego, CA, 2010, San Diego State University.
7. Clayton LA, Stamper MA, Whitaker BR, et al: Mycobacterium abscessus pneumonia in an atlantic bottlenose dolphin (*Tursiops truncatus*). *J Zoo Wildl Med* 43(4):961–965, 2012.
8. Colegrove KM, St Leger JA, Raverty S, et al: *Salmonella newport* omphaloarteritis in a stranded killer whale (*Orcinus orca*) neonate. *J Wildl Dis* 46(4):1300–1304, 2010.
9. Dailey MD: Parasitic diseases. In Dierauf LA, Gulland FMD, editors: *CRC handbook of marine mammal medicine*, ed 2, Boca Raton, FL, 2001, CRC Press.
10. Daly A, Luke Mooney L, et al: Catheter fixation in bottlenose dolphins (*Tursiops truncatus*). In *Proceedings of the 44th Annual Conference, International Association for Aquatic Animal Medicine*, Sausalito, CA, 2013, IAAAM.
11. Delaney MA, Terio KA, Colegrove KM, Briggs MB, Kinsel MJ: Occlusive fungal tracheitis in 4 captive bottlenose dolphins (*Tursiops truncatus*). *Vet Pathol Online* 50(1):172–176, 2013.
12. Dold C, Ridgway S: Cetaceans. In West G, Heard D, Caulkett N, editors: *Zoo animal and wildlife immobilization and anesthesia*, 2007, pp 185–196.
13. Dover SR, Van Bonn W: Flexible and rigid endoscopy in marine mammals. In Dierauf LA, Gulland FMD, editors: *CRC handbook of marine mammal medicine*, ed 2, Boca Raton, Fla., 2001, CRC Press.
14. Dubey JP, Mergl J, Gehring E, et al: Toxoplasmosis in captive dolphins (*Tursiops truncatus*) and walrus (*Odobenus rosmarus*). *J Parasitol* 95(1):82–85, 2009.
15. Dunn JL, Buck JD, Robeck TR: Bacterial diseases of cetaceans and pinnipeds. In Dierauf LA, Gulland FMD, editors: *CRC handbook of marine mammal medicine*, ed 2, Boca Raton, Fla., 2001, CRC Press.
16. Durden WN, St Leger J, et al: Lacaziosis in bottlenose dolphins (*Tursiops truncatus*) in the Indian River Lagoon, Florida, USA. *J Wildl Dis* 45(3):849–856, 2009.
17. Goertz CEC, Frasca S, et al: Brucella sp. vertebral osteomyelitis with intercurrent fatal *Staphylococcus aureus* toxigenic enteritis in a bottlenose dolphin (*Tursiops truncatus*). *J Vet Diagn Invest* 23(4):845–851, 2011.
18. Gonzalez AF, Lopez A, Benavente P: A multiple gestation in a *Delphinus delphis* stranded on the north-western Spanish coast. *J Mar Biol Ass UK* 79:1147–1148, 1999.
19. Harms CA, Maggie RG, et al: Bartonella species detection in captive, stranded and free-ranging cetaceans. *Vet Res* 39:59, 2008.
20. Houser DS, Moore PW, et al: Relationship of blood flow and metabolism to acoustic processing centers of the dolphin brain. *J Acoust Soc Am* 128:1460, 2010.
21. Johnson SP, Venn-Watson SK: Use of phlebotomy treatment in Atlantic bottlenose dolphins with iron overload. *J Am Vet Med Assoc* 235(2):194–200, 2009.

22. Johnson SP, Ferrara S, et al: Ultrasound-guided percutaneous transhepatic catheterization in the bottlenose dolphin (*Tursiops truncatus*). In *Proceedings of the 41st Annual Conference. International Association for Aquatic Animal Medicine*, Vancouver, Canada, 2010, pp 38.

23. Lacave G, et al: Prediction from ultrasonographic measurements of the expected delivery date in two species of bottlenosed dolphin (*Tursiops truncatus* and *Tursiops aduncus*). *Vet Rec* 154(8):228–233, 2004.

24. Maggi RG, Raverty SA, et al: Bartonella henselae in captive and hunter-harvested beluga (*Delphinapterus leucas*). *J Wildl Dis* 44(4):871–877, 2008.

25. Mazzaro LM, Johnson SP, Fair PA, et al: Iron indices in bottlenose dolphins (*Tursiops truncatus*). *Comp Med* 62(6):508–515, 2012.

26. Melero M, Rubio-Guerri C, et al: First case of erysipelas in a free-ranging bottlenose dolphin (*Tursiops truncatus*) stranded in the Mediterranean Sea. *Dis Aquat Organ* 97(2):167–170, 2011.

27. Mikaelian I, Boisclair J, et al: Toxoplasmosis in beluga whales (*Delphinapterus leucas*) from the St. Lawrence estuary: two case reports and a serologic survey. *J Comp Pathol* 122:73–76, 2000.

28. Miller WG, Adams LG, et al: Brucella-induced abortions and infection in bottlenose dolphins (*Tursiops truncatus*). *J Zoo Wildl Med* 100–110, 1999.

29. Muñoz PM, García-Castrillo G, Lopez-Garcia P, et al: Isolation of *Brucella* species from a live-stranded striped dolphin (*Stenella coeruleoalba*) in Spain. *Vet Rec* 158(13):450–451, 2006.

30. Nollens HH, Rivera R, et al: New recognition of *Enterovirus* infections in bottlenose dolphins (*Tursiops truncatus*). *Vet Microbiol* 139(1–2):170–175, 2009.

31. Nollens HH, Wellehan JFX, et al: Characterization of a parainfluenza virus isolated from a bottlenose dolphin (*Tursiops truncatus*). *Vet Microbiol* 128(3):231–242, 2008.

32. Norman SA, Goertz CEC, et al: Seasonal hematology and serum chemistry of wild beluga whales (*Delphinapterus leucas*) in Bristol Bay, Alaska, USA. *J Wildl Dis* 48(1):21–32, 2012.

33. O'Brien JK, Robeck TR: The relationship of maternal characteristics and circulating progesterone concentrations with reproductive outcome after natural breeding and artificial insemination, with and without ovulation induction, in the bottlenose dolphin (*Tursiops truncatus*). *Theriogenology* 78:469–482, 2012.

34. O'Brien JK, Robeck TR: Development of sperm sexing and associated assisted reproductive technology for sex pre-selection of captive bottlenose dolphins (*Tursiops truncatus*). *J Reprod Fertil Dev* 18:319–329, 2006.

35. O'Brien JK, Robeck TR: The value of ex situ Cetacean populations in understanding reproductive physiology and developing assisted reproductive technology for ex situ and in situ species management and conservation efforts. *Intl J Comp Psychol* 23:227–248, 2010.

36. O'Brien JK, Steinman KJ, Robeck TR: Application of sperm sorting and associated reproductive technology for wildlife management and conservation. *Theriogenology* 71:98–107, 2009.

37. O'Brien JK, Steinman KJ, et al: Semen collection, characterisation and artificial insemination in the beluga (*Delphinapterus leucas*) using liquid-stored spermatozoa. *J Reprod Fertil Dev* 20:770–783, 2008.

38. Osborn S, Dalton L, et al: Management of twin pregnancy and perinatal concerns in a Beluga (*Delphinapterus leucas*). *J Zoo Wildl Med* 43(1):193–196, 2012.

39. Ramirez K.: *Animal training: successful animal management through positive reinforcement*. Chicago, 1999, *Shedd Aquarium Society*.

40. Reidarson TH: Cetaceans. In Fowler M, Miller RE, editors: *Zoo and wild animal medicine V*, 2003, Elsevier.

41. Reidarson TH: Hematology of marine mammals. In Weiss DJ, Wardrop KJ, editors: *Schalm's Veterinary Hematology*, ed 6, Hoboken, New Jersey, 2010, Wiley-Blackwell, pp 950–957.

42. Reidarson TH, Jim McBain J, et al: Morbillivirus infection in stranded common dolphins from the Pacific Ocean. *J Wildl Dis* 34(4):771–776, 1998.

43. Reidarson TH, McBain JF, et al: Mycotic diseases. In Dierauf LA, Gulland FMD, editors: *CRC handbook of marine mammal medicine*, ed 2, Boca Raton, Fla., 2001, CRC Press.

44. Resendes AR, Almeria S, et al: Disseminated toxoplasmosis in a Mediterranean pregnant Risso's dolphin (Grampus griseus) with transplacental fetal infection. *J Parasitol* 88(5):1029–1032, 2002.

45. Rivera R, Nollens HH: Characterization of phylogenetically diverse astroviruses of marine mammals. *J Gen Virol* 91(1):166–173, 2010.

46. Robeck TR, Atkinson SKC, Brook F: Reproduction. In Dierauf LA, Gulland FMD, editors: *CRC handbook of marine mammal medicine*, ed 2, Boca Raton, Fla., 2001, CRC Press.

47. Robeck TR, Curry BE, McBain JF, Kraemer DC: Reproductive biology of the bottlenose dolphin (*Tursiops truncatus*) and the potential application of advanced reproductive technologies. *J Zoo Wild Medicine* 25(3):321–336, 1994.

48. Robeck TR, Gili C, Doescher BM, et al: Altrenogest and progesterone therapy during pregnancy in bottlenose dolphins (*Tursiops truncatus*) with progesterone insufficiency. *J Zoo Wild Med* 43(2):296–308, 2012.

49. Robeck TR, Montano GA, et al: Evaluation of deep intra-uterine artificial insemination using cryopreserved sexed spermatozoa in the bottlenose dolphin (*Tursiops truncatus*). *Anim Reprod Sci* 139:168–181, 2013.

50. Robeck TR, Nollens HH: Hematologic and serum biochemical parameters reflect physiological changes during gestation and lactation in killer whales (*Orcinus orca*). *Zoo Biol* 2013; In Press.

51. Robeck TR, Steinman KJ, et al: Deep intra-uterine artificial inseminations using cryopreserved spermatozoa in beluga (*Delphinapterus leucas*). *Theriogenology* 74:989–1001, 2010.

52. Robeck TR, Steinman KJ, et al: Reproductive physiology and development of artificial insemination technology in killer whales (*Orcinus orca*). *Biol Reprod* 71(2):650–660, 2004.

53. Schaefer AM, Goldstein JD, et al: Antibiotic-resistant organisms cultured from Atlantic bottlenose dolphins (*Tursiops truncatus*) inhabiting estuarine waters of Charleston, SC and Indian River Lagoon, FL. *EcoHealth* 6(1):33–41, 2009.

54. Schaefer AM, Reif JS, et al: Serological evidence of exposure to selected viral, bacterial, and protozoal pathogens in free-ranging Atlantic bottlenose dolphins (*Tursiops truncatus*) from the Indian River Lagoon, Florida, and Charleston, South Carolina. *Aquat Mamm* 35(2):163–170, 2009.

55. Schmitt TL, Sur RL: Treatment of ureteral calculus obstruction with laser lithotripsy in an Atlantic bottlenose dolphin (*Tursiops truncatus*). *J Zoo Wildl Med* 43(1):101–109, 2012.

56. Schwacke LH, Hall AJ, et al: Hematologic and serum biochemical reference intervals for free-ranging common bottlenose dolphins (Tursiops truncatus) and variation in the distributions of clinicopathologic values related to geographic sampling site. *Am J Vet Res* 70(8):973–985, 2008.

57. Sklansky M, Levine G, et al: Echocardiographic evaluation of the bottlenose dolphin (*Tursiops truncatus*). *J Zoo Wildl Med* 37(4):454–463, 2006.

58. Smith CR, Jensen ED, et al: Fetal omphalocele in a common bottlenose dolphin (*Tursiops truncatus*). *J Zoo Wildl Med* 44(1):87–92, 2013.

59. Smith CR, Solano M, et al: Pulmonary ultrasound findings in a bottlenose dolphin *Tursiops truncatus* population. *Dis Aquat Organ* 101(3):243, 2012.

60. Spaulding M, O'Leary MA, John Gatesy J: Relationships of Cetacea (Artiodactyla) among mammals: increased taxon sampling alters interpretations of key fossils and character evolution. *PLoS ONE* 4(9):e7062, 2009.

61. Spotte SH: Sterilization of marine mammal pool waters: theoretical and health considerations. No. 1797. *US Dept of Agriculture* 1991.

62. St. Leger J, Wu G, et al: West Nile virus infection in killer whale, Texas, USA, 2007. *Emerg Infect Dis* 17(8):1531–1533, 2011.

63. St. Leger J, Begeman L, et al: Comparative pathology of nocardiosis in marine mammals. *Vet Pathol* 46:299, 2009.

64. Stone BM, Blyde DJ, et al: Fatal cetacean morbillivirus infection in an Australian offshore bottlenose dolphin (*Tursiops truncatus*). *Aust Vet J* 89(11):452–457, 2011.

65. Sweeney JC, Stone R, et al: Comparative survivability of Tursiops neonates from three US Institutions for the decades 1990–1999 and 2000–2009. *Aquatic Mammals* 36(3):248–261, 2010.

66. SYMMERS W: A possible case of Lobo's disease acquired in Europe from a bottle-nosed dolphin (*Tursiops truncatus*). *Bull Soc Path Exot* 76:777–784, 1983.

67. Van Bonn W, Jensen ED, Brook F: Radiology, computed tomography and magnetic resonance imaging. In Dierauf LA, Gulland FMD, editors: *CRC handbook of marine mammal medicine*, ed 2, Boca Raton, Fla., 2001, CRC Press.

68. Van der Toorn JD: A biological approach to dolphinarium water purification: I. Theoretical aspects. *Aquatic Mammals* 13(3):83–92, 1987.

69. Venn-Watson S, Smith CR, Jensen ED: Assessment of increased serum aminotransferases in a managed Atlantic bottlenose dolphin (*Tursiops truncatus*) population. *J Wildl Dis* 44(2):318–330, 2008.

70. Venn-Watson SK, Forrest I, Townsend FI, et al: Hypocitraturia in common bottlenose dolphins (*Tursiops truncatus*): assessing a potential risk factor for urate nephrolithiasis. *Comp Med* 60(2):149, 2010.

71. Venn-Watson S, Daniels R, Smith C: Thirty year retrospective evaluation of pneumonia in a bottlenose dolphin *Tursiops truncatus* population. *Dis Aquat Organ* 99(3):237, 2012.

72. Venn-Watson S, Rivera R, et al: Exposure to novel parainfluenza virus and clinical relevance in 2 bottlenose dolphin (*Tursiops truncatus*) populations. *Emerg Infect Dis* 14(3):397, 2008.

73. Venn-Watson S, Smith CR, et al: Physiology of aging among healthy, older bottlenose dolphins (*Tursiops truncatus*): comparisons with aging humans. *J Comp Physiol B* 181(5):667–680, 2011.

74. Venn-Watson S, Smith CR, et al: Use of a serum-based glomerular filtration rate prediction equation to assess renal function by age, sex, fasting, and health status in bottlenose dolphins (*Tursiops truncatus*). *Mar Mammal Sci* 24(1):71–80, 2008.

75. Wünschmann A, et al: Disseminated panniculitis in a bottlenose dolphin (*Tursiops truncatus*) due to *Mycobacterium chelonae* infection. *J Zoo Wildl Med* 39(3):412–420, 2008.

CHAPTER **44**

Pinnipedia

William George Van Bonn

GENERAL BIOLOGY

Pinnipedia is a suborder of carnivorous mammals found exclusively in aquatic habitats. The suborder includes three recognized extant families: Odobenidae (walrus), Otoriidae (sea lions and fur seals), and Phocidae (true seals). Members of this suborder are easily recognized by their general body shape and the morphology of the appendages that are adapted to the aquatic environment. Both thoracic and pelvic appendages are modified for effective locomotion in water and take the form of flippers. In otoriids, the thoracic appendages are the dominant ones and also allow the animals to support the weight of the trunk on land and effectively "walk," whereas the phocids do not; and odobenids, although able to support their trunks with the forelimbs, are less agile. Members of this suborder are found around the entire globe, including the Arctic and Antarctic regions. One genus, *Pusa* (which includes the Ladoga ringed seal, the Saimaa ringed seal, and the Baikal seal) has established a niche in fresh water habitats, whereas the remainder is marine. The smallest pinniped, *Pusa sibirica* (the Baikal seal), which weighs about 45 kilograms (kg) when full grown, grows to about 1 meter (m) long; the largest, *Mirounga leonina* (the male Southern elephant seal), grows to about 5 m long and weighs up to 3200 kg.[4] Many pinnipeds are typically found foraging and resting in and near the relatively shallow waters of the littoral zone; others spend most of their lives as pelagic animals, and still others are pagophilic (ice loving).

Many members of this suborder have been exploited by humans for centuries. Several are now extinct, and many more have been hunted to near extinction. Notably, the Northern elephant seal population was estimated at only around 20 individuals at the end of the 1890s.[5] This severe population reduction is thought to have contributed to significant loss of genetic diversity and is clinically important.

Rates of congenital defects in Northern elephant seals are highest compared with any other of the pinniped species presented to rehabilitation facilities in North America (Figure 44-1), presumably as a result of defect heritability and lack of genetic diversity.[68] A study of tissues collected from 371 stranded California sea lions (*Zalophus californianus*) found that sick animals have higher-than-normal parental relatedness, suggesting that these animals too have been impacted by human exploitation.[1] Recently, low major histocompatibility complex (MHC) allelic diversity was shown to be a strong predictor of pup survival in the gray seal (*Halichoerus grypus*) on the Isle of May, in the United Kingdom.[15]

The most endangered of the current extant species are the Mediterranean monk seal (*Monachus monachus*), the Hawaiian monk seal (*Monachus schauinslandi*), and the Caspian seal (*Pusa caspica*). Data are deficient, and for a number of other species, no status determination may be made at this time.[38] At the time of writing this chapter, approximately 1100 individual Hawaiian monk seals were estimated to make up the entire population, which is declining at a rate of approximately 4% per year.[53] In contrast, many other pinniped populations are thriving and increasing in numbers and resulting in conflict with human interests or activities. This, at times, results in harassment, injury, or death of animals. Negative human interactions (fishing gear or trash entanglement, gunshots, boat strike, etc.) account for as much as 8% to 10% of the cases admitted to rehabilitation centers in North America annually.

In their natural habitats, pinnipeds share with humans many risk factors for diseases, and many are thus excellent sentinel species used in efforts toward better understanding of several diseases, including domoic acid intoxication, leptospirosis, urogenital carcinoma, and malnutrition.[3,28,56] Pinnipeds possess exquisite anatomic,

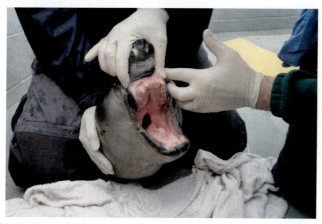

FIGURE 44-1 Restrained Northern elephant seal pup. Note cleft hard palate and position of restrainer's hands and knees.

physiologic, and behavioral adaptations to the aquatic environment. These adaptations such as gas management during diving, thermoregulation, and environmental vigilance are fascinating from a comparative perspective. In addition, pinnipeds are generally easy to train for operant conditioning, and many are capable of complex behavioral modification, including learned behaviors conducive to human endeavors such as performance or utility work. As a result, pinnipeds frequently present to clinical veterinarians and require health assessments, medical care, or support during investigations.

General descriptions of the unique aspects of anatomy, physiology, and behavior important to clinical care and management of the most commonly clinically encountered pinnipeds, as well as typical patient presentations, comprise the remainder of this chapter. Much of the information included here is derived from the experiences of the author and colleagues at The Marine Mammal Center (TMMC) in Sausalito, California, and elsewhere, and a fair amount of personal clinical opinion is also included. TMMC typically treats around 600 to 800 marine mammals annually, the vast majority being California sea lions, elephant seals, and harbor seals. This chapter material should provide the general practitioner of zoologic medicine with enough information to make sound diagnostic and treatment plans for the most commonly encountered pinniped patients and health problems.

UNIQUE ANATOMY

General

All pinnipeds are generally fusiform in body shape with variations in the morphology of the head and appendages. The appendages are adapted to aquatic mobility and thermoregulation, being flattened with little or no individualization between digits. The proximal bones of the pelvic appendage (femur, patella, tibia, and fibula) are incorporated within the trunk at the level of the pelvis, leaving only the tarsus, metatarsus, and phalanges to serve as the hind flipper. Similarly, the proximal caudal vertebrae of the tail are incorporated into the trunk at the pelvis, and only a relatively short, protruding tail is present. Vibrissae and eyes are the prominent features of the head. Male elephant seals and hooded seals have prominent saccular adaptations to the nasal passages, and male walruses have diverticulae of the oropharynx. In all probability, these adaptations are important in acoustic or visual signaling during male-associated reproductive behavior. Pinniped kidneys are discretely multireniculated, composed of multiple functional subunits, presumably an adaptation to life in a hypertonic environment.[58] All pinnipeds are also monogastric, with very long small intestines (averaging 25 times the body length for elephant seals). The ratio of small intestine length

to body length tends to be higher than in most terrestrial herbivores. This anatomic feature is most likely related to the relative high body mass, high energy requirements, diet content, and motility rate of the digesta.[33] Pinniped dentition is polyphydont and heterodont, although deciduous teeth are resorbed prior to or at birth, and the permanent dentition erupts shortly after birth.

Phocids

Phocids lack external pinnae and are unable to rotate their pelvic appendages (hind flippers) underneath their trunk and therefore are unable to "walk" on land. The pelvic appendages are the primary means of generating locomotory force in the water. The animal splays the digits and oscillates the paired hind flippers laterally to create forward thrust. Unilateral hind flipper amputees do well, but bilateral hind flipper amputees may have a significant disability and reduced chance of thriving in the wild.

Nails are prominent on all flippers. Nails may be traumatized, may be prone to nail-bed infections, and may be the source of injury to in-contact animals' eyes. Co-housed seals will frequently "swat" at each other with fore flippers, and this may easily cause corneal injuries. Reducing animal density in enclosures will generally prevent this.

Although phocids do not have pinnae, those that have been examined have a unique anatomy to the external auditory canal. The canal is surrounded by a rich vascular plexus. Presumably, this arrangement aids in protecting the ear canal and the tympanum from pressures at depth during dives.[62,73] At TMMC, a considerable decrease has been observed in cases of otitis externa in seals housed with access to deeper pools compared with those housed with access to only shallow pools. Providing access to deeper pools and encouraging dive behavior by placing novel objects on the pool floor appear to have been contributing factors in the reduction of cases. The hypothesis is that animals that dive more activate dynamic changes in the plexus more frequently, thus causing a "flushing" action and promoting ear canal health.

Thermal insulation in phocids is provided by adaptations of the skin (epidermis, dermis, hypodermis) and subcutaneous adipose stores rather than by the pelage. Species variation exists between the amount of lipids incorporated into the skin itself rather than deposited subcutaneously. As a result, skin thickness, compared with the subcutaneous fat thickness of seals, varies, and this may be clinically significant when surgical incision of the skin is indicated.

Phocids possess remarkable vascular adaptations to diving. The spinal cord is surrounded by a prominent extradural vascular sinus. Using Doppler transducers, flow within this structure has been shown to be quite variable, rostral at times and caudal at others.[55] Clinically, it appears that blood sometimes pools at this site with little circulatory refresh. This is important to keep in mind, as this site is also the most easily accessible for peripheral blood collection in phocid seals. On occasion, clinical chemistry and blood gas results may be impacted by the flow dynamics at this site. The author and his colleagues have infused euthanasia solution at this site with no effect until it was followed by a large bolus of fluids. Phocids also have prominent abdominal venous plexuses that drain to a large "hepatic sinus" and then to the thoracic vena cava. At the diaphragm, a muscular sphincter appears to "meter out" blood as cardiac preload during dives. This is augmented by sympathetically mediated splenic contraction during dives. Venous partial pressure of oxygen may actually exceed arterial partial pressure of oxygen at times as a result of the unique ability of these animals to "shunt" blood to metabolically active tissues.[67]

Phocid males do not have a scrotum of any significance; the testes are contained within the inguinal region and may be difficult to locate by palpation.

Otariids

Sea lions and fur seals are quite similar to each other in overall body shape. They possess pinnae, and the dominant appendages are the

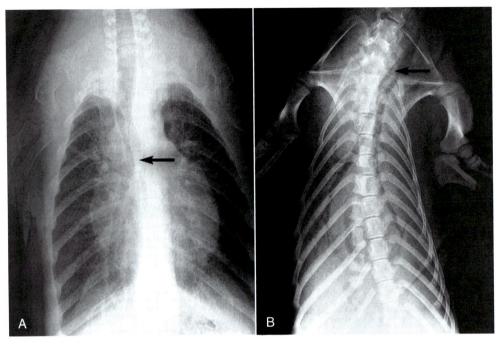

FIGURE 44-2 Dorsoventral projection digital radiographs. **A,** Northern elephant seal pup. **B,** California sea lion yearling thoraxes. Arrows indicate location of respective carinae.

thoracic appendages, which flex laterally at the carpus to provide for locomotion on solid surfaces. Otariids do often "drag" their hind flippers when moving quickly; it would seem a more effective method for higher speeds on land. Amputation of pelvic appendages causes no significant disability, but amputation of a fore flipper is not recommended. Although arthrodesis of the carpal joint has been effective, an individual without a fore flipper would be significantly impaired on land and in water.

Closer inspection reveals the difference between the pelages of sea lions and fur seals. Sea lions have a short, stout, slick hair coat that lies flat against the skin when wet. Fur seals have a highly specialized hair coat with prominent guard and secondary hairs that trap air and is an important means of thermoregulation. Fur seals thus need to "groom" and may be seen lolling at the water surface, rolling and rubbing, as sea otters do. Sea lions rely primarily on subcutaneous adipose tissue to provide insulation.

With practice, the dentition of California sea lions can be used to distinguish between "pups" (animals less than 1 year old) and "yearlings" (animals between 1 and 2 years of age). During the first year of life, the prominent maxillary tooth is the corner incisor, which has the appearance of a canine tooth and can easily be confused with it. During the second year of life, the canine tooth erupts beyond the corner incisor and becomes the dominant tooth in the arcade.

The carina of otariids is located near the level of the thoracic inlet, not over the base of the heart as in phocids (Figure 44-2). This may lead to bronchial intubation during anesthesia if caution is not used. At the other end of the sea lion, the perineum and distal anus are made up of multiple folds of loose tissue, presumably to assist in preventing water intrusion during dives. This may make it difficult to collect samples or insert instruments into the rectum, and care must be taken to avoid causing trauma. Conscious individual animals often are more resistant to attempts to pass something per rectum than to blood sampling.

Nails are present on all flippers but are much reduced on the fore flippers. Otariids also possess a prominent hepatic sinus, but the abdominal plexuses are not nearly as significant as in phocids.

Obenids

Walruses are distinct in their bulk and mass. The morphology and use of their appendages is different from those of phocids and otariids and may be thought of as being intermediate between the two. All flippers are apparently important for effective mobility on land and in water. They are able to support their forequarters with the thoracic flippers and can rotate the pelvic appendages underneath, although they are not nearly as agile on solid surfaces as their smaller "cousins" are.

Their hair coat is sparse, and they rely on massive investment of adipose within the modified skin and subcutaneous tissues for insulation. Maxillary canine teeth are the dominant teeth and are known as *tusks*. Tusks are the prominent features of walruses, apparently important in social and other behaviors, and often presented as clinical concerns.[72]

Walruses appear to be more prone to gastrointestinal (GI) obstructions compared with other pinnipeds. The pyloric outflow tracts of otariids and phocids are remarkably small in diameter. This is probably useful to prevent indigestible objects such as stones, squid beaks, fish otoliths, and so on from passing into the intestines from the stomach. These objects are often incidentally seen within the lumen of the stomach during endoscopic examination or at necropsy. However, in walruses, intestinal foreign body entrapment requiring enterotomy has been reported. Walruses appear to have a propensity to ingest anything accessible in a controlled environment.[52,72]

SPECIAL HOUSING REQUIREMENTS

All pinnipeds require access to water and dry haul-out areas to rest. In the United States, the specifications for enclosure space provisions in permanent collections are mandated by law (the Animal Welfare Act) and include specific formulas based on average adult body length for the species and number of individuals housed within the enclosure. Standards for temporary housing of animals in rehabilitation settings have been developed by the National Oceanic and

Atmospheric Administration (NOAA) Fisheries, and these standards contain useful information regarding the special housing requirements for this taxon.[23] In the author's opinion, it would be difficult to provide an animal too much dry haul-out space or too much water to swim in. Pinnipeds tend to be gregarious, often associating in groups, particularly when hauled out. The tendency for direct contact between hauled-out individuals seems to vary with species. California sea lions are often observed resting while in contact, even on top of one another. Harbor seals, in contrast, appear to desire a gap between each other and, as mentioned earlier, will often "swat" at each other if they get too close. Interestingly, weather conditions may impact the distance between individuals. During rain, resting sea lions have been observed to separate, leaving some space between each other. Sea lions, in particular, appear to enjoy climbing up on structures and will often be seen resting on pool walls, transport crates, shelves, and almost anything that allows them purchase to climb.

Access to water is critical. These animals behaviorally thermoregulate. They are adapted to maintain body temperature while spending much of their lives in the perennial "heat sink" of the ocean. Core body temperature of most is approximately 37° C. Even in "warmer" water environments, the water temperature is lower than core body temperature, and the thermal conductivity of water is about 25 times that of air. Thus, the insulation and circulatory adaptations discussed above are designed to maintain core body temperature; *when the animal is out of the water, the risk of hyperthermia is always present.* A sea lion that has restricted access to water and is producing metabolic heat because of muscular activity such as pacing or struggling against restraint may quickly develop heat prostration. When in doubt, the animal should be cooled off with a dousing of water. It is very difficult to get a pinniped too cold or too wet. Emaciated young animals are an exception to this rule (animals under anesthesia are another). This special class of patients lacks the insulation, is often metabolically challenged, may have immature physiologic mechanisms for thermoregulation and is thus prone to hypothermia when ambient air temperatures are low, particularly if the animals are wet. Protection from the elements must be provided for this special class of patients. Thermal stress risks are the opposite for older animals in fair to good body condition. This author is aware, some concern is felt that a wet animal will heat up faster than a dry one. Recommendations have been made to avoid wetting the animals when they are lying in the sun. These recommendations have been based on published observation that a wet hair coat will be darker in coloration compared with a dry one and thus will absorb more solar radiation.[40] This report did not take into account evaporative cooling or measure core temperatures or any thermal flux from the animals themselves; rather, it was focused on enclosure design. The authors of that paper also made several assumptions based on measures from terrestrial animals. Pinnipeds are *not* terrestrial animals. Individual pinnipeds often appear to be less anxious and more comfortable when in water. Animals transported from one location to another unfamiliar location will often stay in the water almost exclusively (sometimes swimming for days) until they become comfortable in the new surroundings. Wetting an animal will also often stimulate defecation. If physiologically stable, young orphans should be exposed to water following feeding to encourage normal GI motility. Adult sea lions with reduced appetites may sometimes be enticed to eat by directing a steady stream of water from a hose to the face.

Ocular disease is one of the most common presenting complaints of pinniped patients in managed collections, leading to a large number of challenging medical treatments and complicated surgical procedures, sometimes with less-than-desirable outcomes. Protection from exposure to solar radiation is probably significant with regard to the ocular health of pinnipeds. Evidence that keratopathies and secondary intraocular disease are associated with solar radiation exposure is increasing. Captive pinnipeds that did not have access to shade were almost 10 times as likely to develop lens luxations, cataracts, or both compared with those provided shade.[21] From an

empirical perspective, this makes sense. Pinniped eyes, as is the case with all marine mammal eyes, are particularly adapted for low-light visual acuity. These animals forage in the water column, some at great depths with low ambient light. When the animals are kept away from these depths and fed in air, as is often the case with collection animals, their eyes are exposed to more solar radiation than in their natural habitat. Husbandry conditions are a likely contributing factor, so preventive measures should be a priority. Provision of shade; darkened, nonreflective surfaces; feeding underwater; and stringent attention to water quality must be considered in a preventive medicine plan for pinnipeds. In one published study of 111 captive pinnipeds, 48.6% had lens disease, cataracts, or both.[11] Another study documented ocular pathology in 81.5% of 27 captive pinnipeds and only 35% of wild submitted ones.[49] The conclusion was that diseases of the eye are "common" in wild and captive pinnipeds, although a higher prevalence exists in captive populations. However, a retrospective search of the medical records of documented pathology from 10,919 California sea lions presented to TMMC revealed only 272 (2.5%) results with recorded ocular disease. This topic has received considerable attention in the literature (refer to the discussion by Gage in the seventh edition of this text).

Water quality also has a powerful impact on overall pinniped health and welfare. These animals evolved over millions of years to spend most of their waking hours (and many of their sleeping hours) in the sea, a thick soup of microbial life that has evolved over billions of years; the so-called "rare biosphere." This biomass is immense; 98% of the primary production of the oceans and the mediation of all biogeochemical processes in the oceans are accounted for by these microbes.[60] Pinnipeds are merely visitors to this microbial world, but they visit often. They bathe in it, bask in it, swallow it, cover their bodies with it, soak their mucous membranes in it, even inhale it. They have successfully established biologic mechanisms to live in harmony with it, most of the time. It is all about balance. When conditions tip the balance in favor of the microbes, disease may result. The clinical veterinarian will do well to keep in mind the triad of factors that influence the development of disease: the host, the agent, and the environment. Numerous reports of microbial surveillance in free-ranging animals and those that have presented as patients have been published. In a study of healthy pinnipeds off the California coast directed at detection of *Salmonella* spp., 21% of California sea lion pups and 87% of Northern elephant seal pups were culture positive for *Salmonella* spp.[63] What is really needed for effective management of pinniped health is better understanding of the influences on the aquatic system that favor the microbes, and pressures on even the natural system appear to be increasing. Perhaps this is the explanation for the observation that blooms of diatoms responsible for the production of domoic acid and the resulting intoxication in animals appear to be increasing in frequency and magnitude off the coastal North American Pacific.[41]

More importantly for clinical veterinarians, artificial habitats may *always* be expected to place some selection pressures on the microbial ecology of the water within. Alterations of the abiotic water parameters are often performed with the presumed aim of creating a "healthier" environment for inhabitants. In the United States, the water quality of permanent marine mammal enclosures is mandated by the Animal Welfare Act of 1972, as amended and promulgated by the Animal and Plant Health Inspection Service of the United States Department of Agriculture (USDA). With respect to the microbial content of water, the mandate states: "The coliform bacteria count of the primary enclosure pool shall not exceed 1000 MPN (most probable number) per 100 milliliters (mL) of water."[9] This is, in fact, a fairly easy standard to meet through oxidation, as detailed in an instructional pamphlet published by the USDA titled "The Sterilization of Marine Mammal Pool Waters."[61] However, this author argues that in all things, artificial and controlled environments should aim to mimic the natural environment, whenever possible, and that excessive oxidation may work against this goal. The author's experience with both natural and artificial systems has provided strong evidence for just how different the aquatic microbial ecology is between the two types. Evidence also indicates that these differences are manifested clinically as animal health issues. The author has suggested that this situation is similar to the "Hygiene Hypothesis," as discussed in human medicine, and it has been termed the "Aquatic Animal Hygiene Hypothesis."[8,70] While many pinnipeds have been, and some continue to be, housed in fresh water systems, the author and colleagues believe that this is not the most appropriate environment for a marine mammal and that it undoubtedly places some significant physiologic stress on the animals. Much work is needed to revise water quality standards for marine mammals using science-based, sound data.

FEEDING

Pinnipeds are carnivorous and largely piscivorous, although most species have been documented to eat prey items other than fish. Walruses are well known to forage in the benthos for a variety of crustaceans and other invertebrates, making use of their prominent vibrissae and perhaps their tusks as well. Stomach contents and scats of phocids and otariids often contain remnants of invertebrates as well. Squids, octopoids, and crustaceans are commonly consumed, in addition to fishes of all sorts. In permanent collections, most pinnipeds are fed diets similar to those of cetaceans (dolphins and whales), generally a teleost fish–based ration comprising commercially available "bait" species such as herring (Clupeidae), mackerel (Scombridae), and smelt (Osmeridae). Squids are often included, but other invertebrates are offered on occasion, except to walruses. Captive pinnipeds appear to do well on these diets, and, in contrast to captive cetaceans, diseases with a presumed iatrogenic nutritional etiology have not been reported, with the exception of vitamin deficiencies. Thiamin deficiency was experimentally induced in seals in studies conducted 40 years ago and is still a concern today.[13,24] Over 30 years ago, vitamin E deficiency was experimentally induced in harp seals.[20] In addition, the interaction of vitamin A supplementation on vitamin E levels has been investigated in captive fur seals.[45] As a result, most facilities supplement rations fed to pinnipeds, with multivitamins, especially thiamin and vitamin A and E, at levels based on these original studies.

Free-ranging wild pinnipeds do not consume supplements at all. Fat-soluble vitamins are abundant in marine fishes. One kilogram of herring may be expected to provide approximately 2000 international units (IU) of vitamin A, 8000 IU of vitamin D, and 40 to 60 IU of vitamin E, and marine mammals are expected to have a high capacity for storage of fat soluble vitamins.[74] So, if fresh-frozen, properly handled fish products are the base of the diet, supplementation may not be required at all, at least not daily. Proper handling of food fishes must include attention to time–temperature profiles. As a general rule, the shorter the time the product is held and the colder the temperature it is held at, the higher is the expected quality and the lower is the likelihood of nutrient degradation, particularly fat-soluble vitamin oxidation. It is this concern about degradation that apparently drives supplementation—not recognized deficiencies or toxicoses. All food handling from producer source selection, shipping, storage, "breakout," feeding, and cleanup should be subjected to thorough oversight and review. A hazards analysis and critical control point (HACCP) approach, as used for human food service safety, is a wise approach and may, in fact, reduce the costs of future problems significantly. The advantage of reducing supplementation costs to one seventh of current costs by decreasing supplementation to once-weekly from once-daily is quite obvious. The responsible clinician should have a plan to monitor animal health status when any such changes are implemented.

The scientific literature is full of publications on the energetics of marine mammals, including investigations of hypothetical prey changes in association with species decline. One may easily find numerous formulas to calculate caloric requirements of various classes of marine mammals. The caloric content of individual lots of fish fed is also easily calculated from a simple proximate analysis of a sample, and many facilities use caloric density of fish lots to determine ration formulation. Practically, feeding decisions may be simplified by monitoring body weights. Assuming that the handling has been proper and monitored, if a variety of items expected to be found in the animals' natural diet (a variety of fish types and perhaps an invertebrate or two) are fed, the diet may be expected to be balanced. If the fed diet meets energy requirements, the animals will grow or gain weight, depending on their stage of nutrition and health status. If not, the animals will lose weight or not grow. Therefore, an accurate means of monitoring body condition is essential. Regular body weights will suffice in most instances, although more detailed assessments, including ultrasonographic determination of "blubber" thickness or thermographic profiles over time may be useful in some animals. The clinician should also remember that a "lag time" often occurs with any ration change. An animal that has had an increase of caloric intake may not show any weight gain for a week or two and likewise an animal that has had a reduction in intake may not lose weight for a week or two.

Fasting in pinnipeds presents the clinical veterinarian with some unique concerns. Like other marine mammals, pinnipeds are well known to "mask" signs of pathology, appearing normal in spite of significant underlying disease. Appetite and attitude are often the first to change in an ill animal. In general, any collection animal that refuses food without an obvious explanation should be evaluated for a medical disorder. A reduction in appetite may be the only indication of serious illness. However, pinnipeds do fast at times during states of normal health. Elephant seal weanlings fast for 4 to 6 weeks following the departure of the dam prior to initiating foraging. They survive this entire period without any oral intake, neither food nor water, after which they "switch modes" to foraging and begin to seek and perhaps find solid foods to sustain themselves. Animals of this age group are frequently presented for rehabilitation and present a challenge in determining whether they should be fed or not. To date, no practical and specific biomarker of physiologic status that indicates the fasting or foraging stage has been recognized. Plasma hormone levels and fatty acid profiles have been investigated, and ratios of serum blood urea nitrogen (BUN) to creatine (Cr) have showed some promise but have not held up in clinical experience. Intact adult pinniped males will often go "off feed" during times of rut behavior and may not eat for weeks at a time. The clinician faced with a pinniped that refuses food must carefully weigh all the evidence at hand and, when in doubt, pursue an investigation that includes at a minimum a complete blood cell (CBC) count and a serum chemistry profile. Although pinnipeds appear to be exceptionally adept at metabolic water production via oxidative phosphorylation of fats, fresh water should be made available at all times.

Neonates present another challenge to the clinical veterinarian. Preweaned orphans require milk protein replacement and are usually gradually transitioned to a fish-based diet. Numerous references, recipes, and sources of practical information are available for the reader to consider when adopting a strategy for the situation at hand. Here only a few important considerations (in the author's opinion) to be made when formulating a plan will be discussed. It must be kept in mind that these animals are predominantly piscivorous. Protein sources other than fish are not optimal, although some have a strong record of being used with success. Pinniped milk, like the milk of other marine mammals, is virtually devoid of carbohydrates. In fact, marine mammals really never ingest oral carbohydrates, so their inclusion in the fed diet is unnatural. Disorders of GI motility are not uncommon in artificially reared neonate seals and sea lions. Diarrhea, ileus, atony, and impaction have all been noted clinically. Carbohydrates included in the artificial diet have long been suspected to cause these problems. The microbial flora establishing itself in neonates, along with the brush border enzymes and anything else influenced by the biochemical milieu, may be disturbed by exposure to carbohydrate.

In health, pinnipeds acutely switch from suckling to solids without a transitional time of premasticated, regurgitated gruels fed by a parent, as in so many piscivorous birds. Young animals go from sucking milk one day to, in the case of phocids with a minimalistic maternal investment, fasting for a while, to eating solid fish. During attempts to artificially rear them at TMMC, often out of necessity, during a transition period gruel or "fish mash"—an unnatural diet—has been incorporated. Solid fish are generally swallowed whole or with little chewing in the normal weaned animal. The stomach is muscular and serves to masticate the food. Tube feeding gruel, although often necessary, may lead to motility disorders.

Lastly, "hand rearing" neonates increases the risk of abnormal socialization of the pup. For this reason, in rehabilitation facilities, most neonates are tube fed rather than trained to suckle a bottle delivered by hand. This is not a problem, of course, for animals destined to be placed in collections.

RESTRAINT AND HANDLING

Physical Restraint

Inappropriate physical restraint of a pinniped is very dangerous for the personnel involved. These animals are agile, quick, and strong. They communicate with each other often by biting; they cannot effectively kick or scratch. Observing a couple of bull elephant seals or adult California sea lion males sparring for territory helps one realize how powerful and dangerous they can be. When the sheer mass attained by a mature male Steller sea lion or elephant seal is considered, it is easy to realize that safe, simple physical restraint of these animals is impossible. Even the smaller fur seals are notoriously quick in their movements and may bite even without provocation.

Appropriate physical restraint is safe and effective. In rehabilitation or field settings, when working with wild animals, barriers in the form of "crowding boards" or fence panels are often used to "herd" animals from place to place. Tarps or umbrellas may also be perceived as visual menaces by animals on beaches and rookeries. Most seals and sea lions, when given the opportunity to move away from such barriers will do so. Only when cornered, with no option to escape, will larger animals challenge the barriers; handlers should therefore be prepared to meet this challenge. "Boarders" should always use care to avoid having their hands, fingers, and toes being exposed and injured by a bite or being crushed between the board and other solid object.

In permanent collections, animals are often trained to participate in husbandry tasks, including veterinary procedures. Otariids are frequently trained to climb on to a "stand" or platform or lie on a deck and "target," with the nose on a manipulanda or the handler's hand. Well-acclimated animals accustomed to these activities will often allow considerable manipulation and inspection, holding of flippers, opening of mouths, abdominal palpation, and veinipuncture. These "medical behaviors" are often favorite demonstrations at display facilities, illustrating to viewers the importance placed on animal care. However, caution should be used when relying on "medical behaviors." Even the best-trained and most docile of individuals may be unpredictable and uncooperative when ill, the very time a thorough examination is most important. And even when not ill, these animals can be unpredictable. The author has seen, highly trained, highly reliable sea lions savagely bite familiar handlers who simply were not paying total attention to the animal.

In situations where the required clinical information or patient inspection cannot be accomplished by simple observation from a distance or with trained cooperation of the animal, some sort of restraint is needed. For animals weighing less than 30 kg of body weight, with the aid of boarders, an experienced restrainer may wrap a towel about the animal's head to block its vision and the ability to bite. The animal may then be pinned to the deck by grasping at the base of the skull, straddling the animal, and holding the fore flippers

against the trunk with the thighs, knees, and shins so that the animal cannot gain purchase or stand. It is often useful to wet only the ends of the towel, providing weight that will facilitate wrapping the towel around the animal's head. If the towel is not wet, the animal may often toss it easily; if the entire towel is wet, it may be difficult to achieve an effective wrap. Once the animal is immobilized in this fashion, the towel is removed from the nares and care taken to ensure the animal is breathing effectively. This method may be used in otariids and phocids alike (see Figure 44-1). Otariids are much more agile and apt to pose a bite hazard, whereas phocids often thrash the hind flippers back and forth with gusto. Additional restrainers to assist with fore flipper positioning or hind end control will often be needed with larger individuals or those that are healthier. Conversely, malnourished, stranded neonatal seals and sea lions alike may often be safely restrained by one person experienced in the use of this technique.

As the size of the patient increases or the overall condition of the animal improves, it is more difficult and dangerous to restrain it. Animals weighing up to 70 or 80 kg (or larger ones by experienced personnel) may still be effectively restrained without chemical agents. For these animals, the most effective means, in the author's experience is a small mesh conical net designed to fit over the animals head with space only for the muzzle to protrude (Figure 44-3). These nets are tossed over the animal, again with the help of boarders or, in the case of animals on the beach, with a net frame and handle. As the animal moves into the net, the net diameter narrows until only the muzzle of the animal is exposed and the fore flippers are effectively pinned against the trunk. Experienced personnel may grasp the back end of the net, take several wraps to further tighten the net against the fore flippers, and immobilize the animal effectively by lifting the back end. Additional restrainers may then assist in pinning the animal against the deck, again paying close attention to effective breathing in the animal. Many simple procedures and sample collections may be conducted in this manner. If further restraint is needed, the animal may then be anesthetized safely with an inhalant agent delivered via a face mask. This method has proven so effective in the author's experience that it has replaced the use of "Ridgway-Simpson"–style squeeze cages that were once popular.

Chemical restraint is indicated if the patient is too large or obstreperous to safely restrain in a conical net.

Chemical Restraint

With growing experience and success over the past few decades, chemical restraint of pinnipeds, including general anesthesia, has improved in effectiveness and safety. A robust and growing number of excellent reference resources are now available, and the reader is encouraged to consult these when planning a sedation or anesthesia procedure.[6,31,32,37,43] Table 44-1 lists the current chemical induction protocols routinely used in otariids and phocids at TMMC. Current best practices continue to change rapidly with continued experience and retrospective analyses of past procedures.[64] A review of the literature and consultation with experienced practitioners will help obtain useful recommendations, for example, with regard to the use of atropine, the value of end-tidal carbon dioxide ($ETCO_2$) that would indicate controlled ventilation, and so on. The clinician is always responsible for making adjustments to plans in response to information at hand and literature review, keeping in mind that statistical significance does not always imply clinical significance or effectiveness. This appears to be particularly important when using injectable chemical agents in larger free-ranging otariids, using techniques such as remote delivery via darting. In the author's experience, the differing responses to these combinations appear to be associated with the level of awareness or preexisting anxiety in the animal. Doses effectively inducing a deep sedation or a light plane of anesthesia in an animal that was darted while asleep and did not perceive a threat when roused by the dart, may not be as effective in a same-sized animal that is aroused or anxious before or during

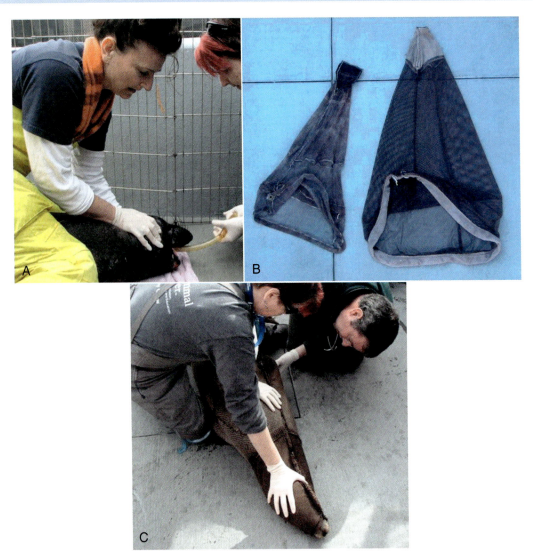

FIGURE 44-3 Pinniped restraint options. **A,** Manual restraint of Northern elephant seal for tube feeding. **B,** Conical nets used for net restraint. Width of base of larger net is approximately 1.3 meter. **C,** Adult female California sea lion restrained in conical net for physical assessment.

TABLE 44-1

Preferred Chemical Restraint Protocols for Otariid and Phocid Patients by Size

Body Mass	Family	Protocol
≤30 kilograms (kg)	Otariidae	Towel and mask with isoflurane in oxygen; intubate and assist or control ventilation, as needed
	Phocidae	Midazolam + butorphanol 0.1 milligram per kilogram (mg/kg) + 0.1 mg/kg combined intravenously (IV) OR Diazepam 0.1–0.2 mg/kg, IV OR Tiletomine/zolazepam 0.8 mg/kg, intramuscularly (IM) or IV Supplement isoflurane in oxygen by mask; intubate and control; or assist ventilation, as needed
>30 ≤80 kg	Otariidae	Conical net and mask with isoflurane in oxygen; intubate and assist; or control ventilation, as needed OR Midazolam + butorphanol 0.1–0.25 mg/kg + 0.1–0.25 mg/kg, IM; followed by net and mask induction; intubate and ventilate, as needed
	Phocidae	Tiletomine/zolazepam 0.8–1.0 mg/kg, IM or IV; supplement isoflurane and oxygen by mask; intubate and assist or control ventilation, as needed
>80 kg	Otariidae	Midazolam + butorphanol + medetomidine 0.1 mg/kg + 0.15 mg/kg + 0.035 mg/kg, IM Follow by mask induction; intubate and assist or control ventilation, as needed
	Phocidae	Tiletomine/zolazepam 0.8–1.0 mg/kg, IM or IV; supplement isoflurane and oxygen by mask; intubate and assist or control ventilation, as needed

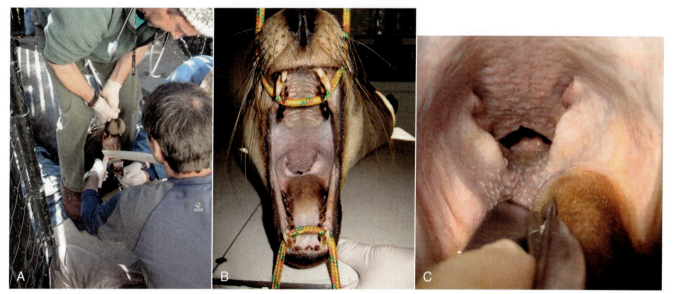

FIGURE 44-4 Endotracheal intubation, adult California sea lion. **A,** Optimal position. Note assistant straddling animal's neck and strap behind maxillary canines. **B,** View of oral cavity with cord positioned behind maxillary and mandibular canines. **C,** View of oropharynx. Note laryngoscope depressing tongue and small epiglottis visible just ventral to margin of soft palate. Tonsils are visible lateral to hard palate.

the darting. The known or expected physiologic status of the animal must also be taken into account. Caution must be used if the animal is in poor condition. Hand injection or using a pole syringe device is often easily accomplished and may be more reliable than remote delivery via darting, particularly in phocids. Although darting has proven very useful and effective, substantial variation in dart delivery seems to exist. Induction times and responses tend to be longer and less predictable when the thigh muscles are used compared with the muscles of the neck and shoulders. It is the author's hypothesis that this has to do with the presence of more fascial planes between the numerous muscle bodies of the thigh compared with the larger mass of muscles of the pectoral girdle and neck. More controlled studies are required to investigate additional drug combinations and delivery techniques.

In the author's experience, the two biggest risks during chemical sedation and anesthesia of pinnipeds are airway maintenance and control of body temperature. During induction and recovery, it is imperative that the airway be maintained and monitored. The pinniped has robust distensible pharyngeal soft tissue that may easily obstruct and occlude the glottis when the animal's level of awareness is diminished. If the animal gets into a position that may cause airway obstruction, it should be roused or repositioned immediately. On more than one occasion, sea lions have suffocated during induction in a transport or restraint cage because they folded up against the side. When manually restraining animals during induction, it must be ensured that nothing compresses the pharynx or trachea and that the airway is clear. The optimal position for the head and neck is extension with the mouth open. This position also facilitates endotracheal (ET) intubation (Figure 44-4). A rope or cord loop is placed around the maxilla behind canine teeth and another around the mandible again caudal to canine teeth to hold the head and neck straight out and the mouth open. With larger animals on the deck, it may be necessary to straddle the neck first and have the animal facing the intubator. A laryngoscope may be used to depress the base of the tongue to visualize the glottis. In some smaller animals, particularly phocids, it may not be possible to visualize the glottis, and the tube is best guided by a gloved hand through the pharynx and an extended finger inserted into the glottis. The bevel of the ET tube

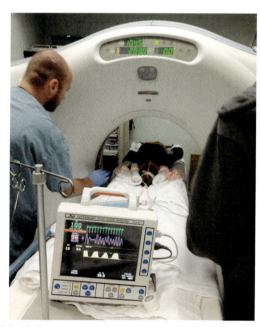

FIGURE 44-5 Patient monitor attached to yearling California sea lion undergoing computed tomography scan of head and neck. Animal is spontaneously ventilating and in sternal recumbency.

is oriented vertically, in line with the glottis, and the insertion is timed with a breath. A gentle rotation of the tube as it is advanced will often help in its proper positioning. The cuff should be positioned just beyond the laryngeal cartilages, keeping in mind that the otariid carina is at the thoracic inlet.

The patient's vital signs should be monitored during the anesthesia period as in any terrestrial species. Airway gasses, core temperature, capillary oxygen saturation, and electrocardiography (ECG) are routinely included (Figure 44-5). $ETCO_2$ partial pressures will frequently be higher than expected in similar-sized terrestrial animals; values into the 70 to 80 millimeters of mercury (mm Hg) range are not uncommon in uncomplicated anesthesia events. The clinician should resist the temptation to drive these down but rather watch trends over time closely and ensure that ventilation–perfusion mismatch is not developing from positional atelectasis. Otariids will usually spontaneously ventilate well and may be easily and effectively maintained by periodically assisting a breath and "sighing" to a positive pressure of 20 to 25 mm Hg. However, obese animals often do not effectively ventilate and should be controlled with mechanical means. Healthy pinniped lungs tolerate higher positive inspiratory pressures than by those of terrestrial animals. They are normally exposed to incredible transthoracic pressures during diving. Caution should be used in animals with presumed pulmonary parenchymal disease such as verminous pneumonia, as bullae, mediastinal and subcutaneous emphysema, and, less frequently, pneumothorax may be induced.

Core body temperature of pinnipeds under general anesthesia will generally trend close to ambient temperature. Thus, in a typical surgical suite on a stainless steel table, the animals will tend to become hypothermic. The smaller the animal and the poorer the body condition, the more likely it is that clinically significant hypothermia may develop. Supplemental heat with a circulating water blanket under the animal or a warm air blanket covering the animal should be provided. Caution should be exercised in the use of hot water bottles. The glaborous skin of the flippers does not tolerate heat from standard hot water bottles or warmed intravenous fluid bags, and serious thermal burns to flippers have been caused by their use.

In contrast, larger animals and obese animals may develop hyperthermia, particularly if exposed to the hot sun. An adult male sea lion lying on a dark rocky beach in the mid-day sun is prone to a hyperthermic event. Caution should also be exercised during magnetic resonance imaging (MRI) of these larger or overconditioned animals, as they do sometimes get heated because of the magnet.

ECG signals from unipolar limb leads are easily obtained to monitor heart rate and rhythm with standard equipment. Alligator-style clips may be applied in the axillae and a reference ground at the pelvic limbs. Wetting the clips with alcohol or saline facilitates good electrode contact. Adhesive contacts may be used but offer no real advantage. The clinician should be aware that only heart rate and rhythm information may be interpreted from the signals. Waveforms are typical but amplitude varies with lead placement, patient positioning, and thoracic excursions. If cardiac contractility or chamber size is in question, diagnostic ultrasonography should be employed to evaluate the heart.

With practice, vascular pressures may be directly monitored by catheter placement into a jugular vein (central venous pressure) or radial artery (mean arterial pressure) with ultrasonographic guidance; however, placement is often challenging and may take as long as the surgical or diagnostic procedure, requiring the general anesthesia. Diagnostics and surgery should never be delayed simply to place catheters. Indirect pressure monitoring has not proven useful to date.

During the recovery period, a pinniped patient should be allowed to regain a high level of awareness prior to extubation. A vigorous response to airway stimulation by a slight manipulation of the tube is recommended prior to removing the tube. After the patient is extubated, airway patency and effective ventilation must be ensured. It is often useful to stimulate the animal during the recovery period from time to time by grasping the nose or "tweaking" the vibrissae until unsafe to do so. Spraying the animal with a robust stream of water, focusing on the nose and face, will also assist in helping patients recover from general anesthesia or deep sedation.

SURGERY

Common

This author is unaware of any comprehensive review of surgical cases or the indications for surgery in pinnipeds. Surgical techniques reported in the scientific literature are heavily biased toward field techniques for research purposes such as biopsies and transmitter implantation rather than on clinical case management. Typical or routine surgical procedures are expected to vary with institutional mission and animal use. In permanent collections, elective (nondiagnostic or therapeutic) surgeries are limited. Some facilities routinely castrate male pinnipeds, and this may be the most common elective surgical procedure performed. The author's preferred method for bilateral orchidectomy is a single prescrotal incision and closed technique as described for domestic dogs. Methods for both subcutaneous and intraabdominal device implantation, including observations of species differences in results, have been described.[26,36]

Various non-elective surgical procedures for diagnostic or therapeutic purposes have been reported in the literature or described in conference proceedings. Ophthalmic surgery and dental surgery are the most commonly performed surgical procedures in most permanent collections, followed by biopsy of masses and other lesions. In rehabilitation settings, it appears that surgical incision and drainage of abscesses, with or without indwelling drain placement, is very common, along with debridement of traumatic wounds (shark bite wounds, blunt force trauma, gunshot trauma, conspecific trauma, etc.). Numerous orthopedic surgeries have been performed, but in the author's experience, most orthopedic surgeries are salvage procedures such as amputations and arthrodeses. Indications for GI surgeries are fewer than in terrestrial animals. The most common appears to be foreign body removal. Most GI foreign bodies do not pass the gastric pylorus, as discussed previously (the walrus, again, the exception here) and may be retrieved under endoscopic guidance per os, precluding the need for laparotomy or laparoscopy. However, laparoscopy and laparotomy are easily performed on most small pinnipeds by using methods described for dogs, and although indications for each exist, a laparoscopic approach is preferred when possible. This author has successfully performed biopsy of the diaphragm, liver, kidney, intraabdominal lymph nodes, neoplastic masses, and other lesions under laparoscopic visualization in both phocid and otariid patients.[7]

Special Considerations

The application of fundamental techniques in veterinary surgery is well suited to pinniped surgery, and the surgeon should strive to optimize these aspects of every procedure.

Because these animals are adapted to an aquatic environment, a few special considerations are worth noting. The application of postoperative bandages—to facilitate tissue stabilization and hemostasis or to reduce dead space by compression—is occasionally helpful but must be weighed against the disadvantages of bandaging a pinniped. Overnight bandaging should be considered when hemostasis or dead space reduction is required, for example, following major amputations; however, in general, providing access to water as soon as possible following surgery is preferred over "dry docking" the animal. These animals appear to be most comfortable and rest best when allowed access to water. If restricted from water, they frequently appear anxious and do not rest, which increases the risk of heat prostration. They also are prone to soiling the surgical incision sites with feces and urine; if the animal is misted or hosed to provide cooling, the bandages become wet anyway. It is often very difficult to fashion a bandage that will effectively stay dry and stay in place on an animal's appendage or trunk. Veterinary ophthalmologists and dentists will frequently recommend "dry docking" the animal for up to several weeks postoperatively. In this author's experience, complications of wound healing are much reduced when animals are allowed access to water within 24 hours of surgery, if not immediately.

Closure methods and suture materials to facilitate primary intention closure are entirely the surgeon's preference. All available materials appear to be well tolerated by most pinnipeds. The author generally elects to use a monofilament absorbable material in most tissues and layers, including the skin, as these may be left in place. Pinnipeds appear to possess a remarkable propensity for wound healing. Major soft tissue wounds that do not allow for primary

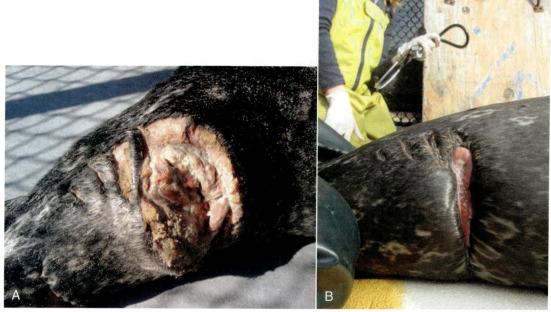

FIGURE 44-6 Juvenile harbor seal with typical shark bite trauma. **A,** At admission. B, Just prior to discharge 7 weeks later.

intention healing in other animals often fare remarkably well in pinnipeds when left to heal by secondary intention, which often includes significant loss of soft tissue, even that resulting in bone exposure. When in doubt, conservative reconstruction and diligent monitoring for complications should always be considered before more radical attempts at repair or euthanasia. Massive soft tissue injury will often granulate, contract, remodel and reepithelialize at an impressive rate (Figure 44-6).

PHARMACEUTICALS

More investigations have been conducted on the pharmacokinetics of persistent organic pollutants and biotoxins in marine mammals than on medications used in clinical treatment. The literature on clinical pharmacokinetics and pharmacodynamics in pinnipeds is woefully sparse. As a result, almost all drug use in these animals is extrapolated from data or experience gained with other species, and "response to therapy" is often the best the clinician can do. Adverse effects, sometimes fatal, have been seen, and usually these are not published. The wise practitioner will consult the literature, even though it is sparse, and consult with colleagues when deciding on a drug treatment plan.

Fortunately, in most cases, pinnipeds appear to at least tolerate drugs, doses, schedules, and routes of administration based on recommendations for dogs. Exceptions do exist, particularly vasoactive drugs such as phenothiazine derivatives and α_2-agonists, which appear to interfere with the complex physiology associated with hemostasis during dives. These must be used with extreme caution and close patient monitoring. Azole antifungals have also been implicated in a fatal hepatopathy of a California sea lion treated with a dosage schedule presumably extrapolated from guidelines for dosages for domestic dogs.[21] Extrapyramidal side effects of the major tranquilizer haloperidol were noted in several collection sea lions being treated for chronic regurgitation.[57]

PHYSICAL EXAMINATION AND DIAGNOSTICS

The physical assessment of a pinniped patient begins with thorough observation from a distance. What is the animal's overall appearance? What is its body condition? Does it respond to stimuli, both auditory and tactile? (Response to auditory stimuli may be useful as an indicator of prior domoic acid intoxication.[12]) Are any swellings or discharges apparent? Can the animal bear weight on all extremities? Is any asymmetry in gait present? Significant observed concerns are useful to target additional inspection under restraint, manual or chemical, as needed. *Care should be taken to ensure a thorough inspection and to avoid overlooking something important.*

The consistency of feces from healthy pinnipeds is quite variable. Stool is not regularly solid or liquid but may be both. Defecation is frequently stimulated when the animal enters the water or is sprayed or misted with a hose. The diagnosis of diarrhea may be difficult and should not be based on fecal consistency alone.

Auscultation is of limited sensitivity and specificity compared with those in most terrestrial animals. Animals with significant pulmonary disease may have presumably normal lung sounds. True adventitial sounds are much less common in pinnipeds than in terrestrial animals. Care should be taken to evaluate air movement in all quadrants and symmetry between one hemi-thorax and the other, but if pulmonary pathology is suspected, diagnostic imaging should be considered. Radiographic references are now available for several species and anatomic regions.[17,50]

Careful attention should be paid when attempting to palpate the lymph nodes of otariid patients. Submandibular, superficial cervical, axillary and popliteal nodes may often be palpated with practice and are often involved in lymphadenopathies. Palpation of the sublumbar lymph nodes should be attempted. They are generally not palpable if normal but are often involved early in cases of metastatic urogenital carcinoma. External genitalia should be inspected, including extending the penis from within the sheath to look for plaques that may be indicative of early neoplastic lesions. It is possible to palpate some abdominal structures of tractable or sedated sea lions and fur seals: both kidneys, the caudal margin of the liver, and sometimes a turgid urinary bladder. Pregnancy and neoplastic masses, both primary and metastatic, may often be identified with careful palpation. In contrast, it is usually not possible to effectively palpate the abdomen of phocids.

Following a thorough observation and direct inspection, obtaining whole blood for routine hematology and clinical chemistry is most valuable for assessing the health status of any marine mammal. These animals are very good at masking signs of illness. Hematology and chemistry results are invaluable for decision making and may be the only real objective data easily obtained. Numerous available references describe expected parameter values, vascular access sites, and methods for routine blood sampling.

If an effective clinical plan—diagnostic, therapeutic, or both—cannot be made with the results of observation, inspection, CBC count, and chemistry panel, diagnostic imaging is usually the next step.

DISEASE

General

Common things occur commonly but in pinniped medicine common things vary with environment. Typical concerns and illnesses seen in a rehabilitation facility are almost never seen in collections. Collection animals tend to experience longer life spans and develop age-associated disease conditions not often seen in rehabilitation settings. Dermatopathies and ocular diseases appear to have a higher prevalence in collections, likely because of environmental conditions such as water quality and exposure to ultraviolet radiation. In managed collections, many skin conditions that are deemed insignificant in free-ranging animals create concern in animal care staff or visitors and are brought to the attention of the attending clinician. The desire and need for a diagnosis should be weighed against potential health risks and behavioral disruption caused by diagnostic and treatment plans.

Infectious and Parasitic Diseases

Wild pinnipeds have co-evolved with a myriad disease agents and parasites with infectious potential; however, the presence of an agent does not mean disease. Balance in the host–agent–environment triad is the normal situation. When this balance is upset, disease may result. A few agents and diseases are frequently seen in rehabilitation centers and frequently cause concern to collection managers, and these warrant a brief mention.

Viral Diseases

Caliciviruses are ubiquitous in the marine environment, and many serovars have been reported. In otariids, caliciviral disease varies, depending on the strain, from mild GI signs to severe vesicular stomatitis and dermatitis of the glaborous skin of the appendages. Abortion and encephalitis have also been reported. Morbidity is moderate and mortality low. Isolates from clinical cases were experimentally transmitted to swine and caused a disease indistinguishable from vesicular exanthema of swine.[69] Managers of collections that include otariids and swine should be aware of this.

Phocine distemper virus (PDV) has caused very large, very-well-documented epizootics in seals in Europe. Phocids have been experimentally infected with canine distemper virus (CDV) and vaccinated against this pathogen as well. PDV has been documented to cause disease in harbor seals in the northeast United States and the Gulf of St. Lawrence in Canada.[19] CDV in one captive born California sea lion in Europe has been reported. CDV infection was confirmed in that animal by immunohistochemistry and real-time polymerase chain reaction (RT-PCR), although the authors speculated that it may have been an incidental finding.[2] Serologic surveys have detected anti-morbilliviral antibodies from pinnipeds from the Antarctic to the Canadian arctic. As many as 50% of sampled fur seals on the Pribilof Islands tested were seropositive (Gulland, personal communication). Morbilliviral nucleic acid identified as PDV has been detected in sea otters in Alaska.[25] To this author's knowledge, serologic evidence from the eastern Pacific, including the California coast of the United States and Baja Mexico, is sparse, and no clinical morbilliviral disease has been reported from this region. Considering the high resident population of (presumably susceptible) marine mammals in this area, the introduction of morbilliviruses could precipitate a devastating epizootic.

Phocine herpesviruses appear to be ubiquitous in the environment, and essentially all free-ranging seals, sea lions, and walrus

seroconvert. These viruses have been associated with outbreaks of central nervous system disease or adrenal disease in rehabilitation facilities.[35]

Influenza A viruses have caused significant epizootics in seals along the Northeastern coast of the United States. Subtypes H7N7, H4N5, H4N6, H3N3, and, most recently, H3N8 have been identified in these seals. Much attention has been focused on the seal as a potential intermediary host in the transmission of the highly pathogenic avian influenza virus from avian hosts to humans, particularly the H3N8 strain isolated in the most recent and unusual mortality event in New England.[54]

Poxvirus infections causing typical lesions are common in young pinnipeds presented to rehabilitation facilities. The verrucous lesions are generally self-limiting and are unusual in mature animals. West Nile virus and eastern equine encephalitis virus infections have been documented in captive harbor seals.[16,46]

A number of other viruses have been isolated from pinniped samples or identified through immunologic or metagenomic methods. Some of the viruses thus identified are adenoviruses, anelloviruses, coronavirus, astroviruses, and parvoviruses. The clinical significance of finding these viruses is often inconclusive. Very likely, disease associated with these viruses is multi-factorial, and additional risk factors are unknown. A recent metagenomic exploration of the fecal virome of rehabilitating California sea lions characterized previously undescribed ribonucleic acid (RNA) and deoxyribonucleic acid (DNA) viruses, including sapeloviruses, sapoviruses, noroviruses, and bocaviruses.[42]

Bacterial Diseases

Leptospirosis is well known as being endemic in California sea lions along the California coast and continues to intrigue disease ecologists. Factors that contribute to periodic epizootic outbreaks from background prevalence are still not completely understood and are under intense investigation. Clinical disease in these animals is most often due to infection with a *L. interrogans pomona* servovar with a genotype that appears to be unique to sea lions.[75] Clinical signs are attributed to acute interstitial nephritis. Early and aggressive fluid and antibiotic therapies have resolved clinical disease in many animals. Rates and periodicity of shedding in free-ranging subclinical or recovered "carrier" animals are currently being sought through field investigation.

Tuberculosis is a widely recognized contagious zoonotic disease of otariid pinnipeds, resulting from infection with *Mycobacterium pinnipedii*. Cases have been reported from Australia, Europe, New Zealand, and South America and include outbreaks and in which the pathogen spread from pinnipeds to Malayan tapirs (*Tapirus indicus*), bactrian camels, (*Camelus bactrianus bactrianus*), and crested porcupines (*Hystrix cristata*). Additional species reported to have been experimentally infected with *M. pinnipedii* include guinea pigs, rabbits, a Brazilian tapir (*Tapirus terrestris*), a llama (*llama glama*), a western lowland gorilla (*Gorilla gorilla gorilla*), and two feline species (*Panthera uncia, Panthera pardus orientalis*). Transmission to humans in zoologic settings has also been documented.[39] Mycobacteriosis in pinnipeds appears to be absent at present in North America. One case report described a mycobacterial infection in a captive California sea lion; however, the isolate was identified as *M. smegmatis*.[29] The obvious implications of this disease should be considered when making management and husbandry decisions.

Infection with marine origin *Brucella* sp. has received a lot of scientific attention recently. Evidence of exposure to or infection with *Brucella* sp. in marine mammals appears to be widespread and global in distribution, although the clinical significance is unknown. Marine mammal biovars of *Brucella sp.* are genetically distinct from terrestrial biovars. Cases of human brucellosis caused by marine origin isolates have been documented.[66] Clinical disease in pinnipeds appears to be less common than in cetaceans; however, this disease may have an impact on conservation efforts. For example, during development of a competitive enzyme-linked immunosorbent assay (cELISA) for marine origin *Brucella* sp. antibodies, 16 of 28 (57%) Hawaiian monk seal samples were interpreted as positive, but interpretation of assay results continues to be hindered by sensitivity and specificity information that is limited and difficult to deduce.[47]

The potential fecal pathogens *Salmonella* spp. and *Campylobacter* spp. have been isolated from many free-ranging and stranded pinnipeds along the coasts of California and Scotland. In one study, 87% of elephant seal pups sampled harbored *Salmonella* spp.[63] *Salmonella* spp. also isolated from the feces of 2 of 13 sampled South American sea lions (*Otaria flavescens*) without clinical signs of disease.[65] Clinical disease in pinnipeds due to infection with these agents appears to be rare, however, they could serve as sources for zoonotic transmission.

Recently, a case of wound infection in a rehabilitating harbor seal caused by methicillin-resistant *Staphylococcus aureus* (MRSA) was documented.[22]

A *Mycoplasma* species has been identified as responsible for soft tissue and joint infections in numerous sea lions.[30] Disease caused by infection with this organism sometimes has an insidious onset and often involves the connective tissues of the appendages. This disease is not responsive to cell wall–inhibiting antibiotics, which are frequently used as first-choice agents to treat many wound and soft tissue infections. Mycoplasmal infection should be considered in nonresponsive cases of presumed soft tissue infection.

Fungal Diseases

Mycotic disease appears to be of lower prevalence in most pinniped populations than in other marine mammal species. In rehabilitation facilities, evidence of fungal dermatopathy is often seen in California sea lions. The lesions are multi-focal maculae characterized by discrete circular hyperpigmentation and patchy alopecia of differing diameters. Less commonly, active lesions and a pronounced suppurative inflammation of the skin are seen. Cytology and culture of these active lesions have identified a *Trychophyton* of unknown species. Attempts to type this fungus are currently ongoing.

Disseminated infection with *Coccidiodes immitis* is also regularly seen along the California coast of the United States, and risk of exposure to humans should always be considered. This organism has been declared a *select agent* by the USDA, and infectious arthroconidia have been detected in tissues from necropsy specimens.

Many other sporadic disseminated fungal infections and dermatopathies have been reported, often presumably exacerbated by environmental conditions, antibiotic therapy, or immunosuppression.[34]

Protozoal Diseases

A large and growing body of evidence suggests exposure to, infection with, and disease caused by protozoan parasites in free-ranging and captive pinnipeds. Otariids, phocids, and obenids all appear to be susceptible to infection with *Toxoplasma*, *Neosporia*, and *Sarcocystis* spp.[18] Antemortem diagnosis is supported by serologic assays and biopsy, and several successfully treated confirmed cases have been reported.[7] Recently, several novel coccidian organisms have been identified in the intestinal tracts of California sea lions. Both sexual and asexual coccidian stages were identified in enterocytes, suggesting that sea lions may be definitive hosts and that these organisms may be pathogenic in other pinniped species.[10]

Metazoal Diseases

Cestodes, nematodes, trematodes, and acanthocephalans are routinely found in free-ranging pinnipeds. The pathology associated with these taxa is quite varied. Verminous pneumonia is a widespread, well-recognized, and debilitating condition in many young pinnipeds. In contrast, ova, larvae, or adults are often found incidentally during diagnostic workups. The astute clinician will evaluate the weight of evidence that these organisms are involved in the disease process against the potential for an adverse response to treatment. Anthelmentic administration to an animal in poor condition with a substantial lungworm burden, for instance, may incite a fatal inflammatory response. In rehabilitation settings, animals destined for release will be reexposed and presumably reinfected following treatment. The goal again is to "tip-the-balance" in favor of the patient when the parasites are a significant part of the disease process—not to completely eliminate the burden. When animals are destined to move from the wild to a permanent collection, consideration should again be given to the risks versus the benefits of therapy. The life cycles of many of these parasites have not been confirmed, but most are likely indirect and require an intermediate host. When animals in collections are fed previously frozen food items, metazoan parasites are presumed killed, so these animals will not be reinfected. If no intermediate host is present in the system the animals are housed in, the infection will likely resolve over time and with appropriate immune response of the host. Anthementic treatment coincident with the stressor of a recent environmental change may be deleterious or even fatal.

Consider the common filarid nematode of California sea lions, *Acanthocheilonema odenhali*. Microfilariae of this worm are frequently found in blood samples from animals presenting for rehabilitation. The adults live in the fascial planes and subcutis of the neck and axillae and do not cause disease. The microfilaria may reportedly be discriminated from those of the potentially pathogenic *A. spirocauda* and *Dirofilaria immitis*; however, in clinical practice, this is difficult and impractical.[14] To this author's knowledge, disease caused by *D. immitis* has never been reported in a free-ranging pinniped and infection with *A. odenhali* is common. The decision to pursue accurate identification of the microfilaria (they appear to cross-react with some commercially available assays for *D. immitis* but not all) or to pursue clearance of the microfilaria with a microfilaricide should be made on the basis of associated risks.

Noninfectious Diseases

Most potential noninfectious causes of morbidity and mortality have been discussed in preceding sections of this chapter. It is worth reiterating a few points here. Risks inherent with disturbances of thermoregulation are constantly present in pinniped patients. The likelihood of hyperthermia or hypothermia should always be evaluated and a means for prevention or response incorporated into the diagnostic or treatment plan.

Malnutrition is perhaps the single most common reason for pinniped patients to present to rehabilitation centers. Not enough is known about the optiml carbohydrate-free artificial ration to use in various stages of treatment. "Gastric mastication" may be an important factor in normal digestion and assimilation in these animals. Anything artificial the patient is exposed to during rehabilitation, including the physical environment, pharmaceuticals, and rations, may put artificial selection pressure on the microbiome and may interrupt normal physiochemical development as well. Despite these challenges, many animals have recovered with supportive care and assist-feeding with a variety of ration recipes in use.

Entanglements with or ingestions of human-made debris are a common problem. Frequently, the entanglement is around the neck and has been present for some time before the animal is reported. These animals tend to be otherwise healthy, often ostracized by conspecifics and wary of predators. As a result, they may be difficult and dangerous to capture until they are so debilitated that their prognosis is poor. Remote sedation with new drug cocktails is showing great promise of helping these animals.[48]

Intestinal foreign bodies are uncommon. If an object passes through the pyloric sphincter, it may pass all the way to the anus, except in the walrus. Gastric foreign bodies are not uncommon but are rarely emergencies. Pinnipeds, like most cetacean species, appear to be able to voluntarily induce emesis and "purge" the stomach periodically. Emesis may sometimes be induced with gastric irritants such as hydrogen peroxide or mustard slurries but less reliably than in canine patients. Endoscopic retrieval is indicated if the object is likely to cause physical damage or toxicosis. Terminal fishing tackle, hooks, lines, and sinkers may pose unique challenges, depending on their location and degree of embedding. Radiography should be performed on any animal seen with external terminal tackle attached to evaluate for the presence of swallowed tackle as well.

Behavioral abnormalities are sometimes significant medical problems. The ability of pinnipeds to induce voluntary emesis appears to be exploited by some individual animals and comprise a displacement behavior that may frustrate keepers, trainers, and caregivers alike. It may also be confused with significant occult medical problems.[71] Stereotypical swim patterns sometimes lead to patchy alopecia or excoriations. Patchy alopecia has also been a feature of some unusual morbidity and mortality in free-ranging animals with unknown etiology.[44] Chewing on or gnawing at enclosure structures has led to significant dental disease in many captive-born pinnipeds.

Neoplasia affects both free-ranging and captive pinnipeds. Urogenital carcinoma affects approximately 1 of 6 adult California sea lions necropsied at TMMC and is a discrete disease syndrome in stranded sea lions. Several risk factors for this disease have been identified, and an international consortium is investigating the etiopathogenesis that includes both infectious and noninfectious factors.[59] Clinical signs include varying degrees of posterior paresis to paralysis and perineal edema. Sublumbar lymphadenopathy is often detected early in the course. No treatment is available. Collection animals are infrequently affected by this carcinoma, although wild-origin animals have developed the disease in captivity. Other neoplasms affecting pinnipeds are scattered types and sporadic in nature.

Toxicoses

The most significant clinically recognized toxicosis of pinnipeds is domoic acid intoxication of free-ranging animals off the California coast. This harmful algal toxin mimics the neurotransmitter glutamate and is biomagnified up the food web. Acute and chronic forms of the intoxication are recognized, and clinical signs at presentation range from subtle behavioral deficits to status epilepticus. Treatment is supportive. Epileptic animals are not candidates for release from rehabilitation centers; they do not make attractive display animals and are generally euthanized. In utero exposure and intoxication of the pups of pregnant dams may lead to serious neurodevelopmental disorders. Pups presumably exposed in utero have developed seizure disorders later in life, and some evidence indicates that the hypothalamic–pituitary–adrenal axis is disrupted in intoxicated animals.[27] It is possible that many yearling-class pinnipeds that present to rehabilitation facilities have cognitive or other neurologic deficits as a result of in utero exposure to domoic acid and that this has contributed to their failure to thrive. Some of these animals end up in managed collections, and a careful history should be taken by the attending veterinarian.

Recognition that these animals are excellent sentinels of the health of the oceanic and near-shore ecosystems has led to numerous investigations into the relationship between contaminant burdens and morbidity or mortality. The scientific literature contains numerous publications that examine the possible connection between burdens of heavy metals, organochlorines, endocrine disruptors, and other anthropogenic contaminants and everything from dermatopathies, reproductive failure, neoplasia, neurologic deficits, and death. Reports of clinical intoxications of collection animals are, in contrast, uncommon. Exposure to toxicants used in pest control programs or to potentially toxic items that are inadvertently introduced into exhibits, such as lead objects or zinc containing coins, should be considered in cases of suspected intoxication.

REPRODUCTION

For a thorough description of pinniped reproduction, consult available references (specifically the excellent text *Biology of Marine Mammals* by Reynolds and Rommel [eds.][58]). Only brief comments considered salient to typical collection and rehabilitation medicine are mentioned here. Not all species have been studied in any detail, but wild pinnipeds generally display a strong population synchrony in reproductive events, and photoperiod is likely a strong influence of timing. All pinnipeds exhibit delayed implantation, and as a result,

diagnosis of pregnancy may be difficult in early gestation. Pregnancy usually results in only one offspring; twins are rare. In managed collections, the reduction of environmental and nutritional stressors may lead to earlier reproductive maturity than in the wild. Two-year old sea lions have sired pups. Contraception may be accomplished by surgical, social grouping, or chemical means. The use of depot formulations of gonadotropin-releasing hormone (GnRH) analogs in adult pinnipeds has resulted in local site reactions. Surgical contraception in females by laparoscopic ovariectomy is feasible in most species but is not commonly performed. The application of advanced reproductive technologies such as hormonal control of cycles and artificial insemination appears to be uncommon in pinnipeds, with the possible exception of walruses. Some work has been done by at least one group to manipulate both male and female reproductive cycles of walruses with the aim of increasing pregnancy rates.[51]

PREVENTIVE MEDICINE

Periodic regular health assessments, including routine CBC counts with differentials and serum chemistry profiles, may detect the onset of some disease conditions at an early stage; however, more often, observations made by caregivers are the first indication of medical problems. Open and frequent communication among keepers, trainers, animal care staff, and the veterinary team is critical to early detection of health problems. All instances of unexplained change in body condition, behavior, appetite, or attitude should be evaluated.

As mentioned earlier, providing an optimal physical environment, with special attention to the water quality and to the specialized anatomic, behavioral, and physiologic adaptations of these animals to the aquatic environs is arguably the most important preventive measure that should be taken in managed collections. Particular attention should be paid to the risks associated with restraint and confinement, namely, hyperthermia and asphyxiation, especially during transportation of pinnipeds from one location to another.

Some institutions have elected to vaccinate pinnipeds against rabies, WNV, and CDV with commercially available vaccines, and most administer a heartworm preventive agent when *D. immitis* infection is endemic in dogs in the area.

ACKNOWLEDGMENT

The author thanks the many colleagues, students, and volunteers at TMMC, who have imparted knowledge during their most excellent animal care. Specific thanks to veterinary student Trica Fleming for surgery literature review and to my wife Anna for editorial oversight of manuscript preparation.

REFERENCES

1. Acevedo-Whitehouse K, Gulland F, Greig D, et al: Disease susceptibly in California sea lions. *Nature* 422:35, 2003.
2. Barrett T, Wohlsein P, Bidwell CA, et al: Canine distemper virus in a California sea lion (*Zalophus californianus*). *Vet Rec* 154:334, 2004.
3. Bejarano AC, Gulland FMD, Rowles TK, et al: Production and toxicity of the marine biotoxin domoic acid and its effects on wildlife: A review. *Human Ecol Risk Assess* 14:544, 2008.
4. Berta A: Pinnipedia: Overview. In Perrin WF, WÜrsig B, Thewissen JGM, editors: *Encyclopedia of marine mammals*, San Diego, CA, 2002, Academic Press.
5. Bonnel ML, Selander RK: Elephant seals genetic variation and near extinction. *Science* 184:908, 1974.
6. Brunson DB: Walrus. In West G, Heard D, Caulkett N, editors: *Zoo animal and wildlife immobilization and anesthesia*, Ames, IA, 2007, Blackwell Publishing.

7. Carlson-Bremer DP, Gulland FMD, Johnson CK, et al: Diagnosis and treatment of *Sarcocystis neurona*- induced myositis in a free-ranging California sea lion. *J Am Vet Med Assoc* 24:324, 2012.

8. Carmack TB, Van Bonn W, Poll C: Potential implications of the hygiene hypothesis on cetacean management systems. *Proc Int Assoc Aquat Anim Med* 38:156, 2007.

9. CFR Title 9, Chapter I, Subchapter A, Part 3, Subpart E, Section 3.106 (online): http://www.law.cornell.edu/cfr/text/9/3.106. Accessed November 6, 2012.

10. Colegrove KM, Grigg ME, Carlson-Bremer D, et al: Discovery of three novel coccidian parasites infecting California sea lions (*Zalophus californianus*), with evidence of sexual replication and interspecies pathogenicity. *J Parasitol* 97:868, 2012.

11. Colitz CMH, Saville WJA, Renner MS, et al: Risk factors associated with cataracts and lens luxations in captive pinnipeds in the United States and the Bahamas. *J Am Vet Med Assoc* 237:429, 2010.

12. Cook P, Reichmuth C, Gulland FMD: Rapid behavioral diagnosis of domoic acid toxicosis in California sea lions. *Biol Lett* 7:596, 2011.

13. Croft LA, Gearhart SA, Hyem K, et al: Thiamine deficiency in a collection of Pacific harbor seals (*Phoca vitulina*). *Proc Int Ass of Aquat Anim Med* 42:160, 2011.

14. Dailey M: Parasitic diseases. In Dieruaf LA, Gulland FMD, editors: *CRC handbook of marine mammal medicine*, ed 2, Boca Raton, FL, 2001, CRC Press.

15. de Assunção-Franco M, Hoffman JI, Harwood J, et al: MHC genotype and near-deterministic mortality in grey seals. *Sci Rep* 2:659, 2012.

16. Del Piero F, Stremme DW, Habecker PL, et al: West Nile flavivirus polioencephalomyelitis in a harbor seal (*Phoca vitulina*). *Vet Pathol* 43:58, 2006.

17. Dennison SE, Forrest L, Gulland FMD: Normal thoracic radiographic anatomy of immature California sea lions (*Zalophus californianus*) and immature Northern elephant seals (*Migounga angustirostris*). *Aquatic Mammals* 35:36, 2009.

18. Dubey JB, Zarnke R, Thomas NJ, et al: *Toxoplasma gondii, Neospora caninum, Sarcocystis neurona,* and *Sarcocystis canis*-like infections in marine mammals. *Vet Parasitol* 116:275, 2003.

19. Duignan J, Sadove S, Saliki JT, et al: Phocine distemper in harbor seals (*Phoca vitulina*) from Long Island New York. *J Wildl Dis* 29:465, 1993.

20. Englehart FR, Geraci JR: Effects of experimental vitamin E deprivation in the harp seal, *Phoca groenlandica*. *Can J Zool* 56:2186, 1978.

21. Field CL, Tuttle AD, Sidor IF, et al: Systemic mycosis in a California sea lion (*Zalophus californianus*) with detection of cystofilobasidiales DNA. *J Zoo Wildl Med* 43:144, 2012.

22. Fravel V, Van Bonn W, Rios C, et al: Methicillin-resistant *Staphylococcus aureus* in a Harbor seal (*Phoca vitulina*). *Vet Rec* 169:155, 2011.

23. Gage L, Whaley JE: Policies and best practices marine mammal, stranding response, rehabilitation and release: http://www.nmfs.noaa.gov/pr/pdfs/health/rehab_standards.pdf. Accessed November 6, 2012.

24. Geraci JR: Experimental thiamine deficiency in captive harp seals, *Phoca groenlandica*, induced by eating herring, *Clupea harengus*, and smelts, *Osmerus mordax*. *Can J Zool* 50:179, 1972.

25. Goldstein T, Mazet JAK, Gill VA, et al: Phocine distemper virus in northern sea otters in the pacific ocean Alaska, USA. *Emerg Infect Dis* 15:925, 2009.

26. Green JA, Haulena M, Boyd IL, et al: Trial implantation of heart rate data loggers in pinnipeds. *J Wildl Manage* 73:115, 2010.

27. Gulland FMD, Hall AJ, Greig DJ, et al: Evaluation of circulating eosinophil count and adrenal gland function in California sea lions naturally exposed to domoic acid. *J Am Vet Med Assoc* 241:943, 2012.

28. Gulland FMD, Hall AJ: Is marine mammal health deteriorating? Trends in the global reporting of marine mammal disease. *ECO Health* 4:135, 2007.

29. Gutter AE, Wells SK, Spraker TR: Generalized mycobacteriosis in a California sea lion (*Zalophus californicus*). *J Zoo Anim Med* 18:118, 1987.

30. Haulena M, Gulland FMD, Lawrence JA, et al: Lesions associated with a novel *Mycoplasma* sp. in California sea lions (*Zalophus californianus*) undergoing rehabilitation. *J Wildl Dis* 42:40, 2006.

31. Haulena M, Heath B: Marine mammal anesthesia. In Dieruaf LA, Gulland FMD, editors: *CRC handbook of marine mammal medicine*, ed 2, Boca Raton, FL, 2001, CRC Press.

32. Haulena M: Otariid seals. In West G, Heard D, Caulkett N, editors: *Zoo animal and wildlife immobilization and anesthesia*, Ames, IA, 2007, Blackwell Publishing.

33. Helm J: Intestinal length of three California pinniped species. *J Zool Lond* 199:287, 1983.

34. Higgins R: Bacteria and fungi of marine mammals: A review. *Can Vet J* 41:105, 2000.

35. Himworth CG, Haulena M, Lambourn DM, et al: Pathology and epidemiology of phocid herpesvirus-1in wild and rehabilitating harbor seals (*Phoca vitulina richardsi*) in the northeastern Pacific. *J Wildl Dis* 46:1046, 2010.

36. Horning M, Haulena M, Tuomi P, et al: Intraperitoneal implantation of life-long telemetry transmitters in otariids. *BMC Vet Res* 4:51, 2008.

37. Huuskonen V, Hughes L, Bennett R: Anaesthesia of three young grey seals (*Halichoerus grypus*) for fracture repair. *Irish Vet J* 64:3, 2011.

38. International Union for the Conservation of Nature: The IUCN Red List of Threatened Species: http://www.iucnredlist.org/search. Accessed November 6, 2012.

39. Jurczynski K, Lyashchenko KP, Gomis D, et al: Pinniped tuberculosis in Malayan tapirs (*Tapirus indicus*) and its transmission to other terrestrial mammals. *J Zoo Wildl Med* 42:222, 2011.

40. Langman VA, Rowe M, Forthman D, et al: Thermal assessment of zoological exhibits I: Sea lion enclosure at the Audubon zoo. *Zoo Biol* 15:403, 1996.

41. Lefebvre KA, Robertson A: Domoic acid and human exposure risks: A review. *Toxicon* 56:218, 2010.

42. Li L, Shan T, Wang C, et al: The fecal viral flora of California sea lions. *J Virol* 85:9909, 2011.

43. Lynch M, Bodley K: Phocid seals. In West G, Heard D, Caulkett N, editors: *Zoo animal and wildlife immobilization and anesthesia*, Ames, IA, 2007, Blackwell Publishing.

44. Lynch M, Kirkwood R, Gray R, et al: characterization and causal investigations of an alopecia syndrome in Australian fur seals (*Arctocephalus pusillus doriferus*). *J Mammol* 93:504, 2012.

45. Mazzaro LM, Dunn JL, Furr HC, et al: Study of vitamin A supplementation in captive northern fur seals (*Callorhinus ursinus*) and its effect on serum vitamin E. *Marine Mammal Sci* 11:545, 1995.

46. McBride MP, Sims MA, Cooper RW, et al: Eastern equine encephalitis in a captive harbor seal (*Phoca vitulina*). *J Zoo Wildl Med* 39:631, 2008.

47. Meegan J, Field C, Sidor I, et al: Development, validation, and utilization of a competitive enzyme-linked immunosorbent assay for the detection of antibodies against *Brucella* species in marine mammals. *J Vet Diagn Invest* 22:856, 2010.

48. Melin SR, Haulena M, Van Bonn W, et al: Reversible immobilization of free-ranging adult male California sea lions (*Zalophus californianus*). *Marine Mammal Sci* 29:529, 2013.

49. Miller S, Colitz CMH, St. Ledger J, et al: A retrospective survey of the ocular histopathology of the pinniped eye with emphasis on corneal disease. *Vet Ophthalmol* 16:1, 2012.

50. Montie EW, Pussini N, Schneider GE, et al: Neuroanatomy and volumes of brain structures of a live California sea lion (*Zalophus californianus*) from magnetic resonance images. *Anat Rec* 292:1523, 2009.

51. Muraco HS, Coombs LD, Procter DG, et al: Taking control of pacific walrus (*Odobenus rosmarus divergens*) reproduction: Achieving a pregnancy in a 16-year-old nulliparous walrus through the use of reproductive technology. *Proc Int Assc of Aquat Anim Med* 42:184, 2011.

52. Murnane RD, Kinsel MJ, Briggs MB: *Clostridium perfringens* type-A induced myositis with probable toxemia in an adult walrus (*Odobenus rosmarus*). *Proc Int Assc of Aquat Anim Med* 28:139, 1997.

53. National Marine Fisheries Service: *Recovery plan for the Hawaiian monk seal (Monachus schauinslandi)*, Silver Spring, MD, 2004, National Marine Fisheries Service.

54. NOAA Fisheries Office of Protected Resources: http://www.nmfs.noaa.gov/pr/health/mmume/pinniped_northeast2011.htm. Accessed October 18, 2012.

55. Nordgarden U, Folkow LP, WallØe L, et al: On the direction and velocity of blood flow in the extradural intravertebral vein of harp seals (*Phoca groenlandica*) during simulated diving. *Acta Physiol Scand* 168:271, 2000.

56. Reddy ML, Dieruaf LA, Gulland FMD: Marine mammals as sentinels of ocean health. In Dieruaf LA, Gulland FMD, editors: *CRC handbook of marine mammal medicine*, ed 2, Boca Raton, FL, 2001, CRC Press.

57. Reidarson T, McBain J, St. Leger J, et al: Side effects of haloperidol (Haldol™) to treat chronic regurgitation in California sea lions. *Proc Int Ass of Aquat Anim Med* 35:124, 2004.

58. Reynolds JE, Rommel SA: *Biology of marine mammals*, Washington, DC, 1999, Smithsonian Institution.

59. Sea lion Cancer Consortium: http://www.smru.st-andrews.ac.uk/slicc/. Accessed November 6, 2012.

60. Sogin ML, Morrison HG, Huber JA, et al: Microbial diversity in the deep sea and the underexplored "rare biosphere". *Proc Natl Acad Sci* 103:12115, 2006.

61. Spotte S: *Sterilization of marine mammal pool waters: Theoretical and health considerations.* USDA Animal and Plant Health Inspection Service Technical Bulletin No. 1797, 1991.

62. Stenfors LE, Sadé J, Hellström S, et al: How can the hooded seal dive to a depth of 1000 m without rupturing its tympanic membrane? A morphological and functional study. *Acta Otolaryngol* 121:689, 2001.

63. Stoddard RA, De Long RL, Byrne BA, et al: Prevalence and characterization of *Salmonella* spp. among marine animals in the Channel Islands, California. *Dis Aquat Org* 81:5, 2008.

64. Stringer EM, Van Bonn W, Chinnadurai S, et al: Risk factors associated with perianesthetic mortality of stranded free-ranging California sea lions (*Zalophus californianus*) undergoing rehabilitation. *J Zoo Wildl Med* 43:233, 2012.

65. Sturm N, Abalos P, Fernandez A, et al: *Salmonella* enteric in pinnipeds. Chile [letter]. *Emerg Infect Dis* 17:2377, 2011.

66. The Center for Food Security and Public Health, Iowa State University: Brucellosis in marine mammals (serial online): http://www.cfsph.iastate.edu/DiseaseInfo/disease.php?name=brucellosis-marine&lang=en. Accessed November 6, 2012.

67. Thornton SJ, Spielman DM, Pelc NJ, et al: Effects of forced diving on the spleen and hepatic sinus in northern elephant seal pups. *Proc Natl Acad Sci* 98:9413, 2001.

68. Trupkiewicz JG, Gulland FMD, Lowenstein LJ: Congenital defects in Northern elephant seals stranded along the central California coast. *J Wildl Dis* 33:220, 1997.

69. Van Bonn W, Jensen ED, House C, et al: Epizootic vesicular disease in captive California sea lions. *J Wildl Dis* 36:500, 2000.

70. Van Bonn W, LaPointe A, Svienty C, et al: Further exploration of the aquatic animal hygiene hypothesis. *Proc Int Assoc Aquat Anim Med* 39:11, 2008.

71. Van Bonn W, Ridgway SH, Williams BH: Chronic refractory emesis associated with a colonic lesion in a California sea lion (*Zalophus californianus*). *J Zoo Wildl Med* 26:286, 1995.

72. Walsh MT, Andrews BF, Antrim J: Walruses. In Dieruaf LA, Gulland FMD, editors: *CRC handbook of marine mammal medicine*, ed 2, Boca Raton, FL, 2001, CRC Press.

73. Welsch U, Riedelsheimer B: Histophysiological observations on the external auditory meatus, middle, and inner ear of the Weddell seal (*Leptonychotes weddelli*). *J Morphol* 234:25, 1997.

74. Worthy G: Nutrition and energetics. In Dieruaf LA, Gulland FMD, editors: *CRC handbook of marine mammal medicine*, ed 2, Boca Raton, FL, 2001, CRC Press.

75. Zuerener RL, Alt DP: Variable nucleotide tandem-repeat analysis revealing a unique group of *Leptospira interrogans* serovar *pomona* isolates associated with California sea lions. *J Clin Microbiol* 47:1202, 2009.

CHAPTER **45**

Sirenia

Michael T. Walsh and Martine de Wit

The Florida manatee (*Trichechus manatus latirostris*), a member of the Trichechidae family of the order Sirenia, will be used to illustrate topics in Sirenia medicine and surgery for this chapter. When possible, the Antillean manatee (*Trichechus manatus manatus*) and the Amazonian manatee (*Trichechus inunguis*) will be included, although material on these and the West African manatee (*Trichechus senegalensis*) is sparse. Data will be used from the only surviving member of the family Dugongidae, the Dugong (*Dugong dugon*), with the help of colleagues in Australia.

Sirenia are found in over 80 countries and territories throughout the tropical and subtropical latitudes.[29] These marine mammal herbivores inhabit coastal waters and river systems. Their range is generally restricted by water temperatures, and both dugongs and Florida manatees, which are at their outer range for comfort, may migrate to warmer water during their respective winter periods.

There has been a great increase in effort in all Sirenia species to collect ecologic and health information as habitats are placed under continuing pressure from anthropogenic and natural factors. The natural history, ecology, and genetic background of these species is covered in a number of publications, and the interested reader is referred to these for additional information.[2,9,29,35,36,45] A valuable source of information on Sirenia is available online in an extensive bibliography compiled by Daryl P. Domning, *Bibliography and Index of the Sirenia and Desmostylia* (http://www.sirenian.org/biblio/).[14] Additional material (and useful videos) on Sirenia health will be available to the reader in the future at http://aquaticanimalhealth.org/multimedia.html.

CLINICALLY IMPORTANT ANATOMY

Anatomy investigations may be traced back to the 1870s.[33] Sirenians are fusiform in shape with very sensitive facial hairs and prehensile capability to acquire vegetation for ingestion. The eyes are generally small, and the external auditory meatus is about 1 millimeter (mm) in diameter along the side of the skull. The variation in the angle of the rostral portion of the skulls between manatees and dugongs is based on their feeding habits. The dugong has prominent incisor teeth (tusks) present in both genders. Sirenia pectoral flippers are flattened laterally and medially, have three to four nails, and may assist in maneuvering, pulling along the bottom during feeding, and tactile contact between animals, including manipulation of females by males whose flippers are longer and rougher medially to hold on during breeding activity. The nipples are placed in the axillary region, as in elephants, and testes are internal. The tail or paddle is round in manatees, and the dugong tail is shaped like that of a dolphin, with symmetrical fluke blades extending laterally from the vertebral attachment. Each lung consists of an elongated single lobe placed in its own pleural cavity created by a midline connection of the hemi-diaphragms to the vertebral bodies. The cranial 70% of each manatee lung attaches medially at the vertebrae. The heart is cranioventral to the pleural cavities and separated from the abdominal cavity by a transverse septum. The liver and intestinal tract lie ventral to the hemi-diaphragms. Manatees are hindgut fermenters, and the gastrointestinal (GI) tract may make up to 23% of an animal's body weight,[37] exhibiting a number of unique features. The stomach is a single C-shaped sac and has a digestive cardiac gland. The duodenum has three portions, including the enlarged duodenal ampulla, the two duodenal diverticula, and the post-ampulla duodenum. The cecum is rounded with two accessory sacs, giving it a rabbit-ear appearance. The kidneys are multilobulated, retroperitoneal, and caudal to the lungs. The vulva is located just anterior to the anus with a circular rim of tissue. The distal portion of the vagina is vertical, with the urethral opening located deep and inaccessible for catheterization unless the animal is heavily sedated. The penile opening is located on the ventral midline and is anterior toward the umbilicus. Vascular access for catheterization is hampered by the presence of vessel bundles in the accessible areas of the flipper and the caudal intervertebral area.

VETERINARY INTERACTION WITH SIRENIA

A number of book chapters and articles cover a range of Sirenia health issues, treatments, and pathologic findings[7,34,42,45] Veterinary involvement with manatees occurs in rescues, research-based health assessments, health assessments of animals being monitored after release, rehabilitation, long-term management in aquaria and zoologic institutions, and necropsies. The chapter will focus on these areas, with references provided where the authors do not have first-hand knowledge of the activity described.

Rescue, Transport, and Rehabilitation

Manatees and dugongs may require intervention for a number of diseases and anthropogenic challenges.[24] First response is usually performed by state or facility personnel with experience in manatee capture and transport. Facility veterinarians may be present for the operation or are in contact with rescuers by phone. The most common reasons for rescue and rehabilitation include cold stress, orphaned calves, other natural disease (reproductive complications, biotoxins, infectious disease, noninfectious disease), watercraft injuries, entrapment, and other human-related etiologies such as entanglement or ingestion of fishing gear. Observation of the ill or injured manatee's behavior prior to capture may be very helpful in understanding the cause of the problem and preparing for transport and therapy. New availability of above-water and underwater cameras placed at winter congregation sites may improve access for visual evaluation of ill and injured animals at specific sites. Cardiopulmonary compromise from pneumonia, fractures, pneumothorax, or pyothorax may require special handling to decrease further damage. If pneumothorax and broken ribs are suspected, attempts should be made to reduce further damage to the lung and the surrounding tissue from manipulation, loading, and transport.

Critical Care Facility Medicine and Management

At the critical care facility, manatees undergo a visual inspection of body condition, eyes, oral cavity, wounds or lesions, and respiratory rate and quality, heart rate, and oral temperature are recorded. Thin or emaciated animals should have a blood sample taken early in the evaluation to include complete blood cell count (CBC), chemistries, spun packed cell volume (PCV), total protein levels, and glucometer glucose levels before placing the animal in water. CBC count and chemistry values are listed in Table 45-1 and 45-2.[22,23] Standard blood sampling for manatees is from the interosseous space between the radius and the ulna, which may be approached medially or laterally. The site is visually defined by flexing the carpal joint and noting the elbow joint and then palpating the caudal edge of the radius between the joints. The medial insertion site may strike the median nerve and create discomfort in and resistance from the animal after multiple blood samples. The lateral approach may result in less discomfort but the vessel location is (goes) deeper, and redirection of the needle or obtaining large volumes is more difficult. Small calves may be bled with 25- to 23-gauge needles with small extension sets; however, rapid clotting may occur, so having (using) preheparinized syringes may help avoid sample loss. One-inch (25-mm), 20-gauge needles with extension sets are used in juveniles. Blood samples may be obtained from adults with 1.5-inch (38-mm) 20- to 18-gauge needles attached to extension sets, which helps avoid needle displacement when the animal moves. Cytology and cultures of lesions may help guide therapy. Absence or presence of a scant amount of dry, hard feces may suggest dehydration and constipation. Hypoglycemic animals should receive glucose supplementation and oral fluids, and a constipated animal's oral fluid should be lubricated with mineral oil prior to release of the animal into a pool. Gavage hydration or feeding is always done last to avoid possible complications related to handling and regurgitation. Additional diagnostic techniques may be delayed, and the priority should be to place the animal back into water after an extended transport.

Radiography may be indicated for evaluation of a number of conditions. Rib fractures, pneumothorax, and spinal and head injuries are common indications for imaging. Care should be taken, as rolling the animals to place the films, lifting the animal in a stretcher, or struggling of an animal may all exacerbate existing damage.

Acclimation, Pain, and Anxiety

Dehydration, in-water support, constipation, pain, adjusting to a foreign environment, strange food and how it is presented, all of these affect recuperation and should be addressed. Noise and human presence should be minimized. Alleviation of discomfort and anxiety is especially important in the first few days after injury. Opioids are generally avoided because of their effect on intestinal motility. Ketoprofen has been used for its analgesic effects for up to 5 days, but care should be taken to ensure that the animals are being properly hydrated to avoid adverse effects on kidneys. Gastric ulcer formation may be promoted with the use of nonsteriodal anti-inflammatory drugs (NSAIDs) in juveniles and leads to a decrease or lack of improvement in appetite. Histamine-2 (H2+) blockers and coating agents may help mitigate ulcer development and treat lesions that are already present.

If necessary, barriers should be erected to maintain distance between humans and new arrivals, especially adult animals that are less adaptable to change. Sinking the food trays into the water mimics common feeding methods in the wild; additional food should be left in the pool at night, as some animals are more likely to eat at that time. Although manatees do not travel in tight groups or pods, they do respond positively to company, which may promote eating and relieve anxiety. Age, gender separation, and reproductive activity may negatively influence appetite and behavior.

Oral valium may be used to alleviate anxiety and enhance appetite in new arrivals. The dosage is started low (15 to 20 milligrams [mg] for a 450-kilogram [kg] animal, twice a day [BID], when

TABLE 45-1

Hematologic Results for Free-Ranging and Captive Manatees (*Trichechus manatus*)*

Analyte	Free-Ranging (*n* = 52)	Captive (*n* = 62)	*P* Value
Hematocrit, liter per liter (L/L)	0.351 (0.289–0.435)	0.350 (0.277–0.461)	0.731
Hemoglobin, gram per liter (g/L)	112 (94–135)	112 (86–149)	0.784
Red blood cell count (×10^{12}/L)	2.76 (2.17–3.39)	2.81 (2.30–3.51)	0.366
Mean corpuscular volume, (fL)	128 (114–140)	124 (105–140)	0.003
Mean corpuscular hemoglobin, picogram (pg)	40.8 (36.6–44.9)	40.0 (32.9–44.3)	0.015
Mean corpuscular hemoglobin concentration (g/L)	320 (280–354)	320 (294–336)	0.973
Red cell distribution width (%)	16.2 (13.9–22.8)	16.6 (13.5–21.4)	0.139
Platelets (×10^9/L)	242 (111–424)	274 (137–507)	0.051
Mean platelet volume (fL)	6.44 (5.02–8.49)	6.40 (5.19–8.80)	0.625
White blood cell count (×10^9/L)	5.98 (2.77–13.50)	6.64 (2.85–14.2)	0.070
Bands (×10^9/L)	0.02 (0–0.22)	0.02 (0–0.16)	0.912
Heterophils (×10^9/L)	2.33 (0.77–6.53)	3.25 (1.40–8.50)	<0.001
Lymphocytes (×10^9/L)	2.90 (1.01–7.20)	2.71 (0.83–8.50)	0.811
Monocytes (×10^9/L)	0.51 (0.08–1.70)	0.56 (0.07–2.80)	.537
Eosinophils (×10^9/L)	0.20 (0–1.23)	0.09 (0–0.41)	<0.001
Basophils (×10^9/L)	0.04 (0–0.27)	0.03 (0–0.14)	0.138
Nucleated red blood cell (×10^9/L)	0.02 (0–0.21)	0.04 (0–0.25)	0.028
Reticulocytes, manual (×10^9/L)†	51 (16–96)	74 (0–127)	0.076
Reticulocytes, automated (×10^9/L)‡	17 (7–45)	21 (3–39)	0.424
Heinz bodies (%)§	8.2 (0.6–22.3)	7.0 (0–15)	0.181
Plasma proteins (g/L)	80 (69–93)	81 (70–92)	0.641
Fibrinogen (g/L)	2.24 (1.00–5.00)	3.23 (1.00–6.00)	0.002

*Data are mean (minimum–maximum). Data for small calves were not included. Except for reticulocytes, *P* values were determined by comparing location (free-ranging versus captive) and age of blood sample (fresh versus day old) using a two-way ANOVA (analysis of variance) with the Tukey test for group comparisons. Only fresh blood samples were analyzed for reticulocyte counts, so *P* values were determined for free-ranging versus captive animals using a *t*-test.
†*n* = 17 free-ranging, 15 captive
‡*n* = 10 free-ranging, 9 captive
§*n* = 28 free-ranging, 40 captive
Table reproduced with permission from Harvey JW, Harr KE, Murphy D, et al: Hematology of healthy Florida manatees (*Trichechus manatus*) *Vet Clin Pathol* 38(2):183–193, 2009.

tubing) and adjusted according to the animal's response. This may also improve cooperation with intubation for administration of fluids and food, treatment of wounds, and blood sampling and avoid handling-associated tissue damage from fractured ribs and pneumothorax.

Restraint, Sedation, and Anesthesia

Physical restraint may pose some danger to animals and handlers, so only trained personnel should be involved. Minimal restraint is often needed for procedures that involve wound care, blood sampling, and gavage feeding. Sedation may be required for biopsies or minor procedures or to avoid causing additional injury to a trauma patient. Sedation may be achieved through a number of approaches (Table 45-3). Heavy sedation and anesthesia require intubation and monitoring as in other species. Intubation may be achieved under heavy sedation, with additional masking, as needed. The tube is placed through the nasal cavity under the guidance of a bronchoscope. The trachea is short (often less than 10 centimeters [cm]), so confirming placement of the tube with the scope helps avoid intubating and ventilating only one lung instead of both.

Diet

Wild manatees eat a wide variety of fresh water and marine vegetation, including sea grasses and algae.[25-27] It is often challenging to provide food close to wild vegetation in facilities because of a wide variation in caloric requirements dictated by injury, age, and size. Compared with adults, juveniles are more likely to begin eating readily in a new rehabilitation environment. Manatees with severe injury or cold stress may require a marked increase in caloric needs, which lettuce cannot provide. Manatees should have a variety of greens available, when possible, and wild vegetation is preferred, although it is difficult to acquire in adequate volume.

Determination of food volume should be based on weights, measured regularly during therapy or when monitoring growth. Rough guidelines that manatees require 10% of their body weight in food underestimate the caloric need for rapidly growing animals with poor forage and overestimate the requirements of inactive adults. Supplementation with gruel formulas is beneficial in the treatment of emaciated or badly injured animals. A gruel made of 720 grams (g) of leaf eater monkey chow, 600 g of spinach, and 400 milliliters (mL) of water results in approximately 1080 calories per liter (L). Generally, the strength of the gruel is started at 25% to avoid gastric damage from increased acidity and then increased over 4 to 6 days. Anorexia or decreased appetite in new arrivals may be associated with illness, dehydration, constipation, intestinal disease, anxiety, discomfort, isolation, hormonal cycles in females, gastric ulcers, noise, human activity, unknown foods, and adaptation difficulty.

TABLE 45-2

Plasma Clinical Biochemistry Analytes in Free-Ranging and Captive *Trichechus Manatus*

Analyte	Free-Ranging	Captive	*P* Value
Sodium, millimole per liter (mmol/L)	150 (143–158)	150 (142–161)	$P = 0.30$
Potassium (mmol/L)	4.9 (3.8–6.3)	4.8 (3.5–6.7)	$P = 0.23$
Chloride (mmol/L)	93 (78–106)	86 (71–98)	$P < 0.001$
Total carbon dioxide (mmol/L)	27 (4–41)	40 (14–54)	$P < 0.001$
Anion gap (mmol/L)	39 (15–59)	28 (5–46)	$P < 0.001$
Lactate (mmol/L)	13 (1–30)	4 (1–24)	$P = 0.002$
Calcium (mmol/L)	2.6 (2.0–3.7)	2.8 (2.2–3.4)	$P = 0.03$
Phosphate (mmol/L)	1.9 (1.1–2.7)	1.6 (1.1–2.9)	$P = 0.03$
Magnesium (mmol/L)	1.9 (1.2–3.1)	1.4 (0.7–1.9)	$P < 0.001$
Urea (mmol/L)	2.1 (0.4–4.3)	4.6 (1.8–8.9)	$P < 0.001$
Creatinine, micromole per liter (μmol/L)	128 (53–336)	194 (115–345)	$P < 0.001$
Bilirubin (μmol/L)	1.7 (0–5.1)	1.7 (0–8.6)	$P = 0.88$
Glucose (mmol/L)	4.6 (2.3–9.9)	4.4 (1.9–8.6)	$P = 0.82$
Cholesterol (mmol/L)	3.0 (2.1–7.3)	3.5 (1.9–7.6)	$P = 0.91$
Triglycerides (mmol/L)	0.9 (0.3–2.2)	0.8 (0.3–1.6)	$P = 0.04$
ALP, unit per liter (Unit/L)	86 (39–192)	122 (51–242)	$P < 0.001$
GGT (Unit /L)	31 (9–47)	46 (11–99)	$P < 0.001$
ALT (Unit /L)	18 (5–48)	17 (1–94)	$P = 0.52$
AST (Unit /L)	9 (4–26)	9 (3–37)	$P = 0.60$
CK (Unit /L)	190 (51–2966)	261 (64–3348)	$P = 0.64$
Total protein, gram per liter (g/L)	76 (64–90)	80 (71–93)	$P < 0.001$
Albumin (g/L)	34 (25–46)	39 (33–47)	$P < 0.001$
Total globulins (g/dL)	41 (33–54)	43 (32–58)	$P = 0.96$
A/G ratio	0.86 (0.61–1.31)	0.89 (0.58–1.33)	$P = 0.006$
Haptoglobin (g/L)	1.5 (0.3–2.5)	0.9 (0.2–2.1)	$P = 0.04$
SAA, milligram per liter (mg/L)	11 (<10–50)	13 (<10–49)	$P = 0.91$

*Values are medians with minimum and maximum values in parentheses. The total number of manatees analyzed for a majority of analytes was 112, but lesser numbers were analyzed for total carbon dioxide and anion gap (98), cholesterol, albumin, globulin, and A/G ratio (86), ALT, AST, and haptoglobin (72), and lactate (61). Albumin and total globulins were determined using plasma protein electrophoresis. Data for small calves were not included. *P* values were determined by comparing location and age classes using a two-way ANOVA (analysis of variance) with the Tukey test used for comparison of free-ranging and captive animals.
A/G ratio, Albumin/globulin ratio; *ALP*, alkaline phosphatase; *ALT*, alanine aminotransferase; *AST*, aspartate aminotransferase; *CK*, creatine kinase; *GGT*, γ-glutamyl transferase; *SAA*, serum amyloid A.
Table reproduced, by permission of Allen Press, from Harvey JW, Harr KE, Murphy D, et al: Clinical biochemistry in healthy manatees (*Trichechus manatus latirostris*). *J Zoo Wildl Med* 38:269–279, 2007.

Environmental Parameters for Facility Sirenia

Manatee facilities should allow for a range of temperatures from 26°C (78°F) to 30°C (86°F). Wild individuals do encounter colder and warmer temperatures, but these are meant to be tolerated as seasonal fluctuations and are not ideal for health. Manatees may shiver or become compromised when temperatures drop below 21°C (70°F). In the winter, springs provide relief from surrounding cold water with temperatures around 23°C (73°F), but they are not inhabited year round.

It may be beneficial for manatees to have access to both fresh water and water with varying salinity, since it appears that the skin exfoliates after shifting between salt water and fresh water, which could avoid retained skin with fungal, algal, or bacterial growth. Chlorine and ozone, used for water disinfection, have caused corneal damage.

CATEGORIES OF ILLNESS AND INJURY

Neonatal, Maternally Dependent Calves

Orphans may present as a result of complications from maternal factors, including maternal injury, death, illness, maternal inexperience, or disinterest. Environmental changes such as extended or severe cold stress may result in calf deterioration, abandonment, and death. Calves may suffer from complications related to prematurity, inanition, poor adaption, watercraft injury, and infection such as omphalitis, which includes hypoglycemia, dehydration, constipation, enterocolitis, and pneumatosis intestinalis.[41] Congenital defects in rescued calves have included ectrodactyly of the pectoral flippers digits, atresia ani, and omphalocele or exteriorization of the intestinal tract at the umbilicus.[43] Facility requirements for orphan care include 24-hour husbandry care, staff trained in feeding techniques that

TABLE 45-3

Analgesic, Anesthetic, and Reversal Agents for the Florida Manatee (*Trichechus manatus latirostris*)

Agent	Use	Dosage	Comments
Atipamezole	Reversal	1 mg/20 mg xylazine, intravenously (IV)	For xylazine reversal[34]
		1 mg/2 mg detomidine, IV	For detomidine reversal[34]
		5 mg/1 mg detomidine, intramuscularly (IM)	For detomidine reversal
Butorphanol	Sedative, analgesic	0.01–0.025 mg/kg, IV	In combination with diazepam for mild painful procedures, anesthetic induction; give butorphanol 10 minutes prior to diazepam[34]
		0.005–0.01 mg/kg	In combination with detomidine for minor surgical procedures or anesthetic induction[34]
		0.0086 mg/kg	In combination with detomidine for heavier sedation, +/– intubation
		0.04–0.06 mg/kg	With midazolam 0.1 mg/kg, IM, for anesthesia induction or for short procedures involving fractious individuals (Walsh, unpublished data)
		0.1 mg/kg	With midazolam 0.1 mg/kg, IM, for anesthesia induction in severely fractious individuals, results in very deep sedation, use with caution (Walsh, unpublished data)
Detomidine	Sedative	0.005–0.01 mg/kg	Moderate sedation; beware of narrow therapeutic index; cardiac and blood pressure effects not noted
		0.025–0.005 mg/kg	In combination with butorphanol, excellent analgesia and muscle relaxation; beware of narrow therapeutic index
		0.0086 mg/kg	In combination with butorphanol for heavier sedation, +/– intubation[34]
Diazepam	Sedative	0.02–0.035 mg/kg, IV	For nonpainful diagnostics[34]
		0.01–0.025 mg/kg, IV	In combination with butorphanol for mild to moderate painful procedure[34]
		0.066 mg/kg, IM	For tranquilization, lasts 60–90 minutes[7]
Flumazenil	Reversal	1 mg/10–20 mg midazolam or diazepam, IV	Reversal for midazolam or diazepam[34]
		Equal volume as midazolam, IM	Reversal for midazolam, may require redosing after long procedure[42]
		Equal volume diazepam, IM	Reversal for diazepam[7]
Isoflurane	Anesthetic	0.5–5%	Similar settings as in domestic animals[42]
Ketoprofen	Analgesic	1–2 mg/kg, IM	Analgesia for severe abdominal pain. *Authors' note*: Caution in dehydrated animals; side effects not well documented in this species (Ray Ball, personal communication)
Lidocaine 2%	Analgesic	Local infusion to effect	Local analgesia
Meperidine	Sedative, analgesic	Upto 1 mg/kg, IM	In combination with midazolam for more painful procedures or anesthetic induction[42]
		0.5–1 mg/kg, IM	Sedation or analgesia for minor surgical procedures[7]
Midazolam	Sedative	0.02–0.05 mg/kg, IM	Mild to moderate sedation[34]
		0.045 mg/kg, IM	Sedation for 60–90 minutes; may also be used in conjunction with meperidine for more painful procedures or anesthetic induction[42]
		0.05–0.072 mg/kg	Sedation for 20–30 minutes at peak effect for endoscopy, freeze branding, or noninvasive procedures (Ray Ball, unpublished data)
		0.08 mg/kg	Anesthetic induction, intubation[42]
		0.1 mg/kg	Anesthetic induction, in combination with butorphanol (Walsh, unpublished data)
Naltrexone	Reversal	1–2 mg/1 mg butorphanol, IV or IM	Reversal for butorphanol[34]
		Equal volume dose, IM	Reversal for meperidine
Xylazine	Sedative	0.05–0.1 mg/kg, IM	Moderate sedation; beware of narrow therapeutic index[34]
Xylocaine 1%	Epidural anesthetic	Dose not noted, epidural	Used in one case for vertebral fracture surgery[7]
Yohimbine	Reversal	1 mg/5–10 mg xylazine, IV	Reversal for xylazine[34]
		2–3 mg/1 mg detomidine, IV	Reversal for detomidine[34]
		IM at the above dosages	Reversal for xylazine, detomidine

Reproduced by permission of Blackwell Publishing, from Chittick EJ, Walsh MT: Sirenians (manatees and dugongs). In West G, Heard D, Cauklett N (eds): *Zoo and wildlife immobilization and anesthesia.*, 2008, Blackwell. References modified to fit chapter.

TABLE 45-4

Selected Infectious Diseases of Sirenia by Species and Reference

Leptospirosis	Toxoplasma gondii	Cryptosporidium	Papilloma virus (TMPv)	Morbillivirus	Mycobacterium
Tml[13,19]	Tml[4,11]	Tmm[3]	Tml[6,15,44]	Tml[16]	Tml[38]
Tmm[39]	Tmm[30,39]	Tmi[3]		Tmm[39]	Tmi[31]
	Tmi[30]	Dd[32]			

Florida manatee: Tml, *Trichechus manatus latirostris*.
Antillean manatee: Tmm, *Trichechus manatus manatus*.
Amazonian manatee: Tmi, *Trichechus manatus inunguis*.
Dugong: Dd, *Dugong dugon*.

emphasize bottle adaption and monitoring, and veterinary staff trained in neonatal critical care. Hypoglycemia should be considered in any neonatal manatee and therapy started immediately.

Infectious Disease

Several authors have described cases and investigations of manatee pathology and infectious disease.[10,12,17,18] Natural parasitic infections involving nematodes, cestodes, and trematodes have been well described.[1,40] Parasite infestations may reach a level of clinical concern in emaciated sub-adults. Both nematode and trematode infestations have been treated with fenbendazole (10 to 15 mg/kg, orally [PO], once) and praziquantel (10 to 20 mg/kg, PO). Detection of infectious disease other than those caused by parasites in Sirenia has been limited, but some are listed in Table 45-4.

Intoxication

Brevetoxin associated with red tide (*Karenia brevis*), a dinoflagellate more commonly found in the Gulf of Mexico, is a common natural mortality factor in manatees.[5] Clinical signs include neurologic compromise, lethargy, incoordination, and seizures. Serologic tests for the *K. brevis* toxin may confirm red tide intoxication, in addition to the presence of increased dinoflagellate counts in water samples.

Treatment focuses on prevention of drowning. Generally, affected manatees are propped up on foam to keep their heads above water for 24 to 48 hours and closely observed. Some medications such as NSAIDs and atropine have been used. Recovery is generally rapid.

Reproduction

Female manatees mature between 3 and 5 years, whereas dugongs start to mature at 10 years.[28,45] Facilities should recognize that reproductive maturation may be more related to biologic size associated with available nutrition than to chronologic age, so reproductive capability may be variable. Gestation lasts about 12 to 14 months in manatees and 13 months in dugongs. Calves nurse from 1 to 2 years, which appears to be dependent on individual needs. Reproductive complications have included fetal death, abortion secondary to trauma and handling in the last trimester, and dystocia. Dystocia treatment has included calf extraction under sedation and cesarean removal in one individual. Female manatees maintained without males may undergo behavioral changes during estrus that include spin swimming, isolation, abdominal flexion, decreased appetite, and other complications. Fatal myopathy has been diagnosed in female manatees presumably associated with exhaustion caused by extensive mating pursuit by males.

HUMAN INTERACTION

Human interaction includes any human activity that results in injury or death and primarily involves watercraft trauma, entanglement in fishing gear, ingestion of fishing gear, and gate and dam lock injury.

Surviving watercraft trauma and entanglement may result in scars that are tracked by the Manatee Individual Photo Identification System (MIPS) maintained by the U.S. Geological Survey (USGS) Sirenia Project in collaboration with the Florida Fish and Wildlife Conservation Commission and the Mote Marine Laboratory.

WATERCRAFT INJURY

Watercraft injuries are one of the largest categories of reasons for rescue and of mortality and may be caused by recreational boats as well as commercial platforms, including working barges, tugs, or cruise ships. Boat injury may result in a range of abrasions, lacerations, blunt trauma, or combinations of all three. External skin and soft tissue damage may not be indicative of the degree of internal damage, but abnormal or asymmetrical buoyancy may indicate the anatomic sites involved.

Blunt Trauma and Pneumothorax

The presence of external wounds in animals with abnormal buoyancy is highly suggestive of traumatic pneumothorax. Excessive intestinal gas may occur from enterocolitis or constipation and mimic the signs of pneumothorax. Radiography is the most common diagnostic method, although handling animals with fractured ribs may cause further damage. Ultrasonography may detect the presence of an extended air pocket but is not definitive. Radiography may be followed by tapping the distended chest to drain air or may be used without prior diagnostics in cases when diagnostic equipment is not available, although caution is advised. CBC count and chemistries may be nondiagnostic for the presence of severe inflammation or infection, but serum amyloid may detect elevated inflammation.[20,21]

Severe unilateral pneumothorax associated with large pulmonary punctures or tears may require the use of flotation jackets to equalize the animal in the water column. This also acts as rib support and requires handlers to be cautious with restraint. Flotation jackets may assist with stimulating appetite by decreasing anxiety in the animal and reduce struggling in the water to right itself to breathe. Some manatees may require time to adapt to the jacket application. Manatees may also be placed in shallow water to facilitate self-righting, but this costs energy and effort and may result in angulation of the pectoral flippers from constant contact with the pool bottom. Therapy for pneumothorax varies widely among clinicians. The chest may be tapped with 7.5- to 12.5-cm, 18- to 16-gauge needles to treat pneumothorax and to estimate the severity of the leak based on refill time after removal of air. Most animals do respond to conservative therapy with tapping of the chest and removal of air once a week till resolution. Chest drains have had mixed results, since they maintain a lung laceration or puncture in an open position in a breath holder. Wound resolution may, in fact, be promoted by initially avoiding expansion of a collapsed lung with a tear. Animals not responding after 4 to 6 weeks may have a large opening in the lung tissue, which requires further evaluation. Interventional thoracoscopy and surgical repair have been attempted, although this is still under development and not widely applied.

Blunt trauma may result in head injury, spinal injury, and abdominal soft tissue damage, including organ fracture. Spinal damage and chronic pyothorax may result in negative buoyancy, although the injured animal may learn to partially regain control of buoyancy.

Propeller Wounds

Propeller trauma often results in a number of (injuries in) evenly spaced parallel lines, ranging from abrasions to deep lacerations. In addition to rib transection, propellers may cause massive soft tissue loss, including lung exteriorization, tail removal, abdominal compromise, and immediate death. Animals may present with a mixture of propeller lacerations and blunt trauma.

Wound treatment in rehabilitation may be challenging because of wound severity, adaptation times for adequate caloric intake, and exposure to fecal contaminants in pools and to resident bacteria. Wound care should include visual inspection each day, use of tissue disinfectants during the pregranulation phase, proper debridement and timing, anti-infective compounds, and bandaging to protect wounds and to maintain cleanliness after application. Large adjustable body wraps made of wet suit material work well to cover and protect wounds.

Fishing Gear

The presence of commercial and recreational fishing gear in manatee habitats may result in ingestion of fishing gear, including lines, hooks, lures (tackles), and netting material. Ingestion of hooks may cause perforation of the GI system, leading to peritonitis and death. Hooks have also been found lodged in the caudal pharynx, resulting in excessive respiratory noise. Gill nets are illegal in Florida, but animals may become entangled in seines, hoop nets, shiner nets, and crab pot and fish trap lines.[8] Floating and sinking lines involve polyester, nylon, polypropylene ropes or lead line ropes. Line entanglement is increased in incidence in areas with concentrated fishing activity. Studies involving lines and manatee behavior show that these animals are curious and that tactile manipulation of the vertical lines may lead to entanglement.[21] In both rope and monofilament line entanglements, the drag created by the line or attached gear promotes embedding of the line and pulls it through tissue, including bone, and this complicates surgical removal. In flipper entanglements, the axial path left by the line is usually replaced by scar tissue.

Health Assessments

Additional health information is gathered on wild manatees through organized health assessments. These events involve biologists, veterinarians, and scientists, who gather information on individual and population parameters at multiple sites in Florida, Puerto Rico, and South America.

REFERENCES

1. Beck C, Forrester DJ: Helminths of the Florida manatee *Trichechus manatus latirostris*, with a discussion and summary of the parasites of Sirenians. *J Parasitol* 74(4):628–637, 1988.
2. Blanchard W: Dugong strandings, veterinary conservation biology: Wildlife health and management in Australia—marine mammal strandings. *Proc Tarongo Zoo* 2001.
3. Borges JCG, Alves LC, Faustino MAG, et al: Occurrence of *Cryptosporidium* spp. in Antillean manatees (*Trichechus manatus*) and Amazonian manatees (*Trichechus inunguis*) from Brazil. *J Zoo Wildl Med* 42(4):593–596, 2011.
4. Bossart GD, Mignucci-Giannoni AA, Rivera-Guzman AL, et al: Disseminated toxoplasmosis in Antillean manatees (*Trichechus manatus manatus*) from Puerto Rico. *Dis Aquat Org* 101:139–144, 2012.
5. Bossart GD, Baden DG, Ewing RY, et al: Brevetoxicosis in manatees (*Trichechus manatus latirostris*) from the 1996 epizootic: Gross, histologic,

6. Bossart GD, Ewing RY, Lowe M, et al: Viral papillomatosis in Florida manatees (*Trichechus manatus latirostris*). *Exp Mol Pathol* 72:37–48, 2002.
7. Bossart GD: Manatee. In Dierauf LA, Gulland FMD, editors: *Handbook of marine mammal medicine*, Boca Raton, FL, 2001, CRC Press.
8. Bowles AE, Yack T, Alves C, et al: *Experimental studies of manatee entanglement in crab traps* (Abstract). Fifteenth Biennial Conference on the Biology of Marine Mammals, Greensboro, NC, 2003.
9. Bryden M, Marsh H, Shaughnessy P: *Dugongs, whales, dolphins and seals: A guide to the sea mammals of Australasia Sydney sea mammals of Australia*, St. Leonards, Australia, 1998, Allen and Unwin.
10. Buergelt CD, Bonde RK, Beck CA, et al: Pathologic findings in manatees in Florida. *J Am Vet Med Assoc* 11:1331–1334, 1984.
11. Buergelt CD, Bonde RK: Toxoplasmic meningoencephalitis in a West Indian manatee. *J Am Vet Med Assoc* 183:1294–1296, 1983.
12. Buergelt CD: Observations on manatee mortality in northern Florida—a necropsy survey. *Proc Int Assoc Aquatic Anim Med* 1(1):28–29, 1984.
13. Cornide RI: Anticuerpos leptospirales en suero sanguíneo del manatí (*Trichechus manatus L.*). *Acad Cienc Cuba Inst Zool Misc Zoologica* 18:1, 1984.
14. Domning DP: *Bibliography and index of the Sirenia and Desmostylia*: http://www.sirenian.org/biblio Accessed 4-15-13.
15. Dona MG, Rehtanz M, Adimey NM, et al: Seroepidemiology of TmPV-1 infection in captive and wild Florida manatees (*Trichechus manatus latirostris*). *J Wildl Dis* 47:673–684, 2011.
16. Duigan PJ, House C, Walsh MT, et al: Morbillivirus infection in manatees. *Marine Mammal Sci* 11:441–451, 1995.
17. Forrester DJ, White FH, Woodard JC, et al: Intussusception in a Florida manatee. *J Wildl Dis* 11:566–569, 1975.
18. Frye FL, Herald ES: Osteomyelitis in a manatee. *J Am Vet Med Assoc* 155:1073–1076, 1969.
19. Geraci JR, Arnold J, Schmitt BJ, et al: *A serologic survey of manatees in Florida*. In 13th Biennial Conference on the Biology of Marine Mammals, Wailea, Maui, HI, 1999, Society for Marine Mammology.
20. Harr K, Harvey J, Bonde R, et al: Comparison of methods used to diagnose generalized inflammatory disease in manatees (*Trichechus manatus latirostris*). *J Zoo Wildl Med* 37:151–159, 2006.
21. Harr KE, Rember R, Ginn PE, et al: Serum amyloid A (SAA) as a biomarker of chronic infection due to boat strike trauma in a free-ranging Florida manatee (*Trichechus manatus latirostris*) with incidental polycystic kidneys. *J Wildl Dis* 47:1026–1031, 2011.
22. Harvey JW, Harr KE, Murphy D, et al: Clinical biochemistry in healthy manatees (*Trichechus manatus latirostris*). *J Zoo Wildl Med* 38:269–279, 2007.
23. Harvey JW, Harr KE, Murphy D, et al: Hematology of healthy Florida manatees (*Trichechus manatus*). *Vet Clin Pathol* 38(2):183–193, 2009.
24. Florida Fish and Wildlife Conservation Commission: Manatee Rescue Program: http://myfwc.com/research/manatee/rescue-mortality-response/rescue/rescue/. Accessed 4-30-13?
25. Ledder DA: *Food habits of the West Indian manatee* (Trichechus manatus latirostris) *in South Florida* (M.S. thesis), Coral Gables, FL, 1986, University of Miami.
26. Lefebvre LW, Reid JP, Kenworthy WJ, et al: Characterizing manatee habitat use and seagrass grazing in Florida and Puerto Rico: Implications for conservation and management. *Pacif Conserv Biol* 5:289–298, 2000.
27. Lefebvre LW, Powell JA: *Manatee grazing impacts on sea grasses in Hobe Sound and Jupiter Sound in Southeast Florida during the winter of 1988–89*, Final Report to the U.S. Marine Mammal Commission, Washington, D.C., Contract #T62239152, 1990.
28. Marmontel M: *Age determination and population biology of the Florida manatee,* Trichechus manatus latirostris (unpublished Ph.D. dissertation), Gainesville, FL, 1993, University of Florida.
29. Marsh H, O'Shea TJ, Reynolds JE, III: *Ecology and conservation of Sirenia, dugongs and manatees. Conservation Biology* 18, Cambridge, U.K., 2012, Cambridge University Press.

and immunohistochemical features. *Toxicol Pathol* 26:276–282, 1998.

30. Mathews PD, da Silva VMF, Rosas FCW, et al: Occurrence of antibodies to *Toxoplasma gondii* and *Leptospira* spp. In manatees (*Trichechus inunguis*) of the Brazilian Amazon. *J Zoo Wildl Med* 43(1):85–88, 2012.

31. Morales P: The life and death of an Amazon manatee. *IAAAM Proc* 43–47, 1986.

32. Morgan UM, Xiao L, Hill BD, et al: Detection of the *Cryptosporidium parvum* "human" genotype in a dugong (*Dugong dugon*). *J Parasitol* 86:1352–1354, 2000.

33. Murie J: On the forma and structure of the manatee (*Manatus americanus*). *Trans Zool Soc Lond* 8(3):127–202, 1872.

34. Murphy D: Sirenia. In Fowler ME, Miller RE, editors: *Zoo and wild animal medicine*, ed 5, St. Louis, MO, 2003, Elsevier Science.

35. Reep RL, Bonde RK: *The Florida manatee biology and conservation*, Gainesville, FL, 2006, University Press of Florida.

36. Reynolds JE, III, Odell DK: *Manatees and dugongs*, New York, 1991, Facts on File, Inc.

37. Reynolds KA, Rommel SA: Structure and function of the gastrointestinal tract of the Florida manatee, *Trichechus manatus latirostris*. *Anat Rec* 245:539–558, 1996.

38. Sato T, Shibuya H, Ohba S, et al: Mycobacteriosis in two captive Florida manatees (*Trichechus manatus latirostris*). *J Zoo Wildl Med* 34(2):184–188, 2003.

39. Sulzner K, Kreuder Johnson C, Bonde RK, et al: Health Assessment and seroepidemiologic survey of potential pathogens in wild Antillean manatees (*Trichechus manatus manatus*). *PLoS ONE* 7(9):e44517, 2012.

40. Upton SJ, Odell DK, Bossart GD, et al: Description of the oocysts of two new species of *Eimeria* (Apicomplexa: Eimerūdae) from the Florida manatee, *Trichechus manatus* (Sirenia: Trichechidae). *J Eukaryot Microbiol* 36:87–90, 1989.

41. Walsh MT, Bossart GD, Young WG, et al: Omphalitis and peritonitis in a young West Indian manatee (*Trichechus manatus*). *J Wild Dis* 23(4):702–704, 1987.

42. Walsh MT, Bossart GD: Manatee medicine. In Miller RE, Fowler ME, editors: *Zoo and wildlife medicine*, Philadelphia, PA, 1999, Saunders.

43. Watson AG, Bonde RK: Congenital malformations of the flipper in three West Indian manatees, *Trichechus manatus*, and a proposed mechanism for development of ectrodactyly and cleft hand in mammals. *Clin Orthop Relat Res* 202:294–301, 1986.

44. Woodruff RA, Bonde RK, Bonilla JA, et al: Molecular identification of a papilloma virus from cutaneous lesions of captive and free ranging Florida manatees. *J Wildl Dis* 41:437–441, 2005.

45. Woods R, Ladds P, Blyde D: Dugongs. In Vogelnest L, Woods R, editors: *Medicine of Australian mammals*, Collingwood, Victoria, Australia, 2008, CSIRO Publications.

CHAPTER 46

Canidae

Luis R. Padilla and Clayton D. Hilton

GENERAL BIOLOGY

The family Canidae currently includes 35 species of dogs, wolves, coyotes, jackals and foxes[39] (Table 46-1), and a larger number of subspecies whose status is under constant revision. All members are part of the subfamily Caninae, which is the only extant group of three subfamilies in the fossil record of this family. Evidence suggests that the Eastern wolf should be considered a distinct wolf species (*Canis lycaon*) that is more closely related to the red wolf (*C. rufus*) than to the gray wolf of which it has been historically considered a subspecies (*C. lupus lycaon*).[21] The most common canid, the domestic dog, derived from the gray wolf (*C. lupus*) through close association and interactions with humans approximately 12,000 years ago. The dingo and the New Guinea singing dog are considered feral populations of domestic dogs that have reverted to a wild status and are thus considered subspecies of *C. lupus*.

Canidae is one of the most geographically widespread carnivore families; at least one wild species is present on each continent, except Antarctica. The red fox, which is present on five continents, and the gray wolf, present on three, span some of the largest geographic ranges of any terrestrial mammal. Canids have diversified to inhabit a wide variety of habitat types. Species occur in desert environments, savannas, tropical and temperate forests, coastal areas, and arctic environments. Individual species range in size from members of the *Vulpes* genus weighing 1 kilogram (kg) or less, to subspecies of the gray wolf exceeding 60 kg. Sexual dimorphism occurs in a majority of species, and males are typically larger. Some species are solitary, some form monogamous or seasonally monogamous pairs, whereas others have large, complex packs of multiple generations within a social unit. Large packs of some species make formidable and efficient units capable of preying on larger animals and fending off predators. Many smaller canids forage for prey alone, in pairs, or in small groups. Some species such as the coyote (*C. latrans*) exhibit extreme social flexibility, being capable of existing as solitary individuals, in pairs, or in large complex packs.

A large proportion of the recognized wild canid species currently face the threat of extinction,[39] and numerous subspecies are at risk even when the species may be stable as a whole. Many populations have been extirpated from portions of their historic range. Persecution by humans, the introduction of diseases from domestic dogs, habitat disturbance, and hybridization with domestic or wild canids pose significant threats to the continued survival of many species. At least one species (the Falkland Island wolf, *Dusicyon australis*) has become extinct within the last 150 years (in 1876) as a result of direct human pressure.

UNIQUE ANATOMIC FEATURES

Canids exhibit characteristic skull features, including the medial position of the internal carotid artery between the entotympanic and petrosal arteries, loss of the stapedial artery, and an inflated entotympanic bulla divided by a partial septum. The insertion point of the digastric muscle is widened in several canid taxa, forming a subangular lobe on the horizontal ramus of the mandible, which has been

TABLE 46-1

Canid Species and Population Status[39]

Common Name	Latin Name (Number of Subspecies)	Adult Weight Range (kg)	Status / Population Trend (IUCN Red List)*
Bat-eared fox	*Otocyon megalotis* (2)	3.2–5.4	Least Concern / Unknown
Raccoon dog	*Nyctereutes procyonoides* (6)	2.9–12	Least Concern / Stable
Channel Island fox	*Urocyon littoralis*	1.4–2.5	Critically Endangered / Decreasing
Gray fox	*Urocyon cinereoargenteus* (16)	2–5.5	Least Concern / Stable
Arctic fox	*Alopex lagopus*	2.4–5.4	Least Concern/ Stable
Indian fox	*Vulpes bengalensis*	1.8–3.2	Least Concern / Decreasing
Blanford's fox	*Vulpes cana*	0.8–1.5	Least Concern / Unknown
Cape fox	*Vulpes chama*	2–4.2	Least Concern / Stable
Corsac fox	*Vulpes corsac*	1.6–3.2	Least Concern / Unknown
Tibetan fox	*Vulpes ferrilata*	3–4.6	Least Concern / Unknown
Kit fox	*Vulpes macrotis* (8)	1.6–2.7	Least Concern / Decreasing
Red fox	*Vulpes vulpes*	3.6–8.7	Least Concern / Stable
Swift fox	*Vulpes velox*	1.6–2.5	Least Concern / Stable
Ruppell's fox	*Vulpes rueppelli*	1–2.3	Least Concern / Unknown
Pale fox	*Vulpes pallida* (5)	2–3.6	Least Concern / Unknown
Fennec fox	*Vulpes zerda*	0.8–1.9	Least Concern / Unknown
Dhole	*Cuon alpinus* (9–11)	10–20	Endangered / Decreasing
Side-striped jackal	*Canis adustus*	7.3–12	Least concern / Stable
Golden jackal	*Canis aureus*	6.5–9.8	Least Concern / Increasing
Black-backed jackal	*Canis mesomelas* (6)	5.9–12	Least Concern / Stable
Coyote	*Canis latrans* (19)	7.7–16	Least Concern / Increasing
Gray wolf	*Canis lupus* (13)	20–60†	Least Concern / Stable‡
Red wolf	*Canis rufus*	20–35	Critically Endangered / Increasing
Ethiopian wolf	*Canis simensis*	11–20	Endangered / Decreasing
African wild dog	*Lycaon pictus*	19–35	Endangered / Decreasing
Maned wolf	*Chrysocyon brachyurus*	18–32	Near threatened / Unknown
Bushdog	*Speothos venaticus*	5–8	Threatened / Decreasing
Short-eared dog	*Atelocynus microtis*	9–10	Near Threatened / Declining
Culpeo (Andean fox)	*Pseudalopex culpaeus* (6)	4–11	Least Concern / Stable
Darwin's fox	*Pseudalopex fulvipes*	2–4	Critically Endangered / Decreasing
Chilla	*Pseudalopex griseus* (4)	2.5–5	Least Concern / Stable
Pampas fox	*Pseudalopex gymnocercus* (3)	4.2–5.9	Least Concern / Increasing
Sechuran Desert fox	*Pseudalopex sechurae*	2.6–4.2	Near Threatened / Unknown
Hoary fox	*Pseudalopex veturus*	2.5–4	Least Concern / Unknown
Crab-eating fox	*Cerdocyon thous*	5–7	Least Concern / Stable

*International Union for the Conservation of Nature: *IUCN Red List of Threatened Species. Version 2012.2.* www.iucnredlist.org. Accessed February 1, 2013.
†Significant size variation occurs between subspecies of *Canis lupus*.
‡Status reflects species as a whole; the status of individual subspecies is at varying risks of extinction, and populations are not stable.

hypothesized to be a functional adaptation for rapid jaw movement.[3] The subangular lobe is prominent in foxes with complex molars, including the genera *Urocyon*, *Otocyon*, and *Cerdocyon*, and in raccoon dogs (*Nyctereutes* spp.).[42] The dental formula of Canidae is incisors (I) 3/3, canines (C) 1/1, premolars (P) 4/4, molars (M) 2/2 in all but three genera (*Speothos*, *Cuon*, and *Otocyon*). Although not unique among carnivores, the maxillary fourth premolar and the mandibular first molar of canids are modified to oppose each other and maximize the shearing efficiency when biting into prey. The modified teeth are termed *carnassial* or *sectorial teeth*.

Specialized lateral nasal glands provide moisture for evaporative cooling during panting, which is the primary heat loss mechanism in canids. Sweat glands are only present in the footpads and are not significant to heat dissipation. Cutaneous muscles may control the pelage and serve an important thermoregulatory role. Seasonal molt of the pelage of temperate species is an important adaptation to coping with temperature extremes. Canids have four digits in each of the hindlimbs and five in each of the forelimbs, although the first digit may be rudimentary. The African wild dog (*Lycaon pictus*) is the exception, with only four digits on each limb.

Many of the larger canids are adapted for traveling long distances as they forage or chase prey, and during seasonal migrations. These species have significant aerobic and anaerobic capabilities for running at high speeds over long distances while chasing prey. Canids have refined senses of hearing, smell, and vision, which are key to maintenance of complex social systems, communication between conspecifics, and maintaining territories. Olfactory cues from urine, feces, and anal and supracaudal glands have an important role in canid social interactions.

The supracaudal gland, commonly called the *tail gland* or the *violet gland* because of its production of volatile terpenes similar to those produced by flowers in the Violaceae family, is a specialized scent gland located on the dorsal surface of the tail. The tail gland is located at the level of the seventh to ninth caudal vertebrae and is most developed in solitary fox species (such as Artic, red, and corsac foxes), less developed in jackals,[38] and absent in African wild dogs.[18] Powerful hair erector muscles associated with the tail gland contract to release a lipoprotein onto the surface of the skin,[38] which plays a role in species and individual recognition.

The raccoon dog (*N. procyonoides*) and other species may undergo a period of seasonal torpor or hibernation, characterized by decreased basal metabolic rates and lower levels of cortisol, insulin, and thyroid hormones.[23] The African wild dog lacks variation at the major histocompatibility complex (MHC), which is a fundamental component of the immune response of all vertebrate species and may be the result of population bottlenecks experienced by this species.[24]

SPECIAL HOUSING REQUIREMENTS

In a family with a broad range of body sizes, occupying all possible habitats and maintaining a diversity of social systems, it is nearly impossible to standardize the ideal housing requirements for all species. Guidelines for captive housing space have been established for most canid species by the Association of Zoos and Aquariums.[35] An ideal enclosure takes into account overall holding area, size of the social group being housed, reproductive status of the group, and complexity of the area to elicit and maintain species-appropriate behaviors. The shape of an enclosure must allow animals to fully use the space, allow for proper interindividual distances, and provide flexibility in managing social groups, whose hierarchy and dynamics may change over time. Complex environmental features in enclosures stimulate the natural display of species-appropriate behaviors and likely minimize stress levels. Features in enclosures should allow for social species housed in groups to separate themselves, as needed, in cases of aggression and for packs to display a healthy behavioral repertoire. Gunnite and concrete wall enclosures may create undesirable acoustics that may be disturbing to many canids. Visual barriers and natural plantings provide cover and shade and also serve to muffle unwanted sounds.

Enclosures should not have sharp corners, as these may facilitate upward propulsion and climbing. Animals running along a fence line may reach a corner and may jump upward and fall or do back flips, often injuring themselves. Sharp corners may be difficult for individuals to maneuver when running and may result in traumatic injuries to the skull, face, or neck. Spiral hindlimb fractures occurring in wolves jumping straight up in a corner and landing on one leg have been documented. Additionally, sharp corners may create conditions that provide a subordinate or incompatible individual with no means of escaping an aggressor.

Enclosures should incorporate a holding space and additional holding areas for temporary holding or transfer. For large canids, where single-sex group of two animals or a nonbreeding pair is housed, the primary enclosure should be 5000 square feet (465 square meters [m²]), and an additional 1000 square feet (93 m²) per additional animal.[35] Maned wolves (*Chrysocyon brachyurus*) in this social setting require more space (10,000 square feet [930 m²]). Enclosures housing two large canids or a nonreproductive pair should have at least two holding pens of 200 square feet (19 m²) each.[35]

Large canids housed as a single generation per breeding enclosure should have 10,000 square feet (930 m²) and at least three holding pens of 200 square feet (19 m²) each.[35] Enclosures intended to serve as multigenerational breeding areas need a minimum of 10,000

square feet (930 m²), plus a secondary enclosure of 5000 square feet (465 m²) and at least three holding pens of 200 square feet (19 m²) each. Enclosures holding groups for potential reintroduction to the wild need larger areas (20,000 square feet [1,860 m²]) plus a secondary enclosure of 5000 square feet (465 m²), and at least three holding pens of 200 square feet (19 m²) each, and special attention must be paid to the management practices and location of the enclosures to maintain wild behaviors and avoid imprinting on humans.[35]

Minimum space recommendations for small canids vary by species and social structure. Primary enclosure areas should be at least 6.5 feet (ft.) × 6.5 ft. × 5 ft. tall (2 m × 2 m × 1.5 m) for one or two animals, 10 ft. × 10 ft. × 5 ft. tall (3 m × 3 m × 1.5 m) for three animals, and 13 ft. × 13 ft. × 5 ft. tall (4 m × 4 m × 2 m) for family groups with up to five offspring. These guidelines are currently under revision, but these dimensions should be exceeded, whenever possible, and attention paid to the space layout, complexity, and social needs of the species. Minimum housing guidelines set for domestic dogs by the Animal Welfare Act of the U.S. Department of Agriculture (USDA), section 3.6(c)(1), are not sufficient for all wild canids and should be exceeded.

Canids are proficient diggers and skilled jumpers. When fences are used, fence posts should be buried properly to secure them. These "dig barriers" should be 6 to 12 inches underground and extend 3 feet toward the center of the enclosure to prevent a prolific digger from tunneling under it.[35] Buried concrete barriers may be used underground instead of fencing. Enclosure perimeter barriers should be of appropriate height to prevent an animal from jumping over, and the top could be angled or covered to discourage animals from obtaining footing on the wall and propelling themselves upward. A containment height of 8 ft. is recommended for most large canids as long as the surface does not allow climbing.

Many species may tolerate a wide range of ambient temperatures, but small canids may be less tolerant of temperature extremes when housed outside of their natural climate and require special attention. Tropical species such as maned wolves, bushdogs, and African wild dogs are less tolerant of cold temperatures compared with temperate species of similar size. Species housed outdoors should have access to dry den structures and bedding, as well as shelters that individuals may choose to use for protection from the wind or rain. A periparturient dam should have multiple choices of warm and dry whelping boxes, and attention should be paid to the breeding season and the time of year, as some species will give birth during the colder months in temperate areas.

FEEDING

The diets of wild canids range from omnivory to strict carnivory, and some species consume primarily insectivorous or piscivorous diets. Bushdogs (*Speothos venaticus*), dholes (*Cuon alpinus*), and African wild dogs are highly carnivorous, whereas bat-eared foxes (*Otocyon megalotis*) are almost exclusively insectivorous in the wild. The Ethiopian wolf (*Canis simensis*) is adapted to a diet that is based almost exclusively on rodents, and maned wolves are the most omnivorous of the large canids. The proportion of dietary components varies seasonally among omnivorous species, depending on prey or plant abundance and the breeding season.

The daily caloric need of a large canid (22–32 kg) has been estimated at 1300 to 1800 kilocalories (kcal) metabolizable energy (ME) per day in a thermoneutral environment under moderate activity.[35] Caloric needs should be adjusted on the basis of the life stage of the animal, activity and thermoregulatory needs, and body condition. As a general guideline, the daily ME requirements of adult domestic dogs have been estimated at 50 to 65 kcal/kg of body weight, approximately 120 kcal/kg for growing puppies, 200 kcal/kg for lactating females, and as high as 450 kcal/kg for heavy working dogs.

Canid diets typically contain 20% to 28% protein, 5% to 18% fat, and 2% to 4% crude fiber.[35] This formula is derived from domestic dog requirements. Although it is recognized that species-specific differences exist with regard to some of these needs, objective information is lacking for most species' needs. Canine diets based on raw meat are commercially available and form the basis of captive diets for some species, whereas others may be maintained on dry kibble. Dietary intolerance manifested by gastrointestinal (GI) disturbances, skin reactions, poor pelage, and cachexia have been reported in individuals that are maintained on cereal-based or highly processed grain diets. Omnivorous canids probably require high amounts of dietary fiber and may benefit from the addition of natural fiber sources to their diet, including produce and fruit.

Whole prey items (rodents, rabbits, chickens) or partial carcasses (bones, ox tails, legs, deer) are used to supplement captive diets, but they must be taken into account when calculating overall dietary needs and should not be offered to the degree whereby they offset a balanced diet. Feeding whole or partial carcasses of wild or domestic ungulates often is used to stimulate pack behaviors and for social enrichment. Caution should be exercised to ensure that the carcasses are fresh, free of parasitic or other diseases, and harvested by using methods that do not contain harmful substances (such as lead shot, euthanasia solution, nonsteroidal anti-inflammatory drugs [NSAIDs], or toxins). Additional caution should be exercised in areas where prion diseases (such as bovine spongiform encephalopathy [BSE] or chronic wasting disease [CWD]) are present, since carnivore species may be susceptible to prion-associated neurologic disease. The USDA Animal Welfare Act (Section 13, 9 CFR, Subsection F, Section 3.129) specifically discourages feeding roadkill to large felids but outlines guidelines for proper handling if it must be fed. The same guidelines are applicable to canids. If whole carcasses are fed to animals intended for reintroduction, only carcasses from natural prey species should be offered, and domestic animal carcasses should never be offered, as canids will likely learn to recognize the species offered as possible prey items.[35]

It has been suggested that the maned wolf has lower animal protein needs compared with other canids.[35] Scat studies of wild maned wolves suggest that plant material may account for 50% of their diet, with small mammals, insects, and birds accounting for the rest.[8] Taurine levels should be monitored in captive maned wolves, and supplementation may be necessary on an individual basis.[8] A soy-based pelleted diet has been commercially developed specifically for captive maned wolves, and preliminary results of experimental feeding show improved fecal consistency and body condition scores.

RESTRAINT AND HANDLING

Small canids may be restrained manually or with the use of nets. The use of leather gloves is recommended, but these do not provide full protection against significant bite injuries to a handler. A towel may be used to temporarily immobilize a small canid, and the head may be restrained through the towel by placing a hand behind the head while supporting the body with the other hand. Muzzles designed for domestic dogs may be used for handler protection when handling, and soft cloth rope or cotton roll gauze may be used as an impromptu muzzle. Muzzles must be monitored so that placement allows for normal breathing and avoidance of hyperthermia and should only be used for short periods. Canids may be conditioned for restraint in squeeze cages, and relatively simple ones may be designed and built if none is commercially available. Animals also may be trained for voluntary restraint and to accept injections.

Hyperthermia is a common phenomenon seen in restrained canids, and body temperatures reaching or exceeding 40° C (104° F) warrant intervention. Persistent or prolonged hyperthermia may have a fatal outcome and has been documented in some species, notably dholes. Treatment with intravenous cool fluids and external cooling is warranted to combat hyperthermia, but this should be done slowly and while continuing to monitor body temperature. Sedatives are indicated in the management of stress-related hyperthermia. Some canids are prone to developing exertional myopathies after prolonged restraint, and if the clinician suspects it, supportive treatment should be instituted immediately.

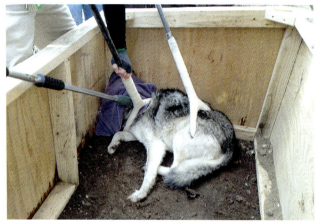

FIGURE 46-1 **Physical restraint of an adult male Mexican gray wolf (*Canis lupus baileyi*).** The individual has been prompted to enter a wooden den box with a hinged top. A restraint pole has been placed on the neck and a towel has been placed over the head while two "Y"-shaped padded poles are placed over the shoulders and hips to prevent the animal from rolling, jumping, or backing up. This mode of restraint provides safe access for limited examinations and performing minor medical procedures. (Photo courtesy of Luis R Padilla, Endangered Wolf Center, Eureka, MO.)

Maned wolves may be physically restrained.[15] Confined gray wolves and red wolves may be physically restrained by experienced crews by using "catch" poles and "Y"-shaped padded poles. A team of people may enter an enclosure and exploit these species' typical aversion to humans, forming a line and funneling the animal into either a corner of an enclosure or a den box. When approached, the animals will often cower, allowing for restraint with a catch pole placed loosely around the neck. Rigid but padded "Y"-shaped poles may be gently, but firmly, placed over the hips and shoulders to prevent an animal from jumping back or rolling while restrained by the catch pole (Figure 46-1). This type of restraint may be used for limited examinations, ultrasonography, blood collection, vaccination, or administration of intravenous injections. This technique is less effective and potentially dangerous when attempting to restrain hand-raised animals and individuals that have no aversion to humans, as they may resist restraint or attempt to attack when cornered and is not recommended for other large canid species (such as African wild dogs). Chemical restraint is recommended for prolonged or invasive procedures involving most large canids.

Trapping is a tool used for the management, relocation, and study of wild canid populations. Box traps have been successfully used for trapping wild canids and are considered more humane and less stressful than other alternatives[47] but are less effective for capturing the majority of wild canid species. Foothold traps (metal "jaw" traps and cable "noose" restraint devices)[6] are used to capture wild canids, specifically wolves, foxes, and dholes, although their use has been outlawed in some countries. Traps should be properly padded and inspected to ensure proper functioning and minimal risk to the animal. Every consideration should be made for humane usage and exclusion of nontarget species. Foothold traps may cause injuries to the feet, legs and teeth,[32] and individuals may develop hyperthermia or myopathy if restraint is prolonged. When initially restrained, some animals may actively dig and pull against the trap and may self-mutilate in trying to escape. If multiple traps are set within a short distance, an animal may be caught in more than one trap, or the mechanism may close around nontarget body parts as the animal rolls, pulls, and tries to escape from the primary restraint. The use of remote monitoring devices (e.g., motion sensors, cameras, and remote alarms that link to personal communication devices) has greatly improved the ability to minimize restraint time, and their use

TABLE 46-2

Select Injectable Anesthetic Combinations Applicable to Canid Species

Species	Suggested Combination
Arctic fox (*Alopex lagopus*)	Ketamine (2.5 mg/kg), Medetomidine (0.05 mg/kg) IM[6]
	Tiletamine-zolazepam (10 mg/kg) IM[6]
Golden jackals (*Canis aureus*)	Ketamine (1.8–2.4 mg/kg), medetomidine (0.09–0.11 mg/kg) IM[15]
	Medetomidine (0.07–0.1 mg/kg), midazolam (0.39–0.55 mg/kg) IM[15]
Coyotes (*Canis latrans*)	Ketamine (4 mg/kg), xylazine (2 mg/kg) IM[6]
	Ketamine (3–4 mg/kg), medetomidine (0.04–0.07 mg/kg) IM
	Telazol (10–11 mg/kg) IM[6]
Gray wolves (*Canis lupus*)	Ketamine (3–4 mg/kg), medetomidine (0.06–0.08 mg/kg) IM[6]
	Medetomidine (0.04 mg/kg), butorphanol (0.4 mg/kg), ketamine (1 mg/kg) IM
	Ketamine (5–10 mg/kg), midazolam (0.1–0.4 mg/kg) IV (after manual restraint)
	Ketamine (4–10 mg/kg), xylazine (1–3 mg/kg) IM[6]
	Telazol (10–13 mg/kg) IM (for helicopter captures)[6]
Red wolves (*Canis rufus*)	Ketamine (2 mg/kg), medetomidine (0.02 mg/kg), butorphanol (0.2 mg/kg) IM6
	Medetomidine (0.04 mg/kg), butorphanol (0.4 mg/kg) IM, supplement with IV diazepam (0.2 mg/kg) or ketamine (1 mg/kg)[6]
	Telazol (5–10 mg/kg) IM[6]
Ethiopian wolves (*Canis simensis*)	Telazol (2–7 mg/kg) IM[23]
Maned wolf (*Canis brachyurus*)	Medetomidine (0.04 mg/kg), butorphanol (0.4 mg/kg) IM
	Dexmedetomidine (0.02 mg/kg), butorphanol (0.4 mg/kg) IM
	Ketamine (2.5 mg/kg), medetomidine (0.08 mg/kg) IM[23]
	Ketamine (6–9 mg/kg), xylazine (0.5–2 mg/kg) IM[23]
	Telazol (3–5 mg/kg)[23]
Dhole (*Canis alpinus*)	Telazol (2 mg/kg), ketamine (2 mg/kg)
	Telazol (4 mg/kg)[16] to (10 mg/kg)[6] IM
African wild dog (*Lycaon pictus*)	Medetomidine (0.04–0.06 mg/kg), butorphanol (0.18–0.3 mg/kg), midazolam (0.18–0.4 mg/kg) IM[11]
	Ketamine (1.5 mg/kg)[18] to (5 mg/kg)[6], medetomidine (0.04 mg/kg)[18] to 0.1 mg/kg)[6] IM
	Telazol (1–4 mg/kg) IM (wild animals may be more sensitive)[23]
Chilla (*Pseudalopex griseus*)	Ketamine (2.5–3.1 mg/kg), medetomidine (0.05–0.06 mg/kg) IM[1]
	Ketamine (9.3–17.7 mg/kg), xylazine (1.2–2.0 mg/kg) IM[1]
	Telazol (1.6–8 mg/kg) IM[1]
Bushdog (*Speothos venaticus*)	Ketamine (5 mg/kg), medetomidine (0.05 mg/kg) IM[7]
	Telazol (3 mg/kg), ketamine (3 mg/kg) IM[7]
	Telazol (10 mg/kg) IM[23]
Red fox (*Vulpes vulpes*)	Ketamine (4 mg/kg), medetomidine (0.02 mg/kg), butorphanol (0.04 mg/kg) IM[23]
	Ketamine (25–30 mg/kg), midazolam (0.6 mg/kg) IM[23]
	Telazol (4–10 mg/kg) IM[23]

Note: Medetomidine and dexmedetomidine should be antagonized with atipamezole. Xylazine may be antagonized with yohimbine or atipamezole.

is reccommended.[22] The use of tranquilizer trap devices has been considered for the capture of some canid species.[37]

A large number of anesthetic protocols have been used for the chemical restraint of canid species.[1,7,11,13,19,23,46] Table 46-2 summarizes some species-specific suggested anesthetic protocols, but readers should consult a more thorough source[23] for specific considerations. In addition, some of these protocols have been used extensively in other canid species despite lack of documentation in the peer-reviewed literature, and clinicians should use a solid understanding of drug mechanisms and sound judgment to extrapolate and use in appropriate situations.

Small canids may be anesthetized with gas anesthetic agents after restraint by hand or confinement in an anesthetic chamber. An injectable tiletamine–zolazepam combination is often used for canid anesthesia because of a relatively wide safety margin, although dose-dependent, prolonged, and rough recoveries are common. Combinations of ketamine with an α_2-adrenergic agonist (xylazine, medetomidine, or dexmedetomidine) have the advantage of reversibility despite concerns with spontaneous arousals and hypertension in many individuals. Variations on combinations of α_2-adrenergic agonists, opioids, and benzodiazepines provide deep sedation and immobilization and reversibility in most species, although anesthetic induction times may be longer than those seen with ketamine-based combinations.

SURGERY

Common surgical problems in nondomestic canids include the repair of lacerations or traumatic wounds, including wounds to the tongue, cheek, or teeth, and orthopedic injuries. Dehiscence of the body wall has been frequently seen after abdominal surgeries in wild canids, and some species will subsequently cannibalize their own internal organs. Good surgical technique, proper pain management, and postoperative restrictions will limit automutilation of the surgical site. Social species such as bushdogs and wild dogs may be particularly challenging, as isolation often leads to increased pacing and activity, and an animal isolated for prolonged periods may not be allowed back into a social group. Alternatively,

TABLE 46-3

Reference Ranges: Hematologic Parameters of Select Canid Species

Parameter	Gray Wolf (*C. lupus*)[18]	Maned Wolf (*C. brachyurus*)[18]	African Wild Dog (*L. pictus*)[18]	Arctic Fox (*A. lagopus*)[18]	Crab-Eating Fox (*C. thous*)[25]
Erythrocytes ($\times 10^6/\mu$L)	5.72–8.36	4.47–6.37	6.84–8.86	7.7–10.1	3.05–6.08
PCV (%)	39.7–56.5	34.3–47.5	38.5–48.7	41.7–54.3	28–53
Hemoglobin (g/dL)	13.3–19.7	11.3–15.9	14.4–17.2	13.7–17.3	10–18.1
MCV (fL)	63.4–78	68.4–83.2	50.8–60.8	49.4–57.8	79.1–100
MCH (pg)	22–27	23.2–28.2	17.5–21.7	16–19.6	26.0–34.9
MCHC (g/dL)	30.5–37.3	31.1–36.1	32.8–37.2	29.6–35.6	30.2–38.5
Leukocytes (/ µL)	6,546–12,868	6,580–14,360	7,340–14,480	3,170–9,350	3,400–23,200
Neutrophils (/ µL)	4353–9719	3669–10,481	5334–11,262	1035–5333	1,460–12,990
Banded neutrophils (/ µL)	0–198	0–395	0–288	0–266	0–700
Lymphocytes (/ µL)	737–2403	1029–3343	570–2724	665–3849	210–3,990
Eosinophils (/ µL)	0–661	0–617	0–658	0–628	270–3,940
Monocytes (/ µL)	0–468	0–334	0–462	0–248	40–2,550
Basophils (/ µL)	0–55	0–79	0–99	0–194	0–520
Platelets ($\times 10^3/$ µL)	166–336	145–285	254–626	225–467	*

*Low value of range published likely not normal based on published average of 233.27 +/– 112.63 $\times 10^3/\mu$l.

fL, Femtoliters; *g/dL*, gram per deciliter; *MCH*, mean corpuscular hemoglobin; *MCHC*, mean corpuscular hemoglobin concentration; *MCV*, mean corpuscular volume; *PCV*, packed cell volume; *pg*, picogram.

reintegration into a social group too soon after a surgical procedure may lead to excessive grooming, licking, or biting at the incision site by conspecifics.

A simple interrupted pattern is the preferred method of abdominal wall closure for most wild canid species.[18] A simple continuous pattern has been advocated as a dependable, time-efficient method of closure of the rectus sheath in domestic dogs with no difference in complications when compared with a simple interrupted pattern,[20] but simple continuous closure of the body wall is not the preferred method in nondomestic canids because of concerns about rapid dehiscence if a knot fails or is chewed at by an individual. Subcuticular skin closure will discourage the grooming or scratching of external sutures.

Cystotomy may be necessary for removal of stones in maned wolves affected by cystinuria, a relatively common condition in this species. In these cases, medical management must accompany surgical intervention, as they are likely to recur. Urethral obstruction may be a life-threatening condition, and the management of these cases may require perineal urethrostomies when medical management is not sufficient. Marsupialization of the bladder to the ventral body wall has been used to establish patency and drainage in cases of extreme, repeated urinary tract obstruction, but this approach only should be used as a last resort. Risks may be life threatening and include repeated urinary tract infections, dermatitis, and urine scalding at the stoma site, dehiscence and detachment of the bladder from the body wall, and possible peritonitis.

Gastric dilatation with volvulus (GDV) and gastric dilatation (GD) without volvulus have been documented in deep-chested canids such as maned, red, and gray wolves. GDV is an acute, life-threatening condition and often is recognized on postmortem examination following unexpected and sudden death. The antemortem diagnosis of GDV and GD is made on the basis of clinical signs and appearance and confirmed by radiography. The predisposing factors in these species are unknown, but the same risk factors as in domestic dogs have been considered, including the protein source of the diet, the kibble size, the amount of food offered, and the individual's age. Feeding an animal shortly after an anesthetic event has been anecdotally linked to GDV. Prompt recognition is vital to survival, and surgical intervention is the only way to correct GDV.

Ovariohysterectomies and castrations are performed for management and contraceptive reasons and for managing reproductive disorders, including pyometra and reproductive tract neoplasms. A reversible vasectomy technique has been documented in bushdogs, and the technique is applicable to other canid species.[7]

PHYSICAL EXAMINATION AND DIAGNOSTICS

The domestic dog is an appropriate model for the physical examination of all canid species. Baseline clinical parameters are similar to those of the domestic dog, although species-specific ranges are available for many species (Tables 46-3 and 46-4).[18,25,35]

DISEASE

Infectious Disease

Canids are susceptible to all diseases of domestic dogs, and special attention is given in this chapter to those of particular importance. Three viral diseases are of outmost importance because of their impact on wild canid populations: rabies, canine distemper, and canine parvovirus.

Rabies is a zoonotic disease caused by a lyssavirus in the Rhabdovirus family. Domestic and wild canid species are geographic reservoirs that maintain species-associated strains that may affect all mammalian species. The distinction between domestic and wild canid rabies may be blurred in areas where domestic canid strains are present but may be maintained by wild canid populations.[36] For instance, a domestic dog strain of rabies has been transmitted by coyotes in south Texas (United States) and Mexico.[5] Rabies has been a continued epizootic threat to the survival of the Ethiopian wolf[33,40] and the African wild dog,[12] and many other canid populations are at risk, specifically following the introduction or spread of domestic dog strains.[33] Jackals often are affected by canine rabies in Africa,[36] but jackals are capable of maintaining rabies cycles independently of domestic dogs.[48] Fluctuations in populations of fox species and raccoon dogs may be attributed to rabies epizootics, even though these species are reservoir hosts for specific strains throughout their range. Oral vaccination of wildlife using recombinant vaccines has been an effective rabies control strategy in certain parts of the world,

TABLE 46-4

Reference Ranges: Serum Biochemical Parameters of Select Canid Species

Parameter	Gray Wolf (*C. lupus*)[3]	Maned Wolf (*C. brachyurus*)[3]	African Wild Dog (*L. pictus*)[3]	Arctic Fox (*A. lagopus*)[3]	Crab-Eating Fox (*C. thous*)[22]
Total protein (g/dL)	5.5–6.9	5.4–7.0	5.5–6.5	5.7–7.1	4.6–9.4
Albumin (g/dL)	3.0–3.8	2.7–3.5	2.8–3.6	3.0–3.8	2–6.2
Globulin (g/dL)	2.1–3.3	2.4–3.8	2.5–3.3	2.3–3.9	1.9–7.5
Calcium (mg/dL)	9.2–10.8	9.1–10.5	9.3–10.9	8.3–11.1	
Phosphorus (mg/dL)	2.2–5.4	3.3–8.5	2.6–6.4	2.1–5.1	
Sodium (mEq/L)	144–154	141–149	144–152	144–154	
Potassium (mEq/L)	4.1–5.1	4.3–5.3	3.9–4.7	4.1–5.3	
Chloride (mEq/L)	112–120	110–118	112–120	108–118	
Creatinine (mg/dL)	0.7–1.7	0.9–1.7	0.9–1.5	0.7–1.1	0.5–1.5
Urea nitrogen (mg/dL)	14–32	14–32	15–33	7–39	22–87
Cholesterol (mg/dL)	118–248	203–571	199–311	151–223	
Glucose (mg/dL)	91–157	90–140	113–181	109–189	

g/dL, Gram per deciliter; *mEq/L*, milliequivalent per liter; *mg/dL*, milligram per deciliter.

and individuals under human care often are immunized with injectable killed rabies vaccine products.

Canine distemper virus (CDV) poses a worldwide threat to canid populations. Natural epizootics occur in wild populations, but the periodic introduction and maintenance of this virus in domestic dogs poses a threat to endangered species such as African wild dogs and Ethiopian wolves.[44,45] CDV infection has occurred in African wild dogs despite vaccination.[48] Vaccine-induced CDV infection has occurred or been suspected following the use of modified-live vaccines in canid species, including gray foxes (*Urocyon cinereoargenteus*),[14] African wild dogs,[9] and bushdogs.[26]

Canine parvovirus is very common in serosurveys of wild canid populations and is a likely factor in juvenile mortality in some species. Parvovirus has caused significant morbidity and mortality in captive animals, with notable cases in bushdogs.[17] Vaccination using modified live vaccines has raised concerns about causing disease in some species and is not recommended for vaccination of maned wolf pups until protective titers are present after using a killed parvovirus vaccine.[35]

Canine adenovirus causes hepatitis in domestic dogs and may affect all canid species. In some species, the disease has a clinical presentation similar to that of canine distemper and has been dubbed "fox encephalitis" because of the predominance of neurologic signs.

All bacterial diseases of domestic dogs may affect their nondomestic counterparts. Brucellosis and leptospirosis have been of concern in certain coyote populations, and numerous strains of leptospira organisms have been suspected in individual infections. Serosurveys of coyote and swift fox (*Vulpes velox*) populations within the geographic range of *Yersinia pestis* (plague) have suggested that infection is common within the endemic range and may play a role in the epidemiology of their disease by carrying flea vectors.

Neorickettsia helminthoeca is a rickettsial organism that causes salmon poisoning in canids. The organism is transmitted by *Nanophyetus salmincola*, an intestinal fluke of canids in the northwestern United States and southwestern Canada.[18] Canids become infected by ingesting fish or amphibians with encysted metacercariae, although the flukes themselves do not cause clinical disease. *Anaplasma phagocytophilum* has been reported as the cause of acute respiratory disease, lethargy, and neurologic signs in captive maned wolves at one facility in Virginia (eastern United States), although seroprevalence in that population suggests that infection is also possible without overt clinical signs.[30]

All known parasitic diseases of domestic dogs are likely to affect wild canids within a certain geographic range. *Giardia*, *Cryptosporidium*, *Eimeria*, and *Isospora* are often seen in nondomestic canids; clinical signs are similar to those seen in domestic dogs and are most significant in juveniles. Babesiosis has been reported in maned wolves in the United States[31] and in South America.[4]

Roundworms, hookworms, and whipworms affect all canids and are suspected to be pathogenic in pups, but clinical disease is often absent in adults. *Dirofilaria immitis* (the cause of heartworm disease) may affect all canid species, although it has been suspected that other parasites may cause cardiac infections. Cardiac ultrasonography detected adult nematodes, suggesting the presence of heartworms in the right pulmonary arteries of two maned wolves that had been prophylactically treated with ivermectin (0.2 mg/kg, orally [PO], monthly) for 2 years prior to detection. Neither wolf showed signs of clinical infection, and blood-based screening tests had been negative for both animals.[10] Trichinosis has been diagnosed in wild Arctic foxes (*Alopex lagopus*), and infection is often attributed to feeding on polar bear carcasses.

Spirocerca lupi is a parasite of canids that may be found in the gastric, esophageal, or aortic wall and usually requires a coprophagous arthropod as an intermediate host, but many species may serve as paratenic hosts. Aortic aneurysms and acute death have been associated with parasitism by *S. lupi* in bushdogs[34] and wild coyotes, and may occur in other canids.

Nematodes from the respiratory tract (*Angiostrongylus vasorum*, *Eucoleus aerophilus*, *Crenosoma vulpis*) commonly affect wild canids.[28,29] The renal parasite *Dioctophyma renale* has been documented in maned wolves, bushdogs, raccoon dogs, coyotes, jackals, red and gray wolves, and foxes.[18] The intermediate host is an aquatic oligochete, although canids get infected when consuming piscean, amphibian, or invertebrate paratenic hosts in the endemic geographic areas. The adult worms usually are found in the right kidney, which often becomes nonfunctional. Diagnosis may be made by ultrasonography or by the presence of ova shed in the urine.

Hepatozoonosis affects coyotes in North America, but recent studies suggest that a great diversity of *Hepatozoon* species occur throughout the range.[41] Encephalitozoonosis is an important disease affecting wild and farmed foxes worldwide and has been reported in African wild dog pups.[45]

Wild canids are reservoirs for two genera of cestodes (*Taenia* and *Echinococcus*), which are significant zoonotic parasites and a risk to other mammalian species.[18] Clinical disease is rare in the canid hosts, but the eggs are shed in canid feces and ingested by an intermediate or aberrant host where clinical signs may occur. Three *Echinococcus* species (*E. granulosus, E. multilocularis,* and *E. vogeli*) maintain their cycles through a definite canid host and its herbivorous prey (rodents, rabbits, sheep, goats, deer, camels, macropods). *Dipylidium caninum* may affect wild canid species, and transmission usually occurs by ingestion of fleas.[18]

Pancreatic flukes (*Eurytrema procyonis*) have been documented in maned wolves in the Midwestern United States[15] and in foxes throughout the United States. Clinical signs are associated with maldigestion and include weight loss and poorly formed stools.

Many ectoparasites (fleas, ticks, chiggers, and lice) are known to affect canids. They may be a significant cause of anemia in juveniles and neonates and may serve as vectors of tick-borne diseases (anaplasmosis, babesiosis, ehrlichiosis, borreliosis).

Noninfectious Diseases

Inflammatory bowel disease (IBD) is a common cause of chronic GI disease (vomiting and diarrhea), weight loss, poor pelage, and overall malaise in several large canid species (notably maned wolves and gray wolves). Hypoproteinemia, specifically hypoalbuminemia, is a significant component of the disease, often leading to ascites. Profound hypoalbuminemia and ascites are poor prognostic indicators. IBD is an inflammatory cell infiltration of the lamina propria (typically lymphocytes, plasma cells, eosinophils, macrophages, and neutrophils), but the predominance of each cell type may correspond to slightly different disease characterization, prognosis, and treatment needs. The term "IBD" should never be used to characterize clinical signs, as these are shared with other conditions. Differential diagnoses include other malabsorption diseases, pancreatic disease (exocrine insufficiency), parasitic and infectious diseases (viruses and bacterial overgrowth), enterocolitis, dietary intolerance, and neoplastic disease. IBD is not synonymous with dietary intolerance or a food allergy to a dietary component.

The etiology of IBD is typically unknown but is believed to involve impaired immunoregulation in the response of gut-associated lymphoid tissue to antigenic stimuli. Bacteria in the gut lumen and parasitic or dietary agents may serve as antigenic initiators to an excessive, chronic gut immune inflammatory response. A presumptive diagnosis of IBD often is made on the basis of clinical signs after excluding other differential diagnoses, but a confirmatory diagnosis requires gut biopsies. Primary treatment modalities mimic those used in IBD in domestic dogs and require supportive care based on the severity of signs and clinical pathology findings. Immunomodulation (either through corticosteroids, immunosuppressive agents, or sulfasalazine), dietary modification (hypoallergenic diets, easily digestible diets), antibiotics (to decrease bacterial overgrowth), and supportive care (fluids, possibly colloids in cases of hypoproteinemia) are the main components of therapy. Supplementation of cobalamine and folate may be beneficial.

Cystinuria is a prevalent condition in maned wolves, both in human care and in the wild, and may have a genetic basis.[15] Cystinuria is often subclinical,[15] but the precipitation of calculi in the urinary tract may have life-threatening consequences if urinary obstructions occur. Obstructions are more likely to occur in males (because of the size and length of the urethra) than in females, although cystinuria occurs equally in both sexes. The persistence of cystine crystals in the urinary tract may predispose to urinary tract infections. Long-term (likely lifelong) medical therapy is essential to managing cystinuria. Surgery is indicated in cases of urethral obstructions that cannot be relieved or when large calculi (stones) are present. Medical therapy is aimed at affecting the solubility of cystine to prevent crystal precipitation and stone formation and reducing the concentration of cystine in the urine. Urine alkalinization has been a mainstay of medical management, as urine pH affects the solubility of cystine. Potassium citrate is the preferred urine alkalinization agent. Sodium bicarbonate has been used as a urinary alkalinization agent, but it is not preferred, since sodium intake increases cystine excretion. Dietary manipulation, specifically decreasing

sodium intake and reducing protein from animal sources (which are higher in sulfur-containing amino acids), is a theoretical means to reducing cystinuria but has not been systemically tested in maned wolves. Tiopronin has been used as a pharmacologic means of modifying the cystine molecule into a more soluble form in domestic dogs[16] and has shown some success in maned wolves despite the high cost, low availability in the United States, and potential side effects with long-term use. Other thiol-based agents such as D-penicillamine have been used with some success in maned wolves with cystinuria. Close monitoring of maned wolves for stranguria is an essential part of the routine care of this species.

Pododermatitis may cause significant morbidity in canids[35] and is an important disease in neonates. Because of their predisposition to dig, many canids suffer traumatic lesions to their pads, including abrasions, pad or nail avulsions, and lacerations. Wounds may become infected, often leading to pododermatitis. Neonates housed on rough surfaces or den boxes may dig or repeatedly push aside bedding material, leading to lesions that often get infected because of the limited mobility of the neonates. *Staphylococcus* spp. and gram-negative bacteria often invade pododermatitic lesions and likely reflect contamination from the adjacent skin or of enteric origin. Interdigital dermatitis and edema have been seen in maned wolves, Mexican gray wolves, fennec foxes (*Vulpes zerda*), and other species. Although the etiology is unknown, tissues between the digits and pads on the plantar surface become erythematous, abraded, and moist. Some of these lesions may be the result of excessive moisture leading to dermatitis and resolve with appropriate disinfection and oral antimicrobials. In some instances, biopsy of nonhealing lesions has been suggestive of an auto-immune component and has responded to treatment with oral prednisone in addition to antibiotics.

A few cases of progressive retinal atrophy have been documented in red and gray wolves.[35] Gingival hyperplasia (proliferative gingivitis) may occur as a result of chronic gingivitis and dental disease and has been documented in maned wolves of all ages. A genetic predisposition is also possible.

Prolonged, cyclic exposure to endogenous steroids associated with the obligate hormonal pseudopregnancy that follows ovulation in female canids has been associated with uterine pathology, including the cystic endometrial hyperplasia–pyometra complex. Progressive uterine growth, infertility, infections, neoplasms, and mammary proliferation have been linked to the use of steroid contraceptives and are not recommended for long-term contraception. Specifically, the use of melengestrol acetate implants for contraception has been associated with endometrial hyperplasia, hydrometra, fibrosis, adenomyosis, and uterine mineralization.[27]

Although all canids are predisposed to the same neoplasms as their domestic canine counterparts, cranial, oral, or facial squamous cell carcinomas seem to be disproportionately common in Mexican gray wolves (*Canis lupus baileyi*). Dysgerminomas have been often reported in maned wolves.[15]

REPRODUCTION

The reproductive system of canids is unique among mammals. Most canids exhibit monogamy, exceptionally long proestrous and diestrous phases, a copulatory lock, behavioral suppression of mating in the subordinate young within a social group, and obligate pseudopregnancy in subordinate females.[2] Most wild canids are seasonal breeders, but notable exceptions exist in the small or tropical canids such as bushdogs, in which the females do not have a rigid, single breeding cycle.[8] Some species may naturally exhibit seasonality in the wild, but not in captivity, and the seasonality of tropical species may be dependent on prey cycles, which follow seasonal rainfall.[2] Mounting evidence suggests that some species, notably the smaller canid species, likely have induced estrus cycles.[3] The copulatory lock is an important mechanism in canid mating behavior, and it may be extremely prolonged in some species such as the fennec fox, with a mean duration of almost 2 hours.[43]

TABLE 46-5

Reproductive Parameters of Select Canid Species

Species	Reproductive Cycle	Gestation (days)	Litter Size
Bat-eared fox (*Otocyon megalotis*)	Monestrus	60–70	2–6
Fennec fox (*Vulpes zerda*)	Monestrus	50–53	1–5
Bushdog (*Speothos venaticus*)	Monestrus or polyestrus	65–70	1–6
Maned wolf (*Canis brachyurus*)	Monestrus	63–67	2–5
Dhole (*C. alpinus*)	Monestrus, possibly seasonally polyestrus	60–62	2–7
African wild dog (*Lycaon pictus*)	Monestrus	69–72	2–20
Red wolf (*C. rufus*)	Monestrus	60–63	4–5
Coyote (*C. latrans*)	Monestrus	60–63	1–18
Mexican gray wolf (*C. lupus baileyi*)	Monestrus	60–63	4–5

Pseudopregnancy is the term used to refer to the prolonged luteal phase following ovulation in canids, which often may be as long as pregnancy. In a pack setting, the hormonal changes associated with pseudopregnancy likely prepare subordinate females to assist in the communal rearing of offspring, and some females may even lactate.[2] Table 46-5 summarizes the reproductive features of select species.

PREVENTIVE MEDICINE

Preventive medicine guidelines for captive canids may follow the same basic principles of domestic dog medicine, and no single protocol is likely to be applicable to all situations. Standardized quarantine guidelines have been established for large canids.[35] Routine prophylaxis against *Dirofilaria immitis* (heartworm) should be considered mandatory in all endemic areas where canids are managed. Routine prevention against ectoparasites is recommended, and most commercially available products used for tick and flea management in domestic dogs may be used in wild species of canids.

Vaccination protocols (Table 46-6) must be designed on the basis of diseases present in the geographic location and the risk of exposure. Rabies, canine distemper, and parvovirus are the "core" diseases affecting canids and deserve special consideration when developing vaccination protocols. Multivalent vaccines have been used in many canid species without adverse effects and are widely available commercially, but some veterinarians prefer to use monovalent products to minimize the risk of possible effects. Modified-live vaccines must be used with caution, as vaccine-induced diseases (distemper and parvovirus) have been seen in some species.[9,14,26] Genetically modified canary-pox vectored vaccines are a safe alternative and are commonly used since they cannot induce disease.

TABLE 46-6

Suggested Vaccine Protocols for Nondomestic Canids

Disease	Vaccine Type	Frequency	Notes
Canine distemper virus (CDV)	All canids: Recombinant canary pox vectored vaccine[a] Modified live vaccines recommended for Mexican gray wolves (*Canis lupus baileyi*)[b] and red wolves (*C. rufus*)[c]	Begin at 6–9 weeks, booster every 2–3 weeks until 16–20 weeks, then yearly or check titers (Rodden AZA)	Recombinant canary pox vectored vaccine[a] is safe, cannot induce CDV disease, and is recommended for all susceptible exotic carnivores[a]
Rabies	All canids: Killed virus vaccine[d,e]	Administer at 16 weeks, booster at 1 year of age, then annually[d] or every third year,[e] depending on product used	A recombinant canary-pox vectored vaccine[f] is available and may be used at veterinarian's discretion, especially for small canids, then booster yearly
Parvovirus	Killed vaccine safest Modified live vaccine used in red wolves,[g] gray wolves,[c] and adult maned wolves Maned wolves should be vaccinated with a killed vaccine product[h] until protective titers (>80) are present, then boostered with a modified live vaccine to avoid vaccine-associated disease	Begin at 6–9 weeks, booster every 2–3 weeks until 16–20 weeks, then yearly or check titers	Concerns with vaccine-induced disease in canids when using modified-live products, and strategy used for maned wolves may be appropriate for other species

Products available in the United States:
[a]Merial, PUREVAX: ferret distemper vaccine.
[b]Schering-Plough Galaxy D: modified live distemper vaccine.
[c]Pfizer Animal Health Vanguard 5: modified live modified live distemper, canine adenovirus type 1 and 2, parainfluenza and parvovirus vaccine.
[d]Merial IMRAB 1: rabies vaccine
[e]Merial IMRAB 3: rabies vaccine
[f]Merial PUREVAX: feline rabies vaccine
[g]Merial RECOMBITEK: modified live canine parvovirus vaccine.
[h]Fort Dodge FeloVax PCT: killed feline panleukopenia vaccine, includes feline rhinotracheitis and feline calicivirus.

Vaccination against coronavirus, Lyme disease, and leptospirosis should be considered if warranted by local disease risks. It must be noted that despite their taxonomic proximity to domestic dogs, all vaccines used in nondomestic canids are considered "off label."

ACKNOWLEDGMENT

This chapter is dedicated to Dr. Holly Reed, friend and former veterinary advisor to the Red Wolf Species Survival Plan, and we honor her positive attitude, knowledge, passion, and dedication to advancing canid and conservation medicine.

REFERENCES

1. Acosta-Jamett G, Astorga-Arancibia F, Cunningham AA: Comparison of chemical immobilization methods in wild foxes (*Pseudalopex griseus* and *Pseudalopex culpaeus*) in Chile. *J Wildl Dis* 46(4):1204–1213, 2010.
2. Asa CS, Valdespino C: Canid reproductive biology: An integration of proximate mechanisms and ultimate causes. *Am Zool* 38:251–259, 1998.
3. Asa CS, Bauman JE, Coonan TJ, et al: Evidence of induced estrus or ovulation in a canid, the Island fox (*Urocyon littoralis*). *J Mammal* 88(2):436–440, 2007.
4. Cansi ER, Bonorino R, Mustafus VS, et al: Multiple parasitism in wild maned wolf (*Chrysocyon brachyurus*, Mammalia: Canidae) in Central Brazil. *Comp Clin Pathol* 21(4):489–493, 2012.
5. Clark KA, Neill SU, Smith JS, et al: Epizootic canine rabies transmitted by coyotes in south Texas. *J Am Vet Med Assoc* 204(4):536–540, 1994.
6. Darrow PA, Skirpstunas RT, Carlson SW, Shivik JA: Comparison of injuries to coyote from 3 types of cable foot-restraints. *J Wildl Manag* 73(8):1441–1444, 2009.
7. DeMatteo K, Silber S, Porton I, et al: Preliminary tests of a new reversible male contraceptive in bush dog, *Speothos venaticus*: Open-ended vasectomy and microscopic reversal. *J Zoo Wildl Med* 37(3):313–317, 2006.
8. DeMatteo KE, Porton IJ, Kleiman DG, et al: The effect of the male bush dog (*Speothos venaticus*) on the female reproductive cycle. *J Mammal* 87(4):723–732, 2006.
9. Durchfield B, Baumgartner W, Herbst W, Brahm R: Vaccine-associated canine distemper infection in a litter of African hunting dogs (*Lycaon pictus*). *Zentralbl Vet B* 37(3):203–212, 1990.
10. Estrada AH, Gerlach TJ, Schmidt MK, et al: Cardiac evaluation of clinically healthy captive maned wolves (*Chrysocyon brachyurus*). *J Zoo Wildl Med* 40(3):478–486, 2009.
11. Fleming GJ, Citino SB, Bush M: Reversible anesthetic combination using medetomidine-butorphanol-midazolam in in-situ African wild dogs (*Lycaon pictus*). *Proc Am Assoc Zoo Vet* 214–215, 2006.
12. Gascoyne SC, Lavrenson MK, Lelo S, et al: Rabies in African wild dogs (*Lycaon pictus*) in the Serengeti region, Tanzania. *J Wildl Dis* 29(3):396–402, 1993.
13. Grassman L, Janecka J, Austin S, et al: Chemical immobilization of free-ranging dhole (*Cuon alpinus*), binturong (*Arctictis binturong*), and yellow-throated marten (*Martes flavigula*) in Thailand. *Eur J Wildl Res* 52(4):297–300, 2006.
14. Halbrooks RD, Swango LJ, Schnurrenberger PR, et al: Response of gray foxes to modified live-virus canine distemper vaccines. *J Am Vet Med Assoc* 179(11):1170–1174, 1981.
15. Hammond EE: Medical management of maned wolves (*Chrysocyon brachyurus*). In Miller RE, Fowler M, editors: *Fowler's zoo and wild animal medicine: Current therapy*, vol 7, St. Louis, MO, 2012, Saunders, pp 451–457.
16. Hoppe A: Cystinuria in the dog: Clinical studies during 14 years of medical treatment. *J Vet Int Med* 15(4):361–367, 2001.
17. Janssen DL, Bartz CR, Bush M, et al: Parvovirus enteritis in vaccinated juvenile bush dogs. *J Am Vet Med Assoc* 181(11):1225–1227, 1982.
18. Kennedy-Stoskopf S: Canidae. In Fowler ME, Miller RE, editors: *Fowler's zoo and wild animal medicine*, ed 5, St. Louis, MO, 2003, Saunders.
19. King R, Lapid R, Epstein A, et al: Field anesthesia of golden jackals (*Canis aureus*) with the use of medetomidine-ketamine or medetomidine-midazolam with atipamezole reversal. *J Zoo Wildl Med* 39(4):576–581, 2008.
20. Kummeling A, van Sluijs FJ: Closure of the rectus sheath with a continuous looped suture and the skin with staples in dogs: Speed, safety, and costs compared to closure of the rectus sheath with interrupted sutures and the skin with a continuous subdermal suture. *Vet Quart* 20(4):126–130, 1998.
21. Kyle CJ, Johnson AR, Patterson BR, et al: Genetic nature of eastern wolves: Past, present, and future. *Conserv Gen* 7:273–287, 2006.
22. Larkin RP, VanDeelen TR, Sabick RM, et al: Electronic signaling for prompt removal of an animal from a trap. *Wildl Soc Bull* 31(2):392–398, 2003.
23. Larsen RS, Kreeger TJ: Canids. In West G, Heard D, Caulkett N, editors: *Zoo animal and wildlife immobilization and anesthesia*, Ames, IA, 2007, Wiley-Blackwell.
24. Marsden CD, Mable BK, Woodroffe R, et al: Highly endangered African wild dogs (*Lycaon pictus*) lack variation at the major histocompatibility complex. *J Hered* 100(S1):S54–S65, 2009.
25. Mattoso CRS, Catenacci LS, Beier SL, et al: Hematologic, serum biochemistry and urinary values for captive Crab-eating Fox (*Cerdocyon thous*) in São Paulo state, Brazil. *Pesq Vet Bras* 32(6):559–566, 2012.
26. McInnes EF, Burroughs RE, Duncan NM: Possible vaccine-induced canine distemper in a South American bush dog (*Speothos venaticus*). *J Wildl Dis* 28(4):614–617, 1992.
27. Moresco A, Munson L, Gardner IA: Naturally occurring and melengestrol acetate-associated reproductive tract lesions in zoo canids. *Vet Pathol* 46(6):1117–1128, 2009.
28. Morgan ER, Tomlinson A, Hunter S, et al: *Angiostrongylus vasorum* and *Eucoleus aerophilus* in foxes (*Vulpes vulpes*) in Great Britain. *Vet Parasitol* 154(1–2):48–57, 2008.
29. Nevárez A, López A, Conboy G, et al: Distribution of *Crenosoma vulpis* and *Eucoleus aerophilus* in the lung of free-ranging red foxes (*Vulpes vulpes*). *J Vet Diagn Invest* 17(5):486–489, 2005.
30. Padilla LR, Bratthauer A, Ware LH, et al: *Anaplasma phagocytophilum* infection in captive maned wolves (*Chrysocyon brachyurus*) at the Smithsonian Conservation Biology Institute. *Proc Am Assoc Zoo Vet* 162, 2010.
31. Phair KA, Carpenter JW, Smee N, et al: Severe anemia caused by babesiosis in a maned wolf (*Chrysocyon brachyurus*). *J Zoo Wildl Med* 43(1):162–167, 2012.
32. Phillips RL, Gruver KS, Williams ES: Leg injuries to coyotes in three types of foothold traps. *Wildl Soc Bull* 24(2):260–263, 1996.
33. Randall DA, Williams SD, Kuzmin IV, et al: Rabies in endangered Ethiopian wolves. *Emerg Infect Dis* 10(12):2214–2217, 2004.
34. Rinas M, Nesnek R, Kinsella JM, DeMatteo KE: Fatal aortic aneurysm and rupture in a neotropical bush dog (*Speothos venaticus*) caused by *Spirocerca lupi*. *Vet Parasitol* 164(1–2):347–349, 2009.
35. Rodden M, Siminski P, Waddell W: *AZA canid TAG: Large canid (Canidae) care manual*, Silver Spring, MD, 2012, Association of Zoos and Aquariums.
36. Sabeta CT, Bingham J, Nel LH: Molecular epidemiology of canid rabies in Zimbabwe and South Africa. *Virus Res* 91(2):203–211, 2003.
37. Sahr DP, Knowlton FF: Evaluation of tranquilizer trap devices (TTDs) for foothold traps used to capture gray wolves. *Wildl Soc Bull* 28(3):597–605, 2000.
38. Shabadash SA, Zelikina TI: The tail gland of canids. *Biol Bull Russian Acad Sci* 31(4):367–376, 2004.
39. Sillero-Zubiri C, Hoffmann M, Macdonald DW: *Canids: foxes, wolves, jackals and dogs. Status survey and conservation action plan*, Cambridge, U.K., 2004, IUCN/SSC Canid Specialist Group.
40. Sillero-Zubiri C, King AA, Macdonald DW: Rabies and mortality in Ethiopian wolves (*Canis simensis*). *J Wildl Dis* 32(1):80–86, 1996.
41. Starkey LA, Panciera RJ, Paras K, et al: Genetic diversity of *Hepatozoon* spp. in coyotes from the South Central United States. *J Parasitol* 99(2):375–378, 2013.

42. Tedford RH, Tayler BE, Wang X: *Phylogeny of the Caninae (Carnivora: Canidae): The living taxa.* In *American Museum Novitates 3146,* New York, 1995, American Museum of Natural History.

43. Valdespino C, Asa CS, Bauman JE: Estrous cycles, copulation and pregnancy in the fennec fox (*Vulpes zerda*). *J Mammal* 83(1):99–109, 2002.

44. Van de Bildt MWG, Kuiken T, Visee AM, et al: Distemper outbreak and its effect on African wild dog conservation. *Emerg Infect Dis* 8(2):211–213, 2002.

45. Van Heerden J, Bainbridge N, Burroughs RE, et al: Distemper-like disease and encephalitozoonosis in wild dogs (*Lycaon pictus*). *J Wildl Dis* 25(1):70–75, 1989.

46. Ward DG, Blyde D, Lemon J, Johnston S: Anesthesia of captive African wild dogs (*Lycaon pictus*) using a medetomidine-ketamine-atropine combination. *J Zoo Wildl Med* 37(2):160–164, 2006.

47. White PJ, Kreeger TK, Seal US, Tester JR: Pathological responses of red foxes to capture in box traps. *J Wildl Manag* 55(1):75–80, 1991.

48. Zulu GC, Sabeta CT, Nel LH: Molecular epidemiology of rabies: Focus on domestic dogs (*Canis familiaris*) and black-backed jackals (*Canis mesomelas*) from northern South Africa. *Virus Res* 140(1–2):71–78, 2009.

CHAPTER 47

Felidae

Nadine Lamberski

BIOLOGY

The family Felidae consists of at least 36 wild cat species. These felids are morphologically similar with rounded, flat faces, facial whiskers, large eyes, and large ears. They have the widest range of body sizes of all living carnivore families, weighing 1 kilogram (kg) to 300 kg. They occupy diverse habitats and are distributed naturally throughout the world except Antarctica and Australia, where they have been introduced by humans.

Felid taxonomy has been intensively studied and yet remains controversial. The number of genera recognized is variable. Although in the past four genera were lumped together, currently at least 12 genera are recognized based on several studies of morphology and genetics.[31] Taxonomy and biostatistics for felids may be found in Table 47-1.

STATUS AND CONSERVATION

Wild felids are predators requiring large areas of habitat with suitable prey density. Human population growth has negatively impacted both these requirements, resulting in a decline in all felid species worldwide in range and number. Felidae are among the most threatened groups of mammals. Larger species are heavily persecuted because of the danger they pose to humans and livestock. Small cat species are also persecuted and are harvested for the fur trade. The International Union for the Conservation of Nature (IUCN) Red List designates 29 of 36 wild felid species as having a decreasing population trend. Nearly 50% of all felid species are listed in the top three threatened categories, and seven of these species are listed as Critically Endangered or Endangered. Felids characterized as threatened are those that appear to be naturally rare with limited distribution or those that have become threatened because of human factors. The Iberian lynx, listed as Critically Endangered, fits into both categories and may become the first cat species to become extinct in modern times.[23,31]

UNIQUE ANATOMY AND SPECIAL PHYSIOLOGY

The anatomy of nondomestic felids is similar to that of the domestic cat. Sexual dimorphism is limited with males generally 5% to 10% larger than females. There are 28 or 30 teeth with the following dental formula: incisors (I) 3/3, canines (C) 1/1, premolars (P) 2-3/2, molars (M) 1/1. The incisors are small and are used for nipping flesh from carcasses. Canines are long with a length-wise groove in the enamel and are used to kill prey. The fourth upper premolars (carnassial teeth) are used to slice meat. The reduced dentition allows for a reduced length of the skull and mandibles, which improves efficiency of the muscles that close the jaw. Cats have a more powerful bite relative to muscle mass than any other carnivore except mustelids. Because of their carnivorous diet, cats have a shorter digestive tract with a smaller cecum and a short large intestine.[31]

The forelimbs are used for locomotion and prey capture. To grasp prey, supination of the paw is needed. This increased mobility of the elbow and wrist joints affects running. Canids run faster as they have stiffer forelimbs. The hindlimbs are the propulsers, and the reduction or loss of a clavicle increases stride length. Cats are digitigrade, with five toes in the front and four in the back. The first digit on the front foot is the dewclaw. All felids have retractable claws, the exception being the cheetah, in which retraction is less developed. Cheetahs lack the fleshy sheath protecting the claw.[31]

A key characteristic that was used to separate the big cats (Pantherinae) from the small cats (Felinae) is the presence of an elastic ligament in the hyoid apparatus below the tongue, which was thought to allow the big cats to roar but not purr. Conversely, the bony hyoid of the small cats was thought to allow them to purr but not roar. More recent studies comparing the hyoid structure and vocal abilities dispute this correlation. It has been found that the main difference between the roaring, nonpurring cats and the others was the presence of long, fleshy, elastic vocal folds within the larynx

TABLE 47-1

Taxonomy and Biostatistics

Category*	Native Region	Genus and Species	Common Name	Longevity (Years)	Adult Mass (kg)	Gestation (Days)
		GENUS FELIS				
LC	Europe, Africa, Asia	F. silvestris	Wild cat	19	5.0–8.0	64–67
LC	North Africa to Indochina, Sri Lanka	F. chaus	Jungle cat	20	3.0–16	63–66
NT	North Africa, Arabia, Asia	F. margarita	Sand cat	13.9	2.75	67
VU	South Africa	F. nigripes	Black-footed cat	12	1.3–2.3	63–68
		GENUS OTOCOLOBUS				
NT	Iran to China	O. manul	Pallas cat	16	2.5–4.5	66–75
		GENUS LYNX				
LC	North America	L. canadensis	Canada lynx	17	8.0–18.0	62–74
LC	Europe, Asia	L. lynx	Eurasian lynx	24	18.0–30.0	67–74
CR	South Europe	L. pardinus	Iberian lynx	13	9.0–27.0	60
LC	North America	L. rufus	Bobcat	32	4.0–18.0	60–70
		GENUS CARACAL				
LC	Africa, Arabia, Asia	C. caracal	Caracal	17	9.0–18.0	78–81
NT	West Africa, Central Africa	C. aurata	African golden cat	21	5.5–16.0	75
		GENUS LEPTAILURUS				
LC	Africa	L. serval	Serval	23	7.0–18.0	66–77
		GENUS PARDOFELIS				
VU	South Asia, Southeast Asia	P. marmorata	Marbled cat	12	2.0–5.0	66–82
EN	Borneo	P. badia	Bornean bay cat	No data	3.0–4.0	70–75
NT	Southeast Asia	P. temminckii	Asian golden cat	23	9.0–16.0	91–95
		GENUS PRIONAILURUS				
LC	South Asia, East Asia	P. bengalensis	Leopard cat	17	3.0–7.0	65–72
VU	India, Sri Lanka	P. rubiginosa	Rusty-spotted cat	18	0.9–1.6	65–70
EN	South Asia, Southeast Asia	P. viverrinus	Fishing cat	17	5.0–16.0	63–70
EN	Borneo, Sumatra, Malaya	P. planiceps	Flat-headed cat	14	1.5–2.5	56
		GENUS LEOPARDUS				
NT	Central America, South America	L. colocolo	Pampas cat	16	3.0–7.0	80–85
LC	North America, Central America, South America	L. pardalis	Ocelot	20	8.0–18.0	79–82
NT	Central America, South America	L. wiedii	Margay	24	2.6–4.0	76–84
VU	Central America, South America	L. tigrinus	Little spotted cat or oncilla	23	1.5–3.0	74–76
NT	South America	L. geoffroyi	Geoffroy's cat	23	2.0–5.0	72–78
VU	South America	L. guigna	Kodkod or guiña	14	2.0–2.5	72–78
EN	South America	L. jacobita	Andean mountain cat	16.5	4.0	No data
		GENUS PUMA				
LC	North America, Central America, South America	P. yagouaroundi	Jaguarundi	15	3.5–10	70–75
LC	North America, Central America, South America	P. concolor	Puma	24	29.0–100.0	90–96
		GENUS NEOFELIS				
VU	Asia	N. diardi	Sunda clouded leopard	11	15.0–30.0	85–95
VU	Asia	N. nebulosa	Clouded leopard	20	15.0–23.0	85–93
		GENUS PANTHERA				
EN	Asia	P. uncial	Snow leopard	21	25.0–75.0	90–103
EN	Asia	P. tigris	Tiger	26	65.0–306.0	93–112
NT	Africa, Asia	P. pardus	Leopard	27	23.0–91.0	90–105
NT	South America, Central America	P. onca	Jaguar	28	30.0–121.0	93–105
VU	Africa, Asia	P. leo	Lion	27	120.0–250.0	100–120
		GENUS ACINONYX				
VU	Africa, Middle East	A. jubatus	Cheetah	20	35.0–72.0	90–95

*CR, Critically Endangered; EN, Endangered; VU, Vulnerable; NT, Near Threatened; LC, Least Concern.

of big cats that resonate to produce a roar. Smaller cats and cheetahs have simpler vocal folds that only allow purring.[31]

Nondomestic felids appear to have an AB blood group system similar to that described in domestic cats. Cross-matching of donor and recipients using standard techniques is important before the administration of transfusions or blood products.[36]

SPECIAL HOUSING REQUIREMENTS

Minimum husbandry guidelines for keeping small (weighing less than 10 kg) and large felids in captivity are available through the Association of Zoos and Aquariums (AZA, www.aza.org) and include recommendations on minimum size specifications, barrier height and width, temperature, humidity, lighting, ventilation, interindividual distances, and sanitation. Additional enclosure features recommended may vary by species and include a vertical component, elevated resting platforms, a heat source, shade, logs or wooden posts to sharpen claws, a visual barrier for cats to hide behind, a den or secure area, varied topography, water features for bathing and swimming, and a shift or secondary holding area to safely move animals from their primary enclosure for cleaning, feeding, or medical procedures. To reduce the incidence of osteoarthritis and pad ulceration, large felids should not be housed for long periods on concrete. Natural substrates or platforms with some flexibility that may be cleaned and disinfected should be provided.[36]

Appropriate safety precautions must be designed into the enclosure and holding facilities to ensure employee and guest safety. These include, but are not limited to, using materials of sufficient strength, covering all openings with mesh or heavy glass, and ability to view all the cats within an enclosure from a safe position. Safety gates provide secondary containment if an animal escapes from the primary holding area. Flares, fire extinguishers, and sound generators may be placed throughout the work area to deter attacks. Keepers may be required to carry pepper spray and communication radios while working with large felids. Escape drills should be held routinely.[36]

FEEDING

The diet of wild felids varies, depending on their sizes. The large cats such as lions and tigers prey on very large mammals, with only two to three species making up the bulk of their diet. Medium-sized felids such as the puma, the snow leopard, and the leopard eat smaller prey but a larger number of different species. The small felids prey on mammals, birds, reptiles, amphibians, and insects. All wild cats hunt and kill their own prey, but some will scavenge opportunistically.[31]

Felids require a much higher proportion of protein in their diet compared with any other mammal, 12% for domestic cats compared with 4% for domestic dogs.[31] In captivity, a formal nutrition program is recommended to meet the nutritional and behavioral needs of all species. Diets should be developed on the basis of the recommendations of nutritionists such as the European Association of Zoos and Aquaria (EAZA) Nutrition Group or the Association of Zoos and Aquarium (AZA) Nutrition Advisory Group (NAG). The AZA-NAG feeding program guidelines suggest a feeding strategy that includes providing a diet that is nutritionally balanced, that reasonably stimulates natural feeding behaviors, that the animal consumes consistently, and that meets the above criteria and is practical and economical to feed. Domestic cats generally require 80 to 90 kilocalories per kilogram of body weight (BW) per day (kcal/kg/day) to meet metabolic requirements. Diet quantity needs to be altered on the basis of the animal's body condition, life stage, and environmental factors. Amounts of feed may also be based on the National Research Council recommendation of 55 to 260 kcal/BW$^{0.75}$ (Requirements for Domestic Dogs and Cats, National Research Council [NRC], 2006).

Most captive felids are fed commercial meat-based complete diets, so additional vitamin or mineral supplements, including calcium and taurine, should not be necessary. Techniques for proper

thawing of frozen diets prior to feeding may be found in the U.S. Department of Agriculture (USDA) guidelines on handling of frozen and thawed meat and prey items fed to captive exotic animals (http://www.nal.usda.gov/awic/pubs/meatprey.pdf). Commercial diets may be supplemented with good-quality carcasses or whole-prey items. If muscle meats or organ meats make up the bulk of the diet, additional supplementation, including calcium, may be necessary. The majority of felids are able to handle the large concentrations of microorganisms present in raw meat. However, guidelines of appropriate bacterial concentrations in received commercial products need to be established for each institution, and commercial products should be tested on a regular basis. Bones may be offered to some species on fast days or twice weekly to promote oral health and to provide enrichment. Fresh water should be made available at all times.

The diet should be analyzed routinely for nutritional content, bacterial contamination, and the presence of foreign material. Several cases of ethylene glycol toxicity from contaminated meat have been reported. The source of the diet components also should be investigated to prevent the transmission of diseases such as spongiform encephalopathies.[36]

RESTRAINT AND HANDLING

Many felids, particularly cheetahs, leopards, lions, and tigers, may be trained to cooperate with veterinary procedures. Behaviors that are particularly helpful include shifting into transport crates, obtaining regular body weights, close visual inspection and oral examination, measurement of temperature, heart rate, and blood pressure, administration of injections or other medications, positioning for abdominal ultrasonography for pregnancy monitoring, and collecting blood or other biologic samples.

Felids less than 10 to 15 kg in body mass may be restrained safely in a net for short procedures such as administration of injections. Heavy gloves may be used, but most felids are capable of biting through them. The majority of cats are darted or confined to a small area or restraint device and hand injected. Commercial squeeze cages are available for restraining and transporting larger felids and work best when incorporated into holding facilities (LGL Animal Care Products, Inc., Bryan, TX; Research Equipment Company, Bryan, TX).[36]

ANESTHESIA

A variety of drug combinations have been used safely to induce anesthesia in felids (Table 47-2). In general, smaller species require a higher dosage of anesthetics compared with larger species on the basis of kilogram of body weight, and free-living individuals may require higher dosages compared with their captive counterparts. The drug combinations most often used include a dissociative (ketamine or tiletamine), and an α_2-agonist (xylazine, medetomidine, or dexmedetomidine), benzodiazepine (diazepam, zolazepam, or midazolam), opioid (butorphanol), or a combination of these. These drugs may be antagonized with yohimbine (0.04 to 0.3 milligram per kilogram [mg/kg], intramuscularly [IM] or intravenously [IV; slow]), atipamezole (0.1 to 0.45 mg/kg, IM), naltrexone (0.05–0.25 mg/kg, IM or IV), and flumazenil (0.01–0.02 mg/kg, IV or IM). Tiletamine and zolazepam (Telazol, Fort Dodge, Fort Dodge, IA) may be used safely in many felids but should be used with caution in tigers. Adverse reactions, including death and neurologic disease (seizures, ataxia), have been anecdotally reported; but controlled studies are lacking. Regurgitation or vomiting during induction or recovery may occur when α_2-agonists are used. Food should be withheld from adult felids for 12 to 24 hours and water for several hours prior to anesthesia to decrease the chances of regurgitation and aspiration during induction and recovery. Species-specific protocols have been reported.[5,10,18,28,29,38]

Anesthesia may be maintained with supplemental ketamine (IV or IM), propofol (IV), or inhalant anesthesia (sevoflurane, isoflurane,

TABLE 47-2

Combinations of Injectable Anesthetic Agents Used in Felids

Generic Name	Dose (mg/kg)	Route	Antagonist	Comments
Ketamine	0.2–2.0	IV or IM	N/A	Not recommended if used alone, best for supplementation or maintenance of anesthesia
Ketamine Xylazine	3.0–10.0 0.3–1.0	IM	N/A Yohimbine	May need to use higher dosages than those listed for small felids
Ketamine Medetomidine (or dexmedetomidine)	2.0–6.0 0.03–0.07 (0.015–0.035)	IM IM	N/A Atipamezole	Supplements may be needed after 45–50 minutes
Ketamine Midazolam	5.0–10.0 0.1–0.3	IM IM	N/A Flumazenil	Use in small felids or debilitated cats Flumazenil may not be necessary
Ketamine Midazolam Butorphanol	3.0–5.0 0.1–0.3 0.1–0.4	IM IM IM	N/A Flumazenil Naltrexone	Use in small felids or debilitated cats Not recommended for healthy large felids Flumazenil may not be necessary
Tiletamine Zolazepam	1.6–4.2 or up to 11.0 in small felids (combined)	IM	N/A	Prolonged recovery Use with caution in tigers Can reduce dosage by adding ketamine or medetomidine
Medetomidine (or dexmedetomidine) Butorphanol Midazolam	0.03–0.04 (0.015–0.02) 0.1–0.4 0.1–0.3		Atipamezole Naltrexone Flumazenil	Spontaneous recoveries after 40–50 minutes Supplements needed for procedures >30 minutes Flumazenil may not be necessary
Ketamine Medetomidine (or dexmedetomidine) Butorphanol Midazolam	1.0–2.0 0.03–0.04 (0.015–0.02) 0.1–0.4 0.1–0.3	IM or IV IM IM IM	N/A Atipamezole Naltrexone Flumazenil	Ketamine may also be given intravenously soon after induction May get spontaneous arousal Flumazenil may not be necessary

IV, Intravenously; *IM,* intramuscularly; *N/A,* not applicable; dosages for antagonists listed in text of chapter.

or halothane). Rapid administration or high doses of ketamine (IV) may induce seizures. Rapid administration of propofol (IV) may result in apnea. Supplemental oxygen is recommended when using injectable anesthetic agents. This may be delivered through the nares, via a face mask, or through endotracheal intubation. Endotracheal intubation is strongly recommended, especially for procedures lasting more than 30 minutes.

Additional anesthetic complications include hypoxia, hypoventilation, hyperventilation, apnea, hypotension, hypertension, bradycardia, arrhythmias, seizures, hypothermia, hyperthermia, and cardiac arrest. Arousal may occur after 40 to 50 minutes when medetomidine is used as the primary anesthetic drug in combination with low doses of ketamine or with a combination of midazolam and butorphanol. This may occur with few premonitory signs, so the clinician must be prepared by having intravenous ketamine or propofol readily available or have an inhalant anesthetic available to maintain anesthesia. A recovery crate should be available in the same room where the procedure is performed if the animal has been removed from its enclosure. This greatly improves safety if there is spontaneous arousal of the animal or a rapid recovery is needed.

VENIPUNCTURE

Venipuncture sites are similar to those of domestic felids. Blood samples may be obtained from the medial and lateral saphenous, jugular, cephalic, or femoral veins. Lateral tail veins may be accessed in larger felids and are located at the 2 o'clock and 10 o'clock positions. This is a particularly useful site if the cat is confined in a squeeze cage. Reference ranges for hematologic and biochemical values for a variety of captive felid species are provided by the International Species Information System (ISIS): Physiologic values in captive wildlife (ISIS, 2002; Apple Valley, MN).

DISEASES

Felids are susceptible to many infectious and noninfectious diseases. Table 47-3 lists several felid species and the common diseases observed in captivity. Some conditions in captive animals may have a genetic predisposition or may be precipitated by chronic stress. Stress causes a reduced immune response that increases susceptibility to infectious diseases and may be associated with noninfectious diseases such as gastritis and AA-amyloidosis in cheetahs. Stress also has an adverse effect on reproduction and results in a higher tendency for self-mutilation or overgrooming.[33] Treatment modalities for the diseases below may be extrapolated from domestic feline medicine.

Infectious Diseases

Felids are susceptible to the same infections carried by domestic cats. They are also susceptible to diseases transmitted by other animals, for example, viral diseases such as canine distemper, rabies, and avian influenza; bacterial infections that cause tularemia (caused by *Francisella tularensis*) or tuberculosis (caused by *Mycobacterium bovis*); and protozoal diseases such as toxoplasmosis (caused by *Toxoplasma gondii*).[6,7,9,16,22,35] Many infections are zoonotic; therefore, good hygiene practices are essential when working with felids. It is also very important to limit exposure of captive felids to feral and domestic cats and dogs, free-living carnivores, bats, rodents, and other small mammals. The common viral diseases in felids are summarized in Table 47-4. *Helicobacter* gastritis may be a significant bacterial infection that results in regurgitation, vomiting, weight loss, and ill thrift. Although all felids may be affected, the clinical disease is most often observed in cheetahs. Management of this condition is well documented in the literature. Additional bacterial diseases include those caused by *Mycoplasma* spp. and *Chlamydophila psittaci*, which are part of the feline respiratory disease complex, and

TABLE 47-3

Common Diseases for Select Species*

Species	Common Infectious Diseases	Common Noninfectious Diseases
Lion	—	Biliary cysts or tumors Spondylosis Lymphoma Pyometra
Tiger	—	Biliary cysts or tumors Spondylosis Chronic renal disease
Jaguar	—	Ovarian and mammary cancer
Clouded leopard	—	Neoplasia especially pheochromocytomas
Cheetah	*Helicobacter* gastritis Herpesvirus dermatitis	Renal secondary amyloidosis Glomerulosclerosis Veno-occlusive disease
Snow leopard	Papillomavirus associated squamous cell carcinoma	Veno-occlusive disease
Fishing cat	—	Transitional cell carcinoma
Black-footed cat	—	Renal amyloidosis, gastrointestinal amyloidosis, or both
Pallas' cat	Toxoplasmosis Herpesvirus infection	—

*K. Terio, unpublished data.

enterocolitis caused by *Campylobacter* spp. *Salmonella* spp. may cause disease but is often passed in the feces of asymptomatic animals secondary to a raw food diet. All felids are susceptible to infections by dermatophytes, especially *Microsporum canis* and *M. gypseum*. Treatment with griseofulvin resulted in toxicity with bone marrow suppression and death in cheetahs.[36] Coccidioidomycosis (caused by *Coccidioides immitis*) has been reported in nondomestic felids in regions of the world where this pathogenic fungus resides in the soil (southwestern United States and northern Mexico). Bovine spongiform encephalopathy (BSE) has been reported in felids in Europe.[27] The cats had been fed cattle carcasses or animal products, including blood and bone meal produced in BSE endemic areas.

Significant protozoal infections include coccidiosis (caused by *Eimeria* spp.) and giardiasis (caused by *Giardia* spp.). These may result in severe enteritis, especially in kittens. Many healthy felids are seropositive for *Toxoplasma gondii* antibodies. Kittens and immunocompromised animals may develop acute generalized toxoplasmosis. High neonatal mortality in Pallas' cats from toxoplasmosis has hampered conservation efforts. Prophylactic treatment of breeding animals and neonates is recommended. *Cytauxzoon felis* is a protozoan that infects blood cells.[4,12,24,41] It is transmitted by the lone star tick (*Amblyomma americanum*). The natural reservoir is the bobcat that becomes a persistent carrier after developing mild or subclinical infection. The disease may be fatal in untreated domestic cats, and a fatal infection in a white tiger has been reported. *Babesia felis*, originally identified in wild cats from Sudan, has been reported sporadically from various countries.[1,4,20,24,41] South Africa appears to be the only country where feline babesiosis is a significant clinical

entity. The infection is assumed to be tickborne, but the vector has not been identified. Concurrent infections may contribute to clinical disease. Ascarids (*Toxocara* and *Toxascaris*) are common in captive animals and may be difficult to eliminate. The ova are highly resistant in the environment. Repeated testing and treatment of animals while in quarantine may prevent the introduction of ascarids into exhibits. In chronically infected cats, routine treatment may be needed to limit worm burdens. Disease caused by *Dirofilaria immitis* (heartworm) has been diagnosed in a black-footed cat.[8] Prophylactic treatment is recommended in endemic areas.

Noninfectious Diseases

Noninfectious diseases are often related to husbandry, diet, or breeding management. Obesity is a significant cause of morbidity in captive felids and may predispose to metabolic conditions such as diabetes mellitus. "Stargazing" has been associated with hypovitaminosis A in young lions.[39] Common dental diseases include gingivitis, calculus accumulation, fractured canines, and fractured molars. Focal palantine erosions have been reported in 15 wild and captive species but is more prevalent in captive animals.[42] Degenerative joint disease and spondylosis are common in geriatric felids, especially the larger species.[19] Chronic renal failure is common in geriatric felids.[37] Renal amyloidosis is particularly common in black-footed cats and cheetahs.[34] Veno-occlusive disease is a slowly progressive liver disease, which results in the fibrosis of the hepatic sinusoids or veins and eventually occlusion of the vessels. It has been reported in cheetahs and snow leopards. Myelopathy has been diagnosed in cheetahs in Europe, and leukoencephalopathy has been diagnosed in cheetahs in North America.[27] Pyometra has been reported in lions, tigers, and a leopard.[21] Lions seem to be at an increased risk for developing pyometra compared with other species. Ovariohysterectomy may be warranted in nonbreeding female lions. The use of progestin-based contraceptives has been associated with endometrial hyperplasia and uterine and mammary adenocarcinoma. Nonsteroidal anti-inflammatory drugs (NSAIDs) should be used cautiously. Aspirin, acetaminophen, and ibuprofen may cause toxicity, and caution is advised when using other formulations such as carprofen, deracoxib, naproxen, etodolac, and indomethacin. Meloxicam has been used in nondomestic felids with no reported adverse effects.[25] Barbiturate and thiafentanil toxicity has been reported in felids fed carcasses of animals that had been euthanized or anesthetized with these agents.

REPRODUCTION

Felidae exhibit a high degree of variability in estrus cycle characteristics, including duration. All felids have induced ovulations, but some have spontaneous ovulations. The occurrence varies across species and between individuals within a species. It occurs frequently in clouded leopards, fishing cats, and margays but rarely in cheetahs, tigrinas, and ocelots. Pallas' cats are very sensitive to photoperiod; tigers, clouded leopards, and snow leopards are moderately affected; and ocelots, tigrinas, margays, lions, leopards, and fishing cats are not influenced by photoperiod. Clouded leopards and Pallas' cats exhibit seasonality in gonadal activity, but margays, cheetahs, and oncillas cycle year round. Suppressed ovarian activity and estrus occurs in cats housed in a group (e.g., cheetahs). All cats have a zonal placentation.[2,3]

Many felid species do not reproduce well in captivity. Assisted reproductive techniques such as artificial insemination are important for managing zoo species.[14,32] This technique is challenged by the variable responses to ovulation induction therapies. Fecal cortisol may be measured and reflects the adrenal status and stress levels of animals managed under different husbandry conditions. These data improve the understanding of how social and environmental factors affect the well-being and reproductive fitness of animals. Contraception of felids is sometimes necessary to facilitate management needs or because of concerns over the health of the animals.

TABLE 47-4

Selected Viral Diseases of Felids

Disease	Etiology	Epizootiology	Signs	Diagnosis	Management
Feline panleukopenia virus (FPV)	Parvovirus	Highly contagious virus shed in all secretions and excretions Shed in feces up to 6 weeks after recovery Illness lasts 5–7 days Mortality is highest in cats <5 months of age	Can be subclinical Peracute cases referred to as *fading kittens* Acute cases show fever, depression, anorexia, and dehydration Vomiting and diarrhea may be present	Presumptive diagnosis based on panleukopenia Confirm by demonstrating FPV antigen in feces Test kits for canine parvovirus antigen may detect FPV antigen during the acute phase	Virus is resistant to inactivation Can survive >1 year in a suitable environment Virus is inactivated by 6% household bleach (sodium hypochlorite) Vaccination using inactivated or killed virus recommended Late pregnancy booster with killed vaccine recommended for cheetahs
Feline rhinotracheitis or feline herpes virus (FHV)	Feline herpesvirus I	Highly contagious Virus shed in saliva and ocular and nasal secretions Easily spread by fomites High morbidity, low mortality Cheetahs and Pallas' cats very susceptible Often self-limiting and may resolve in 14–28 days Can have co-infections with calicivirus, *Chlamydophila psittaci*, *Mycoplasma* spp., or both	Serous ocular discharge, conjunctivitis, blepharospasm, sneezing, and nasal discharge Secondary bacterial infections may occur Keratitis may be seen, especially in kittens Ulcerative dermatitis is common in cheetahs Kittens may develop acute severe infections that lead to blindness or pneumonia	Presumptive diagnosis based on clinical signs, especially in cheetahs[40] Swabs of conjunctiva, nasal, or oropharyngeal region for viral isolation (VI), polymerase chain reaction (PCR), or fluorescent antibody (FA) Immunohistochemical staining (IHC) or VI of tissues	Skin lesions may respond to cryotherapy Use of modified-live virus vaccines may induce the disease in nondomestic felids Only killed vaccines should be used Vaccination will not prevent infection but may decrease severity Cats may become chronic carriers with intermittent shedding of virus Virus viable in environment for 72 hours after a shedding animal has been removed
Feline calicivirus (FCV)	Calicivirus[13]	Highly contagious Virus is shed in saliva and nasal secretions Can also be spread by fomites High morbidity, variable mortality Uncomplicated cases may resolve within 2 weeks Can have co-infections with herpesvirus, *Chlamydophila psittaci*, *Mycoplasma* spp., or both	Sneezing, ocular and nasal discharge, and oral ulcers of the gingiva and tongue Can have pulmonary involvement Secondary bacterial infections	Oropharyngeal and conjunctival swabs of lesions for VI or real time reverse transcriptase PCR (qRT-PCR) Affected tissues for VI, qRT-PCR, IHC, or FA	Use of modified-live virus vaccines may induce the disease in nondomestic felids Only killed vaccines should be used Vaccination will not prevent infection but may decrease severity Virus may survive up to 14 days on inanimate objects Recovered animals may shed virus for months to years

Feline coronavirus (FCoV) has two forms: feline enteric coronavirus (FeCV), which infects the intestines, and the fatal feline infectious peritonitis virus (FIPV), which causes the disease feline infectious peritonitis (FIP)	Coronavirus group 1	Highly contagious among cats in close contact Shed in feces of healthy cats Shedding frequency varies from rare, intermittent, or persistent (best documented in cheetahs) Also reported in domestic cats, African lion, mountain lion, leopard, lynx, jaguar, European wildcat, sand cat, serval, caracal, and Pallas' cat Transmitted by the fecal–oral route through direct contact or by fomites Signs of FeCV can last 2–5 days The more severe FIP form is fatal Most deaths in domestic cats 3–16 months of age, uncommon after 5 years	FeCV may be subclinical or may result in mild diarrhea that may be chronic Signs of FIP are fever, vomiting, diarrhea, and modified transudate effusions with high protein content. Development of FIP depends on two host factors: virus mutation and low immunity FIP is not considered directly transmissible from cat to cat but outbreaks with increased mortality from FIV do occur in groups of unrelated domestic cats in shelters and catteries	Shedding is detected by PCR of feces (three samples a month apart recommended for domestic cats, 5 samples within 30 days for cheetahs)[11] Serologic tests do not differentiate between the two forms of the disease Titers >1:1600–3200 are suggestive of FIP False-positive titers may result in cats recently vaccinated (<4 months) Antibody testing is only useful as a screening tool to detect presence or absence of virus in a collection, recognize potential carriers or shedders when introducing new cats into an antibody-negative collection, and as an aid in the clinical diagnosis of FIP IHC on effusions or lesions is the current gold standard for FIP diagnosis	Cats that recover remain carriers Prevention is by limiting exposure to infected cats and their feces Most cats develop an immune response when exposed and recover Vaccination results in variable efficacy and is not sufficient to control outbreaks of FIP Virus is readily inactivated by detergents and disinfectants but may survive up to 2 months in a dry environment
Feline immunodeficiency virus (FIV)	Lentivirus	Virus shed in saliva. Primary mode of transmission is bites More prevalent in males Most infections reported in older captive animals Reported in free-living puma and bobcats Endemic in certain lion populations in eastern and southern Africa	Most often asymptomatic in nondomestic felids, but may include oral cavity disease, anemia, skin infections, weight loss, vomiting, diarrhea, or neurologic disease	Presence of serum antibodies (Western blot or enzyme-linked immunosorbent assay [ELISA]) Western blot available for domestic cats, cougars, and African lions and may be more sensitive than domestic cat FIV based ELISA Isolation of virus from blood cells and saliva PCR developed for lions	Routine testing recommended Segregate positive cats Infection is lifelong Vaccination available, but may not be necessary if able to prevent exposure to feral cats FIV is labile outside the host and is readily inactivated by common disinfectants
Feline leukemia virus (FeLV)	Retrovirus	Virus may be found in saliva, tears, urine, semen, vaginal fluids, and feces Oronasal contact with saliva or urine is the most common mode of transmission Vertical transmission possible Transmitted to nondomestic cats by contact with or ingestion of domestic feral cats Persistently viremic cats develop fatal diseases Reported in cheetah, Iberian lynx, leopard cat, European wildcat, and cougar	Typically asymptomatic and transient in nondomestic felids Infected cats may experience a prolonged period of clinical latency Immunosuppression, anemia, chronic inflammatory conditions, enlarged lymph nodes, secondary infections, persistent fever, lymphoid or myeloid tumors, or reproductive problems Progressive infection or regressive infection are the outcomes reported in domestic cats	Serologic antigen tests available include immunofluorescent antibody (IFA) or ELISA, false-positives and false-negatives occur Confirmatory test with VI or real time PCR (qPCR) (blood, bone marrow, and tissues)	Routine testing recommended Segregate positive cats Some cats are able to clear the virus, but others remain persistently viremic Vaccination available, but may not be necessary if able to prevent exposure to feral cats Virus unstable outside host, but may survive for up to a week in dried biologic deposits Virus inactivated by detergents and common disinfectants

Continued

TABLE 47-4

Selected Viral Diseases of Felids—cont'd

Disease	Etiology	Epizootiology	Signs	Diagnosis	Management
Feline papillomavirus	Papillomavirus	Species and site-specific infections Reported in domestic cats, Asian lion, bobcats, Florida panther, clouded leopard, Canadian lynx, and snow leopards[1E-30]	Proliferative lesions in the skin or oral cavity Papillomas in snow leopards may undergo malignant transformation to squamous cell carcinoma	PCR of excised lesion developed for snow leopards	Routine screening for skin and oral lesions Remove using surgical excision, laser surgery, or cryosurgery and prevent virus from contacting adjacent tissue Vaccine for snow leopards under development
Canine distemper virus (CDV)	Morbillivirus	Highly contagious Aerosolization of respiratory exudate or contact with other body excretions and secretions Vaccine-induced disease using modified-live virus reported in other carnivores but not felids Not all felids develop disease Mortality reported in captive lions, tigers, leopards, and a jaguar and in free-living lions, lynx (Canadian and Iberian), and bobcats	Infections may be subclinical or fatal. Respiratory, gastrointestinal, integumentary, and central nervous system signs Hyperkeratosis of foot pads and myoclonus	Immunofluorescence of conjunctival scrapings, or buffy coat smears Paired sera by viral neutralization or IFA test. ELISA may detect immunoglobulin G (IgG) and IgM. Antibodies in cerebrospinal fluid (CSF) may be more rewarding than serum Viral isolation, qRT-PCR, or IHC of tissues	Exclude potential reservoirs (domestic dogs, raccoons) Vaccinate susceptible felids using recombinant vaccine
Rabies virus	Lyssavirus	Bites of infected animals (carnivores or bats) Contact of saliva with mucous membranes or open wounds Aerosol in an enclosed environment Fatal disease within 2–7 days of illness	Salivation, abnormal behavior (aggression) or neurologic signs (paresis, seizures)	Recommend euthanasia and shipment of head to a qualified laboratory for FA or VI Serology used to monitor response to vaccination	Reportable disease Zoonotic disease Vaccination recommended Limit exposure to wild carnivores and bats Lyssaviruses are not stable in the environment and are inactivated by common disinfectants
Avian influenza (AI)	Type A influenza virus, subtype H5N1, further classified as highly pathogenic (HPIA) or low pathogenic (LPAI) according to its virulence in poultry	Transmission occurs through the respiratory and oral routes Reported in domestic cats, tigers, leopards, and Asiatic golden cats Direct contact with affected birds or were fed raw poultry Cat-to-cat transmission has been documented	Fever, respiratory distress, severe pneumonia, rapid death Neurologic signs (circling, ataxia) may be observed Subclinical infections also occur	Oropharyngeal, nasal and/or rectal swabs or fecal samples for RT-PCR and/or VI Postmortem samples of lung and mediastinal lymph nodes for VI or RT-PCR	Reportable disease Zoonotic disease Each institution should have a highly pathogenic avian influenza (HPAI) preparedness protocol Do not feed poultry products to nondomestic felids especially in countries with known or potential outbreaks Virus is sensitive to standard disinfectants Virus may persist in cool aquatic environments (>100 days) or indefinitely if frozen

The AZA Wildlife Contraception Center (2012) makes the following recommendations for felid contraception:

1. Gonadotropin-releasing hormone (GnRH) agonists are considered the safest reversible contraceptives, but dosages and duration of efficacy are not well established for all species (caution has to be exercised in their use in lions because of prolonged response with questionable reversibility at certain doses). Side effects are generally similar to those associated with gonadectomy, especially the potential for weight gain.
   - Suprelorin (deslorelin) implants (female or male)
   - Lupron® Depot injection (female or male)
2. Ovariohysterectomy or ovariectomy (females) or castration (males) may be considered if permanent sterilization is an option.
3. In felids, progestin contraceptives are associated with progressive uterine growth that may result in infertility, infections, and sometimes uterine cancer; mammary tissue stimulation may result in cancer. If a progestin is used, treatment should only be short term and should be started before any signs of proestrus. Progestins should not be used in pregnant animals.

PREVENTIVE MEDICINE

Routine Health Examination

Routine, periodic, or opportunistic health examinations should be part of the preventive medicine protocol for felids. Many institutions perform examinations under anesthesia every 2 to 4 years, but this frequency is dependent on the individual animal's age, life stage, health status and medical history, and species and the resources and philosophy of the holding institution. Animals that are trained as part of an operant conditioning program may be visually examined, have blood collected, and receive vaccinations without anesthesia or the need for remote delivery equipment. These examinations may be substituted for one under anesthesia in many cases if dental examination and prophylaxis and thorough palpation are deemed unnecessary. Routine health examination should include an assessment of body condition, body weight determination, complete physical examination, evaluation for ectoparasites (ticks, fleas, flies), blood collection for complete blood cell (CBC) count with manual differential and hemoparasite examination, serum biochemical panel, and serum for banking. Recommended serologic tests include those for feline leukemia virus (FeLV) and feline immunodeficiency virus (FIV). Additional tests that may be necessary based on species, geographic location, or potential for disease exposure include those for *Toxoplasma gondii,* feline coronavirus (FCoV), and canine heartworm (*Dirofilaria immitis*). Serologic tests to monitor response to vaccination may be useful for feline parvovirus (FPV), especially in cheetahs, and for the rabies virus.[26] Vaccine titers for feline herpesvirus (FHV) or feline calicivirus (FCV) are predictive of protection, except for highly susceptible species such as cheetahs. If a cheetah has a low or negative titer to FPV or FHV, more frequent vaccination should be considered. Urinalysis should be performed, if possible. Survey radiography and abdominal ultrasonography may be valuable if resources are available to establish reference information or to diagnose occult conditions. Fecal examination for parasites is recommended at this time if a regular program for parasite surveillance (once to twice yearly) is not already in place.

Vaccination

Vaccination protocols for carnivores have been recently reviewed.[17] Vaccines recommended are divided into core vaccines (recommended for all felids) and noncore vaccines (optional, depending on the specific disease risk of the species and institution, not generally recommended). Vaccine-associated sarcomas have rarely been reported in nondomestic felids. Because of the lack of serologic studies and difficulty in performing challenge experiments on nondomestic felids, specific information on the length of protection from vaccination is lacking. Specific recommendations for vaccination frequency cannot be made, although most institutions vaccinate adults every 1 to 3 years using the core vaccines. Core vaccines include rabies (killed, e.g., Imrab 3, Merial; or recombinant canarypox-vectored, e.g., PureVax Rabies, Merial) and feline panleukopenia, calicivirus, herpesvirus (killed, e.g., Fel-O-Vax PCT Plus, Boehringer Ingelheim). Noncore vaccines that should be considered only in species at risk include canine distemper virus (CDV) (recombinant canarypox-vectored, PureVax Ferret Distemper, Merial) and FeLV (killed).

Preshipment Evaluation and Quarantine

Animals that are being shipped to a new institution should be evaluated using the procedures described earlier. The preshipment examination and test results allow the receiving institution to discuss disease risks associated with the acquisition in advance with animal managers. Results should be compared with the results of the quarantine examination at the receiving institution. Examination and testing during the quarantine period provides vital information following the stress of shipment and change in environment. Biologic samples should be stored for future testing or studies, as needed.

Quarantine should occur in an off-exhibit area away from other animals, especially other carnivores (collection and free-living). Dedicated tools and equipment and personal protective equipment (removable outer wear, gloves) should be used. If dedicated footwear is not an option, a footbath may be used. Quarantine period for all felid species is typically 30 days, but this may vary depending on the source of the cat or institutional practices.

REFERENCES

1. Bosman AM, Venter EH, Penzhorn BL: Occurrence of *Babesia felis* and *Babesia leo* in various wild felid species and domestic cats in Southern Africa, based on reverse line blot analysis. *Vet Parasitol* 144(1–2):33–38, 2007.
2. Brown JL, Graham LH, Wielebnowski N, et al: Understanding the basic reproductive biology of wild felids by monitoring of faecal steroids. *J Reprod Fertil Suppl* 57:71–82, 2001.
3. Brown JL: Female reproductive cycles of wild female felids. *Anim Reprod Sci* 124(3–4):155–162, 2011.
4. Cunningham M, Yabsley MJ: Primer on tick-borne diseases in exotic carnivores. In Miller RE, Fowler ME, editors: *Fowler's zoo and wild animal medicine current therapy*, vol 7, St. Louis, MO, 2012, Saunders, pp 458–464.
5. Curro TG, Okeson D, Zimmerman D, et al: Xylazine-midazolam-ketamine versus medetomidine-midazolam-ketamine anesthesia in captive Siberian tigers (*Panthera tigris altaica*). *J Zoo Wildl Med* 35(3):320–327, 2004.
6. Daoust PY, McBurney SR, Godson DL, et al: Canine distemper virus-associated encephalitis in free-living lynx (*Lynx canadensis*) and bobcats (*Lynx rufus*) of eastern Canada. *J Wildl Dis* 45(3):611–624, 2009.
7. de Camps S, Dubey JP, Saville WJ: Seroepidemiology of *Toxoplasma gondii* in zoo animals in selected zoos in the midwestern United States. *J Parasitol* 94(3):648–653, 2008.
8. Deem SL, Heard DJ, LaRock R: Heartworm (*Dirofilaria immitis*) disease and glomerulonephritis in a black-footed cat (*Felis nigripes*). *J Zoo and Wildl Med* 29(2):199–202, 1998.
9. Deem SL, Spelman LH, Yates RA, et al: Canine distemper in terrestrial carnivores: A review. *J Zoo Wildl Med* 31(4):441–451, 2000.
10. Fahlman A, Loveridge A, Wenham C, et al: Reversible anaesthesia of free-ranging lions (*Panthera leo*) in Zimbabwe. *J S Afr Vet Assoc* 76(4):187–192, 2005.
11. Gaffney PM, Kennedy M, Terio K, et al: Detection of feline coronavirus in cheetah (*Acinonyx jubatus*) feces by reverse transcription-nested polymerase chain reaction in cheetahs with variable frequency of viral shedding. *J Zoo Wildl Med* 43(4):776–786, 2012.
12. Garner MM, Lung NP, Citino S, et al: Fatal cytauxzoonosis in a captive reared white tiger (*Panthera tigris*). *Vet Pathol* 33(1):82–86, 1996.
13. Harrison TM, Sikarskie J, Kruger J, et al: Systemic calicivirus epidemic in captive exotic felids. *J Zoo Wildl Med* 38(2):292–299, 2007.
14. Herrick JR, Campbell M, Levens G, et al: In vitro fertilization and sperm cryopreservation in the black-footed cat (*Felis nigripes*) and sand cat (*Felis margarita*). *Biol Reprod* 82(3):552–562, 2010.

15. Joslin JO: Viral papilloma and squamous cell carcinomas in snow leopards (*Uncia uncia*). In *Proceedings of the American Association of Zoo Veterinarians*, New Orleans, LA, 2000, pp 155–157.

16. Keawcharoen J, Oraveerakul K, Kuiken T, et al: Avian influenza H5N1 in tigers and leopards. *Emerg Infect Dis* 10(12):2189–2191, 2004.

17. Lamberski N: Updated vaccination recommendations for carnivores. In Miller RE, Fowler ME, editors: *Fowler's zoo and wild animal medicine current therapy*, vol 7, St. Louis, MO, 2012, Saunders, pp 442–450.

18. Langan JN, Schumacher J, Pollock C, et al: Cardiopulmonary and anesthetic effects of medetomidine-ketamine-butorphanol and antagonism with atipamezole in servals (*Felis serval*). *J Zoo Wildl Med* 31(3):329–334, 2000.

19. Longley L: Aging in large felids. In Miller RE, Fowler ME, editors: *Fowler's zoo and wild animal medicine current therapy*, vol 7, St. Louis, MO, 2012, Saunders, pp 465–469.

20. Marcos RA, Adania CH, Teixeira RHF, et al: Molecular and serological detection of *Babesia* spp. in neotropical and exotic carnivores in Brazilian zoos. *J Zoo Wildl Med* 42(1):139–143, 2011.

21. McCain S, Ramsay E, Allender MC, et al: Pyometra in captive large felids: A review of eleven cases. *J Zoo Wildl Med* 40(1):147–151, 2009.

22. Meli ML, Simmler P, Cattori V, et al: Importance of canine distemper virus (CDV) infection in free-ranging Iberian lynxes (*Lynx pardinus*). *Vet Microbiol* 146(1–2):132–137, 2010.

23. Nowell K: Cats on the 2009 red list of threatened species. *Cat News* 51:31–33, 2009.

24. Penzhorn BL, Schoeman T, Jacobson LS: Feline babesiosis in South Africa: A review. *Ann New York Acad Sci* 1026:183–186, 2004.

25. Ramsay EC: Use of analgesics in exotic felids. In Miller RE, Fowler ME, editors: *Zoo and wild animal medicine current therapy*, vol 6, Philadelphia, PA, 2008, Saunders, pp 289–293.

26. Risi E, Agoulon A, Allaire F, et al: Antibody response to vaccines for rhinotracheitis, caliciviral disease, panleukopenia, feline leukemia, and rabies in tigers (*Panthera tigris*) and lions (*Panthera leo*). *J Zoo Wildl Med* 43(2):248–255, 2012.

27. Robert N: Neurologic disorders in cheetahs and snow leopards. In Miller RE, Fowler ME, editors: *Zoo and wild animal medicine current therapy*, vol 6, Philadelphia, PA, 2008, Saunders, pp 265–271.

28. Rockhill AP, Chinnadurai SK, Powell RA, et al: A comparison of two field chemical immobilization techniques for bobcats (*Lynx rufus*). *J Zoo Wildl Med* 42(4):580–585, 2011.

29. Stegmann GF, Jago M: Cardiopulmonary effects of medetomidine or midazolam in combination with ketamine or tiletamine/zolazepam for the immobilisation of captive cheetahs (*Acinonyx jubatus*). *J S Afr Vet Assoc* 77(4):205–209, 2006.

30. Sundberg JP, Van Ranst M, Montali R, et al: Feline papillomas and papillomaviruses. *Vet Pathol* 37(1):1–10, 2000.

31. Sunquist ME, Sunquist FC: Family Felidae (cats). In Wilson DE, Mittermeier RA, editors: *Handbook of the mammals of the world*, vol 1, Barcelona, Spain, 2009, Lynx Edicions, pp 54–168.

32. Swanson WF: Application of assisted reproduction for population management in felids: The potential and reality for conservation of small cats. *Theriology* 66(1):49–58, 2006.

33. Terio KA, Marker L, Munson L: Evidence for chronic stress in captive but not free-ranging cheetahs (*Acinonyx jubatus*) based on adrenal morphology and function. *J Wildl Dis* 40(2):259–266, 2004.

34. Terio KA, O'Brien T, Lamberski N, et al: Amyloidosis in black-footed cats (*Felis nigripes*). *Vet Pathol* 45(3):393–400, 2008.

35. Thiry E, Addie D, Belák S, et al: H5N1 avian influenza in cats. ABCD guidelines on prevention and management. *J Feline Med Surg* 11(7):615–618, 2009.

36. Wack RF: Felidae. In Miller RE, Fowler ME, editors: *Zoo and Wild Animal Medicine*, vol 5, St. Louis, 2003, WB Saunders, pp 491–516.

37. Wack RF: Treatment of chronic renal failure in nondomestic felids. In Miller RE, Fowler ME, editors: *Zoo and wild animal medicine current therapy*, vol 6, Philadelphia, PA, 2008, Saunders, pp 462–465.

38. Wenger S, Buss P, Joubert J, et al: Evaluation of butorphanol, medetomidine and midazolam as a reversible narcotic combination in free-ranging African lions (*Panthera leo*). *Vet Anaesth Analg* 37(6):491–500, 2010.

39. Wenker CJ, Robert N: Stargazing in lions. In Miller RE, Fowler ME, editors: *Fowler's zoo and wild animal medicine current therapy*, vol 7, St. Louis, MO, 2012, Saunders, pp 470–476.

40. Witte CL, Lamberski N, Rideout BR, et al: Development of a case definition for clinical feline herpesvirus infections in cheetahs (*Acinonyx jubatus*) housed in zoos. *J Zoo Wildl Med* 2013 (accepted).

41. Yabsley MJ, Murphy SM, Cunningham MW: Molecular detection and characterization of *Cytauxzoon felis* and a *Babesia* spp. in cougars from Florida. *J Wild Dis* 42(2):366–374, 2006.

42. Zordan M, Deem SL, Sanchez CR: Focal palatine erosion in captive and free-living cheetahs (*Acinonyx jubatus*) and other felid species. *Zoo Biol* 31(2):181–188, 2012.

CHAPTER 48

Mustelidae

George V. Kollias and Jesus Fernandez-Moran

NATURAL HISTORY, ANATOMY, AND PHYSIOLOGY

Recent studies have revealed that the Musteloidea emerged approximately 32.4 to 30.9 million years ago in Asia. During the Oligocene, musteloids diversified into four primary divisions: Mephitidae, Ailuridae, Procyonidae, and Mustelidae. Mustelidae arose approximately 16.1 million years ago. The early offshoots largely evolved into the ecologic niches of badgers and martens, whereas later divergences have adapted to other niches, including those of weasels, polecats, minks, and otters.[35]

Extant mustelids are classified in the order Carnivora, suborder Caniformia, family Mustelidae, and subfamily Mustelinae and

Mephitinae. The family Mustelidae currently includes 25 recent genera and approximately 67 species of terrestrial carnivores or piscivores inhabiting all continents except Australia and Antarctica and are also absent in New Guinea, Madagascar and Antarctica. They have been introduced into New Zealand. In the course of evolution, several behavioral adaptations and many physical features have developed, as some species live mainly in the ground (stoat, weasel, polecat) or even partially underground (badger), whereas others are active also above the ground in trees (pine marten). Some have selected marine or fresh water as their preferred habitats most or part of the time (mink, river otter, sea otter).

Included in this family are the smallest living carnivore, the common or least weasel, and the largest representatives, the giant and sea otters in water and the wolverine on land. Mustelid body weights range from under 70 grams (g) (least weasel at 19 centimeters [cm] long) to 45 kg (sea otter at 190 cm long).

The family Mustelidae includes five subfamilies. The weasel-like carnivores (*Mustelinae*) represent the group with the greatest number of species, comprising 10 genera with approximately 33 species including weasels (11 species), polecats (3 species), minks (2 species), grison (1 species), and wolverine (1 species). The subfamily Mellivorinae is represented by only a single species, the honey badger or ratel (*Mellivora capensis*). Subfamily Melinae includes five genera in eight species of badgers represented in Africa, Asia, South America, or wide ranges of northern Eurasia and North America. Skunks (subfamily Mephitinae, recently elevated to Family Mephitidae) are exclusively common in North America. Otters (subfamily Lutrinae) are small to large forms that show the most highly developed adaptations to marine life of all mustelids. They lead an amphibious life and feed mainly on fish or crustaceans. Most mammologists recognize four genera and 13 species.[30]

Most mustelids have a highly flexible spinal column; the limbs are comparatively short, ending in feet with five digits, and they walk either digitigrade or plantigrade. The claws are not (or only partly) retractable. Mustelids lack the clavicle and cecum. They present the typical carnivore dentition with number of teeth varying from 28 to 40. Developed canine (C) teeth are always present and the last premolar (P) in the upper jaw and the first molar (M) in the lower jaw jointly form the "crushing shears" for processing food. The dental formula of weasels is incisors (I) 3/3, C 1/1, P 3/3, M 1/2 on the upper and lower jaws. In the wolverine the formula is I 3/3, C 1/1, P 4/4, M 1/2 upper and lower. Eurasian badger formula is I 3/3, C 1/1, P 4/4, M 1/2 upper and lower, and in the members of the *Lutra* and *Lontra* genera the formula is I 3/3, C 1/1, P 3-4/3, M 1/2 upper and lower. The pine marten has a dental formula of I 3/3, C 2/1, P 4/4, M 1/2 upper and lower (40 teeth total), which is different from that of other mustelids. Glands may be located in various regions of the body surface. The paired anal glands produce odorous secretions characteristic of the species and used for marking their habitat, sometimes for generations. Some species may spray these secretions over long distances as a method to discourage or harm enemies.

In otters, the mandibular salivary glands and lymph nodes lie in the angle of the mandible, whereas the retropharyngeal nodes lie dorsolateral and slightly caudal to the larynx. The thyroid glands of otters are also different from those of other mustelids in that they are long, flat, and tapering, with no isthmus, and closely attached to the trachea. The heart of otters is usually globular with a thick-walled left ventricle and a thin-walled right ventricle. The shape of the heart and thickness of the ventricles should not be confused with ventricular hypertrophy. Otters have a seven-lobed liver. A common hepatic and cystic bile duct joins the duodenum adjacent to the pancreatic duct. The kidneys of otters, like those of cows and cetaceans, are multilobulated. The lungs of otters and badgers are composed of two lobes on the left, three lobes on the right, and an intermediate lobe where the right bronchus terminates.[5,15]

Mustelids are predominantly solitary, sexually dimorphic mammals (males are 25% larger than females). Smaller mustelid species have high metabolic rates. Males and females come together only during the reproductive period, and social communities generally include the mother and offspring. Table 48-1 summarizes the biologic data of selected mustelids.

Members of the family range from the International Union for the Conservation of Nature (IUCN) status Endangered (black-footed ferret) to Near Threatened (wolverine) to IUCN status Least Concern (badger).

Unique Aquatic Adaptations

The family Mustelidae contains numerous fully terrestrial species, two that are semi-aquatic (minks), and a number that are amphibious to fully aquatic (the *Lutrinae*). The latter have adaptations for the aquatic habits that may be relevant for the clinical management. Underwater vision presents challenges for the mammalian eye: the need for increased sensitivity to light, accommodation of the spectral shift toward the blue-green wavelengths, and modification of the ocular focusing capacity because of refractive differences compared with those in air. Different adaptations for these challenges have been proposed, although visual acuity in water is somewhat reduced in some otter species (i.e., Asian small-clawed otter). Little is known of the importance, sensitivity, and mechanisms of hearing in otters, in the aquatic or the terrestrial environment. Olfaction has been retained as an important sense for aquatic mustelids, largely but not exclusively in support of their activities on land. However, evidence suggests that otters have less complex scent production capacities compared with terrestrial mustelids and that scent production capacity in sea otters may be more poorly developed and less important than in other otter species. These changes probably have resulted from the increased importance of vision and the reduced importance of olfaction in the aquatic environment. The long, lean body of Mustelinae species makes them vulnerable to rapid heat loss on land and in the water. Insulation in aquatic mustelids is achieved by means of a dense underfur that prevents water penetration to the skin while providing buoyancy. Because fur is an efficient insulator, furred aquatic mammals require some means of thermoregulation; in sea otters, thermoregulation is conducted through the enlarged rear flippers. In otters and minks, swimming is the primary means of locomotion. These species demonstrate many adaptations that enhance swimming performance and reduce energy expenditure while in the water: body streamlining, large, specialized plantar surfaces for propulsion, and the ability to remain submerged for extended periods. However, most otters, unlike most aquatic mammals, are capable of quadrupedal locomotion on land, and this is why they are considered morphologically intermediate between terrestrial and aquatic mammals.[12]

OUTDOOR AND INDOOR ENVIRONMENTS

Most species tolerate a wide range of temperature ranges. Temperate and cold-adapted species held outdoors need protection from sunlight when the temperature exceeds 50°F (10°C). Tropical species require heated shelters when ambient temperatures drop below 69°F (20°C). Animals kept indoors should not be exposed to temperatures exceeding 78°F (25°C). It is important to be aware that required temperature ranges vary among individuals as well as between species, so individual animals should be given the opportunity to select a comfortable ambient temperature from a gradient provided in the enclosure. Humidity for indoor enclosures should range from 30% to 70% but may be higher for tropical species. The amount of time individuals held indoors are exposed to light should replicate the natural photoperiod of their native environment, particularly for those species that are expected to reproduce in captivity. Currently, data on the effects of varying light intensity or type of light (fluorescent versus natural) on reproductive behavior are not available; however, a correlation exists between the onset of estrus in northern mustelid species.[4] Indoor exhibits should have a negative air pressure of five to eight air changes per hour (for odor control) of non-recirculated air; however, this is not necessarily a requirement and recirculated air may be used in some cases.

TABLE 48-1
Biologic Information of Selected Species of Mustelids

Scientific Name	Common Name	Weight	Geographic Distribution	Distinguishing Features	Life Span	Food
Mustela nivalis	Common weasel Least weasel	Female (F): 30–120 grams (g) Male (M):36–250 g	North Africa, Western Europe, Eastern Siberia; Japan, Alaska, and Northeastern USA, (New Zealand)	Smallest species of family Body size and fur color highly varying	About 1 year	Burrowing voles, true mice, birds, frogs, lizards
Mustela erminea	Ermine, Stoat, Short tail weasel	F: 85–200 g M: 200–310 g	Europe-Eastern Siberia, Japan, Alaska, Northern Greenland, Northern USA, (New Zealand)	Summer fur cinnamon-brown or even yellow on back; underside white	About 1 year	Burrowing voles, true mice, hares, birds, eggs, lizards, frogs
Mustela putorius	European polecat	F: 650–820 g M: 1000–1500 g	Europe	Ancestor of domestic ferret, *M. putorius furo*, facial mask	5–6 years, 10 years and more in isolated cases	Small rodents, rabbits, hares, birds, eggs, frogs, snakes, insects
Mustela nigripes	Black footed ferret		Alberta to northern Texas	Facial mask; black limbs	12 years	Prairie dogs and other small rodents, birds
Mustela lutreola	European mink	400–1200 g	Western Siberia, Eastern Europe, (Western Europe)	Polecat-like; long vibrissae on snout	7–10 years	Mouselike rodents, fishes, crayfish, mollusks, birds, amphibians, reptiles
Mustela vison	American mink	500–2300 g	Canada, USA, (Iceland, north and central Europe, Siberia)	Sparse white spots on chin and ventrum, otherwise very similar to European mink	8–10 years	Same as European mink
Vormela peregusna	Marbled polecat	370–715 g	Southeastern Europe to western China	Spotted back, large ears	8 years	Gerbils, jumping mice, susliks, hamsters, and other rodents
Poecilogale albinucha	White-naped weasel	F: 230–290 g M: 280–380 g	South Africa to Zaire, Uganda	White neck; stripes on back	5 years	Small rodents, birds, snakes, grasshoppers and other insects
Ictonyx striatus	Zorrila or African striped polecat	420–1400 g	Senegal, Ethiopia, and South Africa	Stripes on back; squirts secretion from anal glands for defense	13 years	Small rodents, birds, eggs, insects
Martes martes	Pine marten	F: 800–1300 g M: 1200–1600 g	Western Europe to Western Siberia	Summer fur thin and short, winter fur thick and long	15 years	Mouselike rodents, squirrels, hares, rabbits, birds, eggs, reptiles, amphibians, insects, fruits, berries, nuts
Martes foina	Stone marten or beech marten	F: 1100–1500 g M: 1700–2400 g	Western Europe to Himalayas, and Altai	Similar to pine marten, but heavier, shorter limbs, white throat spot	Unknown	Similar to pine marten
Martes americana	American marten	F: 600–775 g M: 700–1300 g	Canada, north USA	Similar to pine marten; irregular cream to orange spots on throat and chest	17 years	Similar to pine marten
Eira barbara	Tayra	4–6 kilograms (kg)	Northeastern Mexico to Argentina	Dark brown to black body	18 years	Guinea pigs, harelike rodents, birds, reptiles, insects, honey, fruits

Mellivora capensis	Ratel	7–13 kg	Some animals completely black; forelimbs muscular, with strong claws	Northern India to Arabia, Africa, and south of Sahara	Unknown	Small rodents, birds, eggs, lizards, snakes, turtles, frogs, insects, honey, berries, fruits, roots
Meles meles	Badger	7–13 kg in summer; 15–25 kg in fall	Silvery gray back and flanks; throat, chest, belly and legs black or brown	Europe, Japan, and southern China	16 years	Mouselike rodents, small birds, eggs, frogs, lizards, insects, snails, earthworms, fruits, nuts, berries
Taxidea taxus	American badger	6–8 kg in summer; 8–12 kg in fall	Thick dense fur; predominantly gray black with white stripe from nose to root of tail; dark, oblong cheek spot	Southwestern Canada to central Mexico	16 years	Small mammals, birds, eggs, reptiles, insects, invertebrates
Mephitis mephitis	Stripped skunk	1.2–2.5 kg; in the fall up to 5.3 kg	Black, with mostly two white lateral stripes; spray secretion from anal glands up to 6 m with accurate aim into eyes of attacker	Southern Canada to northern Mexico	10 years	Small rodents, birds, eggs, insects, worms, fruits, berries, corn
Lutra lutra	Eurasian otter	5–12 kg	Shiny dark brown or chestnut brown back; fingers and toes joined by swimming membranes	Eurasia, North Africa, Sri Lanka, Taiwan, Sumatra, Java	22 years	Fishes, crustaceans, clams, frogs, small rodents, worms
Lontra canadensis	Nearctic river otter	3.4–15.4 kg	Head blunt, small, flat bullous nose; small eyes; interdigital webs	Canada, USA	14 years in wild; 16–18 years in captivity	Fish (primarily), crustaceans (cray fish); amphibians; insects, birds, mammals
Pteronura brasiliensis	Giant otter	22–32 kg	Very dark fur; chin, throat, and chest have cream-colored spots; flattened tail; swimming membranes	Venezuela to Argentina	13 years	Fishes, crustaceans, other aquatic animals
Enhydra lutris	Sea otter	F: 36 kg M: 46 kg	Largest mustelid by weight; light brown to nearly black pelage; interdigital webs	Bering Sea to California	In wild 22 years (females) 15 years (males)	Generalist predator; decapod crustaceans, gastropod and bivalve mollusks, echinoderms
Gulo gulo	Wolverine	10–20 kg	Bushy tail; long flowing fur; thick, strong paws; partly retractable claws	Scandinavia, Siberia, Alaska, Canada, Western USA	18 years	Rodents, harelike rodents, reindeer, elk, carcasses, ground-nesting birds, berries

Items in parenthesis refer to areas where a particular species as been introduced.

Fresh drinking water should be provided at all times. Nonfiltered water, contained in pools or moats and used for swimming, should be changed on a regular basis. Even if water is filtered, it should be completely changed periodically. Mustelids should not be given access to pools that have recently been treated with chlorine (levels should be <0.5 parts per million [ppm]). For otters that normally inhabit fresh or brackish water environments, dissolved nutrients should be monitored and water changes performed, as appropriate. It is suggested that the coliform level not exceed 400 colony forming units per milliliter (CFU/mL) (water with a level of 100 CFU/mL is reported to be safe for humans). Filtration should be used in closed pools for otter. Sand filters, pool pumps, charcoal filters, and ozone pressure sand filters have all been used effectively. Drain outlets and filter and skimmer inlets should be covered to prevent furnishings from obstructing them or from otters getting stuck in them. Natural flow-through systems work well in otter exhibits. Water flowing in must be clean and pollutant free. All uneaten food items should be removed from pools on a daily basis. Because minks are highly susceptible to methyl mercury toxicity, pools need to be maintained at a neutral or basic pH (acidic pH enhances methylation of mercury).

Controlling of sounds and vibrations that may be detected by mustelids is important to their well-being. Anecdotal reports of loud noises and vibrations of certain amplitude affecting parturition and early kit rearing in mustelids have been published.[3,4]

Habitat Design and Containment

Exhibits should be designed to satisfy the physical, social, behavioral, and psychological needs of the species while closely replicating their habitat in the wild. Enclosure size for arboreal and terrestrial mustelids is based on species' and individual needs (e.g., juveniles versus adults versus geriatric animals). Exhibits that are provided extensive enrichment and are structurally varied may be smaller than exhibits lacking these characteristics. (Note that enrichment items must be chosen carefully, since many mustelid species are prone to chewing and ingesting enrichment parts, putting them at risk of gastrointestinal [GI] foreign body obstruction). Recommended exhibit sizes are based on species size, behavioral repertoire, home range size, daily movements, and activity patterns. Detailed information is given in the Mustelid (Mustelidae) and Otter (Lutrinae) Care Manuals provided by the Association of Zoos and Aquariums, Small Carnivore Taxon Advisory Group.

Animal and human safety must be kept in mind when designing and building mustelid exhibits. Additionally, mustelids are not well suited for free-ranging exhibits because of their uncanny ability to escape. Exhibits must be designed to prevent them from digging, jumping, climbing, or swimming out of enclosures. Outdoor exhibits should have containment perimeters, tops and hotwire 3 to 5 feet (ft.; 1–1.52 meters [m]) installed above ground level to prevent them from climbing and falling. For burrowing species (e.g., badgers), the bottom of the containment fence may need to be buried to a sufficient depth and angled toward the center of the exhibit to prevent escape. For amphibious species (e.g., otters), optimal land-to-water ratios are species dependent. These ratios may need to be changed as exhibit size increases or decreases (e.g., smaller exhibits will require a higher land area proportion within the ratio).[3,4]

FEEDING AND NUTRITION

Within the *Mustelidae* family, food habits vary significantly. Some are strict carnivores (ferrets, weasels, polecats, etc.), some are omnivorous (skunks, badgers or tayras), and some are piscivorous (fish and crustacean eaters such as otters) (see Table 48-1). Mustelids have a relatively simple stomach and a short GI tract and, as mentioned above, no cecum. The more omnivorous species have flattened molars. Captive mustelid species are fed on a great variety of items: commercial dry dog food, mink food, and cat food, and cereal diets mixed with meat, fresh or frozen fish, shellfish, crabs, and crayfish. Fruits, vegetables (carrots, lettuce, green beans, cucumber, collard greens, kale, potatoes, among others), eggs, and live or killed food items (crickets, mealworms, mice, prairie dogs) have also been incorporated into captive diets. Target dietary nutrient values for mustelids are based on several sources. The cat is typically the model species used to establish nutrient guidelines for strict carnivorous animals. The National Research Council (NRC, 2006, for dogs and cats), and Association of American Feed Control Officials (1994, for cats) have provided recommendations. A limited amount of information has been provided by the NRC publication on mink and foxes, which represents the requirements of another mustelid species (Table 48-2). The complete dietary requirements of domestic ferrets are still unknown, so no one particular diet is currently being recommended over another. In the ferret and mink diet, the protein should be of high quality and easily digestible because of their short GI transit time of 3 to 4 hours. Generally, most mustelids need a diet high in good-quality meat protein and fat and low in complex carbohydrates, inclusive of sugars, and fiber. High levels of protein from plant sources have been associated with urolithiasis in mustelids and are therefore undesirable. Food should be offered at least twice a day, and water must be available at all times. When developing appropriate dietary management plans for a specific mustelid species, the following should be considered: feeding ecology, target nutrient values, food items available at zoos, and information collected from diets offered by institutions successfully maintaining and breeding for the species.

RESTRAINT AND HANDLING

Even though some captive mustelids may be gentle with their keepers, all members of this family may be handled with nets, snares, or squeeze cages. Caution must be used while managing wild mustelids, as they have needle-sharp teeth and are agile and aggressive and may inflict severe bites. They are also potential vectors of rabies, so they should be handled with caution. Leather gloves should be used by operators when handling any kind of mustelid, whatever the size. The ferret is best restrained when grasped above the shoulders, with one hand gently squeezing the forelimbs together and the thumb under the animal's chin. Minks are grasped by the tail with one hand, while the other hand grasps the animal behind the neck, with the thumb and finger around the head. Polecats, ermines, weasels, and martens are better restrained initially with a net when an injection has to be administered by hand. Skunks defend themselves by spraying the secretions of the anal sacs, and they may bite as well. The defensive position assumed by a threatened skunk is hindquarters facing the enemy, feet planted firmly on the ground, and tail straight up in the air. They should be captured with a net from behind a shield of glass or plastic, or the handler should wear goggles and protective rain gear. Larger mustelids such as otters, badgers, and wolverine may be placed in a small squeeze cage for manual injection of a tranquilizer or directly injected by means of a pole syringe or a blowpipe.[16]

Mustelids are susceptible to stress caused by improper handling and transport. Fresh water and marine otters are particularly susceptible to stress-associated exertional myopathy. Different techniques have been developed for safe management of this species. Only trained personal should handle mustelids, and usually, a combination of physical restraint and chemical restraint is advocated to reduce stress and avoid capture myopathy. The duration of restraint should be brief, and care should be taken to avoid trauma to the oral cavity and limbs. As mentioned above, sea otters are extremely susceptible to stress caused by improper handling and transporting. Different techniques have been developed for the safe management of this species.[19,24]

Chemical Restraint

Different drugs have been used extensively for the chemical immobilization of mustelids. In most species, dissociative-benzodiazepine–α_2-agonists combinations have been used and are highly recommended for induction or short-term anesthesia. Ketamine in

TABLE 48-2

Nutrient Requirements and Target Nutrient Ranges for Selected Carnivore Species

Nutrient	Cat* (National Research Council [NRC], 1986)	Dog* (NRC, 1974)	Mink† *Mustela vison*	Artic Fox‡ *Vulpes vulpes* (NRC, 1982)	Asian Small-Clawed Otter§ *Aonyx cinerea*
Protein %	24	22	38 (23.9)	24.7	24–32.5
Fat %	—	5	—	—	15–30
Vitamin A, international unit per gram (IU/g)	3.3	5.0	5.93	2.44	3.3–10
Vitamin D (IU/g)	0.5	0.5	—	—	0.5–1.0
Vitamin E, milligram per kilogram (mg/kg)	30	50	27	—	30–120
Thiamin (mg/kg)	5.0	1.0	1.3	1.0	1–5
Riboflavin (mg/kg)	4.0	2.2	1.6	3.7	3.7–4.0
Pantothenic acid (mg/kg)	5.0	10.0	8.0	7.4	5–7.4
Niacin (mg/kg)	40.0	11.4	20.0	9.6	9.6–40
Pyridoxine (mg/kg)	4.0	1.0	1.6	1.8	1.8–4
Folacin (mg/kg)	0.80	0.18	0.5	0.2	0.2–1.3
Biotin (mg/kg)	0.07	0.1	0.12	—	0.07–0.08
Vitamin B_{12} (mg/kg)	—	0.022	—	—	0.02–0.025
Calcium %	0.8	1.1	0.40 (0.3)	0.6	0.6–0.8
Phosphorous %	0.6	0.9	0.40 (0.3)	0.6	0.6
Potassium %	0.4	0.6	—	—	0.2–0.4
Sodium %	0.05	—	—	—	0.04–0.6
Magnesium %	0.04	0.04	—	—	0.04–0.07
Iron (mg/kg)	80	60	—	—	80–114
Zinc (mg/kg)	50	50	—	—	50–94
Copper (mg/kg)	5.0	7.3	—	—	5.0–6.25
Iodine (mg/kg)	0.35	1.54	—	—	1.4–4.0
Selenium (mg/kg)	0.1	0.11	—	—	—

*National Research Council: *Nutrient requirements of dogs and cats.* Washington, DC, 2006, National Academy Press.

†Growing and weaning to 13 weeks. Numbers between parentheses are for maintenance (from National Research Council: *Nutrient requirements for minks and foxes.* Washington, DC, 1982, National Academy Press).

‡National Research Council: *Nutrient requirements for minks and foxes.* Washington, DC, 1982, National Academy Press).

§Maslanka CS: Asian small-clawed otters: Nutrition and dietary husbandry. In: *Nutrition Advisory Group handbook,* 1999.

combination with midazolam, diazepam, xylazine, medetomidine, or acepromazine (*caution:* hyperthermia or hypothermia) to improve muscle relaxation. Xylazine, medetomidine, or dexmedetomidine combined with ketamine has been recommended to improve muscle relaxation, and both combinations may be reversed with atipamezole (2.5 milligram [mg] per 5 mg medetomidine, and 1 mg per 8–12 mg xylazine).[2,13,27] Tiletamine–zolazepam is another option. Doses ranging from 2.2 to 22 mg/kg have been reported for numerous species of mustelids; higher doses result in prolonged recovery. In otters, the usage of a low dose of tiletamine–zolazepam to achieve anesthetic induction, and supplementation with isoflurane or ketamine (5 mg/kg) for maintenance, has been advocated. Flumazemil (0.05–0.1 mg/kg) may be used to antagonize the zolazepam portion of this combination to hasten recovery, but its usage has not been reported in mustelids other than the Nearctic river otter.[38] Drugs and dosages commonly used to provide chemical restraint and sedation in selected mustelids are listed in Table 48-3. These combinations usually provide short periods of chemical restraint (30–45 minutes). If longer periods of anesthesia are needed, inhalation anesthetics (isoflurane and sevoflurane) delivered via an induction chamber, mask, or endotracheal tube is efficient, although the results of chamber induction with inhalation agents may vary and cause excitement in some species. Otters hypoventilate during inhalation anesthesia and require assisted ventilation to prevent hypoxemia and hypercarbia.[26]

Whenever possible, the following parameters should be recorded when immobilizing or anesthetizing a mustelid: actual weight, relative oxyhemoglobin saturation (clamp located on tongue, lips, ears, toes), heart and respiratory rates, and rectal temperature. Possible anesthetic complications include respiratory depression (apnea, bradypnea, tachypnea, hypoxemia), hyperthermia, hypothermia, bradycardia, tachycardia, poor myorelaxation, and excitability during recovery. Hypoventilation has been reported to be a cause of mortality in otters with the use of inhalation anesthesia. During recovery from anesthesia, animals should be kept in a quiet, dark denning box or cage or in a confined area to facilitate smooth recovery from anesthesia.[26]

DIAGNOSTICS

Blood may be collected from various sites; the technique and site chosen depend on the species, how much blood is needed, and operator preference. Sites include the jugular vein, cranial vena cava, ventral coccygeal artery, median caudal vein, lateral saphenous vein,

TABLE 48-3

Drugs and Dosages Recommended for Immobilization of Selected Mustelids

Species	Recommended Anesthetic Combination (milligram per kilogram [mg/kg])	Comments/Alternative
American badger	Tiletamine-zolazepam (4.4)	Ketamine (15), xylazine (1)
American river otter	Ketamine (8–12) + midazolam (0.25–5) / Ketamine (3) + medetomidine (0.030) (atipamezole)	Ketamine (10–12) + diazepam (0.3–5) / Tiletamine–zolazepam (4) + flumazenil (0.08)Respiratory depression may occur
Asian small-clawed otter	Ketamine (15–18) + midazolam (0.75–1)	Ketamine (4–5) + medetomidine (0.1–0.12) (atipamezole) Respiratory depression may occur
Black footed ferret	Ketamine (3) + medetomidine (0.075) (atipamezole)	Ketamine (15) + diazepam (0.1)
Ermine and weasel	Ketamine (5) + medetomidine (0.1) (atipamezole)	Ketamine (3)/ Tiletamine-zolazepam (11–22)
Eurasian badger	Ketamine (5–10) + medetomidine (0.05–0.1) (atipamezole)/ tiletamine–zolazepam (10)	Ketamine (10–16) + xylazine (2–6)/ medetomidine (0.04) + tiletamine–zolazepam (2.5)
Eurasian otter	Ketamine (5) + medetomidine (0.5) (atipamezole)	Ketamine (15) + diazepam (0.5) Respiratory depression may occur
Ferret	Ketamine (10–30) + xylazine (1–2) or diazepam (1–2) or acepromazine (0.05–0.3)	Tiletamine-zolazepam (22) Recovery time may be prolonged
Giant otter	Ketamine (8.5–10.6) + xylazine (1.5–2)	Prolonged recovery
Marten	Ketamine (10) + medetomidine (0.2) (atipamezole)	Ketamine (60) + xylazine (12)
Mink	Tiletamine–zolazepam (15) / Ketamine (40) + xylazine (1)	Ketamine (5) + medetomidine (0.1) (atipamezole)
Ratel (honey badger)	Tiletamine–zolazepam (2.2)	Ketamine (6) + xylazine (0.5)
Sea otter	Butorphanol (0.5)/ oxymorphon (0.3)	Fentanyl (0.3) + azaperone (0.25) *Caution:* Numerous reports of fatal complications
Stripped skunk	Tiletamine–zolazepam (10)	Ketamine (15) + acepromazine (0.2)
Tayra	Tiletamine–zolazepam (3.3)	
Wolverine	Ketamine (5–8) + medetomidine (0.1–0.15)	Ketamine (20) + acepromazine (0.2)

cephalic vein, and femoral vein. Published reference ranges for hematologic and serum biochemistry analyses for selected mustelids are listed in Tables 48-4 and 48-5. Techniques for urine collection, urinary catheterization, splenic and bone marrow aspiration, placement of intravenous and intraosseous catheters, administration of fluids, and blood transfusion have been described for ferret and may be useful when treating other mustelids.[33] A technique of mandibular salivary gland biopsy for rabies testing has been developed in Nearctic river otters.[39] Other diagnostic techniques such as ultrasonography, electrocardiography, radiography, and auscultation are applicable but vary for each species.

DISEASES

Viral and Bacterial Diseases

The following viral diseases have been reported in mustelids: Aleutian mink disease (plasmacytosis), influenza, canine distemper, rabies, rotavirus diarrhea, infectious canine hepatitis, pseudorabies (Aujeszky disease), transmissible mink encephalopathy, mink enteritis, epizootic catarrhal enteritis of ferret (coronavirus) feline panleukopenia, canine parvovirus, feline leukemia, Powassan virus disease (arbovirus), herpes, and necrotizing encephalitis (herpes simplex).[18,21–23]

The following bacteria have been identified as pathogenic in mustelids: *Helicobacter mustelae, Desulfovibrio* spp., *Campylobacter jejuni, C. coli, Salmonella* spp., *Clostridium perfringens* type A, *C. botulinum, C. welchii, Mycobacterium* spp., *Actinomyces* spp., *Pseudomonas aeruginosa, P. putrefaciens* (also known as *Shewanella putrefaciens*), *Streptococcus* spp., *Staphylococcus* spp., *Erysipelothrix rhusiopathiae, Escherichia coli, Klebsiella pneumoniae, K. oozaenae, Bordetella bronchiseptica, Listeria monocytogenes, Yersinia pestis, Y. ruckeri, Bacillus*

anthracis, Brucella abortus, Pasteurella multocida, P. pseudotuberculosis, Francisella tularensis, Leptospira spp., *Bacteroides melanigenicus, Proteus vulgaris, P. mirabilis,* and *Plesiomonas shigelloides.*

Fungal diseases are rarely reported in mustelids, but those cited include histoplasmosis, cryptococcosis, blastomycosis, coccidiomycosis, mucormycosis (*Absidia corymbifera*), adiaspiromycosis (*Emmonsia crescens*), and dermatomycosis (*Microsporum* sp. and *Trichophyton* sp.).

Table 48-6 contains information about some common infectious diseases reported in mustelids.

Parasitic Diseases

Although not generally associated with disease, numerous external and internal parasites have been identified in both wild and captive mustelids. Table 48-7 includes data on selected parasites reported to cause disease in mustelids. Parasitic diseases are also important for wild animals undergoing translocation because of the immune suppression possibly induced by stress.[22,25]

Ectoparasites

External parasites reported to affect mustelids include the following: fleas (*Ctenocephalides canis, C. felis, Pulex irritans, Nosopsyllus fasciatus, Ceratophyllus gallinae, Chaetopsylla globiceps, Parceras melis, Spilopsyllus cuniculi, Monopsyllus sciurorum*), ticks (*Ixodes ricinus, I. bansksi, Amblyomma americanum, Dermacentor variabilis*), lice (orders Mallophaga, and Anoplura), demodectic mange (*Demodex* sp.), sarcoptic mange (*Sarcoptes scabiei*), ear mites (*Otodectes cynotis*), myiasis (*Cuterebra* spp., and *Wohlfahrtia vigil*), Guinea worm (*Dracunculus insignis*), filarial dermatitis (*Filaria taxidae*). Mite, tick, and flea treatments include concurrent treatments of the environment and the animals. Topical treatment should include those approved for use in

TABLE 48-4

Reference Range for Hematologic Parameters of Selected Mustelid Species[a]

North American Parameter*	Nearctic river otter	Eurasian otter	Mink†	Striped skunk	Ferret	European polecat‡	Striped skunk‡
Erythrocytes ×10⁶/microliter (μL)	6.10–14.50	5.2–7.8	8.07 ± 0.67	6.8–12.2	6.35–11.2	8.39 ± 1.86	8.08 ± 0.68
PCV (%)	32.2–60.8	37.8–69.1	45.9 ± 3.1	42–61	36.7–54.9	43.6 ± 8.7	43.0 ± 6.5
Hemoglobin, gram per deciliter (g/dL)	10.4–19.0	11.0–19.9	15. 6 ± 1.1	15–18	11.1–17.1	14.3 ± 2.7	13.4 ± 1.1
MCV, (fL)	38.3–49.0	60.7–105.2	56.9 ± 1.9	—	45.6–54.7	52.1 ± 407	53.0 ± 2.6
MCH, picogram (pg)	11.3–15.8	16.3–26.9	—	—	14.0–17.6	17.3 ± 1.2	17.0 ± 0.4
MCHC (%)	27.8–39.2	24.6–30.9	34.0 ± 0.52	—	30.7–32.9	33.2 ± 1.9	31.8 ± 1.2
WBC (10³/μL)	4.7–33.2	3.1–19.2	6.49 ± 2.02	4-0–19	2.0–9.8	6.20 ± 2.36	8.01 ± 3.12
Neutrophils (10³/μL)	3.0–28.2	1.41–12.86	2.64 ± 1.27	—	0.62–3.33	2.88 ± 1.63	4.22 ± 2.43
Band neutrophils (10³/μL)	0–0.48	0–1.8	0.008 ± 0.020	—	—	0.09 ± 0.05	0.22 ± 0.38
Lymphocytes (10³/μL)	0.12–4.95	0.58–3.84	3.12± 1.05	—	—	2.98 ± 1.73	3.08 ± 1.65
Eosinophils (10³/μL)	0–1.83	0–1.39	0.47 ± 0.44	—	—	0.24 ± 0.19	0.18 ± 0.08
Monocytes (10³/μL)	0–2.38	0–0.99	0.19 ± 0.13	—	0.18–0.90	0.15 ± 0.11	0.16 ± 0.07
Basophils (10³/μL)	0–0.21	0–0.18	0.05 ± 0.54	—	0.01–0.10	0.10 ± 0.07	0.0 ± 0.0
Platelets (10³/μL)	298–931	178–777	729.58 ± 125.40		277–882	303 ± 133	437 ± 0.0
Reticulocytes (%)	—	—	2.1 ± 0.9	—	1–12	—	—

*Values are presented as a range or mean plus-or-minus standard deviation.
†Values for mink refer to although no statistical differences were determined between male and female minks.
‡International Species Information System: *Physiological data reference values*. Apple Valley, MN, 2002, ISIS.
MCH, Mean corpuscular hemoglobin; *MCHC*, mean corpuscular hemoglobin concentration; *MCV*, mean corpuscular volume.

TABLE 48-5

Reference Ranges for Serum Biochemical Parameters for Selected Mustelid Species

North American Parameter*	Nearctic River Otter	Eurasian Otter	Mink	Striped Skunk†	Ferret	Pine Marten	European Polecat†
Total protein, gram per deciliter (g/dL)	5.7–9.0	6.0–7.7	5.94 ± 0.31	6.2 ± 1.2	5.1–7.4	6.1 ± 7	5.7 ± 8
Albumin (g/dL)	2.4–4.1	1.25–3.6	2.98 ± 0.14	—	2.6–4.1	3.0 ± 4	3.3 ± 0.4
Globulin (g/dL)	2.9–5.8	2.7–4.8				3.1 ± 4	2.4 ± 0.7
Calcium (mg/dL)	6.8–10.0	5.2–10.3	9.54 ± 0.39	2.43 ± 0.23	8.0–11.8	9.2 ± 1.6	9.12 ± 0.92
Phosphorus (mg/dL)	3.2–8.3	4.2–8.7	5.29 ± 0.79	1.74 ± 0.61	4.0–9.1	4.95 ± 0.92	6.19 ± 1.70
Sodium, milliequivalent per liter (mEq/L)	136–158	142–158	153.7 ± 1.3	149 ± 7	137–162	155 ± 3	152 ± 6
Potassium (mEq/L)	3.5–5.3	3.9–5.7	4.34 ± 0.23	4.8 ± 0.7	4.3–7.7	4.0 ± 0.2	4.7 ± 0.6
Chloride (mEq/L)	94–121	102–125	114.5 ± 1.7	110 ± 6	102–125	126 ± 1	116 ± 8
Creatinine (mg/dL)	0.4–0.8	0.7–1.0	0.71 ± 0.08	1.09 ± 0.80	0.2–0.9	0.79 ± 0.18	0.49 ± 0.20
Urea nitrogen (mg/dL)	17–56	17.3–68.1	15.2 ± 5.6	33.9 ± 32.9	10–45	31.64 ± 11.2	12.5 ± 3.99
Cholesterol (mg/dL)	63–279	95–220		172.4 ± 103.8	64–296	176.9 ± 23.0	191.9 ± 52.6
Glucose (mg/dL)	56–225	51–400	125.8 ± 18.7	124.8 ± 62.9	62.5–207	314.5 ± 70.90	106.9 ± 28.9
SERUM ENZYMES							
Lactic acid dehydrogenase, international unit per liter (IU/L)	36–10,820	555–3,620	—	581 ± 323	—	1,875 ± 520	474 ± 403
Alkaline phosphatase (IU/L)	29–282	9.0–199	71.6 ± 56.9	70 ± 57	9–120	77 ± 29	64 ± 79
Gamma-glutamyl transferase (IU/L)	8–38	—	—	2 ± 3	—	—	10 ± 8
Creatine kinase (IU/L)	67–1,300	26–1,794	—	895 ± 252	—	555 ± 234	379 ± 384
Alanine aminotransferase (IU/L)	46–990	34–307	—	120 ± 98	82–289	173 ± 44	102 ± 56
Aspartate aminotransferase (IU/L)	34–1,260	71–328	67.0 ± 13.7	75 ± 22	28–248	159 ± 18	74 ± 28

*Values are presented as a range or mean plus-or-minus standard deviation.
†International Species Information System: *Physiological data reference values*. Apple Valley, MN, 2002, ISIS.

TABLE 48-6

Selected Infectious Diseases of Mustelids

Disease	Causative Agent	Epizootiology	Clinical Signs	Diagnosis	Management	Species Reported
Viral canine distemper	Canine distemper virus (Paramyxoviridae)	Transmission of the virus is most commonly accomplished by aerosol exposure or direct contact with conjunctival and nasal exudates, urine, feces, and skin	Weight loss, anorexia, hyperemia of the face and ears, hyperkeratosis of the nasal planum and footpads, and oculonasal discharge	Histopathology, immunofluorescent antibody (IFA) test on conjunctival smear	Vaccination with canary-pox recombinant canine distemper virus subunit vaccine (Purevax, Merial)	Domestic ferret, black footed ferret, American and Eurasian badger, weasel, striped skunk, Eurasian and American mink, sable, stone and pine marten, polecat, weasel, Nearctic river and Eurasian otter
Influenza	Orthomyxoviridae (several strains)	Transmission by inhalation of aerosol droplets	Sneezing, conjunctivitis, unilateral otitis, fever, photophobia	Clinical signs, presence of hemagglutination-inhibiting (HI) antibodies (hemagglutination inhibition test)	Prevention of exposure of susceptible animals to infected individuals (animals or caretakers) Antihistamine, antivirals, and antibiotics may be used	Domestic ferret and mink
Aleutian disease and plasmacytosis	Parvoviridae	Infected animals may serve as potential source of infection	Weight loss, hypergammaglobulinemia, reproductive failure, hemorrhagic enteritis, and immune-mediated glomerulonephritis	Hypergammaglobulinemia usually greater than 20% of total serum protein IFA test, counter immunoelectrophoresis test	No vaccine is available	Typically a disease of farm-raised mink, but has been found in feral mink, domestic ferret, and striped skunk
Ferret kit disease	Rotavirus	Affects kits May become enzootic in the facility	Watery diarrhea, anorexia, and lethargy	Negatively stained virus particles identified in fresh feces	Subcutaneous electrolyte solutions and oral antibiotics (spectinomycin, amoxicillin, and trimethoprim-sulfa)	Ferret
Bacterial salmonellosis	Salmonella newport, S. typhimurium, S. scholerasuis, S. anatum, S. enteritidis, S. kentucky, S. hadar	Salmonella spp. have been isolated in a number of clinically normal animals Associated to feeding with uncooked meat	Hemorrhagic enteritis, dehydration, loss of body weight, fever, and lethargy	Fecal culture	Supportive care and antibiotics	Many mustelids
Tuberculosis	Mycobacterium spp. (M. bovis, M. avium-intracellulare, M. tuberculosis)	Usually infected by eating Mycobacterium-contaminated meat	Weight loss, enlarged lymph nodes, chronic respiratory disease, mastitis	Direct examination of tissue, culture	Evaluate zoonotic potential in case of treatment	Mink, ferret, otters, and Eurasian badger

Disease	Etiologic agent	Comments	Clinical signs	Diagnosis	Treatment	Species affected
Campylobacteriosis	*Campylobacter jejuni, C. coli*	Ferrets may be asymptomatic carriers; Raw meat diets may predispose mink to infection	Fever, leukocytosis, abortion, diarrhea	Fecal culture	Antimicrobials (erythromycin, amoxicillin and others)	Ferret, mink
Botulism	Type A, B, C, E; *Clostridium botulinum*, and *C. perfringens* type A, *C. welchii*	Caused by eating uncooked or contaminated meat; Associated with capture stress in wild otters	Animals are found dead or with paralysis, and dyspnea before dying; Enterotoxemia, acute gastric distention, cyanosis	Fecal Gram stain, toxin assay	Prevention and treatment difficult; Aggressive therapy	Otters, black-footed ferret
Pneumonia	*Pseudomonas aeruginosa, P. putrefaciens, S. zooepidemicus, S. pneumoniae, E. coli, Klebsiella pneumoniae, Bordetella bronchiseptica, Listeria monocytogenes*	Concurrent infection with calicivirus or picornavirus may predispose animal to infection	Dyspnea, cyanotic mucous membranes, increased lung sounds, nasal discharge, fever, lethargy, and anorexia	Clinical signs, complete blood count results (leukocytosis), culture, and cytologic findings	Supportive care, antimicrobial therapy according to test results; Antibiotics to consider include trimethoprim-sulfa, and cephalosporins	Most mustelids
Anthrax	*Bacillus anthracis*		Acute death, with blood draining from body cavities	Staining smears of peripheral blood, postmortem lesions	Penicillin: streptomycin	Eurasian badger, honey badger, and mink
Fungal dermatomycosis	*Microsporum* sp. and *Trichophyton* sp.	Transmitted by direct contact or via fomites and is associated with overcrowding and exposure to cats	Skin and hair lesions similar to those reported in other species	Clinical signs are suspicious but diagnosis is made on the basis of a mycotic culture	Topical treatment with keratolytic shampoos, povidone-iodine scrubs, and antifungal medications (itraconazole, ketoconazole)	Most species

TABLE 48-7

Selected Parasitic Diseases of Mustelids

Parasite	Location in Host	Clinical Signs	Diagnosis	Management	Species Reported
Toxoplasma gondii	Multiple organs (disseminated)	Elevated rectal temperature, lymphadenitis, splenomegaly, myocarditis, pneumonitis, hepatitis, encephalitis	Serologic	Prevention Avoid contact with feline species and feline feces Treatment with pyrimethamine and sulfamerazine, others	Skunk, ferret, weasel, polecat, otters
Lung worms (*Crenosoma* spp., *Perostrongylus* spp., *Filaroides* spp., *Skrjabingylus* spp.)	Lung and sinus	Cachexia, anemia, coughing, dyspnea, depression, nasal discharge, and neurologic signs	Finding the ova or first stage infective larvae in fecal samples	Use of appropiate anthelmintic drug (ivermectin, fenbendazole, mebendazole)	Mink, skunk, sable, Eurasian badger, otter, ermine
Kidney worm (*Dioctophyma renale*)	Kidney (usually right kidney)	Weight loss, hematuria, polyuria, renal colic, and trembling	Finding of characteristic ova in urine, radiography or ultrasonography	Surgical treatment (removal of the parasitized kidney), fluid and antibiotic therapy	Mink, otter, weasel, ermine, marten, fisher, grison
Sarcoptic mange (*Sarcoptes scabiei*)	Skin (especially head and neck)	Scab formation around head and neck, tail, and feet In advanced cases, the entire body may be involved	Finding the mites in skin scraping or biopsy Diagnostic treatment with ivermectin	Ivermectin (0.3–0.4 milligram per kilogram [mg/kg]) as a single injection, or 0.2 mg/kg, orally (PO) every other day for 2 weeks if severe; antibiotics for secondary infection	Most mustelids
Fleas (most often *Ctenocephalides* sp.)		May be asymptomatic, pruritus and flea allergy dermatitis, with chronic scratching and rubbing Severe infestation may lead to debilitation by exsanguination	Visualization of fleas or flea defecations	Affected animals and enclosures should be repeatedly treated with suitable insecticides (pyrethrins, fibronil, imidacloprid [use small cat/kitten vial/dose], lufenuron)	Most mustelids

cats (pyrethrin powders and sprays and others). Organophosphates and carbamates should be used with caution, as safe protocols for mustelids have not been established.

Internal Parasites

Protozoal infection include *Giardia* spp., *Isospora* spp., *Eimeria* spp., *Sarcocystis* spp., *Toxoplasma gondii*, *Neospora caninum*, *Sarcosporidium* sp., *Besnoitia* spp., *Hepatozoon* spp., *Pneumocystis carinii*, *Trypanosomiasis cruzi*, *Cryptosporidium* spp.[40]

Helminths reported from mustelids in both zoos and from the wild include: lung flukes (*Paragonimus westermani* and *P. kellicotti*), intestinal fluke (*Nanophyetus salmincola*, *Troglotrema acutum*), liver flukes (*Fasciola hepatica*), Acanthocephala (*Corynsoma semerme*, *C. strumosum*, *Macracanthorhynchus ingens*), tapeworms (*Taenia* sp., *Monordotaenia* sp., *Oschmarenia* sp.), trichinosis (*Trichinella* sp.), lung worms (*Skrjabingylus* spp., *Crenosoma* spp., *Perostrongylus* spp., and *Filaroides* spp.), heartworms (*Dirofilaria* spp.), ascariasis (*Ascaris* spp., *Baylisascaris devosi*, *Toxocara canis*), *Dioctophyma renale*, *Dracunculus* spp., *Strongyloides* spp., *Capillaria hepatica*, *Uncinaria* sp., *Euyhelmis squamula*, *Aonthotheca putorii*, *Eucoleus* sp., *Pearsonema plica*, *Molineus patens*, and *Mastophorus muris*.

Table 48-8 lists common drugs and doses used for controlling parasitic diseases in mustelids.

Noninfectious Diseases

The following have been reported to affect wild and domestic mustelids (Table 48-9). Renal calculi (calcium oxalate and urate calculi) were detected in 66.1% of the captive North American adult population of Asian small-clawed otters that had been imaged or necropsied, and prevalence in wild-born otters was 76.7%. The captive diet appears to be a contributing factor to urolith formation and progression.[32] Other medical problems associated with nutrition and feeding practices in mustelids are hypovitaminosis A; vitamin E, thiamin, (Chastek disease), calcium, vitamin D, zinc, and biotin deficiencies; zinc toxicity; nutritional secondary hyperparathyroidism (NSH); fibrous osteodystrophy; gastric trichobezoars; dental disease (dental calculus, gingivitis, and periodontal disease); gastric and duodenal ulceration; and gastric dilatation and torsion.[34,36]

Metabolic Diseases

Urolithiasis (magnesium ammonium phosphate, calcium oxalate, calcium urate, calcium phosphate, and ammonium urate uroliths), hypocalcemia, pregnancy toxemia, agalactia, hyperestrogenism, hormonal alopecia, idiopathic hypersplenism, gastric dilatation and torsion (possibly associated with *Clostridium welchii*), dental and skeletal anomalies, periodontal disease, amyloidosis, hyperadrenocorticism (ferret), insulinoma (ferret), diabetes mellitus (ferret), fatty

TABLE 48-8

Parasiticides Recommended for Mustelids

Generic Name	Dosage (milligram per kilogram [mg/kg])	Route of Administration	Comments
Amprolium	19, every 24 hours	Orally (PO)	Coccidia
Carbaryl (0.5%) shampoo		Weekly for 3 weeks	Mange
Fenbendazole	50, for 3–5 days	Oral	Alternatively 20 mg/kg for 5 days
Fipronil	1 pump of spray or $\frac{1}{6}$–$\frac{1}{2}$ of cat dose every 60 days	Topical	Flea adulticide
Ivermectin	0.2–0.5, repeat every 2 weeks if needed	Subcutaneous (SC) or PO	0.006 mg/kg, PO, monthly for heartworm prevention Ectoparasites and endoparasites
Levamisole	10	PO or SC	May be toxic at higher dosages
Mebendazole	50 mg/kg q12h × 2 days	PO	Nematodes
Metronidazole	15–20, every 12 hours for 2 weeks	PO	Protozoa: *Clostridium* spp.
Pyrethroids		—	Ectoparasites
Praziquantel	5–25, repeat in 2 weeks	PO or SC	Cestodes and trematodes
Propoxur	—	Topical	Ectoparasites
Pyantel pamoate	5–60, repeat in 14 days OR 4.4 mg/kg q2 weeks	PO	Nematodes
Sulfadimethoxin	20–50, every 12–24 hours	PO	Antiparasitic, coccidian antimicrobial
Thiacetarsemide	2.2, every 12 hours for 2 days	Intravenously (IV)	Heartworm adulticide Follow 3–4 weeks later with ivermectin Caution must be used

liver, cardiovascular calcification, osteomalacia, and degenerative joint disease.[11,37]

Neoplasia

Over 50 different neoplasms have been reported in the domestic ferret. Although no current consensus exists on the cause of the high prevalence of neoplasia in ferrets, several theories have been proposed: genetic predisposition, early neutering of ferrets at 5 to 6 weeks of age, lack of natural photoperiod or exposure to natural sunlight, diet, and infectious agents. However, neoplasms are not common in species other than ferrets and include: seminoma, leiomyoma, adenocarcinoma, pheochromocytoma, teratoma, lymphosarcoma, anal sac carcinoma, lymphoreticular tumor, bronchoalveolar carcinoma, thyroid carcinoma, malignant melanoma, and a tumor resembling Hodgkin disease.[6,7]

Miscellaneous Diseases

Reproductive toxicity (including decreased baculum weight, cryptorchidism, cystic vas deferens) in European otters exposed to polychlorinated biphenyls and polychlorinated dibenzo-p-dioxins; organophosphate and carbamate intoxication; mortality associated with melarsomine and petroleum residues; mercury toxicity; secondary exposure to rodenticide; shock; exertional myopathy (capture myopathy); trauma; intestinal volvulus; pneumoperitoneum; uterine torsion; interspecific aggression (especially following introductions); behavior problems (self-mutilation); cystic kidneys; dilated cardiomyopathy; cor pulmonale; intervertebral disk disease; osteoarthritis; tail alopecia syndrome; overgrowth of claws; oral, gastric, and intestinal foreign bodies; gastric and intestinal ulcers; pyometra; capture related injuries (mostly digit and tooth damage); pulmonary silicosis; fibrocartilaginous emboli; trauma (mostly associated with gunshots, vehicle encounters, and from traps); and hydrocephalus in European otter cubs have all been reported.[9,14,17,24,31]

REPRODUCTION

Important variations exist in the reproductive cycles among mustelids. Some data for representative species are listed in Table 48-10.

Most mustelids are seasonal breeders, with the sea otter and the Eurasian otter being exceptions. The duration of the breeding season may vary from 1 month (African striped weasel) to 12 months (Eurasian badger). Some mustelids are polyestrous, and others are monoestrous. The duration of estrus ranges from 3 to 5 days to 5 to 8 weeks. Most males that have been studied have active spermatogenesis for only about 3 to 4 months in a year, although exceptions such as the Eurasian badger do exist. Mustelids may be either induced or spontaneous ovulators.

Many mustelids exhibit delayed implantation: sea otters, Nearctic river otters, hog badgers, American and Eurasian badgers, ratels, striped skunks, western spotted skunks, wolverines, all martens, ermines, long tail weasels, minks, and marbled polecats. In those species, embryo development proceeds to the blastocyst stage and then ceases. This period of blastocyst dormancy is called diapause and varies from a few weeks in minks and striped skunks to almost a year in the Eurasian badgers. Extensive studies have been conducted on the mechanisms that control embryonic diapause in three species of mustelids: minks (*Mustela vison*), Eurasian badgers (*Meles meles*), and western spotted skunks (*Spilogale gracilis*). Numerous investigators have speculated on the ecologic significance and selective pressures that might have favored the development of delayed implantation.[29]

Changes in photoperiods are known to alter the secretion of pituitary hormones and thus the onset and duration of breeding, puberty, and timing of implantation. In this way, photomanipulation has been used in some species. Adequate numbers of animals should be maintained for mating, but compatibility does not ensure reproductive success. If copulation or gestation does not occur, different pairings should be tried, but in some cases, animals that are not compatible during most of the year will often breed if introduced during estrus. For this, determining when females are in estrous may be crucial. Various methods for estrus detection have been proposed in different species, including behavioral changes, vulvar swelling, vaginal cytology, and fecal and urinary hormone analyses. In males, the testes enlarge during the breeding season. Pregnancy may be determined by urinary progesterone and conjugated estrogen levels, palpation, radiography (end of gestation period), and ultrasonography.[4]

TABLE 48-9

Selected Noninfectious Diseases of Mustelids

Disease	Etiology	Signs	Management	Prevention	Species Reported
Exertional myopathy	Often, associated to recently immobilized, captured, and transported wild animals	Vary with species. Elevated body temperature, depression, lack of response to the environment, ataxia, weakness, dark colored urine, elevated renal and muscular serum enzymes	Treatment is rarely successful. Selenium or vitamin E preparations given subcutaneously or intramuscularly, sodium bicarbonate balanced electrolyte solution, and nonsteroidal anti-inflammatories	Improve methods of capture or restraint. Reduce stress and hyperthermia during animal handling	Badger, otter, black footed ferret
Urolithiasis	Magnesium ammonium phosphate, calcium oxalate, calcium urate, calcium phosphate, and ammonium urate. Primary cause unknown. Diet (?)	Normally unnoticeable. Abdominal radiography and ultrasonography are the most important diagnostic tools. Signs may be similar to those in dogs and cats	In some cases, surgery or lithotripsy may be considered	—	Mink, ferret, Eurasian otter, small-clawed otter
Petroleum pollution	Spilled petroleum oils (crude or fuel)	Animals look wet and chilled. Lethargy, dermatitis, conjunctivitis, respiratory distress, dehydration, malnutrition, anemia, thermoregulatory dysfunction, diarrhea, and neurologic signs	Primarily symptomatic. Warm intravenous, intraosseous, subcutaneous isotonic fluids, glucose, antibiotics, and glucocorticoids. Good ventilation, flushing the eyes. Hand or tube feeding may be required. Monitor blood parameters	—	Any aquatic mustelid may be affected
Polychlorinated biphenyls (PCBs)	Accumulation of high level of PCBs, especially by fish eating species	Anorexia, bloody stools, hepatic liver, kidney degeneration, gastric ulcers, decreased baculum weight, feminization of males. Population declines, reproductive complications and kit mortality	—	—	Effects diagnosed in mink, Eurasian otter, polecat; may affect any piscivore species
Amyloidosis	Deposition of amyloid (17 different proteins) either locally or systemically	Relate to the specific sites of amyloid deposition. Histologic evaluation of tissues obtained by biopsy or at necropsy	Usually progressive. Treatment unsuccessful. In humans, some trials include antibiotics, colchicine, and dimethyl sulfoxide	—	Beech marten, pine marten, mink, wolverine, Asian small-clawed otter
Thiamine deficiency	Thiaminase present in some fish (especially carp, bullhead, smelt, herring)	Anorexia, salivation, ataxia, incoordination, pupillary dilation, and sluggish reflexes	Parenteral thiamine administration	Supplement with thiamine in piscivores species	Mink and otter. May be a problem in piscivores species
Self-mutilation	Agitation, cutaneous excoriation, hair loss, cutaneous hemorrhage, secondary bacterial infection	Observation, physical examination, skin scrapings for cytology, etc.	Buspirone 10 milligram per kilogram (mg/kg), orally (PO) twice daily for 18 months	Proper housing, diet, species pairings	American badger

TABLE 48-10

Some Reproductive Characteristics of Selected Mustelids

Parameter	Badger (American/ Eurasian)	Ferret, Black-Footed Ferret	Marten (Pine/Stone)	Mink (American; Eurasian)	Otter (Nearctic River; Eurasian)	Giant Otter	Skunk (Striped; Spotted)	Tayra	European Polecat	Common Weasel/Ermine	Wolverine
Gestation	8 months; 9-12 months	41-42 days; 42-43 days	9 months	40-70 days; 35-72 days	245-365 days; 63-63 days	65-70 days	In South, 59-77 days; in North, 230-350 days	63-70 days	40-42 days	34-37 days; 10 months	7-9 months
Delayed implantation	Yes	No	Yes	Yes	Yes/no	No	No/yes	No	No	No/yes	Yes
Litter size	1-7; 1-6	1-18; 1-6	2-5/2-7	3-10; 2-7	2-5; 2-4	1-5	2-10/2-9	2	4-6	4-7; 4-8	2-3
Mass at birth	90-98 grams (g); 5-85 g	8-10 g; unknown	30 g	6-12 g; unknown	100-120 g	170-230 g	32-35;22 g	75-95 g	7-12 g	0.9-2.3/2.6-4.2 g	80-100 g
Weaning	3 months	6-8 weeks; unknown	4 months	3 months	3-4 months	3-4 months	2 months	Unknown	1 month	60 days; unknown	3 months
Sexual maturity	1 year	4-8 months in first year	28 months	In first year	23-27 months; in 2-3 years	Unknown	10 months in first year	1.5-2 years	In first year	115-1150 days; unknown	In 2-3 years
Type estrus*	M; P	P; M	M; —	P; —	M; P	—	M; P	P	—; M	—; M	P
Teats (pairs)	4; 3	2	2	4	—; 2-3	—	5-7; 5	—	3-5	5; 4-5	2

*M, Monoestrous; P, polyestrous.

In ferrets, continued high levels of estradiol from persistent estrus may lead to alopecia and bone marrow suppression, resulting in pancytopenia and even death, so nonbreeding females should be neutered.

Contraception

No specific recommendations for contraception exist for mustelids, and ovariohysterectomy, vasectomy, and castration are currently the safest permanent sterilization procedures of birth control. Melengestrol acetate hormone implants have been used successfully to prevent conception in mustelids. These should be removed after 2 years for one pregnancy, if possible, and are not recommended for more than a total of 4 years. The human contraceptive implant Norplant contains levonorgestrel, a synthetic progestin, and has been used to prevent pregnancy in the striped skunk. Depo-Provera injection (5 mg/kg every 2 months) has also been used. Although no data exist for mustelids, progestin contraceptives may be associated to progressive endometrial hyperplasia, resulting in infertility, infections, and sometimes uterine cancer in other carnivores. Deslorelin implants (gonadotropin-releasing hormone [GnRH] analogue) have been used as an alternative to melengestrol acetate.[1]

PREVENTIVE MEDICINE

Many of the clinical and surgical procedures used in dogs and cats are applied to mustelids. Specialized surgical procedures have been developed for some mustelid species.[20,28,38] Periodic examinations should include the following:

- Checking transponders and tattoos, and reapplication, if necessary
- Checking baseline physiologic parameters (weight, breeding status)
- Examination of the oral cavity
- Evaluation of the reproductive tract, whole body radiography
- Collecting blood for hematologic and biochemical evaluation
- Checking for heartworm in endemic areas using a heartworm enzyme-linked immunosorbent antigen assay test
- Serum banking
- Performing fecal examination for internal parasites (and administering anthelmintics, if necessary). Table 48-8 lists some of the antiparasitic drugs commonly used to treat mustelids. Other drugs (e.g., antibiotics) are dosed at rates for ferrets, dogs, and cats.[8]
- Updating vaccinations

Few viral diseases have been reported in mustelids, except ferrets, although they have been routinely vaccinated against a wide variety of viral diseases. Mustelids have varying susceptibility (species and exposure dependent) to feline panleukopenia, canine distemper, rabies, and leptospirosis.[10] Most authors recommend vaccination of mustelids against rabies and canine distemper. Safety and efficacy of modified live canine distemper vaccinations in exotic species of carnivores has been historically problematic because vaccine-induced distemper has occurred (e.g., a modified-live virus derived from chick embryo cell culture caused the death of four female black-footed ferrets [*Mustela nigripes*], or protection was not achieved). In the past, killed distemper vaccines have not provided longstanding protection in most species. A recombinant canarypox-vectored canine distemper vaccine (Purevax, Merial, Athens, GA) has been shown to be safe and efficacious and is the best choice for general mustelid protection against canine distemper virus.[41] If an alternative modified-live canine distemper vaccine is used, it should be given separately and not in multiple forms, since immunosuppression and other untoward vaccine interactions might lead to disease. Ferret or mink cell culture-derived modified-live vaccines should *never* be used in mustelids. A modified-live canine distemper vaccine of primate kidney tissue cell origin, Onderstepoort type, is available in the United States (Galaxy D; Schering-Plough Animal Health Corporation, Omaha, NE) and has been proven to be safe and efficacious in hybrid black-footed ferrets and Siberian polecats. The only vaccine approved by the U.S. Department of Agriculture (USDA) for ferrets,

Fervac-D (United Vaccines, Madison, WI), which is an egg-adapted strain, has induced anaphylactoid and anaphylactic reactions in some mustelids, so its use is not recommended.

Vaccination schedules for nondomestic species are extrapolated from studies of the domestic dog. Neonates receiving colostrum should be vaccinated every 3 to 4 weeks between 6 and 16 weeks of age. Colostrum-deprived neonates should be given two vaccinations administered at a 3- to 4-weeks interval and starting at 2 weeks of age because maternal antibodies acquired in utero may be absent by 4 to 6 weeks of age. Data on maternal antibody interference with vaccination in ferrets suggest that a final canine distemper vaccine should be administered after 10 weeks of age.

If an animal has an adverse reaction to canine distemper vaccine, an antihistamine (e.g., diphenhydramine hydrochloride, 0.5–2 mg/kg, intravenously [IV] or intramuscularly [IM]) or, for severe reactions, epinephrine (20 microgram per kilogram [μg/kg], IV, IM, subcutaneously [SC], or intratracheally [IT]) should be administered and supportive care provided.

Mustelids are also vaccinated with a killed rabies vaccine (Imrab), although the efficacy of this vaccine has not been proven in exotic mustelids. Rabies should be given at 16 weeks of age to animals at risk of contracting rabies and given boosters annually thereafter.

ACKNOWLEDGMENT

The authors acknowledge Helena Marques, Elena Rafart, Hugo Fernandez, Carlos Feliu, Jon Arnemo, Marie-Pierre Ryser-Degiorgis, Lucy Spelman, Jordi Ruiz, Rafael Cebrian, Jose Domingo, Victor Bonet, Willem Schaftenaar, and Eric Miller for assistance with the preparation of this chapter.

REFERENCES

1. Association of Zoo and Aquariums Wildlife Contraception Center: www.aza.org/wildlife-contraception-center.
2. Arnemo JM, Moe RO, Søli NE: Immobilization of captive pine martens (*Martes martes*) with medetomidine-ketamine and reversal with atipamezole. *J Zoo Wildlife Med* 25:548–554, 1994.
3. Association of Zoos and Aquariums: *Association of Zoo and Aquarium, Small Carnivore Tag 2009. Otter (Lutrinae) care manual*, Silver Spring, MD, 2009, Association of Zoos and Aquariums, pp 5–18.
4. Association of Zoos and Aquariums: *Association of Zoo and Aquarium, Small Carnivore Tag 2010. Mustelid (Mustelidae) care manual*, Silver Spring, MD, 2009, Association of Zoos and Aquariums, pp 5–20, 2010.
5. Baitchman E, Kollias GV: Clinical anatomy of the North American river otter (*Lontra canadensis*). *J Zoo Wildl Med* 32(4):473–483, 2000.
6. Bartlett SL, Imai DM, Trupkiewicz JG, et al: Intestinal lymphoma of granular lymphocytes in a fisher (*Martes martes*). *J Zoo Wildl Med* 41:309–315, 2010.
7. Bunting EM, Garner MM, Abou-Madi N: Proliferative thyroid lesions and hyperthyroidism in captive fishers (*Martes martes*). *J Zoo Wildl Med* 41:296–308, 2010.
8. Carpenter JW, Marion CJ: *Exotic animal formulary*, St. Louis, MO, 2013, Saunders, pp 561–594.
9. Cooper JE: Other mustelids. In Mullineaux E, Best D, Cooper JE, editors: *British Small Animal Veterinary Association manual of wildlife casualties*, Quedgeley, Gloucester, 2003, British Small Animal Veterinary Association, pp 147–151.
10. Deem SL, Spelman LH, Yates RA, Montali RJ: Canine distemper in terrestrial carnivores: A review. *J Zoo Wildl Med* 31:441–451, 2000.
11. Elhensheri M, Linke RP, Blankenburg R, et al: Idiopathic systemic AA-amyloidosis in a skunk (*Mephitis mephitis*). *J Zoo Wildl Med* 43:181–185, 2012.
12. Estes JA: Adaptations for aquatic living by carnivores. In Gittleman JL, editor: *Carnivore behavior, ecology, and evolution*, vol II, New York, 1996, Cornell University Press, pp 242–282.
13. Fahlman A, Arnemo JM, Persson J, et al: Capture and medetomidine-ketamine anesthesia of free-ranging wolverines (*Gulo gulo*). *J Wildl Dis* 44:133–142, 2008.

14. Fairbrother A, Locke LN, Hoff GL: *Noninfectious diseases of wildlife*, Ames, IA, 1996, Iowa State University Press, p 219.

15. Fernandez-Moran J: Mustelidae. In Fowler ME, Miller RE, editors: *Zoo and wild animal medicine*, ed 5, Philadelphia, PA, 2003, Saunders, pp 501–516.

16. Fowler ME: *Restraint and handling of wild and domestic animals*, ed 3, Ames, IA, 2008, Wiley-Blackwell, pp 280–283.

17. Gage LJ: Use of buspirone and enrichment to manage aberrant behavior in an American badger (*Taxidea taxus*). *J Zoo Wildl Med* 36:520–522, 2005.

18. Graham E, Lamm C, Denk D, et al: Systemic coronavirus-associated disease resembling feline infectious peritonitis in ferrets in the UK. *Vet Rec* 171:200–201, 2013.

19. Hartup BK, Kollias GV, Jacobsen MC, et al: Exertional myopathy in translocated river otters from New York. *J Wild Dis* 35(3):542–547, 1999.

20. Hernandez-Divers SM, Kollias GV, Abou-Madi N, et al: Surgical technique for intraabdominal radiotransmitter placement in North American river otters (*Lontra canadensis*). *J Wildl Med* 32(2):202–205, 2001.

21. Keller SM, Gabriel M, Terio KA, et al: Canine distemper in an isolated population of fishers (*Martes pennanti*) from California. *J Wildl Dis* 48:1034–1041, 2012.

22. Kimber KR, Kollias GV: Infectious and parasitic diseases and contaminated-related problems of North American river otters (*Lontra canadensis*): A review. *J Zoo Wildl Med* 31:45–472, 2000.

23. Kimber KR, Kollias GV, Dubovi EJ: Serologic survey of selected viral agents in recently captured wild North American river otters. *J Zoo Wildl Med* 31(2):168–175, 2000.

24. Kimber K, Kollias GV: Evaluation of injury, severity, and hematological and plasma biochemistry values for recently captured North American river otters (*Lontra canadensis*). *J Zoo Wildl Med* 3693:371–384, 2005.

25. Kollias GV: Health assessment, medical management, and prerelease conditioning of translocated North American river otters. In Fowler ME, Miller RE, editors: *Zoo and wild animal medicine*, Philadelphia, PA, 1999, Saunders, pp 443–448.

26. Kollias GV, Abou-Madi N: Procyonids and mustelids. In West G, Heard D, Caulkett N, editors: *Zoo animal and wildlife immobilization and anesthesia*, Ames, IA, 2007, Blackwell Publishing, pp 419–427.

27. Kreeger TJ, Arnemo JM, Raath JP: *Handbook of wildlife chemical immobilization*, Ft. Collins, CO, 2002, Wildlife Pharmaceuticals, Inc.

28. McEwen MM, Moon-Masset PF, Butler FC, et al: Polymerized bovine hemoglobin (oxyglobin solution) administration in two river otters (*Lontra canadensis*). *Vet Anesth Anal* 28:214–219, 2001.

29. Mead RA: The physiology and evolution of delayed implantation in carnivores. In Gittleman JL, editor: *Carnivore behavior, ecology, and evolution*, vol II, New York, 1996, Cornell University Press, pp 437–464.

30. Melquist WE, Polechia PJ, Toweill D: River otter (*Lontra canadensis*). In Feldman GA, Thompson BC, Champman JA, editors: *Wild mammals of North America—biology, management and conservation*, ed 2, Baltimore, MD, 2003, The Johns Hopkins University Press, pp 708–734.

31. Neifer DL, Klein EC, Calle PP, et al: Mortality associated with melarsomine dihydrochloride administration in two North American river otters (*Lontra canadensis*) and a red panda (*Ailurus fulgens fulgens*). *J Zoo Wildl Med* 33:242–248, 2002.

32. Petrini KR, Lulich JP, Treschel L, Nachreiner RF: Evaluation of urinary and serum metabolites in Asian small-clawed otters (*Aonyx cinerea*) with calcium oxalate urolithiasis. *J Zoo Wildlife Med* 30:54–63, 1999.

33. Quesenberry K, Carpenter JW: *Ferrets, rabbits, and rodents*, ed 3, St. Louis, MO, 2012, Elsevier.

34. Righton AL, St. Leger JA, Schmitt T, et al: Serum vitamin A concentrations in captive sea otters (*Enhydra lutris*). *J Zoo Wildl Med* 42:124–127, 2011.

35. Sato JJ, Welsan M, Prevosti F, et al: Evolutionary and biogeographic history of weasel-like carnivorans (*Musteloidea*). *Mol Phylogenet Evol* 63:745–757, 2012.

36. Simpson VR, King MA: Otters. In Mullineaux E, Best D, Cooper JE, editors: *British Small Animal Veterinary Association manual of wildlife casualties*, Quedgeley, Gloucester, 2003, British Small Animal Veterinary Association, pp 137–146.

37. Simpson VR, Tomlinson AJ, Molenaar FM, et al: Renal calculi in wild Eurasian otters (*Luta lutra*) in England. *Vet Rec* 169:49, 2011.

38. Spelman LH: Otter anesthesia. In Fowler ME, Miller RE, editors: *Zoo and wild animal medicine: Current therapy*, ed 4, Philadelphia, PA, 1999, Saunders, pp 436–443.

39. Tocidlowski ME, Harms CA, Summer PW, Summer PW: Technique of mandibular salivary gland biopsy in river otters (*Lutra lutra*). *J Zoo Wildlife Med* 30:252–255, 1999.

40. Van Der Hage MH, Dorrestein GM: *Neospora caninum*: myocarditis in a European pine marten (*Martes martes*). In *Proceedings of the 4th scientific meeting, European association of Zoo and Wildlife Veterinarians*, Heidelberg, Germany, 2002, p 217.

41. Wimsatt J, Biggins D, Innes K, et al: Evaluation of oral and subcutaneous delivery of an experimental canary pox recombinant canine distemper vaccine in the Siberian polecat (*Mustela exermanni*). *J Zoo Wildl Med* 34:25–35, 2003.

CHAPTER 49

Procyonids and Viverids

Edward Ramsay

BIOLOGY

Members of the families Procyonidae and Viveridae are small- and medium-sized, mainly nocturnal members of the order Carnivora. Although the two groups are taxonomically distant, they share susceptibilities to several important infectious diseases and are handled similarly by veterinarians. Only a few procyonid and viverid species are commonly exhibited by zoos or kept as pets.

Procyonids are arctoid or canoid carnivores, more closely related to canids than felids; all but one species, the red panda, are native to the temperate and tropical New World (Table 49-1). Raccoons are the best known and most widely distributed member of this family. In addition to their distribution in their native North and Central Americas, feral raccoon populations have been established in Japan and Eurasia. The raccoon has been the best studied member of the

TABLE 49-1

Biologic Data for the Family Procyonidae

Scientific Name	Common Name	Weight (kilogram)	Geographic Distribution
Procyon lotor	Raccoon	2–12	North America to Panama
Nasua nasua	Coatimundi	3–6	Arizona, United States to Argentina
Potos flavus	Kinkajou	1.4–4.6	Southern Mexico to Central Brazil
Olingo gabbii	Olingo	0.9–1.5	Central America to Northern South America
Bassariscus astutus	Ringtail cat, cacomistle	0.8–1.4	Western United States to Southern Mexico
Ailurus fulgens	Red panda	4–8	Himalayas to Northern Myanmar, Central China

TABLE 49-2

Biologic Data for Selected Members of the Family Viveridae

Scientific Name	Common Name	Weight (kilogram)	Geographic Distribution
Arctictis binturong	Binturong	9–14	Southeast Asia
Genetta spp.	Genets	1–3	Southern Europe, Africa, and the Middle East
Paradoxurus hermaphrodites	Common palm civet	1.5–4.5	Southern and Southeast Asia
Cynictis penecillata	Yellow mongoose	0.4–0.8	Southern Africa
Suricata suricatta	Meerkat, suricate	0.6–1.0	Southern Africa
Cryptoprocta ferox	Fossa	7–12	Madagascar
Mungos mungo	Banded mongoose	1.0–1.2	Sub-Saharan Africa
Helogale parvula	Dwarf mongoose	0.23–68	Eastern and Southern Africa

Procyonidae family because of its almost ubiquitous presence in a wide variety of rural and suburban habitats.

Other members of family Procyonidae are the arboreal kinkajous and olingos, the diurnal coatimundis, and the secretive ringtail cats. Red pandas are an exceptional species in this family—they are the only strictly herbivorous members of the family, and their taxonomy has been a subject of debate. The species has been variously assigned to its own family (family Ailuridae), grouped with the giant panda in the family Ailuropodidae, and assigned to the family Procyonidae. It is the only procyonid native to the Old World, living in the mountainous regions of Nepal, northern Southeast Asia, and central China.

Members of the family Viveridae are feloid carnivores; they are more closely related to felids than to canids and are predominantly forest dwellers. The family contains approximately 36 genera and 70 species, and most are small and nocturnal. They are widely distributed in the temperate and tropical regions of Eurasia and throughout Africa (Table 49-2). Mongooses have been introduced to the Pacific and Caribbean islands for pest control but are now considered a detrimental introduced species. Few members of this family are routinely exhibited outside of their range states. The diurnal, social meerkat is the most widely exhibited viverid species. Banded and dwarf mongooses are also popular exhibit animals, mostly in Europe. The binturong is the largest viverid and is frequently kept in captivity.

UNIQUE ANATOMY AND PHYSIOLOGY

Most procyonids and viverids have elongated, slender bodies and long tails. Kinkajous and binturongs have prehensile tails. Both families are anatomically conservative, quadripedal mammals, with most species having five digits per limb. Several species in both families have semi-retractable claws. The digitigrade viverids have a "waltzing trot" gait, whereas plantigrade species such as the binturong have a more shuffling gait.

The soles of red pandas' feet are covered with hair and possess a central pad scent gland that may be mistaken for a skin lesion. The red panda forelimb also possesses an enlarged radial sesamoid bone, termed the "panda's thumb." This bone is slightly movable and is used to grasp and hold bamboo, their principle food.

Kinkajous have a long, narrow tongue adapted to eating fruit and honey. Procyonids, including the red panda, lack a cecum, whereas the viverids, with the exception of *Nandinia* spp., have a cecum. Male

viverids possess a baculum, and gender identification is not difficult in these animals, with the exception of the immature female fossa (*Cryptoprocta ferox*). The young female fossa undergoes a period of masculination during when the animal has an elongated clitoris, which contains an os clitoris, and may have scrotumlike swellings. The os penis disappears at maturity.

A notable anatomic feature of the viverids is their enlarged perianal scent glands. These glands vary in size and complexity among the species. The glands' secretions are used to mark territories and may also be used as a defense. The perianal glandular secretion from the genera *Civetticits*, *Viverra*, and *Viveriricula* is known as "civet" and is used in the manufacture of perfume and medicines.

SPECIAL HOUSING REQUIREMENTS

All procyonid and most viverid species are good climbers and should be housed in enclosures with climbing structures. Most are hardy animals and adapt to a variety of climates, but the tropical species should be provided with indoor enclosures and heat during harsh winters. The red panda is native to high mountain habitats, so enclosures should be provided with cool areas or air conditioning in regions with hot, humid summers. Pregnant and parturient red pandas should have a variety of denning boxes, as some females frequently move cubs between boxes.

Many mongooses are good burrowers and will spend considerable time digging. Natural substrate should be provided for these species.

FEEDING

Procyonids are generally omnivorous, eating a wide variety of food items. Commercial dog kibble is the basis of most captive raccoon diets and is given along with a variety of fruits and vegetables. Obesity caused by overeating and lack of exercise is also a common problem in captive raccoons. The kinkajou is mainly frugivorous but also eats insects and small vertebrates. The ringtail cats are the most carnivorous of the procyonids, and the red panda eats almost exclusively bamboo in the wild. In captivity, red pandas are typically fed a mixture of commercial "primate" biscuits, fruits, vegetables, and bamboo. If at all possible, bamboo should make at least 50% of the

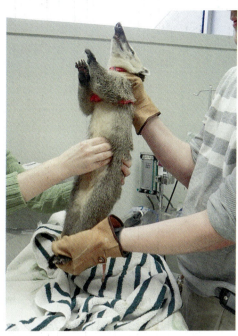

FIGURE 49-1 Hand restraint and examination of an adult coatimundi. (Photo courtesy of Cheryl Greenacre.)

TABLE 49-3

Chemical Restraint Agents and Intramuscular Dosages for Procyonids and Viverids

Species	Induction Agents	Reversal Agents
Raccoon	20 ketamine mg/kg + 4 xylazine mg/kg	Yohimbine 0.125 mg/kg
	3 mg/kg tiletamine and zolazepam + 2 mg/kg xylazine	
Coatimundi	20 mg/kg ketamine + 1 mg/kg xylazine	Yohimbine 0.125 mg/kg
Kinkajou	5.5 mg/kg ketamine + 0.1 mg/kg medetomidine	Atipamizole 0.5 mg/kg
Olingo	5 mg/kg tiletamine and zolazepam	
Red panda	6.6 mg/kg ketamine + 0.08 mg/kg medetomidine	Atipamizole 0.4 mg/kg
Binturong	2 mg/kg ketamine + 0.04 mg/kg medetomidine + 0.2 mg/kg butorphanol	Atipamizole 1.0 mg/kg
	19.7 mg/kg ketamine + 1.3 mg/kg xylazine	Yohimbine 0.125 mg/kg
	2 mg/kg tiletamine and zolazepam	
Civet	4.4–8.8 mg/kg ketamine	
	10–15 mg/kg ketamine + 0.5–1.5 mg/kg xylazine	Yohimbine 0.125 mg/kg
	4.4–8.8 mg/kg tiletamine and zolazepam	
Genet	5.7 mg/kg ketamine + 9.8 mg/kg xylazine	
Mongoose	6 mg/kg ketamine + 6 mg/kg xylazine	Yohimbine 0.125 mg/kg
	4.4–5.5 mg/kg tiletamine and zolazepam	
Fossa	10.5–20 mg/kg ketamine + 2.5–5.0 mg/kg xylazine	Yohimbine 0.125 mg/kg
	5 mg/kg ketamine + 0.1 mg/kg medetomidine	Atipamizole 0.5 mg/kg

mg/kg, Milligram per kilogram.
From references 9, 21, 29, 31, and 33.

diet. Viverids are mostly carnivorous but, depending on the species, will eat varying amounts of vegetable matter. The binturong is the most frugivorous member of this family.

RESTRAINT AND HANDLING

Captive procyonids and viverids may be trained to enter tubes or small kennels for capture and transport. Some small species may be briefly restrained with nets and heavy gloves, but chemical restraint is necessary to safely perform physical examinations and diagnostic procedures (Figure 49-1). The largest issue surrounding restraint of meerkats, and possibly other small, social viverids, is aggression associated with reintroduction of animals into a group, especially if they had been kept separate from the group overnight. Several strategies have been employed, including ensuring return of an immobilized individual to the group the same day, immobilizing several members of the colony at the same time (not just the animal requiring medical attention), and dusting animals to be reintroduced and others in the colony with talcum powder.

CHEMICAL RESTRAINT, ANESTHESIA, AND SURGERY

Most studies of procyonid and viverid immobilization have used a combination of a dissociative agent (ketamine or tiletamine) and either an α_2-adrenergic agonist (xylazine or medetomidine) or a benzodiazepine (zolazepam) injected intramuscularly (Table 49-3). With the disappearance of medetomidine from the North American market, dexmedetomidine has been substituted into protocols at approximately 50% the dosage of medetomidine. The wide range of dosages listed for immobilizing members of both families most likely reflects differences in immobilization of captive and free-living (trapped) animals.

Chamber induction with isoflurane in oxygen is also a widely used induction protocol for all species weighing less than 10 kilograms (kg). Anesthesia is typically maintained by inhalation agents such as isoflurane following endotracheal intubation. Surgical

procedures are performed similar to protocols used for domestic carnivores.

DIAGNOSTICS

Physical examination, radiology, and other diagnostic procedures are similar to those performed in domestic carnivora. Blood samples may be obtained from the jugular, cephalic, femoral, or saphenous vein, but obtaining blood samples from obese individuals may be difficult. Hematology and clinical chemistry values for procyonid and viverid species are generally similar to those for dogs and cats, with a few exceptions (Tables 49-4 and 49-5). Red pandas commonly have lower serum or plasma sodium concentrations (130–135 milliequivalents per liter [mEq/L]) and chloride concentrations (100–105 mEq/L) than those seen in domestic carnivores. In the author's experience, healthy red pandas also may have low hematocrits (30%–35%). Enzyme activities for aspartate aminotransferase (AST), alanine aminotransferase (ALT), lactate dehydrogenase (LDH), and creatinine kinase (CK) are generally greater in procyonids and viverids than those observed in domestic carnivores (see Table 49-5). The cause for this is unclear but may be a result of the procyonids

TABLE 49-4

Hematology of Selected Members of the Families Procyonidae* and Viveridae

	Raccoon	Kinkajou	Red Panda	Slender-Tailed Meerkat	Binturong
RBC (10^6/μL)	8.74 ± 1.2	8.76 ± 2.6	8.49 ± 1.2	9.56 ± 1.5	7.49 ± 1.5
Hemoglobin (g/dL)	12.2 ± 1.5	14 ± 2.8	12.3 ± 1.7	13.0 ± 1.9	16.4 ± 7.4
Hematocrit (%)	36.8 ± 5.4	40.5 ± 8.1	39.3 ± 5.1	41.0 ± 6.2	45.9 ± 8.5
MCH (pg/cell)	14.2 ± 1.4	17 ± 4.4	14.9 ± 1.7)	13.7 ± 1.4	21.7 ± 1.9
MCHC (g/dL)	32.9 ± 2.2	35.3 ± 3.0	31.6 ± 3.2	31.6 ± 2.7	36.5 ± 15.3
MCV (fL)	42.8 ± 5.2	48.8 ± 14.2	46.3 ± 5.2	43.5 ± 3.4	62.9 ± 7.8
WBC (10^3/μL)	9.84 ± 4.1	8.41 ± 3.1	7.42 ± 3.0	6.65 ± 3.6	12.7 ± 5.0
Segs (10^3/μL)	4.84 + 3.7	4.76 ± 2.3	3.79 ± 2.5	4.39 ± 3.0	7.65 ± 4.0
Bands (10^3/μL)	0.44 ± 0.7	0.08 ± 0.01	0.16 ± 0.5	0.12 ± 0.12	0.11 ± 0.36
Lymphocytes (10^3/μL)	3.94 ± 2.0	2.85 ± 1.5	3.1 ± 2.0	2.07 ± 1.4	3.68 ± 2.3
Monocytes (10^3/μL)	0.33 ± 0.3	0.27 ± 0.2	0.27 ± 0.3	0.22 ± 0.2	0.57 ± 0.5
Eosinophils (10^3/μL)	0.78 ± 0.5	0.64 ± 0.7	0.15 ± 0.2	0.13 ± 0.1	0.41 ± 0.6
Basophils (10^3/μL)	0.06 ± 0.04	0.1 ± 0.06	0.13 ± 0.11	0.08 ± 0.01	0.05 ± 0.14
Platelet count (10^3/μL)	470 ± 160	449 ± 76	576 ± 189	389 ± 169	333 ± 115

*Values are means ± standard deviations.[16]

fL, Femtoliter; g/dL, gram per deciliter; MCH, mean corpuscular hemoglobin; MCHC, mean corpuscular hemoglobin concentration; MCV, mean corpuscular volume; μL, microgram; pg, picogram; RBC, red blood cells; Segs, neutrophils; WBC, white blood cells.

TABLE 49-5

Clinical Chemistry Reference Values for Selected Procyonids and Viverids*

	Raccoon	Kinkajou	Red Panda	Slender-Tailed Meerkat	Binturong
Glucose, milligram per deciliter (mg/dL)	65 ± 22	99 ± 36	124 ± 39	122 ± 33	127 ± 63
BUN (mg/dL)	20 ± 7	13 ± 5	27 ± 9	25 ± 7	18 ± 10
Creatinine (mg/dL)	0.9 ± 0.2	0.6 ± 0.2	0.9 ± 0.2	0.9 ± 0.3	1.3 ± 0.4
Uric acid (mg/dL)	1.2 ± 0.5	0.8 ± 0.4	1.2 ± 0.9	0.7 ± 0.4	1.2 ± 0.9
Calcium (mg/dL)	9.0 ± 0.7	9.3 ± 0.7	9.1 ± 0.9	9.7 ± 0.9	10.0 ± 0.9
Phosphorus (mg/dL)	4.7 ± 1.2	5.2 ± 1.1	4.7 ± 1.1	5.3 ± 1.3	5.6 ± 1.9
Sodium, milliequivalent per liter (mEq/L)	146 ± 4	141 ± 4	134 ± 5	149 ± 5	141 ± 5
Potassium (mEq/L)	4.3 ± 0.4	4.6 ± 0.5	4.4 ± 0.6	4.2 ± 0.4	4.8 ± 0.5
Chloride (mEq/L)	110 ± 3	105 ± 3	103 ± 5	114 ± 7	104 ± 5
Iron, microgram per liter (μg/dL)	146 ± 29	278 ± 0	150 ± 91	218 ± 136	190 ± 93
Magnesium (mg/dL)	3.05 ± 0.07	2.95 ± 0.35	2.34 ± 0.54	2.5 ± 1.12	2.97 ± 0.27
Bicarbonate, millimole per liter (mmol/L)	21 ± 0	25 ± 4.2	16.3 ± 4.4	18.0 ± 0	17.3 ± 0.8
Cholesterol (mg/dL)	211 ± 63	106 ± 50	199 ± 59	369 ± 139	74 ± 31
Triglycerides (mg/dL)	33 ± 17	36 ± 20	41 ± 23	41 ± 33	108 ± 54
Total protein, gram per deciliter (g/dL)	7.2 ± 0.7	8.0 ± 0.8	6.6 ± 0.7	6.6 ± 0.9	7.2 ± 0.7
Albumin (mg/dL)	3.4 ± 0.3	4.0 ± 0.4	3.20.5	3.3 ± 0.5	4.2 ± 0.6
Globulins (mg/dL)	3.7 ± 0.7	3.8 ± 0.7	3.3 ± 0.7	3.3 ± 0.8	2.9 ± 0.5
AST, international unit per liter (IU/L)	85 ± 26	195 ± 72	70 ± 37	91 ± 38	39 ± 20
ALT (IU/L)	121 ± 36	49 ± 45	69 ± 58	104 ± 62	21 ± 27
Total bilirubin (mg/dL)	0.2 ± 0.1	0.3 ± 0.2	0.2 ± 0.1	0.3 ± 0.2	0.3 ± 0.2
Amylase, unit per liter (Unit/L)	3119 ± 917	4468 ± 2191	914 ± 670	552 ± 330	1674 ± 398
ALP (IU/L)	60 ± 31	58 ± 30	28 ± 21	36 ± 32	190 ± 197
LDH (IU/L)	1299 ± 673	336 ± 344	506 ± 602	623 ± 215	341 ± 353
CPK (IU/L)	306 ± 198	402 ± 365	286 ± 306	350 ± 307	509 ± 754
GGT (IU/L)	4 ± 2	6 ± 4	3 ± 3	4 ± 3	4 ± 3
TT4 (μg/dL)	2.4 ± 0.4	na	7.3 ± 18.3	na	0.5 ± 0

*Values are mean ± standard deviation.[16]

ALP, Alkaline phosphatase; ALT, alanine aminotransferase; AST, aspartate aminotransferase; BUN, blood urea nitrogen; CPK, creatinine phosphokinase; GGT, glutamyltransferase; LDH, lactate dehydrogenase; na, not available TT4, total thyroxine.

and viverids being restrained and immobilized prior to the blood samples being obtained.

INFECTIOUS DISEASES

Serologic evidence of a wide range of infectious diseases has been documented in wild procyonids and viverids. For example, diseases and agents that have been identified by serology or isolation in raccoons but have not been reported to cause clinical disease include *Borrelia burgdorferi*, *Brucella* spp., Aleutian mink disease virus, *Ehrlichia chaffeensis*, hemorrhagic disease of deer, and raccoon poxvirus.[37] A number of other diseases or agents have caused clinical disease in raccoons, including leptospirosis, pseudorabies virus, canine adenovirus, *Salmonella* spp., snowshoe hare virus, St. Louis encephalitis virus, Tyzzer's disease, and yersiniosis, but these are rarely seen in captive animals.

Several important diseases commonly cause clinical disease in procyonids and viverids and merit discussion. One of these, canine distemper, may infect most, if not all, procyonids and viverids. The disease is best described in raccoons, and epizootics of canine distemper regularly occur in wild North American populations. Distemper has also been reported in coatimundis, kinkajous, red pandas, palm civets, and binturongs.[3,35,37] Vaccine-induced canine distemper has been seen in kinkajous and red pandas vaccinated with modified-live virus domestic dog distemper vaccines.[2,18]

Clinical signs in raccoons resemble those seen in domestic dogs but commonly include diarrhea in addition to upper respiratory signs. Hyperkeratosis of foot pads ("hard pad") is also a typical sign. Canine distemper in raccoons seems to progress to central nervous system (CNS) disease more rapidly than in domestic dogs. This is important, as distemper-induced neurologic signs in raccoons are indistinguishable from signs of rabies, and rabies may only be ruled out after death. Wild raccoons may act as vectors for both distemper and rabies to susceptible captive animals such as red pandas. Pathologic lesions of distemper in raccoons are similar to those seen in distemper-infected dogs. On the other hand, masked palm civets with canine distemper showed neurologic lesions but no GI lesions.[35]

Rabies is endemic in the wild raccoon population in eastern United States. The disease was disseminated by relocation of raccoons from southern United States to the upper Atlantic seaboard states for hunting, and the range extended rapidly. Extensive oral vaccination campaigns have been undertaken to limit the westward extention of raccoon rabies. Rabies is rare in captive raccoons, most likely because of their being protected from wild vector species.

Parvovirus infections have also been recognized in raccoons and many viverids, but the taxonomy of the etiologic agents has been the subject of some debate. Early raccoon cases were thought to be caused by feline parvovirus (feline panleukopenia virus) or "raccoon parvovirus."[37] However, recent outbreaks in wild raccoons in southeastern United States have been caused by canine parvovirus 2.[1] Morbidity was largely restricted to juveniles and neonates, and mortality was high. Serologic evidence of parvovirus infections has been observed in red pandas, but clinical disease has not been described in this species. Feline parvovirus has caused deaths in Asian palm civets.[6]

Several viral diseases of viverids have caused more limited outbreaks. Recently, pandemic flu (H1N1) caused clinical disease in a binturong.[34] An outbreak of cowpox virus in captive banded mongoose showed high morbidity (100%) and mortality (30%), and the virus was later transmitted to humans.[22] Masked palm civets (*Paguma larvata*) were found to be serologically positive for the coronavirus that caused severe acute respiratory syndrome (SARS) in people and were implicated as the source of the infection in humans. Experimental infection of palm civets resulted in clinical disease, suggesting that civets were not natural reservoirs for this agent. Subsequent investigations have shown that fruit bats are the natural reservoirs for this agent.[24]

In young red pandas, dermatophytosis is an important disease.[19] The disease is uniformly caused by *Microsporum gypseum* and

typically affects cubs less than 4 months of age. Signs include small areas of hair loss and crusting on the face, limbs, chest, and tail. Pruritus may be present. The lesions on the face and paws are usually not severe and respond to clipping, cleaning, and application of topical antifungal agents. Infections on the chest or tail may be severe and may progress rapidly to a purulent lesion covered with a crust ("kerion"). Lesions in these areas require more aggressive treatment. In addition to local treatment of lesions, as described above, systemic antifungal agents such as itraconazole (5–10 milligrams per kilogram [mg/kg], orally [PO], every 12–24 hours [q12–24h]), should be considered.

Tyzzer disease is a systemic infection caused by *Clostridium piliformis* and has been reported in two red pandas.[23] This species may be especially susceptible to this bacterium.

Vaccination

Procyonids and viverids may be safely vaccinated with a canarypox-vectored canine distemper vaccine manufactured for domestic ferrets (Purevax, Merial, Duluth, MN). The immunogenicity of this vaccine has been shown in mustelids and giant pandas. Although challenge studies have not been performed in procyonids or viverids, the author is unaware of clinical distemper in any of animals vaccinated with this product. Protocols for vaccination are similar to those for domestic dogs.

Captive procyonids and viverids may be vaccinated with a killed rabies virus vaccine. Recommendations regarding vaccination for parvovirus infection are more variable. Raccoons and palm civets should definitely be vaccinated, with a killed virus vaccine, if available. Vaccination of other procyonids and viverids for parvovirus is the decision of the attending clinician. Routine vaccination of red pandas against canine or feline parvovirus is not recommended at the time of writing this text.

Parasites

The most important parasite of the procyonids is the zoonotic ascarid *Baylisascaris procyonis*, which infects raccoons and kinkajous. This worm is rarely symptomatic in procyonids, but it may cause severe morbidity in humans and other hosts (e.g., parrots) because of larval migrans. *Baylisascaris* larva may cause impaired vision and blindness if it migrates to the eye in humans. Neurologic signs and even death may occur in people and other species if larvae migrate through the CNS. Most people affected by CNS larval migrans are children under 5 years of age or mentally impaired individuals with a propensity to geophagia.

Only a few cases of canine heartworm infections have been reported in raccoons, and they appear to be aberrant hosts for this parasite. Red pandas, however, do appear to be susceptible to infection with the canine heartworm *Dirofilaria immitis*. The infection is usually asymptomatic and typically discovered by routine serologic screening. In areas with significant incidence of canine heartworm, most zoos put their red pandas on a routine heartworm prevention program. A monthly oral dose of ivermectin (0.05 mg/kg) is used at the author's zoo, throughout the year. Treatment of occult heartworm infections with melarsomine, at the recommended canine regimen, has been fatal in red pandas. No data could be found on canine heartworm infection in other procyonids or viverids.

Tetrapetalonema sp. and *Paragonimus* sp. have been identified in captive binturongs in India. Coccidiosis (presumptively *Eimeria procyonis*) and encephalitis induced by *Sarcocystis neurona* have also been reported in raccoons.[11]

In meerkat colonies, outbreaks of toxoplasmosis and microsporidiosis have been reported. Toxoplasmosis was characterized by respiratory distress and rapid death. *Toxoplasma gondii*-like organisms were found widely disseminated in the tissues at necropsy.[17] Toxoplasmosis has also been reported in raccoons, commonly as a concurrent infection with canine distemper. Microsporidiosis has caused neurologic signs and high mortality in meerkats. The outbreak was caused by an agent structurally similar to *Nosema cuniculi*.

TABLE 49-6

Neoplasms Identified in Members of the Families Procyonidae and Viveridae

Scientific Name	Common Name	Neoplasm(s)	Source(s)
Procyon lotor	Raccoon	Pancreatic adenoma	10
		Astrocytoma	13, 26
		Thyroid adenocarcinoma with pulmonary metastases	27, 38
Procyon cancrivorus	Crab-eating raccoon	Nasal carcinoma	25
Nasua narica	White-nosed coatimundi	Nasal carcinoma	25
		Uterine adenocarcinoma	5
Nasua nasua	Ring-tail coatimundi	Nasal carcinoma	25
Potos flavus	Kinkajou	Nasal carcinoma	25
Bassariscus astutus	Ringtail cat	Nasal carcinoma	25
Ailurus fulgens	Red panda	Granulosa cell tumor	7
		Squamous cell carcinoma	32
		Thryoid carcinoma	32
		Hepatocarcinoma	32
		Lymphoma	32
		Myelogenous leukemia	32
		Lymphoid leukemia	32
Civettictis civetta	African civet	Hepatic carcinoma	25
Viverra zibetha	Large Indian civet	Urinary bladder carcinoma	25
Genetta genetta	Genet	Nasal carcinoma	25
		Liver carcinoma	25
		Cecal carcinoma	25
Genetta tigrina	Genet	Cholangiocarcinoma	36
Nandinia binotata	African palm civet	Hepatic angioma	28
		Hepatocellular carcinoma	28
		Lung carcinoma	25
Paguma larvata	White-whiskered palm civet	Lymphosarcoma	25
Arctogalidia trivirgata	Small-toothed palm civet	Hepatocellular carcinoma	36
Arctictis binturong	Binturong	Renal adenocarcinoma	20
		Hepatocellular carcinoma	20
		Pancreatic islet carcinoma	20
		Adenoma of colon	7
		Mammary adenocarcinoma with metastases	7
		Sarcomatoid renal carcinoma	4
		Cholangiocellular carcinoma	30
Fossa fossa	Fanaloka	Squamous cell carcinoma	28
Paradoxurus hermaphrodites	Indian palm civet	Pancreatic adenocarcinoma	7
Viverra tangalunga	Civet	Pulmonary carcinoma	7
Suricata suricatta	Meerkat	Nasal squamous cell carcinoma	15
Herpestes ichneumon	Grey mongoose	Lung carcinoma	25
Cryptoprocta ferox	Fossa	Adrenal adenocarcinoma	28
		Hepatocellular carcinoma	28

NONINFECTIOUS DISEASES

Poor hair coat is a common condition in captive red pandas and occasionally in raccoons. Animals seem to have partial seasonal sheds or patchy hair coats, with hair loss usually starting in the caudal half of the body and extending to the tail. Dermatophytes have not been found in these animals. Hypothyroidism has been reported in one red panda, but thyroid hormone concentrations in most of these animals are within the reference intervals for domestic dogs and cats. In the majority of these cases, the problem seems to be seasonal and requires no treatment.

Osteoarthritis is commonly seen in older procyonids, and chronic renal disease is frequently observed in aged red pandas. Hypertrophic cardiac disease has been reported in kinkajous and binturong.[8,14] Pancreatitis and trichobezoars have been observed in meerkats.

Thyroid pathology has been reported at an unusual frequency in raccoons.[38] Early reports were from captive animals from Germany, but a recent report is of captive animals in North America.[27] One European study identified 77.5% of the raccoons necropsied as having thyroid lesions, almost half of which (15 of 31) were thyroid adenocarcinomas.[38] Other thyroid lesions included follicular hyperplasia (7 of 31), follicular adenomas (4 of 31), and colloid goiters (4 of 31). No thyroid pathology was found at necropsy of feral raccoons captured in the same region of the captive animals. The feral animals were, however, considerably younger than the captive animals examined. One North American raccoon with thyroid carcinoma was obese and had a palpable cervical mass when examined.[27] The animal's total thyroxin (TT4) concentrations were within domestic carnivore reference intervals; thus this neoplasm was considered nonfunctional and similar to the thyroid carcinomas seen in domestic dogs. Another captive North American raccoon was obese, and a cystic thyroid gland was discovered during an attempt at jugular venipuncture. This animal had an increased TT4 concentration, and an excisional thyroid biopsy revealed adenomatous hyperplasia. The thyroid disease in this animal closely resembled that seen in older domestic cats. This animal's hyperthyroidism remained even after surgery and was successfully managed for years with a topical methimazole gel.[27]

Numerous neoplasms have been described in procyonids and viverids (Table 49-6), but as noted above, thyroid neoplasms in raccoons are notable. A large number of nasal carcinomas described in procyonids and genets are all from a group of animals housed in the same building at the Philadelphia Zoo and was, no doubt, likely the result of an environmental issue.[25]

REPRODUCTION

Temperate region species such as raccoons are seasonal animals, with breeding taking place in the late winter or early spring. Tropical species may be nonseasonal or have a seasonality based on rainfall rather than photoperiod. Red pandas in the Northern hemisphere mate in January or February and typically have their young in June or July. Breeding strategies in viverids are varied. Banded mongoose have an unusual strategy of synchronized parturition, where all young in a colony are born within a very short period.

Cystic endometrial hyperplasia has been seen spontaneously in raccoons and in a coati implanted with synthetic progestins.[5,12] Ovariohysterectomy and castration are the contraceptive methods with the best efficacy and the least adverse effects. A current area of investigation in procyonid contraception is use of gonadotropin-releasing hormone (GnRH) implants.

REFERENCES

1. Allison AB, Harbison CE, Pagan I, et al: Role of multiple hosts in the cross-species transmission and emergence of a pandemic parvovirus. *J Virol* 86:685, 2012.
2. Bush M, Montali RJ, Brownstein D, et al: Vaccine-induced distemper in a lesser panda. *J Am Vet Med Assoc* 169:959, 1976.
3. Chandra AMS, Ginn PE, Terrell SP: Canine distemper virus infection in binturongs (*Arctictis binturong*). *J Vet Diagn Invest* 12:88, 2000.
4. Childs-Sanford SE, Peters RM, Morrisey JK: Sarcomatoid renal cell carcinoma in a binturong (*Arctictis binturong*). *J Zoo Wildl Med* 36:308, 2005.
5. Chittick E, Rotstein D, Brown T, et al: Pyometra and uterine adenocarcinoma in a melangesterol actetate-implanted captive coati (*Nasua nasua*). *J Zoo Wildl Med* 32:245, 2001.
6. Demeter Z, Gál J, Palade EA, Rusvai M: Feline parvovirus infection in an Asian palm civet (*Paradoxurus hermaphrodites*). *Vet Rec* 164:213, 2009.
7. Effron M, Griner L, Benirschke K: Nature and rate of neoplasia found in captive wild mammals, birds, and reptiles at necropsy. *J Natl Cancer Inst* 59:185, 1977.
8. Eschar D, Peddle GD, Briscoe J: Diagnosis and treatment of congestive heart failure secondary to hypertrophic cardiomyopathy in a kinkajou (*Potos flavus*). *J Zoo Wildl Med* 41:342, 2010.
9. Fournier P, Founrier-Chambrillon C, Vié J-C: Immobilization of wild kinkajous (*Potos flavus*) with medetomidine-ketamine and reversal with atipamizole. *J Zoo Wild Med* 29:190, 1998.
10. Fox H: *Disease in captive wild mammals and birds*, Philadelphia, PA, 1923, JB Lippincott, Co.
11. Hamir AN, Dubey JP: Myocarditis and encephalitis associated with *Sarcocystis neurona* infection in raccoons (*Procyon lotor*). *Vet Parasitol* 95:335, 2001.
12. Hamir AN: Spontaneous lesions in aged captive raccoons (*Procyon lotor*). *J Am Assoc Lab Anim Sci* 50:322, 2011.
13. Hamir AN, Picton R, Bythe LL, et al: Astrocytoma with involvement of medulla oblongata, spinal cord, and spinal nerves in a raccoon (*Procyon lotor*). *Vet Pathol* 45:949, 2008.
14. Hollamby S, Simmons H, Bell T, et al: Myocardial necrosis in a captive binturong (*Arctictis binturong*). *Vet Rec* 154:596, 2004.
15. Howard LL, Lafortune M, Tocidlowski M, et al: Therapy for nasal squamous cell carcinoma in a slender-tailed meerkat (*Suricata suricatta*). *Proc Am Assoc Zoo Vet, Am Assoc Wildl Vet, Am Zool Assoc/NAG Joint Conf* 141, 2007.
16. International Species Information System: *ISIS normal values, MedArks Program*, http://www2.isis.org/support/MEDARKS.aspx. Accessed February 11, 2013.
17. Juan-Salles C, Prats N, Lopez S, et al: Epizootic disseminated toxoplasmosis in captive slender-tailed meerkats (*Suricata suricatta*). *Vet Pathol* 34:1, 1997.
18. Kazacos KR, Thacker HL, Shivaprasad HL, et al: Vaccination-induced distemper in kinkajous. *J Am Vet Med Assoc* 179:1166, 1981.
19. Kearns KS, Pollock CG, Ramsay EC: Dermatophytosis is red pandas (*Ailurus fulgens fulgens*): A review of 14 cases. *J Zoo Wildl Med* 30:561, 1999.
20. Klaphake E, Shoieb A, Ramsay EC, et al: Renal adenocarcinoma, hepatocellular carcinoma, pancreatic islet cell carcinoma in a binturong (*Arctictis binturong*). *J Zoo Wildl Med* 36:127, 2005.
21. Kreeger TJ, Arnemo JM: *Handbook of wildlife chemical immobilization*, ed 3. Shanghai, China, 2007, Sunquest.
22. Kruth A, Straube M, Kuczka A, et al: Cowpox virus outbreak in banded mongooses (*Mungos mungos*) and jaguarundis (*Herpailurus yagouaroundi*) with a time-delayed infection to people. *PLoS* 4:e6683, 2009.
23. Langan J, Bemis D, Harbo S, et al: Tyzzer's disease in a red panda (*Ailurus fulgens fulgens*). *J Zoo Wildl Med* 31:558, 2000.
24. Li W, Shi Z, Yu M, et al: Bats are natural reservoirs of SARS-like coronaviruses. *Science* 310:676, 2005.
25. Lombard LS, Witte EJ: Frequency and types of tumors in mammals and birds of the Philadelphia Zoological Gardens. *Cancer Res* 19:127–141, 1959.
26. Maurer KE, Nielsen SW: Neurologic disorders in the raccoon in Northeastern United States. *J Am Vet Med Assoc* 179:1095, 1981.
27. McCain SL, Allender MC, Bohling MW, et al: Thyroid neoplasia in captive raccoons (*Procyon lotor*). *J Zoo Wildl Med* 41:121–127, 2010.
28. Montali RJ: An overview of tumors in zoo animals. In Montali RJ, Migaki G, editors: *The comparative pathology of zoo animals*, Washington, DC, 1980, Smithsonian Institution Press.
29. Moresco A, Larsen RS: Medetomidine-ketamine-butorphanol anesthetic combinations in binturongs (*Arctictis binturong*). *J Zoo Wildl Med* 34:346, 2003.
30. Nashiruddullah N, Chakraborty A: Spontaneous neoplasms in captive wild carnivores of Assam State Zoo. *Ind J Vet Pathol* 27:39, 2003.
31. Palomares F: Immobilization of common genets, *Genetta genetta*, with a combination of ketamine and xylazine. *J Wildl Dis* 29:174, 1993.
32. Philippa J, Ramsay EC: Captive red panda medicine. In Glatson A, editor: *The red panda: Biology and conservation of the first panda*, Amsterdam, The Netherlands, 2010, Elsevier.
33. Schaftenaar W: A short note on the immobilization of the red panda (*Ailurus f. fulgens*). In Glatston AR, editor: *The red or lesser panda studbook*, Rotterdam, The Netherlands, 1993, Rotterdam Zoo.
34. Schrenzel MD, Tucker TA, Stalis IH, et al: Pandemic (H1N1) 2009 virus in 3 wildlife species, San Diego, California, USA. *Emerg Infect Dis* 17:747, 2011.
35. Takayama I, Kubo M, Takenaka A, et al: Pathological and phylogenetic features of prevalent canine distemper viruses in wild masked palm civets in Japan. *Comp Immunol Microbiol Infect Dis* 32:539, 2009.
36. Wadsworth PF, Jones DM, Pugsley SL: Primary hepatic neoplasia in some captive mammals. *J Zoo Anim Med* 13:29, 1982.
37. Williams ES, Barker IK: *Infectious diseases of wild mammals*, ed 3, Ames, IA, 2001, Iowa State Press.
38. Wisser J: Zumm vorkommen von thyreopathien bei waschbaeren (*Procyon lotor*). *Verh ber Erkrg Zootierre* 37:435, 1995.

CHAPTER 50

Ursidae

Darin M. Collins

BIOLOGY

Bears are mammals within the order Carnivora of the divergent family Ursidae and are geographically widespread within North and South Americas, Europe, and Asia. Within Ursidae, eight species of bears exist in three different subfamilies: Ursinae, Tremarctinae, Ailuropodinae (Table 50-1). The recognition of the giant panda (*Ailuropoda melanoleuca*) as an early divergent from the bear family is now accepted. The subsequent phylogenetic divergence of the spectacled bear (*Tremarctos ornatus*) to the giant panda, and the grouping of the brown bear (*Ursus arctos*) and the polar bear (*Ursus maritimus*) have been accepted. Bears occupy a wide range of ecologic niches from the arctic ice to the tropical rainforests. Wild bears are generally diurnal but may be active during the night (nocturnal) or twilight (crepuscular). Bears have an excellent sense of smell and some are very adept climbers and swimmers.

All bears have been threatened by human encroachment into their habitats and the illegal trade of bears and bear parts, including the Asian bear bile market. One of the greatest threats to bears is human-imposed environmental alterations such as global warming, chemical pollution, and deforestation. Current and future global climate changes are expected to pose greater risks, particularly for the polar bear, because of their reproductive life history traits, including seasonality. Consequently, six of eight species are currently facing the risk of extinction, with the International Union for the Conservation of Nature and Natural Resources (IUCN) classifications ranging from Endangered to Vulnerable. The IUCN lists all bears except the brown bear and the American black bear as vulnerable or endangered, with the brown bear at risk of extirpation in many range countries. The long-term conservation of small, isolated, and increasingly human-impacted bear populations will require innovative, pragmatic, and site-specific approaches.

UNIQUE ANATOMY

Common characteristics of bears include a large body with stocky legs, a long snout, plantigrade paws with five non-retractile claws, a short tail, and relatively small eyes. Bears generally have brown, black, or white fur of variable length. Many species have white or yellow crescent-shaped markings on the chest thought to be a social signal that may be best seen when bears stand bipedally, as during aggressive encounters or during periods of alert. Bears may become bipedal opportunistically and have been known to carry their young in this way in captivity. The mammae are pectoral. The gastrointestinal (GI) tract is simple. The distal segment of the intestine is marked only by a change in mucosa, and no cecum is present. Kidneys are lobular or reniculate in structure. In place of a renal pelvis, the major calyces drain the minor calyces of each reniculus and join at the proximal end of the ureter.

Unique intraoral epipharyngeal pouches occur in bears as bilateral tubular diverticulations of the caudodorsal pharyngeal wall, which are lined with a respiratory-like epithelium and a thick layer of elastic fibers that suggest a role in phonation.[61] Bears vocalize using grunts, growls, moans, tongue clicks, blowing, and teeth clacking, and giant panda vocalizations are described more as bleats, barks, and honks. The nursing sound of bear cubs is described as a pulsed "humming" vocalization and thought to be a comfort sound that might stimulate milk release by the lactating female.[12]

The giant panda possesses a larger radial sesamoid bone compared with that found in other bear species. This specialized bone articulates with the radial carpal and first metacarpal bone and supports the associated pad and muscle attachments. Such an adaptation provides for the gripping mechanism created by the opposing pads of the other four digits during flexion to manipulate objects such as bamboo.

Bears generally have elongated crushing premolar (P) and molar (M) teeth with a dental formula: incisors (I) 3/3, canines (C) 1/1, P 4/4, M 3/3. In the giant panda it is: I 3/3, C 1/1, P 4/4, M 2/2. Patterns of craniodental variation in the skulls of bears, as relating to their diet and feeding behavior, reflect dietary adaptations of teeth and the biomechanical properties of the skull, jaw, and related musculature.[52] As carnivores, polar bears are distinguished by molar size reduction, flexible mandibles, relatively small carnassial blades, and rounded canines. In contrast, giant pandas, as herbivores, have large molar grinding areas, rigid mandibles, large carnassial blades, and relatively reduced canines. The insectivorous sloth bear has only four upper incisors, with the sizes of post-canine teeth being reduced, and a vaulted hard palate to facilitate feeding by suction. The remaining species, which are omnivores, have a dental morphology intermediate between those of carnivorous and herbivorous species, with mediolaterally compressed, bladed canine teeth and relatively large molar grinding surfaces. Sloth bears and sun bears have soft tissue adaptations related to their insectivorous diet, including long tongues and flexible nares, with reduced hair on the muzzle.

SPECIAL PHYSIOLOGY

Physiologically, bears are remarkable mammals. Wild bears in the Northern Hemisphere during winter months will experience a period of dormancy or torpor, similar to hibernation, a unique state of energy conservation in response to harsh climatic conditions and food scarcity. This dormancy is characterized by inactivity and a lowered metabolic rate, prolonged complete or partial cessation of food and water intake, and absence of defecation or urination, with the possibility of arousal when disturbed. The body temperature of bears does not decrease dramatically during denning. The majority of the energy to support these activities is derived from lipid stores. Pregnant females will also give birth and lactate during this dormancy period. In polar bears, only the pregnant female will undergo this winter denning, and polar bears of either sex may go into torpor during the arctic summer when food is scarce. In captivity, most temperate species lay down fat in the autumn, and winter seasonal food intake is typically decreased with periods of decreased physical activity. This seasonal period of dormancy may be induced in captivity by a controlled decrease of food and hydration and by lowering the ambient temperature.[50] Hibernating brown bears evaluated by ultrasonography showed heart rates that were significantly lowered from active to hibernating states, with no difference in diastolic and stroke volume parameters.[41] Observed changes in reduced atrial chamber function were proposed as the major adaptation during hibernation; this adaptation allows the myocardium to conserve energy, avoid chamber dilation, and remain healthy during this prolonged period of extremely low heart rates. Urea is hydrolyzed, and nitrogen is processed into amino acids, which enter protein synthesis pathways at an accelerated rate.[26] As a result, blood urea does not build up despite the absence of urination. These changes occur independent of gender and reproductive or lactational status.

TABLE 50-1

Biologic Information of Bears, Order Carnivora, Family Ursidae

Scientific Name	Common Name	Adult Mass (kg; Male/Female)	Geographic Distribution
Ursus americanus	American black bear	60–225/40–150	North America
Ursus thibetanus	Asiatic black bear	110–150/65–90	Central, Eastern, and Southeastern Asia
Ursus arctos	Brown or grizzly bear	150–750	Europe, Asia, and North America
Ursus maritimus	Polar bear	400–500/150–300	Artic regions of Eastern Asia and North America
Helarctos malayanus*	Sun bear	27–65	Southeast Asia
Melursus ursinus	Sloth bear	55–145	Southern Asia
Tremarctos ornatus	Spectacled bear	140/60	Andes mountains of South America
Ailuropoda melanoleuca	Giant panda	75–160	Central China

*Sun Bears on Borneo (*Helarctos malayanus euryspilus*) are sufficiently different from those on the Asian mainland and Sumatra, representing the typical form (*H. m. malayanus*), to warrant subspecific differentiation.[38]

Delayed implantation, or *embryonic diapause*, is a reproductive strategy used by bears whereby the embryo (blastocyst) does not immediately implant in the uterus and is maintained in a state of suspended dormancy. *Obligate diapause* is also known as *seasonal delayed implantation* and is a mechanism that allows mammals to time the birth of their offspring for favorable environmental conditions. Little to no development takes place while the embryo remains within the uterine lumen and unattached to the uterine wall. As a result, the normal gestation period may be extended for a species-specific period. Although much of the molecular regulation involved in activating dormant blastocysts has been characterized, little is still known about the initiation of embryonic diapause, and the conditions which enable a blastocyst to remain dormant.

HOUSING REQUIREMENTS

Careful consideration should be given to habitat and off-exhibit housing design to meet the physical, social, behavioral, and psychological needs of the bear species being housed. Bears should be displayed, whenever possible, in exhibits replicating their wild habitat and in numbers sufficient to meet their social and behavioral needs. With the aid of innovative exhibit designs, different feeding strategies, appropriate use of environmental enrichment, and the development of a cooperative husbandry training program, all bear species may be housed in a dynamic and stimulating environment that maximizes their welfare and decreases the potential for the development of stereotypical behaviors.

Given the polar bear's threatened status under the U.S. Marine Mammal Protection Act, additional laws, regulations, and standards of care must be followed.[36] Institutions should be familiar with these regulations, have access to the documents containing these regulations, and, where appropriate, fully comply with the standards of care detailed within them. Regulations pertaining to polar bear captive housing are also contained within the U.S. Department of Agriculture (USDA) Animal Welfare Act (AWA) and the Manitoba Polar Bear Protection Act (PBPA).[1,44] Institutions seeking to acquire or holding polar bears from the Manitoba region are subject to the regulations stated in the PBPA, with the caveat that all institutions housing polar bears should be aware of and consider the management and housing approaches described.

The USDA AWA Animal Welfare Regulations mandate that polar bear primary enclosures housing polar bears consist of a pool of water, a dry resting and social activity area, and a den.[1] Minimum specifications for each enclosure feature are stated within the AWA Regulations. For example, the pool of water should have a minimal horizontal dimension of not less than 2.44 meters (m; 8 feet [ft.]) and a surface area of at least 8.93 square meters (96.0 square feet) with a minimum depth of 1.52 m (5 ft.), excepting entry and exit areas. A pool of this size should be adequate for two polar bears. Records must be kept of water quality assessments, with weekly water samples required for coliform counts and daily samples for measuring pH and any chemical additives used to maintain water quality standards. Water quality records must be maintained for 1 year documenting the time of sample collection, with the results being made available for USDA inspection purposes when requested. USDA regulations require that visual health inspections of polar bears be conducted by the institution's animal care staff at least every 6 months and that a general overall visual health assessment be made and recorded in each animal's health record.

Males and females of all bear species may typically be housed together through the year, with males routinely denied access to females prior to denning for the birth of cubs. Decisions to introduce bears for breeding are based on the temperaments of individual bears, with careful consideration being given to signs of progressive, positive, affiliative interactions observed. Facilities should allow for a range of physical contact situations, beginning with limited physical contact through smaller mesh to widely spaced bars that allow the bears to physically reach through and touch each other. Bear introductions may be aggressive, so full contact introductions should be coordinated with veterinary staff members present or immediately available. Cubbing dens, which are appropriately sized according to species, are confined spaces that are adjacent to larger holding areas in which the female may move around and give birth. Remote monitoring of the den via low-level lighting video cameras and microphones, with remote temperature sensors is recommended. Accommodations for supplemental heat are not typically required inside the den, as heavy bedding may provide for any necessary insulation for the female and the cubs.

FEEDING

Diet formulations should address the bear's nutritional needs, feeding ecology, and individual and natural histories to ensure that species-specific feeding patterns and behaviors are stimulated. In the wild, most bear species are opportunistic omnivores consuming a wide variety of food items depending on seasonal abundance; dietary niche specializations rely on variable seasonal availability of insects, fruits, and plants. The polar bear is mostly carnivorous with occasional consumption of plant matter and the giant panda feeds almost entirely on bamboo, but the remaining six species are classified as omnivorous. The giant panda is a strict herbivore, existing on a diet of bamboo and, unlike most herbivores, does not rely on microbial breakdown of plant material. Bamboo shoots and roots make up most of the diet, and the panda is adapted to consume large quantities of this poor protein source. The sloth bear and the sun bear are adapted to insectivory and feed on termites and other insects in the wild. In captivity, sloth bears and sun bears are typically fed diets similar to those of other bear omnivorous species.

In captivity, bears are typically fed mixtures of commercial dog food, carnivore-based diets, and produce. Institutions should determine seasonal diet changes on the basis of regular visual assessment of body condition, body weight trends, and activity of the bears. Obesity may be a common nutritional problem in captive bears. Body condition scoring is a subjective assessment of the relative amount and distribution of body fat to muscle and provides for a common language when monitoring body weight and condition over time. A useful standardized fat index for body scoring polar bears used by field biologists has validated scores against actual body weights.[56]

Feeding schedules to facilitate shifting or other management needs should be supplemented by irregularly timed feeding opportunities and placing foods in novel locations within the exhibits. Scatter feeding, feeding smaller amounts more often, and using enrichment devices that dispense food or live insects may decrease stereotypical behaviors and provide important physical activity and psychological enrichment. The caloric content for the amounts of enrichment foods such as skins and bones with marrow should be factored into the overall diet.

All new diet items should be monitored closely when first provided. The food type, presentation, and order of offering may have implications for dental health in bears when considering how to minimize the organic buildup that may contribute to dental health issues. Food items that are soft should be fed first and items such as bones, fish, or those with hair and skin should be offered last to help remove soft and sticky foods from teeth. Synthetic hard bones, ice blocks, and hard frozen food items may contribute to tooth damage, and their use should be monitored.

The proper handling and processing of meat and fish products and meat processed on site must follow all USDA standards.[9,10] Because of the presence of fish in many polar bear diets, institutions may supplement polar bear diets with thiamin and vitamin E. This perceived need for supplementation is based on the knowledge that thiamin and vitamin E are broken down in stored, frozen fish. Supplementation of thiamin and vitamin E is based on diets that contain greater than 30% fish. If the diet contains less than 30% fish, then other nonfish food items may be providing the needed nutrients. A safe approach is to supplement the fish portion of the diet at 30 milligrams (mg) thiamin and 100 international units (IU) vitamin E per kilogram of frozen fish.

RESTRAINT AND HANDLING

Bears should be considered dangerous and typically require chemical immobilization for safe handling and physical examination. Bear cubs weighing less than 25 kg may be physically restrained with nets or blankets for limited physical examination. Training may facilitate diagnostic examinations, and bears may be trained for nonpainful and minimally painful veterinary procedures such as venipuncture, injections, ultrasonography, inspection of teeth and feet, radiography, and wound cleaning, without the need for anesthesia or physical restraint.[6,29,37]

Chemical Restraint

Captive bears are not prone to complications during anesthesia because of proven chemical restraint agents, typically known medical histories, and reliable body weight estimates. A careful visual examination should be performed prior to any anesthesia event. Bears are usually isolated individually into separate enclosures without climbing structures prior to chemical immobilization. Bears are monogastrics and may be prone to vomiting upon induction or regurgitation during anesthesia. Recommended food and water fasting times for healthy bears is 12 hours. Providing honey as a distraction technique used for darting or hand injections may facilitate calm inductions. Volume limitations for darting may necessitate the use of potent drug combinations for larger brown bears and polar bears. Many bear species demonstrate seasonal variation in body weight with the deposition of a thick layer of fat over the hindquarters during the winter months, making the shoulder area the preferred location for dart placement. Polar bears may have a thick layer of fat at any time of the year, and the shoulder or neck may be targeted and longer needles used for intramuscular injections.

A variety of agents, combinations, and dosages have been used to immobilize captive and wild bears effectively (Table 50-2).[2,5,7,34,48] The selection of induction agents is typically based on volumes accommodated by the darting systems available. Considerable variations in the doses and combinations of induction agents used for wild bears, compared with those used in captive bears, tend toward increased doses used in wild bears to compensate for unknown weights and to increase the odds of a quick induction. Most immobilization regimens have consisted of a combination of a dissociative agent and an α_2-agonist or benzodiazepine.

Lyophilization of ketamine and its reconstitution at a concentration of 200 milligrams per milliliter (mg/mL) permits the immobilization of larger specimens with most darting systems. Ketamine (2.2 milligrams per kilogram [mg/kg], intramuscularly [IM]) may be used to supplement any immobilization regimen if anesthesia time needs to be prolonged. A combination of tiletamine and zolazepam is also used commonly to immobilize bears. This combination has the advantages of being more potent, on a milligram-per-kilogram basis, than ketamine and being available in a powder form. The combination may be reconstituted with variable quantities of diluent, or another immobilization agent, providing effective doses in small volumes. Flumazenil used to reverse the zolazepam effects of this combination may reduce the anesthesia recovery time.

Medetomidine and xylazine are commonly used as α_2-agonists in combination with a dissociative agent for immobilizing bears to achieve a reliable state of analgesia. Both have advantages as they are commercially available in concentrated forms for dart delivery, are reversible with yohimbine, tolazoline, or atipamezole, and are nonnarcotic drugs. Medetomidine is 10% more potent than xylazine and has a higher α_2-agonist receptor affinity that produces sedation and analgesia. Spontaneous muscle contractions and partial arousal may be seen in some animals sedated with medetomidine.

Etorphine and carfentanil, ultrapotent opioids, have been used variably to immobilize a number of bear species.[23] The advantages of these opioids are the small doses and thus small volumes required and their effects being fully reversible with opioid antagonists. The disadvantages of opioids are profound respiratory depression and concerns about the risk for accidental injection of the personnel involved. Both these disadvantages have resulted in limited use of opioids in bears. Carfentanil, as an induction agent, is mixed with honey or syrup and given slowly to increase mucosal absorption; it has also been administered orally for transmucosal absorption to immobilize black, brown, polar, and spectacled bears.[47] An opioid antagonist is delivered via darting, 20 to 25 minutes after carfentanil administration, in conjunction with a combination of a dissociative agent and α_2-agonist for sustained immobilization.

For prolonged procedures, inhalation anesthetic agents may be used. Young animals may be induced via a face mask. An endotracheal tube typically is placed, with the bear in ventral, dorsal, or lateral recumbency, and is used to maintain anesthesia. Throughout the interval of anesthesia maintenance, measurement of vital signs and full physiologic monitoring, including electrocardiography (ECG), pulse oximetry, evaluating end-tidal carbon dioxide, and tracking blood pressure noninvasively using a cuff around a forelimb, are continuously performed. Body temperature monitoring is vital in the larger species, as hyperthermia may occur. Recovery should be monitored closely, and antagonists should always be used, if available.

DIAGNOSTICS

The use of positive reinforcement training may enable many nonpainful and minimally painful veterinary procedures such as

TABLE 50-2

Chemical Restraint Agents Used for Captive Bears

Generic Name	Trade Name	Dose (mg/kg, IM)*	Reversal Agent/Dose (mg/kg, IM)*	Source	Comments and References
Tiletamine–zolazepam	Telazol	3–9	Flumazenil 0.01 mg/kg, IV	T = Fort Dodge F = Romazicon, Genentech USA	All species Flumazenil typically delivered after 30 minutes of anesthesia time Typical prolonged recovery time
Tiletamine–zolazepam Medetomidine	Domitor	0.5–2 0.01–0.06	Flumazenil Atipamezole 0.2 mg/kg, IV	A = Antisedan, Pfizer	
Tiletamine–zolazepam Ketamine	Ketaset		Flumazenil	K = Fort Dodge	All species Use ketamine to reconstitute Telazol Ketamine reduces typical prolonged recovery time of Telazol
Ketamine		5–10	None		Ketamine used alone rarely used
Ketamine Xylazine	Rompun	4–11 0.6–0.11	Yohimbine 0.11 mg/kg, IV, or Tolazoline 2–4 mg/kg, IV/IM	K = Fort Dodge Y, T = Lloyd Laboratories	Xylazine may induce respiratory depression, monitor closely
Ketamine Medetomidine		1.5–3 0.02–0.04	Atipamezole		Medetomidine induced hypotension controlled by 50% reversal given
Ketamine Medetomidine Midazolam	Versed	2.5–4 0.035–0.075 0.05–0.09	Flumazenil		Used successfully in sloth bears, spectacled bears, American black bears, and polar bears
Ketamine Midazolam		2.5–4 0.05–0.09	Flumazenil		
Ketamine Diazepam	Valium	5–7 0.13	Flumazenil		
Etorphine	Immobilon	0.02–0.06		E = Wildlife Pharmaceuticals	Reported use in American black bears, brown bears, and polar bears[7]
Carfentanil	Wildnil	5.4–7.6 µg/kg 6.8–18.8µg/kg PO†	Naltrexone 100:1	C = Wildlife Pharmaceuticals	Reported use in American black bears, brown bears and polar bears[7]
Carfentanil Xylazine		1.2 µg/kg 0.3	Naltrexone 100:1		Reported use in American black bears, brown bears and polar bears[7]
Carfentanil Xylazine		0.012 0.3	Naltrexone 100:1		Reported use in American black bears, brown bears and polar bears[7]

*All immobilization agents are given as intramuscular dosages unless otherwise indicated.
†Delivered for oral–transmucosal absorption.
IM, Intramuscularly; *IV*, intravenously; *µg/kg*, microgram per kilogram; *mg/kg*, milligram per kilogram.
Fort Dodge Animal Health; Fort Dodge, Iowa; Lloyd Incorporated; Shenandoah, Iowa; Pfizer, Inc.; Exton, Pennsylvania; Genentech USA, Inc., San Francisco, CA; Wildlife Pharmaceuticals, Inc.; Fort Collins, Colorado.

inspection of teeth and feet, radiography, ultrasonography, cleaning of wounds, injections, and blood sampling, without the need for anesthesia or physical restraint. Diagnostic procedures for bears are generally similar to those used for domestic dogs and easily adapted for use in bears. Blood is readily obtained from the jugular vein or the cephalic vein in neonates and adults. The jugular and femoral veins are useful for large-volume blood collection. Catheter placement and stabilization during procedures is most suitable in the cephalic or lateral saphenous vein. The dorsal venous plexus of the forepaws is superficial and of sufficient size to allow for

TABLE 50-3

Reference Values for Hematological Parameters for Selected Members of the Family Ursidae

Parameter	American Black Bear*	Brown Bear*	Polar Bear*	Sun Bear*	Sloth Bear*	Spectacled Bear*	Giant Panda*
Red blood cell count ($\times10^6$/µL)	7.49 (4.81–9.88)	6.33 (4.32–8.35)	6.83 (4.53–8.67)	5.97 (4.42–7.88)	5.85 (4.39–7.38)	8.46 (6.50–10.44)	6.25 (4.57–7.73)
Hematocrit (%)	45.0 32.3–57.5	45.8 (32.6–57.6)	44.0 (30.5–55.6)	41.3 (30.8–53.9)	44.9 (35.5–53.2)	41.2 (30.7–52.5)	35.3 (26.8–43.5)
Hemoglobin (g/dL)	15.7 (11.2–19.7)	16.4 (12.1–21.1)	15.6 (11.3–19.3)	14.5 (10.5–19.1)	15.7 (11.1–19.3)	14.6 (11.2–18.1)	12.6 (9.5–15.4)
MCV (fL)	59.8 (50.7–67.9)	72.6 (62.1–81.9)	64.9 (56.4–73.1)	70.0 (61.0–81.1)	76.5 (68.6–84.6)	48.2 (36.0–57.2)	58.3 (51.4–64.9)
MCH (pg)	21.0 (17.3–23.8)	26.1 (21.3–29.7)	23.0 (20.2–25.3)	24.6 (21.4–27.2)	27.2 (24.3–30.6)	17.2 (14.4–19.4)	20.3 (18.6–22.0)
MCHC (g/dL)	35.0 (31.0–38.8)	36.0 (32.6–39.5)	35.3 (31.6–39.0)	35.0 (28.0–39.8)	34.9 (30.7–40.4)	35.4 (29.6–42.2)	35.2 (31.0–39.0)
White blood cell count ($\times10^3$/µL)	8.20 (4.26–15.17)	8.04 (4.03–14.18)	9.23 (4.77–15.91)	10.52 (5.84–17.43)	11.46 (5.30–22.14)	6.34 (3.59–10.34)	7.87 (2.41–12.43)
Neutrophils ($\times10^3$/µL)	5.32 (2.36–9.83)	5.33 (1.96–10.05)	6.28 (2.30–11.37)	7.45 (3.47–13.74)	8.39 (3.62–18.09)	4.36 (1.23–7.53)	4.54 (0.00–9.75)
Band neutrophils ($\times10^3$/µL)	0.04 (0.02–0.09)	0.04 (0.01–0.08)	0.04 (0.02–0.10)	0.05 (0.03–0.12)	0.06 (0.03–0.12)	0.03 (0.01–0.05)	0.74 (0.00–0.64)
Lymphocytes ($\times10^3$/µL)	1.70 (0.40–3.52)	1.55 (0.33–4.28)	1.51 (0.50–3.39)	1.92 (0.44–4.49)	1.64 (0.33–3.43)	1.27 (0.34–3.12)	1.69 (0.15–3.16)
Eosinophils ($\times10^3$/µL)	0.750 ± 1.035 (0.012–8.979)	579 (44–1639)	688 (82–2230)	549 (69–1877)	1027 (125–3949)	398 (51–1220)	353 (0–913)
Monocytes ($\times10^3$/mL)	331 (56–943)	434 (65–1218)	553 (109–1464)	503 (91–1384)	494 (106–1303)	184 (45–521)	370 (0–814)
Basophils ($\times10^3$/µL)	38 (0–105)	—	—	—	—	122 (0–303)	—
Platelets ($\times10^3$/µL)	390 (112–687)	352 (115–595)	407 (169–649)	518 (167–871)	487 (207–799)	515 (166–840)	552 (331–787)

*Data from From Teare JA, ed: 2013, "Ursus_americanus_ Ursus_arctos_ Ursus maritimus_ Helarctos_malayanus_ Melursus_ursinus_Tremarctos _ornatus_Ailuropoda_melanoleuca_No_selection_by_gender__All_ages_combined_Standard_International_Units__2013_CD.html" in ISIS Physiological Reference Intervals for Captive Wildlife: A CD-ROM Resource., International Species Information System, Bloomington, MN.
MCV, Mean corpuscular volume; *MCH*, mean corpuscular hemoglobin; *MCHC*, mean corpuscular hemoglobin concentration.

venipuncture, even in the awake bear when training for voluntary venipuncture.

Whole body radiography, including head, thoracic, abdominal, and extremity views, is challenging in larger bears because of size, as multiple exposures to cover the entire area are usually necessary and anesthesia time to procedures is increased. Baseline radiographic examinations are recommended during the quarantine period and during examination of otherwise healthy bears. It is challenging to ensure that the x-rays penetrate the abdomen of an adult polar bear or brown bear to obtain high-quality, diagnostic films. Ultrasonography in larger patients is challenging but is easier and routinely performed in the smaller species. Endocavitary probes are commonly used rectally for imaging the reproductive tract. Joints and teeth are also common sites radiographed in bears.

Hematology (Table 50-3) and serum biochemistry (Table 50-4) reference values for bears have been determined through compilation of MedARKS records from multiple institutions. In general, no remarkable differences exist between species of bears, and the reference values follow trends seen in other carnivores and domestic dogs.

DISEASES

In one North American study of 50 institutions, in which the morbidity and mortality rates of bears in captivity were compiled and analyzed, integumentary diseases (54 of 512), gastrointestinal diseases (45 of 512), and ocular diseases (17 of 512) comprised the largest proportion of diseases in the adult age group.[4] Skin diseases predominately were of a parasitic or fungal etiology. GI disease, including neoplasia, GI volvulus, inflammatory bowel disease, and GI obstructions, was another major disease category reported.

Infectious Diseases

A number of infectious agents have been reported to affect bears (Table 50-5). Antibodies to a wide variety of viruses (avian influenza virus, bluetongue virus, canine parvovirus, and Eastern, Western, and Venezuelan equine encephalitis viruses) have been detected in bears, without associated clinical disease.[6] Canine adenovirus 1 (CAV-1), the agent for infectious canine hepatitis (ICH), has been isolated from captive American black bears exposed to canids.[8]

TABLE 50-4

Reference Values for Serum Biochemical Parameters for Selected Members of Family Ursidae

Parameter	American Black Bear*	Brown Bear*	Polar Bear*	Sun Bear*	Sloth Bear*	Spectacled Bear*	Giant Panda*
Total protein (g/dL)	7.5 (5.9–8.9)	7.3 (5.7–8.9)	7.9 (5.5–9.9)	7.2 (6.2–8.2)	7.0 (5.8–8.3)	7.5 (6.0–8.7)	6.3 (5.3–7.3)
Albumin (g/dL)	4.0 (1.9–5.3)	4.0 (2.6–5.3)	4.0 (3.0–5.0)	3.3 (2.6–4.3)	3.6 (2.0–4.6)	4.1 (3.0–4.9)	3.4 (2.6–4.4)
Globulin (g/dL)	3.4 (2.0–5.3)	3.3 (2.2–4.9)	3.9 (2.0–6.4)	3.9 (2.8–5.0)	3.5 (2.6–5.0)	3.4 (2.3–4.5)	2.7 (1.1–4.7)
Calcium (mg/dL)	9.3 (7.9–10.7)	9.6 (8.1–11.1)	9.2 (7.9–10.8)	9.3 (8.2–10.7)	9.3 (8.2–10.7)	9.2 (8.0–10.4)	9.1 (7.4–10.7)
Phosphorus (mg/dL)	5.8 (4.2–8.7)	5.4 (3.8–8.7)	6.3 (4.4–9.6)	5.3 (3.8–7.7)	5.4 (3.5–8.8)	4.8 (2.9–6.7)	5.2 (3.5–6.8)
Sodium (mEq/L)	139 (132–148)	137 (129–146)	139 (129–150)	139 (132–148)	139 (130–147)	139 (131–151)	129 (121–136)
Potassium (mEq/L)	4.6 (3.8–5.6)	4.5 (3.9–5.2)	4.3 (3.5–5.3)	4.6 (3.8–5.4)	4.4 (3.6–5.3)	4.1 (3.2–5.0)	5.2 (4.1–6.3)
Chloride (mEq/L)	103 (96–111)	103 (97–110)	104 (95–113)	108 (101–117)	108 (102–115)	104 (96–112)	99 (92–105)
Creatinine (mg/dL)	1.9 (0.7–3.2)	1.6 (0.4–3.3)	1.2 (0.5–2.1)	1.4 (0.7–2.3)	1.9 (0.8–3.0)	1.7 (0.9–2.5)	1.2 (0.6–1.7)
Urea nitrogen (mg/dL)	17 (6–30)	19 (7–35)	20 (5–40)	17 (8–32)	18 (8–34)	13 (5–23)	16 (2–27)
Cholesterol (mg/dL)	277 (150–451)	269 (184–425)	300 (180–434)	244 (136–376)	232 (142–317)	357 (235–505)	195 (80–289)
Glucose (mg/dL)	101 (47–189)	119 (62–205)	120 (68–198)	95 (55–158)	98 (52–185)	95 (49–183)	77 (21–125)
Total bilirubin (mg/dL)	0.2 (0.0–0.6)	0.2 (0.0–0.6)	0.2 (0.0–0.6)	0.2 (0.0–0.5)	0.2 (0.0–0.4)	0.2 (0.0–0.6)	0.1 (0.0–0.2)
Direct bilirubin (mg/dL)	0.0 (0.0–0.2)	0.0 (0.0–0.1)	0.1 (0.0–0.2)	0.1 (0.0–0.2)	—	0.0 (0.0–0.1)	—
Indirect bilirubin (mg/dL)	0.2 (0.0–0.5)	0.1 (0.0–0.3)	0.1 (0.0–0.3)	0.1 (0.0–0.3)	—	0.1	—
Alanine aminotransferase (IU/L)	47 (42–205)	49 (17–118)	33 (12–69)	54 (20–115)	25 (11–43)	30 (8–70)	72 (23–119)
Aspartate aminotransferase (IU/L)	95 (42–205)	83 (35–153)	75 (34–153)	105 (49–205)	101 (43–151)	36 (11–74)	66 (4–116)
Alkaline phosphatase (IU/L)	29 (5–87)	39 (7–114)	51 (11–150)	69 (21–175)	26 (8–72)	40 (13–105)	142 (28–229)

*Data from From Teare JA, ed: 2013, "Ursus_americanus_ Ursus_arctos_ Ursus maritimus_ Helarctos_malayanus_ Melursus_ursinus_Tremarctos _ornatus_Ailuropoda_melanoleuca_No_selection_by_gender__All_ages_combined_Standard_International_Units__2013_CD.html" in ISIS Physiological Reference Intervals for Captive Wildlife: A CD-ROM Resource., International Species Information System, Bloomington, MN.

Exposure of brown bears and polar bears to CAV-1 has also been reported.[35,46] Clinical signs include anorexia, lethargy, hindlimb ataxia, seizures, paralysis, corneal opacity, and death despite prior vaccination. Those that survived the infection had neurologic signs and lethargy for nearly 3 months. Serologic examination of wild North American brown bears shows 12% to 16.5% of the samples to be positive for ICH antibodies. Antibodies to ICH have been found in captive and giant pandas in China. Exposures to domestic dogs are suspected as one potential source of ICH viral exposure. Two cases of CAV-1 also occurred 5 years apart in two captive Malayan sun bears.[20] Although the two cases did not overlap in the lifetimes of these bears, each did have contact with an asymptomatic conspecific that shared the same exhibit. Skunks and raccoons observed within and near the exhibit were suspected as sources of infection.

Canine distemper virus (CDV), a member of the genus *Morbillivirus*, has been reported in bears.[11] Antibodies to morbillivirus have been found in polar bears, brown bears, and American black bears but without evidence of clinical disease. Canine distemper is reported to have caused the death of three neonate polar bears and a spectacled bear at a European zoo. In contrast to other members of this family, the giant panda appears uniquely susceptible to CDV.[29]

Equine herpesvirus 9 (EHV-9) was identified in a captive polar bear with a progressive encephalitis with the source being traced to Grevy's zebras, a potential equid reservoir species.[53] In this case,

TABLE 50-5

Selected Infectious Diseases of Bears

Disease	Causative Agent	Species Affected	Clinical Signs	Management
VIRAL				
Pseudorabies	Suid herpesvirus type 1	Polar, Asiatic black, American black, and brown bears	Death, tremors, incoordination, and aggression	Acyclovir
West Nile virus disease	West Nile virus	Polar and American black bears	Neurologic deficits	Prevention: vaccination
Equine herpesvirus	EHV-1, EHV-9	Polar and American black bears	Death, seizures	Supportive care Pest control Eliminate shared water sources
Rabies	Rabies virus	Polar and American black bears	Paralysis and aggression	Prevention: vaccination
Infectious canine hepatitis	Canine adenovirus type 1	American black bears and brown bears		None
Canine distemper	Canine distemper virus	Giant panda, polar, and spectacled bears	Polar bear: none	Prevention: vaccination
BACTERIAL				
Yersiniosis	*Yersinia enterocolitica*	Giant panda	Diarrhea	—
Listeriosis	*Listeria* sp.	Giant panda and brown bear	Variable	—
Campylobacteriosis	*Campylobacter jejuni*	Giant panda	Hemorrhagic diarrhea	Ampicillin
Dermatophilosis	*Dermatophilus Congolensis*	Polar bear	Dermatitis	Tetracycline
FUNGAL				
Blastomycosis	*Blastomyces dermatitidis*	Polar bear	Pleuritis and pneumonia	Itraconazole
PARASITIC				
Toxoplasmosis	*Toxoplasma gondii*	Brown bear	Death; lethargy, anorexia, diarrhea	Sulfamerazine and pyrimethamine

EHV-9 infection induced muscle tremors that advanced to generalized seizures and were refractory to treatment; ultimately, this polar bear was euthanized.[14] The polar bear had no direct contact with the animal point source. A recombinant zebra herpesvirus induced a fatal encephalitis in captive polar bears at a different institution.[22] Immunohistochemistry with a polyclonal antibody reactive to several equine herpesviruses was positive within the affected areas of the brain and a polymerase chain reaction (PCR) test conclusively demonstrated the presence of only EHV-9. An asymptomatic infection in one polar bear with the EHV-1 recombinant zebra virus was described in this same report. An EHV-1 infection related to domestic horse strains was also shown to cause fatal encephalitis in American black bears.[62] Fatal herpesvirus encephalitides derived from interspecies transmission underscores the need for extreme caution when placing zebras or other equine species near bears or having the same staff members caring for both species. Rodent pests such as mice and rats may also be vectors for this herpesvirus transmission between species. Among the closest relatives of EHV-1 and EHV-9 in the genus Varicellovirus is pseudo-rabies virus (suid herpesvirus 1), which causes Aujeszky disease.[3] This pathogen of pigs is reported to have infected bears also.[43,54] Bears should never be fed pig meat, and caution must be exercised when feeding carcasses from any hoof-stock source.

A novel gammaherpesvirus, Ursid herpesvirus 1, was identified in 4 sun bears with oral squamous cell carcinoma. Squamous cell carcinoma should be an important consideration in a clinical setting when a sun bear presents for oral lesions including erythematous macules, ulcers, or plaques, particularly if nonresponsive to treatment or if recurrent. The association between the herpesvirus and squamous cell carcinoma is unknown.[34a]

Tuberculosis is reported as a rare disease of carnivores, including bears.[6] Illegally held sloth bears that were confiscated by wildlife authorities in India and moved to rehabilitation centers have been reported to have died from *Mycobacterium bovis* infection, as confirmed at necropsy and by histopathology of caseated nodules within the lungs.[24,49] Clinical signs such as anorexia, persistent cough, nasal discharge, weakness, and progressive loss of weight were observed before the death of these bears. Zoonotic transmission from human handlers or infected meat was speculated to be the origin of the infection.

A geriatric polar bear euthanized for an acute-onset, progressive, nonambulatory paraparesis was found to be positive for West Nile virus (WNV) antibodies by serum neutralization assay, competitive enzyme-linked immunosorbent assay (ELISA), and plaque reduction neutralization assay.[15] In the spleen, WNV was detected by immunohistochemistry and real-time PCR (RT-PCR) test. Antibodies to WNV have been documented in apparently healthy free-ranging European brown bears in Croatia and American black bears in New Jersey in the United States. Vaccination of captive bears against WNV might be indicated in high-risk regions.

Two sun bears were diagnosed with salmon poisoning following fecal examination for ova of *Nanophyetus salmincola*, the trematode vector of *Neorickettsia helminthoeca*, the rickettsial organism that causes salmon poisoning disease.[19] Both bears exhibited acute onset of vomiting, mucoid diarrhea, lethargy, and anorexia approximately 1 week after eating live trout. Both bears responded to treatment with oxytetracycline, doxycycline, and praziquantel and returned to normal within 1 week. Fecal shedding of ova began 4 days after the onset of clinical signs and ceased 9 days later. Salmon poisoning disease may develop outside the geographic range in which the causative organism is endemic as a result of the transplantation of infected fish for sport fishing. Thorough freezing of fish kills the flukes and prevents transmission.

Parasitic Diseases

A wide variety of other parasitic infections, including those with cestodes, trematodes, acanthocephalans, and *Dirofilaria*; toxoplasmosis; trichinellosis; infestation by lice, fleas, and ticks have been recorded in bears; and gastrointestinal nematode infections are very common in bears.[6,48,51] Ascarid infections are very common and may cause diarrhea and anorexia. The nematode *Baylisascaris transfuga* is nearly 15 centimeters (cm) long, and heavy infestations may cause intestinal obstruction and overall poor body condition. Anthelmintics are effective, but reinfection is common. Ascarid ova are not destroyed by routine cleaning and disinfection, and the ova within soil environments will remain infective for several years.

American black bears may be infected with the canine heartworm *Dirofilaria immitis*, but clinical disease has not been reported. Whether bears are suitable hosts for *D. immitis* is still being debated. Bears also have their own species of filarid worm, *Dirofilaria ursi*, which lives in subcutaneous tissues and is considered nonpathogenic.

Trichinella infections in bears have received considerable attention because many bear species are hunted by local people, and raw or undercooked meat may be consumed. Trichinosis has been seen in captive polar bears obtained from the wild with encysted *Trichinella* organisms that appeared as small, white granules on the ventral surface of the tongue.

Skin diseases predominately have parasitic and fungal etiologies. Mange has been identified as a cause of alopecia and dermatitis in wild and captive bears. Mite infections are most commonly reported in American black bears and polar bears, with audycoptic and sarcoptic mange being considered particularly important. Audycoptic mange as a result of *Ursicoptes americanus* mites causes alopecia, pruritus, and crusting, and sarcoptic mange may cause pruritus, alopecia, pustular dermatitis, and crusting and thickening of the skin.[6] Treatment of audycoptid mange with ivermectin has not been routinely successful; amitraz, as a spray or sponge-on dip, is recommended. Demodicosis has been described in wild American black bears and in giant pandas. Dermatophilosis caused by *Dermatophilus congolensis* has been reported in multiple polar bears at a single institution.[42] In these cases, the organism was resistant to penicillin, and oral tetracycline and chloramphenicol, along with topical treatments, were required to resolve the infections.

Noninfectious Diseases

Skin conditions, particularly hair loss and rough hair coats, are encountered frequently in captive bears, especially polar bears and spectacled bears. In spectacled bears, a generalized seasonal alopecia syndrome with progressive symmetrical alopecia, severe pruritus, seborrhea sicca, and lichenification of the skin has been observed predominately in females.[28,58] Skin biopsy samples from female bears with different stages of hair loss were examined by histopathology, and telogenic, atrophic hair follicles, perifollicular fibrosis, and severe yeast infections with perivascular dermatitis and a mixed infiltration of mast cells, eosinophils, and lymphocytes were diagnosed. Alopecia, however, could not be determined. The severe yeast infection in multiple animals most likely developed secondary to the underlying alopecia and inflammatory alterations. Genetics or social stress etiologies were also speculated as etiologies. In one case, intradermal allergen skin testing with an allergy vaccine was successful in resolving the seasonal itching and associated alopecia in a female spectacled bear.[27]

Alopecia is one of the more commonly reported conditions in polar bears. Atopic dermatitis and alopecia have been reported in polar bears.[25] Nutritional issues are not considered a primary factor in these cases of alopecia. Factors more often responsible for hair loss include seasonal allergies, ectoparasites, trauma from rubbing or self-inflicted because of stress, water quality issues, and imbalances

of reproductive hormones. The green discoloration of the hair coat is a unique condition of captive polar bears. This color change is caused by the growth of a cyanophyte, or blue-green, algae, within the unpigmented, hollow shafts of the guard hairs. A yellow discoloration caused by sebaceous secretions may also occur. The hair shafts of the affected bear have many lateral ducts connected to the medulla. These lateral ducts are not present in unaffected bears, and it is not clear whether these lateral ducts are the cause or the result of the algal infection. Control measures have included salt-water treatments and peroxide baths for the polar bears, and water treatment measures designed to reduce the presence of algae in the water.

In all bear species, but most notably in polar bears, skin conditions may include pododermatitis of the foot pads. These lesions range from nonspecific inflammation of the plantar surface to networks of fistulous tracts on the dorsal surface of the foot. Foot pads may become dry and cracked, with deep fissures that bleed from the combined effects of pacing and wear on concrete surfaces. Contributing factors to these conditions include warm environmental temperatures, constantly moist environments, poor sanitation, residual chemical disinfectant irritants, abrasive and hard substrates, and trauma. Some conditions may be responsive to a change in husbandry practices and a simple course of antibiotics, but in other cases, bears may require immobilization for diagnostic assessments and treatment. Training bears for paw presentation may be valuable for diagnostic procedures, as it minimizes the need for immobilization.

Dental pathology is common in captive bears and may be a precursor to secondary abscessation and systemic bacterial infections of the facial bones, myocardium, or kidneys. In one study, over 70% of captive bear skulls studied had broken or open-tipped canine teeth.[31] Primary dental disease syndromes are fractured teeth, caries, periodontal disease, and dark discolored teeth resulting from dental trauma. Calculus deposition and periodontal disease are best minimized and managed through dietary and husbandry measures. Fractured and excessively worn teeth, especially enamel erosion on the lingual surface of canine teeth, are common in bears that compulsively bite and chew on cage bars. Dental fractures may occur as a result of trauma during conspecific aggression. Canine teeth fractures or excessive wear expose the pulpal cavity, which allows for ascending infections to the tooth apex, causing apical tooth root abscesses and alveolar osteomyelitis. Maintenance of tooth structure and integrity through endodontic treatments is the preferred treatment option and is preferred over extraction. Training bears for intraoral visual examinations of teeth is helpful to visually assess for dental disease and for evaluating extraoral fistulous draining tracts, which may be the first observed symptom of a chronic problem. Skulls of an adult polar bear, a brown bear, and a North American black bear were scanned with computed tomography (CT) and are available from the digital morphology website (http://www.digimorph.org) as models for craniodental anatomical review.[13]

Degenerative joint disease, osteoarthritis, and the associated gradual loss of mobility in older bears are indications for routine evaluations to maintain a good quality of life for captive bears. Bears are generally long-lived species in captivity, and geriatric disease considerations are common. Captive bears of all species will commonly live into their late 30s, some living up to 40 years or more.[31] These bears become less active, sleep more, climb less, and are generally slower or more irritable around conspecifics. In animals that are overweight, additional stress is placed on diseased joints, so dietary intake and body weight should be monitored closely. Two brown bear littermates with neurologic signs were diagnosed, with magnetic resonance imaging (MRI), to have cranial thoracic myelopathy spinal cord compressions following an acute onset of progressive paraparesis and proprioceptive ataxia.[59] Reduced activity and steroid therapy were palliative, and ultimately both bears were euthanized. Paralysis was diagnosed, with MRI, in a geriatric North American black bear with thoracic spondylosis deformans, intervertebral disk disease, and myelomalacia, with dorsal and ventral compression of the thoracic spinal cord.[32]

Suspected or diagnosed degenerative joint disease will require pain management with no single therapy typically providing complete pain relief. Non-prescription neutraceutical therapies are a good initial therapy with supplements containing polysulfated glycosaminoglycans, such as chondroitin sulfate, that reduce the collagen degradation in the effected joints. Glucosamine sulfate, an amino monosaccharide, may provide for cartilage maintenance and help to repair joint damage. Non-steroidal anti-inflammatory drugs (NSAID) are very effective in the treatment of arthritic pain. Carprofen, meloxicam, celecoxib, and tepoxalin may be used depending on individual response to treatment. Suggested drug doses for use in bears are modeled from dogs.

Tramadol, a noncontrolled drug, is used in a similar manner as codeine to treat moderate to severe pain. Tramadol may be used in combination with both nonsteroidal anti-inflammatory drugs (NSAIDs) and steroids. Gabapentin is effective in the control of chronic or neurogenic pain and may be used to control otherwise refractory pain.

In captive bears, neoplasms commonly involving the hepatobiliary, GI, and integumentary systems have been reported.[5,48] The etiologies are likely to be multifactorial as in other species, with advanced age being a risk factor. Genetic predisposition and captive diet influences have been suggested as causes for the significantly large incidence of hepatobiliary neoplasms in bears, with a disproportionate number being reported in sloth and sun bears. These tumors appear to originate in the gallbladder or the bile duct and in advanced stages will metastasize to the omentum, pancreas, liver, and lungs. Clinical signs and clinicopathologic changes associated with these neoplasms have been variable. Bears typically exhibit nonspecific weakness, lethargy, vomiting, and weight loss for months. Physical examination, radiography, and ultrasonography have revealed hepatomegaly, abdominal distension, ascites, and icterus. Euthanasia usually is elected because of the advanced stage of the lesions at the time of diagnosis.

Oncology treatment regimens involving surgical reduction, chemotherapeutics, and radiation therapy have been successful in bears. An adult, female Malayan sun bear was diagnosed with squamous cell carcinoma of the rostral mandible and was treated with surgical bilateral mandibulectomy followed by intralesional and perilesional cisplatin injections and radiation therapy. Recovery and postoperative adaptions by the patient were perceived as good, with no recurrence of neoplasia for 3 years.[40] Transitional cell carcinoma of the urinary bladder in an adult spectacled bear was successfully treated with wide-margin mass resection surgery and postoperative oral piroxicam treatments.[39]

REPRODUCTION

Most species of bears exhibit a reproductive strategy that includes a highly defined breeding season, delayed implantation, and an obligate pseudo-pregnancy period of high progesterone after estrus, whether nonpregnant or pregnant. Postpartum estrus does not occur in bears. Wild bear species in temperate regions mate during periods of increasing day length and increased food supply in the spring. Implantation of the blastocyst is delayed until pregnant females initiate denning prior to winter in those species that hibernate. The implantation of the embryo is regulated by the photoperiod. The timing of estrus and parturition in captive bears is indistinguishable from their wild counterparts despite relatively constant and ample food being provided, indicating that both facultative seasonality and obligate seasonality in bears are not merely responses to acute changes in food availability. A comparison of documented birth and estrus dates among all bear species revealed that the temporal distribution of birth is more seasonally restricted than that of estrus, with the exception being the sun bear, for which both captive and wild populations give birth through the year.[55] Ultrasonography was used to characterize giant panda fetal development in 13 giant panda pregnancies, with correlates to fetal development and to the physiologic changes in the female during pregnancy, to confirm delayed

implantation.[64] The reproductive biology of the tropical sun bear appears unique, with no apparent delayed implantation, and this species appears capable of initiating an estrus in the event of the early loss of a cub.[18] Sun bears are polyestrous, nonseasonal breeders, have a captive tendency toward spring and summer estrous cycles, are more behaviorally intense, and have a higher probability of conception.[17]

The corpus luteum becomes dormant following ovulation, allowing the females to re-enter estrus after conception. Because of embryonic diapause, the cumulative embryos all implant at the same time and comprise a single litter.

The temporal distribution of births varies little by latitude among the five species that reside primarily within the Arctic or temperate zones.[55] Four species give birth in winter, whereas the giant panda gives birth in the late summer. The lack of latitudinal variance in the timing of birth and estrus among the Arctic or temperate species provides strong evidence for their classification as obligate seasonal breeders. Sloth bears and spectacled bears as tropical zone endemic species housed in zoos in the northern hemisphere also adhere to a winter birth season. The season of birth in the southern hemisphere is shifted by 6 months from that in the northern hemisphere for all captive seasonal bears. A split parturition with confirmed identical paternity in a captive brown bear involving two cubs born initially followed by a third cub 17 days later has been reported.[60] Multiple paternity of litters has been documented by genetic studies in wild American black bears.[33] The American black bear was described as a model species for oocyte recovery and maturation for endangered bear species.[30]

Bear cubs are small at birth relative to the size of adult bears, and dystocias are rare. Cubs are born altricial, with females displaying a high level of behavioral investment in the offspring while still in the den. Mating behaviors in compatible bears is ritualistic with scent marking and vocalizations, males following females, and periods of body contact until the female is receptive, whereupon multiple copulations are normal. In captivity, there are multiple reports about interspecific hybridization.

In male bears, the function and composition of the testes are dynamic, undergoing seasonal changes in volume, histoarchitecture, steroidogenesis, and spermatogenesis. Spermatogenesis, testicular size, and serum testosterone begin to increase in the winter and remain increased through the breeding season. A number of captive and field studies have documented most of these parameters for the three species found in North America. Male American black bears and polar bears show low levels of serum testosterone and decreased spermatogenesis during the late summer and fall.

Pregnancy Diagnosis

Pregnancy may typically be diagnosed in bears on the basis of serum or fecal progesterone levels.[21,43] Pseudo-pregnancy has been described in several bear species and giant pandas. Late in gestation, approximately during the last month, pregnancy may be diagnosed by using transrectal or transcutaneous ultrasonography.[57] Pregnancy has been difficult to detect in giant pandas because the females gain little weight and their fetuses develop relatively late in gestation.[30]

Contraception

For female bears, the AZA Wildlife Contraception Center recommends the gonadotropin-releasing hormone (GnRH) agonists Suprelorin (deslorelin) implants, or Lupron Depot (leuprolide acetate) as safer alternatives for reversible contraception. Dosages and duration of efficacy for both agents have not been systematically evaluated for all species, and side effects such as weight gain and mood alteration may vary greatly between individuals. A drawback of these products is that time of reversal cannot be controlled. Neither the implant (Suprelorin) nor the depot vehicle (Lupron) may be removed to shorten the duration of efficacy to time reversals. The most widely used formulations are designed to be effective for either 6 or 12 months, but these are, for the most part, minimum durations and may be longer in some individuals. Permanent contraception by castration of males or ovariohysterectomy in females is a commonly used option.

PREVENTIVE MEDICINE

With good husbandry and dietary and veterinary care bears in captivity generally remain healthy. Routine visual and physical examinations are key to a comprehensive preventive medicine program for bears at all life stages. Such evaluations are made in conjunction with animal shipments, during quarantine, and on a periodic, routine basis. Physical examination should include systematic assessment protocols such as abdominal ultrasonographic evaluation and dental cleaning and prophylaxis, as well as assessment of reproductive soundness and collection of morphometric data. Trending the same type of data consistently over time is invaluable in tracking the health of an individual bear. Routine fecal screening and prophylactic anthelmintic treatment with fenbendazole or pyrantel pamoate, at dosages used for domestic dogs, may be used two to four times annually. Bears in areas endemic for the mosquito-transmitted canine heartworm *Dirofilaria immitis* may benefit from prophylactic treatment.

Quarantine procedures should include a 30-day period of housing away from other collection animals. This controlled time for close observation, diet acclimation, and at least one physical examination under anesthesia should follow the same systematic approach as that for routine annual assessments. The scope of the quarantine evaluation may be reduced if pretransfer physical examination and sample collection have been performed by the previous holding facility.

Vaccination

Few vaccines are recommended or used in captive bears. Immunization with a killed-virus rabies vaccine may be warranted if bears are kept in an endemic area where local wildlife might gain access to the enclosure. Given the rarity of clinical disease and the limited exposure of most captive bears to canids, routine vaccination for ICH is not warranted. Captive giant pandas are usually vaccinated for canine distemper. Captive giant pandas have also been vaccinated, at various institutions, with killed-virus canine and feline parvovirus vaccines. Other ursids typically are not vaccinated for CDV or parvoviruses. In all bears, it is advisable to monitor antibody titers to ensure adequate immune responses to vaccinations and track exposure to those diseases for which vaccines are unavailable or not used. Such titers may be analyzed from blood samples taken during routine and quarantine examinations.

BEHAVIORAL MEDICINE

An evolving behavioral enrichment and training program for bears is essential and assists in developing a positive relationship between animal care staff and the animal. Teaching bears how to problem solve, increasing their level of activity, and making training a positive, enriching experience are important parts of the process. Bears may demonstrate abnormal behaviors in captivity, including stereotypical behaviors such as pacing, head swaying and rolling, paw sucking, and regurgitation with reingestion. Pharmacological intervention may be required. Fluoxetine has been used in both brown bears (0.62 mg/kg, orally [PO], daily)[63] and polar bears (at 1 mg/kg, PO, daily)[45] to manage stereotypical pacing without adversely affecting normal behaviors. In the brown bear, increased environmental enrichment was augmented with the administration of fluoxetine, which was discontinued 2 weeks after pacing ceased following 6 months of treatment. The pacing behavior did not resume within the 1-year period reported. Zuclopenthixol has been used successfully to reduce aggressive interactions in two group-housed male Asiatic black bears (at a dose of 0.3–0.5 mg/kg, PO, once daily), based on evidence extrapolated from other species.[2] No negative side effects were reported.

GERIATRIC MEDICINE AND QUALITY-OF-LIFE CONSIDERATIONS

Euthanasia is an unpopular, but often necessary, quality-of-life decision in the management of bears with terminal disease or chronic mobility issues, when treatment options are limited because of the large body size of bears. The bear's quality of life should always be the primary consideration, and preemptive euthanasia is preferable to collapse or to chronic pain caused by inadequate management options. A system of scoring pain evaluations, discomfort levels, and overall physical condition and resultant quality of life of geriatric zoo animals offers a tool to support the decision making for timing the euthanasia of geriatric bears.[16]

REFERENCES

1. Animal Welfare Regulations, 2005. Animal Welfare Act, 7 U.S.C. 9 CFR Chapter 1, Subchapter A, Parts 1–4.
2. Arnemo JM, Brunberg S, Ahlqvist P, et al: Reversible immobilization and anesthesia of free-ranging brown bears (*Ursus arctos*) with medetomidine–tiletamine–zolazepam and atipamezole: A review of 575 captures. In *Proceedings of the AAZV AAWV, NAZWV Joint Conference*, 2001, pp 234–236.
3. Banks M, Monsalve Torraca LS, Greenwood AG, et al: Aujeszky's disease in captive bears. *Vet Rec* 145:362–365, 1999.
4. Blake CN, Collins D: Captive ursids: results and selected findings of a multi-institutional survey. In *Proceedings of the AAZV Annual Conference*, 2002, pp 21–26.
5. Bourne DC, Cracknell JM, Bacon HJ: Veterinary issues related to bears (Ursidae). *Intl Zoo Yb* 44:16–32, 2010.
6. Bourne DC, Vila-Garcia G: *Wildpros bears: Health and management*, London, U.K., 2007, Wildlife Information Network. http://www.wildlife information.org. Accessed February 1, 2013.
7. Caulkett NA, Cattett MRL, Caulkett JM, et al: Comparative physiologic effects of Telazol, medetomidine, ketamine and medetomidine-telazol in captive polar bears (*Ursus maritimus*). *J Zoo Wildl Med* 30:504–509, 1999.
8. Collins JE, Leslie P, Johnson D, et al: Epizootic of adenovirus infection in American black bears. *J Am Vet Med Assoc* 185:1430–1431, 1984.
9. Crissey SD, Slifka KA, Shumway P, et al: *Handling frozen/thawed meat and prey items fed to captive exotic animals: A manual of standard operating procedures*, Beltsville, MD, 2001, U.S. Department of Agriculture, Agricultural Research Service, National Agricultural Library.
10. Crissey SD: *Handling fish fed to fish-eating animals: A manual of standard operating procedures*, Beltsville, MD, 1998, U.S. Department of Agriculture, Agricultural Research Service, National Agricultural Library.
11. Deem SL, Spelman LH, Yates RA, et al: Canine distemper in terrestrial carnivores: A review. *J Zoo Wildl Med* 31(4):441–451, 2000.
12. Derocher AE, Van Parijs SM, Wiig O: Nursing vocalization of a polar bear cub. *Ursus* 21:189–191, 2010.
13. DigiMorph.org: The Digital Library of Morphology, The University of Texas at Austin. http://www.digimorph.org. Accessed February 1, 2013.
14. Donovan TA, Schrenzel MD, Tucker T, et al: Meningoencephalitis in a polar bear caused by equine herpesvirus 9 (EHV-9). *Vet Pathol* 46:1138–1143, 2009.
15. Dutton CJ, Quinnell M, Lindsay R, et al: Paraparesis in a polar bear (*Ursus maritimus*) associated with West Nile Virus infection. *J Zoo Wildl Med* 40:568–571, 2009.
16. Föllmi J, Steiger A, Walzer C, et al: A scoring system to evaluate physical condition and quality of life in geriatric zoo mammals. *Anim Welfare* 16:309–318, 2007.
17. Frederick C, Hunt KE, Kyes R, et al: Reproductive timing and aseasonality in the sun bear (*Helarctos malayanus*). *J Mammal* 93:522–531, 2012.
18. Frederick C, Kyes R, Hunt K, et al: Methods of estrus detection and correlates of the reproductive cycle in the sun bear (*Helarctos malayanus*). *Theriogenology* 74:1121–1135, 2010.
19. Gai J, Marks SL: Salmon poisoning disease in two Malayan sun bears (*Helarctos malayanus*). In *Proceedings of the AAZV, AAWV AZA/NAG Joint Conference*, 2005, pp 175–176.

20. Goodnight AL, Emanuelson K: Two cases of canine adenovirus type 1 infection in Malayan sun bears (*Helarctos malayanus*). In *Proceedings of the AAZV Annual Conference*, 2012, p 77.
21. Göritz F, Hildebrandt TB, Jewgenow K, et al: Transrectal ultrasonographic examination of the female urogenital tract in nonpregnant and pregnant captive bears (Ursidae). *J Reprod Fertil Suppl* 51:303–312, 1997.
22. Greenwood AD, Tsangaras K, Ho SYW, et al: A potentially fatal mix of herpes in zoos. *Curr Biol* 22:1–5, 2012.
23. Haigh JC, Lee LJ: Scheweinsburg RE: Immobilization of polar bears with carfentanil. *J Wildl Dis* 19:140–144, 1983.
24. Harish BR, Chandranaik BM, Venkatesh MD, et al: Tuberculosis in sloth bears (*Melurus ursinus*). *Indian J Vet Pathol* 27(2):129–130, 2003.
25. Harper J: Inhalant allergic dermatitis in a polar bear. In *Proceedings of the AAZV Annual Conference*, 1988, pp 97–98.
26. Hellgren EC: Physiology of hibernation in bears. *Ursus* 10:467–477, 1998.
27. Howard LL, Shepard SE, Fadok V: Oral allergy vaccine for treatment of seasonal pruritus in a spectacled bear (*Tremarctos ornatus*). In *Proceedings of the AAZV AAWV Joint Conference*, 2010, p 163.
28. Jäger K, Langguth S, Einspanier A, et al: The alopecia-syndrome of spectacled bears (*Tremarctos ornatus*) what do we know, what may we do? *J Comp Pathol* 148:90, 2013.
29. Janssen DL, Morris P, Sutherland-Smith M, et al: Medical management of captive adult and geriatric giant pandas. In Wildt DE, Zhang A, Zhang H, et al, editors: *Giant pandas: Biology, veterinary medicine and management*, Cambridge, U.K., 2006, Cambridge University Press.
30. Johnston LA, Donoghue AM, Igo W, et al: Oocyte recovery and maturation in the American black bear (*Ursus americanus*): A model for endangered ursids. *J Exp Zoo* 269:53–61, 1994.
31. Kitchener AC: The problems of old bears in zoos. *Int Zoo News* 51:282–293, 2004.
32. Knafo SE, Divers SJ, Rech R, et al: Magnetic resonance imaging diagnosis of intervertebral disc disease and myelomalacia in an American black bear (*Ursus americanus*). *J Zoo Wildl Med* 43:397–401, 2012.
33. Kovach AI, Powell RA: Influence of body size on mating tactics and paternity in male black bears (*Ursus americanus*). *Can J Zoo* 81:1257–1268, 2003.
34. Kreeger TJ: *Handbook of wildlife chemical immobilization*, Laramie, WY, 1997, International Wildlife Veterinary Services.
34a. Lam L, Garner M, Miller C, et al: A novel gammaherpesvirus found in oral squamous cell carcinomas in sun bears (*Helarctos malayanus*). *J Vet Diagn Invest* 25:99–106, 2013.
35. Kritsepi M, Rallis T, Psychas V, et al: Hepatitis in a European brown bear with canine infectious hepatitis-like lesions. *Vet Rec* 139:600–601, 1996.
36. Marine Mammal Commission: *Marine Mammal Protection Act (2007). The Marine Mammal Protection Act of 1972 As Amended 2007*, Compiled and annotated by the Marine Mammal Commission. Bethesda, MD, 2007, Marine Mammal Commission.
37. Martinez G: Bear training: A tool that improves care. *Shape Enrich* 15(2):9–10, 2006.
38. Meijaard E: Craniometric differences among Malayan sun bears (*Ursus malayanus*) evolutionary and taxonomic implications. *Raffles Bull Zoo* 52:665–672, 2004.
39. Murray S, Sanchez CD, Siemering GH, et al: Transitional cell carcinoma of the urinary bladder in a spectacled bear (*Tremarctos ornatus*). *Vet Rec* 158:306–307, 2006.
40. Mylniczenko ND, Manharth AL, Clayton LA, et al: Successful treatment of mandibular squamous cell carcinoma in a Malayan sun bear (*Helarctos malayanus*). *J Zoo Wildl Med* 36:346–348, 2005.
41. Nelson OL, Robbins CT: Cardiac function adaptations in hibernating grizzly bears (*Ursus arctos horribilis*). *J Comp Physiol* 180(3):465–473, 2010.
42. Newman MS, Cook RW, Appelhof WK, et al: Dermatophilosis in two polar bears. *J Am Vet Med Assoc* 167:561–564, 1975.
43. Palmer SS, Nelson RA, Ramsay MA, et al: Annual changes in serum sex steroids in male and female black (*Ursus americanus*) and polar (*Ursus maritimus*) bears. *Biol Reprod* 38:1044–1050, 1988.
44. *Polar Bear Protection Act*, 2002. PBPA, C.C.S.M. c. p 94.
45. Poulsen EM, Honeyman V, Valentine PA, et al: Use of fluoxetine for the treatment of stereotypical pacing behavior in a captive polar bear. *J Am Vet Med Assoc* 209:1470–1474, 1996.
46. Pursell AR, Stuart BP, Styer E, et al: Isolation of an adenovirus from black bear cubs. *J Wildl Dis* 19:269–271, 1983.
47. Ramsay EC, Sleeman JM, Clyde VL: Immobilization of black bears (*Ursus americanus*) with orally delivered carfentanil citrate. *J Wildl Dis* 31:391–393, 1995.
48. Ramsay EC: Ursidae and hyenidae. In Fowler ME, Miller RE, editors: *Zoo and wild animal medicine*, ed 5, St. Louis, MO, 2003, Saunders.
49. Rishikesavan R, Sha AA, Chandranaik BM, et al: Study on prevalence of tuberculosis in rescued captive sloth bears (*Melursus ursinus*). *J Vet Pub Health* 1:53–54, 2008.
50. Robbins CT, Ben-David M, Fortin JK, et al: Maternal condition determines birth date and growth of newborn bear cubs. *J Mammal* 93:540–546, 2012.
51. Rogers LL, Rogers SM: Parasites of bears: A review. In *Proceedings of the Third International Conference on Bears*, 1976, pp 411–430.
52. Sacco T, Valkenburgh BV: Ecomorphological indicators of feeding behavior in the bears (Carnivora: Ursidae). *J Zool Lond* 263:41–54, 2004.
53. Schrenzel MD, Tucker TA, Donovan TA, et al: New hosts for equine herpesvirus 9. *Emerg Inf Dis* 14:1616–1619, 2008.
54. Schultze AE, Maes RK, Taylor DC: Pseudorabies and volvulus in a black bear. *J Am Vet Med Assoc* 189:1165–1166, 1986.
55. Spady TJ, Lindburg DG, Durrant B: Evolution of reproductive seasonality in bears. *Mammal Rev* 37:21–53, 2007.
56. Stirling I, Thiemann GW, Richardson E: Quantitative support for a subjective fatness index for immobilized polar bears. *J Wildl Mgt* 72(2):568–574, 2008.
57. Sutherland-Smith M, Morris PJ, Silverman S: Pregnancy detection and fetal monitoring via ultrasound in a giant panda (*Ailuropoda melanoleuca*). *Zoo Biol* 23:449–461, 2004.
58. Sutherland-Smith M, VanHorn R, Owen M, et al: Skin conditions in captive Andean spectacled bears (*Tremarctos ornatus*). In *Proceedings of the AAZV AAWV Joint Conference*, 2009, pp 47–48.
59. Thomovsky SA, Chen AV, Robert GR, et al: Spinal cord compression in two related (*Ursus arctos horribilis*). *J Zoo Wildl Med* 43:588–595, 2012.
60. Ware JV, Nelson OL, Robbins CT, et al: Split parturition observed in a captive North American brown bear (*Ursus arctos*). *Zoo Biol* 31:255–259, 2012.
61. Weissengruber GE, Forstenpointner G, Kubber-Heiss A, et al: Occurrence and structure of epipharyngeal pouches in bears (Ursidae). *J Anat* 198:309–314, 2001.
62. Wohlsein P, Lehmbecker A, Spitzbarth I, et al: Fatal epizootic equine herpesvirus 1 infections in new and unnatural hosts. *Vet Microbiol* 149:456–460, 2011.
63. Yalcin E, Aytug N: Use of fluoxetine to treat stereotypical pacing behavior in a brown bear (*Ursus arctos*). *J Vet Behav Clin Appl Res* 2:73–76, 2007.
64. Zhang H, Li D, Wang C, et al: Delayed implantation in giant pandas: The first comprehensive empirical evidence. *Reproduction* 138:979–986, 2009.

CHAPTER 51

Hyaenidae

William Kirk Suedmeyer

BIOECOLOGY

The family Hyaenidae diverged from the family Viveridae 24 million years ago at the beginning of the Miocene period.[5] The family comprises four species in three genera (Table 51-1). The spotted hyena is the most commonly encountered species in the wild; aardwolves, and striped hyenas, and brown hyenas are rarely encountered because of their smaller size, nocturnal habits, and solitary nature. Hyenas as a group communicate through vocalizations, body posture, and scent marking, the last of which is highly developed in the brown hyena and consists of two components, which dry to different colors and consistency on prominent vegetation (Figure 51-1).

Brown hyenas are nocturnal, solitary animals that travel 25 to 40 kilometers (km) per night in search of food. They live in small clans composed of several females, males, and offspring. Clans are rather female bonded, and females are believed to be related (Wiesel, personal communication). Nomadic males are believed to maintain genetic diversity by ranging across clan territories. Males and females are morphologically similar. All clan members participate in communal raising of offspring. Although they are predominantly scavengers, brown hyenas actively hunt and consume Cape fur seal pups (*Arctocephalus pusillus*) along the Namibian coast.[24] In more arid areas, brown hyenas also consume plant material such as Tsama (*Citrullus lanatus*) and gemsbok cucumbers (*Acathosicyos naudinianus*).[15] Diamond mining, vehicular trauma, and human encroachment threaten existing populations of the brown hyena. Estimates of population size range from 5000 to 8000 in the wild and an estimated 800 to 1000 individuals in Namibia. Brown hyenas are not housed in North American zoos and are rarely exhibited in international zoos.

Spotted hyenas live in large maternally dominated clans composed of multiple related individuals. Males emigrate and become nomadic, breeding across neighboring clans.[3] Offspring are raised by the maternal adult. The genitalia of both sexes appear similar; the female exhibits a peniform clitoris; the vagina has fused with the urethra into a common urogenital tract and terminates in a phallic opening.[12,16] Modification of the labia has developed into a false scrotum, containing organized adipose tissue. This modification of the reproductive tract is under the androgenizing effects of androstenedione.[8] This modification appears to enforce maternal dominance of clan society.[15] Females of this species are larger than their male counterparts. Spotted hyenas are well known to scavenge carcasses from lions but will also actively hunt prey as big as zebras.[5] Spotted hyenas are not known to eat herbage. Hunting, human encroachment, and vehicular trauma contribute to declining populations across their range. Current estimates place the wild population between 27,000 and 47,000 individuals.[13] The spotted hyena is occasionally exhibited in North American zoos.

Aardwolves are uniquely adapted to a diet consisting nearly exclusively of harvester termites (*Trinervitermes* and *Hodotermes* sp.). These termites are nocturnal, providing ideal foraging opportunities for the aardwolf. Occasional consumption of rodents, carrion, and eggs has been documented.[5] Aardwolves are solitary, nocturnal foragers and seem to be monogamous. Offspring are raised by both parents. Underground burrows are frequently used for raising cubs or providing shelter during daylight hours. Territorial boundaries are marked, as in other hyenas, through anal gland secretions placed on prominent vegetation. Scent marked areas increase in density around dens and latrines. Aardwolves prefer open dry areas with short grass, especially overgrazed farmland.[5] Population estimates are not available, but aardwolves are widely distributed and are thought to be common, but rarely seen animals. No significant threats to the population seem to exist, although wire snares, hunting, and human encroachment may impact local aardwolf densities. Aardwolves are occasionally exhibited in North American zoos.

Striped hyenas are the most widely distributed hyena, preferring dense, arid, mountainous scrub woodland, and thornveld.[5] Striped hyenas are strictly nocturnal, mostly solitary animals but have been observed in small family groups when foraging. Adult and sub-adult animals participate in caring for offspring in communal dens. Nomadic males are believed to maintain genetic diversity by ranging across clan territories. Males and females are morphologically similar. All clan members participate in communal raising of offspring. Although these hyenas are predominantly scavengers, striped hyenas actively hunt and consume flying insects, small rodents, and birds and capture larger prey such as Cape hares (*Lepus capensis*) and bat-eared foxes (*Otocyon megalotis*).[5] Like the brown hyena, striped hyenas occasionally eat fruit, specifically the desert date (*Balanites* sp.).[5] The world population is estimated at 5000 to 10,000 individuals.[7] None of the hyena species is considered endangered or threatened.

ANATOMY

Hyenas, with the exception of the aardwolf, are powerful animals; the well-developed forelimbs, shoulders, and neck provide ample power to dismember prey animals much larger in size than themselves. The relatively weak hindlimbs sustain long distance loping, which is advantageous when hunting faster, but less so when hunting prey with endurance or distance scavenging. The jaws of the brown, spotted, and striped hyenas are very powerful, able to crush most long bones of large prey items. The brown hyena is also able to break ostrich (*Struthio camelus*) eggs, whereas the spotted hyena cannot.[1] The dental formula of the hyenas is: incisors (I) 3/3, canines (C) 1/1, premolars (P) 4/3, and molars (M) 1/1,[17] whereas that of the aardwolf which is uniquely adapted to an insect diet, is: I 3/3, C1/1, P 3/2-1 and M 1/1-2.[13] All hyenas have four digits on the forelimbs and hindlimbs, with the exception of the aardwolf, which has five digits on the forelimbs and four on the hindlimbs. The pelage is a mix of spots, stripes, and muted shades of brown and black; long and shaggy in the aardwolf, brown (Figure 51-2), and striped hyenas and short and sparse in the spotted hyena (Figure 51-3). Scent marking is the most important form of communication among hyenas. The anal glands are highly developed and large in each species and secrete a pheromone-laced sebaceous paste on prominent vegetation. Scent marking is used to define territories, signal potential mates, and identify conspecific and contraspecific individuals.[5,17]

REPRODUCTION

Hyena reproduction relies on complex social structures.[5,17] Specific reproductive data are provided in Table 51-2.[7] Dystocia has been documented in captive spotted hyenas, all of which were surgically corrected.[4] Other reproductive tract abnormalities are not reported in the literature but likely are similar to the problems in domestic dogs and cats.

509

TABLE 51-1

Natural History and Taxonomy of the Hyaenidae

Common Name	Scientific Name	Adult Weight (kilograms)	Current Distribution
Brown hyena	*Hyena brunnea*	34–43	Arid areas of Southern Africa
Spotted hyena	*Crocuta crocuta*	40–90	Sub-Saharan Africa
Aardwolf	*Proteles cristatus*	9–14	Eastern and Southern Africa
Striped hyena	*Hyaena hyaena*	25–55	Northern, Eastern, and Western Africa; portions of Central and Southern Asia

TABLE 51-2

Reproductive Data for Hyaenidae[7]

Parameter	Aardwolf	Spotted Hyena	Brown Hyena	Striped Hyena
Sexual maturity	Unknown	2–3 years	2–3 years	2–3 years
Seasonality	Unknown	Year-round	Year-round	Year-round
Gestation	90–110 days	110 days	92–100 days	88–92 days
Litter size	1–5	1–3	1–5	1–5
Weaning age	6 weeks	6 months–1 year	3–4 months	3–4 months

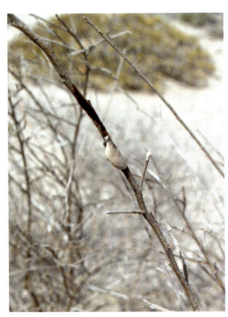

FIGURE 51-1 Two- toned paste mark of the brown hyena (*Hyena brunnea*).

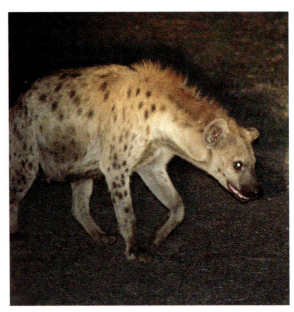

FIGURE 51-3 A female spotted hyena (*Crocuta crocuta*). Note the shorter pelage compared with that of the brown hyena.

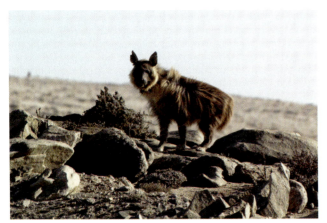

FIGURE 51-2 A brown hyena (*Hyena brunnea*) in Namibia. This animal fed through the night and into the early morning hours, which is unusual for this nocturnal animal.

HUSBANDRY

Hyenas are intelligent, destructive animals that need secure caging. The nocturnal, secretive nature of hyenas presents unique challenges for exhibit in captivity. The complex social structure of the spotted and brown hyena dictates that these animals be housed in compatible groups. All hyenas should be provided with adequate space, dens, and stimulating enrichment to prevent stereotypical behavior; they should be given opportunities to participate in training programs, which have been developed for captive spotted hyenas in a number of institutions. Captive hyenas fare well on commercial meat-based diets supplemented with nutritionally sound dog food and large bones. Aardwolves have been maintained on ground meat, milk, eggs, and supplemental vitamins[7,18] but may benefit from specialized insectivore diets.

RESTRAINT

All species of hyena require chemical restraint for examination. In general, remote delivery systems work well, although smaller

TABLE 51-3

Immobilizing Agents for Restraining Hyenas

Species	Immobilizing Agent	Dosage (mg/kg)	Reversal Agent (mg/kg, IM)
All	Tiletamine/zolazepam	5	None
All	Ketamine/xylazine	8–10/0.5–1.0	Yohimbine 0.11–125
Aardwolf	Ketamine/acepromazine	15/0.3	None
Spotted hyena	Etorphine/xylazine	0.05/0.63	Naltrexone 100 mg per 1 mg etorphine and Yohimbine 0.125
	Ketamine/xylazine	13.2/6.3	Tolazoline 3.7 or yohimbine 0.125
Brown hyena	Ketamine/medetomidine*	2–3/0.035–0.045	Atipamezole 5× mg amount of medetomidine
	Ketamine	15	None

*Field immobilization agents in the author's experience.
IM, Intramuscularly; *mg/kg*, milligram per kilogram.

individuals may be hand-injected through the use of a standard restraint device. The drugs of choice when immobilizing hyenas are listed in Table 51-3.[4,7,10,14,15,20] Hyenas should be administered injections into the shoulders, forelimbs, or neck, whenever possible.

Field Immobilization of the Brown Hyena in Southern Namibia

Field immobilization techniques for the brown hyena are rarely reported in the literature.[15] A working knowledge of the natural history and behavior of this animal facilitates its successful capture. The brown hyena is a nocturnal, silent, solitary forager.[15] However, large carcasses attract several hyenas. As opposed to the spotted hyena, brown hyenas generally feed singly, rather than in groups, even on larger carcasses. Individuals wait in the distance until the conspecific finishes (Wiesel, personal communication). In most instances, black-backed jackals (*Canis mesomelas*) arrive at the bait first; vocalization of larger groups of jackals may attract hyenas to the site. Jackals will commonly signal a hyena's approach by nervously looking in the direction of the hyena.

Camouflage, a low-profile silhouette, and absolute stillness are required for success of immobilization of hyenas. Use of advanced lighting, in the form of infrared technology, facilitates darting. Commercially available remote delivery systems work well, and dart placement is paramount to success. A well-placed dart in the neck or shoulder affords consistent success. A combination of ketamine (2–3 milligrams per kilogram [mg/kg]) with medetomidine (0.035–0.045 mg/kg) is effective within 3 minutes and causes recumbency of the animal within 7 minutes on average.[22] This combination provides rapid smooth induction, good muscle relaxation, stable heart rate and rhythm, slight to moderate pytalism, and 40 to 50 minutes of stable anesthesia. Pulse oximetry trends are undetectable initially (Figure 51-4) but elevate to the mid-90th percentile 20 to 30 minutes after induction without supplementary oxygen,[22] although supplemental oxygen is advisable, if available. Regurgitation is common upon reversal in field situations; this is likely caused by ingestion of bait just prior to immobilization. Application of a bland ophthalmic ointment protects the eyes during times of blowing sand and debris. Covering the eyes and placing plugs in the ear canal also assists in providing consistent recumbency (Figure 51-5). On occasion, an anesthetized hyena may require 30 to 40 mg of supplemental ketamine administered intramuscularly to facilitate completion of medical procedures. Reversal is achieved with atipamezole at five times the dose of medetomidine. Atipamezole given intramuscularly produces reliable recovery within 5 to 10 minutes. Blepharospasm, followed by purposeful movement of the head and cervical spine, is an indication of impending recovery. In general, the hyena ambulates away with mild ataxia, which rapidly resolves to normal ambulation within an additional 3 to 5 minutes. It is important to wait at least

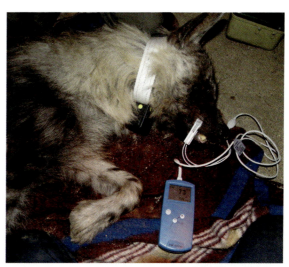

FIGURE 51-4 A female brown hyena (*Hyena brunnea*) anesthetized with ketamine and medetomidine. Note the low pulse oximetry reading.

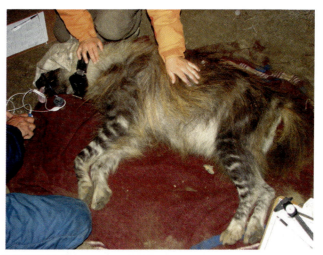

FIGURE 51-5 An anesthetized female brown hyena (*Hyena brunnea*). Note the substrate barrier and covered eyes. The animal also has aural plugs to decrease auditory stimulation.

TABLE 51-4

Select Hematologic Reference Values for Hyaenidae

Parameter	Aardwolf	Spotted Hyena	Striped Hyena
Packed cell volume %	21.8–55.8 (42.4)	29.9–54.1 (42.3)	27.0–57.6 (41.0)
Red blood cell ×10^6/microliter (µL)	4.95–10.62 (7.84)	5.08–9.83 (7.56)	4.35–9.77 (7.06)
Hemoglobin, gram per deciliter (g/dL)	7.8–18.7 (13.8)	9.3–18.5 (14.0)	– (13.6)
Mean corpuscular volume, ? (fL)	45.3–64.3 (55.0)	46.3–63.9 (56.8)	– (57.7)
Mean corpuscular hemoglobin, picogram (pg)	15.0–20.8 (17.9)	15.7–21.4 (18.8)	– (19.6)
Mean corpuscular hemoglobin concentration (g/dL)	28.1–36.4 (32.5)	29.7–37.3 (33.2)	– (33.5)
Leukocytes ×10^3/µL	2.35–13.11 (8.21)	6.28–19.59 (11.98)	5.30–15.34 (10.52)
Neutrophils ×10^3/µL	1.40–8.75 (5.30)	3.71–15.29 (8.62)	3.00–11.65 (7.50)
Band neutrophils ×10^3	0.00–0.07 (0.04)	0.03–0.14 (0.06)	0.00–0.50 (0.14)
Lymphocytes ×10^3/µL	0.01–3.79 (2.08)	0.59–6.35 (2.45)	0.00–4.31 (2.19)
Eosinophils ×10^3/µL	0–537 (238)	0–1684 (667)	—
Monocytes ×10^3/µL	0–806 (369)	79–1550 (483)	0–1179 (484)
Basophils ×10^3/µL	– (163)	0–285 42)	—
Platelets ×10^3/µL	– (222)	72–466 (267)	—

From Teare JA, ed: 2013, *Proteles cristata, Crocuta crocuta, Hyaena hyaena*, No selection by gender. All ages combined. Standard International Units. 2013 CD.html in ISIS Physiological Reference Intervals for Captive Wildlife: A CD-ROM Resource., International Species Information System, Bloomington, MN.
Values listed as reference intervals with mean listed in parentheses.

TABLE 51-5

Select Biochemical Values for Hyaenidae

Parameter	Aardwolf*	Spotted Hyena*	Striped Hyena*	Brown Hyena†
Total protein, gram per deciliter (g/dL)	4.4–7.0 (5.7)	5.7–8.4 (6.8)	– (6.0)	5.8 + 0.6 (3.5–7.0)
Albumin (g/dL)	2.0–3.7 (2.9)	1.9–3.4 (2.6)	– (2.4)	2.6 + 0.4 (1.5–3.3)
Globulin (g/dL)	1.6–3.9 (2.8)	2.9–5.7 (4.1)	– (3.6)	3.3 + 0.5 (1.7–4.4)
Total bilirubin, milligram per deciliter (mg/dL)	0.1–0.9 (0.3)	0.0–0.4 (0.2)	– (0.2)	0.1 + 0.1 (0.0–0.4)
Direct bilirubin (mg/dL)	0.0–0.2 (0.0)	0.0–0.2 (0.0)	—	0.0 + 0.0 (0.0–0.2)
Indirect bilirubin (mg/dL)	– (0.1)	0.0–0.3 (0.1)	—	0.0 + 0.0 (0.0–0.3)
Aspartate aminotransferase, international unit per liter (IU/L)	14–151 (89)	51–139 (87)	32–108 (73)	44 + 34 (10–145)
Alanine aminotransferase (IU/L)	45–247 (115)	50–206 (105)	– (49)	29 + 22 (8–103)
Alkaline phosphatase (IU/L)	0–32 (14)	13–75 (32)	0–86 (37)	96 + 56 (22–245)
Glucose (mg/dL)	57–181 (108)	67–262 (143)	34–192 (116)	87 + 43 (3–172)
Cholesterol (mg/dL)	82–365 (233)	103–355 (220)	125–327 (231)	207 + 90 (73–356)
Urea nitrogen (mg/dL)	14–48 (28)	15–43 (25)	13–29 (21)	35 + 11 (18–66)
Creatinine (mg/dL)	0.6–2.2 (1.4)	0.8–2.4 (1.5)	0.4–1.7 (1.1)	1.0 + 0.2 (0.4–1.4)
Calcium (mg/dL)	8.5–11.6 (9.8)	8.6–11.8 (10.1)	8.8–11.6 (10.2)	9.3 + 1.5 (5.1–11.0)
Phosphorous (mg/dL)	2.8–10.4 (5.2)	2.1–5.4 (3.6)	– (4.8)	5.3 + 1.2 (2.1–7.8)
Sodium, milliequivalent per liter (mEq/L)	135–152 (144)	131–155 (145)	– (146)	145 + 13.5 (76–154)
Chloride (mEq/L)	100–118 (109)	103–127 (115)	– (116)	110 + 11.9 (53–124)
Potassium (mEq/L)	3.7–5.9 (4.9)	3.9–5.3 (4.5)	– (4.3)	4.5 + 0.5 (2.5–5.3)

*From Teare JA, ed: 2013, *Proteles cristata, Crocuta crocuta, Hyaena hyaena*, No selection by gender. All ages combined. Standard International Units. 2013 CD.html in ISIS Physiological Reference Intervals for Captive Wildlife: A CD-ROM Resource., International Species Information System, Bloomington, MN.
Values listed as Reference Intervals with mean listed in parentheses.
†Wild normals N = 30.[25] Values listed as mean +/– standard deviation with minimum and maximum values listed in parentheses.

50-60 minutes from induction, if possible, before reversal to achieve an uncomplicated, smooth recovery. It is advisable to monitor the hyena until complete recovery as black-backed jackals (*Canis mesomelas*) or other brown hyenas may injure the hyena until it is fully recovered.[22] Recovery without reversal is prolonged, up to 90 minutes in undisturbed individuals.

MEDICAL CONDITIONS

Infectious diseases of concern in hyenas are few. Rabies has been documented in wild spotted hyenas[3,15] but not in brown hyenas, possibly because of their solitary nature. Canine distemper virus (CDV) has been documented in asymptomatic and symptomatic wild spotted hyenas; the symptoms were associated with an outbreak in African lions.[2,9] Animals exhibited epiphora and nasal discharge, hematochezia, ataxia, lethargy, and respiratory distress.[9] Feline calicivirus, feline herpesvirus, canine parvovirus or feline panleukopenia, feline immunodeficiency virus, and feline coronavirus were detected in wild spotted hyenas in the Masai Mara of Kenya over an 8-year period.[11] In a serosurvey of 30 brown hyenas in Namibia from 1997 to 2010, 43% of adult hyenas were seropositive for CDV, as opposed to none of the sub-adults.[25] Additional sampling for canine parvovirus, feline panleukopenia virus, rabies, *Ehrlichia canis*, and *Neorickettsia risticii* were negative in these same animals. Fecal direct flotation for ova and parasite examination of numerous stool samples collected from latrines and individual wild brown hyenas in 2011 were surprisingly scant; only one sub-adult demonstrated infection with low levels of coccidea.[25] Numerous ectoparasites and endoparasites of *Hyaenidae* have been reported in the literature,[18] and captive individuals should be screened and treated routinely for clinical parasitemia. Cardiomyopathy caused by *Trypanosoma cruzi* has been documented in an aardwolf.[6] *Dirofilaria* sp. parasites have not been reported in the literature. Intraspecific aggression, resulting in traumatically induced wounds are common in hyenas and occasionally need medical care.[4,23] Hyenas are well known for ingestion of foreign bodies, so appropriate measures should be taken to prevent ingestion.[1,7] Pacing on hard substrates predispose to ulceration of digital pads,[23] so appropriate substrate and proper management should be provided to prevent stereotypical behaviors leading to this condition.

DIAGNOSTIC SAMPLING AND TREATMENT

Techniques for diagnostic sampling are identical to those performed in domestic dogs and cats. Reference values for select hematologic and biochemical values are presented in Tables 51-4 and 51-5. Treatment with pharmaceutical agents is extrapolated from that for domestic dogs and cats. No drugs or pharmacokinetically studied medications have been approved for use in Hyaenidae.

PREVENTIVE CARE

On the basis of the apparent susceptibility of hyenas to CDV, it may be advisable to vaccinate hyenas against canine distemper using a recombinant canarypox vectored or killed vaccine.[4,18] Although exposure to canid and felid viruses is prevalent in wild populations of spotted hyenas, clinical disease has not been documented.[11] Rabies vaccination with a killed product may be advisable in endemic areas. Rabies has been documented in wild spotted hyenas.[3,15]

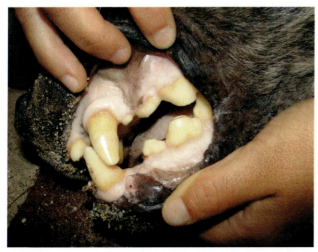

FIGURE 51-6 An anesthetized female brown hyena (*Hyena brunnea*). Note the worn teeth of this younger animal.

Routine examination is advisable to include specific evaluation of dental arcades; hyenas routinely damage their teeth (Figure 51-6), although infections are rare.

PEDIATRICS

Hand rearing of cubs is occasionally necessary and has been achieved by using commercially available kitten formulas.[4] Hand-reared animals are tractable and nonaggressive, although removing food or enrichment from an individual is not advisable.[4,19,21] Vaccination schedules generally follow those for domestic dogs and cats at 2,3, and 4 months of age,[4] using the canine distemper and rabies vaccines mentioned earlier. One author advises the use of killed canine parvovirus vaccination.[4]

ACKNOWLEDGMENTS

The author thanks the tireless efforts of Dr. Ingrid Wiesel of the Brown Hyena Project in Luderitz, Namibia, for increasing our knowledge of the brown hyena.

REFERENCES

1. Agnew DW, Barbiers RB, Poppenga RH, Watson GL: Zinc toxicosis in a captive striped hyena (*Hyena hyena*). *J Zoo Wildl Med* 30:432–434, 1999.
2. Alexander KA, Kat PW, Frank LG, et al: Evidence of canine distemper virus infection among free-ranging spotted hyenas (*Croctua croctua*) in the Masai Mara, Kenya. *J Zoo Wildl Med* 26:201–206, 1995.
3. Alexander KA, Mbugua P, Frank L, et al: Rabies in the spotted hyena (*Crocuta crocuta*): An unprovoked attack on a human settlement in the Masai Mara in Kenya. In *Proceedings of the annual conference of the American association of zoo veterinarians*, 1993, p 389.
4. Berger DMP, Frank LG, Glickman SE: Unraveling ancient mysteries: Biology, behavior and captive management of the spotted hyena (*Crocuta crocuta*). In *Proceedings of the joint conference of the American association of zoo veterinarians and the American association of wildlife veterinarians*, 1992, pp 139–147.
5. Estes RD: *The behavior guide to African mammals*, Los Angeles, CA, 1992, University of California Press, pp 323–348.
6. Fletcher KC, Hubbard GB: Fatal cardiomyopathy caused by *Trypanosoma cruzi* in an aardwolf. *J Am Vet Med Assoc* 187:1263–1264, 1985.
7. Fowler ME, editor: *Zoo and wild animal medicine*, Philadelphia, PA, 1978, Saunders, pp 647–649.
8. Glickman SE, Frank LG, Davidson JM: Androstenedione may organize or activate sex reversed traits in female spotted hyenas. In *Proceedings of the National academy of sciences*, 1987, pp 3444–3447.
9. Haas L, Hofer H, East M, et al: Canine distemper virus infection in Serengeti spotted hyaenas. *Vet Microbiol* 49:147–152, 1996.
10. Hahn N, Parker JM, Timmel G, et al: In West G, Heard D, Caulkett N, editors: *Zoo animal and wildlife immobilization and anesthesia*, Ames, IA, 2007, Blackwell Publishing, pp 437–442.
11. Harrison TM, Mazet JA, Hollekamp KE, et al: Exposure of spotted hyenas (*Crocuta crocuta*) to feline and canine viruses in the Masai Mara National Reserve, Kenya. In *Proceedings of the annual conference of the American association of zoo veterinarians*, 2002, p 10.
12. Hayssen V, van Tienhoven A: *Asdell's patterns of mammalian reproduction: A compendium of species-specific data*, Ithaca, NY, 1993, Cornell University Press, pp 293–295.
13. International union for conservation of nature (IUCN): *Hyena specialist group*, Gland, Switzerland, 2012, IUCN.
14. Kreeger TJ, Arnemo JM: *Handbook of wildlife chemical immobilization*, ed 3, Hacienda Heights, CA, 2007, Sunquest Printing, pp 156, 221–222.
15. Mills MGL: *Kalahari hyenas: Comparative behavioral ecology of two species*, Caldwell, NC, 2003, Blackburn press, pp 27, 146, 174, 187–204.
16. Neaves WB, Griffin JE, Wilson JD: Sexual dimorphism of the phallus in spotted hyaena (*Croctua croctua*). *J Reprod Fertil* 59:509–513, 1980.
17. Nowak RM: *Walker's mammals of the world*, vol II, ed 5, Baltimore, MD, 1991, John Hopkins University Press, pp 1177–1184.

18. Ramsay EC: Ursidae and Hyaenidae. In Fowler ME, Miller RE, editors: *Zoo and wild animal medicine*, St. Louis, MO, 2003, Elsevier Science, pp 534–538.
19. Reiger I: Report on rearing of striped hyenas *Hyaena hyaena*. *Vierteljahrsschrift der naturforschenden Gesellschaft Zurich* 124:169–184, 1979b.
20. Richardson PRK, Anderson MF: Chemical capture of the aardwolf *Proteles cristatus*. In McKenzie AA, editor: *The capture and care manual: Capture, care, accommodation and transportation of wild African animals*, Pretoria, South Africa, 1993, South African Veterinary Foundation, pp 244–246.
21. Schulz WC: Breeding and hand rearing Brown hyenas, *Hyena brunnea*, at Okahandja ZooPark, South West Africa. *Int Zoo YB* 6:173–176, 1966.
22. Suedmeyer WK: Brown hyena (*Hyaena brunnea*) ecology, anesthesia and preliminary ophthalmic evaluation in Namibia, Africa. In *Proceedings of the joint conference American association of zoo veterinarians and the American association of wildlife veterinarians*, 2010, pp 38–39.
23. Wallach JD, Boever WJ: *Diseases of exotic animals*, Philadelphia, PA, 1983, Saunders, pp 535–547.
24. Wiesel I: Killing of cape fur seal (*Arctocephalus pusillus pusillus*) pups by brown hyenas (*Parahyaena brunnea*) at mainland breeding colonies along the coastal Namib desert. *J Acta Ethologica* 13(2):93–100, 2010.
25. Zimmerman D, Wiesel I, Suedmeyer WK, Hernandez Y: Biomedical survey of brown hyenas (*Hyena brunnea*) in Namibia. In *Proceedings of the annual conference of the American association of zoo veterinarians*, 2011, p 57.

CHAPTER **52**

Tubulidentata (Aardvark)

Peter E. Buss and Leith C.R. Meyer

GENERAL BIOLOGY

The aardvark (*Orycteropus afer*) is nocturnal, fossorial, and myrmecophagous and is the only living representative of the order Tubulidentata, belonging to the superorder Afrotheria.[5] The aardvark's tooth is unique in that each molar consists of fused, elongated, hexagonal, perpendicular, dentine columns surrounded by a layer of cementum.[13] This structure gives rise to the order's name: the Latin *tubuli*, tube, and *dentis*, tooth. The common name, aardvark, is derived from two Afrikaans words, *aarde*, earth, and *vark*, pig.[3] Fossil records indicate that aardvarks once existed in Europe and Asia; however, their current distribution is restricted to sub-Saharan Africa.[5] They are found over a wide range of habitats, from semi-arid zones to tropical rainforests, but are totally absent from deserts.[3,12,14]

Aardvarks are solitary and almost exclusively nocturnal, but wild individuals may be observed feeding before sunset during winter. They are efficient burrowers, digging in search of either food or shelter. Burrows provide a microhabitat that is thermally buffered from external ambient extremes (heat and cold) and has a higher relative humidity.[16] Vocalization is restricted to a vigorous snuffling and the occasional grunt or a rare bleat.[3,13] Life expectancy is 10 years in the wild and early 20s in captivity; a single individual is reported to have lived to 29 years of age.[3]

UNIQUE ANATOMY

Aardvarks have evolved anatomic adaptations that allow them to feed on ants and termites.[9,12,13] Long, sharp claws combined with an inability to supinate the wrist provides strength for digging. The radius is shorter than the humerus, and webbing between the digits assists in burrowing.[12] The aardvark's head is elongated and narrow, with a long (25–30 cm), sticky vermiform tongue.[9,12,13] Aardvarks have an excellent sense of smell and hearing. However, their eyesight is poor.[3,12,13]

The skin is thick, with a sparse covering of hair and no subcutaneous fat layer, possibly making the aardvark susceptible to temperature fluctuations.[3,9] Adult body mass is 40 to 65 kilograms (kg), with total body length up to 200 centimeters (cm) and shoulder height of 65 cm. Males are heavier and slightly larger than the females.[3,13,15]

The adult dental formula is: incisors (I) 0/0, canines (C) 0/0, premolars (P) 2/2, molars (M) 3/3, although variations may occur, as in four to seven teeth in the mandible. Teeth lack enamel and grow continuously.[3,13] The stomach is muscular and gizzard-like for grinding up food ingested with sand and soil, and a large cecum is present, which is unusual for an insectivore.[3,13]

Both male and females have a distinct genital eminence that may be confused with a scrotum. Unlike in other Afrotheria, which are testicond, in the aardvark, testes are descended but ascrotal.[2] The penis is soft, short, and shaped like a truncated cone, and the vulva is a long cleft with a large heart shaped clitoris behind the center of the genital eminence. The genitalia and a pair of genital scent glands are visualized by opening a sphincter-like fold of integument.[7,13]

PHYSIOLOGY

Body temperature in the aardvark varies between 34° C to 37° C and is regulated, in part, through the use of burrows. However, aardvarks appear to be susceptible to hypothermia as they return to their burrows once temperatures fall below 2° C.[12,13] Aardvarks drink infrequently and seem able to obtain all their water requirements from their prey.[12]

SPECIAL HOUSING REQUIREMENTS

Aardvarks are best displayed in a nocturnal exhibit with reversed day and night periods.[1,3] The enclosure should be concrete or metal lined to prevent the animals from burrowing out; they should be devoid of sharp edges to prevent tongue injuries and have a substrate of soil, woodchips, or shavings.[1,9] Moats are to be avoided as aardvarks are good swimmers.[1] In the wild, aardvarks are solitary animals;

however, in zoos, they are frequently exhibited in groups of two to four animals and any combination of sexes. Pregnant females are separated shortly before or after parturition.[3]

Indoor temperatures are best kept between 20° C to 27° C and the relative humidity above 70%.[1,3,16] Low humidity may lead to drying and cracking of the skin, especially in young animals.[9] In most zoos, a sleeping box or a den with a sand or straw substrate is provided.[1]

As aardvarks are prone to stereotypical behavior, environmental enrichment is essential, and it may include scatter feeding, the use of hole feeders, and substrates for digging.[1,3]

FEEDING

The natural diet of aardvarks consists almost exclusively of ants and termites; a small proportion may include seeds, fly and scarab beetle pupae, and wild cucumber (*Cucumis humifructus*).[6,10,13,14,17] A substitute high-protein, low-carbohydrate diet, with added vitamin and minerals, is fed as a thick soupy gruel to captive animals.[9] The ingredients may include ground beef, chicken, or horse meat, commercial dog or cat food, mealworms, eggs, oatmeal, corn flakes, milk, low-fat curd cheese, and a variety of fruit and vegetables. Mazuri Insectivore Diet is used at many facilities.[3]

RESTRAINT AND HANDLING

Manual restraint of adult aardvarks is not recommended, as these animals are extremely powerful. Neonates and juveniles may be physically restrained but should be sedated once they become heavier than 10 kg to prevent injuries to the animal and to the personnel.[4] Light-weight darts are effective for drug delivery in both wild and captive animals. Darts with barbed (2-millimeter [mm]) needles are required; otherwise they tend to bounce out of the skin (L. Meyer, personal communication).[4] Captive animals should be fasted prior to drug administration.[15] Free-ranging animals are best approached on foot, keeping an optimal darting distance of 10 to 15 meters (m) (L. Meyer, personal communication). A combination of ketamine and medetomidine, with atipamezole, is currently one of the most widely used protocols for the chemical immobilization of both captive and restrained free-ranging individuals.[4,9,11] Some of the combinations that have been used are ketamine (3 mg/kg) + medetomidine (0.08 mg/kg) reversed with atipamezole (0.4 mg/kg);[11] ketamine (4.3–8.2 mg/kg) + detomidine (0.09–0.18 mg/kg) reversed with atipamezole (0.05–0.09 mg/kg);[15] ketamine (10 mg/kg) + xylazine (1–1.5 mg/kg);[14] ketamine (15–20 mg/kg) + midazolam (0.28–0.68 mg/kg);[4] ketamine (10.6 mg/kg) + diazepam (0.26 mg/kg);[1] and tiletamine/zolazepam (4–5 mg/kg) reversed with flumazenil (0.01 mg/kg);[4] all these drugs are administered intramuscularly. Administering the antidote at approximately 30 to 40 minutes after induction, once most of the ketamine has been redistributed or metabolized, results in smoother recoveries.[4,9,15] Recently, the addition of midazolam (0.25 mg/kg) to ketamine and medetomidine (3.8 mg/kg and 0.1 mg/kg, respectively) has been successfully used in unrestrained free-ranging individuals (L. Meyer, personal communication). Depth of anesthesia may be increased and maintained with volatile inhalation anesthetics, either via a face mask or endotracheal intubation.[4] Intubation may be challenging but is facilitated if the animal is placed in sternal recumbency, with the head extended and the tongue exteriorized; intubation may be done either blindly or by using a long-bladed laryngoscope (L. Meyer, personal communication).[4] Anesthetic monitoring should include normal cardiorespiratory monitoring along with the use of a pulse oximeter, with the probe placed on the tongue, and recording of body temperature. Blood pressure may be determined with a cuff placed on the distal hindlimb or tail or by catheterization of an auricular artery for continuous direct assessment (L. Meyer, personal communication).[4,15] Depending on the duration of anesthesia, animals should be maintained on only oxygen for up to 20 minutes at the end of the procedure.[11] Diazepam (10 mg, orally [PO], once a day) is effective in treating captive animals that pace excessively following an anesthetic episode.[4]

PHYSICAL EXAMINATION AND DIAGNOSTICS

Blood samples may be collected from the cephalic, femoral, medial saphenous, ventral tail, or facial vein for hematology and biochemical analysis. Normal reference values have been previously reported for captive animals (Table 52-1).[9] More recently, blood chemistry values have been determined in seven free-ranging aardvarks captured in South Africa by using chemical restraint (L. Meyer, personal communication). Mean values (standard deviation [SD]) were as follows:

Calcium = 8.91 (1.36) milligrams per deciliter (mg/dL)
Phosphorus = 4.56 (0.42) mg/dL
Sodium =138.86 (13.13) millimoles per liter (mmol/L)
Potassium = 4.83 (1.77) mmol/L
Blood urea nitrogen = 24.86 (3.53) mg/dL
Total bilirubin = 0.29 (0.04) mg/dL
Alkaline phosphatase = 34.43 (8.62) international units per liter (IU/L)
Alanine aminotransferase = 29.71 (7.65) IU/L
Amylase = 52.14 (12.10) IU/L
Total protein = 5.39 (0.85) grams per deciliter (g/dL)
Globulin = 0.87 (0.34) g/dL
Albumin = 4.49 (0.61) g/dL

DISEASES

No infectious diseases are unique to aardvarks. Most captive individuals die from degenerative illnesses associated with old age.[1,3] Recorded medical conditions include arthritis in limb joints, decubital ulcers, fractures of the digits, conjunctivitis, hepatitis, osteomyelitis of the jaw, skin irritations, intestinal abscesses, fecal impactions, peritonitis, pneumonia, bronchitis, gastric ulcers, arterial aneurism, uterine leiomyoma, colitis, aural hematomas, scent gland impaction, and dermatitis.[1,3,9] Dental disease is the most common condition in captive animals. Tooth root abscesses occur predominantly in the mandible and present as firm painful swellings. Maxillary abscesses may cause a discharging rhinitis. Treatment may be challenging because of the small mouth and elongated oral cavity, and a buccostomy may be required for access to teeth. Curettage of infected or necrotic bone may cause significant hemorrhage with a risk of airway obstruction.[4,9] A variety of oral and parenteral antibiotics have been administered to aardvarks, using standard mammalian dosages.[9] A variety of benign nematodes, protozoa, and ectoparasites have been identified in the aardvark; control has been with standard parasiticides.[9]

REPRODUCTION

In the wild, the aardvark male remains with the female for a short period during mating.[3] Intromission is brief and lasts for less than 1 minute.[13] Recent studies suggest that the gestation period is closer to 8 months (248 days) than the earlier cited 7 months.[8] Aardvarks are monotocous, with twins seldom being born. Neonatal aardvarks weigh approximately 1.7 kg (range 1.3–1.9 kg), are naked, and have their eyes open.[3,13] The youngster becomes independent at about 6 months, reaching sexual maturity at 2 years. In captivity, females generally give birth once a year.[3]

In captivity, a large percentage of offspring have been hand raised.[1] Low doses of oral diazepam (0.25–0.45 mg/kg, once daily [SID] or twice daily [BID]) have been used successfully in females to allow their offspring to nurse, with gradual tapering of the dose.[4] A number of commercially available milk formulas, including dog and sow milk substitutes, with added vitamin and calcium supplements, have been used in hand-rearing. Initially, the formula is diluted with water (3 : 1) and gradually increased in strength over several months. It has been suggested that neonates should receive

TABLE 52-1

Reference Hematology and Biochemistry Values for Aardvark

Parameter	Mean (Reference Interval)	Parameter	Mean (Reference Interval)
Hemoglobin (g/dL)	13.7 (9.2–17.9)	Ca (mg/dL)	9.8 (7.9–11.4)
Hematocrit (%)	39.6 (27.8–50.8)	P (mg/dL)	6.0 (0.0–10.6)
MCV (fL)	121.7 (105.9–136.1)	Na (mEq/L)	148 (139–156)
MCH (pg)	42.4 (36.2–49.2)	K (mEq/L)	4.2 (3.1–5.3)
MCHC (g/dL)	35.0 (30.9–38.8)	Cl (mEq/L)	110 (99–122)
Platelet count (×10³/μL)	269 (7–496)	BUN (mg/dL)	22 (0.0–37)
Segmented Neutrophils (×10³/μL)	4.30 (0.0–8.27)	Creat (mg/dL)	1.9 (0.5–3.1)
Neutrophilic band cells (×10³/μL)	0.03 (0.01–0.06)	Tot bili (mg/dL)	0.3 (0.0–0.7)
Leukocytes (×10³/μL)	7.70 (0.69–13.68)	Gluc (mg/dL)	88 (38–136)
Erythrocytes (×10³/μL)	3.22 (2.11–4.22)	Chol (mg/dL)	70 (0.0–154)
Lymphocytes (×10³/μL)	1.96 (0.0–4.31)	Triglyceride (mg/dL)	42 (0.0–101)
Monocytes (cells /μL)	342 (0.0–884)	CPK (IU/L)	124 (0.0–267)
Eosinophils (cells /μL)	598 (0.0–1581)	ALP (IU/L)	205 (0–703)
Basophils (cells /μIL)	369 (0.0–884)	ALT (IU/L)	54 (2–96)
		AST (IU/L)	32 (0.0–63)
		GGT (IU/L)	4 (0.0–13)
		Amylase (IU/L)	82
		TP (g/dL)	5.8 (4.4–7.7)
		Glob (g/dL)	2.8 (1.8–3.9)
		Alb (g/dL)	3.0 (1.6–4.6)

From Teare JA, ed: 2013, "*Orycteropus afer* No selection by gender All ages combined Conventional American Units 2013 CD. Html" in ISIS Physiological Reference Intervals for Captive Wildlife: A CD-ROM Resource, International Species Information System, Bloomington, MN.

only a 5% dextrose solution for the first 24 to 48 hours. *Lactobacillus acidophilus* and *L. bulgaricus* added to the formula will assist in establishing normal gut flora. Hand-raised aardvarks are fed four to six times a day and 12% to 14% of their body weight in a 24-hour period.[1,9]

ACKNOWLEDGMENTS

The author would like to thank Dr. Genny Dumonceaux, Palm Beach Zoo, Florida, for providing an update of medical conditions recorded in captive aardvarks in the United States.

REFERENCES

1. Goldman CA: A review of the management of the aardvark (*Orycteropus afer*) in captivity. *Int Zoo Yb* 24/25:286, 1986.
2. Kleisner K, Ivell R, Flegr J: The evolutionary history of testicular externalization and the origin of the scrotum. *J Biosci* 35:1, 2010.
3. Knöthig J: Biology of the aardvark (*Orycteropus afer*) (student thesis), Heidelberg, Germany, 2005, University of Heidelberg.
4. Langan JN: Tubulidentata and Pholidota. In West G, Heard D, Caulkett N, editors: *Zoo animal and wildlife immobilization and anesthesia*, Ames, IA, 2007, Blackwell Publishing.
5. Lehmann T: Plio-pleistocene aardvarks (Mammalia, Tubulidentata) from East Africa. *Foss Rec* 11:67, 2008.
6. Milton SJ, Dean WR: Seeds dispersed in dung of insectivores and herbivores in semi-arid southern Africa. *J Arid Environ* 47:465, 2001.
7. Pocock RI: Some external characteristics of *Orycteropus afer*. *Proc Zool Soc* XLVI:46, 1924.
8. Reason R, Gierhahn D, Schollhamer M: Gestation in aardvarks (*Orycteropus afer*) at Brookfield Zoo, IL. *Int Zoo Yb* 39:222, 2005.
9. Stetter DS: Tubulidentata (Aardvarks). In Fowler ME, Miller RE, editors: *Zoo and wild animal medicine*, Philadelphia, PA, 2003, Saunders.
10. Taylor WA, Lindsey PA, Skinner JD: The feeding ecology of the aardvark *Orycteropus afer*. *J Arid Environ* 50:135, 2002.
11. Taylor WA, Skinner JD: Activity patterns, home ranges and burrow use of aardvarks (*Orycteropus afer*) in the Karoo. *J Zool Lond* 261:291, 2003.
12. Taylor WA, Skinner JD: Adaptations of the aardvark for survival in the Karoo: A review. *Royal Soc S Afr* 59:105, 2004.
13. Taylor WA: Tubulidentata, Orycteropodidae (Grey, 1821), Aardvark. In Skinner JD, Chimimba CT, editors: *The mammals of southern African subregion*, Cambridge, 2005, Cambridge University Press.
14. Van Aarde RJ, Willis CK, Skinner JD, et al: Range utilization by the aardvark, *Orycteropus afer* (Pallas, 1766) in the Karoo, South Africa. *J Arid Environ* 22:387, 1992.
15. Vodicka R: Chemical immobilization of captive aardvark (*Orycteropus afer*). *J Zoo Wildl Med* 35:544, 2004.
16. Whittington-Jones GM, Bernard RTP, Parker DM: Aardvark burrows: A potential resource for animals in arid and semi-arid environments. *Afr Zool* 46:362, 2011.
17. Willis CK, Skinner JD, Robertson HG: Abundance of ants and termites in the False Karoo and their importance in the diet of the aardvark *Orycteropus afer*. *Afr J Ecol* 30:322, 1992.

CHAPTER 53

Proboscidea

Ellen Wiedner

GENERAL BIOLOGY

As the largest extant land mammal, the elephant is characterized not only by great size but also by extraordinary intelligence, complex social behavior, and its remarkable nose, capable of uprooting large trees or grasping single grains of rice. Over the past 4000 years, elephants have been worshipped as gods, used as work animals and beasts of war, and admired in zoos and circuses. However, elephants now face an uncertain future. The growing demand for ivory has decimated herds in both Africa and Asia, and human–elephant conflicts, ongoing habitat loss, demand for bush meat (African elephants), skewed sex ratios because of ivory poaching (Asian elephants), and politics have caused further massive losses of elephant populations. The captive population is not self-sustaining, and the extinction of elephants—a horrific thought—could become a reality in the not-so-distant future.

Elephants are an ancient species that are placed in superorder Afrotheria, clade Paenungulata, order Proboscidea. Probscideans first appeared in Africa during the early Cenozoic period, approximately 60 million years ago, but these early ancestors were not much larger than a golden retriever and bore little resemblance to modern elephants. Characteristics such as gigantism, the long dexterous trunk, and the distinctive tusks and molars evolved over millions of years as the group migrated into Europe, Asia, India, and the Americas. The taxonomy and classification of the proboscidea continue to be debated, but currently only modern elephants (*Loxodonta* and *Elephas*), mastodons (*Mammut*), and mammoths (*Mammuthus*) are placed together in the family Elephantidae. Woolly mammoths (*M. primigenius*), the last of the ancestral elephants, became extinct 5000 to 10,000 years ago. The closest living relatives to elephants are other members of the Paenungulata: the order Sirenia (manatees and dugongs), and the order Hyracoidea (rock hyraxes). Evidence for these relationships may be found in the fossil record, in genetic and immunologic studies, and in comparative anatomic data.[56]

Today, two genera of elephants are recognized, *Loxodonta* and *Elephas*. Genus *Loxodonta*, the African elephant, includes two species: *L. africana*, the African savanna elephant, and *L. cyclotis*, the forest elephant, although *L. cyclotis* is not universally accepted. Genus *Elephas*, the Asian elephant, includes a single species, *E. maximus*, but some zoologists recognize a variety of subspecies, including *E. m. sumatranus*, *E. m. indicus*, and *E. m. maximus*. This too is controversial.[56] Both *L. africana* and *E. maximus* share the same number of diploid chromosomes ($n = 56$). In nature, the two species are so geographically separated that interbreeding is impossible. However, one known African–Asian hybrid was born in captivity, the calf "Motty," born at the Chester Zoo in 1978, to an Asian elephant mother and an African elephant father. Motty lived less than 2 weeks before dying of necrotizing enterocolitis, but was confirmed to be a hybrid with testing of tissues samples.[31] Table 53-1 provides a comparison of African and Asian elephants.

Elephants are long lived, often reaching their 40s in the wild and their 50s and 60s in captivity.[72] They are a herd species, with an intricate social structure and multiple communication systems. These systems include complex vocalizations, infrasound (sound below the range of human hearing),[23] and chemical signaling via hormones, proteins, and volatile compounds released in urine, feces, breath, and secretions from specialized glands such as the temporal gland, a unique Proboscidean apocrine gland located on each side of the head. These bioactive compounds transmit information about the individual's reproductive status, territory, and dominance and likely about other aspects of elephant society both within and without the herd.[50]

Elephant habitats are highly varied. For African elephants, this includes environments that range from hot deserts to savannas, as well as dense forests and wetlands at a variety of altitudes. Asian elephants are found in similarly diverse habitats that also include shrub land, wet and dry forests, evergreen and deciduous woods, and degraded areas. The International Union for Conservation of Nature (IUCN) Red List of Threatened Species classifies *Loxodonta* as vulnerable but comments that the status is regionally variable. Asian elephants are classified as endangered. Both species are listed in the Convention on International Trade in Endangered Species I (CITES I) Appendix.

UNIQUE ANATOMY

From one end to the other, the elephant's anatomy is highly unusual, starting with the proboscis—or trunk—which is the obvious example. Thickly muscled, extremely flexible, and complexly innervated, the trunk is comparable to a hand. In fact, the fingerlike appendages on the distal trunk (single in *Elephas*, double in *Loxodonta*) are densely packed with Pacinian corpuscles and vibrissae, which enable both refined grasping of small objects and discrimination of diverse sensory stimuli.[50] Since the elephant is unable to lower its head to the ground while in a standing position and has little movement of its neck compared with other species, the trunk is essential for bringing food and water to the mouth. Elephants also use the trunk as a weapon, to toss dirt and sand on their backs, to spray water, and for communication with herdmates both by tactile means and by bringing chemically active substances to the vomeronasal organ located on the dorsal surface of the mouth.[51]

The tusks are upper incisors, present in both genders of African elephants but only in males in Asian elephants. Female Asian elephants often have rudimentary tusks called *tushes*. Tusks grow continuously throughout an elephant's life. For a very brief period after they erupt through the sulcus, they are covered in shining white enamel. When the enamel is shed, what remains underneath is the off-white dentine, the substance known as "ivory." Primary dentine is on the outside of the tusk. Secondary dentine is laid down within the pulp cavity; thus, the diameter of the elephant tusk increases from the interior.[16] The great preference for elephant ivory over that of other species is because of several unusual characteristics. First, elephant ivory is softer than most other ivories; second, it cracks less easily, and, finally, in cut section, its arrangement of overlapping dentine tubules creates subtle checkerboard effects. These are called *Shreger patterns* and are unique to the proboscideans. They give elephant ivory its great beauty when carved.[58]

Tusks grow approximately 18 centimeters (cm) a year and, in large African males, may reach more than 3 meters (m) in length and 70 to 100 kilograms (kg) in weight.[58] In the center of the tusk is the pulp cavity, which is filled with blood vessels, nerves, and growing cells. Over time, as the tusk elongates, the most distal part of the pulp cavity becomes compressed and atrophied. On cross-section, this atrophied tissue may be seen as a black dot in the center of the tusk and should not be confused with the actual pulp cavity.

The absence of tusks (natural tusklessness) is a female sex-linked trait. When wild populations of either Asian or African elephants are

TABLE 53-1

Comparison of African and Asian Elephants[56]

Parameter	*Loxodonta*	*Elephas*
Weight	4000–7000 kilograms (kg)	2000–5500 kg
Height	~4 meters (m)	2–3.5 m
Dorsum	Upward slope toward rump	Downward slope toward rump or no slope
Head	Single large bulge on forehead	Two large bulges on forehead Forehead concavity develops with age
Ears	Very large and hang below neck	Smaller
Molars	Diamond shaped occlusal surface	Narrow loops on occlusal surface
Tusks	Tusks present in both sexes	Tusks only in males Females have vestigial tusks (tushes) or none

heavily poached for ivory, this trait emerges. When poaching decreases, tusklessness diminishes.[59] In most of Asia, tuskless males are called "makhnas."

The molar formula is: incisors (I) 1/0, canines (C) 0/0, premolars (P) 3/3, molars (M) 3/3, although some authors consider all cheek teeth to be molars, which would change the formula to: I 1/0, C 0/0, PM 0/0, M 6/6.[37] However, all of these six cheek teeth are not present at the same time in the mouth but erupt successively over the course of the animal's life. At any moment in time, usually only two functioning molars are present in any quadrant of the jaw. New molars are formed in alveolar pockets at the back of each jaw and are composed of compressed plates of enamel-wrapped dentine (called *laminae* or *lamellae*), which are joined together with cementum. Over time, old worn molars move forward in the jaws, dissolve their roots, and fall out of the mouth to be replaced by newly formed molars that have advanced cranially from the alveolar pockets to come into wear. This continuous process bears some resemblance to an escalator's motion. Techniques to determine an elephant's age by analysis of the wear and number of dental lamellae have been described but involve a large margin of error. Some elephants are not toothless at death, even if they live to an advanced age because molars 6 (M6), the last molars, are not always shed, although they may become extremely worn and fragmented.[37]

Neonates may be born with M1 and M2. If not present at birth, M1 and M2 usually erupt shortly thereafter and are shed by age 2 or 3 years.[37] Milk tusks (also known as *tushes*) on young elephants, which sometimes never erupt, are resorbed and replaced by permanent tusks between 6 months and 1 year.

Elephants do not have lacrimal puncta, lacrimal glands, or a nasolacrimal drainage system. Nevertheless, elephants do produce tears from multiple adnexal glands which, because of the absence of the duct system, regularly—and normally—run down the side of the face from the medial canthus.[74]

The pleura of elephants is represented by thick, diffuse connective tissue that attaches to ribs, diaphragm and lungs and obliterates the pleural space. This tissue is simply pleural membranes that became adhered and thickened, a phenomenon that occurs in utero, early in gestation. Containing mostly collagen fibers and having a slippery, compliant consistency, it slides and moves and still acts functionally as a pleural membrane. Although these unusual pleura attach the lungs to the chest wall, they do not appear to hamper chest wall excursions.[64] The thorax is also the site of two mammary glands; elephants have breasts, not an udder.

The heart may weigh more than 20 kg in an adult elephant. The cranial vena cava is paired, and the caudal vena cava is single. Numerous arteriovenous anastomoses as well as arterial and venous plexuses may be found throughout the body.[45] The veins have multiple valves that likely cause some of the difficulties can be experienced when drawing blood. These valves, plexuses, and anastomoses are related to the complex—and poorly understood—hydraulics involved in moving the massive blood volume around the elephant's body.

Elephants lack a gallbladder but have a duodenal pouch that connects both the biliary and pancreatic ducts.[45] The liver is unusual in that it produces C_{27} bile alcohols rather than bile acids, a characteristic shared with other Paenugulates as well as with some cartilaginous fish. Unlike bile acids, which lose their taurine conjugate when bacteria bind to them, bile alcohols lose a sulfate conjugate. This characteristic renders them insoluble across lipid bilayer membranes and traps them within the bile ducts. These trapped bound bile alcohols are believed to predispose elephants to cholelith formation.[2]

Elephants are hind gut fermenters with a simple stomach. The small intestines terminate at a large sacculated, conical cecum, which, in turn, connects to a partially sacculated large intestine. Microbial fermentation of feed begins in the small intestine, peaks in the cecum, and continues in the colon. Elephants have short intestines and rapid gut transit times, which lead to lower digestibility coefficients compared with those in domestic hoofstock and are a measure of the amount of nutrition taken in from a particular feed.[14]

Elephant kidneys are reniculate and are composed of 6 to 10 lobes, some of which may be fused. In most adult elephants, urine does not concentrate significantly, even if the animals have not drunk water for a while; this may be explained, in part, by the anatomy of the kidney, which includes small or absent renal papillae and minimal contact between urine and the outer renal medulla at the calyx.[66]

The elephant's foot is adapted to support its great weight. The circumference of the forefeet is greater than that of the hindfeet. Foot anatomy is similar in both Asian and African elephants, although minor differences exist in appearance with regard to the number of toenails. The nails are not weight bearing and grow less than 1 cm per month. They are connected to the underlying phalanger by laminae.[46]

All feet have five digits regardless of the number of nails present. By convention, the digits are numbered DI through DV, with the most medial digit always being DI. Each digit consists of three (sometimes two) phalanxes and one metacarpal or metatarsal. DIII is the longest. Because of the vertical arrangement of the metacarpals, they provide equal weight support at the front of the body, whereas the metatarsals are more horizontally organized, resulting in the majority of weight being carried by DII, DIII, and DIV.[46] The bones of the feet sit atop a digital cushion composed of fat and connective tissue, which acts as both shock absorber and fluid pump.[8] With every step the elephant takes, the cushion compresses and deforms outwardly causing the circumference of the foot to expand. Additionally, compression of the cushion helps push blood from the feet back to the heart, another hydraulic adaptation. A cartilaginous prepollux and prehallux in the forefeet and hindfeet, respectively, create subcompartments within the cushion and also act as struts for the foot.[46] The bottom of the foot, sometimes called the *slipper*, consists of the sole (the underside of the toes) and pad (the underside of the foot) and is composed of horny, keratinized tissue. This keratinized material grows from an underlying germinal epithelium, which, in turn, sits atop the sensitive corium. The slipper is quite thin, rarely more than 4 to 12 millimeters (mm) thick, and is usually corrugated in adults.[8] (Figure 53-1).

SPECIAL HOUSING REQUIREMENTS

Elephants are herd animals and generally require contact with other elephants. Housing should provide space for social interactions and

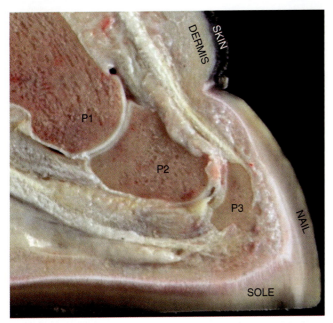

FIGURE 53-1 Sagittal section through the foot of an Asian elephant, showing the alignment of the three phalangeal bones with the nail as well as the thinness of the sole. (Photograph courtesy of Dr. Ramiro Isaza. The increase in nail thickness from top to bottom can also be seen.)

also room to separate the elephants that are not getting along with the others or for medical reasons. Housing may be as simple as a basic shelter offering protection from the elements in warm climates or a sophisticated modern barn with a temperature-controlled environment and hydraulic gates. Good ventilation, ability to thoroughly clean the facility, and construction materials that cannot be destroyed by the elephants are of paramount importance.

A variety of flooring surfaces has been used in elephant housing, but it remains unclear what type of floor is best. Smooth floors, roughened floors, deep sand pits, and specialized polymers have all been used. In some facilities, elephants have pulled up and ingested newly installed floors, so durability is an important consideration.

Outdoor facilities may consist of multiple yards or a single communal yard. Generally, female elephants share paddocks, whereas each male is kept separately. Some facilities have incorporated all of their elephants, young, old, male, and female into herds that share a yard. Because elephants protect their skin by throwing dirt and sand on their backs, access to these materials is necessary. Swimming pools, waterfalls, and ponds are enjoyed by elephants but should be easy to clean and quickly drainable in case of emergency. Pools do not need to be deep, and, in fact, many elephants enjoy playing in just a few inches of water. Filtration systems must be installed out of reach of the elephants.

The size of the yard needed is debatable. The majority of wild elephants, both African and Asian, tend not to move around very much at all, maxing out at 5 to 10 km per day.[40] The only elephants that have been shown to walk long distances, up to 30 miles per day, is a unique group of African elephants living in the extremes of the Namib desert where drought and inadequate food sources make the terrain inhospitable.[62] However, regular exercise does benefit captive elephants as it decreases foot problems, improves heart health, and provides enrichment. Thirty minutes of exercise per day is likely a reasonable goal that may be achieved by walking the animals, encouraging a variety of stretching moves, or both.[65]

Healthy elephants may be acclimated to a wide range of temperatures. Elephants living in northern climates will often freely choose to play in snow and even break ice on ponds to go swimming. Precipitation, wind chill, and scarcity of sunshine may, however, decrease the tolerance levels of the elephants for cold weather. In

very hot environments, appropriate shade structures and water are obviously important, as is sand or dirt for dust bathing.

Toys and enrichment devices should be too big to be swallowed, difficult to destroy, and of sufficient interest to the elephants. Heavy large plastic balls, rubber motorcycle and truck tires, and knotted firehose have been used. Several facilities have installed fake trees where food items are hidden so that elephants spend time searching for them.

Facilities that house bull elephants have additional safety considerations. All institutions holding elephants require adequate perimeter fencing and containment, but those with bulls need containment that should withstand the aggressive behavior of a male in "musth" (a period of hormone-induced aggression). An elephant restraint device (ERD) is recommended and even required at facilities accredited by the Association of Zoos and Aquariums (AZA). An ERD is a large chute that enables restricted contact and close-up handling of any elephant. ERDs come in a variety of configurations, but all permit access to the feet, legs, and head of the elephant via movable gates and may be adjusted to hold elephants of different sizes for the duration of a particular procedure. Some ERDs have a scale built into the floor so that the elephant may be weighed each time it enters the device. Others have incorporated tilt tables. In Asia, elephant camps often have wooden stocks, built of large tree trunks that function like an ERD. Whatever the conformation of the ERD, the elephant needs to be conditioned to it and trained to go in and out reliably.

Breeding facilities need to baby-proof their barns and yards. As Rudyard Kipling noted, little elephants have " 'satiable curiosity." Considerations include keeping the calf from escaping, since calves may wiggle through very small vertical gaps. Pools may need to be lowered or emptied until it has been ascertained that the calf can swim.

FEEDING

In the wild, elephants are browsers and grazers, demonstrating great diversity and selectivity in the foods they eat. They tend to feed throughout the day, rather than eat discrete meals. In general, the natural diet for both African and Asian elephants contains high amounts of fiber and relatively low amounts of protein (8% to 12%). Wild elephants eat approximately 1.2% to 1.9% of their body mass in feed volume daily. Currently, their daily energy requirements are unknown.[27,65]

Captive elephants in Asia are commonly fed palm leaves, bark, rice, tamarind, balls of salt, and green fodder and may be routinely released into nearby forests to browse. Captive elephants in the western hemisphere are typically fed diets of hay, browse, pellets, grains, fruits, vegetables, and miscellaneous items, ranging from bread to beet pulp. Some facilities provide pasture access to their animals. Many North American facilities successfully feed their elephants hay and browse diets without adding commercial pellets, which tend to be low in fiber and high in protein.[65] Regular forage analysis by a reputable laboratory is strongly encouraged because hay quality and nutrients may vary. Weighing feedstuffs and standardizing the diet are also recommended. Feed needs to be stored properly, away from weather and vermin. Caretakers should be educated about hay quality, nontoxic species of browse, and appropriate storage procedures. Variability in browse may provide enrichment, high amounts of fiber, and appropriate abrasiveness for teeth.

Regular weighing of elephants should be part of all captive programs. The use of weight tapes has been described in elephants, but a scale provides better accuracy. Published guides to elephant body condition scoring are available but often fail to describe overweight elephants or acknowledge variations in body type. Accurate assessment of body condition requires gaining experience with different elephant body types as well as typical changes in shape over an elephant's life. With advancing age, gravity and conformation may cause significant alterations in appearance that should not be confused with pathology.[65]

Obesity in captive elephants is linked to various health problems, including reproductive abnormalities, heart disease, and osteoarthritis. Several institutions have successfully put their elephants on a diet by feeding lower-energy forages, increasing browse, and eliminating pellets and other concentrates. Gradual weight losses of 450 kg have been achieved in elephants over an 8- to 12-month period.[27,65]

Like all animals, elephants require adequate amounts of clean water. Although elephants have been reported to drink vast quantities of water at a single time (up to 100 liters [L]) and over the course of the day (up to 225 L), most elephants do not drink this much and will vary their intake. Some will go several days without drinking without ill effects.[65] Nevertheless, in captivity, refusal to drink is often an early sign of illness and should be evaluated. Some facilities offer water on a continuous basis; others provide water to their elephants at specific times of the day. Either system is appropriate as long as keepers have the ability to observe intake. If this is not possible, urine output should be noted. This too may vary by individual.[65]

RESTRAINT AND HANDLING

Working with elephants requires consideration for the safety of the animal, the handler, and the facilities. Nobody should ever go up to an elephant without the express permission and assistance of an experienced handler who is familiar with the animal. Elephants are hierarchical and generally ignore the commands of those they do not know. Because of their strength, speed, and intelligence, they may also be extremely dangerous.

Safety is of paramount concern in an elephant barn. Any work with captive elephants uses training in conjunction with two different methods of handling: (1) nonrestricted contact, in which the elephant and the handler share space, and (2) restricted contact, in which the elephant and the handler do not share space or, if they do share space, the elephant is tethered. The use of either restricted or nonrestricted contact requires adequate training of both elephant and handler. In range countries, captive animals are handled almost entirely in nonrestricted contact. Circuses and organizations that use performing elephants also rely extensively on nonrestricted contact. Zoologic and breeding facilities generally use a combination of techniques that depend on the situation, the animal, and the experience of the handlers. The AZA has mandated the use of restricted contact in all AZA-accredited facilities in North America by 2014, with exceptions made for specific situations requiring direct access to the elephants. Training for these exceptions is also needed.

Tools used for elephant restraint include leg restraints or tethers and a guide, formerly known as an *ankus* or *bullhook*. The guide is a stick, made of metal, wood, or fiberglass with a prong at the end. The prong is tapered into a point that may push or pull at skin but not so sharp that it breaks the skin. The guide has been highly politicized by some who maintain that its only purpose is to beat and abuse elephants. It goes without saying that this is an entirely inappropriate use of this—or any—tool. In truth, the guide acts as an extension of the human arm to enable the handler to direct the animal to move in a desired direction. The AZA, the Elephant Managers Association (EMA) and the American Veterinary Medical Association (AVMA) all recognize the guide and tethers as appropriate tools in elephant management.

Typically, elephants are trained for a variety of minor medical and husbandry procedures. However, elephants are sometimes not cooperative when they are ill. In other situations, young elephants may not be reliably trained, and bull elephants, whether in musth or not, may be unpredictable. In these situations, chemical restraint or general anesthesia may be helpful. For surgical procedures, chemical restraint with analgesia is a necessity.

Chemical restraint may be achieved by standing sedation or general anesthesia in lateral recumbency, with or without gas anesthesia. It is necessary to remember that elephants often have unexpected responses to anesthetic agents, which have to be used with great care and sensitivity; chemical restraint therefore has to be approached as both art and science. Discussing protocols beforehand with veterinarians experienced in sedating and anesthetizing elephants is recommended. Elephants sometimes go down into sternal or even lateral recumbency with a standing sedation protocol. Facilities should prepare in advance for this possibility by having reversal agents available and should perform the procedure at a location where the animal may go down without getting injured.

Drugs typically used for standing sedation including α_2-agonists, often combined with butorphanol. Azaperone has been used as a short-acting tranquilizer both by itself and with butorphanol added. Ultrapotent narcotics are typically used for general anesthesia.[21] Etorphine is preferred over carfentanil. Both halothane and isoflurane have been used to maintain anesthesia following endotracheal intubation. Various local anesthetics have been used in elephants. Use of adequate local anesthesia may sometimes decrease or obviate the use of other sedatives. However, infiltration of the drug may be extremely difficult because of the thickness of the skin. Some of these agents may, however, work well on mucous membranes.[21] Table 53-2 lists drugs and doses for sedation and immobilization of elephants. Box 53-1 lists reversal agents. The reader is strongly encouraged to consult some of the recent textbooks and literature on elephant sedation and anesthesia prior to any sedation procedure.

Obtaining the accurate weight prior to drug administration facilitates safer anesthesia. In wild elephants, this is obviously not possible. Overdosing of drugs given for standing sedation is certainly a risk factor for an elephant falling. In wild animals, higher doses are used because the animals are less calm to begin with. However, underdosing is equally disadvantageous as it may cause excitement, incoordination, and ataxia. Frequent redosing may be dangerous and result in unwanted effects.

Drug delivery may be performed by hand injection in a well-trained elephant or with darting equipment. Drugs should be delivered into the triceps, upper muscles of the thighs, or gluteal muscles using long needles (at least 5 cm) to ensure intramuscular administration. Pole syringes or jab sticks should not be used in elephants that are not enclosed within an ERD, since they may turn quickly and grab the device from the handler. Wild elephants are typically darted using power-charged projectors, often from a helicopter.[21]

For elective surgeries, elephants should be fasted 24 to 48 hours prior to anesthesia, and water should be withheld for 24 hours. Appropriate padding is needed to prevent peripheral nerve damage and compartment syndrome while the elephant is in lateral recumbency. Multiple large and thick mattresses or specially crafted waterbeds may be used. Bolsters or large inner tubes should be placed between the legs.[18]

In a captive setting, elephants may be trained to lie down on command. If so, anesthetic drugs may be directly injected in the awake, recumbent animal, which avoids the elephant falling and being injured during induction. If this is not possible, a system of ropes or a sling may be used to pull the elephant into recumbency.[76] Site hazards such as moats, pools, and parked equipment should be evaluated beforehand and altered, if needed.[18]

BOX 53-1 Reversal Agents for Sedatives Used in Elephants

Drug	Dose*
Naloxone[21]	0.004
Naltrexone[21]	50–100 mg naltrexone per 1 mg opioid
Naltrexone[63]	2.0–3.5
Atipamazole[63]	0.1–0.16
Tolazoline[21]	0.5
Yohimbine[21]	0.073–0.098

*Dose mg/kg unless otherwise stated.

TABLE 53-2

Doses for Sedating and Immobilizing Elephants

Drug	Dose*	Species†	Route	Notes
Azaperone[21]	0.024–0.038	E.m.	Intramuscularly (IM)	Short-acting tranquilizer
Azaperone[21]	0.056–0.107	L.a.	IM, intravenously (IV)	Short-acting tranquilizer
Carfentanil[21]	0.002–0.004	E.m.	IM	Immobilization agent
Carfentanil[21]	0.0013–0.0024	L.a.	IM	Immobilization agent
Detomidine plus Butorphanol[47]	0.013–0.02 0.013–0.02	L.a.	IM	Standing sedation
Detomidine plus Butorphanol[63]	0.02–0.03 0.02–0.03	E.m. young calf	IM	Standing sedation, but may cause very young elephants to lie down
Etorphine[21]	0.002–0.004	E.m.	IM	Immobilization agent
Etorphine[21]	0.0015–0.003	L.a.	IM	Immobilization agent
Medetomidine[21]	0.003–0.005	E.m.	IM	Sedative
Xylazine[21]	0.04–0.08	E.m.	IM	Sedative
Xylazine[21]	0.08–0.1	L.a.	IM	Sedative
Xylazine plus Butorphanol[21]	Xylazine: 0.035–0.16; Butorphanol[21]: 0.005–0.036	L.a.	IM or IV	Can give separately with xylazine IM first followed by butorphanol, IV, 20 minutes later, or together IV
Xylazine plus Ketamine[21]	Xylazine: 0.1, Ketamine 0.3–0.7	E.m.	IM	

*Doses are in milligram per kilogram (mg/kg) unless otherwise stated.
†E.m., *Elephas maximus*; L.a., *Loxodonta africana*.

Following induction, intubation may be done using a 30- to 50-mm internal diameter (ID) cuffed endotracheal (ET) tube in an adult, a 12- to 16-mm ID tube in a newborn calf. The elephant's mouth may be pulled open with cotton ropes and a bite block placed between the upper and lower molars on one side of the jaw prior to intubation. Another technique is to place a strap around the lower jaw and attach it to a rope running between the animal's front legs.[76] Intubation is done blindly with the use of a 2-m stylet or an equine stomach tube used as a guidewire. With one's gloved arm inserted into the back of the throat, the soft palette is pushed upward to access the epiglottis. The ET tube is then slipped over the stylet or tube into the trachea. The external portion of the ET tube may be taped to the trunk.[18,76]

A single large animal ventilator may be adequate in a young calf. Multiple large animal ventilators may be attached together in parallel to provide adequate tidal volume in adults. A few elephant-specific ventilators are also available, some of which have been developed for field use.[76]

Monitoring of the animal under anesthesia may include pulse oximetry, capnography, electrocardiography (ECG), blood gas analysis, and blood pressure measurement. Hypotension may be significant in anesthetized elephants. Pharmaceutical agents that have been used to combat this problem include ephedrine and dobutamine. Circulatory support may also be provided with intravenous fluids. Hypertension and pulmonary edema ("pink foam syndrome") have been reported in wild African elephants following opiate anesthesia, but adding azaperone to the etorphine in a dart may be protective.[76]

In the past, complications reported with elephant anesthesia were numerous and included injury during induction, including tusk and bone fractures, respiratory and lactic acidosis, apnea, bloat, hypotension and hypertension, nerve damage, prolonged recovery, cardiac arrhythmias, hypoxemia and death.[18,76] In recent years, with the increased experience of veterinarians in the use of a variety of anesthetic drugs and protocols, elephant anesthesia has continued to improve in safety.

SURGERY

Surgery on elephants is often fraught with complications. Even a seemingly minor procedure such as suturing a laceration has the potential to go drastically wrong because elephants tend to open incision sites, destroy suture lines, eat bandages, and pack dirt, mud, and other debris into wounds. Conservative treatment such as cold hosing and flushing, use of topical therapies, and systemic antimicrobials often is surprisingly successful in healing even large skin wounds.

Abdominal surgeries such as cesarian sections and colic surgeries on adult elephants have been unsuccessful because of difficulties in obtaining adequate access to surgical sites as well as in manipulating the massive viscera. In addition, the thickness and toughness of the skin make both opening and closing incisions extremely difficult. Other complications include incisional dehiscence and surgical infection.[70] However, cesarian sections done for the purpose of removing dead calves are no longer performed because no animal has survived the procedure and also, more remarkably, because several pregnant elephants at multiple institutions have kept dead, full-term calves in their uterus for years without becoming septic. When the calves were finally passed, the bodies were neither mummified nor macerated.[28]

In the past several years, laparoscopic tools have been constructed specifically for vasectomies on wild African elephants. Multiple adult bulls were vasectomized without complications with the use of a sling to maintain the anesthetized animals in the vertical position.[61] Vestibulotomy, or episiotomy, in which a large incision is made below the rectum to remove a dead calf from the birth canal, is another surgical reproductive procedure, which, however, has frequently resulted in poorly healing or nonhealing incisions.[28]

The most commonly performed surgeries in elephants are dental surgeries. Procedures on fractured tusks include extraction, pulpotomy, and pulpectomy. These entail general anesthesia and specially crafted, elephant-sized dental equipment, along with experienced personnel.[16] However, conservative therapy with antibiotics and flushing and radiography to monitor progress have sufficed for some animals with broken tusks, even though the pulp cavity was open. One tusk extraction was performed by using rubber elastic bands that were advanced proximally, a little at a time each day, up the tusk of an unanesthetized elephant. This resulted in progressive loss of alveolar bone so that the tusk dropped from the sulcus in less than 1 month.[60]

Impacted molars usually require surgery. Molar disease may cause anorexia or colic because of difficulty masticating food. Molar removal is complicated, however, sometimes necessitating cutting the tooth into sections prior to removal. An experienced elephant dentist should be consulted about complex dental issues.

Several procedures formerly done with some frequency are now rarely performed or not at all. An example is surgical castration of adult bulls, which was found not to decrease or only minimally decrease aggressiveness or musth. Surgical artificial insemination (AI) is also infrequently performed because of the growing experiences and success of zoo veterinarians with endoscopic AI.

Uncommonly performed surgeries in elephants include esophagostomy, tail amputation, trunk reattachment (unsuccessful), fracture repairs, biopsies of various tissues and organs, cataract surgery, umbilical hernia repair, temporal gland extirpation, and tumor removal.

Elephant necropsies warrant mention here. They may be difficult, time consuming, and emotionally taxing but may add greatly to general knowledge about elephants as well as about specific issues in a collection of animals. Necropsy guidelines may be found on the AZA website. Having an experienced pathologist available for consultation and preferably direct assistance may be very helpful. A team approach is needed for an elephant necropsy. These include individuals to do the actual gross dissection, heavy machinery operators, and personnel to label and process tissue, sharpen knives, and record data. Prior to starting, the team should discuss how detailed the necropsy will be, review safety protocols for large cutting tools and heavy equipment, and discuss record keeping, sample collection, and submission. Disposal of the carcass should be determined in advance, whether it should be field burial or cremation.

Another consideration at a necropsy is potential exposure to tuberculosis (TB) or other zoonotic diseases. Personal protective equipment includes gowns, gloves, boots, face shields, and respirators specifically designed to protect against aerosolized microorganisms (N 95 facemasks at a minimum). Surgical masks are not appropriate protection. Typically, the thorax is opened last, and if suspicious granulomatous lesions are present anywhere in the respiratory tract, the number of personnel is minimized, protective gear is donned, and power tools are avoided to decrease possible aerosolization. Multiple samples should be collected quickly and packaged securely. Any further manipulation of the carcass should be done only as needed for disposal and with minimal exposure of tissue.

PHARMACEUTICALS

Scant pharmacologic studies have been performed in elephants, so clinicians are often left to extrapolate doses for elephants from those published for domestic hoofstock. Three techniques have been described: linear scaling, metabolic scaling, and allometric scaling. The first two techniques are seldom appropriate for elephants and have the most potential to result in significant overdoses and toxicity. Linear scaling simply inserts the weight of an elephant into a milligram-per-kilogram (mg/kg) dose established for another species. This method assumes that the pharmacokinetics are identical between the two species and that a linear scaler is adequate. As a result, linear scaling tends to vastly overdose larger animals.

The metabolic scaling technique factors in a physiologic estimate such as metabolic rate. Because the scalar is nonlinear, the dosage estimates may be more accurate for larger animals, but identical pharmacokinetics between both species are still assumed. However, several papers have demonstrated that elephant pharmacokinetics are different from horse or cow pharmacokinetics and that this technique also fails to predict accurate dosages.

The last technique, allometric scaling, is probably the most appropriate with regard to elephants but requires having pharmacokinetic data from multiple species about drug half-life, clearance, and volume of distribution which may be plotted against body weight. Drugs most appropriate for allometric scaling are those that have blood flow–dependent clearance. This includes only a select few drugs, primarily antibiotic agents.

Even when pharmacokinetic studies are done in elephants, they do not address pharmacodynamic issues, that is, how the drug behaves in the body—its efficacy, safety, and toxicity. In fact, many pharmaceutical agents cannot be safely extrapolated for use in elephants for reasons that include differences in elephant liver and kidney physiology, drug conjugation mechanisms, and underlying metabolism. An excellent discussion of the issues involved in drug dose extrapolation to elephants may be found in the article by Hunter and Isaza.[32]

Elephants may be medicated through a variety of routes. Oral administration is ostensibly the most straightforward technique, but elephants are highly sensitive to unpleasant tastes and may refuse medications or spit them back out, even if mixed into pleasant-tasting substances such as honey or syrup. Elephants may be trained to use a bite block, but the author has had the experience of medicating an elephant orally with a bite block, watching the animal seeming to swallow and even eat hay for over 2 hours, and then surreptitiously spitting out the entire dose of pills in a corner of her pen.

Intramuscular injections into the triceps or thigh muscles also require training. Repeated administration of drugs intramuscularly (IM) is apt to be painful and result in abscess or scar tissue formation. This is a concern if long-term therapy is needed. The use of longer-acting formulations of various antibiotics may be considered, although they too may cause large swellings at the site of injection.

Intravenous administration of drugs should be avoided unless an intravenous catheter has been placed either in an ear or saphenous vein. Several elephants have sloughed off large portions of their ears because of intravenous drugs leaking extravascularly. In addition, it is not always easy to distinguish between an artery and a vein in the ear, and some of the ear sloughing has been the result of vessel misidentification. Intravenous catheters, however, may be tricky both to place and to maintain in elephants and are subject to thrombosis, hematoma formation, thrombophlebitis, and loss of patency. Elephants also remove them with their trunks. Giving large volume of fluids via intravenous catheter for circulatory support is often difficult as well. Furthermore, because elephant serum osmolarity is extremely low, all commercially available fluids are hyperosmotic to the serum. This has unknown clinical significance.[25] Subcutaneous administration into the folds of the neck is a possibility, but very few drugs have been evaluated using this route.

Another route of drug administration in elephants is via the rectum. The elephant rectum is highly absorptive, and if the elephant is trained for allowing rectal ultrasonography, rectal drug administration may also be done. Prior to drug administration, feces should be manually evacuated from the rectum. The drug should be mixed with warm water until dissolved in a large dosing syringe with a piece of soft rubber tubing attached. The syringe with attached tubing should be deposited into the rectum as far as the arm can reach before depressing the plunger. In addition, large volumes of plain water may also be given rectally for circulatory support. Elephants appear to absorb what they need by this method and excrete the rest. Rectal fluids may be given using a bilge pump or a garden hose turned to a moderate rate and a lukewarm temperature. Fluids should be turned off if the elephant strains, and turned back on when the rectum relaxes. Retention may be aided by holding the tail down firmly after administration.[67]

Table 53-3 lists drugs used in elephants in which the pharmacokinetics were studied. Numerous reports exist of empirical dosing. For the reasons cited earlier, caution is advised.

TABLE 53-3

Selected Pharmaceutical Agents Studied in Elephants

Drug	Species*	Dose†	Route	Notes
ANTIBIOTICS				
Amikacin[42]	L.a.	6.0–8.0	Intramuscularly (IM) q24h	Tested in 2 healthy elephants
Amoxicillin[55]	E.m.	11.0	IM, q24h	Tested in 5 healthy elephants
Ampicillin[53]	E.m.	8.0	Orally (PO), q8or 12h	Single dose tested in 3 healthy elephants
Ceftiofur (short acting)[15]	E.m.	1.1 1.1	IM, q8 or 12h IV, q24h	Tested in 4 healthy elephants
Ceftiofur (long acting)[1]	E.m.	6.6	Subcutaneously (SC), q7-10d	Tested in 11 healthy elephants
Enrofloxacin[54]	E.m.	2.5	PO, q24h	Tested in 6 healthy elephants
Metronidazole[24]	E.m.	15.0	Rectally, q24h	Tested in 1 sick elephant
Oxytetracycline (long acting)[12]	L.a.	18.0	IM, q48h	Tested in 18 healthy elephant calves
Benzathine Penicillin G and Procaine Penicillin[55]	E.m.	4,545.0 international units per kilogram (IU/kg)	IM, q24, 48, or 96h	Dosing regimen dependent on organisms targeted Aqueous suspension used Tested in 5 healthy elephants
Trimethoprim sulfa[49]	L.a.	22.0	PO, q12h	Tested in 3 elephants
NONSTEROIDAL ANTI-INFLAMMATORIES				
Ibuprofen[6]	E.m.	6.0	PO, q12h	Single dose trial of 10 healthy elephants
Ibuprofen[6]	L.a.	7.0	PO, q12h	Single dose trial of 10 healthy elephants
Ketoprofen[33]	E.m.	1.0–2.0	PO, or IV q24 or 48h	Single dose trial of 5 healthy elephants
Phenylbutazone[7]	E.m	3.0	PO, q48h	Single dose trial of 8 healthy elephants
Phenylbutazone[7]	L.a.	2.0	PO, q24h	Single dose trial of 10 healthy elephants
OTHER AGENTS				
Famiciclovir[10]	E.m.	8.0–15.0	PO or rectally, q8h	
Ivermectin[22]	L.a.	0.2–0.4	PO	Single dose trial of 6 healthy elephants

*E.m., *Elephas maximus*; L.a., *Loxodonta Africana*.
†Doses are in mg/kg unless otherwise stat

PHYSICAL EXAMINATION AND DIAGNOSTICS

Prior to any physical examination, the veterinarian and handlers should discuss what needs to be done, for which procedures the elephant is trained, and in which portions of the examination, if any, the elephant needs to be in an ERD. Records, including weight and nutritional data, as well as recent test results should be reviewed. The examination starts by observation of the elephant from a distance. The elephant's interactions with herdmates and behavior in its environment should be noted. Both wild and captive elephants are in almost constant motion, which is natural behavior that should not be equated with stereotypy. These motions include ear flapping, tail swishing, and shifting weight from one leg to another. They are related to temperature, communication with conspecifics, or simply movement of blood from the periphery to the heart.

The examiner should note gait, which is a four-beat, evenly spaced, ambling walk but may also be a very fast walk. Elephants do not trot, pace, canter, or gallop. At higher speeds, elephants look like they are bouncing on coiled springs, which tends to be how young calves move. The backbone is flexible, and movement of the spine and evenness of gait should be noted. Lame elephants do not exhibit a head nod or a hip hike as do horses, and determining which leg is lame may be surprisingly difficult at times. Conformation should be noted, including varus or valgus deformities, which may be subtle or severe, whether one leg is shorter than another, and general proportions.

Close-up evaluation starts with an assessment of the skin. African elephants usually have more wrinkles compared with Asian elephants. However, as Asian elephants age, their skin depigments irregularly on the edges of the ears, down the center of the trunk, and often on the body and legs as well, making the animal look as though it has pink freckles. In range countries, these are considered marks of distinction.

Lumps and bumps on older elephants may become quite large but are rarely of medical significance. Asian elephants frequently develop verrucous, barnacle-like growths on their trunks and legs. These are normal. Large fibromas and hygromas on the body may be distinguished by ultrasonography. Bumps should be noted, measured, and monitored, but most of these lesions are benign, particularly if longstanding, and should not be routinely opened because of the likelihood of iatrogenically creating a difficult-to-treat infection. Large vulval papillomas occur commonly in old elephants. These are unsightly but benign. Bumps, nodules or vesicles appearing acutely on mucous membranes, however, warrant prompt investigation.

Dark circles around the eyes of elephants are often noted in warm weather and are caused by secretions from glands in these areas. As noted earlier, elephants do not have a nasolacrimal system, so tears constantly drain down skin grooves along the sides of the face. Blepharospasm, not tearing, is a more reliable indicator of ocular disease. Fluid drainage from the temporal glands may also be seen. This drainage may occur in males and females of either species. In an adult male, however, temporal gland drainage usually indicates musth and suggests that continuing the examination close to the animal is unsafe.

If the elephant is trained, the handler should ask the animal to lift each foot in turn to permit examination of the pad and sole. The pad is often smooth in younger animals and becomes roughened and ridged with age. Cracked, overgrown, or misshapen nails should be

BOX 53-2 Normal Vital Parameters for Adult Elephants

Temperature:	36–37°C (97°F–99°F)
Respiratory rate, standing:	10–12 breaths per minute
Respiratory rate, sleeping:	4–5 breaths per minute
Heart rate, standing:	25–35 beats per minute
Heart rate, recumbent:	30–50 beats per minute

noted. Cuticles should be neatly trimmed although some elephants find this uncomfortable. If so, mild cuticle overgrowth is acceptable. Hangnails should be trimmed.

Normal values for temperature, pulse and respiration are given in Box 53-2. To obtain body temperature, a thermometer should be placed in the center of a freshly passed fecal ball. The center of a fecal ball is marginally hotter than actual body temperature but provides a more accurate temperature reading than inserting the thermometer into the rectum. The consistency of the fecal ball should also be noted. African elephant manure is usually softer than Asian elephant manure, which tends to be firm and fibrous. Large undigested pieces of hay or extremely large fecal balls may indicate dental disease or other gastrointestinal (GI) issues. Nursing calves tend to have "milk stool," which is quite soft and yellow and should not be confused with diarrhea.

A pulse rate may be determined by placing the fingers on an auricular artery. Auscultation of the heart is generally possible only on elephants weighing less than 2270 kg (5000 pounds [lb]). The elephant should be asked to lift the front leg ("salute position"), and the stethoscope should be placed behind the elbow. Respiratory rate may be measured by feeling air currents at the end of the trunk. Thoracic movements from breathing are generally subtle in elephants. The clinician should try to assess the odor of the air coming from the trunk, since elephants with pneumonia sometimes have a fetid smell coming from their trunks. Both African and Asian elephants often develop varying degrees of trunk paralysis with age. The cause of this is unknown.

The elephant should be asked to open its mouth. It is extremely difficult to visualize the lower molars, but the upper molars can usually be seen. The surface of the tongue and the hard and soft palettes should be checked for ulcers, vesicles, or injury. Some elephants with elephant endotheliotropic herpesvirus (EEHV) have presented with oral ulcers or vesicles, but many have not. Elephants with severe dental disease often have halitosis. Elephants do bite, so putting the hand in the elephant's mouth is discouraged.

Diagnostics performed in elephants include blood work, typically a complete blood cell (CBC) count and serum chemistry, along with urinalysis. In elephants, assessing trends over time is often more helpful than evaluating a single sample, and regular sampling is optimal. Blood may be drawn from the veins on the back or front of the ear, with the elephant standing or in lateral recumbency. In cold weather, the veins may be extremely difficult to locate. Exercising the elephant or using a hair dryer or warm compress on the ear may help raise the veins. Blood may also be taken from the cephalic vein on the proximal medial forelimb or the medial saphenous vein, distal on the hindlimb. For either of these, a bungee cord or inflated bicycle inner tube used as a tourniquet may help raise the veins, which are deep and require the needle to be placed into the skin perpendicularly. A larger needle should be used to avoid lysing the massive erythrocytes. Hematologic and serum chemistry values are given in Tables 53-4 and 53-5.

Elephants have the largest red blood cell (RBC) of all mammals, elephants and somewhat lower cell counts compared with other species.[11] Reticulocytes do not normally appear in peripheral blood. The erythrocyte sedimentation rate in elephants is the fastest among those of all mammals, but how it changes in disease is unknown. Elephants have heterophils, rather than neutrophils, as well as eosinophils and basophils. They also have lymphocytes and two types of

TABLE 53-4

Complete Blood Count Values in Elephants*

Parameter	Loxodonta	Elephas
White blood cells (×10³ cells /µl)	9.83 (9.56)	12.29 (11.81)
Red blood cells (×10⁶ cells /µl)	2.93 (2.90)	2.91 (2.86)
Hemoglobin (g/dL)	12.8 (12.8)	12.1 (12.0)
Hematocrit (%)	37.0 (36.9)	35.6 (35.0)
MCV (fL)	125.5 (125.6)	122.3 (122.8)
MCH (pg)	44.1 (44.1)	41.7 (42.0)
MCHC (g/dL)	35.1 (35.0)	34.1 (34.4)
Segmented neutrophils [heterophils] (×10³/µl)	3.34 (3.03)	3.6 (3.09)
Lymphocytes (×10³/µl)	4.14 (3.81)	3.53 (2.74)
Monocytes (cells/µl)	2050 (1559)	4780 (5287)
Eosinophils (cells/µl)	175 (130)	293 (233)
Basophils (cells/µl)	135 (105)	121 (115)
Platelets (×10³/µl)	381 (313)	447 (411)

*Values given are mean (median).
From Teare JA, ed: 2013, "Elephas maximus. No selection by gender. All ages combined. Standard International Units. 2013 CD.html" and "Loxodonta africana. No selection by gender. All ages combined. Standard International Units. 2013 CD.html" in ISIS Physiological Reference Intervals for Captive Wildlife: A CD-ROM Resource., International Species Information System, Bloomington, MN.

monocytes. One type of monocyte is unsegmented and visually identical to the monocytes of any other mammalian species. The other is bilobed, sometimes trilobed. Whether functional differences exist between these two cell types is unknown.[11] Monocytes often increase during inflammation or infection. Band heterophils, even in very small numbers, may indicate severe inflammation. The caveat is that the large size of elephant erythrocytes and the two types of leukocytes have been known to confound automatic blood analyzers. Validation of these machines should be performed in advance, and a blood smear should be manually read by an experienced clinical pathologist.

On the serum chemistry, elephants demonstrate lower sodium and chloride values compared with other species. Serum osmolarity is significantly lower than in other species.[25] Total protein is usually high, consisting primarily of globulins. Elephants have blood groups and preformed blood group antibodies. They should be cross-matched in advance if the need for a transfusion arises.[67]

Amylase is always high, which is likely a function of the testing methodology rather than a reflection of pancreatic function. Liver enzyme alterations are difficult to interpret because their specificity and relationship to hepatobiliary disease is unknown. The clinician is reminded that elephants do not produce bile acids; currently, no liver function tests are validated in elephants. Blood urea nitrogen (BUN) and creatinine are generally low.

Urine may be obtained by free catch, and typically a cup is attached to a broom handle and held under the elephant. Normal urine varies in color from pale yellow to dark orange and is highly crystalline and generally alkaline. Transient glycosuria and ketonuria may occur in otherwise healthy animals. Specific gravity tends around 1.020, but very elderly elephants often produce hyposthenuric urine, which likely represents a degree of renal disease. Here, too, trends over time are useful. Urine culture is difficult to interpret, since contamination from normal bacterial flora inside the urogenital canal occurs during voiding. Elephant urine cannot be used to confirm prerenal, renal, or postrenal azotemia because in elephants, normally urine is not significantly concentrated even if the animal is dehydrated.[66] Oddly, newborn elephants often pass extremely concentrated urine initially after birth, but within 24 hours, the specific

TABLE 53-5

Biochemistry Blood Values in Elephants*

Parameter	Loxodonta	Elephas
Glucose (mg/dL)	85 (85)	87 (86)
Blood urea nitrogen (mg/dL)	9 (9)	12 (12)
Creatinine (mg/dL)	1.3 (1.3)	1.5 (1.5)
Uric acid (mg/dL)	0.2 (0.1)	0.2 (0.2)
Calcium (mg/dL)	10.9 (10.8)	10.6 (10.5)
Phosphorus (mg/dL)	4.9 (4.8)	4.8 (4.7)
Sodium (mEq/L)	129 (129)	131 (130)
Potassium (mEq/L)	4.8 (4.7)	4.6 (4.6)
Chloride (mEq/L)	89 (89)	91 (91)
Total protein (g/dL)	7.8 (7.8)	8.1 (8.2)
Albumin (g/dL)	3.1 (3.2)	3.2 (3.2)
Globulin (g/dL)	4.6 (4.6)	4.8 (4.8)
Fibrinogen (mg/dL)	264 (255)	389 (400)
Alkaline phosphatase (IU/L)	96 (88)	115 (101)
Lactate dehydrogenase (IU/L)	937 (984)	411 (336)
Aspartate aminotransferase (IU/L)	20 (18)	19 (18)
Alanine aminotransferase (IU/L)	8 (5)	9 (6)
Creatine kinase (IU/L)	223 (199)	177 (145)
Gamma-glutamyltransferase (IU/L)	10 (10)	6 (6)
Amylase (IU/L)	1798 (1214)	2247 (1008)
Lipase (IU/L)	9 (6)	17 (23)
Bilirubin, Total (mg/dL)	0.2 (0.2)	0.2 (0.2)
Bilirubin, Direct (mg/dL)	0.1 (0.1)	0.1 (0.1)
Bilirubin, Indirect (mg/dL)	0.1 (0.1)	0.1 (0.1)
Cholesterol (mg/dL)	72 (70)	42 (42)
Triglyceride (mg/dL)	60 (53)	50 (44)
Bicarbonate (mEq/L)	25.6 (26.0)	24.9 (25.0)
Magnesium (mg/dL)	2.23 (2.30)	2.17 (2.14)
Iron (ug/dL)	80 (80)	63 (62)
Carbon dioxide (mEq/L)	25.4 (25.5)	24.7 (25.0)
Progesterone (ng/mL)	0.43 (0.30)	0.34 (0.25)

*Values given are mean (median).
From Teare JA, ed: 2013, "Elephas maximus. No selection by gender. All ages combined. Standard International Units. 2013 CD.html" and "Loxodonta africana. No selection by gender. All ages combined. Standard International Units. 2013 CD.html" in ISIS Physiological Reference Intervals for Captive Wildlife: A CD-ROM Resource, International Species Information System, Bloomington, MN.

gravity drops to a level comparable with that of adults (Wiedner, unpublished).

Other diagnostics may be challenging in elephants. In some cases, this is because normal values have not been established for the species or tests have not been adequately validated. In other cases, the size of the animal or safety issues preclude diagnostic testing. Most require training the animal in advance to tolerate the procedure. In some cases, anesthesia is necessary.

Rectal examination and rectal ultrasonography may be performed in smaller animals. Transabdominal ultrasonography may help assess intestinal motility and intestinal wall thickness.[70] Drenching the elephant's skin with water before placing the gel-covered ultrasound probe on it often improves the image. Gastric endoscopy on smaller animals may be performed with the animals under sedation or anesthesia.

ECG may be performed in standing and recumbent animals but requires modifications to the leads so that they may be attached to the thick skin of the elephant. ECG measurements and values have been reported, and use of Lead 1 is recommended. Sinus arrhythmia and U-waves are normal in elephants. Values of cardiac enzymes such as troponin isoenzymes have not yet been validated.[5]

Both direct and indirect ophthalmology may be performed. Ocular disease is common in elephants, and fluorescein staining is important in checking for ulcers. Elephants must be trained to tolerate light being shined into their eyes because they would otherwise shut their lids tightly in response. Auriculopalpebral nerve blocks are not possible because the nerves are too deep. Transpalpebral ultrasonography is a noninvasive way to examine all parts of the eye.[4] Schirmer tear strips may be used to evaluate tear production. Conjunctival samples may be obtained by placing a sterile swab into the medial canthus of the eye and gently rubbing the conjunctiva with the swab.[74]

The respiratory tract may be difficult to evaluate. Auscultation is not helpful in adult animals, but may be useful in calves. A 3-m endoscope may be used to evaluate the length of the trunk; sedation or anesthesia is needed. Blood gas analysis and pulse oximetry are commonly performed in anesthetized elephants but are difficult to perform stallside. The trunk wash, usually used for TB detection (discussed later), may also be used for bacterial culture in suspected cases of pneumonia; performed correctly, it represents the microbiota of the lower respiratory tract. A caveat with regard to interpretation is that the elephant trunk is normally filled with numerous organisms, some of which may be pathogenic but may not be causing disease in the animal. These may contaminate the trunk wash.

A properly performed trunk wash requires the participation of a trained elephant, although trunk washes have been obtained from wild elephants placed under anesthesia.[36] Sterile saline (60 milliliters [mL]) is instilled into one nostril of the trunk with a dosing syringe. Then the handler lifts the trunk tip high in the air and places a 1-quart plastic zipper bag over the end of the trunk. The trunk is lowered, and the elephant is given a command to exhale forcefully. Ideally, 65% to 70% of the original 60 mL of saline will be recovered, along with visible mucus. The amount of dirt in the sample may be reduced by doing the trunk wash first thing in the morning before the elephants leave the barn. Special procedures may be needed for bull elephants that will not tolerate handling of their trunks. These include training the male to inhale and exhale saline from pipes or sinks built into the ground. After the saline is exhaled into the container, the bull is removed from the enclosure so that the sample may be recovered.

Both radiography and ultrasonography may be used in elephants. Reproductive ultrasonography (discussed later) is used extensively in captive breeding programs to monitor pregnancy and assess reproductive tract health. Ultrasonography of the abdomen and thorax may be performed in young animals, although sedation may be required beforehand. However, in adult elephants, even the lowest-frequency ultrasound probes seldom provide adequate depth of penetration to allow clear visualization of internal organs.[70]

Radiography of elephant feet may be performed by using either plain film or digital systems. Because of the shape of the elephant's foot, two orthogonal views are not possible. Thus, the angle of the x-ray beam used to take foot films should be consistent. A tripod and mounted protractor may improve repeatability. Great variation may occur in the shape of the third phalanx of each digit, so it is important not to confuse normal changes with pathology. The last phalanx is often saucer shaped and may have multiple sites of ossification. These should not be confused with osteomyelitis or fracture, respectively. The last phalanx may also be absent, which may be normal.[57]

Radiography of bones proximal to the foot require a high power x-ray generator. In elephants, the ulna is much larger than the radius. The chest and abdomen may only be radiographed successfully in calves. The tusks of elephants may be radiographed to identify the pulp cavity prior to trimming the tusk tips.

Thermography has also been attempted in elephants, but very little hard data is available on its use. Computed tomography (CT) and magnetic resonance imaging (MRI) have been used for anatomic studies on cadaver legs and heads.

DISEASE

Elephants are susceptible to a variety of infectious and noninfectious diseases, but recognizing that they are even sick may be difficult. Elephants often hide signs of illness until the disease has progressed significantly. Subtle signs of illness include decreased appetite, changes in manure or urine production, changes in herd interactions, difficulty rising, refusal to lie down, yawning, biting the trunk, standing or lying down in odd positions, and stretching. Elephants are thought not to be able to cough or vomit because of their anatomy. Close familiarity with the animal is necessary to recognize mild changes in behavior, and veterinarians should strive to communicate closely with keepers who are generally the eyes and ears of the elephant barn.

Infectious Disease

EEHV is arguably the most serious disease threat to elephants, both wild and captive. EEHV may cause acute hemorrhagic disease, with a mortality rate of approximately 85%, if untreated. Young Asian elephants between the ages of 1 and 4 years are most commonly affected, but cases have also occurred in African elephant calves, and in adults of both species. Multiple species of EEHV have been identified; those most commonly associated with severe disease are variants of EEHV-1, namely, EEHV-1a and EEHV1b. However, all elephants may carry multiple species and strains of EEHV—including EEHV-1—and yet never develop clinical disease.

EEHV is not a disease of captivity. Although the epidemiology is still under investigation, it is known that the viruses are routinely shed in respiratory, conjunctival, and vulval secretions of asymptomatic elephants, suggesting they are endemic in all elephants.[26] Hemorrhagic disease caused by EEHV has been confirmed in wild elephants in multiple Asian range countries. In Africa, hemorrhagic disease has not yet been confirmed, but various species and strains of EEHV have been recovered from the skin and pulmonary nodules of asymptomatic wild elephants.[52] The cohabitation of *Loxodonta* and *Elephas* in captivity does not appear to be a risk factor, as previously thought. The pathophysiology leading to sporadic outbreaks of hemorrhagic disease is unknown.

Phylogenetic analyses suggest that the EEHVs are as ancient as elephants themselves, and have evolved in conjunction with the Elephantidae. The EEHVs are β-herpesviruses in the genus *Probiscivirus*; however, elephants are also hosts to multiple ancient γ-herpesviruses, which are not associated with hemorrhagic disease. Although the index case of EEHV occurred in a young Asian elephant at the Smithsonian's National Zoo in 1995, testing of historical blood samples from elephants that died acutely has identified cases of EEHV-associated disease occurring much earlier. These findings indicate that the disease has been present in elephant populations for a long time but has been recognized only recently.[52] Several elephants with vague signs of colic and anorexia have tested positive with the polymerase chain reaction (PCR) for various species of EEHV, but it is unclear whether EEHV caused the signs or opportunistically appeared secondarily to another disease process. It is also possible that EEHV may cause different syndromes, only one of which is hemorrhagic disease.

Early signs of hemorrhagic EEHV-associated disease are nonspecific, with lethargy being most commonly reported. The disease progresses quickly, with animals dying within 24 to 72 hours of initial presentation. Some animals have developed oral ulcerations, but many have not. Cyanosis and edema of the tongue and head appear to be late stage signs. Lameness, heart murmurs, heart arrhythmias, and sleepiness have also been reported.[52]

The viruses target vascular endothelial cells, causing leakage of blood and plasma into the extravascular space. Most elephants appear to die of circulatory shock rather than blood loss.[67] At necropsy, widespread hemorrhage and petechiation of multiple organs are seen, along with hemopericardium, cerebral bleeding, and cerebral edema. Histopathologic findings include intranuclear viral inclusion bodies, as well as necrosis and edema in multiple blood vessel walls.[51] Viral deoxyribonucleic acid (DNA) may be confirmed in multiple organs. Clinical pathology findings include severe thrombocytopenia, anemia, hypoproteinemia, and a left shift.[67]

Currently, antemortem diagnosis may only be done by PCR assay of whole blood. Results take a minimum of 24 hours, and only a few laboratories worldwide are able to perform this test. Because of the rapid progression of the disease, most clinicians choose to start treatment on the basis of suspicion of EEHV-associated disease and before confirmation of infection. Aggressive therapy is thought to have dropped the mortality rate since 2009 significantly. Early, aggressive fluid therapy appears to be essential. The use of antivirals, usually famciclovir (oral or rectal) and, at least one institution, ganciclovir, as well as nursing care, including nasal oxygen supplementation, antibiotics, and antioxidants, are typically used.[67]

At the time of this writing, none of the EEHVs have been successfully grown in cell culture despite intensive efforts to do so. This has hampered studies of pathophysiology as well as research focused on antiviral choice and vaccine development.

TB, in contrast, is generally diagnosed in adult elephants, more often in Asian elephants than in African elephants. It is commonly caused by *Mycobacterium tuberculosis*, but several cases of *M. bovis* have also been reported. Single cases of *M. szulgai*, *M. avium*, and *M. elephantis*, all of which are atypical mycobacteria, have been recorded as well. The disease is uncommon in the United States, where the median point prevalence of *M. tuberculosis* in Asian elephants between 1997 and 2011 is calculated at 5.1% and at 0% in African elephants.[17] The point prevalence in other countries is unknown. Latency is suspected to occur in elephants.

Definitive diagnosis of TB is through culture. In elephants, the gold standard antemortem test is the trunk wash, described earlier. PCR test, high-performance liquid chromatography (HPLC), and DNA sequencing have been used for mycobacterial identification. Strain genotyping is performed with spoligotyping, variable number tandem repeat (VNTR) sequences, restriction fragment length polymorphisms (RFLP), and whole or partial genome analysis. Other diagnostic tests are nondiagnostic (purified protein derivative [PPD] skin test) or cannot be done (chest radiography) in elephants. Tests of cell-mediated immunity, the more relevant branch of acquired immunity for intracellular pathogens such as mycobacteria, have been minimally investigated for use in pachyderms. These include the interferon-gamma (IFN-γ) test and T-cell proliferation assay. Although culture of trunk washes is 100% specific, it is not particularly sensitive, since infected elephants may shed the TB bacteria infrequently.

In human-to-human transmission of TB when active pulmonary disease is present, the risk of infection is proportional to the degree of closeness and length of exposure.[29] Small, enclosed spaces with shared ventilation and prolonged or repeated exposure increase the likelihood of transmission of *M. tuberculosis* organisms.[29] It is probable that the occupational health risk of individuals such as veterinarians and handlers who work closely with TB-positive elephants is similar to the risks associated with human-to-human transmission. In a few cases, handlers of TB-positive elephants have converted to latent reactors on the PPD skin test. However, the risk of an elephant transmitting the infection to a member of the general public during a circus performance, elephant ride, or outdoor viewing at a zoo is considered negligible. First, *M. tuberculosis* is inactivated by sunlight and other ultraviolet (UV) light.[29] Second, no evidence suggests that *M. tuberculosis* is spread through fomites or contaminated surfaces or over long distances by wind currents.[29]

Serologic tests, including the Stat-Pak, Multi-Antigen Print Immunoassay (MAPIA) and Dual Path Platform test (DPP), are used as screening tests but are not confirmatory tests and should not be used as definitive regulatory tests. Serologic tests have been associated with high numbers of false-positives and poor intertest agreement.[43] In 2011, the World Health Organization (WHO) stated that serologic tests are unsuitable for the diagnosis of tuberculosis in humans.[75] It is hoped that this will also be recognized in the veterinary community because positive TB serology has been used to make treatment and euthanasia decisions for zoo animals in several cases where the animal, in fact, did not have the disease.[9,73]

In the United States, testing and treatment protocols for elephants with TB have been created by the U.S. Department of Agriculture (USDA) and may be found on the USDA website. These protocols mandate a multidrug regimen to be administered over 15 to 18 months. The drugs include isoniazid (INH), rifampin, pyrazinamide, and ethambutol. Other drugs such as fluoroquinolones and amikacin may be substituted in specific situations. Serum drug levels established for treated elephants are transposed from the levels recommended for humans with TB. However, both the pharmacodynamics and pharmacokinetics of the antituberculous drugs in elephants are different from those in humans. Severe side effects and suspected fatalities have occurred in elephants treated with these protocols.[68,73] These problems suggest that human serum levels are toxic for elephants. Isoniazid is particularly problematic as a first-line drug against TB, since it has an extremely narrow margin of safety and is quite hepatotoxic. Adverse effects of INH seen in elephants resemble those reported in domestic farm animals more than those reported in humans. They include colic, depression, inappetence, and fetid, scant, and black feces.[68] As in humans, however, elevations in hepatocellular enzymes are common.[68] INH doses and frequency of administration may be altered if toxicity occurs, and several treated elephants have tolerated prolonged INH dosing intervals.

Most elephants with TB do not show clinical signs. In only a very few end-stage cases, lethargy and weight loss have occurred. Without specific clinical signs, monitoring the progress of antituberculosis treatment in elephants is difficult. From an evidence-based perspective, three factors may be monitored during TB treatment: (1) whether or not the animals are shedding, which may be determined from trunk wash cultures; (2) measurement of blood levels of antituberculosis medications to determine if bactericidal doses are being given (based on in vitro testing), and (3) clinical evidence of drug-induced toxicity, which, if identified, should prompt decreasing that medication's dosage or discontinuing it entirely.

Anthrax (*Bacillus anthracis*) has been reported in wild and captive elephants of both species. The disease is zoonotic, and cases of human anthrax have occurred as the result of individuals handling elephant tusks with surface contamination by anthrax spores. Sudden death is the most typical presentation, but colic, diarrhea, weakness, petechiation and hemorrhage, and convulsions may occur. Diagnosis, which is seldom made with antemortem examination, is through blood culture. The carcasses of affected animals need to be burned, and insect control is required to prevent further spread. Oral vaccines have been preventive in elephants.[19]

Encephalomyocarditis virus (EMC) is a cardiovirus (family Picornaviridae), which has caused sporadic outbreaks in captive and wild African and Asian elephants worldwide. Rodents are the reservoir hosts, and transmission is by the fecal–oral route. Elephant-to-elephant transmission does not occur. Sudden death is the most common presentation. In milder cases, the heart may be damaged, and survivors often have weakened hearts. However, some animals remain asymptomatic even with active infection. Diagnosis is usually made at necropsy from viral culture of tissue. Necropsy findings that should increase suspicion of EMC include hydropericardium, white streaks throughout the myocardium, and myocardial degeneration seen histopathologically. Electron microscopy sometimes identifies viral particles in heart tissue. Inactivated vaccines have been specially produced for affected facilities and used during outbreaks. Routine vaccination against EMC, however, is uncommon.[19]

Foot and mouth disease (FMD), caused by an aphthovirus (family Picornaviridae), is thought to have affected wild and captive Asian and African elephants. Transmission is by direct contact, inhalation of aerosolized virus, fomites, and contaminated feed and water.

Affected elephants present with anorexia, vesicles on mucosal surfaces, trunk exudate, and swelling of the feet. Lameness is common, and in severe cases, the nails and the slipper slough off. The oral lesions may cause anorexia because of pain. FMD is reportable, and suspected cases must be quarantined until diagnosis is confirmed via electron microscopy, serology, viral culture, or PCR assay. Treatment is supportive. Some countries have specific requirements for euthanasia or vaccination.[19]

Multidrug resistant *Staphylococcus aureus* (MRSA) has been the cause of morbidity and mortality in calves in the United States and Europe. The animals typically present with localized skin pustules, along with diarrhea and depression. Diagnosis is by bacterial culture. Both zoonotic and reverse zoonotic transmission have occurred. Treatment requires antibiotics, supportive therapy, and increased hygiene and sanitation.[35]

Acute pasturellosis, also called *hemorrhagic septicemia*, is caused by *Pasturella multocida* and has been reported in Asian range countries, where it is thought to be contracted from domestic cattle. Is it suspected, however, that some of these cases, which were diagnosed entirely on clinical appearance, may actually be EEHV deaths. Transmission is via inhalation, ingestion, and contaminated wounds. Affected elephants present with anorexia, yawning, high fevers, hot painful lymph nodes, dyspnea, diarrhea, or sudden death. Diagnosis is by bacterial culture. Treatment is with antibiotics but excellent sanitation is needed as well. Cattle vaccines have been used in elephants in several countries.[19]

Elephantpox, caused by an orthopoxvirus (family Poxviridae), is associated with rodent vectors, which may also be reservoirs. Transmission occurs via direct contact with the virus on fomites or other infected animals. Like other poxviruses, elephantpox causes localized or generalized vesicles on the skin and mucous membranes, inflammation of affected tissue, and signs of systemic disease including fever and anorexia. The disease may be fatal. Pox vesicles are large, measuring up to 2 cm in diameter and are often yellowish. They eventually coalesce, become necrotic, and slough. In some elephants, nails and slippers slough off. Secondary bacterial infections are common. Necropsy findings include lesions on internal organs and mucous membranes. Intracytoplasmic inclusion bodies (Bollinger bodies) may be seen on light microscopy, and viral particles on electron microscopy. No specific treatment is available except for nursing care. Some animals require antibiotics and analgesics. Rodent control is necessary to control and eliminate outbreaks. Vaccination using vaccinia strains has been successfully employed during outbreaks. The disease is thought to be zoonotic.[19]

Several cases of rabies, reported in Asian elephants in range countries, is caused by a lyssavirus (family Rhabdoviridae). Affected animals display a variety of neurologic signs, as well as ptyalism, anorexia, and excessive vocalization. The disease is virtually always fatal and is spread through saliva from the bites of infected animals. Diagnosis is only possible at necropsy. Vaccination appears to be protective.[34]

Salmonella spp. is anecdotally more likely to affect African elephants than Asian elephants. Transmission is by the oral–fecal route, and elephants tend to show classic signs such as diarrhea, colic, depression, and anorexia. Other signs include sepsis, abortion, vaginal discharge, and death. Diagnosis usually requires multiple fecal cultures. Septic animals will be positive on blood culture. The PCR test may indicate the presence of the organism but not whether it is actively being shed. Strain identification may be useful. Antibiotics do not stop fecal shedding and are controversial in treating this disease, but if young animals are involved, antibiotic therapy may be necessary to control secondary infections. Aggressive fluid therapy is usually necessary, and hygiene and sanitation should be strictly maintained. Salmonella is zoonotic.[19]

Tetanus has been reported in multiple elephants. Following wound contamination by *Clostridium tetani*, tetanospasmin, the toxin that causes the classic signs of tetanus, including trismus, hyperesthesia, muscle spasms, and a sawhorse stance, is elaborated by the bacterium. Death results from respiratory failure. Affected elephants have been treated with high doses of penicillin, tetanus antitoxin, and supportive care, but the fatality rate is high. Regular vaccination with tetanus toxoid appears protective.[41]

Noninfectious Disease

Elephants are also subject to a wide variety of noninfectious diseases affecting various organ systems. Dental disease has already been mentioned. Elephants also develop a host of ophthalmologic problems, including cataracts, superficial and deep corneal abscesses, and retinal disease. Any of these conditions may result in blindness. Parasitic ocular disease is well documented in wild elephants. Elderly elephants often show evidence of corneal degeneration. The cause is unknown, but topical application of nonsteroidal anti-inflammatories and calcium EDTA (ethylenediaminetetraacetic acid) solution has been helpful.

Both atherosclerosis and arteriosclerosis occur in wild African elephants. Coronary infarctions, aneurisms, and cardiomyopathy have been reported in both Asian and African elephants. Congenital cardiac abnormalities have been reported in calves.[5]

GI disease in elephants includes surgical and medical colics. Surgical colics include a variety of strangulating obstructions. Unfortunately, because of the current impossibility of successfully performing abdominal surgeries on adult elephants, these have all been fatal. Noninfectious causes of medical colics include sand, feed, and fecal impactions; esophageal obstructions (choke); and foreign body ingestion. Cholelithiasis, pancreatic malabsorption, and carcinomatosis have also caused GI disease in elephants. Unlike horses, elephants tend to show subtle signs of abdominal discomfort. Postural changes and straining may sometimes be seen in younger animals, but adults often simply go off feed and act depressed. Diagnosis may be as difficult as treatment, but assessment of vital signs and blood work, along with rectal and transabdominal ultrasonography may be helpful.[67]

Renal disease occurs with some frequency in elephants. Urolithiasis and nephrolithiasis resulting in dysuria and even obstruction have been reported. Medication-induced nephrotoxicity, pyelonephritis, and acute and chronic renal failure also occur. Diagnosis involves urinalysis, blood work, and rectal ultrasonography of the urogenital tract. On smaller animals, transcutaneous ultrasonography may be possible for visualizing the kidneys.[66]

Neoplasia appears to be common in older elephants, although infrequently reported in the literature. Uterine leiomyomas, are common in older nulliparous Asian cows.[28] These tumors may get quite large with necrotic centers that may break off and pass down the urogenital canal. As a result, they are a frequent cause of non–kidney-related hematuria.[66]

Foot problems occur in both wild and captive elephants, both Asian and African. Any part of the foot may be affected and problems range from mild to life threatening. Lameness is not always present. Cracks in the nails may be superficial or deep. Superficial cracks often require little or no treatment, but deeper cracks generally require paring. Since deep cracks contact sensitive corium underneath, they tend to be more painful. Spraying a topical anesthetic into the crack before trimming may improve comfort. The edges of the crack should be gently beveled to help take the pressure off the area and prevent further cracking. The black tract within the crack should be carefully cleaned out. Since the toenails grow only from the nail bed at the top, and nails grow downward at a rate of 0.5 to 1.0 cm month, a large crack may take several months to completely disappear.

Other issues with the toenails include infections, swollen digital sweat glands, or formation of exuberant granulation tissue, colloquially known as "crab meat." This proliferative, primarily epithelial tissue may be very difficult to control, but cryotherapy has been successful in several cases. Trimming the tissue with a knife tends to cause pain and is bloody.[77]

The sole and pad of the foot may develop bruises, abscesses, or punctures. Tetanus prophylaxis is necessary if punctures are noted, or if a foreign body is embedded in the foot. Bruising may occur from stepping on a sharp object, but the actual bruise may not become visible until several days after the incident causing the bruise. If the elephant is foot sore, analgesics are recommended. Infections or wounds in the slipper may become serious medical situations. Occasionally, elephants are placed into specially made boots to protect the foot while it is healing. Although slipper abscesses need to be opened and cleaned out, overly aggressive trimming and paring should be avoided, and the clinician is reminded that the pad is less than 1 cm thick.

Osteoarthritis, or degenerative joint disease, is common in older elephants, both captive and wild. The causes of arthritis are debatable—and sometimes controversial—but conformation, history of injury, and obesity are likely contributors. Treatments have included analgesics, gentle exercise if not too painful for the animal, softer substrates, and weight loss in overweight animals to decrease stress on joints. Nutraceuticals have been used empirically. Very little data exists in support or against them.[65]

Parasitic Disease

Parasitic infections of elephants are common in range countries, but rare in the western hemisphere. Ectoparasites include biting lice (but not sucking lice), ear mites, and multiple tick species, one of which, *Amblyoma tholloni*, is a vector for *Ehrlichia ruminatum* (heartwater disease). Interestingly, none of the mange mites (*Psoroptes*, *Chorioptes*, and *Sarcoptes*) has been reported on elephants. Ectoparasites may be associated with dermatitis and pruritus often behind the ears and at the base of the tail. Heavily infested animals often act agitated.[20]

Of the protozoans, only *Trypanosoma evansi*, has been associated with clinical disease in elephants. *Cryptosporidium parvum* has been thus far identified only in asymptomatic African elephants. Two piroplasms, *Babesia* spp. and *Nutallia loxodontis*, have been documented but also without disease association; although many elephants have high titers to *Toxoplasma gondii*, the test is not validated in elephants, and its significance is unknown.[20]

Parasites most often causing clinical disease are nematodes and trematodes. *Fasciola* spp. has caused both acute and chronic diseases in elephants, as have nematodes belonging to numerous phylogenetic groups. Signs of intestinal parasitism in elephants are no different from those in other animal groups and include diarrhea, weight loss and, in some cases, anemia and hypoproteinemia.[20]

Diagnosis of intestinal nematodes is obtained through performance of direct fecal smear, centrifugation, or flotation. Although many different anthelmintics have been used in elephants empirically, only ivermectin has been investigated pharmacokinetically.[22]

TOXICITIES

The majority of toxicities reported in elephants have occurred following toxic plant ingestion, some of which were accidentally fed to elephants by keepers who either did not recognize what they were feeding or did not notice the plant mixed into normal, nontoxic browse. Sadly, too often it has been reported in the media that elephants in range countries are often deliberately poisoned by poachers. Strychnine, arsenic, and other heavy metals are typically used. A variety of poisons are used to coat arrows and spears used for killing elephants in both Asia and Africa. Both accidental and deliberate poisonings have occurred in association with insecticide-contaminated well water or with organophosphate-spiked watermelons.[13]

Poisoned elephants often seek water because of great thirst caused by the poisoning and to deter flies that they have become too weak to swat away. Management of poisoned animals in the field is generally not possible because many of the toxins have no antidote, and by the time the animal is found, it is past the point of recovery. Unfortunately, lack of available analytical laboratories and difficulties in transporting samples to them also hinder field investigations of suspected poisonings.[13]

REPRODUCTION

The reproductive tract of the male elephant is characterized by intraabdominal testes that sit caudal to the kidneys. Each testicle has a central artery that radiates smaller arteries outwardly. Although a pampiniform plexus to cool the testicles—and sperm—is absent, elephants still manage to maintain an intratesticular temperature of 94° F to 97° F, the same as that found in scrotal testes. Another peculiarity is that unlike other mammals, elephants do not have a true epididymis, and the primary site of sperm storage is the ampulla, one of four paired accessory sex glands. The other accessory sex glands are the prostates, seminal vesicles, and bulbourethral glands. These may be visualized by using rectal ultrasonography, except for the bulbourethral glands, which may be viewed via transdermal ultrasonography slightly below the anus. Each of the accessory sex glands provides different and specific nutrients to the ejaculate. The S-shaped penis has levator muscles that elevate the vulva into position prior to penile penetration and ejaculation.[30]

Musth is a complex hormonal phenomenon that occurs annually in adult Asian and African bulls. Because it is not seasonal, musth is not considered a rut, although it is associated with increased aggression and breeding, as well as with changes in androgen secretion. Testosterone levels often increase 20-fold, and the androstenedione-to-testosterone ratio changes. However, musth still occurs in castrated males and, thus, may be associated with other unknown factors.[50] During musth, a complex array of chemical compounds are released from the breath, urine, and temporal glands, conveying the status of the musth male to conspecifics.[50]

Musth males are dangerous and unpredictable, and anyone who works with elephants should be able to recognize the phenomenon. Temporal gland secretion, visible as dark liquid tracts on the sides of the face is a prime sign. Perineal swelling, constant dribbling of urine, and a fetid odor are other signs. The stance of a musth male is also different, with the head being held more erect and the ears extended. Characteristic vocalizations called "musth rumbles" may be heard. Brain chemistry is thought to be affected during musth, and bulls may appear dazed and unresponsive. At the height of musth, males often stop eating and will lose large amounts of weight. In this condition, they also will not breed, another way in which musth differs from rut.[50]

Young sexually immature males sometimes secrete a sweet-smelling liquid from their temporal glands; this is referred to as a "honey musth" or "moda musth." Studies on these fluids indicate that they too contain a complex mixture of pheromones.[50]

A number of facilities are opting to increase reproductive efficiency in their herds via AI. Semen is typically collected by manual rectal massage in a trained bull secured in an ERD. Electroejaculation, which requires sedation or anesthesia, is performed only rarely. Ejaculation occurs in multiple aliquots that may vary considerably in quality. Semen quality, motility, and concentration collected from manual rectal massage may also vary on a day-to-day basis from a single bull, and its unpredictability adds another challenge for AI.[38] After collection, sperm viability may deteriorate rapidly within 12 hours of collection, and the use of different semen extenders and novel freezing protocols to improve and extend semen quality is an area of active research.[38] Although semen from both African and Asian elephants has been successfully frozen, pregnancies from frozen semen are extremely rare.

The urogenital canal of the female elephant, also called the *vestibule*, measures 1 to 1.4 m in length and opens between the hind legs. The clitoris is located distally. At the level of the anus, the urogenital canal curves sharply into the pelvis. Both the urethral opening and vagina are found in the cranial portion of the urogenital canal. Lateral to the vagina are two blind pouches. The vagina leads into the cervix, characterized by longitudinal folds. The ovaries are small, and the uterus is bicornuate and short bodied. Most of the reproductive tract may be visualized by rectal ultrasonography, but a probe extender may be required to examine the most cranial portions.[30]

During copulation, semen is deposited in the urogenital canal and not into the vagina. The hymen is equivalent to a one-way valve and does not rupture until a calf is delivered through it. These characteristics—the great length of the urogenital canal and the blind pockets of the vagina—create technical challenges during AI.

The estrous cycle lasts approximately 15 to 16 weeks and consists of an 8- to 12-week luteal phase followed by a 4- to 6-week follicular (or interluteal) phase. Progestogen levels are high during the luteal phase and low during the follicular phase. Cycle length may vary between cows but usually is consistent for an individual. During the follicular phase, two luteinizing hormone (LH) peaks occur, approximately 3 weeks apart. Ovulation occurs following the second LH peak. The significance of the first, nonovulatory LH peak is still debated. By monitoring the estrous cycle, both natural breeding in captive environments, and AI may be correctly timed. Typically, the female is inseminated the day of and the day after the second LH peak. In captive natural breeding situations, the male and female elephants are housed together on these days.[30]

Acyclicity is a significant problem in African and Asian elephants in North America. Rising incidence of reproductive tract pathology, including uterine leiomyomas, vestibular cysts and polyps, ovarian cysts, and endometrial hyperplasia, indicates an aging population.[30] Population modeling of captive elephants in North America suggests that the birth rate is too low to be self-sustaining for either species.[71] Ironically, contraception of wild African elephants as an alternative to culling is an important area of research. The long-term effect of vasectomy on elephant overpopulations in Africa has yet to be determined, but contraceptive vaccines for females are also being tested, including a porcine zona pellucida vaccine and melengestrol acetate (MGA) implants.[28]

Sexual maturity occurs in elephants between the ages of 4 and 12 years. Earlier onset of sexual maturity may be associated with better nutrition. In areas with high levels of poaching, the mean age of first-time mothers among wild elephants decreases. Because of decreased fertility, difficulty maintaining pregnancy, and increased risk of dystocia, it is recommended that captive elephants have their first offspring at a young age. Although elephants have an approximately 4- to 6-year intercalf interval, they may continue bearing calves well into middle age.[28]

Gestation ranges between 21 and 24 months, the average being 659 days. The embryo undergoes delayed implantation.[30] 5α-reduced-pregnane, rather than progesterone, is the primary progestogen in elephants, but standard progesterone assays using feces, urine, serum, and saliva have been used to monitor estrus cycles because of cross-reactivity with 5α-reduced-pregnane and other progestogens. Because placentation is zonary and endotheliochorial,[30] calves are born immune competent with antibodies received transplacentally.[48]

Elevated serum progestogen beyond the normal 12-week luteal period indicates pregnancy. These levels stay increased until 3 to 5 days (rarely longer) before parturition. After 6 months of gestation, an elevated prolactin level may also confirm pregnancy. Rectal ultrasonography may detect an embryo by 8 to 9 weeks, and transabdominal ultrasonography may be used to visualize the fetus after 40 weeks of gestation. During pregnancy, however, at certain periods, it may be extremely difficult to visualize the fetus. If progestogen levels are appropriately elevated and the elephant is otherwise healthy, the inability to find the fetus on ultrasonography is likely not a concern and another examination may be scheduled for a future date. Between 30 and 60 weeks of gestation, fetal sex in Asian elephants may be determined by measuring testosterone levels in the cow's blood.[30] Testosterone measurement has not been reliable in *Loxodonta* for sex determination.

Signs of impending parturition are variable and include breast development, mild contractions, increased discomfort, and passage of a mucosal plug. Birth usually occurs within 24 hours of the passage of the plug and within 2 hours of rupture of the fetal membranes. Progestogens drop to baseline usually within 5 days of birth. Cervical dilation may be monitored by rectal ultrasonography. In specific situations, in which the calf is confirmed to be appropriately positioned in the birth canal, and the cervix is dilated, oxytocin, vigorous rectal massage, or both may stimulate labor. A large bulge underneath the tail usually becomes visible shortly before the calf is born. Both anterior and posterior presentations are normal. Often, the presentation may be determined by the direction of the toenails as seen on rectal ultrasonography.[30]

Cows give birth standing, so the calf drops to the floor. The amniotic sac usually breaks by itself. In the wild, the herd matriarch may be seen to push aside the new mother to tend to the newborn herself. In captivity, inexperienced cows are sometimes overly aggressive toward their offspring, and many facilities routinely restrain a cow during birth in such a way that she is free to move, kick, and labor, but the newborn may be taken out of reach after birth until the mother's behavior toward the calf may be assessed. This period also allows veterinary personnel to evaluate the calf's health and well-being.

The placenta, weighing between 15 and 24 kg, is usually passed within 4 to 12 hours after birth, but delays of up to several months have occurred in some cases. Placental retention sometimes, but not always, results in metritis.[39] The veterinarian should weigh and examine the placenta. It is normal for the chorioallantoic membranes to be covered with white "buttons"; these are called "verrucae" and are simply connective tissue surrounding a mesh of minute blood vessels.[3]

In the author's experience, most calves have been seen to be able to sit in a sternal position within 5 to 10 minutes of birth and to stand within 10 to 30 minutes. Many calves have slightly cyanotic membranes initially, which become pink within 10 to 20 minutes. A suckle reflex is usually present at birth, and nursing commences within 2 to 12 hours after birth. Surprisingly, a few calves suckled for the first time approximately 24 hours after birth without any ill effects. Normal heart rate at birth is between 60 and 90 beats per minute and normal respiratory rate is between 60 and 80 breaths per minute, rapidly declining to 30 to 50 breaths per minute (and slower when sleeping). Urine and meconium are typically passed within the first 6 hours.

The umbilicus usually breaks very close to the calf's abdomen and dries up over 24 to 48 hours. Often, considerable swelling around the umbilicus remains for the first few days of life. Although this may be normal, a variety of umbilical problems have occurred in elephant calves, including hernias, fistulas, patent urachus and prolonged bleeding from umbilical vesicles. Thus, the abdomen should be visually evaluated and palpated and ultrasonography performed, if needed. If umbilical bleeding appears excessive, suturing may be necessary. Both surgical and nonsurgical management of umbilical hernias are possible.[69]

Birth weights have ranged between 59 and 181 kg (130 and 400 lb), but the average weight is generally around 113 kg (250 lb). Larger calves are associated with increased risk of dystocia. The majority of fetal growth occurs at the end of gestation, and pregnant cows should not be overfed. After birth, the calf should be weighed regularly to make sure that nursing is adequate. Calves often lose 10% of their body weight in their first week of life before starting to gain at a rate of 0.5 to 2 kg per day.[65] Both oxytocin and domperidone have been given to postparturient cows for milk let-down.

Calves typically suckle vigorously—with loud slurping sounds—for short periods several times a day. Between nursing sessions, they often sleep. Elephant milk is low in protein but varies considerably in fat and total solids during lactation.[44] Creating appropriate and adequate formulas for orphaned calves has been difficult. The available commercial formulas have required supplementation with vitamins and fats and have been associated with diarrhea and inadequate weight gain in several cases. Raising orphans or rejected neonates has been very difficult.

Calves typically urinate a minimum of twice a day and pass feces at least once daily. A normal calf is active, vocal, and curious about its environment. Calves that seem "not right," even in minor ways, need a thorough medical evaluation.

PREVENTIVE MEDICINE

In the elephant barn, preventive medicine requires a team approach to keep animals healthy and identify problems early, in conjunction with an understanding of the laws and regulations associated with elephant health care. Elephants are regulated by numerous government agencies, at the international, national, and local levels. Caretakers need to develop an understanding of the mandates associated with the elephants in their care and always support the best interests of the animals.

Daily examination by keepers involves inspection of the skin, eyes, mouth, feet, consistency of feces, and eating and drinking behaviors. Foot trimming should be performed, as needed.

Current recommendations for elephants in North America include annual rabies vaccine and tetanus toxoid.[34,41] Tetanus toxoid, however, is recommended for all elephants worldwide, and additional vaccines may be warranted in particular areas of the world. Fecal screening to identify parasites should be done annually in North America and Europe and more often in range countries.

Animals should be weighed, either with a scale or a weight tape, at least once a year, ideally more frequently. Foot radiography should be performed annually. CBC count, blood chemistry, and urinalysis should also be performed at least once a year and preferably more often.

The USDA mandates an annual trunk wash, consisting of three samples within a 7-day period or more often, depending on the TB status of the herd. In addition, a serologic blood test for TB must be done under supervision at the time of the trunk wash. The trunk wash should be securely packaged and sent for culture to appropriate laboratories. The most current regulations and protocols may be found in the "Elephant TB Guidelines" listed on the USDA or USAHA websites.

Some facilities do additional screening for EEHV and other diseases. Reproductive system examinations, including rectal ultrasonography to assess the integrity of the tract, hormone analyses, and breeding soundness examinations are also recommended for adult elephants. For facilities that belong to the AZA, a list of annual testing recommendations is available.

REFERENCES

1. Adkesson MJ, Junge RE, Allender MC, et al: Pharmacokinetics of a long-acting ceftiofur crystalline-free acid formulation in Asian elephants (*Elephas maximus*). *Am J Vet Res* 73:1512–1518, 2012.
2. Agnew DW, Lee H, Shoshani J: The elephants of Zoba Gash Barka, Eritrea: Part 4. Cholelithiasis in a wild African elephant (*Loxodonta africana*). *J Zoo Wildl Med* 36:677–683, 2005.
3. Allen WR: Ovulation, pregnancy, placentation and husbandry in the African elephant (*Loxodonta africana*). *Philos Trans R Soc London [Biol]* 361:821–834, 2006.
4. Bapodra P, Bouts T, Mahoney P, et al: Ultrasonographic anatomy of the Asian elephant (*Elephas maximus*) eye. *J Zoo Wildl Med* 41:409–417, 2010.
5. Bartlett SL, Abou-Madi N, Kraus MS, et al: Electrocardiography of the Asian elephant (*Elephas maximus*). *J Zoo Wildl Med* 40:466–473, 2009.
6. Bechert U, Christensen JM, Finnegan M: Pharmacokinetics of orally administered ibuprofen in elephants. In *Proceedings of the American Association of Zoo Veterinarians*, 2003.
7. Bechert U, Christensen JM, Nguyen C, et al: Pharmacokinetics of orally administered phenylbutazone in African and Asian elephants (*Loxodonta africana* and *Elephas maximus*). *J Zoo Wildl Med* 39:188–200, 2008.
8. Benz A, Zenker W, Hildebrandt TB, et al: Microscopic morphology of the elephant's foot. *J Zoo Wildl Med* 40:711–725, 2009.
9. Bouts T, Vordermeier M, Flach E, et al: Positive skin and serologic test results of diagnostic assays for bovine tuberculosis and subsequent isolation of *Mycobacterium interjectum* in a pygmy hippopotamus (*Hexaprotodon liberiensis*). *J Zoo Wildl Med* 40:536–542, 2009.

10. Brock AP, Isaza R, Hunter RP, et al: Estimates of the pharmacokinetics of famciclovir and its active metabolite penciclovir in young Asian elephants (*Elephas maximus*). *Am J Vet Res* 73:1996–2000, 2012.

11. Brown IRF, White PT: Elephant blood haematology and chemistry. *Comp Biochem Physiol B* 65:1–12, 1980.

12. Bush M, Stoskopf MK, Raath JP, et al: Serum oxytetracycline concentrations in African elephant (*Loxodonta africana*) calves after long-acting formulation injection. *J Zoo Wildl Med* 31:41–46, 2000.

13. Cheeran JV: Poisons and the Pachyderm—a field guide for responding to poisoning in Asian elephants. In Menon V, Ashraf NVK, Panda PP, Gureja N, editors: *Conservation References Series Wildlife Trust of India*, New Delhi, India, 2007, WTI.

14. Clauss M, Steinmetz H, Eulenberger U, et al: Observations on the length of the intestinal tract of African *Loxodonta africana* (Blumenbach 1797) and Asian elephants *Elephas maximus* (Linné 1735). *Eur J Wildl Res* 53:68–72, 2006.

15. Dumonceaux G, Isaza R, Koch DE, et al: Pharmacokinetics and I.M. bioavailability of ceftiofur in Asian elephants (*Elephas maximus*). *J Vet Pharmacol Ther* 28:441–446, 2005.

16. Fagan DA, Oosterhuis JE, Roocroft A: Significant dental disease in elephants. *Verhandlung bei Erkrankungen Zootiere* 39:125–134, 1999.

17. Feldman M, Isaza R, Prins C, et al: Point prevalence and incidence of *Mycobacterium tuberculosis* complex in captive elephants in the United States. *Vet Quart* 33:25–29, 2013.

18. Fowler ME: Problems with immobilizing and anesthetizing elephants. In *Proceedings of the AAZV*, 1981, pp 87–91.

19. Fowler ME: Infectious diseases. In Fowler ME, Mikota SK, editors: *Biology, medicine and surgery of elephants*, Ames, IA, 2006, Blackwell Publishing.

20. Fowler ME: Parasitic diseases. In Fowler ME, Mikota SK, editors: *Biology, medicine and surgery of elephants*, Ames, IA, 2006, Blackwell Publishing.

21. Fowler ME, Mikota SK, Steffey EP: Chemical restraint and general anesthesia. In Fowler ME, Mikota SK, editors: *Biology, medicine and surgery of elephants*, Ames, IA, 2006, Blackwell Publishing.

22. Gandolf AR, Lifschitz A, Stadler C, et al: The pharmacokinetics of orally administered ivermectin in African elephants (*Loxodonta africana*): Implications for parasite elimination. *J Zoo Wildl Med* 40:107–112, 2009.

23. Garstang M: Long-distance, low-frequency elephant communication. *J Comp Physiol [A]* 190:791–805, 2004.

24. Gulland FMD, Carwardine PC: Plasma metronidazole levels in an Indian elephant (*Elephas maximus*) after rectal administration. *Vet Rec* 120:440, 1987.

25. Hall NH, Isaza R, Hall JS, et al: Serum osmolality and effects of water deprivation in captive Asian elephants (*Elephas maximus*). *J Vet Diag Invest* 24:688–695, 2012.

26. Hardman K, Dastjerdi A, Gurrala R, et al: Detection of elephant endotheliotropic herpesvirus type 1 in asymptomatic elephants using TaqMan real-time PCR. *Vet Rec* 170:205, 2012.

27. Hatt J-M, Clauss M: Feeding Asian and African elephants *Elephas maximus* and *Loxodonta africana* in captivity. *Int Zoo YB* 40:88–95, 2006.

28. Hermes R, Goeritz F, Streich WJ, et al: Assisted reproduction in female rhinoceros and elephants—current status and future perspective. *Reprod Domestic Anim* 42:33–44, 2007.

29. Heymann D: *Control of communicable diseases manual*, ed 19, Washington, DC, 2008, American Public Health Association.

30. Hildebrandt TB, Goeritz F, Hermes R, et al: Aspects of the reproductive biology and breeding management of Asian and African elephants *Elephas maximus* and *Loxodonta* africana. *Int Zoo YB* 40:20–40, 2006.

31. Houck ML, Kumamoto AT, Gallagher DS, Jr, et al: Comparative cytogenetics of the African elephant (*Loxodonta africana*) and Asiatic elephant (*Elephas maximus*). *Cytogenet Cell Genet* 93:249–252, 2001.

32. Hunter RP, Isaza R: Concepts and issues with interspecies scaling in zoological pharmacology. *J Zoo Wildl Med* 39:517–526, 2008.

33. Hunter RP, Isaza R, Koch DE: Oral bioavailability and pharmacokinetic characteristics of ketoprofen enantiomers after oral and intravenous administration in Asian elephants (*Elephas maximus*). *Am J Vet Res* 64:109–114, 2003.

34. Isaza R, Davis RD, Moore SM, et al: Results of vaccination of Asian elephants (*Elephas maximus*) with monovalent inactivated rabies vaccine. *Am J Vet Res* 67:1934–1936, 2006.

35. Janssen D, Lamberski N, Dunne G, et al: Methicillin-resistant *Staphylococcus aureus* skin infections from an elephant calf,– San Diego, California, 2008. *MMWR Morb Mortal Wkly Rep* 58:194–198, 2009.

36. Janssen DL, Oosterhuis JE, Fuller J, et al: Field technique: A method for obtaining trunk wash mycobacterial cultures in anesthetized free-ranging African elephants (*Loxodonta africana*). In *Proceedings of the AAZV, AAWV, WDA Joint Conference*, San Diego, California, 2004.

37. Johnson OW, Buss IO: Molariform teeth of male African elephants in relation to age, body dimensions, and growth. *J Mammal* 46:373–384, 1965.

38. Kiso WK, Brown JL, Siewerdt F, et al: Liquid semen storage in elephants (*Elephas maximus* and *Loxodonta africana*): Species differences and storage optimization. *J Androl* 32:420–431, 2011.

39. Lamberski N, Oosterhuis JE, Zuba JR, et al: Treatment of a retained placenta in a primiparous African elephant (*Loxodonta africana*), In *Proceedings of the AAZV, AAWV Joint Conference*, Tulsa, Oklahoma, 2009.

40. Leighty KA, Soltis J, Wesolek CM, et al: GPS determination of walking rates in captive African elephants (*Loxodonta africana*). *Zoo Biol* 28:16–28, 2009.

41. Lindsay WA, Wiedner E, Isaza R, et al: Immune responses of Asian elephants (*Elephas maximus*) to commercial tetanus toxoid vaccine. *Vet Immunol Immunopathol* 133:287–389, 2010.

42. Lodwick LJ, Dubach JM, Phillips LG, et al: Pharmacokinetics of amikacin in African elephants (*Loxodonta africana*). *J Zoo Wildl Med* 35:367–375, 1994.

43. Lyaschenko KP, Greenwald R, Esfandiari J, et al: Field application of serodiagnostics to identify elephants with tuberculosis prior to case confirmation by culture. *Clin Vacc Immunol* 19:1269–1275, 2012.

44. Mainka SA, Cooper RM, Black SR, et al: Asian elephant (*Elephas maximus*) milk composition during the first 280 days of lactation. *Zoo Biol* 13:389–393, 1994.

45. Miall LC, Greenwood F: *Anatomy of the Indian elephant*, London, U.K., 1878, MacMillan and Company.

46. Miller CE, Basu C, Fritsch G, et al: Ontogenetic scaling of foot musculoskeletal anatomy in elephants. *J Royal Soc Interface* 5:465–475, 2008.

47. Neiffer DL, Miller MA, Weber M, et al: Standing sedation in African elephants (*Loxodonta africana*) using detomidine-butorphanol combinations. *J Zoo Wildl Med* 36:250–256, 2005.

48. Nofs SA, Atmar RL, Keitel WA, et al: Prenatal passive transfer of maternal immunity in Asian elephants (*Elephas maximus*). In *Proceedings of the Elephant Endotheliotropic Herpesvirus Conference*, Houston, TX, 2013.

49. Page CD, Mautino M, Derendorf HD, et al: Comparative pharmacokinetics of trimethoprim-sulfamethoxazole administered intravenously and orally to captive elephants. *J Zoo Wildl Med* 22:409–416, 1991.

50. Rasmussen LEL, Krishnamurthy V: How chemical signals integrate Asian elephant society: The known and the unknown. *Zoo Biol* 19:405–423, 2000.

51. Rasmussen LEL, Munger BL: The sensorineural specializations of the trunk tip (finger) of the Asian elephant, *Elephas maximus*. *Anat Rec* 246:127–134, 1996.

52. Richman LK, Hayward GS: Elephant Herpesviruses. In Fowler ME, Miller RE, editors: *Fowler's zoo and wildlife medicine*, vol 7, St. Louis, MO, 2012, Saunders.

53. Rosin E, Schultz-Darken N, Perry B, et al: Pharmacokinetics of ampicillin administered orally in Asian elephants (*Elephas maximus*). *J Zoo Wildl Med* 24:515–518, 1993.

54. Sanchez CR, Murray SZ, Isaza R, et al: Pharmacokinetics of a single dose of enrofloxacin administered orally to captive Asian elephants (*Elephas maximus*). *Am J Vet Res* 66:1948–1953, 2005.

55. Schmidt MJ: Penicillin G and amoxicillin in elephants: A study comparing dose regimens administered with serum levels achieved in healthy elephants. *J Zoo Anim Med* 9:127–136, 1978.

56. Shoshani J, Tassy P: Advances in proboscidean taxonomy and classification, anatomy and physiology, and ecology and behavior. *Quaternary Int* 126–128:5–20, 2005.

57. Siegal-Willott J, Isaza R, Johnson R, et al: Distal limb radiography, ossification, and growth plate closure in the juvenile Asian elephant (*Elephas maximus*). *J Zoo Wildl Med* 39:320–334, 2008.

58. Sperber GH: Tusks. *J Dental Assoc* 5:257–268, 1976.

59. Steenkamp G, Ferreira SM, Bester MN: Tusklessness and tusk fractures in free-ranging African savanna elephants (*Loxodonta africana*). *J S Afr Vet Assoc* 78:75–80, 2007.

60. Steiner M, Gould AR, Clark TJ, et al: Induced elephant (*Loxodonta africana*) tusk removal. *J Zoo Wildl Med* 34:93–95, 2003.

61. Stetter M, Hendrickson DA: Laparoscopic surgery in the elephant and rhinoceros. In Fowler ME, Miller RE, editors: *Fowler's zoo and wildlife medicine*, vol 7, St. Louis, MO, 2012, Saunders.

62. Viljoen PG: Spatial distribution and movements of elephants (*Loxodonta africana*) in the northern Namib Desert region of the Kaokoveld South West Africa/Namibia. *J Zool* 219:1–19, 1989.

63. Weber M, Junge R, Black P, et al: Management of critical juvenile Asian elephants (*Elephas maximus*). In *Proceedings of the AAZV*, 2009, pp 82–83.

64. West JB: Why doesn't the elephant have a pleural space? *News Physiol Sci* 17:47–50, 2002.

65. Wiedner E: Elephant nutrition: Feeding your herd for optimum health. In Olson D, editor: *Elephant husbandry resource manual*, ed 2, In press, American Association of Zoos and Aquariums.

66. Wiedner E, Alleman RA, Isaza R: Urinalysis in Asian elephants (*Elephas maximus*). *J Zoo Wildl Med* 40:659–666, 2009.

67. Wiedner E, Howard LL, Isaza R: Treatment of elephant endotheliotropic herpesvirus (EEHV). In Fowler ME, Miller RE, editors: *Fowler's zoo and wildlife medicine*, vol 7, St. Louis, MO, 2012, Saunders.

68. Wiedner E, Schmitt DL: Preliminary report of side effects associated with drugs used in the treatment of tuberculosis in elephants. In *Proceedings of the International Elephant Foundation*, Orlando, FL, 2007.

69. Wiedner EB, Gray C, Rich P, et al: Nonsurgical repair of an umbilical hernia in two Asian elephant calves (*Elephas maximus*). *J Zoo Wildl Med* 39:248–251, 2008.

70. Wiedner EB, Peddie J, Peddie LR, et al: Strangulating intestinal obstructions in four captive elephants (*Elephas maximus* and *Loxodonta africana*). *J Zoo Wildl Med* 43:125–130, 2012.

71. Wiese RJ: Asian elephants are not self-sustaining in North America. *Zoo Biol* 19:299–309, 2000.

72. Wiese RJ, Willis K: Calculation of longevity and life expectancy in captive elephants. *Zoo Biol* 23:365–373, 2004.

73. Wilson E, Mikota S, Bradford JP, et al: Seropositive, culture negative tuberculosis in an Asian elephant (*Elephas maximus*). In *Proceedings of the AAZV, AAWV Joint Conference*, South Padre Island, TX, 2010.

74. Wong MA, Isaza R, Cuthbert JK, et al: Periocular anterior adnexal anatomy and clinical adnexal examination of the adult Asian elephant (*Elephas maximus*). *J Zoo Wildl Med* 43:793–780, 2012.

75. World Health Organization: *Commercial serodiagnostic tests for diagnosis of tuberculosis policy statement*, Geneva, Switzerland, 2011, World Health Organization, pp 26.

76. Zuba JR, Oosterhuis JE: Anesthetic complications and clinical intervention in opioid anesthetized captive elephants. In *Proceedings of the AAZV Conference*, Oakland, CA, 2012, pp 1–6.

77. Zuba JR, Oosterhuis JE, Pessier AP: The toenail "abscess" in elephants: Treatment options including cryotherapy and pathologic similarities with equine proliferative pododermatitis (canker). In *Proceedings of the Association of Zoo Veterinarians Conference*, Tampa, FL, 2006.

CHAPTER 54

Hyrocoidea (Hyraxes)

Julie E. Napier

BIOLOGY

The hyrax is a unique animal and the only one in the order Hyrocoidea. The one recognized family, Procaviidae, consists of three species: (1) the cape or rock hyrax (*Provacia capensis*), (2) the gray or yellow-spotted hyrax (*Heterohyrax* sp.), and (3) the tree or bush hyrax (*Dendrohyrax* sp.) (Table 54-1). Although the hyrax looks more like a rodent or a rabbit, its closest living relatives are the elephant, as well as the manatee and dugong, both of which are marine mammals. Hyraxes may be found throughout southwest Asia and most of Africa.[22] The rock hyrax is the most widely held species in zoologic institutions.

UNIQUE ANATOMY

Hyraxes are stout, squat animals with short legs (Figure 54-1). They have a double coat, with a finer under layer and coarser outer layer, and a scent gland on the back covered in longer hairs (see Table 54-1). They have a cleft upper lip, short round ears, and guard hairs around the snout. The deciduous dental formula for the hyrax is:

incisors (I) 2/2, canines (C) 1/1, premolars (P) 4/4, for a total of 28 teeth. The permanent dental formula is: I 1/2, C 1/1, P 4/4, molars (M) 3/3 for a total of 38 teeth. Hyrax teeth, which are adapted for eating grasses, have high crowns and relatively short roots. The two upper incisors, used for grooming, are elongated and tusklike in appearance and are often mistaken for canines.

These animals are plantigrade, with four digits on the front feet that look like hooves and three digits on the hindfeet. The second digit on the hindfoot has a long claw, also used for grooming. The other two digits are hooflike in appearance as well. The soles of the feet are rubbery in texture, which gives these animals traction on smooth, uneven, or steep surfaces. The only location of sweat glands in this species is the plantar surface of the feet.[4]

The hyrax's digestive system is adapted to handle relatively low-quality food. A simple stomach has glandular and nonglandular sections, a tubular small intestine, and a large intestine that is almost as long as the small intestine. The large intestine is unique to this species. It starts with a cecumlike sac, which has a narrow connecting colon with thick walls and a second connecting colon with wide,

TABLE 54-1

Biologic Information on the Hyrax

Scientific Name	Common Name	Adult Mass (kg)	Geographic Distribution	Identification
***PROCAVIA* SPP.** P. ruficeps P. capensis P. habessinica P. johnstoni	Rock hyrax, rock dassie, rock rabbit	Both sexes: 1.8–5.4	Southwestern and northeastern Africa, Syria, Lebanon, Israel, Jordan, Sinai, southeastern Arabian Peninsula Habitat: rock boulders in arid to alpine zones of Mt. Kenya	Black, brown, yellow, or orange hairs over dorsal gland; head and body length 44–54 centimeters (cm); round head and short muzzle, diurnal[22]
Heterohyrax brucei	Bush hyrax, gray hyrax, yellow-spotted hyrax, Bruce's hyrax, rock rabbit	Both sexes: 1.3–2.4	Southern Algeria, southeastern Egypt to central Angola and northeastern South Africa; east central Zaire Habitat: rock boulders and hollow trees in arid zones	Yellow or reddish hairs over dorsal gland; head and body length 32–47 cm; no external tail; narrow head and short muzzle; and are diurnal[3]
***DENDROHYDRAX* SPP.** D. arboreus D. validus D. dorsalis	Tree hyrax	Both sexes: 1.7–4.5	Forest zone from Gambia to Uganda and extreme northwestern Angola, eastern Zaire and central Kenya to east South Africa, Tanzania and the islands of Zanzibar, Pemba, and the Kenya coast Habitat: evergreen forests to rock boulders	White to yellow hair over dorsal gland; head and body length 32–60 cm; tail length is 10–30 millimeters (mm); crowns of molars lower in tree hyrax than in the other genera; nocturnal[3]

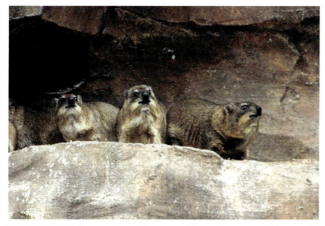

FIGURE 54-1 Group of rock hyraxes (*Procavia capensis*) housed in a zoologic facility.

thin walls. The second portion of the colon is where the primary absorption of water and volatile fatty acids takes place. The two connecting colons are followed by a colonic sac with two appendages that ends with a distal colon. The hindgut is important for microbial digestion.[1,10,17] The hyrax does not have a gallbladder. The testicles of the male are intraabdominal and are attached to the posterior pole of the kidney. Females have four mammae and a duplex uterus.

The eye of the hyrax is unique, as a portion of the iris above the pupil bulges slightly into the aqueous humor to cut off light directly above the animal.[17]

SPECIAL HOUSING REQUIREMENTS

The hyrax is a poor thermoregulator, and its body temperature fluctuates in relation to the environment, so it is important to provide a shelter with relatively stable environmental temperatures and humidity. Hyraxes spend many hours basking in the sun and will often huddle in groups when temperatures start to drop. These animals are reluctant to emerge if the weather is cold or rainy, but they may also seek shelter in extreme heat from the sun. They should have a heated area or shelter provided if they are exhibited outdoors.

In spite of their build, hyraxes are quick, agile, and adept at climbing. A variety of surfaces should be provided for this activity. They are also capable of jumping up to 1.5 meters (m) so enclosures should be designed accordingly. These animals are quite fastidious and prefer to use a designated area for urinating and defecating, so their exhibit should contain a sandy area for these purposes so that it may be cleaned daily.

FEEDING

In the wild, the hyrax is a facultative grazer, feeding on anything from succulents to lower-quality fibrous foods. They spend less than an hour a day eating. The relatively long transit time for digestion, coupled with a low nitrogen requirement, enables this animal to survive periods of poor diet and low protein availability.

The hyrax has an effective calcium absorption mechanism in the alimentary canal. The majority of excess calcium is excreted in urine, as in the rabbit, guinea pig, and other rodents. This may give the hyrax urine a chalky appearance. Hemosiderosis has been a concern in the hyrax, so low-iron diets are recommended.[3,6] A 2004 study found that hyraxes fed a low-fiber diet were more likely to be affected by pancreatic islet fibrosis (PIF).[8]

Most zoologic institutions feed hyraxes once a day and offer either some type of pelleted herbivore feed or primate biscuits with a variety of vegetables and greens, a small amount of fruit and some type of hay ad libitum.[17] Water is consumed, when available, but is not generally needed. The hyrax efficiently metabolizes water by producing highly concentrated urine, having low evaporative water loss because of the low metabolic rate, and minimal fecal water loss. Consequently, water demand may usually be met in the diet. This species is not known to exhibit coprophagy as adults, but juveniles will eat or may be fed feces to stimulate the appropriate bacteria for a diet high in fiber.[17]

HANDLING AND RESTRAINT

Some animals, especially those that have been hand raised, will adjust to handling by humans. However, most hyraxes are caught by using a strong hoop net and heavy leather gloves. Care must be taken to avoid causing injury and stress to the animals. Hyraxes may also be run into a crate or trained to go into one.

TABLE 54-2

Chemical Restraint Agents Used for the Hyrax*

Generic Name	Trade Name and (Source)	Dosage	Reversal Agent, (Trade Name and Source)	Dosage
INDIVIDUAL AGENTS				
Acepromazine	PromAce (Boehringer Ingelheim Vetmedica, Inc.), AceproJect (Butler Schein)	0.5–1.0 milligram per kilogram (mg/kg), intramuscularly (IM)	None	0.0.1–0.2 mg/kg slow IV to effect
Diazepam	Valium (Roche)	1–5 mg/kg, IM	Flumazenil (Romazicon, Roche)	
Isoflurane	IsoFlo (Abbott) Aerrane (Anaquest) Isovet (Schering/Plough)	3%–5% induction; 1%–2% Maintenance	None	
Ketamine	Ketaset, Vetalar (Fort Dodge)	20–50 mg/kg, IM	None	
Medetomidine	Domitor (Pfizer)	0.25 mg/kg, IM	Atipamezole (Antisedan, Pfizer)	5× mg total of medetomidine, IM
Midazolam	Versed (Roche)	1–2 mg/kg, IM	Flumazenil (Romazicon)	0.01–0.2 mg/kg slow IV to effect
Propofol	Diprivan (Zeneca Pharmaceuticals)	7.5–15.0 mg/kg, intravenously (IV) (slow bolus over 5 minutes)	None	
Sevoflurane	SevoFlo (Abbott Animal Health) Ultane (Abbott)	3%–8% induction; 1%–4% Maintenance	None	
Tiletamine–zolazepam	Telazol (Fort Dodge)	5–25 mg/kg, IM	Flumazenil for zolazepam, (Romazicon)	0.01–0.2 mg/kg, slow IV to effect
Xylazine	Rompun (Bayer)	1–5 mg/kg, IM	Yohimbine (Antagonil, ZooPharm, Yobine, Lloyd)	0.2–1.0 mg/kg, IM or IV
COMBINATION AGENTS				
Ketamine–diazepam, followed by isoflurane	Ketoset or Vetalar–Valium	5–30 mg/kg and 1–3 mg/kg, IM	None Flumazenil (Romazicon)	0.01–0.2 mg/kg, slow IV to effect
Ketamine–xylazine	Vetalar–Rompun	30–40 mg/kg and 3–5 mg/kg, IM	None Yohimbine (Antagonil, Yobine)	0.2–1.0 mg/kg, IM or IV
Ketamine–acepromazine	Ketoset or Vetalar–PromAce	40 mg/kg and 0.5–1.0 mg/kg, IM	None None	
Ketamine–medetomidine	Ketaset or Vetalar–Domitor	5 mg/kg and 0.35 mg/kg, IM	None Atipamezole (Antisedan)	5× mg total of medetomidine

*Use lower end of dose range for debilitated, geriatric, or obese animals for optimal results.

ANESTHESIA AND SURGERY

Inhalant anesthesia, specifically isoflurane, is the most common form of anesthesia used in this species. After manual restraint by running the animal from a crate into an induction chamber or by placing a plastic bag over the crate itself, the anesthetic is most often administered via a face mask. It may be challenging to intubate the hyrax, but if intubation is elected, a 4- or 5-millimeter (mm) endotracheal tube may be used.[12] Injectable anesthetics may also be used (Table 54-2). The most common reasons for anesthesia are surgery or treatment for trauma, caused either by conspecifics or falls, and for dental disease.

DIAGNOSTICS

Venous access sites for this species include the jugular and the femoral veins. Boxes 54-1 and 54-2 list the hematologic and serum chemistry reference ranges, respectively, for the rock hyrax. Annual

examinations may include, but are not limited to, blood work; a dental examination and tooth trims, as needed; routine fecal checks for parasites; fecal or rectal culture; nail trims, as needed; and radiography. Vaccinations are given to this species for rabies and tetanus. The necropsy database for hyraxes includes four cases of tetanus as probable cause of death.[17]

DISEASES

A number of disease processes and health concerns affect the hyrax. Some health issues stem from behavior related to stress, quarantine, lack of enrichment, or isolation. These include overgrooming, alopecia, and intermittent diarrhea. Some problems, including hemosiderosis, pancreatic islet fibrosis, prolapsed rectum (caused by large amounts of produce in relation to other diet items), steatitis, and obesity, may possibly be related to nutrition, as previously mentioned.

BOX 54-1 Reference Ranges for Hematologic Parameters of the Hyrax

Parameter	Rock Hyrax (Adult)*
WBC (×10³/microliter [µL])	4800–29,900
RBC (×10⁶/µL)	4.25–9.07
Hemoglobin, gram per deciliter (g/dL)	7.4–15.5
Hematocrit (%)	24.0–51.2
MCH, picogram per cell (pg/cell)	15.6–24.5
MCHC, gram per deciliter (g/dL)	20.0–44.2
MCV, femtoliter (fL)	48.3–69.9
Neutrophils (×10³/µL)	3720–22,100
Band neutrophils (×10³/µL)	1360–8970
Lymphocytes (×10³/µL)	7160–20,100
Monocytes (×10³/µL)	1–5989
Eosinophils (×10³/µL)	1–8237
Basophils (×10³/µL)	67–411
Nucleated RBCs/100 WBCs	0–1
Platelets (×10³/µL)	96–695
Plasma protein (g/dL)	5.0–8.1

*Values are given as minimum to maximum.
MCH, Mean corpuscular hemoglobin; *MCHC,* mean corpuscular hemoglobin concentration; *MCV,* mean corpuscular volume; *RBC,* red blood cell; *WBC,* white blood cell.

BOX 54-2 Reference Ranges for Serum Biochemical Parameters of the Hyrax

Parameter	Rock Hyrax (Adult)*
Glucose, milligram per deciliter (mg/dL)	20–287
Urea nitrogen (mg/dL)	6–62
Creatinine (mg/dL)	0.5–2.8
Uric acid (mg/dL)	0.1–3.0
Calcium (mg/dL)	7.8–14.9
Phosphorus (mg/dL)	1.9–8.6
Sodium, milliequivalent per liter (mEq/L)	139–158
Potassium (mEq/L)	2.6–5.4
Chloride (mEq/L)	97–120
Magnesium (mg/dL)	1.4–2.6
Cholesterol (mg/dL)	42–312
Triglyceride (mg/dL)	19–223
Total protein, gram per deciliter (g/dL)	3.8–8.1
Albumin (g/dL)	2.8–6.2
Globulin (g/dL)	0.4–3.9
Aspartate aminotransferase, international unit per liter (IU/L)	0–126
Alanine aminotransferase (IU/L)	2–84
Total bilirubin (mg/dL)	0.1–1.8
Direct bilirubin (mg/dL)	0.0–0.1
Indirect bilirubin (mg/dL)	0.1–1.2
Amylase, unit per liter (Unit/L)	1555–3985
Alkaline phosphatase (IU/L)	60–366
Lactic acid dehydrogenase (IU/L)	162–1310
Creatine kinase (IU/L)	317–2826
Total carbon dioxide (mEq/L)	11.0–30.0
Gamma-glutamyltransferase (IU/L)	0–103
Lipase (Unit/L)	6–43

*Values are given as minimum to maximum.

Infectious Diseases

Bacterial Diseases

Bacterial diseases that may affect the hyrax include mycobacteriosis, which has been reported in this species in the United States, Australia, Canada, Europe, and South Africa. In all cases, both in captivity and in the wild, the isolated organism was either typical or atypical *Mycobacterium tuberculosis* complex (MTBC).[5,11,13,15] A particular variant of MTBC, called the "dassie bacillus" was identified in 1958.[21] It has low virulence in rodent species, rabbits, and guinea pigs. Clinically, this disease has presented as lameness, pneumonia, mild weight loss, and reproductive abnormalities. On gross necropsy, granulomas may be seen in the lungs, spleen, kidneys, and liver. Acid-fast bacilli have been seen on histopathology. A multidrug treatment protocol may be implemented, but the prognosis is poor; generally, the disease leads to death or euthanasia. Currently, no effective antemortem diagnostic tool is available for this species.

Yersiniosis was a significant problem in one captive colony in the United Kingdom over a 4-year period. Increased rodent control and an autogenous killed vaccine, administered annually following the deaths in the collection for several years thereafter, prevented deaths from this disease process.[2]

A list of antibiotics recommended for the hyrax is provided in Table 54-3.

Viral Diseases

Oral and tongue lesions, including glossitis and ulceration, along with intranuclear inclusion bodies noted in the tissues, have been seen in the hyrax. The general aspects of this presentation have been attributed to a suspected herpesvirus.[4,10]

A novel α-herpesvirus was identified in 2009 in a rock hyrax group (*P. capensis*) from a closed collection in a zoo. Clinical presentation, which was generally acute, included blepharoconjunctivitis (Figure 54-2) and blisterlike lesions on the tongue, mouth, and face (Figure 54-3). Molecular characteristics tentatively support the inclusion of this α-herpesvirus in the genus *Simplexvirus.* Disease caused by this organism did not respond to treatment. Ultimately, seven juveniles and three adults died or were euthanized.[7] After this outbreak ended, additional deaths have not been seen in the collection.

Fungal Diseases

Ulcerative lesions of the squamous epithelium of the tongue, gingiva, esophagus, and stomach of a number of hyraxes have contained large numbers of *Candida* organisms. Spores were generally restricted to the mucosa and rarely seen in the submucosa. It is unknown if this was the primary pathogen or if the clinical presentation stemmed from the α-herpesvirus with the fungus being an opportunistic invader.

Parasitic Diseases

Grassinema procavia is a small, white nematode, which is approximately 3 mm in length and may be found in the alimentary canal of the hyrax, especially in the stomach. It is easily missed but should be strongly considered as a cause when gastric ulceration is present. Animals may be tested for the presence of this parasite with the use of gastric lavage. This intestinal parasite and others may be treated with anthelmintics. Effective sanitation and prevention of fecal contamination of food and water help to manage this problem.

A case of generalized demodecosis in hyrax was reported in 2010.[18] Three juvenile siblings presented with hemorrhagic areas with scabbing, purulent material in the hair and nonpruritic, nonalopecic mildly encrusted skin nodules, particularly affecting the dorsum, head, and rear legs. Skin biopsies were performed, and samples were submitted for parasitologic identification and electron microscopy. Fusiform mites consistent with *Demodex* sp. were also identified. This mite is being described and named as a new species of *Demodex.* The animals in this clinical case were treated successfully with avermectin.

Cutaneous leishmaniasis has been reported in hyraxes, which are a suspected natural reservoir for this disease. Causative agents in this species include *L. aethiopica* and *L. tropica.* The high rates of infection

TABLE 54-3

Systemic Antibiotics Recommended for the Hyrax*

Generic Name	Trade Name	Dosage	Route of Administration†	Interval
Amikacin	Amiglyde-V (Fort Dodge)	2–10 mg/kg	SC, IM, or IV	Every 8–24 hours
Cefpodoxime Proxetil	Simplicef (Pfizer)	5–10 mg/kg	PO	Every 24 hours for 7–10 days
Ceftiofur crystalline free acid	Excede (Pfizer)	6.6 mg/kg	IM	Every 7 days
Ceftazidime	Fortaz (GlaxoWellcome)	40 mg/kg	IM, IV	Every 8–hours
Chloramphenicol	Chloromycetin (Parke-Davis)	30–50 mg/kg	SC, IM, or IV	Every 8–12 hours
Ciprofloxacin	Cipro (Schering Plough)	5–15 mg/kg	PO	Every 12 hours
Doxycycline	Vibramycin (Pfizer)	2.5–5 mg/kg	PO	Every 12 hours
Enrofloxacin	Baytril (Bayer)	5–20 mg/kg	PO, SQ, IM, or IV	Every 12 hours
Gentamicin	Gentamax (Butler, Phoenix Pharmaceuticals)	2–4 mg/kg	SC, IM, or IV	Every 8–24 hours
Metronidazole	Flagyl (Pfizer)	20–40 mg/kg	PO	Every 12 hours for 3–5 days
Oxytetracycline	Terramycin (Bio-Ceutic)	10–15 mg/kg	SC or IM	Every 24 hours
Penicillin G benzathine–penicillin G procaine	Flo-Cillin (Fort Dodge)	20,000 80,000 IU/kg	IM or SC	Every 48 hours
Penicillin G procaine	Pfizerpen (Roerig)	20,000–60,000 IU/kg	SC or IM	Every 24 hours
Tetracycline	Achromycin-V (Lederle)	50 mg/kg	PO	Every 8–12 hours
Trimethoprim–sulfadiazine	Tribrissen (Schering-Plough)	30 mg/kg	SC	Every 12–24 hours
Trimethoprim–sulfamethoxazole	Bactrim (AR Scientific)	15–30 mg/kg	PO	Every 12 hours

*The potential exists for antibiotic-induced enterotoxemia following administration of some antimicrobial agents; appetite and fecal character must be monitored closely during and following therapy; concurrent probiotic therapies may be indicated. Parenteral antibiotic therapies are preferred over oral therapy. Repeated subcutaneous injections may cause sloughing. Alternative injection sites should be used.
†All aminoglycosides administered intravenously should be diluted with saline or sterile water at 4 mL/kg and delivered over 20 minutes.
IM, Intramuscularly; *IU/kg*, international unit per kilogram; *IV*, intravenously; *mg/kg*, milligram per kilogram; *PO*, orally; *SC*, subcutaneously.

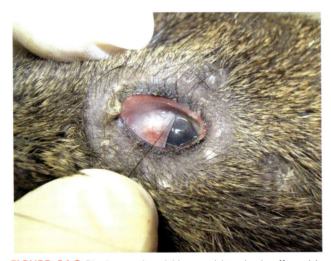

FIGURE 54-2 Blepharoconjunctivitis noted in animals affected by the novel α-herpesvirus.

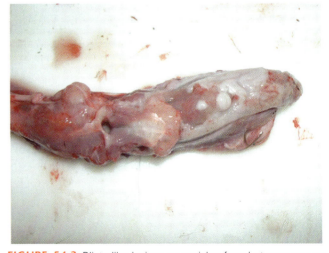

FIGURE 54-3 Blisterlike lesions or vesicles found at necropsy on the tongue of a hyrax affected by the novel α-herpesvirus.

and exposure in hyraxes, especially to *L. tropica*, supports their involvement in the transmission cycle of this parasite and their potential role as a reservoir for disease in humans. The vector in natural ranges for free-ranging hyraxes is the sandfly. This disease may be diagnosed by analysis of blood smears or ulcerative lesions of affected animals.[4,14,19]

A list of parasiticides recommended for hyrax are listed in Table 54-4.

Noninfectious Diseases

Iron overload has been reported on numerous occasions in the hyrax. The causes are most likely multifactorial and are thought to include diet and genetics. Hemochromatosis associated with severe degenerative changes in the liver has been reported in the rock hyrax.[16] Animals generally present with anorexia caused by gastric enteritis and hemorrhage. Minimizing concurrent parasitic loads and bacterial infections may help manage this problem. Hemosiderosis

TABLE 54-4

Parasiticides Recommended for the Hyrax

Generic Name	Trade Name	Dosage	Route of Administration	Comments/Used Against
Amprolium, 9.6%	Corid (Huvepharma)	1 mL/7 kg every 24 hours	PO	Coccidia
Carbaryl, 5% powder		Dust lightly once per week	Topical	Ectoparasites
Doramectin	Dectomax (Pfizer)	0.2 mg/kg	SC, IM	Ectoparasites
Fenbendazole	Panacur (Intervet)	25–50 mg/kg every 24 hours for 3–5 days	PO	Roundworms
Ivermectin	Ivomec (Merial)	0.2 mg/kg repeat 7–14 days	PO, SC	Gastrointestinal nematodes; lungworms
Praziquantel	Droncit (Bayer)	5–10 mg/kg; repeat in 10 days	PO, SC, or IM	Tapeworms
Pyrethrins	—	Apply to effect	Topical	Fleas
Sulfadimethoxine	Albon (Pfizer)	25–50 mg/kg every 24 hours for 10 days	PO	Coccidia

IM, Intramuscularly; *IV*, intravenously; *mg/kg*, milligram per kilogram; *mL/kg*, milliliter per kilogram; *PO*, orally; *SC*, subcutaneously.

and PIF, as mentioned previously, have also been seen in this species and may be contributing causes to another problem, diabetes mellitus (DM).[9] Clinical signs include a rough haircoat, formed but soft feces, weight loss, and a persistent hyperglycemia. PIF with concurrent DM is usually found at necropsy.[8]

Pregnancy toxemia has occurred in primarily older females, around 8 to 9 years of age. Dystocia and stillbirths are quite common in hyraxes. The rock hyrax studbook, updated through October 2012, estimates that abortion, stillbirths, and neonatal deaths account for approximately a third of the deaths with known diagnoses in the population.[17]

Dental disease, caused by age-related changes such as excessive wear or dental fractures, is common in older animals. Extractions or root canals should be performed, as indicated, with concurrent administration of appropriate antibiotics.[10]

Aggression-related trauma is very common in hyraxes. Fighting is generally caused by issues related to behavioral hierarchy and group social structure. Care should be taken to maintain an appropriate group size for the space available to avoid crowding, especially among males.[4,10,17] Overcrowding may also cause food competition and lead to malnutrition and chronic weight loss.[4,10]

A disease process called *hyracoidea stress syndrome* was identified in a European journal in 2009.[20] A 3-year study on 37 animals concluded that environmental stress factors led to respiratory and nervous symptoms just before death. Cold temperatures leading to pneumonia, gastric ulcerations, and damage to endocrine glands, specifically the pituitary, thyroid, and adrenal glands, were determined to be the primary cause of this syndrome. This study concluded that because of the very low numbers of *Grassinemia procavia* in each individual, this organism was not the primary cause of death but rather an incidental finding.

REPRODUCTION

Rock hyraxes are karyotype 2n with 54 chromosomes. They reach sexual maturity at 16 to 17 months of age and at approximately 1.5 kg body weight. Females are monestrous, seasonal breeders, becoming receptive in the spring and summer months, primarily from April to July in the Northern hemisphere and in November and December in South Africa.[4,10] The uterus is bicornuate, forming a Y-shape, and placentation is hemochorial, villous, and zonary.[10] The testes of the males increase in size during the breeding season. Hyraxes have a polygamous mating system.[4,17] For successful breeding in captivity, an isolated nest box packed with hay and a supplemental heat source should be provided, and the holding area or exhibit should be checked for any areas where youngsters could

escape or fall. Isolated females and young should be returned to the group as soon as possible.

Pregnancy may be detected through abdominal palpation or ultrasonography. The gestation period is 201 to 245 days, and a litter may range from 1 to 6 offspring. In captivity, the mean size of a litter is 2.6. Newborns are precocious and weigh 170 to 240 grams (g). The young have been seen nibbling on grasses and solid food as early as 4 days; they are usually weaned around 6 weeks of age, weighing approximately twice their birthweight.[17]

Numerous methods of birth control have been tried in this species, including melengestrol acetate and deslorelin implants, tubal ligation, and porcine zona pellucida vaccination with varying success.[17] Castration has been performed, with few complications, on aggressive or nonbreeding males.

REFERENCES

1. Björnhag G, Becker G, Buchholz C, et al: The gastrointestinal tract of the rock hyrax (*Procavia habessinica*). 1. Morphology and motility patterns of the tract. *Comp Biochem Physiol* 109A:649–654, 1994.
2. Chitty J: Disease syndromes in the rock hyrax (*Procavia capensis*). In *Proceedings of the American Association of Zoo Veterinarians*, Los Angeles, CA, 2008, pp 30–32.
3. Clauss M, Paglia DE: Iron storage disease in captive wild mammals: The comparative evidence. *J Zoo Wildl Med* 43:S6–S18, 2012.
4. Collins D: Hyracoidea (Hyraxes). In Fowler ME, Miller RE, editors: *Zoo and wild animal medicine*, ed 5, St. Louis, MO, 2003, Saunders, pp 550–558.
5. Cousins DV, Peet RL, Gaynor WT, et al: Tuberculosis in imported hyrax (*Procavia capensis*) caused by an unusual variant belonging to *Mycobacterium tuberculosis* complex. *J Zoo Wildl Med* 42:135–145, 1994.
6. Frye FL: Iron storage disease (hemosiderosis) in an African rock hyrax (*Provacia capensis*). *J Zoo Wildl Med* 13:152–156, 1982.
7. Galeota JA, Napier JE, Armstrong DL, et al: Herpesvirus infections in rock hyraxes (*Procavia capensis*). *J Vet Diagn Invest* 21:531–535, 2009.
8. Gamble KC, Garner MM, Krause L, et al: Pancreatic islet fibrosis in rock hyraxes (*Procavia capensis*), Part 1. *J Zoo Wildl Med* 35:361–369, 2004.
9. Garner MM, Gamble KC, Raymond JT, et al: Pancreatic Islet fibrosis in rock hyrax (*Procavia capensis*), Part 2: Pathology, immunohistochemistry, and electron microscopy. *J Zoo Wildl Med* 35:280–291, 2004.
10. Griner LA: Hyraxes (Hyrocoidea). In Fowler ME, editor: *Zoo and wild animal medicine*, ed 2, Philadelphia, PA, 1986, Saunders, pp 600–603.
11. Gudan A, Artuković B, Cvetnić Ž, et al: Disseminated tuberculosis in hyrax (*Procavia capensis*) caused by *Mycobacterium africanum*. *J Zoo Wildl Med* 39:386–391, 2008.

12. Horne WA, Loomis MR: Elephants and hyrax. In West W, Heard D, Caulkett N, editors: *Zoo animal and wildlife immobilization and anesthesia*, Ames, IA, 2007, Blackwell Publishing, pp 519.

13. Lutze-Wallace C, Turcotte C, Glover G, et al: Isolation of a *Mycobacterium-microti*-like organism from a rock hyrax (*Procavia capensis*) in a Canadian zoo. *Vet J* 47:1011–1013, 2006.

14. Morsy TA, al Dakhil MA, el Bahrawy AF: Natural leishmania infection in rock hyrax, *Procavia capensis*, trapped in Najran, Saudi Arabia. *J Egypt Soc Parasitol* 27:75–81, 1997.

15. Parsons S, Smith SG, Martins Q, et al: Pulmonary infection due to the dassie bacillus (*Mycobacterium tuberculosis* complex sp.) in a free-living dassie (rock hyrax-*Procavia capensis*) from South Africa. *Tuberculosis (Edinb)* 88:80–83, 2008.

16. Rehg BJ, Strandberg J, Montali R: Hemochromatosis in the rock hyrax. In Montali RJ, Migaki G, editors: *The comparative pathology of zoo animals*, Washington, DC, 1980, Smithsonian Institution Press, pp 1287–1292.

17. Strode Y: *Rock hyrax Procavia capensis 2012 husbandry resources*, Peoria, IL, 2012, Peoria Zoo.

18. Takle GL, Suedmeyer WK, Mertins JW, et al: Generalized demodecosis in three sibling juvenile hyraxes (*Preocavia capensis*). *J Zoo Wildl Med* 41:496–502, 2010.

19. Talmi FD, Jaffe CL, Nasereddin A, et al: Leishmania tropica in rock hyraxes (*Procavis capensis*) in a focus of human cutaneous leishmaniasis. *Am J Trop Med Hyg* 82:814–818, 2010.

20. Tamam AS, El-Mahdy MM: Hyrocoidea stress syndrome in rock hyrax (*Procavia capensis*). *Euro J Sci Res* 32:128–134, 2009.

21. Wagner JC, Buchanan G, Bokkenheuser V, et al: An acid fast bacillus isolated from the lungs of cape hyrax, *Procavia capensis* (Pallus). *Nature* 181:284–285, 1958.

22. Walker EP: Hyrocoidea. In Nowak R, editor: *Mammals of the world*, vol 2, ed 5, Baltimore, MD, 1991, Johns Hopkins Press, pp 1287–1292.

CHAPTER 55

Rhinoceridae (Rhinoceroses)

Michele A. Miller and Peter E. Buss

BIOLOGY

Rhinoceroses (rhinos) are among the most primitive of the world's large mammals, and in prehistoric times were common large herbivores in North America. Five extant species exist in four genera; in Africa, the white (*Ceratotherium simum*) and black (*Diceros bicornis*) rhinos and in Asia, the Sumatran (*Dicerorhinus sumatrensis*), Indian (*Rhinoceros unicornis*), and Javan (*Rhinoceros sondaicus*) rhinos. The Sumatran rhino is the most primitive and predates the extinct woolly rhino (*Coelodonta antiqitatis*), which inhabited in northern Europe and Asia during the last Ice Age.

African rhinos live in habitats that are related to dietary requirements; the white rhino requires relatively flat terrain with areas of short grass, whereas the black rhino prefers areas with shrubs and young trees. The Javan rhino inhabits lowland coastal forests rather than the more mountainous inland areas. Sumatran rhinos are found in areas of dense primary rain forest. Indian rhinos exist across a wide range of habitats, including marshes, alluvial plains, grasslands, and aril forests. All species of rhino require regular access to water. They need to drink daily or every second day, as they are hindgut fermenters with relatively fast gut transit times which reduce the time for water resorption from the feces.[35] Rhinos wallow in mud pools to cool off during the heat of the day and to help keep their skin free of external parasites.

Habitat loss and severe poaching has led to the devastation of rhino populations. Current worldwide population estimates (2012) are 35 to 44 Javan, 152 to 199 Sumatran, 3270 Indian, 4837 black, and 20,143 white rhinos (International Rhino Foundation; www.rhinos.org). In contrast, in the 1970s, the black rhino population in Africa was approximately 65,000.[22]

UNIQUE ANATOMY

Rhinos have a barrel-shaped torso; short, thick legs and broad feet with three weight-bearing digits; and an elongated, bulky skull. The soles of the feet have a large pad to cushion the weight of the animal. The most distinctive feature of rhino is the presence of a single horn (*Rhinoceros* sp.) or a pair of horns (*Ceratotherium*, *Diceros*, and *Dicerorhinus*) that are composed of tubular hairlike keratin filaments, which are outgrowths of the skin. The horn is relatively easy to displace, since it is not attached to the skull but rather set on bony protuberances.[35] African rhinos lack both incisors and canine teeth: incisors (I) 0, canines (C) 0, premolars (P) 3–4, molars (M) 3; in contrast, the Asian species have incisors: I 1/1–2, C 0, P 3–4, M 3).[28] Hypertrophied and tusklike lateral lower incisors are characteristic of the three Asian rhinos, with only members of the genus *Rhinoceros* having a pair of small central incisors. The black, Sumatran, and Javan rhinos are browsers with prehensile upper lips, which assist in grasping the plants that they consume. White and Indian rhinos have wide, flat lips for grazing.

The rhino's skin is thick, and in the white rhino, it may reach a thickness of 5 centimeters (cm), with a thick vascular dermis covered by an epidermis 1 millimeter (mm) thick.[35] All rhinos have skinfolds, although these are more pronounced in the Asian species, with the Indian rhino being best known for the exaggerated armorlike plates. The Sumatran rhino is unique, having a distinctive shaggy coat of hair with particularly hairy ears and a tuft of long hair at the tip of the tail.

SPECIAL HOUSING REQUIREMENTS

Enclosures for all rhino species need to be sturdy and constructed of concrete, large-diameter wooden or metal poles or of more natural materials such as rocks; however, it should ensure that the animals cannot climb over or become entrapped within the enclosures. Spacing between vertical bars should be 0.5 m. If calves are present, chains or cables should be added. When horizontal poles are used, a potential for horn avulsion or climbing exists.

Substrate should be textured to minimize slipping yet not abrade foot pads. Most indoor stalls are made of concrete to facilitate cleaning. Natural substrate used in outdoor enclosures or pens should allow adequate drainage and cleaning or be periodically changed to prevent buildup of parasites, pathogens, or excessive moisture.

All rhinos must be provided with access to pools and wallows. The access and depth of the pool should be sufficient to encourage use and allow complete submersion, especially for Indian and Sumatran rhinos. Enclosure items such as scratching posts, rocks, and vegetation promote natural, species-specific behaviors but should be designed to avoid head or limb entrapment or horn rubbing or avulsion.

Rhinos may be acclimated to cold and inclement weather if provided access to shelter during wet and windy conditions. However, supplemental heat (to maintain 13°C) should be provided in cold climates when temperatures consistently drop below 10°C. Ill, old, or young animals may need higher temperatures.

Of the four rhino species, white rhinos are the most social and usually housed in groups. Black rhinos are more solitary but have been housed in small family groups in captivity. Indian rhinos are mostly solitary. Therefore they should be kept as individual animals except in very large spaces. Sumatran rhinos should also be housed individually and only introduced for breeding purposes. Significant aggression during breeding may occur with black, Indian, and Sumatran rhinos, and adequate space should exist to prevent cornering of animals.

FEEDING AND NUTRITION

Feeding strategies differ by species. Black and Sumatran rhinos are browsers, white rhinos are considered grazers, and Indian rhinos are classified as intermediate feeders. Studies on digestibility in captive rhinos show that the horse is a useful model for the development of diets for Indian and white rhinos but not for black rhinos.[7] Captive black rhinos appear to receive higher proportions of concentrates compared with other species and would benefit from higher proportion of browse.

In captivity, a rough guideline for diet quantity is 1% to 3% body weight as fed, with no more than one third of total calories obtained from pellets.[22] Energy management for weight control is especially important in Indian rhinos; 0.5% to 1.1% body weight in dry matter (DM) is adequate in this species.[9] Grass hay should be fed to white and Indian rhinos, whereas a grass–legume mixture or a legume–browse mixture is used for black and Sumatran rhinos. Alfalfa fed as exclusive forage may lead to mineral imbalances, colic, and diarrhea. Black rhinos appear to have higher calcium (Ca) and magnesium (Mg) absorption compared with horses and higher fecal losses of sodium (Na) and potassium (K).[7] Therefore, excessive mineral supplementation should be avoided. Natural browses appear to be limited in Na, phosphorus (P), zinc (Zn), and selenium (Se). Appropriate Ca:P ratio should also be monitored, since low phosphorus values have been associated with poorly defined syndromes, including dermatologic and hematologic disorders, in black rhinos.[10]

Vitamin E deficiency has been linked to health issues, especially in black rhinos. Therefore, the contents of the diet should be analyzed to ensure a sufficient concentration (150–200 international units per kilogram [IU/kg] DM).[22]

Black and Sumatran rhinos are susceptible to iron storage disorder in captivity, so a high-fiber, low-iron diet should be provided to these species. A low-iron herbivore pellet, in addition to browse, fed to captive black rhinos resulted in a decrease in serum ferritin levels.[27] Low-iron diets consisting of browse, long-stem forage, and low-iron pellets (iron [Fe] ≤350 parts per million [ppm]) is recommended for browser rhino species (Valdes E, personal

communication). Citrus and other produce containing vitamin C may enhance iron absorption and should be minimized in the diets of these species.

Analyses of rhino milk have shown that it is lower in total solids compared with the milk of most ungulates (8.2%–8.8%). The relative composition is high in sugars (63%–82% of total solids), with 14%–28% protein and low fat (2.6%–6.8% of total solids).[3] Formulas used for hand-raising rhinos are based on cows' milk or commercial formulas (ZooLogic Milk Matrix 20/14, PetAg, Inc., Hampshire, IL). Lactase (Lactaid) has been useful as a milk additive in these cases. Indian, white, and black rhino calves have been successfully hand-reared with these formulas.

In neonates that have not received colostrum, bovine or equine colostrum should be fed at a 50% dilution to provide immunoglobulins if rhino colostrum is unavailable. Addition of 10% colostrum to the formula for up to 1 month is recommended for local gastrointestinal (GI) immunity.[3] Feeding for the first 3 days is 10% of body weight (kg) divided into seven feedings, with an increase to 15%–20% on day 4 through 6 months of age. At 6 months through the start of weaning at 1 year, a constant volume of 11 kg of formula at each of three feedings should be offered. Calves should be weighed regularly and gain 1 to 2 kg/day.

RESTRAINT AND HANDLING

Physical Restraint

Chutes for rhinos may be simple free-stall designs, in which an individual animal is trained to enter voluntarily and poles or bollards allow protected contact. More sophisticated designs include hydraulic or movable walls, head restraints, and access doors for examinations and minor medical or reproduction-related procedures. Ideally, the design should be incorporated into the facility so that the animal has to pass through and it is not a dead-end. Successful use of these devices usually requires operant conditioning of the rhino, the use of tranquilization or sedation, or a combination.

Chemical Restraint

This section will focus on restraint of captive rhinos. Excellent sources of information on the immobilization of free-ranging rhinos are available.[5,35] The two techniques used are standing restraint and recumbent immobilization.

For captive rhinos, drug delivery usually requires use of darting equipment. Depending on the situation, pole syringes with robust needles or hand-injection in conditioned animals may be used. Most darting systems may be used in captive situations, as long as a robust needle (minimum 40–60 mm × 2 mm needle) is used to penetrate the thick skin and deliver the drug intramuscularly. Nylon darts (Teleinject, Daninject) are preferred in these situations, since they cause less trauma compared with metal darts. Ideal sites for drug injection are just caudal to the ear on the lateral cervical area, upper caudal hindlimb, shoulder, or nuchal hump in the white rhino. However, any site may be used if the dart is placed perpendicular to the skin and is adequate to penetrate muscle.

Depending on the animal's health status, the environment, and the procedure planned, food and water should be withheld prior to the procedure, at least overnight, although regurgitation and aspiration are infrequent complications in rhinos.

Procedures should be planned for the coolest time of day, preferably early mornings. Rapid induction and minimal excitement further decrease the risk of hyperthermia. Rectal enemas, evaporative cooling with sprayers and fans, or cold water baths for small individuals are warranted if the rectal temperature is greater than 39°C, although complete anesthetic reversal should be performed immediately if the temperature reaches 41°C or above.[5]

Rhinos are prone to developing myopathy and neuropathy after prolonged recumbency. Inflated truck inner tubes, heavy mats, or padding may be used under pressure points to prevent radial nerve paralysis and other neuropathies if the procedure is to take place on a hard surface.

The optimal body position is still being debated. Lateral recumbency is often preferred, since it provides optimal circulation to the limbs; however, sternal recumbency may allow better ventilation. If the animal needs to be in sternal recumbency for the procedure, it is ideal to roll the animal into lateral recumbency, whenever possible, to ensure adequate peripheral circulation. Limbs should be "pumped" about every 20 minutes to promote perfusion of muscles.[35]

It is imperative that immobilized rhinos be closely monitored to minimize complications. Hypoxia, hypercapnia, and hypertension are commonly associated with the use of potent opioids in rhinos.[22,33-] Accurate weight or estimated weight facilitates optimal drug calculation and prevents drug overdosing or underdosing and associated problems.

Pulse oximetry is useful for monitoring trends in hemoglobin oxygen saturation. Sites for placement include the ear pinnae (scraping of the skin surface may sometimes provide more accurate readings), mucosal folds of the prepuce, vulva, and rectum; and sensor pads placed side by side in the conjunctival sac, gingival mucosa, nasal mucosa, and inside the rectum, vagina, or prepuce. Ideally, readings should be greater than 90%, but interpretation must be made in conjunction with the color of the mucous membranes and blood and other clinical signs. Capnography may be used by placing a small-animal endotracheal tube inside a nostril in nonintubated rhinos. Direct and indirect blood pressure may be measured by using either an arterial catheter in the medial auricular artery or a blood pressure cuff at the base of the tail, respectively.

Standing sedation should only be attempted after proper consideration of animal and staff safety. In captive rhinos, standing chemical restraint has historically been performed using low doses of the potent opioid etorphine. However, variable responses may lead to recumbency. More recently, butorphanol, alone or in combination with azaperone or α_2-agonists (detomidine, medetomidine), has been successfully used. In the author's experience, a combination of etorphine (1 mg /1000 kg), butorphanol (10 mg butorphanol to 1 mg etorphine), and azaperone (20 mg standard dose, intramuscularly [IM]) has been effective in "walking" captive white rhino, with the use of a white flag as a target to bring the rhino from the holding facility to the crate. Once in the crate, the animal will remain standing and tolerate minor procedures. Chemical restraint may be partially to fully reversed with naltrexone (40–100 mg naltrexone:1 mg etorphine or 1–2.5 mg naltrexone:1 mg butorphanol) with or without atipamezole (5 mg atipamezole:1 mg α-$_2$-agonist), depending on the drug combination chosen (Box 55-1).[22,33,35]

Potent opioids are the primary drugs used for general anesthesia in rhinos. Etorphine is mostly commonly used, although carfentanil (in some species, this has been suggested to cause excitable inductions) and, more recently, combinations of etorphine and thiafentanil have also been administered to rhinos. Opioids are typically combined with azaperone, α_2-agonists, or acepromazine to decrease complications. Hyaluronidase may be included to increase absorption and decrease induction time. To deepen the anesthesia or for prolonged procedures, supplemental doses of etorphine, ketamine, propofol, or inhalant anesthetics have been used. Midazolam, diazepam, and guaifenisen infusion may provide additional muscle relaxation. Suggested doses for recumbent immobilization in captive rhinos are given in Box 55-2.[5,22,33–35,41]

White rhinos and, to a lesser extent, Indian rhinos appear to be more sensitive to the effects of opioids compared with black rhinos and exhibit muscle tremors, limb paddling, hypoxia, hypercapnia, and hypertension.[33,35] Butorphanol has been administered to antagonize respiratory depressive effects in white rhino (10–20:1 mg butorphanol to etorphine ratio); however, it may also lighten

---

BOX 55-1 Standing Chemical Restraint Doses for Adult Captive Rhinoceros[22,33,35]

Black Rhino
- 0.5–0.85 milligram (mg) etorphine, intramuscularly (IM)
- Doses as low as 0.25 mg used to walk rhino into crate
- 25–50 mg butorphanol, IM or intravenously (IV)
- 20–30 mg butorphanol + 20–50 mg detomidine, IM

White Rhino
- 0.8–1.5 mg etorphine, IM
- 50–70 mg butorphanol + 100 mg azaperone, IM
- 1.1 mg etorphine + 5 mg acepromazine + 15 mg detomidine + 15 mg butorphanol, IM
- 120–150 mg butorphanol + 5–7 mg medetomidine, IM (give 1–2 mg nalorphine, IV, to keep standing)

Indian Rhino
- 100 mg butorphanol + 100 mg azaperone, IM
- 0.5–1.5 mg etorphine, IM

Sumatran Rhino
- 25–40 mg butorphanol, IM
- 120–150 mg butorphanol + 5–7 mg medetomidine, IM (use 1–2 mg nalorphine, IV to keep standing)
- 0.8–1.5 mg etorphine, IM

BOX 55-2 Recumbent Immobilizing Doses for Adult Captive Rhinoceros[5,22,33–35,41]

Black Rhino
- 1.5–2 mg etorphine + 2–3 milligrams (mg) medetomidine, intramuscularly (IM)
- 2.5–3 mg etorphine + 20–60 mg azaperone, IM
- 1.5–2mg etorphine + 2–3 mg medetomidine + 1 gram per liter (g/L) ketamine in 5% guaifenisen drip
- 0.7–1.2 mg carfentanil ±10 mg midazolam
- 70–120 mg butorphanol + 100–160 mg azaperone, IM
- 120–150 mg butorphanol + 5–7 mg medetomidine, IM

White Rhino
- 1.2 mg carfentanil, IM
- 2–3 mg etorphine + 20–40 mg azaperone, IM
- 120–150 mg butorphanol + 5–7 mg medetomidine, IM ± 5% guaifenisen drip
- 70–120 mg butorphanol + 100–160 mg azaperone, IM

Indian Rhino
- 3.5–3.8 mg etorphine + 14 mg detomidine + 400 mg ketamine, IM
- 2.5 mg etorphine + 10 mg acepromazine, IM
- 0.7–1 mg carfentanil, IM
- 120 mg butorphanol + 80 mg detomidine, IM

Sumatran Rhino
- 30–50 mg butorphanol + 50–60 mg azaperone, IM
- 1 mg etorphine + 60 mg azaperone, IM
- 10 mg butorphanol + 10 mg detomidine IM, wait 20 min then 1.2 mg etorphine + 5 mg acepromazine, IM

the plane of anesthesia.[21] It should be used with caution in black rhinos, since they appear to be more sensitive and may suddenly get to their feet.[35] Other partial opioid agonist–antagonists are routinely used in the field and may be adapted for captive rhinos, when available (e.g., nalbuphine). Butorphanol–azaperone and butorphanol–medetomidine or detomidine combinations have successfully induced recumbency in captive Sumatran, Indian, and white rhinos.[34,35,41]

Oxygen supplementation by intratracheal intubation or nasal insufflation (flow rates of 15–30 liters per minute [L/min]) may increase oxygen saturation values.[24] Doxapram has been administered for apnea in rhinos but may only provide short-term relief. Partial or complete reversal should be considered in severe cases of hypoxia.

On some occasions other than medical procedures, rhinos may need to be sedated, as for crating and transport. For short-duration tranquilization or sedation, benzodiazepines (2–6 hours; adult doses: midazolam 5–50 mg, IM; diazepam 10–30 mg, IM) and azaperone (2–4 hours; 80–200 mg, IM) are useful choices in rhinos. Long-acting neuroleptics (LANs) are typically administered in free-ranging rhinos after capture for transport and boma acclimation, although they have also been used in captive rhinos for longer-duration tranquilization. Zuclopenthixol acetate (Clopixol-Acuphase) at doses of 60 to 200 mg lasts 3 days, and perphenazine enanthate (Trilafon-LA) does not take effect for 12 to 18 hours but lasts 7 to 10 days (100–200 mg, IM).[5]

SURGERY

Most surgical procedures involve the skin, eyes, digits, and horn, including treatments for corneal ulcers, cataracts, pododermatitis, wounds, and tumors. Because of the thickness and inelasticity of the rhino skin, suturing of wounds often results in dehiscence, so unless necessary, wounds are often left to heal by secondary intention. Use of wire sutures, stents, and mattress patterns may improve closure of the rhino skin. Surgical management of horn and integument problems, including tumors, may be achieved with the use of operant conditioning, standing sedation, or full immobilization.

Surgical treatment of ocular problems, including corneal ulcers and cataracts, is fairly common. Management of pododermatitis by surgical debridement has also become a more routine procedure, especially in Indian rhinos. Treatment of osteomyelitis in a black rhino, involving surgical debridement and vacuum-assisted closure, has been recently described.[16] Surgical repairs of rectal prolapse in black and Indian rhinos and patent urachus in a white rhino calf have been reported. Although most abdominal surgeries are unsuccessful, an adult white rhino has survived an exploratory celiotomy.[40] Laparoscopic techniques for rhinos are still in their developmental stages but have been successfully used for reproductive procedures such as uterine biopsy and oocyte retrieval.[18]

OTHER PHARMACEUTICALS

With the exception of studies on anesthetics and a few vaccines, no pharmacokinetic trials in rhinos have been performed. Most clinicians use the horse as the model to determine drug dosages, especially for antibiotics and antiparasitics. Commonly used antibiotics include oral trimethoprim–sulfadiazine equine formulations, parenteral large-animal cephalosporins, and oral fluoroquinolones. Antiparasitics are not routinely required in captive rhinos, but oral and injectable ivermectin; oral fenbendazole, pyrantel pamoate, and niclosamide; and pour-on acaricides, including flumethrin 0.5%, have been used in rhinos.[22] Nonsteroidal anti-inflammatories are frequently prescribed for analgesia.

PHYSICAL EXAMINATION AND DIAGNOSTICS

Rhinos should be trained to permit sample collection and clinical examination. Resting values for heart rate, respiratory rate, temperature, and other values have been obtained for nonrestrained black and white rhinos. The various species appear to be similar with regard to heart rates (30–40 beats per minute) and respiratory rates (6–12 breaths per minute). Rectal temperatures are typically 34.5° C to 37.5° C, although temperatures may be higher in anesthetized rhinos (37° C–39° C) because of exertion or muscle tremors.[22,35] Limited information on electrocardiography (ECG) values in rhinos is available.[19] Indirect blood pressure has been measured in unsedated black and white rhinos by using a human blood pressure cuff around the base of the tail. Mean values reported for unanesthetized white rhinos are 160 +/−2.9 millimeters of mercury (mm Hg; systolic), 104 +/−2.3 mm Hg (diastolic), and 124 +/−2.2 mm Hg (mean blood pressure).[6] In anesthetized animals, etorphine may cause hypertension, but some authors have observed more variable mean blood pressure values (107–280 mm Hg) depending on the drugs used and when measurements were taken.

Hematologic and biochemical parameters have been published (Tables 55-1 through 55-3).[14,22] Although most values may be interpreted as being similar to other perissodactyls, total protein and globulins tend to be higher and sodium and chloride lower than in domestic horses. Hypophosphatemia (low blood phosphorus) is a recognized problem in captive black rhinos, with levels dropping below 1 milligram per deciliter (mg/dL). Low serum phosphorus has been linked to hemolytic anemia and other blood disorder syndromes.[10,22] Supplemental doses of elemental phosphorus (preferably chelated) (10 to 24 g, orally [PO], once daily [SID]) are used in black rhinos until normal serum levels are reestablished, as reported anecdotally (Valdes E, personal communication). In critical cases, intravenous sodium or potassium phosphate may be administered at 14.5 millimoles per hour (mmol/hr), but serum calcium should be carefully monitored.

Venipuncture may be routinely performed on awake captive rhinos with the use of conditioning of the animal, restraint devices, or both. The most commonly used sites for blood collection are the auricular vein, radial vein (inside the forelimb crossing the carpus), and metacarpal vein (lower inside forelimb). The ventral tail (coccygeal) vein has also been used, particularly in Sumatran rhinos, and the blood collection technique is similar to that used in domestic cattle. Arterial access is available for blood gas sampling from the medial auricular artery. Rhino blood cells resemble those of domestic horses. Nucleated red blood cells (RBCs) and reticulocytes may be observed in anemic animals. Blood smears should be carefully screened for the presence of hemoparasites, especially in recently captured or imported animals.

Urinalysis panels in captive rhinos are similar to those for horses, with the large numbers of calcium carbonate crystals creating a normal milky yellow appearance of urine. Calcium oxalate, phosphate, and ammonium crystals may also occur, depending on the diet. Occasionally, dark discoloration of urine, which is associated with the pigmentation of certain browse species, may be mistaken for blood or myoglobin (e.g., ash, mulberry). Normal values for the different rhino species have been published and typically are pH of 8.0 to 8.7 and specific gravities of 1.010 to 1.030.[15]

Because of the rhino's size, cerebrospinal fluid (CSF) collection has not been successful except in a few rhino calves.[22] Therefore, extrapolation of normal values from domestic horses and other perissodactyls should be used for interpretation.

Incorporation of scales into rhino facilities has permitted monitoring of body weights and physical condition. Average ranges for adult body weights for each of the rhino species are as follows: black rhino 800–1350 kg, white rhino 1800–2200 kg, Indian rhino 1800–2200 kg, and Sumatran rhino 600–800 kg.[22]

Radiography of the distal extremities, skull, horn, and, in calves, thorax has become more routine and useful with digital technology. Thermography is also available in many institutions. Localization of inflammation associated with acute lameness, laminitis, abscesses, and changes in skin temperature associated with dermatologic conditions may all be detected by using this tool. Fluoroscopy has also been used for skull and horn imaging to

TABLE 55-1

Mean Hematology Values in Rhinos (±SD)[14]

Parameter	Black Rhino	White Rhino	Indian Rhino	Sumatran Rhino
White blood cell (WBC) × 10³/microliter (µL)	8.42 (2.48)	9.30 (2.46)	7.20 (1.33)	8.27 (1.55)
Red blood cell (RBC) ×10⁶/µL	4.01 (0.88)	5.77 (1.28)	6.43 (0.86)	5.32 (1.09)
Hemoglobin, gram per deciliter (g/dL)	12.0 (2.0)	13.8 (3.8)	13.4 (1.5)	12.4 (1.6)
Hematocrit %	33.4 (5.7)	36.9 (9.3)	37.0 (4.6)	36.9 (4.2)
Mean corpuscular volume, (fL)	85.7 (9.0)	63.8 (7.8)	57.8 (4.9)	71.5 (11.2)
Mean corpuscular hemoglobin, picogram per cell (pg/cell)	30.5 (3.3)	23.5 (1.9)	21.3 (3.0)	23.9 (3.8)
Mean corpuscular hemoglobin concentration (g/dL)	35.7 (2.7)	37.9 (7.3)	36.3 (3.2)	33.5 (2.1)
Platelets ×10³/µL	284 (83)	378 (103)	178 (53)	198 (135)
Nucleated RBC/100 WBC	0	1 (1)	0	—
Reticulocytes %	1.6 (2.9)	—	—	—
Neutrophils ×10³/milliliter (mL)	5.24 (2.18)	5.42 (2.05)	5.13 (1.24)	4.86 (1.16)
Lymphocytes ×10³/mL	2.48 (1.1)	2.35 (1.15)	1.74 (0.67)	2.52 (0.90)
Monocytes ×10³/mL	0.43 (0.32)	0.65 (0.55)	0.22 (0.15)	0.36 (0.22)
Eosinophils ×10³/mL	0.25 (0.22)	0.54 (0.59)	0.32 (0.31)	0.37 (0.21)
Basophils ×10³/mL	0.17 (0.09)	0.10 (0.05)	0.13 (0.05)	0.08 (0.01)
Neutrophilic bands ×10³/mL	0.27 (0.35)	0.71 (1.18)	0.22 (0.20)	0.31 (0.24)

TABLE 55-2

Mean Blood Chemistry Values in Rhinos (±SD)[14]

Parameter	Black Rhino	White Rhino	Indian Rhino	Sumatran Rhino
BUN (mg/dL)	13 (3)	16 (3)	3 (2)	6 (2)
Creatinine (mg/dL)	1.1 (0.2)	1.8 (0.4)	1.3 (0.2)	0.9 (0.1)
Uric acid (mg/dL)	0.5 (0.2)	0.9 (0.8)	0.3 (0.2)	—
Bilirubin (mg/dL)	0.3 (0.1)	0.3 (0.3)	0.4 (0.3)	0.2 (0.1)
Glucose (mg/dL)	69 (21)	97 (39)	82 (25)	76 (13)
Cholesterol (mg/dL)	102 (37)	93 (26)	53 (21)	48 (21)
CPK (IU/L)	255 (248)	409 (722)	260 (203)	617 (398)
LDH (IU/L)	595 (427)	537 (320)	267 (149)	231 (38)
Alkaline Phosphatase (IU/L)	80 (55)	92 (51)	80 (41)	17 (6)
ALT (IU/L)	16 (7)	16 (9)	7 (7)	6 (3)
AST (IU/L)	85 (27)	71 (25)	61 (27)	39 (9)
GGT (IU/L)	27 (18)	19 (14)	18 (16)	6 (2)
Total protein (g/dL)	7.6 (0.9)	8.5 (1.0)	7.5 (0.9)	7.5 (0.4)
Globulin (g/dL) (electrophoresis)	4.9 (0.9)	5.3 (0.8)	4.5 (0.7)	3.8 (0.7)
Albumin (g/dL) (electrophoresis)	2.6 (0.4)	3.2 (0.5)	2.9 (0.5)	3.6 (0.6)
Fibrinogen (mg/dL)	104 (195)	101 (241)	350 (84)	324 (85)

ALT, Alanine aminotransferase; *AST*, aspartate aminotransferase; *BUN*, blood urea nitrogen; *CPK*, creatine phosphokinase; *GGT*, gamma-glutamyltransferase; *g/dL*, gram per deciliter; *IU/L*, international unit per liter; *LDH*, lactate dehydrogenase; *mg/dL*, milligram per deciliter.

detect dental, jaw, and horn problems, including fractures and neoplasia.

DISEASES

Infectious Diseases

Mycobacterium bovis and *M. tuberculosis* have caused infections in captive rhinos.[22] Although not currently reported in free-ranging rhinos, *M. bovis* infection was recently reported in a black rhino brought into captivity in South Africa.[12] Initial infection may be asymptomatic or result in progressive weight loss and emaciation, with coughing and dyspnea occurring in the terminal stages. Nasal discharge may be present but is inconsistent. Most infections are pulmonary. Antemortem testing includes intradermal tuberculin test, tracheal lavage, gastric lavage, or both for mycobacterial culture, and serologic tests. Retrospective analyses of sera from *M. tuberculosis*-infected black rhinos, with the use of ElephantTB Stat-Pak (Chembio Diagnostic Systems Inc., Medford, NY), have shown positive results.[11] Treatment with isoniazid, rifampin, ethambutol, and pyrazidamide has been attempted. However, assessment of a successful response is limited.

Mycobacterium avium subspecies *paratuberculosis* has recently been isolated from a wild-caught black rhino with diarrhea and

TABLE 55-3

Mean Serum Mineral Values and Blood Gases in Rhinos (±SD)[14]

Parameter	Black Rhino	White Rhino	Indian Rhino	Sumatran Rhino
Calcium (mg/dL)	12.7 (1.0)	11.8 (0.9)	11.4 (0.8)	13.3 (1.1)
Phosphorus (mg/dL)	4.8 (1.1)	4.0 (0.9)	4.0 (0.9)	3.7 (0.7)
Sodium (mEq/L)	133 (3)	134 (5)	132 (3)	133 (4)
Potassium (mEq/L)	4.7 (0.6)	4.7 (0.8)	4.1 (0.4)	4.6 (0.6)
Chloride (mEq/L)	96 (0.3)	95 (4)	91 (3)	100 (3)
Bicarbonate mEq/L	23.3 (4.2)	18 (0)	27.0 (0)	—
Carbon dioxide (mEq/L)	25.4 (9.9)	25.3 (8.8)	27.3 (3.7)	22.8 (2.4)
Iron (µg/dL)	227 (66)	176 (67)	152 (70)	—
Magnesium (mg/dL)	3.34 (3.45)	118.2 (232.5)	7.95 (8.56)	—

mEq/L, Milliequivalent per liter; *mg/dL*, milligram per deciliter; *µg/dL*, microgram per deciliter.

weight loss. After a course of antimycobacterial drugs, clinical signs resolved, and fecal cultures were negative.[4]

Salmonella infection may cause enteritis and fatal septicemia in captive and newly captured wild rhinos. In a retrospective survey of captive black, white, and Indian rhinos in the United States, 11% demonstrated positive cultures, usually associated with clinical signs. Research has shown that asymptomatic black rhinos may carry and intermittently shed *Salmonella* in their feces.[23] Clinical infection may occur secondary to transport, changes in diet, immobilization, concurrent disease, or exposure to a large number of organisms. Lethargy, anorexia, signs of colic, diarrhea, and death may be observed. Successful treatment using trimethoprim–sulfamethoxazole and supportive care is possible if initiated early. However, treatment of asymptomatic animals is not recommended.

Leptospirosis usually presents with depression and anorexia. Other signs may include hemolytic anemia (not present in all cases), hemoglobinuria, colic, and development of skin ulcers. Abortion has also been linked to infection with leptospirosis in an Indian rhino.[22] Fatality rates are high in clinically affected black rhinos, although successful treatment with trimethoprim–sulfamethaxozole and ceftiofur has been reported.[29] Diagnosis is based on high antibody titers (microagglutination test [MAT]) and confirmed by detection of leptospiral organisms in urine or tissues (through immunofluorescent antibody [IFA] test or, more recently, polymerase chain reaction [PCR] test). Low levels of antibodies have been observed in free-ranging and nonvaccinated black rhinos without evidence of disease. Preventive measures include annual vaccination of black and possibly Indian rhinos with a multivalent large animal product, rodent and wildlife control programs, and good husbandry to minimize contamination of feed and water.

Fatal gastroenteritis caused by *Clostridium* infection has occurred in adult white rhinos. Neosporosis has also been documented in a white rhino calf.[42] Colitis of unknown etiology and secondary endotoxic shock led to the death of an adult black rhino. *Escherichia coli*, *Campylobacter coli*, and *Pseudomonas* sp. have caused enteritis in hand-reared rhinos.

Encephalomyocarditis virus (EMCV) infection usually results in acute death from myocarditis. Diagnosis is usually based on isolation of the virus from heart, spleen, or other tissues at necropsy. Prevention should target rodent control in endemic areas.

Fungal pneumonia is usually caused by *Aspergillus* sp. and is primarily observed in black rhinos that have had concurrent disease and broad-spectrum antibiotic or corticosteroid therapy. Clinical signs may include weakness, weight loss, epistaxis, or other signs consistent with pneumonia. Diagnosis is challenging, although serology and bronchoscopy, with cytology and fungal culture, may be useful. Long-term treatment with antifungal drugs (e.g., itraconazole) is expensive and has unknown efficacy.

Death caused by anthrax has been observed in wild rhinos and has been implicated in a die-off of several Javan rhinos in the Ujon Kulan National Park. Most cases result in sudden death. Foamy discharge from the mouth and nostrils may be seen and can appear similar to EMCV infection. Diagnosis is based on identification of anthrax bacilli in blood or tissue smears. Vaccination of ranched rhinos has been used in some endemic areas of Africa, since rhinos have been infrequently affected during outbreaks. Black rhino in the Etosha National Park, Namibia, have been vaccinated for more than 30 years.[39]

Isolated cases of rabies and tetanus have been documented in rhinos.[22] Antibodies to West Nile virus (WNV) have been detected in black, white, and Indian rhinos in endemic areas of the United States. Black rhinos and Indian rhinos have been vaccinated with a commercial equine product without any apparent adverse effects. In the author's limited experience, black rhinos appear to develop some humoral response to vaccination, although in one study, Indian rhinos did not develop significant titers. Infections with eastern equine encephalitis virus (EEEV), western equine encephalitis virus (WEEV), or Venezuelan equine encephalitis virus (VEEV) have not been reported in any of the rhino species.

Antibodies to African horse sickness, Akabane, bluetongue, epizootic hemorrhagic disease of deer (EHD), Wesselbron, and Rift Valley fever viruses have been detected during serosurveys of free-ranging African rhinos, although no association with disease has been established.[20,22]

Parasitic Diseases of Rhinoceroses

Internal Parasites

A variety of parasites, including nematodes (*Chabertia*, *Necator*, *Bunostomum* spp.), trematodes (*Paramphistomum* sp.), cestodes (*Anoplocephala* sp., hydatid cyst), and protozoa (*Balantidium coli*), have been found in wild-caught Indian rhinos. *Balantidium* has also been reported in white rhino.[31] Larvae of *Gyrostigma* sp., the rhinoceros bot fly, are commonly found in the stomachs of free-ranging black rhinos. Over 40 species of helminths have been identified in African rhinos, the majority being nematodes. Although most are asymptomatic, some such as *Diceronema versterae* may cause tumorlike lesions in the stomach. The most abundant species is a small pinworm, *Probstmayria*, found in the cecum and colon of black rhinos.[31] Trematodes and cestodes (*Anoplocephala* sp.) are also found in African rhinos. Tapeworms, coccidia, and, occasionally, strongyles are found in captive rhinos, although they are rarely a cause of disease.

Tsetse flies transmit trypanosomes that may lead to serious consequences, such as fatal infection or abortion, in naïve black and white rhinos that are translocated from a tsetse-free area.[31] Hemoparasites (*Babesia bicornis*, *Theileria bicornis*, *Theileria equi*) have been observed in free-ranging African rhinos. *T. equi* is relatively common in white rhinos, but neither *Theileria* sp. appear to cause disease. However, *B. bicornis* and *T. bicornis* have been associated with increased mortality in black rhinos stressed by capture and transport.[30]

External Parasites

Skin ulcers in free-ranging black rhinos have been associated with a filarial parasite, *Stephanofilaria dinniki*, presumed to be transmitted by a blood-sucking arthropod. Recently, an outbreak of filariasis in both white and black rhinos occurred in the Meru National Park, Kenya, and lesions resolved after treatment with ivermectin and long-acting amoxicillin.[26]

In free-ranging African rhinos, tick infestation is common and includes *Rhipicephalus*, *Dermacentor*, *Ambylomma*, and *Hyalomma* species. Since these ticks are vectors for a number of diseases, treatment of recently captured or newly imported rhinos with acaricides is usually required for movement.

Noninfectious Diseases

Injuries such as skin lacerations, punctures, abrasions, and other wounds are common in both captive and free-ranging rhinos. Common sense application of wound treatment principles apply, although the thick skin of the rhino does not lend itself to primary closure, and abscesses have a tendency to undermine the integument along fascial planes.

Horn avulsion, cracks, or other trauma may be self-induced as a result of acute or chronic rubbing, damage from the enclosure, or intraspecific fighting. Laminitis and neoplasia may also affect the horn. Treatment may involve debridement, antibiotics, wound treatment, and fly control. Dermatitis, especially in Indian and Sumatran rhinos, may be caused by inadequate access to wallows and pools. Exfoliative dermatitis has been reported in a captive white rhino. *Malassezia pachydermatis* and *Candida parapsilosis* were identified in black rhino with dermatitis and successfully treated using natamycin solution.

Neoplasia is relatively uncommon in rhinos. Cases of squamous cell carcinoma (various locations) in white, black, and Indian rhinos, cutaneous melanoma in black and Indian rhinos, and isolated cases of thyroid carcinoma, hepatocellular carcinoma, and acute lymphoblastic leukemia in black rhinos have been reported.

Although all species of rhino are susceptible to developing pododermatitis caused by inappropriate substrate, long-term indoor housing in northern climes, limited access to a pool, or other husbandry conditions in captivity, the Indian rhino appears to be more susceptible to chronic foot problems.[1] Management of the condition includes improvements in husbandry and in medical and surgical interventions. Medical treatment may be in the form of oral antimicrobial medication and topical use of copper sulfate and oxytetracycline. Regular hoof trimming and surgical debridement of necrotic lesions, along with use of collagen products for granulation tissue stimulation, may lead to improvement in appearance and comfort of the animal. In addition to the factors mentioned above, nutritional imbalances (e.g., zinc) have also been investigated. Black rhinos develop laminitis that may or may not be related to idiopathic hemorrhagic vasculopathy syndrome (IHVS). Frequent foot trimmings, analgesics, and antibiotics are needed to manage this condition, as with laminitis in domestic horses.

Corneal trauma and secondary infection may result in corneal ulceration and perforation. Corneal ulcers may become severe in Indian rhinos. Surgical management of a melting corneal ulcer with the use of a conjunctival graft has been described in one case. Exposure keratitis is a relatively common problem for captive Sumatran rhinos. Medical and surgical treatments are similar to those for equine corneal conditions.

Noninfectious causes of GI problems in rhinos may be a result of dental problems, dietary changes, dehydration, ingestion of foreign material (i.e., sand), changes in GI motility because of inflammation, neoplasia, or inadequate dietary fiber. Gastric ulcers have been observed on gastroscopy and at necropsy in rhinos that have received long-term nonsteroidal anti-inflammatory therapy, have concurrent disease, or are undergoing a stressful condition. Gastroprotectants such as omeprazole, histamine 2 (H_2)-blockers, or sucralfate have been used in rhinos both prophylactically and therapeutically, although treatment depends on a specific diagnosis.

Since 2001, chronic glomerulonephritis, renal failure, or both have been recognized as a contributing cause of death in at least seven black rhinos. Significant changes in blood urea nitrogen (BUN)

and creatinine values or in urinalysis were not always evident in these cases, making diagnosis difficult until necropsy. In contrast, two white rhinos (aged >40 years) developed progressive chronic renal failure characterized by uremia, isosthenuria, and hypercalcemia. Nutritional management with the use of a high-energy, low-protein feed (Equine Senior, Purina Mills, St. Louis, MO) appeared to stabilize both animals (Ferrell S, Radcliffe R, personal communication).

Toxicities

Seven fatalities occurred among a group of 20 black rhinos captured and housed in bomas constructed with creosote-treated wood in Zimbabwe. The presumptive cause of death was liver dysfunction caused by creosote toxicosis. Exposure of all rhino species to creosote-treated housing materials should be avoided. Free-ranging white rhinos have succumbed to blue-green algae toxicity (*Microcystis* spp.). Periodic algal blooms occur in water bodies with high organic matter and low water levels following dry summers and abnormally warm falls in the Kruger National Park.

Three black rhinos died from suspected vitamin D toxicosis caused by an accidental incorporation of high levels of vitamin D in the commercial black rhino pellet.[13] Caution should be used when treating with high dosages of cocciodiostats such as salinomycin, which have been reportedly toxic to rhinos.[22] An apparent adverse drug reaction to firocoxib in a white rhino resulted in a generalized vesiculobullous dermatitis.[37] Food items to be avoided in rhino diets include kale, onions, red maple (*Acer rubrum*), and members of *Brassica* plants because of their predisposition to cause hemolysis.[22]

Diseases of Unknown Etiology in Black Rhinos

Skin disease may be the most common health problem in black rhinos, with over 50% having at least one episode during their lifetime. Several distinct syndromes have been reported in captive rhinos.

Superficial necrolytic dermatopathy has also been called *ulcerative skin disease*, *vesicular* or *ulcerative dermatopathy*, and *mucosal* or *cutaneous ulcerative syndrome*.[25] Initial signs are epidermal plaques or vesicles that progress to ulcers, often over the pressure points, ear margins, coronary bands, and tail tip. Oral or nasal ulcers may develop concurrently. The affected rhinos may also be anorexic, depressed, and lame, have oral or nasal bleeding, and lose weight. These animals may have decreased albumin and hematocrits. In most cases, the skin lesions are associated with other concurrent health issues, including GI and respiratory diseases. Management includes symptomatic treatment. If the lesions become extensive, the condition may be fatal. Treatment with cryotherapy and steroids has been successful. Lesions may resolve spontaneously.

Eosinophilic granuloma syndrome usually presents with oral and nasal nonhealing ulcers and granulomas, which may lead to epistaxis or oral bleeding.[32] Cytology shows a predominance of eosinophils associated with lysis of collagen and mineralization. Although the lesions may resolve spontaneously, usually over 1 to 7 months, they may recur. Treatment has included the administration of corticosteroids, local cryotherapy, or laser therapy. Eosinophilic granulomas in wild rhinos are typically associated with *Stephanofilaria dinniki*.

A rare single case of primary vitiligo has been reported in a black rhino. The condition began around the nares at 2 years of age and progressed to include multiple areas without any evidence of other syndromes.[38]

All rhino species appear to accumulate dental tartar in captivity, especially if they are not given access to hard or coarse food items. However, black rhinos appear to develop severe proliferative gingivitis, not always directly associated with the degree of accumulation of calculus.[2,39] Like horses, rhinos also develop dental points that may eventually create clinical problems with prehension as they age and require periodic dental floats.

Cases of hemolytic anemia in the captive black rhino population appear to be decreasing since the peak occurrence in the 1990s. Of the 47 known occurrences, a high mortality rate (75%) was observed among the 39 animals that had been affected.[6] Possible etiologies include a hereditary deficiency of glucose-6-phosphate dehydrogenase (G-6-PD) leading to decreased RBC adenosine triphosphate (ATP) levels, hypophosphatemia, and hypovitaminosis E.[22] Leptospirosis is a known cause of hemolytic anemia in this species but was not associated with all cases. Management of this syndrome includes intravenous or oral supplementation of phosphorus, supplementation of vitamin E, prophylactic antibiotics for secondary infections, and whole blood transfusion in severe cases.

IHVS in black rhinos is characterized by severe limb, facial, and neck swelling associated with a nonhemolytic anemia. Additional signs include lethargy, respiratory stridor, laminitis and nail sloughing, aural hematomas (swelling of the ears), and oral or skin ulcers. The syndrome presents acutely without any known cause, and recurrent episodes are likely. The fatality rate is high, but a number of animals have recovered with antibiotic and nonsteroidal anti-inflammatory therapy with fatty acid and phosphorus supplementation, and topical treatment of lesions. Between 1995 and 2007, 13 black rhinos were documented to have been affected, often with recurrent episodes. The majority of cases occurred during the cooler months (October–March) in animals that lived in Texas or the southern United States. It has been proposed that the syndrome is an immune-mediated vasculitis, similar to equine purpura hemorrhagica. A possible association with *Streptococcus* sp. infection has been observed. Treatment is supportive.

Iron storage disorder (ISD) results in significantly higher tissue iron and serum ferritin levels in captive black and Sumatran rhinos than those measured in wild or recently captured animals. Levels appear to increase with time in captivity. In contrast, values for ferritin and tissue iron do not appear to be elevated in captive white or Indian rhinos.[8,22] Although hemolytic anemia, vitamin E deficiency, and hereditary disorders have all been proposed as potential causes, it is now believed to be related to dietary factors in the captive browser species. Hemosiderosis (tissue iron accumulation) is a common finding in multiple organs in black rhinos, although inflammation and lesions associated with these changes are infrequently observed (hemochromatosis). A recent fatality in a captive Sumatran rhino was associated with multi-organ hemochromatosis. Recommendations to minimize accumulation and reduce iron load include low iron diets, provision of browse, therapeutic phlebotomy (regular large-volume blood collection), and treatment with iron-chelating agents in those individuals with suspected clinical disease.

Leukoencephalomalacia, a severe neurologic disease caused by necrosis of the cerebrum, was diagnosed in four female black rhino calves; three became comatose within 1 to 7 days of signs and eventually died. Some investigators hypothesize that the cause may be related to dam age (mean 17.3 years) or excessive maternal iron.[22] Research has focused on possible congenital or hereditary causes of encephalomalacia. No known treatment exists.

REPRODUCTION

Female Anatomy and Reproduction

Specific reproductive parameters are provided in Table 55-4.[18,22] The female reproductive anatomy is similar in all species, with a bicornuate uterus, which has a short body and long tubular horns. Ovaries are found caudal to the kidneys but typically cranial to the last rib. The cervix is a thick, fibrous structure containing a complex system of folds. Wrinkling of the vagina may make visualization of the cervical os difficult. A hymen may be present in nonbred females. Two mammary glands are positioned in the inguinal region.

Estrus cycles are variable among the species, with the longest occurring in the Indian rhino at 43 to 48 days, although the white rhino has been reported to have cycle lengths of 31 to 35 or 66 to 70, which may be caused by fetal resorption.[18] Ovarian activity and pregnancy may be monitored with transrectal ultrasonography and fecal, urinary, or serum hormone assays. Because of the risk of fetal resorption, early pregnancy should be confirmed starting at 2 weeks with ultrasonography. Embryonic vesicles may be visualized as early as 15 days following ovulation. Late pregnancy may be monitored with transabdominal ultrasonography of the flank region. Early embryonic loss has been documented in wild and captive black, white, and Sumatran rhinos.[18] Black and Sumatran rhinos have been successfully treated for early fetal resorption with oral progestin.

Although dystocia is relatively uncommon in rhinos, it does occur in all captive species.[18] If dystocia occurs, oxytocin (100 IU) may be effective if no signs of labor are observed for 4 to 6 hours after rupture of fetal membranes. Otherwise a fetotomy is indicated and has been successfully performed. Cesarean section is not an option in rhinos.

Signs of impending birth include increase in teat size and mild vaginal prolapse up to 30 days prior to calving. Dramatic changes in mammary size, restlessness, change in appetite, and relaxation of

TABLE 55-4

Reproductive Parameters in Rhinoceros[18,22]

	Black Rhino	White Rhino	Indian Rhino	Sumatran Rhino
Age at Puberty*	F: 4–7 years M: 7–10 years	F: 6–7 years M: 10–12 years	F: 5–7 years M: 10 years M	F&M: 7–8 years
Estrus cycle	21–27 days	31–35 or 66–70 days	43–48 days	21–25 days
Gestation length	465–475 days	485–518 days	462–489 days	475–510 days
Intercalving interval	2.5–4 years	2–3 years	3 years	3–4 years
Estrus determination†	Ultrasonography – ovulatory follicle (5.0 cm)	Ultrasonography – ovulatory follicle (3.2–3.5 cm)	Ultrasonography – ovulatory follicle (10–12 cm)	Ultrasonography – ovulatory follicle (2–2.5 cm)
Pregnancy diagnosis	Urine: PdG, second half of gestation, pregnanetriols Fecal: 20 α-protagestagen and 20 keto-protagestagen after 60 days; PdG last half of gestation	Urine: PdG Fecal: pregnanetriols, progesterone	Urine: PdG after 3 months	Fecal: progesterone

*In captivity, onset of puberty may be earlier; 3.5–5.5 years in females and 5.5–9 years in males.
†Specific urinary, fecal, and serum hormone assays have been developed to detect pregnancy in each rhino species.
PdG, Pregnanediol-glucuronide.

pelvic ligaments may be observed within 48 hours of birth. Calving should occur rapidly (1–3 hours) with the placenta passed within 6 to 7 hours.[18]

Reproductive system problems are relatively common in captive rhinos. Disorders occur with greater frequency in nulliparous females and increase with age.[18] Ovarian and paraovarian cysts have been diagnosed with ultrasonography in white rhinos. Black and white rhinos typically have cystic hyperplasia of the uterus, and Asian species have neoplastic changes. Leiomyomas are the most common tumor found in these species, although adenoma and adenocarcinoma have also been reported in white rhinos.

Assisted reproduction has advanced rapidly in rhinos. The ability to induce ovulation, time artificial insemination (AI), and use both fresh and cryopreserved semen has resulted in the conception of seven rhinos by AI, with five live births.[18] With the use of in vitro fertilization technology, the first rhino embryo has been produced.[17]

Male Anatomy and Reproduction

Testes are located along the dorsal preputial fold either adjacent to the inguinal rings or with the caudal aspect protruding between the rear legs and positioned horizontally in the body. The scrotum is more obvious in the Asian species. Accessory sex glands in male rhinos are similar in all four species and include vesicular glands, bulbourethral glands, and a prostate.[18] The penis is curved backward unless erect which allows urination for territorial marking. Lateral projections are found on the glans penis. Semen collection attempts in rhinos have been historically inconsistent, although development of a rhino-specific probe has resulted in more reliable results by electroejaculation.[36] Rhino semen characteristics for all four species have been published.[18] Techniques for cryopreservation of semen from white, Sumatran, and Indian rhinos have been successfully developed and used for AI.

The penis may be traumatized by injuries from mating or masturbation. Testicular fibrosis is a common finding in older males and may be detected by ultrasonography as hyperechoic spots, although it typically does not cause changes in semen quality. Testicular neoplasia, typically seminoma, has been observed in black and white rhinos and may be diagnosed with ultrasonography and biopsy. Hemicastration may be curative. Epididymal cysts (Sumatran and white rhinos), hematoma, or seroma may also be differentiated with ultrasonography and fine-needle aspiration. These conditions may have variable effects on sperm production.

PREVENTIVE MEDICINE

Annual vaccination for leptospirosis is recommended in black rhinos and possibly Indian rhinos. The animal should be observed for 30 minutes following vaccination because isolated cases of anaphylatic-like reactions have been reported. Vaccination for rabies, tetanus, arboviruses (EEEV/WEEV/WNV) may be considered if the area is considered endemic or increased risk factors are involved. Prior to vaccination, serologic screening for leptospirosis (multiple serovars), and WNV is recommended. Other vaccination regimens depend on regional requirements and exposure risks (consider multivalent vaccination for clostridial diseases).

ACKNOWLEDGMENT

The authors wish to thank their many colleagues, especially Drs. Scott Citino, Eric Miller, Pete Morkel, Robin Radcliffe, Terri Roth, and Eduardo Valdes, for providing information and advice used in the preparation of this manuscript.

REFERENCES

1. Atkinson MW, Hull B, Gandolf AR, et al: Long-term medical and surgical management of chronic pododermatitis in a Greater one-horned rhinoceros (*Rhinoceros unicornis*): A progress report. In Schwammer HM, editor: *Proceedings of the International Elephant and Rhino Research Symposium*, Vienna, Austria, 2002.
2. Beagley JC, Lowder MC, Langan JN, et al: Dental conditions of captive black rhinoceros (*Diceros bicornis*). In *Proceedings of the AAZV AAWV Joint Conference*, South Padre Island, TX, 2010, pp 138.
3. Blakeslee T, Zuba JR: Hand-rearing rhinoceroses. In Gage L, editor: *Hand-rearing wild and domestic mammals*, Ames, IA, 2002, Iowa State University Press.
4. Bryant B, Blyde D, Eamens G, et al: *Mycobacterium avium* subspecies *paratuberculosis* cultured from the feces of a Southern black rhinoceros (*Diceros bicornis minor*) with diarrhea and weight loss. *J Zoo Wildl Med* 43:391, 2012.
5. Burroughs R, Hofmeyr M, Morkel P, et al: Chemical immobilization—individual species requirements. In Kock MD, Burroughs R, editors: *Chemical and physical restraint of wild animals: A training and field manual for African species*, Greyton, South Africa, 2012, International Wildlife Veterinary Services.
6. Citino SB, Bush M: Reference for cardiopulmonary physiologic parameters for standing, unrestrained white rhinoceros (*Ceratotherium simum*). *J Zoo Wildl Med* 38:375, 2007.
7. Clauss M, Castell JC, Kienzle E, et al: Mineral absorption in the black rhinoceros (*Diceros bicornis*) as compared with the domestic horse. *J Anim Physiol Anim Nutr* 91:193, 2007.
8. Clauss M, Paglia DE: Iron storage disorders in captive wild mammals: The comparative evidence. *J Zoo Wildl Med* 43:S6, 2012.
9. Clauss M, Polster C, Kienzle E, et al: Energy and mineral nutrition and water intake in the captive Indian rhinoceros (*Rhinoceros unicornis*). *Zoo Biol* 24:1, 2005.
10. Dennis PM, Funk JA, Rajala-Schultz PJ, et al: A review of some of the health issues of captive black rhinoceroses (*Diceros bicornis*). *J Zoo Wildl Med* 38:509, 2007.
11. Duncan AE, Lyashchenko K, Greenwald R, et al: Application of Elephant TB STAT-PAK and MAPIA (multi-antigen print immunoassay) for detection of tuberculosis and monitoring of treatment in black rhinoceros (*Diceros bicornis*). *J Zoo Wildl Med* 40:781, 2009.
12. Espie IW, Hlokwe TM, Gey van Pittius NC, et al: Pulmonary infection due to *Mycobacterium bovis* in a black rhinoceros (*Diceros bicornis minor*) in South Africa. *J Wildl Dis* 45:1187, 2009.
13. Fleming GJ, Citino SB: Suspected vitamin D$_3$ toxicity in a group of black rhinoceros (*Diceros bicornis*). In *Proceedings of the AAZV, NAG Joint Conference*, Minneapolis, MN, 2003, pp 34.
14. Flesness N: *Normal hematological values*, Apple Valley, CA, 2002, International Species Inventory System.
15. Haffey MB, Pairan RD, Reinhart PR, et al: Urinalysis in three species of captive rhinoceros (*Rhinoceros unicornis, Dicerorhinus sumatrensis,* and *Diceros bicornis*). *J Zoo Wildl Med* 39:349, 2008.
16. Harrison TM, Stanley BJ, Sikarskie JG, et al: Surgical amputation of a digit and vacuum-assisted-closure (V.A.C.) management in a case of osteomyelitis and wound care in an eastern black rhinoceros (*Diceros bicornis michaeli*). *J Zoo Wild Med* 42:317, 2011.
17. Hermes R, Goritz F, Portas TJ, et al: Ovarian superstimulation, transrectal ultrasound-guided oocyte recovery, and IVF in rhinoceros. *Theriogenology* 72:959, 2009.
18. Hermes R, Hildebrandt TB: Rhinoceros theriogenology. In Miller RE, Fowler ME, editors: *Fowler's zoo and wild animal medicine: Current therapy*, ed 7, St. Louis, MO, 2012, Saunders.
19. Jayasinge JB, Silva V: Electrocardiographic study on the African black rhinoceros. *Br Vet J* 128:X, 1972.
20. Miller M, Buss P, Joubert J, et al: Serosurvey for selected viral agents in white rhinoceros (*Ceratotherium simum*) in Kruger National Park, 2007. *J Zoo Wildl Med* 42(29), 2011.
21. Miller M, Buss P, Joubert J, et al: Use of butorphanol during immobilization of free-ranging white rhinoceros (*Ceratotherium simum*). *J Zoo Wildl Med* 44:55, 2013.
22. Miller RE: Rhinoceridae (Rhinoceroses). In Fowler ME, Miller RE, editors: *Zoo and wild animal medicine*, ed 5, St. Louis, MO, 2003, Saunders.
23. Miller M, Schille B, Pancake C: *Salmonella* surveillance in a herd of asymptomatic captive black rhinoceros (*Diceros bicornis*) using fecal culture and PCR. *J Zoo Wildl Med* 39:56–60, 2008.

24. Morkel PvdB, Radcliffe RW, Jago M, et al: Acid-base balance and ventilation during sternal and lateral recumbency in field immobilized black rhinoceros (*Diceros bicornis*) receiving oxygen insufflation: A preliminary report. *J Wildl Dis* 46:236, 2010.

25. Munson L, Miller RE: Skin diseases of black rhinoceroses. In Fowler ME, Miller RE, editors: *Zoo and wild animal medicine*, ed 4, Philadelphia, PA, 1999, Saunders.

26. Mutinda M, Otiende M, Gakuya F, et al: Putative filariosis outbreak in white and black rhinoceros at Meru National Park in Kenya. *Parasit Vect* 5:206, 2012.

27. Mylniczenko ND, Sullivan KE, Corcoran ME, et al: Management strategies of iron accumulation in a captive population of black rhinoceroses (*Diceros bicornis minor*). *J Zoo Wildl Med* 43:S83, 2012.

28. Nardelli F: *The rhinoceros: A monograph*, London, U.K., 1988, Basilisk Press.

29. Neiffer DL, Klein EC, Wallace-Switalski C: *Leptospira* infection in two black rhinoceroses (*Diceros bicornis michaeli*). *J Zoo Wildl Med* 32:476, 2001.

30. Nijhof AM, Penzhorn BL, Lynen G, et al: *Babesia bicornis* sp. nov. and *Theileria bicornis* sp. nov.: Tick-borne parasites associated with mortality in the black rhinoceros (*Diceros bicornis*). *J Clin Microbiol* 41:2249, 2003.

31. Penzhorn BL, Krecek RC, Horak IG, et al: Parasites of African rhinos: A documentation. In Penzhorn BL, Kriek NPJ, editors: *Proceedings of the Symposium on Rhinos as Game Ranch Animals*, Pretoria, Republic of South Africa, 1994.

32. Pessier AP, Munson L, Miller RE: Oral, nasal, and cutaneous eosinophilic granulomas in the black rhinoceros (*Diceros bicornis*): A lesion distinct from superficial necrolytic dermatitis. *J Zoo Wildl Med* 35:1, 2004.

33. Portas TJ: A review of drugs and techniques used for sedation and anaesthesia in captive rhinoceros species. *Austr Vet J* 82:542, 2004.

34. Radcliffe RW, Citino SB, Dierenfeld ES, et al: *Intensive management and preventative medicine protocol for the Sumatran rhinoceros* (*Dicerorhinus sumatrensis*): *Scientific report prepared for the International Rhino Foundation*, Yulee, FL, 2002, International Rhino Foundation.

35. Radcliffe RW, Morkel PvdB: Rhinoceros anesthesia. In West G, Heard D, Caulkett N, editors: *Zoo animal and wildlife immobilization and anesthesia*, Ames, IA, 2007, Blackwell Publishing.

36. Roth TL, Stoops MA, Atkinson MW, et al: Semen collection in rhinoceroses (*Rhinoceros unicornis, Diceros bicornis, Ceratotherium simum*) by electroejaculation with a uniquely designed probe. *J Zoo Wildl Med* 36:617, 2005.

37. Stringer EM, DeVoe RS, Linder K, et al: Vesiculobullous skin reaction temporally related to firocoxib treatment in a white rhinoceros (*Ceratotherium simum*). *J Zoo Wildl Med* 43:186, 2012.

38. Takle GL, Suedmeyer WK, Garner MM: Vitiligo in a sub-adult eastern black rhinoceros (*Diceros bicornis michaeli*). In *Proceedings of the AAZV, AAWV, AZA/NAG Joint Conference*, Knoxville, TN, 2007, pp 243.

39. Turnbull PC, Tindall BW, Coetzee JD, et al: Vaccine-induced protection against anthrax in cheetah (*Acinonyx jubatus*) and black rhinoceros (*Diceros bicornis*). *Vaccine* 22:3340, 2004.

40. Valverde A, Crawshaw GJ, Cribb N, et al: Anesthetic management of a white rhinoceros (*Ceratotherium simum*) undergoing an emergency exploratory celiotomy for colic. *Vet Anaesth Analg* 37:280, 2010.

41. Walzer C, Goritz F, Hermes R, et al: Immobilization and intravenous anesthesia in a Sumatran rhinoceros (*Dicerorhinus sumatrensis*). *J Zoo Wildl Med* 41:115, 2010.

42. Williams JH, Espie I, van Willpe E, et al: Neosporosis in a white rhinoceros (*Ceratotherium simum*) calf. *Tydskr S Afr Vet Ver* 73:38, 2002.

CHAPTER 56

Tapiridae

Dawn M. Zimmerman and Sonia Hernandez

GENERAL BIOLOGY

Tapiridae are a family in the order Perissodactyla that comprises odd-toed ungulates, including horses and rhinoceroses. Tapiridae were once a large group of Neotropical browsers, which largely disappeared at the end of the Pleistocene period;[39] currently, four extant species of Tapiridae remain (Table 56-1). Baird's tapir (*Tapirus bairdii*), the lowland tapir (*T. terrestris*), and the mountain tapir (*T. pinchaque*) are the only New World perissodactyls of Central and South Americas, isolated geographically from the Malayan tapir of Southeast Asia (*T. indicus*).[17] The Malayan tapir has fewer chromosomes compared with South American tapirs (karyotype 2n = 52, compared with 76 and 80) and shares fewer homologies with the American species.[23] No hybridization has been described. A fifth living species of Tapirus with the proposed name of T. kabomani has recently been described in the Amazon, sympatric with T. terrestris.[13a]

Tapirs are primarily crepuscular or nocturnal and are almost exclusively solitary, apart from mother–offspring pairs. Their life span is approximately 25 years in the wild and 35 years in captivity.[55,57] As adults, they have few natural predators but are hunted by humans for their meat and hide. Loss of their preferred habitat of old growth forests has further isolated already small populations of wild tapirs, resulting in population decline and reduced genetic variability. The lowland tapir is classified as Vulnerable by the International Union for the Conservation of Nature (IUCN) and CITES Appendix II, whereas Baird's, Malayan, and mountain tapirs are classified as Endangered by the IUCN and CITES Appendix I.[25] All four species are listed as endangered under the Endangered Species Act. According to the IUCN, less than 5000 Baird's tapirs and less than 2500 mountain tapirs remain in the wild.[25]

UNIQUE ANATOMY

The Malayan tapir is the largest species (>300 kilogram [kg]), and the mountain tapir is the smallest (approximately 150–200 kg) (Table 56-2). Females are often larger than males, with no other apparent sexual dimorphism.[49] Except for the longer, woolly fur of the mountain tapir, tapirs have short hair coats, ranging in color from dark brown or reddish-brown to black. The coat of infant tapirs is

TABLE 56-1

Biologic Information of the Four Extant Tapir Species

Genus and Species	Common Name	Weight (kilogram [kg]; average adult male / female)[68]	Visual Description[28]	Geographic Range[68]	IUCN Conservation Status / CITES Listing
Tapirus bairdii	Baird's or Central American tapir	180–270 / 225–340	Dark brown with tan cheek and throat patches	Southern Mexico to Northern Colombia and Ecuador west of the Andes	Endangered / CITES I
Tapirus indicus	Malayan or Asian tapir	295–385 / 340–430	Black with a caudodorsal white saddle-shaped marking	Southern Burma, Malay Peninsula, southeastern Thailand and Sumatra	Endangered / CITES I
Tapirus pinchaque	Mountain or wooly tapir	135–225 / 160–250	Dark brown to black; thick bristly fur and white lips	The Andes central mountains from northwest Venezuela, Colombia and Ecuador, to northwestern Peru	Endangered / CITES I
Tapirus terrestris	Lowland, Brazilian, or South American tapir	160–250 / 180–295	Brown in coloration with a prominent sagittal crest under a short black mane	Colombia and Venezuela to northern Argentina and southern Brazil	Vulnerable / CITES II

TABLE 56-2

Physiological Parameters and Vital Signs for Adult Tapirs

Parameter (units)	Baird's Tapir	Malayan Tapir	Mountain Tapir	Lowland Tapir
Head-body length (centimeters [cm])[47]	200–230	250–300	180–200	191–242
Shoulder height (cm)[47]	~120	100–130	80–90	83–118
Life span (years)[55,57]	~25 in wild; ~35 in captivity			
Chromosome number[23]	80	52	76	80
Dental formula[1]	Incisors 3.1, canines 4.3, premolars 3.1, molars 3–4.3 = 42–44 teeth			
Vertebral formula[57]	7 cervical 26 thoracic 4 lumbar 6 sacral 5 caudal			
Rectal temperature (° C/° F)[24,38]	36.3–37.2° C 97.3–99° F			
Heart rate (beats per minute [beats/min]) Anesthetized[2] Resting[38]	52 ± 9 (6) 45			
Respiratory rate (beats/min; under anesthesia)[16]	8–21			
Systolic blood pressure (mm Hg; under anesthesia) Invasive[2] Noninvasive[16]	94 ±18–114 ±13 (6) 99–202	n/a	n/a	n/a
Diastolic blood pressure (mmHg; under anesthesia) Invasive[2] Noninvasive[16]	58 ± 18–74 ± 11 (6) 46–118	n/a	n/a	n/a
Mean blood pressure (mmHg; under anesthesia) Invasive[2] Noninvasive[16]	74 ± 17–87 ± 13 (6) 66–127	n/a	n/a	n/a
Newborn calf weight (kg)	~5–8[3,68]	~10[3,68]	4–7[47]	3.2–5.8[57]

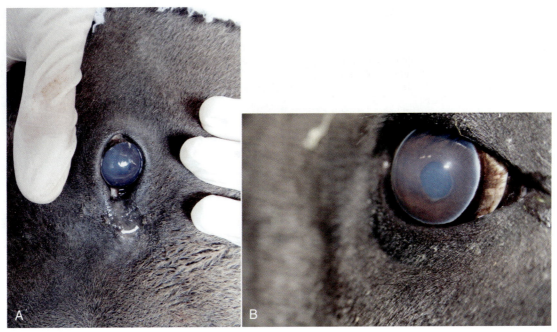

FIGURE 56-1 Corneal cloudiness in two lowland tapirs. (Courtesy of Maria Fernanda Gondim and Dorothée Ordonneau.)

a distinct white or yellow striped and spotted pattern to camouflage them against predation. This coloration gradually fades around 5 to 6 months, with adult coloration developing by 12 months of age.[47] Tapirs have monocular vision and poor eyesight but good olfactory and auditory senses. All species have brown eyes, often with a bluish cast to them, which is described as corneal cloudiness of unknown etiology and is most commonly found in Malayan tapirs (Figure 56-1). This condition has never been definitively diagnosed in wild individuals and may be associated with excessive exposure to light or trauma in captivity.[26]

The most notable morphologic feature of the tapir is the muscular proboscis, an extension of the upper lip and nose into a mobile, tactile soft tissue structure devoid of an internal skeleton, making the skull of tapirs unique among perissodactyls.[73] Three-dimensional computed tomography (CT) modeling of the skull and images of sinus anatomy are available.[13] They have four hooflike nails on the front feet and three on the hind feet. The ancestral front fourth digit, retained from the earliest perissodactyls, is small and does not touch the ground. The tapir foot posture is plantigrade, with splayed toes that help them walk on soft muddy ground. Their mesaxonic limb structure distributes most of their body weight on the third digit.[47] The vertebral formula, reported only for lowland tapirs, is 7 cervical, 26 thoracic, 4 lumbar, 6 sacral, and 5 caudal, totaling 48 vertebrae.[57] The radius and ulna are separate, and the fibula is complete.[47,55] Tapirs exhibit brachyodont, or low-crowned, teeth that lack cement, which is thought to be an adaptation to a diet of soft forest vegetation. Their dental formula is: incisors (I) 3.1, canines (C), 4.3, premolars (P) 3.1, molars (M) 3 to 4.3 (the first premolar may be absent), totaling 42 to 44 teeth. Tapirs have chisel-shaped incisors with enlarged maxillary third incisors, small maxillary canines, and lophodont cheek teeth. Permanent dentition develops by 30 months of age.[55]

The internal anatomy of the tapir is analogous to the domestic horse (*Equus ferus caballus*).[27] Tapirs have guttural pouches located in the pharyngeal region lateral to the hyoid bones.[28,34] The kidneys are nonlobulated, and the cortex makes up 71% to 80% of the renal mass.[40] Females have a bicornuate uterus, epitheliochorial placentation, and a single pair of mammary glands. In males, the testes are located cranioventral to the external anal sphincter within a slightly pendulous scrotum[62] but may retract into the inguinal canal in lateral recumbency. The penis is directed caudally and capable of spraying urine at distances of 5 meters (m).[28,34] Tapirs are monogastric hindgut fermenters, with a large cecum and colon, where all alloenzymatic digestion occurs. Nonglandular squamous epithelium lines the cardia of the stomach, and the remaining gastric epithelium is glandular, especially toward the pylorus.[57] The cecum has four fibrous taeniae creating sacculations, and the distal colon has no mesenteric attachments. Like other perissodactyls, tapirs lack a gallbladder. Malayan tapirs normally have anatomic fibrous connective tissue between the visceral and parietal pleurae, as in the elephant, which could be mistaken for adhesions secondary to pleural disease at necropsy.[28,33] This homogeneous pleural space connective tissue is not observed in the other three species, which exhibit the mesothelial serous membranes typical of other mammals.[27]

SPECIAL HOUSING REQUIREMENTS

Proper environmental management of captive tapirs may prevent some of the more common medical problems observed in captivity. Tapirs are typically maintained in outdoor enclosures with an indoor night den. Minimum recommendations include 600 square feet of outdoor space per animal, with off-exhibit individual enclosures measuring a minimum of 12 × 15 feet (180 square feet) or 16 × 16 feet for a female and calf.[68] Two-meter high barriers are necessary, as tapirs reportedly climb well.[68] In the wild, forested habitat provides safe harbor for hiding or resting;[46,68] therefore, artificial habitats should offer adequate vegetation as visual barriers to decrease stress associated with captivity.[41] Adult tapirs generally tolerate temperatures from just above 0°C (32°F) to 38°C (100°F),[68] but calves should not be exposed to temperatures below 10°C (50°F) until three months of age.[1] Even within these temperature ranges, tapirs should be shielded from prolonged exposure to direct sunlight, rain, or wind. At least 25% of outdoor habitats should be shaded, as ocular pathologies and dermatopathies have been associated with exposure to excessive sunlight (Figures 56-1 and 56-2).[27] Hard (cement or packed earth) and rough floor surfaces should be avoided in artificial habitats, as they lead to foot problems and chronic lameness (Figure 56-3). Substrates and bedding should be chosen with caution because some substances (e.g., sand and pine shavings) may cause colic and intestinal impaction if ingested, especially in

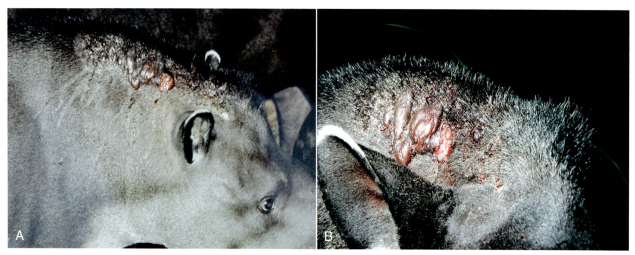

FIGURE 56-2 Vesicular dermatopathy in a lowland tapir, showing the classic presentation of raised, blood-filled vesicles that rupture leaving sanguinous discharge over the withers. (Courtesy of Mitch Finnegan.)

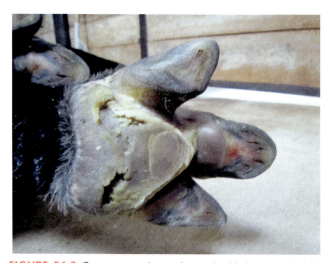

FIGURE 56-3 Overgrown sole causing embedded stones, bruising of the toes, and lameness in an 11-year-old mountain tapir. (Courtesy of Liza Dadone.)

newborns.[27] As with other species, coarse hay has been linked with lumpy jaw.[68] Wild tapirs inhabit aquatic and riparian regions, therefore a large water source should be provided in captivity for bathing, temperature regulation (cooling), copulation, and defecation. Pools should be large enough for multiple tapirs to submerge; a depth of 4-6 feet with a 1:8 slope is recommended.[68] Tapirs almost always defecate while standing in water, and lack of access to water has been associated with an increased incidence of rectal prolapse.[68]

Crowded conditions in captivity may cause chronic stress and abnormal or aggressive social interactions. When considering the addition of conspecifics, enclosure size as well as individual behaviors must be taken into consideration. In particular, aggressive interactions among males may be prevented by separating immature males from adult males at 12 months of age.[68] Although tapirs have been successfully integrated into Neotropical and Asiatic multispecies exhibits, caution should be exercised with regard to integration, as tapirs have been known to eat birds.[68] Tapirs may be extremely aggressive and have been known to inflict serious harm on keepers and other tapirs.

FEEDING

In the wild, tapirs consume a wide variety of woody and nonwoody plant taxa, feeding on various plant parts, including leaves, fruits, grasses, and twigs.[46,47] Captive diet recommendations are based on known nutrient requirements of the domestic horse,[68] which includes 70% roughages (legume hay, commercial produce, and browse) and 30% concentrates (commercial herbivore pellet).[68] Roughage should comprise high-quality alfalfa hay (>15.9% crude protein; <42.8% neutral detergent fiber) or grass hay (>9.8% crude protein; <67.4% neutral detergent fiber).[68] Roughage maintains normal gastrointestinal (GI) function, and decreased dietary fiber is linked to problems such as rectal prolapse.[27,68] Commercial produce and browse should also be offered, although the latter is lacking in most captive diets.[65] Concentrates used to complement nutrition from roughages include high-fiber herbivore pellets with 12% to 18% crude protein.[68] Fruits, greens, and root vegetables may be offered in limited quantities. It is important to use these foods sparingly, as excess starch and sugar may contribute to dental disease and obesity,[27] which may exacerbate foot, hoof, and chronic joint problems. Tapirs should not be fed directly off the ground, as this may lead to ingestion of foreign bodies and reinfection with parasites.[68]

Wild tapirs are known to seek out salt accumulations or natural mineral licks,[47] but mineral supplementation is not necessary in captive individuals with a balanced diet. However, a salt block may be offered as a supplement or enrichment. No known species-specific trace mineral requirements exist; however, copper and zinc levels should not be lower, and iron not higher, than that recommended for horses.[10] Tapirs are highly efficient in calcium absorption, an adaptation to the high calcium-to-phosphorus (Ca : P) ratios of their natural diet; therefore, alfalfa hay is adequate.[10] Iron storage disease is prevalent in tapir species. Although a dietary cause has not been identified,[6] pelleted compound feeds often contain high levels of iron (Fe),[9] and elevations of vitamin C from high fruit intake may promote GI iron absorption.[15] Captive tapirs reportedly have much lower serum copper concentrations compared with wild tapirs (Patrícia Medici, personal communication)[26] as well as domestic horses,[27] although no known pathologies have been reported.

Daily food intake for an adult tapir should be 4% to 5% of body weight,[68] although pregnant or lactating females and young calves may require a higher intake. Ideal body condition scores in tapirs are maintained at the presumed maintenance energy requirement for hindgut fermenting herbivores (digestible energy [DE] intakes of 0.6 megajoules/dietary energy [DE]/kg$^{0.75}$/day).[12] In the wild, tapirs are continuous feeders, spending up to 90% of their active hours foraging,[47] necessary to acquire adequate nutrition with their limited stomach capacity.[69] Overconsumption at one feeding, especially of nonfibrous foods, may contribute to GI problems (colic, volvulus, torsion, impaction, obstruction, obstipation) or founder.[26-28] Enteroliths of vivianite and newberyite structure have been reported, in contrast to the struvite composition normally found in horses.[54] To prevent enterolith formation, dietary recommendations for captive tapirs promote carbohydrate fermentation while minimizing protein fermentation in the large intestine.[54]

RESTRAINT AND HANDLING

Tapirs have traditionally been managed through "direct contact"; however, reports of severe or lethal injuries to caretakers highlight the risks of manual restraint. The current Association of Zoos and Aquariums (AZA) standards recommend that tapirs be managed with "protected contact."[1] The only acceptable type of physical immobilization, which requires training, is the use of a large animal chute.[28] Depending on the disposition of individual animals, some tapirs may be trained with positive reinforcement to be moved, to be prompted to present body parts, and to stand still for biologic sample collection or intravenous catheterization. Tapirs may also be "scratched-down" to lateral recumbency, with a coarse horse brush or outdoor broom used to stroke the animal's dorsum, neck, and the lateral and abdominal walls. Although some have used "scratch-downs" for physical examination, administration of injections, and even repeated blood collection,[28] the level of immobilization induced by this "state" should not be exaggerated.[35]

The recent increase in use of α_2-adrenergic agonists, alone or in combination with other drugs, has decreased the need for ultrapotent narcotics such as etorphine and carfentanil. The preferred anesthetic protocol depends on both the environmental setting (i.e., captive or free-ranging) and the individual's disposition. It is important to establish a quiet environment while working with these animals. If stress is unavoidable (i.e., transport, trauma, or disease), preanesthetic medication is recommended. The success of some anesthetic protocols used for free-ranging tapirs depends on the animal's degree of relaxation.[16,20] Tapirs often retreat into water when threatened, so this should be taken into consideration during immobilizations. It is recommended that the animal be fasted for 24 hours to minimize the potential for regurgitation and minimize the pressure on the diaphragm from the GI tract. Protocols should emphasize maintenance of euthermia, through the heating of enclosures in cold climates or cooling the animal in hot weather. Because tapirs are tropical animals that are rarely exposed to full sunlight, they should not be immobilized in full sun.

Preanesthetic agents such as xylazine and butorphanol have been used in tapirs successfully.[20] An estimated dosage of butorphanol (0.15–0.25 milligram per kilogram [mg/kg]) combined with xylazine (0.3–0.5 mg/kg) delivered intramuscularly (IM) produces sufficient immobilization. Alternatively, detomidine (0.06 mg/kg) combined with butorphanol (0.15–0.2 mg/kg) has been used successfully in captive Baird's tapirs.[62] It is worth noting that these dosages are less than those required to achieve recumbency in domestic horses. For example, a sick adult lowland tapir was successfully sedated with only 5 mg detomidine hydrochloride and 10 mg butorphanol.[59] Anesthetic induction is typically achieved by hand or remote delivery of intramuscular (free-ranging and captive) or intravenous injection (captive animal previously sedated or conditioned). Factors influencing the choice of induction protocol are provided in Table 56-3. Intravenous induction with propofol or ketamine is possible in trained or sedated individuals. Standing sedation with xylazine, alternative α_2-agonist combinations, or azaperone (1 mg/kg) may be used for short, less invasive procedures (e.g., skin biopsy, blood collection, portable radiography, etc.).[26] Following anesthetic induction, tapirs adopt a saw-horse position, drop their heads, drool, and may lose control of their proboscis; then they progress to a sitting-dog position before achieving recumbency. Isoflurane is the most

common inhalant used to maintain anesthesia in tapirs. Intravenous guaifenesin in a dextrose solution has been used safely in a small number of Baird's tapirs (L. Padilla, personal communication) to increase relaxation, depth, and duration of anesthesia following induction with other agents. At rates used in horses, intravenous guaifenesin provided similar anesthetic effects as well as dose-dependent and rate-dependent respiratory depression. Since guaifenesin susceptibility varies among equid species,[44] it should be used in tapirs with extreme caution until additional research has been conducted. Constant rate infusions of propofol have been reported in tapirs,[20] and small boluses have been used as supplements to maintain or reach deeper planes of anesthesia.

Tapirs may be maintained in sternal or lateral recumbency once anesthetized; however, the latter position allows for better ventilation and minimizes the potential for neuropathies. A blindfold should be applied to the eyes and gauze placed in the ears to minimize external stimuli—which is particularly important when using α_2-agonists, opioids, or both to minimize premature arousal. At the minimum, heart rate, peripheral pulse strength, respiratory rate, and body temperature should be monitored regularly during the anesthetic period (see Table 56-2). The reader is directed to other sources for in-depth discussion of monitoring equipment and techniques recommended in tapirs.[22] Hypoxemia has been reported,[16] so supplemental oxygen is recommended, at least intranasally at 10 to 15 liters per minute (L/min). Improved oxygen saturation and ventilation may be accomplished in the field with a demand valve driven by 100% oxygen or a manual resuscitator bag with supplemental oxygen attachment. Blind intubation of tapirs is relatively simple (adult tapir: 16–20 mm internal diameter endotracheal tube); thus tracheal insufflation of oxygen or positive pressure ventilation (20–30 centimeters of water [cm H_2O]) are reasonable means to address hypoxemia.

Protocols that include α_2-adrenergic agonists are typically antagonized well and yield smooth, uneventful recoveries. In captivity, animals should be maintained in a quiet, dark enclosure until they recover fully. Tapirs recovering from anesthesia exhibit ear twitching, tongue retraction, twitching of the proboscis, and rapid return to sternal recumbency. From sternal recumbency they may first sit on their hindquarters or stand fully. Physical restraint is not recommended once a tapir stands. Anecdotal evidence suggests that tapirs may experience "renarcotization" hours after reversal of α_2-agonists medetomidine or detomidine, which may be circulating longer than their antagonists.

SURGERY

The basic recommendations and techniques in equine surgery apply to tapirs. Padding should be used if prolonged recumbency is expected. Standard equine surgical instruments, approaches, and techniques are used in the tapir. Preemptive analgesia and postsurgical pain management is recommended. Few surgical procedures have been reported: rectal prolapse repair,[66] management of an abdominal abscess,[36] and mass resection, with or without biopsy.[32,50] Dental extraction and castration are probably the most common procedures performed. Mandibular fracture fixation is the only orthopedic surgery reported in tapirs.[67]

OTHER PHARMACEUTICALS

Most pharmaceutical therapeutics and dosages are extrapolated from equine medicine. Antibiotics commonly used include ceftiofur, long-acting penicillins, and trimethoprim–sulfonamide combinations. Injection site abscesses are not uncommon. When injecting medications and treating abscesses, note that skin thickness may be up to 2.5 centimeters (cm) along the back of the head and neck. Oral nonsteroidal anti-inflammatory drugs (NSAIDs) and Cosequin at equid dosages are often used for treating arthritis in tapirs.[70] Although therapeutic regimens for vesicular dermatopathy rarely provide earlier resolution, treatment has included topical antiseptics and antibiotics, systemic antibiotics in severe cases, and NSAIDs for

TABLE 56-3

Summary of Protocols Used to Immobilize Free-Ranging Tapirs

Species	Animal Status	Anesthetics	Comments
Tapirus pinchaque	Captive	Carfentanil (5.4 microgram per kilogram [μg/kg]), ketamine (0.26 milligram per kilogram [mg/kg]) and xylazine (0.13 mg/kg,) intramuscularly [IM]) Reversal: yohimbine (0.2 mg/kg, intravenously [IV]); and naltrexone (100–200 mg/kg, half IV, half subcutaneously [SC])	Six immobilizations of tapirs (1 female, 3 males; 1 juvenile male immobilized 3 times) for footwork, gastrointestinal endoscopy, reproductive surgery[52]
Tapirus indicus	Captive	Butorphanol (0.15 mg/kg) and detomidine (0.05 mg/kg) OR xylazine (0.3 mg/kg, all IM); use ketamine if needed (0.5 mg/kg, IV) Reversal: naloxone and yohimbine (0.2–0.3 mg/kg, IV)	Nineteen immobilizations of Malayan and mountain tapirs[28]
Tapirus bairdii	Captive	Butorphanol (0.15–0.2 mg/kg) and detomidine (0.06 mg/kg); ketamine (1–2 mg/kg) was used to reach or maintain recumbency and light anesthesia Boluses of propofol (0.2–2.0 mg/kg per bolus) were used to effect as needed	Report of 11 males anesthetized for semen collection by electroejaculation in three captive institutions in Panama,[16] but authors (personal communication) report similar usage in similar number of females has the same effects, and that anesthesia was antagonized with naltrexone and yohimbine
Tapirus indicus	Captive	Butorphanol (80 mg, IM) and Xylazine (120 mg total, IM) OR detomidine (12 mg total, IM) Reversal: naltrexone (200 mg total, IM), tolazoline (1400 mg total, IM)	Estimated body weight 340 kg; repeated immobilizations of light anesthesia for diagnosis and treatment of oral squamous cell carcinoma[50]
Tapirus terrestris	Captive	Detomidine (0.03mg/kg, orally [PO]), 20 minutes later, carfentanil (1.85 μg/kg, PO)	One animal repeatedly immobilized for wound management; variety of combinations of α_2-agonist or etorphine or carfentanil were used but eight immobilizations with detomidine/carfentanil, PO, were most useful.[60]
Tapirus bairdii	Attracted wild tapirs to bait stations	Total dosage for a 200–300 kg animal: 40–50 mg of butorphanol and 100 mg of xylazine in the same dart Additional ketamine (187 ± 40.86 mg/animal) or constant rate infusion of propofol (50–200 mcg/kg/min), administered IV Reversal: Naltrexone 50 mg, with 1200 mg of tolazoline in the same syringe IM; no sooner than 30 minutes from last administration of ketamine	Administered to animals from a tree blind via a dart The animals had been habituated to come to bait for several days and thus were relatively calm when darted[16]
Tapirus terrestris	Tapirs were captive, semi-captive or wild	Ketamine (3.5–4 mg/kg) and xylazine (2–2.2 mg/kg) IM, supplemented with ketamine (1.4 mg/kg) IM Reversal: Tolazoline (4 mg/kg)	Administered using darts projected by a blowpipe, or IV using syringe[4]
Tapirus terrestris	Wild tapirs captured in pens or pit-falls	Butorphanol tartrate (0.15 mg/kg) with medetomidine (0.03 mg/kg) IM, in same dart Reversal: Atipamezole (0.06 mg/kg) with naltrexone (0.6 mg/kg) in same syringe, IV	Adequate immobilization for radio collaring, and biologic sampling[71]
Tapirus terrestris and *Tapirus pinchaque*	Wild tapirs captured in pens or pit-falls, or immobilized by dart	Dosages were calculated using allometric scaling: ketamine (0.62–0.41 mg/kg) and atropine (0.025–0.04 mg/kg), and tiletamine-zolazepam (1.25–083 mg/kg), and romifidine (0.05–0.03 mg/kg) OR detomidine (0.06–0.04 mg/kg) OR medetomidine (0.006–0.004 mg/kg) in the same dart Reversal: atipamezole (0.06 mg/kg)	Medetomidine produced best results obtaining good muscular relaxation and more stable cardiopulmonary parameters[43]

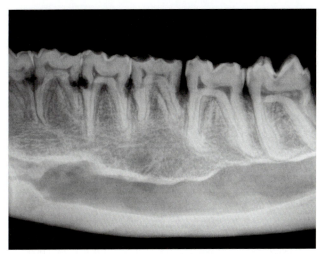

FIGURE 56-4 Dental radiograph of a Malayan tapir, exhibiting radio-lucencies correlating to resorptive lesions at the cementoenamel junction. (Courtesy of Mads Bertelsen.)

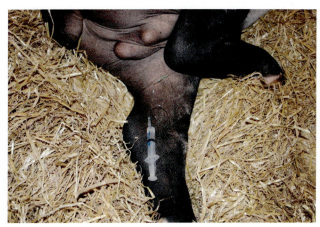

FIGURE 56-5 Demonstration of phlebotomy technique using the medial saphenous vein during a scratch-down procedure. (Courtesy of Mads Bertelsen.)

neuromuscular signs.[14] Iron dextran may be administered prophylactically (10 mg/kg, IM) if iron deficiency anemia is of concern in captive neonates.[19] Fluorouracil has been used in tapirs for the successful treatment of corneal papillomas[30] and oral squamous cell carcinoma,[50] with no adverse drug effects.

PHYSICAL EXAMINATION AND DIAGNOSTICS

Physical examinations may be performed during scratch-down procedures or immobilizations. Emphasis should be placed on dental, ophthalmic, and hoof or foot pad examination.[27,28] Dental radiography and foot radiography may be important diagnostic tools (Figure 56-4). Rectal palpation may be difficult and may be limited to the caudal abdomen because of the tight anal sphincter.[37] Blood may be collected from the marginal auricular, cephalic, medial carpal, or medial saphenous veins during scratch-down procedures (Figure 56-5) and from the carpal or jugular veins during immobilizations. A complete blood cell (CBC) count, including fibrinogen, and a serum chemistry panel should be performed, and banking a minimum of 10 milliliters (mL) of serum in either a −70° C (−94° F) freezer or a frost-free −20° C (−4° F) freezer is recommended.[68] Although not validated for tapirs, laboratory tests for equine diseases are thought to be credible.[68] Serum ferritin concentrations may be most useful for diagnosis of iron storage disease, as ferritin assay is reportedly the single most reliable noninvasive indicator of total body iron stores, and species-specific reagents are available for tapirs at the Laboratory of Comparative Hematology, Kansas State University College of Veterinary Medicine.[58] Table 56-4 provides hematology and chemistry values for all four tapir species.[28] Values are similar to those of the horse and other perissodactyls, and no significant differences have been reported between tapir species.[26] Urine may be collected via catheterization;[28] it must be noted that tapir urine may normally be cloudy or chalky because of calcium excretion observed in most perissodactyls.[28] Hypercalcemia and hypertension have been associated with chronic renal disease in tapirs.[31]

No validated reliable antemortem test for tuberculosis (TB) in tapirs is available, and a combination of diagnostic techniques is recommended.[29] An intradermal test may be performed using 0.1 mL purified protein derivative (PPD) of *Mycobacterium bovis* in regions where the skin is thin and pliable such as the inguinal area near the nipples, the axillary area, or perineum.[27,51] A high number of false reactions have been reported in tapirs,[51] in which case additional diagnostics should be considered (comparative intradermal test with bovine and avian tuberculin; thoracic radiography; and nasal, gastric,

tracheal, or bronchoalveolar lavage to obtain fluid for cytology, culture, and polymerase chain reaction [PCR] testing). Adjunct testing with the enzyme-linked immunosorbent assay (ELISA) and multi-antigen print immunoassay (MAPIA), which uses recombinant antigens to *M. tuberculosis* and *M. bovis*, has shown some diagnostic potential.[27,29] In addition, a point-of-care lateral flow immunochromatographic rapid test assay, the Elephant TB STAT-PAK (Chembio Diagnostic Systems, Inc., Medford, NY), detects immunoglobulin M (IgM) and IgG antibodies against *M. tuberculosis* and *M. bovis*. This test is now recommended for TB testing in elephants, has been used in rhinoceros, and may prove useful in tapirs.[37]

Imaging diagnostics include general radiography (with a minimum 300 milliamperes [mA] capacity machine for thoracic images),[28] transabdominal or transrectal ultrasonography (the latter often with a transvaginal transducer),[63] endoscopy,[5] flexible bronchoscopy,[28] and echocardiography. Thermography may be useful as an adjunct procedure in the diagnosis of musculoskeletal disorders (Figure 56-6).

DISEASES

General

Mortalities in wild tapirs from infectious disease are rarely reported, possibly because of an extended evolutionary history that allowed for adaptation to common infectious agents. However, conditions in captivity such as exposure to dusty substrates, more frequent contact with conspecifics, and contact with novel species have resulted in mortalities.

Infectious Disease

Both salmonellosis and campylobacteriosis have been reported in tapirs in captivity presumably from exposure to conspecifics or rodents actively shedding the bacteria. *Salmonella typhimurium* was associated with fatal septicemia in a lowland tapir, and *S. poona* was isolated from a neonatal Baird's tapir with acute GI distress.[64] *Mycobacterium bovis* sporadically affects captive tapirs,[28] and at least one report of *M. tuberculosis* presumed to be anthropozoonotic has been reported.[53] Mycobacteriosis is a protracted disease that causes weight loss and progressive respiratory disease. Coughing and weight loss may also be caused by *Coccidiodes immitis* and should be suspected in endemic regions. Tapirs appear particularly prone to developing "lumpy jaw" as a result of molar apical abscesses. A variety of bacteria have been isolated from these lesions, including *Corynebacterium pyogenes*, ß-hemolytic *Streptococcus*, *Actinomyces* spp., *Necrobacillus* spp., *E. coli*, and *Mycobacterium* spp. Unvaccinated tapirs are

TABLE 56-4

Hematology and Serum Chemistry Values of Tapirs by Species [reference interval; mean (n)].[67]

Parameter (units)	Baird's Tapir	Malayan Tapir	Mountain Tapir	Lowland Tapir
Hematocrit (%)	23.6–43.5; 32.4 (218)	21.8–48.3; 35.6 (403)	21.1–43.8; 32.3 (62)	27.5–58.0; 39.7 (161)
Leukocytes (*10³/µl)	3.89–13.23; 7.42 (204)	4.10–14.44; 8.12 (332)	3.05–8.36; 5.76 (60)	4.34–16.67; 9.14 (139)
Neutrophils (*10³/µl)	1.94–8.96; 4.57 (204)	2.40–9.36; 5.26 (330)	1.34–6.20; 3.81 (60)	2.46–11.99; 5.43 (139)
Lymphocytes (*10³/µl)	0.36–5.54; 2.54 (202)	0.54–4.93; 2.15 (329)	0.84–2.44; 1.67 (60)	1.06–5.76; 2.80 (139)
Monocytes (cells/µl)	52–592; 213 (157)	58–851; 306 (303)	0–282; 142 (55)	0–543; 241 (116)
Eosinophils (cells/µl)	44–559; 191 (144)	45–664; 230 (214)	0–380; 157 (44)	30–1578; 510 (120)
Basophils (cells/µl)	—	0–221; 102 (52)	—	—
Band Neutrophils (*10³/µl)	0.01–0.06; 0.03 (194)	0.01–0.11; 0.04 (298)	0.01–0.04; 0.02 (51)	0.01–0.08; 0.04 (131)
Total Protein (g/dL)	5.5–8.4; 7.1 (170)	5.4–8.4; 6.8 (321)	5.5–7.6; 6.6 (58)	5.1–8.4; 6.8 (147)
Fibrinogen (mg/dL)	250 (32)	0–806; 384 (90)	—	—
Albumin (g/dL)	1.7–4.3; 3.0 (172)	1.6–4.1; 3.0 (317)	2.2–4.3; 3.1 (60)	1.8–4.1; 3.0 (142)
Globulin (g/dL)	1.2–5.4; 3.8 (172)	1.1–5.1; 3.6 (314)	2.0–4.5; 3.3 (59)	2.2–5.3; 3.9 (141)
Sodium (mEq/L)	126–144; 134 (184)	127–144; 134 (329)	126–143; 135 (65)	127–144; 135 (132)
Chloride (mEq/L)	91–106; 98 (185)	87–103; 95 (320)	95–108; 102 (59)	93–107; 99 (124)
Potassium (mEq/L)	2.9–5.1; 4.0 (195)	2.9–5.4; 4.1 (330)	3.1–4.6; 3.9 (65)	2.6–5.0; 3.9 (133)
Calcium (mg/dL)	9.1–12.2; 10.8 (198)	8.6–15.3; 11.3 (346)	9.0–12.2; 10.5 (64)	8.4–12.1; 10.5 (154)
Phosphorus (mg/dL)	4.1–8.6; 5.8 (146)	3.0–8.5; 5.5 (334)	2.6–6.7; 4.7 (65)	3.2–7.8; 5.1 (145)
Bicarbonate (mEq/L)	—	18.4–32.2; 25.2 (66)	—	—
Carbon Dioxide (mEq/L)	18.2–30.2; 24.2 (108)	18.5–35.3; 26.8 (131)	—	17.1–34.2; 24.7 (44)
Iron (µg/dL)	205 (31)	52–292; 170 (57)	—	—
Magnesium (mg/dL)	—	0.87–2.53; 1.69 (93)	—	—
Blood Urea Nitrogen (mg/dL)	5–16; 10 (196)	5–20; 11 (348)	2–16; 10 (58)	5–16; 8 (154)
Creatinine (mg/dL)	0.6–1.6; 1.1 (189)	0.8–2.3; 1.4 (343)	0.4–1.4; 0.9 (57)	0.7–1.9; 1.2 (140)
Total Bilirubin (mg/dL)	0.4–1.8; 0.8 (190)	0.1–1.3; 0.5 (322)	0.0–1.2; 0.6 (56)	0.1–1.3; 0.5 (147)
Glucose (mg/dL)	60–162; 100 (188)	63–157; 104 (349)	67–139; 104 (60)	62–160; 100 (151)
Cholesterol (mg/dL)	94–257; 180 (140)	93–237; 155 (293)	70–168; 121 (55)	99–374; 199 (125)
Triglyceride (mg/dL)	0–100; 52 (67)	8–76; 32 (126)	—	0–79; 41 (75)
Amylase (IU/L)	0–4958; 2354 (54)	0–4084; 2106 (96)	—	2452 (33)
Lipase (IU/L)	—	0–43; 14 (51)	—	—
Creatine Phosphokinase (IU/L)	116–423; 247 (135)	115–506; 259 (211)	39–384; 223 (51)	16–236; 136 (73)
Lactate Dehydrogenase (IU/L)	0–2178; 949 (89)	0–1762; 756 (108)	—	0–1164; 639 (69)
Alkaline Phosphatase (IU/L)	26–663; 195 (179)	4–51; 20 (292)	6–133; 73 (55)	8–77; 28 (143)
Alanine Aminotransferase (IU/L)	6–31; 16 (167)	2–27; 11 (236)	—	0–20; 9 (112)
Aspartate Aminotransferase (IU/L)	53–201; 116 (188)	62–275; 136 (318)	16–58; 40 (53)	32–124; 74 (138)
Gamma Glutamyltransferase (IU/L)	0–33; 17 (111)	2–65; 21 (197)	5–32; 20 (49)	0–34; 15 (69)

From Teare JA, ed: 2013, "Tapirus_bairdii/indicus/pinchaque/terrestris_No_selection_by_gender__All_ages_combined_Standard_International_Units__2013 _CD.html" in ISIS Physiological Reference Intervals for Captive Wildlife: A CD-ROM Resource., International Species Information System, Bloomington, MN.

susceptible to infection with *Clostridium* spp. Specifically, *C. tetani* produces muscle stiffness, hemoglobinuria, and death. Antibodies against various *Leptospira* serovars have been documented in tapirs.[21,41,45,46] Evidence of clinical disease from infection with *Leptospira interrogans* serovar *pomona* was described in a female lowland tapir sympatric with cattle and horses in the Brazilian Pantanal.[41]

Morbidity and mortality caused by herpesvirus, encephalomyocarditis virus, and foot-and-mouth disease virus have been reported in captive tapirs.[28] In a health evaluation of 23 captive *T. bairdii* in Panama, 21% were seropositive for Venezuelan encephalomyelitis H1 virus, 47% for vesicular stomatitis, and 13% for West Nile virus (WNV), although none of the animals demonstrated clinical signs. Furthermore, antibodies against equine herpesvirus (types 1, 2 and 4), equine influenza virus, and equine rhinovirus (types 1 and 2) were detected in these individuals.[61] Although some institutions

choose to vaccinate against encephalitides and antibodies have been detected in wild tapirs, morbidity from equine encephalitis viruses have not been definitively diagnosed.[21,42,46] One report documented mortality in Malayan tapirs as a result of herpesvirus infection;[18] however, the type of herpesvirus was not determined.

Parasitic Disease

Tapirs are susceptible to a variety of ectoparasites and endoparasites.[28,41] Tapirs are parasitized by several species of ticks, which are known vectors of a wide variety of rickettsial and hemoparasitic diseases. To date, no reports of rickettsial disease in tapirs have been published, but an intraerythrocytic parasite resembling *Babesia equi* was found in a recently imported Malayan tapir manifesting clinical signs of anemia and icterus.[1] It would be wise to monitor imported animals. Both amebic meningoencephalitis and schistosomiasis have

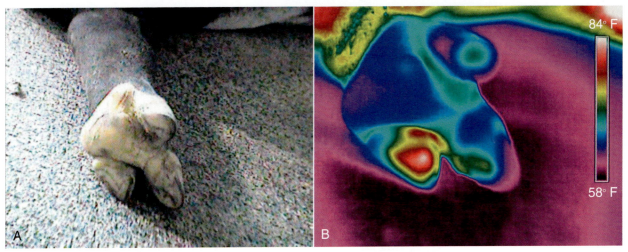

FIGURE 56-6 Thermography of the left rear foot of a captive tapir imaged during a scratch-down procedure (**B**), indicating a heat signature at the lateral toe which corresponded with a sub-solar abscess (**A**).

been reported in tapirs.[28] Watery diarrhea caused by *Cryptosporidium* was reported in tapirs at the Shanghai Zoo; the molecular characterization of the parasite demonstrated a 99% identity with *Cryptosporidium suis*.[8] *Balantidium* and *Giardia* are considered normal enteric flora, but they have also been suspected as a cause of intermittent watery diarrhea.[1]

Noninfectious Disease

The majority of noninfectious diseases of tapirs involve the GI system and includes colic, rectal prolapse (as a result of colonic impactions), and enteroliths.[28] With advances in the nutrition and husbandry of tapirs, these syndromes appear to be declining. A syndrome termed "vesicular dermatitis," which is characterized by skin vesicles on the dorsal skin with bloody discharge,[14] (see Figure 56-2) continues to affect captive tapirs, and its etiology has not been definitively determined. Ideally, skin biopsies of affected areas should be collected and preserved in 10% buffered formalin for histopathologic examination. The condition may be associated with a fluctuation in hormones in females and typically resolves spontaneously. Plantar dermatitis and ulceration are usually caused by inappropriate, hard substrates. Some evidence suggests that the iron levels in captive tapirs are significantly higher than in their free-ranging counterparts and may result in hemochromatosis.[11]

See Table 56-5 for clinical signs and potential etiologies commonly seen or previously reported in tapirs in the United States.

PREVENTIVE MEDICINE

Development of a preventive medicine protocol for tapirs should follow the same logic as that for other animals; this includes an understanding of the relevant infectious diseases and clinical syndromes, risk assessment that considers contact with other species (including domestics), and consideration of region-specific and institution-specific problems. For example, the majority of clinical problems seen in tapirs in South America[56] are related to husbandry or nutrition, whereas the only comprehensive review of tapir mortalities in North American zoologic institutions indicates that infectious diseases are more common.[26] Three types of health examinations are recommended for tapirs: (1) pre-shipment or quarantine examinations, (2) regular (annual or opportunistic) health examinations, and (3) neonatal examinations. Quarantine protocols should include 30 days in isolation, during which a minimum of a complete physical examination, basic blood work, three serial fecal examinations for parasites, fecal culture, and TB testing should be performed. Collection of appropriate biologic samples to test for relevant

pathogens is also recommended, either used for immediate analysis or preserved for future testing. The Tapir Specialist Group provides a comprehensive report on recommendations for reintroduction protocols.[48]

Vaccination

Tapir immunization protocols and immunologic responses have not been thoroughly evaluated but have been adapted from similar species.[34,64,56] Inactivated vaccines are often recommended to avoid the possibility of vaccine-induced disease.[56] Vaccination against tetanus[64] and other clostridial diseases are strongly recommended, particularly where domestic ungulates are present in the proximity of tapir enclosures.[56] Equine encephalomyelitis virus (EEV) and WNV vaccination is recommended for endemic areas.[34,64] Vaccination against infectious bovine rhinotracheitis is recommended for endemic areas and if the risk of infection from contact with domestic cattle is high.[56] Rabies vaccination may be indicated. Encephalomyocarditis virus (EMCV) infection has been reported occasionally in zoos in warm climates, some resulting in deaths, but no vaccine is available; therefore, the main prevention is maintenance of appropriate hygiene, feeding practices, and pest control.

REPRODUCTION

Tapirs reach sexual maturity generally between 2 and 4 years of age, although the timing varies.[68] Females have bred as young as 13 months of age in captivity; therefore, the general recommendation is to separate them from unwanted breeding males from the age of 15 months.[3,68] Tapirs are nonseasonal breeders. Estrus cycle length varies from 1 to 3 months but is generally considered to be monthly on the basis of progesterone levels.[7,35] Vulvar swelling, white and stringy mucous discharge, urine dribbling, and increased vocalization, as well as low progesterone levels may signify the onset of estrus.[35] Estrus lasts 1 to 4 days,[3,7] during which multiple copulations may occur. Injuries during breeding do occur.[68]

Tapir gestation lasts 13 to 14 months, generally 390 to 410 days.[47,55] Female tapirs may resume estrus at an average of 16 (9–27) days after parturition; therefore, the inter-birth interval may be as short as 14 months.[7,47] Pregnancy is often difficult to determine, as the body weight of pregnant tapirs may only increase by about 10%.[47] Pregnancy diagnosis methods include blood serum hormone concentration and ultrasonography. Progesterone levels vary but appear to be quite low in the luteal phase and pregnancy; however, progesterone values higher than 2.5 nanograms per milliliter (ng/mL) are suggestive of pregnancy. Confirmation of pregnancy is

TABLE 56-5

Clinical Signs and Potential Etiologies Commonly Seen or Previously Reported in American Tapirs

Clinical Sign or Problem	Possible Etiologies	Comments
Colic	1. Bacterial enterocolitis 2. Intestinal accidents (e.g., volvulus, torsion, intussuception) 3. Sand or foreign body impaction 4. Inappropriate diet	Important to quickly differentiate medical from surgical problems
Corneal cloudiness	1. Excessive light exposure 2. Trauma 3. Bacterial infection	Etiology not definitively known Most common in *Tapirus indicus* Can be associated with corneal ulceration
Death, neonatal	1. Failure of passive transfer or septicemia 2. Hypothermia 3. Drowning or trauma	Neonatal mortality will be high unless a suitable birthing environment is available
Death, sudden	1. Encephalomyocarditis virus 2. Intestinal accidents	—
Dermatitis, general	1. Sarcoptic mange 2. Dermatophyte (*Microsporum* sp.) 3. Ectoparasites 4. Bacterial dermatitis	Both reported in Europe
Diarrhea, chronic vomiting	1. Inappropriate diet 2. Bacterial or protozoal enteritis 3. Eosinophilic enterocolitis	Minimize fruit in diet Bacterial enteritis most frequently caused by *Salmonella, Campylobacter* Chronic cases may require endoscopic gastrointestinal biopsies and other diagnostics
Dorsal skin vesicles and sloughs or collapsing	1. Vesicular skin disease	Cause of this syndrome unknown
Dyspnea or coughing	1. Pulmonary tuberculosis 2. Bacterial pneumonia 3. Coccidioidomycosis 4. Laryngeal abscess 5. Foreign bodies	These signs may be indicative of life-threatening disease
Lameness, acute	1. Overwear of foot pads 2. Overactivity during introduction 3. Hard substrate 4. Laminitis 5. Plantar dermatitis and trauma 6. Capture myopathy	Severe pad ulcerations may develop when animals become overactive A hard substrate or continuously wet concrete will precipitate foot problems
Lameness, chronic	1. Degenerative joint disease (DJD) 2. Chronic foot pad ulcers or dermatitis	DJD common in older animals and carries worse prognosis than foot pad problems
Mandibular swelling	1. Molar apical abscess 2. Mandibular osteomyelitis 3. Neoplasia 4. Trauma	Difficult to treat successfully and may become chronic May cause death
Nasal discharge	1. Guttural pouch infection 2. Bacterial rhinitis 3. Pneumonia 4. Foreign bodies	Nasal discharge may indicate more serious lower airway disease
Rectal prolapse	1. Diet, stress 2. Unknown 3. Absence of water body	Not commonly reported anymore Possibly as a result of improved diets
Vaginal discharge Cloudy, chalky urine	1. Normal: 2–3 weeks before parturition 2. Genitourinary tract infection or estrus; normal urinary calcium excretion 3. Leiomyosarcoma 4. Metritis	Best differentiated by urinalysis or cytology
Weight loss, chronic	1. Renal failure 2. Dental disease 3. Tuberculosis 4. Chronic bacterial pneumonia	Pulmonary tuberculosis has been frequently reported in the literature

Adapted from references 28 and 41.

achieved by observing increasing progesterone values in three serial tests over 15 days[7] or via urinary and fecal hormone analyses.[28] Fetal viability and development may be assessed by measuring serum hormone levels or by ultrasonography. In lowland tapirs, serum progesterone concentrations increase and decrease throughout gestation with minimum values of 2.67 ng/mL during the first period of gestation and maximum values of 22.6 ng/mL during the last period.[63] Serum estrogen remains fairly constant at 20 to 30 picograms per milliliter (pg/mL), increasing just prior to parturition.[63] Transabdominal and rectal ultrasonography are useful starting at 30 to 45 days of gestation. Fetal growth may be monitored through serial measurements of total body length, cranial (biparietal) diameter, thoracic diameter, and abdominal diameter (at gastric axis level).[1,27,49]

Signs of impending parturition vary. Both serum progesterone and serum estrogen reach their highest concentration 7 to 10 days prior to parturition and rapidly drop just hours before parturition.[49,63] Estrogen concentrations in Baird's tapirs were 85 to 131 pg/mL,[7] higher than those seen in the lowland tapir at 14 to 34.6 pg/mL.[63] Significant serum cortisol changes do not appear to precede parturition, at least in lowland and Baird's tapirs, and may not contribute to initiation of labor.[7,49,63] Enlarged mammary glands and vulvar edema may be observed approximately 2 weeks prior to parturition.[68] Mammae may begin to secrete colostrum 7 days prior to parturition, and vaginal mucoid discharge may be observed 2 days prior to parturition. Dystocia, vaginal prolapse, and metritis have been reported. Females should be separated from males prior to parturition. Depending on the housing situation and individual personalities of the tapirs, the male is commonly reintroduced when the calf is 1 to 3 months old.[63,68] Although young tapirs are strong swimmers, neonates may drown, so pools should be drained. Tapirs undergo a short labor period of 2 hours and usually give birth to a single calf, which is born head first. Twinning is rare.[47] Tapir calves are fairly small at birth, with average weights between 3 and 11 kg.[3,47,68] Healthy calves should be able to stand within 2 hours of birth, and nursing should commence within 5 hours.[68] Tapir dams nurse their calves in lateral recumbency, at 10- to 15-minute intervals approximately 5 to 10 times per day.[68] If the calf fails to nurse or the female is inexperienced, it may be possible to scratch down the dam onto her side and place the calf on the nipple or manually milk the colostrum to bottle feed to the calf.[3] Neonatal examinations should be performed 1 to 3 days after birth. Hand rearing has been successful in cases of maternal neglect or death. Transfaunation may be necessary to encourage growth of normal flora in hand-reared tapirs.[27] Aspiration pneumonia has been reported in bottle-fed neonates.[41]

Tapir calves grow rapidly, with body weight doubling within the first 2 to 3 weeks.[68] The growth rate of mother-reared calves was reported at 1.33 kg/day from ages 0 to 29 days.[26] As early as 1 to 2 weeks of age, calves begin to take solid food. Weaning occurs by 4 to 6 months of age, but young tapirs will continue to nurse as long as milk is available.[57] Calves are usually independent of their mothers by 18 months of age, when fully grown.[47] Neonatal mortality may be high and is dependent on a suitable birthing environment.[28] Neonates should be housed at 21°C to 29°C (70°F–85°F), and the floor should be bedded or padded for insulation and traction.[68] Most common causes of neonatal death are stillbirth, drowning, hypothermia, failure of passive transfer, septicemia, maternal neglect, and intraspecific or interspecific trauma.[41,68] Other mortalities reported were caused by necrotizing bacterial enteritis, cecocolic tympany, atresia ani, and primiparous female's failure to nurse. Iron deficiency anemia has also been documented and may be a predisposing factor for neonatal septicemias.[19] Neonatal isoerythrolysis was suspected in two Baird's calves from the same dam and sire.[72]

Contraception methods include physical separation, castration, and pharmaceutical agents. The most common contraceptives used in tapirs are medroxyprogesterone acetate injections (Depo-Provera, Upjohn) administered at 5 mg/kg every 3 months and porcine zona

pellucida (PZP) vaccination used short term for 2 to 3 consecutive years. After PZP use for 3 years, discontinuation will allow the female to regain fertility within 1 to 4 years, otherwise the continuation of PZP use every other year will render the female infertile in 5 to 7 years (Kimberly Frank, personal communication). Melengesterol acetate (MGA), deslorelin implants and oral altrenogest (Regu-Mate 0.044 mg/kg/day) are also effective. Complications observed include abscessation at PZP injection sites and rejection of MGA implants. Recommendations from the AZA Wildlife Contraception Center may be found at the website (http://www.stlzoo.org/animals/scienceresearch/contraceptioncenter/contraceptionrecommendatio/contraceptionmethods/perissodactyls/).

Little information is available regarding the prevalence and causes of reproductive failures. The maximum age for reproductive success is approximately 15 to 20 years for both males and females;[47] however, the oldest tapir to give birth was a lowland tapir at 28 years of age.[57] Reproductive senescence in older nulliparous females as well as asymmetric reproductive aging is thought to occur at least in Malayan tapirs (Thomas Hildebrandt, personal communication). Spermatozoa collection (via electroejaculation) and cryopreservation in the Baird's tapir has been demonstrated,[62] but not successful artificial insemination of tapirs.

ACKNOWLEDGMENT

The authors would like to thank Michele Stancer, Dr. Patricia Medici, Dr. Don Janssen, Dr. Viviana Quse, Dr. Drury Reavill, Dr. Mike Garner, Dr. Mads Bertelsen, Dr. Mitch Finnegan, Maria Fernanda Gondim, Dr. Dorothée Ordonneau, Dr. Liza Dadone, and the Tapir Specialist Group.

REFERENCES

1. AZA Tapir TAG: *Tapir (Tapiridae) care manual*, Silver Spring, CO, 2013, Association of Zoos and Aquariums.
2. Bailey JE, Foerster SH, Foerster CR: Evaluation of oscillometric blood pressure monitoring during immobilization of free-ranging Baird's tapirs (*Tapirus bairdii*) in Costa Rica. *Vet Anaesth Analg* 28(2):97–110, 2001.
3. Barongi RA: Husbandry and conservation of tapirs. *Intl Zoo YB* 32:7–15, 1993.
4. Blanco MP, Blanco MVJ: Anesthetic protocols used on *Tapirus terrestris* in Venezuela. In IUCN, IUCN/SSC-TSG, AZA, Houston Zoo, CI, editors: *Conference report of the Second International Tapir Symposium*, Panama City, 2004.
5. Bonar CJ, Lewandowski AH, Skowronek AJ: Embryonal rhabdomyosarcoma in an immature Baird's tapir (*tapirus bairdii*). *J Zoo Wildl Med* 38(1):121–124, 2007.
6. Bonar CJ, Trupkiewicz JG, Toddes B, et al: Iron storage disease in tapirs. *J Zoo Wildl Med* 37(1):49–52, 2006.
7. Brown JL, Citino SB, Shaw J, et al: Endocrine profiles during the estrous cycle and pregnancy in the Baird's tapir (*Tapirus bairdii*). *Zoo Biol* 13(2):107–117, 1994.
8. Chen SH, Ai I, Cai YC, et al: Diagnosis of *Cryptosporidium suis* infection of Baird's tapir. *J Animal Vet Advances* 11:627–630, 2012.
9. Clauss M, Hummel J, Eloff P, et al: Sources of high iron content in manufactured pelleted feeds: A case report. In Fidgett A, Clauss M, Eulenberger K, et al, editors: *Zoo animal nutrition*, vol III, Furth, Germany, 2006, Filander Verlag.
10. Clauss M, Lang-Deuerling S, Kienzle E, et al: Mineral absorption in tapirs (*Tapirus* spp.) as compared to the domestic horse. *J Anim Physiol Anim Nutr* 93(6):768–776, 2009.
11. Clauss M, Paglia DE: Iron storage disorders in captive wild mammals: The comparative evidence. *J Zoo Wildl Med* 43(3 Suppl):S6–S18, 2012.
12. Clauss M, Wilkins T, Hartley A, et al: Diet composition, food intake, body condition, and fecal consistency in captive tapirs (*Tapirus* sp.) in UK Collections. *Zoo Biol* 27:1–13, 2009.
13. Colbert M: Tapirus indicus, Digital Morphology: http://digimorph.org/specimens/Tapirus_indicus/. Accessed January 13, 2013.

13a. Cozzuol MA, Clozato CL, Holanda EC, et al: A new species of tapir from the Amazon. *J Mammalogy* 94(6):1331–1345, 2013.

14. Finnegan M, Munson L, Barrett S, et al: *Vesicular skin disease of tapirs. Proceedings of the American Association of Zoo Veterinarians,* St. Louis, MO, 1993.

15. Fleming DJ, Tucker KL, Jacques PF, et al: Dietary factors associated with the risk of high iron stores in the elderly Framingham Heart study cohort. *Am J Clin Nutr* 76:1375–1384, 2002.

16. Foerster SH, Bailey JE, Aguilar R, et al: Butorphanol//xylazine/ketamine immobilization of free-ranging Baird's tapirs in Costa Rica. *J Wildl Dis* 36(2):335–341, 2000.

17. Garcia MJ, Medici EP, Naranjo EJ, et al: Distribution, habitat and adaptability of the genus *Tapirus. Integrat Zool* 7:346–355, 2012.

18. Göltenboth R, Busch W, Jenschke J, et al: Herpesvirus infection in an Indian tapir (*Tapirus indicus*) and in a black rhinoceros (*Diceros Bicornis*). In *Proceedings of the American Association of Zoo Veterinarians,* Puerto Vallarta, Mexico, 1996.

19. Helmick KE: Iron deficiency anemia in captive Malayan tapir calves (*Tapirus indicus*). In *Proceedings of the American Association of Zoo Veterinarians,* Tulsa, OK, 2009.

20. Hernandez-Divers S, Bailey JE, Aguilar R, et al: Butorphanol/Xylazine/ Ketamine Immobilization of Free-ranging Baird's Tapirs in Costa Rica. *J Wildl Dis* 36(2):335–341, 2001.

21. Hernandez-Divers SM, Aguilar R, Leandro-Loria D, Foerster CR: Health evaluation of a radio collared population of free-ranging Baird's tapirs (*Tapirus bairdii*) in Costa Rica. *J Zoo Wildl Med* 36:176–187, 2005.

22. Hernandez-Divers SM, Bailey J: Tapirs. In West G, Heard D, Caulkett N, editors: *Zoo animal and wildlife immobilization and anesthesia,* Ames, IA, 2007, Blackwell Publishing.

23. Houck ML, Kingswood SC, Kumamoto AT: Comparative cytogenetics of tapirs, genus *Tapirus* (Perissodactyla, Tapiridae). *Cytogenet Cell Genetics* 89:110–115, 2000.

24. International Species Information Systems (ISIS): *Reference ranges for physiological values in captive wildlife,* Apple Valley, CA, 2002, ISIS.

25. International Union for the Conservation of Nature: *Red List of Threatened Species, 2008, Version 2012.2:* www.iucnredlist.org. Accessed December 27, 2012.

26. Janssen DL, Rideout BA, Edwards ME: Medical management of captive tapirs (*Tapirus* sp.). In *Proceedings of the American Association of Zoo Veterinarians,* Puerto Vallarta, 1996.

27. Janssen DL, Rideout BA, Edwards MS: Tapir medicine. In Fowler ME, Miller RE, editors: *Zoo and wild animal medicine,* ed 4, Philadelphia, PA, 1999, Saunders.

28. Janssen DL: Tapiridae. In Fowler ME, Miller RE, editors: *Zoo and wild animal medicine: Current therapy,* ed 5, Philadelphia, PA, 2003, Saunders.

29. Jurczynski K, Lyashchenko KP, Gomis D, et al: Pinniped tuberculosis in Malayan tapirs (*Tapirus indicus*) and its transmission to other terrestrial mammals. *J Zoo Wildl Med* 42(2):222–227, 2011.

30. Karpinski LG, Miller CL: Fluorouracil as a treatment for corneal papilloma in a Malayan tapir. *Vet Ophthalmol* 5(3):241–243, 2002.

31. Keller DL, Highland MA, Clyde VL, et al: Epistaxis secondary to suspected hypertension in Malayan tapirs (*Tapirus indicus*) with hypercalcemic chronic renal disease. In *Proceedings of the American Association of Zoo Veterinarians,* Kansas City, MO, 2011.

32. Kidney BA, Berrocal A: Sarcoids in two captive tapirs (*Tapirus bairdii*): Clinical, pathological and molecular study. *Vet Dermatol* 19(6):380–384, 2008.

33. Kono N, Shitsiri S, Hiramatsu H, et al: Some findings in thoracic cavities of Malayan tapirs (*Tapirus indicus*). *J Jpn Assoc Zool Gard Aquariums* 31:11–13, 1989.

34. Kuehn G: Tapiridae. In Fowler ME, editor: *Zoo and wild animal medicine,* ed 2, Philadelphia, PA, 1986, Saunders.

35. Kusuda S, Ikoma M, Morikaku K, et al: Estrous cycle based on blood progesterone profiles and changes in vulvar appearance of Malayan tapirs (*Tapirus indicus*). *J Reprod Develop* 53(6):1283–1289, 2007.

36. Lambeth RR, Dart AJ, Vogelnest L, et al: Surgical management of an abdominal abscess in a Malayan tapir. *Aust Vet J* 76(10):664–666, 1998.

37. Lecu A, Ball R: Mycobacterial infections in zoo animals: Relevance, diagnosis and management. *Int Zoo Yb* 45:183–202, 2011.

38. Lee AR: *Management guidelines for the welfare of zoo animals: Tapirs,* London, 1993, The Federation of Zoological Gardens of Great Britain and Ireland.

39. Lessa EP, Fariña RA: Reassessment of extinction patterns among the late Pleistocene mammals of South America. *Palaeontology* 39:651–662, 1996.

40. Maluf NS: The kidney of tapirs: A macroscopical study. *Anat Rec* 231(1):48–62, 1991.

41. Mangini PR, Medici EP, Fernandessantos RC: Tapir health and conservation medicine. *Integrat Zool* 7:331–345, 2012.

42. Mangini PR, Medici EP: Sanitary evaluation of wild populations of *Tapirus terrestris* in Pontal do Paranapanema region, São Paulo state, Brazil. Book of Abstracts, First International Tapir Symposium 3–8, 2001: http://www.tapirs.org. Accessed December 27, 2012.

43. Mangini PR, Velastin GO, Medici EP: Protocols of chemical restraint used in 16 wild *Tapirus terrestris. Arch Vet Sci Curitibita* 6:6–7, 2001.

44. Matthews NS, Taylor TS, Hartsfield SM: Anaesthesia of donkeys and mules. *Equine Vet Educ* 9(4):198–202, 1997.

45. May JA, Jr: *Avaliação de parâmetros fisiológicos e epidemiológicos da população de anta-brasileira* (Tapirus terrestris Linnaeus, 1758) *na Mata Atlântica do Parque Estadual Morro do Diabo, Pontal do Paranapanema, São Paulo* (MSc thesis), São Paulo, Brazil, 2011, Universidade de São Paulo.

46. Medici EP: *Assessing the viability of lowland tapir populations in a fragmented landscape,* (Ph.D. dissertation), Canterbury, U.K., 2010, Durrell Institute of Conservation and Ecology (DICE), University of Kent.

47. Medici EP: Family Tapiridae (Tapirs). In Wilson DE, Mittermeier RA, editors: *Handbook of the mammals of the world,* vol 2, Barcelona, Spain, 2011, Lynx Edicions.

48. Medici P, Mangini PR, da Silva AG, et al: *Guidelines for Tapir re-introductions and translocations,* 2008, IUCN/SSC Tapir Specialist Group.

49. Medici P, Mangini PR, Perea JAS, editors: *Tapir field veterinary manual,* 2009, IUCN/SSC Tapir Specialist Group (TSG) Veterinary Committee.

50. Miller CL, Templeton RS, Karpinski L: successful treatment of oral squamous cell carcinoma with intralesional fluorouracil in a Malayan tapir (*Tapirus indicus*). *J Zoo Wildl Med* 31(2):262–264, 2000.

51. Miller MA: Current diagnostic methods for tuberculosis in zoo animals. In Fowler ME, Miller RE, editors: *Zoo and wild animal medicine,* ed 6, St. Louis, MO, 2008, Saunders.

52. Miller-Edge M, Amsel S: Carfentanil, ketamine, xylazine combination (CKX) for immobilization of exotic ungulates: clinical experience in bongo (*Tragelaphus euryceros*) and mountain tapir (*Tapirus pinchaque*). In *Proceedings of the American Association of Zoo Veterinarians,* Pittsburg, PA, 1994, pp 192–195.

53. Murakami PS, Monego F, Ho JL, et al: Detection of RD[RIO] strain of *Mycobacterium tuberculosis* in tapirs (*Tapirus terrestris*) from a zoo in Brazil. *J Zoo Wildl Med* 43(4):872–875, 2012.

54. Murphy MR: Tapir (*Tapirus*) enteroliths. *Zoo Biol* 16(5):427–433, 1997.

55. Nowak RM: *Walker's mammals of the world,* ed 6, Baltimore, MD, 1999, Johns Hopkins Press.

56. Nunes ALV, Mangini PR, Ferreira JRV: Perissodactyla Family Tapiridae: Capture methodology and medicine. In Fowler ME, Cubas ZS, editors: *Biology, medicine and surgery of South American wild animals,* Ames, IA, 2001, Iowa State University Press.

57. Padilla M, Dowler RC: *Tapirus terrestris. Mammalian Species* 481:1–8, 1994.

58. Paglia DE: Recommended phlebotomy guidelines for prevention and therapy of captivity-induced iron-storage disease in rhinoceroses, tapirs and other exotic wildlife. In *Proceedings of the American Association of Zoo Veterinarians,* San Diego, CA, 2004.

59. Peters A, Raidal SR, Blake AH, et al: Haemochromatosis in a Brazilian tapir (*Tapirus terrestris*) in an Australian zoo. *Aust Vet J* 90(1–2):29–33, 2012.

60. Pollock C, Ramsay E: Serial immobilization of a Brazilian tapir (*Tapirus terrestris*) with oral detomidine and oral carfentanil. *J Zoo Wildl Med* 34(4):408–410, 2003.

61. Pukazhenthi BS, Padilla LR, Togna GD, et al: *Biomedical survey of Baird's tapir (Tapirus bairdii) in captivity in Panama*, Book of Abstracts, Fourth International Tapir Symposium 26, 2008, IUCN/SSC Tapir Specialist Group. [Cited 10 Jan 2011.] http://www.tapirs.org. Accessed December 27, 2012.

62. Pukazhenthi BS, Togna GD, Padilla L, et al: Ejaculate traits and sperm cryopreservation in the endangered Baird's tapir (*Tapirus bairdii*). *J Androl* 32(3):260–270, 2011.

63. Quse VB, Francisco E, Gachen G, et al: Hormonal and ultrasonography studies during the pregnancy of lowland tapir. In *Proceedings of the Second International Tapir Symposium*, Panama City, Panama, 2004.

64. Ramsay EC, Zainuddin Z: Infectious diseases of the rhinoceros and tapir. In Fowler M, editor: *Zoo and wild animal medicine: Current therapy*, ed 3, Philadelphia, PA, 1993, Saunders.

65. Rose PE, Roffe SM: A case study of Malayan tapir (*Tapirus indicus*) husbandry practice across 10 zoological collections. *Zoo Biol* 32(3):347–356, 2013epub 10.1002/zoo.21018, 2012.

66. Satterfield W: Internal fixation of a rectal prolapse in a Malayan tapir. In *Proceedings of the American Association of Zoo Veterinarians*, Houston, TX, 1971.

67. Schnieder HJ, Franz W, Audort F, et al: Medical treatment of a mandibular fracture through osteosynthesis in a lowland tapir (*Tapirus terrestris*). *Erkrankungen Zootiere* 28:195–199, 1986.

68. Shoemaker AH, Barongi R, Flanagan J, et al: *Husbandry guidelines for keeping tapirs in captivity*, 2006, Tapir Specialist Group.

69. Stevens CE: *Comparative physiology of the vertebrate digestive system*, New York, 1988, Cambridge University Press.

70. Stringfield CE, Wynne JE: Nutraceutical chondroprotectives and their use in osteoarthritis in zoo animals. In *Proceedings of the American Association of Zoo Veterinarians*, Columbus, OH, 1999.

71. Velastin GO, Mangini PR, Medici EP: Utilização de associação de tartarato de butorfanol e cloridrato de medetomidina na contenção de *tapirus terrestris* em vida livre—relato de dois casos. In *Anais XXVIII Congresso da Sociedade de Zoológicos do Brasil* 1:T063, 2004.

72. Wack RF, Jones AA: Suspected neonatal isoerythrolysis in two Baird's tapirs (*Tapirus bairdii*). *J Zoo Wildl Med* 28(3):285–289, 1997.

73. Witmer LM, Sampson SD, Solounias N: The proboscis of tapirs (Mammalia: Perissodactyla: a case study in novel narial anatomy. *J Zool* 249(3):249–267, 1999.

CHAPTER **57**

Equidae

Donald L. Janssen and Jack L. Allen

GENERAL BIOLOGY

Equidae, Tapiridae, and Rhinocerotidae are families within the mammalian order Perissodactyla and are distinguished from the family Artiodactyla by their foot morphology and digestive system. Equidae is a small family that includes the horses, wild asses, and zebras. The taxonomy of nondomestic Equidae is somewhat dynamic and subject to change. The International Union for the Conservation of Nature (IUCN) Equid Specialist Group lists seven species and numerous subspecies of the single genus *Equus*[18] (Table 57-1). Most species are at risk of extinction today. The genus *Equus* first appeared during the Pliocene Age and was once widespread in grassland and desert habitats through North America, Asia, Africa, and Europe. The current distribution is over open habitats of eastern and southern Africa and regions of Asia. This pattern of significantly reduced distribution from former times is a pattern seen among all perissodactyls. Modern equids tend to live in harsh, dry lands, and many occupy grasslands shared by nomadic peoples. Wild equids generally are polygynous and highly social.[18]

UNIQUE ANATOMY

The structure and anatomy of the members of Equidae are quite similar to those of the domestic horse. Nondomestic equids are most easily distinguished by their external appearance. Table 57-1 gives brief descriptions of the distinguishing characteristics of each species. The Przewalski horse is most noted for its horselike appearance. The

Asian and African wild asses are distinguished by the solid and subtle color patterns on their bodies and legs. The various zebra species have distinct striping patterns and characteristics that differentiate them by species and even as individuals.

The internal anatomy of equids is analogous to that of the domestic horse and other Perisodactyla species. Equids are bulk-feeding herbivores with large body mass. The dental formula is: incisors (I) 3/3, canines (C) 1/1, premolars (P) 3-4/3, molars (M) 3/3) for a total of 40 to 42 teeth. The canine teeth are vestigial or absent in females. Their cheek teeth have high crowns and relatively short roots (hypsodont). Their gastrointestinal (GI) anatomy has a structure and function designed for hindgut fiber fermentation, with a relatively small stomach and large cecum and colon. The foot posture is unguligrade, bearing weight on one functional digit. Minor differences exist in external foot anatomy in nondomestic equids compared with domestic horses. In general, nondomestic horses have smaller feet compared with domestic horses. Specifically, the Przewalski horse's hoof is the most similar to the domestic horse but a little smaller. The foot has a strong and robust appearance, with the ratio of frog to sole being identical to that of domestic horses. The Grevy zebra's foot is similar to that of a mule or donkey and is narrower and more upright than that of domestic horses. The frog-to-sole ratio is less than that in the domestic horse. The mountain zebras have a smaller foot than the Grevy zebra but otherwise similar. The African wild asses' feet are similar to those of zebras but are less robust in appearance. The Asian wild asses' feet are similar to those of the African asses except that they have a more robust structure.

TABLE 57-1

Biologic Information of Selected Nondomestic Equids, Order Perissodactyla, Family Equidae[18]

Scientific Name	Common Names	Weight (adults, kilograms)	Geographic Distribution	Karyotype 2n =	Distinguishing Characteristics
HORSES					
Equus przewalskii	Przewalski horse Mongolian wild horse	200–350	Mongolia (reintroduced)	66	Brown in color with dorsal stripe and erect mane Robust shape with thick, short neck
WILD ASSES					
Equus africanus (2 ssp.)	Somali and Nubian wild asses	250–300	Ethiopia, Somalia	62–64	Buff-gray with black leg stripes
Equus hemionus (5 ssp.)	Asiatic wild ass, kulan, onager	200–250	Mongolia	55–56	Sandy yellow with white underside and dorsal stripe
Equus kiang (3 ssp.)	Eastern, Western, and Southern kiang	250–4003	Central Asia, northern India	51–52	Chestnut color with white underside
ZEBRAS					
Equus zebra Equus hartmannae[35]	Cape mountain zebra Hartmann zebra	200–260	Southern Africa	32	Dewlap; "gridiron" pattern on croup
Equus grevyi[13]	Grevy zebra	350–450	Kenya, Ethiopia	46	Tightly packed, narrow stripes
Equus burchelli[19] (5 ssp.)	Plains or Burchell zebra	175–275	Southeastern Africa	44	Broad body stripes

SPECIAL HOUSING REQUIREMENTS

Most equids are managed in a similar way in zoos. Equids are generally hardy and withstand normal to severe temperature variations as long as shelter and protection from wind and sun are available. Equids acclimated to the southern California climate do well in temperatures ranging from 0°C to over 38°C. Grevy zebras are reported to be less cold tolerant in zoos compared with other zebras.[13] Shelter should be provided to keep food dry and to provide shade. Although wild equids may go without water for long periods in the wild, they drink water when it is accessible, so they should have a constant supply of fresh water when managed in zoos. Periodic hoof trimming is needed in some individuals and under certain management conditions. Some species of equids (e.g., mountain zebras and Przewalski horses) seem to require more frequent hoof trimming compared with others. Przewalski horses, for example, may require trimming every 6 to 9 months.[37]

Some interactions and introductions among equids may be quite violent and aggressive, resulting in injuries from kicking or from bite wounds on the neck or tail area. Several cases of infanticide have been documented in wild equids.[16] Care should be exercised when introducing a male to a new herd or a pregnant female to a new stallion. Stallions may be aggressive toward new foals, so mares that are close to foaling should be separated from stallions. Stallions may also be aggressive toward keepers, and extreme caution should be used when working around them.[37]

FEEDING

All equids are bulk-feeding grazers, feeding primarily on grass and roughage. In the wild, grass constitutes over 90% of the common zebra's diet. They may resort to some browsing and digging of plant materials in the dry periods. Grevy zebras reportedly eat some browse in the wild.[19] As with other perissodactylids, equids are hind gut fermenters and have a large cecum and colon. In general, nondomestic equids have no specialized feeding requirements and may be fed like domestic equines. Specifically, feeding a diet combining high-fiber pellets and grass hay to nonruminant grazers in zoos is recommended. The pellet serves as a source of nutrients and may be designed to compensate for specific regional dietary deficiencies or

for deficiencies in the hay. In regions where enteroliths are a problem, reducing or eliminating alfalfa in the pellet or hay source is advisable. Pellet and hay may be fed at a ratio of approximately 50% pellet to 50% hay. Intake should be about 1.5% to 3.0% body weight.[25] In group-housed animals, adequate feeders are necessary to avoid competition from dominant animals. Salt and trace mineral blocks may be used if the pelleted diet cannot be specially formulated. Feeding of produce is not recommended, since readily fermentable substances may lead to digestive upset. Often, these items are desired for behavioral husbandry or enrichment. It is recommended that produce be offered at no more than 2% to 5% of the diet on a dry-matter (DM) basis.[25] The document "Nutrient Requirement for Horses," from the National Research Council (NRC) may be consulted for specific nutrient and energy requirements for maintenance, growth, gestation, and lactation.[14]

Obesity may be a problem in nondomestic equids maintained in zoo environments. Encouraging exercise and restricting the amount of pelleted feed may help. A body scoring system may be used to track body condition and used as an objective assessment of obesity.[11,14]

RESTRAINT AND HANDLING

Physical restraint is not often practical in adult equids because of their size and strength. Newer hydraulic hugger restraint chutes do make it possible to restrain nondomestic equids, usually with the aid of chemical restraint (Table 57-2). Blood sampling and other minor procedures are then possible.[21] Animal care staff must work cautiously around any nondomestic equid because they may startle and bolt unexpectedly into solid obstacles, which may result in fatal neck or head injuries.

Chemical Restraint

Several authors provide regimens for successful chemical restraint of equids under both captive and free-ranging conditions (see Table 57-2). Acepromazine granules and oral haloperidol are effective for oral sedation to aid in acclimation to new housing or for transport. Injectable short-acting sedatives such as xylazine, acepromazine, and butorphanol may be used. Long-acting neuroleptic sedatives may be used as injectable drugs, sometimes in combination and staged to

TABLE 57-2

Chemical Restraint Agents Used in Equids

Species	Drug	Dose	Reversal Agent	Comments	Reference
SEDATION					
Grevy zebra Burchell zebra	Detomidine Butorphanol	0.10 milligram per kilogram (mg/kg), intramuscularly (IM) 0.13 mg/kg, IM, 10 minutes later	Atipamezole 2 mg per 1 mg detomidine, intravenously (IV) Naltrexone 0.1 mg/kg, IV	Median doses for 70 standing procedures. Some required supplements with etorphine or acepromazine	Hoyer[21]
	Acepromazine granules	0.5 to 1.5 mg/kg, orally (PO)		Granules mixed into moistened feed Used to aid transport	Walzer[42]
Przewalski horse	Perphenazine Haloperidol	0.5 mg/kg, IM 0.3 mg/kg, PO		Given to facilitate establishment of a bachelor herd	Atkinson[7]
Grevy zebra Przewalski horse	Haloperidol injection	0.2–0.35 mg/kg, IM		8–18 hours duration	Walzer[43]
Burchell zebra	Zuclopenthixol	50–100 mg/adult, IM		3–4 days duration	Walzer[43]
Burchell zebra	Perphenazine	100–200 mg/adult, IM		10 days duration	Walzer[43]
IMMOBILIZING AGENTS/COMBINATIONS					
Mongolian wild horse	Carfentanil	0.020 mg/kg	Naltrexone at 50:1, IV	No renarcotization in 18 study animals	Allen[4]
Mongolian wild horse	Medetomidine Ketamine	0.09 mg/kg 2.1 mg/kg	Atipamezole 0.19 mg/kg, IV	Mean dosages for 11 mature horses	Matthews[29] [31]
Hartmann mountain zebra	Carfentanil	0.011 mg/kg	Naltrexone or nalmefene at 50:1, IV	No renarcotization in 12 study animals	Allen[2]
Grevy zebra	Etorphine Acepromazine	5 mg initial 14 mg in 4 hours 15 mg total	Diprenorphine 14 mg, IV	Prolonged anesthesia for cesarean section	Bristol[12] [33]
Grevy zebra	Etorphine Detomidine Acepromazine	4.6 mg 15.2 mg 10 mg		Mean values for series of 20 animals during cardiac evaluation Initial doses only, supplements also given	Adin[1]
Grevy zebra	Etorphine Detomidine Acepromazine	0.01–0.017 mg/kg 0.03–0.04 mg/kg 0.02–0.04 mg/kg	Naltrexone 100:1, IV	Used for free-ranging animals	Walzer[43]
Persian onager	Carfentanil	0.055 mg/kg	Naltrexone 50:1, IV		Allen[3]
Eastern kiang	Carfentanil	0.044 mg/kg	Naltrexone 50:1, IV		Allen[3]
Somali wild ass	Carfentanil	0.046 mg/kg	Naltrexone 50:1, IV		Allen[3]

achieve the desired length of sedation. Haloperidol is a short-acting agent and has a relatively rapid onset of 5 to 10 minutes and a duration of 8 to 18 hours. Zuclopenthixol is a medium-acting drug and has an onset of action in 1 hour and a duration of action of about 3 to 4 days. Finally, perphenazine is a long-acting drug that has an onset of action in 12 to 16 hours and duration of 10 days.[43] These drugs may occasionally cause extrapyramidal signs such as hyperexcitability and incoordination. A detailed review of long-acting neuroleptic tranquilizers in equids is provided elsewhere.[43]

For full immobilization, opioid narcotics are the primary agents available. Etorphine is the most commonly used agent because of its familiarity, availability, and reliability in most species of equids. It is most often used in combination with α_2-agonists, ketamine, phenothiazine tranquilizers, or a combination of these agents. Carfentanil has also been used with the Przewalski horse and Hartmann mountain zebras (see Table 57-2). In the authors' experience, carfentanil has been less consistent and more unpredictable in onagers, kiangs, and Somali wild asses. Carfentanil is largely ineffective and thus not a good choice for anesthetizing Grevy zebras. Another narcotic

opioid, thiafentanil (A3080), shows promise for anesthetizing nondomestic equids.

Opioids generally cause significant muscle rigidity. When opioids are used alone, the animals often will not become recumbent on their own and may require "casting" to achieve recumbency. This may be avoided by using α_2-agonists prior to or along with administration of the opioid. Supplemental drugs such as guaifenesin (5% solution given intravenously [IV] to effect) or propofol (1% solution 3 to 5 mg/kg, IV, to effect) may be used to provide sufficient relaxation during field procedures. Relaxation is important to allow adequate ventilation depth, tidal volume, and intubation, if desired. Renarcotization following etorphine anesthesia and diprenorphine reversal has been shown to range from approximately 5% to 10%.[5] A review of alternative non-narcotic anesthetic agents for chemical immobilization of equids covered several drug categories, including α_2-agonists, benzodiazepines, butyrophenones, and others, which might be useful if potent opioid narcotics are not available.[30]

Besides the chemical agents themselves, several other factors need to be considered when immobilizing nondomestic equids. A well-thought-out plan is critical for success. Some factors to consider include (1) obtaining an accurate body weight, (2) work with experienced or trained support staff, (3) precise dart placement, (4) advantages and disadvantages of preanesthetic medications, (5) the prevalence of renarcotization in the species, and (6) a safe, appropriate area for recovery. Although regurgitation is not a risk, food and water must be withheld for 18 to 24 hours prior to a planned procedure to reduce GI volume. During hot weather, it is probably best to provide water during the fasting period. Anesthetic drugs may be administered with a variety of remote delivery devices. If the horse is nervous and excited prior to darting, achieving the desired effect of the anesthetic drugs may be made more difficult. Dart location is ideally in a large muscle mass such as the gluteals, shoulder, or neck region, but areas of fat should be avoided. Horses generally do well in lateral recumbency when under anesthesia and do not need to have the head elevated. Blindfolds and ear plugs are useful to decrease stimulation. It is recommended that supplemental oxygen be provided via a mask or a nasal cannula, at a flow rate of 6 to 10 liters per minute (L/min). At a minimum, anesthesia monitoring should include heart rate and rhythm, rate and depth of ventilations, and oxygen saturation by pulse oximetry. Using a veterinary clip sensor, pulse oximetry is usually successful on the tongue, ear pinna (clipped and scraped of superficial pigment), vulva, prepuce, or eyelid (reflectance sensor).

Once equids are immobilized with chemical restraint, many minor procedures such as physical examination, diagnostic sampling, hoof care, and assisted birthing may be performed. For prolonged procedures such as dental work, radiography, extensive diagnostics, and abdominal surgery, general anesthesia and additional monitoring are recommended. Isoflurane works well for maintenance of inhalation anesthesia in equids. Mechanical ventilation is recommended. Intermittent intravenous propofol may be used to extend the anesthesia. Performing endotracheal intubation is straightforward in nondomestic equids. Blind intubation, as in the domestic horse, is the usual method. Direct visualization of the larynx is not difficult with proper positioning and the use of a long laryngoscope blade. With either technique, it is important to have the animal adequately relaxed and its neck fully extended in the dorsal direction. Indirect blood pressure may be measured with an appropriate-sized cuff placed around the metacarpal or metatarsal area. Arterial samples for blood gas determination may be obtained from the facial artery or the intermediate branch of the caudal auricular artery. End-tidal carbon dioxide (CO_2), a direct arterial line in the facial artery for direct blood pressure, and electrocardiography (ECG) are also useful in monitoring horses under prolonged anesthesia. ECG parameters in Grevy zebras have been described elsewhere.[32]

SURGERY

As in the domestic horse, acute abdominal discomfort is not uncommon in nondomestic equids. Some cases require surgery. Enterolith-associated colic requiring rapid surgical intervention has been reported.[20] See Table 57-7.

OTHER PHARMACEUTICALS

Other pharmaceuticals used in domestic horses may also be indicated in nondomestic equids. When a nondomestic equid is hospitalized, is a new arrival into quarantine, or is under other short-term stress, it is good practice to provide oral omeprazole using the equine dose.

PHYSICAL EXAMINATION AND DIAGNOSTICS

Most diagnostic techniques used for horses may be adapted for use in nondomestic equids. Blood is most commonly collected from the jugular vein. Alternative sites include the cephalic vein, the medial saphenous vein, and the transverse facial venous sinus. Catheter placement is most suitable in the jugular vein. Urine may be collected with direct catheterization by using techniques and catheters designed for domestic horses. Urine often is cloudy and chalky in appearance because of normal urinary calcium excretion seen in most Perissodactyla species.

Thoracic and abdominal radiography may be a challenge in adult equids simply because of their size. Multiple exposures may need to be taken systematically to cover the entire field to identify, for example, enteroliths.[20] Feet and dental structures are other sites most frequently radiographed in equids. Upper GI tract endoscopy requires the use of long, flexible endoscopes up to 3 m in length. Rectal palpation is generally more difficult than in the domestic horse because of the necessity for recumbency and the smaller size of the nondomestic equids. Diagnosis of intestinal disease using paracentesis is limited by the need for the animal to be in the standing position.

HEMATOLOGY

Hematologic parameters are similar in most nondomestic equids.[42] Reference ranges for selected hematologic parameters are summarized in Table 57-3. Reference ranges for selected biochemical parameters are summarized in Table 57-4.

DISEASES

Infectious Disease

Selected infectious diseases in nondomestic equids are summarized in Table 57-5. Nondomestic equids are generally hardy, and relatively few infectious diseases have been reported in the literature. In general, disease susceptibility is likely similar to that in domestic horses. Infectious disease risk should be considered during translocation and reintroduction programs. The readers are referred to other texts for a review of disease concerns with regard to these programs and a comprehensive list of infectious diseases reported in zoo and free-ranging nondomestic equids.[36]

Equine herpesviruses (EHV) have received attention recently, and the susceptible host range for these viruses may be wider than previously thought. Zebras have been shown to be asymptomatic reservoir hosts for some EHVs affecting zoo animals, including polar bears, Thomson gazelles, and a reticulated giraffe.[17,39] Preventative measures should be put in place to minimize the risk of cross-infection, including fomite transmission from known reservoir hosts such as zebras and susceptible hosts such as polar bears.

Anthrax has become a threat to populations of free-ranging Grevy zebras in Africa. One study documented a local population decline among this endangered zebra. Both mature and immature animals were affected. Drought and other adverse environmental conditions were predisposing factors. It is thought that dry conditions could promote trauma in the oral cavity, which increases the risk of acquiring anthrax spores.[24,31] Widespread vaccination, supported by local governments and conservation organizations, has been used in an effort to control outbreaks.

The systemic fungal disease coccidioidomycosis has been reported in Przewalski horses in California, where *Coccidioides immitus* is endemic. Infections caused by this organism are usually asymptomatic and resolve spontaneously. Immunosuppression increases the risk of disseminated infections in humans and domestic animals. Coccidioidomycosis was the leading cause of death in a population of Przewalski horses, likely from poor immune response to *C. immitus*.[40] Use of management strategies that reduce stress in the herd may be helpful in preventing this disease.

Parasitic Diseases

Selected parasitic diseases of nondomestic equids are summarized in Table 57-6. The protozoal disease piroplasmosis has been identified as a possible cause of mortality in reintroduced Przewalski horses in Mongolia. *Babesia caballi* and *Theileria equi* are probably endemic throughout Asia. During reintroductions of Przewalski horses from

TABLE 57-3

Reference Range for Hematologic Parameters in Wild Equids

Parameter	Przewalski Horse Mean ± Standard Deviation	African Wild Ass Mean ± Standard Deviation	Onager Mean ± Standard Deviation	Common Zebra Mean ± Standard Deviation	Mountain Zebra Mean ± Standard Deviation	Grevy Zebra Mean ± Standard Deviation
Erythrocytes ($\times 10^6$/microliter [µL])	8.7 ± 1.6	6.7 ± 1.4	8.1 ± 0.7	10.5 ± 2.3	10.8 ± 1.6	10.2 ± 2
Hemoglobin, gram per microliter (g/µL)	14.4 ± 2.3	12.9 ± 2.4	18.0 ± 1.9	14.6 ± 2.2	157 ± 17	153 ± 19
Hematocrit (%)	42 ± 6	37 ± 6	50 ± 5	42 ± 6	0.44 ± 0.05	0.44 ± 0.05
Mean corpuscular volume, femtoliters (fL)	48.4 ± 6	56.5 ± 6	62 ± 4	41.3 ± 7	42.6 ± 5	44.3 ± 6
Mean corpuscular hemoglobin (g/µL)	17.5 ± 2	19.6 ± 2	22.2 ± 1.4	14.4 ± 3	14.6 ± 1.9	15.4 ± 2
Mean corpuscular hemoglobin concentration (g/µL)	34.4 ± 3.9	34.7 ± 2.9	36.2 ± 2.2	34.6 ± 3.8	351 ± 21	348 ± 24
Leukocytes ($\times 10^3$/µL)	7.9 ± 2.5	9.2 ± 3.2	10.2 ± 2.9	8.8 ± 2.7	9.7 ± 2.5	8.7 ± 2.3
Segregated neutrophils ($\times 10^3$/µL)	4.3 ± 1.6	4.2 ± 1.6	7.3 ± 3	5.6 ± 2.3	5.8 ± 2.3	5.7 ± 2
Lymphocytes ($\times 10^3$/µL)	3 ± 1.6	4.5 ± 2.3	2.4 ± 1.2	2.9 ± 1.7	3.2 ± 1.3	2.6 ± 1.3
Monocytes ($\times 10^3$/µL)	0.3 ± 0.25	0.4 ± 0.3	0.5 ± 0.3	0.3 ± 0.2	0.3 ± 0.2	0.24 ± 0.2
Eosinophils ($\times 10^3$/µL)	0.2 ± 0.2	0.3 ± 0.3	0.17 ± 0.1	0.12 ± 0.1	0.21 ± 0.2	0.2 ± 0.18
Basophils ($\times 10^3$/µL)	0.06 ± 0.1	0.12 ± 0.07	0.01 ± 0.03	0.05 ± 0.09	0.1 ± 0.04	0.11 ± 0.07
Neutrophilic bands ($\times 10^3$/µL)	0.1 ± 0.14	0.4 ± 1.0	0.005 ± 0.02	0.13 ± 0.16	0.25 ± 0.29	0.47 ± 1.4
Platelet count ($\times 10^9$/µL)	0.14 ± 0.06	0.24 ± 0.08	0.18 ± 0.07	0.22 ± 0.08	0.18 ± 0.14	0.22 ± 0.08
Nucleated red blood cells (/100 white blood cells)	0.0	0.0	3 ± 1	2 ± 9	0.0	1 ± 1
Reticulocytes (%)	0.0	0.0	—	0.0	—	0.0

From Walzer C. Equidae. In Fowler ME, Miller RE (eds): *Zoo and Wild Animal Medicine*, 5th ed. St. Louis, MO, 2003, Saunders, pp. 578–586.

TABLE 57-4

Selected Reference Ranges for Serum Biochemical Parameters for Wild Equids

Parameter	Przewalski Horse Mean ± Standard Deviation	African Wild Ass Mean ± Standard Deviation	Onager Mean ± Standard Deviation	Common Zebra Mean ± Standard Deviation	Mountain Zebra Mean ± Standard Deviation	Grevy Zebra Mean ± Standard Deviation
Total protein, gram per deciliter (g/dL)	6.7 ± 0.7	6.5 ± 0.8	6.9 ± 0.9	6.3 ± 0.8	6.5 ± 0.7	6.5 ± 0.6
Globulin (g/dL)	3.4 ± 0.6	3.3 ± 0.7	3.1 ± 0.8	3.1 ± 0.7	3.1 ± 0.5	2.9 ± 0.6
Albumin (g/dL)	2.3 ± 0.28	2.3 ± 0.28	2.6 ± 0.42	2.3 ± 0.28	2.4 ± 0.284	2.5 ± 0.35
Fibrinogen, gram per liter (g/L)	300 ± 140	250 ± 130	250 ± 130	250 ± 150	290 ± 160	75 ± 130
Calcium, milligram per deciliter (mg/dL)	11.2 ± 0.8	11.6 ± 0.8	11.6 ± 0.8	10.8 ± 0.8	10.0 ± 0.8	10.4 ± 0.8
Phosphorus (mg/dL)	4.0 ± 0.9	4.3 ± 1.6	4.3 ± 1.2	5.3 ± 1.6	4.0 ± 1.5	5.3 ± 1.2
Sodium, milliequivalent per liter (mEq/L)	137 ± 3	136 ± 4	138 ± 4	137 ± 4	136 ± 3	137 ± 4
Potassium (mEq/L)	4.6 ± 0.6	4.3 ± 0.4	4.4 ± 1.3	4.1 ± 0.6	4.5 ± 0.8	4.1 ± 0.4
Chloride (mEq/L)	97 ± 4	102 ± 4	99 ± 5	99 ± 4	99 ± 5	99 ± 4
Iron (mg/dL)	147.9 ± 53	125 ± 42	158 ± 63	189 ± 77		128 ± 58
Creatinine (mg/dL)	1.27 ± 0.30	1.17 ± 0.30	1.65 ± 0.39	1.84 ± 0.48	1.95 ± 0.39	1.95 ± 0.39

Continued

TABLE 57-4

Selected Reference Ranges for Serum Biochemical Parameters for Wild Equids—cont'd

Parameter	Przewalski Horse Mean ± Standard Deviation	African Wild Ass Mean ± Standard Deviation	Onager Mean ± Standard Deviation	Common Zebra Mean ± Standard Deviation	Mountain Zebra Mean ± Standard Deviation	Grevy Zebra Mean ± Standard Deviation
Blood urea nitrogen (mg/dL)	17.14 ± 3.93	14.89 ± 5.06	21.92 ± 2.1	17.14 ± 5.90	19.10 ± 7.87	17.98 ± 0.39
Total bilirubin (mg/dL)	1.24 ± 0.58	0.18 ± 0.12	0.41 ± 0.18	0.58 ± 0.41	0.53 ± 0.29	0.89 ± 0.71
Glucose (mg/dL)	169.2 ± 48.6	106.2 ± 39.6	162 ± 73.8	158.4 ± 46.8	169.2 ± 57.6	176 ± 59.4
Cholesterol (mg/dL)	81.2 ± 15.47	92.81 ± 27.07	100.54 ± 15.47	139.21 ± 54.14	104.41 ± 15.47	108.28 ± 27.07
Triglyceride (mg/dL)	35.4 ± 17.7	123.9 ± 70.8	97.35 ± 35.4	70.8 ± 79.65	53.1 ± 53.1	44.25 ± 35.4
Creatine kinase, unit per liter (Unit/L)	454 ±375	337 ± 427	157 ± 18	309 ± 303	432 ± 531	263 ± 285
LDH (Unit/L)	494 ± 233	310 ± 163	731 ± 454	604 ± 463	518 ± 215	498 ± 355
AP (Unit/L)	179 ± 84	196 ± 129	197 ± 254	272 ± 440	141 ± 52	275 ± 195
ALT (Unit/L)	13 ± 10	15 ± 20	15 ± 12	15 ± 12	7 ± 5	19 ± 15
AST (Unit/L)	347 ± 125	328 ± 124	411 ± 149	303 ± 125	375 ± 131	344 ± 129
GGT (Unit/L)	23 ± 19	34 ± 20	42 ± 35	48 ± 35	34 ± 19	43 ± 24
Amylase (Unit/L)	7 ± 8.5	10.5 ± 12.2	4.2 ± 1.6	9.9 ± 10.9	41 ± 29	13.7 ± 16.3
Lipase (Unit/L)	5.6 ± 2.5	3.9 ± 2.5	—	4.4 ± 3.6	3 ± 3	3.3 ± 3.9
Total T-3, nanogram per deciliter (ng/dL)	—	52.1 ± 6.5	—	—		—
Total T-4 (ng/dL)	—	27.97 ± 27.20	—	13.21 ± 0.78	29.49 ± 0	—

From Walzer C. Equidae. In Fowler ME, Miller RE (eds): *Zoo and Wild Animal Medicine*, 5th ed. St. Louis, MO, 2003, Saunders, pp. 578–586.

TABLE 57-5

Selected Infectious Diseases Reported in Nondomestic Equids

Disease	Etiology	Epizootiology	Signs	Diagnosis	Management
VIRAL					
Equine herpesvirus[10]	EVH-1 EHV-4	Presumably exposure from infected equids	Respiratory, epizootic abortions, neurologic	Histopathology, isolation	Vaccination
Equine herpesvirus[39]	EHV-9	Grevy zebra asymptomatic reservoir species	No signs in zebras; progressive encephalitis in a polar bear	Intranuclear inclusion bodies, polymerase chain reaction (PCR)	Minimize direct animal-to-animal and fomite transmission
Equine herpesvirus[17]	EHV-1 and EHV-9	Recombination of zebra EHV-1 and EHV-9	No signs in zebras; nonsuppurative encephalitis in a polar bear	Histopathology, PCR	Minimize direct animal-to-animal and fomite transmission
Rabies[23]	Rabies virus (lyssavirus)	Tourist exposure of infected zebra foal	Neurologic signs in zebra	Rabies antigen detected by direct fluorescent antibody	Postexposure prophylaxis in tourists
Sarcoids[26, 27]	Bovine papillomavirus (BPV) type 1	Presumed similar to disease in domestic horses	Masses in inguinal region and on nose	Histopathology, PCR	Reduce exposure risk Treated with surgical excision, 5-fluorouracil, allogenous vaccine, or a combination[39]
BACTERIAL					
Tetanus[34]	*Clostridium tetani*	Reported associated with hoof abscesses in Somali wild ass	Tonic spasms and hyperesthesia	Clinical signs and evidence of recent trauma	Active immunization with tetanus toxoid

TABLE 57-5

Selected Infectious Diseases Reported in Nondomestic Equids—cont'd

Disease	Etiology	Epizootiology	Signs	Diagnosis	Management
Anthrax[31]	Spores of *Bacillus anthracis*	Outbreaks related to drought conditions in Grevy's zebra in Kenya	Sudden death in healthy animal	Blood smears, PCR	Mass vaccination of zebra has helped to control outbreaks
Mycobacteriosis[15]	*Mycobacterium avium hominissuis*	Presumed to be alimentary route transmission; ubiquitous organism	Progressive loss of condition, liver disease in a kiang	Histopathology, culture	Not known
FUNGAL					
Coccidioidomycosis[40]	*Coccidioides immitus*	Exposure in endemic regions exacerbated by immunosuppression	Weight loss; respiratory signs; disseminated disease	Bronchial wash, histopathology	Caution with bachelor herds, reduce herd stressors

TABLE 57-6

Selected Parasitic Disease Reported in Nondomestic Equids

Parasitic Disease	Etiology	Transmission	Clinical Signs	Diagnosis	Comments
Piroplasmosis[38]	*Theileria equi* or *Babesia caballi*	Ixodid tick vector	Erythrolysis, fever, anemia, icterus, hemoglobinuria	Giemsa-stained blood smears; complement fixation (CF), immunofluorescent antibody (IFA)	Prevention and control through tick prevention and chemoprophylaxis with imidocarb
Equine protozoal myeloencephalitis[28]	*Sarcocystis neurona*	Feces from definitive host opossum	Ataxia and weakness	Histology, immunohistochemistry	Possibly associated with immunosuppression from severe gastrointestinal (GI) parasitism
Internal parasites[34]	*Parascaris equorum* *Strongylus* spp. *Strongyloides* spp. *Oxyuris* spp.	Direct		Fecal parasitologic examination	*P. equorum* particularly pathogenic in zebra foals[15]

outside this endemic area, increased susceptibility was demonstrated. This was thought to be caused by the lack of acquired immunity against the protozoa and the fact that these animals were transported to the endemic area at an age when juvenile innate resistance factors had already been lost.[38]

Noninfectious Disease

Selected noninfectious diseases of nondomestic equids are summarized in Table 57-7. One of the most significant noninfectious diseases in the authors' experience is enterolithiasis.[20] This disease most often manifests as acute onset of colic. Diagnosis is confirmed by radiographic examination performed with the animal under anesthesia, in lateral recumbency, with the use of the four-quadrant approach described for domestic horses. Rapid surgical intervention is often indicated for enterolith-associated colic. Reducing dietary alfalfa, because of its excessive magnesium content, may be useful to prevent enteroliths.[14] Radiography may be used as the cornerstone of a preventive screening program as well.[20]

Hoof problems commonly occur, especially in large collections of nondomestic equids. Routine hoof trimming may be necessary in some species and under some management conditions. The mountain zebras, for example, seem to require more frequent hoof trims compared with other species, especially when housed on soft or sandy soil. Hoof abscesses should be suspected when a horse

becomes severely and suddenly lame. In most cases, rapid action to anesthetize the horse and drain the abscess is indicated. These abscesses usually heal without complications, if addressed quickly.

REPRODUCTION

Reproductive characteristics of nondomestic equids are summarized in Table 57-8. As all equids have a similar reproductive biology, the domestic horse is a good model. Equids are seasonally polyestrous, with estrous behavior recurring until conception or the end of the breeding season. In temperate regions, seasonality is determined primarily by photoperiod. In tropical species, seasonal birth peaks relate to other environmental factors such as the rainy season. Assays of steroid hormones in urine and feces may be used for determination of endocrine cycles and pregancy.[6,33] Immunocontraception using porcine zona pellucida has been used extensively and successfully in feral and some nondomestic horses.[22] For current contraception recommendations, consult the Association of Zoos and Aquariums (AZA) Wildlife Contraception Center.[8]

PREVENTIVE MEDICINE

Any routine procedure that requires anesthesia and restraint may provide an opportunity to perform a preventive medicine

TABLE 57-7

Selected Noninfectious Diseases Reported in Nondomestic Equids

Disease or Syndrome	Etiology	Prevalence	Signs	Management
Colic[7]	Intestinal accidents Sand impactions Enterocolitis	Occasional problem	Abdominal pain, distress, recumbency, shock	Important to be able to differentiate surgical from medical problems
Enteroliths[14,20]	Diet of alfalfa hay Struvite stones	Predominantly kiangs, Somali wild ass Regional problem	Acute, severe abdominal discomfort	Rapid surgical intervention Radiography: four-quadrant abdomen Prevention: dietary changes
Equine degenerative myeloencephalopathy[14,41]	Vitamin E deficiency	Reported in Przewalski's horses, zebras, kulans	Hindlimb incoordination in foals	Oral vitamin E supplementation
Laminitis[14]	Consumption of carbohydrate-rich feed	Occurs rarely; reported in Przewalski horse	Lameness	Avoid rich pasture and carbohydrate-rich feeds
Hoof abscesses[34]	Wounds, cracks, bruises	More common in Somali wild asses	Sudden, severe lameness relieved by drainage of abscess	Avoid extreme wet or dry conditions Treat with drainage
Red maple leaf toxicity[44]	Gallic acid in dry or wilted leaves	Reported in Grevy zebra	Methemoglobinemia; hemolytic anemia	No *Acer* sp. trees should be planted in or around housing areas

TABLE 57-8

Reproductive Characteristics of Non-Domestic Equids[6]

Parameter	*Equus hemionus*	*Equus africanus*[34]	*Equus przewalskii*	*Equus burchelli*[19]	*Equus grevyi*[13]	*Equus zebra*[35]
Breeding age	Mares = 24 months; Males = 26–30 months[37]	2.5–3 years	Females = 24 months; Males = 5 years	Males = 4.5 years Females = 1.5–2 years	Females = 3–4 years Males = 4 years	Female = 26 months Male = 42–54 months
Estrous cycle length	—	—	24 days[6]	19–33 days	19–33 days	—
Foaling interval	2 years[37]	—	—	14 months	13–27 months	13–69 (median = 25) months
Postpartum estrus (foal heat)	17–18 days[6]	5–14 days	—	8–10 days	9–14 days	—
Duration of copulation	—	—	—	—	3–10 minutes	—
Gestation	12 months[37]	12.5–13.5 months	11–12 months	12 months	12–14 months	12 months
Lactation length	—	—	—	Up to 16 months	9 months	10–20 months
Progesterone (ng/mL) Nonpregnant pregnant	—	—	—	—	—	<0.6 0.5–2.444
Placentation[9,45]			Epitheliochorial			

examination. Health monitoring may be performed as part of a quarantine examination, preshipment examination, opportunistically (e.g., during a hoof trim), or as needed, depending on the animal's age, health status, or other factors. For animals housed in large herds, the herd history may be reviewed for medical problems and causes of mortality.

Preshipment testing is recommended for any equid relocation. Relocation may include zoo or free-ranging transfers such as reintroduction, translocation, and relocation from one institution or field site to another. The following guidelines are recommended to aid in decision making by veterinarians, together with animal managers and biologists, when planning the safe transfer of a nondomestic equid: (1) fecal sample for parasites; (2) fecal culture; (3) blood sample for complete blood cell (CBC) count, serum chemistries, and serum archive; (4) vaccination, if indicated regionally (e.g., tetanus toxoid, rabies, etc.); and (5) a physical examination—particularly oral and hoof inspections and hoof trims. Quarantine of individuals should be performed before exposure to other animals at the new location. The risk of disease transmission should be factored into any preshipment or translocation strategy. Specific recommendations for disease screening and biomedical precautions to implement prior to translocation are available.[36,41]

ACKNOWLEDGMENT

The authors thank their colleagues Michael Schlegel, Randy Rieches, and David Heiar for their substantial contributions to this chapter.

REFERENCES

1. Adin DB, Maisenbacher HW, Ojeda N, et al: Cardiac evaluation of anesthetized Grevy's zebras (*Equus grevyi*). *Am J Vet Res* 68(2):148–152, 2007.
2. Allen J: Immobilization of Hartmann's mountain zebras (*Equus zebra hartmannae*) with carfentanil and antagonism with naltrexone or nalmefene. *J Zoo Wildl Med* 25(2):205–208, 1994.
3. Allen JL: Anesthesia of nondomestic horses with carfentanil and antagonism with naltrexone. In *Proceedings American Association of Zoo Veterinarians*, Houston, TX, 1997, pp 126.
4. Allen JL: Immobilization of Mongolian wild horses (*Equus przewaslskii przewalskii*) with carfentanil and antagonism with naltrexone. *J Zoo Wildl Med* 23(4):422–425, 1992.
5. Allen JL: Renarcotization following etorphine immobilization of nondomestic equidae. *J Zoo Wildl Med* 21(3):292–294, 1990.
6. Asa C: Equid reproductive biology. In Moehlman PD, editor: *Equids: Zebras, asses, and horses. Status Survey and Conservation Action Plan*, Gland, Switzerland; and Cambridge, UK, 2002, IUCN/SSC Equid Specialist Group, pp 113–117.
7. Atkinson MW, Blumer ES: The use of a long-acting neuroleptic in the Mongolian wild horse (*Equus przewalskii przewalskii*) to facilitate the establishment of a bachelor herd. In *Proceedings American Association of Zoo Veterinarians*, Houston, TX, 1997, pp 199–200.
8. AZA Contraception Center: Equids—contraception recommendations: http://www.stlzoo.org/animals/scienceresearch/contraceptioncenter/contraceptionrecommendatio/contraceptionmethods/perissodactyls/. Accessed February 1, 2013.
9. Benirschke K: Comparative placentation. 2012: http://placentation.ucsd.edu/homefs.html. Accessed January 22, 2013.
10. Blunden AS, Smith KC, Whitwell KE, et al: Systemic infection by equid herpesvirus-1 in a Grevy's zebra stallion (Equus grevyi) with particular reference to genital pathology. *J Comparat Pathol* 119(4):485–493, 1998.
11. Bray RE, Edwards MS: Application of existing domestic animal condition scoring systems for captive (zoo) animals. In Edwards MS, Schlegel ML, Bray RE, editors: *Proceedings of the Nutrition Advisory Group Fourth Conference on Zoo and Wildlife Nutrition*, Lake Buena Vista, FL, 2001, Nutrition Advisory Group, pp 25.
12. Bristol DG, Smith J, Silberman MS: Acepromazine and etorphine for prolonged anesthesia of a zebra. *J Am Vet Med Assoc* 185(11):1439–1440, 1984.
13. Churcher C: *Equus grevyi. Mammal Species* 453:1–9, 1993.
14. Committee on Nutrient Requirements of Horses: Donkeys and other equids. In *Nutritional requirements of horses*, ed 6, Washington, DC, 2007, National Academies Press, pp 268–279.
15. Dagleish MP, Stevenson K, Foster G, et al: *Mycobacterium avium* subsp. *hominissuis* infection in a captive-bred kiang (*Equus kiang*). *J Comparat Pathol* 146(4):372–377, 2011.
16. Feh C, Munkhtuya B: Male infanticide and paternity analyses in a socially natural herd of Przewalski's horses: Sexual selection? *Behav Proc* 78(3): 335–339, 2008.
17. Greenwood AD, Tsangaras K, Ho SYW, et al: A potentially fatal mix of herpes in zoos. *Curr Biol* 22(18):1727–1731, 2012.
18. Groves CP: Taxonomy of living Equidae. In Moehlman P, editor: *Equids: Zebras, asses, and horses. Status Survey and Conservation Action Plan*, Gland, Switzerland; and Cambridge, UK, 2002, IUCN/SSC Equids Specialist Group, pp 94–107.
19. Grubb P: *Equus burchelli. Mammal Species* 157:1–9, 1981.
20. Howard L: Management of enterolithiasis in Somali wild ass (*Equus africanus somalicus*) at the San Diego Wild Animal Park. In Baer CK, editor: *Proceedings AAZV, AAWV, WDA Joint Conference*, Oakland, CA, 2004, American Association of Zoo Veterinarians, pp 113–117.
21. Hoyer M, De Jong S, Verstappen F, et al: Standing sedation in captive zebra (*Equus grevyi* and *Equus burchellii*). *J Zoo Wildl Med* 43(1):10–14, 2012.
22. Kirkpatrick JF, Rowan A, Lamberski N, et al: The practical side of immunocontraception: Zona proteins and wildlife. *J Reproduct Immunol* 83(2):151–157, 2009.
23. Lankau EW, Montgomery JM, Tack DM, et al: Exposure of US travelers to rabid zebra, Kenya, 2011. *Emerg Infect Dis* 18(7):1202–1204, 2012.
24. Lelenguyah G: Drought, diseases and Grevy's zebra (*Equus grevyi*) mortality—the Samburu people perspective. *Afr J Ecol* 50:371–376, 2012.
25. Lintzenich B, Ward A: Hay and pellet ratios: Considerations in feeding ungulates. In Nutrition Advisory Group, editor: *Nutrition Advisory Group Handbook, Fact Sheet 006.*, 1997, Nutrition Advisory Group, pp 1–12. http://www.nagonline.net/Technical%20Papers/NAGFS00697Hay_Pellets-JONIFEB24,2002MODIFIED.pdf.
26. Löhr CV, Juan-Sallés C, Rosas-Rosas A, et al: Sarcoids in captive zebras (*Equus burchellii*): Association with bovine papillomavirus type 1 infection. *J Zoo Wildl Med* 36(1):74–81, 2005.
27. Marais HJ, Page PC: Treatment of equine sarcoid in seven Cape mountain zebra (*Equus zebra zebra*). *J Wildl Dis* 47(4):917–924, 2011.
28. Marsh A, Denver M, Hill F: Detection of *Sarcocystis neurona* in the brain of a Grant's zebra (*Equus burchelli bohmi*). *J Zoo Wildl Med* 31(1):82–86, 2000.
29. Matthews NS, Petrini KR, Wolff PL: Anesthesia of Przewalski's horses (*Equus przewalskii przewalskii*) with medetomidine/ketamine and antagonism with atipamezole. *J Zoo Wildl Med* 26(2):231–236, 1995.
30. Morris PJ: Evaluation of potential adjuncts for equine chemical immobilization. In *Proceedings Joint Meeting AAZV/AAWV*, vol 2, Oakland, CA, 1992, American Association of Zoo Veterinarians, pp 211–223.
31. Muoria PK, Muruthi P, Kariuki WK, et al: Anthrax outbreak among Grevy's zebra (*Equus grevyi*) in Samburu, Kenya. *Afr J Ecol* 45(4):483–489, 2007.
32. Myers DA, Citino S, Mitchell MA: Electrocardiography of Grevy's zebras (*Equus grevyi*). *J Zoo Wildl Med* 39(3):298–304, 2008.
33. Ncube H, Duncan P, Grange S, et al: Pattern of faecal 20-oxopregnane and oestrogen concentrations during pregnancy in wild plains zebra mares. *Gen Comparat Endocrinol* 172(3):358–362, 2011.
34. Pagan O, Von Houwald F, Wenker C, et al: Husbandry and breeding of Somali wild ass *Equus africanus somalicus* at Basel Zoo, Switzerland. *Int Zoo YB* 43(1):198–211, 2009.
35. Penzhorn B: Equus zebra. *Mammal Species* 134:1–7, 1988.
36. Radcliffe R, Osofsky S: Disease concerns for wild equids. In Moehlman P, editor: *Equids: Zebras, asses, and horses. Status Survey and Conservation Action Plan*, Gland, Switzerland; and Cambridge, UK, 2002, IUCN/SSC Equid Specialist Group, pp 124–153.
37. Rieches RR: *Housing standards for a select group of wild equids at the San Diego Zoo Safari Park (unpublished)*, 2012, pp 35.
38. Rüegg SR, Torgerson PR, Doherr MG, et al: Equine piroplasmoses at the reintroduction site of the Przewalski's horse (*Equus ferus przewalskii*) in Mongolia. *J Wildlife Dis* 42(3):518–526, 2006.
39. Schrenzel MD, Tucker T, Donovan T, et al: New hosts for equine herpesvirus 9. *Emerg Infect Dis* 14(10):1616–1619, 2008.
40. Terio KA, Stalis IH, Allen JL, et al: Coccidioidomycosis in Przewalski's horses (*Equus przewalskii*). *J Zoo Wildl Med* 34(4):339–345, 2003.
41. Walzer C, Baumgartner R, Robert N, et al: Medical aspects in Przewalski horse (*Equus przewalskii*) reintroduction to the Dzungarian Gobi, Mongolia. In *Proceedings AAZV and IAAAM Joint Conference*, New Orleans, LA, 2000, American Association of Zoo Veterinarians, pp 17–21.
42. Walzer C: Equidae. In Fowler ME, Miller RE, editors: *Zoo and wild animal medicine*, ed 5, St. Louis, MO, 2003, Saunders, pp 578–586.
43. Walzer C: Non-domestic equids. In West G, Heard D, Caulkett N, editors: *Zoo and wildlife immobilization and anesthesia*, Ames, IA, 2007, Blackwell Publishing, pp 523–531.
44. Weber M, Miller RE: Presumptive red maple (*Acer rubrum*) toxicosis in Grevy's zebra (*Equus grevyi*). *J Zoo Wildl Med* 28(1):105–108, 1997.
45. Westlin-van Aarde LM, Van Aarde RJ, Skinner JD: Reproduction in female Hartmann's zebra, Equus zebra hartmannae. *J Reprod Fertil* 84(2):505–511, 1988.

CHAPTER 58

Suidae and Tayassuidae (Wild Pigs, Peccaries)

Meg Sutherland-Smith

BIOLOGY

The families Suidae (swine) and Tayassuidae (peccaries) are nonruminating ungulates belonging to the Suina clade or suborder within the order Artiodactyla.[49] Fossil records show suids appearing around 35 million years ago (upper Eocene era) in the part of the world now known as Thailand.[49] Of the family Suidae, Suinae is the only extant subfamily. The characteristics of suid molars have resulted in dividing the subfamily into different tribes.[49] The Hippohyini originated in Asia and have hypsodont dentition. Swine species from Africa with hypsodont dentition are in the Phacocherini tribe. The Suini tribe comprises members of the genus *Sus*. The Potamochoerini tribe includes the genera *Hylochoerus* and *Potamochoerus*. Molecular studies of *Babyrousa* spp. have yielded conflicting results, with some placing them in a separate tribe, Babirusina. Depending on the source, 14 to 19 species of suids exist (Table 58-1).[15,32,35,49] Recent references have given species designation to the subspecies of *Babyrousa babirussa*.[15,49] The natural range of the Suidae family spans across Europe, Africa, Asia, and East Indies. Evidence to support any wild suids having originated in the Americas is lacking. They were introduced by humans into the Americas and into Australia, New Zealand, and New Guinea. Ancestors of extant peccaries are thought to have dispersed into the New World from eastern Asia. Currently, three species of peccary range from Southwestern United States to South America (Table 58-2).[15,28,35,49]

Wild suids and peccaries have poor vision but good hearing and a keen sense of smell. They are known for their rooting behavior. Despite their short limbs they are good runners and jumpers, and some are adept swimmers. Bornean bearded pigs have been recorded as swimming 45 kilometers (km), and babirusas have been observed swimming underwater.[49] In general, wild suids and peccaries live in social groupings, although breeding males become solitary after the breeding season. Wild suid females and their offspring live in herds known as *sounders*. Suids are quite vocal, and peccaries make a characteristic clacking sound with their teeth. Wild suid and peccary populations are primarily threatened by habitat destruction through human encroachment and hunting.[14,35,49] Isolated island populations are particularly susceptible. The International Union for the Conservation of Nature (IUCN) status of selected species is provided in Table 58-3.[18]

UNIQUE ANATOMY

Suids are a diverse group ranging in size from 6 to 200 kilograms (kg). They are characterized as having a stout, barrel-shaped body, with a large head and short limbs relative to body size. The peccary has a piglike shape; however, the limbs are long and slender with small hooves. In addition, peccaries only have one dewclaw on the hindlimbs, and hindlimb dewclaws are generally lacking in Chacoan pecarries.[49] Suid males are generally larger than females; however, little size dimorphism exists between sexes in peccaries.[14,32,49] The pelage of wild suids varies from being sparse in the babirusa to being entirely covered with coarse bristly hair in the wild boar. Peccaries have a dense covering of long, coarse bristles, which makes it difficult to estimate body condition, especially during piloerection.

In the genus *Sus*, except for *Sus scrofa*, all adult males have three pairs of fleshy protuberances on the face ("warts"). Warthogs also possess these characteristic facial structures. Wild suids may possess a variety of scent glands, including preputial, anal, metacarpal, mandibular, salivary, Harderian, eyelid, genal, and preorbital glands.[35,49] Pecarries possess a unique dorsal rump scent gland located on the midline, approximately 15 centimeters (cm) cranial to base of the tail.[14,32,49] The author has also observed a prominent papillae adjacent to the first and second maxillary molars, which are presumed to be of salivary origin in Chacoan peccaries (Figure 58-1).

The suid skull is unique in that it possesses an elongated flange of bone originating from the zygomatic root referred to as the *prezygomatic shelf*.[49] This shelf of bone separates the muscles of mastication from the muscles involved in snout movement. This adaptation is thought to facilitate rooting behavior. The disklike shape of the snout, the terminally placed nostrils, which are capable of closing, and the presence of a prenasal bone within the cartilaginous disk of the snout are also adaptions for rooting behavior.[32,35,49] The prenasal bone can be seen radiographically. Babirusas tend to root in soft, moist soils, hence their rostral bone is not as well developed as in other suids or is absent.[35,49] The rostrum of the Chacoan peccary is reported to have a more complex internal anatomy compared with other peccaries, and this is theorized to be an adaptation to living in dusty, xeric conditions.[49]

Another distinguishing feature of wild suids is their large canines. The orientation of canines in several species allows these teeth to grow upward and outward and thus capable of inflicting serious damage. In most species, the tusks of the males are larger than those of the females except in the warthog, in which both sexes have large tusks. The babirusa is known for its peculiar tusk arrangement. The alveoli of the upper canines rotate during development such that these teeth grow upward through the rostrum and spiral caudally.[49] The lower canines also grow in a spiral shape. Canines are markedly reduced or absent in female babirusas. In peccaries, canines point straight down, which allows interlocking. This arrangement facilitates stabilization of the jaw when the animal is cracking hard seeds between the other teeth.[14,49]

The dentition of suids has been used in their taxonomic classfication.[49] The desert warthog differs from other suids but is similar to other ungulates in that it does not have upper incisors. Smaller species of pigs have molars with high pointed cusps; these species tend to forage on forest vegetation and fruit, whereas larger species have dentition better suited for tougher forages, with thick enamel and conical premolars.[49] Similarly, because their natural diet is composed primarily of cactus, Chacoan peccaries have higher-crowned molars versus the lower-crowned molars of the other peccary species.[32,49]

Except for the babirusa, suids have a simple stomach. The stomach of the babirusa is bigger and has a large diverticulum.[22,32,35,49] The pH in a large area of mucus-producing cardiac glands (5.3–6.4) is able to support microbial fermentation.[22,23] Hence the babirusa is characterized as a nonruminant foregut fermenting frugivore and concentrate selector.[22–24] The ultrastructure of the babirusa stomach has been extensively studied.[23] Foregut fermentation is also reported

TABLE 58-1

Biologic Information for Selected Species of Pigs[15,32,35,49]

Common Name	Scientific Name	Body Weight (adults, in kilograms)	Geographic Distribution	Dental Formula (incisors, canines, premolars, molars)	Longevity (years)
Buru babirusa	*Babyrousa babyrussa*	Up to 90	Indonesia, Buru, and Sulu Islands	2/3, 1/1, 2/2, 3/3	Up to 24
Bola Batu babirusa	*Babyrousa bolabatuensis*	Up to 90	Indonesia, Lembeh	2/3, 1/1, 2/2, 3/3	Up to 24
Malenge babirusa	*Babyrousa togeanesis*	Up to 90	Malenge Island	2/3, 1/1, 2/2, 3/3	Up to 24
North Sulawesi babirusa	*Babyrousa celebensis*	Up to 90	Northern Sulawesi	2/3, 1/1, 2/2, 3/3	Up to 24
Giant forest hog	*Hylochoerus meinertzhageni*	130–275	Congo basin, parts of west and east Africa	3/3, 1/1, 4/4, 3/3	—
Common warthog	*Phacochoerus africanus*	50–100	Sub-Saharan Africa	1/3, 1/1, 3/2, 3/3	12–15
Desert warthog	*Phacochoerus aethiopicus*	—	Eastern Ethiopia, northern Kenya, Somalia	—	—
Pygmy hog	*Porcula salvanius*	6–10	Bhutan, southern Nepal, northern India	3/3, 1/1, 4/4, 3/3	10–12
Red River hog	*Potamochoerus porcus*	50–120	Western Africa, Congo basin	3/3, 1/1, 4/4, 3/3	10–15
Bushpig	*Potamochoerus larvatus*	50–120	Eastern and southern Africa	3/3, 1/1, 4/4, 3/3	10–15
Wild boar	*Sus scrofa*	50–200	Europe, N. Africa, Asia; introduced into N. America, Australia, New Zealand, New Guinea	3/3, 1/1, 4/4, 3/3	15–20
Palawan pig	*Sus ahoenobarbus*	—	Philippines	—	—
Bearded pig	*Sus barbatus*	100–200	Malaysia, Sumatra, Borneo	3/3, 1/1, 4/4, 3/3	—
Heude pig	*Sus bucculentus*	—	Vietnam, Laos	—	—
Visayan warty pig	*Sus cebifrons*	—	Philippines	—	—
Celebes or warty pig	*Sus celebensis*	—	Indonesia	—	—
Oliver warty pig	*Sus oliveri*	—	Philippines	—	—
Philippine warty pig	*Sus philippensis*	—	Philippines	—	—
Javan warty pig	*Sus verrucosus*	Up to 185	Java, Bawean	3/3, 1/1, 4/4, 3/3	—

Data modified from Morris and Shima.[28]

TABLE 58-2

Selected Biological Data for Peccaries[14,15,28,49]

Common Name(s)	Scientific Name	Weight (adults, in kilograms)	Geographic Distribution	Dental Formula (incisors, canines, premolars, molars)	Chromosomes (2n)	Longevity (years)
Collared peccary/ Javelina	*Pecari tajacu*	15–35	Southwest United States to Argentina	2/3, 1/1, 3/3, 3/3	30	16–24
White-lipped peccary	*Tayassu pecari*	27–40	Mexico to Argentina	2/3, 1/1, 3/3, 3/3	26	15–21
Chacoan peccary/ Tagua	*Catagonus wagneri*	30–43	Argentina, Bolivia, Paraguay	2/3, 1/1, 3/3, 3/3	20	At least 9

Data modified from Morris and Shima.[28]

TABLE 58-3

IUCN Conservation Status of Selected Species

IUCN Red List Classification	Genus and Species
Critically Endangered	*Porcula salvanius, Sus cebifrons*
Endangered	*Babyrousa togeanensis, Catagonus wagneri, Sus oliveri, Sus verrucosus*
Near Threatened	*Sus celebensis, Tayassu pecari*
Vulnerable	*Sus ahoenobarbus, Sus barbatus, Sus phillipensis*
Of Least Concern	*Hylochoerus meinertzhageni, Phacochoerus aethiopicus, Phacochoerus africanus, Potamochoerus larvatus, Potamochoerus porcus, Sus scofa, Pecari tajacu*

IUCN, International Union for the Conservation of Nature.

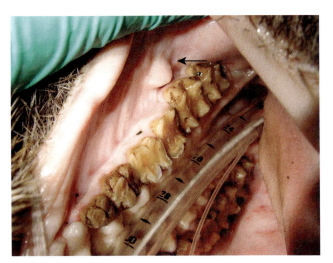

FIGURE 58-1 Presumed salivary papilla (*arrow*) in a Chacoan peccary (*Catagonus wagneri*).

in peccaries, which have a four-chambered stomach: two nonglandular blind sacs, a nonglandular gastric pouch, and a glandular hind stomach.[14,32,49] Unlike pigs, peccaries do not have a gallbladder.[14]

SPECIAL HOUSING REQUIREMENTS

The natural behaviors of wild suids and peccaries should be taken into account for appropriate exhibit specifications. The opportunity to root and dig should be provided without disrupting the structural integrity of the enclosure. These behaviors may also result in damage to indoor facilities such as padded barn floors. Animals should be given access to mud wallows, where appropriate, and kept free from fecal and urine contamination. Nesting is a common behavior, and animals should be provided bedding materials for nesting. Other considerations for housing suids and peccaries include escape potential, substrate, and intraspecific aggression. Pigs are quite capable of either jumping (both vertically and horizontally) or digging their way out of an enclosure if given the opportunity. Substrate should not be abrasive as running, pacing, or both may cause excessive hoof wear, and enclosures should be evaluated for other potential sources of foot trauma. When running along chainlink fence lines animals may traumatize the lateral dewclaws. Usually, a dominance hierarchy in social groupings exists, hence visual barriers to help divert aggression are recommended. Animals should have access to shade and, depending on the climate, protection from harsh weather.

A recent study from Brazil evaluated enclosures of three different sizes for housing collared peccaries.[30] Behavioral observations were performed, and the authors concluded that a minimum of approximately 200 square meters (m²) per animal of space resulted in the least agonistic behaviors. They also found that shelter use increased with allocation of more space, which supported earlier findings regarding the importance of shelters in peccary husbandry.[43]

Pigs are considered fourth in intelligence of animals behind primates (human and nonhuman), dolphins, and elephants; therefore they require a stimulating environment.[49] They are quick learners and have sophisticated problem-solving abilities. Environmental and behavioral enrichment should be part of any program managing suids or peccaries. Many useful resources for enrichment are available.[10,47]

FEEDING

In general, wild suids and peccaries, which are considered omnivores, consume such things as leaves, grasses, young saplings, seeds, roots, tubers, fruits, fungi, eggs, invertebrates, carrion, and small vertebrates.[14,32,35,49] In the wild, cactus also makes up a significant portion of the diet for the Chacoan peccary and, to a lesser extent, the white-lipped peccary.[14,49] The natural biology of the various species also reveals the opportunistic nature of pig foraging based on seasonal availability.[24] Some authors have considered wild suids more herbivorous, with species occupying nutritional niches.[8,24] Warthogs have been classified as grazers and forest hogs as browsers. *Hylochoerus, Potomachoerus* sp., *Sus scrofa, Sus barbatus,* and possibly the warty pigs have been considered more frugivorous.[8,24] The exact nutritional requirements of wild suids are not well-defined.[24] In general, diets fed to wild suids and peccaries in captivity consist of a complete pelleted herbivore ration, with varying amounts of fruits, vegetables, browse, and hay. A study evaluated the apparent digestibility of different macronutrients in warthogs, red river hogs, warty pigs, and babirusa.[8] No difference in protein digestibility was observed between the species, including peccaries when comparing with prior literature. Despite differences in gastric anatomy, neither peccaries nor babirusa had more efficient fiber digestion. Hemicellulose was digested more efficiently than cellulose by red river hogs, babirusas, and peccaries, whereas warthogs were capable of efficiently digesting both hemicellulose and cellulose. Therefore, dietary items high in hemicellulose would be appropriate for most wild suids, whereas incorporating items such as grass hays that have higher cellulose content would be appropriate for warthogs.

In captivity, wild suids are prone to obesity, which may interfere with reproduction and exacerbate musculoskeletal conditions such as osteoarthritis. Routine weight monitoring is recommended. Feeding strategies should be incorporated that minimize the impact of social domination by one individual or a few and food-motivated aggression.

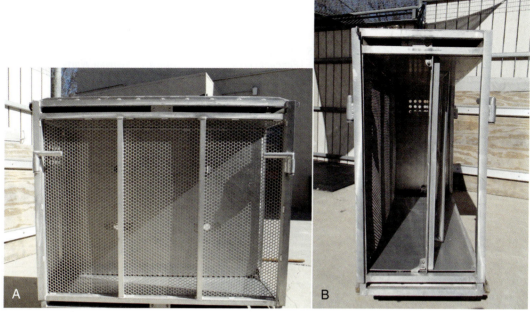

FIGURE 58-2 A, Metal squeeze chute or crate used for anesthetic induction of small- to medium-sized suids and peccaries. **B,** End-on view illustrating squeeze mechanism.

RESTRAINT AND HANDLING

In general, physical restraint is not recommended in wild suids or peccaries. Most individuals struggle violently, and no part of the body is easily held. A cornered pig may become quite aggressive, and its tusks are capable of inflicting significant injury. Attempting to restrain a nondomestic pig by the hind leg, as is done with domestic swine, is not recommended because it may result in injury to the animal. Some individual animals will remain very flighty in captivity, whereas others become quite tractable. Operant conditioning in these animals may facilitate close visual inspection and limited palpation. Some animals go into lateral recumbency when scratched with a broom or scrub brush. In animals with formidable tusks, such evaluations should be done in a protected contact situation. Piglets and infant peccaries may be manually restrained for minor procedures.

Chemical Restraint

Although immobilization in suids may be challenging, it is recommended for a thorough examination and for diagnostic procedures. Most wild suids have a thick layer of subcutaneous fat. Deposition of immobilizing agents into this fat layer may interfere with drug absorption, which would create a less than ideal immobilization. Peccaries generally do not have large subcutaneous fat reserves.[14,32] Some animals may become quite excited during immobilization. Although exotic species do not have the genetic defect that causes malignant hyperthermia in domestic swine, they are quite susceptible to hyperthermia because of their inability to sweat and the likelihood of extreme muscle exertion during an immobilization, especially in escape scenarios.[27] Excessive running, lengthy inductions, and violent recoveries are also risk factors for exertional myopathy. Foot trauma may also occur with excessive running on hard surfaces. When darting an animal in a group, precautions need to be taken to avoid causing trauma to conspecifics.

In addition to remote delivery via dart systems, squeeze chutes or crates may be used for hand injections. Figure 58-2 shows a metal squeeze crate used for hand injections in small- to medium-sized animals at the author's institution. Peccaries, warty pigs, and medium-sized red river hogs are transferred into the squeeze apparatus from a transport crate. This system works well and keeps animals confined during induction.

Fasting times of 12 to 24 hours have been recommended; however, hypoglycemia has been observed in some fasted pigs, especially in *Potamochoerus* sp. and *Sus celebifrons*, at the author's institution.[5,26,28,33,48] Therefore, fasting times have been reduced to 3 to 6 hours for all suids and peccaries. In addition, blood glucose is monitored during immobilization and hypoglycemia treated, as needed. Problems secondary to a short fasting interval, for example, vomiting or gas distension of the gastrointestinal tract, have not been encountered.

Chemical immobilization protocols for swine and peccaries have been reviewed recently (Table 58-4).[33] Multiple drug combinations have been used successfully. In addition, the author has added ketamine at 0.5 to 1 milligram per kilogram (mg/kg) with or without azaperone (0.25–1.3 mg/kg) to medetomidine–butorphanol–midazolam combinations. This has helped minimize some of the unpredictability in the response of wild suids to immobilizing agents. Azaperone (0.5–1.5 mg/kg, intramuscularly [IM]) has also been administered to anesthetized swine prior to recovery from anesthesia in case of concern about a possible violent recovery or excitability in the postrecovery period. Attempts to handle an animal before immobilizing agents have reached their full effect or the need for additional dosing in an animal may result in significant stimulation, which may override the drug effects and prolong induction.

For neurolepsis, the author's institution has used a protocol of diazepam and amitriptyline (0.5 mg/kg each, orally [PO], twice daily [BID]) to help reduce excitability during shipment or other relocation events. Dosages may be adjusted upward or downward based on the individual responses. Azaperone (1–2 mg/kg, IM) has been used to facilitate animal introductions.

ANESTHESIA AND SURGERY

General anesthesia is indicated for prolonged or invasive procedures. The most common conditions that require surgical intervention in nondomestic suids and peccaries are trauma and dystocias. These are managed with standard veterinary techniques.

TABLE 58-4

Reference Range for Hematologic Parameters (Adults) in Selected Species

Parameter	Red River Hog (*Potamochoerus porcus*)*	S. African Warthog (*Phacochoerus africanus*)†	Babirusa (*Babyrousa babyrussa*)†	Visayan Warty Pig (*Sus celebrifons*)*	Collared Peccary (*Tayassu tajacua*)†
Erythrocytes × 10⁶/microliter (μL)	5.08–8.86	4.73–10	4.56–10.5	4.8–9.7	4.89–9.58
Packed cell volume (%)	31.3–56.5	27.4–60	28.8–54.3	30.9–53.2	26–53
Hemoglobin, gram per deciliter (g/dL)	1.36–16.2	9.4–16.2	9.1–17.6	9.9–15.9	9.4–18
Mean corpuscular volume, (dL)	17.5–69.9	39.4–71.7	51.5–93.8	25.9–69.6	43.8–92
Mean corpuscular hemoglobin, picogram (pg)	16.3–23.3	10.2–23.9	15.7–28.1	14.2–22.3	16–23.4
Mean corpuscular hemoglobin concentration, (g/dL)	28.6–36.8	25.8–36.8	26.3–35.7	0.6–33.2	21.5–36.4
Leukocytes/μL	4500–1800	4.1–15,000	3500–17,800	5900–23,300	2900–22,600
Neutrophils/μL	2745–12060	614–10,300	714–12,100	2599–18,407	1800–15,100
Band neutrophils/μL	87–424	86–801	57–595	83	44–5420
Lymphocytes/μL	391–5610	224–7840	755–9870	1328–7520	414–8100
Eosinophils/μL	45–1761	23–1357	44–1176	59–352	33–528
Monocytes/μL	213–1980	47–1053	38–1780	112–1066	33–1668
Basophils/μL	67–200	0–340	11–540	54–264	44–225
Platelets ×10³/μL	0.176–499	120–732	36–784	0.194–296	106–255
Plasma protein (g/dL)	5.7–9.5	ND	ND	ND	ND
Fibrinogen, milligram per deciliter (mg/dL)	200–500	ND	0–700	100–600	200–300

*Zoological Society of San Diego, San Diego Zoo Department of Pathology, Clinical Pathology Laboratory.
†International Species Information System, August 2002.
ND, No data.

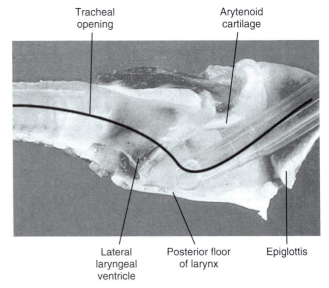

FIGURE 58-3 Laryngeal anatomy of a domestic pig. (From Thurmon, JC, Tranquilli WJ, Benson GJ: *Lumb and Jones veterinary anesthesia*, 3rd ed. Baltimore, MD, 1996, Williams & Wilkins.)

Intubation may be difficult in suids. Laryngeal access is problematic because of their inability to open their mouths widely, their long rostrum, and the narrow oropharyngeal space.[33,48] In addition, a straight path from the epiglottis to the trachea does not exist because of the laryngeal anatomy (Figure 58-3).[33,48] A long laryngoscope blade and stylet facilitate intubation. If a stylet is used, precautions need to be taken so to avoid trauma to the larynx. Once within the larynx, the endotracheal tube should be rotated 180 degrees to reach the tracheal opening. Threading an endoscope through the endotracheal tube may facilitate passage into the trachea. Laryngospasm may also complicate intubation. The use of benzodiazepines has been noted to significantly reduce jaw tone, which may facilitate easier intubation. In peccaries, however, intubation is generally not difficult, as the mouth can be opened widely to gain adequate access to the larynx and a more direct path exists from the epiglottis into the trachea. Intubation may be done in lateral, sternal, or dorsal recumbency, but sternal recumbency is generally recommended.

Anesthesia monitoring is similar as for other ungulates. Inhalant or injectable agents may be used to maintain anesthesia. If venous access is available, propofol is an option for the use of injectable anesthetics.

DIAGNOSTICS

Anesthesia is generally required for most diagnostic procedures. Standard techniques used in domestic swine and other ungulates may be applied in wild suids and peccaries. Similar to domestic swine venipuncture may be difficult in exotic species. Vascular access sites include the saphenous vein, femoral vein, cephalic vein, coccygeal vein, and aural vein, as well as the cranial vena cava, which is used in the traditional technique. The cranial vena cava is, however, not routinely used at the author's institution. A technique for jugular venipuncture has been described.[33] A needle greater than 1.5 inches in length is inserted cranially and slightly medially into jugular furrow. Ultrasonography may facilitate localization of jugular veins, which are buried within the musculature of the neck. The saphenous vein in peccaries is prominent as it courses over the cranial aspect of the proximal tibia and is easily accessed.[25] For low-volume infusions, the aural vein, if present, may be catheterized. Catheters may also be placed in the cephalic and saphenous veins; however, a blind stick may be necessary, as the veins are not always visible. Hematology and serum biochemistry data for selected species are summarized in Tables 58-5 and 58-6.

DISEASES

Infectious Disease

Nondomestic suids and peccaries are susceptible to many of the same diseases as domestic swine and ungulates. These include leptospirosis, pasteurellosis, rabies, salmonellosis, and tuberculosis. Diagnosis and treatment are similar as for other species. A thorough review of infectious and parasitic diseases was previously compiled and is presented in Tables 58-7 and 58-8.[28]

Necrotizing enteritis caused by *Clostridium perfringens* was reported in collared peccaries and white-lipped peccaries from a facility in Brazil.[6] Lethargy and inappetence were followed by death within 24 hours in seven animals. Crowded housing conditions were thought to have played a role in the disease outbreak.

Feral swine have been a concern for the domestic swine industry because of the risk of disease transmission.[36,37,51] Similarly, local feral swine may also act as a source of disease for exotic suids located in rural areas. Brucellosis was diagnosed in a group of red river hogs at a facility in Florida. Through testing of serum banked from the originating institution and genotyping of the *Brucella* isolate, it was determined that local feral swine were the likely source of the infection (Janssen, personal communication, 2012).

Postweaning multisystemic wasting syndrome (PMWS) emerged in the domestic swine industry in the mid-1970s, and porcine circovirus 2 (PCV2) was discovered to be associated with the syndrome.[50] An illness in a 10-month old red river hog in a facility in England fitted the criteria for PMWS. The hog died following a course of

Text continued on p. 581

TABLE 58-5

Reference Ranges for Serum Biochemical Parameters for Selected Species

Parameter	Red River Hog (*Potamochoerus porcus*)*	S. African Warthog (*Phacochoerus africanus*)†	Babirusa (*Babyrousa babyrussa*)†	Visayan Warty Pig (*Sus celebrifons*)*	Collared Peccary (*Tayassu tajacua*)†
Total protein (g/dL)	5.2–9	5.2–7.0	6.0–9.1	4.7–7.2	5.8–8.9
Albumin (g/dL)	2–5	3.3–4.1	3.3–5.7	4–5.7	3.1–4.7
Calcium (mg/dL)	7.5–10.60	9.0–14.4	8.8–11.9	7.6–10.2	8.0–12.2
Phosphorus (mg/dL)	3.1–8	3.4–11.8	3.2–8.3	3.5–8.4	3.5–8.3
Sodium (mEq/L)	130–150	131–154	134–154	134–144	134–160
Potassium (mEq/L)	2.7–6.0	3.4–6.9	3.5–5.5	3.2–4.9	3.5–5.5
Chloride (mEq/L)	92–115	90–110	94–112	99–109	93–115
Creatinine (mg/dL)	0.5–1.6	1.2–3.9	0.7–2.1	0.9–1.6	1.0–2.3
Urea nitrogen (mg/dL)	8.5–22.9	5–8	6–31	8–22.6	11–23
Cholesterol (mg/dL)	57–151	48–340	25–136	16–89	53–166
Glucose (mg/dL)	50–171	39–250	24–192	63–154	76–258
Total carbon dioxide (mmol/L)	8–40	18–36	13–45	21–41	8–40
ALP (IU/L)	2.2–186	11–1283	12–209	20–299	7–293
ALT (IU/L)	23–349	12–231	19–64	41–189	11–104
AST (IU/L)	6–296	7–156	4–60	7–76	18–82
GGT (IU/L)	7–123	25–145	39–137	30–65	0–21
Amylase (U/L)	9.2–3052	23–1898	60–914	778–1994	25–158
CPK (IU/L)	179–1344	227–3356	127–656	251–1893	99–2447
Uric acid (mg/dL)	0.1–3.2	0–0.3	0–1.3	0.1–1.4	0.1–0.4

*Zoological Society of San Diego, San Diego Zoo Department of Pathology, Clinical Pathology Laboratory.
†International Species Information System, August 2002.
ALP, alkaline phosphatase; *ALT,* alanine aminotransferase; *AST,* aspartate aminotransferase; *CPK,* creatine phosphokinase; *g/dL,* gram per deciliter; *GGT,* gamma glutamyltransferase; *IU/L,* international unit per liter; *mEq/L,* milliequivalent per liter; *mg/dL,* milligram per deciliter; *mmol/L,* millimole per liter.

TABLE 58-6

Common Immobilization Protocols Used in Nondomestic Suids and Peccaries[33]

Drug Combination	Dose (mg/kg)	Species Documented	Comments	References
Ketamine (K)	20 (K)	Collared peccaries	Not recommended as first choice for immobilization Recoveries may be prolonged and violent Fatality associated with ambient temperature	16
Ketamine (K)/tiletamine–zolazepam (TZ)/medetomidine (M)	3.9(K)/0.63(TZ)/0.03(M)	Chacoan peccaries	Prolonged recoveries despite medetomidine reversal with atipamezole, residual ataxia	45
Tiletamine–zolazepam (TZ)	2–5 (TZ)	Multiple species	Smooth induction, poor muscle relaxation, prolonged recoveries might be rough Duration of recovery is dose dependent	1,5
	2.18 (TZ)	Chacoan peccaries	Prolonged recoveries, poor relaxation	
Tiletamine–zolazepam (TZ)/xylazine (X)	2.35 (TZ)/2.35 (X)	Collared peccaries	Prolonged recoveries, but study did not antagonize xylazine Fatality associated with double dose	13
	1.23 (TZ)/1.23 (X)	White-lipped peccaries	Dose of 1.51 TZ and 1.51 X not successful in collared peccaries	39
	1.2–2.1(X)/1.8–3.3 (TZ)	Babirusa	(X) administered as premedicant, followed by TZ 20 min later Antagonism with 0.14 mg/kg yohimbine and 1 mg flumazenil for every 20 mg zolazepam Bradycardia seen in some cases	19
	3 (TZ)/0.5 (X)	Warthogs	Recoveries > 90 min	42
	3.3 (TZ)/1.6 (X)	Feral pigs		46
Tiletamine–zolazepam (TZ)/ romifidine (R)	3–6 (TZ)/0.1 (R)	Wild pigs	—	40
Tiletamine–zolazepam (TZ)/ butorphanol (B)	1.46 (TZ)/0.14 (B)	White-lipped peccaries	Similar doses ineffective for collared peccaries	39
	1.26 (TZ)/0.36 (B)	Babirusa	Reverse with naltrexone, poor overall relaxation	34
Medetomidine (M)/butorphanol (B)/ midazolam (Mz)	0.04–0.07 (M)/0.15–0.3 (B)/0.08–0.3 (Mz)	Multiple species	Bradycardia, hypoxemia reported Antagonize with atipamezole, naloxone or naltrexone, and flumazenil Lower dose range used in calm, captive individuals	28
Detomidine (D)/butorphanol (B)/ midazolam (Mz)	0.12 (D)/0.3 (B)/0.3 (Mz)	—	—	29
Xylazine (X)/butorphanol (B)/ midazolam (Mz)	2–3 (X)/0.3–0.4 (B)/0.3–0.4 (Mz)	—	—	29
Detomidine (D)/butorphanol (B)/ tiletamine–zolazepam (TZ)	0.12 (D)/0.3 (B)/0.6 (TZ)	—	—	29

TABLE 58-7

Selected Infectious Diseases of Wild Swine and Peccaries[12,20,31,36]

Disease	Etiology	Epizootiology	Signs	Diagnosis	Management
African swine fever	Asfivirus (Asfarviridae)	Wild boar, feral swine Giant forest hog, bushpig, warthog have inapparent infections Peccaries are not susceptible	Acute form: inappetence, fever, leukopenia, hemorrhagic syndrome Chronic form: respiratory signs, abortion	CF, ELISA, TEM, immunoperoxidase staining, DNA-hybridization Most useful is direct immunofluorescence and hemagglutination	Vaccines are experimental Test and slaughter is the accepted management method Avoid swill (garbage) feeding any swine
Classical swine fever (hog cholera)	Pestivirus (Togaviridae)	All swine species affected Peccaries are mildly affected	Fever, rapid death, hemorrhagic syndrome in highly susceptible species Infertility, abortions mummified fetuses with mild viral strains	During outbreaks, direct FA for viral antigen and using conserved epitopes on frozen pharyngeal tonsil is the method of choice Virus isolation, ELISA, virus neutralization are available	Vaccination limits the use of diagnostics Vaccines are available for domestic swine C strain vaccine in widest use for domestic swine Test and slaughter of affected animals is widely practiced for control of outbreaks Avoid swill feeding any swine
Canine distemper virus	Morbillivirus Paramyxoviridae	Collared peccaries	Encephalitis	Serum neutralization	Thought to be enzootic in free-ranging collared peccaries in southern Arizona
Encephalomyocarditis	Cardiovirus (Picornaviridae)	Wild boar and domestic swine affected Unknown effects in other swine species Rats and mice thought to be primary reservoirs	Reproductive failure, high preweaning mortality, fever, malaise, dyspnea, inappetence, syncope, rapid death	Histopathology of heart lesions is suggestive Virus isolation from heart muscle of young/newborn swine Antibody titers are most useful from fetal serum	Inactivated vaccine is available for domestic swine use in the United States Active vermin control program in endemic areas
Foot-and-mouth disease (FMD)	Aphthovirus (Picornaviridae)	Feral pig, wild boar, giant forest hog, bushpig, warthog, babirusa affected Peccaries mildly affected Highly contagious in aerosols, fomites direct contact	Vesicles on lips, oral cavity, coronary bands, soreness, inappetence, malaise	Virus isolation CF, antigen capture, animal inoculation, from vesicles; serology for precipitating antibodies, neutralizing antibodies Vaccinates may be differentiated from wild type infections with ELISA by using baculovirus-expressed FMD nonstructural proteins 3D, 2C	Test and slaughter is currently or historically used to eradicate the disease Inactivated vaccine available

Continued

TABLE 58-7

Selected Infectious Diseases of Wild Swine and Peccaries—cont'd

Disease	Etiology	Epizootiology	Signs	Diagnosis	Management
Pseudorabies	Alphaherpesvirus (Herpesviridae)	Feral swine, wild boar, giant forest hog, bushpig, warthog, peccary susceptible	Peripheral neuritis, pruritus, encephalitis, convulsions, especially in young animals Older animals generally show respiratory signs often mistaken for influenza Causes abortion in sows Signs are species and viral strain dependent, varying from inapparent infection to high mortality	Direct FA detection in tonsillar tissue or virus isolation of brain, spleen, or lung are methods of choice Serodiagnosis by serum neutralization, latex agglutination, ELISA, CF, immunodiffusion, indirect immunofluorescence have all been used but have limited value in diagnosis	Modified-live, inactivated, and gene-modified vaccines are available and are effective in domestic swine
Rinderpest	Morbillivirus (Paramyxoviridae)	All swine and peccaries are susceptible Asian swine (*Sus scrofa*) are especially sensitive, followed by African species European species (*Sus scrofa*) are more resistant Some swine species have subclinical infections Peccaries are also susceptible to canine distemper virus	Enteritis, fever, malaise, vomiting, epistaxis, oral, perineal vesicles, hemorrhagic diarrhea, in severe cases Inapparent signs, abortion, mild dermatitis, malaise in milder cases	Electron microscopy, immunofluorescence staining of tissues, immunoperoxidase staining of tissues, PCR, ELISA, agar-gel immunodiffusion, counterimmunoelectrophoresis, passive hemagglutination	Vaccination of endemic nidus areas with perimeter serosurveillance zones is recommended in the Global Rinderpest Eradication Program (GREP)
Swine vesicular disease	Enterovirus (Picornaviridae)	Feral swine and wild boar are affected No data on African swine or peccaries Virus is long-lived in the environment	Oral and foot vesicles indistinguishable from FMD	Virus isolation, test animal inoculation, ELISA, serum neutralization, antigen precipitation, and CF are available	Prevention is primarily through banning of swill feeding
Swine influenza	Type A influenza virus (Orthomyxoviridae)	Feral swine and wild boar affected No data on African swine or peccaries	Pneumonia, conjunctivitis, rhinitis, inappetence, weight loss High morbidity, low mortality in domestic swine	Virus isolation or viral antigen (serum ELISA), immunofluorescent staining of lung or nasal preps, PCR, enzyme immunoassay membrane test are applicable	Good biosecurity practices offer the best prevention
Tranmissible gastroenteritis (TGE)	Coronavirus (Coronaviridae)	Feral swine, wild boar are affected No data on other swine or peccaries	Vomiting, diarrhea, weight loss, dehydration High morbidity and mortality in very young swine Coronavirus was seen in EM of diarrhea samples from red river hog piglets (*Potamochoerus porcus*)	Most common method is immunofluorescent staining or immunoperoxidase staining of intestinal mucosal scrapings, ELISA of cell culture media inoculated with gut samples from affected animals; fecal nucleic acid hybridization probe detection, TEM, virus isolation	Vaccination with modified-live and inactivated vaccines in young swine has been used to help prevent TGE in domestic swine

Disease	Etiologic Agent	Epidemiology	Clinical Signs	Diagnosis	Treatment/Control
Vesicular exanthema	Calicivirus (Caliciviridae)	Feral swine, wild boar, and peccaries reported susceptible No data for African swine species Typically virus is spread through swill feeding in domestic species	Oral and foot vesicles indistinguishable from FMD	Virus isolation, serum neutralization	Avoid swill feeding Practice good biosecurity with new additions
Vesicular stomatitis	Vesiculovirus (Rhabdoviridae)	Feral swine, wild boar, and peccaries susceptible Transmission by sandflies (*Lutzomyia shanoni*) and black flies also (*Simulium* sp.) is reported as the primary route of transmission	Oral and foot vesicles indistinguishable from FMD	Virus isolation, serum neutralization, ELISA CF; ELISA on epithelial and vesicular fluid or tissue samples	Vaccine is generally not used in domestic swine Avoidance of infected domestic and wild animals is reported as the default preventive measure
Brucellosis	*Brucella suis*	Feral swine and wild boar affected Biovar 1 most significant Biovars 2 and 3 are reported as significant regionally Spread is mainly venereal	Abortion, infertility, posterior paralysis, lameness, undulating pyrexia	Lymph node culture is best diagnostic Serology (plate agglutination) to detect antibodies is most practical	For domestic swine, whole herd slaughter and replacement with SPF animals has been the most successful practice Testing and removing affected animals from herds has been the least effective strategy
Colibacillosis	*Escherichia coli*	Associated with severe diarrhea/death in red river hog piglets Reported in feral swine, wild boar, African swine, peccaries	Enterotoxemia, diarrhea, dehydration, acidosis, metabolic crisis, death	Culture of feces and characterization of colonies for enterotoxigenic properties Sensitivity to antimicrobials aids in treatment	Fluids, antibacterials, supportive therapy for affected cases Colostral *E.coli* vaccination of dams appears to be protective
Erysipelas	*Erysipelothrix rhusiopathiae*	Feral swine, wild boar, African swine species affected No data for peccaries Many wild animals are reservoirs	Septicemia, fever, malaise, diamond skin lesions Acute, subacute, and chronic forms are described in domestic swine	Culture of blood, joint fluids, and other body fluids	Penicillin is historic drug of choice Tetracycline, chlortetracycline, lincomycin, and tylosin are effective Hyperimmune serum treatment Prevention with attenuated bacterial vaccines and bacterins are available Concomitant attenuated vaccine with antibiotic therapy is not recommended

CF, Complement fixation; *DNA*, deoxyribonucleic acid; *ELISA*, enzyme-linked immunosorbent assay; *FA*, fluorescent antibody; *PCR*, polymerase chain reaction; *TEM*, transmission electron microscopy.
Data modified from Morris and Shima.[28]

TABLE 58-8

Selected Parasitic Diseases of Swine and Peccaries[11,36,44]

Disease	Etiology	Location in Host		Diagnosis	Management
		Adult	**Immature**		
Nasal bots	*Rhinoestrus* sp.	Nasopharynx	Nasopharynx Life cycle is known only for the horse	Morphology of bots and larvae	Organophosphates or macrocyclic lactones reported to be effective
Sarcoptic mange	*Sarcoptes scabei* Transmission is via direct contact of affected skin, and indirect contact with mites in environment	Skin	Skin	Microscopic inspection of skin scrapings	Biosecurity protection of large herds from exposure is invaluable Treatment of individual cases with avermectins at weekly intervals will resolve active cases Ivermectin at 500 µg/kg, PO, q7d, resolved cases of sarcoptic mange in red river hogs over a 6-month period
Sucking lice	*Hematopinus suis* Sucking louse of feral and domestic swine *Pecaroecus javalii* Sucking louse of peccaries Direct life cycle May cause decreased activity, retarded development, and hematologic changes in young swine	Skin	Skin	Morphology	Topical acaricides Doramectin (pour-on) is reported effective against many parasites in domestic swine
Biting lice	*Pecaroecus javalii* (collared peccary)	Skin	Skin		
Ticks	*Amblyomma inoratum, Dermacentor halli, Haemaphysalis leporispalustris* (peccaries) *Ixodes scapularis, Amblyomma americanum, cajennense, maculatum; Dermacentor albipictus, D. andersoni, D. varibilis* *Ornithodoros coriaceus, truicata, puertoricensis, tahale, dugesi* are potential vectors of African swine fever *Ornithodoros moubata* is the primary vector of African swine fever in Africa	Skin, multifocal dermatitis	Skin	Morphology	Destruction of animal bedding or nesting materials where adults breed, topical insecticides, systemic or topical avermectins

Ascarids	*Ascaris suum*	Small intestines; usually no disease results	Direct life cycle; Hepatotracheal larval migration	Egg or adult morphology	Elimination of adults through anthelminthic treatment of new acquisitions in quarantine (FBZ, AVE, PIP, PRT, LVM, DCV, TBZ); Periodic anthelminthic treatment of infested herds
Strongyloidiasis (threadworm)	*Strongyloides ransomi*	Small intestine, producing diarrhea, dehydration	Eggs hatch into infective larvae and/or free-living adults that mate, thereby giving rise to more infective larvae; Larvae mature into adults in small intestine; Percutaneous larval and transcolostral infestation occur	Egg or adult morphology	Anthelminthic treatment (LVM, TBZ, AVE)
Nodular worms	*Oesophagostomum* sp.	Cecum or colon, producing parasitic mucosal nodules	Eggs hatch in the environment, developing to infective, ensheathed L3, which may survive in the environment for up to 12 months	Egg or adult morphology, parasitic nodules in cecum, colon, rectum	Anthelminthic treatment (FBZ, AVE, DCV, LVM, PRT, PIP), housing on fallow substrate
Lungworms	*Metastrongylus* sp.	Lungs; adults and eggs found in the bronchioles mainly of diaphragmatic lobes	Earthworms are intermediate hosts for L1-L3	Egg or adult morphology, verminous pneumonia in severe cases	Anthelminthic treatment (FBZ, AVE, LVM)
Trichinosis	*Trichinella* sp.	Larval cysts within skeletal muscle, adults in small intestine	Ingestion of infested meat containing encysted larvae	Adult and larval morphology	Public health significance; Avoidance of uncooked skeletal muscle; Trichinosis is a cosmopolitan concern
Stomach worms	*Hyostrongylus* sp.	Stomach, usually incidental; Heavy infestation may result in gastritis	Stomach	Egg or adult morphology	Anthelminthic treatment (DCV, FBZ, TBZ, PRT, AVE)
Thick stomach worm	*Ascarops* sp. *Physocephalus* sp.	Stomach	Dung beetles are intermediate hosts	Egg or adult morphology	Anthelminthic treatment (FBZ, DCV)

Continued

TABLE 58-8

Selected Parasitic Diseases of Swine and Peccaries—cont'd

Disease	Etiology	Location in Host		Diagnosis	Management
		Adult	**Immature**		
Thorny-headed worm	*Macrocanthorhynchus hirudinaceus*	Ileum, producing parasitic mucosal nodules, but rarely results in disease Mucosal perforation and peritonitis occasionally results	Intermediate hosts are beetle grubs Infestation via ingestion of grubs carrying larval stages	Egg or adult morphology	
Kidney worm	*Stephanurus dentatus*	Kidneys primarily, also perirenal fat, ureters, lumbar muscles, spinal cord, lungs	Eggs passed in urine primarily in the morning Eggs hatch and develop in environment to L3 Infestation occurs via ingestion of larvae, earthworms harboring infective larvae, or by percutaneous penetration by larvae	Egg or adult morphology	Avoidance of infective larvae is essential Affected animals are housed on concrete that is cleaned regularly to remove voided eggs. PRT, FBZ effective
Cysticercosis	*Echinococcus granulosus*	Intestines (canids)	Multiple organ cysts	Morphology of cysticerci	Albendazole and/or praziquantel may be of some benefit
	Taenia acinonyxi	Intestines (cheetah, leopard)	African swine are intermediate hosts		
	Taenia multiceps	Intestines (canids)	*Sus scrofa* is intermediate host		
	Taenia regis	Intestines (lion, leopard)	Warthogs, bushpigs are intermediate hosts		
	Taenia solium	Intestines (human)	*Sus scrofa* is an intermediate host		
Trematodiasis	*Fascioloides magna*	Liver Variable lesions from mild fibrosis of migratory tracts to severe cirrhosis	Snails	The diagnosis typically is made at necropsy	Treatment of larvae with rafoxanide or triclabendazole Treatment of adults with oxyclozanide or triclabendazole
Lancet fluke	*Dicrocoelium dendriticum*	Wild hogs Causes liver damage, cirrhosis, cholangitis, regional cholestasis, and anemia	Two intermediate hosts Snails eat eggs; cercariae develop in the lungs Expelled cercariae eaten by ants and develop into metacercariae Ants ingested by definitive host, adults develop in the liver	Morphology of eggs or adults	Praziquantel and benzimidazoles may be helpful to treat liver flukes

AVE, Avermectins; *DCV*, dicloros; *FBZ*, fenbendazole; *LVM*, levamisole; *PIP*, piperazine; *PRT*, pyrantel; *TBZ*, thiabendazole.
Data from Morris and Shima.[28]

profuse diarrhea and weight loss. An enterophathogenic *Escherichia coli* and PCV2 were isolated from the hog. The source of the PCV2 was not identified.

In recent years, research has focused on influenza viruses. Domestic swine are of interest because of their ability for gene reassortment with the avian, human, and swine influenza viruses. They may also be infected by various influenza viruses and the risk exists for influenza viruses to be transmitted among exotic swine species, their caretakers, and the visiting public.

Neoplasia

Reports of neoplasia in exotic swine are sparse. Neoplasia is generally seen in older animals. The following neoplasms were reported at necropsy in exotic suids at the author's institution: intestinal lymphosarcoma and intestinal carcinoma in two Bornean bearded pigs, each 11 years of age; squamous cell carcinoma involving the prepuce and multiple carcinomas in warthogs aged 10 and 13 years, respectively; reproductive neoplasia in four wild boars, ages 12 to 17 years: (1) testicular malignant seminoma, (2) uterine leiomyosarcoma, (3) uterine adenocarcinoma, and (4) uterine sarcoma; pharyngeal squamous cell carcinoma in an 18-year-old babirusa; and carotid body tumor in a 10-year-old red river hog.

Dentistry

Dental problems are not uncommon in wild suids and peccaries: fractured or avulsed canines, periodontal disease, and dental abscesses are seen. Figure 58-4 shows a Visayan warty pig with a mandibular canine fractured at the gumline. An endodontic procedure consisting of a vital root canal was performed, and the canine continued to grow normally. A nylon screw was used to successfully cap a tooth defect in a babirusa.[38] Sites of tusk avulsions generally granulate with wound care and antimicrobial therapy. Some animals may need periodic tusk trimming. Dental attrition and uneven wear are expected findings in aging suids and peccaries (Figure 58-5). Some species in the wild have been noted to only have canines and caudal molars.[32] Floating dental points is performed, as needed. Periodontal disease is managed through regular prophylaxis, dental extractions, as needed, and antimicrobial therapy. Pulsatile low-dose doxycycline (0.3 mg/kg, PO, BID, for 1–3 months, rotating on and off therapy) has been used for adjunct management of periodontal disease in suids and tassysuids.[4] Diets high in simple sugars may predispose these animals to periodontal disease. Routine dental care should be a part of suid and peccary preventive health care.

Disorders of the Feet

Trauma, especially to the feet, is common in exotic swine and peccaries.[41] The delicate nature of the suid and peccary hoofs compared with those of other ungulates makes them more susceptible to abrasive wear. Some animals may need periodic hoof trims, depending on the substrate used and activity levels (Figure 58-6). Excessive sole wear and hoof trauma may occur from digging, running, or pacing on hard or abrasive surfaces (Figure 58-7, A and B). Any lame suid or peccary should be carefully monitored and examined if lameness does not resolve within a few days. If left untreated, sole erosions and hoof defects may progress to infection of soft tissues and osteomyelitis. Hoof acrylics may be used to repair defects once the tissue has become healthy (Figure 58-8). Vettec hoof care products (Vettec Hoof Care Products, Oxnard, CA, www.vettec.com) are commonly used at the author's institution. Hoof acrylics are also used prophylactically to create protective toe caps when the animals are likely to pace excessively (e.g., during relocations). These products have also been used on the bottoms of bandages to extend bandage wear. Behavioral conditioning to facilitate inspection of feet is helpful to monitor hoof conditions.

Miscellaneous Conditions

Although pigs are quite hardy, they are still susceptible to hyperthermia, exertional myopathy, or both. Possible scenarios include stormy

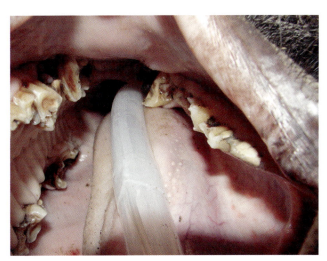

FIGURE 58-5 Dental attrition and wear in a wild boar.

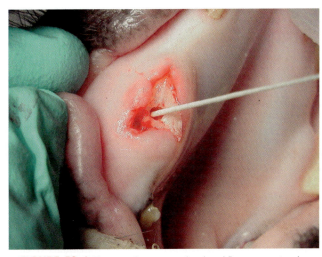

FIGURE 58-4 Fractured upper canine in a Visayan warty pig.

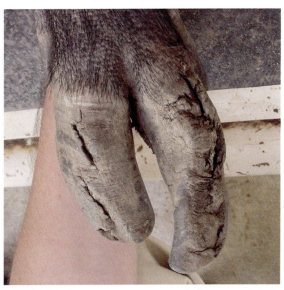

FIGURE 58-6 Overgrown hooves in a Bornean bearded pig.

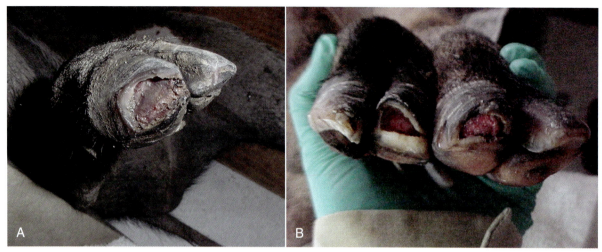

FIGURE 58-7 **A,** Toe tip trauma in a Visayan warty pig. **B,** Toe tip defects in a red river hog.

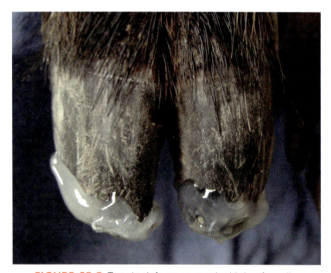

FIGURE 58-8 Toe tip defects covered with hoof acrylic.

anesthetic induction or recovery, escape, excessive chasing by enclosure mates, and conspecific aggression. In addition, suids are prone to gastric ulceration. Prophylactic treatment with gastroprotectants is recommended when animals are stressed such as by relocation, hospitalization, anorexia, or social aggression.

A pheochromocytoma was found at necropsy in a 14-year-old male warthog that had been evaluated for epistaxis.[9] No lesions were present in the nasal cavity. On the basis of blood pressure readings and epinephrine norepinephrine ratios, the epistaxis was presumed secondary to the pheochromocytoma.

REPRODUCTION

Compared with other ungulate species, gestation is shorter in wild suids, and they are considered the only true multiparous group of the artiodactylids.[35] Because of this, the young are smaller relative to the size of the dam. Males actively court females. Females develop vulvar swelling and urinate frequently when in estrus. The uterine horns of the warthog and babirusa are reported to be smaller than those in other suid species, and this is attributed to be the reason for their smaller litters.[49] Peccary uterine horns are shorter than those of suids.[14] The penis is curved in a sigmoid shape, and the ends have

a corkscrew appearance, correlating with the shape of the cervix.[49] A summary of reproductive parameters for select species are summarized in Table 58-9.

Fecal hormones to characterize reproductive biology were evaluated in red river hogs, babirusas, and warthogs.[3] Researchers found that estrus cycles could be monitored using 20 α-OH- and 20-oxopregnane assays. In contrast, estrogens and androgens were not useful in characterizing follicular activity during estrus. The duration of the estrus cycle was approximately 35 days for all three species in this study. During the second half of pregnancy, estrogens and 17-oxo-androstanes were elevated.

Use of ultrasonography to diagnose and monitor pregnancy in both awake and anesthetized babirusa has been reported.[17] Uterine changes were noted at 28 to 32 days of gestation. Ventral midline transabdominal ultrasonography was superior to rectal ultrasonography in visualizing fetal structures. During weekly ultrasonographic examinations, fetuses were detected at 38 days of gestation. Cranial measurements, done weekly, revealed a linear growth pattern. The authors documented resorption of one of three fetuses in each of three pregnancies.

Suids also differ from other artiodactylids in that they show nesting behavior prior to parturition. They generally do not clean their young after birth. Except for the *Babirusa* sp., *Phacochoerus* sp., and *Hylochoerus* sp., piglets are born with horizontal stripes.[32,35,49] Similar to other artiodactylids, placentation is epitheliochorial, so neonates are dependent on nursing for transfer of maternal immunity. At the author's institution, pregnant suids are vaccinated, where feasible, against colibacillosis. In captivity, promiscuous suckling has been observed in white-lipped peccaries but not in collared peccaries.[49]

Most newborn piglets are not able to fully thermoregulate, so protection from the elements and supplemental heat are needed, depending on weather circumstances. Infanticide and cannibalism of young have been reported in pigs and peccaries and are not uncommon in exotic swine species in zoos as well. Neonatal mortality comprises a large proportion of swine and peccary mortality at the author's institution. Trauma accounts for a majority of cases, followed by infectious etiologies. When the young start to sample solids, creep feeders may have to be provided to allow the young access to food without interference from adult animals.

Melengesterol acetate implants, gonadotropin-releasing hormone (GnRH) inhibitors, and medroxyprogesterone injections have been used in females for contraception. Information on the most current contraceptive recommendations for swine and peccaries may be found through the Association of Zoos and Aquariums' Wildlife Contraception Center.[2]

TABLE 58-9

Reproductive Parameters in Selected Species of Pigs and Peccaries[7,14,21,32,35,49]

Parameter	Red River Hog (*Potamochoerus Porcus*)	Babirusa (*Babyrousa Babyrussa*)	Bearded Pig (*Sus Barbatus*)	Common Warthog (*Phacochoerus Africanus*)	Collared Peccary (*Tayassu Tajacu*)	Chacoan Peccary (*Catagonus Wagneri*)
Karyotype (2n)	34	38	36–40	34	30	20
Age at sexual maturity	3 years	In captivity as early as 5–10 months	10–20 months	18–20 months	8–10 months	1–2 years
Details of estrous cycle	Seasonal?	Polyestrous, may have two litters per year; urinary hormones. 28–42 day estrous cycle	Breed through year, two litters per year	Seasonal polyestrous; estrus lasts 72 hours approximately every 6 weeks	Polyestrous; 27–28 day estrous cycle; 1- to 5-day estrus (5.7 day mean)	Breed through year
Gestation	127 days	155–175 days (163 day mean)	160 days	160–170 days	140–150 days (142 day mean)	~150 days
Litter size	1–8 (usually 3–4)	1–3 (usually 2)	8–10	1–8 (usually 2–3)	1–3 (usually 2)	1–4 (usually 2)
Number of mammae	3 pairs	2 pairs	6 pairs	2 pairs	2 pairs	4 pairs
Weaning	—	26–32 weeks	5–6 weeks	24–25 weeks	6 weeks	—

Data modified from Morris and Shima.[28]

ACKNOWLEDGMENT

The author wishes to recognize Dr. Pat Morris for his valuable contributions to the field of exotic swine medicine. The author also thanks Dr. Pat Morris for his input into this chapter, as well as the San Diego Zoo Global library staff for their assistance with references.

REFERENCES

1. Allen JL: Immobilization of Chacoan peccaries (*Catagonus wagneri*) with a tiletamine hydrochloride/zolazepam hydrochloride combination. *J Wildl Dis* 28:499–501, 1992.
2. Association of Zoos and Aquariums, Contraceptive Advisory Group: http://www.stlzoo.org/animals/scienceresearch/contraceptioncenter/. Accessed 2/1/2013.
3. Berger EM, Leus K, Vercammen P, et al: Fecal steroid metabolites for non-invasive assessment of reproduction in common warthogs (*Phacochoerus africanus*), red river hogs (*Potamochoerus porcus*) and babirusa (*Babyrousa babyrussa*). *Anim Reprod Sci* 91:155–171, 2005.
4. Bicknese BJ, Fagan DA, Lamberski N: "Cyclic" regime of low-dose doxycycline to treat periodontal disease in a Chacoan peccary (*Catagonus wagneri*), red pandas (*Ailurus fulgens*), and bat-eared foxes (*Otocyon megalotis megalotis*). In *Proceedings of the American Association of Zoo Veterinarians*, Los Angeles, CA, 2008.
5. Calle PP, Morris PJ: Anesthesia for nondomestic suids. In Fowler ME, Miller RE, editors: *Zoo and wild animal medicine*, ed 4, Philadelphia, PA, 1999, Saunders.
6. Carvalho MAG, Santos PS, Nogueira SSC, et al: Necrotic enteritis in collared (*Pecari tajacu*) and white-lipped (*Tayassu pecari*) peccaries. *J Zoo Wildl Med* 42:732–734, 2011.
7. Chaudhuri M, Carrasco P, Kalk P, et al: Urinary oestrogen excretion during oestrus and pregnancy in the Babirusa. *Int Zoo Yb* 29:188–192, 1990.
8. Clauss M, Nijboer J, Loermans JH, et al: Comparative digestion studies in wild suids at Rotterdam Zoo. *Zoo Biol* 27:305–319, 2008.
9. Cole G, Suedmeyer WK, Johnson G: Pheochromocytoma in an African warthog (*Phacochoerus aethiopicus*). *J Zoo Wildl Med* 39:663–666, 2008.
10. Disney's Animal Kingdom: www.animalenrichment.org. Accessed 2/1/2013.
11. Durden LA: Lice. In Samuel WM, Pybus MF, Kocan AA, editors: *Parasitic diseases of wild mammals*, ed 2, Ames, IA, 2001, Iowa State University Press.
12. Fowler ME: Husbandry and diseases of captive wild swine and peccaries. *Rev Vet Tech Off Int Epizootiol* 15:141–154, 1996.
13. Gabor TM, Hellgren EC, Silvy JH: Immobilization of collared peccaries (*Tayassu tajacu*) and feral hogs (*Sus scrofa*) with Telazol® and xylazine. *J Wildl Dis* 33:161–164, 1997.
14. Gottdenker N, Bodmer R: Peccaries. In Hutchins M, editor: *Grzimek's animal life encyclopedia*, vol 16, ed 2, Detroit, MI, 2004, Gale.
15. Grubb P: Artiodactyla. In Wilson DE, Reeder DM, editors: *Mammal species of the world: A taxonomic and geographical reference*, ed 3, Baltimore, MD, 2005, The John Hopkins University Press.
16. Hellgren EC, Lochmiller RL, Amoss MS, et al: Endocrine and metabolic responses of the collared peccary (*Tayassu tajacu*) to immobilization with ketamine hydrochloride. *J Wildl Dis* 21:417–425, 1985.
17. Houston EW, Hagberg PK, Fisher MT, et al: Monitoring pregnancy in babirusa (*Babyrousa babyrussa*) with transabdominal ultrasonography. *J Zoo Wildl Med* 32:366–372, 2001.
18. International Union of Conserving Nation: Red List, http://www.iucnredlist.org. Accessed 2/1/2013.
19. James SB, Cook RA, Raphael BL, et al: Immobilization of babirusa (*Babyrousa babyrussa*) with xylazine and tiletamine/zolazepam and reversal with yohimbine and flumazenil. *J Zoo Wildl Med* 30:521–525, 1999.
20. Karesh WB, Uhart MM: Health evaluation of white lipped peccary populations in Bolivia. In *Proceedings of the American Association of Zoo Veterinarians*, Omaha, NB, 1998.
21. Kemp Y: Growth and development in captive Bornean bearded pigs, *Sus barbatus*, at the San Diego Zoo. *Zool Garden NF* 70:73–92, 2000.
22. Leus K, Goodall GP, Macdonald AA: Anatomy and histology of the babirusa (*Babyrousa babyrussa*) stomach. *C R Acad Sci Paris* Ser III 233:102, 1999.
23. Leus K, Macdonald AA, Goddall G, et al: Light and scanning microscopy of the cardiac gland region of the stomach of the Babirusa (*Babyrousa babyrussa*—Suidae, Mammalia). *C R Biologies* 327:735–743, 2004.
24. Leus K, Macdonald AA: From babirusa (*Babyrousa babyrussa*) to domestic pig: The nutrition of swine. *Proc Nutr Soc* 56:1001–1012, 1997.
25. Lochmiller R, Hellgren E, Robinson R, Grant W: Techniques for collecting blood from collared peccaries, *Dicotyles tajacu*. *J Wildl Dis* 20:47–50, 1984.

26. Mercado JA, Morris PJ: Comparative serum glucose levels in sedated Suidae and Tayassuidae. In *Proceedings of the American Association of Zoo Veterinarians*, Los Angeles, CA, 2006.

27. Moon PF, Smith LJ: General anesthetic techniques in swine. *Vet Clin North Am Food Anim Pract* 12:663–691, 1996.

28. Morris P, Shima A: Suidae and Tayassuidae. In Fowler M, Miller E, editors: *Zoo and wildlife medicine*, ed 5, St. Louis, MO, 2003, Saunders.

29. Morris PJ, Bicknese EL, Janssen DL, et al: Chemical immobilization of exotic swine at the San Diego Zoo. In *Proceedings of the American Association of Zoo Veterinarians*, Columbus, OH, 1999.

30. Nogueira SS, Silva MG, Dias CT, et al: Social behaviour of collared peccaries (*Pecari tajacu*) under three space allowances. *Anim Welfare* 19:243–248, 2010.

31. Noon TH, Heffelfinger JR, Olding RJ, et al: Serologic survey of antibodies to canine distemper virus in collared peccary (*Tayassu tajacu*) populations in Arizona. *J Wild Dis* 39:221–223, 2003.

32. Nowak R: *Walker's mammals of the world*, vol 2, ed 6, Baltimore, MD, 1999, Johns Hopkins University Press.

33. Padilla LR, Ko JCH: Non-domestic suids. In West G, Heard D, Caulkett N, editors: *Zoo animal and wildlife immobilization and anesthesia*, Ames, IA, 2007, Blackwell Publishing.

34. Padilla LR: Immobilization of babirusa (*Babyrousa babyroussa*) using a butorphanol-tiletamine-zolazepam combination. In *Proceedings of the American Association of Zoo Veterinarians*, San Diego, CA, 2004.

35. Powell DM: Pigs. In Hutchins M, editor: *Grzimek's animal life encyclopedia*, vol 16, ed 2, Detroit, MI, 2004, Gale.

36. Roberts DC: Disease transfer from wild to domestic pigs. In Leman AD, Straw BE, Mengeling WL, editors: *Diseases of swine*, ed 7, Ames, IA, 1992, Iowa State University Press.

37. Sandfoss MR, DePerno CS, Bets CW, et al: A serosurvey for *Brucella suis*, classical swine fever, porcine circovirus type 2, and pseudorabies virus in feral swine (*Sus scrofa*) of Eastern North Carolina. *J Wildl Dis* 48:462–466, 2012.

38. Schaftenaar W: Treatment of a fractured tusk in a male babirusa (*Babyrousa babyrussa*) using a polyoxymethylene bolt. *J Zoo Wildl Med* 22(3):364–366, 1991.

39. Selmi AL, Mendes GM, Figueiredo JP, et al: Chemical restraint of peccaries with tiletamine/zolazepam and xylazine or tiletamine/zolazepam and butorphanol. *Vet Anesth Analg* 30:24–29, 2003.

40. Siemon A, Siesner H, vin Hegel G: Die Verwendung von Tiletamine/Zolazepam/Romifidine zur Distansimmobilization von Wildschweinen. *Tierarztl Prax* 20:55–58, 1992.

41. Singleton C, Morris P: Survey of foot problems in a collection of captive exotic swine. In *Proceedings of the American Association of Zoo Veterinarians*, Tampa, FL, 2006.

42. Sonntag S, Hackenbroich C, Boer M, et al: Tiletamine-zolazepam-xylazine immobilization in warthogs (*Phacochoerus aethiopicus*). In *Proceedings European Association of Zoo and Wildlife Veterinarians*, Ebeltoft, Denmark, 2004.

43. Sowls LK: *Javelinas and other peccaries: Their biology, management, and use*, ed 2, Tucson, AZ, 1997, University of Arizona Press.

44. Straw BE, Allaire SD, Mengeling WL, Taylor DJ, editors: *Diseases of wild swine*, ed 8, Ames, IA, 1999, Iowa State University Press.

45. Sutherland-Smith M, Campos JM, Cramer C, et al: Immobilization of Chacoan peccaries (*Catagonus wagneri*) using medetomidine, Telazol®, and ketamine. *J Wildl Dis* 40:731–736, 2004.

46. Sweitzer RA, Ghneim GS, Garnder AI, et al: Immobilization and physiological parameters associated with chemical restraint of wild pigs with Telazol® and xylazine hydrochloride. *J Wildl Dis* 33:198–205, 1997.

47. The shape of enrichment: www.enrichment.org. Accessed 2/1/2013.

48. Thurmon JC, Tranquilli WJ, Benson GJ: *Lumb and Jones veterinary anesthesia*, ed 3, Baltimore, MD, 1996, Williams & Wilkins.

49. Wilson DE, Mittermeir RA, editors: *Handbook of mammals of the world*, vol 2, Barcelona, Spain, 2011, Lynx Edicions.

50. Woodger NGA, Hosegood OM: PMWS associated with diarrhoea and ill thrift in a captive red river hog (*Potamochoerus porcus*). *Vet Rec* 168:512, 2011.

51. Wu N, Abril C, Thomann A, et al: Risk factors for contacts between wild boar and outdoor pigs in Switzerland and investigations on potential Brucella suis spill-over. *BMC Vet Res* 8:1–12, 2012.

CHAPTER **59**

Hippopotamidae (Hippopotamus)

Chris Walzer and Gabrielle Stalder

BIOLOGY

Today, two extant species of the Hippopotamidae coexist within two genera: (1) the small and rare pygmy hippopotamus (*Choeropsis liberiensis*, previously *Hexaprotodon liberiensis*) native to the forests of West Africa, and (2) the far larger, more widespread, and common hippopotamus (*Hippopotamus amphibius*). The geographic distribution of the common hippopotamus today is restricted to sub-Saharan Africa, where it inhabits rivers, lakes, and wetlands.

In 2006, this species was included for the first time in the International Union for the Conservation of Nature (IUCN) Red List of Threatened Species and was listed as Vulnerable to Extinction.[31] The common hippopotamus is listed in Appendix II of the Convention on International Trade in Endangered Species of Wild Fauna and Flora.[9] The wild population is rapidly dwindling, with a 30% decrease in the past decade. In some countries such as the Democratic Republic of Congo, the wild population has diminished by as much as 95%.[36] Unfortunately, there are very few recent surveys of hippopotamus ("hippo") populations and, therefore, a significant uncertainty concerning the momentary situation exist.

As its name indicates, the *common hippopotamus* has an amphibious lifestyle, gregariously resting in shallow water during the day and emerging at night to feed solitarily. Common hippos live in loose, social, polygynous groups of females with offspring and territorial males, based on mating territoriality. Spreading its dung by tail wagging while defecating, a behavior more commonly observed in males, is believed to have a signaling function, rather than a territorial one. Although conflicts are highly ritualized and usually restricted to threat displays, fierce territorial fights may occur when a bachelor challenges a territorial male. These territorial fights, which usually occur in the water, may result in considerable trauma and even death caused by the huge canines.

Similar to its larger relative, the pygmy hippo is facing a considerable population decline in the wild and is currently listed as Endangered on the IUCN Red List of Threatened Species.[31] The pygmy hippo is listed in Appendix I of the Convention on International Trade in Endangered Species of Wild Fauna and Flora.[9] The species occurs in four African countries, namely, Sierra Leone, Guinea, Côte d'Ivoire, and Liberia, where the largest populations are found. Because of its secluded and nocturnal lifestyle, not much is known about the ecology of the species. The pygmy hippo is less gregarious compared with the common hippo and is usually found either solitary or in pairs. The few studies indicate that the pygmy hippo retreats into swamps, river banks, and heavily forested habitat during daytime and that it shows a strong affinity to water and is therefore found close to rivers or streams.[39,60]

Both species are long lived, with reported ages of 35 to 50 years (61 years reported in a captive animal) in the common hippo, and up to 55 years in the pygmy hippo.[45,72] Weights range up to 2500 kg in the female and 3000 kg in the male common hippos, with a tendency to be higher in captivity; and around 160 to 350 kg in the pygmy hippo.

UNIQUE ANATOMY

Compared with its larger relative, the common hippo, which is designed to support its enormous body weight (the scapula is oriented vertically and forms a vertical column with the limb bones; the pelvis is oriented at a 45-degree angle), the skeleton of the pygmy hippo is built slightly lighter.[45] The shape of the skull and the position of the eyes differ among the species, according to their individual lifestyles. In the common hippo, the eyes face forward, whereas in the pygmy hippo, the skull is proportionally smaller and rounder, with the orbits positioned laterally. In the common hippo, the brain case is extremely small compared with the head, which should be taken into account when euthanasia performed with a rifle is considered. The jaw of the common hippo is capable of a 150-degree opening, which is less in the pygmy hippo.

Hippos are considered pseudoruminants, as they have a complex four-chambered stomach structure with a ruminant-type digestion, although they do not ruminate. As in ruminants, fermentation occurs mainly in the forestomachs, which contain a rich ciliate fauna. Cecum and gallbladder are missing. However, necropsy reports have described a structure that contains bile and have reported it as "gallbladder-like."[45] In contrast to other species of artiodactyls, hippos have four functional toes with nail-like hooves on the end of the toes.

Both hippo species show marked physiologic adaptations for a (semi-)aquatic life style. Accordingly, the external sensory organs are positioned high on the head.[5] The skin is thick, lacks sebaceous glands, and retains few hairs. Muscular valves close the ears and nostrils during diving. Recently, the hippo has been identified as the artiodactyl sister group of cetaceans.[2]

The unique morphology and the physiology of the hippo may constitute a challenge during medical procedures. The thick skin and the dense subcutaneous tissue may impede darting and the resorption and distribution of drugs. Difficulties caused by their large size, dive response, arousal during anesthesia, and limited vascular access have been previously reported.[45,56,68]

Furthermore, knowledge gaps with regard to the anatomy and location of specific organs such as the testes have led to intrasurgical difficulties.[15,56] A decade ago, it was already realized that more research is required before surgical castration of the male hippo can

be recommended.[45] The location of the testes in the hippo is still described as "internal" in analogy to cetaceans that have true intraabdominal testes. However, in the hippo, the testes are actually partially descended and remain in the inguinal canal.[71] A scrotum, as such, is not developed in the hippo. The hippo evolving between land and water appears, in contrast to true terrestrial mammals, to have partially retracted testes.[14]

Dental Formula

The dental formula of the common hippo is: incisors (I) 2/2, canines (C) 1/1, premolars (P) 3-4/3-4, molars (M) 3/3; and that of the pygmy hippo is: I 2/1, C 1/1, P 3/3, M 3/3. The tusklike canines are used for fighting, and the enlarged incisors grow continuously. In males, canines are twice as long as in females and are kept sharpened by constant wear against the shorter upper canines. The low crowned molars are used for mastication of food.

SPECIAL PHYSIOLOGY

The unique skin of the hippo, consisting of a thin epidermis and a thick dermis with dense subcutaneous and fat tissue, characterizes both species. Subepidermal capillary loops, considered to play an important role in thermoregulation, have a diameter 20 times larger and density three times higher than in other mammals and were recently described in the integument of the common hippo.[43] Furthermore, these capillaries are uniquely adapted for high blood pressure, allowing for efficient blood vessel–based heat transfer to the periphery.[43]

No sebaceous or sweat glands exist, but large, subdermal mucous glands secrete a thick, oily red fluid—the so called "blood sweat" or "red sweat."[21] The secretions are believed to protect the thin epidermis against water loss, sunburn, and infections.

Hippos have an exceedingly good predisposition for wound healing.[41] Good wound healing is clearly necessary for the common hippo, as territorial fighting results in wounds of significant size and number.[10] One possible explanation for the good wound healing properties is the particular "red sweat" observed in this species. The pigments responsible for the color have been described as hipposudoric acid (the red pigment) and norhipposudoric acid (the orange pigment).[27] The red pigment has been shown to have significant bacteriocidal activity by inhibiting the growth of pathogenic bacteria such as *Pseudomonas aeruginosa* and *Klebsiella pneumonia*.[61] Similarly, the closest relatives of the common hippo, cetaceans, also have an epidermal defense mechanism against bacteria, fungi, algae, and ectoparasites.[42]

SPECIAL HOUSING REQUIREMENTS

Common Hippo

Because of their size and strength, the common hippo requires robust housing and adequate barriers. Many existing barriers in zoos are very low and could easily be scaled by adult hippos. The animals are generally not considered to be frost resistant, although they are found in Africa at higher altitudes (1500–2000 m above sea level) with cool night temperatures and have been held in zoologic collections in Europe in subzero conditions. However, for animal welfare reasons, they should be provided with heated interior enclosures in temperate climates. Room temperature is suggested to range from 16° C to 20° C. The animals need interior and exterior pools, which should have a depth of at least 2.5 m so that the animals can remain totally submerged.[45,55] Additional shallower areas in the pools have been shown to be beneficial for the resting behavior.[1] Extensive filtering is needed to provide conditions for underwater viewing. Furthermore, the animals require adequate areas to rest and shaded areas in the outside enclosures. The interior enclosure design should allow for easy separation of individuals and removal of individuals from the pool for medical interventions. Naturalistic exhibits have been suggested to enhance animal welfare and provide the public with a clearer view of the lifestyle of the hippo.[1]

Pygmy Hippo

The pygmy hippo has similar enclosure requirements as the common hippo. Although smaller, this species is reported to be far more aggressive toward conspecifics and humans.[55] Adequate separation of individuals is generally necessary and must be considered when designing an enclosure. Some individuals will need to be housed separately to prevent fighting. It has been suggested that females be kept dry prior to parturition to allow a slow introduction of the calf to the water environment.[45] Several descriptions of pygmy hippo enclosures are provided at the website of zoolex.org (http://www.zoolex.org 2013).

FEEDING

Both hippo species are easy to keep in captivity and usually pose few veterinary problems related to feeding. Disorders associated with the GI tract are mainly reported to be foreign body ingestion leading to obstruction of the small intestine.[16] Hippos are considered strict herbivores, although cases of carnivory in the wild common hippo have been reported.[12] Common hippos are described as exclusive grazers with a capacious foregut fermentation system.[65] Interestingly, this species is reported to have a comparatively low food intake and also short feeding times.[7] The diet of an adult common hippo should consist of some 30 to 45 kilograms (kg) of a mixture of good-quality grass, clover, lucerne, and green maize. Additionally, various vegetables may be provided. In winter, the grass may be replaced with good-quality hay and silo.[55] The few studies on pygmy hippos

suggest that the diet in this species contains ferns, herbs, leaves, and fruits, with grass playing a minor role.[29] In captivity, a wide range of vegetables and fruits may be provided, along with high-quality hay. It is important to note that both hippo species are reported to have unusually low metabolic rates, and therefore the provision of energy-dense pelleted foods should be considered carefully in view of the species' proneness to obesity.[64]

RESTRAINT AND HANDLING

Physical restraint and handling are difficult in both hippo species, as they are extremely dangerous. Especially, the common hippo, because of its weight, size, sharp canine teeth, and the often-aggressive demeanor, may easily inflict fatal injuries. For any procedures that require closer contact with the animal, additional chemical restraint is recommended (Tables 59-1 and 59-2).

To avoid anesthesia, which is associated with challenges in both species, training for minor examinations or procedures (e.g., oral examination) may be implemented.

ANESTHESIA AND SURGERY

The common hippo (*Hippopotamus amphibius*) is difficult to anesthetize, and in the past, procedures were associated with high mortality. Both the unique morphology and the physiology of the hippo constitute anesthetic challenges.

Because of the strength, body size, and weight of the hippo, several facts should be considered during preanesthetic planning.

TABLE 59-1

Chemical Restraint Agents Used for Common Hippos

Generic Name	Trade Name	Dosage (milligram per kilogram [mg/kg]) (adult total dose)	Reversal Agent (mg/kg)	Comments
Etorphine[56]	M99	0.001–0.005 (2–6)	Diprenorphine 2–3.2 ×M99dose Naltrexone 100× M99 dose	Fatal complications with high dosages of M99 (up to 7–12 mg)[32]
Etorphine/xylazine[45,56]	M99/Rompun	0.001–0.005 (2–6)/ 0.067–0.083 (100) (2–6/100–150)	Naltrexone 100× M99 dose/ Yohimbine 0.1–0.3	Fatal complications with high dosages of M99 (up to 7–12 mg)[32]
Ketamine/ medetomidine[45,68]	Ketasol, Ketanest/ Dormitor, Zalopine	1/0.06–0.08 1.5/0.067 (900/40)–600 kg	Atipamezole 2–5× Med. dose	
Detomidine/ butorphanol[13,45,47]	Domosedan, Domidine/Butomidor	0.02–0.06/0.1–0.2 0.05/0.15 (100/300 for est. weight of 2270 kg) (40/60 for est. weight of 950 kg) (30/90)–550kg	Yohimbine 0.1–0.3 or Atipamezole 5× Det. dose Naltrexone 0.4–0.6	Caution: Arousal due to stimulation
Butorphanol/azaperone/ Medetomidine[18]	Butomidor/Stresnil/ Dormitor, Zalopine	0.1–0.12/0.05–0.10/ 0.04–0.05	Atipamezole 2× Med. dose Naltrexone 2× But dose	Caution: Arousal due to stimulation
Tiletamin-Zolazepam/ Ketamin[50]		3/1		Profound sedation
Azaperone[45]	Stresnil	(400–800)		Sedation only
Acepromazine[45]		0.2		Oral administration; mild sedation
Diazepam (Miguel Cesares, personal communication)		0.2		Oral administration; mild sedation

Adapted from Miller M: Hippopotamidae (hippopotamus). In Fowler ME, Miller RE, editors: Zoo and wild animal Medicine, ed 5, Philadelphia, 2003, WB Saunders.

TABLE 59-2

Chemical Restraint Agents Used for Pygmy Hippos

Generic Name	Trade Name	Dosage (milligram per kilogram [mg/kg]) (adult total dose)	Reversal Agent (mg/kg)	Comments
Carfentanyl/xylazine[45]	Carfentanyl/Rompun	0.0075/0.05 (1.5/10)	Naltrexone 100× Carfentanyl dose Yohimbine (Antagonil) 0.1–0.3	
Etorphine-acepromazine/ [xylazine][45,52]	Immobilon/ Rompun	2.45 LAI/10/ [150 mg] 0.011–0.017/0.046–0.2 (2–3/10)	Diprenorphine 2–3× etorphine dose	
Etorphine/xylazine[17,44,45,46,52]	M99/Rompun	0.009–0.014/0.46–0.69 (2–3/100–150) (5/10)	Naltrexone 100× M99 dose Yohimbine (Antagonil) 0.1–0.3	
Ketamine/xylazin[33,52]	Ketasol, Ketanest/ Rompun	5–8/1.4–1.6 (1100–1800/300) 10–15/2		
Medetomidine/ketamine[3]	Dormitor, Zalopine/ Ketasol, Ketanest	0.08/1.2		Isoflurane maintenance
Medetomidine/ butorphanol[44,45]	Dormitor, Zalopine/ Butomidor	0.034–0.09/0.184–0.19 (12/80) 0.036/0.2 0.09/0.18 (22.5/45)	or Atipamezole (Antisedan) 5× Medetomidine dose/ naltrexone 3× Butorphanol dose	Sedation only; possible arousal due to stimulation
Tiletamine/zolazepam[45]	Telazol/Zoletil	2.2–3.5 (500–1000)		
Detomidine/butorphanol[44,45]	Domosedan, Domidine/ Butomidor	0.04–0.06/0.1–0.2 0.02–0.06/0.1–0.2 best combination: 0.05/0.15	Yohimbine (Antagonil) 0.1–0.3 or Atipamezole (Antisedan) 5× Detomidine dose/ naltrexone 0.4–0.6	Doses for heavy sedation/light anesthesia Potential arousal due to stimulation; may require supplemental drugs
Midazolam[44,45]		0.1 (25)		Premedication, mild sedation
Diazepam/detomidine[73]		0.5/0.044	Yohimbine 0.11	Oral administration as premedication
Ketamine/butorphanol[73]		1.25/0.0184		Induction after premedication with (diazepam/detomidine); supplemental doses of ketamine, butorphanol and detomidine

Adapted from Miller M: Hippopotamidae (hippopotamus). In Fowler ME, Miller RE, editors: Zoo and wild animal Medicine, ed 5, Philadelphia, 2003, WB Saunders.

The area where anesthesia will be administered should be easily accessible and adequate for darting of the animal. For the safety of the animals and the personnel, working space and escape routes should be secure. As the animals are difficult to move once in anesthesia, devices for moving the animal, such as ropes, winches, or cranes, should be readily available.

Fasting the hippos 24 to 48 hours and restricting their water intake for 12 to 24 hours before anesthesia are recommended by some authors to reduce the volume of gut content and, thus, the pressure on the diaphragm during recumbency.[40,44,45,56] However, other authors have successfully anesthetized hippos with fasting of the animals for only some 12 hours.[68]

Anesthetic agents may be applied manually in trained animals, but usually pole syringes, anesthetic pistols, or guns are used. Especially in large adult animals, only the area caudal to the ear or the medial and caudal aspects of the hind leg are recommended sites for injection, as the dense subcutaneous tissue and fat of several centimeters thickness will impede darting and the resorption in other areas. In juvenile or smaller animals, other sites may be used for injection. To penetrate the skin and the fat layer, long, reinforced, nonbarbed needles of 60 to 100 millimeters (mm) length are recommended.

The literature and reports on anesthesia of hippos are rare. Very early reports on capture and chemical restraint provide descriptions of field captures in which various muscle relaxants such as succinylcholine chloride,[53,70] varying combinations of phencyclidine hydrochloride with α_2-agonists, acepromazine, or ethorphine,[59,69,76] or fentanyl-acepromazine were used.[25] These historical immobilizations in the field often resulted in drowning of animals, as hippos tend to retreat into water when threatened. This fact should be kept in mind when considering anesthesia, and access to pools should be blocked to prevent accidental drowning.

The use of detomidine–butorphanol and medetomidine–butorphanol–azaperone (BAM) combinations have been described.[8,13,19,47] Spontaneous arousal of animals following stimulation makes these protocols only suitable for sedation and very minor or nonsurgical procedures.

The most commonly used anesthetic is the potent opioid etorphine, sometimes in combination with xylazine or acepromazine.[40,45,56,69] Reported complications with these opioid-based anesthetic combinations include apnea, cyanosis, bradycardia, and fatal respiratory arrest.[44] In a retrospective study, 6 of 16 immobilizations were shown to have resulted in complications from bradypnea and apnea. In 3 of 4 cases, these respiratory complications were successfully resolved with the administration of doxapram, a respiratory stimulant. In the same study, only 2 of 16 procedures provided an anesthetic depth sufficient for surgical interventions.

The successful use of a medetomidine–ketamine combination in 10 adult male hippos undergoing castration has been reported.[68] In this study, self-limiting apnea was observed in 5 of 10 animals. The authors considered this a physiologic process related to the dive response in this semi-aquatic species, as no intervention was necessary, and vital parameters remained unchanged throughout.

The literature on anesthesia in the pygmy hippo is scarce. Various case reports provide brief descriptions of anesthetic protocols.[4,17,20,35,46] Anesthesia in this species has been described in more detail elsewhere.[3,33,34,44,45,52,73]

The protocols used are similar to the ones used in the common hippo. Etorphine, alone or in combination with acepromazine; azaperone; propionylpromazine; or xylazine were used most commonly. The use of ketamine in combination with α_2-agonists has been reported.[33] Ketamine and medetomidine (with isoflurane maintenance) has been successfully used in the pygmy hippos.[3,4,35] Combinations of detomidine or medetomidine with butorphanol have been described, but as in common hippos, pygmy hippos also showed arousal because of stimulation.[44,45] Ketamine–butorphanol combination is reported to be used for anesthesia induction.[44,45] Midazolam–zolazepam–tiletamine combination has been used for mild sedation in this species.

Although difficult, anesthesia monitoring is crucial for successful anesthesia in hippos. The most serious adverse effects of anesthesia in hippos include hypopnea or apnea, bradycardia, and hyperthermia. This is especially true with regard to long procedures with poor oxygen saturation. Respiratory rate may be assessed directly by observing thoracic excursions or indirectly with a respirometer, capnography (side or mainstream), or observation of the rebreathing bag when the animal is intubated.

Endotracheal tubes of 24 to 30 mm are recommended for an adult hippo.[40,45,47] To keep the hippo's mouth open and to safely intubate, a mouth gag (e.g., wood block) may be used. Because of the pygmy hippo's smaller, more caudal pharynx and smaller trachea, intubation is reported to be more difficult than in the common hippo and is usually performed by manual palpation with a tube size of 14 mm for an adult pygmy hippo.[17,44,73] Heart rate may be auscultated in smaller animals or by pulse oximetry (with the probe attached to the tongue, inside lip, eyelid, ear [after removing the corneal layer of the skin] vulva, prepuce).[45,68] Doppler ultrasonography (with probes placed on the cornea),[45] or palpation of an artery (sublingual artery) may also be used (Stalder, personal communication). Electrocardiography (ECG) is generally difficult to perform under routine anesthesia. Saturation of peripheral oxygen (SpO$_2$) may be measured by pulse oximetry at the same locations as stated for the heart rate or by blood gas analysis (saturation of arterial oxygen [SaO$_2$]). Oxygen supplied by nasal insufflation or via a tube with a flow rate of up to 15 liters per minute (L/min) is recommended to improve oxygen saturation.[40,68] The use of a Hudson demand valve may be useful in view of the very low respiratory rate in anesthetized hippos.

Arterial access is generally difficult, but blind puncture of the ventromedial tail artery is possible.[68] Several venipuncture sites have been used in the hippo (ventral tail vein, sublingual vein, cephalic vein, medial vein at the antebrachium, or the palmar digital vein, caudal on the lower limb, medial saphenous and plantar digital vein, auricular vein).[45,47,68] Intravenous catheterization is usually difficult. The thickness of the skin may necessitate a cut-down procedure or the use of ultrasonography to locate the veins. On the legs, the veins are extremely thin walled and collapse easily, so these veins are less suitable for catheterization.

Especially during longer procedures, body temperature should be closely monitored, as hippos could become hyperthermic. Water should be available to keep the skin moist and support thermoregulation. A cold-water rectal enema may also be used to decrease body temperature.

SURGERY

Surgical procedures are not commonly performed in hippos. Case reports describe treatment for dermatitis, skin biopsy and wound debridement, tusk trim, and removal of a perineal mass in the common hippo,[8,13] as well as treatments for rectal and uterine prolapses, hernia umbilicalis, removal of an oral mass and tusk trim, and cesarian section in pygmy hippos.[17,20,46,73] A recent study reported castration in 10 common hippos.[71]

DIAGNOSTICS

Physical examination and obtaining of samples for diagnostics in nonsedated hippos are generally difficult because of the nature of the animals. In sufficiently conditioned animals and in facilities with well-designed restraint devices, superficial examination and evaluation and, in some cases, palpation of the oral cavity, eyes, skin, and feet or other superficial structures may be performed.

Sampling of urine may be easily performed using a collecting vessel attached to a pole as the urine stream is usually discharged caudally. Bone marrow biopsy or collection of cerebrospinal fluid is usually performed only during necropsy.

Blood sampling, in most cases, requires sedation or anesthesia. For venipuncture sites, see Chapter 59 Hippopotamidae - Anesthesia and Surgery. Because of the constraints in collecting blood samples from nonsedated animals, reference values are derived mainly from ill or chemically restrained animals. No adequate values are available for the common hippo (Andrew Teare, ISIS, personal communication, 2013). It must be kept in mind that the values provided for the pygmy hippo are derived from sample sizes greater than 10 but less than 50 and do not fulfill American Society for Veterinary Clinical Pathology (ASVCP) criteria (Andrew Teare, ISIS, personal communication, 2013). Hematology and serum biochemistry data are summarized in Tables 59-3 and 59-4.

DISEASES

Hippos usually pose few veterinary problems with respect to diseases. Clinical examination and diagnostics are challenging, as they require training or chemical restraint in most cases.

TABLE 59-3

Reference Ranges for Hematologic Parameters for the Pygmy Hippo

Parameter	Units	Range
White blood cell count	*10^3 cells per microliter (cells/µL)	6.10–26.60
Red blood cell count	*10^6 cells/µL	3.11–7.25
Hemoglobin	Gram per deciliter (g/dL)	10.8–17.9
Hematocrit	%	18.0–55.0
Mean corpuscular volume	Femtoliter (fL)	57.9–80.3
Mean corpuscular hemoglobin	Picogram (pg)	20.1–26.2
Mean corpuscular hemoglobin concentration	g/dL	32.0–35.7
Segmented neutrophils	*10^3 cells/µL	3.40–24.5
Neutrophilic band cells	*10^3 cells/µL	0.03–1.37
Lymphocytes	*10^3 cells/µL	0.38–5.20
Monocytes	cells/µL	102–1290
Eosinophils	cells/µL	74–1560

TABLE 59-4

Reference Ranges for Serum Biochemical Parameters for the Pygmy Hippo

Test	Units	Range
Glucose	Milligram per deciliter (mg/dL)	32–193
Blood urea nitrogen (BUN)	mg/dL	10–47
Creatinine	mg/dL	0.5–2.7
BUN : Creatine ratio		8.9–33.3
Uric acid	mg/dL	0.0–1.2
Calcium	mg/dL	8.7–14.3
Phosphorus	mg/dL	4.4–11.4
Calcium : Phosphorus ratio		1.1–2.8
Sodium	Milliequivalent per liter (mEq/L)	139–156
Potassium	mEq/L	3.5–8.4
Sodium : Potassium ratio		18.6–41.4
Chloride	mEq/L	94–115
Total protein	Gram per deciliter (g/dL)	5.5–10.2
Albumin	g/dL	3.4–5.9
Globulin	g/dL	1.7–5.6
Alkaline phosphatase	International unit per liter (IU/L)	19–309
Lactate dehydrogenase	IU/L	2–867
Aspartate aminotransferase	IU/L	16–493
Alanine aminotransferase	IU/L	8–51
Creatine kinase	IU/L	21–274
Gamma-glutamyltransferase	IU/L	6–189
Total bilirubin	mg/dL	0.3–2.5
Cholesterol	mg/dL	17–155
Carbon dioxide	mEq/L	12.4–31.0

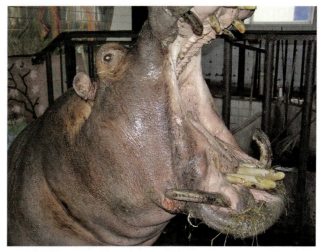

FIGURE 59-1 An ingrown canine in a common hippopotamus. Tusks are easily shortened using a Gigli wire-saw or adapted power tool. (Photo courtesy of Dr. Frank Göritz.)

Infectious Disease

Descriptions of infectious diseases in captive hippos consist mostly of individual case reports. Large disease outbreaks are restricted to the wild population. Anthrax (*Bacillus anthracis*) is the single most significant pathogen associated with high mortalities and periodic outbreaks in the wild hippopotamus.[30] Bacterial infections include tuberculosis, salmonellosis, and pasteurellosis,[45] and fatal *E. coli* septicemia and *Clostridium perfringens* type A infection have been reported in juvenile hippos.[16,37] Several serotypes of *Salmonella* have been isolated from asymptomatic animals as well as animals with clinical signs such as lethargy, anorexia, or GI-colic.[45]

β-hemolytic and γ-non-hemolytic streptococcal infections are the most common reported bacterial infections in captive animals, with a clinical spectrum ranging from frequently occurring skin infections resulting in severe dermatitis[8,67] to rarer cases of vasculitis, osteomyelitis, placentitis, mastitis, or septicemia, sometimes resulting in fatalities.[45] These skin infections are commonly associated with opportunistic co-infections by organisms such as *Morganella morganii*, *Klebsiella pneumonia*, *Citrobacter freundii*, *Enterococcus faecalis*, *Serratia liquifaciens*, and *Proteus vulgaris* and tend to persist but respond to aggressive antibiotic treatment with sulfamethoxazole and trimethoprim, amoxicillin, pentoxifylline, cephalosporins. Furthermore, seasonally recurring dermatopathies, similar to *Streptococcus* infections have been reported, but these could not be attributed to a specific pathogen.[28] Antibody titers to tetanus virus, *Brucella*,

and *Leptospira* have been reported in the wild common hippopotamus.[45] *L. icterohaemorrhagiae* infection in a zoo animal led to a fatal outcome in a pygmy hippo.[11]

Antibodies to bovine herpesvirus 2 (BHV2), rinderpest virus, infectious bovine rhinotracheitis virus (IBR), and contagious bovine pleuropneumonia virus have been found in wild common hippos.[14,26,54] A fatal encephalomyocarditis virus (EMCV) infection in a pygmy hippo was reported from an Australian zoo.[58]

Parasitic Disease

A wide range of parasites have been found in free-ranging hippos. These include platyhelminthes (e.g., Fasciolidae, Schistosomatidae, Taenidae), nematodes (e.g., Trichostrongylidae, Filariidae, Ascarididae), and protozoans (e.g., Coccidia, *Trypanosoma*). Additionally, antibodies to *Toxoplasma gondii* and the isolation of *Trypanosoma brucei*, *T. congolese*, and the malaria parasite *Hepatocystis hippopotami* have been demonstrated in the wild common hippo.[14,22] Ectoparasites such as ticks (*Amblyomma tholloni*, *Rhipicephalus simus*) and leeches (*Limnatis nilotica*) have been described.

Intestinal parasites (e.g., Ascaridae, Capillariidae, Strongyloididae, Strongylidae, Ancylostomatidae) have been sporadically described in captive animals but are usually not associated with clinical symptoms and are easily treated with anthelmintics commonly used in large animals.[45] A case of coccidial infection of the placenta leading to premature expulsion of the fetal membranes in a captive common hippo has been recently described.[38]

Noninfectious Disease

Noninfectious diseases have been reported on a single case basis in the two hippo species. These diseases are mostly similar to those found in domestic equids and ungulates and have been listed previously.[16,45]

Canines and incisors grow continuously in hippos and may reach impressive lengths. Tusk fractures and abnormal growth are a frequent finding in the common hippo. In both species, abnormal length of teeth may constitute a problem. These dental abnormalities may lead to oral lesions, penetrating wounds, and persisting fistulas. Tusks are easily shortened by using a Gigli wire-saw or various adapted power tools (Figure 59-1).[16]

In the pygmy hippo, polycystic kidney disease (PKD) has been reported on several occasions.[3,48,57] Various clinical signs have been reported in conjunction with PKD, including inter alia, anorexia, polydipsia, polyuria, and hind leg weakness.[57] If PKD is suspected, ultrasonography should be performed.

REPRODUCTION

Females

Determining the sex of the hippo from a distance may represent a challenge. The vulva is difficult to visualize, as it lies hidden in the perineal folds. The common hippo reproduces well in captivity. Sexually mature at 3 years, females can have up to 25 calves during their estimated 40-year life span. Gestation lasts 240 days, and postpartum estrus in this species contributes to very short intercalving periods of 1.5 to 2 years.[74] An enzyme immunoassay to determine progestagens in feces and serum is available.[24] Hippos are polyestrous and have an estrous cycle length of 30 days.[24] This impressive reproductive potential poses significant challenges in captivity, since the holding capacity of facilities is limited. As a consequence, research into hippo reproduction is primarily focused on endocrine events and methods of contraception in females.[23,24,49,74,75]

Contraception of the female hippo is possible with the use of synthetic progestins such as melengestrol acetate (MGA) in the feed. The Contraception Advisory Group (CAG) presently suggests 2 to 3 mg/day/animal. Alternatively, medroxyprogesterone acetate (MPA) (800 mg every 6 weeks, intramuscularly [IM]), may be used (http://www.stlzoo.org/animals/scienceresearch/contraceptioncenter/contraceptionrecommendatio/contraceptionmethods/artiodactyls/). The disadvantages of these methods are that they have to be administered on a regular basis. The duration of efficacy for MGA is most probably only 24 hours, so it must be administered daily, and MPA injections must be repeated every 6 weeks.[51]

Males

Contributing to the difficulty in sexing hippos is the barely visible prepuce located on the ventral midline. Zoologic institutions must consider castration to control population growth and to minimize male-to-male aggression. Information on castration of hippos is limited in the peer-reviewed veterinary medical literature, and only very limited information in the gray literature is available. In the past, procedures have often failed because of anesthesia-related problems, knowledge gaps concerning the anatomy of the male reproductive tract, and intrasurgical difficulties in locating the testis (Klarenbeek, personal communication, 2008).[15,56] The location of the testes in the hippo is still often described as "internal" in analogy to cetaceans, which have true intraabdominal testes. However, in the hippo, the testes are actually partially descended and remain in the inguinal canal.[14,71] A scrotum, as such, is not developed in the hippo. Possibly the first successful castration of a male hippo (estimated weight 1000 kg) was performed at the Auckland Zoo in 1993.[6] In 1994, in Amsterdam, a hippopotamus had one testis removed, and in a subsequent procedure the epididymis was amputated from the second testicle.[15] A castration is mentioned in a review paper on anesthesia in the hippo.[56] In Emmen Zoo, two sub-adult male hippos were successfully castrated (Klarenbeek, personal communication, 2008).

For castration, the hippo is rolled into a right lateral recumbent position. The dorsal hind leg is secured with a rope and slightly raised to provide access to the inguinal region for castration. Testes are not externally visible or manually palpable, and the location is highly variable, both on a horizontal and vertical plane, and varies some 40 cm in depth. Presurgical, transcutaneous ultrasonography is necessary to locate the testes in the inguinal region. Subsequently, the skin is incised just ventral of the located testes. If the testes cannot be located following incision, the ultrasonographic examination is repeated in the incision with the use of a sterile cover on the ultrasound probe. The surgical technique is a species-specific modification of standard equine castration techniques.[66] The most important difference to the various reported equine procedures is the actual location of the testes. Correct positioning of the dorsal leg in lateral recumbency is essential because when the leg is raised too high, the testes retract into the inguinal fold. Another factor of major difference from the equine procedure is the very short spermatic cord of the common hippo, which does not allow the testes to be

exteriorized. The entire procedure is necessarily performed at a depth of 20 to 30 cm inside the surgical wound. This is a particular surgical challenge and considerably complicates the intervention.[71]

Semen has been successfully collected from the pygmy hippopotamus with the use of electroejaculation and preserved for up to 7 days.[62] It has previously been shown that epididymal sperm extraction in the common hippopotamus is feasible, and this can supplement a castration procedure.[63] However, more work is needed on cryopreservation of the hippo semen so that the survival of the male gametes is improved.[63]

ACKNOWLEDGMENT

The authors would like to dedicate this chapter to the memory of Dr. Greg Fleming, who shared so many insights into hippo anesthesia (and equally fabulous stories) with us in the past years.

REFERENCES

1. Blowers TE, Waterman JM, Kuhar CW, et al: Female Nile hippopotamus (*Hippopotamus amphibius*) space use in a naturalistic exhibit. *Zoo Biol* 31:129–136, 2012.
2. Boisserie JR, Fisher RE, Lihoreau F, et al: Evolving between land and water: Key questions on the emergence and history of the Hippopotamidae (Hippopotamoidea, Cetancodonta, Cetartiodactyla). *Biol Rev* 86:601–625, 2011.
3. Bouts T, Hermes R, Gasthuys F, et al: Medetomidine-ketamine-isoflurane anaesthesia in pygmy hippopotami (*Choeropsis liberiensis*)—a case series. *Vet Anaesth Analg* 39:111–118, 2012.
4. Bouts T, Vordermeier M, Flach E, et al: Positive skin and serologic test results of diagnostic assays for bovine tuberculosis and subsequent isolation of Mycobacterium interjectum in a pygmy hippopotamus (*Hexaprotodon liberiensis*). *J Zoo Wildlife Med* 40:536–542, 2009.
5. Caskey R: Animal adaptations to environmental influences. *Bios* 1:52–63, 1930.
6. CBSG: World's first hippo castration. *CBSG News* 2:24, 1993.
7. Clauss M, Streich WJ, Schwarm A, et al: The relationship of food intake and ingesta passage predicts feeding ecology in two different megaherbivore groups. *Oikos* 116:209–216, 2007.
8. Clyde VL, Wallace RS, Pocknell AM: Dermatitis caused by group G beta-hemolytic *Streptococcus* in Nile hippos (*Hippopotamus amphibius*). In *Procedures of the American Association of Zoo Veterinarians*, Omaha, USA, 1998, pp 221–225.
9. *Convention on International Trade in Endangered Species of Wild Fauna and Flora (CITES)*, Geneva, Switzerland, 2013, CITES.
10. Cowan De F, Thurlbeck WM, Laws RM: Some diseases of the hippopotamus in Uganda. *Pathol Vet* 4:553–567, 1967.
11. Cracknell JM, Stidworthy M, Holliman A: Leptospirosis in a pygmy hippopotamus (*Choeropsis liberiensis*). In *Procedures of the American Association of Zoo Veterinarians*, Kansas City, USA, 2011, pp 35–37.
12. Dudley JP: Reports of carnivory by the common hippo *Hippopotamus Amphibius*. *S Afr J Wildl Res* 28:58–59, 1998.
13. Dumonceaux G, Citino SB, Burton M: Chemical restraint and surgical removal of a perineal mass from a Nile hippopotamus (*Hippopotamus amphibius*). In *Procedures of the American Association of Zoo Veterinarians*, New Orleans, USA, 2000, pp 288–290.
14. Eltringham SK: *The Hippos: Natural history and conservation*, London, U.K., 1999, Academic Press.
15. Erken A, Klaver P, Frankenhuis MT: Castration and sterilisation of an adult male hippopotamus. *Erkrankungen der Zootiere* 36:333–335, 1994.
16. Eulenberger K: Flusspferde. In Göltenboth R, Klös H-G, editors: *Krankheiten der Zoo- und Wildtiere*, Berlin, Germany, 1995, Blackwell Wissenschafts-Verlag.
17. Flach EJ, Furrokh IK, Thornton SM, et al: Caesarean section in a pygmy hippopotamus (*Choeropsis liberiensis*) and the management of the wound. *Vet Rec* 143:611–613, 1998.
18. Fleming GF, Walzer C: Compare and contrast two successful anesthetic protocols in the Nile hippopotamus (*Hippopotamus amphibius* app.). In

American Association Zoo Veterinarians Annual Conference, Oakland, USA, OCT 21-26, 2012.

19. Fleming GJ, Citino SB, Hofmeyr M, et al: Reversable chemical restraint of Nile hippopotomus (*Hippopotamus amphibious* spp.). In *Procedures of the American Association of Zoo Veterinarians*, South Padre Island, USA, 2010, p 205.

20. Franz W, Heymann H, Zscheile D: Immobilisierung und Nabelbruchoperation beim Zwergflusspferd (*Choeropsis liberiensis*). *Verhber Erkrg Zootiere* 20:197–200, 1978.

21. Galasso V, Pichierri F: Probing the molecular and electronic structure of norhipposudoric and hipposudoric acids from the red sweat of *Hippopotamus amphibius*: A DFT investigation. *J Physic Chem A* 113:2534–2543, 2009.

22. Garnham PCC: A malaria parasite of the hippopotamus. *J Eukaryot Microbiol* 5:149–151, 1958.

23. Graham LH, Reid K, Webster T, et al: Endocrine patterns associated with reproduction in the Nile hippopotamus (*Hippopotamus amphibius*) as assessed by fecal progestagen analysis. *Gen Comp Endocrinol* 128:74–81, 2002.

24. Graham LH, Webster T, Richards M, et al: Ovarian function in the Nile hippopotamus and the effects of Depo-Provera administration. *Reprod Suppl* 60:65–70, 2002.

25. Haigh JC: Fentanyl based mixtures in exotic animal neuroleptanalgesia. In *Procedures of the American Association of Zoo Veterinarians*, St. Louis, USA, 1976, pp 164–180.

26. Hamblin C, Hedger RS: Prevalence of neutralizing antibodies to bovid herpesvirus 2 in African wildlife. *J Wildl Dis* 18:429–436, 1982.

27. Hashimoto K, Saikawa Y, Nakata M: Studies on the red sweat of the *Hippopotamus amphibius*. *Pure Appl Chem* 79:507–517, 2007.

28. Helmick KE, Rush EM, Ogburn AL, et al: Dermatopathy in captive hippopotamus (*Hippopotamus amphibius*). In *Procedures of the American Association of Zoo Veterinarians*, Knoxville, USA, 2007, p 92.

29. Hentschel K: Untersuchungen zu Status, Ökologie und Erhaltung des Zwergflusspferdes (*Choeropsis liberiensis*) in der Elfenbeinküste (Dissertation), Braunschweig, Germany, 1990, Technische Universität Carolo-Wilhelmina.

30. Hugh-Jones ME, de Vos V: Anthrax and wildlife. *Revue Scientifique Et Technique De L'Office International Des Epizooties* 21:359–383, 2002.

31. International Union for the Conservation of Nature: IUCN Red List—Common Hippopotamus (*Hippopotamus amphibius*), Cambridge, UK, 2013, IUCN.

32. Jarofke D, Klös HG: Immobilisierung und Krankheiten von Flußpferden (*Hippopotamus amphibius*). Auswertung einer Umfrage bei mehr als 100 Zoologischen Gärten. *Verhber Erkrg Zootiere* 25:389–403, 1983.

33. Jarofke D, Klös HG: Immobilisierung und Krankheiten von Zwergflusspferden. *Verhber Erkrg Zootiere* 24:361–374, 1982.

34. Jarofke D: Hippopotamidae (Hippopotamus). In Fowler ME, editor: *Zoo and wild animal medicine: Current therapy*, Philadelphia, PA, 1993, Saunders.

35. Johnston NW: Atraumatic malocclusion in two pygmy hippos (*Choeropsis liberiensis*). *J Vet Dent* 19:144–147, 2002.

36. Kaboza Y, Debonnet G: Conserving biodiversity in times of conflict. In *International Conference on Promoting and Preserving Congolese Heritage: Linking biological and cultural diversity*, Paris, France, 2004, The World Heritage Center—UNESCO, pp 109–114.

37. Kim YS, Kim BS, Shin NS: *Clostridium perfringens* type A infection in a hippopotamus (*Hippopotamus amphibious*): A case report. *Korean J Vet Public Health* 30:244, 2006.

38. Kuttin ES, Loupal G, Köhler H, et al: Über eine Plazentarkokzidiose bei einem Flußpferd (*Hippopotamus amphibius*). *Zentralblatt für Veterinärmedizin Reihe B* 29:153–159, 1982.

39. Lang EM: *Das Zwergflußpferd: Choeropsis Liberiensis*, Wittenberg Lutherstadt, Germany, 1975, Ziemsen.

40. Loomis MC, Ramsay EC: Anesthesia for captive Nile hippopotamus. In Fowler ME, Miller RE, editors: *Zoo and wild animal medicine: Current therapy*, Philadelphia, PA, 1999, Saunders.

41. Luck CP, Wright PG: Aspects of the anatomy and physiology of the skin of the hippopotamus (*H. amphibius*). *Q J Exp Physiol Cogn Med Sci* 49:1–14, 1964.

42. Meyer W, Seegers U: A preliminary approach to epidermal antimicrobial defense in the Delphinidae. *Mar Biol* 144:841–844, 2004.

43. Meyer W: A special construction of subepidermal capillary loops in the hippopotamus (*Hippopotamus amphibius*). *Zool Sci* 29:458–462, 2012.

44. Miller M: Hippopotami. In West G, Heard D, Caulkett N, editors: *Zoo animal and wildlife immobilization and anesthesia*, Ames, IA, 2007, Blackwell Publishing.

45. Miller M: Hippopotamidae (Hippopotamus). In Fowler ME, Miller RE, editors: *Zoo and wild animal medicine: Current therapy*, Philadelphia, PA, 2003, Saunders.

46. Miller RE, Boever WJ: Repair of a rectal stricture and prolapse in a pygmy hippopotamus (*Choeropsis liberiensis*). *J Zoo Anim Med* 14:63–66, 1983.

47. Morris PJ, Bicknese B, Janssen DL, et al: Chemical restraint of juvenile East African river hippopotamus (*Hippopotamus amphibius kiboko*) at the San Diego Zoo. In Heard D, editor: *Zoological restraint and anesthesia*, Ithaca, NY, 2001, International Veterinary Information Service.

48. Nees S, Schade B, Clauss M, et al: Polycystic kidney disease in the pygmy hippopotamus (*Hexaprotodon Liberiensis*). *J Zoo Wildlife Med* 40:529–535, 2009.

49. Owen-Smith RN: *Megaherbivores: The influence of very large body size on ecology*, Cambridge, UK, 1988, Cambridge University Press.

50. Ozturk H, Cihan H, Erginoglu D, et al: Chemical immobilisation of a common hippopotamus with zolezepam-tiletamine and ketamine combination. In *Proceedings of the International Conference on Diseases of Zoo and Wild animals*, Lisbon, Spain, 2011.

51. Patton ML, Jöchle W, Penfold LM: Contraception in ungulates. In Asa CS, Porton IJ, editors: *Wildlife contraception: Issues,methods, and application*, Baltimore, MD, 2005, John Hopkins University Press.

52. Pearce PC, Gustavo C, Gulland F, et al: Immobilization of a pygmy hippopotamus (*Choeropsis liberiensis*). *J Zoo Anim Med* 16:104–106, 1985.

53. Pienaar UDV: The field-immobilization and capture of hippopotami (*Hippopotamus Amphibius Linnaeus*) in their aquatic element. *Koedoe* 10:149–157, 1697.

54. Plowright W, Laws RM, Rampton CS: Serological evidence for the susceptibility of the hippopotamus (*Hippopotamus amphibius Linnaeus*) to natural infection with rinderpest virus. *J Hygiene* 62:329–336, 1964.

55. Puschmann W, Zscheile D, Zscheile K: *Säugetiere*, Frankfurt, Germany, 2009, Wissenschaftlicher Verlag Harri Deutsch.

56. Ramsay EC, Loomis MR, Mehren KG, et al: Chemical restraint of the Nile hippopotamus (*Hippopotamus amphibius*) in captivity. *J Zoo Wildlife Med* 29:45–49, 1998.

57. Raymond JT, Eaton KA, Montali RJ: A disease in captive pygmy hippopotamuses (*Choeropsis liberiensis liberiensis*) anatomically resembling polycystic kidney disease. In *Procedures of the American Association of Zoo Veterinarians*, New Orleans, USA, 2000, p 302.

58. Reddacliff LA, Kirkland PD, Hartley WJ, et al: Encephalomyocarditis virus infections in an Australian zoo. *J Zoo Wildlife Med* 28:153–157, 1997.

59. Reed GT: Immobilization of two captive adult nile hippo (*Hippopotamus amphibius*). In *Procedures of the American Association of Zoo Veterinarians*, Knoxville, USA, 1978, pp 150–153.

60. Robinson PT: The status of the pygmy hippopotamus and other wildlife in West Africa (M.S. thesis), East Lansing, MI, 1970, Michigan State University.

61. Saikawa Y, Hashimoto K, Nakata M, et al: Pigment chemistry: The red sweat of the hippopotamus. *Nature* 429:363, 2004.

62. Saragusty J, Hildebrandt TB, Bouts T, et al: Collection and preservation of pygmy hippopotamus (*Choeropsis liberiensis*) semen. *Theriogenology* 74:652–657, 2010.

63. Saragusty J, Walzer C, Petit T, et al: Cooling and freezing of epididymal sperm in the common hippopotamus (*Hippopotamus amphibius*). *Theriogenology* 74:1256–1263, 2010.

64. Schwarm A, Ortmann S, Hofer H, et al: Digestion studies in captive Hippopotamidae: A group of large ungulates with an unusually low metabolic rate. *J Anim Physiol Anim Nutr* 90:300–308, 2006.

65. Scotcher JSB, Stewart DRM, Breen CM: The diet of the hippopotamus in Ndumu Game Reserve, Natal, as determined by faecal analysis. *S Afr J Wildl Research* 8:1–11, 1978.

66. Searle D, Dart AJ, Dart CM, et al: Equine castration: Review of anatomy, approaches, techniques and complications in normal, cryptorchid and monorchid horses. *Aust Vet J* 77:428–434, 1999.

67. Spriggs M, Reeder C: Free contact" behavioral conditioning allowing diagnosis and treatment of dermatitis in a 59-year-old nile hippopotamus (*Hippopotamus amphibious*). In *Procedures of the American Association of Zoo Veterinarians*, South Padre Island, USA, 2010, p 147.

68. Stalder GL, Petit T, Horowitz I, et al: Use of a medetomidine-ketamine combination for anesthesia in captive common hippopotami (*Hippopotamus amphibius*). *J Am Vet Med Assoc* 241:110–116, 2012.

69. Stoskopf MK, Bishop L: Immobilization of two captive adult Nile hippos (*Hippopotamus amphibious*). *Am Assoc Zoo Vet* 9:103–107, 1978.

70. Van Niekerk JW, Pienaar UDV: Adaptations of the immobilizing technique to the capture, marking and translocation of game animals in the Kruger National Park. *Koedoe* 5:137–143, 1962.

71. Walzer C, Petit T, Stalder GL, et al: Surgical castration of the male common hippopotamus (*Hippopotamus amphibius*). *Theriogenology* doi: 10.1016/j.theriogenology.2013.10.018.2013.

72. Weigl R: *The living collections of the world: A list of mammalian longevity in captivity*, Stuttgart, Germany, 2005, E. Schweizerbart'sche.

73. Weston HS, Fagella AM, Burt L, et al: Immobilization of a pygmy hippopotamus (*Choeropsis liberiensis*) for the removal of an oral mass. In *Procedures of the American Association of Zoo Veterinarians*, Puerto Vallarta, Mexico, 1996, pp 576–581.

74. Wheaton CJ, Joseph S, Reid K, et al: Body weight as an effective tool for determination of onset of puberty in captive female Nile hippopotami (*Hippopotamus amphibious*). *Zoo Biol* 25:59–71, 2006.

75. Wheaton CJ, Joseph S, Reid K, et al: Suppression of ovulation in nile hippopotamus (*Hippopotamus amphibious*) using melengestrol acetate-treated feed or high dose depo-provera injection. *Zoo Biol* 26:259–274, 2007.

76. York W: Case report: Immobilization of a hippo. In *Procedures of the American Association of Zoo Veterinarians*, Houston, USA, 1972, pp 256–258.

CHAPTER **60**

Camelidae

P. Walter Bravo

BIOLOGY

Camelid evolution began in western North America, 40–50 million years ago. Old World camels (OWCs) crossed the Bering Strait land bridge during a glacial period in the Pleistocene Epoch, approximately three million years ago. Likewise, New World camelids (NWCs) traveled south across the Central American land bridge around the same time. Both OWCs and NWCs continued evolving in harsh, but differing, environments. The two environments had a common characteristic of sparse, poor-quality forage for at least part of the year. See Table 60-1 for additional information.

Camels have been domesticated for 4500 to 5000 years and NWCs up to 7000 years ago. No truly wild dromedary camels, *Camelus dromedarius* exist, but a sizable population of feral camels exists in the outback of central and Western Australia, a result of escape or purposeful release of camels imported into Australia during the 20th century. A small population (<1000) of wild Bactrian camels, *Camelus Bactrianus ferus*, exists in the Gobi desert of Mongolia.[5]

Present South American camel (SAC) wild species are the guanaco (*Lama guanicoe*) and the vicuña (*Vicugna vicugna*). Domestic species are the llama (*Lama glama*), and the alpaca (*Vicugna pacos*). Recent studies on the phylogenetics of SACs on mitochondrial deoxyribonucleic acid (DNA) strongly indicate that the alpaca evolved from the vicuña and the llama from the guanaco.[6] All camelids share the same number of chromosomes (2n = 74). SACs may interbreed naturally and with artificial insemination, producing fertile offspring. Likewise, camel species also interbreed. Hybrids of a dromedary male and a guanaco female have been produced with artificial insemination.

UNIQUE ANATOMY AND PHYSIOLOGY

In camelids, a foregut fermentation system and a rumination cycle evolved in parallel with the digestive systems of ruminants. It appears that the common ancestor of both lines had a simple stomach. Camelids have a three-compartment stomach (C-1, C-2, C-3), and the compartments are not analogous to the four compartments of the ruminant.[5] All of the compartments of the camelid stomach have a glandular epithelium. Numerous other morphologic differences of the digestive system affect the diagnosis, treatment, surgery, and management of diseases in SACs. A greater omental sling is absent. The spiral colon has five coils.

The dental formula for both Bactrian and dromedary camels is incisors (I) 1/3, canines (C) 1/1, premolars (P) 3/2, molars (M) 3/3. The upper incisor has migrated caudally and become caniniform. The first premolars of the upper and lower jaws have migrated rostrally and have also become caniniform. This array of canine teeth (three in each upper jaw and two in each lower jaw), coupled with the unique ability of the camel to open the mouth widely, provides the camel with a formidable tool for offensive and defensive behaviors, so handlers should be continually alert.[2]

The dental formula for NWCs is I 1/3, C 1/1, P 1-2/1-2, M 3/3. The upper incisor has migrated caudally to become caniniform. The canine teeth of the llama male are large and saber shaped and may be used to inflict lacerations on other male llamas and humans. The incisors of alpacas and vicuñas have an open pulp cavity and continue to grow similarly to rodents.

Camelids have a fiber coat that is harvested and manufactured into garments. The finest fibers, with a diameter of 15 microns, are from the coat of the vicuña. The finest camel fiber is shorn from

TABLE 60-1

Biologic Information of Old World Camels and New World Camelids: Suborder Tylopoda, Family Camelidae

Scientific Name	Common Name	Weight (adults, kilograms [kg])	Geographic Distribution	Identification
Camelus dromedarius	Dromedary	660–1430	Middle East, North Africa, southern Asia	Single hump, color varies from nearly white to dark brown
Camelus bactrianus	Bactrian camel	990–1520	China, southern Russia, central Asia	Two humps, heavy fiber, short ears
Camelus bactrianus ferus	Wild Bactrian camel	Unknown	Gobi Desert, Mongolia	Two small humps
Lama guanicoe	Guanaco	100–120	Peru, Bolivia, south to Tierra del Fuego	Basic body color is light to dark reddish brown above, whitish hair below White extends up behind the fore legs and in the front of the rear leg, around the perineum, inside of legs, and up the bottom of the neck Head, face, and ears are dark gray to black
Vicugna vicugna	Vicuña	38–42 Height at withers 85–90 cm, at rump 90–94 cm	High Andes of Peru, Bolivia, Chile, and Argentina	The basic body color is a yellowish light brown The white in front of the rear limbs may extend to the top of the back White bib on the chest No sexual dimorphism in color or size
Lama glama	Llama	113–250	Throughout Peru, Bolivia, northern Chile, and Argentina	Numerous solid colors from white to black Multicolors (pinto, appaloosa) also seen
Vicugna pacos	Alpaca	55–90	Similar to llama	22 solid colors recognized, ranging from white to black

Bactrian camel yearlings (16–18 microns). The fiber diameter of the alpaca is 21 to 22 microns and llamas, guanacos and adult camels may reach 31 to 35 microns.

Camelids have two digits on each foot (digits 3 and 4), with a nail, not a hoof, at the tip of each digit. The nail is attached to the corium of P3 by means of numerous lamellae. In the SAC, P-2 and P-3 lie in a horizontal plane just dorsal to a tubular fibroelastic digital cushion. In the camel, P-3 is horizontal, but P-2 is at approximately a 35-degree angle with the ground and P-1 is at 55 degrees, when the foot is flat on the ground but not weight bearing. When weight is applied, the angles become more acute as the digital cushion is compressed. In camelids, separate digital cushions for each digit are present ventral to the articulation between P-1 and P-2 and occupying the caudal half of the foot. Each digital cushion consists of a central mass of adipose tissue surrounded by a thick capsule of fibroelastic connective tissue. The digital cushion gives this suborder of artiodactylids the name of *Tylopoda* (padded foot). The entire ventral surface of the camel foot is covered by a thick, cornified, but pliable sole or slipper. In SACs, the slipper is on each digit.[3]

Male dromedary camels have a palatine diverticulum ("dulaa"), which is an expandable diverticulum present on the ventral median aspect of the soft palate and which protrudes from the mouth when the animals are angry, agitated, frustrated, in rut, or sexually stimulated. *Dulaa* is an Arab word meaning "balloon-like structure." Bactrian camel males and females, as well as dromedary males castrated before or near puberty, do not extrude the dulaa.[5]

Camels are uniquely adapted for dealing with heat and dehydration. Camels are able to endure a diurnal fluctuation of body temperature, from 36.5°C to 42°C (97.7°F to 107.6°F), allowing them to avoid losing moisture through sweating during the day and becoming chilled in the cool desert night. Other species cannot tolerate such a fluctuation. Camels are able to sustain a 25% body weight loss as a result of dehydration without observable ill effects. Furthermore, they are able to rehydrate immediately when given free access to water. The elliptical erythrocyte of camels is able to swell to 240% of normal without rupturing. Other moisture-conserving adaptations include reabsorption of water from the bladder and concentration of urine to a thick syrup consistency before excretion. Also, feces are passed so desiccated that it may be used for fuel immediately.

When other lactating mammalian species are starved and lack sufficient water intake, their milk becomes more concentrated and diminishes in quantity. Even though a camel may be on a poor ration and may be dehydrated, its milk actually becomes less concentrated, allowing camel calves to obtain necessary fluids and be nourished at the same time.

NWCs are adapted to cool weather and are not heat tolerant. Special care must be given them in hot, humid climates to prevent heat stress.

HOUSING

Camelids may be housed as other domestic livestock species, taking into consideration that dromedaries are adapted to hot desert environments and Bactrian camels are adapted to cool to cold desert environments. NWCs require minimal housing. They should be provided with protection from inclement weather, particularly harsh winds in extremely cold climates; however, these animals are often seen standing or recumbent in rain or snow storms, even when shelter is available.

Guanacos and vicuñas are social animals and generally tolerate close association with others of their own kind. Adult breeding males should not be kept in the same enclosure to avoid fighting among males.

FEEDING AND NUTRITION

OWCs and NWCs have no unique nutrient requirements. They may be maintained on a diet of good-quality grass hay or mixed grass and legume hay. Supplemental feeding with concentrates is usually not necessary except for growing juveniles, working animals, and lactating females. Vitamin and mineral supplements are appropriate for specific regions. Numerous feeding regimens are used worldwide, indicative of the adaptability of these animals to available feed. Camelids consume approximately 1% to 2% of their body weight in dry matter when consuming good-quality forage. A maintenance diet should contain 10% to 14% crude protein and 50% to 55% total digestible nutrients (TDNs). During late gestation or heavy lactation, females should consume 60% to 65% TDNs.[5]

Camelids that eat only native pasture plants may experience fluctuation of body weight. During the dry season animals may lose weight that in other domestic animals could be fatal. NWCs have a feast or famine cycle. With the abundance of grass and shrubs available in the rainy season, an NWC will gain significant weight by storing adipose tissue in muscles and retroperitoneal tissue in the abdomen. During the dry season, NWCs alter their metabolism to use up the stored fat. Management of NWCs maintained in zoos or kept as livestock in non-native countries may not have this normal cycle and may become obese with constant access to feed.

It is important to monitor body weight periodically or perform a body condition evaluation in managed herds. Body condition is assessed by feeling the muscles over the withers and over the ribs. The accumulation of fat between both the forelimbs and hindlimbs should also be taken into consideration. The scoring is performed on the basis of either a 5-point or 10-point system. Low numbers indicate poor condition, medium-range numbers are considered normal, and high numbers indicate overconditioning or obesity.

RESTRAINT

A camelid's response to restraint varies with its age and stage of life. Camelids have been domesticated for thousands of years and are easily managed if they are accustomed to handling by people. Training has become important in the management of camelids and may obviate some of the following procedures. Improperly trained adult camelids (some zoo camels, privately owned camelids, feral camels) may inflict serious to fatal injuries on an unsuspecting handler. Even well-trained adult males may become belligerent and dangerous while in rut.[4]

Camelid offensive and defensive behaviors include spitting, biting, and kicking. Spitting, which involves spewing the contents of the first compartment of the stomach, is aimed at people or other camelids when the animals become angry or frustrated. Biting may be dangerous, especially when a male camel bites, clamps on, and shakes its head, causing considerable contusions and severe lacerations. In camels, all four feet and legs may become formidable weapons. The front legs may strike out in any direction. The rear legs have the ability to reach forward to the extent of scratching the head. Thus, no place is safe around an untrained camel, compared with, say, a horse (at the side of the withers).

NWCs also spit and kick. Their kick involves a sweep forward and outward, similar to the kick of a bovine species. Other aggressive behaviors include charging and bumping. If a human victim is knocked down, which is most likely to happen, an aggressive camelid may stomp on the person as on another camelid knocked down during a fight. Llamas and alpacas may also bite, but do so rarely.

The degree of psychological restraint that may be employed depends on taming and training. Camelids exhibit emotions by body language, particularly through its ear and tail positions. Ear position is not as apparent in camels as it is in llamas or alpacas because the ears of camels are not as long or as expressive, but they do reflect mood. The farther the ears are pulled toward the rear, the higher is the degree of agitation. The tail of an agitated camelid is elevated. Vocalization is an indication of a camelid's displeasure. Restraint of even a mild degree is likely to elicit a long, complaining roar in a camel or a scream in an NWC.

It is wise to take advantage of the social behavior of camelids and move them as a group to a smaller enclosure, through the alley way, and to the box stall or catch pen. This is particularly important when handling alpacas.

Positioning a camel in sternal recumbency ("kushing") provides an opportunity to closely examine or collect specimens for laboratory tests without risk of being kicked or struck. Either a leather strap or rope is used to place a simple or figure-of-8 loop around the front limb when the leg is flexed at the knee (carpus). If only the simple loop is used around the front leg, the camel may be able to rise to its knees. Most camels are trained to allow hindlimb physical restraint, in which a person on either side of the camel brings a soft cotton rope up behind the hindlimbs below the fetlock as the camel is being directed to kush (lie down). Once the camel is recumbent, the rope is placed medial to the stifles and tied tightly over the back behind the hump. Rising on the forelimbs is prevented by placing a loop over a flexed limb, extending the rope over the top of the neck and securing the opposite foreleg in the same manner.

The method of catching a camelid and controlling the head depends on the experience and usual practice of the personnel involved. Camelids may be roped with a lariat, but the roper needs to be highly skilled. A loop may be placed around the neck to pull the head toward a barrier, thus allowing placement of some type of halter.

Numerous types of chutes and stocks have been used to restrain camelids. One design may be constructed next to a barn or solid wall. A heavy post is set approximately 45 centimeters (cm; 1.5 feet) from another post positioned next to the wall. A 2.5-cm (1-inch) thick sheet of marine plywood—1.2 meters m (4 feet) by 2.4 m (8 feet)—is fixed on the post with heavy bolt hinges. Another post may be attached on the inside of one post to narrow the openings in enclosures for smaller camelids. A post set 60 cm (2 feet) in the front of the shoulder posts allows the animal to be tied, thus restricting backward movement. Once the camelid is tethered, the gate(s) may be swung closed, restricting side motion. Bales of hay or straw may be placed behind the camelid if a rectal examination is necessary.

Even the best-designed stock or chute is useless if the camelid will not enter it or cannot be led into it. Placement of the stock or chute in relation to the corral design is the key. If the chute is located in an area that is strange to a camel, or if a camel has not been trained to walk into the chute, handlers will be unable to force an adult camel to enter. Chutes for handling llamas or alpacas are available commercially in a variety of designs.

Chemical Restraint

Generally, it is not necessary to sedate trained camelids for routine diagnostic procedures. When dealing with camels having had little or no taming or training and if chutes or stocks are not available for physical restraint, it may be necessary to administer a tranquilizer or chemical immobilizing agent before procedures. Numerous agents have been administered to camelids for this purpose (Table 60-2). Availability, cost, and experience in using the agent may dictate the choice of agent.[5]

As noted, camelids are able to regurgitate stomach contents easily, so passive regurgitation during immobilization is a common hazard. A mature camelid should be fasted for 36 hours prior to performing any elective procedure. Water should be withheld for 10 to 12 hours. Even this partial emptying of the first compartment of the stomach does not guarantee that regurgitation will not occur. If at all possible, the camelid should be kept in the sternal position; if lateral recumbency is required, the camelid should be placed on its right side to allow for eructation of gas. The neck should be slightly elevated, and

TABLE 60-2

Chemical Restraint Agents Used in Camelids

Generic Name	Trade Name	Dose (milligram per kilogram, intramuscularly [mg/kg, IM])	Reversal Agent/Dose (mg/kg)
Xylazine hydrochloride (HCl)	Rompun[1,7]	0.1–0.4	Yohimbine (Antagonil[8], yobine[5]) 0.125–0.25 mg/kg Tolazoline HCl (Tolazine[5]) 0.5–5 mg/kg
Xylazine/butorphanol	Rompun/torbugesic[3]	0.2/0.05	Tolazoline 0.5–5 mg/kg
Butorphanol tartrate	Torbugesic	0.05–0.1	Naloxone (Narcan[8]) 0.1–0.25 mg/kg, intravenously (IV), plus 0.04–0.07, subcutaneously (SC)
Diazepam	Valium[4]	0.05–0.3	Flumazenil (Mazicon[4]) 1–2 mg/kg, IM
Midazolam HCl	Versed[4]		Flumazenil
Acepromazine maleate	Promace[3]	0.05–0.1	None
Propionylpromazine	Combelen[1]	0.03–0.2	None
Xylazine/ketamine	Rompun/Vetelar[3]	0.25–0.4/2–3	Tolazoline for xylaxine
Xylazine/ketamine/butorphanol	Rompun/Vetelar/Torbugesic	0.1/2–3/0.05–0.1	Tolazoline for xylazine
Meditomidine/Ketamine	Domitor[2]/Vetelar	0.06–0.08 /2–4	Atipamesole for meditomidine, 4 to 5 times dose of meditomidine, 0.1–0.15 mg/kg, IV, rest SC
Tiletamine/zolazepam	Telazol[3]/Zoletil	2–3	Flumazenil for zolazepam
Diazepam/ketamine	Valium/Vetelar	0.2–0.3/5–6	Flumazenil for diazepam

1. Bayer, P.O. Box 390, Shawnee, KS, 66201.
2. Farmos Pharmaceuticals, P.O. Box 425, SF, 20101, Turku, Finland.
3. Fort Dodge Laboratories, P.O. Box 518, Fort Dodge, IA, 50501.
4. Hoffman-La Roche, Nutley, NJ, 07110.
5. Lloyd Laboratories, P.O. Box 86, Shenandoah, IA, 51601.
6. Pfizer Inc., 812 Springdale Drive, Exton, PA 19341.
7. VEDCO, Route 6, Box 35A, St Joseph, MO 64504.
8. Wildlife Pharmaceuticals, 1401 Duff Dr., Fort Collins, CO 80524.

the muzzle should be allowed to drop so that if regurgitation occurs, the ingesta can flow out of the mouth rather than pooling in the pharynx and subsequently being inhaled into the trachea.

Drugs may be administered with standard equipment used to immobilize wild animals. In a confined space, a stick-pole syringe is ideal. A blow gun is very useful, but the maximum volume may be too low for larger camels.

ANESTHESIA AND SURGERY

Anesthesia for short procedures may be achieved through an extension of immobilization with injectable agents. Inhalation anesthesia is recommended for prolonged surgery. Isoflurane, sevoflurane, and halothane are suitable agents, but isoflurane and sevoflurane provide more rapid induction and recovery.

Disorders requiring surgery in OWCs include superficial and deep abscesses, skin lacerations, salivary fistula, prolapsed palatine diverticulum, esophageal obstruction (choke), gastric foreign bodies, intestinal obstruction, rectal prolapse, scrotal bite wounds, hematoma of testicle, preputial prolapse, phimosis, paraphimosis, urethral obstruction, perineal laceration, corneal laceration, eye enucleation, and fractures of long bones.[9] A special fracture, which has a high prevalence in male camels, is fracture of the mandible. This condition is diagnosed and managed in the same way as in livestock and horses, taking into consideration variation in anatomy. Additional surgeries reported include dental surgery for avulsion of the incisors, castration, cryptorchid castration, cesarean section, and ovariohysterectomy.

Disorders of NWCs that require surgery, in addition to those reported in camels, include retained deciduous incisors, alveolar abscesses, hernias, atresia ani, prolapse of the vagina, persistent hymen, uterine torsion, uterine rupture, urinary bladder rupture, patent urachus, carpal flexor contraction, and angular limb deformity. Additional surgeries reported include disarming canine teeth, trimming incisors, extraction of cheek teeth, tracheostomy, laparotomy, gastroenterotomy, vasectomy, and limb amputation.

DIAGNOSTIC PROCEDURES

In camels, venous blood may be collected from the jugular vein or the lateral thoracic vein. In SACs, several sites may be used. Most commonly, the jugular vein is accessed high on the neck behind the ramus of the mandible or low, medial to the ventral processes of fifth and sixth cervical vertebrae. Blood may also be collected from the brachial vein on the anterior aspect of the forearm or the middle ventral tail vein. In NWCs, the tail vein is superficial, rather than deep, next to the coccygeal vertebrae, as it is in cattle. The needle is inserted through the skin, and negative pressure is established on the syringe plunger, which is inserted deeper. Other blood collection sites include the lateral vein on the pinna of the ear and the saphenous vein on the medial aspect of the stifle of a lateral recumbent SAC. A syringe with a 20-gauge (G), 1.5-inch needle is enough for blood collection, even in a large llama or camel. The placement of a jugular catheter for intravenous administration is done using a 16-G or 18-G catheter. For crias, a 20-G catheter is suitable. After insertion of the catheter, a butterfly connector is attached, and the intravenous line may be left in place and secured to the neck with elastic bandage. The author has maintained the same catheter for 14 days. Tables 60-3 and 60-4 provide information on the hematologic parameters and serum biochemistry for camelids.

TABLE 60-3

Hematologic Parameters in Camelids

Parameter/Units Conventional/US	South American Camelids				Racing Camels		Bactrian Camels		Parameter/Unit (International/SI)
	<6 Months		Adults		Adults		Adults		
	US	SI	US	SI	US	SI	US	SI	
Erythrocytes/ 10^6/mm^3	9.6–17.2	9.6–17.2	10.5–17.2	10.5–17.2	7.5–12.0	7.5–12.0	10.2–13.2	10.2–13.2	Erythrocytes, 10^{12}/L
Hemoglobin, gram per deciliter (g/dL)	10.1–18.1	101.0–181.0	11.9–19.4	119.0–194.0	12.0–15.0	120.0–150.0	11.72–13.68	117.0–137.0	Hemoglobin, g/L
Packed cell volume (PCV) (%)	24.0–28.5	24.0–28.5	27.0–45.0	27.0–45.0	26.0–38.0	26.0–38.0	36.5–42.7	36.5–42.7	PCV,L/L
Mean corpuscular volume (MCV)/microliter (µL)	21.5–29.0	21.5–29.9	22.2–29.9	22.2–29.9	26.0–34.0	26.0–34.0			MCV, Femtoliter (fL)
Mean corpuscular hemoglobin (MCH)/microgram (µg)	9.0–11.9	9.0–11.9	10.1–12.7	10.1–12.7					MCH, picogram (pg)
Mean corpuscular hemoglobin concentration (MCHC), (g/dL)	39.4–44.9	39.4–44.9	39.3–46.8	39.3–46.8					MCHC, g/L
Leukocytes/ 10^3/mm^3	7.1–22.9	7.1–22.9	8.0–21.4	8.0–21.4	6.0–13.5	6.0–13.5	10.0–15.8	10.0–15.8	Leukocytes, 10^9/L
Neutrophils % Band neutrophils %	34.9–63.0		41.7–72.9		50.0–60.0		28.0–83.0		Neutrophils, % Band neutrophils, %
Lymphocytes %	18.3–41.9		9.2–25.2		30.0–45.0		19.0–56.0		Lymphocytes, %
Monocytes %	0–5.2		0–4.6		2.0–8.0		0–7.0		Monocytes, %
Eosinophils %	0–9.5		2.2–21.4		0–6.0		0–18.0		Eosinophils, %
Basophils %	0–1.0		0–14.0		0–2.0		0–3.0		Basophils, %
Thrombocytes 10^3/mm^3	268–912	268–913	200–600	200–600	200–700	200–700			Thrombocytes
Reticulocytes/ % of red blood cells (RBCs)	0–7.5		0–0.4						Reticulocytes, % of RBCs

From Fowler ME: *Medicine and surgery of camelids.* Ames, IA, 2010, Wiley-Blackwell.

TABLE 60-4

Selected Serum Biochemistry Parameters in Camelids

Parameter/Units Conventional/US	South American Camelids				Racing Camels		Bactrian Camels		Parameter/Unit (International/SI)
	<1 Year		Adults		Adults		Adults		
	US	SI	US	SI	US	SI	US	SI	
Total protein, gram per deciliter (g/dL)	4.9–7.1	49.0–71.0	5.1–7.8	40.0–78.0	5.7–7.5	57.0–75	5.47–7.37	54.7–73.7	Total protein, g/L
Albumin, g/dL	3.4–4.5	34.0–45.0	3.1–5.2	31.0–52.0	3.0–4.3	30.0–43.0	3.66–5.3	36.6–53.0	Albumin, g/L
Fibrinogen, milligram per deciliter (mg/dL)	100.0–400		100.0–500.0		250.0–400.0		268.0		Fibrinogen, mmol/L
Urea nitrogen, mg/dL	12.0–28.0	4.28–18.0.	9.0–34.0	3.21–12.14	3.0–21.0	1.07–7.5	12.3–17.7	4.38–6.33	Urea nitrogen, mmol/L
Creatinine, mg/dL	1.3–2.4	114.9–212.2	1.4–3.2	123.8–282.9	0–2.2	0–194.5	0.2–4.0	17.7–35.4	Creatinine, mmol/L
Glucose, mg/dL	108.0–156.0	5.99–8.66	74.0–154.0	4.11–8.55	0–110.0	3.89–6.11	37.0–67.0	2.05–3.72	Glucose, mmol/L
Calcium, mg/dL	8.6–10.7	2.15–2.68					2.2–2.68	0.60–0.67	Calcium, mmol/L
Phosphorus, mg/dL	5.1–10.2	1.65–3.29	2.6–7.3	0.84–2.36	3.5–6.0	1.13–1.94	1.6–2.0	0.52–0.68	Phosphorus, mmol/L
Sodium, millimole per liter (mmol/L)	149.0–153.0	149.0–153	148.0–158.0	148.0–158.0	150.0–160.0	150.0–160.0	129.0–161.0	129.0–161.0	Sodium, mmol/L
Chloride, milliequivalent per liter (mEq/L)	102.0–114.0	102.0–114.0	102.0–120.0	102.0–120.0	90.0–110.0	90.0–110.0			Chloride, mmol/L
Potassium, mEq/L	4.4–7.0		3.7–6.1		3.5–5.5		6.0–6.1		Potassium, mmol/L
Magnesium, mg/dL	2.0–2.3		2.0–3.5				1.8–2.9		Magnesium, mmol/L
Iron, mg/dL	70.0–148.0		70.0–148.0				49.0–57.0		Micromole per liter (µmol/L)

From Fowler ME: *Medicine and surgery of camelids.* Ames, IA, 2010, Wiley-Blackwell.

Blood may be collected from an SAC cria by a single person straddling the sternally recumbent cria. The operator's left arm holds the neck of the cria against his or her left leg. The left thumb presses the lower jugular vein and the right hand is free to place the needle into the vein.

Cardiac assessment and auscultation of lung sounds requires a stethoscope placed on the lower thorax in the relatively fiberless area just caudal to and above the elbow. Other diagnostic procedures similar to those used on cattle or horses may be performed.

DISEASES

Infectious Disease

Common infectious diseases of camels include enterotoxemia (*Clostridium perfringens*, C and D), salmonellosis, colibacillosis, paratuberculosis, tuberculosis, camel pox, and contagious ecthyma. Occasional infectious diseases include botulism, anthrax infection, hemorrhagic diathesis (*Bacillus cereus)*, hemorrhagic septicemia (*Pasteurella multocida)*, leptospirosis, tetanus, rabies, influenza, foot-and-mouth disease, opportunistic gram-negative infections (*Proteus* spp., *Enterobacter aerogenes, Klebsiella pneumoniae*, and *Campylobacter* spp.), dermatophylosis (*Dermatophylus congolensis*), and papillomatosis. Encephalomyocarditis has been diagnosed only rarely in dromedaries.[5,7]

SACs have only one unique infectious disease, mycoplasmosis, which is caused by *Mycoplasma hemolamae*; this disease was previously thought to be a parasitic disease caused by *Eperythrozoon* spp. but is now classified as having a bacteriologic etiology. The clinical syndrome varies from nonclinical anemia to severe anemia. The pathogen is transmitted by blood sucking arthropods.

Viral diseases are not common in camelids, but Eastern equine encephalomyelitis, West Nile virus disease, and rabies have been reported. Also, equine herpes virus, type 1, has been reported to have caused blindness and encephalitis in llamas and alpacas. The following bacterial diseases may be regionally prevalent: enterotoxemia (*C. perfringens*, type A, type C, and type D), colibacillosis (*Escherichia coli*), and actinomycosis. Common fungal infections include dermatophytosis (ringworm, *Trichophyton verrucosum, Microsporum* spp.) and coccidioidomycosis (*Coccidioides immitus*).

Additional uncommon bacterial diseases include botulism, tetanus, malignant edema (*Clostridium septicum*), brucellosis (*Brucella melitensis*), necrobacillosis (*Fusobacterium necrophorum*), corynebacteriosis (*Corynebacterium pseudotuberculosis*), staphylococcosis, and infection with the anaerobe *Bacteroides fragilis*. Cryptococcosis has been reported in a vicuña. Opportunistic gram-negative organisms such as *Pseudomonas* spp. and *Klebsiella* spp. may also cause infection. Uncommon viral diseases include rabies, vesicular stomatitis, contagious ecthyma, equine herpesvirus type 1, and Borna disease. Tables 60-5 and 60-6 provide more details on selected diseases.

Diseases rarely reported and to which the NWCs have a high level of resistance include foot-and-mouth disease, bovine virus diarrhea, Johne disease (*Mycobacterium paratuberculosis*), and tuberculosis (*Mycobacterium bovis* and *Mycobacterium* spp).[2]

Parasitic Disease

The management of parasitism is important in camelids. Tables 60-7 and 60-8 provide some details on selected important parasites.

Noninfectious Disease

Selected noninfectious diseases in camelids are listed in Table 60-9.

PREVENTIVE MEDICINE

The parasite load of camelids should be monitored and managed appropriately. Immunizations vary with locality but should include protection against tetanus, leptospirosis, enterotoxemia types D and C, and rabies.

REPRODUCTION

The female camelid is an induced ovulator. No true estrous period exists. The follicular cycle of NWCs and OWCs follow a similar pattern. In NWCs, follicles grow and regress in an average time of 10 to 12 days, with ovaries alternating, in 85% of the cases, for presence of mature follicles. Studies of ovarian follicle dynamics with the use of laparoscopy and ultrasonography, correlated with hormone concentrations, revealed that follicles grow, mature, and regress in an overlapping wavelike pattern (follicular wave). Estrogen levels from follicular activity are generally high enough to stimulate a female NWC to be receptive to a male unless she is pregnant or has recently bred.

The reproductive cycle of the camel is similar to that of the NWC, with one notable exception. In the camel, the follicular waves are spaced further apart, which allows estrogen levels to diminish and sexual receptivity to cease for a few days. This pause in sexual receptivity seems to mimic the estrous cycle of most other mammals. However, ovulation does not occur without copulation.[1,3,5]

During copulation, the female SAC is in sternal position, and copulation lasts for about 20 minutes. Ovulation occurs 24 to 36 hours after copulation. Implantation occurs by 20 to 22 days after copulation.[2,5] The corpus luteum is present and functioning during the entire pregnancy period. Fetus is usually located in the left uterine horn, but the placenta spreads into both uterine horns. The placenta is diffuse and epitheliochorial.[1,5,8] Normal delivery of the SAC fetus is rapid, lasting no more than 10 minutes.

The placenta is usually expelled within 2 hours following parturition. Resumption of ovarian follicular activity begins a week after parturition, but uterine involution takes 14 to 21 days. Camelids have a fourth fetal membrane that arises from the epidermis of the fetus in late pregnancy. This thin epidermal membrane is unique to camelids. It envelops the fetus but is attached at body orifices and at the coronary band of the toenails. Its precise function is unknown.

The penis in the male camelid has a sigmoid flexure, similar to that of a bull or ram. The prepuce is directed caudally in a nonsexually aroused male. Urine is directed caudally without extrusion of the penis. The scrotum of camelids is nonpendulous, and closely opposed to the body just ventral to the ischial arch.

Male NWCs have no breeding season and will mate any time when nonpregnant females are available. Male OWCs have a defined breeding period, called *rut*, which is an androgen-driven seasonal change, recognized by the secretion of a foul-smelling brownish liquid from the poll glands. While urinating, the camel spreads his hindlimbs and flips his tail up and down, throwing urine up and over the back. Accumulation of dirt in the urine-soaked hair fibers may produce a heavily-odoriferous crust on the back. At the same time, saliva, whipped into froth, starts to flow from the mouth, and the dulaa is extruded. All the while, the male grinds its teeth and emits a gurgling or blubbering roar. This behavior is most often exhibited when another male is near, but the display may be used around people when the camel is agitated.

Semen deposition occurs within the uterine horns, and the male begins to ejaculate after passage of the penis through the cervix of the female. Ejaculation is a continuous process, with no pelvic thrust as in rams or bulls; however, the male repositions the penis intermittently within both uterine horns while ejaculating. Semen is thick and gelatinous in appearance. Camelids do not have seminal vesicles. Spermatozoa are trapped with the seminal plasma; the presence of this plasma makes it difficult to evaluate semen. See Table 60-10 for more information on the reproductive characteristics of camelids.

ACKNOWLEDGMENTS

The author is indebted to Dr. Murray Fowler for his contribution to this chapter.

TABLE 60-5

Selected Infectious Diseases of Old World Camels

Disease	Etiology	Epizootiology	Signs	Diagnosis	Management
Viral camelpox	Poxviridae, *Orthopoxvirus cameli*	Most common viral disease of both Bactrian and dromedary camels Not found in the United States or Australia Not a zoonosis Spread by direct contact and insects	Incubation 9–13 days Pustules on nostrils, lips, eyelids, and oral and nasal mucosa Severe cases have fever, diarrhea, anorexia, depression, eruptions over entire body	Enzyme-linked immunosorbent assay (ELISA), monoclonal antibody panels, deoxyribonucleic acid (DNA) restriction enzyme analysis, and dot blot assay	Vaccines now being used
Papillomatosis (warts)	Papoviridae, *Papillomavirus* spp.	Spread by direct contact through lacerations and abrasions	Epidermal proliferation (warts) Uncommon	Pedunculated warts differentiate from pox and contagious ecthyma Histopathology, electron microscopy.	Usually self-limiting, autogenous vaccines used
Bacterial pseudotuberculosis, caseous lymphadenitis	*Corynebacterium pseudotuberculosis* Other organisms may be isolated, including: *Staphylococcus aureus, Corynebacterium pyogenes, Rhodococcus equi, Escherichia coli*	Spread by ingestion, inhalation, and direct contact with wounds	Common and widespread Lymph node abscessation Deep abscesses rare in camels Abscesses are not hot, but may cause soreness Swelling may be preceded by edema	Signs, culture, and sensitivity	Usually sensitive to penicillin, but the antibiotic may not reach the organisms Isolation of the affected animal is appropriate, but seldom practical
Hemorrhagic diathesis or hemorrhagic disease	*Bacillus cereus* toxin	*B. cereus* is usually considered nonpathogenic but has been associated with food poisoning in humans A toxic syndrome is seen only in racing camels fed green alfalfa	Fever, anorexia, agranulocytosis, atony of stomach compartment 1, colic, cough, blood on feces, swollen submandibular lymph nodes, recumbency May develop central nervous system disturbance, lacrimation, and hypersalivation	History (fresh alfalfa, racing camel) Hemorrhages of serosa and mucosae of abdominal and thoracic organs Hepatopathy, pronounced agranulocytosis	Avoid manure fertilized alfalfa Sanitation

TABLE 60-6

Selected Infectious Diseases of New World Camelids

Disease	Etiology	Epizootiology	Signs	Diagnosis	Management
Enterotoxemia	*Clostridium perfringens*, type A	Ingestion	Sudden death, colic recumbency, bloat, depression, anorexia, convulsions, coma, opisthotonos	Monoclonal antibody panel, polymerase chain reaction (PCR), history, lesions	Correct environment Intensive supportive care Antibiotics for secondary infection
Retinal degeneration	*Equine herpesvirus*, type 1	Transmission unknown	Blindness, nonresponsive pupils, encephalitis	Clinical examination, retinal degeneration	Blindness is permanent Vaccination in face of an epizootic
Coccidioidomycosis, valley fever	Coccidioides immitus	*C. immitis* is a soil fungus found in certain desert soil types If the soil is disturbed, arthroconidia become windborne and inhaled, then convert to the yeast form	Dyspnea, and variable, depending on where the organism disseminates Dermatitis	Culture, cytology, agar gel immunodiffusion (AGID), complement fixation (CF)	Prognosis poor, amphotericin B and other fungicidal antibiotics

TABLE 60-7

Selected Parasitic Diseases of Camels

Disease	Etiology	Location in Host		Diagnosis	Management
		Adult	**Immature**		
Nagana, trypanosomiasis	*Trypanosoma brucei*	Peripheral blood, lymph nodes, liver	Intermediate host is the tsetse fly (*Glossina*)	Observation of the trypansomes in peripheral blood, lymph nodes, liver Serologic testing	Control insects Treatment with trypanocides
Surra, trypanosomiasis	*Trypanosoma evansi*	Peripheral blood, parenchymal organs	No intermediate host needed Biting flies are mechanical vectors	Observation of trypanosomes in peripheral blood Clinical signs (fever, depression, weakness, edema, pulmonary edema, anemia, emaciation)	Control insects Treatment with trypanocides
Nasal bot	*Cephalopina titilator*	Free-flying fly	Nasal pharynx and nasal cavity	Clinical signs, endoscopy	Ivermectin
Whipworms	*Trichuris* spp.	Cecum and colon	Larvae in wall of anterior small intestine	Fecal flotation	Aggressive anthelmintic administration

TABLE 60-8

Selected Parasitic Disease Challenges of New World Camelids

Parasite	Etiology	Location of the Adult in Host	Clinical Signs	Diagnosis	Management
Deer nasal bots	*Cephenemyia* spp.	Nasopharyngeal granulomas	Sneezing, coughing, noisy breathing, exercise intolerance	Radiography, endoscopy	Double dose of ivermectin
Spinose ear tick	*Otobius megnini*	External ear canal, perianal region	Head shaking, scratching, exudation from the ear	Observation of ticks in the ear canal, and around tail	Acaricide, removal of ticks
Mange mites	*Sarcoptes scabei* *Chorioptes* sp. *Psoroptes* sp.	In or on the skin	Alopecia, crusts, thickening of the skin	Skin scrapings	Insecticides
Lice	*Damalinia breviceps* *Microthoracis cameli*	On the skin	Alopecia, pruritus	Direct visualization, skin scrapings	Insecticides

TABLE 60-8

Selected Parasitic Disease Challenges of New World Camelids—cont'd

Parasite	Etiology	Location of the Adult in Host	Clinical Signs	Diagnosis	Management
Thread-necked strongyle	*Nematodirus battus*	Small intestine	Diarrhea	Fecal flotation, ova are large	Anthelmintics
Meningeal worm	*Parelaphostrongylus tenuis* White-tailed deer is definitive host Intermediate hosts are terrestrial snails	Spinal cord, brain	Lameness, ataxia, stiffness, circling, blindness, hypermetria, paresis, paralysis, abnormal head position	Signs, history of exposure to white-tailed deer Eosinophils in cerebrospinal fluid	Anthelmintics monthly during the snail season
Whipworms	*Trichuris tenuis* *Trichuris ovis*	Colon, cecum	Weight loss, diarrhea, anemia	Fecal flotation, ova have double operculae	Anthelmintics, high doses (2–3×), repeated every 3 weeks

TABLE 60-9

Selected Noninfectious Diseases of New World Camelids

Disease	Etiology	Prevalence	Signs	Management
Myopathy, nutritional	Selenium or vitamin E deficiency	Regionally common with supplementation	Dyspnea, inability to eat, stiffness, paresis, paralysis	Supplement the diet, Selenium or vitamin E injections
Rickets	Vitamin D deficiency and hypophosphatemia	Regionally common	Lameness, reluctance to run and play, cessation of growth, excessive recumbency, standing humpbacked, swollen carpi and tarsi	Vitamin D injections, oral dosage with vitamin D paste
Hyperthermia	High ambient temperatures and humidity, excessive exercise in hot climates	Unfortunately quite common in many of the contiguous states, especially the southern tier of states	Elevated body temperature, depression, convulsions, colic, increased heart rate	Rapid cooling with cold-water enemas, fluids to counter hypotension
Hypothermia	Primarily a neonatal problem caused by low ambient temperatures Premature crias especially vulnerable	Common in northern states without proper protection at the time of birth	Low body temperature, depression, coma, decreased cardiac output	Immerse in warm water, hot-water bottles, heat lamps

TABLE 60-10

Reproductive Characteristics of Camelids

Parameter	Llama/Alpaca	Dromedary Camel	Bactrian Camel
Karyotype (2n)	74	74	74
Puberty, age (years)	≥1	3–4	2–3
Follicular cycle (days)	12–20	26	28
Receptivity detection	Accepts the male	Becomes restless, bleats, attracted to male, moves tail up and down, accepts copulation	Becomes restless, bleats, attracted to male, moves tail up and down, accepts copulation
Duration of copulation	5–55 minutes	7–22 minutes	1–6 minutes
Gestation, days	335–350	365–410	374–419
Pregnancy determination	Rectal palpation, ultrasonography, progesterone level	Holds tail horizontal or curled up over back, rectal palpation, ultrasonography, progesterone	Holds tail horizontal or curled up over back, rectal palpation, ultrasonography
Placentation	Diffuse epitheliochorial	Diffuse epitheliochorial	Diffuse epitheliochorial
Semen volume	0.8–4 mL		1.0–12.5
Size of spermatozoa	49 +/− 2 total length, head 5.3 µm	51 +/− 1, head 6.6 µm	43 +/− 2, head 6 µm

REFERENCES

1. Bravo PW: *The reproductive process of South American camelids*, Salt Lake City, UT, 2002, Seagull Printing USA.
2. Fowler ME: Camelids. In Fowler ME, editor: *Zoo and wild animal medicine*, ed 2, Philadelphia, PA, 1986, Saunders, pp 969–981.
3. Fowler ME: Reproductive anatomy and physiology of camels. In Fowler ME, editor: *Zoo and wild animal medicine*, ed 3, Philadelphia, PA, 1993, Saunders, pp 525–531.
4. Fowler ME: Restraint of camelids. In Fowler ME, editor: *Restraint and handling of wild and domestic animals*, ed 2, Ames, IA, 1995, Iowa State University Press, pp 279–287.
5. Fowler ME: General biology and evolution. In Fowler ME, editor: *Medicine and surgery of camelids*, ed 3, 2010, Wiley-Blackwell Publication.
6. Kadwell M, Fernandez M, Stanley HF, et al: Genetic analysis reveals the wild ancestors of the llama and the alpaca. *Proc Roy Soc Lond B Biol* 268:2575–2584, 2001.
7. Manefield GW, Tinson AH: *Camels—a compendium. Series C, No. 22, The T.G. Hungerford Vade Mecum Series for Domestic Animals*, Sydney, Australia, 1996, University of Sydney Post Graduate Foundation in Veterinary Science.
8. Olivera L, Zago D, Leiser R, et al: Placentation in the alpaca (*Lama pacos*). *Anat Embryol* 207:45–62, 2003.
9. Ramadan RO: *Surgery and radiology of the dromedary camel*, Al Asha, Kingdom of Saudi Arabia, 1994, College of Veterinary Medicine, King Faisal University. Published by the author.

CHAPTER **61**

Giraffidae

Mads F. Bertelsen

BIOLOGY[15,47]

Two species exist within the artiodactylid family of Giraffidae; the giraffe (*Giraffa camelopardalis*) and the okapi (*Okapia johnstoni*). Giraffids first arose eight million years ago during the Miocene period, and fossil evidence suggests that the family was once much more extensive, with over 10 fossil genera described.

Up to nine races or subspecies of giraffe have been described, although genetic research and the fact that distinct morphologic distinctions between groupings exist despite the lack of physical boundaries have led some authorities to consider several distinct species. The subspecies most commonly held by zoos are the reticulated giraffe (*Giraffa camelopardalis reticulata*), the Rothschild giraffe (*G.c. rothschildi*), and the Masai giraffe (*G.c. tippelskirchi*). Once widespread across the African continent, giraffes are now largely confined to national parks and game farms in eastern and southern Africa, with scattered populations in west Africa.

Because of its height, the giraffe has access to browse unavailable to other species and thus may coexist with grazers and smaller browsers and even livestock. Adult giraffes are rarely preyed upon by predators, but calf mortality is high. Giraffes are sociable animals usually found in dynamic, ever-changing groups, the most stable of which are those composed by mothers and their young. Subadult males are social, whereas mature males become more solitary.

With an estimated 80,000 animals left in the wild, the giraffe is classified by the International Union for the Conservation of Nature (IUCN) as a species "Of Least Concern." However, several of the subspecies are now considered "Endangered" (e.g., West African and Rothschild). At least 2000 giraffes are maintained in captivity, making the captive population self-sustaining.

Discovered by science only as recently as 1901, the okapi was the last large African mammal species to be described. The okapi is now endemic to the Democratic Republic of the Congo in central Africa, where they inhabit dense damp forests on both sides of the Congo River. Okapis are diurnal and live alone, in pairs, or in small family groups, but relatively little is known about their social structure, largely because of their remote habitat and timid nature.

Estimated remaining wild population is between 10,000 and 35,000, and the fate of these animals is closely linked to the unstable political climate of the region. The okapi is listed as "Near Threatened" by the IUCN but is not listed on the Convention on International Trade in Endangered Species (CITES) Appendix. With less than 200 animals in captivity, the okapi population is considered fragile.

UNIQUE ANATOMY[15,47]

Giraffe

With a height of up to more than 5 meters (m), giraffes are characterized by their extremely long necks and long legs, with considerably longer forelimbs than hindlimbs. The head is fairly small, with two horns or ossicones and a central osseous protuberance, which is particularly developed in the males. The tongue is long and flexible, its distal 20 cm pigmented. Mature males weigh 850 to 1950 kilograms (kg) and females 700 to 1200 kg. The internal anatomy of giraffes is analogous to that of the domestic cow and other artiodactylids. The dental formula for giraffes is incisors (I) 0/3, canines (C) 0/1, premolars (P) 3/3, molars (M) 3/3, for a total of 33. Often, the gallbladder is absent, although it occurs in some individuals. Two jugular veins run immediately under the skin on either side of the ventral neck.

The skin varies in thickness from being thin on the ears and medial aspects of the legs to being thick along the neck and lateral body. The thick skin aids in edema prevention in the lower leg and forms a dermal armor for protection against predators or fighting with conspecifics. The dark patches of the skin have been suggested to have a thermoregulatory role in acting as regions where heat loss to the environment is enabled by selective vasodilation.

The relative lung mass as well as volume is only approximately 60% of that of other mammals, and the lung volume-to-body mass ratio decreases during growth.[43] The extremely long trachea has a diameter significantly narrower than in similar-sized mammals, so the dead space volume, although greater than in most species, is not as large as could be expected and is compensated for by a slightly larger tidal volume.[43]

Previously described as extraordinarily large, the giraffe heart has a relative weight of approximately 0.5% of body weight, which is essentially identical to that of other mammals.[42] The basis for the massive blood pressure generated is smaller ventricular radii and an unusually thick left ventricular wall with oblique muscle fibers. The giraffe vein has a venous valve layout similar to that in other large mammals, and no arterial valves exist.[49]

Okapi

The okapi reaches a head-to-body length of 200 to 210 cm and a shoulder height of 150 to 170 cm and has a body weight of 200–300 kg. Females are larger than males. The eyes and ears are large, and the tongue long enough to reach the ear base. Males have a pair of short-haired ossicones that are directed backward. The body is short and compact with a sloping back, as in the giraffe, but the neck is much shorter. Available information on okapi anatomy and physiology is limited, but the dental formula and internal anatomy resemble those of the giraffe.

UNIQUE PHYSIOLOGY[6,29,42,43,49]

To compensate for the hydrostatic challenge of perfusing the brain, the giraffe heart generates a blood pressure twice that of other mammals, and its cardiovascular anatomy and physiology have been subject to considerable speculation and myths. Both stroke volume and cardiac output are lower than in similar-sized mammals. Blood volume is unusually low, and compliance of the vascular system is also low. The peculiar vascular anatomy—with narrow, rigid veins with low compliance in the legs and large, compliant veins in the neck region—gives rise to an interesting and nonintuitive physiologic phenomenon.[6] When the head of the anesthetized giraffe is lowered, blood pressure at head-level briefly spikes, before returning to much lower values. The lowering of the blood pressure coincides with pooling of blood in the compliant jugular veins, giving rise to a decreased cardiac preload and consequently lower systemic blood pressure (Frank-Starling mechanism). As a consequence of this mechanism, the arterial pressure at head level is maintained at or near 100 millimeters of mercury (mm Hg), and the central blood pressure is directly proportional to the position of the head relative to the heart. Because of the high arterial pressures and the hydrostatic pressure, the arterial pressure in the lower leg may exceed 450 mm Hg. Edema in this region is prevented through a gravity-suit-like fascia and skin, prominent lymphatics, and well-developed valves in veins and lymphatics, as well as an abrupt narrowing of the arterial lumen at the level of the elbow or stifle.

The giraffe kidney experiences much higher pressures compared with the human kidney and appears to cope with this through a fibrous capsule and an increased interstitial pressure of about 30 to 40 mm Hg. This means that normal kidney perfusion depends on a mean arterial pressure of at least 130 mm Hg.

Similar to camels, the giraffe is capable of varying the body temperature within a couple of degrees Celsius, saving energy otherwise needed for increasing the temperature at night and cooling during daytime.

SPECIAL HOUSING REQUIREMENTS[9]

Giraffes may learn to lower their heads to walk through doors only slightly higher than their withers; however, stressed or sedated animals will often not do this, which necessitates high doors for a giraffe house.

Soft flooring and lack of exercise may lead to overgrowth of feet and the need for trimming, so the giraffe should be encouraged to walk on abrasive surfaces. Coarse gravel may be used on top of concrete to provide traction and wear. Neonates require sure footing and do best when born on pasture or a thick layer of bedding to prevent splaying.

Giraffes have a high surface-to-volume ratio and are adapted to tropical climates. In moderate climates, they may be maintained in outdoor enclosures year-round. In temperate climates, access to stables heated to the range of 18°C to 24°C (65°F–75°F) must be provided, and in subzero temperatures, outdoor access should be restricted.

Both okapis and giraffes are prone to sterotypies, particularly those involving the tongue, and it is important to incorporate in enclosure design pulleys and other systems to provide browse and enrichment items at head level. When designing facilities for giraffids, the logistics of loading and unloading animals should also be considered. Ideally, narrow walkways leading to an appropriate docking ramp for transport vehicles should be incorporated into the design.

FEEDING

Both giraffes and okapis are selective browsers seeking out the high-nutrient components of plants such as fresh leaves and buds. In the wild, giraffes mainly feed on Acacia species, and the natural diet of the okapi includes a variety of species. In an attempt to avoid negative energy balance, captive diets have traditionally contained high levels of protein (15%–20%) and starch (20%–30%). Based on wild diets, current recommendations include crude protein levels of only 10%–14%, starch levels below 5%, fat 2%–5%, and high amounts of fiber (minimally 25% acid detergent fiber) all based on a dry-matter basis.[58] Care should be taken to keep calcium levels high and phosphorus levels low. The new diet regimens have recently been shown to lead to increased serum levels of magnesium as well as n3 and n6 fatty acids and decreased levels of phosphorus and saturated fatty acids[36,41] so that blood nutrient profiles more closely match those of free-ranging giraffe.[36]

The importance of browse, for both the nutritional value and the behavioral well-being of animals, cannot be overstated and browse should be provided to the greatest extent possible, but good-quality hay and alfalfa as well as silage may be substituted. Surplus buds and twigs from rose growers have been used successfully in okapis.[59] The precise mineral and vitamin requirements of giraffids have not been established, but animals should have access to trace mineral salt blocks, and copper supplementation should be considered if deficiencies are suspected.

RESTRAINT AND HANDLING

Giraffes may be quite tame and may become habituated to some manipulation, including blood sample collection and light hoof trimming; however, many individuals do not respond well to this approach. The safest nonchemical method for collecting routine samples and closely examining animals is to accustom them to a chute during daily routines. Forced physical restraint without specialized stalls or chutes is likely to be unsuccessful and dangerous. Giraffes may deliver a formidable kick with all four legs in essentially any direction. In tall narrow chutes, with secure footing for personnel as well as animals, giraffes may be physically restrained for minor procedures such as injections, blood collections, tuberculosis testing and so on, but the risks involved for the animal as well as the staff should be kept in mind. Okapis respond well to training and positive reinforcement and poorly to physical restraint.

Once they get started, giraffes have the tendency to keep walking along hallways and so on, which may be exploited for crating or loading into vehicles. A curtain with a weight at the bottom, which will fall from a horizontal position to a vertical position behind the animal when released, may be helpful to encourage the animal to take that last step into an unknown crate.

CHEMICAL RESTRAINT

Giraffe anesthesia remains a challenge because of considerations of size as well as the peculiar anatomy and physiology of these animals; however, several good protocols and excellent information resources are now available.[12]

Standing Sedation

Standing sedation may work well, but ataxia may develop, so it is important to be prepared for the animal to go down unexpectedly. A chute or restraint device is ideal, but a large door that can close off a triangular space may provide a similar confined area. Several drug combinations have been used with success for procedures such as clinical examinations, hoof trimming, reproductive manipulation, minor surgery, and catheter placement (Table 61-1).

Immobilization and Anesthesia

Two main schools in giraffe anesthesia exist: (1) opioid-based protocols[7,11,66,67] and (2) ketamine, combined with high-dose medetetomidine.[8,39] The latter approach has been popular over the past decade because of the avoidance of an opioid component and relatively smooth inductions; however, it may result in hypertension and tachypnea, and re-sedation from medetomidine as the reversal agent wears off is a real concern. The opioids, however, may induce excitation and hyperthermia if underdosed and result in hypoventilation when used in high dosages. A compromise, which involves incorporating opioids, ketamine, and α_2-agonists in one protocol, appears to be the best solution so far.[11,24] Refer to Table 61-1 for suggested protocols.

The giraffe has traditionally been considered one of the most challenging animals to anesthetize, and most problems arise during induction and recovery. The key to success is careful planning and the availability of trained personnel and necessary equipment. The ideal induction occurs in a well-designed restraint device, which may be opened fully once the animal is recumbent. The second-best solution is a chute-system, where a halter may be placed on the sedated giraffe prior to induction, which will allow control of the head via a rope and pulley. The third-best option is to place a loop of thick rope around the base of the neck of the sedated animal and "walk" the animal to an open area with no obstacles, where it is made to walk in circles, with one to three handlers holding the rope. The animal is then tripped with another rope while still awake enough to maintain some control of the head during the fall. If neither of these options are available, the animal may be allowed to become recumbent in a padded stall or at least in an area without major obstacles. In either case, it is crucial to gain control of the animal's head as soon as it becomes recumbent, as most injuries occur when the heavily sedated giraffe attempts to stand and falls again.

For anesthetic induction in okapi, a padded restraint device is the safest option, but a quiet stall with sure footing will suffice. With opioid-based protocols, induction may sometimes result in excitement or tumbling. A staged approach, in which sedatives are allowed to set in for 15 to 20 minutes prior to opioid administration, is preferable, and once the opioid takes effect, two experienced helpers may use mild physical restraint with mattresses or boards to prevent injury.[12]

Regurgitation under anesthesia may be a concern in both giraffes and okapis, but particularly in the latter. The frequent early reports of regurgitation in okapis sedated with Immobilon (etorphine and acepromazine) was attributed to etorphine but likely largely was a reaction to acepromazine, which this author considers contraindicated in okapis. In animals fed mainly hay and pelleted feed, withholding food and water for 12 hours prior to a planned procedure is sufficient, but in animals eating large amounts of fresh browse, a 24-hour period is advisable. To minimize pulmonary compromise and ventilation–perfusion mismatch, a sternal position is preferable, when feasible, but giraffes generally do well in lateral recumbency for shorter periods. To reduce the risk of regurgitation and to stabilize blood pressure (see Unique Physiology section), the head should be elevated 80 to 150 cm above heart level. The neck should be kept as straight as possible, and placement of a padded board or ladder under the shoulder and onto bales of straw or similar material works well for this purpose.

Performing endotracheal intubation is straightforward in giraffes. Direct visualization of the larynx is possible with the use of a long laryngoscope blade, and insertion of a relatively thin catheter to subsequently guide the endotracheal tube is a good option.[12] However, in giraffes larger than 350 to 400 kg, the fastest approach is to manually insert a stomach tube or similar device into the trachea and then thread the endotracheal tube over that. Appropriate endotracheal tube sizes are 20 to 25 millimeters (mm) for okapis and juvenile giraffes and 25 to 30 mm for adult giraffes.

Hypoventilation is often a concern, and oxygen should be provided, whenever possible. A Hudson demand valve or similar device will provide the animal with oxygen and allow intermittent ventilation, as needed. Even in animals breathing well, a "sigh" every 2 to 5 minutes appears to be beneficial to avoid alveolar closing and shunting. In animals not intubated, supplemental oxygen via a deep nasal cannula and flowing at one liter per 100 kilograms per minute is recommended.

For recovery, a quiet area with good footing should be provided. Adequate space should be available for the animal to swing its head forward as it gets onto its hindfeet, and obstacles should be removed to avoid injury if the animal falls over. Reversal agents may be given intramuscularly or intravenously (IM or IV), depending on the situation. The goal is to get the animal into sternal recumbency, with strong spontaneous ventilation as fast as possible, and to then keep it there as long as possible, ideally for 10 to 15 minutes. Keeping the animal blindfolded during this time helps prevent its attempts to stand prematurely. Doxapram (0.1 mg/kg, given rapidly IV) may be used to stimulate animals that are reluctant to get up.[24]

Capture[12,63]

The immobilization of free-ranging giraffes for capture purposes has little in common with controlled anesthesia for longer procedures in captive animals. The approach currently employed by most successful capture crews relies on massive dosing with potent opioids (etorphine, carfentanil, thiafentanil, or a combination) to reduce the time from darting to recumbency and subsequent skilled handling of the awake, but physically restrained, animal.[63] The giraffe is darted from the ground or, more commonly, from a helicopter, and typically the animal goes down within minutes, although some animals need to be cast with ropes. Soon after the giraffe becomes recumbent, it is blindfolded, ears plugged, and haltered and reversal agents are administered. Once the animal stands again after a few minutes, it is led with ropes into an open trailer used to be transported to a larger contained trailer that accommodates several animals. Refer to Table 61-1 for doses. Other methods incorporating ketamine, with or without medetomidine, to reduce the opioid dosage result in longer induction times but more controlled immobilization.[8,11] Recently, mass capture using a funnel system has been employed successfully for translocations.

Longer Procedures and Monitoring

Once immobilized, many minor procedures—such as diagnostic sampling, foot care, and assisted calving—may be performed. Supplementation is rarely necessary for the first 45 minutes, but after that, periodic intravenous ketamine (0.2 mg/kg) or etorphine or thiafentanil (0.5 microgram per kilogram [μg/kg]) may be used. However, for longer procedures, a continuous infusion of one or more of these drugs or in combination with guaifenesin is preferable, and additional monitoring is recommended. Inhalation anesthesia with isoflurane is another option, but reduced blood pressure and ataxia following recovery are potential concerns.

At a minimum, monitoring should include heart rate and rhythm, rate and depth of ventilations, and oxygen saturation by pulse oximetry. Indirect blood pressure may be measured with an appropriately sized blood pressure cuff placed around the tail base. Measurements may not be accurate but will provide a trend to help guide supplementary drug administration, fluid therapy, and head positioning. To ensure kidney perfusion, the mean arterial pressure should be maintained above 130 mm Hg. As mentioned under "Unique Physiology," lowering of the head will result in pooling of blood in the jugular veins and reduced blood pressure. Therefore,

TABLE 61-1

Protocols for Chemical Restraint Used in Giraffidae*

Generic Name	Dosage	Reversal Agent/Dosage	Reference/Comment
GIRAFFE STANDING SEDATION			
Xylazine (X)	0.1–0.2 milligram per kilogram, intramuscularly (mg/kg, IM)		Mild sedation (e.g., to allow calf to nurse)[19]
Azaperone (Aza)/ detomidine (D)	Aza: 0.2–0.5 mg/kg, IM D: 15–30 µg/kg, IM	Yohimbine 0.1–0.2 mg/kg, IV/IM; or atipamezole 0.01–0.05 mg/kg, IV/IM	[9,12] For deeper sedation, add butorphanol 10–25 µg/kg
Detomidine/ acepromazine (Ace)/ butorphanol (B)/ methadone (Met)	D: 30–40 µg/kg Ace: 15–25 µg/kg B: 20–30 µg/kg Met: 20–30 µg/kg	Atipamezole 0.03–0.06 mg/kg, IM/IV Naltrexone 40–60 µg/kg, IM/IV	[24] For deeper sedation, add xylazine 20–50 µg/kg
GIRAFFE ANESTHESIA†			
Xylazine/etorphine (E)/ ketamine (K) (etorphine may be replaced with carfentanil)	X: 0.05–0.1 mg/kg E: 5–8 µg/kg K: 0.5–1 mg/kg	Atipamezole 0.05 mg/kg, IM/IV Naltrexone 0.3 mg/kg, IM/IV	[24] Allow 10–20 minutes after xylazine before giving etorphine and ketamine
Medetomidine (Med)/ ketamine	Med:40–60 µg/kg, IM K: 1.0–1.5 mg/kg, IM (approximately equal to M: 150 µg + K 3/centimeters (cm) of shoulder height)	Atipamezole 0.05–0.15 mg/kg IV/IM	[8,39] Tachypnea common High potential for re-sedation from medetomidine Re-dose atipamezole at 4 hours, and if needed again at 8 hours
Thiafentanil/ketamine/ medetomidine	T: 5–6 µg/kg Med: 8–13µg/kg K: 0.6–1 mg/kg	Atipamezole 0.05 mg/kg Naltrexone 0.2 mg/kg	[5,11] Beware of potential re-sedation from medetomidine
GIRAFFE CAPTURE			
Etorphine or thiafentanil or 1:1 mix.	10–14 mg/sub-adult 14–15 mg/adult cow Up to 18 mg/adult bull	Naltrexone 0.3–0.4 mg/kg	[63] Immediate reversal required!
Thiafentanil/ketamine/ medetomidine	T: 6–10 µg/kg Med: 10–14 µg/kg K: 0.5 mg/kg	Atipamezole 0.05 mg/kg Naltrexone 0.2–0.3 mg/kg	[11] Beware of potential re-sedation from medetomidine
OKAPI STANDING SEDATION			
Xylazine/butorphanol	X: 0.4–0.8 mg/kg, IM B: 80–200 µg/kg, IM	Yohimbine 0.1–0.2 mg/kg, IV/IM; or atipamezole 0.05–0.1 mg/kg, IV/IM	[12] If indicated, reverse butorphanol with naltrexone 1–2 times dose of butorphanol, IM/IV
Detomidine/butorphanol	D: 40–100 µg/kg, IM B: 80–200 µg/kg, IM	Yohimbine 0.1–0.2 mg/kg, IV/IM; or atipamezole 0.05–0.1 mg/kg, IV/IM	[12] If indicated, reverse butorphanol with naltrexone 1–2 times dose of butorphanol, IM/IV
Xylazine/ketamine	X:0.4–0.6 mg/kg, IM K: 0.4–0.6 mg/kg, IM	Yohimbine 0.1–0.2 mg/kg, IV/IM; or atipamezole 0.03–0.6 mg/kg, IV/IM	[64] Normally, the animal will stay standing, but may lie down
Detomidine/butorphanol/ acepromazine/ midazolam (Mid)	D: 40–60 µg/kg B: 40–60 µg/kg Ace: 30–40 µg/kg Mid: 30–40 µg/kg	Atipamezole 0.03–0.06 mg/kg, IM/IV Naltrexone 40–60 µg/kg, IM/IV	[24]
OKAPI ANESTHESIA†			
Carfentanil/xylazine	X: 0.12 mg/kg C: 5 µg/kg, IM	Naltrexone 0.5 mg/kg, IM	[12] Allow 10–20 minutes after xylazine before giving C Add azaperone 50 mg/adult in stressed animals
Etorphine/xylazine 1:1	X: 0.1–0.2 mg/kg, IM E: 8–15 µg/kg, IM	Atipamezole 0.05 mg/kg, IM/IV Naltrexone 0.2–0.3 mg/kg, IM/IV	Allow 10–20 min after xylazine before giving etorphine Do not use Immobilon because of risk of regurgitation from acepromazine
Medetomidine/ketamine	Med: 60–120 µg/kg, IM K: 1–3 mg/kg, IM	Atipamezole 0.3–0.6 mg/kg, IV/IM	[12,45,64]

*Refer to text for details.
†Provide oxygen via deep nasal cannula or intubate.

lifting the head will typically result in an increase in blood pressure. Invasive blood pressure monitoring or arterial samples for blood gas determination are most easily obtained from the dorsal auricular artery. End-tidal carbon dioxide, functional oxygen saturation (pulse oximetry), and electrocardiography are also useful in monitoring prolonged anesthesia in giraffes.[12]

Long-Acting Tranquilizers

In both species, mild sedation for transport or introductions may be achieved with zuclopenthizole acetate (0.5 mg/kg IM, lasting 3 days) or zuclopenthixole decanoate (2 mg/kg IM, lasting 21 days).[24] In giraffes, haloperidol (15–20 mg/female, 20–30 mg/male IM, lasting 12–24 hours) is useful for loading, as animals will often start walking in 15–20 minutes.

SURGERY

Because of size considerations and the challenges of obtaining minimal ataxia during recovery, only a rather limited array of surgical interventions have been reported in giraffes. Tongue tip amputation, partial mandibular resection, mandibular ostrosynthesis, arthroscopy, arthrotomy, tenotomy, and castration have all been successfully performed.[5,55] Although cesarian sections have been performed, abdominal surgery in giraffes is generally challenging because of the short body making access difficult. A laparoscopic approach has been suggested,[53] but its application would likely be limited. Several cases of colonic obstruction have been documented, and aggressive supportive care and early surgical intervention have been advocated.[16] A glue-on hoof block was successfully used to treat a distal phalangeal fracture.[33]

For the okapi, which is a much better surgical candidate,[57] procedures have included fracture repair, rectal prolapse reduction, rumenotomy and abomasotomy for foreign body retrieval, and surgery for umbilical hernias.

DIAGNOSTICS

Most diagnostic techniques used for other large ungulates may be adapted for use in giraffids. Blood is readily obtained from the jugular vein or other sites such as the lateral saphenous vein. As mentioned previously, giraffes may be trained to accept blood sampling, typically from the jugular vein. In tractable okapis, blood may sometimes be drawn from an auricular vein using a butterfly needle.

Indwelling catheters may be placed in the same locations, but long-term catheter maintenance is difficult in conscious adult animals.

Urine may be collected from female animals by direct catheterization by using techniques and catheters designed for cows. In males, urinary catheters may be placed only with extreme difficulty because of the long and narrow urethra and sigmoid flexure, so urine is usually collected opportunistically.

Radiography of the head, neck, and limbs is straightforward, but thoracic radiography is a challenge in giraffes simply because of their size.

Hematology (Table 61-2) and serum biochemistry (Table 61-3) reference values for giraffes and okapis were determined through compilation of MedARKS records from multiple institutions.[62]

INFECTIOUS DISEASE

In general, infectious diseases are not a major concern in giraffids maintained in captivity. Overall giraffids are susceptible to most diseases of domestic ruminants, but while several individual cases of infectious diseases have been reported, no real patterns or extreme susceptibilities exist.

Bacterial Diseases

Reported bacterial diseases include salmonellosis, paratuberculosis, brucellosis, anthrax, actinomycosis, listeriosis, Q-fever, and *Mycoplasma*-associated polyarthritis.[9,14,27] Both *Mycobacterium bovis* and *M. tuberculosis* have caused tuberculosis (TB) in giraffes. Intracutaneous TB testing appears to be sensitive and may be supplemented by serologic testing. Enteritis caused by *Escherichia coli* or *Clostridium perfringens* appears to occur with some frequency in okapis.[17,57] *Anaplasma marginale* infection appears to be a common subclinical infection in free-ranging giraffe.[46] Similarly, giraffes may be healthy carriers of *Ehrlichia* (*Cowdria*) *ruminantium* transmitted with *Amblyomma* sp. and do not develop clinical disease following artificial infection.[51]

Otitis, involving various bacteria and fungi, was seen in several okapis in one collection but not in 15 others, and environmental factors were suspected.[2]

Viral Diseases

Viral diseases reported in giraffes and okapis include rinderpest, to which giraffes are very susceptible,[9] malignant catarrhal fever, foot-and-mouth disease, encephalomyocarditis, and lumpy skin disease.

TABLE 61-2

Reference Ranges for Hematological Parameters for Giraffidae from Composite MedARKS records[62]

Parameter	Unit	Giraffe Mean ± Standard Deviation	Okapi Mean ± Standard Deviation
Leukocytes or white blood cell count	10^9/liter (L)	12.6 ± 4.8 (479)	8 ± 3 (91)
Neutrophils: bands	10^9/L	0.86 ± 1.2 (181)	0.11 ± 0.1 (14)
Neutrophils: segmented	10^9/L	9.2 ± 4.2 (446)	5.1 ± 2.5 (81)
Lymphocytes	10^9/L	2.3 ± 1.4 (451)	2.4 ± 1 (81)
Eosinophils	10^9/L	0.40 ± 0.40 (266)	0.16 ± 0.11 (32)
Monocytes	10^9/L	0.41 ± 0.37 (370)	0.29 ± 0.31 (70)
Basophils	10^9/L	0.29 ± 0.22 (255)	0.15 ± 0.09 (18)
Hematocrit or packed cell volume	Liter per liter (L/L)	0.35 ± 0.06 (550)	0.36 ± 0.08 (92)
Erythrocytes or red blood cell count	10^{12}/L	10.5 ± 2.4 (350)	10.0 ± 2.7 (80)
Hemoglobin	Gram per liter (g/L)	119 ± 18 (376)	124 ± 27 (90)
Mean corpuscular hemoglobin	Picogram per cell (pg/cell)	11.7 ± 2.7 (340)	12.7 ± 1.7 (79)
Mean corpuscular hemoglobin concentration	g/L	348 ± 35 (373)	347 ± 29 (89)
Mean corpuscular volume	Femtoliters (fL)	34.1 ± 8.4 (346)	36.7 ± 4.1 (78)
Platelets	10^{12}/L	0.42 ± 0.17 (93)	0.38 ± 0.11 (20)

Note: Values represent mean ± standard deviation (n).

TABLE 61-3

Reference Ranges for Serum Biochemical Parameters for Giraffidae Based on Composite MedARKS records[62]

Parameter	Unit	Giraffe Mean ± Standard Deviation	Okapi Mean ± Standard Deviation
Total protein	Gram per liter (g/L)	74 ± 14 (312)	71 ± 10 (77)
Albumin	g/L	31 ± 5 (282)	31 ± 8 (61)
Globulin	g/L	42 ± 14 (280)	40 ± 10 (59)
Fibrinogen	g/L	2.3 ± 1.8 (135)	0.4 ± 0.9 (33)
Glucose	Millimole per liter (mmol/L)	7.7 ± 3.3 (434)	7.2 ± 2.4 (83)
Alanine aminotransferase	Unit per liter (Unit/L)	13 ± 11 (237)	17 ± 20 (73)
Alkaline phosphatase	Unit /L	522 ± 476 (388)	397 ± 547 (77)
Aspartate aminotransferase	Unit /L	96 ± 55 (393)	66 ± 36 (77)
Creatine phosphokinase	Unit /L	1356 ± 1677(198)	615 ± 612 (77)
Gamma glutamyltransferase	Unit /L	61 ± 82 (207)	58 ± 101 (57)
Lactate dehydrogenase	Unit /L	864 ± 650 (235)	522 ± 296 (41)
Blood urea nitrogen	mmol/L	7.1 ± 2.5 (417)	7.5 ± 2.9 (80)
Creatinine	Micromole per liter (µmol/L)	159 ± 44 (373)	194 ± 71 (39)
Iron	µmol/L	16.7 ± 12.5 (28)	25.1 ± 9 (14)
Calcium	mmol/L	2.50 ± 0.45 (404)	2.58 ± 0.40 (80)
Phosphorus	mmol/L	3.0 ± 0.8 (372)	2.6 ± 0.7 (74)
Magnesium	mmol/L	1 ± 0.2 (63)	1 ± 0.3 (7)
Potassium	mmol/L	4.8 ± 0.6 (379)	5.0 ± 0.5 (77)
Sodium	mmol/L	145 ± 4 (381)	142 ± 5 (76)
Chloride	mmol/L	104 ± 6 (358)	103 ± 6 (74)
Triglyceride	mmol/L	0.45 ± 0.3 (245)	0.37 ± 0.3 (35)
Bilirubin: Total	µmol/L	17 ± 15 (377)	7 ± 5 (75)

Note: Values represent mean ± standard deviation (n).

A rotavirus was commonly involved in diarrhea in okapi calves in the 1980s and 1990s[56,57] but appears less prevalent now. Another rotavirus closely related to bovine rotavirus was recently isolated from a giraffe calf with diarrhea.[44] Similarly, a coronavirus closely related to bovine coronavirus was isolated from several giraffes with diarrhea.[30] None of these infections appear to be of particular concern.

Equine herpes virus types 1 and 9 were found to cause severe nonsuppurative meningoencephalitis in giraffes, and it was suspected that the infection originated from zebras sharing the enclosures.[31,35]

Bovine papillomavirus (BPV-1 and -2) was identified in multifocal to coalescing nodular and occasionally ulcerated lesions of the head, neck, and trunk of two giraffes.[68] Lesions were similar to equine sarcoids and locally invaded the subcutis but did not appear to metastasize. A pestivirus related to bovine viral diarrhea (BVD) virus has been isolated from a giraffe but appears to have little clinical significance.[28]

An outbreak of papules, vesicles, and pustules in several okapi caused by an orthopoxvirus was described in the early 1970s[70] but has not been of major concern since then. A single case of bluetongue has been described in an okapi, while the giraffe does not appear to be susceptible. Vaccination appears effective and may be considered for okapi kept in endemic areas.

Parasitic Diseases

Multiple parasites have been described in both giraffes and okapis; however, none constitute major problems in captive animals. Giraffes appear to be susceptible to many of the parasites of domestic ruminants,[21] and both species respond well to treatment with anthelmintics used in domestic cattle. As with any species, these drugs should be used prudently, and resistance has proven to be a concern, as evidenced by the report of giraffe-derived *Haemonchus contortus* resistant to benzimidazoles, imidazothiazoles, and macrocyclic lactones.[22] Orally administered copper oxide wire particles provide an alternative treatment to traditional anthelmintics and have been used successfully as part of an anthelmintic strategy in several institutions.[22]

Originally identified in a fatal case, a *Cytauxzoon* sp. was retrieved from several normal free-ranging giraffes.[37] In contrast, novel species of *Babesia* and *Theileria* were identified in the blood of young semi–free-ranging giraffes and were suspected to be the cause of death in these animals.[48]

Other parasites reported in giraffes include multiple tick species, *Rhinoestrus* sp., *Sarcoptes scabei*, *Thelazia gulosa*, *Capillaria* sp., *Camelostrongylus mentulatus*, *Trichostrongylus axei*, *Ostertagia ostertagi*, *Teladorsagia circumcincta*, *Teladorsagia trifurcata*, *Monodontella giraffae*, *Marshallagia marshalli*, *Trichostrongylus vitrinus*, *Trichostrongylus colubriformis*, *Spiculopteragia asymmetrica*, *Trichuris giraffae*, *Parabronema skrjabini*, *Skrjabinema* sp., *Haemonchus mitchelli*, *Echinococcus* sp., *Cryptosporidium parvum*, *Giardia* sp., and *Hepatozoon* sp.[3,4,9,21,57]

NONINFECTIOUS DISEASE

Noninfectious problems are probably more prevalent than infectious disease in captive giraffids, and several "syndromes" are seen with some frequency. Congestive heart failure of unknown etiology has been diagnosed in several adult female okapis in a single collection.[1] Clinical signs were managed with oral furosemide and enalapril. Interestingly, myocardial hypertrophy or ventricular dilation was a frequent finding in a survey of postmortem findings.[17]

Both species are susceptible to overgrown hooves in captivity mainly because of lack of movement, dry environments, and shortage of sufficiently abrasive surfaces. Apart from simple overgrowth, excessively steep stance, crossing over of cleats, and flaring hoof walls are the most common problems in okapis, whereas in giraffes crossing over of the cleats is the problem most commonly encountered. The hoof horn, particularly of giraffes, is extremely hard, and the use of power tools will significantly facilitate corrective trimming.

Gastrointestinal Disorders

Colic without specific etiology is seen with some frequency in okapis, and intestinal stasis following anesthetic events has been anecdotally reported.[64] Intestinal volvulus has been seen in both juvenile and adult okapis.[17]

Colonic obstruction with phytobezoars or fecal matter was documented in three giraffes[16] and has also been seen in okapis. The spiral colon appears to be particularly prone to these obstructions, and unless diagnosed and resolved early, these obstructions hold a poor prognosis.[16] In okapis, excessive maternal grooming of calves may lead to anal trauma and stricture.[59]

Giraffids, like other browsing ruminants, have lower chewing efficiency compared with grazers, and the feeding of traditional "grazer diets" leads to significantly larger mean fecal particle size in captive giraffes than in free-ranging giraffes.[32] It has been speculated that this deficient particle size reduction could contribute to potential clinical problems such as gastrointestinal blockage and bezoar formation.

Acute Mortality Syndrome

Acute mortality syndrome was a major cause of death in captive giraffes for decades,[34] but the frequency has decreased in recent years, largely because of improved feeding practices. Many animals died without any history of illness, others after a mild or short-term illness or stressful incident. Emaciation with serous atrophy of fat is the key pathologic finding, often accompanied by pulmonary edema, petechial hemorrhages, intestinal ulceration, and myocardial degeneration.[13] Essentially, this "syndrome" appears to be simply caused by a negative energy balance, either from insufficient nutrition[13] or poor dental health,[18] and the "last straw" or event triggering death may be hypothermia or stress.[34,54] Similar pathologic findings are observed in winter in free-ranging giraffes at the southern margin of their distribution and are interpreted as starvation. A similar phenomenon appears to exist in the okapi, and emaciation with serous atrophy of fat was noted in 17 of 134 okapi postmortem reports reviewed.[17]

Urolithiasis

Urolithiasis occurs with some frequency in captive giraffes, and some uroliths have been diagnosed as carbonate or apatite with a shell of struvite.[69] In a recent survey, 6 of 43 zoos reported a history of urolithiasis.[61] High dietary phosphorus content and a high level of concentrate relative to hay (>1) may be contributing factors to urolith formation.[61]

Chronic Interstitial Nephritis

Renal tubular atrophy, with conical and medullary interstitial fibrosis and severe thickening of the basement membranes of atrophic tubules, has been described in several okapis.[25,26] Focal glomerular atrophy, probably secondary to ischemic collapse of the glomerular capillary tuft, was also observed. Although the etiologies and pathogenesis of these nephropathies are unclear, primary damage of the tubular epithelium appears to be the most likely cause, and toxicity from ingested plant material, possibly willow (*Salix* sp.), has been proposed as an etiologic factor.[26]

Glycosuria

Asymptomatic glycosuria is very prevalent in adult captive okapis,[20,23] whereas animals tested at the Epulu station (Democratic Republic of Congo) were nonglucosuric.[20] The etiology is unknown; animals have normal serum levels of insulin, glucose, and fructosamine, and no correlation with stress or dietary glucose content has been found.[65]

Neoplasia

Neoplasia is not frequently seen in giraffids. Neoplasms reported in giraffes include embryonal rhabdomyosarcoma, pelvic chondrosarcoma causing dystocia, umbilical cord teratoma, verrucous squamous cell carcinoma, and glioneuronal hamartoma in the mesencephalic aqueduct. Findings in okapis include luteoma, ependymoma, and phechromocytoma.

REPRODUCTION[10]

Giraffids are considered nonseasonal breeders, with a short cycle of approximately 15 days and a comparatively long gestation of 420 to 468 days in the giraffe and 414 to 491 days in the okapi. Females attain sexual maturity at an age of about 20 months. Under zoo conditions, both species may live up to an age of well over 30 years. Reproduction is discussed in Table 61-4.

The female giraffid has a bicornuate uterus. In the male, the testes are scrotal, and the penis is fibroelastic and has a long urethral process resembling that of a goat. Interestingly, three variations of chromosome numbers have been identified in the okapi (44, 45, 46).[52] The reduction of 46 chromosomes to 45 is the result of a Robertsonian translocation between chromosomes 8 and 21. Individuals with 45 and 46 have both reproduced successfully in mixed karyotype pairs. Females are nonseasonal breeders and come into estrus at 15-day intervals. Estrus behavior is fairly subtle and consists of mild mucus production and vulvar flaring. Breeding normally is uneventful, with copulation lasting only seconds.

Pregnancy may usually be detected visually about half way through. In trained animals, ovarian cycles and pregnancy may be monitored with transrectal ultrasonography.[40] In pregnant giraffes,

TABLE 61-4

Reproductive Characteristics of Giraffids[9,10,38,40]

Parameter	Giraffe	Okapi
Karyotype (2n)	30	44, 45, or 46[52]
Puberty, age (years)	Female at 3–4 Male at 4–5	Females at 2.5 Males at 2–4
Estrus cycle (days)	14–15	15–16
Luteal phase	8	11
Follicular phase	6	5
Duration of copulation	Few seconds	Few seconds
Gestation	420–468 days	414–491 days
Pregnancy determination	Urinary/fecal PdG	Urinary/fecal PdG
Placentation	Cotyledonary placentation	Cotyledonary placentation
Urinary pregnanediol-3-glucuronide (PdG), nanogram per milliliter (ng/mL) Nongravid:		
Follicular	3.6 ± 7 ng PdG/mg Cr	1.9 ± 0.1 ng PdG/mg Cr
Luteal	30.9 ± 1.7 ng PdG/mg Cr	27.2 ± 3.9 ng PdG/mg Cr
Gravid	Persistent luteal levels >250 ng PdG/mg Cr in late gestation	Persistent luteal levels With levels >100 ng PdG/mg Cr
Semen volume	4–6 mL	Unknown

the corpus luteum (CL) reaches a diameter significantly larger (40 mm) than during the cycle (33 mm), and follicular activity may still be present.[40] Transabdominal ultrasonography may detect later stage pregnancy. Pregnancy may also be detected by means of urinary and fecal steroid analysis.[38,60]

Predicting the time of birth precisely is difficult in giraffes. The udder typically, but not always, becomes enlarged in the last few weeks prior to parturition. Vulvar edema and a mucoid discharge may precede parturition by a few days. If possible, the female should be isolated from the herd shortly before parturition and remain separate with the calf for at least 24 hours, but if adequate space is available, the female may simply give birth while with the herd. Giraffids usually give birth to a single calf; however, twinning does occur. In the okapi, several twin pregnancies have ended in stillbirths.[59] Labor is usually short (3–6 hours), and the healthy calf should be standing within an hour or so of birth. The birthing environment is important for neonatal survival. A proper substrate of compacted soil, rubber pads, or straw bedding is important to prevent hypothermia and splaying. Nursing should start within the first few hours after birth. First-time mothers may be nervous and may at first refuse to allow the calf to suckle. They usually relax after a few hours, but mild sedation has been necessary in several instances.[19]

Neonatal examinations are useful for assessing the general health of the neonate and determining the success of immunoglobulin transfer from the dam. Normal birth weight is approximately 60 kg in the giraffe and 15 to 30 kg for okapis.

An okapi that experienced five abortions because of deficient placental progestagen production was treated with altrenogest in a subsequent pregnancy and carried the fetus to term.[60]

Retained placenta occurs with some frequency in both species, particularly when the calf is stillborn or dies within the first day. Ideally, as much of the placenta should be removed as possible, but cases have been managed with only supportive therapy, including antibiotics.[59]

Contraception

In some cases, preventing reproduction in giraffes is desirable. Surgical castration is an effective, although nonreversible, means of contraception in male giraffes. Open castration using an emasculator and ligation has been advocated, but partial or complete scrotal closure is probably a superior technique.[5]

For contraception in females, melengestrol acetate (2–3 mg/kg/day) administered in the feed, or the progesterone-derivative medroxyprogesterone acetate (Depo-Provera, Pfizer Animal Health), (450–800 mg/female, every 6 weeks) have been the traditional pharmaceutical means of contraception; however, the gonadotropin-releasing hormone (GnRH) agonist deslorelin (Suprelorin, Peptech Animal Health/Virbac) administered as implants has recently proven to be superior and effective for more than a year.[50] It is suggested to check the current recommendations of the Contraceptive Advisory Group before initiating contraception.

PREVENTIVE MEDICINE

Preventative measures in giraffids include regular inspections of feet and provision of abrasive surfaces. If necessary, routine foot care should be provided, ideally through use of training. Regular screening for intestinal parasites and deworming, if indicated, should be part of the strategy, and regular weighing of animals is highly recommended.

Routine vaccination is seldom performed, but vaccines against rabies, clostridial diseases, and bluetongue, as well as rotavirus and coronavirus, are sometimes used.

Preshipment testing is recommended for any giraffe relocation, but specific tests to be performed depend on local conditions. The following are recommended guidelines to aid in decision making when planning the safe transfer of a giraffe or okapi: (1) fecal sample for parasites, particularly nematodes; (2) fecal culture, especially for *Salmonella*; (3) tuberculin skin testing and auxiliary TB tests; (4) blood sample for complete blood cell (CBC) count and serum chemistries; (5) physical examination, including foot inspection. Intracutaneous TB testing may be performed in the eyelids, as in primates, to avoid the need for a second restraint of the animal.

Quarantine of individuals should be performed before exposure to animals at the new location.

ACKNOWLEDGMENTS

The author thanks Mira Strøm Braten, Carsten Grøndahl, Sander Hofman, Kristin Leus, Torsten Møller, Willem Schaftenaar, and Francis Vercamen for their contributions to this chapter.

REFERENCES

1. Aitken-Palmer C, Citino S: Cardiopulmonary disease in okapi (*Okapia johnstoni*). In *Proceedings of the American Association of Zoo Veterinarians*, Kansas City, MO, 2011, p 84.
2. Allender MC, Langan J, Citino S: Investigation of aural bacterial and fungal flora following otitis in captive okapi (*Okapia johnstoni*). *Vet Dermatol* 19:95–100, 2008.
3. Benirschke K: General survey of okapi pathology. *Acta Zool Pathol* 71:63–78, 1978.
4. Bertelsen MF, Østergaard K, Monrad J, et al: Monodontella giraffae infection in wild-caught southern giraffes (*Giraffa camelopardalis giraffa*). *J Wildl Dis* 45:1227–1230, 2009.
5. Borkowski R, Citino S, Bush M, et al: Surgical castration of subadult giraffe (*Giraffa camelopardalis*). *J Zoo Wildl Med* 40:786–790, 2009.
6. Brøndum E, Hasenkam JM, Secher NH, et al: Jugular venous pooling during lowering of the head affects blood pressure of the anesthetized giraffe. *Am J Physiol Regul Integr Comp Physiol* 297:R1058–R1065, 2009.
7. Bush M, Ensley PK, Mehren K, et al: Immobilization of giraffes with xylazine and etorphine hydrochloride. *J Am Vet Med Assoc* 169:884–885, 1976.
8. Bush M, Grobler DG, Raath JP, et al: Use of medetomidine and ketamine for immobilization of free-ranging giraffes. *J Am Vet Med Assoc* 218:245–249, 2001.
9. Bush M: Giraffidae. In Fowler ME, Miller RE, editors: *Zoo and wild animal medicine*, ed 5, St. Louis, MO, 2003, Saunders, pp 625–633.
10. Calle PP, Raphael BL, Loskutoff NM: Giraffid reproduction. In Fowler ME, editor: *Zoo and wild animal medicine: Current therapy*, ed 3, Philadelphia, PA, 1993, Saunders, pp 549–554.
11. Citino SB, Bush M, Lance W, et al: Use of thiafentanil (A3080), and ketamine for anesthesia of captive and free-ranging giraffe (*Giraffa camelopardalis*). In *Proceedings of the American Association of Zoo Veterinarians*, Tampa, FL, 2006, pp 211–213.
12. Citino SB, Bush M: Giraffidae. In West G, Heard D, Caulkett N, editors: *Zoo animal and Wildlife immobilization and anesthesia*, Ames, IA, 2007, Blackwell, pp 595–605.
13. Clauss M, Rose P, Hummel J, et al: Serous fat atrophy and other nutrition-related health problems in captive giraffe—an evaluation of 83 necropsy reports. In *Proceedings of the European Association of Zoo and Wildlife Veterinarians*, Budapest, Hungary, 2006, pp 233–235.
14. Cranfield MA, Eckhaus BA, Valentine JD, et al: Listeriosis in Angolan giraffes. *J Am Vet Med Assoc* 187:1238–1240, 1985.
15. Dagg AI, Foster JB: *The giraffe: Its biology, behavior, and ecology*, New York, 1976, Van Nostrand Reinhold Co.
16. Davis MR, Langan JN, Mylniczenko ND, et al: Colonic obstruction in three captive reticulated giraffe (*Giraffa camelopardalis reticulata*). *J Zoo Wildl Med* 40:181–188, 2009.
17. EAZWV Students, Clauss M: Evaluation of Okapi (*Okapia johnstoni*) necropsy reports and studbook data as part of the EAZWV summer school. In *Proceedings of the European Association of Zoo and Wildlife Veterinarians*, Leipzig, Germany, 2008, pp 323–327.
18. Enqvist KE, Chu JI, Williams CA, et al: Dental disease and serous atrophy of fat syndrome in captive giraffes (*Giraffa camelopardalis*). In *Proceedings of the American Association of Zoo Veterinarians*, Minneapolis, MN, 2003, pp 262–263.

19. Fischer MT, Miller RE, Houston EW: Serial tranquilization of a reticulated giraffe (*Giraffa camelopardalis reticulata*) using xylazine. *J Zoo Wildl Med* 28:182–184, 1997.

20. Fleming GJ, Citino SB, Petric A: Glucosuria in captive okapi (*Okapia johnstoni*). *J Zoo Wildl Med* 37:472–476, 2006.

21. Garijo MM, Ortiz JM, Ruiz de Ibáñez MR: Helminths in a giraffe (*Giraffa camelopardalis giraffa*) from a zoo in Spain. *Onderstepoort J Vet Res* 71:153–156, 2004.

22. Garretson PD, Hammond EE, Craig TM, et al: Anthelmintic resistant *Haemonchus contortus* in a giraffe (*Giraffa camelopardalis*) in Florida. *J Zoo Wildl Med* 40:131–139, 2009.

23. Glatston AR, Smit S: Analysis of the urine of the okapi (*Okapia johnstoni*). *Acta Zool Pathol Antverp* 75:49–58, 1980.

24. Grøndal C, Bertelsen MF: Unpublished data.

25. Haenichen T, Rietschel W: Post mortem findings in the okapi. *Verhandlungsbericht Erkrankungen der Zootiere* 40:99–105, 2001.

26. Haenichen T, Wisser J, Wanke R: Chronic tubulointerstitial nephropathy in six okapis (*Okapia johnstoni*). *J Zoo Wildl Med* 32:459–464, 2001.

27. Hammond EE, Miller CA, Sneed L, et al: Mycoplasma-associated polyarthritis in a reticulated giraffe. *J Wildl Dis* 39:233–237, 2003.

28. Harasawa R, Giangaspero M, Ibata G, et al: Giraffe strain of pestivirus: Its taxonomic status based on the 5′-untranslated region. *Microbiol Immunol* 44:915–921, 2000.

29. Hargens AR, Millard RW, Pettersson K, et al: Gravitational haemodynamics and oedema prevention in the giraffe. *Nature* 329:59–60, 1987.

30. Hasoksuz M, Alekseev K, Vlasova A, et al: Biologic, antigenic, and full-length genomic characterization of a bovine-like coronavirus isolated from a giraffe. *J Virol* 81:4981–4990, 2007.

31. Hoenerhoff MJ, Janovitz EB, Richman LK, et al: Fatal herpesvirus encephalitis in a reticulated giraffe (*Giraffa camelopardalis reticulata*). *Vet Pathol* 43:769–772, 2006.

32. Hummel J, Fritz J, Kienzle E, et al: Differences in fecal particle size between free-ranging and captive individuals of two browser species. *Zoo Biol* 27:70–77, 2008.

33. James SB, Koss K, Harper J, et al: Diagnosis and treatment of a fractured third phalanx in a Masai giraffe (*Giraffe camilopardalis tippelsckrchi*). *J Zoo and Wildlife Med* 31:400–403, 2000.

34. Junge RE, Bradley TA: Peracute mortality syndrome of giraffe. In Fowler ME, editor: *Zoo and wild animal medicine: Current therapy*, ed 3, Philadelphia, PA, 1993, Saunders, pp 547–549.

35. Kasem S, Yamada S, Kiupel M, et al: Equine herpesvirus type 9 in giraffe with encephalitis. *Emerg Infect Dis* 14:1948–1949, 2008.

36. Koutsos EA, Armstrong D, Ball R, et al: Influence of diet transition on serum calcium and phosphorus and fatty acids in zoo giraffe (*Giraffa camelopardalis*). *Zoo Biol* 30:523–531, 2011.

37. Krecek RC, Boomker J, Penzhorn BL, et al: Internal parasites of giraffes (*Giraffa camelopardalis angolensis*) from Etosha National Park, Namibia. *J Wildl Dis* 26:395–397, 1990.

38. Kusuda S, Morikaku K, Kawada K, et al: Excretion patterns of fecal progestagens, androgen and estrogens during pregnancy, parturition and postpartum in okapi (*Okapia johnstoni*). *J Reprod Dev* 53:143–150, 2007.

39. Lamberski N, Newell A, Radcliffe RW: Thirty immobilizations of captive giraffe (*Giraffa camelopardalis*) using a combination of medetomidine and ketamine. In *Proceedings of the American Association of Zoo Veterinarians*, Omaha, NB, 2004, pp 118–120.

40. Lueders I, Hildebrandt TB, Pootoolal J, et al: Ovarian ultrasonography correlated with fecal progestins and estradiol during the estrous cycle and early pregnancy in giraffes (*Giraffa camelopardalis rothschildi*). *Biol Reprod* 81:989–995, 2009.

41. Miller M, Weber M, Valdes EV, et al: Changes in serum calcium, phosphorus, and magnesium levels in captive ruminants affected by diet manipulation. *J Zoo Wildl Med* 41:404–408, 2010.

42. Mitchell G, Skinner JD: An allometric analysis of the giraffe cardiovascular system. *Comp Biochem Physiol A Mol Integr Physiol* 154:523–529, 2009.

43. Mitchell G, Skinner JD: Lung volumes in giraffes, Giraffa camelopardalis. *Comp Biochem Physiol A Mol Integr Physiol* 158:72–78, 2011.

44. Mulherin E, Bryan J, Beltman M, et al: Molecular characterisation of a bovine-like rotavirus detected from a giraffe. *Vet Res* 4:46, 2008.

45. Murison PJ, Jones A, Redrobe S: Repeated anaesthesia in an Okapi (*Okapia johnstoni*). *Vet Anaesth Analg* 39:449–450, 2012.

46. Ngeranwa JJ, Shompole SP, Venter EH, et al: Detection of Anaplasma antibodies in wildlife and domestic species in wildlife-livestock interface areas of Kenya by major surface protein 5 competitive inhibition enzyme-linked immunosorbent assay. *Onderstepoort J Vet Res* 75:199–205, 2008.

47. Nowak RM: Artiodactyla: Family Giraffidae. *Walker's mammals of the world*, ed 6, Baltimore, MD, 1999, Johns Hopkins University Press, pp 1284–1289.

48. Oosthuizen MC, Allsopp BA, Troskie M, et al: Identification of novel Babesia and Theileria species in South African giraffe (*Giraffa camelopardalis, Linnaeus, 1758*) and roan antelope (*Hippotragus equinus, Desmarest, 1804*). *Vet Parasitol* 163:39–46, 2009.

49. Østergaard KH, Bertelsen MF, Brøndum ET, et al: Pressure profile and morphology of the arteries along the giraffe limb. *J Comp Physiol [B]* 181:691–698, 2011.

50. Patton ML, Bashaw MJ, del Castillo SM, et al: Long-term suppression of fertility in female giraffe using the GnRH agonist deslorelin as a long-acting implant. *Theriogenology* 66:431–438, 2006.

51. Peter TF, Anderson EC, Burridge MJ, et al: Demonstration of a carrier state for *Cowdria ruminantium* in wild ruminants from Africa. *J Wildlife Dis* 34:567–575, 1998.

52. Petit P, de Meurichy W: On the chromosomes of the okapi, Okapia johnstoni. *Ann Genet* 29:232–234, 1986.

53. Pizzi R, Cracknell J, Dalrymple L: Postmortem evaluation of left flank laparoscopic access in an adult female giraffe (*Giraffa camelopardalis*). *Vet Med Int* ID:789465, 2010.

54. Potter JS, Clauss M: Mortality of captive giraffe (*Giraffa camelopardalis*) associated with serous fat atrophy: A review of five cases at Auckland Zoo. *J Zoo Wildl Med* 36:301–307, 2005.

55. Quesada R, Citino SB, Easley JT, et al: Surgical resolution of an avulsion fracture of the peroneus tertius origin in a giraffe (*Giraffa camelopardalis reticulata*). *J Zoo Wildl Med* 42:348–350, 2011.

56. Raphael BL, Sneed L, Ott-Joslin J: Rotavirus-like infection associated with diarrhea in okapi. *J Am Vet Med Assoc* 189:1183–1184, 1986.

57. Raphael BL: Okapi medicine and surgery. In Fowler ME, Miller RE, editors: *Zoo and wild animal medicine: Current therapy*, ed 4, Philadelphia, PA, 1999, Saunders, pp 646–650.

58. Schmidt D, Barbiers R: *Giraffe nutrition workshop proceedings*, 2005, Lincoln Park Zoo. http://www.petfoods.com.mx/PetFoods/Herbivoros _files/Giraffe%20Workshop%20Proceedings%202005.pdf. Accessed December 20th, 2013.

59. Schaftenaar W: Unpublished data.

60. Schwarzenberger F, Rietschel W, Matern B, et al: Noninvasive reproductive monitoring in the okapi (*Okapia johnstoni*). *J Zoo Wildl Med* 30:497–503, 1999.

61. Sullivan K, van Heugten E, Ange-van Heugten K, et al: Analysis of nutrient concentrations in the diet, serum, and urine of giraffe from surveyed North American zoological institutions. *Zoo Biol* 29:457–469, 2010.

62. Teare JA: *ISIS reference ranges for physiological values in captive wildlife* [electronic resource], Apple Valley, MN, 2002, International Species Information System.

63. Van Niekerk C: Unpublished data.

64. Vercammen F: Unpublished data.

65. Vercammen F, Stas L, Bauwens L, et al: Long-term assessment of the dietary influence on glucosuria in okapi (*Okapia johnstoni*). In *Proceedings of the American Association of Zoo Veterinarians*, Kansas City, MO, 2011, p 13.

66. Vogelnest L, Ralph HK: Chemical immobilisation of giraffe to facilitate short procedures. *Aust Vet J* 75:180–182, 1997.

67. Wiesner H, von Hegel G: Zur Immobilisation on Giraffen [The immobilization of giraffes]. *Tierarztl Prax* 17:97–100, 1989.

68. Williams JH, van Dyk E, Nel PJ, et al: Pathology and immunohistochemistry of papillomavirus-associated cutaneous lesions in Cape mountain zebra, giraffe, sable antelope and African buffalo in South Africa. *J S Afr Vet Assoc* 82:97–106, 2011.

69. Wolfe BA, Sladky KK, Loomis MR: Obstructive urolithiasis in a reticulated giraffe (*Giraffa camilopardalis reticulata*). *Vet Rec* 146:260–261, 2000.

70. Zwart P, Gispen R, Peters JC: Cowpox in okapis Okapia johnstoni at Rotterdam zoo. *Br Vet J* 127:20–24, 1971.

CHAPTER 62

Tragulidae, Moschidae, and Cervidae

Nicholas J. Masters and Edmund Flach

Deer have been known to, and hunted by, human beings for millennia, and the annual cycle of antler growth has long been a source of fascination and folklore. Currently, veterinarians may work with deer and their relatives in zoos, in farms, and in the wild, with an increasing involvement in conservation programs for endangered deer species (both in situ and ex situ). Many names have been given to age or sex categories of deer of different species, but to avoid confusion, the authors refer to adult males as *stags*, adult females as *hinds*, and juveniles as *calves*. This chapter focuses on seasonal species kept in zoos in Europe and North America, but a useful reference to neotropical species has recently been published.[15]

GENERAL BIOLOGY

The taxonomy of the chevrotains—or mouse deer (Family Tragulidae), musk deer (Moschidae), and true deer (Cervidae)—has changed over recent years, but in the recent revision by Groves and Grubb,[26] all have been classified as members of the suborder Ruminantia within the order Artiodactyla. The 10 species in the three genera of Tragulidae are sufficiently distinct to have a separate infraorder (Tragulina) from all other ruminants (Percora). The general consensus is that seven Moschus species (Moschidae) exist, but numbers of species and genera within Cervidae vary among texts.[26,27,42,57,72] The authors have followed the classification of Wilson and Mittermeier (2010)[72] and have placed 53 species in 18 genera, with Hydropotes included in the suborder Capriolinae (Table 62-1).

All deer and their relatives are herbivorous, but they may be browsers, grazers, or intermediate feeders (see Feeding). Body mass tends to be greater in males, although exceptions (e.g., some Tragulidae) do exist. Social structure varies from solitary existence to herd living. The group, as a whole, is extremely widespread, from the arctic tundra to tropical forests, and deer are arguably the most successful ungulates. Despite this, many species and subspecies are declining in population because of exploitation by humans, habitat loss, and environmental threats (see Table 62-1). One species, the Père David deer (*Elaphurus davidianus*), has become extinct in the wild, but the species has been reintroduced in China, thanks to long-term captive programs.

UNIQUE ANATOMY

The chevrotains (Tragulidae) have many ruminant features such as a four-chambered stomach (with a poorly developed omasum), no upper incisor teeth, and incisor-like lower canines, but they also resemble pigs and hippopotami in having four toes with supporting bones, as well as incomplete fusion of the third and fourth metacarpals and metatarsals.[42,57] Members of this family lack antlers and have elongated upper canines as in musk deer and Chinese water deer (*Hydropotes inermis*) and, like musk deer, also possess a gallbladder and lack preorbital scent glands. However, they do possess a chin gland.

Musk deer (Moschidae) lack antlers, have a gallbladder, and possess just one pair of mammary glands. They have no facial glands but have caudal glands ventral to the tail and well-developed preputial or musk glands, from which the commercially valuable musk

is obtained. Moschidae used to be included as a subfamily in Cervidae but has now been raised to family status.[26,72]

The defining characteristic of the true deer (Cervidae) is the possession of antlers (Figure 62-1). Males of all species, except the Chinese water deer, grow antlers each year before the breeding season and lose them later. In the species that comprises the reindeer, or caribou (*Rangifer tarandus*), both sexes have antlers. The size and complexity of antlers increases with distance from the equator, as climatic and nutritional conditions become more exacting. Hinds select males that can thrive best in the environment, and the choice of a female may be the most important factor for the evolution of large antlers. Antler growth occurs annually under hormonal control. The antlers arise from the frontal bones and skin and, until fully grown, they are covered with a highly vascularized and sensitive skin known as *velvet*. As the mating season approaches, the testosterone level rises, the antlers harden, and the velvet dries. Stags may rub their antlers against objects to remove the flaking velvet. After the mating season, the testosterone level declines, and a layer of bone-dissolving cells invades the base of the antlers, causing them to fall off. Each year, the size and, in some species, the complexity of antlers increase until full maturity. Antler growth has a less well-defined seasonality in tropical and subtropical zones.

Deer possess a range of specialized scent glands, most commonly preorbital in location but also occurring on the limbs. Deer have no gallbladder, and female deer have two pairs of inguinal mammary glands. The skeleton has evolved for running and jumping, with reductions of the ulna and the fibula, loss of the first digit, reductions of digits II and V, and fusion of the third and fourth metacarpals and metatarsals to form cannon bones. The location of the vestigial metacarpal bones II and V (splint bones) is the basis for differentiation of the subfamily Cervinae (proximal or plesiometacarpalian) from the Capreolinae (distal or telemetacarpalian). The Chinese water deer has been placed in the subfamily Capreolinae, as it is telemetacarpalian and is phylogenetically very close to the roe deer (*Capreolus capreolus*); this is based on mitochondrial cytochrome analysis,[60] which suggests that the loss of antlers is a secondary characteristic.

SPECIAL HOUSING REQUIREMENTS

The majority of deer species may be kept in natural-ground paddocks bounded by fences or walls that may have to be 2.5 to 3 meters (m) high for the larger species and well buried. High-tensile steel netting 1.8 to 2 m high, with posts 5 to 8 m apart, commonly is used for farming red deer (*Cervus elaphus*) and fallow deer (*Dama dama*), but chain-link fencing and electric fencing also may be used. With any form of fencing comes the risk that stags may get their antlers caught. Cattle grids may be used to stop deer exiting enclosures via roadways, but they should be at least 2 m (preferably 3 m) wide. Shelters should be sufficient for the number of animals, and some should be partially enclosed. Trees and shrubs help provide windbreaks and cover but must be protected from bark-stripping and extensive browsing. Dead trees and logs act as rubbing posts when stags are losing their velvet.

611

TABLE 62-1

Basic Biologic Information and Conservation Status of Tragulidae, Moschidae, and Cervidae[72]

Scientific Name (number of species)	Common Name(s)	Weight Range (kg)	Distribution	Species and Subspecies of Conservation Concern
TRAGULIDAE				
Hyemoschus (1)	Water chevrotain	7–16	C and W Africa	—
Moschiola (3)	Chevrotain	2.4–3	SC and SE Asia	—
Tragulus (6)	Mouse deer	1.5–4.5	SC and SE Asia	Balabac mouse deer (*T. nigricans*) EN
MOSCHIDAE				
Moschus (7)	Musk deer	6–17	Asia	All EN (6) or VU (1)
CERVIDAE				
Capreolinae				
Alces (1)	Moose (Eur. elk)	280–600	Circumpolar	—
Blastocerus (1)	Marsh deer	70–130	S. America	VU
Capreolus (2)	Roe deer	17–50	Eurasia	
Hippocamelus (2)	Taruka, huemel	45–75	S. America	S Andean huemel (*H. bisulcus*) EN N Andean huemel (*H. antisensis*) VU
Hydropotes (1)	Chinese water deer	11–15	SE Asia	VU
Mazama (10)	Brocket	8–35	C and S America	Five species VU
Odocoileus (2)	Mule and white-tailed deer	25–130	Americas	—
Ozotoceros (1)	Pampas deer	22–40	S America	—
Pudu (2)	Pudu	5–14	S America	Both VU
Rangifer (1)	Reindeer (caribou)	55–170	Circumpolar	—
Cervinae				
Axis (4)	Axis deer (chital), hog deer	30–110	SE & S Asia	Bawean deer (*A. kuhlii*) CR Calamian deer (*A. calamianensis*) EN Hog deer (*A. porcinus*) VU
Cervus (5)	Red deer (Am. Elk), sika deer	20–400	Eurasia, N Africa, America	White-lipped deer (*C. albirostris*) VU
Dama (2)	Fallow deer	35–140	Asia	Persian fallow (*D. mesopotomica*) EN
Elaphodus (1)	Tufted deer	17–30	S Asia	—
Elaphurus (1)	Père David deer	140–220	E Asia	EW
Muntiacus (11)	Muntjac	12–35	SE and S Asia	Giant muntjac (*M. vuquangensis*) EN Black muntjac (*M. crinifrons*) VU
Rucervus (2)	Barasingha, brow-antlered (Eld's) deer	60–200	S Asia	Brow-antlered (*R. eldii*) EN Barasingha (*R. duvaucelii*) VU
Rusa (4)	Javan (rusa) and sambar deer	40–350	SE and S Asia	Phillipine spotted (*R. alfredi*) EN Others VU

C, Central; *CR*, critically endangered; *E*, east; *EN*, endangered; *EW*, extinct in the wild; *N*, north; *S*, south; *VU*, vulnerable; *W*, west.

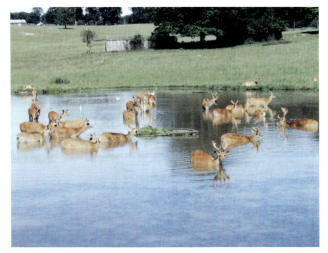

FIGURE 62-1 Swamp deer, or barasingha (*Rucervus duvaucelii*), in a large, drive-through, mixed-species enclosure.

Small, tropical species cannot be kept outdoors all year in a temperate climate and require heated housing. Many zoos keep chevrotains in nocturnal houses with reversed lighting.

FEEDING

All chevrotains and deer (musk and true) are herbivorous, but they range from species that inhabit forests and bush, for example, musk, muntjac (*Muntiacus* species), brocket (*Mazama* species), roe deer, and moose (*Alces alces*), which are browsers on dicotyledonous plant material (leaves and twigs of trees and shrubs, as well as herbs and forbs), to grazers such as fallow deer and Père David deer, which feed on monocotyledonous plant material (primarily the leaves or blades of grass). The majority of species are intermediate or mixed opportunistic feeders. The feeding habits are reflected in gastrointestinal (GI) anatomy and physiology; thus, the greater the proportion of grass and roughage in the natural diet (the grazers), the greater is the retention time of fiber in the rumen and the less frequently the animal needs to feed.[31] Grazing species also have hypsodont dentition (high-crowned teeth) adapted to abrasive wear, whereas browsers have brachyodont (low-crowned) dentition for attritional wear.[35] Browsers may produce tannin-binding and similar proteins in their saliva to neutralize the secondary compounds present in woody plants.[12] Unfortunately, the feeding of browsers in captivity has traditionally been problematic, with many species avoiding grass and grass-based forage and therefore ingesting higher proportions of concentrate pellets. This is suspected to have led to cases of chronic ruminal acidosis and ill-thrift, for example, "wasting syndrome complex" in moose,[12] and a decreased relative life-expectancy in captivity in relation to grazing species.[53] Ruminal acidosis may also be seen in wild deer that ingest large quantities of supplementary food.[63] Deer in seasonal climates, especially browsers, build up body fat during spring and summer (or wet season) to provide energy for the rut and winter (or dry season) when the quantity and nutrient quality of plants is low.

Feeding in captivity is based on management goals. For deer farmers, supplementing pasture grazing so that animals meet target weights is important, as is keeping the breeding stags and hinds in good condition for rutting or mating, pregnancy, and lactation. In zoos and deer parks, slower growth is acceptable, or even preferred, but supplementary feeding may be necessary during the winter or dry season and also for pregnant and lactating hinds and their calves. In the temperate areas of the northern hemisphere, grass paddocks and an appropriate stocking density provide energy and protein for grazing species in spring and summer, with hay offered during the fall and winter seasons and low-protein concentrates (maximum 12%) only offered if the hay is of poor quality. Indeed, excess feeding of pregnant Père David hinds may result in dystocia caused by oversized calves. Intermediate or mixed deer species require hay during the fall and winter seasons, plus additional concentrates (maximum 14% crude protein). Root crops have been used successfully for winter feeding of farmed deer. Browsers should receive a browser-specific concentrate diet (high-fiber and low-energy diet, preferably with beet pulp as a pectin source to avoid grains) plus browse (fresh, dried, or ensiled), with or without alfalfa (lucerne).[12] Easily digested energy sources such as starch are not necessary and should be avoided.[47] If the natural pattern of reduced appetite during the winter season is followed, deer may lose up to 10% of body weight because of higher energy demands (thermoregulation, activity). This weight is regained in the spring season, with juveniles especially showing a compensatory growth spurt. Deer overwintered indoors will have much lower energy requirements, so supplementary feeding may be greatly reduced.

Nutrient requirements, including minerals and vitamins, for selected deer have been published,[56] but in general, commercial cattle salt or mineral blocks are suitable, with the addition of specific minerals and vitamins if local grazing or the forage fed are deficient.

RESTRAINT AND HANDLING[20,22,29,68]

Behavioral Restraint

Captive artiodactyls, including deer, can be habituated to routine management practices and, with appropriate handling facilities and expertise (see below), it is possible to undertake simple veterinary procedures, including venipuncture, vaccination, and physical examination within restraint devices.

Physical Restraint

The correct use of appropriate physical restraint may be the safest and most efficient way to handle wild, zoo, and game-farmed deer for management, treatment, diagnostic, and research purposes, but good planning and teamwork are essential to prevent capture stress and subsequent myopathy.

Small deer may be confined in padded boxes, entrapped with the use of net-guns, or driven into collapsible nets for manual capture. However, they should only be restrained in lateral recumbency for short periods of 15 minutes or less; any longer procedure would require sedation or anesthesia. Hobbles may be applied to the

ipsilateral forelimbs and hindlimbs at the level of the metacarpophalangeal joint for safety, and the use of blindfolds may calm the animal.

Sophisticated handling systems have been designed to be used in farmed species to allow deer to be moved, separated, loaded for transport, and restrained for management and veterinary procedures.[28] Typically, collecting funnels from paddocks lead to chutes and yards with smooth, solid walls (e.g., plywood attached to metal frames), sufficiently high to prevent animals from jumping out and with viewing holes so that deer and handlers are able to see and be aware of each other. Wild deer may be encouraged into the funnels by regular feeding or by driving (e.g., by helicopter). Once inside, deer may be separated and channeled into different raceways from sorting pens that are covered to be kept dark, especially when dealing with nervous species. Particular consideration should be paid to the specific flight distances of the species to be handled. Deer held in crushes (manual or hydraulic) with a drop floor may be examined and many minimally invasive procedures carried out without causing undue stress. Male cervids and both sexes of reindeer should not be restrained when antlers are in growth because of the potential for major blood loss and severe pain associated with trauma. Once hardened, the antlers should be removed if the stags (or reindeer hinds) are to go through a handling system.

Chemical: Anesthesia

Deer are prone to capture myopathy, hyperthermia and trauma, so any anesthetic procedure should be carefully planned, taking into account the method of capture, ambient temperature, physiology of species, and clinical condition of the individual. Table 62-2 lists dose rates of commonly used chemical restraint agents, some for specific species. The data are taken from a variety of sources, from different conditions, which explains the wide ranges shown. Captive deer often have drug requirements very different from those of free-ranging animals, so this must be taken into consideration.[11] Ideally, therefore, advice should be sought from those regularly immobilizing the species of interest, and doses should be tailored to each circumstance.

Sedation alone may be unrewarding in deer, except in tamer animals such as reindeer, when an α_2-agonist such as xylazine may be injected intravenously (IV). Relatively high doses of xylazine may be administered intramuscularly (IM) to produce recumbent sedation. Excited animals may overcome the drug's sedative effects, so stimulation must be minimized during induction; the animal should be left alone until recumbent and then approached cautiously and quietly to be blindfolded. For longer or painful procedures, an intravenous bolus of ketamine (1 milligram per kilogram [mg/kg]) may be given, with additional intravenous boluses (1–2 mg/kg) as required. However, intubation and inhalation anesthesia are preferred.[11] Diazepam may be given orally (PO) before a stressful situation, but the effect of this drug is variable.

Xylazine and ketamine are still a useful combination for the immobilization of small deer. For example, an adult Chinese water deer requires approximately 1.5 milliliters (mL) of the "Hellabrun" mixture (125 mg/mL xylazine plus 100 mg/mL ketamine). Darting medium- and large-sized deer with an opioid agent is more economical and practical; etorphine hydrochloride (HCl), carfentanil citrate, or, most recently, thiafentanil oxalate, is used usually in combination with an α_2-agonist to reduce excitation, muscle tremors, and respiratory depression.[74] The choice of opioid primarily depends on availability, but all opioids can be antagonized. However, re-narcotization may occur some hours after reversal because of the shorter duration of action of some antagonists compared with the opioid drug. Animals should be monitored for 72 hours with administration of further doses of the antagonist, if necessary. Compared with the other opioids, thiafentanil oxalate has the advantages of more rapid induction (reducing chase time), equal or greater potency, and a shorter half-life, thus reducing the likelihood of re-narcotization.[39] The combination of medetomidine and ketamine is increasingly preferred because of the inherent risks in the use of opioids, and the

TABLE 62-2

Chemical Restraint Agents Used for Tragulidae, Moschidae, and Cervidae

Agent	Species	Dosage*	Reversal Agent and Dosage
Diazepam	All	0.5–2.0 milligram per kilogram (mg/kg), IV or oral[18]	Flumazenil 0.04–0.15 mg/kg
Xylazine	All White-tailed deer and mule deer Wapiti/North American elk (*Cervus canadensis*) Red deer	0.4–8.0 mg/kg, IM (½ dose IV)[18] 2.0–3.0 mg/kg, IM[10] 1.0 mg/kg, IM[10] 0.5–1.0 mg/kg, IM[11]	Yohimbine 0.10–0.20 mg/kg (half IM/half IV), or Atipamezole 0.04–0.8 mg/kg, IV (i.e., 0.1 mg/mg xylazine)
Etorphine/acepromazine	All	0.02–0.05 mg/kg; and 0.08–0.2 mg/kg, IM[18]	Diprenorphine 0.027–0.066 mg/kg, IV
Etorphine/acepromazine/xylazine	All	0.01–0.06 mg/kg; 0.04–0.24 mg/kg; and 0.25–0.60 mg/kg, IM[18]	Diprenorphine for etorphine, 0.013–0.08 mg/kg, IV Yohimbine or atipamezole for xylazine
Carfentanil	All	0.006–0.03 mg/kg, IM[18]	Diprenorphine 0.06–0.3 mg/kg, or naltrexone 0.06–0.3 mg/kg
Carfentanil/xylazine	Wapiti/North American elk	0.01 mg/kg; and 0.1 mg/kg, IM[52]	Naltrexone for carfentanil
Thiafentanil	White-tailed deer Moose	3 mg total dose[39] 10 mg total dose[39]	Naltrexone 10 mg/mg thiafentanil, IM
Thiafentanil/xylazine	Wapiti/North American elk Mule deer	12–15 mg thiafentanil, and 50 mg xylazine, IM[39] 10–12 mg thiafentanil; and 100 mg xylazine, IM; or 0.15–0.20 mg/kg thiafentanil and 100 mg xylazine, IM[39]	Naltrexone for thiafentanil
Xylazine/ketamine	All White-tailed deer and mule deer Wapiti/North American elk	0.5–23 mg/kg and 2.7–18.7 mg/kg IM[18] 2.0 mg/kg, and 3–4 mg/kg IM[10] 1.0 mg/kg, and 3–4 mg/kg IM[10]	Yohimbine or atipamezole for xylazine
Medetomidine/ketamine	All Red deer Moose Reindeer/caribou	0.05–0.10 mg/kg and 0.8–3.2 mg/kg, IM[18] 0.11 mg/kg; and 2.2 mg/kg, IM[3] 0.06 mg/kg, and 1.5 mg/kg IM[4] 0.1 mg/kg, and 2.5 mg/kg IM[2]	Atipamezole 0.25–0.5 mg/kg, split IV and IM (i.e., 5 mg/mg medetomidine)
Tiletamine/zolazepam	All	2.9–20 mg/kg, IM (33 mg/kg, IM, for fallow)[18]	Flumazenil, 0.11–0.77 mg/kg
Tiletamine/zolazepam/xylazine	White-tailed deer and mule deer Moose	4.4 mg/kg; and 2.2 mg/kg, IM[54] 3.0 mg/kg; and 1.5 mg/kg, IM[11]	Yohimbine or atipamezole for xylazine
Tiletamine/zolazepam/medetomidine	All Fallow deer	0.7–1.3 mg/kg, and 0.08–0.12 mg/kg IM[18] 1.0 mg/kg, and 0.1 mg/kg IM[17]	Flumazenil 0.03–0.1 mg/kg Atipamezole 0.4–0.6 mg/kg, split IV and IM
Butorphanol/azaperone/medetomidine (BAM)	White-tailed deer and mule deer Wapiti/North American elk	0.58 mg/kg; and 0.37 mg/kg; and 0.19 mg/kg, IM[9] 0.11 mg/kg; and 0.07 mg/kg; and 0.05 mg/kg, IM[9]	Atipamezole 3.0 mg/mg medetomidine; and naltrexone 50 mg/ butorphanol 30 mg, IM

*IV, Intravenously; IM, intramuscularly.

lower required dose of ketamine compared with the xylazine–ketamine mixture.[33] The tiletamine–zolazepam combination results in a long recovery period, unless the zolazepam is reversed with flumazenil. Alternatively, as flumazenil is expensive, a lower dose of tiletamine–zolazepam may be used with xylazine or medetomidine, and recovery, after reversal of the α_2-agonist, is much quicker. This combination is reported to be ideal for the immobilization of fallow deer.[17] Since 2008, the combination of butorphanol, azaperone, and medetomidine (BAM) has been frequently used in hoofstock. Hyperthermia is avoided, and excellent respiration and good muscle relaxation are achieved. Reversal following injections of atipamezole (3 mg/1 mg medetomidine) and naltrexone (50 mg/30 mg butorphanol) is usually complete within 10 minutes. Over 1000 white-tailed deer (*Odocoileus virginianus*) have been anesthetized successfully with BAM, but results in fallow deer have been disappointing.[9]

After induction, deer should be positioned in sternal recumbency, with the neck extended but the nose pointing slightly toward the ground, to maintain a patent airway and to reduce the likelihood of aspiration of any regurgitated ruminal contents and development of ruminal tympany. Ideally, deer should be intubated (see below) and given supplemental oxygen; if not, oxygen may be provided via nasal insufflation (to the level of the medial canthus of the eye). In either case, oxygen flow is adjusted to maintain saturation of peripheral oxygen (SpO_2) of 95% or greater. Intubation may be difficult in deer because of the depth of the larynx, the narrowness of the buccal cavity, and the long and mobile epiglottis but is facilitated by correct positioning, the use of a long laryngoscope, a stylet to stiffen the endotracheal tube, and increasing anesthetic depth with an intravenous bolus of ketamine (1–2 mg/kg) or propofol (2–4 mg/kg).

For elective inhalation anesthesia, food should be withheld for 24 to 36 hours and water for 12 hours prior to induction. The principles of anesthesia and monitoring are the same as for domestic ruminants. At the end of all procedures during which the animal was intubated, extubation, with the cuff still partially inflated, should only be performed once the swallowing reflex has returned. When reversing α_2-agonists, the appropriate agents should be divided and half-doses given IM and IV.[10]

Capture myopathy is a potentially life-threatening complication of anesthesia that may present in acute, subacute, or chronic forms. Treatment is based around the correction of shock and acid–base balance, the maintenance of normothermia, and oxygenation. Results are generally unrewarding, so prevention is better and is achieved by ensuring that the animals are not deficient in vitamin E and selenium and by minimizing the duration of chase and restraint.[11,59]

Chemical: Neuroleptics

Two classes of human antipsychotic drugs (butyrophenones and phenothiazines) have been used as tranquilizers in wild animals since the 1980s for loading, transportation, and acclimatization. These drugs reduce dopamine neurotransmission, which minimizes stress and reduces the risk of trauma and capture myopathy. However, extrapyramidal side effects may occur. The butyrophenones azaperone and haloperidol, injected IM or IV, are shorter-acting (up to 72 hours), and azaperone (0.2 mg/kg) may be given immediately after anesthetic reversal for short translocations (<6 hours). The phenothiazines are slower in onset but longer-acting and may only be given IM.[25] Zuclopenthixol acetate (1 mg/kg) has been shown to reduce flight distance and stress and increase water and food consumption.[61] Zuclopenthixol acetate lasts up to 4 days, perphenazine enanthate up to 10 days, and pipothiazine palmitate up to 21 days, with their time to onset of action correspondingly long. Therefore, they are often used in combination.

SURGERY

Common procedures that require anesthesia are the amputation of antlers, investigation of lameness or preventive hoof work, treatment of dystocia, and, if necessary, cesarean section. These and other surgical procedures are the same as performed in domestic ruminants. Local anesthesia may be useful to produce "ring block" and effective analgesia for the removal of antlers in velvet (either complete, or partial following traumatic injury), and this is preferable to antler pedicle compression.[34]

PHYSICAL EXAMINATION AND DIAGNOSTICS

The diagnostic process for investigating disease in chevrotains, musk deer, and true deer is no different from that in other ruminants but takes into account the unique anatomic and physiologic features mentioned earlier. Blood samples usually are collected from the jugular vein or the ventral coccygeal vein. Tables 62-3 and 62-4 list selected hematologic and biochemical parameters. Interpretation of results should take into consideration the method of capture,[46] handling, time delays after collection,[41] and also differences between sexes and age categories.[64]

DISEASE[6,14,15,18,23,55,73]

Infectious Microbial Diseases

Table 62-5 outlines the major microbial infectious diseases, but two diseases deserve further discussion.

Chronic wasting disease (CWD), a unique transmissible spongiform encephalopathy (TSE), has emerged as an important health problem in free-ranging and captive cervid populations in North America,[51] including mule deer (*Odocoileus hemionus*), white-tailed

Text continued on p. 621

TABLE 62-3

Reference Ranges for Hematologic Parameters of Selected Tragulidae, Moschidae, and Cervidae

Parameter	Tragulus napu	Moschus moschiferus*	Odocoileus virginianus	Pudu puda	Rangifer tarandus	Axis axis	Cervus elaphus	Muntiacus reevesi
Red blood cell count ($\times 10^6$/microliter (µL))	61.9–168.3	10–12	8.2–15.8	7.8–11.0	8.8–11.6	7.4–15.7	6.6–10.6	8.6–21.9
Hemoglobin, gram per deciliter (g/dL)	11.0–15.6	14–18	11.5–16.7	12.6–17.6	13.5–20.1	10.6–19.4	10.8–18.2	11.7–17.7
Hematocrit (%)	37.6–59.6	39–51	31.2–49.4	35.4–51.8	38.8–55.2	31.4–57.0	31.7–50.1	33.1–50.5
Mean corpuscular volume (fL)	2.5†–46.3	36–42	24.1–47.3	41.2–53.0	42.4–52.6	23.4–57.4	40.4–58.4	12.2–54.8
Mean corpuscular hemoglobin, picogram (pg)	0.8†–14.3	13–15	8.3–16.3	14.0–19.0	15.3–18.7	8.0–20.4	14.0–20.6	4.6–19.2

Continued

TABLE 62-3

Reference Ranges for Hematologic Parameters of Selected Tragulidae, Moschidae, and Cervidae—cont'd

Parameter	Tragulus napu	Moschus moschiferus*	Odocoileus virginianus	Pudu puda	Rangifer tarandus	Axis axis	Cervus elaphus	Muntiacus reevesi
Mean corpuscular hemoglobin concentration (g/dL)	21.8–32.6	33–39	32.8–37.8	30.3–38.3	31.8–38.4	27.2–40.4	31.0–38.0	31.2–40.0
White blood cell count (×10³/µL)	5.32–16.36	1–5	1.82–5.26	4.91–10.19	2.41–8.51	2.16–6.40	2.43–6.85	2.63–8.13
Segmented neutrophils (×10³/µL)	1.73–7.37	0.2–1.8	0.50–3.58	1.43–4.66	0.68–5.42	0.37–4.54	0.97–4.51	1.07–5.40
Lymphocytes (×10³/µL)	2.29–7.79	0.5–2.5	0.54–1.91	2.08–5.70	0.55–3.22	0.62–2.40	0.50–2.35	0.63–3.23
Monocytes (×10³/µL)	0.05†–1.20	0.1–0.3	0.01†–0.26	0.09–0.63	0.00–0.43	0.00†–0.32	0.02–0.35	0.00†–0.40
Eosinophils (×10³/µL)	0.09–0.92	0.0–0.1	0.0–0.54	0.06–0.68	0.03–0.78	0.00†–0.29	0.00†–0.88	0.00†–0.27
Basophils (×10³/µL)	0.00†–0.44	0.0–0.1	0.01–0.08	0.04–0.16	0.00–0.23	0.01–0.06	0.00†–0.21	0.01–0.11
Platelets (×10³/µL)	No data	23–277	287–583	115–435	275–521	26–570	83–509	160–422

Note: Data from ISIS[32] except where marked *.
*Data from San Diego Zoo Global clinical data.
Range = one standard deviation below to one above the mean, except where the standard deviation was larger than the mean (marked †), in which case the lower value is the minimum value in the dataset. Data submitted by between 10 and 40 collections, depending on species.

TABLE 62-4

Reference Ranges for Biochemical Parameters of Selected Tragulidae, Moschidae, and Cervidae

Parameter	Tragulus napu	Moschus moschiferus*	Odocoileus virginianus	Pudu puda	Rangifer tarandus	Axis axis	Cervus elaphus	Muntiacus reevesi
Total protein, gram per deciliter (g/dL)	6.2–8.0	6–7	5.1–7.1	6.7–9.1	5.7–8.1	5.8–7.2	5.8–7.4	5.4–7.2
Globulin (g/dL)	2.4–4.6	—	2.3–4.7	3.3–5.7	2.5–4.3	2.7–3.9	2.2–3.8	2.1–3.5
Albumin (g/dL)	3.2–4.8	4–5	1.9–3.5	2.7–3.9	2.8–4.2	2.7–3.9	2.9–4.3	2.7–4.3
Calcium, milligram per deciliter (mg/dL)	9.2–11.2	7–9	8.0–9.8	8.1–10.3	8.9–10.9	8.0–10.2	8.5–10.5	8.3–10.7
Phosphorus (mg/dL)	4.7–9.9	4–8	5.9–10.9	7.8–12.2	5.4–9.4	5.9–10.7	5.5–9.7	7.4–12.2
Sodium, milliequivalent per deciliter (mEq/L)	142–156	145–155	140–148	145–155	139–149	141–151	139–147	144–158
Potassium (mEq/L)	3.5–5.7	3–5	3.4–5.2	4.8–7.0	3.8–5.6	4.7–6.7	4.2–5.4	4.6–7.4
Chloride (mEq/L)	103–113	108–117	97–109	95–105	95–105	99–107	98–106	101–113
BUN (mg/dL)	20–34	30–48	17–37	24–40	20–56	19–31	17–33	22–38
Creatinine (mg/dL)	0.7–1.3	0.9–1.5	1.1–2.1	0.8–1.4	1.1–2.1	1.5–2.5	1.2–2.6	0.9–1.7
Glucose (mg/dL)	78–168	120–230	83–201	74–126	69–175	87–269	112–214	93–237
Cholesterol (mg/dL)	17–61	—	45–85	54–114	46–90	83–155	37–81	86–158
CPK, international unit per liter (IU/L)	35–651	150–690	58†–1599	79†–1445	11†–773	8†–1876	38†–515	97†–2444
LDH (IU/L)	702–1982	760–1295	370–1030	234–1204	244–994	48–1702	157–947	56–2736
AP (IU/L)	48–300	7–730	0†–443	31–1187	8†–774	11†–641	7†–469	18†–568
ALT (IU/L)	8–20	7–40	26–66	40–76	7–77	16–46	11–67	13–49
AST (IU/L)	27–117	395–955	11–337	88–160	47–127	28–140	38–96	41–249
GGT (IU/L)	9–33	17–35	32–122	21†–254	1†–263	6†–298	11–77	6†–306
Amylase, unit per liter (Unit/L)	28–110	50–90	34†–709	45–389	13†–216	5†–2981	25–127	24–204
Fibrinogen (mg/dL)	61–361	—	0†–216	51–367	61–463	69–483	65–615	99–363

ALT, Alanine aminotransferase; *AP,* alkaline phosphatase; *AST,* aspartate aminotransferase; *BUN,* blood urea nitrogen; *CPK,* creatinine phosphokinase; *GGT,* gamma glutamyltransferase; *LDH,* lactic acid dehydrogenase.
Note: Data from ISIS[32] except where marked *.
*Data from San Diego Zoo Global clinical data.
Range = one standard deviation below to one above the mean, except where the standard deviation was larger than the mean (marked †), in which case the lower value is the minimum value in the dataset. Data submitted by between 10 and 40 collections, depending on species.

TABLE 62-5

Selected Infectious Diseases of Tragulidae, Moschidae, and Cervidae

Disease	Causative Agent	Epizootiology	Signs	Diagnosis	Management
PRION					
Chronic wasting disease (CWD)[8,30,51]	CWD prion; single or multiple strains of cervid-associated proteinaceous infectious agent	Poorly understood, suspect fecal-oral route Incubation period at least a year	Depression, subtle behavioral changes, ataxia, head tremor, hyperexcitability or esthesia, abnormal tongue movement and swallowing and progressive weight loss	History of contact with deer from CWD areas; clinical signs; histopathologic lesions; immunohistochemistry	No treatment Cull and restock, but may be unsuccessful Avoid movement of deer from CWD areas Vaccination in the future?
VIRAL					
Bluetongue[44,66,69]	Bluetongue virus; an orbivirus with at least 24 serotypes described	Endemic in tropics and subtropics *Culicoides* spp. vectors Recent emergence of BTV8 in northwest Europe with overwintering and seasonal pattern of disease Cervids known to be susceptible	Hemorrhage and ulceration of the muzzle, oral cavity and teats, epiphora and periocular inflammation, transient but severe corneal edema, limb edema	History and clinical signs, histopathologic examination, PCR test and serologic examination	Vector control, restriction of live ruminant movements, vaccination
Deer alpha-herpesviruses[37]	Cervine herpesvirus 1 and 2, plus other α-herpesviruses	Direct or indirect transmission via body secretions	Pyrexia and conjunctivitis with or without corneal opacity and nasal discharge Usually resolves	Clinical signs, virus isolation, serology (multiple ruminant herpesviruses), and immunofluorescence (multiple α-herpesvirus antigens	No treatment; antibiotics to treat secondary bacterial infections
Epizootic hemorrhagic disease of deer (EHD)	EHD virus	Transmitted by vectors, usually *Culicoides* spp. White-tailed deer are susceptible, red and fallow deer appear resistant	Pyrexia, mucopurulent nasal discharge, swollen tongue, subcutaneous edema, and death	Widespread hemorrhages at necropsy, histopathologic examination, virus isolation, and serologic examination	Serological test before importing deer
Foot-and-mouth disease (FMD)[62]	FMD virus	Aerosol transmission primarily; also indirect transfer and ingestion Disease progression and transmission risk varies between species	Anorexia, lethargy, copious salivation and nasal discharge associated with mucosal vesicles and erosions; lameness with digital lesions Disease varies across species (e.g., North American elk appears resistant)	History and clinical signs; virus detection (electron microscopy, isolation and PCR) from vesicles or pharyngeal swabs; serologic examination	In FMD-free countries, cases and in-contact animals are culled, but wild deer are not normally included In enzootic areas, deer may be vaccinated

Continued

TABLE 62-5

Selected Infectious Diseases of Tragulidae, Moschidae, and Cervidae—cont'd

Disease	Causative Agent	Epizootiology	Signs	Diagnosis	Management
Malignant catarrhal fever (MCF)[36,40,70]	MCF-associated γ-herpesviruses: ovine herpesvirus 2 (OvHV-2), alcelaphine herpesvirus 1 (AHV-1), caprine herpesvirus 2 (CpHV-2), and possibly other related viruses	Direct or indirect contact with sheep, goats, or wildebeest at or around parturition, or with their young. At least 17 deer species susceptible in captivity, but Père David deer particularly so	Sudden death; dysentery, oculonasal discharge and erosions, corneal opacity or edema with fibrin clots in the anterior chamber, and neurologic signs. Or subacute, nonfatal disease with anorexia, depression, hematuria, weight loss, and chronic dermatitis	Generalized lymphadenopathy at necropsy. Lymphoid infiltration and vasculitis on histopathologic examination, plus presence of MCF virus DNA detected by PCR	Keep susceptible deer species away from sheep, goats, and wildebeest, and avoid indirect contact. Serologic surveys just indicate exposure
BACTERIAL					
Anthrax[16]	*Bacillus anthracis*	Ingestion of spores, enteritis, and bacteremia; contamination of soil with resistant spores after death. Certain deer appear to be highly susceptible	Sudden death or peracute pyrexia, dehydration, and diarrhea or constipation, collapse, and death	History of previous cases. Check suspect cases for presence of organism in blood film. If necropsied, the carcass is toxemic: blood oozing from orifices, bloody fluid in body cavities with or without engorged spleen. Culture and/or PCR by veterinary authorities	Treat with intravenous penicillin in epizootic. Identify and fence contaminated pastures and waterways. Vaccination is possible
Brucellosis[58,67]	*Brucella* species	Ingestion of organism from abortions or calving; directly or indirectly	Abortions; birth of weak calves; swellings of joints and tendon sheaths	Clinical signs; serologic examination; culture	Cull infected animals. Vaccinate against *Brucella abortus* strain 19 or RB51
Clostridial blackleg	*Clostridium chauvoei*	Contamination of deep anaerobic wounds	Sudden death or peracute stiffness, anorexia, depression, collapse, and death	History; severe muscle necrosis; presence of *C. chauvoei* in smears, FA test, or culture	Reduce stocking density and rest contaminated pastures. Avoid sudden changes in diet. Vaccinate with multivalent clostridial vaccine
Clostridial enterotoxemia	*Clostridium perfringens* type D	Fecal–oral transmission, especially on heavily stocked pasture; triggered by change in nutrition, especially low-to-high plane	Sudden death or peracute disease: profound depression and rapid collapse and death	History and clinical signs; toxemic carcass with straw-colored fluid in body cavities, pulpy kidneys, and glucose in the urine; ε-toxin in the intestinal contents (ELISA or mouse inoculation)	Treat as for blackleg
Clostridial gas gangrene/ malignant edema	*Clostridium* spp.	Contamination of wounds; more likely with heavily contaminated pasture and in stags during rut	Sudden death or peracute fever, depression, collapse, and death	History; muscle necrosis with gas extending from wound site; presence of *Clostridium* species in smears (FA) or culture	Treat as for blackleg. Reduce the incidence of traumatic injuries

Disease	Etiologic Agent	Epidemiology	Clinical Signs	Diagnosis	Treatment/Prevention
Johne disease[13,43,45]	*Mycobacterium avium paratuberculosis* (MAP), multiple strains. The organism may persist in the environment for more than a year.	Fecal–oral transmission, normally in first 6 months of life, or in utero. Bacteria survive >1 year in environment. Long prepatent phase; systemic disease in adults. All species are susceptible	Affected animals >1 year old, usually much older. Loss of body condition/wasting, poor coat, occasionally diarrhea. Captive cervids appear to deteriorate more rapidly than free-ranging	Clinical signs, necropsy findings: thickening of terminal ileum with erosions, petechiae and white foci, enlargement of mesenteric nodes; histopathology; detection of MAP by acid-fast stains, PCR, culture, serology	Treatment impractical and unrewarding. Infection-free herd: strict quarantine and testing of all incoming deer. Infected herd: test feces and sera, and cull positives, or vaccinate calves before 48 hours old
Lumpy jaw	*Actinomyces bovis*	Organism survives in environment. Entry is through buccal mucosa	Swelling of mandible and/or maxilla with granulomata, pus-filled tracts, and sinuses	Clinical signs. Organism found in pus. Stained smears (sulfur granules) or culture	Treat with antibiotics. Provide local debridement and cleaning
Meningoencephalitis	Bacteria and fungi, including *Listeria monocytogenes*, *Streptococcus*, *Staphylococcus*, and *Actinomyces* species	Ingestion and hematogenous spread to brain, or direct entry from trauma, especially to antler	Pyrexia, neurologic signs, recumbency, and death	Clinical signs; edema and hemorrhage in brain; histopathologic lesions; culture of relevant organism	Give broad-spectrum antibiotics and nurse animal to health
Necrobacillosis	*Fusobacterium necrophorum*	Organism survives in environment. Enters through mucosae of mouth, umbilicus, rumen, interdigital skin, etc.	Variable; swollen jaw, lameness, depression, and anorexia with or without death	Clinical signs: necrotic lesions with foul smell; presence of organism in smears or on culture	Give local and systemic antibiotics. Provide local debridement. Reduce stocking density, avoid muddy areas in paddocks, and reduce injuries to the mouth, feet, etc.
Neonatal enteritis	*Escherichia coli*, *Clostridium perfringens*, and *Salmonella* species, plus *Rotavirus* and *Cryptosporidium parvum*	Fecal–oral transmission. Increases in incidence with contamination, increased stocking density, and/or failure of colostrum transfer	Acute diarrhea in first few days of life; dehydration and death	History and clinical signs; fecal culture	Treat with fluids with or without antibiotics if appropriate. Reduce stocking density. Allow hinds plenty of areas for calving

Continued

TABLE 62-5

Selected Infectious Diseases of Tragulidae, Moschidae, and Cervidae—cont'd

Disease	Causative Agent	Epizootiology	Signs	Diagnosis	Management
Pasteurellosis	*Pasteurella multocida; Mannheimia haemolytica*	Aerosol transmission; clinical disease often associated with other factors; respiratory form with other pathogens; septicemic form after stress	*P. multocida:* suppurative bronchopneumonia with or without rhinitis: nasal discharge, dullness, anorexia, pyrexia, tachypnea/dyspnea *M. haemolytica:* septicemia: sudden death or acute depression and pyrexia	History and clinical signs; auscultation of pneumonic lungs; necropsy findings; culture from lungs or blood	Treat cases with antibiotics, keep warm and well-ventilated, and treat other infections Reduce overcrowding and stress Give prophylactic antibiotics before transport
Salmonellosis	*Salmonella* species	Fecal–oral transmission, but disease usually secondary to stress and overcrowding	Anorexia and listlessness with or without dysentery, recumbency, and death	History and clinical signs; enteritis, widespread congestion, and necrosis; culture	Provide oral rehydration and antibiotics (based on culture/sensitivity) Reduce stress
Tetanus	*Clostridium tetani*	Spores in deep anaerobic wounds germinate and produce toxin May follow castration or velvet harvest	Stiffness, muscle tremors, spasms, hyperesthesia, drooling saliva, recumbency, and death	Clinical signs; presence of a deep wound and organism	Treat with penicillin and antitoxin with or without sedation Vaccinate with tetanus toxoid
Tuberculosis (TB)[48,49,71]	*Mycobacterium bovis, M. tuberculosis* complex (MTC)	Transmitted in aerosols and other secretions, especially when crowded and confined	Variable; localized lymph node swelling, acute respiratory distress with or without death, weakness, and chronic emaciation	Antemortem testing: multi-modal approach, and cautious interpretation Clinical and necropsy findings; detection of *M. bovis* by acid-fast and immunohistochemical stains, PCR, and culture ("gold standard"); tuberculin skin test, antigen-stimulation tests, and serologic tests for herds	Maintain herd TB-free Testing and culling positive animals to establish TB-free status Only import animals from other TB-free herds, and continue to isolate and test
Yersiniosis	*Yersinia pseudotuberculosis*	Fecal–oral transmission carried and excreted by many wild mammals and birds Survives in wet and cold Affects calves in first winter or when stressed such as by handling and change in diet	Sudden death or anorexia and green watery diarrhea with or without blood; dehydration and death Outbreaks with high mortality seen in cervids	History and clinical signs; necropsy: hemorrhagic gastroenteritis and edematous mesenteric lymph nodes, culture and PCR	Treat with antibiotics and fluids Reduce stress Vaccine available in some countries

ELISA, Enzyme-linked immunosorbent assay; *FA,* fluorescent antibody; *PCR,* polymerase chain reaction.

deer, and moose. Although vertical transmission is experimentally possible, fecal–oral transmission is the likelier natural mode, with movement of infected animals being the main cause of geographic spread. Clinical signs are subtle and nonspecific, so diagnosis relies on finding spongiform lesions in histologic sections of the brain or by using positive immunohistochemistry on brain and lymphoid tissues for CWD-associated prion protein (PrP).[51] Enzyme-linked immunosorbent assay (ELISA) has been used for field screening, but treatment and vaccination are still in development.

Cervid tuberculosis (TB) continues to be an important disease in captive and free-ranging populations worldwide, with *Mycobacterium bovis* isolated from a range of cervid species.[49] Intradermal TB testing is fraught with problems, and certain species, including reindeer, commonly show nonspecific reactions.[49] Serologic testing has shown promise but still has to be developed and validated.[71] Zoological institutions should perform regular TB testing on all cervids, including all incoming animals, using tuberculin skin testing in combination with at least one ancillary test. Any animal with suspicious clinical signs should be investigated thoroughly with the use of radiography, bronchial lavage for acid-fast stain, culture and polymerase chain reaction (PCR) test, blood sampling for immunoassays, and possibly lymph node biopsy for acid-fast stain, histology, culture, and PCR.[49]

Parasitic Diseases

Table 62-6 lists the most important parasitic diseases of deer. However, this list is far from exhaustive; for example, deer also may be hosts to lice (e.g., *Damalinia* sp.), ticks, mange mites (e.g., *Sarcoptes* and *Demodex* sp.), and keds, the populations of all of which may increase greatly during winter if the herd has limited shelter. Clinical signs include pruritus and hair loss, and in the chronic forms of mange, skin thickening also may occur. Tick-bite toxicosis has been described.

Noninfectious Diseases

Deer tolerate the climates in their natural habitats, but temperate species are susceptible to hyperthermia during summer in Australia, whereas tropical species lose condition and may die during extended cold and wet weather in the United Kingdom. Suitable, and sufficient, shelters are essential in both cases. Hypothermia or exposure is a common cause of neonatal mortality among tropical species in the United Kingdom, unless they are managed to prevent winter births, whereas starvation or maternal neglect, predation, and neonatal septicemia are more common causes of death among temperate species.

Deer often suffer from traumatic injuries. During rut, stags commonly receive puncture wounds to the face, neck, forelimbs, and thorax, but hinds also may be injured. Wild deer are commonly hit by motor vehicles and may need to be euthanized because of severe injuries. Captive deer hurt themselves running into fences when startled or during poorly executed capture procedures. Capture myopathy is a common sequel to physical capture and other stressful events (see Restraint and Handling), and in extreme cases, deer die rapidly from capture stress. Survivors may suffer from myopathy, with or without nephritis, and hemoglobinuria for 24 to 48 hours and take weeks to recover. Lameness may follow fighting or be caused by infections such as *Fusobacterium necrophorum* infection or by laminitis, solar bruising (if animals are brought onto concrete yards from grass), or interdigital foreign bodies.

Deer may be affected by many of the same nutritional diseases as those seen in domestic ruminants. Energy deficiency is common in temperate region winters because of reduced intake and increased demands, and exotic species will require supplementation. Native species may cope well unless they have additional energy demands, for example, heavy GI parasitism. In contrast, in reindeer, which naturally survive long periods without food, maintaining normal feeding over winter has been implicated in poor fertility. Accidental overfeeding of grains may cause rumen overload and acidosis, and any sudden change of diet may trigger clostridial disease. A high-protein diet is also one possible cause of abomasal and duodenal ulcers. These are reported primarily from farmed deer, and other suggested causes include stress, ingestion of sharp roughage, erosion or infection of parasite nodules, and fungal toxins.

Copper deficiency may lead to many of the same clinical signs as in cattle and sheep, but proving the cause is often difficult. Pasture copper levels may be low, or the deficiency may be secondary to high concentrations of other elements (molybdenum, sulfur, or iron), to heavy gastrointestinal helminth infestations, or both. Enzootic ataxia is recognized in deer, usually in yearlings and adults. Excess magnesium has been associated with urinary stone formation. Deer fed on apparently balanced, high-quality feeds may suffer from hypocalcemia and hypomagnesemia, likely caused by chronic subclinical ruminitis and the resultant impaired mineral absorption. In these animals, muscle fasciculations and tetany often occur after anesthesia and should not be confused with re-narcotization. Other signs include dystocia, weak calves, laminitis, abnormal hoof growth, and poor coat and body condition.[50] Selenium deficiency in farmed deer may occur in areas where sheep also are affected. Deer show ill-thrift and have a pale, unkempt coat. In contrast, deer appear to be less susceptible than sheep to cobalt deficiency.

Although deer are selective feeders, cases of oak poisoning (*Quercus* species) have been reported after heavy falls of acorns, and oilseed rape (*Brassica napus*), ragwort (*Senecio jacobaea*), and foxglove (*Digitalis purpurea*) have caused deaths of deer in the United Kingdom. Mycotoxicosis, caused by ingestion of tall fescue (*Festuca arundinacea*) infected by the endophytic fungus *Acremonium coenophialum* is suspected to be the cause of fat necrosis (which may resemble neoplasia), reported in swamp deer (barasingha, *Rucervus duvaucelii*), brow-antlered or Eld deer (*Rucervus eldii*), and Javan deer (*Rusa timorensis*). Liver failure and facial eczema were reported in fallow deer, but not in red deer, that ingested sporodesmin, present in the spores of the fungus *Pithomyces chartarum*.

A large number of neoplasms have been described previously.[1]

DIFFERENTIAL DIAGNOSIS

Sudden death may be caused by microbial infections such as malignant catarrhal fever (MCF), clostridial diseases, pasteurellosis (particularly following transport or other stress), and yersiniosis (especially in weaned calves). Anthrax may occur sporadically, but in some areas, it may be a frequent, often seasonal problem. Nonmicrobial causes include heavy lungworm infestations, overwhelming liver fluke infection (especially in roe deer), and acute stress or peracute capture myopathy. Loss of condition may be caused by tuberculosis or paratuberculosis (Johne disease) and by chronic parasitism (especially liver fluke or GI nematodiasis), malnutrition (e.g., copper deficiency), or chronic wasting disease. Individual animals may lose condition with many infectious and noninfectious diseases, including neoplasms.

Signs of respiratory disease are seen with bacterial, viral, and fungal pneumonias, heavy *Dictyocaulus* infestations, nasal bots, neoplasms, or as part of generalized infections such as tuberculosis and MCF. Inhalation pneumonia may occur in bottle-fed calves or following regurgitation in immobilized animals. Chronic pleurisy or pleuropneumonia may be sequelae to trauma to the thorax, especially fighting injuries and road traffic accidents.

Green, watery diarrhea, possibly with blood, is seen commonly in cases of acute yersiniosis. Similar soft or watery feces also may be a sign of GI nematodiasis, particularly when the animals are also losing weight and have fecal soiling around the anus, tail, and hindlegs. Dysentery may be a feature of MCF and enterotoxemia, although death often occurs before changes in feces occur, and of shock-induced hemorrhagic enteritis. Chronic cases of paratuberculosis may include intermittent diarrhea, but this is less characteristic than the severe loss of condition. Similar, but usually more subtle, signs are a feature of copper deficiency. Diarrhea is also a presenting sign of bovine viral diarrhea. The disease is uncommon in deer, but cases with lameness, weakness, and dehydration, but not oral ulceration,

TABLE 62-6

Selected Parasitic Diseases of Tragulidae, Moschidae, and Cervidae

Disease	Causative Agent	Location In Host		Diagnosis	Management
		Adult	**Immature**		
Babesiosis[7,75]	*Babesia capreoli, B. odocoeli, B. venatorum* (EU1), and possibly *B. divergens*	Tick vector: *Ixodes ricinus* (*B. capreoli* and *venatorum*), *I. scapularis* (*B. odocoeli*)	Erythrocytes	History of movement of susceptible deer to enzootic area; clinical signs; serologic examination; Giemsa stained blood smears; PCR	Treat with babesiocidal drugs. Maintain enzootic stability
Cerebrospinal and tissue nematodiasis	*Elaphostrongylus cervi, Parelaphostrongylus tenuis,* and *P. andersoni,* and *Pneumostrongylus tenuis*	Muscle fascia and meninges of brain and spinal cord	Intermediate hosts: slugs and snails. Larvae are ingested from infected pasture, penetrate intestinal wall, and migrate to the muscles and central nervous system	Nervous signs and death in susceptible species; first-stage larvae in feces; usually subclinical in natural host species	Treat with anthelmintics
Deer warble[65]	*Hypoderma diana* and *H. tarandi*	Free-living. *H. tarandi* naturally infects reindeer but may infect red deer	Larvae migrate through body, develop in spinal canal, and finish growth in subcutaneous tissues of back; they pupate on the ground	Clinical signs: swellings along back; identification of larvae	Treat with avermectins or organophosphates
Gastrointestinal parasitism	Abomasal: ostertagids such as *Ostertagia* spp., *Spiculopteragia* spp., and *Haemonchus* spp. and *Trichostrongylus axei*	Abomasum	Eggs passed in feces and three larval stages free-living on pasture. Ingested by the host, with further larval development in the abomasal or intestinal walls	History of pasture use. Clinical signs: reduced weight gain or loss of body condition. Diarrhea not always present. Fecal egg count (FEC) often but not always raised (e.g., abomasitis from type II ostertagiasis). Elevated plasma pepsinogen (abomasal damage only). Parasitic nodules in abomasum and high worm counts	Treat individual and herd with anthelmintics. Monitor herd FEC, and treat when FEC rises above a threshold or routinely at preparturition (hinds), growing period (calves), and prewinter (all). Reduce stocking density, or move to clean pasture in early summer
	Small intestine: other *Trichostrongylus* spp., *Bunostomum, Nematodirus,* and *Cooperia* spp. plus coccidia	Small intestine	Bunostomum may penetrate the skin and migrate through the body. Coccidial sporozoites develop in resistant oocysts that are ingested	As above	As above
	Large intestine: *Oesophagostomum* and *Trichuris* spp.	Large intestine	*Trichuris* larvae develop in resistant eggs that are ingested	As above	As above
Liver fluke	*Fascioloides magna* and *Fasciola hepatica*	Liver	Liver. Immature stages in snails	History of access to snail habitats; loss of condition and signs of liver failure; ova in feces	Treat with anti-trematode drugs. Fence off snail habitats
Lungworm	*Dictyocaulus* species	Bronchial tree	Ova are coughed up the trachea, swallowed, and passed in feces. Immature larvae on pasture are ingested. Migration occurs from gastrointestinal tract through liver to lungs	Clinical signs: reduced appetite, loss of weight and condition; tachypnea or dyspnea, often not coughing; larvae in feces. Adults found during necropsy	Monitor fecal larval count and treat with anthelmintics if positive. Provide routine worming of hinds prepartum and young calves
Nasal bots	*Cephenemyia* species	Nasal cavities and pharyngeal pockets	Nasal cavities	Snoring respiration; often subclinical	Treat with avermectins
Nodular verminous pneumonia	Protostrongylids such as *Varestrongylus capreoli, V. sagittus,* and *Muellerius* species	Lungs	As for *Dictyocaulus,* but slugs and snails act as intermediate hosts	Larvae in feces. Nodules in lungs found during necropsy. Adult worms present	Usually subclinical, but, if a factor in disease, treat with anthelmintics

have been reported. Neonatal enteritis is a frequent problem among farmed deer and is caused by the same pathogens as in domestic ruminants, particularly *Escherichia coli*, rotavirus, and *Cryptosporidium parvum*. *Campylobacter jejuni* is sometimes found in fecal samples from calves dying after the neonatal period, but the significance is not clear.

Neurologic signs in deer may be caused by tetanus, bacterial meningoencephalitis (especially listeriosis), MCF, chronic wasting disease, cerebrospinal nematodiasis, the enzootic ataxic form of copper deficiency, capture myopathy, louping ill, cerebrocortical necrosis (thiamine deficiency), and rarely, neoplasms.

Keratoconjunctivitis sometimes occurs as an outbreak in farmed deer, particularly following mixing and overcrowding. Infectious causes such as *Moraxella bovis* and *Listeria monocytogenes* may be found, but often no pathogen is predominant, although subconjunctival antibiotic injections are reported to be highly effective. Predisposing factors include a dusty environment, flies, and larvae of the nasal bot (*Cephenemyia* species).

TREATMENT

Few drugs are licensed for use in deer, but many products for domestic ruminants have been used safely and effectively. The following antibiotics have been given to deer at cattle dose rates and routes of administration: amoxicillin, amoxicillin–clavulanic acid, cephalexin, co-trimazine, enrofloxacin, marbofloxacin, oxytetracycline, and benzyl penicillin sodium. For the treatment of nematode infections, fenbendazole, albendazole, oxfendazole, levamisole, doramectin, and moxidectin may be used at cattle dose rates, but ivermectin is safe and may be more effective at 0.4 mg/kg body mass, or double the cattle dose rate. Other parasiticides recommended for use at domestic ruminant dose rates include nitroxynil, closantel, clorsulon (with ivermectin), and triclabendazole for trematode infections, imidocarb for babesiosis, diclazuril for coccidiosis, and permethrin and amitraz for ectoparasitism.

PREVENTIVE MEDICINE

Good management is at the heart of preventive medicine. Enclosures for captive deer should meet the behavioral and physiologic needs of the species held (see Special Housing Requirements). Herd size and composition should be maintained according to the enclosure size and type to minimize the risk of contamination by infectious organisms, allow regeneration of vegetation, and prevent stress and aggression within the group. Thus, a carrying capacity should be set for the enclosure and excess animals culled. In particular, in groups with a stag, harem, and calves, subadult males should be removed

before they start to threaten the stag's position, unless this natural behavior, as well as the likelihood of injuries, is accepted and sufficient land is available for the coexistence of bachelor groups. Immunocontraception with porcine zona pellucida (PZP) and, more recently, gonadotropin-releasing hormone (GnRH) vaccines has been employed successfully to control reproduction in deer.[24,38] Feeding (including access to vegetation within the enclosure) should meet the physiologic needs of all individuals in the herd (including calves and subdominant animals) and should be performed in such a way that all individuals have access to feeds.

Health monitoring should include regular population counts, assessment of body condition and signs of ill-health, routine fecal parasite screening, and necropsy following any unexplained deaths. It may be helpful to weigh and examine calves if caught for eartagging and to take opportunistic diagnostic samples (feces, blood) whenever an individual is restrained for any procedure. Routine anthelmintic treatment should be based on a knowledge of the resident helminths and their life-cycles (see Disease) and also the susceptibility of the species, as many deer harbor GI nematodes without showing clinical signs.[19] However, this situation may change if the stocking density is too high or in a deer farming situation. Alternative parasite control strategies will be increasingly necessary to address concerns of anthelmintic resistance.[21] Vaccinations (e.g., multivalent clostridial vaccine) should be similarly based on knowledge of local disease risk and species susceptibility. However, unlike anthelmintic treatments, which may be given orally (most efficiently if added to the concentrate pellet), vaccinations need to be injected by hand or dart, so good handling and restraint facilities are essential.

Any animals to be imported should be tested for evidence of infectious disease (particularly helminths and chronic bacterial infections such as tuberculosis) before transport and should undergo a period of quarantine after arrival, during which they are monitored for signs of disease and the presence of pathogens.

REPRODUCTION

Breeding in deer originating from temperate regions of the world is seasonal (Table 62-7).[5] Rut occurs in the fall season, followed by mating as individual hinds come into estrus. Gestation lasts over winter in the large species, and calves are born in spring. One exception is the roe deer, in which pregnancy lasts about 5 months. Rut takes place in summer, but the fertilized ovum does not implant until the shortest day of the year, so that the calf is born in spring.

Reproduction is triggered by the shortening day length, which stimulates the pineal gland to initiate one or two silent ovulations, followed by regular estrus cycles over the next 4 to 6 months. More commonly, mating at the first or second cycle results in pregnancy.

TABLE 62-7

Reproductive Characteristics of Selected Cervidae

Parameter	Fallow Deer	Axis Deer	Red Deer	Moose	Reindeer
Puberty (age)	12–24 months	<12 months	12–24 months	12–24 months	12–24 months
Estrus cycle (days)	21–23	27–30	18–20	24–27	24
Gestation (days)	225–234	229	223–238	227–239	210–238
Pregnancy determination	Plasma progesterone >4 ng/mL after breeding season	—	Plasma progesterone >4 ng/mL after breeding season	—	—
Placentation	Syndesmochorial	Syndesmochorial	Syndesmochorial	Syndesmochorial	Syndesmochorial
Progesterone (ng/mL)	Estrus 1–2, luteal phase	—	Estrus 1–2, luteal phase	—	—
Nongravid	2–4		2–4		
Gravid	4–10		4–10		

ng/mL, Nanogram per millilter.

Ovulation occurs approximately 24 hours after the onset of estrus. Pregnancy usually is detected by testing plasma progesterone (greater than 4 nanograms per milliliter [ng/mL]) after the breeding season, but avoiding stress is important because the adrenal gland also may secrete progesterone. In the male, the shortening day length also stimulates luteal hormone secretion, which, in turn, activates testicular development, spermatogenesis, and secretion of testosterone. The increase in testosterone is responsible for antler mineralization and other secondary sexual characteristics. Stags continue to be fertile in early spring until testicles regress and antlers are shed.

Tropical deer show little or no seasonality and may breed throughout the year. When moved to a temperate region, some remain aseasonal (e.g., Reeve muntjac, *Muntiacus reevesi*), others show a wide breeding season (e.g., axis deer [chital, *Axis axis*] in Australia), and a few such as the Javan deer exhibit reverse seasonality: spring rut and conception; and fall or winter calving.

The reproductive biology of the chevrotains is poorly understood. They are solitary except at breeding times. In the male, the penis is spiral shaped at the tip, and the scrotum is poorly defined. Gestation is approximately 5 months in the Asian species and 6 to 9 months in the water chevrotain (*Hyemoschus aquaticus*), and usually a single calf is produced. Postpartum estrus and mating usually occurs after 1 or 2 days. The young are weaned at 3 months of age and reach sexual maturity at 4 to 5 months (greater mouse deer, *Tragulus napu*) or 10 months (water chevrotain).[5]

ACKNOWLEDGMENT

We should like to thank Marcus Clauss for many helpful comments, and Tracy Clippinger for ideas and references.

REFERENCES

1. Alexander TL, Buxton D: *Management and diseases of deer: A handbook for the veterinary surgeon*, ed 2, London, U.K., 1994, Veterinary Deer Society/British Veterinary Association.
2. Arnemo JM, Aanes R, Oystein OS, et al: Reversible immobilization of free-ranging Svalbard reindeer, Norwegian reindeer and woodland caribou: A comparison of medetomidine-ketamine and atipamezole in three subspecies of Rangifer tarandus. In *Proceedings of the Wildlife Disease Association Conference*, 2000, Grand Teton National Park, WY, pp 49–50.
3. Arnemo JM, Moe R, Soli NE: Chemical capture of free-ranging red deer (*Cervus elaphus*) with medetomidine-ketamine. *Rangifer* 14:123–127, 1994.
4. Arnemo JM, Soveri T, Soli NE: Immobilization of free-ranging moose (*Alces alces*) with medetomidine-ketamine and reversal with atipamezole. In *Proceedings of the Joint Conference of the American Association of Zoo Veterinarians and the Association of Reptilian Amphibian Veterinarians*, Pittsburg, PA, 1994, pp 197–199.
5. Asher GW, Fisher MW: Reproductive physiology of farmed red deer (*Cervus elaphus*) and fallow deer (*Dama dama*). In Renecker LA, Hudson RJ, editors: *Wildlife production: Conservation and sustainable development (miscellaneous publication 91-6)*, Fairbanks, AL, 1991, Agricultural and Forestry Experimental Station, pp 474–484.
6. Audigé L, Wilson PR, Morris RS: Disease and mortality on red deer farms in New Zealand. *Vet Rec* 148:334–340, 2001.
7. Bonnet S, Jouglin M, L'Hostis M, et al: *Babesia* sp. EU1 from roe deer and transmission within *Ixodes ricinus*. *Emerg Infect Dis* 13:1208–1210, 2007.
8. Browning SR, Mason GL, Seward T, et al: Transmission of prions from mule deer and elk with chronic wasting disease to transgenic mice expressing cervid PrP. *J Virol* 78:13345–13350, 2004.
9. Bush M, Citino SB, Lance WR: The use of butorphanol in anesthesia protocols for zoo and wild mammals. In Fowler ME, Miller RE, editors: *Zoo and wild animal medicine: Current therapy*, ed 7, Philadelphia, PA, 2012, Saunders, pp 596–603.
10. Caulkett NA: Anesthesia for North American cervids. *Can Vet J* 38:389–390, 1997.
11. Caulkett N, Haigh JC: Deer (Cervids). In West G, Heard D, Caulkett N, editors: *Zoo animal and wildlife immobilization and anesthesia*, Ames, IA, 2007, Blackwell Publishing Ltd., pp 607–612.
12. Clauss M, Dierenfeld ES: The nutrition of "browsers." In Fowler ME, Miller RE, editors: *Zoo and wild animal medicine: Current therapy*, ed 6, Philadelphia, PA, 2008, Saunders, pp 444–454.
13. de Lisle GW, Yates GF, Montgomery H: The emergence of *Mycobacterium paratuberculosis* in farmed deer in New Zealand-A review of 619 cases. *N Z Vet J* 51:58–62, 2003.
14. Duarte JMB, Merino ML, Gonzales S, et al: Order Artiodactyla, family Cervidae (deer). In Fowler ME, Cubas ZS, editors: *Biology, medicine and surgery of South American wild animals*, Ames, IA, 2001, Iowa State University Press, pp 402–422.
15. Duarte JMB, Gonzalez S: *Neotropical cervidology: Biology and medicine of Latin American deer*, Brazil/Gland, Switzerland, Funep, 2010, Jabotical/IUCN.
16. Fasanella A, Palazzo L, Petrella A, et al: Anthrax in red deer (*Cervus elaphus*), Italy. *Emerg Infect Dis* 13:1118–1119, 2007.
17. Fernandez-Moran J, Palomeque J, Peinado VI: Medetomidine/tiletamine/zolazepam and xylazine/tiletamine/zolazepam combinations for immobilization of fallow deer (*Cervus dama*). *J Zoo Wildl Med* 31:62–64, 2000.
18. Flach E: Cervidae and tragulidae. In Fowler ME, Miller RE, editors: *Zoo and wild animal medicine*, ed 5, St. Louis, MO, 2003, Elsevier Science, pp 634–648.
19. Flach E: Gastrointestinal nematodiasis in hoofstock. In Fowler ME, Miller RE, editors: *Zoo and wild animal medicine: Current therapy*, ed 6, Philadelphia, PA, 2008, Saunders, pp 416–422.
20. Fletcher J: Handling farmed deer. *In Pract* 17:30–37, 1995.
21. Fontenot DK, Miller JE: Alternatives for gastrointestinal parasite control in exotic ruminants. In Fowler ME, Miller RE, editors: *Zoo and wild animal medicine: Current therapy*, ed 7, Philadelphia, PA, 2012, Saunders, pp 581–588.
22. Fowler ME: *Restraint and handling of wild and domestic animals*, ed 2, Ames, IA, 1995, Iowa State University Press, pp 288–292.
23. Fowler ME, Boever WJ: Cervidae. In Fowler ME, editor: *Zoo and wild animal medicine*, ed 2, Philadelphia, PA, 1986, Saunders, pp 981–985.
24. Gionfriddo JP, Denicola AJ, Miller LA, et al: Efficacy of GnRH immunocontraception of wild white-tailed deer in New Jersey. *Wildl Soc Bull* 35:142–148, 2011.
25. Grimm KA, Lamont LA: Clinical pharmacology. In West G, Heard D, Caulkett N, editors: *Zoo animal and wildlife immobilization and anesthesia*, Ames, IA, 2007, Blackwell Publishing Ltd, pp 3–36.
26. Groves C, Grubb P: *Ungulate taxonomy*, Baltimore, MD, 2011, John Hopkins University Press.
27. Grubb P: Order Artiodactyla. In Wilson DE, Reeder DM, editors: *Mammal species of the world: A taxonomic and geographic reference*, ed 3, Baltimore, MD, 2005, Johns Hopkins University Press, pp 637–722.
28. Haigh JC: The use of chutes for ungulate restraint. In Fowler ME, Miller RE, editors: *Zoo and wild animal medicine: Current therapy*, ed 4, Philadelphia, PA, 1999, Saunders, pp 657–662.
29. Haigh JC, Hudson RJ: *Farming wapiti and red deer*, St. Louis, MO, 1993, Mosby.
30. Hibler CP, Wilson KL, Miller MW, et al: Field validation and assessment of an enzyme-linked immunosorbent assay for detecting chronic wasting disease in mule deer (*Odocoileus hemionus*), white-tailed deer (*Odocoileus virginianus*), and Rocky Mountain elk (*Cervus elaphus nelsoni*). *J Vet Diagn Invest* 15:311–319, 2003.
31. Hofmann RR: Digestive physiology of the deer: Their morphophysiological specialisation and adaptation. In Fennessy PF, Drew KR, editors: *Biology of deer production*, Wellington, New Zealand, 1985, Royal Society of New Zealand Press, pp 393–407.
32. International Species Information System (ISIS), Teare JA, editor: *Reference ranges for physiological values in captive wildlife: 2002 edition.*, Apple Valley, MN, 2002, ISIS.
33. Jalanka HH, Roeken BO: The use of medetomidine, medetomidine-ketamine combinations, and atipamezole in nondomestic mammals: A review. *J Zoo Wildl Med* 21:259–282, 1990.
34. Johnson CB, Wilson PR, Woodbury MR, et al: Comparison of analgesic techniques for antler removal in halothane-anaesthetized red deer

(*Cervus elaphus*): Electroencephalographic responses. *Vet Anaesth Analg* 32:61–71, 2005.

35. Kaiser TM, Brasch J, Castell JC, et al: Tooth wear in captive wild ruminant species differs from that of free-ranging conspecifics. *Mammal Biology* 74:425–437, 2009.

36. Keel MK, Patterson JG, Noon TH, et al: Caprine herpesvirus-2 in association with naturally occurring malignant catarrhal fever in captive sika deer (*Cervus nippon*). *J Vet Diagn Invest* 15:179–183, 2003.

37. Keuser V, Schynts F, Detry B, et al: Improved antigenic methods for differential diagnosis of bovine, caprine, and cervine alphaherpesviruses related to bovine herpesvirus 1. *J Clin Microbiol* 42:1228–1235, 2004.

38. Kirkpatrick JF, Lyda RO, Frank KM: Contraceptive vaccines for wildlife: A review. *Am J Reprod Immunol* 66:40–50, 2011.

39. Lance WR, Kenny DE: Thiafentanil oxalate (A3080) in nondomestic ungulate species. In Fowler ME, Miller RE, editors: *Zoo and wild animal medicine: Current therapy*, ed 7, Philadelphia, PA, 2012, Saunders, pp 589–595.

40. Li H, Dyer N, Keller J, et al: Newly recognized herpesvirus causing malignant catarrhal fever in white-tailed deer (*Odocoileus virginianus*). *J Clin Microbiol* 38:1313–1318, 2000.

41. Lux Hoppe EG, dos Santos Schmidt EM, Zanuzzo FS, et al: *azoubira* (Fischer, 1814) (Cervidae: Odocoileinae). *Comp Clin Pathol* 19:29–32, 2010.

42. Macdonald D: *The new encyclopaedia of mammals*, Oxford, U.K., 2001, Oxford University Press, pp 500–513.

43. Mackintosh CG, Labes RE, Griffin JFT: The effect of Johne's vaccination on tuberculin testing in farmed red deer (*Cervus elaphus*). *N Z Vet J* 53:216–222, 2005.

44. Maclachan NJ, Drew CP, Darpel KE, et al: The pathology and pathogenesis of bluetongue. *J Comp Pathol* 141:1–16, 2009.

45. Manning EJB, Sleeman JM: Johne's disease and free-ranging wildlife. In Fowler ME, Miller RE, editors: *Zoo and wild animal medicine: Current therapy*, ed 7, Philadelphia, PA, 2012, Saunders, pp 628–635.

46. Marco I, Lavin S: Effect of the method of capture on the haematology and blood chemistry of red deer (*Cervus elaphus*). *Res Vet Sci* 66:81–84, 1999.

47. McClusker S, Shipley LA, Tollefson TN, et al: Effects of starch and fibre in pelleted diets on nutritional status of mule deer (*Odocoileus hemionus*) fawns. *Anim Physiol Anim Nutr* 95:489–498, 2011.

48. Miller JM, Jenny AL, Payeur JB: Polymerase chain reaction detection of *Mycobacterium tuberculosis* complex and *Mycobacterium avium* organisms in formalin-fixed tissues from culture-negative ruminants. *Vet Microbiol* 87:15–23, 2002.

49. Miller MA: Current diagnostic methods for tuberculosis in zoo animals. In Fowler ME, Miller RE, editors: *Zoo and wild animal medicine: Current therapy*, ed 6, St. Louis, MO, 2008, Saunders, pp 10–19.

50. Miller MA, Weber M: Hypocalcemia, hypomagnesemia, and rumenitis in exotic ruminants. In Fowler ME, Miller RE, editors: *Zoo and wild animal medicine: Current therapy*, ed 6, St. Louis, MO, 2008, Saunders, pp 404–407.

51. Miller MW: Chronic wasting disease of cervid species. In Fowler ME, Miller RE, editors: *Zoo and wild animal medicine: Current therapy*, ed 6, St. Louis, MO, 2008, Saunders, pp 430–437.

52. Moresco AM, Larsen RS, Sleeman JM, et al: Use of naloxone to reverse carfentanil citrate-induced hypoxemia and cardiopulmonary depression in rocky mountain wapiti. *J Zoo Wildl Med* 32:81–89, 2001.

53. Müller DWH, Bingaman Lackey L, Streich WJ, et al: Relevance of management and feeding regimens on life expectancy in captive deer. *Am J Vet Res* 71:275–280, 2010.

54. Murray S, Monfort SL, Ware L, et al: Anesthesia in female white-tailed deer using telazol and xylazine. *J Wildl Dis* 36(4):670–675, 2000.

55. Mylrea GE, English AW: The diseases of farmed deer in New South Wales, Australia. In Renecker LA, Judson RJ, editors: *Wildlife production: Conservation and sustainable development (miscellaneous publication 91-6)*, Fairbanks, AL, 1991, Agricultural and Forestry Experimental Station, pp 421–428.

56. National Research Council (NRC): *Nutrient requirements of small ruminants. Sheep, goats, cervids and New World camelids*, Washington, DC, 2007, National Academy of Science Press.

57. Novak RM: *Walker's mammals of the world*, vol 2, ed 6, Baltimore, MD, 1999, Johns Hopkins University Press, pp 1081–1132.

58. Olsen SC, Fach SJ, Palmer MV, et al: Immune responses of elk to initial and booster vaccinations with *Brucella abortus* strain RB51 or 19. *Clin Vaccine Immunol* 13:1098–1103, 2006.

59. Paterson J: Capture myopathy. In West G, Heard D, Caulkett N, editors: *Zoo animal and wildlife immobilization and anesthesia*, Ames, IA, 2007, Blackwell Publishing Ltd., pp 115–121.

60. Randi E, Mucci N, Pierpaoli M, et al: New phylogenetic perspectives on the Cervidae (Artiodactyla) are provided by the mitochondrial cytochrome b gene. *Proc R Soc Lond B* 265:793–801, 1998.

61. Read M, Caulkett NA, McCallister M: Evaluation of zuclopenthixol acetate to decrease handling stress in wapiti. *J Wildl Dis* 36:450–459, 2000.

62. Rhyan J, Deng M, Wang H, et al: Foot-and-mouth disease in North American bison (*Bison bison*) and elk (*Cervus elaphus nelsoni*): Susceptibility, intra- and interspecies transmission, clinical signs, and lesions. *J Wildl Dis* 44:269–279, 2008.

63. Ritz J, Hofer K, Hofer E, et al: Forestomach pH in hunted roe deer (*Capreolus capreolus*) in relation to forestomach region, time of measurement and supplemental feeding and comparison among wild ruminant species. *Eur J Wildl Res* 59:505–517, 2013.

64. Rosef O, Nystøyl HL, Solenes T, et al: Haematological and serum biochemical reference values in free-ranging red deer (*Cervus elaphus atlanticus*). *Rangifer* 24(2):79–85, 2004.

65. Samuelsson F, Nejsum P, Raundrup K, et al: Warble infestations by *Hypoderma tarandi* (Diptera; Oestridae) recorded for the first time in West Greenland muskoxen. *Int J Parasitol Parasites Wildl* 2:213–216, 2013.

66. Sanderson S: Bluetongue: Lessons from the European outbreak 2006–2009. In Fowler ME, Miller RE, editors: *Zoo and wild animal medicine: Current therapy*, ed 7, Philadelphia, PA, 2012, Saunders, pp 573–580.

67. Seleem MN, Boyle SM, Sriranganathan N: Brucellosis: A re-emerging zoonosis. *Vet Microbiol* 140:392–398, 2010.

68. Shury T: Capture and physical restraint of zoo and wild animals. In West G, Heard D, Caulkett N, editors: *Zoo animal and wildlife immobilization and anesthesia*, Ames, IA, 2007, Blackwell Publishing Ltd., pp 131–144.

69. Van Rijn PA, Heutink RG, Boonstra J, et al: Sustained high-throughput polymerase chain reaction diagnostics during the European epidemic of Bluetongue virus serotype 8. *J Vet Diagn Invest* 24:469–478, 2012.

70. Vikøren T, Li H, Lillehaug A, et al: Malignant catarrhal fever in free-ranging cervids associated with OvHV-2 and CpHV-2 DNA. *J Wildl Dis* 42:797–807, 2006.

71. Waters WR, Palmer MV, Bannantine JP, et al: Antibody responses in reindeer (*Rangifer tarandus*) infected with *Mycobacterium bovis*. *Clin Diagn Lab Immunol* 12:727–735, 2005.

72. Wilson DE, Mittermeier RA: *Handbook of the mammals of the world*, vol 2, Barcelona, Spain, 2010, Lynx Edicions, pp 320–443.

73. Wilson PR: Diseases of farmed deer. In *Proceedings No. 72. Deer Refresher Course*, Sydney, Australia, 1984, Post-graduate Committee in Veterinary Science: University of Sydney, pp 505–529.

74. Wolfe LL, Lance WR, Miller MW: Immobilization of mule deer with thiafentanil (A-3080) or thiafentanil plus xylazine. *J Wildl Dis* 40:282–287, 2004.

75. Zintl A, Finnerty EJ, Murphy TM, et al: Babesias of red deer (*Cervus elaphus*) in Ireland. *Vet Res* 42:7, 2011.

CHAPTER 63

Bovidae (Except Sheep and Goats) and Antilocapridae

Barbara A. Wolfe

GENERAL BIOLOGY

Formerly classified in the order Artiodactyla, even-toed ungulates have been reclassified, on the basis of recent molecular evidence, to the order Cetartiodactyla, which includes the families Cetacea, Hippopotamidae, Camelidae, Suidae, Tayassuidae, Tragulidae, Moschidae, Cervidae, Giraffidae, Bovidae, and Antilocapridae.[23] The last six of these families belong to the suborder Ruminantia. Antilocapridae consists of a single species, the pronghorn *Antilocapra americana*, whereas Bovidae consist of eight subfamilies: Aepycerotinae, Alcelaphinae, Antilopinae, Bovinae, Cephalophinae, Caprinae, Hippotraginae, and Reduncinae. General taxonomy and characteristics of Antilocapridae and Bovidae are listed in Table 63-1.

Antilocapridae

Pronghorns (*Antilocapra americana*) are the sole species of the family Antilocapridae and are distinct from cervids and antelopes in that they possess forked horns, which are shed annually.[1] Five subspecies exist: *A.a. anteflexa, A.a. oregona, A.a. mexicana, A.a. peninsularis,* and *A.a. sonoriensis*. Ranging throughout western North America from northern Mexico to southern Canada, pronghorn are found in open areas of prairies and deserts, eating primarily forbs, browse, and grasses. The Sonoran and Peninsular subspecies are considered Endangered according to federal classification. Although extremely fast runners, they are not agile jumpers, and local populations have been fragmented by fencing.[57] They are extremely fractious, are prone to stress hyperthermia, and may be difficult to maintain in captivity.[10] Pronghorns are fall breeders, producing twins in spring, and are the only known ungulates to exhibit multiple paternity.[7]

Bovidae

The diverse family Bovidae consists of 143 known species, ranging in size from the 3-kilogram (kg) royal antelope to the 1200-kg gaur. Bovids are found across all of mainland Africa and in 30 countries in Europe, the Middle East, and Asia. Four subfamilies exist only in the African continent; none is native to Australia or Antarctica; and only bison (*Bison bison*) are native to the Americas.

UNIQUE ANATOMY

Bovid species are characterized by the presence of horns composed of keratinized sheaths covering a bony prominence of the frontal bone, which are never shed. All males, and the females of some genera, possess horns. Only *Tetracerus quadricornis*, the four-horned antelope, possesses more than two horns. Most bovid horns continue to grow throughout life and are unbranched, varying in shape from short spikes to long, curved, and spiraled structures.

Bovids and pronghorns are true ruminants, possessing four specialized stomach chambers. Pronghorns and other primarily grazing species have a large, stratified rumen, a smaller reticulum, a well-developed omasum, a larger abomasum, and roughly twice the relative intestinal length (25–30 times body length) of browsing species. This anatomy is adapted for digestion of large amounts of cellulose. Browsers have a smaller rumen, with evenly distributed, dense ruminal papillae, and tend to have comparatively larger salivary glands and livers compared with grazers.[51] A gallbladder is usually present in bovids, and the kidneys may or may not be lobulated.[10] Reproductive anatomy is similar to that of domestic cattle in most bovids, with the exception that females of some species such as the Hippotraginae demonstrate duplex uteri, in which the cervix is bifurcated, creating a physical separation between the uterine horns with no uterine body.

Bovid and pronghorn species lack upper incisors and canines. The dental formula is: incisors (I) 0/3, canines (C) 0/1, premolars (P) 3/3, molars (M) 3/3, to a total of 32. Scent glands vary in size and location and may be found in the subauricular, prefrontal, forehead, submandibular, inguinal, interdigital, metacarpal, and preputial regions.

Bovids have an unguligrade stance, walking on well-developed hooves on the third and fourth digits of each foot. The second and fifth digits, if present, are called *dewclaws*. The hooves of each species have a characteristic size and shape adaptively suited to their habitat.

MANAGEMENT AND HUSBANDRY

Population Management

The 21st century has brought a grim outlook to the conservation of nondomestic bovid species. Ever-increasing human populations and their livestock encroaching on natural habitats, agriculture, transportation infrastructure, and fencing are some of the factors causing disruption of habitat and migration and are decreasing population size and genetic diversity across the taxon. In captivity, a loss of nearly 1000 spaces for antelope between 1999 and 2011 and a predicted decline in future space are reported by the Association of Zoos and Aquariums (AZA) Antelope Taxon Advisory Group.[2] Of the 82 species of ungulates in AZA collections, 42% are in decline or have a negative growth rate. Few sustainable bovid populations—those that are able to persist indefinitely without supplementation—exist, either in the wild or in captivity. Over 25% of antelope species are threatened by extinction, three exist in populations of fewer than 500 individuals, and many are not represented by captive populations, all of which increases the risk of extinction.[34] Recent recommendations to manage antelope in larger, less intensively managed groups have been based on (1) the difficulty of maintaining genetic diversity in small, isolated captive populations; (2) the risk of transporting animals for breeding purposes; (3) advanced methodology in genetics and population modeling; and (4) the relative success of large-landscape game ranches in population management.[34,57]

Special Housing Requirements

Pronghorns in the wild are accustomed to wide open spaces in arid regions and may tolerate wide temperature fluctuations. They often do not thrive in captivity and are compromised by high humidity, unnatural social structure, novel stimuli, and enclosed spaces. They are more likely to crawl under fencing than to jump over fencing 1.5 meters (m) or higher, but until accustomed to an enclosure, this fractious species should have visible sight barriers and minimal obstacles near fence lines to reduce trauma. A shelter that does not restrict view may be preferred by pronghorns over an enclosed barn.[10] In captivity, they benefit behaviorally from frequent human proximity from a young age to maintain tractability. Pronghorns are

TABLE 63-1

Taxonomy and General Characteristics of the Family Bovidae[1,26,41]

Genus (# Species)	Common Name	Adult Weight (kilograms)	Female Sexual Maturity (months)	Gestation Length (months)	Lifespan (years)	Feeding Strategy	IUCN Status
SUBFAMILY AEPYCEROTINAE							
Aepyceros	Impala	40–80	18–24	6.5–7	15	I	LC
SUBFAMILY ALCELAPHINAE							
Alcelaphus	Hartebeest	120–200	18–30	8		G	LC
Beatragus	Hirola (Hunter's hartebeest)	80–118	—	7.5–8	—	G	CE
Connochaetes (2)	Black, blue wildebeest	110–180	18–30	8–8.5	20	G	LC
Damaliscus (3)	Topi, tsessebe; blesbok/bontebok	75–160; 55–80	18–30	7.5–8.5	12–17	G	LC
SUBFAMILY ANTILOPINAE							
Ammodorcas	Dibatag	22–35	12–18	6–7	10–12	B	VU
Antidorcas	Springbok	30–45	6–9	5.5–6	20	I	LC
Antilope	Blackbuck	25–35	18–24	5–6	10–12	I	NT
Dorcatragus	Beira	9–11.5	—	6	—	I	VU
Eudorcas (4)	Mongalla, red-fronted, Red, Thompson gazelle	25–30	9	6	14.5	G	LC; VU; DD; NT
Gazella (10)	Arabian, Indian, Queen of Sheba, Cuvier, Dorcas, mountain, slender-horned, Saudi, Speke, goitered gazelles	15–25	7–12	6–7	12	I	DD; LC; EX; EN; VU; VU; EN; EX; EN; VU
Litocranius	Gerenuk	30–50	12–18	6.5–7	10–12	B	NT
Madoqua (4)	Kirk, Gunther's, silver, Salt's dik-dik	2.2–7	6–8	5–6	10	I	LC
Nanger (3)	Dama (Addra, Mhorr), Grant, Soemmerring gazelles	35–75	6–18	6–6.5	12–14	I; B; G	CE; LC; VU
Neotragus (3)	Suni; pygmy/royal antelope	1.5–6	12–18	6	6–10	B	LC
Oreotragus	Klipspringer	10–18	12	7	15	I	LC
Ourebia	Oribi	15–20	9	6.5–7	14	I	LC
Procapra (3)	Mongolian gazelle	20–29	18–24	6.1	7	G	LC
	Tibetan/Przewalski gazelles	13–32	12–24	5.5–6	8	I	NT; EN
Raphicerus (3)	Steenbok; Grysbok	7–23	6–9	5.5–6	8–12	I	LC
Saiga	Saiga	20–50	8	4.5	6–10	B	CE
SUBFAMILY BOVINAE							
Bison (2)	American; European	545–1,000	24–36	8–10	25–27	G; I	NT; VU
Bos (5)	Gaur; banteng; kouprey	600–1,000	24–36	9–9.5	20–30	G; I; I	VU; EN CE
	Yak	305–820	72	8.5	23	G	VU
	Auroch	—	—	—	—	—	EX
Boselaphus	Nilgai	120–240	18	8	21	I	LC
Bubalus (3)	Indian (Asian) water buffalo	800–1,200	18	10–11	25	I	EN
Bubalus	Anoa; tamaraw	200–300	24–72	9–10.5	20–25	I; G	EN; CE
Pseudoryx	Saola	80–100	Not available	7.5–8	8–9	B	CE
Syncerus	African buffalo	300–900	36–60	11.5	18–20	G	LC
Tetracerus	Four-horned antelope	15–25	—	7.5–8	10	I	VU
Tragelaphus (9)	Greater kudu; bongo; mountain nyala	120–400	14–36	7–9	15–23	I	LC; NT; EN
	Lesser kudu; bushbuck; Nyala; Sitatunga	25–140	9–36	6–8	12–19	I	NT; LC; LC; LC
	Common, giant eland	300–1,000	14–36	9	25	I	LC

Continued

TABLE 63-1

Taxonomy and General Characteristics of the Family Bovidae—cont'd

Genus (# Species)	Common Name	Adult Weight (kilograms)	Female Sexual Maturity (months)	Gestation Length (months)	Lifespan (years)	Feeding Strategy	IUCN Status
SUBFAMILY CEPHALOPHINAE							
Cephalophus (15)	Bush, black, zebra, red-flanked, yellow-backed duiker	7–80	—	—	—	B	CE
	Abbott, Jentink duikers	50–80	—	8	21	B	E
Philantomba	Blue, Maxwell duikers	4–10	0.9–12	6–7.5	10–12	I; B	LC
Sylvicapra	Common duiker	10–20	9–10	6–7	14	B	LC
SUBFAMILY HIPPOTRAGINAE							
Addax	Addax	60–125	18	8.5	19	I	CE
Hippotragus	Bluebuck	—	—	—	—	—	EX
	Roan, sable antelope	190–300	24–36	9	17	I; G	LC
Oryx (4)	Arabian oryx	65–70	18–24	8.5–9	20	I	VU
	Beisa oryx; gemsbok	150–240	18–24	8.5–10	18–22	I	NT; LC
	Scimitar-horned oryx	180–200	18–24	8–8.5	20	I	EW
SUBFAMILY REDUNCINAE							
Kobus (5)	Kob; red lechwe; Nile lechwe; Puku	50–130	18–24	7–9	15–21	G	LC; LC; EN; NT
	Waterbuck	150–250	12–16	8.5–9	18	I	LC
Pelea	Rhebok	18–30	14	7	8–10	I	LC
Redunca (3)	Southern, mountain, Bohor reedbuck	40–95	12	7.75	16	G	LC

B, Browser; CE, critically endangered; EN, endangered; EW, extinct in the wild; EX, extinct; G, grazer; I, intermediate; LC, least concern; NT, near threatened; VU, vulnerable.

relatively tolerant of species with which they have historically grazed (bison, elk, and deer); however, interspecific aggression has been documented.[10]

Housing and husbandry practices for antelope and cattle species vary widely, depending on management goals, climate, and available space. Fences and bomas may be constructed of a variety of materials and should be a minimum of 2.5 m (8 feet) in height and designed with the species size, temperament, and jumping ability in mind. Fences with sight barriers are beneficial in management areas to prevent trauma and between adjacent enclosures to prevent aggression and fence damage. Electric wires may be useful for keeping animals away from fence lines but may also present an entrapment and trauma risk through horn entanglement. Space and temperature recommendations are listed in Table 63-2. Some species may experience regular hoof problems when housed on substrates to which they are not adapted. For example, hoof abscesses may be common in desert species exposed to muddy conditions for prolonged periods. Indoor substrates should be considered with regard to hoof hardness and wear to minimize trimming and hoof lesions.

Shelter conditions should take into account the natural history of the species and ambient conditions. Desert-adapted animals may tolerate high temperatures (≥38°C [100°F]) provided adequate water and shade are available, but most desert and tropical species need to be housed indoors during the cold season in colder regions. Frostbite and ear tip loss are frequently seen at temperatures below 9°C (15°F). Forest and cold-adapted or altitude-adapted species may require more shade during the warm season, and shelters for all species should provide cover and windbreaks facing away from prevailing winds.[10] Forest species such as duikers will benefit from plantings or other structures that support hiding behaviors. Indoor housing should provide temperatures between 10°C and 27°C (50°F–80°F), with adequate ventilation to control humidity and reduce ammonia concentrations.

Nutrition

Feeding the Neonate

Maternal rejection is not uncommon in captive nondomestic ruminants. If a calf cannot be raised by its dam, hand rearing is labor intensive and requires early intervention to provide the calf with the best chance of survival. Neonatal ruminants acquire immune protection passively through ingestion of maternal colostral immunoglobulins (IgG) in the first 24 to 48 hours of life. The calf's ability to absorb antibodies ends approximately 24 hours after the first meal,[15] and failure of passive transfer (FPT) occurs when inadequate levels of IgG are absorbed during this period. Even calves nursing from their dams may experience FPT by ingesting colostrum in inadequate volume or low IgG content, and FPT calves are highly susceptible to disease, often into the postweaning period. The prophylactic use of parenteral antimicrobials in calves with FPT should be considered but must be combined with colostrum replacement and management practices that minimize pathogen exposure. The first choice for colostrum replacement should be oral administration of fresh or frozen intraspecific colostrum, followed by low-temperature pasteurized cow's colostrum, commercial freeze-dried cow's colostrum replacer, and commercial bovine plasma. Feed calves 10% of their body weight in colostrum, or 5 grams per kilogram (g/kg) colostrum replacer, over the first 24 to 48 hours. Tests for FPT are readily available.[56] If passive transfer is inadequate after 48 hours, calves may receive parenteral conspecific plasma or commercial bovine plasma (20–40 milliliters per kilogram [mL/kg]).

Milk composition varies considerably among species, and a formula's composition should mimic that of the dam's milk in protein, carbohydrate, fat, and total solids. Goat's milk is a good choice for many species, alone or in combination with a milk replacer. However, milk may be low in vitamin E, zinc, copper, and iron, necessitating vitamin and mineral supplementation. Probiotics may also be

TABLE 63-2

Recommended Housing Conditions for Selected Species of Antilocapridae and Bovidae*

Common Name	Native Range	Native Climate	Minimum Barrier Height (feet)	Minimum Exhibit Size (square feet)	Minimum Holding Size (square feet)	Temperature (°F)
Pronghorn	Not available	Temperate	8	600	200	45–100
SUBFAMILY AEPYCEROTINAE						
Impala	African	Tropical	8	600	200	45–100
SUBFAMILY ALCELAPHINAE						
Hartebeest, wildebeest, bontebok, blesbok, topi	African	Tropical	8	600	200	45–100
SUBFAMILY ANTILOPINAE						
Dik-dik, royal antelope, steenbok, klipspringer	African	Tropical	8	200	140	45–100
Suni	African	Arid	8	200	140	45–100
Addra, Mhorr, Dorcas, Speke gazelle	African	Arid	8	400	92	45–100
Grant, Thomson's, slender-horned, red-fronted, Soemmerring gazelle	African	Tropical	8	400	92	45–100
Saudi goitered gazelle	Asian	Arid or tropical	8	400	92	45–100
Cuvier gazelle	African	Arid	8	600	92	45–100
Springbok	African	Arid	8	400	140	45–100
Gerenuk	African	Arid	8	400	140	60–100
Blackbuck	Asian	Tropical	8	400	140	45–100
SUBFAMILY BOVINAE						
Common, giant eland	African	Tropical	10	600	200	45–100
Lowland nyala Eastern bongo Lesser, greater kudu Sitatunga	African	Tropical	8	600	200	45–100
Nilgai	Asian	Tropical	8	600	200	45–100
Bushbuck	African	Tropical	8	400	140	45–100
SUBFAMILY CEPHALOPHINAE						
Crowned, Maxwell blue, red-flanked duiker	African	Tropical	8	200	140	45–100
Bay, black duiker	African	Tropical	8	400	140	45–100
Yellow-backed duiker	African	Tropical	8	600	200	45–100
SUBFAMILY HIPPOTRAGINAE						
Roan, sable antelope	African	Tropical	8	600	200	45–100
Addax, gemsbok scimitar-horned, Arabian oryx	African	Arid	8	600	200	45–100
Beisa, fringe-eared oryx	African	Arid or tropical	8	600	200	45–100
SUBFAMILY REDUNCINAE						
Common, Defassa waterbuck Uganda kob red, Nile lechwe	African	Tropical	8	600	200	45–100
Rhebok	African	Tropical	8	400	140	45–100

*Personal communication: D. Beetem and M. Fischer, AZA Antelope Taxon Advisory Group.

beneficial in establishing a healthy rumen flora. Calves should receive 8% to 15% of their body weight in formula every 24 hours, divided into four to six feedings per day. Resources are available to assist with milk replacer formulation and methods of feeding.[48,59]

In the first 2 to 3 weeks of a ruminant's life, milk digestion occurs in the abomasum and small intestine. Milk deposited into the nonfunctional rumenoreticulum during this period is not digested and may lead to rumenitis and septicemia.[15] For this reason, tube feeding or force feeding a calf with a poor suckle response may be harmful. Closure of the esophageal groove is stimulated by suckling and normally prevents this deposition. If tube feeding is necessary in the first weeks of life, a tube passed to the mid-esophagus may stimulate swallowing and closure of the groove. Additionally, oral administration of 10% sodium bicarbonate or 2% to 5% copper sulfate prior to milk feeding may facilitate groove closure for several minutes. By 2 to 3 weeks, the ruminal papillae are stimulated, and the calf begins to take in small amounts of dry feed. Changes in gastrointestinal (GI) flora occur throughout this period and until weaning (around 4 months), often manifesting as changes in fecal consistency.

Feeding the Adult

Many of the common health problems of nondomestic ruminants have recently been associated with direct or indirect dietary causes.[11] Chronic weight loss, rumen acidosis or rumenitis, laminitis, hoof overgrowth, and periodontal disease have all been attributed, at least in part, to historical feeding of all exotic bovids diets designed for domestic cattle. Cattle are grazing species, but many of the nondomestic Bovidae are intermediate or browse feeders. Browsers are adapted to eating the leaves and twigs of woody plants, intermediate feeders to both browse and grasses, and grazers to consuming grasses (see Table 63-1). All of these forages are fermented by the microbes of the ruminoreticulum, which produce fatty acids, providing energy to the ruminant. The grazer rumen is adapted for fermenting the high cellulose content in grasses through prolonged fermentation and particle retention, compared with the smaller, less muscular browser rumen. Consequently, browsers tend to eat less hay and are often fed higher amounts of pelleted concentrate to compensate for low hay consumption. High levels of easily digested carbohydrates such as starch and sugar, often found in pelleted concentrates, are too rapidly fermented in the rumen, leading to rumen acidosis. The ideal rumen pH range is 6.7 ± 0.5, and variation from this results in disturbance of the microflora. Altered and depleted rumen flora decrease the energy delivered to the ruminant, which results in weight loss. In response, many of these animals will receive increased amounts of concentrate, which compounds the problem. Rumen acidosis and resulting rumenitis may also lead to systemic acidosis, mineral imbalances, and laminitis or abnormal hoof growth.

Appropriately formulated pelleted feed for browsers should be based on a high-fiber forage meal such as aspen, alfalfa, soy or sunflower hulls, or cellulose powder, and should contain (1) a high-pectin, low-sugar energy source such as beet pulp; and (2) limited amounts of grain and corn.[11] A low-starch, high-fiber pelleted diet that meets these criteria has been recently formulated for browsing and intermediate ruminants (Wild Herbivore and Wild Herbivore Plus; Mazuri Zoo Feeds, PMI Feeds, St. Louis, MO). The recommended feed intake is 1.5% to 2.5% of body weight per day in addition to ad libitum grass or legume hay, and supplementation with natural nontoxic browse is recommended for all browsers. Grazers are generally fed commercial herbivore pelleted concentrate diet containing 12% to 18% protein and 16% to 25% acid detergent fiber at approximately 1% body weight per day in addition to hay. Salt blocks should be available at all times, and trace mineral salt blocks should be available to herds primarily on pasture or not receiving trace mineral balanced concentrates.

Adult bovids experiencing negative energy balance and weight loss from illness may require nutritional support during treatment. Commercially available products useful for boosting caloric intake include Low Odor MEGALAC Rumen Bypass Fat (Arm & Hammer, Church & Dwight Co., Inc., Princeton, NJ) and Wild Herbivore Boost (Mazuri Zoo Feeds, PMI Feeds, St. Louis, MO). These compromised animals may also benefit from transfaunation with rumen contents collected from a healthy conspecific. Tube feeding ruminants may be challenging because of the consistency and volume of feed they require; a commercial tube-feeding formula is available for herbivores (Critical Care, Oxbow Pet Products, Murdock, NB).[10]

RESTRAINT AND HANDLING

Restraint is an important aspect of medical practice in nondomestic ruminants, requiring careful planning and experience.[21] Because of the size and fractious nature of the species, most wild bovids require restraint for any type of physical examination for the safety of both the animal and the handlers. Capture and restraint of animals in the wild is conducted by a multitude of means, including drive nets, drop nets, net guns, bomas, chutes, traps, and remote injection. Some of these procedures require helicopters and specialized training and are conducted by full-time capture professionals. In zoologic settings, capture and restraint capabilities depend on the facilities

and expertise available, and each procedure conducted must be planned with the animal, handler ability, and equipment in mind.

Restraint may be classified as physical, behavioral, and chemical, and many procedures in these taxa will require some combination of all three methods. Planning for any restraint procedure should take into account the goal, the conditions (e.g., restraint type and capability, ambient temperature, footing, enclosure size), and the temperament of the animal.[9] Restraint planning should also include plans for alternative physical and chemical restraint and emergency release in case of injury, failure of behavioral compliance, or signs of severe distress in the animal. Safety of the personnel and the patient are the primary considerations. Any manipulation of bovids and pronghorns may result in extreme panic, self-injury, capture myopathy (see Noninfectious Disease), and even sudden death, necessitating efficiency of time and force used to achieve the goal of restraint.

Behavioral Restraint

Continuous development of improved behavioral management techniques in captive settings has allowed for procedures that once required anesthesia to be performed with minimal restraint. Some species accustomed to human proximity may be managed to a degree with little or no physical restraint through training of specific behaviors such as placing feet for hoof trimming. Desensitization and operant conditioning may be used to train animals to move calmly to a restraint area, enter a chute or crate, lie down, or tolerate minor procedures, but special attention to the explosive nature of many bovids requires slow, deliberate movements, quiet conditions, and safety precautions. Movement may be aided by careful design and planning of stalls, doors, hallways and chute approach, and the use of baffle boards may protect the handler and assist in movement.

Physical Restraint

Manual Capture and Restraint

Smaller species may be manually restrained by experienced handlers for brief procedures or induction of anesthesia after being caught by hand or with hoop nets. Restraint should be initiated on an isolated animal in a darkened, quiet, obstacle-free enclosure that is small enough to minimize the risk of injury to the animal but large enough to allow free movement and escape of the handlers. A stall with padded walls and hay or straw floor substrate is optimal for animal safety. A minimum of two handlers should perform the capture, depending on the size and temperament of the animal, and the handlers should wear protective clothing, footwear, eyewear and gloves. Hand restraint in bovids under 5 kg may be accomplished by a single handler by quickly lifting the animal, supporting the abdomen and spine against the handler's body, and restraining the head and legs. Restraint of medium-sized animals may be initiated by catching the head and quickly pushing the animal against a wall, pad, or floor with head restraint and placing a knee under the flank, with a second handler restraining the rear legs. Horns may be used for restraint of most species, but young animals or those with thin horns may be prone to horn avulsion. The head and legs should be tightly restrained to prevent the use of horns and hooves, and placement of a hand or a pad between the hocks may help to prevent self-trauma. The duration of physical restraint should be minimized to prevent distress and hyperthermia, and a clear airway and adequate chest excursion should be ensured at all times. Use of a blindfold may reduce struggling. If an animal is to be restrained repeatedly, short pieces of hosing placed on the horn tips improves safety for the handlers. Release should be coordinated such that handlers act quickly and in concert, directing the animal toward a clear path and to an open area that provides the patient with a sense of refuge and minimizes the risk of injury.

Mechanical Restraint

The development of sophisticated chute systems for hoof stock has allowed for the handling of entire herds of nondomestic bovids rapidly and without chemical restraint.[25] Procedures such as venipuncture, vaccination, tuberculin testing, physical examination, treatment of minor conditions, hoof trimming, and reproductive procedures may be conducted without chemical restraint in an effectively designed chute system. In designing a restraint, considerations such as maneuvering animals from a pen into the chute, the ability to stop and sort animals within the system, the inclusion of movable rear walls for pushing resistant animals, the presence of a scale within the system, and multiple exit routes may be critical to creating a process that is efficient and safe, minimizing time and stress to the animals. Desensitizing animals to any chute system by incorporating movement through the system into the animals' regular routine may greatly facilitate restraint. Many facilities housing large numbers of bovid and equid species are now using chute systems to facilitate preventive medicine, reproductive management, research, and extended treatment of animals, while alleviating the need for repeated chemical restraint.

Mechanical restraints are of three basic types: (1) box chutes or stanchions, (2) drop-floor chutes, and (3) crushes or squeeze chutes. Box chutes are the simplest and least expensive of the three, consisting of a simple pass-through enclosure with front and rear sliding barriers to retain the animal temporarily. Rear entry or exit restraints are not recommended for nondomestic bovids, as many of these animals are reluctant to enter an area with no perceived exit.

Drop-floor chutes are available commercially and consist of a ramp leading to, or a recessed area underneath, an adjustable V-shaped chute with sliding front and rear doors. When the animal is secured in the chute, the floor is dropped such that the animal is suspended by the hips and shoulders (Tamer Drop Floor Chute, Fauna Research, Inc., Red Hook, NY). Most bovids will refrain from struggling without foot purchase, allowing short procedures to be conducted. Width settings for each animal should be carefully established with drop-floor chutes to provide proper restraint, while not overly restricting the abdomen and chest, and duration of procedures should be limited to a few minutes. Drop-floor chutes may be portable or permanently installed.

Squeeze chutes vary from simple adaptations to an aisle way to highly adjustable hydraulic systems. Squeeze chutes developed for domestic cattle have been adapted to larger nondomestic bovids such as wild cattle and bison by adding "crash" gates—barred swinging front doors to prevent bypass of the head gate. Hydraulic squeeze chutes, available commercially (e.g., Hydraulic Tamer, Fauna Research, Inc., Red Hook, NY), provide the most flexible and rapid manipulation of large numbers of animals, as they are adjusted remotely while the animal is in the device. The padded walls of this restraint device are moved hydraulically to apply pressure to the hips and shoulders of the animal and may lift—achieving a result similar to a drop-floor chute—or close down over the animal to provide a darkened enclosed space. Doors installed in the restraint walls provide access for examination, treatment, and venipuncture.

Chemical Restraint

When physical and behavioral restraints are inadequate to maintain control of an animal for the length of time or invasive nature of the desired procedure, chemical restraint is necessary as an adjunct or sole method of restraint. Chemical restraint is commonly necessary in the management of nondomestic bovids and carries significant risks because of the fractious nature of the species, the difficulty of drug delivery, and the unique biology of the taxon. Veterinary practitioners caring for nondomestic Bovidae are constantly evaluating and improving protocols for sedation and anesthesia, as sensitivity to different anesthetics among nondomestic bovids tend to be species-specific. Chemical restraint in this taxon has been the subject of many reviews.[3,10,13,29,53]

Tranquilization and Sedation

Chemical restraint may be accomplished by two means: tranquilization and general anesthesia. Increasingly, neuroleptics of the butyrophenone and phenothiazine families have been used to attenuate the stress response in nondomestic ruminants undergoing intensive

TABLE 63-3

Onset and Duration of Action of Selected Neuroleptics Used in Bovidae[16,44]

Drug	Route	Onset	Duration
Azaperone	IV	<10 minutes	≤6 hours
	IM	30 minutes	≤6 hours
Haloperidol lactate	IV	<5 minutes	≤8 hours
	IM	<15 minutes	8–18 hours
Zuclopenthixol acetate	IM	1 hour	3–4 days
Zuclopenthixol decanoate	IM	1 week	10–21 days
Haloperidol decanoate	IM	2–3 days	21–30 days
Perphenazine enanthate	IM	hours	7–10 days
Pipothiazine palmitate	IM	2–3 days	21–28 days
Fluphenazine decanoate	IM	3 days	21–28 days

IM, Intramuscularly; *IV*, intravenously.

management for capture, translocation, isolation, or adaptation to environmental changes.[10,16,44] Licensed for use in humans as antipsychotic agents, these drugs act by blocking D2 dopamine receptors, thereby producing a state of lucid relief from anxiety. Most of the longer-acting formulations have an onset of action of 1 to 3 days, necessitating the addition of short-acting neuroleptics to produce immediate and long-term tranquilization. Table 63-3 lists common formulations and their onset and duration of action, and Table 63-4 lists suggested doses of neuroleptic drugs for tranquilization of pronghorns and bovids. Recommended dosages per kilogram of body weight are inversely proportional to body size. It should be noted that neuroleptic use may improve the ease of captive management of smaller hoof stock by increasing flight distance, but reducing the fear response may have the opposite effect in larger, more aggressive species, resulting in reduced avoidance behavior, reluctance to move, and aggression. Overdosing is known to produce behavioral side effects such as tardive dyskinesia, including abnormal facial and tongue posture, head pressing and other unusual movement patterns, and anorexia. Treatment of clinical signs of overdosing may be accomplished using low doses of xylazine, diazepam, or diphenhydramine.[44]

Induction of General Anesthesia

General anesthesia is induced parenterally by intramuscular or intravenous routes. Intravenous administration may be performed on manually or mechanically restrained animals and provides the advantage of decreased induction and recovery time. However, in larger animals, intravenous administration of a mechanically restrained animal may result in difficulty in removing the rapidly-induced animal from the restraint device. In general, intramuscular induction of an animal with an appropriate regimen in a darkened, quiet enclosure provides a relatively rapid and smooth induction and may minimize the need for anesthetic supplementation because of longer duration of action. Administration of anesthetics intramuscularly (IM) may be conducted by hand, pole syringe, or projectile dart. The use of darts and remote injection systems has been previously reviewed[27] and requires careful planning and experience. Planning an anesthetic event should include considerations such as environmental temperatures, approach, enclosure size, obstacles, and the presence of other animals. Failure to deliver an appropriate dose accurately and quickly to an animal in the wild or in a large enclosure may result in excessive running or pacing injury, capture stress or myopathy, and death. Muscle masses of the rump, shoulder, and neck are preferred sites of remote injection. Failure of induction within an appropriate time (usually 5 to 15 minutes, depending on the regimen) may be caused by many factors, including dart failure,

TABLE 63-4

Suggested Doses of Selected Neuroleptics Used in Adult Bovidae[16,44]

Family	Azaperone	Haloperidol lactate (IM or IV)	Zuclopenthixol acetate	Perphenazine enanthate	Pipotiazine palmitate	Fluphenazine decanoate
Aepycerotinae	0.5	0.2–0.5	1.0	1.0	4.0–4.5	0.5–1.0
Alcelaphinae	0.3–1.0	0.05–0.01	1.0	0.25–1.0	2.0–4.0	0.25–0.5
Antilopinae	0.25–0.5	0.1–1.0	2.0–5.0	1.0–5.0	1.0–2.5	0.5–1.0
Bovinae	0.1–0.5	0.025–0.2	0.3–2.0	0.1–1.0	0.1–1.0	0.25–0.5
Cephalophinae	0.5–1.0	0.25–0.5	—	2.0–5.0	—	—
Hippotraginae	0.5	0.1–0.2	0.5–1.0	0.5–1.0	0.25–0.5	0.25–0.5
Reduncinae	0.5–1.0	0.1–0.2	1.0–2.0	1.0	0.3–2.0	0.25–0.5

Note: All doses are intended for intramuscular use unless indicated.
IM, Intramuscularly; *IV,* intravenously.

inappropriate dosing, and operator error. A partially anesthetized animal is susceptible to capture myopathy, so a decision to repeat induction should be made within 20 minutes of initial dart placement. Supplementation by remote means generally requires a full anesthetic dose, as the animal may be rapidly metabolizing the anesthetic because of stress and activity.

Many anesthetic regimens have been described for pronghorns and bovids,[3,10,29,53] and these regimens generally consist of ultrapotent narcotics (carfentanil, etorphine, thiafentanil), with or without sedatives or tranquilizers (α_2-agonists, butyrophenones), dissociative cyclohexamines (ketamine or tiletamine), or both. The use of the mixed opioid agonist–antagonist butorphanol tartrate as a component of anesthetic cocktails has been recently reviewed.[6] Historically, the ultrapotent opioid (narcotic) agents carfentanil citrate, etorphine, and thiafentanil oxalate have been the primary components of anesthetic cocktails used in nondomestic bovid species for many reasons: (1) Opioid agents have a relatively wide margin of safety for the patient and are highly potent, allowing for small volumes to be contained in remote delivery darts; (2) they are rapid acting and provide an efficient induction and minimize the risk of hyperthermia; and (3) they are reversible. However, ultrapotent opioids are associated with significant side effects such as suppression of respiration and GI motility, poor muscle relaxation, and renarcotization[46] and carry a risk to human safety, as the lethal human dose of some agents is as low as 20 micrograms (μg).[29] Ultrapotent opioids are Schedule II substances controlled by the Drug Enforcement Agency and thereby require the practitioner to possess special licensing and to follow defined possession, storage, and recordkeeping guidelines. Safety protocols and special training for handling narcotics and exposure emergencies must be maintained for all staff involved in ultrapotent narcotic procedures. Carfentanil citrate is the most potent of the three agents. Etorphine and thiafentanil oxalate may produce desirable effects such as improved muscle relaxation and decreased respiratory suppression in some species. Opioids, particularly carfentanil, may produce general anesthesia when administered alone; however, combination with other agents may reduce the narcotic dose, ease induction and recovery, increase muscle relaxation, and decrease respiratory suppression.

The α_2-agonists reported in bovid anesthetic regimens include xylazine, detomidine, and medetomidine. In general, bovids are more sensitive to the α_2-agonists compared with equids, and these agents may improve muscle relaxation, decrease narcotic doses, and ease induction and recovery. In smaller bovids and pronghorns, these drugs may be combined with cyclohexamines, benzodiazepines, butorphanol, or a combination, eliminating the need for an ultrapotent opioid. α_2-agonists, however, require 20 minutes to reach full effect when administered IM; approaching a recumbent animal prior to this time may result in spontaneous recovery and the need to re-administer the induction dose. α_2-agonists—particularly

medetomidine—cause peripheral vasoconstriction, which may result in hypertension, bradycardia, poor mucous membrane color, and second-degree atrioventricular blocks. Use of parasympathomimetics such as atropine or glycopyrrolate to increase heart rate is controversial, as the resulting increased cardiac output may exacerbate hypertension. Medetomidine is available in highly concentrated formulations (Wildlife Pharmaceuticals, Inc., Fort Collins, CO), improving its usefulness for remote delivery in large species.

Dissociative anesthetics include the cyclohexamines ketamine hydrochloride and tiletamine (which is formulated in combination with the benzodiazepine zolazepam). These drugs are rapid acting, carry a high margin of safety, and are often used as adjuncts or supplemental anesthetics either intravenously (IV) or IM at 0.3 to 1.0 mg/kg. However, cyclohexamines are not reversible and thereby may affect duration of and recovery from anesthesia. When ketamine is used as a supplement, antagonism of reversible anesthetics should be delayed until 20 minutes after ketamine administration. This allows for ketamine metabolism and may prevent stormy recovery. Tiletamine, particularly when used without reversal of the zolazepam component (see Table 63-6), may be associated with prolonged recovery.

A partial list of suggested regimens for general anesthesia of bovids and pronghorns by species is presented in Table 63-5, and suggested reversal agents and doses are listed in Table 63-6.

ANESTHESIA AND SURGERY

The risks associated with general anesthesia in any species are confounded in bovids by their physiology, size, and temperament. Measures should be taken during any anesthetic procedure to prevent, identify, and treat hyperthermia, capture myopathy, metabolic derangements, respiratory depression, tympany, circulatory compromise, and regurgitation. Regurgitation is a common reaction to anesthetics and is complicated by positioning and anesthetic-induced ileus and tympany. Consequently, aspiration pneumonia is a significant risk in the unintubated ruminant. Intubation may be performed in most species by using a laryngoscope and a flexible stylet.[3,10] The patient should be at an adequate plane of anesthesia prior to intubation to prevent swallowing and stimulation of regurgitation.[3] Once intubated, the animal should be maintained in ventral or right lateral recumbency to minimize gastric pressure and ease ventilation. The head should be supported, with the nose down to allow regurgitated material to flow from the mouth. Adequate padding should be ensured, especially in heavy-bodied animals, to prevent pressure neuropathy of the limbs. Eye covers and ear plugs are recommended to minimize stimulation during anesthesia.

Intubation offers multiple measures of safety to the anesthetic procedure, including the ability to perform intermittent positive pressure ventilation (IPPV), often necessary to prevent hypoxemia

TABLE 63-5

Combinations of Chemical Restraint Agents Used for Induction of Anesthesia in Selected Species of Antilocapridae and Bovidae*[3,8,10,29,31,53]

	CARF	ETOR	THIA	XYL	MED	DET	KET/AZAP
ANTILOCAPRIDAE							
Pronghorn	0.05			1.0			
		0.1		1.0			
					0.3		
			0.1	0.5			5 K
AEPYCEROTINAE							
Impala	0.02–0.03			± 0.1–0.2			
		0.08–0.10		0.1–0.3			
			0.08				
			0.04	0.5–0.1	Or 0.025–0.05		
					0.20–0.25		3–5 K
ALCELAPHINAE							
Hartebeest	0.01			0.15			
Wildebeest	0.008			0.08			
			0.03	0.1			
Bontebok/blesbok	0.015–0.025			0.2–0.35			1.5–2.5 K
		0.020–0.025		0.2–0.3			0.2–0.3 K
			0.03				0.5 A
					0.05–0.09		1.0–1.3 K
Tsessebe			0.03	0.1			0.3 A
ANTILOPINAE							
Springbok	0.03						
		0.05–0.10		0.15–0.25			
				0.5			9.0 K
Blackbuck	0.05						
		0.1					
					0.25		2.0 K
Addra gazelle	0.015–0.02			±0.20			
		0.03–0.06					
					0.06–0.10		1.8–4 K
Slender-horned gazelle	0.03–0.05			0.10–0.25			
Grant gazelle	0.035						
Thomson's gazelle	0.02–0.03						
		0.05–0.07		0.2–0.45			0.2–0.45 K
Gerenuk					0.06–0.07		1.5–2.0 K
			0.04				3.5 K
Dik-dik		0.01		0.4			
Suni		0.01		0.4			
				0.2–0.4			15 K
Klipspringer		0.01		0.4			
		0.05					
					0.16		2.1 K
Saiga	0.05–0.1						
BOVINAE							
Bison	0.004–0.008			0.05–0.10			
		0.01		0.05			
				0.5–1			4 K
					0.05–0.08		1.5–2.5 K
Gaur, gayal, banteng	0.006–0.01			0.1–0.2			
		0.01–0.02					
Nilgai	0.02						
		0.03					
Anoa	0.008–0.012			0.06–0.12			

Continued

TABLE 63-5

Combinations of Chemical Restraint Agents Used for Induction of Anesthesia in Selected Species of Antilocapridae and Bovidae—cont'd

	CARF	ETOR	THIA	XYL	MED	DET	KET/AZAP
African buffalo	0.005			0.05			
		0.015		0.1–0.15			
			0.01–0.025		±0.05–0.1		
Giant eland	0.008					0.03	
	0.005–0.007			0.05–0.10			
Common eland	0.01–0.016			0.15–0.20			
		0.02		0.40			
			0.03–0.07	0.1			
				0.8			4 K
Nyala	0.015–0.025			0.10–0.25			
		0.04		0.30			
			0.045		0.05		3–4 K
			0.08	0.3			
Sitatunga	0.04			0.3			
Tibetan yak			0.02	0.15			
Bongo	0.01–0.025			0.1–0.25			
	0.01			0.15–0.2			0.5 K
			0.02–0.05	0.05–0.15			
Greater kudu	0.02–0.25			0.2–0.25			
		0.02–0.03		0.2–0.3			
			0.05	0.25			
CEPHALOPHINAE							
Maxwell duiker	0.025						
		0.02		1			
				0.2–0.3			15–25 K
Blue duiker		0.01		0.40			
				0.3			15 K
					0.2		2.2 K
Yellow-backed duiker	0.02–0.03			0.2			
		0.02		1			
Common duiker			0.01–0.02	0.5			
HIPPOTRAGINAE							
Addax	0.025			± 0.15–0.25			
		0.03–0.04				0.02	
					0.05–0.06		1.0 K
Roan	0.015–0.02			0.15–0.2			
		0.025		0.15–0.25			
			0.01–0.02		0.005–0.006		0.3–0.6 K
Sable	0.015–0.02			0.15–0.2			
		0.015–0.025		0.1–0.2			±0.15–0.2 K
			0.03	0.1–0.2			
Scimitar-horned oryx	0.015–0.03			0.15–0.3			
		0.025		0.15			
		0.05			0.005		
Gemsbok	0.01–0.02			0.1–0.2			
		0.03		0.25			
		0.015		0.15–0.25			0.15–0.25 K
			0.02–0.04		0.02–0.04		1.0 K
Arabian oryx	0.03–0.04			0.25			
		0.03–0.04		0.3			
		0.04			0.005		
		0.045–0.05				0.045–0.05	
					0.03–0.06		1.2–2 K

TABLE 63-5

Combinations of Chemical Restraint Agents Used for Induction of Anesthesia in Selected Species of Antilocapridae and Bovidae—cont'd

	CARF	ETOR	THIA	XYL	MED	DET	KET/AZAP
REDUNCINAE							
Waterbuck	0.01–0.025			0.10–0.25			
		0.03		0.25			
			0.03–0.05	0.2			
Red lechwe	0.02						
	0.01			0.1			
			0.02–0.05	0.1–0.4			0.1–0.4 K
Nile lechwe	0.02			0.25			1.0–2.0 K
			0.02				1.5–3.0 K
Uganda kob	0.035			0.35			
Reedbuck			0.05–0.07	0.2			±0.1 A
Rhebok	0.01			0.4			
		0.01		0.4			

AZAP (A), Azaperone; *CARF*, carfentanil citrate; *DET*, detomidine; *ETOR*, etorphine; *KET (K)*, ketamine; *MED*, medetomidine; *THIA*, thiafentanil oxalate; *XYL*, xylazine.
*Doses are intended for intramuscular injection.

TABLE 63-6

Common Antagonists for Anesthetic Drugs Used in Antilocapridae and Bovidae

Anesthetic	Preferred Antagonist	Dosage	Comments
Carfentanil	Naltrexone	100 milligram per milligram (mg/mg) carfentanil, intramuscularly (IM)	May be given partially intravenously (IV)
Etorphine	Naltrexone	50 mg/mg etorphine, IM	May be given partially IV
Thiafentanil	Naltrexone	30 mg/mg thiafentanil, IM	May be given partially IV
Butorphanol	Naltrexone	5 mg/mg butorphanol, IM	
Medetomidine	Atipamezole or tolazoline*	5 mg/mg medetomidine, IM 1 milligram per kilogram (mg/kg), IM	
Detomidine	Atipamezole or tolazoline*	0.1 mg/kg, IM 1 mg/kg, IM	
Xylazine	Atipamezole or tolazoline*	0.1 mg/kg, IM 1 mg/kg, IM	
Tiletamine/ zolazepam	Flumazenil	0.01 mg/kg, IV	Ketamine and tiletamine are not reversible

*Intravenous administration of tolazoline in artiodactyls may cause profound hypotension and death.

caused by apnea or inadequate ventilation. IPPV pressure and volume should be less than 25 millimeters of mercury (mm Hg) and 8 to 12 mL/kg, respectively.[10] In larger animals, the use of a demand valve aids delivery of high volumes of oxygen, ensuring adequate tidal volume.[46] Administration of inhalant anesthetics (isoflurane or sevoflurane) via an endotracheal tube provides control of the duration and depth of anesthesia and may assist in management of hypertension or hypotension.

Depth of anesthesia, cardiovascular parameters, respiration, hydration, and GI motility should be monitored in any ruminant undergoing general anesthesia and surgery. Heart rate should be 40 to 80 beats per minute (beats/min), mucous membranes pink and moist (cyanosis indicates <70% oxygen saturation),[30] and capillary refill time less than 2 seconds. Hemoglobin oxygen saturation as measured by pulse oximetry should be greater than 90%, below which arterial partial pressure of oxygen may be less than 60 mm Hg (normal = 70–100 mm Hg).[30] Proper ventilation should maintain end tidal carbon dioxide (CO_2) levels at less than 60 mm Hg. Hydration may be subjectively measured by skin turgor, corneal and mucous membrane moistness, and ocular retraction. Normal partial pressure of arterial carbon dioxide ($PaCO_2$) is 35 to 50 mm Hg, and normal blood bicarbonate is 20 to 30 millimoles per liter (mmol/L).[10] The conditions of recovery from anesthesia are as important to animal and human safety as those during induction. Prior to reversal of anesthesia, the animal should be removed from inhalant anesthesia and adequately ventilated for at least 5 minutes. Maintenance of minimal levels and progressive reduction of inhalant anesthesia during the procedure, in addition to allowing for metabolism of supplemental injected anesthetics, may improve the quality and speed of recovery. The animal should be supported in ventral recumbency in a quiet, darkened enclosure, if possible. Following administration of the reversal agent, the eye cover and the endotracheal tube may remain in place until a swallow response is detected. Gentle removal of a partially inflated endotracheal tube will help to clear regurgitated materials from the pharynx.

Vascular access of most nondomestic bovids is most easily accomplished following a small cut-down with a large gauge needle or scalpel blade.[3] Relatively common conditions requiring surgery

TABLE 63-7

Adult Reference Ranges for Hematologic Parameters of Select Species of Antilocapridae and Bovidae[49]

Parameter*	Pronghorn	Impala	Brindled wildebeest	Thomson's gazelle	American bison	Common duiker	Scimitar-horned oryx	Common waterbuck
WBC ($\times 10^3$/ microliter [µL])	6.470 ± 4.911 (159)	3.528 ± 1.464 (314)	6.918 ± 2.358 (29)	3.855 ± 2.205 (291)	7.152 ± 3.674 (134)	6.200 ± 2.201 (7)	6.275 ± 2.393 (537)	6.354 ± 3.855 (125)
Neutrophils ($\times 10^3$/µL)	4.879 ± 4.133 (155)	2.028 ± 1.309 (266)	4.174 ± 1.587 (19)	2.623 ± 1.952 (262)	3.544 ± 2.709 (131)	3.154 ± 2.435 (7)	4.179 ± 1.884 (403)	4.170 ± 3.663 (106)
Lymphocytes ($\times 10^3$/µL)	1.085 ± 0.794 (156)	1.342 ± 0.773 (270)	2.490 ± 2.149 (19)	1.188 ± 0.766 (272)	2.867 ± 1.875 (133)	2.989 ± 1.155 (7)	1.393 ± 0.799 (412)	2.114 ± 1.561 (106)
Monocytes ($\times 10^3$/µL)	0.181 ± 0.181 (122)	0.105 ± 0.123 (127)	0.230 ± 0.088 (14)	0.094 ± 0.079 (163)	0.264 ± 0.261 (116)	—	0.132 + 0.185 (347)	0.117 ± 0.129 (59)
Eosinophils ($\times 10^3$/µL)	0.331 ± 0.424 (104)	0.121 ± 0.125 (144)	0.181 ± 0.119 (14)	0.062 ± 0.094 (59)	0.466 ± 0.478 (115)	0.060 ± 0.026 (3)	0.183 ± 0.263 (315)	0.155 ± 0.245 (47)
Basophils ($\times 10^3$/µL)	0.085 ± 0.111 (48)	0.031 ± 0.038 (42)	0.163 ± 0.079 (11)	0.046 ± 0.047 (34)	0.125 ± 0.127 (57)	—	0.022 ± 0.046 (219)	0.085 ± 0.043 (18)
RBC ($\times 10^6$/µL)	10.29 ± 1.83 (71)	12.49 ± 6.59 (262)	10.50 ± 3.64 (22)	10.22 ± 1.62 (280)	8.23 ± 1.72 (105)	11.67 ± 1.22 (7)	8.70 ± 1.94 (486)	10.25 ± 2.52 (118)
Hematocrit (%)	41.1 ± 6.8 (170)	42.0 ± 9.1 (319)	42.4 ± 8.7 (31)	48.7 ± 7.3 (317)	44.1 ± 6.8 (141)	54.3 ± 3.4 (7)	37.6 ± 6.7 (590)	44.6 ± 9.1139)

*Values are reported as mean ± standard deviation (number of samples).
RBC, Red blood cells; *WBC*, white blood cells.

include trauma, abscesses, horn fractures and avulsions, hoof abscesses, castration, vasectomy, herniorrhaphy, ovariectomy, ovariohysterectomy, exploratory laparotomy, and tumor excisions. Less commonly, eye enucleation, cesarean section, and surgical treatment of corneal lacerations and ulcers, cataracts, angular limb deformities, GI or urinary obstructions, umbilical abscess, patent urachus, and rectal, uterine or vaginal prolapse are warranted.[10] Laparoscopy is useful in nondomestic bovids for assisted reproduction, minimally invasive abdominal and thoracic exploratory, biopsy, and endosurgical techniques. In large bovids, laparoscopic procedures may require intubation and positive pressure ventilation because of the pressure of the abdominal viscera on the thoracic cavity when the animal has been secured in dorsal recumbency at a head-down tilt.

DIAGNOSTICS

Diagnostics used in nondomestic bovids and pronghorns are similar to those used in domestic cattle, sheep, and goats. Common sites of vascular access include the jugular, cephalic, medial and lateral saphenous, and ventral tail veins, as well as the auricular, facial, medial tarsal, and digital arteries.[10] Cystocentesis is accomplished most easily with the aid of ultrasonography; normal urine pH is 7 to 9.5 with a specific gravity of 1.020 to 1.050.[10] Cerebrospinal fluid (CSF) may be collected from the lumbosacral cistern or the cisterna magna. The specific gravity of normal bovid CSF is 1.004 to 1.008, with less than 40 mg/dL protein and fewer than three white blood cells (WBCs) per microliter.[10]

Hematologic (Table 63-7) and serum biochemistry (Table 63-8) values of nondomestic bovids may vary within and among subfamilies. Measurement of fibrinogen is generally more useful than a WBC count for assessing inflammation in bovids, and protein electrophoresis may be useful in monitoring chronic inflammation. Serum bile acids are a useful measure for monitoring the course of hepatic disease and its response to therapy.[10]

INFECTIOUS DISEASE

Transboundary Animal Diseases

Animals and animal products are transported globally at an increasing rate every year such that entrance of an animal disease to a country formerly free of the disease is considered more a probability than a possibility.[5] Zoologic veterinarians have an increased opportunity to encounter such diseases and should therefore be aware of clinical signs and appropriate reporting and diagnostic plans in case of a suspected reportable disease. A description of foreign (transboundary) animal diseases, emergency procedures, and disinfectants is available in the publication of the *Committee on Foreign and Emerging Animal Diseases of the United States Animal Health Association*.[5] Notifiable diseases listed by the World Organization for Animal Health (OIE) that may affect or be carried by nondomestic bovids are listed in Table 63-9. Rinderpest, formerly listed as notifiable by the OIE, has been reported to have been eradicated worldwide.[35]

Common Infectious Diseases

Nondomestic bovids are susceptible to virtually all of the common infectious diseases of domestic ruminants. Selected diseases of concern to zoologic species of bovids and pronghorns are listed in Tables 63-10 and 63-11. Bacterial infections are of increasing importance in zoologic species because of multidrug-resistant pathogens.[28] Abscesses and other infections caused by pathogens such as *Arcanobacterium pyogenes*, *Fusobacterium necrophorum*, *Staphylococcus*, *Streptococcus*, *Pseudomonas*, and others may lead to systemic infection and death if not treated to resolution, on the basis of culture and sensitivity testing. Strict sanitation measures in hospital settings are required to prevent frequent infections and development of antibacterial resistance of resident organisms. Hoof infections are particularly common in some species, especially in weather and substrate conditions unnatural to the species[60] and may involve lengthy treatment with systemic antibiotics, regional perfusion, hoof curettage, topical treatment, and protective bandaging. Some animals cannot tolerate long-term confinement to allow healing: once infection is eliminated, hoof deficits may, in some cases, be filled with hoof repair material (which may be impregnated with antibiotics), allowing return of the animal to its home enclosure. These materials are worn away as granulation tissue fills the hoof capsule and results in a normal hoof.

Mycobacterial diseases remain a concern because of the lack of clinical signs in early stages and to the sensitivity and specificity of existing diagnostics. Of most concern are tuberculosis[37] (*Mycobacte-*

TABLE 63-8

Adult Reference Ranges for Serum Biochemical Parameters of Select Species of Antilocapridae and Bovidae[49]

Parameter*	Pronghorn	Impala	Brindled wildebeest	Thomson gazelle	American bison	Common duiker	Scimitar-horned oryx	Common waterbuck
Total protein, gram per deciliter (g/dL)	5.8 ± 1.2 (132)	5.6 ± 0.6 (200)	6.5 ± 0.5 (18)	5.8 ± 0.9 (189)	7.6 ± 1.2 (97)	7.2 ± 0.7 (5)	6.0 ± 0.8 (414)	6.6 ± 1.0 (84)
Albumin (g/dL)	2.8 ± 1.0 (120)	3.3 ± 0.5 (200)	3.9 ± 0.4 (11)	2.9 ± 0.5 (174)	3.6 ± 0.7 (78)	3.3 ± 0.4 (5)	3.3 ± 0.8 (339)	3.1 ± 0.7 (72)
AST, international unit per liter (IU/L)	155 ± 146 (128)	245 ± 124 223	131 ± 88 (21)	185 ± 136 (204)	102 ± 46 (87)	116 ± 27 (6)	106 ± 67 (427)	151 ± 96 (91)
ALT (IU/L)	24 ± 23 (100)	45 ± 20 (195)	106 ± 199 (17)	41 ± 25 (193)	29 ± 18 (52)	11 ± 6 (6)	18 ± 9 (177)	33 ± 19 (94)
ALP (IU/L)	369 ± 412 (104)	241 ± 280 (225)	183 ± 196 (19)	498 ± 841 (219)	98 ± 104 (93)	472 ± 340 (6)	222 ± 347 (427)	281 ± 442 (99)
GGT (IU/L)	—	—	117 ± 19 (12)	—	20 ± 32 (56)	169 ± 64 (3)	25 ± 28 (86)	278 ± 191 (42)
Calcium, milligram per deciliter (mg/dL)	9.4 ± 0.9 (118)	9.8 ± 1.7 (234)	8.1 ± 2.3 (19)	9.3 ± 1.1 (226)	9.3 ± 1.2 (95)	9.4 ± 1.1 (6)	9.4 ± 1.1 (456)	10.6 ± 0.7 (95)
Phosphorus (mg/dL)	8.4 ± 1.5 (113)	7.2 ± 2.0 (228)	6.6 ± 2.2 (15)	6.8 ± 2.3 (216)	7.3 ± 2.7 (88)	6.9 ± 0.8 (6)	6.5 ± 1.9 (432)	7.2 ± 1.9 (87)
Sodium, milliequivalent per liter (mEq/L)	150 ± 4 (119)	150 ± 4 (218)	137 ± 5 (16)	150 ± 5 (216)	141 ± 6 (90)	147 ± 2 (6)	143 ± 4 (436)	147 ± 5 (91)
Potassium (mEq/L)	4.8 ± 0.6118	4.3 ± 0.8 (223)	5.2 ± 1.2 (16)	4.9 ± 1.1 (221)	4.7 ± 0.6 (90)	6.6 ± 1.7 (6)	4.5 ± 0.6 (444)	4.9 ± 0.8 (92)
Chloride (mEq/L)	106 ± 4 (117)	107 ± 4 (223)	95 ± 3 (14)	107 ± 5 (219)	102 ± 4 (84)	105 ± 4 (6)	103 ± 4 (360)	103 ± 6 (91)
Magnesium (mg/dL)	1.73 ± 0.27 (50)	1.65 ± 0.21 (16)	1.05 ± 0.88 (6)	1.95 ± 0.43 (28)	10.39 ± 8.6 (20)	—	1.60 ± 0.61 (32)	2.12 ± 0.62 (14)
Glucose (mg/dL)	136 ± 50 (133)	148 ± 44 (227)	95 ± 46 (21)	143 ± 57 (226)	145 ± 52 (100)	81 ± 32 (6)	174 ± 71 (427)	157 ± 61 (98)
Urea nitrogen (mg/dL)	29 ± 10 (132)	26 ± 8 (233)	20 ± 8 (21)	27 ± 9 (224)	21 ± 7 (98)	26 ± 9 (6)	24 ± 7 (460)	25 ± 7 (98)
Creatinine (mg/dL)	1.1 ± 0.3 (129)	1.7 ± 0.4 (223)	19.5 ± 52.4 (18)	1.6 ± 0.4 (225)	2.6 ± 0.9 (97)	1.3 ± 0.4 (6)	1.6 ± 0.5 (425)	2.2 ± 0.7 (98)

*Values are reported as mean ± standard deviation (number of samples).
ALP, Alkaline phosphatase; ALT, alanine aminotransferase; AST, aspartate aminotransferase; GGT, gamma-glutamyltransferase.

TABLE 63-9

Transboundary Diseases of Importance to Nondomestic Bovids Listed as Notifiable by the World Organization for Animal Health (OIE)*

Disease	Country/Region of Occurrence	Etiology	Transmission	Comments
Anaplasmosis	Tropical or subtropical climates and some temperate regions	*Anaplasma marginale, A. centrale*	Mechanically or biologically by arthropod vectors	
Anthrax	Worldwide	*Bacillus anthracis*	Ingestion, inhalation, fomites	Zoonotic High mortality
Bovine babesiosis	Tropical and subtropical climates worldwide	*Babesia bigemina*	Vectorborne: ticks	Morbidity and mortality vary
Bovine tuberculosis	Worldwide	*Mycobacterium bovis*	Direct contact Inhalation Milk ingestion	Zoonotic
Bovine viral diarrhea	Worldwide	Flaviviridae, pestivirus	Direct contact	Multifactorial disease
Brucellosis	Asia, Middle East, Mediterranean, sub-Saharan Africa, Peru, and Mexico, western United States	*Brucella abortus*	Ingestion of placental tissues, transmammary Contamination of wounds (human)	Causes late term abortion Zoonotic: undulant fever in humans
Contagious bovine pleuropneumonia	Africa	*Mycoplasma mycoides*	Inhalation	Zoonotic
Echinococcosis or hydatidosis	Worldwide	*Echinococcus granulosus* and other spp.	Carnivore-ungulate cestode cycle	Zoonotic Human disease: organ damage and anaphylaxis
Enzootic bovine leukosis	Worldwide, some countries disease free	Retrovirus	Vertical Bloodborne	Subclinical, lymphocytosis, lymphosarcoma
Epizootic hemorrhagic disease	North America, Far East, Mediterranean	Reoviridae, orbivirus	Vectorborne, biting midges	Increasing in host range
Foot-and-mouth disease	Asia, Africa, Middle East, South America	Picornaviridae, aphthovirus	Direct contact—infected animals, fomites, meat and milk, aerosols	Maintained in African buffalo Highly contagious
Heartwater	Africa, Caribbean	*Ehrlichia ruminantium*	Vectorborne: ticks Colostrum Blood inoculation	
Hemorrhagic septicemia	Asia, Africa, S. Europe, and Middle East	*Pasteurella multocida*	Direct contact with infected animals and fomites	
Infectious bovine rhinotracheitis or infectious pustular vulvovaginitis	Worldwide Eradicated in Austria, Denmark, Finland, Sweden, Switzerland, and Norway	α-herpesvirus	Inhalation	Vaccine available, does not completely prevent infection
Lumpy skin disease	Africa, Middle East	Capripoxvirus	Mechanical vector: mosquitoes and flies Direct contact possible	High morbidity and mortality
Paratuberculosis (Johne disease)	Global	*Mycobacterium avium* subsp. *paratuberculosis*	Infected animals shed bacterium in manure, colostrum, and milk	See Table 63-11
Screwworm (New World, Old World)	Central America, Caribbean, South America, Africa, Middle East, Southeast Asia	*Cochliomyia hominivorax* (New world) *Chrysomya bezziana* (Old world)	Blowfly (myiasis)	Zoonotic Eradication efforts focus on release of sterile flies
Q fever	Worldwide, except New Zealand	*Coxiella burnetii*	Ingestion of milk, urine, feces, amniotic fluid, and placenta	Zoonotic Can be transmitted by ticks
Rabies	Global	Rhabdovirus	Saliva of infected animal Possible by inhalation	Zoonotic

TABLE 63-9

Transboundary Diseases of Importance to Nondomestic Bovids Listed as Notifiable by the World Organization for Animal Health (OIE)—cont'd

Disease	Country/Region of Occurrence	Etiology	Transmission	Comments
Rift Valley fever	Africa	Bunyaviridae, phlebovirus	Vectorborne: mosquitoes	Zoonotic: ingestion of meat
Theileriosis	Africa, southern Europe, Asia, Middle East	Protozoan: *Theileria parva, T. annulata*	Vectorborne: Ticks (*Rhipicephalus, Hyalomma*)	East Coast fever Corridor disease
Trichomonosis	Worldwide	Protozoan: *Trichomonas foetus*	Venereal	Causes abortion and infertility
Trypanosomiasis	Africa, Central/S. America	*Trypanosoma brucei, cruzi, evansi*	Vector-borne: tsetse fly Mechanical: biting flies, esp. tabanids	African sleeping sickness, Chagas disease, Surra
Vesicular stomatitis	South and Central America, Western US Endemic in feral pigs on Ossabaw Island, Georgia	Rhabdoviridae, vesiculovirus	Mechanism unclear— transcutaneous, mucosal	High morbidity, low mortality

*From http://www.oie.int/manual-of-diagnostic-tests-and-vaccines-for-terrestrial-animals/. Accessed June 26, 2012.

TABLE 63-10

Identification and Management of Selected Infectious Diseases of Antilocapridae and Bovidae

Disease	Clinical Presentation/Lesions	Diagnosis	Management
Viral enteritis (coronavirus, rotavirus)	Acute diarrhea Dehydration Malabsorption Neonatal death	Fecal electron microscopy Fecal ELISA IFA	Supportive care Colostrum supplementation Vaccination Sanitation
Bacterial enteritis	Diarrhea Depression Dehydration Asymptomatic	Bacterial culture PCR Histopathology	Supportive care Appropriate antibiotics Vaccination Sanitation
Tuberculosis[37]	Lymphadenopathy Wasting Bronchopneumonia or cough Mild or no clinical signs	Histopathology Intradermal tuberculin test (CT for Bovinae, SCT for other bovids)	Routine testing Identify and remove affected animals Prevent introduction Treatment not recommended
Johne disease (paratuberculosis)[12]	Stage I: subclinical Stage II: subclinical, intermittent shedding Stage III: ill-thrift, wasting, diarrhea Stage IV: lethargy, emaciation, diarrhea, intermandibular edema	Difficult in early stages Histopathology (Stage I-IV) Fecal culture (II-IV) PCR (II-IV) ELISA (II-IV) IFN-γ (II-IV)	Routine testing Identify and remove affected animals Prevent introduction
Malignant catarrhal fever (MCF)	Nasal and ocular discharge Lymphadenopathy Diarrhea, anorexia Fever, death	ELISA VN PCR	Prevent contact of potentially affected carriers with susceptible hosts Supportive care Antiviral medications
Meningeal worm	Ataxia, paresis, circling, hypermetria, abnormal head posture, wasting	Clinical signs Histopathology	Reduce exposure to deer; control snails; deworm every 4 to 6 weeks during spring/summer

CT, Caudal tail fold; *ELISA*, enzyme-linked immunosorbent assay; *IFA*, immunofluorescent antibody; *IFN-γ*, interferon-γ; *L3*, third-stage larva; *PCR*, polymerase chain reaction; *SCT*, single cervical test; *VN*, virus neutralization.

TABLE 63-11

Selected Differential Diagnoses for Nondomestic Bovids and Pronghorns

Viral	Bacterial	Parasitic	Fungal
MULTISYSTEMIC DISEASES			
Adenovirus	Anaplasmosis	Besnoitiosis	Aspergillosis
Bluetongue virus	Anthrax	Toxoplasmosis	Blastomycosis
Bovine viral diarrhea	Chlamydiophilosis	Cestodiasis	Candidiasis
Epizootic hemorrhagic disease	Leptospirosis		Coccidioidomycosis
Encephalomyocarditis			Cryptococcosis
Malignant catarrhal fever			
RESPIRATORY SYSTEM DISEASES			
Infectious bovine rhinotracheitis	Mycoplasmosis	Lungworm (*Dictyocaulus,*	Aspergillosis
Parainfluenza (PI-3)	Pasteurellosis	*Protostrongylus)*	
Bovine respiratory syncytial virus			
GASTROINTESTINAL SYSTEM DISEASES			
Coronavirus	*Clostridium perfringens* (A, B, C, E)	Amebiasis	Candidiasis
Rotavirus	Colibacillosis	Coccidiosis	
	Campylobcter jejuni	Cryptosporidiosis	
	Yersinia spp.	Giardiasis	
	Salmonella spp.	Nematodiasis	
		Liver flukes	
		Rumen flukes	
REPRODUCTIVE SYSTEM DISEASES			
Akabane virus	Brucellosis	Neosporosis	
Infectious pustular vulvovaginitis (BHV-1)	Q fever	Trichomoniasis	
	Campylobacter foetus		
INTEGUMENTARY/MUSCULOSKELETAL SYSTEM DISEASES			
Contagious echthyma (parapox)	Actinomycosis	Parafilariasis	Dermatophytosis
Poxvirus	*Corynebacterium*	Scabies	Dermatophilosis
	Pseudomonas spp.	Ticks	Sporotrichosis
	Fusobacterium spp.	Lice	
	Staphylococcus spp.	Warbles, bots, grubs	
	Streptococcus spp.	Screwworm	
	Arcanobacterium pyogenes	Flies	
	Blackleg/gangrene	Sarcocystosis	
	(*Clostridium* spp.)		
NERVOUS SYSTEM DISEASES			
Spongiform encephalopathy*	Listeriosis	Meningeal worm	
Eastern equine encephalitis	Tetanus		
Equine herpesvirus			
Rabies			
CIRCULATORY SYSTEM DISEASES			
	Eperythrozoonosis	Babesiosis	
		Cytauxzoonosis	
		Trypanosomiasis	
		Theileriosis	

*Prion disease.

rium bovis) and Johne disease[12] (*Mycobacterium avium* subsp. *paratuberculosis*) (see Table 63-10).

Transmissible spongiform encephalopathies have been rarely reported in zoo bovids and are suspected to be caused by cross-species transmission of bovine spongiform encephalopathy (BSE).[47]

Emerging Infectious Diseases

Deforestation, altered migration, increased international travel, and globalization of trade are some of the factors leading to the rapid evolution, emergence, and host susceptibility changes of diseases in recent decades. Diseases reported to be emerging in bovids because of increasing prevalence, host susceptibility, or both include Schmallenberg virus infection,[4] bovine besnoitiosis (*Besnoitia* spp.),[19,24] bartonellosis,[33] epizootic hemorrhagic disease (EHD),[18]

Johne disease (*Mycobacterium avium* subsp. *paratuberculosis*), malignant catarrhal fever, and equine herpesvirus infection. Malignant catarrhal fever and equine herpesvirus infection are of particular note because of their uncharacterized host susceptibility and the likelihood of these herpesviruses causing severe clinical disease in nondomestic bovid species.

Malignant Catarrhal Fever

Malignant catarrhal fever (MCF), a γ-herpesvirus of the genus Macavirus, is incompletely characterized and of importance to zoologic and wild bovid species and pronghorns. Currently, 10 viruses have been recognized within the MCF group, six of which are clearly associated with clinical disease.[32] The two most well-documented viruses, sheep-associated (SA-MCF) and wildebeest-associated MCF

(WA-MCF), are caused by ovine herpesvirus 2 (OvHV-2) and alcelaphine herpesvirus 1 (AlHV-1), respectively. Both viruses are carried asymptomatically in the reservoir host species (after which they are named), are pathogenic to other species, and are shed through ocular and oronasal secretions. WA-MCF is generally transmitted by calves from birth up to 4 months of age, but lambs are generally not infected with OvHV-1 until after 2 months of age and shed the pathogen intensively from 6 to 9 months of age. Lambs may, therefore, be separated from dams and raised virus-free.[32] Other described MCF viruses include hippotragine (HipHV-1) and alcelaphine 2 (AlHV-2) MCF, isolated from roan antelopes and hartebeests, respectively, but the epidemiology of these viruses remains poorly understood. Oryxes, ibexes, muskoxen, and aoudads are also known to harbor MCF viruses of unknown pathogenicity. Species susceptible to disease caused by MCF viruses include cattle, bison, deer, and pigs, but sporadic cases of MCF or MCF-like disease in a variety of captive nondomestic bovids have been reported.[22,32] Susceptible hosts may be subclinically or clinically affected. Bison are known to be 1000 times more susceptible, compared with cattle, to clinical SA-MCF,[32] and bongos have been recently reported to acquire fatal MCF from Nubian ibexes.[22,32] The clinical presentation of MCF is variable but usually includes profuse nasal and ocular discharge, corneal opacity, diarrhea, enlarged lymph nodes, fever, anorexia, and often death within 24 to 72 hours. Pathologic findings include lymphoproliferative vasculitis and epithelial necrosis. Identification of clinically relevant reservoir species is complicated by the incomplete characterization of these complex and evolving viruses: serologic tests distinguishing OvHV-2 and AlHV-1, however, are available. In the face of a suspected outbreak in a mixed-species situation, a multiplex PCR is the first choice diagnostic.[32]

Equine Herpesviruses

Equine herpesvirus (EHV-9) has been reported to cause fatal encephalitis in a number of non-equid species, including Thomson's gazelles and blackbucks.[14,55] The epidemiology of this virus outside its natural host has not been completely elucidated; EHV-9 and the closely-related EHV-1 have been transmitted to aberrant hosts both directly and indirectly. This, as well as the potentially wide species susceptibility, has led to recent concern about the zoologic setting creating unnatural proximity among geographically diverse species, encouraging cross-species disease transmission.

PARASITIC DISEASES

Ectoparasites found on nondomestic bovids include sucking and chewing lice; warble and bot flies, ticks, mites, various mosquitoes, biting midges, sand flies, black flies, tabanid flies, louse flies, and muscoid flies. Control of ectoparasites may use multiple methodologies, including life cycle disruption, baiting and trapping, and biologic control agents, although the most commonly used methods are topical and parenteral parasiticides.[10,45]

Protozoal diseases affecting bovids include opportunistic amebiasis, babesiosis, besnoitiosis, coccidiosis (*Eimeria* spp. and *Isospora* spp.), cryptosporidiosis (*Cryptosporidim parvum* and *C. muris*-like sp.), cytauxzoonosis, giardiasis (*Giardia duodenalis*), hepatozoonosis, neosporosis (*Neospora caninum*), sarcocystosis (*Sarcocystis* spp.), theileriasis (*Theileria* spp.), toxoplasmosis (*Toxoplasma gondii*), and trypanosomiasis (*Trypanosoma* spp.).[10,45] Cestodes commonly affecting bovids include *Echinococcus, Moniezia, Taenia,* and *Thysanosoma.* The most common GI nematodes of captive bovids are the *Haemonchus, Ostertagia, Nematodirus, Strongyloides,* and *Trichuris,* although a number of other parasites are found to cause diarrhea, ill-thrift, and anemia.[45] Meningeal worm (*Parelaphostrongylus tenuis*) infestation is a regional disease carried asymptomatically in the subdural sinuses of white-tailed deer and is transmitted to aberrant hosts (nondomestic bovids, cervids, camelids, and goats) through ingestion of third-stage larvae in feces. Larvae migrate in the spinal cord, causing clinical signs and often death. Identification and management are discussed in Table 63-10.

Management of Gastrointestinal Parasites

Effective control programs must be multifactorial, as reliance on parenteral parasiticides has led to widespread anthelmintic resistance.[20] Such programs may be extremely labor intensive and involve (1) routine parasite monitoring, (2) larval drug sensitivity assays, (3) pasture larval counts, and (4) alternatives to pharmaceuticals for parasite control. Nonpharmaceutical strategies for reducing parasite burdens, which are reviewed thoroughly elsewhere,[20, 45,50] include decreasing stocking density, pasture rotation, elevating feed and browse, feeding tannin-containing plants such as sericia lespedeza (*Lespedeza cuneata*) and nematode-trapping fungi,[50] and providing refugia (untreated nonclinical animals) for susceptible parasites to dilute the frequency of resistant alleles.[52] The use of oral copper oxide wire particles (COWP; Copasure, Butler Schein Animal Health, Dublin, OH) is increasing in zoologic institutions with some success.[20] Although dosing for nondomestic artiodactyls has not been thoroughly investigated, the manufacturer's recommended dose of COWP for cattle (70–225 kg) is 12.5 g, and 2 to 6 grams per animal has been reported efficacious and without toxicity in sheep and goats.[50] COWP may be administered in capsules or feed, are effective against abomasal parasites only, and should be limited to no more than every 6 to 12 month usage, with careful monitoring of fecal parasite levels and attention to potential toxicity. Pharmaceutical parasiticides used in nondomestic bovids include albendazole, amprolium, decoquinate, doramectin, eprinomectin, fenbendazole, ivermectin, levamisole, metronidazole, morantel, moxidectin, oxfendazole, praziquantel, pyrantel, selamectin, and sulfa/trimethoprim, with dosages similar to those used in domestic bovids.[10]

NONINFECTIOUS DISEASE

Common noninfectious diseases of wild and captive bovids are characterized as traumatic injuries, congenital and growth disorders, and degenerative; environmental (hypothermia, frostbite); dental (periodontal disease, dental abscessation); GI (choke, foreign bodies, abomasal impaction, rumen acidosis or rumenitis, tympany); metabolic (hypocalcemia/hypomagnesemia, capture myopathy); renal or urinary (urolithiasis, renal failure); toxic; reproductive (abortion, fetal mummification, dystocia); nutritional; and neoplastic diseases.[10] Capture myopathy remains a significant concern in management of nondomestic bovids.

Capture Myopathy

Capture myopathy was first described decades ago and remains a significant concern in pronghorns and bovids under all conditions of management.[42,54] The syndrome is most often associated with prolonged pursuit, capture, restraint, transportation, and high ambient temperatures, although many other stress-inducing factors may precipitate its development. Capture myopathy is most commonly characterized by ataxia, metabolic acidosis, muscle necrosis, and myoglobinuria; however, several closely related syndromes have been described (Table 63-12). In general, the pathophysiology of the disease includes exhaustion of muscular adenosine triphosphate (ATP) (skeletal and cardiac), decreased oxygen delivery to tissues, and increased production of lactic acid leading to muscle necrosis, myoglobin release, and renal failure. Predisposing factors include species (reported to be common in pronghorn, nyala, tsessebe, duiker, roan, hartebeest, eland, springbok, kudu, and impala[17]); environment (high temperature and humidity); capture or restraint; underlying conditions (pregnancy, advanced age); and vitamin E or selenium deficiency. By the time signs of capture myopathy are obvious, treatment is generally unrewarding. Prevention consists primarily of careful restraint planning and includes limiting pursuit to less than 3 minutes; avoiding capture in ambient temperatures over 20° C; reducing visual and auditory stimulation during restraint; minimizing restraint time; and using sedation and general anesthesia, when warranted. If, despite careful planning, an animal becomes highly stressed, hyperthermic, or hypoxemic during capture,

TABLE 63-12

Four Syndromes of Capture Myopathy in Nondomestic Ruminants[42,54]

Syndrome	Conditions	Clinical presentation	Pathologic findings
Capture shock (hyperacute) syndrome	Occurs during or within 6 hours after capture	Ataxia, tachypnea, tachycardia, hyperemic mucous membranes, hyperthermia, weak pulse, sudden death	Pulmonary congestion and edema; intestinal hemorrhage; small areas of necrosis of skeletal and cardiac muscle, brain, liver, adrenal glands, lymph nodes, spleen, pancreas, and renal tubules
Ataxic myoglobinuric (acute) syndrome	Most common syndrome, occurring hours to days after capture	Ataxia, torticollis, myoglobinuria, death with elevated AST, CK, LDH, BUN	Dark colored urine, dark, swollen kidneys, pale streaking of skeletal muscle, renal tubular dilation and necrosis with myoglobin casts
Ruptured muscle (subacute) syndrome	Occurs 24 to 48 hours following capture	Hindquarter weakness, recumbency with extremely elevated AST, CK, LDH BUN may be normal	Subcutaneous hemorrhage of rear limbs, multifocal soft lesions and ruptures in muscles, severe, diffuse skeletal muscle necrosis
Delayed-peracute (chronic) syndrome	Occurs rarely, at least 24 hours but may be up to 30 days following capture	Normal appearance when undisturbed, but acute stress results in attempt to flee followed by ventricular fibrillation and sudden death	No lesions or small pale foci of rhabdomyolysis, particularly in hindlimbs

AST, Aspartate aminotransferase; *BUN*, blood urea nitrogen; *CK*, creatine kinase; *LDH*, lactate dehydrogenase.

treatment may be successfully provided to prevent fatal myopathy. Aggressive fluid therapy and treatment of metabolic acidosis should be initiated as early as possible. Point-of-care analyzers are helpful in evaluating acid–base and electrolyte disturbances and guiding treatment. Sodium bicarbonate administration may be given as a bolus (1–2 milliequivalents per kilogram [mEq/kg]) and re-administered, as indicated by blood gas analysis. In a normal animal, lactate should be less than 2 mmol/L; a lactate value greater than 5 to 6 mmol/L carries a poor prognosis.[30] Administration of corticosteroids, dimethyl sulfoxide (DMSO, 10% in intravenous fluids), or a combination of both may be preferable to nonsteroidal anti-inflammatory drugs (NSAIDs) for the control of inflammation because of the likelihood of renal compromise with NSAIDs and may also protect vascular integrity. Following initial treatment, patients should be kept in a cool, quiet area and monitored closely for adequate renal output (1 mL/kg/hr)[30] for several days.

REPRODUCTION

General characteristics of the bovid reproductive cycle include a 24- to 72-hour estrous period and an 18- to 25-day luteal phase. Male behavior such as following, foreleg kicking, chin resting, and mounting may be good indicators of estrus; however, females will generally only stand to be mounted by a male during peak estrus. Seasonality varies among artiodactyls and may shift to some degree ex situ. Species from higher latitudes tend to be more seasonal compared with tropical species.[58]

Onset of sexual maturity may vary widely within and among species and is influenced by diet and general health (see Table 63-1). In herd settings, the removal of the breeding male may accelerate sexual maturity in young males. Fertility assessment in males is best achieved by microscopic examination of spermatozoa, collected by electroejaculation under general anesthesia. Most healthy bovid species produce highly concentrated spermatozoa with over 50% motile cells. Diagnosis of pregnancy may be made through rectal palpation or ultrasonography in many bovids; however, the risk of anesthesia, if necessary, may outweigh the benefit of early pregnancy diagnosis in many fractious species. Fecal progestin assays, available in many laboratories, provide a means of noninvasive pregnancy diagnosis but require repeated collection of multiple fecal samples over many weeks.[38]

Assisted Reproduction

As the sustainability of nondomestic bovids in captive collections becomes less certain, the development of assisted reproductive techniques becomes more important to species' success because of the potential to facilitate the infusion of new genetics into a herd while eliminating the cost and risk of transportation. These techniques also have the potential advantage of reducing the risk of disease transmission, but international transport of gametes remains challenging because of the risk of transboundary disease transmission.[43] Because assisted reproduction has been widely used in domestic cattle, techniques have been adapted from domestic protocols for many nondomestic species.[39] However, species differences in estrous cycle length, sensitivity to exogenous hormones, and stress response have limited the success of using domestic bovine protocols in bovids. In general, estrus synchronization protocols must be developed through research on each species. To date, estrus synchronization and artificial insemination using frozen-thawed semen have been successful in the eland, banteng, gaur, addax, scimitar-horned oryx, suni, blackbuck, Speke gazelle, Mhorr gazelle, and springbok.[39,43]

Perinatal Care

Neonatal mortality rates among nondomestic bovids are often over 30%. Because management techniques differ significantly between these animals and their domestic counterparts, an understanding of the special needs and risks involved in dam and neonate management may prevent unnecessary problems and losses, as previously reviewed.[56] Housing should provide the opportunity for seclusion, adequate ventilation and drainage, and exposure to sunlight. Species with strong herd instincts may be most successful when housed with conspecifics and in a familiar environment during calving. In temperate areas, careful timing of breeding to favor mild-season calving may also improve neonatal survival. One month prior to expected parturition, the energy ration should be increased and special attention paid to the provision of adequate calcium and minerals, particularly if the regional soil is deficient in specific minerals such as selenium.

TABLE 63-13

Diagnosis and Treatment of Common Conditions in the Sick Neonatal Ruminant

Condition	Diagnostic Findings	Treatment
Hypothermia	Body temperature < 37°C (99°F)	Warm neonate slowly (2°F per hour) using dry circulating air, blankets, heat lamps, and warmed intravenous fluids or warmed oral colostrum.
Hypoglycemia	Blood glucose <60 milligrams per deciliter (mg/dL)	500 milligrams per kilogram (mg/kg) (10 milliliters per kilogram [mL/kg] 5% solution) dextrose intravenously over several minutes Repeated dosing may be necessary Once corrected, maintain glucose administration at least 250 mg/kg/day until neonate accepts food or begin parenteral nutrition
Metabolic acidosis	Base deficit >10 millimoles per liter (mmol/L) Blood pH <7.25	Intravenous sodium bicarbonate (1.3%): Milliequivalent bicarbonate (mEq HCO_3) = Base deficit × body weight × 0.5, or Empirical treatment with 1–2 mEq/kg
Hypoxemia	Saturation of arterial oxygen (SaO_2) <90% Partial pressure of arterial oxygen (PaO_2) <70 mm Hg	Nasal insufflation with 5–10 liters per hour (L/hr) oxygen or ventilation
Septicemia	Blood culture positive Elevated or reduced white blood cell count Fibrinogen > 500 mg/dL >2% band neutrophils	Initiate broad-spectrum intravenous antibiotics Consider plasma transfusion Maintain body temperature, hydration, acid–base balance, and blood glucose Provide adequate nutrition

From Wolfe BA, Lamberski NL: Approaches to management of neonatal nondomestic ungulates. *Vet Clin North Am Exot Anim Pract* 15(2):61–72, 2012.[56]

Impending parturition may be signified by teat and udder enlargement (weeks) and vulvar swelling or relaxation (days) prior to parturition. Dams will often seek isolation and give birth at night. Dystocia is not uncommon, particularly in species of limited genetic diversity, and represents an important risk factor for morbidity and mortality in calves. If birth intervention is required, many dams will not accept an offspring following general anesthesia, resulting in failure of passive transfer (FPT) and the need for hand rearing.

Neonatal Care

Close observation of neonates soon after birth is important to document normal behavior and nursing.[56] Although in many wild cattle and gazelle species, the neonate will stand and follow the dam soon after birth, most other nondomestic ruminants are "hiders" and are left by their mothers to lie motionless for long periods.[58] In these species, finding the neonate and observing nursing may be a challenge. Neonates should be observed nursing within a few hours of birth, and a calf that is weak, unresponsive to stimulation by the dam, unable to stand soon after birth, or fails to nurse warrants evaluation.

Timely intervention is critical, but the decision to treat an unthrifty neonate may be complicated. Maternal neglect is common in dams that are inexperienced or stressed, but when a healthy, experienced dam abandons her offspring, it may point to an underlying problem compromising the viability of the offspring. The costs of committing to treatment and hand rearing, the likelihood of success, and the future of the neonate must all be taken into account in the decision to remove a high-risk neonate from the care of its dam.

Guidelines for the diagnosis and treatment of common neonatal conditions are listed in Table 63-13. Following normal birth, mild metabolic acidosis is common for up to 48 hours. However, severe acidosis may result in weakness, inability to nurse, and FPT. Clearing the airway and providing whole-body and nasal stimulation may stimulate respiration. Neonates born to anesthetized dams may have pharmacologic respiratory depression and should receive specific antagonists. Oxygen therapy has been shown to improve neonatal survival in at-risk domestic calves.[40] Intravenous fluid therapy may improve the chance of survival and provides a means of rapidly treating metabolic abnormalities. Treatment for acidosis with sodium bicarbonate (see Table 63-13) should only be administered after the establishment of a normal breathing pattern and may otherwise exacerbate respiratory acidosis. Provision of an external heat source 24 hours or more after parturition may improve thermoregulation, oxygen saturation, tidal volume, and respiratory rate.[40]

Common causes of illness in neonatal ruminants include acidosis, hypothermia, hypoglycemia, dehydration, pneumonia, and septicemia, each of which may be rapidly fatal.[36] Physical examination findings of hypothermia or hyperthermia, tachycardia, tachypnea, hyperemia or petechiae of mucous membranes, increased capillary refill time, cold extremities, diminished peripheral pulse, and inability to correct hypoglycemia despite treatment are suggestive of septicemia. Supportive treatment for neonatal septicemia should include provision of a clean, warm, lowly lit environment; soft, clean bedding; intravenous fluid supplementation; and plasma transfusion, colostrum supplementation, or milk-based nutritional support, depending on the age and condition of the neonate. Bedding should be changed frequently as septicemic neonates are usually too weak to stand and therefore susceptible to urine scald and corneal irritation or ulceration.

PREVENTIVE MEDICINE

Well-designed preventive medicine protocols, including quarantine, regular disease screening, vaccination, sanitation, and vermin control, are important to the successful maintenance of nondomestic bovid collections. Annual vaccination for diseases of particular concern such as *Clostridium* species and rabies is commonly performed. Regional disease risks should be considered, as vaccination for some diseases following an outbreak may interrupt the disease cycle. Live vaccines should be used with caution in nondomestic ruminants.

ACKNOWLEDGMENTS

The author gratefully acknowledges the assistance of Stephen Fowler, Priya Bapodra, Rae Gandolf, Lana Kelly, Lisa Bigelow, Dan Beetem, and Justin Rosenberg in the preparation of this chapter, and Scott Citino for the chapter in the previous edition.

REFERENCES

1. Animal Diversity: http://animaldiversity.ummz.umich.edu/. Accessed June 13, 2012.
2. Association of Zoos and Aquariums: *AZA Antelope and Giraffe Advisory Group Regional Collection Plan*, ed 5. 2008. http://www.antelopetag.com/regional_collection_plan.htm. Accessed November 11, 2012.
3. Ball RL: Antelope. In West G, Heard D, Caulkett N, editors: *Zoo animal and wildlife immobilization and anesthesia*, Ames, IA, 2007, Blackwell Publishing, pp 613–622.
4. Beer M, Conraths FJ, Van der Peol WHM: Schmallenberg virus—a novel orthobunyavirus emerging in Europe. *Epidemiol Infect* 141(1):1–8, 2012.
5. Brown C, Torres A, editors: *Committee on foreign and emerging animal diseases of the Unites States Animal Health Association*, ed 7, Boca Raton, FL, 2008, Boca Publications Group.
6. Bush M, Citino SB, Lance WR: The use of butorphanol in anesthesia protocols for zoo and wild mammals. In Fowler ME, Miller RE, editors: *Zoo and wild animal medicine: Current therapy*, ed 7, St. Louis, MO, 2012, Saunders, pp 596–603.
7. Carling MD, Wiseman PA, Byers JA: Microsatellite analysis reveals multiple paternity in a population of wild pronghorn antelopes. *J Mammal* 84:1237–1243, 2003.
8. Caulkett N, Haigh JC: Bison. In West G, Heard D, Caulkett N, editors: *Zoo animal and wildlife immobilization and anesthesia*, Ames, IA, 2007, Blackwell Publishing, pp 643–646.
9. Christman J: Physical methods of capture, handling, and restraint. In Kleiman DG, Tompson KV, Baer CK, editors: *Wild mammals in captivity: Principles and techniques for zoo management*, ed 2, Chicago, IL, 2010, University of Chicago Press, pp 39–48.
10. Citino SB: Bovidae (except sheep and goats) and antilocapridae. In Fowler ME, Miller RE, editors: *Zoo and wild animal medicine: Current therapy*, ed 5, St. Louis, MO, 2003, Saunders, pp 649–674.
11. Clauss M, Dierenfeld ES: The nutrition of "browsers." In Fowler ME, Miller RE, editors: *Zoo and wild animal medicine: Current therapy*, ed 6, Philadelphia, PA, 2008, Saunders, pp 444–453.
12. Committee on Diagnosis and Control of Johne's Disease, National Research Council: *Diagnosis and control of Johne's disease*, Washington, DC, 2003, National Academies Press.
13. Curro T: Nondomestic cattle. In West G, Heard D, Caulkett N, editors: *Zoo animal and wildlife immobilization and anesthesia*, Ames, IA, 2007, Blackwell Publishing, pp 635–642.
14. Donovan TA, Schrenzel MD, Tucker T, et al: Meningoencephalitis in a polar bear caused by equine herpesvirus 9 (EHV-9). *Vet Pathol* 46:1138–1143, 2009.
15. Drackley JK: Calf nutrition from birth to breeding. *Vet Clin N Am Food Anim Pract* 24(1):55–69, 2008.
16. Ebedes H: *The use of tranquilizers in wildlife. Department of Agricultural Development, Bulletin No. 423*, Pretoria, South Africa, 1992, Directorate of Agricultural Information.
17. Ebedes H, Van Rooyen J, Du Toit JG: Capturing wild animals. In Bothma JDP, editor: *Game ranch management*, ed 4, Pretoria, South Africa, 2002, Van Schaik Uitgewers, pp 382–430.
18. Eschbaumer M, Wenike K, Batten C, et al: Epizootic hemorrhagic disease virus serotype 7 in European cattle and sheep: Diagnostic considerations and effect of previous BTV exposure. *Vet Microbiol* 159:298–306, 2012.
19. European Food Safety Authority: Bovine besnoitiosis: An emerging disease in Europe. *EFSA J* 8(2):1499, 2010.
20. Fontenot D, Miller J: Alternatives for gastrointestinal parasite control in exotic ruminants. In Fowler ME, Miller RE, editors: *Zoo and wild animal medicine: Current therapy*, ed 7, St. Louis, MO, 2012, Saunders, pp 581–627.
21. Fowler ME: *Restraint and handling of wild and domestic animals*, ed 2, Ames, IA, 1995, Iowa State University Press.
22. Gasper D, Barr B, Li H, et al: Ibex-associated malignant catarrhal fever-like disease in a group of bongo antelope (*Tragelaphus euycerus*). *Vet Pathol* 49:492–497, 2012.
23. Groves CP, Grubb P: *Ungulate taxonomy*, Baltimore, MD, 2011, Johns Hopkins University Press.
24. Gutierrez-Exposito D, Ortega-Mora LM, Gajadhar AA, et al: Serological evidence of *Besnoitia* spp. infection in Canadian wild ruminants and strong cross-reaction between *Besnoitia besnoiti* and *Besnoitia tarandi*. *Vet Parasitol* 190:19–28, 2012.
25. Haigh J: The use of chutes for ungulate restraint. In Fowler ME, Miller RE, editors: *Zoo and wild animal medicine: Current therapy*, ed 4, Philadelphia, PA, 1999, Saunders, pp 657–661.
26. Huffman B: The ultimate ungulate page: Your guide to the world's hoofed mammal species, http://www.ultimateungulate.com. Accessed July 21, 2012.
27. Isaza R: Remote drug delivery. In West G, Heard D, Caulkett N, editors: *Zoo animal and wildlife immobilization and anesthesia*, Ames, IA, 2007, Blackwell Publishing, pp 61–74.
28. Ishihara K, Hosokawa Y, Makita K, et al: Factors associated with antimicrobial-resistant *Escherichia coli* in zoo animals. *Res Vet Sci* 93:574–580, 2012.
29. Kreeger TJ: *Handbook of wildlife chemical immobilization*, Laramie, WY, 1996, International Wildlife Veterinary Services.
30. Lamberski N, Fuller J: Practical aspects of ruminant intensive care. In Fowler ME, Miller RE, editors: *Zoo and wild animal medicine: Current therapy*, ed 7, St. Louis, MO, 2012, Saunders, pp 636–643.
31. Lance WR, Kenny DE: Thiafentanil oxalate (A3080) in nondomestic ungulate species. In Fowler ME, Miller RE, editors: *Zoo and wild animal medicine: Current therapy*, ed 7, St. Louis, MO, 2012, Saunders, pp 589–595.
32. Li H, Cunha CW, Taus NS: Malignant catarrhal fever: Understanding molecular diagnostics in context of epidemiology. *Int J Mol Sci* 12:6881–6893, 2011.
33. Maillard R, Petit E, Chomel B, et al: Endocarditis in cattle caused by *Bartonella bovis*. *Emerg Infect Dis* 13(9):1383–1385, 2007.
34. Mallon D: The current status of antelopes: An overview. In *Antelope conservation in the 21st century: From diagnosis to action*, London, U.K., 2011, Zoological Society of London, pp 3–4. http://static.zsl.org/files/antelope-conservation-in-the-21st-century-abstracts-1674.pdf. Accessed October 13, 2012.
35. Mariner JC, House JA, Mebus CA, et al: Rinderpest eradication: Appropriate technology and social innovations. *Science* 337:130–1312, 2012.
36. Menzies P: Lambing management and neonatal care. In Youngquist RSTW, editor: *Current therapy in large animal theriogenology*, ed 2, St. Louis, MO, 2007, Saunders, pp 680–695.
37. Miller MA: Current diagnostic methods for tuberculosis in zoo mammals. In Fowler ME, Miller RE, editors: *Zoo and wild animal medicine: Current therapy*, ed 6, Philadelphia, PA, 2008, Saunders, pp 10–19.
38. Monfort SL: Non-invasive endocrine measures of reproduction and stress in wild populations. In Wildt DE, Holt W, Pickard A, editors: *Reproduction and integrated conservation science*, Cambridge, U.K, 2003, Cambridge University Press, pp 147–165.
39. Morrow CJ, Penfold LM, Wolfe BA: Artificial insemination in deer and non-domestic bovids. *Theriogenology* 71:149–165, 2009.
40. Nagy DW: Resuscitation and critical care of neonatal calves. *Vet Clin N Am Food Anim Pract* 25:1–14, 2009.
41. Nowak RN, editor: *Walker's mammals of the world*, ed 6, Baltimore, MD, 1999, Johns Hopkins University Press.
42. Paterson J: Capture myopathy. In West G, Heard D, Caulkett N, editors: *Zoo animal and wildlife immobilization and anesthesia*, Ames, IA, 2007, Blackwell Publishing, pp 115–121.
43. Penfold LM, O'Brien J: Importation of nondomestic semen for management of zoological populations using artificial insemination. In Fowler ME, Miller RE, editors: *Zoo and wild animal medicine: Current therapy*, ed 7, St. Louis, MO, 2012, Saunders, pp 604–611.

44. Read M: Long-acting neuroleptic drugs. In Heard D, editor: *Zoological restraint and anesthesia*, Ithaca, NY, 2002, International Veterinary Information Service.

45. Samuel WM, Pybus MJ, Kocan AA, editors: *Parasitic diseases of wild mammals*, ed 2, Ames, IA, 2001, Iowa State University Press.

46. Schumacher J: Side effects of etorphine and carfentanil in nondomestic hoofstock. In Fowler ME, Miller RE, editors: *Zoo and wild animal medicine: Current therapy*, ed 6, Philadelphia, PA, 2008, Saunders, pp 455–461.

47. Sigurdson CJ, Miller MW: Other animal prion diseases. *Br Med Bull* 66:199–212, 2003.

48. Stringfield C, Greene K: Exotic ungulates. In Gage L, editor: *Hand-rearing wild and domestic mammals*, Ames, IA, 2002, Iowa State Press, pp 256–262.

49. Teare JA: *Reference ranges for physiological values in captive wildlife*, Apple Valley, MN, 2010, International Species Information System.

50. Terrill TH, Miller JE, Burke JM, et al: Experiences with integrated concepts for the control of *Haemonchus contortus* in sheep and goats in the United States. *Vet Parasitol* 186:28–37, 2012.

51. Van Soest PJ: *Nutritional ecology of the ruminant*, ed 2, Ithaca, NY, 1994, Cornell University Press.

52. Van Wyk J, Hoste H, Kaplan R, et al: Targeted selective treatment for worm management:—How do we sell rational programs to farmers? *Vet Parasitol* 139:336–346, 2006.

53. West G: Gazelles. In West G, Heard D, Caulkett N, editors: *Zoo animal and wildlife immobilization and anesthesia*, Ames, IA, 2007, Blackwell Publishing, pp 623–628.

54. Williams ES, Thorne ET: Exertional myopathy (capture myopathy). In Fairbrother A, Locke LN, Hoff GL, editors: *Noninfectious diseases of wildlife*, ed 2, Ames, IA, 1996, Iowa State University Press, pp 181–193.

55. Wohlsein P, Lehmbecker A, Spitzbarth I, et al: Fatal epzootic equine herpesvirus 1 infections in new and unnatural hosts. *Vet Microbiol* 149:456–460, 2011.

56. Wolfe BA, Lamberski N: Approaches to management and care of the neonatal nondomestic ruminant. *Vet Clin N Am Exotic Anim Pract* 15(2):265–277, 2012.

57. Wolfe BA, Aguilar RF, Aguirre AA, et al: Sorta situ: The new reality of management conditions for wildlife populations in the absence "wild" spaces. In Aguirre AA, Ostfeld R, Daszak P, editors: *New directions in conservation medicine: Applied cases of ecological health*, New York, 2012, Oxford University Press, pp 576–589.

58. Zerbe P, Clauss M, Codron D, et al: Reproductive seasonality in captive wild ruminants: Implications for biogeographical adaptation, photoperiodic control, and life history. *Biol Rev* 87:965–990, 2012.

59. Zoologic Formulation and Mixing: Pet Ag, Inc., Hampshire IL, http://www.petag.com/PDFs/Zoologic%20Formulations.pdf. Accessed June 28 2012.

60. Zuba JR: Hoof disorders in nondomestic artiodactylids. In Fowler ME, Miller RE, editors: *Zoo and wild animal medicine: Current therapy*, ed 7, St. Louis, MO, 2012, Saunders, pp 619–627.

CHAPTER 64

Sheep, Goats, and Goat-Like Animals

Martha A. Weber

BIOLOGY

Wild sheep and goats belong in the family Bovidae and are grouped in the subfamily Caprinae. The three tribes within the Caprinae are (1) Ovibini (muskox and takin), (2) Rupricaprini (goral, serow, and chamois), and (3) Caprini (sheep, goat, and tahr). Eighty-five species and subspecies are recognized by the International Union for the Conservation of Nature (IUCN); 63% of these are categorized as Near Threatened, Vulnerable, Endangered, or Critically Endangered. Overhunting, habitat loss, and disease transfer from domestic sheep and goats are responsible for many population declines.

Caprinae species are distributed across the northern hemisphere, often in inhospitable environments such as deserts, tundra, mountains, or forests. Generally, both sexes have horns; depending on the species, these may be short and sharp or large and ornate. Marked sexual dimorphism exists in the size and shape of the horns in animals in the tribe Caprini; this is less distinct in the other tribes. Table 64-1 lists characteristics for selected species.

Global climate change may hasten the population decline or extinction of some species. Cold-adapted animals may experience increased stress in the face of local temperature changes. Movement of animals out of their traditional ranges, exposure to novel pathogens as species commingle, and changes in parasite and vector dispersal could all play a role in the development of new epizootic diseases in populations.

SPECIAL HOUSING REQUIREMENTS

Most Caprinae are agile climbers and jumpers. Enclosures and holding areas need adequate moats, fencing, or both to prevent escape. Climbing structures promote natural behaviors and hoof wear in montane species, but it must be ensured that they do not provide a point from which an animal can leap out of the enclosure. Species adapted to northern climates should have access to shade structures and cooling sprays when housed in warm and humid environments.

FEEDING

Caprinae are ruminants and, in the wild, may be grazers, browsers, or generalist herbivores. Diets in captivity generally consist

TABLE 64-1

Selected Species Information for Caprinae

Common Name	Scientific Name	Weight Range (kilograms)	Gestation (days)	Captive Life Span (years)
Takin	*Budorcas taxicolor*	200–400 (male) 150–250 (female)	240–260	12–15
Muskox	*Ovibos moschatus*	180–400	225	18–24
Japanese serow	*Capricornus crispus*	30–130	200	15–20
Goral	*Naemorhedus griseus*	35–45	250–260	12–15
Rocky Mountain goat	*Oreamnos americanus*	70–100 (male) 45–70 (female)	180	15–18
Chamois	*Rupicapra rupicapra, R. pyrenica*	40–50 (male) 30–35 (female)	170	14–20
Aoudad (Barbary sheep)	*Ammotragus lervia*	40–145	160	15–20
Tahr	*Hemitragus, Arabitragus, Nilgiritragus*	50–125 (male) 45–70 (female)	180–190	10–20
Markhor	*Capra falconeri*	80–110 (male) 30–40 (female)	135–170	10–14
Ibex	*Capra ibex, C. nubiana, C. pyrenica*	40–120	150	10–15
Bighorn sheep	*Ovis canadensis*	55–135 (male) 55–90 (female)	175	12–15
Thin horn sheep (Dall sheep)	*Ovis dalli*			
Urial	*Ovis orientalis arkal*	60–100 (male) 40–50 (female)	150–160	12–15
Bharal (Blue sheep)	*Pseudois nayaur*	35–75	160	10–15

of concentrate pellets and grass or alfalfa hay. Salt blocks may be provided. Some species may be sensitive to high levels of dietary copper, so trace mineral blocks should not be used at all or used with caution. Food items should be presented in multiple locations around an enclosure to keep dominant animals from preventing others access to food. Nontoxic browse items may be added to the diet as they are available.

RESTRAINT AND HANDLING

Free-ranging animals may be manually captured with drive nets or box traps. When herding animals, it is important to be aware of hazards such as rock faces, precipices, or water. Prolonged running may induce hyperthermia and capture myopathy. Acepromazine, azaperone, xylazine, and haloperidol have been used, with variable results, to provide sedation for wild chamoises and ibexes that were restrained for several hours after capture.[4,20,22]

Some smaller species in captivity (e.g., urial, goral) may be hand captured and restrained for short procedures (hoof trim, venipuncture, tuberculin testing). Handlers need to take into consideration that the animals may jump, bank off walls, and inflict injury with their horns. The horns of juvenile animals should not be handled for restraint, as the bony core may not be fused to the skull and thus may break. Blindfolding restrained animals may help keep them calm during the procedure. Respiratory rate and body temperature should be monitored during restraint.

Chemical Restraint and Anesthesia

General anesthesia may be used for large species, invasive procedures, or procedures of longer duration. Commonly used chemical restraint agents in Caprinae include opioids, dissociative agents, and α_2-agonists.[5] Opioids used include the ultrapotent narcotic agents

carfentanil, thiafentanil, and etorphine. These agents are highly regulated in some countries and do pose a risk to personnel who may come into contact with the substances. The use of butorphanol, a partial opiate agonist–antagonist, in combination with α_2-agonists, has been reported to result in excellent anesthesia in takins, with a significant decrease in rumen reflux.[23] Reversal of opiate anesthesia is generally achieved using naltrexone administered intramuscularly (IM) or intravenously (IV).

α_2-agonists, including xylazine, medetomidine, and detomidine, have been used in Caprinae. Medetomidine and detomidine bind more specifically to the α_2-receptors than xylazine, resulting in greater potency. Atipamezole is recommended for reversal, although yohimbine or tolazoline may also be used to reverse the effects of xylazine.

The dissociative anesthetic agents ketamine and tiletamine–zolazepam are also commonly used in Caprinae. Good quality anesthesia is usually obtained with these agents, in combination with α_2-agonists or opiates. Ketamine and tiletamine are not reversible, which may be a disadvantage when immobilizing free-ranging specimens. Supplemental ketamine may be given intravenously, either as boluses or a constant rate infusion, to enhance or prolong anesthesia.

Induction doses are generally administered intramuscularly by hand syringe, pole syringe, or projectile dart. If an animal is restrained manually or in a chute intravenous injection may be an option.

Intubation is recommended for all animals that are fully anesthetized to prevent aspiration of refluxed rumen contents. The use of stylets greatly facilitates intubation in species with narrow muzzles. Isoflurane works well to maintain anesthesia for procedures of long duration.

The published literature should be reviewed to identify current dosage recommendations for anesthetic agents and species-specific factors.

TABLE 64-2

Reference Ranges for Hematologic Parameters of Selected Caprinae Species

Parameter	Takin (*Budorcas taxicolor*)	Goral (*Naemorhedus griseus*)	Urial (*Ovis aries arkal*)	Domestic Goat (*Capra hircus*)
Erythrocytes (×10^6/ml)	8.0–14.0	7.8–13.5	10.7–14.5	9.3–14.7
Packed cell volume (%)	25–35	27–45	39–50	26–39
Hemoglobin (g/dl)	9.1–12.3	9.4–15.8	12.3– 5.5	9.2–13.3
Leukocytes (per ml)	4900–12,000	2400–6,300	3500–8000	4500–12,300
Neutrophils (per ml)	3200–8500	1100–3,200	1000–4700	2400–8800
Lymphocytes (per ml)	1500–2500	750–2,500	1000–4000	2100–7300
Monocytes (per ml)	100–300	0–300	0–300	150–400
Eosinophils (per ml)	0–100	0–100	0–200	0–400
Basophils (per ml)	0–50	0–50	0–50	0–200
Platelets (x 10^3/ml)	250–700	250–900	300–750	200–700
Fibrinogen (mg/dl)	100–500	100–500	200–500	250–500

TABLE 64-3

Reference Ranges for Biochemical Parameters of Selected Caprinae Species

Parameter	Takin (*Budorcas taxicolor*)	Goral (*Naemorhedus griseus*)	Urial (*Ovis orientalis*)	Domestic goat (*Capra hircus*)
Glucose, milligram per deciliter (mg/dL)	70–115	95–150	65–130	50–80
Blood urea nitrogen (mg/dL)	19–35	14–25	15–28	15–24
Creatinine (mg/dl)	0.8–2.5	0.7–1.6	0.8–2.2	0.5–1.2
Calcium (mg/dL)	8.1–10.3	8.4–9.2	8.1–10.9	8.8–11.3
Phosphorus (mg/dL)	3.1–5.6	4.7–7.7	5.6–7.7	4.2–8.1
Sodium, milliequivalent per liter (mEq/L)	130–144	144–150	142–156	142–151
Potassium (mEq/L)	4.4–5.8	3.5–5.1	4.5–5.9	4.1–6.3
Chloride (mEq/L)	108–115	100–109	104–115	107–118
Magnesium (mg/dL)	1.9–2.6	1.7–2.1	2.0–3.4	1.8–2.4
Total protein, gram per deciliter (g/dL)	6.4–7.9	6.0–6.8	5.4–7.9	6.7–8.6
Albumin (g/dL)	2.8–3.6	2.5–3.5	2.7–3.7	2.8–3.5

DIAGNOSTICS

Physical examination is performed as in other ruminant species. Body condition should be assessed regularly.

Blood is generally collected from the jugular vein. Hematologic and biochemical parameters for selected species are listed in Tables 64-2 and 64-3. Hematocrit values from automated cell counters are often very low in takins and a spun packed cell volume (PCV) should be measured as well.

Tuberculin testing is performed as for domestic sheep and goats, using 0.1 milliliter (mL) of bovine tuberculin injected intradermally. The test site should be read 72 hours after injection. Specific sites for tuberculin testing have not been officially recognized in these species. Most commonly the injection is performed in a shaved area on the lateral cervical region. Takins may show a nonspecific response to intradermal tuberculin testing. To minimize the number of anesthetic episodes associated with tuberculin testing, it may be appropriate to be prepared to perform a comparative cervical tuberculin test as the initial test.

INFECTIOUS DISEASE

Selected infectious diseases are summarized in Table 64-4.

Malignant catarrhal fever (MCF) is caused by a herpesvirus (ovine herpesvirus-2) carried by some Caprinae species. It does not generally cause disease in the host species but may cause severe, often fatal, disease in other ruminants, especially cervids.[7] Transmission is through contact with aerosols. Young lambs are believed to shed the highest level of viruses. A unique MCF virus, distinct from ovine herpesvirus-2, has been identified in the muskox.[19]

Echthyma (orf) is a highly contagious, zoonotic parapoxvirus, which primarily affects sheep and goats. Infections have been reported in the wild muskox as well as in the captive muskox and the takin.[15,28]

Border disease virus (BDV), a pestivirus, has been reported to cause high mortality in free-ranging chamoises. Affected animals showed weakness, cachexia, alopecia, and abnormal behavior.[3,10]

Other viral infections that may affect Caprinae include bovine viral diarrhea virus, foot-and-mouth disease, rinderpest, vesicular stomatitis, bluetongue, ovine progressive pneumonia, caprine arthritis and encephalitis, and rabies.

Mycobacterium avium ssp. *paratuberculosis*, the causative agent of Johne disease, has been detected in both captive and free-ranging populations of Caprinae.[11] Clinical signs vary by species but may include diarrhea and poor body condition, with granulomatous enteritis seen at necropsy. Culture of fecal samples is necessary for definitive diagnosis.

TABLE 64-4

Selected Infectious Diseases of Caprinae

Disease	Causative Agent	Epizootiology	Signs	Diagnosis	Management
Malignant catarrhal fever	Ovine herpesvirus-2	Spread by aerosols, usually associated with lambs	No disease in carriers May cause severe fatal disease in other ruminants	Serology	Keep Caprinae separated from susceptible species, especially cervids
Contagious echthyma	Parapoxvirus	Spread by direct contact, fomites, insects Zoonotic	Crusting on muzzle and around eyes; papillomatous growths on oral mucous membranes, facial edema May see lesions on udders	Histopathology of lesions Differentiate from vesicular diseases (e.g., foot-and-mouth, bluetongue)	Separate affected animals
Epizootic pneumonia of bighorn sheep	Multifactorial, including *Mycoplasma ovis*, Pasteurellaceae, *Protostrongylus* sp.	Aerosol transmission from carriers	Severe respiratory disease Most marked in naïve populations	Clinical signs, culture, serology, polymerase chain reaction (PCR), histopathology	Maintain separation between bighorn sheep and domestic sheep
Infectious keratoconjunctivitis	*Mycoplasma* spp., *Branhamella* spp., *Moraxella* spp., *Chlamydophila* spp.	Contact with carriers	May range from mild conjunctivitis to corneal perforation and blindness	Clinical signs, culture, PCR	Maintain separation between domestic and wild Caprinae

TABLE 64-5

Selected Parasitic Diseases of Caprinae

Parasite	Clinical Signs	Treatment
Eimeria spp.	Diarrhea, poor weight gain, ill-thrift	Amprolium, sulfadimethoxine, toltrazuril
Trichostrongyles (*Haemonchus contortus*, *Ostertagia* spp., *Trichostrongylus axei*)	Diarrhea, weight loss, anemia, hypoproteinemia	Ivermectin, benzimidazoles, levamisole, copper Development of anthelminthic resistance is likely
Fascioloides magna	Anemia, clotting disorders Marked hepatic damage seen at necropsy	Triclabendazole
Psoroptes ovis	Crusting, hair loss, primarily around ears and face	Ivermectin
Sarcoptes scabei	Alopecia, lichenification, crusting	Ivermectin

Bighorn sheep have long been known to suffer outbreaks of severe respiratory disease following contact with domestic sheep. Pathologic changes may include pneumonia, rhinitis, sinusitis, otitis media, tracheitis, and pleuritis. The etiology of this disease may be complex, with multiple infectious agents implicated as pathogens. Pasteurellaceae (*Mannheimia hemolytica*, *Bibersteinia trehalosi*, *P. multocida*) are frequently isolated from the lungs of bighorn sheep with pneumonia. *Mycoplasma ovipneumoniae* has recently been identified as playing a significant role in disease pathogenesis.[1]

Infectious keratoconjunctivitis has been described in bighorn sheep, chamoises, mouflons, and ibexes. *Mycoplasma* spp., *Branhamella ovis*, *Moraxella* spp., and *Chlamydophila* spp. have all been implicated as possible causative agents.[13,16,21]

Other significant bacterial pathogens reported in Caprinae include *Brucella suis* and *B. melitensis*, *Yersinia pseudotuberculosis*, and *Dichelobacter nodosus*.

PARASITIC DISEASE

Selected parasitic diseases of Caprinae are listed in Table 64-5.

Coccidial infections (*Eimeria* spp.) in lambs and kids may cause significant morbidity with diarrhea, poor weight gain, and general ill-thrift.

Trichostrongyle parasites (*Haemonchus contortus*, *Ostertagia* spp., and *Trichostrongylus axei*) may be a significant problem in captive Caprinae because substantial numbers of ova and larvae may build up on pastures, and the parasites may rapidly develop resistance to anthelminthic agents. *Haemonchus* may cause significant anemia and generalized edema secondary to blood loss. *Ostertagia* and *Trichostrongylus* are more often associated with malabsorption, weight loss, and diarrhea.

Lungworms (*Dictyocaulus* sp., *Muellerius* sp., and *Protostrongylus* sp.) may cause low-grade respiratory disease or pneumonia. *Protostrongylus* spp. have been implicated as pathogens in epizootic pneumonia of bighorn sheep.

Babesia odocoilei is a tickborne, intraerythrocytic parasite of cervids. Two captive muskoxen died following infection with *B. odocoilei*, and two others in the same collection were positive on polymerase chain reaction for the organism but did not develop disease. The affected animals showed lethargy and hematuria and died within 36 to 72 hours of showing clinical disease. The remaining muskoxen were successfully treated with ivermectin milled into a concentrate pellet.[26,27]

Elaeophora schneideri, a parasite of mule deer and black tailed deer, has been found in bighorn sheep and aoudads in the United States.[2,25] Affected animals had crusted skin lesions on the face and ears. Nematodes were found in the animals' carotid arteries, and microfilariae were seen in the skin, nasal lesions, and pulmonary vessels of the bighorn sheep.

Parelaphostrongylus odocoilei is established in many populations of thinhorn sheep, causing granulomatous pneumonia (larvae) and localized myositis (adult parasites).[17]

Fascioloides magna has caused morbidity and mortality in captive muskoxen. Affected animals had grossly apparent hepatic damage with fibrosis and hemorrhage, bile duct hyperplasia, anemia, and peritonitis. Animals with vague signs were treated with triclabendazole, and the clinical signs resolved.[9]

Psoroptes ovis may be a significant problem in free-ranging bighorn sheep and is associated with local population declines. Animals may be checked for infection by swabbing the ears. Ivermectin is effective for treatment of *P. ovis* infection.

Sarcoptes scabei has been documented in the serow, aoudad, blue sheep, chamois, and ibex.[6,8,14,18] Affected animals show varying degrees of alopecia, skin lichenification, crusting, and fissuring. One outbreak in a free-ranging herd of aoudad resulted in a loss of 86% of the affected population.[14]

NONINFECTIOUS DISEASE

Trauma, hoof overgrowth, capture myopathy, hypothermia (lambs), dental disease, foreign body ingestion, trichobezoars, urinary obstruction secondary to calculi, and toxic plant ingestion may affect Caprinae, especially those maintained in captivity.

REPRODUCTION

Some species may display seasonal courtship behaviors.

Contraception in Caprinae has been successful with the use of porcine zona pellucida vaccine.[12] Melengestrol acetate compounded into pelleted feed was used for contraception in a herd of gorals.[24] Treated animals did not calve during the treatment period and did calve during the following season, which indicated that contraception was reversible.

REFERENCES

1. Besser TE, Cassirer EF, Highland MA, et al: Bighorn sheep pneumonia: Sorting out the cause of a polymicrobial disease. *Prev Vet Med* 108:85–93, 2013.
2. Boyce W, Fisher A, Provencio H, et al: Elaeophorosis in bighorn sheep in New Mexico. *J Wildl Dis* 35(4):786–789, 1999.
3. Cabezon O, Velarde R, Mentaberre G, et al: Experimental infection with chamois border disease virus causes long-lasting viraemia and disease in Pyrenean chamois (*Rupicapra pyrenaica*). *J Gen Virol* 92:2494–2501, 2011.
4. Casas-Diaz E, Marco I, Ramon J, et al: Effect of acepromazine and haloperidol in male Iberian ibex (*Capra pyrenaica*) captured by box-trap. *J Wildl Dis* 48(3):763–767, 2012.
5. Caulkett N, Haigh JC: Wild sheep and goats. In West G, Heard D, Caulkett N, editors: *Zoo animal and wildlife immobilization and anesthesia*, Ames, IA, 2007, Blackwell Publishing, pp 629–633.
6. Chen CC, Pei KJC, Lai YC, et al: Participatory epidemiology to assess sarcoptic mange in serow of Taiwan. *J Wildl Dis* 48(4):869–875, 2012.
7. Cooley AJ, Taus NS, Li H: Development of a management program for a mixed species wildlife park following an occurrence of malignant catarrhal fever. *J Zoo Wildl Med* 39(3):380–385, 2008.
8. Dagleish MP, Ali Q, Powell RK, et al: Fatal *Sarcoptes scabei* infection of blue sheep (*Pseudois nayaur*) in Pakistan. *J Wildl Dis* 43(3):512–517, 2007.
9. Enright C: Morbidity and mortality due to *Fascioloides magna* in a captive herd of North American musk ox (*Ovibos moschatus moschatus*).

In *Proceedings of the American Association of Zoo Veterinarians Conference*, Kansas City, KS, 2011, p 121.
10. Fernandez-Sirera L, Riba L, Cabezon O, et al: Surveillance of border disease in wild ungulates and an outbreak in Pyrenean chamois (*Rupicapra pyrenaica pyrenaica*) in Andorra. *J Wildl Dis* 48(4):1021–1029, 2012.
11. Forde T, Kutz S, De Buck J, et al: Occurrence, diagnosis, and strain typing of *Mycobacterium avium* subspecies *paratuberculosis* infection in Rocky Mountain bighorn sheep (*Ovis canadensis canadensis*) in southwestern Alberta. *J Wildl Dis* 48(1):1–11, 2012.
12. Frank KM, Kirkpatrick JF: Porcine zona pellucid immunocontraception in captive exotic species: Species differences, adjuvant protocols, and technical problems. In *Proceedings of the American Association of Zoo Veterinarians Conference*, Milwaukee, WI, 2002, pp 221–223.
13. Giangaspero M, Orusa R, Nicholas RA, et al: Characterization of *Mycoplasma* isolated from an ibex (*Capra ibex*) suffering from keratoconjunctivitis in northern Italy. *J Wildl Dis* 46(4):1070–1078, 2010.
14. Gonzalez-Candela M, Leon-Vizcaino L, Cubero-Pablo MJ: Population effects of sarcoptic mange in Barbary sheep (*Ammotragus lervia*) from Sierra Espuna Regional Park, Spain. *J Wildl Dis* 40(3):456–465, 2004.
15. Guo J, Rasmussen J, Wunschmann A, et al: Genetic characterization of orf viruses isolated from various ruminant species of a zoo. *Vet Microbiol* 99:81–92, 2004.
16. Jansen BD, Heffelfinger JR, Noon TH, et al: Infectious keratitis in bighorn sheep, Silver Bell Mountains, Arizona, USA. *J Wildl Dis* 42(2):407–411, 2006.
17. Jenkins EJ, Hoberg EP, Polley L: Development and pathogenesis of *Parelaphostrongylus odocoilei* (Nematoda: Protostrongylidae) in experimentally infected thinhorn sheep (*Ovis dalli*). *J Wildl Dis* 41(4):669–682, 2005.
18. Leon-Vizcaino L, Cubero MJ, Gonzalez-Capitel E, et al: Experimental ivermectin treatment of sarcoptic mange and establishment of a mange-free population of Spanish ibex. *J Wildl Dis* 37(4):775–785, 2001.
19. Li H, Gailbreath K, Bender LC, et al: Evidence of three new members of malignant catarrhal fever virus group in muskox (*Ovibos moschatus*), Nubian ibex (*Capra nubiana*), and gemsbok (*Oryx gazella*). *J Wildl Dis* 39(4):875–880, 2003.
20. Lopez-Olvera JR, Marco I, Montane J, et al: Effects of acepromazine on the stress response in Southern chamois (*Rupicapra pyrenaica*) captured by means of drive-nets. *Can J Vet Res* 71(1):41–51, 2007.
21. Mavrot F, Vilei EM, Marreros N, et al: Occurrence, quantification, and genotyping of *Mycoplasma conjunctivae* in wild Caprinae with and without infectious keratoconjunctivitis. *J Wildl Dis* 48(3):619–631, 2012.
22. Mentaberre G, Lopez-Olvera JR, Casas-Diaz E, et al: Haloperidol and azaperone in drive-net captured Southern chamois (*Rupicapra pyrenaica*). *J Wildl Dis* 46(3):923–928, 2010.
23. Morris PJ, Bicknese E, Janssen D, et al: Chemical immobilization of takin (*Budorcas taxicolor*) at the San Diego Zoo. In *Proceedings of the American Association of Zoo Veterinarians and International Association of Aquatic Animal Medicine Joint Conference*, New Orleans, LA, 2000, pp 102–105.
24. Patton ML, Aubrey L, Edwards M, et al: Successful contraception in a herd of Chinese goral (*Naemorhedus goral arnouxianus*) with melengestrol acetate. *J Zoo Wildl Med* 31(2):228–230, 2000.
25. Pence DB, Gray GG: Elaeophorosis in Barbary sheep and mule deer from the Texas panhandle. *J Wildl Dis* 17(1):49–56, 1981.
26. Rasmussen JM, Miller JA, Wunschmann A, et al: Babesiosis in a captive herd of musk oxen (*Ovibos moschatus*): Treatment and a novel approach for prevention. In *Proceedings of the American Association of Zoo Veterinarians and Association of Reptile and Amphibian Veterinarians Joint Conference*, Los Angeles, CA, 2008, pp 58–59.
27. Schoelkopf L, Hutchinson CE, Bendele KG, et al: New ruminant hosts and wider geographic range identified for *Babesia odocoilei* (Emerson and Wright 1970). *J Wildl Dis* 41(4):683–690, 2005.
28. Vikoren T, Lillehaug A, Akerstedt J, et al: A severe outbreak of contagious echthyma (orf) in a free-ranging musk ox (*Ovibos moschatus*) population in Norway. *Vet Microbiol* 127:10–20, 2008.

CHAPTER 65

Avian Deflighting Techniques

R. Avery Bennett and Katrin Baumgartner

Over the years, various procedures have been developed to prevent flight in birds, either to improve their quality of life or to prevent their escape from public exhibits.[33] By preventing flight, birds may often be allowed more freedom within the facilities. Birds on display in open-air exhibits may interact with conspecifics and with other species of birds as well as specimens of other taxa, thus creating a more realistic and natural display. Although housing birds in large, enclosed exhibits may also meet these goals, such arrangements tend to be very expensive and may not be an option for all institutions. It may be desirable to only temporarily render the birds unable to fly; however, in open exhibits, it may be more appropriate to take permanent measures to prevent flight. It is ideal to preserve as much as possible of the bird's normal anatomy while taking steps to prevent flight. Unfortunately, most procedures used to deflight birds also change the appearance and function of the wing. In some countries, amputation of any body part of any animal other than for medical reasons is prohibited by law. This limits what procedures may be used to prevent flight even in birds in a zoologic setting.

The majority of the literature regarding techniques for preventing flight involves surgery, and such surgery has reportedly been performed without anesthesia or analgesia.[1] Many of these articles report deaths caused by shock in some patients.

Any procedure that involves incision or transection of tissues must be considered painful and should be conducted under general anesthesia with appropriate postoperative analgesia for 2 to 5 days. In some cases, such as in chicks, a local anesthetic along with an analgesic and appropriate postoperative analgesia may be acceptable.

Most commonly, procedures are only performed on one wing to cause imbalance and thus make flight more difficult.[1,16,34,36] A common comment made in many publications is that surgical deflighting procedures impair the bird's ability to balance and that this may affect the ability of male birds to reproduce. Some reports in the literature describe that a given deflighting procedure does not affect the birds' ability to groom and breed,[1,34] and some others indicate that it does, indeed, affect the ability to breed.[10,28] Interestingly, in one report, the author indicated that pinioning causes imbalance and inhibits breeding, but follicle extirpation, a procedure advocated in the study, does not.[22] Intuitively, it seems that having no primary flight feathers on one wing would have the same effect on balance that pinioning would. The authors of this study were, however, unable to find scientific evidence to support these claims.

Preventing birds from flying has been discussed as a matter related to animal welfare for many years.[17] Some species of birds such as waterfowl, gallinaceous birds, cranes, storks, and flamingos seem to do well even if they cannot fly, whereas other species such as hummingbirds, bee-eaters, swifts, swallows, and some raptors need flight to thrive. Small-sized aviaries expose birds to the risk of wing trauma.

LEGAL ISSUES

In zoologic collections, different deflighting techniques are used to control flight in birds. Some countries have legislation preventing any surgical procedure being performed for nonmedical reasons.

Such legislative regulations are often limiting and not directed specifically toward zoo birds, so in many countries, zoo veterinarians are placed in a legal limbo. Because deflighting, including trimming wing feathers, involves removal of a body part or partial removal or destruction of tissue, the following legislations may be applied to any deflighting technique.

The *German Animal Welfare Law* states in paragraph 6 (1):

The complete or partial amputation of body parts or the complete or partial removal or destruction of organs or tissues of a vertebrate are prohibited.

Because this law pertains to all vertebrates, birds are not exempted from it. The amputation of parts of the body (pinioning), the complete or partial removal of tissue (tenotomy or tenectomy, follicle excision), and the destruction of tissue (laser or cryosurgical follicle ablation), and even flight feather trimming are all considered illegal, and veterinarians performing these procedures may be prosecuted. In Germany, exemptions, even for feather trimming, do not exist.

In Switzerland, legislation specifically against pinioning birds has been enacted.

The *Swiss Animal Welfare Ordinance* states:

Article 20: Prohibited actions in domestic poultry:
b. Trimming of the comb and wattles and the wings.
Article 24: Other prohibited actions:
b. Surgical procedures to make it easier to keep pets, such as resection of teeth, clipping of wings, or removal of secretory glands; procedures to prevent reproduction or the removal of dewclaws, are exempted.

The European Convention for the Protection of Pet Animals was opened for signature in Strasbourg on November 13, 1987, enforced on May 1, 1992. This Convention states: "Surgical operations ... for other non-curative purposes shall be prohibited ...." At present, 15 of the 27 States in the European Union have ratified this Convention and have prohibited cosmetic surgical procedures. In addition, four European states have prohibited these operations, even though they did not ratify the Convention.

In the Swiss and European regulations, pet and poultry are included, but zoo birds are not. Nevertheless, some veterinary authorities in Europe consider deflighting amputation or tissue destruction and a modification of appearance; therefore, it is an illegal procedure. They cite article 10 of the European Convention to prohibit any deflighting techniques other than feather trimming. It has been suggested that these laws be changed with respect to zoo birds.[27]

In the United States, the *Animal Welfare Act* of 1996 regulates the treatment of animals in research institutions and exhibitions. Birds, rats, mice, farm-animals, and cold-blooded animals are excluded from the Animal Welfare Act.[2]

ANATOMY AND PHYSIOLOGY OF THE WING[4,7,38]

The anatomy and physiology of birds have been adapted to allow flight. The bones in the wing include the humerus, ulna, radius,

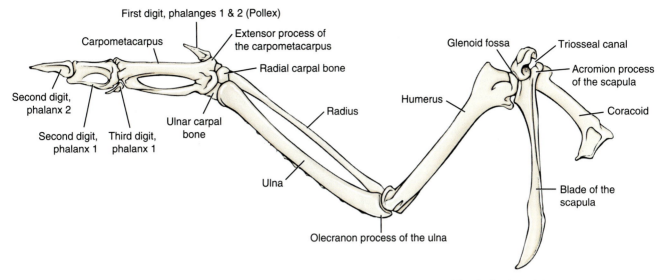

FIGURE 65-1 The osseous anatomy of the wing. (Diagram courtesy of Dr. Stefan Harsch.)

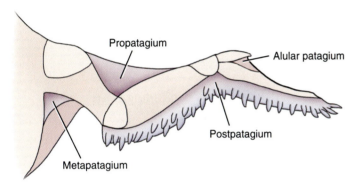

FIGURE 65-2 The four patagia of the wing include the *propatagium*, where the wing and the neck join the thorax; the *postpatagium*, which is located at the caudal angle of the carpus; the *metapatagium* at the caudal junction of the thorax and the wing, and the *alular patagium* between the alula and the carpometacarpus.

radial carpal bone, ulnar carpal bone, carpometacarpus, and bones of the digits of the manus (digitus alularis, digitus major, and digitus minor) (Figure 65-1). The alula (digit II) has one or two phalanges and has an important aerodynamic function.

The wing has four patagia (Figure 65-2).[7] The propatagium is the largest skinfold of the wing, and it fills the angle formed by the partially flexed elbow. It is composed of a network of multiple layers of collagen and elastin, which are suspended between the leading edge and the dorsal antebrachium of the wing.

The primary avian flight muscles are the pectoralis and the supracoracoideus.[12,38] The pectoralis is a large muscle composed of primarily large fibers and is attached to the humerus at the deltopectoral crest. It may make up 35% of the bird's total body weight.[11] This muscle contracts during the downstroke and pronates the wing. The supracoracoideus is a smaller muscle with short fibers and originates from the sternum; its tendon of insertion passes through the triosseal canal to the dorsal surface of the humerus. This muscle elevates and supinates the wing during the upstroke. Both muscles, the pectoralis and the supracoracoideus, accelerate and decelerate the wing across the transition between downstroke and upstroke.[38] The extensor carpi radialis originates from the medial epicondyle of the humerus, extends over the cranial surface of the carpal joint, and ends in the carpometacarpal extensor apophysis. This muscle extends the carpus and advances the primary flight feathers forward. The musculus pollicis brevis inserts craniodorsally on the base of the alula and abducts it or, if the musculus flexor pollicis is relaxed, raises it. The musculus pollicis longus originates on the proximal ventral surface of the ulna and the radius. The tendon of insertion attaches to the

extensor process of the carpometacarpus. This muscle extends the carpus when the elbow is flexed. Two smaller muscles, the triceps brachii and the biceps brachii, control the wing's shape by flexion and extension of the elbow.

ANATOMY AND PHYSIOLOGY OF REMIGES[6]

Feathers have different functions. The contour feathers include the feathers involved in flight (remiges) and the tail (rectrices). Remiges are divided into primary and secondary remiges. The primary remiges insert dorsally from the carpus and distally along the carpometacarpus and phalanges. In most species of birds, 10 primary remiges exist and are numbered from proximal to distal. The secondary remiges insert dorsally along the ulna and are counted from distal to proximal. They vary in number from six in hummingbirds to as many as 40 in some species. The primary and secondary remiges are not fixed rigidly in place, but they are able to twist during flight. The remiges are attached to feather follicles, which are specialized pockets of epidermal and dermal cells from which a new feather grows after the old feather is lost during molt by extrusion of the old feather from its base. When the feather is growing from the papilla of the follicle, it is called a *blood feather* because it has an active blood supply. As the feather matures, it loses its blood supply and becomes hollow. The follicle grips the feather at the calamus (the hollow portion of the feather shaft) by muscular contraction of the follicular muscle and friction.

The main shaft of the feather is the scapus and is divided into the vexillum, or vaned portion, and the calamus, or unvaned portion

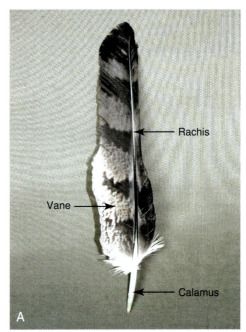

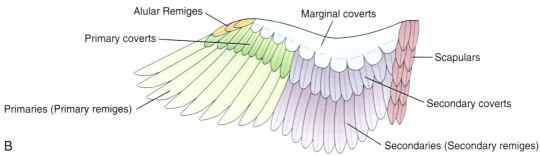

FIGURE 65-3 The main shaft of the feather is the scapus and is divided into the vexillum (vaned portion) and calamus (unvaned portion). The vane is the majority of the feather extending perpendicular to the shaft. The scapus is the central axis of a feather composed of the calamus (unvaned) and the rachis (vaned).

(Figure 65-3). The vane comprises the majority of the feather, extending perpendicular to the shaft. The scapus is the central axis of a feather composed of the calamus and the rachis.[7] The rachis (vaned portion of the scapus) is the solid, long, tubular portion of the shaft distal to the skin and is the continuation of the calamus, which is the hollow, short, tubular, unpigmented end of the mature feather that extends below the level of the skin.

WING FEATHER TRIMMING

The most commonly used method to prevent flight in birds is to cut the remiges and has only a temporary effect.[10,18] The advantages of this method are that it is temporary and nonpainful and therefore does not require anesthesia or analgesia, it is minimally stressful (if not performed in large groups and repeated on a regular basis), and it is inexpensive. However, the fact that it is temporary may also be a disadvantage.[10,33] Feather trimming is usually done on only one wing on the basis of the concept that this will make it more difficult for the birds to fly because the birds are unbalanced. However, in some species, it may be necessary to trim the feathers on both wings to effectively prevent flight.[33] Larger, heavier-bodied birds are more likely to be unable to fly having had only the feathers on one wing trimmed. Trimming the feathers on both wings may be advantageous in allowing the bird to balance better, which may be important in some situations such as during breeding.[18]

The duration of effectiveness depends on the rate of molt in different species. Most birds only molt once a year, and the molt occurs over a relatively brief period. Some birds such as ducks molt twice a year because they develop eclipse plumage during breeding season, and some other species such as cranes only molt every other year.[36] Feather trimming should be postponed until after a molt to minimize the number of times the bird has to be caught to trim remiges.[34] If trimming of flight feathers is used as a method of preventing flight, it is important to monitor the wing for feather regrowth and trim the new feathers once they have regrown into a mature, nonvital feather.

In general, all primary remiges on one wing are cut. Trimming the feathers on the same side for all specimens of one sex and the opposite side for the other sex allows for quick identification of the sex of the bird, even from a distance. When trimming remiges, blood feathers should not be trimmed.[36] Generally, cutting feathers just proximal to the distal tip of the covert feathers, will prevent damage to blood feathers and is considered more cosmetically acceptable because the covert feathers cover the cut ends of the remiges. Birds may also be less likely to chew on cut feathers that are covered by covert feathers. It is considered best to cut each feather individually; cutting only the rachis results in a more cosmetically pleasing appearance because the vane then extends beyond the cut end of the rachis (Figure 65-4). Leaving the first and possibly the second primary flight feathers uncut also produces a more cosmetically acceptable result, but some birds will still be able to fly.[36] In species

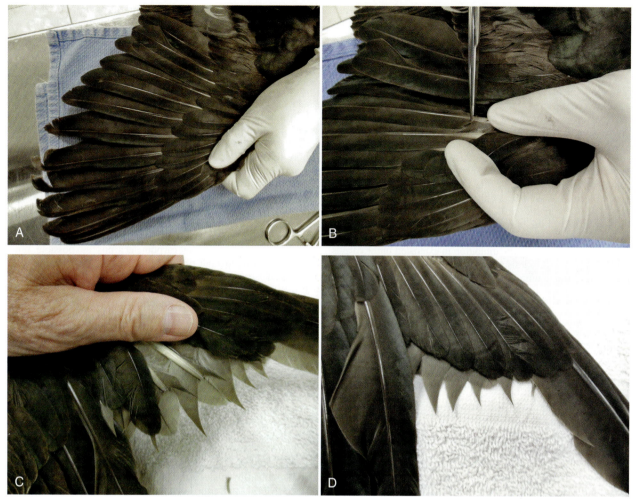

FIGURE 65-4 A, It is best to cut the feathers just proximal to the covert feathers. **B,** When the rachis is cut but the vane is not, the vane extends beyond the cut part. **C,** Birds are then less likely to experience irritation of the cut end. **D,** It is more cosmetically acceptable when the cut ends are not visible when the wing is extended.

that are heavier-bodied, it is preferable to leave these two feathers, as this allows the bird to land more gently. African gray parrots (*Psittacus erithacus*) are prone to developing lesions on the skin over the keel from hitting the substrate hard during attempts to fly after having their feathers trimmed.[10] Some species such as cockatoos are prone to chewing on cut flight feathers, which may lead to self-mutilation.

BRAILING

Brailing was first described in 1930[32] and involves temporarily immobilizing the carpus to prevent flight by using external coaptation. Brailing is applied around the carpus to prevent it from extending, thereby preventing flight. It is usually only applied to one wing.

Historically, brailing has been used primarily to prevent flight in juvenile pheasants prior to placing them into an enclosed flight cage. However, it has also been used to prevent birds from flying or traumatizing themselves during shipment.[1,10,36] Pheasants are often reared for their feathers or for hunting, so amputation and follicle extirpation techniques are not used. Once flight feathers begin to grow in the chicks, which occurs at an early age in pheasants (10–14 days), the brail sling is applied.[36] It is recommended that the sling not be left in place for more than 3 weeks or it may result in wing deformity.[1,36] If it is necessary to prevent flight for a longer period, the brail sling is removed and a slightly longer one applied to the

contralateral wing.[36] This allows the first wing to recover and grow properly. Brailing may also cause damage to growing flight feathers.[13]

RADIAL NEURECTOMY

The radial nerve runs along the medial aspect of the distal humerus and has only skin covering it at this location. Excision of a portion of the radial nerve has been done in an effort to prevent flight in birds by paralyzing the muscles that flex and extend the carpus.[34] Paralysis persists for months, and the wing droops after the procedure. The results are unpredictable, and most sources agree that the procedure does not permanently prevent flight.[1,34,39]

TENOTOMY AND TENECTOMY PROCEDURES

These techniques often result in short-term prevention of flight, but it is likely that even when a portion of a tendon is excised, the severed ends reunite with scar tissue resulting in return of enough function to allow birds to escape.

Tenotomy or Tenectomy of the Extensor Metacarpi Radialis Longus Muscle

In an effort to prevent flight in birds, without removing a portion of the wing for cosmetic reasons, tenotomy of the tendon of the extensor metacarpi radialis longus muscle was performed in 1940.[32] It was theorized that with the cutting of this tendon, birds would no longer be able to extend the carpus enough to be able to fly. In theory, the wing should not droop because it is an extensor of the manus and the flexors remain undamaged. Although the authors reported success with this technique, they noted that it should be done bilaterally and that the birds at the San Diego Zoo were still able to "glide off (a hill) to a lower level." Subsequently, others have recommended partial tenectomy—removing a section of the tendon, rather than just transecting it. However, this has not improved the success rate of deflighting birds.[33,39] Other sources have reported that birds, in fact, do have a wing droop after the procedure.[34,39]

One author suggested that it is important to immobilize the wing for approximately 6 weeks following surgery to allow joint ankylosis.[26] In 452 birds in his study, either tenotomy or tenectomy was performed. In 349 of the birds, the wing was immobilized for 6 weeks, and in 333 of the birds the carpi were fused; and in only 5 of the 103 birds in which the wing was not immobilized, the carpus considered fused. It is likely the inhibition in extension of the carpus resulted from joint arthrodesis rather than from transecting or excising a portion of the tendon.

Tenectomy of the Adductor Pollicis Longus and Brevis

Excision of the tendon of the adductor pollicis longus has been reported to result in an inability to extend the carpus without causing a wing droop.[34] It inhibits take off and gliding and has been recommended in storks and herons. Results are reported to be similar to tenectomy of the extensor metacarpi radialis longus.

Tenectomy of the Supracoracoideus Muscle

The supracoracoideus muscles are located deep to the pectoral muscles along the keel of the sternum. The tendon of insertion passes through the triosseal canal at the shoulder formed by the clavicle, scapula, and coracoid bones attaching on the dorsal tubercle of the proximal humerus. Excision of a portion of this tendon of insertion on the proximal humerus was first reported in 1936 as an experimental procedure;[37] it was investigated more scientifically by Degernes and Feduccia in 2001 as a means to prevent flight in birds while maintaining their normal appearance. The tensor propatagialis pars brevis muscle fibers must be separated longitudinally to access the supracoracoideus tendon, and in some experimental birds, the wrong tissue was transected, which indicates that it is not easy to accurately identify the supracoracoideus tendon.[10]

The procedure did alter wing function by limiting wing extension in all birds, but it did not prevent the birds from flying and gaining altitude. Birds with bilateral supracoracoideus tenectomy had difficulty righting themselves when placed on the back. Most birds eventually regained the ability to right themselves, but one bird was euthanized because it was never able to right itself.

Tenotomy of the Superficial and Deep Pectoralis Muscles

Tenotomy or partial tenectomy of the superficial[10] or deep[28] pectoral muscle has also failed to prevent flight over the long term in birds.[10,34] Tenectomy of the deep pectoralis muscle has been reported to be effective in swans and pigeons, but the dissection is difficult, and birds might regain the ability to fly.[34]

Tenotomy of the Triceps Brachii

Transection of the triceps tendon at the elbow or distal humerus results in a severe wing droop in over 50% of birds, and it is, therefore, not recommended.[34]

PINIONING

Pinioning is the act of surgically removing one pinion joint, the joint of a bird's wing farthest from the body, to prevent flight.[29] It is basically a surgical amputation at the carpus. The procedure is usually only performed on one wing, based on the assumption that this will result in imbalance. The authors have been unable to find reports comparing unilateral pinioning with bilateral pinioning.

Hatchling Birds

Most sources recommend pinioning of hatchling birds between the ages of 3 and 10 days.[31,36] Chicks are allowed to begin eating and adapt to life outside the egg before this potentially painful and stressful procedure is performed. The tip of one wing is cut off with scissors by lifting the alula and positioning the scissor across the carpometacarpus to transect proximal to the major and minor portions to ensure that the follicles of all primary remiges are removed.[36] Topical or injectable local anesthetic should be applied to reduce the pain associated with the procedure, making sure to calculate an appropriate dose, which may be difficult in small chicks. Hemorrhage is minor, and the amputation site heals quickly by secondary intention. The alula is left in an effort to protect the amputation site during healing and after the bird has grown feathers.[33] As much of the caudal aspect of the carpometacarpus as possible must be removed to remove all primary flight feather follicles. If the cut is too distal, some remiges will grow, and the bird may be able to fly.[35] If the cut end extends beyond the alula, it is more prone to trauma and development of a stump granuloma. Chicks under parental care, for example, wading birds, psittacines, and pelicans, may be rejected by the parent after pinioning.[34]

In hatchlings that are slightly older (1–3 weeks), hemorrhage is more likely to be significant. A hemostatic clip may be applied just proximal to the amputation site, as proximal as possible, to preserve the alula.[31,34] The clip is applied at an angle under the alula, from distal to proximal, to allow removal of all of the primary remiges. The clip will provide hemostasis when scissors are used to amputate distal to the clip, and the tissue within the clip will necrose and heal proximal to it. In 8 to 10 days, the clip will fall off.

Adult Birds

In more mature chicks and in adult birds, surgical amputation of the distal wing is performed for pinioning. The goal is to remove the carpometacarpus to which the primary remiges are attached thus preventing birds from flying. General anesthesia and aseptic technique are used.[33,36] Hemostasis is vital and may be achieved using ligatures, hemostatic clips, electrosurgery, laser, or other techniques. Postoperative analgesia should be provided for 3 to 5 days following surgery.

Surgical removal of the carpometacarpus was first reported in 1912.[19] Since then, various procedures for amputation of the wing tip in adult birds have been reported.[1,14,23,33,34,36,39] The procedures include the use of an elastic band to control hemorrhage; a double-action bone cutter to cut just distal to the alula, leaving it to heal by secondary intention;[23] and performing an aseptic surgical disarticulation at the carpus.[39] When the wing is extended, no primary remiges remain, and this is considered unsightly by many.[10,16,33,34] Some have reported leaving the cut end to heal by secondary intention,[1,23,33,34] since not enough soft tissue remains to cover the cut end of the bone. Other authors have reported preserving the skin 1 to 2 cm distal to the carpus, performing a disarticulation at the distal radius and ulna, but preserving the radial carpal bone or transecting the carpometacarpus, and then using the soft tissues to cover the ends of the bones.[14,36,39]

In much of the literature regarding deflighting of birds by amputation of the distal wing, much concern has been expressed about trauma to the stump.[1,33] The bone has very little soft tissue covering it, and when allowed to heal by secondary intention, the scar tissue does not hold up to the trauma well. Birds may traumatize the stump if the enclosure is too small and the wing hits the walls, or they may attempt to fly and hit the stump on the substrate. The risk of stump trauma (lacerations, ulcerations, and granulomas) may be minimized by surgically covering the stump with normal, feathered skin. In addition, the site heals faster with less risk of infection when sutured.[39] Some birds, including pelicans (*Pelecanus sp.*) and ground

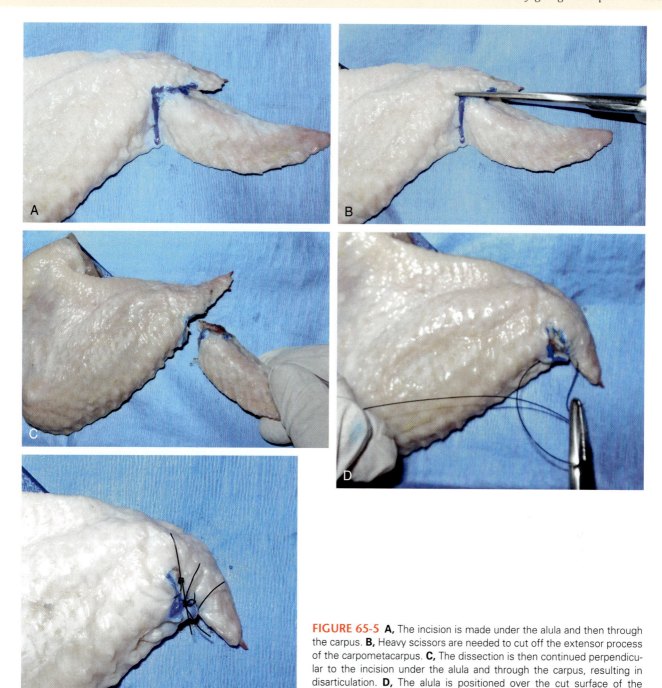

FIGURE 65-5 A, The incision is made under the alula and then through the carpus. **B,** Heavy scissors are needed to cut off the extensor process of the carpometacarpus. **C,** The dissection is then continued perpendicular to the incision under the alula and through the carpus, resulting in disarticulation. **D,** The alula is positioned over the cut surface of the carpus and sutured in place. **E,** The amputation stump is covered with normal, feathered skin and protected by the alular remiges.

hornbills (*Bucorvus leadbeateri*), have pneumatic carpometacarpal bones. In these birds, transected bone must be covered, or the bird may drown from aspiration of water through the exposed cut bone.[14]

One author reported performing pinioning by disarticulation at the carpus (n = 80) or by ostectomy of the carpometacarpus just distal to the articular surface (n = 26) with virtually no complications.[1] Another author performed 4491 deflighting procedures with the use of different techniques and preferred amputation distal to the articular surface of the carpometacarpus to other methods of deflighting birds as being the most reliable and cosmetically acceptable.[34]

One of this chapter's authors (RAB) has developed a modification of the technique reported by Fletcher.[14] The distal wing is amputated

at the carpus, preserving the alula and using it to cover the amputation site (Figure 65-5). With the use of this technique, the end of the wing at the amputation site is not only covered with normal, healthy, feathered skin, but it is also covered by the bone in the alula and the tough alular remiges. After plucking the feathers and preparing the skin for aseptic surgery, an incision is made under or caudal to the alula from distal to proximal to the level of the carpus. Then the incision is continued caudal to the alula at the carpus from dorsal, across the caudal aspect of the joint, then ventrally toward the cranial edge of the joint. The skin should not be cut on the cranial edge near the alula. Sharp dissection is used to disarticulate the carpus at the carpometacarpus, leaving the ulnar carpal and radial carpal bones in place. The extensor process of the carpometacarpus articulates with the alula. A bone cutter or a pair of heavy scissors is used to cut this projection off, leaving it with the alula. If this is removed, the flap created containing the alula will have a very thin base and may necrose. The alula is rotated caudally to cover over the radial and ulnar carpal bones. Suture the skin on the dorsal and ventral aspects of the amputation site. This technique provides a very sturdy stump resistant to environmental trauma.

Severe hemorrhage and shock have been reported as complications from pinioning adult birds,[10,36] and many authors have recommended the use of a tourniquet to control hemorrhage.[1,33,34] A single artery supplies the distal wing—the ventral metacarpal artery, which runs along the ventral aspect of the carpus from cranially at the distal radius and radial carpal bone to the minor portion (metacarpal IV) of the carpometacarpus.[14] Ideally, this is ligated prior to being transected, but if it is accidentally transected, it is fairly easy to identify, clamp, and ligate.[33] A technique to occlude the ventral metacarpal artery prior to transecting it involves passing a suture between the major and minor portions of the carpometacarpus.[14] The venous drainage at this location is not single or discrete. Continuous, slow bleeding may occur but is generally easy to control with digital pressure, electrosurgery, suture pressure, or bandage. It is best to bandage the amputation site to keep it clean and to bandage the wing to the body because many birds will hold the wing drooped because of postoperative pain and discomfort. After 1 to 2 days, the sutured skin incision will have sealed and the pain will have subsided, so bandaging is usually no longer needed.

ARTHRODESIS OF A WING JOINT

Arthrodesis is defined as the artificial induction of joint ossification between two bones via surgery.[3] Generally, to accomplish fusion of two articular bones, the cartilage on the articular surface must be removed and the joint immobilized to allow the bones to heal together as one bone. A cancellous bone graft is also recommended to facilitate bone healing. Once the bones have healed together as one unit, the joint is fixed in the position in which it was immobilized during healing.

Carpus

Carpal arthrodesis has been reported to permanently prevent flight in large birds with a cosmetically pleasing outcome.[33] A surgical approach is made at the carpus to expose the distal ulna, the ulnar carpal bone, and the proximal carpometacarpus. Holes are drilled in the distal end of the ulna, the middle of the ulnar carpal bone, and the proximal end of the carpometacarpus. An orthopedic wire is passed through the three holes and tightened with the carpus in flexion to prevent motion at the carpus. Primary closure eliminates the need for postoperative wound management. No mention is made of removing articular cartilage, although the author claims good results. No long-term outcome was reported, but it would be expected that with cyclic stress, the wire may break and because articular cartilage still exists, fusion of the bones would probably not occur. For this technique to result in arthrodesis, the articular cartilage would have to be removed and the wing immobilized for several weeks.

In another report, the author obliterated the articular cartilage before passing the wire.[34] The wing was kept bandaged for 2 to 3 weeks in an effort to immobilize the joint to allow fusion. Still, the author reported that the procedure yielded unacceptable results in at least 50% of geese on which the procedure was performed. Birds regained the ability to fly after about 3 to 4 weeks, and at that point, the wing was also drooped. This would be expected if the bones had not yet fused, the wire broke, and the joint could once again be extended for flight.

The authors of both articles mentioned above noted that this procedure is difficult and requires some level of surgical expertise. It is not a quick procedure and is only useful in large birds in which the bones are large enough to create holes through which wire may

be passed.[33,34] Additionally, both authors reported that birds have a wing droop at rest after the procedure.

Elbow

Performing elbow arthrodesis immobilizes the elbow preventing flight while maintaining all of the remiges with a cosmetic result.[16] Unilateral arthrodesis of the elbow was performed in nine peafowl, and the birds were able to strut and display normally during courtship; however, they were also able to cross over a 1.3-meter (m) fence.[16]

In this procedure, the medial aspect of the elbow joint is incised and the cartilage removed from the distal humerus and the proximal ulna. The joint capsule is closed and the elbow is placed in a flexed position. A pilot hole is drilled through the distal caudal humerus and into the proximal ulna at the elbow joint. A screw is placed through the distal humerus and into the proximal ulna. The wing is bandaged to the body for 3 weeks.

This procedure is often more time consuming compared with amputation of the distal wing and requires equipment and knowledge for bone screw application. A bone graft was not applied, but arthrodesis was considered complete in 3 weeks.

PROPATAGIECTOMY (PATAGIECTOMY)

Surgical removal of the propatagium, along with sutures passed around the radius and humerus to prevent wing extension, has been successful in preventing flight in birds while maintaining the osseous anatomy and all of the flight feathers.[24,30,34] The propatagium is excised from the carpus to the proximal humerus and to the elbow close to the radius and humerus. The sutures are passed around the humerus and radius and tightened to approximate the incised skin edges. The skin is sutured along the dorsal (lateral) and ventral (medial) aspects of the wing, and the permanently flexed wing is maintained in a "figure-of-8" bandage until the soft tissues have healed. Hemorrhage is generally minor and easy to control.

This technique preserves all of the feathers of the wing and prevents wing extension and flight. The cosmetic results are mixed because even though all of the feathers remain, the wing cannot be extended. Some species such as storks and cranes that have a low body weight and large wingspan are often still able to fly enough to escape.[34] This procedure generally takes more time to complete compared with the techniques used to amputate the wing tip, but because all remiges are still present, the cosmetic results may be worth the effort it takes to perform the procedure.

PRIMARY REMIGE FOLLICLE EXTIRPATION

Extirpation is defined as the complete excision or surgical destruction of a body part.[25] Recently, feather follicle extirpation has been recommended as the method of choice for deflighting birds (WAZA resolution 2005, WAZA Science and Veterinary Committee).[21,22]

Surgical Excision

Surgical excision of the follicles of the primary remiges was first reported in 1940.[32] The skin along the insertion of the primary remiges was removed to include all of the follicles. The wound was left to heal by secondary intention. The procedure was reported to result in "some hemorrhage" and took approximately 1 month for the resulting wound to heal. After the follicles that form the primary remiges are removed, the feathers are not able to regrow, which leaves the wing tip without flight feathers, thus preventing flight. The follicles of the primary remiges are attached to the major portion (metacarpus III) of the carpometacarpus and the major digit (digit III). All of the germinal tissue must be removed, or the feathers will regrow and are generally deformed because of the trauma and partial excision of germinal epithelium. It is recommended that actively growing feathers (blood feathers) not be removed until they have become hollow. In some birds, especially young birds and birds that are actively molting, the feathers may grow back, and a second procedure may be needed to remove regrown feathers.[22]

It is recommended that a tourniquet be placed to minimize hemorrhage; however, if a tourniquet is used, it is important to keep it in place for as short a period as possible. Occlusion of the blood flow to the distal wing may result in avascular necrosis distal to the site of tourniquet application. In large birds, this procedure may be time consuming, and excessive hemorrhage, even with a tourniquet, is still reported as a complication.[22] Other techniques such as electrosurgery should be used, if available, to control intraoperative hemorrhage.

In smaller birds, a single incision is made along the minor portion (metacarpus IV) of the carpometacarpus, providing access to the follicles of all 10 or 11 primary remiges, where they are attached to carpometacarpus. The skin is elevated caudally to expose the follicles, and each follicle is individually elevated to completely excise the germinal tissue. The calami are cut 6 to 8 mm distal to the point of insertion, but below skin level, and that portion of feather is removed along with the follicle. The rest of the feather is left attached to the skin where it exits and the skin is sutured closed. The wing is bandaged for 2 to 3 days. In larger birds, a longitudinal incision is made in the skin over each of the primary remiges individually to provide exposure to the follicle (Figure 65-6). The follicle is elevated and removed, along with 1 cm of the calamus, leaving the portion attached to the skin. One or two sutures are placed in the skin. It has been reported that large and heavy birds such as storks and pelicans may still fly unless the follicles of six coverts are also removed.[22]

The ventral metacarpal artery must be preserved because damage to this vessel may result in avascular necrosis of the wing distal to the point of thrombosis. Reported complications include feather regrowth; excessive hemorrhage, especially in pelicans and flamingos (*Phoenicopterus*); necrosis; and infection.[22] It has been suggested that follicle extirpation does not affect breeding, although this has not been scientifically evaluated.[22] Cosmetically, the wing tip has not been amputated and contains no flight feathers, which some find unsightly.[16,34]

The classical extirpation method has been performed over a long period in over 50 species by zoo veterinarians in Germany with good results, but to a limited extent in some species.[15]

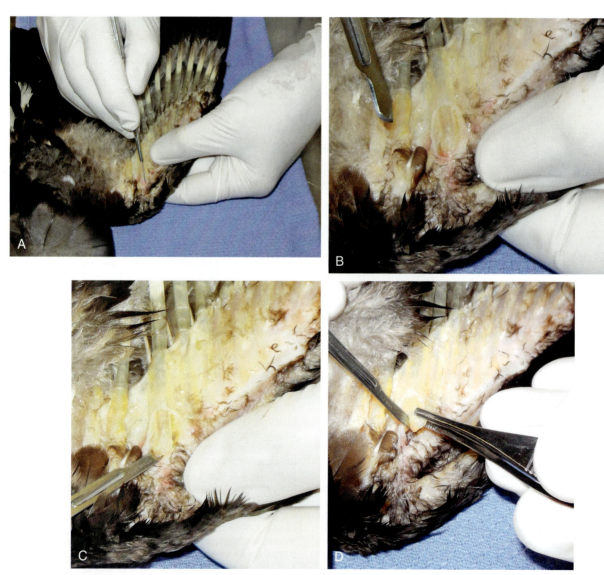

FIGURE 65-6 For remige follicle excision in a large birds, make an incision parallel to the calamus from the insertion on the carpometacarpus about 1 centimeter (cm) long (**A**). Expose the follicle and about 1 cm of calamus (**B**). Elevate the follicle from its attachments (**C**). Expose 5 to 10 millimeters (mm) of the calamus (**D**).   *Continued*

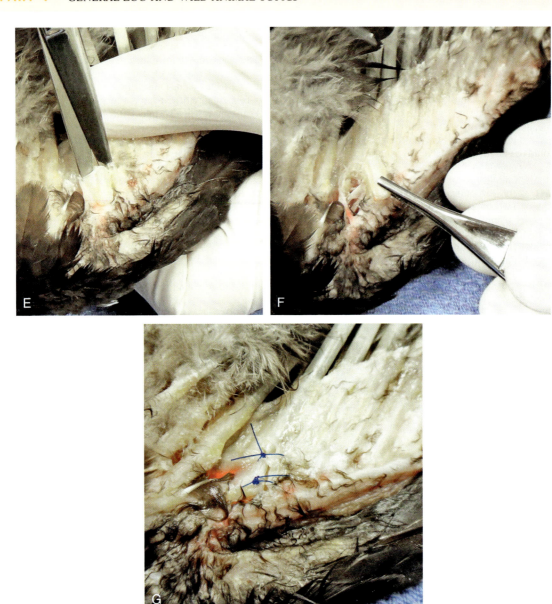

FIGURE 65-6, cont'd Cut the calamus proximal to the skin with heavy scissors (**E**). Discard the piece of calamus with the follicle (**F**). Place one or two sutures in the skin (**G**).

Electrosurgical Fulguration

Electrosurgery refers to the use of electric current passing from a device through the patient and back to the generator. The effect may be to cut tissue, coagulate vessels, or destroy (fulgurate) the tissue. In one report, electrocoagulation was used to destroy feather follicles preventing them from regrowing.[8] The authors of the study reported successfully preventing feather growth and indicated that the degree of flight may actually be controlled by selectively destroying individual follicles. The technique to perform this procedure was, however, not described in the report. Electrosurgical units are available in many institutions, and this procedure warrants further investigation, since cryosurgery and laser units are often not available.

Cryosurgery

Cryosurgery typically involves the use of a cryogen, usually liquid nitrogen, to freeze tissue, which results in necrosis. Most commonly, more than one freeze–thaw cycle are performed to improve the chances of tissue killing. Cryosurgery units are commonly available to veterinarians, but it is difficult to control the amount of tissue frozen by the cryoprobe, and this risks the creation of an open wound as tissues slough.

In one study, cryosurgery was evaluated as a method for feather follicle extirpation in pigeons.[9] The unit was set at −80°C with a probe size 2 mm and each follicle was frozen for 5, 20, or 30 seconds then allowed to thaw for 2 minutes. This freeze–thaw cycle was repeated three times. All of the follicles (n = 10) treated for 5 seconds were all producing new feathers 5 weeks after the procedure; however, none of the follicles (10th primary) treated for 20 seconds regrew feathers (n = 12). Seven of twelve follicles (6th primary) treated for 30 seconds regrew feathers at 5 weeks after the procedure. The authors theorized that the failure in the 5-second group was a result of the cryoprobe being too large to fit into the calamus to the level of the follicle and that using a smaller probe in direct contact with the follicle would likely be more effective. Since cryosurgery units are relatively inexpensive, this technique warrants further investigation.

Laser

A diode laser may be used to extirpate the primary remiges in birds.[5,9,35] Rather than removing the follicle surgically, the heat from the laser light energy results in thermal necrosis of the feather follicle. Lasers may be used to fulgurate tissues where the intention is to cause heat necrosis.

The wavelength of the light beam produced by the diode laser is absorbed by hemoglobin. It passes through other media such as water and air. It has the ability to fulgurate the vascular area of the feather follicle.[9] Following laser extirpation of the feather follicles, the necrotic tissue must heal by invasion of inflammatory cells following the phases of wound healing. If the area of necrosis is small, the bird's body may resorb the necrotic debris, but too much tissue damage results in an open wound.

Pigeons were used as a model to develop a technique using a diode laser to ablate flight feather follicles.[9] In 6 pigeons, the 10 primary remiges of both wings were treated with the diode laser (20 watts [W] for 4 seconds or 10 W for 2 seconds). The one bird that received the high dose (20 W, 4 seconds) developed an area of skin necrosis at one of the laser-treated sites that healed completely in 3 days; histologically, an area of osseous necrosis was observed. The other 5 birds received the lower dose of energy and had mild swelling 24 hours after the treatment but it resolved by 48 hours. Two of 12 feathers were regrowing after the treatment but the method was considered successful.[9]

More recently, one of this chapter's authors (KB) used a diode laser to extirpate remige follicles with improved results. In this method, the relevant feathers are cut at skin level, and any dry material within the shaft is removed with forceps (Figure 65-7). The laser tip is inserted through the hollow calamus. A bare-fiber laser tip is inserted into the cut calamus and moved in small circles with the laser activated at a setting of 3.0 to 3.5 W for different periods. The laser is activated intermittently to allow cooling of the adjacent tissues until the tip is felt to have penetrated the follicle. Depending on the species of bird and the stage of development of the feather, this may take between 20 and 200 seconds in total, including the off intervals, with laser treatment being delivered for a total of 5 to 60 seconds. In young flamingos that have feathers that have recently matured, for example, the procedure is quicker, taking only 3 to 5 seconds (3–17.5 joules [J]). In adult birds of large species with large feathers, it takes more time (up to 200 seconds, 700 J). Growing feathers should be left until they are mature.

The calami of the fulgurated follicles are left and are shed as a result of tissue necrosis. Minor bleeding sometimes occurs during the procedure, and a cotton-tip applicator soaked in a topical hemostatic agent such as policresulen (Lotagen, Essex) may be inserted into the calamus. The swabs are left in the calamus and fall out within 24 hours. No topical medications or bandages are applied to the wing, and no topical or systemic antibiotic treatment is administered. The birds may be taken back to their group immediately after recovering from anesthesia.[20] The first

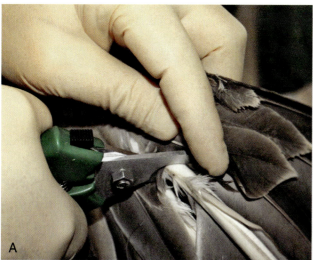
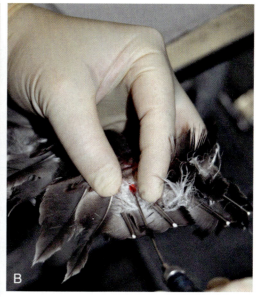
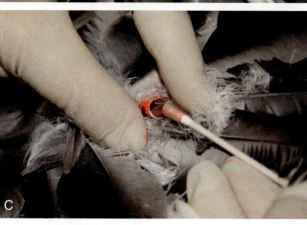

FIGURE 65-7 A, The calamus is cut, allowing the laser tip to be inserted into the calamus down to the follicle. **B,** The tip of the laser is inserted into the calamus onto the follicle and energy delivered to destroy the follicle tissue. **C,** If hemorrhage occurs, insert a cotton-tipped applicator with a hemostatic agent into the calamus down onto the destroyed follicle.

postoperative days meloxicam (Metacam®, Boehringer Ingelheim) is given orally.

This deflighting technique has been used for 3 years in zoo birds with good success. Of 318 follicles ablated with the diode laser using this technique, 18 feathers have regrown, resulting in a 94% success rate. The improved success may be attributed to the lower power setting (3.0–3.5 W) used. It is a quick procedure with a short anesthesia time, bleeding and tissue damage are minimal, no bandaging is needed, and early reintroduction into the group is possible.

CONCLUSION

The decision to use a deflighting technique in a bird must be made carefully, and the goal should be the well-being of the individual. The deprivation of the ability to fly may provide birds with opportunities not possible in aviaries.[17] The behavioral effects of deflighting have not been scientifically studied. Many methods are described in the literature. Veterinarians should choose the procedure most appropriate for the species of bird, the facility, and the equipment available.

ACKNOWLEDGMENT

Dr. Baumgartner would like to thank her collaborators on the laser follicle extirpation technique, Hermann Kempf, Christine Lendl, and Herman Will.

REFERENCES

 1. Acharjyo LN, Ojha SC: Pinioning of wild birds in captivity—a clinical study. *Indian Vet J* 49:720–724, 1972.
 2. Wikipedia online encyclopedia: *Animal Welfare Act*: http://en.wikipedia .org/wiki/Animal_Welfare_Act_of_1966. Accessed February 1, 2013.
 3. Wikipedia online encyclopedia: *Arthrodesis*: http://en.wikipedia.org/wiki/ Arthrodesis. Accessed February 1, 2013.
 4. Baumel JJ, Witmer LM: Osteologia. In Baumel J, Paytner RA, editors: *Handbook of avian anatomy: Nomina anatomica avium*, ed 2, Cambridge, U.K., 1993, Cambridge Club, pp 45–132.
 5. Baumgartner K, Kempf H, Will H, et al: Feather follicle atrophying by laser—an improvement of extirpation for animal welfare reasons. In *Proceedings of the International Conference on Disease of Zoo Wild Animals*, Bussolengo, Italy, 2012, pp 25–28.
 6. Bicudo JE, Buttemer WA, Chappell MA, et al: Introduction—blueprint of a bird (bauplan/ body plan). In Bicudo JE, Buttemer WA, Chappell MA, Pearson JT, Bech C, editors: *Ecology and environmental physiolgy of birds*, Oxford, U.K., 2010, Oxford University Press, pp 1–26.
 7. Cooper JE, Harrison GJ: Dermatology. In Ritchie B, Harrison G, Harrison L, editors: *Avian medicine: Principles and application*, Lake Worth, FL, 1994, Wingers Publishing, pp 607–621.
 8. Cwiertna Z, Frak W: Über einige chirurgische methoden zur flugbeschränkung bei zoovögeln. In *Proceedings 14 Visz*, Hungary, 1972, pp 147.
 9. D'Agostino JJ, Snider T, Hoover J, et al: Use of laser ablation and cryosurgery to prevent primary feather growth in a pigeon (*Columa livia*) model. *J Av Med Surg* 20:219–224, 2006.
10. Degernes LA, Feduccia A: Tenectomy of the supracoracoideus muscle to deflight pigeons (*Columba livia*) and cockatiels (*Nymphicus hollandicus*). *J Av Med Surg* 15(1):10–16, 2001.
11. Dial KP, Kaplan SR, Goslow GE: A functional analysis of the primary upstroke and downstroke muscles in the domestic pigeon (*Columba livia*) during flight. *J Exp Biol* 134:1–16, 1987.
12. Dial KP: Activity patterns of the wing muscles of a pigeon (*Columba livia*) during different modes of flight. *J Exp Zool* 262:357–373, 1992.
13. Ellis DH, Dein FJ: Flight restraint. In Ellis DH, Gee GF, Mirande CM, editors: *Cranes: Their biology, husbandry, and conservation*, Washington, DC, 1996, Hancock House Publisher, pp 241–244.
14. Fletcher KC, Miller BW: A technique for cosmetic pinioning of adult birds. *Vet Med Small Anim Clin* 75:1898–1904, 1980.
15. Gauckler A, Baumgartner K: Die exstirpation der handschwingenpapillen bei wasser- und stelzvögeln. In *21 Arbeitstagung der Zootierärzte im Deutschsprachigen Raum*, Halle, 2001.
16. Gross WB, Alexander J: A surgical method for controlling the flight of peafowl (*Pavo cristata*). *Av Dis* 32:553–555, 1988.
17. Hestermann H, Gregory NG, Boardman WSJ: Deflighting procedures and their welfare implications in captive birds. *Anim Welfare* 10:405–419, 2001.
18. Hillyer EV: Physical examination. In Altman RB, Clubb SL, Dorrestein GM, Quesenberry K, editors: *Avian medicine and surgery*, Philadelphia, PA, 1997, Saunders, pp 139.
19. Hornaday WT, Crandall L: Breeding mallard ducks for profit. *New York State Conserv Dept Bull* 13, 1912.
20. Kempf H, Baumgartner K, Will H, Lendl C: Balanced anaesthesia in pelicans (*Pelecanus* spp.) and cranes (*Grus* spp., *Balearica pavonina*) induced with medetomidin-ketamine-butorphanol. In *Proceedings of the International Conference on Disease of Zoo Wild Animals*, Bussolengo, Italy, 2012, pp 18–22.
21. Krawinkel P, Weber H, Schauerte N, et al: Extirpation of feather follicles—a practical, acceptable and permanent method to prevent zoo birds from flying. In *Proceedings of the meeting of the European Association of Zoo and Wildlife Veterinarians*, 2008, Leipzig, Germany, pp 363–364.
22. Krawinkel P: Feather follicle extirpation: Operative techniques to prevent zoo birds from flying. In Fowler ME, Miller RE, editors: *Zoo and wildlife medicine: Current therapy*, ed 7, St. Louis, MO, 2011, Saunders, pp 275–280.
23. Lewandowski AH, Sikarskie JG: Pinioning: A quick and simple technique. In *Proceedings of the Annual Conference of the American Association of Zoo Veterinarians*, Turtle Bay, HI, 1987, pp 414–415.
24. Mangili G: Unilateral patagiectomy: A new method of preventing flight in captive birds. *Int Zoo YB* XI:252–254, 1971.
25. Merriam Webster Medical Dictionary Online: http://www.nlm.nih.gov/ medlineplus/mplusdictionary.html. Accessed February 1, 2013.
26. Miller JC: The importance of immobilizing wings after tenectomy or tenotomy. *Vet Med Small Anim Clin* 68(1):35–38, 1973.
27. Münker D: Das Flugunfähigmachen von Vögeln. In *TVT Nachrichten 2/2012, Mitteilungen der Tierärztlichen Vereinigung für Tierschutz e.V*, 2012, pp 42–45.
28. Olsen GE: Anseriformes. In Ritchie BW, Harrison GJ, Harrison LR, editors: *Avian medicine: Principles and applications*, Lake Worth, FL, 1994, Wingers, pp 1236–1275.
29. Wikipedia. online encyclopedia: *Pinioning*: http://en.wikipedia.org/wiki/ Pinioning. Accessed February 1, 2013.
30. Robinson PT: Unilateral patagiectomy: A technique for deflighting large birds. *Vet Med Small Anim Clin* 70:143–145, 1975.
31. Robinson PT, Buzikowski RB: Pinioning young birds with hemostatic clips. *Vet Med Small Anim Clin* 70:1415–1417, 1975.
32. Schroeder CR, Koch K: Preventing flight in birds by tenotomy. *J Am Vet Med Assoc* 97:169–170, 1940.
33. Sedgwick CJ: Deflighting pet birds. *Mod Vet Pract* 48:38–40, 1967.
34. Seidel B: Methods of flight prevention in birds. In *Proceedings of the European Chapter of the Association of Avian Veterinarians*, 1991, pp 131–141.
35. Shaw SN, D'Agostino JJ, Davis MR, et al: Primary feather follicle ablation in common pintails (*Anas acuta acuta*) and a white-faced whistling duck (*Dendrocygna viduata*). *J Zoo Wildl Med* 43(2):342–346, 2012.
36. Startup CM: The clipping and pinioning of wings. *J Small Anim Pract* 8:401–403, 1967.
37. Sy M: Functionall-anatomische untersuchungen am vogelflugel. *J Ornithol* 84:199–296, 1936.
38. Tobalske BW: Biomechanichs of flight. *J Exp Biol* 3135–3146, 2007.
39. Williamson WM, Russell WC: Prevention of flight in older captive birds. *J Am Vet Med Assoc* 159(5):596–598, 1971.

CHAPTER 66

The Use of Computed Tomography and Magnetic Resonance Imaging in Zoo Animals

Hanspeter W. Steinmetz and Mariano Makara

The uses of cross-sectional modalities such as computed tomography (CT) and magnetic resonance imaging (MRI) have become more widespread, representing a considerable advancement in the veterinary standard care. CT and MRI have superior diagnostic capabilities than conventional radiography or ultrasonography because of their increased contrast resolution and their tomographic nature. To understand the role of these modalities in the imaging workup, it is essential to first appreciate how these features help overcome the several limitations of conventional radiography or ultrasonography because of its two-dimensional nature and by poor contrast resolution.

COMPUTED TOMOGRAPHY

Equipment and Procedure

CT scanners consist of a scanning gantry, x-ray generator, computer system, and operator's console. The gantry houses the x-ray tube, which produces x-ray photons, and a set of detectors, which collects the information produced after the x-rays interact with the structure under examination. The x-ray tube and the detectors rotate around the patient, generating a series of x-ray projections. A number of these projections are progressively taken from slightly different angles as the tube rotates around the patient. The information collected from these projections is used to generate CT images. The images created are cross-sectional, representing slices of the anatomy at a particular level. The possibility of acquiring cross-sectional images represents a major advantage over conventional radiology. Conventional radiology produces a two-dimensional image from a three-dimensional object, which results in superimposition, which may create confusing opacities that do not represent a structure within the patient. As opposed to radiography, CT examines the tissue in thin sections, or slices, thereby eliminating superimposition.[37,45]

Physics

Anatomic structures in a CT image are displayed by varying shades of gray. The shades of gray depend on the interaction between the x-rays and the patient. The x-rays may either pass through the patient, be redirected (scatter), or be attenuated. The degree of attenuation depends on the x-ray energy and the characteristics of the structure under examination, including its electron density, physical density, thickness, and effective atomic number.[8] After interacting with the patient, x-ray photons strike the detectors. A computer processes the information recorded by these detectors to generate a CT image. By convention, if an object absorbs only a small fraction of the x-ray beam, it will be represented as a black area on the image. If an object absorbs the entire x-ray beam, it will be represented as a white area on the image. Between these extremes, objects with intermediate absorption will be represented by various shades of gray.[45] The amount of the x-ray beam that is absorbed or scattered as it passes through the object is expressed by the linear attenuation coefficient. Because of a higher atomic number and density, the linear attenuation coefficient will be higher for bone than it would be for muscle. In other words, bone allows fewer photons to reach the detectors, resulting in an image with a lighter shade of gray, than that representing muscle. These differences in linear attenuation coefficients between tissues determine the image contrast in CT and conventional radiography. Although the basic principles of CT are similar to those of radiography in that x-rays are used to create an attenuation map of the patient, CT has superior contrast resolution. This may be explained by two mechanisms: (1) optimization of the differences in x-ray attenuation between tissues using computer processing and (2) virtual elimination of scatter radiation.[8,45] This improvement in contrast resolution allows CT to better discriminate between normal or pathologic processes, which is otherwise not possible by conventional radiography.

Image Acquisition and Image Formation

CT image acquisition is dependent on the information acquired by the detectors as they rotate around the patient, creating an attenuation profile of the object from many different angles. For these data to be presented as a diagnostically useful image, the data have to be reconstructed. In loose terms, this process consists of the projection of the attenuation profiles onto a matrix. This process of converting the data from the attenuation profile to a matrix is known as *back projection*.[37]

A CT image is composed of a matrix of thousands of small two-dimensional squares called *picture elements* or *pixels*. Each of these pixels displays information from a small volume element from the patient, also referred to as a *voxel*. The sum of the linear attenuation coefficients along the path of an x-ray beam through multiple voxels is used to calculate the individual contributions from each voxel.[37] The attenuation value of each pixel is then standardized using a scale by which these values may be expressed relative to the attenuation of water. Attenuation values are expressed in Hounsfield units (HU). This scale arbitrarily assigned the number 0 to water, the number 1000 to bone, and the number −1000 to air.[8] Pixels are assigned relative shades of gray based on the HU of the tissues within their voxels. Even though 2000 different shades of gray may be assigned to each of the HU values, the monitor use to show CT images may only display 256 shades of gray. An even more limiting factor is that the human eye can only recognize fewer than 40 shades of gray. To solve this problem, only a certain number of HU values are assigned to a level of gray. The number of these units represented on a specific image is determined by the window width. In other words, the window width will determine the quantity of HU to be displayed on an image. By increasing the window width, more HU values will be assigned a shade of gray. The window level determines the center HU value of the window width. For example, if a window level of 50 is used and the window width is 200, the range of HU values that would be displayed would include −50 to 150 HU. Any structure with a HU of −50 or below would appear totally black, and any structure with a HU of 150 or above would appear totally white. A wide window width is used when studying structures with a wide spectrum of HU, for example, the lung. A narrow window width is used when studying structures with a narrower spectrum of HU, for example, the white and gray matter of the brain or the ventricular system.[8,37,45]

Reconstruction

Other important parameters are the reconstruction filters, which determine the level of edge reinforcement applied while processing raw data. These parameters must be set carefully according to the region of interest. For example, a low-pass filter, commonly known as "standard or soft tissue filter" is recommended when soft tissue contrast must be emphasized, as in brain imaging, which, however, has the disadvantage of creating blurry images. "Bone filters," conversely, maximize spatial resolution but introduce more noise, thus reducing contrast resolution. Such images are sharper but grainier.[37]

MAGNETIC RESONANCE IMAGING

Since the beginning of the new millennium, MRI has become an important diagnostic tool in veterinary medicine. Its excellent contrast resolution allows detailed characterization of soft tissues. MRI is currently the imaging modality of choice for the evaluation of disease processes involving the nervous system and the musculoskeletal system.[21]

Equipment and Procedure

MRI systems may vary in size and shape. Scanners use electromagnets and radio signals to produce cross-sectional images and are composed of a magnet, radiofrequency (RF) generators, gradient coils, and a transceiver. The main coil surrounds the bore (which holds the patient) with a uniform strong magnetic field. Different gradient coils create varying magnetic fields, for example, from top to bottom across the scanning tube (y-coil), from the entrance to the exit of the scanning tube (z-coil), and from left to right across the scanning tube (x-coil). The transceiver sends RF signals to protons and receives signals from them. All of these components interact with a computer, which precisely synchronizes the transfer of energy to the hydrogen protons and processes the response from these protons. This information is then processed and converted into a diagnostically useful image.[21]

During the scanning procedure, which takes approximately 30 to 90 minutes, the patient is placed into the tube in the center of the scanner, which, as noted above, is known as the *bore*, and is about 1 meter (m) in diameter and varies between 1.5 m and 2.5 m in length. Any movement of the patient would alter image quality, so most animals are anesthetized for the procedure.

Physics

The clinical applications of MRI rely on the electromagnetic properties of the hydrogen nucleus. Hydrogen protons spin about their own axis and are oriented in a random fashion within the body. Because of their positive charge, these moving protons possess their own magnetic fields and therefore may be thought of as small bar magnets. When the patient is placed within the bore of an MRI scanner, the magnetic field of the hydrogen protons are forced to align with the uniform magnetic field of the scanner magnet. Some protons align parallel to the main field and others align opposite to it, canceling each other out. A few more protons align with the field rather than in the opposing direction. This number is proportional to the external magnetic field strength. In addition to spinning about their own axis, protons wobble like toy tops. The rate of wobbling is termed *precession*. By applying an RF pulse at the precession frequency, energy may be transferred to the spinning protons. This is the "resonance" part of the MRI.[21] The protons excited by this pulse jump into a higher energy state. When the RF is turned off, the spins begin to return to their lower energy state by two distinct, but simultaneous, processes. At this time, the three gradient coils are turned on and off rapidly,

altering the main magnetic field on a local level; The rising electrical current in the wires of the gradient coils opposing the main magnetic field makes a continual rapid hammering noise; the louder this noise is, the stronger is the main field. When the hydrogen protons slowly return to their natural alignment within the magnetic field, they release the energy absorbed from the RF pulses, and this signal is picked up by the transceiver and sent to the computer system and is converted to a picture.[8,21]

Image Acquisition and Image Formation

The release of energy from spins to their molecular environment is called *T1 relaxation*, and the release of energy by the interaction of spins with each other is called *T2 relaxation*.[21] The rate at which T1 and T2 relaxations occur varies, depending on the tissues under examination. The energy released by these processes is captured by the receiver coil and represents the signal with which computers create a diagnostically useful image. The response of different tissues to this energy stimulus may be manipulated to accentuate the signal they emit by using instrument controls. The MRI system uses injectable contrast agents to alter the local magnetic field in the tissue being examined. Normal and abnormal tissues respond differently, thus giving different signals. Contrast in MRI therefore relies on multiple parameters, including differences in proton density, the response of protons to magnetic and RF fields, and the adjustment of technical parameters. An MRI may display more than 250 shades of gray to depict various tissues.[21]

Image Manipulation

The standard clinical imaging sequences commonly include T2-weighted, short tau inversion recovery (STIR), fluid attenuated inversion recovery (FLAIR), T1-weighted, and postcontrast T1-weighted images.[21] In T2-weighted images, both fat and fluid are displayed as high signal intensity. Bright fluid is a desirable feature, as most disease processes have an increased fluid content. Unfortunately, this increased fluid content is not specific for any particular disease process. Lesions such as tumors, granulomas, abscesses, or edema all display a high signal in T2-weighted MRI scans. In T1-weighted images, fat is hyperintense, and fluid is hypointense. T1-weighted sequences are generally used after the administration of contrast agents. A precontrast T1-weighted sequence is mandatory if a postcontrast T1-weighted sequence needs to be performed. In some cases, breaks in tissue structure such as the blood–brain barrier allow the contrast agent to leak into the tissue and change the relaxation of the tissue, leading to increased signal intensity. STIR is a fluid sensitive sequence similar to the T2-weighted sequence with suppression of the fat signal. Because of this suppression, STIR sequences display fluid associated with lesions as bright images on a dark background. FLAIR sequences are similar to STIR sequences except that they suppress the signal from the cerebral spinal fluid (CSF). Therefore, hyperintense lesions located around the ventricular system are easily detected as they contrast with the black CSF.[21]

SAFETY

According to its frequency (measured in hertz [Hz]) and its ability to ionize an atom or molecule in biologic tissues, electromagnetic (EM) radiation is classified in two categories: ionizing and nonionizing.[25] The term *ionizing radiation* refers to x-rays and γ-rays, which have the ability to produce ionization of the biologic tissues and cell damage. *Nonionizing radiation* in the electromagnetic spectrum refers to static electromagnetic fields, RF, and optical waves.[25]

Although it is well established that ionizing radiation (x-ray, CT) poses risks to animal and human health, mainly because of its ability to ionize tissues, available data on the possible effects of nonionizing radiation on patient and worker safety have not been elucidated.[25] Accidents and noxious effects at the present time are mostly the result of failure to follow safety guidelines.

CT technology uses computer-processed x-rays, similar to conventional radiography. Both techniques have the disadvantage that the x-rays are energetic enough to ionize the deoxyribonucleic acid (DNA) or the surrounding molecules and thus may damage the DNA directly or indirectly. Direct damage occurs when x-rays create ions that physically break one or both of the sugar phosphate or break the base pairs of the DNA.[40] Indirect damage is caused by the creation of radicals in surrounding tissue, which interact with nearby DNA and cause strand breaks or base damage.[7] Most radiation-induced damage is rapidly repaired by various systems within the cell, but DNA double-strand breaks are less easily repaired, and occasional inappropriate repair may lead to induction of point mutations, chromosomal translocations, and gene fusions, all of which are linked to the induction of cancer.[3] The risk increases with radiation dose, longevity of life expectancy, growing stage, and the exposed tissue.

The average yearly medical x-ray dose has been increased considerably in human medicine since CT technology has become more available, and a similar increase is already observed in veterinary medicine or may occur in the near future. Organ doses from CT scanning are larger than those for corresponding conventional radiography. For example, a conventional anterior-posterior abdominal radiographic examination results in an approximately 50 times smaller x-ray dose to the stomach than the corresponding CT scan.[7] For better risk estimation, various quantitative measures have been developed to describe the radiation dose delivered by CT scanning. The most relevant being absorbed dose, organ dose, effective dose, and CT dose index (CTDI).[7] The *absorbed dose* is the energy absorbed per unit of mass (Gray [Gy]). The *organ dose* is the distribution of the dose in the organ and largely determines the level of risk to that organ from the radiation.[7] For risk estimation, the organ dose is the preferred quantity. The *effective dose* (Sievert [Sv]) is used for dose distributions that are not homogeneous; it is designed to be proportional to a generic estimate of the overall harm to the patient caused by radiation exposure. The effective dose allows for a rough comparison between different CT scenarios but provides only an approximate estimate of the true risk. The *CTDI* is the historical measurement (milli-Gray [mGy]) that was used to measure the radiation for a single slice in standard cylindrical acrylic phantoms.[29] The CTDI was used for quality control but is not directly related to the organ dose or risk.[7]

A CT evaluation requires a clear indication and should be planned carefully. The expected information gain should outweigh the risks of potential side effects. The risk depends on various factors such as the growing stage of the patient, the affected organs, and the radiation dose. Compared with adults, growing animals are at greater risk from a given dose of radiation because they are inherently more radiosensitive *and* have more remaining years of life during which a radiation-induced cancer could develop. Most of the other factors are under the control of the radiologist, and ideally, they should be tailored to the type of study being performed and to the particular patient (species, age, size).[31] Radiation doses to particular organs for any given CT study depend on a number of factors. The most important are the number of scans, the scanning time (milliamperes [mAs]), the size of the patient, the axial scan range, the scan pitch (the degree of overlap between adjacent CT slices), the tube voltage in the kilovolt peaks (kVp), and the specific design of the scanner being used.[29] It is always the case that the quality (relative noise) of the CT images decreases as the radiation dose decreases, which means that a tradeoff always exists between the need for low-noise images and the desirability of using low doses of radiation.[45] Reducing the energy dose is important in long-living animals, especially to protect sensible organs such as the thyroid gland, the retina, the lens, or the gonads from the side effects of the x-rays. Repeating a study because of poor quality images results in higher amounts of x-ray exposure compared with an adequate energy setup that produces high-quality images.

No largescale epidemiologic studies of the long-term risks associated with CT in veterinary medicine have been reported so far, so extrapolation from human medicine and conventional radiology has become necessary. Since evidence of an increased risk of cancer from exposure to x-ray has been reported, it is also necessary to use CT technology responsibly and consider all necessary measurements to reduce exposure of animals and employees to x-rays during CT (Box 66-1).

MRI is considered a safe technology without major side effects. Nevertheless, the MRI technology may have some adverse biologic effects, and concerns about it are related to the effects of magnetic fields on patients, equipment, and personnel.[6,12,14,17] Most MRI-related injuries and the few fatalities in human medicine were the result of failure to follow safety guidelines or the result of use of inappropriate or outdated information related to the safety aspects of equipment and biomedical implants. Therefore, it is necessary to continuously revise and enforce the information on biologic effects and safety according to changes that have occurred in MRI technology.

In the proximity of an MRI scanner three electromagnetic fields exist: (1) the static magnetic field, (2) the gradient magnetic field, and (3) the RF field. The most important health hazards arise from the presence of the strong static magnetic field and also from failure to follow basic safety guidelines. We must be aware that the static magnetic field is always present, even when the MRI equipment is shut down. It may attract ferromagnetic metal objects, which may become powerful projectiles and may cause serious injury or even death.[10] The strength of attraction is inversely proportional to the square of the distance. Therefore, all equipment must be tested to ensure that it is safe to use in the MRI room, and all personnel and patients must be screened for ferromagnetic objects before entering. For example, in the current time, many animals are implanted with microchips for identification. Although microchips may contain metal pieces and a sensitive microtransponder, they seem to be safe and remain fully functional after routine MRI scans.[24,38]

Most studies of potential hazards associated with short-term exposure to a strong static magnetic field did not report adverse effects to human health[20] and did not produce any substantial harmful biologic effect.[1,40] Nevertheless, one phenomenon that has been observed is the *magneto-hydrodynamic effect*, which is the result of the blood flow in the heart in a strong magnetic field and leads to an induced current in the heart.[41] The effect may be observed as an elevation of the S-T segment on the patient's electrocardiogram, and the degree of change is directly related to the strength of the magnetic field. Although the effect is not associated with any serious effects and is totally reversible by removing the patient from the magnet, it is imperative that any patient with compromised cardiovascular function be closely monitored with an MRI-compatible pulse oximeter, blood pressure monitor, or both because an elevated S-T segment may be indicative of myocardial infarction, ischemia, or electrolyte imbalance.

In addition, the strong magnetic field may rotate ferromagnetic implants to align them along the magnet's field line. Depending on the strength of the magnetic field, type and location of the implant, physical dimensions and orientation of the implant, and the length of time the implant has been in place, the twisting force may be strong enough to rotate the implant and cause serious injury to the patient.

The gradient magnetic field, which varies at different times, induces an electric current that could stimulate nerves and muscles and is known as *peripheral nerve stimulation (PNS)*.[42] PNS may cause muscle contractions or discomfort to the subjects, depending on whether the stimulated nerve is a sensory nerve or a motor nerve, and result in the subject moving in the scanner.[42] Several in vivo studies have been performed to obtain gradient-induced stimulation thresholds in animals and in humans.[5,20,42] The mean thresholds for PNS in the head and body are similar, and the greatest frequency of reported PNS occurs in these areas.[18] If the stimulation occurs in cardiac muscle, it could, in theory, disrupt the normal cardiac cycle and lead to arrhythmia or even cause ventricular fibrillation.[22] In

BOX 66-1 Safety Considerations for Computed Tomography and Magnetic Resonance Imaging

Computed Tomography (CT)
- Reduced exposure to personnel:
  - Room isolation
  - Limited access
  - Personnel not present during study
  - Marked safety zones
- Reduced exposure to animals:
  - Clear indication
  - Consideration of age
  - Protection of sensitive or growing tissue
  - Avoidance of repeated studies
  - Reduction in scanning time
  - Limited scanning field
  - Limited scan pitch
- Assessment of renal function before using contrast medium

Magnetic Resonance Imaging (MRI)
- Reduced exposure to personnel:
  - Room isolation
  - Limited access
  - Personnel not present during study
  - Marked safety zones
- Labeling of all equipment and use only in safety zones accordingly:
  - "MR safe"
  - "MR conditional"
  - "MR unsafe"
- General health check, questionnaire, pre-MRI examination:
  - Eye injuries (e.g., metal objects)
  - Past surgeries—biomedical implants (e.g., clips)
  - Pacemaker (employees)
- Before entering, checking for ferromagnetic metal objects:
  - Testing all equipment with hand magnet (>3000 Gray)
  - Empty pockets—special MRI working suit
- Monitoring of:
  - Body temperature
  - Cardiovascular function
    - Electrocardiography (elevation S-T segment)
    - Pulse oximeter
    - Blood pressure
- Application of ear plugs (personnel and animals)
  - Acoustic noise up to 140 decibels (dB)

addition, direct stimulation of the retina, the optic nerve, or both may produce what is known as *magnetophosphenes*. Magnetic phosphenes may cause a flashing sensation in the eyes that could affect the work of the medical personnel executing delicate interventional MRI procedures.[37]

The RF field may also heat the metallic implants in the subject's body.[30] Fortunately, most animals have a very efficient thermoregulation system and may adequately respond to temperature increase by increasing capillary flow. But health problems (e.g., cardiovascular disease, hypertension, diabetes, fever, and obesity), old age, or medications (e.g., anesthetics, diuretics, muscle relaxants, and sedatives) may impair the normal cooling mechanisms. Conducting materials close to the patient, for example, the leads of equipment for monitoring physiologic parameters (heart rate, blood pressure, oxygen saturation, and temperature), may lead to local burns. This kind of risk may be more serious in the case of internal biomedical implants (aneurism clips, stents, etc.).[16,26]

In conclusion, although CT and MRI technologies are considered safe, precautionary measures must be taken (see Box 67-1). CT has long-term side effects that induce carcinogenesis, and MRI procedures tend to have immediate side effects seen during the procedure.

INDICATION

Each cross-sectional modality, either CT or MRI, has its own advantages and disadvantages, and the appropriateness choice of either application is based on a strong and clear objective (Table 66-1). In zoologic medicine, many additional factors such us equipment availability, growing stage of the patient, or the required information need to be included into considerations.

CT is usually cheaper, faster, and less noisy than MRI. The CT procedure is relatively easier to perform, and only minor sources of errors need to be considered. Nevertheless, limitations are imposed by the size and weight of an animal. The diameter of the gantry is always the limiting measurement for the size of the animal that needs to be examined, and the length of the tube is considerably

shorter in CT than in MRI. This allows examining larger animals with CT than with MRI, but limitations do exist. Because most scanners are designed for human or domestic animal medicine, attention must be paid to the weight limits of automated examination tables and floor loading capacity. Size and species-specific anatomy might pose additional challenges in positioning the subject for the scanning procedure. CT may be universally used and displays most organs, lymph nodes, vessels, and bones in a reliable manner. Nevertheless, its use requires a clear indication and meticulous planning because of the risks of radiation and the potential adverse effects of the contrast medium. MRI is more complex, with various sequences, different settings, and specific contrast media required for specific examination protocols for specific medical indications. Thus, the strength of MRI is its ability to provide answers for specific questions. But the various settings increase the risk of potential mistakes.

Generally, CT is indicated when ferromagnetic implants are present or when metallic foreign bodies are suspected.[33] The strong electromagnetic field in MRI would interact with these objects and pose an unnecessary risk to these animals. CT has superior contrast resolution when an increased difference in physical tissue density is expected. The different tissue attenuations lead to high contrast details and thus excellent pictures are obtained in a generalized examination of the ear, in patients with multiple trauma, or in animals in which osteolysis, metabolic bone disease, joint luxations or complex, multifragmented fractures are suspected.[2,36] Three-dimensional reconstruction and excellent image quality lead to better localization of pathologic alterations and thus to better treatment preparation and outcome. Moreover, with increasing experience and availability, CT technology will be more and more indicated in specialized examinations in many zoologic species. For example, on the basis of experiences from human nasal surgery, diagnostic imaging technology was adapted to advance the treatment choices for orangutans (*Pongo pygmaeus*, *Pongo abelii*) affected by chronic upper respiratory tract disease.[44] In addition, in the past, diagnoses of dental diseases in rodents and other commonly affected species required several specialized radiographs and, thus, a considerable amount of

TABLE 66-1

General Decision Recommendations for Cross-Sectional Imaging Modalities

	Magnetic Resonance Imaging	**Computed Tomography**
General	Pregnancy	Ferromagnetic implants
	Young animals	Ferromagnetic foreign bodies
	Kidney insufficiency	
Head	Neurologic diseases, when small lesions are suspected or in chronic processes	Initial diagnostic tool for neurologic diseases if trauma and acute bleeding are suspected
	Brain	Skull fractures
	Cranium	Sinus
	Tumors	Ear
	Epilepsy	Dental disease
	Salivary gland (except stones)	
Musculoskeletal system	Occult fractures	Complex, multifragment fractures
	Bone tumors	Polytrauma
	Muscle, cartilage, tendon injury	Osteolysis
	Joint disease	
Thorax	Cardiovascular diseases	Intrapulmonary lesions
Abdomen	Soft tissue tumor staging	Metastasis tumor screening
	Small intestine	Colonoscopy
	Pancreas	Adrenal gland
	Gonads	Kidney stones
	Vessels	Arteriosclerosis

time, but with CT's advanced diagnostic modalities and excellent display of alterations, the decision process for an appropriate prognosis has been made easier today.[9,28] CT is also the diagnostic modality of choice for acute neurologic diseases associated with a history of trauma and the risk of acute bleeding in the proximity of the brain. Standard CT scanning allows for immediately differentiating between intracranial infarction and hemorrhage and thus optimizes emergency care. The numerous anatomic variations in zoologic species often make the interpretation of pulmonary lesions difficult with common diagnostic tools. Considerable improvement in diagnostics with CT has been achieved in reptiles, avian species, and dolphins.[11,23,32] Also, in relatively newer veterinary specializations such as oncology, CT is the modality of choice. Surgical tumor resection planning and screening for tumor metastasis take advantage of the technology with contrast medium.[43] CT is increasingly used also as a sensitive diagnostic tool to diagnose abdominal diseases. Screening for gastrointestinal tumors, search for urolithiasis, or the evaluation of suspected arteriosclerosis are all important indications for the use of CT technology.

MRI shows good contrast between the different soft tissues of the body; it clearly exceeds CT in image resolution, which makes MRI especially useful in imaging the brain, muscles, the heart, and cancers. Generally, MRI use is preferred in pregnant animals or during growth in long-living species because of reduced exposure to ionizing radiation. Thus, MRI has been recommended in addition to ultrasonography to monitor pregnancy and is already used in zoologic medicine, for example, to monitor fetal development in the veiled chameleon (*Chamaeleo calyptratus*) or in chickens.[19,27] Contrast media used in CT have also been shown to impair kidney function. Thus, in animals with moderate or severe renal dysfunction, alternative imaging techniques such as MRI, which may yield the same information without the risks, should be considered.[4] Precautionary measures, including renal blood biochemistry analysis and fluid therapy, are necessary. MRI produces excellent soft tissue contrast, which may be improved even more with contrast medium. Therefore, MRI is used for screening for chronic neurologic disease processes such as tumors or hypovitaminosis A and for research in neurosciences, for example, study of the neurobiology of

birdsongs.[15,35] Difficulties might arise in relatively new, emerging neurologic diseases in zoologic species. For example, although leukoencephalopathy may be diagnosed with MRI in domestic cats,[13] the disease process in cheetahs (*Acinonyx jubatus*) might be suspected clinically before MRI shows unequivocal lesions,[39] but MRI may help ultimately differentiate this disease from other neurologic diseases such as myelopathy.[46] MRI also has application in the diagnosis of musculoskeletal problems. Lameness of unknown origin caused by occult fractures or joint problems may be visualized, which helps determine treatment options.[34,47]

It is, nevertheless, advisable to consider the use of both cross-sectional modalities, for example, in case of neurologic diseases, to differentiate between bony and soft tissue lesions. For example, vertebral fractures are best displayed by CT, whereas spinal cord injuries are better visualized with MRI.

CONCLUSION

The new technology in cross-sectional modalities has already proven its usefulness in zoologic medicine. Most institutions have established relationships with local diagnostic imaging facilities, and others have made substantial investments for on-site equipment. The complementary use of CT, MRI, and other diagnostic modalities helps particularly in the diagnosis of difficult cases. Species, diagnostic equipment availability, and required information will determine the choice of the appropriate diagnostic modality for individual cases.

REFERENCES

1. Abart J, Ganssen A: [Safety aspects in MR imaging]. *Aktuelle Radiol* 5:376–384, 1995.
2. Abou-Madi N, Scrivani PV, Kollias GV, et al: Diagnosis of skeletal injuries in chelonians using computed tomography. *J Zoo Wildl Med* 35:226–231, 2004.
3. Allen CP, Fujimori A, Okayasu R, et al: Radiation-induced delayed genome instability and hypermutation in mammalian cells. In Mittelman D, editor: *Stress-induced mutagenesis*, New York, 2013, Springer.

4. Baerlocher MO, Asch M, Myers A: Contrast-induced nephropathy. *Can Med Assoc J* 182:1445, 2010.

5. Bencsik M, Bowtell R, Bowley RM: Electric fields induced in a spherical volume conductor by temporally varying magnetic field gradients. *Phys Med Biol* 47:557–576, 2002.

6. Boutin RD, Briggs JE, Williamson MR: Injuries associated with MR imaging: Survey of safety records and methods used to screen patients for metallic foreign bodies before imaging. *AJR Am J Roentgenol* 162:189–194, 1994.

7. Brenner DJ: It is time to retire the computed tomography dose index (CTDI) for CT quality assurance and dose optimization: For the proposition. *Med Phys* 33:1189–1190, 2006.

8. Bushberg JT, Seibert JA, Leidholdt EM, et al: *The essential physics of medical imaging*, ed 3, Philadelphia, PA, 2011, Lippincott Williams & Wilkins.

9. Capello V, Cauduro A: Clinical technique: Application of computed tomography for diagnosis of dental disease in the rabbit, guinea pig, and chinchilla. *J Exot Pet Med* 17:93–101, 2008.

10. Chaljub G, Kramer LA, Johnson RF, 3rd, et al: Projectile cylinder accidents resulting from the presence of ferromagnetic nitrous oxide or oxygen tanks in the MR suite. *AJR Am J Roentgenol* 177:27–30, 2001.

11. Clayton LA, Stamper MA, Whitaker BR, et al: *Mycobacterium abscessus* pneumonia in an Atlantic bottlenose dolphin (*Tursiops truncatus*). *J Zoo Wildl Med* 43:961–965, 2012.

12. Colletti PM: Size "H" oxygen cylinder: Accidental MR projectile at 1.5 Tesla. *J Magn Reson Imaging* 19:141–143, 2004.

13. Comito B, Evans J, Tidwell AS, et al: Adult-onset spongiform leukoencephalopathy in 2 ragdoll cats. *J Vet Intern Med* 24:977–982, 2010.

14. Coskun O: Magnetic resonance imaging and safety aspects. *Toxicol Ind Health* 27:307–313, 2011.

15. De Risio L, Beltran E, de Stefani A, et al: Neurological dysfunction and caudal fossa overcrowding in a young cheetah with hypovitaminosis A. *Vet Rec* 167:534–536, 2010.

16. Dempsey MF, Condon B, Hadley DM: Investigation of the factors responsible for burns during MRI. *J Magn Reson Imaging* 13:627–631, 2001.

17. Dempsey MF, Condon B: Thermal injuries associated with MRI. *Clin Radiol* 56:457–465, 2001.

18. Den Boer JA, Bourland JD, Nyenhuis JA, et al: Comparison of the threshold for peripheral nerve stimulation during gradient switching in whole body MR systems. *J Magn Reson Imaging* 15:520–525, 2002.

19. Falen SW, Szeverenyi NM, Packard DS, et al: Magnetic resonance imaging study of the structure of the yolk in the developing avian egg. *J Morphol* 209:331–342, 1991.

20. Formica D, Silvestri S: Biological effects of exposure to magnetic resonance imaging: An overview. *Biomed Eng Online* 3:11, 2004.

21. Gavin PR, Bagley RS: *Practical small animal MRI*, Ames, IA, 2011, Wiley-Blackwell.

22. Glover PM: Interaction of MRI field gradients with the human body. *Phys Med Biol* 54:R99–R115, 2009.

23. Gumpenberger M, Henninger W: The use of computed tomography in avian and reptile medicine. *Semin Avian Exot Pet Med* 10:174–180, 2001.

24. Haifley KA, Hecht S: Functionality of implanted microchips following magnetic resonance imaging. *J Am Vet Med Assoc* 240:577–579, 2012.

25. Hartwig V, Giovannetti G, Vanello N, et al: Biological effects and safety in magnetic resonance imaging: A review. *Int J Environ Res Public Health* 6:1778–1798, 2009.

26. Kanal E, Borgstede JP, Barkovich AJ, et al: American College of Radiology White Paper on MR Safety: 2004 update and revisions. *AJR Am J Roentgenol* 182:1111–1114, 2004.

27. Kummrow MS, Gilman C, Mackie P, et al: Noninvasive analysis of fecal reproductive hormone metabolites in female veiled chameleons (*Chamaeleo calyptratus*) by enzyme immunoassay. *Zoo Biol* 30:95–115, 2011.

28. Lee KJ, Sasaki M, Miyauchi A, et al: Virtopsy in a red kangaroo with oral osteomyelitis. *J Zoo Wildl Med* 42:128–130, 2011.

29. McNitt-Gray MF: AAPM/RSNA physics tutorial for residents: Topics in CT. Radiation dose in CT. *Radiographics* 22:1541–1553, 2002.

30. Nitz WR, Brinker G, Diehl D, et al: Specific absorption rate as a poor indicator of magnetic resonance-related implant heating. *Invest Radiol* 40:773–776, 2005.

31. Paterson A, Frush DP, Donnelly LF: Helical CT of the body: Are settings adjusted for pediatric patients? *AJR Am J Roentgenol* 176:297–301, 2001.

32. Pees M, Kiefer I, Oechtering G, et al: Computed tomography for the diagnosis and treatment monitoring of bacterial pneumonia in Indian pythons (*Python molurus*). *Vet Rec* 163:152–156, 2008.

33. Penninck D, Daniel GB, Brawer R, et al: Cross-sectional imaging techniques in veterinary ophthalmology. *Clin Tech Small Anim Pract* 16:22–39, 2001.

34. Podadera JM, Bell RJ, Dart AJ: Using magnetic resonance imaging to diagnose non-displaced fractures of the second phalanx in horses. *Austral Vet J* 88:439–442, 2010.

35. Poirier C, Vellema M, Verhoye M, et al: A three-dimensional MRI atlas of the zebra finch brain in stereotaxic coordinates. *Neuroimage* 41:1–6, 2008.

36. Raiti P, Haramati N: Magnetic resonance imaging and computerized tomography of a gravid leopard tortoise (*Geochelone pardalis pardalis*) with metabolic bone disease. *J Zoo Wildl Med* 28:189–197, 1997.

37. Romans LE: *Computed tomography for technologists*, Baltimore, MD, 2010, Lippincott Williams & Wilkins.

38. Saito M, Ono S, Kayanuma H, et al: Evaluation of the susceptibility artifacts and tissue injury caused by implanted microchips in dogs on 1.5 T magnetic resonance imaging. *J Vet Med Sci* 72:575–581, 2010.

39. Schulz J, Hammond EE, Haymon M, et al: Magnetic resonance imaging as a method of diagnosing leukoencephalopathy in a cheetah (*Acinonyx jubatus*). *Verh ber Erkrg Zootiere* 41:1–6, 2003.

40. Schwenzer NF, Bantleon R, Maurer B, et al: Detection of DNA double-strand breaks using gammaH2AX after MRI exposure at 3 Tesla: an in vitro study. *J Magn Reson Imaging* 26:1308–1314, 2007.

41. Shellock FG, Crues JV: MR procedures: Biologic effects, safety, and patient care. *Radiology* 232:635–652, 2004.

42. So PP, Stuchly MA, Nyenhuis JA: Peripheral nerve stimulation by gradient switching fields in magnetic resonance imaging. *IEEE Trans Biomed Eng* 51:1907–1914, 2004.

43. Steinmetz HW, Rutten M, Ruess-Melzer K, et al: Clinical course of a malignant peripheral nerve sheath tumor in a Siberian tiger (*Panthera tigris altaica*). *J Vet Diagn Invest* 22:970–975, 2010.

44. Steinmetz HW, Zimmermann N: Computed tomography for the diagnosis of sinusitis and air sacculitis in orangutans. In Miller E, Fowler M, editors: *Zoo and wild animal medicine*, St. Louis, MO, 2012, Saunders.

45. Thrall DE: *Textbook of veterinary diagnostic radiology*, ed 6, St. Louis, MO, 2013, Saunders.

46. Walzer C, Url A, Robert N, et al: Idiopathic acute onset myelopathy in cheetah (*Acinonyx jubatus*) cubs. *J Zoo Wildl Med* 34:36–46, 2003.

47. Weissengruber GE, Fuss FK, Egger G, et al: The elephant knee joint: Morphological and biomechanical considerations. *J Anat* 208:59–72, 2006.

CHAPTER 67

Gout in Exotic Animals

Mary Duncan

Historically, gout has been thought of as inflammatory arthritis that has developed in response to the deposition of urate crystals in the tissue (crystalline arthropathy). Differences have developed in the way the disease is reported in the veterinary and human medical literature, which bears further consideration in the future treatment and care of cases of gout in exotic species. In reptiles, generally, the same small cluster of cases forms the basis of suggested treatments in standard texts. From the position of a pathologist, the condition seems more common than these texts suggest—that cases frequently develop insidiously and that medical treatment is rarely successful.

Urate is derived from the breakdown of purine bases (guanine and adenine), which may originate from nucleic acids of both exogenous and endogenous sources. Dietary nucleic acids (exogenous source) are broken down by pancreatic nucleases into nucleotides, which, in turn, are hydrolyzed to release pyrimidine and purine bases. Mucosal enzymes remove the phosphates and sugars.[4] The degree of purine breakdown varies with species (Figure 67-1 and Box 67-1). Hypoxanthine produced by adenine breakdown may be excreted or converted to xanthine by xanthine oxidase, whereas all guanine breakdown results in xanthine generation, leading to uric acid production (see Figure 67-1). In humans, nonhuman primates, birds, some terrestrial reptiles, amphibians, and insects, uric acid is formed on purine breakdown. Urate salts and uric acid are relatively insoluble. With the enzyme uricase or urate oxidase, other mammals and reptiles break down urates further to allantoin, which is soluble.[13] Guanine is excreted directly by pigs and spiders. Aquatic turtles excrete urea or ammonia. In fish, allantoin is further degraded into allantoic acid and urea. Aquatic invertebrates break down purines to ammonia. Excretion of both ammonia and urea result in the concomitant loss of water, so it is the form of excretion generally seen in semi-aquatic and aquatic species.

Amino acids are also assembled into purine and pyrimidine in the liver for the synthesis of nucleic acids (endogenous nucleic acid production). (Endogenous nucleic acid production is reduced in starvation.) When adenosine triphosphate (ATP) is used to generate energy, adenosine compounds are released.[4] The adenosine is degraded via adenine to uric acid. Net degradation of ATP occurs in acute severe disease events such as infarction or severe tissue hypoxia, seizures, and tumor lysis syndrome (and, in humans, adult respiratory distress syndrome).[4] Fructose phosphorylation in the liver requires abundant ATP; thus, diets high in fructose increase the risk of gout development and cause phosphate depletion.[4] Fructose is the only carbohydrate that has a direct effect on urate metabolism.[4,5] Oxidative phosphorylation is impaired in insulin-resistant individuals, so systemic adenosine levels rise with increased levels of intracellular coenzyme A esters and retention of sodium, urate, and water in the kidney.[4]

Two thirds of urate excretion from the body occurs through the kidneys and the remaining third from the gut.[4] Circulating uric acid (monosodium urate) is filtered out of blood in the renal glomerulus, but nearly all the urate is resorbed in the proximal convoluted tubule, only to be actively secreted back into urine. The importance of the proximal convoluted tubule as a site of drug action becomes clear through these processes. Postsecretory reabsorption of urate is sodium dependent and stimulated by antiuricosuric drugs. (Insulin increases urate reabsorption by stimulating a urate anion exchanger; i.e., it drives circulating uric acid levels up, and the glycosuria seen in diabetes is uricosuric and may reduce the risk of gout.)[13] Urate excretion is altered with renal disease, hypertension, and starvation. (Estrogen has an uricosuric effect and results in higher rates of gout in men than premenopausal women.)[13]

Damage to the renal tissue generally results in increased urate retention, and decreased perfusion leads to decreased urate clearance, for example, with dehydration or renal disease.[9] Nephrotoxic drugs (aminoglycosides, sulfonamides) decrease urate excretion by damaging the renal tissue. The relative decrease in the glomerular filtration rate (GFR) that occurs in hypertension results in decreased urate excretion and increased risk of gout.[4] Diuretics, alcohol intake, and acute diarrhea reduce hydration and so decrease urate excretion.[13] Liver failure decreases the effectiveness of the filtering of blood and results in increased circulating urate levels. In humans, cases of gout are seen in association with diabetes, insulin resistance syndrome, cardiovascular disease, hypertension, nephropathy, and diseases with increased cell turnover (i.e., neoplasia and tissue breakdown), including tumor lysis disease, which is seen in primary leukemias, and lymphoma, and other malignancies.[4,5] An increase in the incidence of gout in humans has been suspected in recent decades and is thought to have coincided with the rise in obesity and insulin resistance syndrome, dietary changes, and an aging population.[4,13]

ETIOLOGY

Primary gout occurs with overproduction of uric acid as an innate metabolic problem, which is generally caused by a defect in the renal urate transporters. Primary gout is the most common form seen in humans and usually has a familial inheritance (e.g., superactivity of the enzyme 5'-phosphoribosyl 1-pyrophosphate synthetase, deficiencies of hypoxanthine-guanine phosphoribosyl transferase, adenine phosphoribosyltransferase or xanthine dehydrogenase).[1,4] An elevated predisposition to gout in the presence of other risk factors such as increased dietary purine is noted in certain groups (e.g., the Maori of New Zealand).[1] Genetic factors resulting in hyperuricemia have not been identified in most urate-excreting species, although certain strains of poultry have been identified to have a simple autosomal recessive gene that causes a defect in the renal tubular secretion of urate.[14]

During evolution, gene mutations in primates resulted in variable activity of the uricase enzyme, depending on species.[1] The retention of these gene mutations suggests that the loss of uricase confers some advantage.[1] Urate may act as a bloodborne antioxidant, removing singlet oxygen and free radicals.[1,4,5] Protection against oxidative damage may be especially important in the nervous system;[5] the metabolic rate of the brain is relatively high, and the higher levels of fatty acids and lipid in the tissue suggest a greater need for defense against lipid peroxidation.[1] Hyperuricemia appears to be protective against some neurodegenerative diseases: Alzheimer disease, Parkinson disease, and amyotrophic lateral sclerosis.[1] Uric acid may be important in the maintenance of blood pressure when diets are very low in salt, acutely through stimulation of the renin–angiotensin system and chronically by producing sensitivity to salt by microvascular and interstitial renal disease.[1] Conversely, in cases of persistent hyperuricemia, hypertension develops.[1]

Secondary gout develops with the loss of balance between uric acid production and excretion, resulting in net underexcretion and eventually hyperuricemia. Excess purine intake results when the

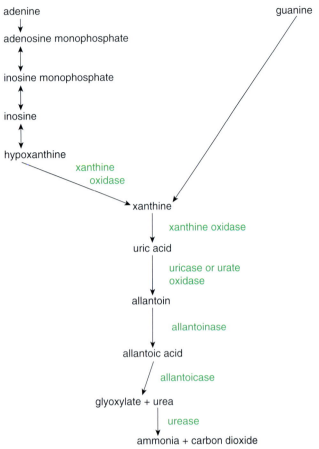

FIGURE 67-1 Purine degradation pathway.

BOX 67-1 Guanine-Derived Purine Excretory Products Depending on Species

Excretory Product	Species Group
Guanine	Pigs, spiders
Urate	Primates, Dalmatian dogs, terrestrial reptiles, birds, some amphibians, insects
Allantoin	Most mammals, aquatic reptiles, mollusks
Allantoic acid	Some fish
Urea	Most fish, amphibians, aquatic turtles
Ammonia	Aquatic turtles and aquatic invertebrates

expected proportion of purine in the diet fed exceeds the amount in the natural diet for a particular species; the most common situation that arises is that of herbivorous reptiles fed a meat-rich diet. In general meat, fish, or shellfish diets have higher levels of purine compared with vegetable-based diets.[3] Availability of water and hydration of the individual further affect purine levels (use of diuretics increases propensity to develop hyperuricemia).[13] The diet provided may have a different percentage of dry matter from that in food naturally available to the species. The bioavailability of purines may vary in the diet of a captive animal relative to the form of its presentation in nature. Exhibit humidity and temperatures may affect uric acid levels.

CLINICAL SIGNS AND DIAGNOSIS

In humans, gout is seen in acute and chronic forms, which are generally preceded by a period of asymptomatic hyperuricemia.[13] The acute form is intermittent and painful, with hyperuricemia, for periods lasting 7 to 10 days.[13] During the intercritical period between attacks, no clinical signs are noted. Hyperuricemia is defined in humans as a serum urate level of greater than or equal to 6.8 milligrams per deciliter (mg/dL).[13] Uric acid levels reflect values at the time of sampling and may not reflect the circulating levels at the time when crystals were deposited. Increased serum urate levels are directly related to the risk of future acute attacks once the diagnosis has been made.

The chronic form of gout is characterized by deposition of crystals as tophi, and this is the form of disease clinically diagnosed in birds and reptiles.[13] The acute form is identified to occur naturally in humans but has been induced experimentally by injecting urate crystals into the joints of other species.[6]

Since primary gout is the most common form seen in humans, a family history may lead to testing and diagnosis prior to the development of clinical signs. In chronically affected humans, application of pressure to gouty joints is painful; over time, joint deformity develops, and reduced movement results. In other species, physical examination of joints that exhibit swelling and visible deposition of white substance and a history with respect to predisposing factors may lead to a diagnosis of chronic gout.

Monosodium urate stones are radiolucent, but addition of a calcium component to the crystals causes radio-opacity, for example, with the addition of calcium oxalate and calcium phosphate. Tophi and renal enlargement may be diagnosed with radiography, ultrasonography, or renal biopsy (snakes may have visible swelling of the caudal coelom). In humans, synovial content is examined by electron microscopy or crystallography to confirm gout, and the crystal diameter is characteristic. Biopsy and cytology may be used to confirm a diagnosis of gout in veterinary cases;[10] cytologically, under polarized light, the crystals have a cross-hatched pattern.[8] Retrospectively, nonspecific symptoms such as anorexia and lethargy may have been noted in cases prior to the development of the joint lesions.

PATHOPHYSIOLOGY

Hyperuricemia occurs with decreased urate or uric acid excretion, as seen with the use of diuretics, renal vasoconstriction, hyperinsulinemia, decreased GFR, and damage to the nephron. Decreased perfusion of the nephron occurs with dehydration and damage to the nephron or reduction in nephron number. Tubular damage may be obstructive or toxic.[14] Obstructive or retrograde tubular damage is seen with ureteral blockage, for example, by ligation, calculus deposition, or squamous epithelial hyperplasia (as may occur with hypovitaminosis A).[14] Increased uric acid production occurs with tissue ischemia, oxidative stress, and alcohol (ethanol) intake. Recently, it has been found that monosodium urate crystals are released from dying cells, acting as a danger signal and leading, in turn, to the release of cytokines (interleukin-1beta [IL-1β]), which activate autoinflammatory pathways.[11]

Urate crystals stimulate both humoral and cell-mediated immunities; they interact with lipid and protein at membranes and cause histamine to be released from mast cells. In acute gout, crystals are coated in protein (opsonization) and cleared by macrophages releasing inflammatory mediators (including IL-1β).[4,13] The complement system is also activated. Synovial lining cells and resident inflammatory cells are stimulated. Neutrophils adhere to the endothelial cells through IL-1 and tumor necrosis factor–alpha (TNF-α). With time, tophi cause cartilage lysis, metalloproteinases are secreted, and chondrocytes are activated.[4] In humans with gout, urate calculi may develop in the renal medulla, which may cause obstruction and pain.

Solubility of urate in synovial fluid is influenced by temperature, pH, cation concentration, articular hydration, and the presence of nucleating agents. When urine pH is reduced, a tendency for urate crystal deposition exists. Nucleating agents, including insoluble collagens, chondroitin sulfate, and nonaggregated proteoglycans, may form a nidus for crystal deposition and growth.[4] (In humans, lesions tend to develop first at the extremities, especially the big toes, which is thought to be associated with a mild reduction in temperatures at the periphery.)

PATHOLOGIC FINDINGS

Acute gout in humans is characterized as a neutrophilic synovitis.[4] Tophi are seen in chronic disease, and these are urate crystals, possibly bundled with a lipid or necrotic core surrounded by inflammatory cells, phagocytes, multinucleate giant cells, and fibroblasts. Over time, tophi may cause chondrolysis, metalloproteinase secretion, and bone erosion.[4] Renal changes are seen in 40% of humans with gout, and these changes include advanced arteriolosclerosis, glomerulosclerosis, interstitial fibrosis, and intratubular crystals.[5] (The microvascular changes may contribute to the development of hypertension.)[5] In uricotelic species, it is customary to refer to the condition as *articular* and *visceral gout* at postmortem examination, although it is probably more correct to refer to visceral gout as *visceral urate deposition*, since generally no tissue reaction occurs with terminal rapid deposition of urate at serosal surfaces (e.g., liver, peritoneum, pericardium).[14] Urate is leached out of tissue during formalin fixation, so a wispy radiating network is all that is seen histologically when the crystals have been lost. Optimally, gout tissue samples would be fixed in alcohol and visualized with the De Galantha staining method, but this is rarely necessary for diagnostic purposes.

DIFFERENTIAL DIAGNOSIS

Pseudogout develops when a crystal other than monosodium urate is deposited at joints. Periarticular calcium hydroxyapatite deposition has been reported in red-bellied, short-necked turtles (*Emydura albertisii*).[15] (Hydroxyapatite crystals are harder to flush from a joint compared with urates.) Calcium pyrophosphate is the usual crystal in pseudogout in humans. Apatite crystals are significantly smaller, nanometers, relative to urate 2 to 20 micrometers μm and pyrophosphate crystals, which are rhombic and 2 to 10 μm.[8] Urate crystals are leached out of formalized samples; conversely, the crystals of hydroxyapatite and pyrophosphate are retained in formalin, and the calcium component may be stained with Alizarin red or von Kossa stains.[8] Nodular bone deposits extend from the subperiosteum with fluorosis (in cattle and guinea pigs fluoride, >3000 parts per million [ppm], was revealed when bone was ashed).[2] Osteophytes may be deposited at the periosteum or endosteum in reptiles with calcium–phosphorus imbalances in nutritional fibrous osteodystrophy. Metastatic calcification of soft tissue may occur with hypervitaminosis D.[2,8] Joint swelling with septic arthritis may be identified with cytologic Gram stain preparations and culture of joint aspirates.[13]

TREATMENT

Circulating uricemia may be reduced in humans simply by a change to a purine-free diet, in particular, with decreased intake of animal-derived protein, and with supportive therapy.[4] Optimizing hydration improves urate excretion. Selection of a diet with lower purine bioavailability and a lower proportion of adenine to guanine will reduce the buildup of uric acid. Humans with hyperuricemia who show no clinical signs generally receive no drug treatments because of the adverse effects of these medications in spite of the risk of development of hypertension, vascular remodeling, and cardiovascular disease.[5,13]

Three main forms of drug treatment are used,[4,13] with dosages extrapolated from those used in humans:

1. *Xanthine oxidase inhibitors (allopurinol, febuxostat):* Xanthine oxidase inhibitors decrease uric acid formation but appear to be relatively ineffective in reptiles and birds.

2. *Uricase or urate oxidase:* Uricase oxidizes uric acid to allantoin (soluble) and is used in the treatment of gout in humans. Some of the available uricase treatments require intravenous administration, which is a limiting factor. Little information is available in the veterinary literature on the use of uricase. (Poultry on a high-protein diet developed hyperuricemia, which was reversed with uricase injection.)[14]

3. *Uricosuric drugs (probenicid, sulfinpyrazone):* Uricosuric drugs promote urate excretion by the kidneys, thus lowering serum uric acid. Probenicid promotes urate excretion in the kidney and inhibits tubular reabsorption; however, its use is contraindicated in humans when urate calculi are present in the tubules, since it leads to further stone formation.[13] (Nephrolithiasis should be suspected in patients with gout with sudden onset flank pain.) Promotion of urate excretion is also contraindicated in those being treated with chemotherapy or radiation therapy for cancer. Tubular urate crystals are frequently seen histologically in birds and reptiles, which suggests that uricosuric drugs may not be the most appropriate form of treatment.

Supportive care in the form of palliative management of the acute attacks and pain should be considered, for example, with colchicine (decreases inflammatory response within 24 hours)[9] or corticosteroids (intraarticular injections are given to humans with only one joint affected by gout).[13] IL-1β antagonists are being studied for treatment in humans.[13] Colchicine blocks IL-1β maturation, reducing inflammation and the development of gout or pseudogout. Resting the joint and application of ice are recommended to relieve swelling in humans with gout.[13]

Surgical removal and flushing of crystals from joints are performed, although some residual changes are frequently seen in the joints,[9] and the underlying hyperuricemia has not been addressed. Many of the treatments used in humans have not been evaluated in other species with regard to severity of disease and the safety and efficiency of the treatments. As urate is excreted by insects, these species (e.g., silkworms) may be used as animal models for treatment trials.[16] Severe gout has a poor prognosis in animals, so humane euthanasia may be considered when management with analgesia, diet, and environment has failed.

PREVENTIVE MEDICINE

Drugs such as diuretics, cyclosporine, tacrolimus, β-blockers, and low-dose salicylate, which increase the tendency for the development of uricemia, should be avoided. Nephrotoxic plants, household items, and drugs such as aminoglycosides and sulfonamides should be avoided, since all of these result in further reduction of uric acid secretion in the tubules. Purine in the diet should be minimized.[3] Increased consumption of meat or seafood increases the risk of development of gout, whereas increase in dairy proteins is protective, as the milk proteins casein and lactalbumin decrease serum uric acid by increasing the amount excreted in the urine (uricosuric effect).[3] Increased purine-rich vegetable protein in the diet has not been shown to increase the risk of gout development.[3] The bioavailability of purines varies, so they are more available from a ribonucleic acid (RNA) source compared with an equivalent deoxyribonucleic acid (DNA) source; purines are more available from ribonucleotides than from nucleic acids and from sources rich in adenine versus those rich in guanine.[3] Scientifically prepared diets that are low in protein and calcium are commercially available for dogs and have been used in reptiles.[12] Optimal ambient temperature is important for metabolism and the maintenance of body functions in reptiles. Adequate hydration is important to maintain renal secretion, thus fluid therapy in uricotelic species should not be neglected.[7] The use of omega-3 fatty acids (lipid products of arachidonic acid metabolism) are used in the treatment of chronic arthritis; however, in cases with concomitant gout, care should be taken to ensure that the patient receives a plant-sourced eicosapentaenoic or docosahexanoic acid rather than the usual fish oil source, which may have higher purine levels.[4]

FURTHER CONSIDERATION

Exotic species with evidence of articular gout should be considered to have chronic disease. Renal disease with urate crystals deposited in renal tubules is often already present. Consequently, the use of uricosuric drugs, which further increase urate excretion, results in further crystal development. Currently, efforts are being made to identify cases earlier in the course of disease and to investigate the use of the appropriate drug types to establish more effective treatments.

REFERENCES

1. Alvarez-Lario B, Macarron-Vicente J: Uric acid and evolution. *Rheumatology* 49(11):2010–2015, 2010.
2. Chiodini RJ, Nielsen SW: Vertebral osteophytes in an iguanid lizard. *Vet Pathol* 20:372–375, 1983.
3. Choi HK, Atkinson K, Karlson EW, et al: Purine-rich foods, dairy and protein intake and the risk of gout in men. *N Engl J Med* 350:1093–1103, 2004.
4. Choi HK: Pathogenesis of gout. *Ann Intern Med* 143:499–516, 2005.
5. Feig DI, Kang D-H, Johnson RT: Uric acid and cardiovascular risk. *N Engl J Med* 359:1811–1821, 2008.
6. Floersheim GL, Brune K, Seiler K: Colchicine in avian sodium urate and calcium pyrophosphate microcrystal arthritis. *Agents Actions* 3(1):20–23, 1973.
7. Frye FL: *Biomedical and surgical aspects of captive reptile husbandry*, Malabar, FL, 1991, Krieger Publishing Company.
8. Jones YL, Fitzgerald SD: Articular gout and suspected pseudogout in a basilisk lizard (*Basilicus plumifrons*). *J Zoo Wild Med* 40(3):576–578, 2009.
9. Mader DR: Gout. In Mader DR, editor: *Reptile medicine and surgery*, ed 2, St. Louis, MO, 2006, Saunders.
10. Martinez-Silvestre A: Treatment with allopurinol and probenecid for visceral gout in a Greek tortoise, *Testudo graeca*. *Bull Assoc Reptil Amphib Vet* 7(4):4–5, 1997.
11. Martinon F, Petrilli V, Mayor A, et al: Gout-associated uric acid crystals activate the NALP3 inflammasome. *Nature* 440:237–241, 2006.
12. Muro Figueres J: Treatment of articular gout in a Mediterranean pond turtle, *Mauremys leprosa*. *Bull Assoc Reptil Amphib Vet* 7(4):5–8, 1997.
13. Neogi T: Gout. *N Engl J Med* 364:443–452, 2011.
14. Siller WG: Renal pathology of the fowl—a review. *Avian Pathol* 10:187–262, 1981.
15. Wenker CJ, Bart M, Guscetti F, et al: Periarticular hydroxyapatite deposition disease in two red-bellied short-necked turtles (*Emydura albertisii*). In *Proceedings of the American Association of Zoo Veterinarians*, Columbus, Ohio, 1999, pp 23–26.
16. Zhang X, Xue R, Cao G, et al: Silkworms can be used as an animal model to screen and evaluate gouty therapeutic drugs. *J Insect Sci* 12(4):1–9, 2012.

CHAPTER **68**

The EAZWV and AAZV Infectious Diseases Notebooks

Jacques Kaandorp

HISTORY AND DEVELOPMENT OF THE EUROPEAN TRANSMISSIBLE DISEASES HANDBOOK

At the 2000 European Association of Zoo and Wildlife Veterinarians (EAZWV) Congress in Paris, the establishment of an Infectious Diseases Working Group (IDWG) within the EAZWV was proposed. In North America, the American Association of Zoo Veterinarians (AAZV) already had an Infectious Disease Committee since the early 1990s. In Europe, this idea for a similar committee emerged when the problems of diagnosing and handling paratuberculosis were discussed in a presentation. It was obvious that commonly agreed recommendations were urgently needed for improved control of the infectious diseases that threatened the European collections. Also, as Europe was becoming more unified, it was necessary to deal with European politics and legislation via international collaboration. The idea to produce a comprehensive document containing disease fact sheets, legislation, laboratories, identifiable diseases, and so on resulted in the IDWG, which led to the production of the first edition

of *The Transmissible Diseases Handbook* in May 2002 under the EAZWV-IDWG umbrella[4] (Figure 68-1).

The foot-and-mouth disease (FMD) outbreak in Europe in 2001 clearly underlined the importance of this initiative and made agreement on European standards a matter of even greater urgency. During this outbreak, the difficulties in controlling diseases in domesticated animals was realized; public opinion, politics, money, limited knowledge of the disease, and lack of agreement on legislation all contributed to this situation. It became obvious that even more misunderstandings would arise when dealing with such diseases in lesser-studied animals, including nondomestic species. In 2006, the highly pathogenic avian influenza spread across Europe and threatened zoo collections. Outbreaks of classic swine fever also occurred. Additionally, blue tongue disease created serious problems in transporting hoof stock and thus jeopardized organized programs for breeding endangered species.[5] African swine fever, West Nile virus (WNV), African horse sickness, and monkeypox also threatened zoologic collections. The severe acute respiratory syndrome (SARS) epidemic (related to an animal coronavirus) confirmed these

EAZWV Transmissible Disease Fact Sheet   Sheet No.

DISEASE NAME

ANIMAL GROUP AFFECTED	TRANS- MISSION	CLINICAL SIGNS	FATAL DISEASE ?	TREATMENT	PREVENTION & CONTROL
					In houses in zoos

Fact sheet compiled by   **Last update**

Fact sheet reviewed by

Susceptible animal groups

Causative organism

Zoonotic potential

Distribution

Transmission

Incubation period

Clinical symptoms

Post mortem findings

Diagnosis

Material required for laboratory analysis

EU Reference Laboratory

OIE Reference Laboratories

Relevant diagnostic laboratories

Treatment

Prevention and control in zoos

Suggested disinfectant for housing facilities

Notification

Guarantees required under EU Legislation

Guarantees required by EAZA Zoos

Measures required under the Animal Disease Surveillance Plan

Measures required for introducing animals from non-approved sources

Measures to be taken in case of disease outbreak or positive laboratory findings

Conditions for restoring disease-free status after an outbreak

Contacts for further information

References

FIGURE 68-1 Template of a European Association of Zoo and Wildlife Veterinarians (EAZWV) *Transmissible Disease Fact Sheet*. Courtesy EAZWV (Courtesy EAZWV [European Association of Zoo and Wildlife Veterinarians]).

points and led to the recognition of the importance of *The Transmissible Diseases Handbook*. The second edition of the *Handbook* was published in 2004, the third edition in 2006, and the fourth edition in 2010; these updates were necessary because of the changes in threatening diseases, the changes in legislation, and the needs and demands for information expressed by its readers.[2,3,4,6] European laws (e.g., the Balai Directive[1]) are still under discussion and in development. Differing opinions (e.g., whether or not to vaccinate against FMD and avian influenza), various levels of veterinary faculties and laboratories, and thus differences in the rates of successful diagnoses, pose further problems for European zoo veterinarians. Since *The Transmissible Diseases Handbook* is a living document and because of all these changes a fifth edition will be produced in 2014.

The IDWG brings together experienced zoo veterinarians and specialists in infectious diseases from several European countries and from around the world. The idea of the Group is to combine knowledge to deal more effectively with future disease outbreaks that may threaten zoo collections. The effort to create a reference manual published under the umbrella of EAZWV was, and still is, an important step in the process of standardization for zoos in Europe, and it should provide a useful tool for zoo practitioners, zoo managers, and European legislative authorities dealing with wildlife and zoo animals.

AAZV AND THE INFECTIOUS DISEASE COMMITTEE

The American Association of Zoo Veterinarians (AAZV) Infectious Disease Committee (IDC) has been very active since its inception. This committee already has its own *Infectious Disease Reviews Notebook* published in the early 1990s. This Notebook contained loose leaf handouts, with descriptions of various diseases important for zoo veterinarians and fact sheets on the diagnostics of important diseases such as tuberculosis. After the second edition of the EAZWV-IDWG *Transmissible Diseases Handbook* was published in May 2004, Dr. Julie Napier, a member of the AAZV and the chair of the IDC at the time, proposed creating a handbook for infectious diseases affecting nondomestic species and wildlife in North America, using the European version as a template (see Figure 68-1).

The difference between the European and American notebooks was that chapters on legislation, laboratories, web links, notifiable diseases, and so on were included in the European *Transmissible Diseases Handbook*, but not in the American equivalent. It was the intent of the IDC that the formatting of its manual would include more in-depth information, including etiologies, clinical signs, and treatment protocols for diseases relevant to the United States, Canada, and Mexico. Following discussions on providing a similar tool for North American veterinarians, it was agreed that the IDC could use the European disease fact sheet as a template, which provided a standardized and unified format. Thanks to the hard work of many people under the leadership of Dr. Julie Napier and Dr. Kathryn Gamble, The first American edition was published in 2011, titled *Infectious Disease Manual 2011*, with the subtitle "Infectious Diseases of Concern to Captive and Free-Ranging Wildlife in North America" (Boxes 68-1 and 68-2). An update of the manual was released at the end of 2013.

PURPOSE AND GOAL OF INFECTIOUS DISEASES NOTEBOOKS

The manuals on transmissible diseases, created by the EAZWV-IDWG and the AAZV-IDC, are not intended to provide extensive descriptions of all transmissible diseases that may occur in zoo collections but are meant as useful reference tools for zoo and wildlife veterinarians encountering such diseases. The handbooks help find answers to the question "What should I do" when an infectious

---

> **BOX 68-1 Table of Contents of the *AAZV Infectious Disease Manual*, 2011.**
>
> Introduction
> Notes from the Editors
> Authors (in alphabetical order)
> Reportable Diseases for the United States, Canada, and Mexico (in alphabetical order)
> Disease Fact Sheets (in alphabetical order)
> Reviewers Disease Fact Sheets (grouped by classification)

AAZV, American Association of Zoo Veterinarians.

> **BOX 68-2 Table of Contents of the EAZWV *Transmissible Diseases Handbook*, Fourth Edition, 2010**
>
> Introduction
> General Considerations
> European Union (data on EU Member States, EU Animal Health Strategy and Animal Health Advisory Committee, EU Animal Health Law, EAZA Position Statement on the Animal Health Strategy for the European Union, OIE)
> Links (EU Veterinary Faculties, Useful [veterinary] Web Links)
> Animal Health Legislation in Europe
> Recommendations for the application of Annex C to the Balai Directive
> Postmortem Procedures
> Guidelines for Cleaning and Disinfection in Zoological Gardens
> Bluetongue in Nondomestic Ruminants: Experiences Gained in EAZA Zoos during the 2007 & 2008 BTV8 and BTV1 Epizootics
> Tuberculosis in Zoo Species: Diagnostic Update and Management Issues
> Vaccination of Nondomestic Avian Species Against Highly Pathogenic Avian Influenza (HPAI) Viruses
> Vaccination of Nondomestic Carnivores: A Review
> List of Laboratories
> Template Fact Sheet
> Fact Sheets (133)

BTV, Blue tongue virus; *EAZA*, European Association of Zoos and Aquaria; *EAZWV*, European Association of Zoo and Wildlife Veterinarians; *EU*, European Union; *OIE*, Office of International Education.

---

disease is suspected. Furthermore, it is critical to standardize surveillance programs for infectious diseases in zoos, especially with regard to inter-zoo exchanges. Both the European and American handbooks assist in overcoming the differences and attaining the required standardization by legislation such as the Balai Directive (92/65/EC) in Europe.[1]

Both manuals are designed to be overviews or reviews and are not scientific textbooks. For detailed information on all diseases, it is necessary to refer to textbooks. The handbooks summarize information related to various diseases: susceptible animals, zoonotic potential, clinical symptoms, pathology, diagnostic methods, qualified laboratories, treatment, prevention, experts who may be consulted, legislation, and relevant literature. The detailed table of contents and the standardized format of the fact sheets should help the reader find information quickly. Most of the fact sheets in both manuals were peer reviewed by two experts, which makes these notebooks accepted reference documents for zoo associations in the respective regions of the world.

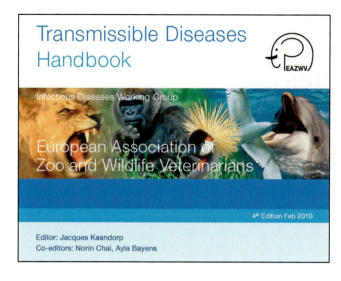

FIGURE 68-2 Front page of the European Association of Zoo and Wildlife Veterinarians, Infectious Diseases Working Group (EAZWV-IDWG) *Transmissible Diseases Handbook*, CD-ROM, fourth edition, 2010. From EAZWV (From EAZWV [European Association of Zoo and Wildlife Veterinarians]-IDWG *Transmissible Diseases Handbook* CD-ROM, fourth edition, 2010.

Both handbooks are intended to be "living" books, as the information presented becomes outdated if revisions are not made regularly. A continuous updating process is therefore maintained to make them reliable and useful tools.

PRINTED BOOK, CD-ROM, ONLINE MATERIAL

For the third and fourth editions, the EAZWV-IDWG moved away from the printed format and chose to publish the material digitally on a CD-ROM (Figure 68-2) or as downloadable material at www.eazwv.org and www.eaza.net. This significantly reduced the costs of production and distribution. Another advantage was the ability to increase the contents, without concerns about number of pages (the second edition was already 662 pages long!). Thus, the third and fourth editions contain more information on legislation and other new topics, thus a lot more pages. A printed version would have become too big and cost-prohibitive in terms of production and distribution. It was also hoped that this format would allow easier global access, which turned out to be the case. The fourth edition, like the previous editions, was distributed to all EAZWV members, all EAZA zoos, Central Veterinary Officers of the 27 EU Member States, the OIE, and the SANCO in Brussels. Another advantage of the book on a CD-ROM is the facility to search and have quick access to chapters and fact sheets (see Figure 68-2).

The first *American Infectious Disease Manual* and its 2013 update may be accessed, free of charge, at the web site of the AAZV (www.aazv.org). Also the Infectious Disease Committee from the AAZV had these documents peer-reviewed by topic experts. It needs to be stressed again that these documents are not intended to be used as exclusive information sources. As in the case of the European documents, they provide quick access to information on specialists, diagnostics, laboratories, and treatment recommendations for the clinician, pathologist, or wildlife biologist who is facing an infectious disease situation and needs information and guidance.

Summarized state regulations for infectious disease concerns are provided, and reminders for reportable situations are also included. During the preparation of the documents, state veterinary authorities were encouraged to be reviewers for their geographic area. Additionally, as in Europe, CDs are provided to the state health authorities and to the United States Department of Agriculture (USDA) Area Veterinarians in Charge (AVICs); it is hoped that this shared information gives a common point of communication among American zoo and wildlife veterinarians battling these infectious diseases on the frontlines. It is important to keep in mind that the fact sheets are not to replace state or federal regulations. As such, they are not legally enforceable documents or required standards of care.

REFERENCES

1. Dollinger P: "Balai" Directive of the European Union: Difficult veterinary legislation. In *Zoo and wild animal medicine: Current therapy*, vol 6, St. Louis, MO, 2008, Saunders, pp 68–74.
2. Kaandorp J: *Transmissible diseases handbook*, IDWG-EAZWV, ed 2, Houten, NL, 2004, Van Setten Kwadraat.
3. Kaandorp J: *Transmissible diseases handbook*, IDWG-EAZWV, ed 4, Hilvarenbeek, NL, 2010, IDWG Secretariat.
4. Ryser M-P: *Transmissible diseases handbook*, IDWG-EAZWV, Berne, CH, 2002, IDWG Secretariat.
5. Sanderson S: Bluetongue: Lessons from the European outbreak 2006–2009. In *Fowler's zoo and wild animal medicine: Current therapy*, vol 7, St. Louis, MO, 2012, Saunders, pp 573–580.
6. Schoemaker N, Kaandorp J, Fernandèz Bellon H: *Transmissible diseases handbook*, IDWG-EAZWV, ed 3, Hilvarenbeek, NL, 2006, IDWG Secretariat.

CHAPTER 69

Update on Iron Overload in Zoologic Species

Linda J. Lowenstine and Iga M. Stasiak

Iron overload (IO), also called *iron storage disease (ISD)* or *iron overload disorder*, was considered rare in veterinary species until the 1970s and 1980s, after which it became increasingly recognized in many taxa of birds and mammals.[37] The current understanding of molecular mechanisms of iron metabolism and of diseases associated with excessive iron accumulation has greatly expanded as a result of research in humans, mice, birds, and bats.[5,24,28,32,40,64] An international workshop highlighted the concern about the impact of ISD on captive management of black rhinoceroses and resulted in the publication of a special issue of *Journal of Zoo and Wildlife Medicine*.[23]

In this chapter, the term *hemosiderosis* refers to an accumulation (overload) of stainable iron without morphologic or biochemical evidence of toxicity, and the term "hemochromatosis" indicates a serious state of iron overload, in which organ damage occurs. In contrast, in human medicine, "hemochromatosis" often refers specifically to primary hereditary iron storage disease. The term "iron overload (IO)" connotes too much iron, whereas ISD connotes disease associated with IO. Hemosiderosis may progress to hemochromatosis. However, very high concentrations of iron may occur without evidence of molecular, cellular, or structural damage if sequestration of toxic, labile free iron by ferritin and hemosiderin is adequate to prevent cell death.[13,32]

Iron overload may be primary (implying a constitutional, genetic propensity to accumulate iron, generally as a result of inability to control intestinal absorption, as in human hereditary hemochromatosis) or secondary to a variety of causes, including excessive enteral or parenteral (e.g., transfusions) intake, diseases of the erythron, liver disease (including intoxications and infections), systemic inflammatory processes (with iron sequestration as an antibacterial defense), stress, chronic renal disease, and malnutrition.[1,61]

The majority of iron in the body is present in hemoglobin in the red blood cells (RBCs) and is recycled from senescent erythrocytes by macrophages in the spleen, bone marrow, and liver.[1,24] Most of the remainder is stored in the cytosol of cells as ferritin, from which it may be readily accessed, or as hemosiderin, which is a less active, aggregated form. Hemosiderin appears as golden brown granules in hematoxylin and eosin (H&E)–stained sections and is confirmed to be iron by blue precipitates formed by Prussian blue techniques (e.g., Perl). Ferritin is not visible with H&E staining but appears as a faint blue "wash" in Prussian blue stains.[3] Hepatocytes are the major site of iron storage in overload states. The shift from ferritin to hemosiderin in hepatocytes may be caused by increasing iron concentrations or by hepatocellular injury, atrophy, or autophagy; thus, increases in stainable granular iron may reflect a relative, rather than absolute, increase in intracellular iron concentration.

REVIEW OF IRON ABSORPTION AND TRANSPORT AND LIVER HANDLING OF IRON

Iron is essential for almost all life forms from prokaryotes to vertebrates, but it is also a toxin. Organisms have thus evolved complex regulatory mechanisms for ensuring enough iron to meet metabolic needs while preventing excessive uptake. Since "off-loading" of body iron is limited, control is primarily at the level of intestinal uptake.

Dietary iron is present in two main forms: *heme* and *non-heme*.[61] Heme-iron is highly bioavailable; it is released by proteolytic digestion of myoglobin and hemoglobin in the small intestine and is the major source of iron in carnivores. Non-heme iron is complexed with organic acids or peptides and is the predominant form of dietary iron available to omnivorous, frugivorous, folivorous, granivorous, and other plant-eating species.[32] In humans, non-heme iron in the oxidized state is reduced and then taken up by the cellular iron importer divalent metal transporter-1 (DMT-1).[23,61] Gastric acid enhances the solubility and absorption of non-heme iron complexes, and dietary vitamin C increases iron absorption by forming highly bioavailable, soluble iron complexes.[1] Iron bioavailability is decreased by iron chelating compounds in the diet.

Within the enterocyte, depending on the metabolic demand, iron is either bound to the iron storage protein, ferritin, in the cytosol or is exported into plasma via ferroportin. Ferroportin, a transmembrane protein and the most important iron exporter, is also expressed in macrophages, hepatocytes, and placental trophoblasts.[5,23,32] Iron not transferred to plasma is sloughed off with exfoliating enterocytes and eliminated through feces. Oxidized iron is taken up by plasma transferrin for distribution throughout the body, and a majority is carried to erythropoeitic cells.

Hepcidin, the key iron regulatory hormone, expressed primarily in the liver, is induced when tissue and plasma iron levels are high.[24] Hepcidin induction results in the internalization and degradation of ferroportin, thus downregulating enteric iron absorption and iron mobilization from cellular stores and causing depletion of the plasma iron pool. Hepcidin production is also induced in inflammatory states and appears to be a key mediator in anemia of chronic disease. Hepcidin is strongly suppressed in states requiring accelerated erythropoiesis.

The active hepcidin peptide appears to be highly conserved among vertebrate taxa with homologous sequences in over 51 different highly diverse species, including fish, amphibians, reptiles, and mammals.[27] However, hepcidin has not been confirmed in birds (pigeons and chickens).

In humans, in a majority of cases, hereditary hemochromatosis is associated with a deficiency in hepcidin because of mutations in the hepcidin (*HAMP*) gene itself or its regulators.[23,61] Investigations of the role of hepcidin in the regulation of iron balance in susceptible exotic species have included genetic studies in rhinoceroses and red deer (*Cervus elaphus*) and experimental studies in bats.[6,23,50,64] Since hepcidin may not be present in birds, other iron-regulatory molecules may be of primary importance. Those identified include DMT1 in chickens and mynahs; ferroportin (Ireg1) in chickens and mynahs; intestinal cytochrome B reductase, serum and ovo-transferrins in chickens; and ferritin in several species.[2,42,43,65]

In mammals, iron crosses the placenta via placental DMT-1, ferroportin, and transferrins, mostly in the late stages of pregnancy.[36] Unless born to an iron-deficient dam, infants are endowed with sufficient iron to carry them through early postnatal life to compensate for the relatively low concentration of iron in milk. This may account for the common finding of hemosiderosis in the livers of neonates of several species of mammals.[37,62] Transfer of iron to the embryos of birds and presumably fish, amphibians, and reptiles occurs through the yolk.

CONSEQUENCES OF IRON OVERLOAD

Unbound iron is cytotoxic and causes peroxidation of membranes, cell death, and organ dysfunction.[3] Cirrhotic liver failure ("pigmentary cirrhosis"), hepatocellular carcinoma, type 2 diabetes ("bronze diabetes"), male sexual dysfunction, arthropathies, and heart disease (cardiomyopathy and fatal dysrhythmias) are consequences of untreated ISD in humans.[3,5,32,61]

IO increases susceptibility to bacterial and fungal infections through direct effects on immune system function and by providing iron for microbial growth.[5,23,67] This is highlighted by deaths caused by sepsis in human hemochromatosis, yersinosis in birds with IO, and, possibly, cases of atypical mycobacteriosis and aspergillosis in black rhinos.[5,13,30,53] Increasing evidence suggests that elevated total body iron stores may be related to the development of metabolic syndrome and type 2 diabetes in humans and, possibly, in bottlenose dolphins and black rhinoceroses, perhaps through endogenous corticosteroid production.[26,37,46,66,75]

DIAGNOSIS

Early diagnosis of ISD poses a challenge, as clinical signs are not specific and often not apparent until disease is advanced. Clinical signs are typically associated with liver failure and ascites, hepatomegaly, weight loss, icterus, anorexia, vomiting (in lemurs), "malaise" (in dolphins) and, in birds, cardiomegaly, dyspnea, coughing, or wheezing.[15,39,63] Liver enzymes are often elevated, and hypoproteinemia ensues as the disease progresses to liver failure. Signs in domestic cattle and red deer include poor hair coat, weight loss in the face of a good appetite, and poor bone quality leading to loss of incisors and fractures in young animals.[31,50] Radiography is useful in identifying hepatomegaly and cardiomegaly in birds with ISD.[30,40] Liver biopsy, for histologic grading of iron accumulation and liver damage, and chemical analysis of iron concentration remain the gold standard for diagnosis of ISD in exotic species.[40,62,71] Because of the invasiveness of liver biopsy, serum "iron analytes" (iron, total iron binding capacity, % transferrin saturation, and ferritin) have been used in humans and mammalian species and have proven useful in the diagnosis, determination of prognosis, and treatment of ISD.[5,14,29,39,53,61,62,70]

Serum ferritin (SF) is considered the best test for noninvasive measurement of body iron status in mammalian species.[12,21,62] In humans, SF level vary with age and gender (males greater than females) and increases in inflammatory processes and conditions such as hyperthyroidism, chronic hepatitis, alcohol-induced liver disease, and neoplasia, which limits its usefulness as a stand-alone test.[5,32,61] In humans, normal values are less than 200 microgram per liter (µg/L) in women and <300 µg/L in men, whereas SF >1000 indicates IO and >5000 indicates ISD.[32] Variation in the molecular structure of ferritin requires species-specific radioimmunoassays, only available for humans, dogs, cats, cattle, horses (used for bats), pigs, rhinoceroses (used for tapirs), lemurs (used for callitrichids), dolphins, and fur seals (Kansas State Veterinary Diagnostic Laboratory, Comparative Hematology, Manhattan, KS).[21,51,62,70]

Serum iron (SI) levels reflect the total amount of iron in blood, including transferrin-bound and non–transferrin-bound iron. In mammalian species and birds, diurnal and seasonal variations exist in SI.[7] Variations occur among closely related taxa, necessitating evaluation of the usefulness of serum iron analyte testing on a species-by-species basis.[70] Total iron binding capacity (TIBC) and the calculated percentage transferrin saturation (%TS) are also used as indicators of body iron stores, with %TS considered more reliable than SI, TIBC, or both. In humans and many mammalian species, transferrin is normally about 30% saturated. TS persistently over

BOX 69-1 Conversion Factors for Comparison of Liver Iron Levels

1 mole of iron (Fe) is 55.85 grams (g) of iron (e.g., 1 micromole per gram [µmol/g] = 55.85 microgram per gram [µg/g])
3.3 g of fresh (wet) liver yields 1 g of liver when dried.
Wet weight (ww) value × 3.3 equals the dry weight (dw) value (or dw value ÷ 3.3 = ww value)
µg/g or mg/kg = parts per million (ppm)

45% strongly suggests hereditary hemochromatosis in humans.[61] A panel consisting of SF, SI, and %TS is recommended for assessment of body iron levels in mammals.

In birds, SI analytes seem to be of little diagnostic value, although relative changes in SI and %TS may be used to monitor treatment.[27,40,69] SF assays are not yet commercially available for avian species, and liver biopsy remains the only reliable antemortem diagnostic test.[13,30,37,40] The use of magnetic resonance imaging (MRI) to assess hepatic and cardiac iron stores is an accepted modality in humans; however, limitations exist.[32,61] In pigeons with experimentally induced IO and hornbills with spontaneous ISD, MRI signal intensity corresponded well with hepatic iron concentration.[38,56]

Liver iron concentration (LIC) may be assessed histologically or analytically. Semi-quantitative assessment of Prussian blue–stained liver sections, using scoring schemes or morphometric techniques, approximates analytic quantification for comparisons of iron levels and assessing response to treatment.[7,8,13,18,54,62,69] Analytic determination of LIC may be performed on fresh, frozen or formalin fixed biopsies or from deparaffinized samples retrieved from tissue blocks. Small volumes of tissue are best measured using atomic absorption spectrophotometry (AAS) or inductively coupled plasma mass spectroscopy (ICP-MS). Iron concentration is expressed as millimoles per gram (mmol/g), micrograms per gram (µg/g), grams per kilogram (g/kg) or milligrams per gram (mg/g) (parts per million [ppm]) on either a wet weight (ww) or dry weight (dw) basis (Box 69-1).

Normal reference ranges for LIC are lacking for most species in zoologic medicine. In humans, the normal is 400 to 2000 µg/g dw in men and 100 to 1600 in women; mild to moderate IO is 3000 to 10,000, and greater than 10,000 indicates potential toxicity. Fibrosis is always present at 22,000 µg/g.[3] The interpretation of LIC in animals is complicated by seasonal variation associated with life history events, for example, reproduction and molting in birds and migration in reindeer.[7,30]

IRON OVERLOAD SYNDROMES IN ZOOLOGIC SPECIES

Amphibians and Reptiles

Hepatocellular hemosiderosis, often with hepatic lipidosis, is not uncommon in amphibians and reptiles and is likely secondary to systemic inflammation or inanition, not caused by a primary susceptibility to ISD.[37] Liver iron reference values are generally lacking, but mean LIC in Chinese alligators (*Alligator sinensus*) was 380 ppm dw.[73]

Birds

Both primary ISD and secondary ISD occur in avian species, with toucans, birds of paradise, mynahs, and starlings considered "susceptible" or "iron sensitive" taxa (Box 69-2).[13,30,37,40] Liver iron concentrations of 6683 to 23,078 µg/g dw, found in clinically normal mynahs, are well above the 487 to 701 in adult chickens and within the range of IO and ISD in humans.[43] A primary genetic basis for iron overload in mynahs (*Gracula religiosa* and *Acridotheres tristis*) is

BOX 69-2 Birds in Which Hepatic Hemosiderosis Is Common on Postmortem Examination

Phoenicopteriformes: Flamingos*
Anseriformes: Eider ducks (associated with reproduction and molt), mallards
Columbiformes: Fruit doves and imperial pigeons
Piciformes:
    Rhamphastidae: Toucans, toucanettes, aracari*
Coriciiformes:
    Coraciidae: Rollers
    Buceriotidae: Hornbills (frugivorous species) *
Cuculiformes:
    Muscophagidae: Turacos and go-away birds
Passeriformes:
    Sturnidae*: Starlings and mynahs
    Paradisaeidae*: Birds of paradise
    Cotingadiae*: Contingas, Capuchin bird, umbrella bird
    Piperidae: Manakins
    Emberizidae: Tanagers and euphonias
    Ptylonorhynchindae: Bower birds*
    Corvidae: Magpies and crows
    Lanidae: Shrikes
Psittaciformes:
    Loridae: Lorys and lorikeets
    Psittacidae: Red-spectacled Amazons

*Hemochromatosis in addition to hemosiderosis.

BOX 69-3 Mammals in Which Hepatic Hemosiderosis Is Common on Postmortem Examination

Marsupials: Neonatal macropods
Insectivora: House shrew
Macroscelidea: Elephant shrews
Rodentia: Naked mole rats,*
    gerbils, prehensile-tail porcupine, kangaroo rat
Lagomorpha: Afghan pika*
Nonhuman primates: Lemurs,* callitrichids, muriquis, zoo-housed western lowland gorillas
Chiroptera: Egyptian fruit bat,* other fruit bat species
Cetacea: California gray whales (migration/fasting), captive bottle-nose dolphins*
Artiodactyla:
    Reindeer (seasonal), Red deer* (diet overload), Salers cattle*
    Bay duiker, dik-dik,
    Bongo (neonatal)*
    Neonatal hemosiderosis: Gazelles, caprines, cervids and ovines
Perissodactyla: Black* and Sumatran rhinos, tapirs,* Persian onagers, horses, donkeys
Afrotheria: African and Asian elephants (secondary, inflammation), Rock hyrax*
Carnivora:
    Procyonids: Red panda, coati mundi*
    Pinnipeds: Harbor seals neonatal hemosiderosis, weanling elephant seals (fasting)
    California sea lions and northern fur seals* (older, captive-housed)
    Felids: Cheetah, snow leopards (veno-occlusive disease)

*Hemochromatosis with liver damage in addition to hemosiderosis.

likely. Compared with collared doves (*Streptopelia decaocto*), mynahs have much higher uptake and retention of dietary iron and demonstrate high levels of expression of the intestinal iron transporters DMT-1 and intestinal Ireg1 (ferroportin).[41,42] This supports a working hypothesis that natural diets for which "sensitive" species have evolved are low in bioavailable iron leading to selection for enhanced iron uptake and storage.[60] However, diets in captivity that provide too much available iron may exacerbate primary ISD, as shown in starlings.[16]

Reports of ISD in psittacines are interesting because this diverse order contains both generalist and specialized feeders. Species that have evolved to use low iron diets would be expected to be more "iron-sensitive" compared with other species. This seems to be the case for lorids, adapted to nectivorous and palynivorous (pollen) diets, and the red-spectacled Amazon (*Amazona pretrei*), adapted to a pine nut diet.[54,68] Liver iron concentration in affected lories was 3500 to 7600 ppm ww (about 11,550 to 25,000 µg/g dw), comparable with LIC in mynahs. A report of two diabetic macaws with ISD parallels the frequent occurrence of diabetes in human hemochromatosis.[22,61]

In flamingos, moderate to marked hepatocellular and Kupffer cell hemosiderosis increases with age and is associated with hepatitis, cirrhosis, and hepatocellular carcinoma in older birds. Concurrent diseases that could drive ISD (e.g. pododermatitis, aspergillosis, and amyloidosis) are present in some, but not all, birds. This species warrants further investigation to determine whether an evolutionary predisposition exists or if ISD is secondary to management.

Hemosiderosis in other orders of birds such as the anseriforms appears to be secondary to intoxications (e.g., lead), infections, captive diets, or seasonal life history events such as molt and reproduction.[30,37] Studies in Eider ducks have indicated that inanition increases LIC; however, in wild black-necked swans (*Cygnus melanocoryphus*), elevated SI in the face of starvation was considered to indicate mobilization and reduction of tissue iron storage.[7,48] In the latter study, serum iron, TIBC, and %TS were used as surrogates for body iron stores but may not accurately reflect LIC.

Mammals

Although hemosiderosis has been reported in many species of mammals, hemochromatosis, as evidenced by fibrotic liver disease, is less common (Box 69-3).[12,31,37] However, other serious adverse effects of IO (e.g., poor bone quality or susceptibility to infections) exist and may occur in taxa without the classic "pigmentary cirrhosis."[12,17,31,50,53]

Chiroptera

Hemochromatosis is the leading cause of morbidity and mortality in captive Egyptian fruit bats (*Rousettus aegyptiacus*).[15,21,35] Isolated cases of ISD in the straw-colored fruit bat (*Eidelon helvum*), long-haired rousette (*Rousettus lanosus*), Indian flying fox (*Pteropus giganteus*), and grey-headed flying fox (*Pteropus poliocephalus*) have been reported.[15,34]

In Egyptian fruit bats, clinical signs characteristic of liver failure are generally not apparent until advanced stages of the disease and include icterus, weight loss and emaciation, weakness, dehydration, and ascites. Hepatomegaly may be detected by radiography or abdominal palpation. Elevated serum iron analytes and bilirubin are also reported.[15]

Gross postmortem findings in affected bats reflect the clinical findings. The liver is often nodular with rounded edges, a dark rusty coloration, a firm texture, and an irregular granular cut surface (Figure 69-1). Histologically, disruption of hepatic architecture occurs, with extensive periacinar and periportal fibrosis bordering foci of nodular regeneration and areas of hepatocellular necrosis (Figure 69-2). Hepatocytes and Kupffer cells contain coarse iron granules, most prominently bordering areas of fibrosis.

In a retrospective study of captive Egyptian fruit bats, bats with hemochromatosis were significantly more likely to develop hepatocellular carcinoma compared with bats with hemosiderosis.[35] Although cardiomyopathy was seen in some bats, this was not significantly correlated with increased cardiac or hepatic iron levels.

The high prevalence of hemochromatosis in one population of Egyptian fruit bats was historically attributed to high levels of dietary iron (400 mg/kg on a dry matter [DM] basis) and vitamin C.[15] Although diet is likely a major factor contributing to ISD, recent research has shown that Egyptian fruit bats may have a limited ability to upregulate expression of hepcidin, which may predispose to iron overload in states of dietary iron excess.[64] This is in contrast to vampire bats (*Desmodus rotundus*), which have an impressive hepcidin upregulation.[64]

Perissodactyls

Iron storage disease has been well defined in the highly endangered black (*Diceros bicornis*) and Sumatran (*Dicerorhinus sumatrensis*)

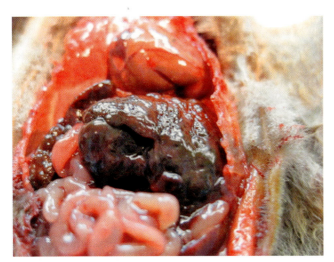

FIGURE 69-1 Liver from an Egyptian fruit bat with hemochromatosis. The liver is dark and enlarged and has rounded edges and an irregular surface.

rhinoceroses.[6,9,12,31,49,53] Although stainable iron is present in hepatocytes, more remarkable accumulations are in phagocytic cells of the liver, spleen, bone marrow, lung, and many other tissues, suggesting a problem in iron mobilization. In the black rhinoceros, iron levels increase with age and time in captivity; holding wild rhinoceroses in bomas for as little as 2 weeks prior to translocation may lead to systemic hemosiderosis and elevation of serum ferritin levels. This rapid development of hemosiderosis might be a result of stress, in addition to diet, since corticosteroids may upregulate intestinal ferroportin.[26] Elevated LIC of 2960 +/− 661 mg/kg ww (~10,000 ppm dw) has been reported in zoo-housed black rhinoceroses, compared with 474 +/− 142 mg/kg ww in recently translocated wild rhinoceroses.

The mechanism underlying development of ISD in rhinoceroses is not clear. Hereditary predisposition has been suggested on the basis of the presence of an S88T polymorphism in the hemochromatosis gene (HFE) of the black rhinoceros. However, this polymorphism is also present in the Indian rhinoceros (*Rhinoceros unicornis*), which only occasionally exhibits ISD.[6,49] It has been suggested that ISD in black rhinoceroses is secondary to "chronic iron intoxication" rather than to a primary hereditary sensitivity.[31,49] The fact that the most affected species (black and Sumatran) are browsers highlights the complexity of developing appropriate diets for captive folivores.[9,10,12,31,53] Whether it is primary or secondary, IO in black rhinoceroses is a serious problem, and the species suffers from several other devastating diseases, some of which (e.g., susceptibility to opportunistic infections and neonatal leukoencephalomalacia) are possibly associated with IO.[53]

Baird, Brazilian, and Malayan tapirs (*Tapirus bairdii, T. terrestris,* and *T. indicus*) are also affected by ISD in captivity, as shown by necropsy data.[4,52] Hematologic evidence for IO is also present, as SI, %TS, and SF levels were all markedly elevated in captive Baird, Malayan, and mountain (*T. pinchaque*) tapirs compared with free-ranging Baird tapirs in indigenous habitats.[52]

Equids (domestic horses, donkeys, and Persian onagers) are reported to develop hepatic hemosiderosis and occasionally hemochromatosis because of dietary iron overload.[8,12,37]

Artiodactyls

Clinical signs of IO in artiodactyls are not restricted to those of liver failure and include loss of weight in spite of good appetite, poor

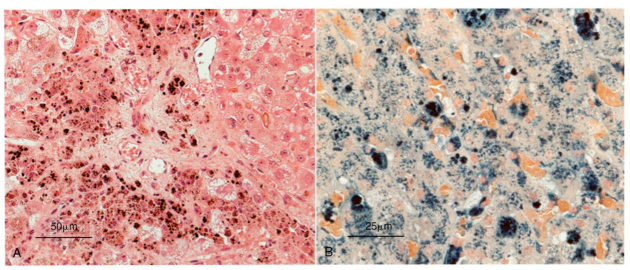

FIGURE 69-2 A, Hematoxylin and eosin (H&E)–stained section of liver from an Egyptian fruit bat with hemochromatosis. Extensive periportal fibrosis, hepatocellular loss, and accumulation of large amounts of coarse hemosiderin granules within hepatocytes and Kupffer cells in the periportal region are seen. **B,** Perl Prussian blue stain showing large amounts of iron within hepatocytes and Kupffer cells.

hair coat, and osteopenia with incisor loss and fractures in young animals.[50] Hepatic hemosiderosis is a seasonal occurrence in reindeer (*Rangifer tarandus*) and is related to winter foraging on mosses high in iron but low in nutritional value. The IO was not caused by starvation alone; reindeer foraging on poor diets low in iron had lower LIC.[7]

Deaths associated with ISD were reported in six related 2-year-old captive red deer bucks.[50] Marked hepatocellular hemosiderosis, hepatocellular necrosis, and fibrosis, as well as hemosiderosis in renal epithelium and myocardium, were found at necropsy, although liver iron concentrations of 1108 to 2275 mg/kg ww (approximately 3656–7508 ppm dw; reference range 100–200), were below levels generally considered hepatotoxic. No differences were found in the HFE gene of affected versus control deer, and dietary IO was likely, as the deer were drinking water from a rusty iron tub.

Hepatocellular hemosiderosis is fairly common in neonatal zoo-housed hoof stock and has been seen in gazelles, caprines, ovines, and cervids; it is considered physiologic rather than pathologic.[36,37] However, death in the first weeks of life associated with neonatal hemochromatosis was described in captive bongos (*Boocercus eury-ceros*) from one collection.

Carnivores

Carnivores would be expected to efficiently control iron absorption, as most of their dietary iron is easily absorbed heme-iron. Nonetheless, hepatic hemosiderosis has been reported in several felids (cheetah, *Acinonyx jubatus*; and snow leopard, *Uncia uncia*), procyonids (red panda, *Ailurus fulgens*; and coati mundis, *Nasua* spp.), and pinnipeds (see below).[12,37] Although classified as carnivores, coatis are, in fact, omnivores, and dietary IO in captivity likely caused the hemosiderosis or hemochromatosis seen at necropsy in 77% of coatis in a retrospective study.[11]

Marine Mammals

Hemosiderosis is common in neonatal pinnipeds dying in rehabilitation and on the rookeries, especially Pacific harbor seals (*Phoca vitulina richardsii*), in which it may represent a normal physiologic finding.[37] Northern elephant seal (*Miruonga agustirostris*) weanlings have abundant hemosiderin in hepatocytes, Kupffer cells, and splenic macrophages, likely associated with their normal post-weaning catabolic state. In yearling California sea lions (*Zalophus californianus* [CSL]), hepatic IO is commonly seen with malnutrition and parasitism. Hepatic IO is rare in adult stranded CSL and is associated with sepsis and parasitism. The marked hepatic hemosiderosis noted in California gray whales (*Eschrichtius robustus*) stranding during migration might be caused by seasonal fasting and changes in diet similar to the situation in reindeer.

In captive marine mammals, marked hepatocellular hemosiderosis and hemochromatosis have been reported in northern fur seals (*Callorhincus ursinus* [NFS]) and CSL, especially in older females. NFS females had significantly higher SF levels compared with males (500 nanograms per milliliter [ng/mL] versus 54 ng/mL) and higher TS (63% for females versus 41% for males), compatible with ISD.[39]

IO was also reported in a managed population of bottlenose dolphins (*Tursiops truncatus*).[66] High SI (>300 μg/dL), high TS (83%–85%) and elevated liver enzymes were used to classify this as hemochromatosis. Liver biopsies confirmed abundant hepatocellular hemosiderin. Hepatic lipidosis, dyslipidemia, and glucose tolerance patterns in this population suggested concurrent metabolic syndrome and ISD.

Nonhuman Primates

Hepatocellular hemosiderosis is commonly seen in lemurs, New World monkeys, colobines, and apes.[12,37] Old World cheek-pouch monkeys (cercopithecines) seem to be more resistant. Huge variation

in LIC was noted in zoo-housed primates, with a high of 16,000 μg/g ww (52,800 dw) in a common marmoset (*Callithrix jacchus*) and a low of 28.4 μg/g ww in a moor macaque (*M. maura*).[47] Marked variation was also noted in SI and %TS in banked serum from a variety of primate species from European zoos; %TS suggestive of ISD (>45%) was found in lemurs, common marmosets, and colobus.[20]

Hemosiderosis and hemochromatosis have been documented in lemurs on the basis of necropsy findings, LIC, and serum analytes.[14,25,55,63,70,71,72] In initial reports, the prevalence of ISD was 69% to 100% in zoo-housed lemurs, and ISD was considered a serious medical issue, especially in ruffed lemurs (*Varieca* sp.) and less so in ring-tailed lemurs (RTL, *Lemur catta*).[63] Severity of ISD increased with age, and liver necrosis and neoplasia were seen. IO was attributed to diet, specifically too much vitamin C and an overall paucity of dietary tannins. In more recent reports, hemosiderosis is considered an incidental finding, with a prevalence of only 32% in a large collection of 12 species of prosimians.[25] Mean LIC ranged from 209 to 2957 ppm ww, with the lowest in RTL and the highest in fat-tailed dwarf lemurs (*Chirogaleus medius*). Examination of an iron analyte panel (SI, TIBC, SF, %TS) in nine species of prosimians showed great interspecies and intraspecies variations.[70] No correlation existed between dietary levels of iron, fiber, or vitamin C and iron analyte values. Serum analytes were compared with liver biopsy LIC in three species of lemurs: RTL; red-ruffed lemur (RRL, *Varecia rubra*) and black lemur (BL, *Eulemur macaco*) from a zoo and a research collection, and ferritin was the only analyte that paralleled LIC in all three.[71] Mean LIC (ppm ww) was 1300 in RT, 3123 in BL, and 4845 in RRL, and SF ranges (ng/dL) were 11 to 242, 59 to 333, and 11 to 195, respectively, in the three species.

Liver neoplasia in prosimians is common and has been attributed to both ISD and a lemur-specific hepadnavirus. However, a review of hepatocellular neoplasms in prosimians found no evidence of a viral etiology.[74] As well, LIC was not significantly different in animals with or without tumors, in contrast to the findings in Egyptian fruit bats.

Hepatocellular hemosiderosis has been considered a common incidental necropsy finding in New World monkeys; however, associated liver disease was demonstrated in several species of callitrichids.[62] Hepatic iron ranged from 40 to 5596 ppm ww (132–18,466 ppm dw). There was positive correlation between LIC, SF (range 36–17,697 ng/dL) and histologic grade of iron accumulation. Serum iron, TIBC, and %TS did not correlate with amount of liver iron. Feeding trials in marmosets showed that a 3.5- to 5-fold increase in dietary iron caused a 10-fold median increase in liver iron; deaths were associated with the high iron diet (500 ppm).[44]

Although not as common in cebids, IO was recently described in captive-housed, endangered muriquis (*Brachyteles* sp.).[57] A hepatic hemosiderosis index (HHI) was determined by histomorphometry. No correlation existed between HHI and age, gender, or time in captivity. A third of the animals died of sepsis, but whether infection caused iron sequestration or the IO increased susceptibility to infection could not be determined. Woolly monkeys (*Lagothrix* spp.) in European zoos might also be susceptible to IO, as shown by serum iron analytes.[20]

Hepatocellular IO is often noted in adult captive western lowland gorillas (*Gorilla gorilla gorilla* [Ggg]) but is infrequent in wild mountain gorillas (*Gorilla beringei beringei* [Gbb]).[37] The median LIC is significantly higher in zoo Ggg than in wild Gbb (5440 ppm dw versus 1280) (LJL, unpublished). These levels are below toxic range, and significance to gorilla health is uncertain.

Miscellaneous Other Mammalian Species

ISD in hyraxes, pikas, gerbils, and other rodents is discussed in detail elsewhere.[12,31,37] Recently, ISD has been reported to be a consistent finding in naked mole rats (*Heterocephalus glaber*), in which both a genetic predisposition and dietary overload are suspected.[17]

PREVENTION AND TREATMENT

Dietary Manipulation

Dietary manipulation, in the form of decreasing iron (<100 ppm DM basis), limiting vitamin C, and/or adding ingredients that bind iron and prevent absorption, is the most important means of preventing IO in zoological species. Iron concentrations as low as 30 ppm DM basis for birds, 50 ppm for rhinoceroses, and 65 ppm for lemurs have been recommended, but it is difficult to formulate balanced diets this low.[10,40,60,72] Hidden sources of extra iron include other minerals such as dicalcium phosphate and drinking water.[16,44,60]

Dietary manipulation may be used to treat IO. Periodic removal of commercial pellets (for 30 days once or twice a year) from the diet decreased iron analytes in birds of paradise.[27] Prevention of iron absorption by intraluminal binding by polyphenols such as tannic acid, in the form of tea (leaves or infusion) or tamarind (pods or juice), has been used in birds, lemurs, and fruit bats.[33,34,58,60,63,72] This was shown to be effective in lemurs by following %TS.[72] However, replacing iron-rich fish by squid and removing vitamin pills with iron and vitamin C from diets of captive otariid seals for several years did not reduce ISD.[39]

Cautions for dietary manipulation include the fact that polyphenols also bind other essential trace minerals and could theoretically cause unintended deficiencies.[60] Specific vitamin C requirements for species at risk must also be considered. Several passerine species cannot synthesize vitamin C, although iron-susceptible families have not been specifically examined.[19] Lemurs may synthesize vitamin C, but New World monkeys, Old World monkeys, apes, and tarsiers cannot.

Treatment

The two main approaches to therapy of ISD are phlebotomy and chelation.[5,61] In humans, removal of 450 to 500 mL of blood (approximately 6–7 mL/kg)—once weekly until serum ferritin is reduced to less than 50 μg/L and once every 3 months thereafter—is suggested as the treatment of choice for primary ISD. Reduction of hematocrit by as little as 5% is therapeutic. Phlebotomy has been used in birds, rhinoceroses, dolphins, and lemurs. The recommendation in mynahs and toucans is 1 to 2 mL/day until borderline anemia or clinical improvement, then weekly until SI is less than 200 mg/mL.[37] Low-iron diet as well as 10 phlebotomy sessions (1% total blood volume every other week) were used successfully in a macaw.[22] In bottlenose dolphins, withdrawing 7% to 17% of estimated blood volume, weekly for 22 to 30 weeks, successfully reduced SI and %TS.[29] For rhinoceroses and tapirs, treatment is recommended if %TS is 65% to 70% and/or SF is greater than 500 ng/mL (means for wild black rhinoceroses: 34%TS and 180 SF).[51] In black rhinoceroses, target volume for removal was 8 to 10 L per phlebotomy session, but actual volumes removed were only 1 to 4 L per session with one to two sessions per month; blood flow, keeper time, and animal cooperation were limiting factors.[45] Phlebotomy at 1% body weight 26 times over 25 weeks significantly improved iron analytes in a black-and-white ruffed lemur (BWRL, *Varecia varigata*) with biopsy-proven hemosiderosis but was not successful in treating a second BWRL with cirrhosis at time of initial presentation.[14]

Chelation may be used alone or in conjunction with phlebotomy. The most commonly used chelating drugs are injectable deferoxamine (DFO) and oral deferiprone.[5] The advantages of chelation are better mobilization of iron from tissues such as heart muscle and not having to induce anemia in cases of RBC disease and transfusion-induced ISD; however, these drugs may be toxic. In chickens and pigeons, gastrointestinal absorption of deferiprone is excellent at a dose of 50 mg/kg; therapeutic plasma concentrations were shown to be maintained for 8 hours.[69] In experimentally induced IO in these species, doses of 50 or 70 mg/kg orally once daily for 6 days significantly reduced liver iron concentration, decreased %TS, and increased iron concentration in excreta, sometimes evidenced by rust-colored urates. Adverse effects included decreased weight gain, decreased serum zinc levels, and 30% mortality in the chickens, possibly from rapid iron depletion. Low-iron diet (<80 ppm) plus DFO (50 mg/kg, intramuscularly [IM] four times in 12 hours for 14 days, 8 times over 20 months) reduced stainable iron in the liver and controlled diabetes in a macaw.[22] Deferiprone (75 mg/kg, orally [PO], once daily for 90 days) significantly decreased biopsy confirmed levels of liver iron in three hornbills with ISD.[56]

In common marmosets with experimentally induced IO, deferiprone was poorly absorbed orally and was given subcutaneously instead.[59] In spite of increased urinary iron excretion, LIC remained high even after 2 years on a low-iron diet and multiple chelation treatments. A combination of chelation (DFO 10 mg/kg, IM, every other day for 4 weeks) and phlebotomy (10 mL/kg, weekly) resulted in decreased SF, TS, SI, bilirubin, and bile acids in a lemur with severe hemochromatosis; however, the animal died of liver failure and hepatocellular carcinoma.[55]

CONCLUSION

In many iron-sensitive species, an evolutionary, genetic basis may exist for increased iron uptake, which may have evolved along with specific dietary ecologies, including frugivory, folivory, gumivory, palynivory, and insectivory. However, in both iron-sensitive and iron-insensitive species, high dietary iron, liver disease, systemic inflammation, metabolic syndrome, and, possibly, stress may drive iron accumulation. Changing diets to better reflect iron concentrations in wild-type diets has been shown to decrease IO in birds, rhinoceroses, and nonhuman primates. Establishing reference ranges for liver iron concentrations and serum iron analytes for more zoo species would facilitate diagnosis and monitoring of treatment in affected individuals.

ACKNOWLEDGMENTS

The authors appreciated all the many other fine publications on iron overload that could not be listed here because of editorial constraints. We also thank Dr. Dale Smith for helpful comments.

REFERENCES

1. Andrews NC: Disorders of iron metabolism. *N Eng J Med* 341:1986–1995, 1999.
2. Bai SP, Lu L, Luo XG, Liu B: Cloning, sequencing, characterization, and expressions of divalent metal transporter one in the small intestine of broilers. *Poult Sci* A87(4):768–776, 2008.
3. Batts K: Iron overload syndromes and the liver. *Mod Pathol* 20:S31–S39, 2007.
4. Bonar DV, Trupkiewicz JG, Toddes B, et al: Iron storage disease in tapirs. *J Zoo Wildl Med* 37(1):49–52, 2006.
5. Beutler E, Hoffbrand AV, Cook JD: Iron deficiency and overload. *Hematol Am Soc Hematol Educ Prog* 1:40–61, 2003.
6. Beutler E, West C, Speir JA, et al: The hHFE gene of browsing and grazing rhinoceroses: A possible site of adaptation to a low-iron diet. *Blood Cells Mol Dis* 27(1):342–350, 2001.
7. Borch-Iohnsen B, Thorstensen K: Iron distribution in the liver and duodenum during seasonal iron overload in Svalbard reindeer. *J Comp Pathol* 141(1):27–40, 2009.
8. Brown PJ, Whitbread TJ, Burden FA, et al: Haemosiderin deposition in donkey (*Equus asinus*) livers: Comparison of quantitative histochemistry for iron and liver iron content. *Res Vet Sci* 90(2):284–287, 2011.
9. Candra D, Radcliff RW, Mohammad Kahn A, et al: Browse diversity and iron loading in captive Sumatran rhinoceroses (*Dicerorhinus sumatrensis*): A comparison of sanctuary and zoological populations. *J Zoo Wildl Med* 43(3):S66–S73, 2012.
10. Clauss M, Dierenfeld E, Goff J, et al: IOD in rhinos—nutrition group report: Report from the nutrition working group of the international workshop in iron overload disorder in browsing rhinoceros (February 2011). *J Zoo Wildl Med* 43(3):S108–S113, 2012.

11. Clauss M, Hänichen T, Hummel J, et al: Excessive iron storage in captive omnivores? The case for the coati (*Nasua* spp.). In Fidgett A, Clauss M, Eulenberger K, editors: *Zoo animal nutrition*, vol III, Fürth, Germany, 2006, Filander Verlag, pp 91–99.

12. Clauss M, Paglia DE: Iron storage disorders in captive wild mammals: The comparative evidence. *J Zoo Wildl Med* 43(3):S6–S18, 2012.

13. Cork SC: Iron storage diseases in birds. *Avian Pathol* 29(1):7–12, 2000.

14. Crawford GC, Andrews GA, Chavey PS, et al: Survey and clinical application of serum iron, total iron binding capacity, transferrin saturation, and serum ferritin in captive black and white ruffed lemurs (*Varecia variegata variegata*). *J Zoo Wildl Med* 36(4):653–660, 2005.

15. Crawshaw G, Oyarzun S, Valdes E, et al: Hemochromatosis (iron storage disease) in fruit bats. In *Proceedings of the Annual Meeting of the Nutritional Advisory Group of the American Zoo and Aquarium Association*, Toronto, Canada, 1995, pp 136–147.

16. Crissey SD, Ward AM, Block SE, et al: Hepatic iron accumulation over time in European starlings (*Sturnus vulgaris*) fed two levels of iron. *J Zoo Wildl Med* 31(4):491–496, 2000.

17. Delaney MA, Nagy L, Kinsel MJ, et al: Spontaneous histologic lesions of the adult naked mole rat (*Heterocephalus glaber*): A retrospective survey of lesions in a zoo population. *Vet Pathol* 50(4):607–621, 2013.

18. Deugnier Y, Turlin B: Pathology of hepatic iron overload. *World J Gastroenterol* 13(35):4755–4760, 2007.

19. Drouin G, Godin JR, Pagé B: The genetics of vitamin C loss in vertebrates. *Curr Genom* 12(5):371–378, 2011.

20. EAZWV: Scientific Writing Experience. Serum iron metabolites in an opportunistic sample of different captive primate species. *Int Zoo YB* 46:195–200, 2012.

21. Farina LL, Heard DJ, LeBlanc DM, et al: Iron storage disease in captive Egyptian fruit bats (*Rousettus ageyptiacus*): Relationship of blood iron parameters to hepatic iron concentrations and hepatic histopathology. *J Zoo and Wildl Med* 36(2):212–221, 2005.

22. Gancz AY, Wellehan JF, Boutette J, et al: Diabetes mellitus concurrent with hepatic haemosiderosis in two macaws (*Ara severa, Ara militaris*). *Avian Pathol* 36(4):331–336, 2007.

23. Ganz T, Nemeth E: Iron homeostasis and its disorders in mice and men: Potential lessons for rhinos. *J Zoo Wildl Med* 43(3 Suppl):S19–S26, 2012.

24. Ganz T, Nemeth E: Hepcidin and iron homeostasis. *Biochim Biophys Acta* 1823(9):1434–1443, 2012.

25. Glenn KM, Campbell JL, Rotstein D, et al: Retrospective evaluation of the incidence and severity of hemosiderosis in a large captive lemur population. *Am J Primatol* 68(4):369–381, 2006.

26. He F, Ma L, Wang H, et al: Glucocorticoid causes iron accumulation in liver by up-regulating expression of iron regulatory protein 1 gene through GR and STAT5. *Cell Biochem Biophys* 61(1):65–71, 2011.

27. Helmick KE, Kendrick EL, Dierenfeld ES: Diet manipulation as treatment for elevated serum iron parameters in captive Raggiana bird of paradise (*Paradisaea raggiana*). *J Zoo Wildl Med* 42(3):460–467, 2011.

28. Hilton KB, Lambert LA: Molecular evolution and characterization of hepcidin gene products in vertebrates. *Gene* 415(1–2):40–48, 2008.

29. Johnson SP, Venn-Watson SK, Cassle SE, et al: Use of phlebotomy treatment in Atlantic bottlenose dolphins with iron overload. *J Am Vet Med Assoc* 235(2):194–200, 2009.

30. Klasing KC, Dierenfeld ES, Koutsos EA: Avian iron storage disease: Variations on a common theme? *J Zoo Wildl Med* 43(3):S27–S34, 2012.

31. Klopfleisch R, Olias P: The pathology of comparative animal models of human haemochromatosis. *J Comp Pathol* 147(4):460–478, 2012.

32. Kohgo Y, Ikuta K, Ohtake T, et al: Body iron metabolism and pathophysiology if iron overload. *Int J Hematol* 88(1):7–15, 2008.

33. Lavin SR: Plant phenolics and their potential role in mitigating iron overload disorder in wild animals. *J Zoo Wildl Med* 43(3 Suppl):S74–S82, 2012.

34. Lavin SR, Chen Z, Abrams SA: Effect of tannic acid on iron absorption in straw-colored fruit bats (*Eidolon helvum*). *Zoo Biol* 29(3):335–343, 2010.

35. Leone AM, Crawshaw GJ, Garner MM, et al: A retrospective study of the lesions associated with iron storage disease in captive Egyptian fruit bats (*Rousettus aegyptiacus*). In *Proceedings of the American Association of Zoo Veterinarians Annual Conference*, Oakland, CA, 2012, p 210.

36. Lipiński P, Styś A, Starzyński RR: Molecular insights into the regulation of iron metabolism during the prenatal and early postnatal periods. *Cell Mol Life Sci* 70(1):23–38, 2013.

37. Lowenstine LJ, Munson L: Iron overload in the animal kingdom. In Fowler ME, Miller RE, editors: *Zoo and wild animal medicine: Current therapy*, ed 4, Philadelphia, PA, 1999, Saunders, pp 260–268.

38. Matheson JS, Paul-Murphy J, O'Brien RT, et al: Quantitative ultrasound, magnetic resonance imaging, and histologic image analysis of hepatic iron accumulation in pigeons (*Columba livia*). *J Zoo Wildl Med* 38(2):222–230, 2007.

39. Mazzaro LM, Dunn JL, St Aubin DJ, et al: Serum indices of body stores of iron in northern fur seals (*Callorhinus ursinus*) and their relationship to hemochromatosis. *Zoo Biol* 23(3):205–218, 2004.

40. Mete A: *Etiology of iron overload in captive birds (PhD thesis)*, The Netherlands, 2005, Utrecht University.

41. Mete A, van Zeeland YR, Vaandrager AB, et al: Partial purification and characterization of ferritin from the liver and intestinal mucosa of chickens, turtledoves and mynahs. *Avian Pathol* 34(5):430–434, 2005.

42. Mete A, Jalving R, van Oost BA, et al: Intestinal over-expression of iron transporters induces iron overload in birds in captivity. *Blood Cells Mol Dis* 34(2):151–156, 2005.

43. Mete A, Hendriks HG, Klaren PH, et al: Iron metabolism in mynah birds (*Gracula religiosa*) resembles human hereditary haemochromatosis. *Avian Pathol* 32(6):625–632, 2003.

44. Miller GF, Barnard DE, Woodward RA, et al: Hepatic hemosiderosis in common marmosets, *Callithrix jacchus*: Effect of diet on incidence and severity. *Lab Anim Sci* 47(2):138–142, 1997.

45. Mylniczenko NE, Sullivan KE, Corcoran ME, et al: Management strategies of iron accumulation in a captive population of black rhinoceroses (*Diceros bicornis minor*). *J Zoo Wildl Med* 43(3 Suppl):S83–S92, 2012.

46. Nielsen BD, Vic MM, Dennis PM: A potential link between insulin resistance and iron overload disorder in browsing rhinoceroses investigated through the use of an equine model. *J Zoo Wildl Med* 43(3 Suppl):S61–S65, 2012.

47. Ninomiya R, Koizumi N, Murata K: Concentrations of cadmium, zinc, copper, iron, and metallothionein in liver and kidney of nonhuman primates. *Biol Trace Elem Res* 87(1–3):95–111, 2002.

48. Norambuena MC, Bozinovic F: Effect of malnutrition on iron homeostasis in black-necked swans (*Cygnus melancoryphus*). *J Zoo Wildl Med* 40(4):624–631, 2009.

49. Olias P, Mundhenk L, Bothe M, et al: Iron overload syndrome in the black rhinoceros (*Diceros bicornis*): Microscopical lesions and comparison with other rhinoceros species. *J Comp Pathol* 47(4):542–549, 2012.

50. Olias P, Weiss AT, Gruber AD, et al: Iron storage disease in red deer (*Cervus elaphus elaphus*) is not associated with mutations in the HFE gene. *J Comp Pathol* 145(2–3):207–213, 2011.

51. Paglia DE: Recommended phlebotomy guidelines for prevention and therapy of captivity-induced iron storage disease in rhinoceroses, tapirs and other exotic wildlife. In *Proceedings of the AAZV, AAWV, WDA Joint Conference*, San Diego, CA, 2004, pp 122–127.

52. Paglia DE, Miller CL, Foerster SH, et al: Evidence for acquired iron overload in captive tapirs (*Tapirus* spp.). In *Proceedings of the American Association Zoo Veterinarians Annual Conference*, New Orleans, LA, 2000, pp 124–126.

53. Paglia DE, Tsu IH: Review of laboratory and necropsy evidence for iron storage disease acquired by browser rhinoceroses. *J Zoo Wildl Med* 43(3 Suppl):S92–S104, 2012.

54. Pereira LQ, Strefezzi Rde F, Catão-Dias JL, et al: Hepatic hemosiderosis in red-spectacled Amazons (*Amazona pretrei*) and correlation with nutritional aspects. *Avian Dis* 54(4):1323–1326, 2010.

55. Sanchez CR, Murray S, Montali RJ: Use of desferoxamine and S-adenosylmethionine to treat hemochromatosis in a red ruffed lemur (*Varecia variegata ruber*). *Comp Med* 54(1):100–103, 2004.

56. Sandmeier P, Clauss M, Donati OF, et al: Use of deferiprone for the treatment of hepatic iron storage disease in three hornbills. *J Am Vet Med Assoc* 240(1):75–81, 2012.

57. Santos SV, Strefezzi R de F, Pissinatti A, et al: Liver iron overloading in captive muriquis (*Brachyteles* spp.). *J Med Primatol* 40(2):129–134, 2011.

58. Seibels B, Lamberski N, Gregory CR, et al: Effective use of tea to limit dietary iron available to starlings (*Sturnus vulgaris*). *J Zoo Wildl Med* 34(3):314–316, 2003.

59. Sergejew T, Forgiarini P, Schnebli HP: Chelator-induced iron excretion in iron-overloaded marmosets. *Br J Haematol* 110(4):985–992, 2000.

60. Sheppard C, Dierenfeld E: Iron storage disease in birds: Speculation on etiology and implications for captive husbandry. *J Avian Med Surg* 16(3):192–197, 2002.

61. Siddique A, Kowdley KV: Review article: The iron overload syndromes. *Aliment Pharmacol Ther* 35(8):876–893, 2012.

62. Smith KM, McAloose D, Torregrossa A, et al: Hematologic iron analyte values as an indicator of hepatic hemosiderosis in Callitrichidae. *Am J Primatol* 70(7):629–633, 2008.

63. Spelman LJ, Osborn KG, Anderson MP: Pathogenesis of hemosideroiss in lemurs: Role of dietary iron, tannin and ascorbic acid. *Zoo Biol* 8(3):239–251, 1989.

64. Stasiak I: *The role of hepcidin in regulation of iron balance in bats (DVSc thesis)*, Guelph, Ontario, Canada, 2012, University of Guelph. http://atrium.lib.uoguelph.ca/xmlui/bitstream/handle/10214/4014/Stasiak_Iga_201209_DVSc.pdf?sequence=7. Accessed December 1, 2012.

65. Tako E, Rutzke MA, Glahn RP: Using the domestic chicken (*Gallus gallus*) as an in vivo model for iron bioavailability. *Poult Sci* 89(3):514–521, 2010.

66. Venn-Watson S, Benham C, Carlin K, et al: Hemochromatosis and fatty liver disease: building evidence for insulin resistance in bottlenose dolphins (*Tursiops truncatus*). *J Zoo Wildl Med* 43(3):S35–S47, 2012.

67. Walker EM, Jr, Walker SM: Effects of iron overload on the immune system. *Ann Clin Lab Sci* 30(4):354–365, 2000.

68. West GD, Garner MM, Talcott PA: Hemochromatosis in several species of lories with high dietary iron. *J Avian Med Surg* 15(4):297–301, 2001.

69. Whiteside DP, Barker IK, Mehren KG, et al: Clinical evaluation of the oral iron chelator deferiprone for the potential treatment of iron overload in bird species. *J Zoo Wildl Med* 35(1):40–49, 2004.

70. Williams CV, Campbell J, Glenn KM: Comparison of serum iron, total iron binding capacity, ferritin, and percent transferrin saturation in nine species of apparently healthy captive lemurs. *Am J Primatol* 68(5):477–489, 2006.

71. Williams CV, Junge RE, Stalis IH: Evaluation of iron status in lemurs by analysis of serum iron and ferritin concentrations, total iron-binding capacity, and transferrin saturation. *J Am Vet Med Assoc* 232(4):578–585, 2008.

72. Wood C, Fang SG, Hunt A, et al: Increased iron absorption in lemurs: Quantitative screening and assessment of dietary prevention. *Am J Primatol* 61(3):101–110, 2003.

73. Xu Q, Fang S, Wang Z, Wang Z: Heavy metal distribution in tissues and eggs of Chinese alligator (*Alligator sinensis*). *Arch Environ Contam Toxicol* 50(4):580–586, 2006.

74. Zadrozny LM, Williams CV, Remick AK, et al: Spontaneous hepatocellular carcinoma in captive prosimians. *Vet Pathol* 47(2):306–311, 2010.

75. Zhao Z, Li S, Liu G, et al: Body iron stores and heme-iron intake in relation to risk of type 2 diabetes: A systematic review and meta-analysis. *PLoS ONE* 7(7):e41641, 2012.

CHAPTER 70

The Journal of Zoo and Wildlife Medicine

R. Eric Miller

With a circulation of nearly 1500 in 2013, the *Journal of Zoo and Wildlife Medicine* (JZWM) is one of the most read international, scientific, peer-reviewed journals that features articles on the diagnosis, treatment surgery, and preventive medicine of zoo animals and free-ranging wildlife. It is the official journal of the American Association of Zoo Veterinarians (AAZV), the European Association of Zoo and Wildlife Veterinarians (EAZWV), the American College of Zoological Medicine (ACZM), the European Association of Zoos and Aquariums (EAZA), and the World Association of Zoos and Aquariums (WAZA).

The JZWM was founded by the AAZV in 1970 titled as the *Journal of Zoo Animal Medicine* and has always been published quarterly. It quickly became a major vehicle for the dissemination of information about zoo animal medicine in North America and later developed an international authorship and readership. It was, and still is,

affectionately known by many as the "giraffe" journal because of the prominent giraffe logo on its cover (Figure 70-1). However, in 1987, the logo was revised, with the addition of more species, including cervid, amphibian, shark, avian, chelonian rhinoceros, primate, and cheetah species (Figure 70-2).

Pages of the early editions were printed and stapled together, and although these editions were simple, they contained an interesting mix of case reports and short studies that served as a primary vehicle for dissemination of information in the growing field of zoo medicine. The four journals have grown from an average of 128 pages per year in 1974 to over 1000 pages in 2012. The JZWM is now organized under the sections Review Articles, Case Series Reports, Brief Communications, and Clinical Challenges. Early editors worked on their own to a great extent and their work was vital to the early and continuing function of the JZWM (Box 70-1). In the 1900s, some

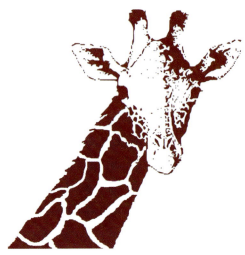

FIGURE 70-1 The original giraffe logo for *the Journal of Zoo Animal Medicine*. (Courtesy of American Association of Zoo Veterinarians.)

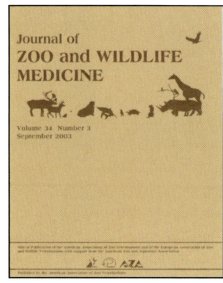

FIGURE 70-2 The current cover design of the *Journal of Zoo and Wildlife Medicine*. (Courtesy of American Association of Zoo Veterinarians.)

BOX 70-1 Editors of the *Journal of Zoo Animal Medicine* and the *Journal of Zoo and Wildlife Medicine*

Joel Wallach, DVM, and Weaver Williamson: 1970–1973
Don Farst, DVM: 1973–1978
Murray E. Fowler, DVM, DACZM, DACVIM, DABVT: 1978–1988
James Carpenter, DVM, DACZM: 1988–1992
Duane Ullrey, PhD: 1992–1995
Wilbur Amand, VMD: 1995–2005
Teresa Y. Morishita, DVM, PhD, DACPV: 2005–Present

---

editions were dedicated to specialty topics, and more recently in 2012, the findings of a workshop on iron storage issues in rhinoceroses were published as a supplement, and more such supplements are anticipated.

In 2010, the *JZWM* became available digitally, which greatly accelerated its dissemination around the world, particularly in countries where publication costs are prohibitive. Translations of *JZWM* abstracts into various languages (Chinese, French, German, Japanese, Portuguese, Russian, Spanish) have been made available online (www.aazv/jzwm). As the translation work is done by volunteers, the availability of materials in some languages has been variable.

As noted, *JZWM* is now the official journal of the AAZV and the EAZWV; in recent years, the *JZWM* has also become the official journal of the ACZM, the EAZA, and the WAZA. In 2010, following many years of negotiations, the EAZWV and the AAZV signed a Memorandum of Understanding, which made the *JZWM* the official joint journal of both organizations, and a membership benefit for each was provided. This increasing international outlook to the *JZWM* is reflected in the primary authorship: In 2012, 53% of the senior authors were non-American, coming from 42 countries across the world. The four countries with the highest totals of submissions were Brazil (21), France (10), South Africa (10), and Spain (8). Also, since 2012, an electronic version of the *JZWM* has been made available to veterinarians in developing countries through a reduced fee program supported by the AAZV and now the EAZWV as well.

The result of all of these efforts is that the *JZWM* has become a vital tool in the advancement of knowledge for zoo and wildlife veterinarians. Institutional or individual subscriptions to the *JZWM* may be made as members of the AAZV, the EAZWV, and the other organizations noted above.

ACKNOWLEDGMENTS

The author wishes to acknowledge Murray Fowler, Rob Hilsenroth, and Teresa Morishita for their contributions to and review of this article and their contributions to the *JZWM*.

CHAPTER 71

A Legal Overview for Zoologic Medicine Veterinarians

Gregory M. Dennis[†] and David S. Miller

This chapter is a general overview of some laws of the United States and other countries, as well as regulations, policies, court decisions, and international treaties for zoologic medicine veterinarians* or others who might want such information as relevant to treating or handling wild or zoo animals. This chapter is not a detailed analysis of each law, regulation, policy, treaty, or court decision pertaining to veterinarians or other persons treating or handling wild or zoo animals.‡ Certain regulations have been fully quoted because an awareness of their precise wording may often be critical to ensure compliance and to support decisions where any misunderstanding or miscomprehension could have legal ramifications.

LEGAL STATUS OF WILD ANIMALS— UNITED STATES

Countries with legal systems rooted in English common law tend to classify animals under two categories: (1) *domitoe naturoe* (domesticated or tame) animals and (2) *feroe naturae* (wild) animals.[1] Unlike domesticated animals, wild animals generally cannot be owned by individuals. Rather, wild animals are considered to be owned by or held in trust by the government for the benefit of its people.[2] Even if an individual captures and keeps a wild animal, the possession is considered only temporary and is lost if the wild animal escapes.[3] Wild animals are generally considered to be owned by the state in which they are located, and occasionally, American federal law may step in and designate certain animals, commonly endangered species, as being under its protection.[4]

INFECTIOUS DISEASE CONTROL— UNITED STATES

Control of infectious diseases has been one of the most important responsibilities of veterinarians. Regulations concerning the prevention of exposure to foreign animal diseases or limiting endemic diseases are generally targeted toward production animals used for food and fiber. However, the potential for these diseases to be transmitted to nondomestic species, particularly free-ranging populations or the potential for nondomestic species to serve as reservoirs and vectors of disease can greatly impact the activities of zoologic

medicine veterinarians, as livestock represent a multibillion dollar international industry with interests that generally supersede the interests of nondomestic species.

The United States Department of Agriculture, Animal and Plant Health Inspection Service, Veterinary Services (APHIS-VS) has the responsibility for safeguarding animal health and other livestock concerns and also regulates veterinary biologics that may be used in the practice of zoologic medicine. The responsibilities of the APHIS-VS include, but are not limited to, establishing policies and practices to limit introduction of foreign animal diseases and coordination of disease control responses with the World Organisation for Animal Health (Office of International Epizootics [OIE]) and other international entities. The APHIS-VS has also established the National Veterinary Accreditation Program (NVAP) as a means of enlisting support among nongovernmental veterinarians for foreign and endemic disease programs, emergency management and disease control programs (e.g., for tuberculosis, brucellosis, and other diseases), and coordination of animal shipping and control of disease among states with varying animal health regulations. Testing and examination of animals for interstate transport is one of the common responsibilities of many zoologic medicine veterinarians. Adherence to legal responsibilities is required for continued or nondisciplined licensure to practice veterinary medicine. Although the NVAP is federally managed, accreditation duties are held at the state level.

Recent changes include online availability of continuing education modules on transmission, recognition, and reporting of exotic and emerging diseases and establishment of Category I (mostly small mammal companion animal species) and Category II (all animals) accreditation levels. Key to NVAP is accredited veterinarians' adherence to the program and the profession's legal responsibilities. The *Code of Federal Regulations* (CFR), having the force of law, is the comprehensive and detailed "rule book," which contains all of the current federal regulations and provides directions for prior versions. In addition to the CFRs, all veterinarians should be aware that besides infectious disease concerns, the OIE's *Terrestrial Animal Health Code 2012* and *Aquatic Animal Health Code 2010* (Boxes 71-1 and 71-2) include veterinary and animal welfare standards that have international ramifications.

ANIMAL WELFARE ACT—UNITED STATES

In 1966, President Lyndon Johnson signed into law the *Animal Welfare Act* (AWA). Since its original enactment, it has been strengthened and expanded. Today, the AWA sets minimum standards for the care and treatment of certain animals: "regulated animals" (or "AWA animals"). The AWA does not cover "nonregulated" animals; however, matters involving nonregulated animals that affect regulated animals might come under the authority of the United States Department of Agriculture (USDA)-APHIS (or, simply, "APHIS") but only to the extent of the affected AWA regulated animals.

Depending on particular circumstances, place of employment, and entity or person to whom veterinary services are being provided, veterinarians may find themselves having to comply with various regulations, policies, and guidelines of APHIS. The two principal

---

*For this chapter, the term "veterinarian" also includes "veterinary doctor," "veterinary medical doctor," "veterinary practitioner," "practitioner of veterinary medicine," "practitioner of veterinary surgery," "veterinary surgeon," and "veterinarian practitioner."

†Deceased.

‡**THIS CHAPTER IS NOT INTENDED TO BE NOR SHOULD IT BE, USED OR RELIED UPON BY ANY PERSON AS LEGAL ADVICE OR AS AN ALTERNATIVE OR SUBSTITUTE FOR LEGAL ADVICE. READERS ARE STRONGLY ENCOURAGED TO CONSULT WITH A LICENSED, REGISTERED, COMPETENT KNOWLEDGEABLE ATTORNEY, LAWYER, COUNSELOR, SOLICITOR, OR LEGAL ADVISOR IN THEIR COUNTRY, PROVINCE, DISTRICT, STATE, OR JURISDICTION ABOUT ANY LEGAL ISSUES, SUBJECTS, OR MATTERS THAT MIGHT BE MENTIONED IN THIS CHAPTER AND/OR ABOUT TREATING OR HANDLING WILD OR ZOO ANIMALS.**

BOX 71-1 Terrestrial Animal Health Code: Article 3.4.6: Veterinarians and veterinary para-professionals

1. *Veterinary medicine/science:* In order to ensure quality in the conduct of veterinary medicine/science, the veterinary legislation should provide a definition of veterinary medicine/science sufficient to address the following;
   a. define the prerogatives of veterinarians and of the various categories of veterinary para-professionals that are recognised by the Member Country;
   b. define the minimum initial and continuous educational requirements and competencies for veterinarians and veterinary para-professionals;
   c. prescribe the conditions for recognition of the qualifications for veterinarians and veterinary para-professionals;
   d. define the conditions to perform the activities of veterinary medicine/science; and
   e. identify the exceptional situations, such as epizootics, under which persons other than veterinarians may undertake activities that are normally carried out by veterinarians.
2. *The control of veterinarians and veterinary para-professionals:* Veterinary legislation should provide a basis for regulation of veterinarians and veterinary para-professionals in the public interest. To that end, the legislation should:
   a. describe the general system of control in terms of the political, administrative and geographic configuration of the country;
   b. describe the various categories of veterinary para-professionals recognised by the Member Country according to its needs, notably in animal health and food safety, and for each category, prescribe its training, qualifications, tasks and extent of supervision;
   c. prescribe the powers to deal with conduct and competence issues, including licensing requirements, that apply to veterinarians and veterinary para-professionals;
   d. provide for the possibility of delegation of powers to a professional organisation such as a veterinary statutory body; and
   e. where powers have been so delegated, describe the prerogatives, the functioning and responsibilities of the mandated professional organisation.

From 2010 ©OIE—Terrestrial Animal Health Code, World Organisation for Animal Health.

BOX 71-2[57,58] Terrestrial Animal Health Code: Article 6.11.2: Zoonotic diseases transmissible from nonhuman primates

"Veterinary Authorities of exporting countries should issue international veterinary certificates only upon presentation of valid *CITES* documentation.

Veterinary Authorities should make sure that the animals are individually identified by approved methods that assure traceability and to avoid transmission of disease (*see* Chapter 4.15: *Hygiene Precautions, Identification, Blood Sampling and Vaccination*[1]).

For reasons of public health, animal welfare and pathogen introduction to wild populations, Veterinary Authorities of importing countries should not authorise the import of non-human primates for the purpose of being kept as pets.

In the case of a non-human primate being imported directly from a country within the natural range of the animal's species concerned, and where only limited diagnostic testing is available, Veterinary Authorities of importing countries should place more emphasis on quarantine procedures and less on veterinary certification. As a matter of principle, limited health guarantees given by the supplier or the Veterinary Authority of the country of origin should not constitute an obstacle to imports, but very strict post import quarantine requirements should be imposed. Particularly, the quarantine should meet the standards set in Chapter 5.9 (*Quarantine measures applicable to non-human primates*[2]), and should be of sufficient length to minimise the risk of transmission of diseases where tests are not readily available or of limited value.

Veterinary Authorities of importing countries may reduce the quarantine requirements for non-human primates imported from premises with permanent veterinary supervision provided that the animals were born or have been kept for at least two years on these premises, are individually identified and accompanied by proper certification issued by qualified officials, and the official certification is supplemented by a complete documentation of the clinical history of each animal and its group of origin.

In cases where it is necessary to import non-human primates which are known or suspected to be carriers of a zoonotic disease, the import should not be restricted by any of these recommendations, provided that the Veterinary Authority of the importing country requires the placing of the animals in an establishment located on its territory which has been approved to receive them and which meets the standards set in Chapter 5.9 (*Quarantine measures applicable to non-human primates*)."

From 2010 ©OIE—Terrestrial Animal Health Code, World Organisation for Animal Health.

regulations that zoological medicine veterinarians must be aware of are as follows:

1. *9 CFR § 2.40 (Dealer and exhibitors [Zoos]:* Attending veterinarian and adequate veterinary care), to-wit:
   "(a) Each dealer or exhibitor shall have an attending veterinarian who shall provide adequate veterinary care to its animals in compliance with this section.
      (1) Each dealer and exhibitor shall employ an attending veterinarian under formal arrangements. In the case of a part-time attending veterinarian or consultant arrangements, the formal arrangements shall include a written program of veterinary care[5] and regularly scheduled visits to the premises of the dealer or exhibitor; and
      (2) Each dealer and exhibitor shall assure that the attending veterinarian has appropriate authority to ensure the provision of adequate veterinary care and to oversee the adequacy of other aspects of animal care and use.
   (b) Each dealer or exhibitor shall establish and maintain programs of adequate veterinary care that include:
      (1) The availability of appropriate facilities, personnel, equipment, and services to comply with the provisions of this subchapter;

   (2) The use of appropriate methods to prevent, control, diagnose, and treat diseases and injuries, and the availability of emergency, weekend, and holiday care;
   (3) Daily observation of all animals to assess their health and well-being; *Provided, however,* That daily observation of animals may be accomplished by someone other than the attending veterinarian; and *Provided, further,* That a mechanism of direct and frequent communication is required so that timely and accurate information on problems of animal health, behavior, and well-being is conveyed to the attending veterinarian;
   (4) Adequate guidance to personnel involved in the care and use of animals regarding handling, immobilization, anesthesia, analgesia, tranquilization, and euthanasia; and
   (5) Adequate pre-procedural and post-procedural care in accordance with established veterinary medical and nursing procedures."

It has been judicially declared that it is not a reasonable interpretation of "adequate veterinary care" in 9 CFR § 2.40 [for APHIS] "to insist that all the animals under such care should have unflaggingly perfect health."[6]

2. *9 C.F.R. § 2.33:* Veterinarians working at research facilities should also be aware of this regulation and its provisions pertaining to the facility's Institutional Animal Care and Use Committee (IACUC).

APHIS does not issue licenses for veterinarians, but much can stem from these regulations, which may impact veterinarians treating or handling AWA-regulated animals and, derivatively, their state licenses to practice veterinary medicine.

Veterinarians treating or handling animals should also be familiar with, among other items, the following:

- 9 CFR § 2.32: Research facilities; Personnel qualifications
- § 2.35: Research facilities; Recordkeeping requirements
- § 2.75: Records; Dealers and exhibitors
- § 2.78: Health certification and identification
- § 2.131: Handling of animals
- § 3.110: Marine mammal; Veterinary care
- 9 CFR Part H: Compliance with Standards and Holding Period [9 CFR §§ 2.100, .101 and .102]
- Animal Care Resource Guide Policies, in particular:
  - Policy # 1: Control of Tuberculosis in Regulated Elephants
  - Policy # 3: Veterinary Care
  - Policy # 4: Necropsy Requirements
  - Policy # 7: Brachiating Species of Nonhuman Primates
  - Policy # 11: Painful and Distressful Procedures
  - Policy # 12: Consideration of Alternatives to Painful / Distressful Procedures
  - Policy # 14: Major Survival Surgery, Dealers Selling Surgically-Altered Animals to Research[7]
  - Animal Care Inspection Guide, Chapter 8.0: Veterinary Care

Veterinarians performing a necropsy on an AWA-regulated animal species when she or he has not previously done a postmortem examination on that species should bear in mind Policy # 4, which requires that necropsy be done "by or under the *direct* supervision of a veterinarian experienced with that species" (*emphasis added*). Unlike state veterinary practice acts or veterinary board regulations, neither the AWA nor its companion CFR defines "direct supervision" or, for that matter, "indirect supervision." Consequently, veterinarians should be aware what is legally required for "direct supervision" in the state in which they are performing such a first-time necropsy. Typically, direct supervision requires the supervising veterinarian to be on the premises.[8] In contrast, indirect supervision commonly entails the supervising veterinarian being readily available, by telephone or other means of immediate communication, or having given either written or oral instructions before leaving the premises.[9] This requirement might be in conflict with regulations mandating necropsy of a captive collection animal.

Maintenance of adequate veterinary medical records is important.[10] This includes a reliable and secure system for backing up and archiving records.[11] Failure to do so may result in USDA-APHIS citations and sanctions. What constitutes "adequate" records is not any one veterinarian's personal opinion about what should be—or should have been—documented but what APHIS' regulations, policies, and inspection guidelines require to be documented.[12] APHIS tends to categorize records into "required" and "recommended."[13] APHIS requires records to be kept for at least 1 year after an animal's death or disposition with research facilities having to keep them for at least 3 years after either occurrence.[14] Necropsy reports are to be kept for at least 3 years following the examination.[15]

Except in the case of marine mammals, APHIS should issue an inadequate recordkeeping citation only in conjunction with related noncompliant items (e.g., animal well-being, etc.). "A lack of any of these records or inadequacy of these records may not be cited as a stand-alone violation."[16] Besides APHIS regulations, other USDA divisions, US-DEA, and state and provincial board regulations also have requirements for documentation. Also, adherence to federal requirements is not a defense to state requirements if the state requires more,[17] and vice versa.

All veterinarians working at an APHIS-licensed facility are subject to the regulations, policies, and guidelines of APHIS. No distinction is made between an employee-veterinarian and a contract or independent-contractor veterinarian except that the latter must sign a written *Program of Veterinary Care* (PVC).[18]

An APHIS regulation[19] appears to prohibit, at least research facilities, from discriminating or taking retaliatory actions against employees, committee members, or laboratory personnel who report to APHIS violations of any regulation or standards. However, under the AWA, court decisions have ruled that regulation does not give the employee the right to sue, as the AWA's purpose is not to protect humans but only animals.[20]

ENDANGERED SPECIES ACT AND RELATED LAWS (UNITED STATES) AND CONVENTION ON INTERNATIONAL TRADE IN ENDANGERED SPECIES OF WILD FAUNA AND FLORA

A foundational purpose of the *Endangered Species Act*[21] (ESA) was, and still remains, the promotion of measures to protect species threatened by immediate or foreseeable extinction.[22] The ESA is administered by the United States Fish and Wildlife Service (FWS) and the National Oceanic and Atmospheric Administration (NOAA), with NOAA being primarily responsible for marine species. Atlantic sturgeon, sea turtles, and other species in marine and fresh water environments are jointly managed by the FWS and the NOAA and other federal agencies with responsibilities for enforcing various statutes, regulations, and international treaties. Threats to a species outside of the United States and its overseas territories or possessions are considered part of a species' rating.

The *Migratory Bird Treaty Act* (MBTA)[23] between the United States and Canada and the *Convention on International Trade in Endangered Species of Wild Fauna and Flora* (CITES), which became effective on July 1, 1975, are internationally significant treaties. CITES signatory nations can still enforce and adopt domestic laws or measures that are stronger or stricter than CITES.

Similar American laws (e.g., *African Elephant Conservation Act*,[24] *Marine Mammal Protection Act*,[25] and *National Environmental Protection Act*[26]) and foreign laws and treaties are in effect, but ESA, MBTA, and CITES are central to the practice of zoologic medicine in the United States. What is shared by these laws and treaties is limitation, with civil and criminal penalties for the taking, possession, and transport of threatened, endangered, or otherwise protected species. These laws and treaties are generally concerned with protecting animals in their natural environments from harvest, transport, euthanasia, handling, or possession of live animals; biomedical sampling or other such activity is highly regulated, so familiarity with client (animal owner/possessor) and veterinary responsibilities for exhibition, research, conservation is critical.

In addition to the above, veterinarians should ensure and maintain compliance with agricultural (e.g., APHIS-VS), human health (e.g., Centers for Disease Control [CDC]), and veterinary public health permits at the state, provincial, national, and international levels, including with aboriginal peoples. Finally, Institutional Animal Care and Use Committees (IACUCs) often have oversight over research and other regulated activities.

LAWSUITS OR LEGAL CLAIMS FOR OR BY ANIMALS

The ESA grants individuals legal standing to file lawsuits to enforce its provisions, and some lawsuits have named an animal, group of animals, or species as plaintiffs or aggrieved parties. Alternatively, a human may be named as a guardian, or guardian ad litem, for an animal, as for a child or mentally incompetent person,[27] or the court may be requested to consider the animal a "legal person."[28] Such legal endeavors in the United States and other countries[29] have largely been rejected by the courts,[30] but they continue to be made.

TERRESTRIAL ANIMAL HEALTH CODE—WORLD ORGANISATION FOR ANIMAL HEALTH

The *Terrestrial Animal Health Code 2012* of the World Organisation for Animal Health (OIE) has established worldwide standards for the improvement of the health and welfare of terrestrial animal (mammals, birds, and bees) and veterinary public health.[31] Rules for safe international trade in terrestrial animals and their products is included within these standards. According to the OIE, the "health measures in the *Terrestrial Code* should be used by the veterinary authorities of importing and exporting countries to provide for early detection, reporting and control agents pathogenic to terrestrial animals and, in the case of zoonoses, for humans, and to prevent their transfer via international trade in terrestrial animals and terrestrial animal products, while avoiding unjustified sanitary barriers to trade."[32] (See Boxes 71-1 and 71-2.)

CONTROLLED SUBSTANCES ACT (CSA)—UNITED STATES; FOOD, DRUG, AND COSMETIC ACT (FDCA)—UNITED STATES; AND LAWS ON FOREIGN CONTROLLED SUBSTANCES, DRUGS, OR DANGEROUS DRUGS

Veterinarians having a U.S. Drug Enforcement Administration (US-DEA) registration in one state may not administer, dispense, or prescribe a controlled substance in another state until they also have US-DEA registration for that state.[33] Also, possessing a US-DEA and/or an American state-controlled substance registration does not mean that a U.S.-licensed veterinarian or any other "practitioner"[34] holding such a registration can carry or import into another country controlled substances, controlled drugs, controlled medications, or dangerous drugs. Nor does a U.S.-DEA registration empower an American veterinarian or any other practitioner to administer, dispense, distribute, or prescribe any controlled substances or other prescription medication[35] in another country.[36] Additionally, a nonprescription over-the-counter (OTC) drug in one country may be deemed a prescription drug, controlled drug, dangerous drug, or banned substance in another.[37]

In summary, American veterinarians[38] or other practitioners have no right or privilege to fail to comply with another nation's drug laws while in that nation,[39] as this may result in severe penalties,[40] including capital punishment.[41] Additionally, a conviction in one country might provide a basis for veterinary disciplinary action in the veterinarian's home country up to and including loss of license or being struck off the roll.[42]

The US-DEA's *Export Waiver for International Humanitarian or Veterinarian Charitable Assistance*—"Medical Missions"—program has no force or effect in any foreign country.[43] That program simply provides a means by which US-DEA registrants may seek a waiver of federal law requirements to legally *export* controlled substances from the United States[44] for use in an international veterinary charitable mission, not for importation of such drugs into a foreign country for their administration, dispensing, or distribution in that country.

APHIS' *Animal Care Resources Guide Policies*, Policy # 3: *Veterinary Care* (March 25, 2011) prohibits the use of expired drugs for AWA-regulated animals. However, APHIS "has no jurisdiction over facilities using expired medical materials for *nonregulated* animals or *nonregulated* activities"[45] (*emphasis added*). Additionally, Policy # 3 states that "[f]or acute terminal procedures, where an animal is put under anesthesia, the research is carried out (surgery or testing of a compound) and the animal is euthanized without ever waking up, medical materials may be used beyond their 'to be used by' date if

such materials use does not adversely affect the animal's well-being or compromise the validity of the scientific study." Regardless of the immediate above, this APHIS policy declares that for all veterinary procedures, expired anesthesia, analgesia, emergency, and euthanasia drugs cannot be used.

MINOR USE AND MINOR SPECIES ANIMAL HEALTH ACT (MUMS)—UNITED STATES

In 2001, the United States enacted the *Minor Use and Minor Special Animal Health Act*, better known as MUMS, with amendments made in 2004.[46] The purpose of *MUMS* is (or, some might say, was) to provide the United States Food and Drug Administration (US-FDA) with a means to provide authorization for drugs for less common species or uses. Even with MUMS, drug availability for zoo and wild animals has remained limited in the United States.

Periodically, the US-FDA, through its Division of Dockets Management, publishes a list of MUMS drugs,[47] as well as drugs that have been removed from the designated list.[48] Veterinarians treating or handling wild or zoo animals should regularly check these lists to determine if a drug is on the MUMS list or has been removed.

COMPOUNDING OF DRUGS—UNITED STATES

Currently, compounding of drugs by American veterinarians is in a state of flux. Some state pharmacy laws still acknowledge that veterinarians can compound drugs in their clinics for the animals they are treating,[49] whereas others do not allow it or are silent on the subject.

Particularly, status of companies doing bulk compounding of prescription (legend or veterinary legend) drugs[50] or controlled substances[51] for veterinarians remains undetermined. Given the uncertainty at the time of this writing, zoo and wildlife veterinarians are strongly encouraged to check with their state veterinary and pharmacy boards and an experienced attorney about compounding of drugs and controlled substances.

OFF-LABEL OR EXTRA-LABEL USE OF CONTROLLED SUBSTANCES—UNITED STATES

Given the limited range of drugs approved for use in animals in the United States, many veterinarians have found that they cannot practice veterinary medicine without off-label or extra-label use of drugs. Although this is common, the US-DEA has not been so flexible toward off-label or extra-label use of controlled substances.[52]

VETERINARIANS UNLAWFULY PRACTICING VETERINARY MEDICINE

As in the case of laws on controlled substances and prescription medicines, possessing a veterinary license from an American state does not mean that such a veterinarian can practice anywhere in the world.[53] Rather, any veterinarian must be compliant with the laws of each nation or jurisdiction in which she or he desires to engage in the practice of veterinary medicine[54] or qualify for an exemption from licensure or temporary licensure or registration of that nation or jurisdiction.[55] Failure to do so may result in significant monetary fines, imprisonment, or both.[56] Veterinary malpractice insurance policies issued in one country are not likely to cover a negligent act or omission in another country.

CONCLUSION

Zoologic medicine veterinarians must be familiar with a number of legal concerns that may impact their professional activities, state licensure, federal and state drug registrations, and participation in accredited programs. Depending on the particular activity, local, state, provincial, and federal laws, regulations, international treaties, court, administrative and disciplinary decisions, and attorney general opinions may be applicable. Most veterinarians are generally familiar with state or provincial veterinary licensure requirements; however, they often must be more knowledgeable about multiple legal requirements, limitations, and restrictions. In addition, the dynamic environment of regulations with regard to animal welfare and drug or controlled substances requires that veterinarians be attentive to legal and regulatory changes. General practice lawyers may not be familiar with many of the veterinary licensure statutes and regulations that exist, and certain legal conundrums may require the expertise of an attorney who is particularly experienced in a given area of law.

REFERENCES

1. E.g., Washington State Dept. of Fisheries v. Public Utility District, 91 Wash.2d 378, 382, 588 P.2d 1146, 1149 (1979).
2. E.g., State of Washington v. Longshore, 97 Wash. App. 144, 150, 982 P.2d 1191, 1195 (1999) aff'd 141 Wash.2d 414, 5 P.3d 1256 (2000).
3. E.g., Wiley v. Baker, 597 S.W.2d 3, 5 (Tex. App. 12th Dist. 1980).
4. E.g., New Mexico v. Morton, 406 F. Supp. 1237 (D.N.M. 1975) aff'd 426 U.S. 529, 545 reh. denied 429 U.S. 873 (1976).
5. See APHIS, Animal Care Inspection Guide, Written Program of Veterinary Care, p. 8.3.1, with form agreement (APHIS Form 7002); Animal Care Resource Guide Policies, Policy # 3: Veterinary Care, Program of Veterinary Care, p. 3.3.
6. Hodgins v. U.S. Dept. of Agriculture, 238 F.3d 421 (Table), 59 Ag. Dec. 534, 2001 WL 1785733, *15 (6th Cir. 2000) appeal after remand 33 Fed. Appx. 784, 2002 WL 649102 (6th Cir. 2002).
7. Depending on the jurisdiction, a veterinarian who surgically alters an animal might find her or himself subject to disciplinary action. E.g., Kansas (USA) Admin. Reg. § 70-8-1(m).
8. E.g., Indiana (USA) Code § 25-38.1-1-7.7, " 'Direct supervision' means a supervisor is readily available on the premises where the animal is being treated."
9. E.g., Indiana Code § 25-38.1-1-9.5, " 'Indirect supervision' means a supervising veterinarian is not on the premises but: (1) is present within the veterinarian's usual practice area; (2) has given written protocols or oral instructions for the treatment of an animal for which a veterinarian-client-patient relationship exists; and (3) is readily available by telephone or other means of immediate communication."
10. E.g., In re: McDonald, Findings of Fact, no. 12, p. 7 (USDA, AWA Docket no. 03-0012, January 4, 2005).
11. E.g., In the Matter of the Arbitration Between Llizo, VMD and The City of Topeka, Kansas, 2011 WL 7139076 (Federal Mediation and Conciliation Service no. 101202-51832-8, July 8, 2010)—"… the City's IT [Information Technology] Department experienced what it described as a 'catastrophic' failure resulting in the loss of two years' of Zoo medical records. There was no explanation of why the backup system failed, but the IT Department acknowledged that it did. The loss of data was clearly not the fault of [the zoo veterinarian], but she was responsible for finding hard copies of the lost data and re-entering them into the Zoo's MedARKS system. Moreover, the data loss occurred … shortly before the unannounced USDA inspections and while the effort at data re-entry was still underway. …"
12. APHIS, Animal Care Inspection Guide, Records: Records Requirements, pp. 7.3.1–7.3.8 and Veterinary Care Records, pp. 8.2.1–8.2.4.
13. Animal Care Inspection Guide, Veterinary Care Records, Required Records, p. 8.2.1 and Recommended Records, p. 8.2.3.
14. Animal Care Inspection Guide, Veterinary Care Records, Availability, p. 8.2.4.
15. Animal Care Inspection Guide, Veterinary Care Records, Necropsy Reports, p. 8.2.3.
16. Animal Care Inspection Guide, Records: Records Requirements, Dealer, p. 7.3.2; Exhibitor, p. 7.3.4; Research Facility, p. 7.3.7; and Veterinary Care Records, p. 8.2.3.
17. E.g., Harrison v. Ohio Veterinary Medical Licensing Bd., 2008 Ohio 6519, ¶ 13 (Ohio App. 10th Dist. 2008) appeal denied 121 Ohio St.3d 1453, 904 N.E.2d 902 (2009).
18. Animal Care Inspection Guide, Written Program of Veterinary Care, p. 8.3.1, with form agreement (APHIS Form 7002). See also, Animal Care Resource Guide Policies, Policy # 3: Veterinary Care, Program of Veterinary Care, p. 3.3.
19. 9 CFR § 2.32(c)(4).
20. E.g., Zimmerman v. Wolff, 622 F. Supp.2d 240, 243–44 (E.D. Pa. 2008)—"courts have uniformly held that the AWA does not create a private cause of action and that Congress intended that only the Secretary of [USDA] be able to enforce the law." See also, Otto v. Hillsborough County, Florida, 2013 WL 2456095, *5 (M.D. Fla. 2013).
21. 16 USC §§ 1531–1544.
22. Cayman Turtle Farms, Ltd. v. Andrus, 478 F. Supp. 125, 129 (D.D.C. 1979).
23. 16 USC §§ 703–712, with § 709 omitted.
24. 16 USC § 4201 et seq.
25. 16 USC §§ 1371–1421h et seq.
26. 16 USC §§ 4321–4347 et seq.
27. Black's Law Dictionary, pp. 774–75 (West, 9th ed. 2009)
28. E.g., Cetacean Community v. Bush, 386 F.3d 1169, 1178 (9th Cir. 2004); Hawksbill Sea Turtle v. Federal Emergency Management Agency, 126 F.3d 461, 466, fn. 2 (3rd Cir. 1997); Veale v. Furness, 2007 WL 54820 report and recommendation adopted, 2007 WL 465405, 2007 U.S. Dist. LEXIS 9276 (D.N.H. 2007); McAdams v. Faulk, 2002 WL 700956, 2002 Ark App. LEXIS 258 (2002) appeal after remand 96 Ark. App. 118, 239 S.W.3d 17 (2006); Bass v. State of Florida, 791 So.2d 1124 (Fla. App. 4th Dist. 2000); Coho Salmon v. Pacific Lumber Co., 30 F. Supp.2d 1231, 1239, fn. 2 (N.D. Cal. 1998); Bobin v. Sammarco, 1995 WL 303632, *2 (E.D. Pa. 1995); Miller v. Peranio, 426 Pa. Super. 189, 627 A.2d 637 (1993); City of Akron v. Tipton, 53 Ohio Misc.2d 18, 559 N.E.2d 1385 (Akron Mun. 1989); Kihlstadius v. Nodaway Veterinary Clinic, 697 F. Supp. 1087 (W.D. Mo. 1988).
29. In April 2007, an Austrian court denied an application to appoint a guardian for a chimpanzee. The court rules that if it appointed a guardian, then this might create a public perception that humans with court-appointed guardians were at the same level as animals. E.g., Chimp Denied Legal Guardian www.nature.com/news/2007/070423/full/news070423-9.html.
30. E.g., International Primate Protection League v. Institute for Behavioral, Inc., 799 F.2d 934 (4th Cir. 1986) cert. denied 481 U.S. 1004 reh. denied 482 U.S. 909 (1987); Oberschlake v. Veterinary Associates Animal Hosp., 151 Ohio App.3d 741, 785 N.E.2d 811 (2nd Dist. 2003); Falls Mills Associates Ltd. v. Maurzo, 13 Conn. App. 119, 534 A.2d 912 (1987); Jones v. Beame, 86 Misc.2d 832, 383 N.Y.S.2d 1004 (1976) rev'd and dismissed 56 App. Div.2d 778, 392 N.Y.S.2d 444 (1977) aff'd 45 N.Y.2d 402, 408 N.Y.S.2d 449, 380 N.E.2d 277 (1978); Jones v. Butz, 374 F. Supp.2d (S.D.N.Y.) aff'd 419 U.S. 806 (1974); Williams v. Michigan Central R.R. Co., 2 Mich. 259, 55 Am. Dec. 59 (1851). See also, American Veterinary Medical Law Association, Ownership of Animals vs. Guardianship of Animals: The Effect of a Change in the Law on Veterinarians in California, Vol. 56, no. 3, California Veterinarian (May–June 2002).
31. More than 175 member countries, including the United States, are members. For a list of member countries see www.oie.int/about-us/our-members/member-countries/.
32. www.oie.int/index.php?id=169&L=0&htmfile=preface.htm See generally, Bamako Declaration: "The Role of Veterinary Statutory Bodies" (Bamako, Mali, April 2011).
33. www.deadiversion.usdoj.gov/21cfr/21usc/index.html.
34. 21 USC § 802(21). Compare, Australia New Zealand Therapeutic Products Authority, Standard for the Uniform Scheduling of Medicines and Poisons, § 101: Definitions; Authorised Prescriber.
35. E.g., Royal College of Veterinary Surgeons (RCVS) Advice Note 27: Overseas Veterinary Surgeons Visiting the UK; Temporary Registration, no. 9 (March 2009).
36. E.g., Kenya Veterinary Surgeons and Veterinary Para-Professional Act, § 14: Definition of "practice"; Zambia Veterinary Surgeons Act, § 2: Definitions.
37. E.g., Zambian Drug Enforcement Commission (DEC) has Detained a Number of Americans for Possession of Benadryl, Zambian Chronicle (January 27, 2009). http://brainsplus.wordpress.com/2009/01/27/zambian-drug-enforcement-commission-dec-has-detained-a-number-of-americans-for-possession-of-benadryl/.

38. E.g., Oklahoma State Bd. of Veterinary Examiners v. Bonham, DVM, Findings of Fact, no. 6, p. 2 (OKBVE no. 98-05-0031, January 21, 1999); United States v. Bonham (D.W.D. Okla. no. 5:98-CR-00087); and Thorpe v. California Bd. of Examiners in Veterinary Medicine, 104 Cal. App.3d 111, 163 Cal. Rptr. 382, 8 A.L.R.4th 206 (4th Dist. 2006).

39. By way of examples only, see Saint Christopher and Nevis Drug (Prevention and Abatement of the Misuse of Drugs) Act, § 1; South Africa Veterinary and Para-Veterinary Professions Act, No. 19 of 1982, § 34: Dispensing of medicine; Zambia Dangerous Drug Regulations, Part I.

40. E.g., Kenya—besides substantial monetary fines, up to life imprisonment. Kenya Narcotic Drugs and Psychotropic Substances (Control) Act 1994, § 4: Penalty for trafficking in narcotic drugs, etc. For non-narcotic drugs, up to 20-years in prison for each violation; Zambia Narcotic Drugs and Psychotropic Drugs Act 1993, Part III: Offences and Penalties, imprisonment from 15-to-25 years per offense.

41. Among such countries are Afghanistan, Bangladesh, Brunei, China, Cuba, Egypt, India, Indonesia, Iran, Iraq, Jordan, Kuwait, Laos, Malaysia, North Korea, Oman, Pakistan, Qatar, Saudi Arabia, Singapore, Somalia, South Sudan, Sudan, Sri Lanka, Syria, Thailand, Taiwan, United Arab Emirates, Yemen and Zimbabwe. According to the Human Rights Watch (HRW) and the International Harm Reduction Association (IHRA), for certain drug offenses, death sentences are mandatory in Brunei, India, Laos, Singapore and Malaysia. India's status is in question in light of a June 2011 court ruling. www.lawyerscollective.org/files/IHRN%20 judgment.pdf.

42. E.g., Nebraska Rev. Stat. § 71-8917(1)(b). See also California Bus. and Prof. Code § 4883(a); 24 Delaware Code § 3316(a)(4); Hawai'i Rev. Stat. § 471-10(b)(9); 255 Illinois Compiled Stat. § 115/25.1(Z); Kansas Stat. Ann. § 47-830(p); North Dakota Century Code § 43-29-14.1(j); Nevada Rev. Stat. § 638.140.4; 59 Oklahoma Stat. Ann. § 698.14a(E)(3); Rhode Island Gen. Laws § 5-25-14(1).

43. www.deadiversion.usdoj.gov/imp_exp/med_missions.htm.

44. See, generally, 21 USC § 953: Exportation of controlled substances.

45. Animal Care Resources Guide Policies, Policy # 3: Veterinary Care, Expired Medical Materials, p. 3.1.

46. E.g., 21 USC §§ 360b, 360ccc, 360ccc-1 and 360ccc-2. See also, 21 CFR, Part 516: New Animal Drugs for Minor Use and Minor Species.

47. 21 CFR § 516.28: Publication of MUMS Drug-Designations.

48. 21 CFR § 516.29: Termination of MUMS Drug-Designations.

49. E.g., Arkansas Code Ann. § 17-92-102(a); Missouri Rev. Stat. § 338.220.4.

50. E.g., United States v. Franck's Labs, Inc., 816 F. Supp.2d 1209 (M.D. Fla. 2011). Note: While this case was on appeal both the government and the compounder dismissed their appeals with the lower court's decision being vacated, as though it had never been issued.

51. E.g., Wedgewood Village Pharmacy v. Drug Enforcement Admin., 370 U.S. App. D.C. 14, 509 F.3d 541 (2007).

52. Ackerman L, editor: *Blackwell's Five-Minute Veterinary Practice Management Consult*, § 11:15: Extra-Label Drug Use, p. 470, col. 2 (2007); Gallagher v. Intermune, Inc., 2005 WL 742434 (E.D. Pa. 2005); and In re: Koller, DVM, 71 Fed. Reg. 66975 (November 16, 2005).

53. E.g., Lawendy v. Connecticut Bd. of Veterinary Medicine, 109 Conn. App. 113, 951 A.2d 13 (2008); Tennessee Bd. of Veterinary Medical Examiners v. Collins (August 24, 2006). https://health.state.tn.us/Downloads/Vet_Min082406.pdf.

54. E.g., Kenya Veterinary Surgeons and Veterinary Para-Professional Act, § 14: Definition of "practice"; Zambia Veterinary Surgeons Act, § 2: Definitions, id., § 7(1)(a) and (b).

55. E.g., South Africa Veterinary and Para-Veterinary Professions Act, No. 19 of 1982, § 22: Unregistered persons shall not practise veterinary or para-veterinary professions; Ghana Veterinary Surgeons Law 1992, § 16: Temporary Register; Kenya Veterinary Surgeons and Veterinary Para-Professional Act, § 16: Temporary Registration of Foreign Veterinary Surgeons. Compare Zambia Veterinary Surgeons Act, First Schedule: Operations, Treatments, Tests, Advice, Diagnosis and Attendance which may be Performed, Given or Provided by Unregistered Persons—no such exemption present. See also, Royal College of Veterinary Surgeons, Advice Note 27: Overseas Veterinary Surgeons Visiting the UK; Temporary Registration (March 2009).

56. Ghana Veterinary Surgeons Law 1992, § 25: Offences and Penalties—Fine of up to approximately US$528,708.14 and/or 2 years imprisonment with a further fine of approximately US$10,574.16 per day for continuing violations; Nigeria Veterinary Surgeons Act 1969, § 15(4) and up to 2 years in prison.

57. www.oie.int/index.php?id=169&L=0&htmfile=chapitre_1.4.15.htm#chapitre_1.4.15.

58. www.oie.int/index.php?id=169&L=0&htmfile=chapitre_1.5.9.htm#chapitre_1.5.9.

CHAPTER 72

Minimally Invasive Surgery Techniques

Romain Pizzi

Minimally invasive surgery (MIS) techniques such as laparoscopic cholecystectomy and appendectomy are used routinely in human surgery in the developed world and are currently regarded as the gold standard for these and numerous other human surgical procedures.[17,32,33,63] They demonstrate notable improvements in rapid recoveries and reduced postoperative pain compared with traditional open surgery. Veterinary MIS techniques also hold the potential for reduced patient morbidity, reduced wound contamination and breakdown, shorter patient recovery periods, and reduced postoperative care requirements.[6,15,25,30,31,35,64] It stands to reason that MIS is likely to hold even greater advantages in captive or free-ranging wildlife than in domestic animals, although the current evidence base is still small.

Although wildlife surgery is a small specialist field, it can still play an important role in zoo and free-ranging wildlife medicine. MIS has obvious welfare advantages for permanent captive wildlife species as well as for free-ranging wildlife species undergoing rehabilitation, potentially shortening the stressful time of treatment in captivity. Wildlife surgery may also play an occasional role in the conservation of endangered species. In critically endangered species, optimal treatment of each remaining individual is important if a species is to survive and maintain reasonable genetic heterogeneity. For example, only four Yangtze giant soft shell turtles (*Rafetus swinhoei*) remain in the world, of which 2 remain in the wild, and one of these last remaining wild turtles recently required capture and surgical treatment for wounds.[3] Similarly, other critically endangered species exist, with small remaining wild populations under 50 individuals. Successful surgical treatment and return to the wild of even a single injured individual in such small critical populations could have an important impact on maximizing the remaining genetic diversity in the population. In these cases, the least invasive method of intervention with the most rapid healing and return to the wild would be ideal.

This chapter will provide a brief overview of current techniques and applications of MIS in wildlife, highlight MIS-specific risks and disadvantages, and discuss some recent developments in human and domestic animal surgery that have relevance or implications for wildlife surgery. Several available texts provide detailed discussions of the basic MIS equipment and instruments needed for most animal species and describe the basic procedures commonly performed in humans, domestic animals, and exotic pets.[10,15,20,26,39,40,60]

OVERVIEW

The term *minimally invasive surgery (MIS)* is generally used to refer to any procedure that is less invasive than open surgery used for the same purpose.[65] Although this has most often been used to refer to rigid endosurgical procedures such as laparoscopy, the term can also be applied to percutaneous interventional techniques.

Laparoscopy, thoracoscopy, and arthroscopy are also alternatively referred to as *minimal access surgery*, *video surgery*, *endosurgery*, and *endoscopic surgery* and, by lay persons and professionals alike, as "keyhole surgery." It appears advisable to avoid the use of the term "keyhole surgery" as some ambiguity surrounds the meaning of this term; for example, it is not uncommon for veterinarians to also refer to open surgery performed through small incisions as "keyhole surgery." Small wounds are a clearly recognizable feature and an obvious benefit, but these small wounds are not the only benefit of this type of MIS. A very notable benefit is the markedly enhanced visualization (helped by the magnification allowed by the endoscope), which, if used correctly, leads to safer and more physiologic surgery. The ultimate aim of all MIS should always be safe, visual physiologic surgery, the added benefit being small wounds. In contrast, very small open abdominal surgery incisions tend to lead to poor visualization and result in unsafe surgery.[40]

Laparoscopy and Coelioscopy

Laparoscopy encompasses MIS procedures in the abdominal cavity. Coelioscopy, which is endoscopy of the coelomic cavity in nonmammalian species, is also commonly referred to as *laparoscopy*, although this usage is not strictly accurate. This is the most widely recognized and the best reported MIS technique in the zoo and wildlife surgical field. It has been applied in mammal species ranging from mice[56] to elephants,[58] as well as in birds, reptiles, amphibians, and fish.[10,39] It has applications in diagnosis, surgery, and assisted reproduction in wildlife. The emphasis in this chapter is on laparoscopy and coelioscopy, as still relatively few reports on the application of other MIS modalities in wildlife have been published.

Thoracoscopy

Thoracoscopy holds potential for further application in zoo animal surgery. Maintenance of postoperative chest drains commonly employed in open thoracotomy procedures is difficult in wildlife patients. Many human surgeons prefer the term *video-assisted thoracic surgery* (VATS) to *thoracoscopy*, which highlights one of the main

benefits that endosurgery brings to thoracic surgery—visualization. Endoscopic visualization allows examination of parts of the pleural cavity, which are difficult to access or see adequately in open thoracotomy procedures. VATS also recognizes that although the majority of a procedure such as a lung lobectomy can be completed thoracoscopically, a mini-thoracotomy is usually still needed for tissue extraction. In laparoscopy, alternatives such as insertion of hand access ports, motorized tissue morcellators, and rip-proof impervious extraction bags allow an entire liver lobe to be broken down with sponge forceps and extracted through a 10- to 15-millimeter (mm) port site.

Currently, published thoracoscopy reports have largely been limited to those on laboratory primates such as macaques[4] and domestic animals.[40] Postmortem thoracoscopic access was assessed in an adult giraffe, but visualization and access were notably limited by the wide, closely spaced ribs that allowed for little angulation of the endoscope and instruments,[44] which is also an issue with other large herbivores and megavertebrates. Access was, however, sufficient for peripheral lung biopsies. Thoracoscopy is not possible in elephants because of the lack of a pleural space.[8]

Vascular ring anomalies such as persistent right aortic arch have been treated in zoo animals such as a tiger by open thoracotomy,[22] and the procedure has been performed in domestic animals via 3-mm thoracoscopy,[40] making this equally applicable in zoo animals not intended for breeding. Esophageal hiatal hernias, diaphragmatic hernias, and chylothorax, reported in zoo species,[19,21,23,29] are amenable to operative thoracoscopy techniques.

The extracorporeal applied Meltzer knot (Figure 72-1), which is an extremely useful technique for performing lung biopsies, also has other MIS and open surgery applications. It can be used in a wide range of taxa and body sizes, in cases where alternatives such as endosurgical staplers cannot be used. It is more cost effective than staplers or commercially available pretied endoloops (Surgitie, Covidien; Endoloop, Ethicon). This also allows surgeons greater choice of suture material and diameter than commercially available endoloops. The author has used this in species ranging from 1 to 650 kilograms (kg), via 3-mm ports and larger ports in thoracoscopy and laparoscopy. A loop with a pretied Meltzer knot is inserted via one port with a knot pusher and grasping forceps inserted via a different port. The forceps end is passed through the loop to grasp the tissue to be ligated for purposes such as biopsy. The tip of the knot pusher is then placed on the tissue where ligation is required, and the suture loop tightened, thus locking the knot. Knot ends of about 1 centimeter (cm) length should be left for safety. The tissue may then be transected. A suture may also be first passed around a fixed structure such as the cystic duct or ligamentum arteriosis before the suture exits from the same port, and the knot is then tied and similarly placed with a knot pusher for ligation.

It is inadvisable for surgeons not already familiar with standard thoracotomy techniques to attempt thoracoscopic procedures. An emergency situation such as intrathoracic hemorrhage is not the time to learn how to perform a thoracotomy. During surgical preparation and draping, the decision to convert to a thoracotomy, if needed, may be determined.

Arthroscopy

Surprisingly few reports of arthroscopic surgery in wildlife species have been published, considering how widespread and established the use of this MIS modality is in domestic animals. Two reports of arthroscopy in giraffe—one of arthroscopic treatment of a metacarpophalangeal joint injury and osteochondral fragment,[50] and the second of exploratory arthroscopy in the femorotibial joint of a giraffe with an avulsion fracture of the peroneus tertius origin—have been published.[49] Arthroscopy has also been reported in the Dromedary camel,[2,36] alpaca, and llama.[37] With the increased longevity of zoo animals and the associated needs for diagnosis and management of geriatric conditions such as osteoarthritis, arthroscopy is likely to be increasingly performed in individual zoo animals in future. Arthroscopy also has a potential role to play in the diagnosis of some

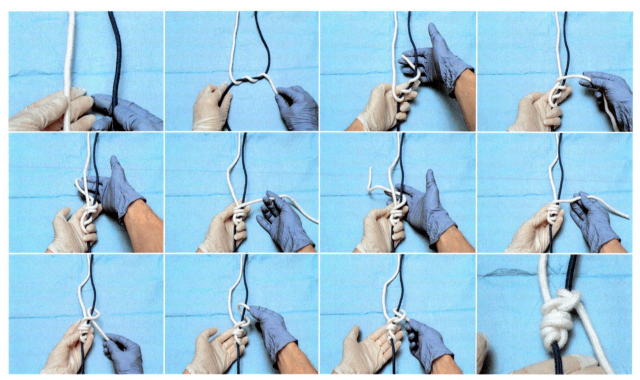

FIGURE 72-1 Method of tying the Meltzer extracorporeal locking knot. This knot is useful for biopsies in laparoscopic and thoracoscopic surgery, as well as for ligation of vascular pedicles and structures. (Copyright Zoological Medicine Ltd.)

dysplastic joint diseases that may have heritable factors, with subsequent implications for captive breeding.

Further studies are needed to clarify optimal safe entry sites in the joints of different species, particularly in species that markedly differ anatomically from domestic animal models and humans. Poor site selection for joint entry or lack of experience in the operators poses the risk of cartilage and joint damage. In larger animals, as in domestic equines, insufflation of the joints with carbon dioxide may be helpful in improving visualization.[51]

Percutaneous Surgical Interventions

Interventional procedures include interventional radiology, interventional cardiology, and ultrasound-guided procedures. Some conditions that were surgically managed previously are increasingly performed via percutaneous techniques, which hold potential applications in wildlife species. These include occlusion of patent ductus arteriosis, balloon valvuloplasty for pulmonic stenosis, cardiac pacemaker implantation, and attenuation of single portosystemic shunts, performed under fluoroscopy. These percutaneous techniques are all based on the Sildinger technique of vascular access.[55] The implantation of a cardiac resynchronization device in a gorilla has been reported,[52,53] and in the future more interventional procedures may be used for managing the health and welfare of nonbreeding great apes, carnivores, and other charismatic exhibit animals.

Ultrasound-guided procedures are also replacing surgical procedures used previously and even other more invasive MIS techniques such as laparoscopy in some applications. Much of the initial research on wildlife laparoscopy was focused on its applications in assisted reproduction, such as examination of ovaries, artificial insemination, and oocyte retrieval.[5,8] These applications of laparoscopy are increasingly being replaced by ultrasonography, transcervical insemination, and transvaginal ultrasound-guided fine-needle techniques. Transrectal ultrasound-guided oocyte recovery has been performed in white and black rhinoceroses,[18] in which, as in other megavertebrates, laparoscopic access to the ovaries is not easily achieved.[44,58]

Other Endosurgical Techniques

Other rigid and flexible endoscopic modalities may be used for both diagnostic and operative applications, although only a small number of reports of their operative use in wildlife have been published. Operative rhinoscopy has been used to remove obstructing nasal polyps in a chimpanzee[12] and a California sea lion.[57] Endoscopy, in conjunction with fluoroscopy, may be used to apply temporary or permanent stents. Urethral stenting, in conjunction with laser lithotripsy, has been used in a bottlenose dolphin[54] and an Asian small-clawed otter.[66] Bilateral urethral stenting in a Guinea baboon has been reported in the management of urethral strictures caused by endometriosis that occurred after an ovariohysterectomy.[9] The author is unaware of any reports of permanent stenting for tracheal collapse in zoo animals, but the technique appears feasible in many mammalian species, should it be needed.

Natural orifice transluminal endoscopic surgery (NOTES) has been investigated for its potential for truly "scarless" surgery in human abdominal surgery. Transvaginal and transgastric cholecystectomies have been performed in humans, as an alternative to laparoscopy or open surgery. However, the use of NOTES in human surgery is still highly controversial and has only been performed in a small number of cases. Besides studies in laboratory animals, NOTES has been investigated experimentally in domestic horses for standing bilateral ovariectomies with reasonable initial technical results.[34] Transvaginal laparoscopy for oocyte retrieval was investigated in a black rhinoceros,[48] as a potential alternative to flank laparoscopy, but the technique was problematic and has been replaced by other less invasive methods such as an ultrasound-guided fine-needle transrectal technique,[18] which appears safer and more feasible.

Cosmesis is the main reason for the development of NOTES in human surgery and is of little concern in wildlife patients. The need for expensive specialist equipment such as double-channel operative flexible endoscopes; difficulties in monitoring surgical entry sites in the stomach, rectum, or vagina postoperatively; increased technical difficulty and increased procedure time; and ongoing controversy over its safety and benefits in humans make it unlikely that NOTES will find much application in wildlife surgery in the near future.

CURRENT KNOWLEDGE

Evidence for the advantages of MIS in domestic animals is increasing,[30] but further research is still needed to better establish an evidence base for the safe, relevant, and ethical application of MIS techniques in captive and free-ranging wildlife patients. The current literature on MIS in wildlife species consists largely of concept trials and case reports and is likely to have an unintentional positive publication bias. Type II error, that is, not meeting sample size requirements, is a particular limitation in surgical trials, even in human medicine.

The large sample sizes needed to demonstrate statistical significance of low-frequency adverse events is problematic in wildlife surgery, with the relatively small numbers of procedures performed. Preemptive power calculations highlight how difficult it would be to perform a randomized controlled trial to demonstrate the reduced complication rates in wildlife MIS compared with open surgical techniques. Demonstration of a 50% reduction in baseline risk from 20% to 10% would require a total study group of 438 individuals. Demonstration of a more modest improvement, or a lower frequency event requires even larger numbers: Demonstration of a 50% reduction in baseline risk from 2% to 1% would require a study group of 5030 individuals; and demonstration of a 10% reduction in baseline risk from 20% to 18% would require a study group of 12,278 individuals.[7] At least for the foreseeable future, the evidence base for wildlife surgery, including MIS, is likely to continue to be based on small feasibility trials, case series, case reports, and anecdotal experience. The profession needs to debate on and determine the ethics of what is not only possible but also reasonable. Increasing surgical capabilities make correction of numerous congenital abnormalities and other previously untreated conditions feasible, but the possibility of unknown heritable components and the implications for the genetic viability of captive populations of endangered animals require consideration.

Cognitive Bias in Wildlife MIS

Cognitive bias caused by heuristics and subsequent errors in decision making need to be recognized in wildlife MIS.[61] Veterinary surgeons able to perform MIS may inadvertently be subject to the risk of "technology bias," or "law of the instrument," which is summed up by Maslow as follows: "If the only tool you have is a hammer, everything looks like a nail."[28] All surgery, even MIS, is invasive and carries risks of adverse consequences for the patient. A 2010 study in the *British Journal of Surgery* found that not only were a significant number of human elective surgery patients not better a year after elective surgery, 17% actually suffered worse pain than before surgery, and 14% had less function than before surgery.[38] This indicates that approximately 1 in 7 human elective surgery patients are, in fact, worse off a year later after the surgery. No comparable veterinary data are available, but it is uncertain whether veterinary surgical patients fare any better. It is strongly recommended that wildlife surgical decisions be routinely discussed with nonsurgical colleagues, to evaluate if a procedure is technically feasible and if it, in fact, is indicated, carries a reasonable likelihood of a successful outcome for the patient, and another equally applicable nonsurgical option is not available. Without this consideration, everything may start to resemble "a chance to cut being a chance to cure," rather than "Primum non nocere" ("First do no harm"). Auditing surgical outcomes is vital to improving surgical skills and reducing complications, as well as to improving future surgical decisions.

MIS being less invasive does not always mean that it is better than open surgery. Recent systematic reviews have found no evidence for better long-term oncologic or functional outcomes among open

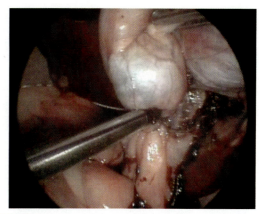

FIGURE 72-2 Ligation of the cystic duct, by means of an extracorporeal Meltzer knot, during laparoscopic cholecystectomy in an Asiatic black bear rescued from illegal bile farming in Vietnam. (Copyright Zoological Medicine Ltd.)

prostatectomy, laparoscopic prostatectomy, and robotic radical prostatectomy in men.[14,24]

Wildlife surgeons may benefit from surgical research into nonpatient factors that affect surgery on humans, domestic animals, and wildlife equally. Even relatively small changes in surgical practice may have a large influence on patient safety and outcomes. Under the World Health Organization (WHO) "Safe surgery saves lives" initiative, the use of a simple surgical checklist in human surgery has been found to reduce surgical complications by more than one third and reduce deaths by almost half.[27] A safety checklist modified for veterinary endosurgery can be downloaded from http://www.veterinarylaparoscopy.com/Vet endosurgery safety checklist.pdf.

Cognitive bias may also lead to the belief that new equipment or additional instrumentation would improve surgical capabilities and the procedures that can be performed, when the procedures may not, in fact, be necessary. The author is aware of several hundred laparoscopic cholecystectomies safely and rapidly performed by experienced surgeons in human medicine working in developing countries, when electrosurgery was not available, simply by careful and meticulous dissection.[59] When performing laparoscopic cholecystectomies in bears (Figure 72-2), self-tied extracorporeal knots may be the only viable option for ligation of the cystic duct, as clips are too small and access for 12-mm diameter endosurgical staplers is insufficient.[45]

In human surgery, some surgeons wish to further improve cosmetic results by reducing the number and diameters of ports used in MIS procedures. This has culminated in the controversial "scarless surgery" approaches of the natural orifice transluminal endoscopic surgery (NOTES) previously mentioned, as well as single incision laparoscopic surgery (SILS). SILS is performed by inserting a single, large, multiple-instrument cannula via the navel, with the resulting umbilical scar remaining hidden after surgery. The improved cosmetic result comes at the cost of several other compromises. The incision and body wall deficits are larger, at least 2 to 3 cm, and carry a greater risk of developing postoperative hernias and other complications. Visualization and instrument angulation are markedly more restricted, with limited ability to mobilize tissues; this results in notable increases in surgery times, requires greater technical skills from the surgeon, and results in increased surgical risks.

Some reported veterinary SILS procedures are only from proof-of-concept technical feasibility studies, without strong evidence regarding patient benefit or safety to justify many applications in wildlife surgery. SILS may perhaps have a role to play in the removal of large, firm organs such as the spleen in carnivores or in nephrectomy, when a morcellator is not available or the tissue is not

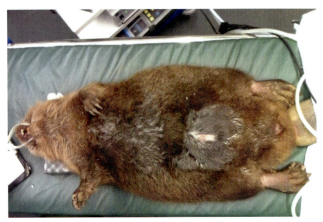

FIGURE 72-3 Small fur clip in a Eurasian beaver for laparoscopy, requiring a return to water within 24 hours of surgery. The author now performs laparoscopy in this species without clipping the fur. (Copyright Zoological Medicine Ltd.)

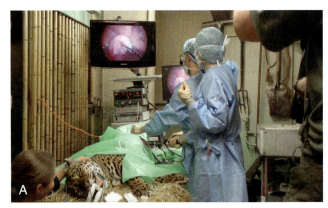

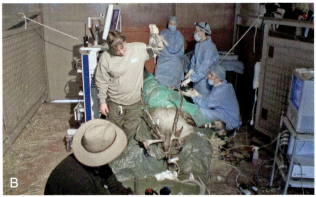

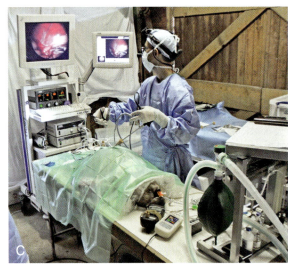

FIGURE 72-4 Minimally invasive surgery carries less risk of postoperative infection when operating in less ideal environments such as (**A**) an off-show area (for a jaguar), (**B**) an enclosure, with hay bales used as a surgery table (for a reindeer), (**C**) a shed in a field as a makeshift operating theater (laparoscopy in a Eurasian beaver). (Copyright Zoological Medicine Ltd.)

amenable to pulping in a rip-proof impervious bag (E-sac, Espiner Medical), followed by suction or piecemeal removal from the exteriorized neck of the bag via a slightly enlarged standard port site wound. In many mammals, a liver lobectomy (performed by means of an extracorporeal knot) can be effectively performed by this means. In wildlife patients, a single, larger wound is generally less desirable than several smaller incisions because of the increased risks of wound interference, complications, and herniation.

Emphasis is commonly placed on the small wounds and reduced postoperative pain in veterinary MIS. However, the enhanced magnified visualization, access to parts of the body and structures difficult to visualize in open surgery, provision of excellent illumination, and ability to perform less traumatic and more physiologic surgery in MIS are also of considerable value to the wildlife surgeon. Reducing the invasiveness of surgical procedures through different MIS techniques should not, however, be accomplished at the cost of increased risks to the patient.[46]

Potential Advantages of MIS in Wildlife

MIS techniques do potentially hold additional advantages when applied to captive and free-ranging wildlife species. In wildlife patients, postoperative care and monitoring is difficult, and it may not be possible to restrict postoperative activity at all.[8,43] In social primates, separation from the group after surgery may adversely affect group stability and behavior and result in fighting and injury or death on reintroduction of the operated individual. Primates undergoing MIS procedures may be more rapidly returned to their normal enclosures and groups, which results in minimal social disruption.[41]

In aquatic species such as pinnipeds, an early postoperative return to the water may be desirable, so small water-resistant wounds are ideal.[47] In these cases, the use of 36-cm length, 3-mm diameter mini-laparoscopy instruments (Logi, Surgical Innovations; MiniLap, Karls Storz), and even 2.3-mm diameter percutaneous needle access instruments (MiniLap, Stryker) are advantageous. In addition, animals such as otters and beavers, which rely on their fur for water proofing and limiting body heat loss, may have surgery with a minimal clip, or even no clipping; thorough cleaning and disinfection of fur, clear adhesive drapes, and care not to inadvertently introduce fur into the incisions at port entry or closure are all important. The author has performed laparoscopy in 25 Eurasian beavers, which were returned with unrestricted access to water within 12 to 24 hours postoperatively, without adverse effects noted[43] (Figure 72-3).

When operating under less than ideal conditions such as in animal enclosures, outdoors, or in makeshift theatres in the field

(Figure 72-4), small MIS wounds help reduce the risks of wound contamination and infection both intra-operatively and postoperatively. Some other general advantages and disadvantages of MIS are listed in Box 72-1.

SPECIFIC RISKS OF MIS

Safe Laparoscopic Access

Despite numerous notable advantages, MIS techniques such as laparoscopy and thoracoscopy carry some injury risks specific to this

BOX 72-1 Benefits and Disadvantages of Minimally Invasive Surgery, Based on Human and Domestic Animal Studies

SOME BENEFITS OF MIS

- Reduced postoperative pain
- Shorter postoperative recovery
- Low dehiscence risk
- Reduced postoperative care requirements
- Magnified visualization of target organs
- Smaller wounds
- Reduced tissue trauma and inflammation
- Accurate minimal hemostasis
- More accurate "physiologic" surgery
- Positive curatorial, keeper, public, and media perception

SOME DISADVANTAGES OF MIS

- Equipment setup cost
- Steep learning curve
- Lack of tactile feedback
- Not suitable for all patients or procedures
- Risk of MIS-specific injuries
- Need for occasional conversion to open surgery
- Increased procedure time and costs for some procedures
- High cost of specific consumables
- Delayed recognition of bowel injury

MIS, Minimally invasive surgery.

type of surgery and must be taken into consideration. The greatest MIS-specific surgical risk is in achieving safe access (entry) at the start of MIS procedures, commonly underestimated by novice surgeons.[31,40] The merits and risks of different abdominal access techniques in both human and veterinary laparoscopy continue to be debated. Despite strongly held personal opinions and experiences, a Cochrane collaboration systematic review found no clear evidence for any one technique being safer than another.[1] It is recognized, however, that adverse events in surgery are underreported in the literature.

Access may be *open* (a small incision into the abdomen, followed by port placement); *blind* (blind entry into the abdomen with a sharp trocar, normally after blind insertion of a Veress needle to insufflate the abdomen); or *optical* (using a laparoscope to assist entry, either with or without prior abdominal insufflation with a Veress needle). Many veterinary surgeons prefer performing MIS with blind access, using a Veress needle or an optical cannula (Ternamian EndoTip, Karl Storz).

In trials with different access techniques, in cadavers as well as in surgeries in a wide range of wildlife species, injuries may occur with any of the techniques, although the incidence and injury type and severity have differed. Even supposedly atraumatic cannulas may cause severe entry injuries. The author caused an inadvertent large bowel puncture with a Ternamian EndoTip (Karl Storz) in an adult chimpanzee as well as a similar injury in a guinea pig. The high incidence and extent of abdominal wall adhesions in chimpanzees makes entry problematic in some individuals, irrespective of the technique selected.

The author's personal preference in the majority of mammals is for a modified open approach to access, through the caudal umbilical scar. This is the thinnest part of the abdominal wall, and entry can normally be achieved even in morbidly obese bears without notable difficulty. Incising through the caudal aspect of the umbilicus also helps avoid inadvertent entry into the often large, fat-filled falciform ligament seen in many carnivores. In the majority of cases, it is possible to make an incision in the linea alba, which is smaller than the cannula to be inserted. The body wall is lifted and the cannula inserted with a blunt-tipped trocar, which results in a gas-tight seal for insufflation. Some surgeons use a conical adaptor or a Hasson cone, which fits into an incision larger than the cannula diameter to

prevent gas leakage and can be sutured in position to the skin or the subcutus. Alternatively, a single suture or a surrounding purse-string suture may be placed for the same purpose, as needed. An exception is in adult pinnipeds, in which the author uses blind access after insufflation with a Veress needle. In reptiles and amphibians, the author favors open access in a paramedian or lateral location, which avoids the ventral midline vein. In birds, open access may similarly be created by means of blunt dissection of the body wall after skin incision, with curved mosquito hemostats.

The National Health System in the United Kingdom requires new general surgeons to use open access for laparoscopy, considering the risks of major vascular trauma from blind entry. Most human surgical authorities recommend open access in patients undergoing laparoscopy during pregnancy as well as in patients with abdominal adhesions or a heavily scarred abdomen from previous surgery. If blind access is used, it is preferable to incise the skin before introduction of a Veress needle or sharp trocars to reduce the force needed for insertion and to reduce the potential of traumatizing underlying organs such as the bowel or the spleen.

It is strongly advised that a brief inspection of the area be performed immediately beneath the initial cannula and the Veress needle, if used, immediately after inserting the laparoscope, as this offers the best chance of detecting any entry injuries to the bowel before they are hidden by organ movement. After this, a brief visual examination of the entire abdomen and organs is performed, irrespective of the target organ and procedure planned, to detect any other unexpected asymptomatic pathology such as neoplasia of the liver. The other ports for instrumentation may then be inserted under visual control with the laparoscope. Transillumination in smaller and medium-sized animals allows better visualization and avoids the subcutaneous vessels, and the laparoscope can be used to visualize and avoid structures such as the bladder and inferior epigastric vessels. A repeat brief visual examination is made of the entire abdomen and organs at the end of the procedure before deflation of the abdomen and port closure, to again check for inadvertent hidden injuries or unexplained hemorrhage.

Other MIS-Specific Risks

Inadvertent bowel injuries incurred during laparoscopy also carry MIS-specific increased risks. Because of the more physiologic nature of MIS, postoperative peritoneal and systemic inflammatory responses are less than in open surgery. This is a benefit under normal conditions, but it is a problem in cases of bowel trauma, as it results in an important delay in the manifestation of clinical signs. This results in a poorer prognosis and higher mortality rate in these cases compared with cases of unrecognized bowel trauma in open surgery, as these injuries are notably further progressed before detection. The most frequent causes of laparoscopic bowel injury in humans are Veress needle punctures, sharp trocar injuries, and thermal injuries from electrosurgical instruments, and the small intestine is most frequently affected.[62]

Thermal injuries to the bowel and other sensitive structures in the vicinity of an operative site (such as nerves, vessels, and spermatic cord in proximity to the internal inguinal ring) may occur irrespective of the electrosurgical modality employed, whether it is a monopolar, bipolar, tissue feedback bipolar (Ligasure, Covidien; Enseal, Ethicon Endosurgery; Thunderbeat, Olympus), or ultrasonic scalpel (Harmonic ACE, Ethicon Endosurgery; Sonicision, Covidien; Sonicbeat/Thunderbeat, Olympus). The tips of all electrosurgical instruments become hot with use and may inadvertently cause thermal injuries to the bowel, which are easily missed if care is not taken. These injuries may result in delayed perforations 24 to 48 hours later, with late onset of clinical signs and a poorer prognosis, as already mentioned.

Monopolar surgery carries further risks related to insulation failures as well as poor contact with the ground plate leading to patient burns. This is a particular risk in small mammals with thick fur, which acts as an insulator, as well as in birds. Radiosurgery frequency units (Surgitron, Ellman International) may help reduce this risk.

Monopolar electrosurgery is still an extremely useful modality despite these risks and remains the mainstay of procedures such as laparoscopic cholecystectomy in humans, but its safe use requires knowledge and understanding of electrosurgical safety principles.

Another MIS specific injury risk is from "out of sight" injuries. These are injuries that occur in the abdomen behind the tip of the endoscope and are hence unseen. In addition to inadvertent thermal injuries from electrosurgical instruments, trauma may occur from nonvisualized instrument entry through ports. This is a particular risk in thoracoscopy with resultant lung puncture, which, if missed, may result in life-threatening postoperative pneumothorax. Should lung puncture be diagnosed during thoracoscopy, an affected section of lung should be ligated with a Meltzer knot suture loop. Prevention of these injuries requires, when possible, insertion of instrument ports away from the surgeon in front of the endoscope port so that instrument entry is best visualized during procedures.

Endoscope Selection

The diameter of the laparoscope selected often on the basis of availability or the advantages of a slightly smaller wound size, but these considerations may not always be applicable. Although smaller-diameter instruments and the resultant slightly smaller wounds are considered advantageous, it is worth considering the trade-off between a small reduction in wound size and light transmission as well as image quality, and the effect of biopsy forceps size on diagnostic tissue yielded, as illustrated in Tables 72-1 and 72-2. It is possible to get fixated on "minimizing" the minimally invasive nature of endosurgery, and it is questionable if reducing the laparoscope diameter to decrease a port site wound by 3 mm offers much physiologic advantage to a medium- or large-sized carnivore or primate in terms of pain and wound healing, especially when compared with

TABLE 72-1

Different Endoscope Diameters and Effect on Endoscope Tip Area

Endoscope Diameter	Surface Area of Endoscope Tip (πr^2)	Percentage Area Compared with 5-mm Endoscope	Percentage Area Compared with 10-mm Endoscope
2.7 mm	23 mm^2	29%	7%
3 mm	28 mm^2	35%	9%
5 mm	79 mm^2	100%	25%
10 mm	314 mm^2	397%	100%

Note: These measurements do not directly equating to illumination and image size, but are adequate to illustrate the concept.
mm, Millimeter; *mm^2*, millimeter squared.

TABLE 72-2

Illustrative Comparisons of MIS Biopsy Sizes

Biopsy Diameter	Illustrative Biopsy Volume (d^3)	Percentage of Volume in Comparison with 5-mm Biopsy Volume
5 mm	125 mm^3	100%
3 mm	27 mm^3	22%
1.7 mm (5Fg)	5 mm^3	4%

These are not actual biopsy forceps sample measurements, and used purely for illustrative purposes to demonstrate the marked reduction in diagnostic sample volume with small changes in instrument diameter.
MIS, Minimally invasive surgery; *mm*, millimeter; *mm^3*, millimeter cubed.

large wounds from open surgery. The selection of a small-diameter laparoscope may result in poor visualization or longer duration of anesthesia to complete a procedure, and smaller-diameter biopsy forceps may result in a missed histopathologic diagnosis. Good visualization is one of the main aims and advantages of endosurgery. Thirty-degree endoscopes have the added advantage of allowing a wider field of view, when rotated, confer the ability to see around corners, are more comfortable to hold for long abdominal procedures, and are essential for adequate visualization during thoracoscopy. Zoom lenses on endoscopy cameras cannot compensate for poor illumination.

Environmental Impact of Disposable Instruments

Increasing numbers of human surgeons and hospitals are attempting to limit or reduce their use of single-use, disposable surgical instruments for environmental reasons, and wildlife veterinary surgeons should ideally aim to do the same. When necessary, many single-use instruments may be sterilized for reuse with ethylene oxide or paraformaldehyde[16,27] to reduce their adverse impact on the environment.

CLINICAL APPLICATIONS OF MIS IN WILDLIFE

Diagnostic Laparoscopy

Diagnostic, or exploratory, laparoscopy and organ biopsy are especially useful in captive wildlife, considering the limitations of other diagnostic modalities in wildlife species and the limited availability and high cost of advanced imaging modalities such as computed tomography (CT) and magnetic resonance imaging (MRI). Laparoscopic biopsy of the liver, pancreas, mesenteric lymph node, kidney, and spleen are all accomplished relatively easily. Organs such as the pancreas ideally require loop ligation. Kidney biopsies in species with a unilobular kidney are performed by Tru-Cut needle biopsy of the cortex, or, in multilobular species such as pinnipeds and cetaceans, via dissection, loop ligation, and resection of a single lobe.[11,47] Mesenteric lymph node biopsy is accomplished by stabilization of the lymph node with forceps, to prevent tearing of the mesentery with loss of the vascular supply to a section of bowel. The lymph node capsule is then incised with scissors, before biopsy forceps are inserted via the incision. This prevents the occurrence of severe crush artifacts. Full-thickness intestinal biopsies can be easily performed as laparoscopy-assisted procedures, in which the section of bowel to be biopsied is exteriorized through an enlarged port site, taking care not to crush the bowel. This serves to isolate the biopsy section outside the abdomen, with minimal risk of abdominal contamination, and facilitates leakage testing before the bowel is returned to the abdomen.

Operative Laparoscopy

The reports of both elective and emergency operative procedures, other than reproduction related, are still relatively few in wild mammals.[5,8,11,13,43,45,47] Many wildlife species not only have differing anatomies from humans and domestic animals but also suffer from very different pathologies and diseases requiring surgery. Available instrumentation and techniques for humans may not be directly applicable to wildlife patients (Figure 72-5).[46] Differences in pathology and anatomy results in the potential for novel applications of MIS techniques that are not indicated in humans or domestic animal species. Applications may even be unique to a particular location. The author has performed a successful laparoscopy-assisted ventriculoperitoneal shunt placement in an adult Asiatic black bear with hydrocephalus, under field conditions in South East Asia (Figure 72-6). The country's legislation prohibited killing of listed wildlife species, including bears, with no legal exception for euthanasia on welfare grounds. The procedure was performed in an effort to improve the individual animal's welfare in the specific rescue center situation. In most countries, this compromised welfare situation likely, and sensibly, would have been resolved by humane euthanasia.

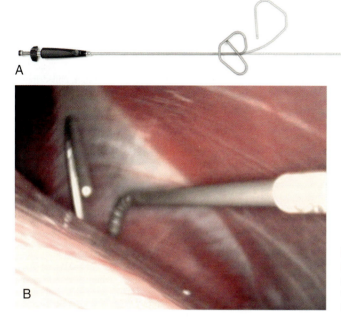

FIGURE 72-5 Use of a 5-mm articulated retractor (LogiFlex, Surgical Innovations) (**A**) to retract the rumen in a reindeer to perform a laparoscopy-assisted cryptorchidectomy. Note the limited space for visualization and working, typical in cases involving recumbent large ruminants (**B**). (Copyright Zoological Medicine Ltd.)

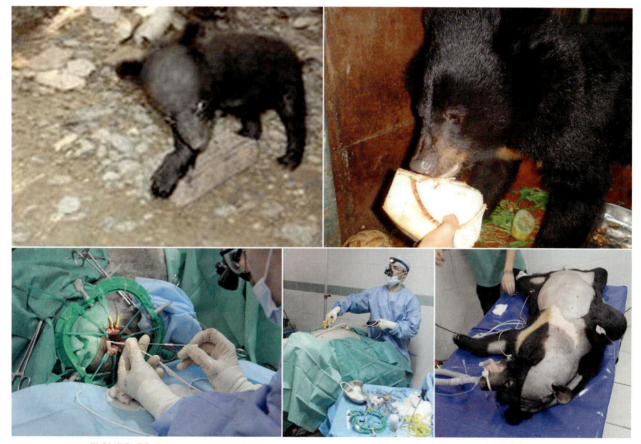

FIGURE 72-6 Laparoscopy-assisted placement of a ventriculoperitoneal shunt for treatment of hydrocephalus in an adult Asiatic black bear in South East Asia. (Courtesy of Matt Hunt, Free The Bears.)

Reproduction Management

The use of laparoscopy in assisted reproductive techniques has been the most reported application in wildlife,[8] although advances in fields such as ultrasonography and endocrinology have reduced its application in more recent times, with the advent of less invasive alternatives such as transcervical and ultrasound-guided needle techniques for insemination and oocyte and embryo collection.[18]

Sterilization via MIS has increased in scope and range of species, with laparoscopic vasectomies having been performed in African elephants.[58] Laparoscopic tubal ligations and laparoscopic vasectomy

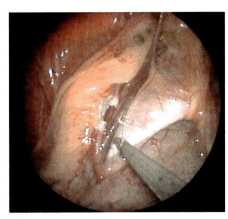

FIGURE 72-7 Laparoscopic vasectomy in a capuchin using 3-mm instrumentation. Note the ease of visualizing the vas in the abdomen. (Copyright Zoological Medicine Ltd.)

are useful in controlling reproduction in captive wildlife. Preservation of gonadal production of hormones results in maintenance of normal behavior and no disruption of social hierarchy, which is particularly useful in large primate groups. Gonadal hormones also maintain normal desirable secondary sexual characteristics such as the mane in lions and the fur colors of gibbon species. This may be altered or lost if animals are castrated or ovariectomized. Laparoscopic vasectomy in primates carries the further advantages of being rapid to perform; the vas is very easily visualized in the abdomen (Figure 72-7), in contrast to open vasectomies; and wound interference is minimal, in contrast to the frequent postoperative wound interference and complications that can occur with open vasectomy.[41,42] Laparoscopic, or laparoscopy-assisted, castration may be performed not only in cryptorchid males.[60] Retraction of testes into the abdomen is possible in some species such as pinnipeds that do not have a true scrotum. The author has castrated a sub-adult California sea lion by using this method.

Tubal ligation cannot be performed in species such as many carnivores, which are prone to developing uterine disorders as a sequela. When ovariectomy is performed in these cases or when alterations in behavior are required, care must be taken in deciding between laparoscopic ovariohysterectomy and laparoscopy-assisted ovariohysterectomy. Despite ovariohysterectomy being a major, more technically demanding procedure, it should be considered in cases with a risk of uterine pathology, for example, older multiparous carnivores, lagomorphs, and some primates at risk of developing endometriosis.

REFERENCES

1. Ahmad G, Duffy JMN, Phillips K, Watson A: Laparoscopic entry techniques. *Cochrane Database Syst Rev* (2):Art. No.: CD006583, 2008. doi: 10.1002/14651858.CD006583.pub2.
2. Ali MM, Abd-Elnaeim M: Arthroscopy of the fetlock joint of the dromedary camel. *Vet Comp Orthop Traumatol* 25(3):192–196, 2012.
3. BBC: 2011. http://www.bbc.co.uk/news/world-asia-pacific-12952474. Accessed February 2013.
4. Bohm RP, Jr, Rockar RA, Ratterree MS, et al: A method of video-assisted thoracoscopic surgery for collection of thymic biopsies in rhesus monkeys (*Macaca mulatta*). *Contemp Top Lab Anim Sci* 39(6):24–26, 2000.
5. Bush M, Seger SWJ, Wildt DE: Laparoscopy in zoo mammals. In Harrison RM, Wildt DE, editors: *Animal laparoscopy*, Baltimore, MD, 1980, Williams and Wilkins, pp 169–182.
6. Case JB, Marvel SJ, Boscan P, Monnet EL: Surgical time and severity of postoperative pain in dogs undergoing laparoscopic ovariectomy with one, two, or three instrument cannulas. *J Am Vet Med Assoc* 239(2):203–208, 2011.
7. Chang DC, Yu PT, Easterlin MC, Talamini MA: Demystifying sample-size calculation for clinical trials and comparative effectiveness research: The impact of low event frequency in surgical clinical research. *Surg Endosc* 27:359–363, 2013.
8. Cook RA, Stoloff DR: The application of minimally invasive surgery for the diagnosis and treatment of captive wildlife. In Fowler ME, Miller RE, editors: *Zoo and wild animal medicine: Current therapy*, ed 4, Philadelphia, PA, 1999, Saunders, pp 30–40.
9. Dallwig RK, Langan JN, Hatch DA, et al: Bilateral hydronephrosis secondary to endometriosis managed by endoscopic ureteral stent placement in a captive Guinea baboon (*Papio papio*). *J Zoo Wildl Med* 42(4):747–750, 2011.
10. Divers SJ: Endoscopy and endosurgery. *Vet Clin North Am Exot Anim Pract* 160, 2010.
11. Dover SR, Van Bonn W: Flexible and rigid endoscopy in marine mammals. In Dierauf LA, Gulland FMD, editors: *CRC handbook of marine mammal medicine: Health, disease, and rehabilitation*, Boca Raton, FL, 2001, CRC Press, p 621.
12. Dumonceaux GA, Lamberski N, Clutter D, et al: Treatment of bilateral nasal polyposis and chronic refractory inhalant allergic rhinitis in a chimpanzee (*Pan troglodytes*). *J Zoo Wildl Med* 28(2):215–219, 1997.
13. Fauquier D, Gulland F, Haulena M, Spraker T: Biliary adenocarcinoma in a stranded northern elephant seal (*Mirounga angustirostris*). *J Wildl Dis* 39(3):723–726, 2003.
14. Ferronha F, Barros F, Santos VV, et al: Is there any evidence of superiority between retropubic, laparoscopic or robot-assisted radical prostatectomy? *Int Braz J Urol* 37(2):146–158, discussion 159–160, 2011.
15. Freeman LJ, editor: *Veterinary endosurgery*, St. Louis, MO, 1999, Mosby, pp xv–xvii.
16. Gracia-Calvo LA, Martín-Cuervo M, Jiménez J, et al: Intra- and postoperative assessment of re-sterilised ligature atlas for orchidectomies in horses: Clinical study. *Vet Rec* 171:2012.
17. Haynes AB, Weiser TG, Berry WR, et al, Safe Surgery Saves Lives Study Group: A surgical safety checklist to reduce morbidity and mortality in a global population. *N Engl J Med* 360(5):491–499, 2009.
18. Hermes R, Goeritz F, Portas TJ, et al: Ovarian superstimulation, transrectal ultrasound-guided oocyte recovery, and IVF in rhinoceros. *Theriogenology* 72(7):958–996, 2009.
19. Hettlich BF, Hobson HP, Ducot TJ, et al: Esophageal hiatal hernia in three exotic felines—*Lynx lynx, Puma concolore, Panthera leo*. *J Zoo Wildl Med* 41(1):90–94, 2010.
20. Hodgson-Moore A, Ragni R: *Clinical manual of small animal endosurgery*, 2012, Wiley-Blackwell Publishing, p 334.
21. Kearns KS, Jones MP, Bright RM, et al: Hiatal hernia and diaphragmatic eventration in a leopard (*Panthera pardus*). *J Zoo Wildl Med* 31(3):379–382, 2000.
22. Ketz J, Radlinsky M, Armbrust L, et al: Persistent right aortic arch and aberrant left subclavian artery in a white Bengal tiger (*Panthera tigris*). *J Zoo Wildl Med* 32(2):268–272, 2001.
23. Kimber K: Diaphragmatic hernias in captive cheetahs (*Acinonyx jubatus*). In *Proceedings of the American Association of Zoo Veterinarians*, 2001, p 151.
24. Kowalczyk KJ, Yu HY, Ulmer W, et al: Outcomes assessment in men undergoing open retropubic radical prostatectomy, laparoscopic radical prostatectomy, and robotic-assisted radical prostatectomy. *World J Urol* 30(1):85–89, 2012.
25. Lhermette P, Sorbel D: An introduction to endoscopy and endosurgery. In *BSAVA Manual of endoscopy and endosurgery*, Gloucester, U.K., 2008, BSAVA, pp 1–10.
26. Lhermette P, Sorbel D: *BSAVA manual of canine and feline endoscopy and endosurgery*, Gloucester, U.K., 2008, BSAVA, p 300.
27. Lubbe AM, Henton MM: Sterilisation of surgical instruments with formaldehyde gas. *Vet Rec* 140:450–453, 1997.
28. Maslow AH: *The psychology of science*, 1966, Harper & Row, p 168.
29. Matheson JS, Gamble KC, Lacasse C: Treatment of unilateral pleural effusion in a black and white ruffed lemur (*Varecia varecia*) with rutin. In *Proceedings of the American Association of Zoo Veterinarians*, 2004, p 601.

30. Mayhew P: Developing minimally invasive surgery in companion animals. *Vet Rec* 169:177–178, 2011.

31. Mayhew PD, Freeman L, Kwan T, Brown DC: Comparison of surgical site infection rates in clean and clean-contaminated wounds in dogs and cats after minimally invasive versus open surgery: 179 cases (2007–2008). *J Am Vet Med Assoc* 240:193–198, 2012.

32. Mclatchie G, Borley N, Chikwe J: *Oxford handbook of clinical surgery*, ed 3, Oxford, U.K., 2007, Oxford University Press, pp 300–303.

33. Mclatchie GR, Leaper DJ: *Operative surgery: Oxford specialist handbooks in surgery*, ed 2, Oxford, U.K., 2006, Oxford University Press, pp 336–341.

34. Pader K, Freeman LJ, Constable PD, et al: Comparison of transvaginal natural orifice transluminal endoscopic surgery (NOTES®) and laparoscopy for elective bilateral ovariectomy in standing mares. *Vet Surg* 40(8):998–1008, 2011.

35. Parkinson TJ: Progress towards less invasive veterinary surgery. *Vet Rec* 171:67–68, 2012.

36. Pearce SG, Hurtig MB: Surgical repair of a ruptured cranial cruciate ligament in a dromedary camel. *J Am Vet Med Assoc* 215(9):1325–1327, 1282, 1999.

37. Pentecost RL, Niehaus AJ, Santschi E: Arthroscopic approach and intraarticular anatomy of the stifle in South American camelids. *Vet Surg* 41(4):458–464, 2012.

38. Peters ML, Sommer M, van Kleef M, Marcus MAE: Predictors of physical and emotional recovery 6 and 12 months after surgery. *Br J Surg* 97:1518–1527, 2010.

39. Pizzi R: Small exotic species endosurgery. In Hodgson-Moore A, Ragni R, editors: *Clinical manual of small animal endosurgery*, 2012, Wiley-Blackwell Publishing, pp 273–306.

40. Pizzi R: Thoracoscopy. In Hodgson-Moore A, Ragni R, editors: *Clinical manual of small animal endosurgery*, 2012, Wiley-Blackwell Publishing, pp 169–208.

41. Pizzi R: Welfare and behavioural advantages of keyhole sterilisation of New world primates. In *Proceedings of the First International New World Primate Symposium*, Warwickshire, U.K., March 17–18, 2012, Twycross Zoo.

42. Pizzi R, Brown D, Girling S: *Minimally invasive vasectomy in primates: Cost-efficacy, welfare, and behavioural advantages*, November 10–11, 2012, British Veterinary Zoological Society, Edinburgh Zoo.

43. Pizzi R, Cracknell J, Carter P: Ante-mortem screening of beavers for *Echinococcus*. *Vet Rec* 170:293–294, 2012.

44. Pizzi R, Cracknell J, Dalrymple L: Postmortem Evaluation of Left Flank Laparoscopic Access in an Adult Female Giraffe (Giraffa camelopardalis). *Veterinary Medicine International* vol. 2010, Article ID 789465, 4 pages, 2010. doi:10.4061/2010/789465.

45. Pizzi R, Cracknell J, David S, et al: Laparoscopic cholecystectomy under field conditions in Asiatic black bears (Ursus thibetanus) rescued from illegal bile farming in Vietnam. *Vet Rec* 169(18):469, 2011. doi: 10.1136/vr.d4985.

46. Pizzi R, Girling S, Bell A, et al: Laparoscopic-Assisted Cryptorchidectomy in an Adult Reindeer (Rangifer tarandus). *Veterinary Medicine International* vol. 2011, Article ID 131368, 4 pages, 2011. doi:10.4061/2011/131368

47. Pizzi R, Seddon C, Liddell C: *Minimally invasive surgical access in grey seals (Halichoerus grypus) and harbour seals (Phoca vitulina)*, Ashford, U.K., April 2011, British Veterinary Zoological Society (BVZS).

48. Portas TJ, Hermes R, Bryant BR, et al: Anaesthesia and use of a sling system to facilitate transvaginal laparoscopy in a black rhinoceros (Diceros bicornis minor). *J Zoo Wildl Med* 37(2):202–205, 2006.

49. Quesada R, Citino SB, Easley JT, et al: Surgical resolution of an avulsion fracture of the peroneus tertius origin in a giraffe (Giraffa camelopardalis reticulata). *J Zoo Wildl Med* 42(2):348–350, 2011.

50. Radcliffe RM, Turner TA, Radcliffe CH, Radcliffe RW: Arthroscopic surgery in a reticulated giraffe (Giraffa camelopardalis reticulata). *J Zoo Wildl Med* 30(3):416–420, 1999.

51. Rossetti RB, Massoco Cde O, Penna AC, Silva LC: An experimental study to compare inflammatory response due to liquid or gas joint distension in horses submitted to arthroscopy. *Acta Cir Bras* 27(12):848–854, 2012.

52. Rush EM, Ogburn AL, Hall J, et al: Surgical implantation of a cardiac resynchronization therapy device in a western lowland gorilla (*Gorilla gorilla gorilla*) with fibrosing cardiomyopathy. *J Zoo Wildl Med* 41(3):395–403, 2010.

53. Rush EM, Ogburn AL, Monroe D: Clinical management of a western lowland gorilla (*Gorilla gorilla gorilla*) with a cardiac resynchronization therapy device. *J Zoo Wildl Med* 42(2):263–276, 2011.

54. Schmitt TL, Sur RL: Treatment of ureteral calculus obstruction with laser lithotripsy in an Atlantic bottlenose dolphin (*Tursiops truncatus*). *J Zoo Wildl Med* 43(1):101–109, 2012.

55. Seldinger SI: Catheter replacement of the needle in percutaneous arteriography: A new technique. *Acta Radiol* 39(5):368–376, 1953.

56. Shapira Y, Katz M, Ali M, et al: Utilization of murine laparoscopy for continuous in-vivo assessment of the liver in multiple disease models. *PLoS ONE* 4(3):e4776, 2009.

57. Sherrill J, Peavy GM, Kopit MJ, et al: Use of laser rhinoscopy to treat a nasal obstruction in a captive California sea lion (*Zalophus californianus*). *J Zoo Wildl Med* 35(2):232–241, 2004.

58. Stetter M, Hendrickson DA: Laparoscopic surgery in the elephant and rhinoceros. In Miller RE, Fowler ME, editors: *Zoo and wild animal medicine: Current therapy*, vol 7, St. Louis, MO, 2011, Saunders, pp 524–530.

59. Svenson O: Are we all less risky and more skillful than our fellow drivers? *Acta Psychol (Amst)* 47(2):143–148, 1981.

60. Tams TR, Rawlings CA: *Small animal endoscopy*, ed 3, St. Louis, MO, 2011, Mosby, p 696.

61. Tversky A, Kahneman D: Judgement under uncertainty: Heuristics and biases. *Science* 185:1124–1131, 1974.

62. van der Voort M, Heijnsdijk EA, Gouma DJ: Bowel injury as a complication of laparoscopy. *Br J Surg* 91(10):1253–1258, 2004.

63. Varma R, Gupta JK: Laparoscopic entry techniques: Clinical guideline, national survey, and medicolegal ramifications. *Surg Endosc* 22(12):2686–2697, 2008.

64. Walsh PJ, Remedios AM, Ferguson JF, et al: Thoracoscopic versus open partial pericardectomy in dogs: Comparison of postoperative pain and morbidity. *Vet Surg* 28:472, 1999.

65. Wickham JE: The new surgery. *Br Med J* 295:1581–1582, 1987.

66. Wojick KB, Gamble KC, Slater O, et al: Bilateral ureteral stent placement and lithotripsy in an Asian small-clawed otter (*Aonyx cinerea*) with nephrolithiasis. In *Proceedings of the American Association of Zoo Veterinarians*, 2009, p 129.

SUGGESTED READING

Abutarbush SM, Carmalt JL: *Endoscopy and arthroscopy for the equine practitioner*, 2008, Teton New Media, p 292.

Barakzai S: *Handbook of equine respiratory endoscopy*, St. Louis, MO, 2006, Saunders, p 144.

Beale BS, Hulse DA, Schultz K, Whitney WO: *Small animal arthroscopy*, St.Louis, MO, 2003, Saunders, p 256.

Brearley MJ, Cooper JE, Sullivan M: *A colour atlas of small animal endoscopy*, 1991, Wolfe Publishing, p 128.

Divers SJ: Endoscopy and endosurgery. *Vet Clin North Am Exot Anim Pract* 160:2010.

Fischer AT: *Equine diagnostic and surgical laparoscopy*, St.Louis, MO, 2001, Saunders, p 365.

Freeman LJ: *Veterinary endosurgery*, St.Louis, MO, 1998, Mosby, p 384.

Harrison RM, Wildt DE: *Animal laparoscopy*, 1980, William and Wilkins, p 256.

Hodgson-Moore A, Ragni R: *Clinical manual of small animal endosurgery*, 2012, Wiley-Blackwell Publishing, p 334.

Lhermette P, Sorbel D: *BSAVA manual of canine and feline endoscopy and endosurgery*, Gloucester, U.K., 2008, BSAVA, p 300.

McCarthy TC: *Veterinary endoscopy for the small animal practitioner*, St.Louis, MO, 2004, Saunders, p 624.

McIlwraith CW, Wright I, Nixon AJ, Boening KJ: *Diagnostic and surgical arthroscopy in the horse*, ed 3, St.Louis, MO, 2005, Mosby, p 480.

Radlinsky M: *Veterinary clinics of North America, small animal practice: Endoscopy*, St.Louis, MO, 2009, Saunders, p 240.

Ragle CA: *Advances in equine laparoscopy*, 2012, Wiley-Blackwell, p 360.

Tams TR, Rawlings CA: *Small animal endoscopy*, St.Louis, MO, 2011, Mosby, p 696.

WEBSITES

www.vetlapsurg.com—the internet portal for all aspects of minimally invasive surgery in all veterinary species, including a numerous videos, pictures, and equipment reviews, and a veterinary endosurgery safety checklist.

www.websurg.com—a human laparoscopic surgery website, with a large number of surgery videos, useful in demonstrating principles and techniques, although the majority of common human procedures are very different from those applicable in veterinary patients.

www.who.int/patientsafety—the World Health Organization site on human surgical patient safety, and the original safe surgery checklist, as well as other useful documents on learning from errors.

CHAPTER **73**

Conservation Medicine to One Health: The Role of Zoologic Veterinarians

Sharon L. Deem

One of the penalties of an ecological education is that one lives alone in a world of wounds.

—Aldo Leopold

The approaches of conservation medicine and One Health are well known to zoologic veterinarians, and, indeed, almost everything we do professionally fits within the objectives of these approaches. However, it is possible that few zoologic veterinarians give sincere thought to the underlying global changes that threaten the conservation of biodiversity and human health and the historical context behind these transformative approaches. In this chapter, both conservation medicine and One Health will be reviewed following a brief overview of current conservation and health challenges, which were the catalyst behind the establishment of both these initiatives. Lastly, the leadership roles of accredited zoos in ex situ and in situ conservation programs and more specifically the role that zoologic veterinarians play within conservation medicine and One Health will be discussed with examples of zoo-led, zoo-supported, and zoo-based projects.

CHALLENGES TO THE CONSERVATION OF BIODIVERSITY AND HUMAN HEALTH

Global challenges that threaten the conservation of biodiversity and the health of *Homo sapiens* are extensive and beyond the scope of this chapter. Briefly, these challenges range from the uncertain, but very real, impacts on species' health exerted by global climate change to the documented increasing interactions among wildlife, domestic animals, and humans, which have resulted in the current concerns regarding emerging infectious diseases (EIDs).

The pressures limiting the long-term survival of many of the wildlife species that zoos are dedicated to conserving are largely human driven (anthropogenic). These pressures include climate change, habitat degradation and fragmentation, introduction of invasive species, trade in wildlife, and exposure to emerging pathogens, all of which are associated with the human population growth, which surpassed 7 billion individuals in 2012. In fact, these anthropogenic changes have led many to contend that planet Earth is presently in a new "Anthropocene" epoch.[5] Simply stated, humans are the drivers of planetary health. According to recent scientific reports, humans have transformed between one third and one half of the land surface and now appropriate over 40% of the net primary terrestrial productivity, consume 35% of the productivity of the oceanic shelf, and use 60% of the freshwater run-off each year.[29,32,36,40] What might these statistics indicate in terms of resource availability and health challenges for the other species that share the planet with humans? Additionally, with the estimated 50% increase in human consumption of animal-based protein by the year 2020, it is inevitable that human use of resources will continue to rise.[12] Lastly, the estimated billions of live wildlife animals and animal products that are traded annually also place heavy burdens that threaten the long-term survival of species.[37] In addition to the direct impacts that wildlife trade places on the conservation of species, are the less apparent, but potentially devastating, impacts associated with cross-species microbial mixing and exposure to novel microbes that further threaten the health of all species, including humans.

Concurrent with the recognition of the new Anthropocene era comes the demonstration by recent analyses that species' extinctions occur at rates of 100 to 1000 times the baseline levels in the pre-agricultural era, with these rates increasing steadily.[31] For example, it is estimated that since 1970, global population sizes of wildlife species have decreased by 30%.[41] With regard to species decline by animal taxa, the species threatened with extinction include 12% of birds, 21% of mammals, 30% of amphibians, and 27% of reef-building corals.[23] Zoologic veterinarians must be cognizant of the current conservation challenges and incorporate this knowledge into health programs directed at the conservation of wildlife species, both ex situ and in situ, while ensuring human public health.

HEALTH CARE FOR SPECIES LIVING IN A WORLD OF WOUNDS

During the last few decades, an increasing focus has been placed on conservation and health approaches, termed *conservation medicine* and *One Health*. These approaches provide the framework for developing the environmental and health solutions necessary to address the above challenges. The shift to embrace more holistic approaches in ecologic studies, conservation projects, and human public health has led to a number of publications that provide definitions and examples of both these approaches.[15,17]

Although often presented as new approaches, these initiatives are built on centuries of collaborative thought guided by principles similar to those that direct much of our conservation medicine and One Health work today. This may have been most eloquently phrased as early as the 1800s by the physician Rudolf Virchow in his statement: "Between animal and human medicine, there is no dividing line—nor should there be." In the 1900s, the term *One Medicine* was coined and signaled the beginnings of the conservation medicine and One Health initiatives.[38] Early leaders of the movement paved the way for the current development of the well-accepted and increasingly practiced approaches of conservation medicine and One Health.

Conservation medicine as an ecologically driven and conservation-minded approach first appeared in the literature in the 1990s.[19] Although a number of definitions for conservation medicine exist, at the core is the realization that the health of environments and the animals and the humans within them are intimately related and that multiple disciplines are required to better understand and manage conservation efforts and disease challenges, which impact all three. Conservation medicine may best be defined as a transdisciplinary approach to study the relationships among the health states of humans, animals, and ecosystems to ensure the conservation of all, including *Homo sapiens*.[1,10,19]

Starting in the 2000s, the One Health initiative has become widely accepted and increasingly driven by the human medical field, although veterinary medicine has embraced this approach as well. As the One Health approach gains momentum, it may be important to consider how it differs from conservation medicine. One Health may be based less on understanding the ecosystems compared with conservation medicine. In fact, an early definition of the One Health concept stated that this initiative aims to merge animal and human health sciences to benefit both.[13] However, as with conservation medicine, a number of recent definitions of One Health do consider ecosystems as important as human and animal health. One unifying theme has been that One Health is a strategy that strives to expand transdisciplinary collaborations and communications to improve health care for humans, animals, and the environment.[17] This defining theme is rather analogous to conservation medicine.

It is easy to appreciate that these approaches have many similarities; both have the objective to improve the health of animals and humans while recognizing the constant interplay and growing interconnections among animals, humans, and ecosystems. In fact, One Health might be viewed as having evolved from conservation medicine, triggered by the growing realization that EIDs in humans are largely of zoonotic origin.[16] One Health initiatives now support the use of animal and human disease models, as well as the use of animals and humans as sentinels for each other to advance the understanding of diseases to benefit *all* animal species and to emphasize the need for preventive measures that minimize the spread of pathogens across species.[34]

It is more important to develop programs that fit into both the conservation medicine and One Health paradigms rather than picking either term for describing a program. Zoologic veterinarians practice both conservation medicine and One Health. However, it is important that all these programs do consider the relationship between the health of animals and that of humans, and how environmental conditions play a vital role in the health of all species. In the years to come, the tougher challenges for effective conservation medicine and One Health approaches may be related to the ethics of efforts with different cost–benefit ratios for the different groups of interest (i.e., animals, humans, and ecosystems). Significant health benefits to one may be at the cost of another. One example may be public health measures that involve large scale culling of wildlife in an effort to protect human health but which may ultimately result in damage to the health of other species, to the ecosystems, and possibly to humans as well. As zoologic veterinarians practicing conservation medicine and One Health, it is important to remain true to the underlying objectives of these transdisciplinary approaches and work to ensure the conservation of biodiversity.

OPPORTUNITIES FOR ZOOLOGICAL INSTITUTIONS

While the number of species threatened by extinction grows daily, accredited zoologic institutions are now being fully recognized as conservation organizations. In this chapter, the word *accredited* will refer to the approximately 218 zoos and aquariums accredited by the Association of Zoos and Aquariums (AZA), other regional zoo organizations, and the approximately 300 organizations accredited by the World Association of Zoos and Aquariums (WAZA). The term *zoologic veterinarian* will refer to zoologic and aquarium veterinarians. Unlike many other conservation organizations, zoos are often seen as organizations that work for species survival and that are dedicated to the long-term conservation of wildlife species. One example is the documentation that of the 68 species which had their conservation threat level reduced by the International Union for the Conservation of Nature (IUCN), the reduction for 17 (25%) of these species was associated with captive breeding efforts at zoologic institutions.[4]

As accredited zoos are being increasingly recognized for their conservation initiatives, it has also become evident that this leadership role of zoos in the conservation of species developed along with advancements in health care that ensured population viability. Veterinary sciences, which were previously overlooked as being instrumental in the role of zoos in the conservation of species, are now seen as imperative for conservation efforts and the long-term survival of populations in zoo collections and of free-living populations.[11,24] In fact, one of the key reasons that zoos are successful conservation organizations is related to the veterinary care provided to animals in collections and to field-based health studies that improve conservation efforts and provide comparative health data for free-living and collection populations.[11] Today, with the push for AZA-accredited zoos to dedicate 3% of their revenue to conservation, the time is right for zoos to also show their leadership roles in conservation medicine and One Health initiatives. In fact, a core objective of a zoo conservation program is often to ensure healthy wildlife populations and ecosystems without compromising the health of humans, and thus the conservation mission of accredited zoos fits perfectly within the objectives of conservation medicine and One Health. Furthermore, to attain accreditation, zoos must have animal care providers and veterinary clinicians on staff. Often zoos also have epidemiologists, nutritionists, reproductive physiologists, pathologists, endocrinologists, geneticists, education specialists, public relations experts, and animal behaviorists on staff, all equipped to advance the conservation medicine and One Health objectives.

Roles of Zoologic Veterinarians in Conservation Medicine and One Health

The education, experiences, and responsibilities of zoologic veterinarians position them as key players in the transdisciplinary approaches of conservation medicine and One Health. In fact, the role of zoologic veterinarians has been well-represented in conservation medicine over the last 15 years and is now also recognized in One Health.[7,10,11,15,39] Zoos today are much more than simple "arks" of protection for threatened and endangered wildlife, and staff provide health care and conduct health studies on animals both within zoo walls (ex situ) and in the wild (in situ).[11] As we move forward and strengthen the efforts of zoologic veterinarians in these initiatives, it will be important to develop strong relationships between successful zoo-based conservation medicine and One Health activities across the entire zoologic community and in the conservation medicine and One Health communities.[7,39]

The significant contributions of zoologic veterinarians to conservation medicine and One Health and the benefits that zoos offer to both biodiversity conservation and human health may be categorized into five roles: (1) providing healthcare for zoologic species, thus ensuring sustainability of biodiversity; (2) conducting studies on diseases of conservation concern; (3) understanding diseases in zoo wildlife as sentinels for emerging diseases of humans and animals in surrounding areas; (4) performing surveillance of diseases in wild animals at the interface of wildlife, domestic animals, and humans; and (5) making contributions to the fields of comparative medicine and the discovery of *all* life forms (Figure 73-1 and Box 73-1).

Providing Healthcare for Zoo Wildlife to Ensure Sustainability of Biodiversity

Accredited zoos have succeeded in their efforts to bring some species back from the brink of extinction for many intersecting reasons. One reason is the advances in veterinary care, including preventive and therapeutic care to minimize the negative impacts of infectious and noninfectious diseases. Similar to public health programs (e.g., vaccination and proper nutrition) that were instrumental in the human population reaching beyond seven billion individuals, these veterinary health care methods have been essential for the propagation of species. Now as wild spaces are being reduced and free-living wildlife often live within habitats that are little more than large zoos, these veterinary advancements, many of which are first developed with zoo collection animals, are also being used for the long-term

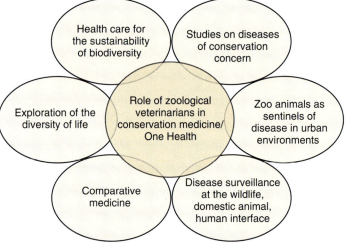

FIGURE 73-1 The roles of zoologic veterinarians in conservation medicine and One Health.

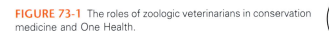

BOX 73-1 The Role of Zoologic Veterinarians in Conservation Medicine and One Health

Role	Examples
Providing health care for zoo wildlife, thus ensuring the sustainability of biodiversity	◆ Captive breeding programs ◆ Reintroduction programs with healthy zoo-bred animals ◆ Veterinary care of zoo animals that serve as healthy ambassadors for public support of conservation
Conducting studies on diseases of conservation concern	◆ Canine distemper virus infection ◆ Chytridiomycosis in amphibians ◆ Diclofenac poisoning ◆ Elephant endothelial herpes virus infection ◆ Tasmanian devil disease
Understanding diseases in zoo wildlife as sentinels for emerging diseases of humans and animals	◆ Avian influenza ◆ *Baylisascaris procyonis* infection ◆ Chronic wasting disease ◆ Tuberculosis ◆ West Nile virus infection

Surveillance of disease in wild animals at the interface of wildlife, domestic animals, and humans	◆ Most accredited zoos fund or conduct health programs throughout the world. A few examples:
	  1. Cleveland Metroparks Zoo
	  2. Global Health Program of Wildlife Conservation Society
	  3. Saint Louis Zoo Institute for Conservation Medicine and WildCare Institute
	  4. San Diego Zoo Global
	  5. Smithsonian National Zoo

Contributing to the field of comparative medicine and the discovery of all life forms	◆ Most accredited zoos work with medical and veterinary universities on comparative medicine projects ◆ Many accredited zoos work with genomic laboratories to better categorize the microbiome

survival of populations in the wild.[11] Lastly, a number of reintroduction programs such as those for black-footed ferrets, red wolves, Hawaiian songbirds, and freshwater mussels have resulted in the propagation of species at accredited zoos and successful placement back in the wild (http://www.aza.org/reintroduction-programs/). The successes of these (and many other) reintroduction programs were only possible when health challenges were appropriately addressed within the reintroduction plans in conjunction with other important program components.

Conducting Studies on Diseases of Conservation Concern

Zoos conduct studies to better understand the clinical impacts, epidemiology, and pathology of diseases that have population impacts and, in some cases, species-level impacts. Diseases in wildlife species have now been documented to impact the survival of species with both population extirpations and even species extinctions.[6,30] Many of the infectious diseases that threaten the long-term survival of wildlife species, including fibropapillomatosis in sea turtles, chytridiomycosis in amphibians, canine distemper in a number of carnivores, and Ebola virus in humans and animals are studied by zoologic health professionals.[6,9] Disease-related conservation challenges are not solely linked to infectious diseases, possibly best exemplified by the near-extinction of three *Gyps* spp. in India associated with the use of an anti-inflammatory drug in livestock.[28] Whether infectious or noninfectious, diseases may have impacts on multiple scales, affecting individuals (fitness costs), populations (population size and connection), communities (changes in species composition), and ecosystems (structure, function, and resilience).[8] The epidemiology, pathology, and clinical implications of many of these significant disease challenges are studied extensively by zoo health professionals, both in situ and ex situ.[25,35] These scientific investigations are often turned into conservation actions implemented by zoos to minimize the negative impacts identified by these studies.

Benefits gained from these zoo-led studies are many and include the sustainability of biodiversity, which may help ensure the continuation of ecosystem services provided by biodiversity such as the prevention of disease. The recently recognized "dilution" effect, in which a larger assembly of species (increased biodiversity), each with different disease susceptibilities, may minimize emerging infectious diseases of humans and other animals, is a great example of how zoo-based studies to better manage diseases of conservation concern may have broad-reaching, cross species health implications.[18]

Understanding Diseases in Zoo Wildlife as Sentinels for Emerging Diseases of Humans and Animals

Animals cared for in accredited zoos include a variety of nondomestic species, with differing susceptibilities to infectious and noninfectious diseases. These zoo animals provide a sentinel system for the regions where they are housed. Animals in accredited zoos receive veterinary care, documented in medical records, and contribute to blood and tissue banks, both of which offer a sustainable epidemiologic monitoring system that may be beneficial for animal and public health. One example is the Lincoln Park Zoo Davee Center for Epidemiology and Endocrinology, which coordinates national efforts of accredited zoos in the United States to serve as sentinels by testing and monitoring for zoonotic disease outbreaks.

A well-known example of zoo animals serving as sentinels is the detection of West Nile virus (WNV) at a zoo in New York State, which led to the zoo community alerting other human and animal health communities to the arrival of this vector-borne pathogen to the New World.[22,33] The network of accredited zoologic parks in the United States and Europe now have surveillance programs for zoonotic pathogens such as avian influenza virus and WNV, linking zoos and effectively covering continents.[3,33] Additionally, many zoos in North America have surveillance programs for urban wildlife on and near zoo grounds for zoonotic pathogens such as rabies virus and *Baylisascaris procyonis*. Lastly, with the sophisticated record keeping capabilities of these institutions, along with the careful pathologic evaluations at necropsy, the ability to better understand trends in

potential noninfectious health concerns shared by animals and humans (e.g., cancers and toxins) is also explored at zoologic institutions. Veterinary staff members at accredited zoos often have ties with doctors in human medicine, thus ensuring communication of comparative findings from zoo animals and human patients in the region. This collaborative work between the human and veterinary medical fields may serve as an early warning system for diseases of concern for both animals and humans.

Surveillance of Disease in Wild Animals at the Interface of Wildlife, Domestic Animals, and Humans

Staff members of accredited zoos conduct conservation studies that give zoos a global footprint. For example, an overlay of 113 WAZA-branded projects with documented biodiversity and emerging disease hotspots demonstrates that this footprint includes regions of significant conservation and human health concerns (Figure 73-2).[14,16,26] The often long-term commitments to field conservation and research from these zoo-led programs provide a means for zoo staff to perform health surveillance studies that may include species of conservation interest and sympatric species. A number of these in situ studies also have a human health component, as many of the pathogens of interest are zoonotic and may spillover and spillback among wild populations, domestic animals, and humans sharing the habitat.[2,20]

Contributing to the Field of Comparative Medicine and the Discovery of All Life Forms

Comparative medicine, a long-established field within both the veterinary and human medical professions, is based on comparisons and contrasts of the anatomy, physiology, and pathophysiology of diseases of humans and other species. Advances in human medicine are largely from comparative studies based on animal models. Today, growing applications of human studies promote understanding of the diseases of animals (e.g., cancers, arthritis) and the use of sentinel animals and humans for the health of each other.[34] The role zoos play in the field of comparative medicine was underutilized in the past; however, it is now being increasingly documented. Zoos and the animals in their care are important in comparative medicine studies and have gained crossover appreciation by both veterinary and human medical professionals and a general nonmedical audience.[27]

In biodiversity conservation, much emphasis has been placed on the long-term survival of vertebrate species, with lesser emphasis on invertebrate conservation and even less on the conservation of microorganisms. However, without microorganisms, biodiversity would not exist. Species are metagenomic in that they are composed of their own gene complements and those of all their associated microbes. Each species—in fact, each individual—is known to have unique "microbiomes." One study of the bacterial 16S ribosomal RNA gene sequences from a variety of zoologic animals demonstrated that host diet and phylogeny both influence bacterial diversity while adding new microbial species to the list of life forms on Earth.[21] Accredited zoos, with their collections of diverse species and their outreach across the globe through studies on free-living wildlife populations, can, and must, contribute to the exploration of the diversity of life at the microbial level.

CONCLUSION

In this chapter, roles that zoologic veterinarians have to contribute within conservation medicine and One Health approaches were discussed. Zoologic veterinarians will continue to serve as key players dedicated to the conservation of biodiversity and as health care providers for animals, ecosystems, and humans. They also will fully participate in conservation medicine and One Health initiatives. In addition to these roles, zoologic veterinarians must be educators, disseminating the message about the health continuum that exists among people, animals, and the ecosystems that support biodiversity.

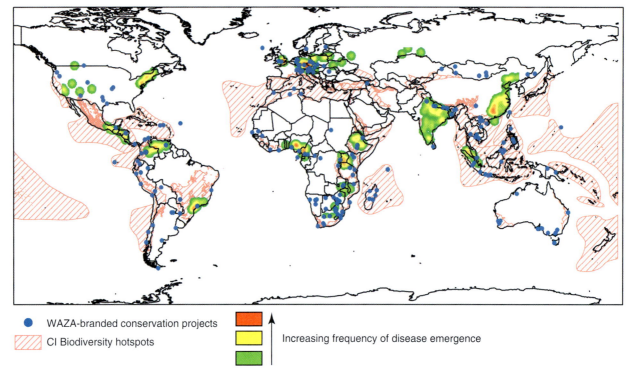

● WAZA-branded conservation projects

▨ CI Biodiversity hotspots

Increasing frequency of disease emergence

FIGURE 73-2 The global footprint of in situ programs branded by the World Association of Zoos and Aquariums, which are found in many of the Earth's biodiversity and emerging disease hotspots. (Map modified from data presented in Myers et al., 2000; Jones et al., 2008; and Gusset and Dick, 2010.)[14,16,26]

During the past decades, as conservation medicine and One Health initiatives gained global support, the conservation and health challenges that engendered these approaches have also continued to grow. The increasing evidence of global climate change impacts, including the hottest year in recorded history for the United States, EID issues with the worst year of human West Nile virus cases in the United States, and the documentation of increases in the illegal trade in wildlife species all clearly demonstrate these challenges. The need for practicing conservation medicine and One Health approaches and bringing these efforts into the mainstream has never been more pressing, and zoologic veterinarians are in a key position to meet this need.

Since the 1990s, ecologists have embraced the conservation medicine movement, with disease ecology recognized as an important new subspecialty within the study of ecology. In the past few years, the human medical establishment has become increasingly aware of the link between human and animal health and the need to approach human health in a more ecologic context. It is imperative that zoologic veterinarians continue to be active participants in these efforts and that they work on projects that ensure the health of all—the animals in their direct care, the humans that interact with these animals, and the habitats that sustain all life on Earth.

REFERENCES

1. Aguirre AA, Ostfeld RS, Tabor GM, et al: *Conservation medicine ecological health in practice*, Oxford, U.K., 2002, Oxford University Press.
2. Bronson E, Emmons LH, Murray S, et al: Serosurvey of pathogens in domestic dogs on the border of Noël Kempff Mercado National Park, Bolivia. *J Zoo Wildl Med* 39:28–36, 2008.
3. Chosy J, Travis D, Nadler Y: Zoos as disease sentinels: Piloting an avian influenza surveillance system in zoological institutions. *J Mol Gen Med* 3:184, 2009.
4. Conde DA, Flesness N, Colchero F, et al: An emerging role of zoos to conserve biodiversity. *Science* 331:1390–1391, 2011.
5. Crutzen PJ: Geology of mankind. *Nature* 415:23, 2002.
6. Daszak P, Cunningham AA, Hyatt AD: Emerging infectious diseases of wildlife–Threats to biodiversity and human health. *Science* 287:443–449, 2000.
7. Deem SL, Dennis P: The role of zoos in One Health. *One Health Newslett* 5:4–7, 2012. http://www.doh.state.fl.us/environment/medicine/One_Health/FallOHNL2012.pdf. Accessed 2/23/2013.
8. Deem SL, Ezenwa VO, Ward JR, Wilcox BA: Research frontiers in ecological systems: Evaluating the impacts of infectious disease on ecosystems. In Ostfeld RS, Eviner VT, Keesing F, editors: *Infectious disease ecology: Effects of ecosystems on disease and of disease on ecosystems*, Princeton, NJ, 2008, Princeton University Press, pp 304–318.
9. Deem SL, Karesh WB, Weisman W: Putting theory into practice: Wildlife health in conservation. *Cons Biol* 15:1224–1233, 2001.
10. Deem SL, Kilbourn AM, Wolfe ND, et al: Conservation medicine. *Ann NY Acad Sci* 916:370–377, 2000.
11. Deem SL: Role of the zoo veterinarian in the conservation of captive and free-ranging wildlife. *Int Zoo Yb* 41:3–11, 2007.
12. Delgado C, Rosegrant M, Steinfeld H, et al: Livestock to 2020: The next food revolution. *Outlook Agric* 30:27–29, 2001.
13. Enserink M: Initiative aims to merge animal and human health science to benefit both. *Science* 316:1553, 2007.
14. Gusset M, Dick G: Building a future for wildlife? Evaluating the contribution of the world zoo and aquarium community to in situ conservation. *Int Zoo Yb* 44:183–191, 2010.
15. Jakob-Hoff R, Warren KS: Conservation medicine for zoo veterinarians. In Miller RE, Fowler ME, editors: *Fowler's zoo and wild animal medicine: Current therapy*, ed 7, St. Louis, MO, 2012, Saunders, pp 15–23.
16. Jones KE, Patel NG, Levy MA, et al: Global trends in emerging infectious diseases. *Nature* 451:990–994, 2008.
17. Kahn LH, Monath TP, Bokma BH, et al: One Health, One Medicine. In Aguirre AA, Ostfeld RS, Daszak P, editors: *New directions in conservation*

medicine: Applied cases of ecological health, New York, 2012, Oxford University Press, pp 33–44.

18. Keesing F, Belden LK, Daszak P, et al: Impacts of biodiversity on the emergence and transmission of infectious diseases. *Nature* 468:647–652, 2010.

19. Koch M: Wildlife, people, and development. *Trop Anim Hlth Prod* 28:68–80, 1996.

20. Leendertz FH, Pauli G, Maetz-Rensing K, et al: 2006. Pathogens as drivers of population declines: The importance of systematic monitoring in great apes and other threatened mammals. *Biol Cons* 131:325–337, 2006.

21. Ley RE, Hamady M, Lozupone C, et al: Evolution of mammals and their gut microbes. *Science* 320:1647–1651, 2008.

22. Ludwig GV, Calle PP, Mangiafico JA, et al: An outbreak of West Nile virus in a New York City captive wildlife population. *Am J Trop Med Hyg* 67:67–75, 2002.

23. Marton-Lèfevre J: Biodiversity is our life. *Science* 327:1179, 2010.

24. Miller RE: Zoo veterinarians—the doctors on the ark? *J Am Vet Med Assoc* 200:642–647, 1992.

25. Munson L, Nesbit JW, Meltzer DG, et al: Diseases of captive cheetahs (*Acinonyx jubatus jubatus*) in South Africa: A 20-year retrospective survey. *J Zoo Wildl Med* 30:342–347, 1999.

26. Myers N, Mittermeier RA, Mittermeier CG, et al: Biodiversity hotspots for conservation priorities. *Nature* 403:853–858, 2000.

27. Natterson-Horowitz B, Bowers K: *Zoobiquity: What animals can teach us about health and the science of healing*, New York, 2012, Random House.

28. Oaks JL, Gilbert M, Virani MZ, et al: Diclofenac residues as the cause of vulture population declines in Pakistan. *Nature* 427:630–633, 2004.

29. Pauly D, Christensen V: Primary production required to sustain global fisheries. *Nature* 374:255–257, 1995.

30. Pedersen A, Jones KE, Nunn CL, Altizer S: Infectious diseases and extinction risk in wild mammals. *Cons Biol* 21:1269–1279, 2007.

31. Pimm SL, Russell G, Gittleman JL, Brooks TM: The future of biodiversity. *Science* 269:347–350, 1995.

32. Postel SL, Daily GC, Ehrlich PR: Human appropriation of renewable fresh water. *Science* 271:785–788, 1996.

33. Pultorak E, Nadler Y, Travis D, et al: Zoological institution participation in a West Nile virus surveillance system: Implications for public health. *Pub Hlth* 125:592–599, 2011.

34. Rabinowitz PM, Conti LA: Sentinel disease signs and symptoms. In Rabinowitz PM, Conti LA, editors: *Human-animal medicine: Clinical approaches to zoonoses, toxicants, and other shared health risks*, Maryland Heights, MO, 2010, Saunders, pp 18–23.

35. Rideout BA, Stalis I, Papendick R, et al: Patterns of mortality in free-ranging California condors (*Gymnogyps californianus*). *J Wildl Dis* 48:95–112, 2012.

36. Rojstaczer S, Sterling SM, Moore NJ: Human appropriation of photosynthesis products. *Science* 294:2549–2552, 2001.

37. Rosen GE, Smith KF: Summarizing the evidence on the international trade in illegal wildlife. *EcoHealth* 7:24–32, 2010.

38. Schwabe C: *Veterinary medicine and human health*, ed 3, Baltimore, MD, 1984, Williams and Wilkins.

39. Vitali S, Reiss A, Eden P: Conservation medicine in and through zoos. *Int Zoo Yb* 45:1–8, 2011.

40. Vitousek PM, Ehrlich PR, Ehrlich AH, Matson PA: Human appropriation of the products of photosynthesis. *Bioscience* 36:368–373, 1986.

41. World Wildlife Fund: Living Planet Index, Report—2010: Biodiversity, biocapacity, and development, http://www.library.drexel.edu/blogs/drexelbioscience/2010/11/30/living-planet-report-2010-biodiversity-biocapacity-development/. 57 pp. Accessed 2/23/2013.

CHAPTER 74

Recent Updates for Antemortem Tuberculosis Diagnostics in Zoo Animals

Alexis Lecu and Ray L. Ball

Tuberculosis (TB) and other mycobacterial diseases remain a difficult issue for veterinarian and zoo stakeholders to deal with. Regulatory requirements may give very broad obligations for prophylactic screening but are rarely precise enough to allow adequate follow-up with every zoo animal. Meanwhile, the risk of silent transmission between zoo animals and humans remains a real concern, as several cases of transmission are still reported every year from zoos and other institutions keeping captive wild animals all over the world.[11,27,42,49,50] Within the last 5 years, more than 19 peer-reviewed publications dealt with single or grouped TB outbreaks in zoo settings, and more than 50 peer-reviewed publications were about the application of diagnostics methods in various wild animal species;[11] this confirms that the research and tools currently available are improving greatly. It is imperative that zoo and wildlife clinicians have a basic understanding and access to these reference materials to choose between all recent methods and apply and interpret them properly. Although mycobacterial diseases will likely remain a challenge because of their complex pathophysiology, the zoo and wildlife practitioner has a larger, developing array of diagnostic options for both TB and non-TB mycobacterial screening. Most of the time, an indirect test alone is meaningless if it is not combined with clinical examination, direct screening, and with another indirect assay. Combinations of tests always improve the accuracy of TB diagnostics, as long as parallel tests that are independent of each other are chosen.

DIRECT TEST

Although culture remains the gold standard to confirm the presence of mycobacteria, several tools are now available to get information indicating the presence of mycobacteria more quickly. Culture may be accelerated with the use of custom broth media associated with automated microbacteriologic detection systems such as the BACTEC Microbacteria Growth Indicator Tube (MGIT), which can produce results in 6 weeks with *Mycobacterium tuberculosis* or *M.bovis*.[19] *Mycobacterium* DNA (deoxyribonucleic acid) sequences may also be revealed by molecular amplification techniques, which are now broadly available and have improved sensitivity values compared with those existing 10 years ago.[24] Genotyping techniques are useful in understanding the epidemiologic origin and transmission of mycobacterial infections,[47,48] and those techniques may sometimes be applied on raw samples (biopsies, fluids), prior to culture results, as long as sufficient mycobacterial DNA quantity is present. Intermittent shedding[38,63] and low amounts of mycobacteria in internal fluids are likely to lower the sensitivity of the test, even if the molecular technique has excellent intrinsic sensitivity. Frequent collection such as repeated trunk washes in elephants[38] is a way to overcome this limitation. The selection of an ideal sample should be based on clinical examination.[34] Direct detection of mycobacteria in peripheral blood is a technique that is used especially for the diagnostic of extrapulmonary disseminated forms of TB.[26] This technique demonstrates a sensitivity of 50% to 80%[7,26] and has been recently applied in deer to investigate *M. bovis* or *M. tuberculosis* infection[4] by using duplex and multiplex polymerase chain reaction (PCR) methods applied on EDTA (ethylenediaminetetraacetic acid) blood samples.

INDIRECT TEST

Cell-Mediated Immunity

One of the most common antemortem indirect tests used over the years is the intradermal tuberculin skin test (TST), but its limitations have been already described in many wildlife species.[9,45] Interferon gamma release assays (IGRAs) are now being used in veterinary medicine[9,34] as an alternative to TST (Table 74-1). These tests measure in vitro cytokine (interferon-gamma [IFN-γ]) production by live lymphocytes contained in a fresh blood sample while exposed to selected mycobacterial antigens. The IGRAs measure the presence of an adaptive immune response to *M. tuberculosis* antigens and are thus only an indirect measure of exposure.[31] The first advantage is that they are in vitro tests, which removes some of the variability of in vivo tests. Secondly, these tests could be further modified to bring more specific information by exposing blood cell samples to selected specific antigens from any *Mycobacterium* species. However, IGRAs have their own limitations that must be kept in mind when ordering them or interpreting their results.[21] The animal IGRAs available commercially (e.g., Bovigam or Primagam) do not have positive controls, so they must then be selected and added into the tests by the operator.[15] The choice of this mitogen will influence the result, as all interpretations of flowcharts are based on comparisons between the amounts of IFN produced by negative controls, antigens, and positive controls. A great discrepancy exists between mitogen stimulation abilities, according to the animal species,[10,64] so the clinician should ask the reference laboratory about the molecule used as positive control or even suggest it according to the literature.

In commercial kits, enzyme-linked immunosorbent assay (ELISA) is used to detect the IFN-γ of cattle (Bovigam) or certain primate species (Primagam). As indicated in Tables 74-2 and 74-3, ELISA may be able to detect IFN-γ from a broader range of species.[33] Moreover, use of a monoclonal IFN antibody designed for the targeted animal species may be used[29,46] within these commercial IGRAs to improve the test quality (Table 74-4). RNA (ribonucleic acid) sequences coding for IFN-γ primers are now available for a wide range of animal species,[6,61] with gene expression in peripheral blood mononuclear cells (PBMCs) of cattle[5] or elephants[58] used to distinguish infected animals from noninfected animals.

TABLE 74-1

Examples of Mitogens to Be Used as Positive Controls for IGRAs in Some Primate Species

	Relative Amount of Gamma Interferon Released By Stimulation of Each Mitogen				
	PHA	ConA	PWM	SEA	SEB
Pan troglodytes	+++	+	+	+	+
Hylobates leucogenys	++	ND	++++	+++	++++
Gorilla gorilla	–	+	++	++	++
Chlorocebus aethiops	–	+	++++	ND	++++
Cecropithecus neglectus	++	++	++	+	+
Trachypithecus auratus auratus	–	++++	+++	++++	++++
Trachypithecus obscures	–	ND	++++	+++	+++
Lemur catta	ND	–	–	–	–
Varecia variegate	–	+	–	–	–
Eulemur fulvus albifrons	+	ND	–	ND	ND
Macaca fascicularis	–	++	–	ND	+
Macaca silenus	+	–	–	–	–
Macaca nemestrina	–	+	+	+	+
Macac mulatta	–	+	ND	ND	+
Mandrillus sphinx	+++	+	+++	ND	+++
Callithrix jaccus	ND	ND	+++	ND	+++
Pongo pygmaeus	++++	++	+++	++++	++++
Saimiri sciureus	+	ND	+++	ND	+++
Ateles geofroyi	–	–	+	+	+
Leontideus rosalia	–	–	+	+	++

ConA, concanavaline A; *IGRA*, interferon gamma release assay; *ND*, not done; *PHA*: phytohemagluttinin; *PWM*, pokeweed; *SEA*, staphylococcal enterotoxin A; *SEB*, staphylococcal enterotoxin A.
+ = Absorbance reading >0.15.
++ = Absorbance reading 0.15–0.50.
+++ = Absorbance reading 0.50–0.75.
++++ = Absorbance reading >0.75.
– = Absorbance reading<0.15.
From Schroeder, B. "Primagam®—The Primate IFN-γ Test." Deutsches Primatenzentrum. Web. Accessed December 23, 2014. <http://www.dpz.eu/fileadmin/content/Infektionspathologie/Bilder/Dokumente/SCHROEDER%20TB%20FORMAT%20Cop_Korr.pdf>

Humoral Immunity

Some animal species seem to present a strong, early, and persistent humoral component of their immune response to mycobacterial infections.[38] Several assays, including lateral flow technology, that may be performed at the zoo premises are now available.[39] Unique or multiplex ELISA or fluorescence polarization assays[46] targeting various mycobacterial surface proteins must be run in a laboratory. Measurement of humoral response requires only serum, which may be obtained from a serum bank, as these antibodies can remain stable in frozen serum for a number of years.[22] When used as such, they could be helpful to trace the epidemiologic origin of TB infection and transmission over time.[2,37]

Serologic tests have several limitations. First, the technique used to reveal antibody must not cross-react with the target animal species. Immunodominant antigens and respective antibody titers may vary according to animal host species, mycobacterial species, and the stage of the mycobacterial infection. Some seroreactive TB antigens are now documented in species such as primates.[65]

Lack of knowledge of precise dominant antigens may be overcome by multiplex tests that assess reactivity to a large panel of antigens at once. This technique is used in all "rapid tests" (STAT PAK and Dual Path Platform DPP), in which a single result, reflected as a test band, may express reactivity to one or several antigens. In other multiplex tests such as ENFERPLEX TB[5,28] or multi-antigen print immunoassays (MAPIA), reactivity to each individual antigen is readable individually.

Boosting Immunologic Answer to Enhance Sensitivity

Stimulation of both cell-mediated immunity and humoral immunity by injection of mycobacterial antigens such as purified protein derivatives (PPDs) or recombinant antigens has been used to elicit a greater reaction to subsequent testing by provoking an anamnestic rise of the immunologic response.[17] Usually, this effect may be detected several days after antigen(s) injection and may last for several weeks. Individuals without TB infection typically do not express this increased response, and the difference between prebooster and postbooster responses should remain within the variability ranges for these animals.[35] This technique has been used to enhance the sensitivity of IGRAs,[52] and serologic assays.[17] However, the real effect of a booster is still being debated by some authors,[62] as an anamnestic rise is not always obviously distinctive from test variability. Moreover, the amount of tuberculin used to launch the booster effect is still rather empiric. A nonspecific inflammatory stimulation caused by the injection of foreign immunostimulant proteins may occur and then mimic an anamnestic rise, producing false-positive results and thus decreasing specificity. This is especially common in cytokines release assays. Therefore, use of the booster effect should be restricted to species for which sufficient knowledge

TABLE 74-2

Summary of Applicable Tests on Zoo and Wildlife Species

Method of Detection	Test	Sample	Species	Pro	Con
Direct cellular immunity	PCR	Fluids (urine, BAL, discharges) Biopsies Histology slides	All	Molecular techniques	Contamination with other environmental mycobacteria
	PCR	Blood		Screens mycobacterial antigens of highly disseminative forms	Mycobacteria itself rarely present within circulation
	Culture	Biopsies, frozen tissues, fluids		Gold standard method Delay could be shortened by use of enhanced methods (see text)	Test turnaround is lengthy
	Stain	Biopsies, fluids		Inexpensive	Limited by intermittent shedding
Indirect cellular immunity	Single tuberculin skin test	Soft, naked or shaved visible skin area. Should not be exposed to high temperature variation or external inflammation causes	NHP, Bo	Reduced cost	Poorer sensitivity and specificity Discrepancy among tuberculin Dosage is often empiric Reading test may require immobilization at 48–72 hours
	Comparative tuberculin skin test		NHP, Bo, Cv	Enhanced specificity: could differentiate *Mycobacterium avium* or non-tuberculosis mycobacterial infection	Reading test may require immobilization at 48–72 hours
	IGRA	Whole fresh (<8 h) blood on heparin	Bo, some OWM, Rh	Marketed for primates and cattle. Cattle test could be used with success in a lot of Bovidae and Giraffidae	Experimental rhinos and felids Not applicable to all primates Short viability of sample
Indirect humoral immunity	ELISA	Serum	Ta, El, Cv, Rh, Bo	Test antibody to broad antigens (filtrate) or very specific ones (ESAT6, CFP10,...) Retrospective analysis	Cross reactivity to non-targeted species may confound results Host must mount humoral response
	Rapid Lateral Flow Assays	Whole blood Serum (fresh or frozen)	Bo, some OWM, El, Rh, Fe, Bo	Field use, results within 20 min Retrospective analysis	Host must mount humoral response

BAL, Bronchoalveolar lavage; *ELISA*, enzyme-linked immunosorbent assay; *IGRA*, interferon gamma release assay; *NHP*, nonhuman primate; *OWM*, Old World monkey; *Bo*, Bovidae; *Cv*, Cervidae; *EL*, elephant; *Fe*, felids; *Pi*, pinnipeds; *PCR*, polymerase chain reaction; *Ta*, tapir; *Rh*, rhinoceros.
From Schroeder B: Presented at Deutsches Primatenzentrum 01.12.2010 PrimagamThe Primate IFN-γ Test, Deutsches Primatenzentrum, Prionics AG; Wagistr 27A, 8952 Schlieren, Switzerland. Accessed December 23, 2013 http://www.dpz.eu/filadmin/content/Infektionspathologie/Bilder/Dokuments/SCHROEDER%20TB%20FORMAT%20Cop_Korr.pdf.

TABLE 74-3

Cross-Reactivity of Two Interferon-Gamma ELISAs

	ELISA	
Species	**"Monkey" Interferon-Gamma**	**"Human" Interferon-Gamma**
Macaca rhesus	+	−
Macaca fascicularis	+	−
Macaca nemestrina	+	−
Papio sp.	+	+
Cercocebus athys	+	ND
Aotus sp.	+	+
Callithrix jacchus	−	+
Saimiri sciureus	ND	+
Pan troglodytes	ND	+

ELISA, Enzyme-linked immunosorbent assay; *ND,* not done.
+ = detection/binding of species interferon.
− = detection failed.
From Mabtech. "Human/Monkey cross-reactivity info." Mabtech AB 2013. Web. Accessed December 23, 2014. <www.mabtech.com/Main/Page.asp? PageId=41>

on IGRA exists and should ideally be performed in association with testing of negative control animals for comparison of effects.

SPECIES UPDATES

Camelids

M. bovis and *M. tuberculosis* are able to infect all camelids, but *M. microti* is of special concern in South American camelids (SACs), as a "llama type" of this *Mycobacterium* species exists. In SACs, a combination of antibody screening and custom-designed IGRA has been used successfully to identify infected animals.[37] It should be noted that the commercial IGRA Bovigam does detect camelid IFN-γ.[16] Neither serologic nor IGRA kits alone seem to have a sensitivity greater than 70%, but combinations of both can be adequate for proper detection of infected animals (Table 74-2).

Elephants

Asian (*Elephas maximus*) and African (*Loxodonta africana*) elephants in captivity are frequently affected by TB and other mycobacterial diseases. In the United States, between 1994 and July 2012, TB was detected in 55 elephants. *M. tuberculosis* was isolated from 51 Asian elephants and 3 African elephants, and *M. bovis* was cultured from one African elephant. Thirty-five cases were diagnosed before death and 20 after death. Elephants are believed to be a species similar to humans in that TB infection may involve a latent stage.[51] Increasing the frequency of trunk washes[38] and using adjusted methods of DNA extraction[60] should be coordinated to enhance the effectiveness of direct screening. Among the current US population of 246 Asian elephants, the estimated prevalence of TB is 18% versus 2% in the

TABLE 74-4

Interferon-Gamma Release Assays and Serologic Assays*

Species	Commercial IGRA Brand Name Mitogen Used Stimulation Antigens (PPD) or (Re)combinant (ESAT6, CFP10)	Experimental IGRA Mitogen Used Stimulation Antigens (PPD) or (Re)combinant (ESAT6, CFP10)	Serologic Assay Comment†
Cattle: Domestic and wild (buffaloes, watusis)	**Bovigam** ConA *Pokeweed* **PPD**		
Giraffes	**Bovigam**[55] ConA *Pokeweed* **PPD**		*ELEPHANT STAT PAK*
Bovinae, including Tragelpahinae	**Bovigam**[55] ConA *Pokeweed* **PPD**		*Elephant TB STAT PAK*[23]
Reduncinae, including *Kobus* sp.	**Bovigam**[55] ConA *Pokeweed* **PPD**		
South American camelids		Based on pan-species IFN-γ ELISA *Pokeweed*[30] **PPD + REC**	**ENFERPLEX** **Vet TB STATPAK** *DPP*[38]
Rhinoceroses		Under development[25]	*Elephant TB STAT PAK*[23] *MAPIA*[23]
Elephants		Under development[53]	**Elephant TB STAT PAK**[12] **ELEPHANT DPP** ® MAPIA[12]

TABLE 74-4

Interferon-Gamma Release Assays and Serologic Assays—cont'd

Species	Commercial IGRA Brand Name Mitogen Used Stimulation Antigens (PPD) or (Re)combinant (ESAT6, CFP10)	Experimental IGRA Mitogen Used Stimulation Antigens (PPD) or (Re) combinant (ESAT6, CFP10)	Serologic Assay Comment†
Baboons	**Primagam** ConA[55] PHA **PPD**		PRIMATB STAT PAK
Macacas	**Primagam** ConA[55] PHA, SEB **PPD**		PRIMATB STAT PAK
Gorillas	**Primagam Quantiferon Gold T SPOT TB**[58] **PPD + REC**		PRIMATB STAT PAK
Orangutans	**Primagam Quantiferon Gold T SPOT TB**[58] **PPD + REC**		PRIMATB STAT PAK
Chimpanzees	**Primagam Quantiferon Gold T SPOT TB**[58] **PPD + REC**		
Pinnipeds			**Elephant TB STAT PAK**[65] **DPP** MAPIA[65]
Tapirs			**Elephant TB STAT PAK**[65] **DPP** MAPIA[65]
Deers		Based on pan-species IFN-γ ELISA or on IFN mRNA sequences detection by PCR *Pokeweed* **PPD + REC**	
Meerkats			**Elephant TB STAT PAK**[62] DPP MAPIA[62]
Felidae		Based on monoclonal lion IFN-γ antibody *PMA*[48] **PPD + REC** Not yet to confirm culture positive animals	**Vet TB STATPAK**[48] *Elephant TB STAT PAK*[73]

*Recently used in several zoo species with confirmation of culture positive findings.
†Bold = commercial; Italic = experimental/out of species range.
ConA, Concanavaline A; *DPP*, dual-path platform; *ELISA*, enzyme-linked immunosorbent assay; *IFN-γ*, interferon-gamma; *IGRA*, interferon-gamma release assay; *IGRA*, interferon gamma release assay; *mRNA*, messenger ribonucleic acid; *PCR*, polymerase chain reaction; *PHA*: phytohemagluttinin; *PPD*, purified protein derivative; *REC*, recombinant.

204 African elephants. With such prevalence, predictive values of serologic assays are high. Seroreactivity usually develops months to years prior to culture-based diagnosis and also wanes gradually in successfully treated elephants[38] and rhinoceroses.[13] This offers a convenient real-time monitoring tool for prognosis and response to treatment as well as detecting recrudescence of infection through a rise in antibody level after post-treatment decline.[38] This monitoring tool is also potentially valuable to examine environmental factors that may have allowed the original infection to occur or factors such as vitamin D deficiency, which may allow a latent infection to become active.[2]

In-house IGRAs using monoclonal IFN antibodies are still under development for elephants.[60] Cellular immunity plays an important role in the physiopathology of TB infection in elephants and may also be assessed by measuring several cytokines in peripheral blood samples.[29]

Nonhuman Primates

In nonhuman primates (NHPs), TB infection is often caused by *M. tuberculosis* and *M. bovis* in Old World monkeys, and New World monkeys may be infected by *M. microti* as well, through transmission via rodents.[18] However, recently discovered species from the TB complex may also infect apes,[8] which suggests a wide sensitivity of NHPs to all mycobacteria from the complex. Active TB and associated shedding of bacteria may be investigated by bronchoalveolar lavage (BAL) sampling, but mouth swabs may also be used as samples to perform culture, stains, and PCR.[66]

Indirect diagnostic of TB in primates historically relies on assessment of cellular immunologic status through an intradermal TST. The intradermal TST is still the most commonly used and the only method approved by Institute of Laboratory Animal Research and the Centers for Disease Control and Prevention (ILAR/CDC) for tuberculosis testing of animals in import quarantine.[58] However, the usual amount of tuberculin used in primate TSTs to elicit proper delayed hypersensitivity reaction is noticeably very high; 2000 tuberculin units of bovine PPD or 1500 units for old mammalian tuberculin, compared with the only 2 tuberculin units of PPD RT23 used in humans. These high doses of antigens could increase interference with the outcome of the test by eliciting a nonspecific local inflammatory process and thus produce false-positive results.

Humoral screening may also be performed in NHPs. A commercial rapid lateral flow test is available (PrimaTB STAT PAK) and was primarily validated for use on rhesus macaques (*Macaca mulatta*), cynomolguses (*Macaca fascicularis*), and African green monkeys (*Cercopithecus aethiops sabaeus*).[36] Application to other nonhuman primates must be done with cautious interpretation of the results, as sensitivity and specificity values are not available for species other than these three validated species. IGRAs have been used in various species of primates, but the parameters of the IGRA should be carefully chosen according to the primate species to be tested. *Mycobacterium* antigens used for stimulation will influence the specificity of the test. The final results may vary according to the chosen combination,[20] so choices have to be made on the basis of current information and cut-offs, based on risk assessment and goals of the screening, have to be defined and known.

Carnivores

In natural settings, carnivores may play a role as either reservoirs or spill-over hosts for mycobacteria, especially badgers[3,10,21] and lions[41] for *M. bovis*. A new species of *Mycobacterium* belonging to the TB complex, *Mycobacterium mungi*, has been recently discovered from TB outbreaks among banded mongooses.[32] Antemortem diagnostic techniques reported to successfully diagnose TB from carnivores are mainly direct ones. BAL,[32] upper respiratory cavity mucosal sampling,[1] or even breathing air analysis[21] have been used to diagnose TB in carnivores. However, it should be noted that in felids, the likelihood of respiratory lesions caused by mycobacterial infections is low.[59]

Specially designed IGRAs have been used in domestic cats[57] and lions.[41] Use of these recently created IGRAs for animals in high-risk environments or within groups of known infected cohorts has been helpful in canids[54] and felids,[57] but IGRAs for some species such as lions are still under development. *M. tuberculosis* infections have already been associated with rapid serologic assays seropositivity in some felids species such as lions[44] and jaguars.[23]

Pinnipeds

Mycobacterium pinnipedii, belonging to the TB complex, is the most common pathogen causing TB in sea lions, seals, and even dolphins. Among those marine animals, the South American sea lion (*Otaria byronia*) seems to be the most at risk, mainly because of sequential importations of infected wild animals in the early 1980s to the 1990s from Chile and Uruguay. The European Association of Zoos and Aquaria (EAZA) Taxon Advisory Group flowchart[14] for the diagnosis of TB in pinnipeds includes direct examination methodologies such as culture, stains, and PCR on BAL fluids, computed tomography (CT), and serologic testing. Feedback from the field seems to suggest that some serological assays such as dual-path platform (DPP) assays have a better sensitivity than STAT PAK. However, none of these tests has been studied with a large enough sample size compared with culture, so the results should be interpreted with caution. Additionally, the aquatic environment of these species is likely to expose them to many environmental (waterborne) mycobacteria, and this may interfere with any outcome of indirect testing. Therefore, a single

seropositivity with one serologic assay should raise concerns and initiate further screening.

Tapirs

TB has been reported in all species of tapirs, both in the wild and in captivity. Their ground foraging behavior places them at risk of contact with mycobacteria in soil and may increase their baseline immune response to antigen stimulation, thus lowering the specificity of indirect tests. Diagnostic flowcharts[55] recommend direct examination methodologies such as BAL fluid culture and PCR, serologic assays such as STAT PAK and ELISA, and skin testing (comparative avian and bovine PPD). Direct examination on swabs and fluids has already been reported to recover *M. tuberculosis* strain from live tapirs.[48]

ACKNOWLEDGMENTS

The authors would like to thank all European Association of Zoo and Wildlife veterinarians; Tuberculosis Working group members; as well as Michelle Miller and Konstantin Lyashchenko, for their tremendous help. Thanks also to Björn Schröder from Prionics.

REFERENCES

1. Alexander KA, Laver PN, Michel AL, et al: Novel *Mycobacterium tuberculosis* complex pathogen *M. mungi*. *Emerg Infect Dis* 16(8):1296–1299, 2010.
2. Ball RL: Preliminary epidemiological findings using serology in an outbreak of Mycobacterium tuberculosis in managed Asian elephants (*Elephas maximus*) at a single facility. In *Proceedings of the Elephant and Rhino Research and Conservation Symposium*, Rotterdam, NL, 2011, pp 45–46.
3. Chambers MA, Waterhouse S, Lyashchenko K, et al: Performance of TB immunodiagnostic tests in Eurasian badgers (*Meles meles*) of different ages and the influence of duration of infection on serological sensitivity. *BMC Vet Res* 5:42, 2009.
4. Chu CS, Yu CY, Chen CT, Su YC: *Mycobacterium tuberculosis* and *M. bovis* infection in Feedlot deer (*Cervus unicolor swinhoei* and *C. nippon taiouanus*) in Taiwan. *J Microbiol Immunol Infect* 45(6):426–434, 2012.
5. Churbanov A, Milligan B: Accurate diagnostics for bovine tuberculosis based on high-throughput sequencing. *PLoS ONE* 7(11):1–9, 2012.
6. Churbanov A, Milligan B: Accurate diagnostics for Bovine tuberculosis based on high-throughput sequencing. *PLoS ONE* 7(11):e50147, 2012.
7. Condos R, McClune A, Rom WN, Schluger NW: Peripheral-blood-based PCR assay to identify patients with active pulmonary tuberculosis. *Lancet* 347(9008):1082–1085, 1996.
8. Coscolla M, Lewin A, Metzger S, et al: Novel *Mycobacterium tuberculosis* complex isolate from a wild chimpanzee. *Emerg Infect Dis* 19(6):969–976, 2013.
9. Cousins DV, Florisson N: A review of tests available for use in the diagnosis of tuberculosis in non-bovine species. *Rev Sci Tech* (International Office of Epizootics) 24(3):1039–1059, 2005.
10. Dalley D, Davé D, Lesellier S, et al: Development and evaluation of a gamma-interferon assay for tuberculosis in badgers (*Meles meles*). *Tuberculosis (Edinb)* 88(3):235–243, 2008.
11. Dassanayake DLB, Jayawardene KLTD, Siribaddana A, Dangolla A: Prevalence of tuberculosis in keepers of captive elephants in Sri Lanka: A preliminary study. In *Proceedings of the Peradeniya University Research Sessions*, Sri Lanka, 2011, p 115.
12. Drewe JA, Dean GS, Michel AL, et al: Accuracy of three diagnostic tests for determining *Mycobacterium bovis* infection status in live-sampled wild meerkats (*Suricata suricatta*). *J Vet Diagn Invest* 21(1):31–39, 2009.
13. Duncan AE, Lyashchenko K, Greenwald R, et al: Application of Elephant TB STAT-PAK assay and MAPIA (multi-antigen print immunoassay) for detection of tuberculosis and monitoring of treatment in black rhinoceros (*Diceros bicornis*). *J Zoo Wildl Med* 40(4):781–785, 2009.
14. EAZWV Infectious Diseases Working Group: Tuberculosis in zoo species: Diagnostic update and management issues. In *Transmissible diseases handbook*, ed 4, 2009, EAZWV.

15. Faye S, Moyen JL, Gares H, et al: Determination of decisional cut-off values for the optimal diagnosis of bovine tuberculosis with a modified IFNγ assay (Bovigam®) in a low prevalence area in France. *Vet Microbiol* 151(1–2):60–67, 2011.

16. García-Bocanegra I, Barranco I, Rodríguez-Gómez IM, et al: Tuberculosis in alpacas (*Lama pacos*) caused by *Mycobacterium bovis*. *J Clin Microbiol* 48(5):1960–1964, 2009.

17. Harrington NP, Surujballi OP, Prescott JF, et al: Antibody responses of cervids (*Cervus elaphus*) following experimental *Mycobacterium bovis* infection and the implications for immunodiagnosis. *Clin Vaccine Immunol* 15(11):1650–1658, 2008.

18. Henrich M, Moser I, Weiss A, Reinacher M: Multiple granulomas in three squirrel monkeys (*Saimiri sciureus*) caused by *Mycobacterium microti*. *J Comp Pathol* 137(4):245–248, 2007.

19. Hines N, Payeur JB, Hoffman LJ: Comparison of the recovery of *Mycobacterium bovis* isolates using the BACTEC MGIT 960 system, BACTEC 460 system, and Middlebrook 7H10 and 7H11 solid media. *J Vet Diag Invest* 18(3):242–245, 2006.

20. Hoby S: Tuberculosis screening of chimpanzees (*Pan troglodytes*) and gorillas (*Gorilla g. gorilla*)—confusion or benefit? In *Proceedings of the International Conference on Diseases of Zoo Wild Animals*, Bussolengo, Italy, 2012, p 108.

21. Jones RM, Ashford R, Cork J, et al: Evaluation of a method to detect *Mycobacterium bovis* in air samples from infected Eurasian badgers (*Meles meles*) and their setts. *Letter Appl Microbiol* 56(5):361–365, 2013.

22. Jurczynski K, Lyashchenko KP, Gomis D, Moisson P: Pinniped tuberculosis caused by *Mycobacterium pinnipedii*: Transmission from aquatic to terrestrial mammals and diagnostic options. In *Proceedings of the AAZV, AAWV, AZA/NAG Joint Conference*, Knoxville, TN, 2007, pp 74–75.

23. Kasputin N, Ball R, Teare A, et al: Tuberculosis diagnosis in jaguar (*Panthera onca onca*) and Addra gazelle (*Gazealla dama ruficollis*) using multiple antigen print immunoassay and rapid lateral flow technology. In *Proceedings of the American Association of Zoo Veterinarians*, Tampa, FL, 2006, pp 257–260.

24. Kay MK, Linke L, Triantis J, et al: Evaluation of DNA extraction techniques for detecting *Mycobacterium tuberculosis* complex organisms in Asian elephant trunk wash samples. *J Clin Microbiol* 49(2):618–623, 2011.

25. Kay MK, Linke L, Triantis J, et al: Evaluation of DNA extraction techniques for detecting *Mycobacterium tuberculosis* complex organisms in Asian elephant trunk wash samples. *J Clin Microbiol* 49(2):618–623, 2011.

26. Khosla R, Dwivedi A, Sarin BC, Sehajpal PK: Peripheral blood based C-PCR assay for diagnosing extra-pulmonary tuberculosis. *Indian J Exp Biol* 47(6):447–453, 2009.

27. Kiers A, Klarenbeek A, Mendelts B, et al: Transmission of *Mycobacterium pinnipedii* to humans in a zoo with marine mammals. *Int J Tuberc Lung Dis* 12(12):1469–1473, 2008.

28. Kim S, Kim YK, Lee H, et al: Interferon gamma mRNA quantitative real-time polymerase chain reaction for the diagnosis of latent tuberculosis: A novel interferon gamma release assay. *Diagn Microbiol Infect Dis* 75(1):68–72, 2013.

29. Landolfi JA, Mikota SK, Chosy J, et al: Comparison of systemic cytokine levels in *Mycobacterium spp.* seropositive and seronegative Asian elephants (*Elephas maximus*). *J Zoo Wildl Med* 41(3):445–455, 2010.

30. Deleted in pages.

31. Lange C, Pai M, Drobniewski F, Migliori GB: Interferon-gamma release assays in the diagnosis of active tuberculosis: Sensible or silly? *Eur Respir J* 33:1250–1253, 2009.

32. Lantos A, Niemann S: Mezõsi L et al: Pulmonary tuberculosis due to *Mycobacterium bovis* subsp. *caprae* in captive Siberian tiger. *Emerg Infect Dis* 9(11):1462–1464, 2003.

33. Lécu A, Riquelme L: Evolution des outils diagnostiques de la tuberculose des espèces sauvages. *Bull Acad Vét Fr* 161:151–158, 2008.

34. Lecu A, Ball R: Mycobacterial infections in zoo animals: Relevance, diagnosis and management. *Int Zoo YB* 45(1):183–202, 2011.

35. Lyashchenko K, Whelan AO, Greenwald R, et al: Association of tuberculin-boosted antibody responses with pathology and cell-mediated

immunity in cattle vaccinated with *Mycobacterium bovis* BCG and infected with *M. bovis*. *Infect Immun* 72(5):2462–2467, 2004.

36. Lyashchenko KP, Greenwald R, Esfandiari J, et al: PrimaTB STAT-PAK assay, a novel, rapid lateral-flow test for tuberculosis in nonhuman primates. *Clin Vaccine Immunol* 14(9):1158–1164, 2007.

37. Lyashchenko KP, Greenwald R, Esfandiari J, et al: Diagnostic value of animal-side antibody assays for rapid detection of *Mycobacterium bovis* or *Mycobacterium* in South American camelids. *Clin Vaccine Immunol* 18(12):2143–2147, 2011.

38. Lyashchenko KP, Greenwald R, Esfandiari J, et al: Field application of serodiagnostics to identify elephants with tuberculosis prior to case confirmation by culture. *Clin Vaccine Immunol* 1:1269–1275, 2012.

39. Lyashchenko KP, Greenwald R, Esfandiari J, et al: Tuberculosis in elephants: Antibody responses to defined antigens of *Mycobacterium tuberculosis*, potential for early diagnosis, and monitoring of treatment. *Clin Vaccine Immunol* 13:722–732, 2006.

40. Maas M, Michel AL, Rutten VPMG: Facts and dilemmas in diagnosis of tuberculosis in wildlife. *Comp Immunol Microbiol Infect Dis* 1–17, 2012.

41. Maas M, van Kooten PJS, Schreuder J, et al: Development of a lion specific interferon gamma assay. *Vet Immunol Immunopathol* 149:292–297, 2012.

42. Michel AL, Huchzermeyer HF: the zoonotic importance if *Mycobacterium tuberculosis*: Transmission from human to monkey. *J South Afr Vet Assoc* 69(2):64–65, 1998.

43. Deleted in pages.

44. Miller M, Joubert J, Mathebula N, et al: Detection of antibodies to tuberculosis antigens in free-ranging lions (*Panthera leo*) infected with *Mycobacterium bovis* in Kruger National Park, South Africa. *J Zoo Wildl Med* 43(2):317–323, 2012.

45. Miller M: Current diagnostic methods for zoo animals. In Fowler ME, Miller RE, editors: *Zoo and wild animal medicine: Current therapy*, ed 6, St. Louis, MO, 2008, Saunders.

46. Morar D, Tijhaar E, Negrea A, et al: Cloning, sequencing and expression of white rhinoceros (*Ceratotherium simum*) interferon-gamma (IFN-gamma) and the production of rhinoceros IFN-gamma specific antibodies. *Vet Immunol Immunopathol* 115(1–2):146–154, 2007.

47. Moser I, Prodinger WM, Hotzel H, et al: *Mycobacterium pinnipedii*: Transmission from South American sea lion (*Otaria byronia*) to Bactrian camel (*Camelus bactrianus bactrianus*) and Malayan tapirs (*Tapirus indicus*). *Vet Microbiol* 127(3–4):399–406, 2008.

48. Murakami PS, Monego F, Ho JL, et al: Detection of RDRIO strain of *Mycobacterium tuberculosis* in tapirs (*Tapirus terrestris*) from a zoo in Brazil. *J Zoo Wild Med* 43(4):872–875, 2012.

49. Murphree R, Warkentin JV, Dunn JR, et al: Elephant-to-human transmission of tuberculosis. *Emerg Infect Dis* 17:366–371, 2009.

50. Obanda V, Poghon J, Yongo M, et al: First reported case of fatal tuberculosis in a wild African elephant with past human-wildlife contact. *Epidemiol Infect* ?:1–5, 2013.

51. Ong BL, Ngeow YF, Razak MF, et al: Tuberculosis in captive Asian elephants (*Elephas maximus*) in Peninsular Malaysia. *Epidemiol Infect* 18:1–7, 2013.

52. Palmer MV, Waters WR, Thacker TC, et al: Effects of different tuberculin skin-testing regimens on gamma interferon and antibody responses in cattle experimentally infected with *Mycobacterium bovis*. *Clin Vaccine Immunol* 13(3):387–394, 2006.

53. Parsons SD, Menezes AM, Cooper D, et al: Development of a diagnostic gene expression assay for tuberculosis and its use under field conditions in African buffaloes (*Syncerus caffer*). *Vet Immunol Immunopathol* 148(3–4):337–342, 2012.

54. Parsons SD, Warren RM, Ottenhoff TH, et al: Detection of *Mycobacterium tuberculosis* infection in dogs in a high risk setting. *Res Vet Sci* 92(3):414–419, 2012.

55. Pollock NR, Macovei L, Kanunfre K, et al: Validation of *Mycobacterium tuberculosis* Rv1681 protein as a diagnostic marker of active pulmonary tuberculosis. *J Microbiol* 51(5):1367–1373, 2013, in Press.

56. Deleted in pages.

57. Rhodes SG, Gunn-Mooore D, Boschiroli ML, et al: Comparative study of IFNγ and antibody tests for feline tuberculosis. *Vet Immunol Immunopathol* 144(1–2):129–134, 2011.

58. Roberts JA, Andrews K: Nonhuman primates quarantine: Its evolution and practice. *ILAR J* 49(2):145–156, 2008.

59. Rüfenacht S, Bögli-Stuber K, Bodmer T, et al: *Mycobacterium microti* infection in the cat: A case report, literature review and recent clinical experience. *J Feline Med Surg* 13(3):195–204, 2011.

60. Rutten VMPG: Development of an interferon-gamma test and serology for tuberculosis in Asian elephants. *J Kasetsart Veterinarians* 16:191, 2006.

61. Sawyer J, Mealing D, Dalley D, et al: Development and evaluation of a test for tuberculosis in live European badgers (*Meles meles*) based on measurement of gamma interferon mRNA by real-time PCR. *J Clin Microbiol* 45(8):2398–2403, 2007.

62. Schiller I, Vordermeier HM, Waters WR, et al: Bovine tuberculosis: Effect of the tuberculin skin test on in vitro interferon gamma responses. *Vet Immunol Immunopathol* 136(1–2):1–11, 2010.

63. Verma-Kumar S, Abraham D, Dendukuri N, et al: Serodiagnosis of tuberculosis in Asian elephants (*Elephas maximus*) in Southern India: A latent class analysis. *PLoS ONE* 7(11):e49548, 2012.

64. Waters WR, Palmer MV, Thacker TC, et al: Blood culture and stimulation conditions for the diagnosis of tuberculosis in cervids by the Cervigam assay. *Vet Rec* 162(7):203–208, 2008.

65. Whelan C, Shuralev E, Kwok HF, et al: Use of a multiplex enzyme-linked immunosorbent assay to detect a subpopulation of *Mycobacterium bovis*-infected animals deemed negative or inconclusive by the single intradermal comparative tuberculin skin test. *J Vet Diagn Invest* 23(3):499–503, 2011.

66. Wilbur AK, Engel GA, Rompis A, et al: From the mouth of monkeys: Detection of *Mycobacterium tuberculosis* DNA from buccal swabs of synanthropic macaques. *Am J Primatol* 74:676–686, 2012.

CHAPTER 75

Updates on West Nile Virus

Tracey McNamara

It has been 13 years since West Nile virus (WNV) first appeared in North America. Although some progress has been made in the understanding of its neurotropism, pathogenicity, modes of transmission, and species susceptibility, many unanswered questions remain about this resourceful and devastating virus. It is not hard to see how much has changed by just looking back at what was believed in 1999. At that time, it was thought that WNV could only be spread through the bite of a mosquito; that it usually caused a mild febrile and self-limiting infection; that only the very young and very old were at risk of developing neuroinvasive disease that affected only the brain; that mammals were dead-end hosts. By 2002, everything that had been said about WNV had to be reevaluated. By then, it had been shown that WNV could, in fact, be spread by many routes other than mosquito bite;[6,7] that even mild infections might not be benign and may cause long-term sequelae such as fatigue and cognitive deficits;[5] that other risk factors might be involved in development of West Nile neuroinvasive disease (WNND); that patients with WNND could also present with poliomyelitis[18] and serious long-term deficits such as Parkinsonism-like disorders;[23] that mammals are not necessarily dead-end hosts and may play a role in the epidemiology of WNV spread; and so on. And we are still learning.

Steele et al.[58] described WNV infection and illness in a number of avian zoo species in 2000 and suggested that species other than crows were susceptible. Although corvids are certainly excellent sentinels for WNV, the list of known susceptible avian species is now lengthy.[29] We also now know that species as diverse as alligators,[36] polar bears,[16] reindeer,[43] harbor seals and gray seals,[15] killer whales,[57] Barbary macaques,[41] and psittacines[44] may succumb to WNV infection. Ducks, which had been believed to be resistant to WNV infection, have also experienced die-offs.[22] Unusual cutaneous lesions were described in American alligators.[36] Species other than crows such as blue jays and sparrows[17,39] have emerged as good indicators of WNV activity. Mammals such as fox squirrels (*Sciurus niger*),[51]

eastern chipmunks (*Tamias striatus*),[48] and eastern cottontail rabbits (*Sylvagus floridanus*)[25] have been found to develop viremias sufficient to infect mosquitoes and may play a role in the epidemiologic spread of WNV in urban environments. WNV infection has also had significant impacts on raptors. Clinical and pathologic findings have been described elsewhere.[32] Raptors also emerged as an excellent surveillance tool. In one study, raptor admissions to rehabilitation clinics took place 14 weeks earlier than other surveillance methods.[34,35] Ophthalmologic lesions were described both in humans[26] and birds,[46] and this led to the development of a rapid, safe sampling method in crows called the "intraocular cocktail" that involves inserting a needle through the cornea and vigorously scraping the intraocular contents, aspirating them, and processing the material for nucleic acid extraction.[30] Feather testing has also proven useful.[35] Mosquito saliva was found to enhance WNV infection in mice bitten by *Culex tarsalis*, which suggests that it exerts a local effect.[62]

Steele et al.[58] also demonstrated abundant WNV antigens in the kidneys and intestinal tracts of infected zoo birds and suggested that direct horizontal transmission might be taking place among birds. Demonstration of antigen in ovarian and testicular tissue also hinted at the possibility of vertical transmission. We now know the virus may be transmitted directly bird to bird.[31] Studies have demonstrated oral and cloacal shedding of WNV,[28] which ultimately led to the development of a rapid diagnostic test used by many zoos and health departments across the nation.[45,59,60] WNV may also be spread via oral transmission,[2,53] via breast milk,[2] via the intrauterine route,[2] and via organ transplantation[9] and blood transfusions. Perhaps the fact that, as shown by experimental studies in primates,[49] hamsters,[70] and mice,[1] WNV may persist for months in infected animals is of greatest concern. Most recently, human studies have confirmed that viral persistence is present years after infection and is associated with the development of chronic kidney disease.[37] What this means for humans or animals has yet to be elucidated, but viral persistence may be associated with well-documented long-term sequelae seen in people.

The majority of recent literature has focused on the molecular biology of WNV. This chapter will summarize some of the recent work in that area, as well as information on viral persistence, long-term sequelae, and recent vaccine efforts.

In the past decade, much has been learned about the structure of the WNV virion. The WNV virion has several key structural proteins: the capsid protein C that binds viral ribonucleic acid (RNA), the premembrane (prM) protein that blocks premature viral fusion; and an E protein that mediates viral attachment, membrane fusion, and viral assembly. The majority of neutralizing antibodies are directed against regions of the E protein, although a subset likely recognizes prM.[52] The virion also has nonstructural proteins that regulate viral transcription and replication and attenuate host antiviral responses.[52] In 2002, a new strain of WNV emerged, but it differed from the NY99 strain in the envelope (E) protein at amino acid 159 (WNV02).[13] This is now the dominant genotype in North America. This single amino acid change has led to increased intensity of transmission of WNV and rapid geographic expansion.[13]

How WNV crosses the blood–brain barrier (BBB) and whether central nervous system (CNS) damage is caused by direct viral infection, indirectly by the host's immune response, or both, is a question that has been the subject of many studies.[8,10,13,19,20,33,52,54–56,66,67] Entry into the CNS is most likely through hematogenous spread with the help of tumor necrosis factor–alpha (TNF-α) and matrix metalloproteinases (MMPs), which increase the permeability of the BBB.[52,66] Adhesion molecules on the vascular endothelium and leukocytes play important roles in controlling entry into the CNS. Intercellular adhesion molecule 1 (ICAM-1) is critical to this process and plays an important role in neuroinvasion in mice.[10] Leukocyte trafficking to the CNS has been linked to the chemokine receptor CCR5, which is upregulated by WNV infection and is associated with CNS infiltration of CD+4 and CD+8 T cells, natural killer cells, and macrophages expressing the receptor.[19] CD+8 cells control infection by producing antiviral cytokines (interferon [IFN] or TNF-α) early in infection or by triggering the death of WNV-infected cells through perforin or FAS ligand–dependent pathways.[56] TNF-related apoptosis-inducing ligand (TRAIL) produced by CD+8 T-cells contributes to disease resolution by helping to clear WNV from the neurons in the CNS.[55] However, WNV has developed strategies for enhancing viral replication in the host by blocking the action of type 1-IFN and evading the antiviral activity of IFN-stimulated genes.[33] Two human genes, *CCR5* and 2′5′ oligoadenylate synthetase (*OAS1b*), have been identified as susceptible loci for WNV infection.

LONG-TERM SEQUELAE

In 1999, WNV was believed to cause a mild, febrile, self-limiting illness in the majority of patients, with a small percentage developing neuroinvasive disease. By 2004, it was recognized that WNV infection could result in a protracted convalescent period with long-term problems with memory; confusion; clinical depression; muscle weakness; tremors; and parkinsonism-like disorders[21,27] 18 months after infection. In a Houston study, 60% of encephalitic patients reported signs 5 years after infection.[65] Patients with a milder form of illness are just as likely to suffer long-term health problems as encephalitis cases.[4] In this study of WN fever, 84% of patients reported persistent fatigue, 59% memory problems, and 49% ongoing muscle weakness. Studies on long-term sequelae in naturally infected animals are not available. It is postulated that long-term sequelae may be a result of viral persistence.

VIRAL PERSISTENCE

In 1983, Pogodina et al.[49] published a study on WNV persistence in primates experimentally infected with several strains of WNV. They found that encephalitis was present in animals with neuroinvasive disease, with only febrile illness, or with asymptomatic infections. This was considered unusual, as most RNA viral infections are transient and are subsequently cleared by the host.[1] Concerned about this possibility, the Department of Pathology at the Bronx Zoo began long-term studies on known positive WNV cases in the zoo collection. In 2000, evaluation of brain tissue from known positive animals suggested that viral persistence might be taking place with the NY99 strain of WNV in naturally infected animals. A symptomatic snow leopard (*Panthera uncia*) and a greater Indian rhinoceros (*Rhinoceros unicornis*) died 3 and 8 months following illness and seroconversion. Both exhibited dramatic lymphoplasmacytic cuffing in the CNS at the time of death. An asymptomatic but seropositive babirousa (*Babyrousa babyrussa*) that died 10 months after seroconversion also had mild to moderate lymphoplasmacytic cuffing in the brain, which suggested that subclinical infections may also produce CNS pathology.

In 2006, WNV was demonstrated in the brain and CSF of an immunocompromised patient 4 months after initial diagnosis and in spite of treatment with IFN, immunoglobulins, and ribavirin. Persistent infection with WNV was demonstrated by the identification of WNV nucleic acid in the brain by reverse-transcriptase polymerase chain reaction (RT-PCR) assay and immunohistochemical demonstration of antigen in tissue.[47] A 2010 study[1] developed a murine model of viral persistence. It found viral persistence in the face of a robust antibody response and in the presence of inflammation in the brain even in subclinical infections and showed that WNV persisted in the CNS and peripheral tissues for up to 6 months following infection in mice with subclinical infections. The authors concluded that the "frequency, duration, and tissue location of WNV persistence are species dependent, probably due to differences in host immunity, severity of disease, initial viral loads and tissue tropism, and cell targets."[1] These studies have raised concerns about the role of viral persistence in the development of the now-recognized long-term sequelae of WNV infection. They also raise concerns about the estimated 1.2 million people with asymptomatic WNV infections in the United States and possible subclinical CNS disease.

The kidney has also been a focus of persistence studies. In 2005, WNV was detected in the urine of a patient with encephalitis 8 days after symptom onset. Viral RNA was detected by RT-PCR.[64] In another 2005 study in hamsters,[63] chronic renal infection and persistent shedding was found in urine up to 8 months after infection. When the isolates that resulted in renal tropism were compared with the wild-type parent virus (NY 385-99), nucleotide changes were found in coding regions, causing amino acid substitutions in the E, NS1, NS2B, and NS5 proteins.[14] A 2012 long-term study of patients in Houston found an association between neuroinvasive WNV infection and the development of chronic kidney disease and suggested that all patients with WNV should have their renal function closely monitored.[33]

It is not known what impact viral persistence may have on zoo species, but many zoo species tested WNV positive on plaque reduction neutralization test (PRNT) or RT-PCR during the national zoological surveillance for WNV project and, like humans, the animals also should have long-term follow-up. Unlike the human medical community, zoo practitioners have ready access to necropsy material for study. The zoo community is in the position to render a great service to public health, given its ability to follow animals over the long term and evaluate them for viral persistence and renal and neuropathology. Tissues should be harvested and frozen at −80°C for virus isolation and RT-PCR from all known WNV-positive birds and mammals at the time of necropsy. Any zoo clinician or pathologist who performs a necropsy on a previously positive animal, especially a long-lived mammal, is urged to contact this author. A grant is in preparation to cover the costs of virus isolation (VI), RT-PCR, histopathology, and immunohistochemistry on WNV survivors.

VACCINATION

A variety of vaccines and vaccine protocols have been used in the Chilean flamingos (*Phoenicopterus chilensis*);[38] red-tailed hawks (*Buteo jamacensis*);[50] Andean condors (*Vulture gryphus*) and Californian condors (*Gymnogyps californicus*);[61] greater one-horned rhinoceros (*Rhinoceros unicornis*);[68,69] sandhill cranes (*Grus canadensis*);[42] black-footed penguins (*Sphenicus demersus*), little blue penguins (*Eudyptula minor*), and American flamingos (*Phoenicopterus ruber*);[40] Humboldt (*Sphenicus humboldti*), Magellanic (*Sphenicus magellanicus*), Gentoo (*Pygoscelis papua*), and Rockhopper penguins (*Eudyptes chrysocome*);[11] and Attwater prairie chickens (*Tympanuchus cupido*)[40] with varying results. In a 2012 study in squirrel monkeys, a measles vaccine expressing the secreted form of WNV envelope glycoprotein induced protective immunity.[3] A 2013 study in captive Nene geese (*Branta sandvicensis*) showed that a vaccine developed for human use (WN-80E) was highly immunogenic and had no adverse biologic effects.[24] A recent paper provides excellent summaries of the current status of vaccine research.[12] *West Nile Encephalitis Virus Infection— Viral Pathogenesis and the Host Immune Response*, edited by Michael S. Diamond, discusses available vaccines, as well as all other aspects of this important virus and must be consulted by anyone interested in WNV.

CONCLUSION

Although some progress has been made in the understanding of WNV, many things still remain unexplained. What the human and animal model studies on viral persistence mean for zoo species is unclear, but ongoing investigation is warranted.

REFERENCES

1. Appler KK, Brown AN, Stewart BS, et al: Persistence of West Nile virus in the central nervous system and periphery of mice. *PLoS ONE* 5:e10649, 2010.
2. Blázquez AB, Sáiz JC: West Nile virus (WNV) transmission routes in the murine model: Intrauterine, by breastfeeding and after cannibal ingestion. *Virus Res* 151:240–243, 2010.
3. Brandler S, Marianneau P, Loth P, et al: Measles vaccine expressing the secreted form of West Nile virus envelope glycoprotein induces protective immunity in squirrel monkeys, a new model of West Nile virus infection. *J Infect Dis* 206:212–219, 2012.
4. Carson PJ, Konewko P, Wold KS, et al: Long-term clinical and neuropsychological outcomes of West Nile virus infection. *Clin Infect Dis* 43:723–730, 2006.
5. Carson PJ, Konewko P, Wold KS, et al: Long-term clinical and neuropsychological outcomes of West Nile virus infection. *Clin Infect Dis* 43:723–730, 2006.
6. Centers for Disease Control and Prevention: Possible West Nile virus transmission to an infant through breast-feeding—Michigan, 2002. *MMWR Morb Mortal Wkly Rep* 51:877–878, 2002.
7. Charatan F: Organ transplants and blood transfusions may transmit West Nile virus. *Br Med J* 325:566, 2002.
8. Cho H, Diamond MS: Immune responses to West Nile virus infection in the central nervous system. *Viruses* 4:3812–3830, 2012.
9. Cushing MM, Brat DJ, Mosunjac MI, et al: Fatal West Nile virus encephalitis in a renal transplant recipient. *Am J Clin Pathol* 121:26–31, 2004.
10. Dai J, Wang P, Bai F, et al: Icam-1 participates in the entry of West Nile virus into the central nervous system. *J Virol* 82:4164–4168, 2008.
11. Davis MR, Langan JN, Johnson YJ, et al: West Nile virus seroconversion in penguins after vaccination with a killed virus vaccine or a DNA vaccine. *J Zoo Wildl Med* 39:582–589, 2008.
12. De Filette M, Ulbert S, Diamond M, et al: Recent progress in West Nile virus diagnosis and vaccination. *Vet Res* 43:16, 2012.
13. Diamond MS: Virus and host determinants of West Nile virus pathogenesis. *PLoS Pathog* 5:e1000452, 2009.
14. Ding X, Wu X, Duan T, et al: Nucleotide and amino acid changes in West Nile virus strains exhibiting renal tropism in hamsters. *Am J Trop Med Hyg* 73:803–807, 2005.
15. Duncan AE, Stremme DW, Murray SZ, et al: Clinical illness in two harbor seals (*Phoce vitulina*) and one grey seal (*Halichoerus grypus*) caused by the West Nile virus. In *Proceedings of the American Association of Zoo Veterinarians*, Minneapolis, Minnesota, 2003.
16. Dutton CJ, Quinnell M, Lindsay R, et al: Paraparesis in a polar bear (*Ursus maritimus*) associated with West Nile virus infection. *J Zoo Wildl Med* 40:568–571, 2009.
17. Gibbs SE, Ellis AE, Mead DG, et al: West Nile virus detection in the organs of naturally infected blue jays (*Cyanocitta cristata*). *J Wildl Dis* 41:354–362, 2005.
18. Glass JD, Samuels O, Rich MM: Poliomyelitis due to West Nile virus. *N Engl J Med* 347:1280–1281, 2002.
19. Glass WG, Lim JK, Cholera R, et al: Chemokine receptor CCR5 promotes leukocyte trafficking to the brain and survival in West Nile virus infection. *J Exp Med* 202:1087–1098, 2005.
20. Glass WG, McDermott DH, Lim JK, et al: CCR5 deficiency increases risk of symptomatic West Nile virus infection. *J Exp Med* 203:35–40, 2006.
21. Hall DA, Tyler KL, Frey KL, et al: Persistent neurobehavioral signs and symptoms following West Nile fever. *J Neuropsychiatry Clin Neurosci* 20:122–123, 2008.
22. Himsworth CG, Gurney KE, Neimanis AS, et al: An outbreak of West Nile virus infection in captive lesser scaup (*Aythya affinis*) ducklings. *Avian Dis* 53:129–134, 2009.
23. Hughes JM, Wilson ME, Sejvar JJ: The long term outcomes of human West Nile virus infection. *Clin Infect Dis* 44(12):617–1624, 2007.
24. Jarvi SI, Hu D, Misajon K, et al: Vaccination of captive nēnē (*Branta sandvicensis*) against West Nile virus using a protein-based vaccine (WN-80E). *J Wildl Dis* 49:152–156, 2013.
25. Jeffrey Root J: West Nile virus associations in wild mammals: A synthesis. *Arch Virol* 148(4):735–752, 2013.
26. Khairallah M, Ben Yahia S, Ladjimi A, et al: Chorioretinal involvement in patients with West Nile virus infection. *Ophthalmology* 111:2065–2070, 2004.
27. Klee AL, Maidin B, Edwin B, et al: Long-term prognosis for clinical West Nile virus infection. *Emerg Infect Dis* 10:1405–1411, 2004.
28. Komar N, Lanciotti R, Bowen R, et al: Detection of West Nile virus in oral and cloacal swabs collected from bird carcasses. *Emerg Infect Dis* 8:741–742, 2002.
29. Komar N: West Nile virus: Epidemiology and ecology in North America. *Adv Virus Res* 61:185–234, 2003.
30. Lim AK, Dunne G, Gurfield N: Rapid bilateral intraocular cocktail sampling method for West Nile virus detection in dead corvids. *J Vet Diagn Invest* 21:516–519, 2009.
31. McLean RG, Ubico SR, Bourne D, Komar N: West Nile virus in livestock and wildlife. *Curr Top Microbiol Immunol* 267:271–308, 2002.
32. Miller ER, Fowler ME: *Fowler's zoo and wild animal medicine: Current therapy*, vol 7, St. Louis, MO, 2012, Saunders.
33. Murray KO, Walker C, Gould E: The virology, epidemiology, and clinical impact of West Nile virus: A decade of advancements in research since its introduction into the Western Hemisphere. *Epidemiol Infect* 139:807–817, 2011.
34. Nemeth N, Kratz G, Edwards E, et al: Surveillance for West Nile virus in clinic-admitted raptors, Colorado. *Emerg Infect Dis* 13:305–307, 2007.
35. Nemeth NM, Young GR, Burkhalter KL, et al: West Nile virus detection in nonvascular feathers from avian carcasses. *J Vet Diagn Invest* 21:616–622, 2009.
36. Nevarez JG, Mitchell MA, Morgan T, et al: Association of West Nile virus with lymphohistiocytic proliferative cutaneous lesions in American alligators (*Alligator mississippiensis*) detected by RT-PCR. *J Zoo Wildl Med* 39:562–566, 2008.
37. Nolan MS, Podoll AS, Hause AM, et al: Prevalence of chronic kidney disease and progression of disease over time among patients

enrolled in the Houston West Nile virus cohort. *PLoS ONE* 7:e40374, 2012.

38. Nusbaum KE, Wright JC, Johnston WB, et al: Absence of humoral response in flamingos and red-tailed hawks to experimental vaccination with a killed West Nile virus vaccine. *Avian Dis* 47:750–752, 2003.

39. O'Brien VA, Meteyer CU, Reisen WK, et al: Prevalence and pathology of West Nile virus in naturally infected house sparrows, western Nebraska, 2008. *Am J Trop Med Hyg* 82:937–944, 2010.

40. Okeson DM, Llizo SY, Miller CL, et al: Antibody response of five bird species after vaccination with a killed West Nile virus vaccine. *J Zoo Wildl Med* 38:240–244, 2007.

41. Ølberg RA, Barker IK, Crawshaw GJ, et al: West Nile virus encephalitis in a Barbary macaque (*Macaca sylvanus*). *Emerg Infect Dis* 10:712–714, 2004.

42. Olsen GH, Miller KJ, Docherty DE, et al: Pathogenicity of West Nile virus and response to vaccination in sandhill cranes (*Grus canadensis*) using a killed vaccine. *J Zoo Wildl Med* 40:263–271, 2009.

43. Palmer MV, Stoffregen WC, Rogers DG, et al: West Nile virus infection in reindeer (*Rangifer tarandus*). *J Vet Diagn Invest* 16:219–222, 2004.

44. Palmieri C, Franca M, Uzal F, et al: Pathology and immunohistochemical findings of West Nile virus infection in Psittaciformes. *Vet Pathol* 48:975–984, 2011.

45. Panella NA, Burkhalter KL, Langevin SA, et al: Rapid West Nile virus antigen detection. *Emerg Infect Dis* 11:1633–1635, 2005.

46. Pauli AM, Cruz-Martinez LA, Ponder JB, et al: Ophthalmologic and oculopathologic findings in red-tailed hawks and Cooper's hawks with naturally acquired West Nile virus infection. *J Am Vet Med Assoc* 231:1240–1248, 2007.

47. Penn RG, Guarner J, Sejvar JJ, et al: Persistent neuroinvasive West Nile virus infection in an immunocompromised patient. *Clin Infect Dis* 42:680–683, 2006.

48. Platt KB, Tucker BJ, Halbur PG, et al: West Nile virus viremia in eastern chipmunks (*Tamias striatus*) sufficient for infecting different mosquitoes. *Emerg Infect Dis* 13:831–837, 2007.

49. Pogodina VV, Frolova MP, Malenko GV, et al: Study on West Nile virus persistence in monkeys. *Arch Virol* 75:71–86, 1983.

50. Redig P, Tully T, Ritchie B, et al: Testing of a DNA-plasmid vaccine for protection against West Nile virus challenge in red-tailed hawks (*Buteo jamaicensis*). In *Proceedings of the Association of Avian Veterinarians*, San Diego, California, 2004.

51. Root JJ, Oesterle PT, Nemeth NM, et al: Experimental infection of fox squirrels (*Sciurus niger*) with West Nile virus. *Am J Trop Med Hyg* 75:697–701, 2006.

52. Samuel MA, Diamond MS: Pathogenesis of West Nile Virus infection: A balance between virulence, innate and adaptive immunity, and viral evasion. *J Virol* 80:9349–9360, 2006.

53. Sbrana E, Tonry JH, Xiao SY, et al: Oral transmission of West Nile virus in a hamster model. *Am J Trop Med Hyg* 72:325–329, 2005.

54. Shrestha B, Gottlieb D, Diamond MS: Infection of neurons by West Nile encephalitis virus. *J Virol* 77(24):13203–13213, 2003.

55. Shrestha B, Pinto AK, Green S, et al: CD8+ T cells use TRAIL to restrict West Nile virus pathogenesis by controlling infection in neurons. *J Virol* 86:8937–8948, 2012.

56. Shrestha B, Samuel MA, Diamond MS: CD8+ T cells require perforin to clear West Nile virus from infected neurons. *J Virol* 80:119–129, 2006.

57. St. Leger J, Wu G, Anderson M, et al: West Nile virus infection in killer whale, Texas, USA, 2007. *Emerg Infect Dis* 17:1531–1533, 2011.

58. Steele KE, Linn MJ, Schoepp RJ, et al: Pathology of fatal West Nile virus infections in native and exotic birds during the 1999 outbreak in New York City, New York. *Vet Pathol* 37:208–224, 2000.

59. Stone WB, Okoniewski JC, Therrien JE, et al: VecTest as diagnostic and surveillance tool for West Nile virus in dead birds. *Emerg Infect Dis* 10:2175–2181, 2004.

60. Stone WB, Therrien JE, Benson R, et al: Assays to detect West Nile virus in dead birds. *Emerg Infect Dis* 11:1770–1773, 2005.

61. Stringfield C, Davis B, Chang G: Vaccination of Andean condors (*Vultur gryphus*) and California condors (*Gymnogyps californianus*) with a West Nile virus DNA vaccine. In *Proceedings of the American Association of Zoo Veterinarians*, Minneapolis, Minnesota, 2003.

62. Styer LM, Lim PY, Louie KL, et al: Mosquito saliva causes enhancement of West Nile virus infection in mice. *J Virol* 85:1517–1527, 2011.

63. Tesh RB, Siirin M, Guzman H, et al: Persistent West Nile virus infection in the golden hamster: Studies on its mechanism and possible implications for other flavivirus infections. *J Infect Dis* 192:287–295, 2005.

64. Tonry JH, Brown CB, Cropp CB, et al: West Nile virus detection in urine. *Emerg Infect Dis* 11:1294–1296, 2005.

65. Voelker R: Effects of West nile virus may persist. *JAMA* 299:2135–2136, 2008.

66. Wang P, Dai J, Bai F, et al: Matrix metalloproteinase 9 facilitates West Nile virus entry into the brain. *J Virol* 82:8978–8985, 2008.

67. Wang Y, Lobigs M, Lee E, et al: CD8+ T cells mediate recovery and immunopathology in West Nile virus encephalitis. *J Virol* 77:13323–13334, 2003.

68. Wolf T, Gandolf A, Dooley J, et al: Evaluation of the efficacy of West Nile virus vaccination in the greater one-horned rhinoceros (*Rhinoceros unicornis*). In *Proceedings of the American Association of Zoo Veterinarians*, Omaha, Nebraska, 2005.

69. Wolf TM, Gandolf AR, Dooley JL, et al: Serologic response to West Nile virus vaccination in the greater one-horned rhinoceros (*Rhinoceros unicornis*). *J Zoo Wildl Med* 39:537–541, 2008.

70. Xiao SY, Guzman H, Zhang H, et al: West Nile virus infection in the golden hamster (*Mesocricetus auratus*): A model for West Nile encephalitis. *Emerg Infect Dis* 7:714–721, 2001.

CHAPTER 76

Use of Ultrasonography in Wildlife Species

Thomas Bernd Hildebrandt and Joseph Saragusty

When a great new technology is invented, the inventors rarely imagine all the different uses that will be found for their invention in the years to come. The pioneers in the field of ultrasound applications, Sir Francis Galton who developed the ultrasonic whistle at the end of the 19th century or Paul Langevin who used it to detect icebergs in 1917, certainly did not anticipate the many industrial and medical uses of ultrasonography today. By definition, *ultrasound* is any sound with frequencies exceeding the upper limit of the human hearing range (maximum 20 kilohertz [kHz]). In the animal kingdom, the capacity for hearing, or the perception of sound, may be as high as about 200 kHz. Known examples are many nocturnal animals such as bats, moths, and other insects and many marine mammals that use sound to locate their prey.

Starting in the 1930s, the role of ultrasonography as a medical treatment tool was established and, in the 1940s, it was also recognized as a diagnostic tool. Gaining acceptance as a noninvasive imaging technology—and thanks to the many technological improvements that facilitated enhancements in sound waves production, reception, processing, and displaying—ultrasonography has become the second most used (after radiography) imaging technology in medicine today. Whereas radiography is known to have adverse effects resulting from radiation exposure, ultrasonography is deemed free of risks at the energies used for diagnostic purposes.[51] Generally, the use of ultrasound in medical applications is a trade-off between penetration depth and resolution. The higher the frequency of the sound produced, the better is the resolution but the lower is the penetration depth, which makes visualization through thick body layers difficult or impossible. Imaging by ultrasonography is also restricted by its very limited penetration through bone structures or gas and the need for proper coupling of the transducer, as coupling may be limited by external structures such as feathers, scales, or fur.

Ultrasonography gained a foothold in veterinary medicine starting in the late 1950s when it was used to estimate fat and muscle thickness.[71] The first peer reviewed report on such use of the technology appeared in 1961,[70] and the first veterinary report appeared a few years later when the technology was used to evaluate pregnancy in ewes.[41] The technology helps in visualizing shape, structure, and size, and identifies pathologic lesions in many body structures, including skin, muscles, tendons, and internal organs. Ultrasonography has many uses in veterinary medicine, ranging from assessment of body fat[24] to searching for pathologies in soft tissues and tendons, but probably the leading application of this technique today is in reproductive medicine.

Ultrasonography was introduced to the field of reproduction management in humans in the late 1950s, thus opening the way to the exploration and characterization of morphologic, biologic, and pathologic processes and to fertility treatment and intervention under the guidance of ultrasound, thereby revolutionizing the entire field. Despite significant advances in ultrasonographic applications in human and veterinary medicine, adoption of this technology has been slow in zoo and wildlife medicine. Probably the first description of its use as a diagnostic tool in zoo animals was in 1978.[56] For a long time, the use of ultrasonography for reproduction management in nondomestic species was sporadic, but over the years, a growing number of ultrasonographic descriptions of various species have been published. Today, this technique has become an indispensable imaging modality in university veterinary hospitals and private clinics, as well as in the veterinary clinics of many zoos.

Various reasons exist for the slow introduction of ultrasonography in the management of nondomestic animals. By definition, species are different from each other in many aspects, including their morphology and specialized structures. For example, significant differences exist in cardiac anatomy and blood flow among the various taxa. Without detailed knowledge of all species, interpretation of body structures seen in each new species may be challenging. Use of carcasses to conduct comparative studies with ultrasonography and conventional anatomic dissection may benefit all. Although some wild animals (e.g., elephants, rhinoceroses, marine mammals) may be trained to allow examination, in the majority of cases, physical restraint, sedation, or anesthesia are required to facilitate safe examination. Effective penetration of ultrasound is limited to certain depths, which makes it often challenging or practically impossible to visualize various internal structures in large-sized animals (e.g., elephants, whales).

In exotic animals, certain specialized structures or features such as the carapace and plastron in tortoises and turtles, feathers and air sacs in birds, scales on many fish and reptilian species, or exoskeleton in many invertebrates may all interfere with the ultrasonographic examination and may require innovative scanning techniques to overcome at least some of these limiting factors that are usually not encountered in human or mainstream veterinary medicine.[24] The unique features that characterize different taxonomic groups with relation to ultrasonographic examination and the different ways this imaging technique may be used when working with zoo and wild animals belonging to these taxa will be discussed in this chapter. Recent developments in ultrasonography and modifications of commercial system configurations, the decrease in machine size that makes it more portable and affordable, and the new methods of examination will all facilitate increased use of this tool for health and reproduction management in wildlife species. Intraoperative ultrasonographic applications will not be discussed in this chapter, besides their value as a diagnostic tool to improve decision quality during surgery.

FISH

One of the main considerations in ultrasonography is the quality of coupling. When used in human or domestic species, for example, coupling gel is required to exclude air from the interface between the transducer and the body. If the fish remains in water (this is highly recommended to reduce the risk for trauma and stress), the water provides excellent coupling conditions, so coupling gel is not needed. Existence of a large body of water around the fish would also make it possible to scan its body without making actual contact with it, by holding the transducer at a distance of as much as 2 centimeters (cm), depending on the frequency used. Naturally, the transducer must be waterproof or otherwise wrapped in a way that will preclude the risk of exposure to water (e.g., by placing it inside a latex glove). Since electricity is involved, especially in devices that are connected to the electricity grid, every precaution should be taken to ensure safety. The need to keep the fish in water also precludes the use of radiography, which is yet another advantage of ultrasonography.

Small fish are normally sedated for the examination, and large ones may be physically restrained. For large fish, transducers of 2 to 5 megahertz (MHz) are usually chosen, and for small fish, 7.5 to 16 MHz would be more appropriate for better visualization of the small body structures. Some fish and elasmobranchs have scales or calcified integument on their body surface (see Figure 76-1, *D*), and these may interfere with the passage of sound waves, resulting in poor visualization. In many of these species, conducting the examination from the ventral surface may produce better results. When this is not sufficient, and when the animal is large enough, transintestinal ultrasonography may be considered. The tissues of fish (skin, muscle) have higher water content compared with tissues in mammals or birds, and this makes the tissues of fish look somewhat different for practitioners who usually work with mammals. It is also important to remember that the velocity of sound wave transmission through muscle decreases with temperature, whereas that in fat increases, so one may distinguish well between muscle and fat at room temperature, but at about 5° C to 11° C, they may look very similar.[59]

Ultrasonography has been used in the fish industry at least since the early 1980s. The main application of this technology has been for the determination of the sex and maturity status of juvenile and adult fish.[55] This has been done in a wide range of fish species such as Coho salmon (*Oncorhynchus kisutch*), cod (*Gadus morhua*), Atlantic salmon (*Salmo salar*), and Pacific herring (*Clupea harengus pallasi*). Other areas in which ultrasonography has been found to be a useful tool include evaluation of ovarian activity and ovulation,[47] health assessment and diagnosis of pathologies,[65] anatomic studies,[14] and, in aquaculture, muscle development evaluation[4] (see Figure 76-1, *A* through *D*).

Assessment of reproductive potential, sexual maturity, and pregnancy has also been done in elasmobranchs (sharks and rays) such as nurse sharks (*Ginglymostoma cirratum*),[7] thornback ray (*Raja clavata*) and small-spotted cat shark (*Scyliorhinus canicula*),[74] and broadnose sevengill sharks (*Notorynchus cepedianus*).[10] Furthermore, ultrasonography has been used for anatomic description and as a diagnostic tool in various species of sharks. Long-term investigations with ultrasonography may also help elucidate unusual phenomena such as intrauterine cannibalism occurring in lamnid sharks.

AMPHIBIANS

For at least three reasons, amphibians are well suited for ultrasonographic examination: (1) They do not have external structures such as fur, feathers, or scales that may impede imaging; (2) their coelom usually contains some fluid that helps enhance the quality of the images. This fluid may increase in volume in diseased animals (see Figure 76-1, *G*); and (3) to varying degrees, depending on the species, they dwell in water, making it possible to scan them while they are submerged in water, as is done in fish. Because of their body sizes, normally transducers ranging from 5 to 16 MHz are used and are placed directly on the animal's skin, in the water without any direct contact with the animal (Figure 76-2, *A*), or in contact with the outside of a water-filled plastic container with the animal in it.[68] When the transducer is applied directly to the skin or from outside the plastic container, coupling gel is required to enhance image quality. Restraining the animals may be achieved through sedation, direct manual restraint, or placement of the animal inside a water-filled plastic container that restricts its ability to move. If cold water is used, this will further reduce the mobility of the animal, but caution should be taken not to chill the animal too much.

When studying an amphibian by using ultrasonography, the amphibian heart, which is composed of two atria and a single ventricle, is a good point to start the examination. It is located at the ventral midline between the front limbs and may easily be identified

because of its pumping activity. Often, the pericardial space contains a moderate amount of fluid, making visualization better. Amphibians lack a diaphragm, so the liver, which, in healthy animals, would have an appearance similar to that in mammals, could be located next to the heart. The gallbladder, which may be as large as the heart, would appear as an anechoic spherical structure near the heart and the liver. Other abdominal organs such as the stomach, gonads, and urinary bladder may also be visualized[29,68] (see Figure 76-1, *E* and *G*). In both caudates and anurans, especially in those in good body condition, unique fat bodies may be visualized within the coelomic cavity. In anurans, these fat bodies appear as fingerlike projections originating from a common stalk stemming from the base of the gonads. These fat bodies would normally appear to be a bit hyperechoic compared with the liver. In salamanders, these fat bodies have a band shape and may be found between the gonads and the kidneys.

The main applications of ultrasonography in amphibians include assessment of the reproductive status,[38] sex determination,[29] evaluation of cardiac activity and blood flow (including the use of Doppler ultrasonography),[8] and health assessment (e.g., parasitic and neoplastic status) and anatomic studies[29,69] (see Figure 76-1, *E* through *G*).

REPTILES

Reptiles are good candidates for ultrasonography. It may be used either as a stand-alone modality or as a complement to radiography, which is used to clearly image the skeleton and the respiratory system, the two body components that ultrasonography cannot image properly. Most reptile species are relatively docile and may be imaged with minimal physical restraint. Some snakes and lizards, however, are less "cooperative" or are poisonous, and special care should be taken to protect the animal and the handler.

Transcutaneous ultrasonography may be problematic in some reptilian species because of the shell or scales that cover their bodies (e.g., Australian bobtail lizard, *Tiliqua rugosa*; or Komodo dragon, *Varanus komodoensis*). Data are scarce with regard to the normal anatomy and architecture of the coelomic cavity and visceral organs in many reptilian species, as well as the way these structures are viewed in ultrasonographic images, so special care should be taken not to mistake, for example, fat structures for other internal organs. This is especially true because many internal organs in reptiles look quite different from those in mammals. Furthermore, the sizes, shapes, and positions of various internal organs may change, depending on the size of the gastrointestinal and reproductive tracts. When possible, comparative studies between ultrasonography and necropsy are highly recommended. Generally, the lungs in reptiles are positioned dorsal to the other coelomic organs, so ultrasonography is best performed from the lateral or ventral aspect at the region where the lungs are located. In turtles, because of their shell, ultrasonography may be conducted from two restricted windows between the carapace and the plastron. From the front of the animal, between the head, front leg, and thorax, one may visualize the heart, liver, and gallbladder. Preferably a small probe (convex or sector scanner) should be used. From the rear of the animal, next to the pelvic region, the visceral organs, including the kidneys, gonads, urinary bladder, intestines, liver, spleen, and so on, may be viewed. The only exception is the pancake tortoise (*Malacochersus tornieri*), in which direct scanning through the soft plastron is possible. In snakes and lizards, especially those that are covered with thick hard scales, the best ultrasonographic visualization may be achieved from the ventral aspect of the animals. For this purpose, a platform or table with openings in it may be designed so that the animal may be placed over it. This will allow for extended duration of examination with minimal need for restraint of the animal.

Smaller animals are best imaged with 7.5 to 16 MHz transducers, and large ones may be better examined with 2.0 to 5.0 MHz probes. Coupling gel should be applied to achieve proper coupling. In some cases, when the ventral and lateral aspects of the animal are covered with very thick scales or scutes that partially or completely block

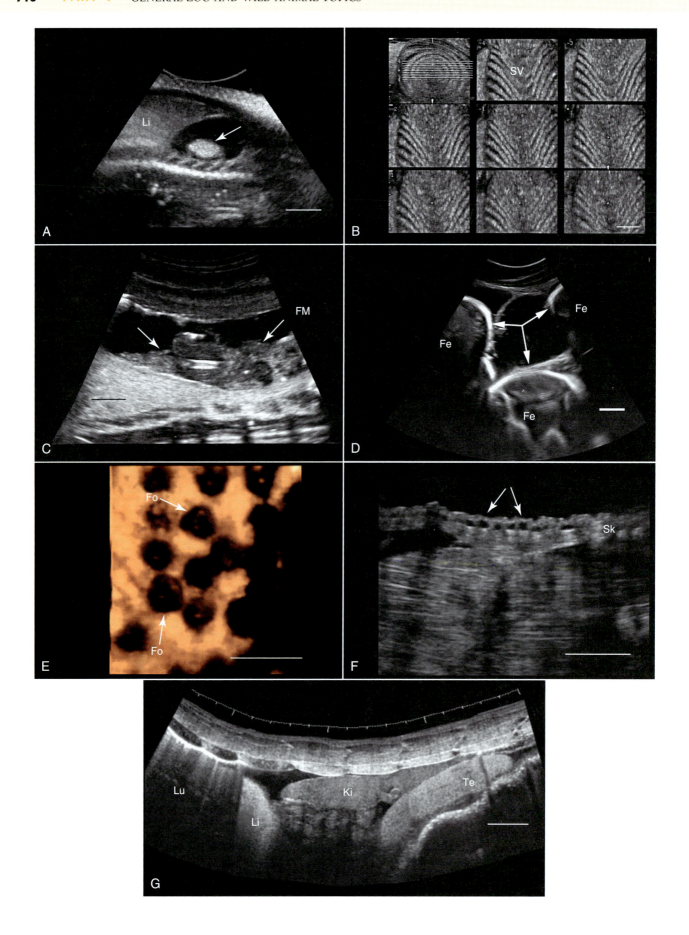

FIGURE 76-1 A, B-Mode sonogram of the liver, and gall bladder that contains a hyperechoic mass (*white arrow*), in a West African lungfish (*Protopterus annectens*). The nature of the lesion (nutritional dysfunction? parasitic product?) has not been diagnosed yet. The wild caught animal was skinnier and smaller than its counterparts. **B,** Three-dimensional ultrasound image of the spiral valve in a black devil stingray (*Potamotrygon leopoldi*) presented in tomographic mode. The unusual sonographic appearance of the modified ileum is normal in rays. Such spiral valves are also found in some shark, skate, and bichir species. As a consequence of the constricting effect the spiral valve has on the lumen of the ileum, rays and sharks cannot pass large hard objects (such as bones) through their lower intestine. Because of its narrow lumen, the spiral valve is often involved in digestive dysfunction in captive elasmobranchs. **C,** B-mode sonogram of the uterine cavity of a black devil stingray (*P. leopoldi*) containing disintegrated fetal material (detritus, *white arrows*) as a result of a failed pregnancy. The caudal part of the liver appears hyperechoic because of the high fat content the liver has in this species. **D,** B-mode sonogram of the uterine cavity of a pregnant lemon shark (*Negaprion brevirostris*) that contained 14 fetuses. Three of them are partially visualized here, along with the fetal membranes (*white arrows*). The surface of the fetal bodies appears surprisingly highly hyperechoic because of the early formation of the typical rough shark skin in these fetuses. The examination was performed directly through the skin on the restraint patient caught in swallow water. **E,** Three-dimensional mode sonogram of an active ovary in an adult female giant salamander (*Andrias davidianus*) containing many large anechoic follicles of approximately 6 millimeters (mm) in diameter with an echogenic center. This reproductive stage is close to egg laying event. **F,** B-mode image of the skin region in an adult male giant salamander (*A. davidianus*). The remarkable fluid-filled skin glands can be easily misinterpreted as follicle formation during sonographic sexing. If a salamander is wrongly handled, it may secrete, within seconds, a sticky, whitish material deriving from these skin glands. **G,** Sonogram of an adult male giant salamander (*A. davidianus*) in panoramic view mode consisting of several single ultrasound images. It allows visualizing a longer region of interest. *From left to right:* The caudal lung field, part of the liver, the elongated kidney, and the cigar-shaped active right testis. A moderate amount of fluid (anechoic region between liver and kidney) is present in the coelomic cavity, which is not unusual in amphibians.

All images were generated using transcutaneous ultrasonography. With the exception of image **C**, all were generated through the water, without direct contact with the animals. Chemical and, in most cases, physical restraint of the patients were not needed. Image **B** was generated using a 6 to 16 megahertz (MHz) transducer, and for all other images, a 2 to 5 MHz transducer was used. White or black bar represents 20 mm. *Fe*, fetus; *FM*, fetal mass; *Fo*, follicle; *Ki*, kidney; *Li*, liver; *Lu*, lung; *Sk*, skin; *SV*, spiral valve; *Te*, testis.

---

ultrasound waves (e.g., *Tiliqua* spp., *Corucia zebrata*), coupling gel may be applied and left for 15 to 30 minutes so that the scales absorb some of the gel for better imaging. The alternative is to submerge the region of interest (excluding the head) in water to improve coupling. Placing the probe between the scales or from a more lateral position may also help. In larger reptiles, a good alternative would be to use specialized transducers that allow for transintestinal endosonography (see Figure 76-2, *C*). By inserting the transducer through the cloaca into the intestine, the entire urogenital tract, intestines, adrenal, and fat bodies may be visualized.[27]

The primary use of ultrasonography in reptiles is probably for the assessment of the reproductive tract and reproductive status (see Figure 76-2, *B*, *C*, and *E*). This was done in a wide variety of terrestrial, marine, and fresh-water reptilian species.[39,60,62] Sex determination in sub-adult or monomorphic reptiles has also been done with the use of ultrasonography, for example, in komodo dragons (*Varanus komodoensis*), white-throated monitors (*Varanus albigularis*), Gila monsters (*Heloderma suspectum*), and beaded lizards (*H. horridum*).[27,52] Ultrasonography has also proven useful for medical diagnosis[45] (see Figure 76-2, *D*), as well as for ultrasound-guided transcutaneous biopsy.[34] Ultrasonography is very useful for anatomic, morphologic, and nutritional studies in reptiles.[27,64]

BIRDS

Birds are normally covered with feathers that have a large volume of air within them. Even with the use of coupling gel, this may hinder clear depiction of the different internal structures. The existence of large air sacs, the very compacted intestines, and the subcutaneous accumulation of fat, as well as the follicles of the feathers may all

further impede transmission of the sound waves. For these reasons, transcutaneous application of ultrasonography is of limited value in birds compared with other vertebrates. When transcutaneous ultrasonography does not provide clear images, transcloacal[23] or transintestinal[15] ultrasonography, using high-resolution miniaturized probes, may be considered. The entire urogenital system, the gonads, and the adrenals may be viewed by the transintestinal technique, and only the caudal part of the genital tract may be viewed by the transcloacal technique (Figure 76-3, *A*). Identifying the inactive ovaries and visualizing the kidneys, which are located next to the vertebral column and hidden by the compacted intestines and the air sacs, may be difficult at times.

In larger species of birds such as penguins, it is also possible to view much of the abdominal cavity by inserting a small ultrasound probe through the esophagus and conducting nonsurgical transgastric ultrasonography (see Figure 76-2, *G* and *H*). This new transgastric examination technique allows fast and accurate evaluation of large parenchymatous organs such as the lungs, liver, spleen, and kidneys with ultrasonography. Such examination is relevant, for example, when aspergillosis is suspected in penguins. In the very large birds such as the ostrich (*Struthio camelus*) or brown kiwi (*Apteryx mantelli*), ultrasonography may easily be used transcutaneously to monitor ovarian activity and development of ova and to view internal organs such as the heart, intestines, liver, and kidneys.[35,72] The gallbladder is available as an anechoic round or oval-shaped landmark dorsal to the right liver lobe in most birds but not in Psittacines and Columbiformes.

To view internal organs by using transcutaneous ultrasonography, the feathers at the ventral midline, just caudal to the sternal keel and cranial to the pubic bones, are parted, and coupling gel is applied.

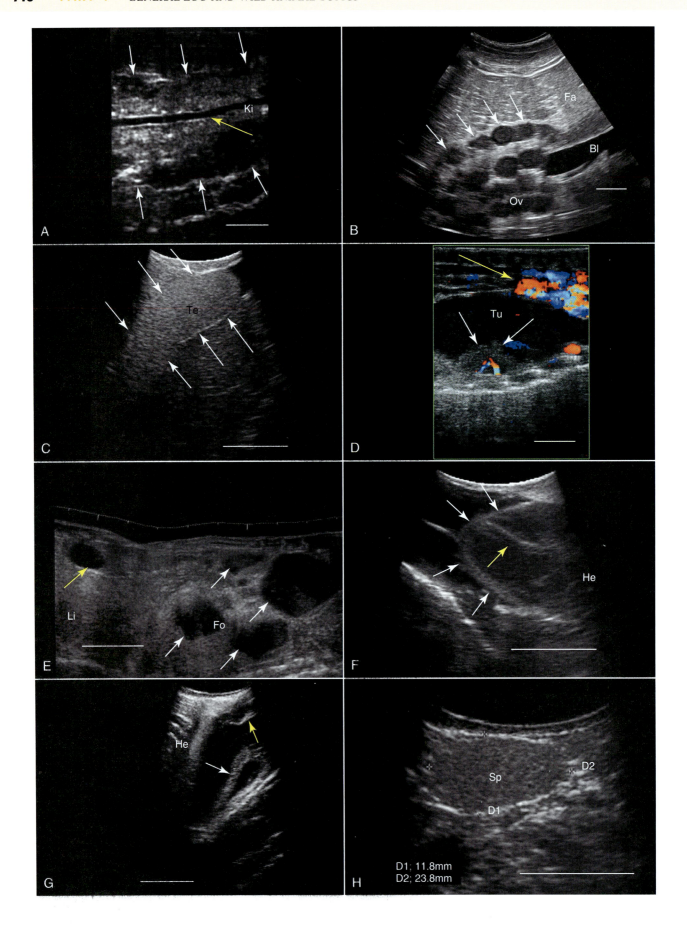

FIGURE 76-2 A, Transcutaneous B-mode image (2 to 5 megahertz [MHz]) of the elongated kidneys (*border marked by white arrows*) separated by a central blood vessel (*yellow arrow*) in an adult hellbender (*Cryptobranchus alleganiensis*). Both kidneys show clear signs of gout (*irregular white dots*) in their parenchyma. The sonogram was generated through the water, without direct contact with the animals. Physical or chemical restraints of the patient were not needed. **B,** Transcutaneous ultrasound image (2 to 5 MHz) showing early development of ovarian follicles in a female Komodo dragon (*Varanus komodoensis*). The partially filled urinary bladder borders the ovary from the caudal aspect. **C,** Because of the ossified scales in the Komodo dragon (*V. komodoensis*), it is not possible to visualize the testes by transcutaneous ultrasonography in this species. The only option for imaging the cigar-shaped testes, located cranioventral to the kidneys, is by transintestinal ultrasonography using a miniaturized transducer (fingertip probe, 7.5 MHz). **D,** Sonogram in color-flow-Doppler mode (6 to 16 MHz, transcutaneous) showing a productive tumor (*white arrows*) with own blood supply, diagnosed in an inland taipan (*Oxyuranus microlepidotus*). The fluid-producing lesion (hypoechoic area above solid tumor tissue) is located near the heart base (*yellow arrow*). **E,** Panoramic view mode sonogram (6 to16 MHz, transcutaneous) showing the coelomic region in a female tuatara (*Sphenodon punctatus*) with an active ovary (*white arrows*). Yellow arrow marks the fluid-filled gall bladder. The patient was physically restrained for the ultrasound assessment. **F,** Transcutaneous B-mode sonogram (7.5 MHz) of a diseased heart in a touraco (*Tauraco leucolophus*). The coelomic cavity is filled with anechoic transudate framing the apex of the heart (*white arrows*). The left and right ventricles are dilated. The yellow arrow points toward the intraventricular septum. Coelomic cavity aspiration was performed under ultrasound guidance to diagnose the origin of the coelomic effusion. **G,** B-mode sonogram (7.5 MHz) of the four-chamber heart view in an anesthetized rockhopper penguin (*Eudyptes chrysocome*) generated by transgastric technique, in which a miniaturized transducer (fingertip probe) is inserted through the open beak into the empty stomach. The white arrow points to the interventricular septum and the right ventricle. The yellow arrow indicates the aortic valve at the heart base. **H,** B-mode sonogram (7.5 MHz) of the egg-shaped spleen in an anesthetized rockhopper penguin (*E. chrysocome*), generated by transgastric ultrasonography. The organ capsule appears hyperechoic, and the parenchyma appears homogeneous and moderately echogenic. The dimension and echographic appearance indicate a healthy organ.

In all images, the white bar represents 20 millimeters (mm).

Bl, bladder; *Fa*, fat; *Fo*, follicle; *He*, heart; *Ki*, kidney; *Li*, liver; *Ov*, ovary; *Sp*, spleen; *Te*, testis; *Tu*, tumor.

The ventral plumage may also be plucked, when needed, to improve coupling. In small bird species, transducers of 7.5 to 16 MHz are used, and 2 to 5 MHz transducers are useful in the large birds. In some species, the available window may be very limited because of caudally extended keel (e.g., Galliformes and Anseriformes). In such cases, a more lateral approach, placing the transducer just caudal to the last rib on the right side, may provide some view of the internal organs. Fasting the birds for several hours (birds of prey even for a day or two) may enhance clarity of the images. Especially in small and unhealthy birds, the cooling effect the coupling gel may have on the bird as well as the stress and respiratory distress that restraint, positioning, and handling may have on the animal are important considerations.

Some of the uses of ultrasonography in birds include monitoring of muscle development and changes with activity and season,[42] ultrasound-guided fine-needle aspiration[54] (see Figure 76-2, *F*), medical evaluation of internal organs,[58] estimating bone mineral density using amplitude-dependent speed-of-sound quantitative ultrasonography and detection of bone pathologies,[13,53] determination of sex in monomorphic species,[23] evaluation of ovarian status,[50] study of the anatomy and morphology of organs,[19] monitoring the development of the cardiovascular system,[49] and endocardiography.[57] In addition, use of ultrasonography for high-resolution eye examination (20 MHz) in raptors and large birds may be helpful for verification of the impact of trauma and identification of neurologic symptoms.

MAMMALS

Almost two decades ago, the vast majority of publications on ultrasonography use in vertebrates were focused on mammals.[17] This is most probably still the case today. Mammals vary significantly in size, ranging from the 1.8-gram (g) Etruscan shrew (*Suncus etruscus*) to the 170-ton blue whale (*Balaenoptera musculus*), and live in a wide variety of environments, that is, air (e.g., bats), water (e.g., marine mammals), and land. In the over 5400 extant mammalian species, a wide variety of anatomic features have evolved, making knowledge gained on one species not always applicable to another in a straightforward manner. The ideal, which is still lacking for many species, is to have a clear anatomic picture of the species involved before attempting to apply ultrasonography. In the absence of such anatomic knowledge or past experience, identification of pathologic changes may not always be possible.

The vast differences among species dictate the selection of ultrasonography technique to be applied and the quality of images obtained. Some species or individuals may be trained to allow ultrasonographic examination without the need for sedation or anesthesia. These include many marine mammals, primates, elephants, and rhinoceroses, among others. Many mammals have fur cover over their bodies. To achieve good coupling during transcutaneous examination, the fur is ideally clipped over the area of interest. If clipping the fur is not an option, soaking it with alcohol and then applying coupling gel may also help obtain acceptable results. The fur in marine mammals is a very important part of their insulation layer, so it is best not to clip it unless absolutely necessary. In such cases, when high-quality transcutaneous imaging cannot be achieved, transrectal examination may provide excellent results for much of the visceral region. Many other marine mammals and a few other mammals such as the naked mole rat (*Heterocephalus glaber*), the naked bat (*Cheiromeles torquatus*), and the common (*Hippopotamus amphibious*) and pygmy (*Choeropsis liberiensis*) hippopotamuses have skin almost devoid of hair, which makes scanning easy. Marine mammals are sensitive to ultrasonic waves and may be trained to accept ultrasonographic examination in water. Their examination

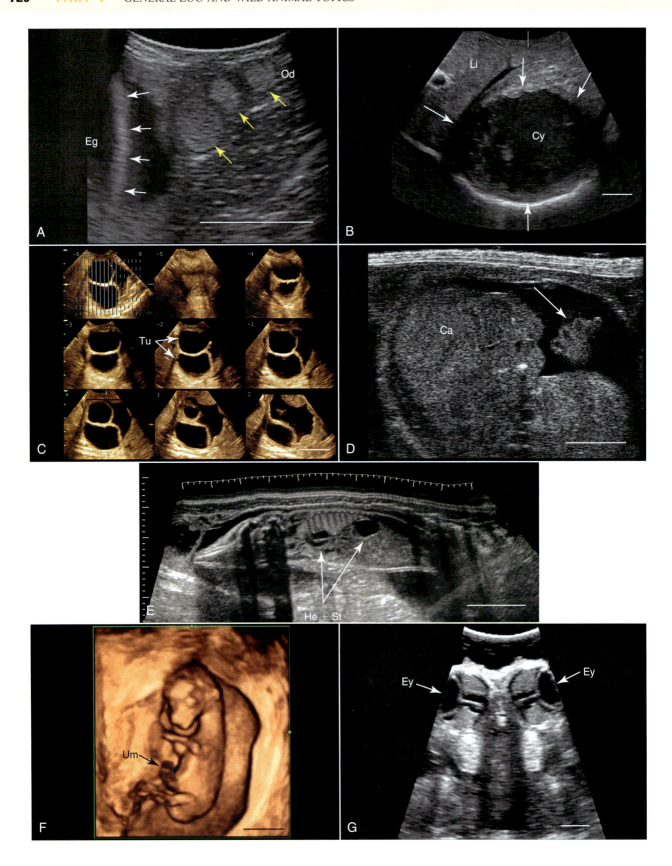

may thus be conducted in a manner similar to that in fish, keeping in mind the size and anatomic differences.

Skin thickness in animals such as rhinoceroses, hippopotamuses, or elephants and fat pads in many marine mammals limit the use of transcutaneous ultrasonography in these animals. The very large body sizes of some mammals also limit the ability to visualize some internal structures, even when using the transrectal ultrasonography approach. Development of special tools and extensions may help,[30] but even these have their limitations with regard to imaging the deep structures in the body. At the other end, the very small mammals

FIGURE 76-3 A, B-mode sonogram (7.5 megahertz [MHz]) of the oviduct in a Humboldt penguin (*Spheniscus humboldti*) visualized by transintestinal ultrasonography via the cloaca. White arrows point at the caudal part of a forming egg surrounded by anechoic oviductal fluid. Yellow arrows indicate three cross-sections of the activated and folded oviduct. **B,** Transcutaneous ultrasound image (B-mode, 2 to 5 MHz) of the central liver lobe of a chimpanzee (*Pan troglodytes*). The lobe is severely altered by an echinococcosis. White arrows mark the border of the parasitic cyst formation; the content in the hydatid cyst has an irregular appearance because of the large number of protoscoleces in it. **C,** Transvaginal three-dimensional ultrasound image presented in tomographic mode (5 to 9 MHz). The sonogram shows an aggressive ovarian tumor in a female Western lowland gorilla (*Gorilla gorilla gorilla*) with several fluid-filled chambers (*white arrows*). **D,** High-frequency ultrasound image (B-mode, 55 MHz) generated with an "ultrasound biomicroscope," which operates with transducer frequencies of up to 70 MHz. The resolution allows counting the fingers (*white arrow*) of a 4-week-old naked mole rat fetus (*Heterocephalus glaber*) in this transcutaneous sonogram. **E,** Panoramic-view-mode sonogram consisting of several single ultrasound images, allowing visualization of a longer region of interest. The image shows a 2-month-old bottlenose dolphin (*Tursiops aduncus*) fetus (2 to 5 MHz, transcutaneous). The calcified fetal skull is causing shadow artifacts. White arrows mark heart and fluid-filled stomach. **F,** Three-dimensional mode sonogram (2 to 5 MHz, transcutaneous) of a 7-week-old Beira antelope (*Dorcatragus megalotis*) fetus. **G,** B-mode sonogram (3.5 MHz) of the eyes region (*white arrows*) in a North Pacific giant octopus (*Enteroctopus dofleini*). Note the clearly visible nervus opticus running from the eyes into the central brain. The image was generated through the water without direct contact with the animal. Physical or chemical restraints of the patient were not needed. In **D,** the white bar represents 2 millimeters (mm), and in all other images, the white or black bar represents 20 mm.

Ca, cranium; *Cy,* cyst; *Eg,* egg; *Ey,* eye; *He,* heart; *Li,* liver; *Od,* oviduct; *St,* stomach; *Tu,* tumor; *Um,* umbilicus.

may be easily studied with normal transducers of 7.5 to 16 MHz or with ultrasound biomicroscopes of 50 to 70 MHz, which may provide excellent images at a resolution of 30 micrometers (μm) or less[61] (see Figure 76-3, *D*). In elephants, rhinoceroses, giraffes, and some other large terrestrial mammals, ultrasonography is usually performed with the animal in the standing position with the use of training of the animal to accept the examination or with sedation. In smaller species, examination would be ideally performed with the animal in dorsal recumbency, which allows easy access to the abdominal area. For cardiac imaging, it is best to turn the animal to left recumbency, with the probe being moved from under the animal, facing up.

The early application of medical ultrasonography in animals was for pregnancy diagnosis in mammals.[41] Today, the leading application for ultrasonography is still in the area of reproduction in wildlife mammalian (and other) species (see Figure 76-3, *C* through *F*). It is used to monitor the urogenital tract in both males[31] and females;[28] identify reproductive tract pathologies;[22] characterize the female reproductive status and elucidate the reproductive cycle pattern through longitudinal studies;[43] assess male reproductive status and collect semen;[26,30] help determine the sex of the fetus[9] as well as that of adult animals in the few monomorphic mammalian species such as beavers, sloths, and the spotted hyena;[33] and determine and monitor pregnancy and fetal development and diagnose embryonic resorption in various species, including the giant panda (*Ailuropoda melanoleuca*), Asian (*Elephas maximus*) and African (*Loxodonta africana*) elephants, snow leopard (*Uncia uncia*), bonobos (*Pan paniscus*), European brown hare (*Lepus europaeus*), and tammar wallaby (*Macropus eugenii*).[11,12,16,25,44,66] Beyond reproductive assessment and monitoring, ultrasonography is highly useful when it comes to the application of assisted reproductive technologies, many of which are performed under the guidance of ultrasound. Ultrasonography plays a paramount role in procedures such as ovum pickup, artificial insemination, and embryo transfer in various species.[21,32]

Ultrasonography is also used in nondomestic mammals for diseases diagnosis and identification of pathologic processes in species such as the cheetah (*Acinonyx jubatus jubatus*),[73] koala (*Phascolarctos cinereus*),[48] and oncilla (*Leopardus tigrinus*).[3] As a specialization within ultrasonography, echocardiography is performed in both adults[63] and fetuses[67] to evaluate the health of the cardiovascular system. Ultrasonography has been used in anatomic studies[2] and for assessing body fat (and, thus, nutritional status) since the 1950s in the cattle and swine industries.

Marine mammals may be considered a specialized group within the mammalian class. The group includes the cetaceans, sirenians, pinnipeds, and fissipeds, the first two being fully aquatic and the last two being semi-aquatic in nature. Handling of the semi-aquatic species for ultrasonographic examination is similar to that of other terrestrial mammals. Many of the seals may be trained to lie on land for the examination, or they may be physically restrained relatively easily for the duration of the examination. Some of the aquatic species may also be trained to present themselves for examination and, at times, also to come on land. Because of the sensitivity of many of these species to ultrasound waves, care should be taken to avoid contact between the transducer and the water, unless the animal has been specifically trained to accept this. As in their terrestrial counterparts, ultrasonography has been used in marine mammals to assess reproductive status in both males[6] and females,[1] study early embryonic development[1] (see Figure 76-3, *E*), identify fetal malformations,[5] and for medical diagnosis.[36] Ultrasonographic evaluation of body condition and nutritional status is performed through measurements of the dermis, epidermis, and blubber. This has been performed in a wide variety of species, including Steller sea lions (*Eumetopias jubatus*), harbor seals (*Phoca vitulina*), and Southern elephant seals (*Mirounga leonine*).

INVERTEBRATES

By definition, *invertebrates* are animals that are not included in the vertebrata subphylum. Generally, very little work has been done and published on the use of ultrasonography in invertebrates. When imaging water-dwelling invertebrates, ultrasonography may be used with the animal submerged in the water, as in the case of fish. Here, too, direct contact of the transducer with the animal's body is not an absolute must (see Figure 76-3, *G*). Because of their relatively small body size, transducers of 5 MHz and above, up to 20 MHz, for normal ultrasonography and further to the ultrasound biomicroscope range of 50 to 70 MHz, are normally used for most species.

As invertebrates lack bones, no interference with ultrasound transmission occurs. However, many invertebrate species (e.g., insects, crustaceans) have an exoskeleton, which significantly limits the available windows for viewing visceral organs. In one study in crustaceans (iridescent swimming crab, *Portunus gibbesii*), the heart and scaphognathites could be easily detected, but other internal organs could not be properly visualized.[20] If exoskeleton is absent, anatomic studies of various body parts may be conducted. Ultrasonography has been used, for example, to study the morphology of the arms,[46] or the brain,[18] in the common octopus (*Octopus vulgaris*) or blood circulation in cuttlefish (*Sepia officinalis*).[37] The heart in invertebrates may also be studied by using Doppler ultrasonography.[40]

CONCLUSION

Advances in ultrasound technology have turned it into a highly accessible, relatively inexpensive, and, in many models, portable imaging tool. Keeping in mind the vast anatomic differences among and within the various taxonomic groups, the technology may be used in the study and management of zoo and wildlife animals in all vertebrates and, to a lesser extent, in invertebrates. Ultrasonography has a wide range of applications related to reproduction assessment and assisted reproduction technologies, disease diagnosis, and physiologic, anatomic, and morphologic studies. Being a real-time, noninvasive and practically risk-free imaging technique, ultrasonography has many advantages over radiography, particularly when soft tissue is the target. The veterinary literature, however, is still lacking in detailed reports on the use of ultrasonography in different taxa. This will certainly change in time as the use of ultrasonography in nondomestic species expands rapidly.

ACKNOWLEDGMENTS

The authors would like to acknowledge and thank Dr. Frank Göritz for his significant contributions to the writing of this chapter.

REFERENCES

1. Adams GP, Ward Testa J, Goertz CEC, et al: Ultrasonographic characterization of reproductive anatomy and early embryonic detection in the northern fur seal (*Callorhinus ursinus*) in the field. *Marine Mammal Sci* 23(2):445–452, 2007.
2. Bapodra P, Bouts T, Mahoney P, et al: Ultrasonographic anatomy of the Asian elephant (*Elephas maximus*) eye. *J Zoo Wildl Med* 41(3):409–417, 2010.
3. Bignardi Jarretta G, Bombonato PP, de Barros Vaz Guimarães MA: Renal ultrasonographic evaluation in the oncilla (*Leopardus tigrinus*). *J Zoo Wildl Med* 35(3):356–360, 2004.
4. Bosworth BG, Holland M, Brazil BL: Evaluation of ultrasound imagery and body shape to predict carcass and fillet yield in farm-raised catfish. *J Anim Sci* 79(6):1483–1490, 2001.
5. Brook F: Ultrasound diagnosis of anencephaly in the fetus of a bottlenose dolphin (*Tursiops aduncas*). *J Zoo Wildl Med* 25(4):569–574, 1994.
6. Brook FM, Kinoshita R, Brown B, et al: Ultrasonographic imaging of the testis and epididymis of the bottlenose dolphin, *Tursiops truncatus aduncas*. *J Reprod Fertil* 119(2):233–240, 2000.
7. Carrier JC, Murru FL, Walsh MT, et al: Assessing reproductive potential and gestation in nurse sharks (*Ginglymostoma cirratum*) using ultrasonography and endoscopy: An example of bridging the gap between field research and captive studies. *Zoo Biol* 22(2):179–187, 2003.
8. Coucelo J, Coucelo J, Azevedo J: Ultrasonography characterization of heart morphology and blood flow of lower vertebrates. *J Exp Zool* 275(2–3):73–82, 1996.
9. Curran S, Ginther OJ: Ultrasonic diagnosis of equine fetal sex by location of the genital tubercle. *J Equine Vet Res* 9:77–83, 1989.
10. Daly J, Gunn I, Kirby N, et al: Ultrasound examination and behavior scoring of captive broadnose sevengill sharks, *Notorynchus cepedianus* (Peron, 1807). *Zoo Biol* 26(5):383–395, 2007.
11. Drews B, Hermes R, Göritz F, et al: Early embryo development in the elephant assessed by serial ultrasound examinations. *Theriogenology* 69(9):1120–1128, 2008.
12. Drews B, Roellig K, Menzies BR, et al: Ultrasonography of wallaby prenatal development shows that the climb to the pouch begins in utero. *Sci Rep* 3:1458, 2013.
13. Fleming RH, Korver D, McCormack HA, et al: Assessing bone mineral density in vivo: Digitized fluoroscopy and ultrasound. *Poult Sci* 83(2):207–214, 2004.
14. Goddard PJ: Ultrasonic examination of fish. In Goddard PJ, editor: *Veterinary ultrasonography*, Wallingford, U.K., 1995, Cab International, pp 289–302.
15. Göritz F, Hildebrandt TB, Hermes R, et al: Immobilisation and transintestinal sonography in cassowary. In *Verhandlungsbericht des 38 Internationalen Symposiums über die Erkrankungen der Zoo- und Wildtiere*, Zurich, Switzerland, 1997, pp 181–186.
16. Göritz F, Hildebrandt TB, Jewgenow K, et al: Transrectal ultrasonographic examination of the female urogenital tract in nonpregnant and pregnant captive bears (Ursidae). *J Reprod Fertil Suppl* 51:303–312, 1997.
17. Göritz F: *Sonographie bei Zoo- und Wildtieren. D.V.M. Dissertation Thesis*, Berlin, Germany, 1996, Free University.
18. Grimaldi AM, Agnisola C, Fiorito G: Using ultrasound to estimate brain size in the cephalopod *Octopus vulgaris* Cuvier in vivo. *Brain Res* 1183:66–73, 2007.
19. Gumpenberger M, Kolm G: Ultrasonographic and computed tomographic examinations of the avian eye: Physiologic appearance, pathologic findings, and comparative biometric measurement. *Vet Radiol Ultrasound* 47(5):492–502, 2006.
20. Haefner PA, Jr: Application of ultrasound technology to crustacean physiology: Monitoring cardiac and scaphognathite rates in Brachyura. *Crustaceana* 69(6):788–794, 1996.
21. Hermes R, Göritz F, Portas TJ, et al: Ovarian superstimulation, transrectal ultrasound-guided oocyte recovery, and IVF in rhinoceros. *Theriogenology* 72(7):959–968, 2009.
22. Hermes R, Hildebrandt TB, Walzer C, et al: The effect of long nonreproductive periods on the genital health in captive female white rhinoceroses (*Ceratotherium simum simum, C.s. cottoni*). *Theriogenology* 65(8):1492–1515, 2006.
23. Hildebrandt T, Pitra C, Sömmer P, et al: Sex identification in birds of prey by ultrasonography. *J Zoo Wildl Med* 26(3):367–376, 1995.
24. Hildebrandt TB, Göritz F: Use of ultrasonography in zoo animals. In Fowler ME, editor: *Zoo and wild animal medicine*, Philadelphia, PA, 1998, Saunders, pp 41–54.
25. Deleted in proof.
26. Hildebrandt TB, Brown JL, Göritz F, et al: Ultrasonography to assess and enhance health and reproduction in giant panda. In Wildt DE, Zhang A, Zhang H, et al, editors: *Giant pandas: Biology, veterinary medicine and management*, Cambridge, U.K., 2006, Cambridge University Press, pp 410–439.
27. Hildebrandt TB, Göritz F, Pitra C, et al: Sonomorphological sex determination in subadult Komodo dragon. In *Proceedings of the annual conference of the American Association of Zoo Veterinarians*, Puerto Vallarta, Mexico, 1996, pp 251–254. (abstract).
28. Hildebrandt TB, Göritz F, Pratt NC, et al: Ultrasonography of the urogenital tract in elephants (*Loxodonta africana* and *Elephas maximus*): An important tool for assessing female reproductive function. *Zoo Biol* 19(5):321–332, 2000.
29. Hildebrandt TB, Göritz F, Schaftenaar W, et al: Sonomorphologische Geschlechtsbestimmung und Einschätzung der reproduktiven Kapazität bei Riesensalamandern (Cryptobranchidae). In *Verhandlungsbericht des 38 Internationalen Symposiums über die Erkrankungen der Zoo- und Wildtiere*, Zurich, Switzerland, 1997, pp 175–180.
30. Hildebrandt TB, Hermes R, Jewgenow K, et al: Ultrasonography as an important tool for the development and application of reproductive

technologies in non-domestic species. *Theriogenology* 53(1):73–84, 2000.

31. Hildebrandt TB, Hermes R, Pratt NC, et al: Ultrasonography of the urogenital tract in elephants (*Loxodonta africana* and *Elephas maximus*): An important tool for assessing male reproductive function. *Zoo Biol* 19(5):333–345, 2000.

32. Hildebrandt TB, Hermes R, Saragusty J, et al: Enriching the captive elephant population genetic pool through artificial insemination with frozen-thawed semen collected in the wild. *Theriogenology* 78(6):1398–1404, 2012.

33. Hildebrandt TB, Pitra C, Göritz F, et al: Sonomorphologische Geschlechtsdiagnose bei der Tüpfelhyäne (*Crocuta crocuta* Erxleben). *Fertilität* 12:46–50, 1996.

34. Isaza R, Ackerman N, Schumacher J: Ultrasound-guided percutaneous liver biopsy in snakes. *Vet Radiol Ultrasound* 34(6):452–454, 1993.

35. Jensen T, Durrant B: Assessment of reproductive status and ovulation in female brown kiwi (*Apteryx mantelli*) using fecal steroids and ovarian follicle size. *Zoo Biol* 25(1):25–34, 2006.

36. Kenny DE, Irlbeck NA, Eller JL: Rickets in two hand-reared polar bear (*Ursus maritimus*) cubs. *J Zoo Wildl Med* 30(1):132–140, 1999.

37. King AJ, Henderson SM, Schmidt MH, et al: Using ultrasound to understand vascular and mantle contributions to venous return in the cephalopod *Sepia officinalis* L. *J Exp Biol* 208(11):2071–2082, 2005.

38. Kouba AJ, Vance CK: Applied reproductive technologies and genetic resource banking for amphibian conservation. *Reprod Fertil Dev* 21(6):719–737, 2009.

39. Lance VA, Rostal DC, Elsey RM, et al: Ultrasonography of reproductive structures and hormonal correlates of follicular development in female American alligators, *Alligator mississippiensis*, in southwest Louisiana. *Gen Comp Endocrinol* 162(3):251–256, 2009.

40. Lewbart GA, Mosley C: Clinical anesthesia and analgesia in invertebrates. *J Exotic Pet Med* 21(1):59–70, 2012.

41. Lindahl IL: Detection of pregnancy in sheep by means of ultrasound. *Nature* 212(5062):642–643, 1966.

42. Lindström A, Kvist A, Piersma T, et al: Avian pectoral muscle size rapidly tracks body mass changes during flight, fasting and fuelling. *J Exp Biol* 203(5):913–919, 2000.

43. Lueders I, Niemuller C, Gray CS, et al: Luteogenesis during the estrous cycle in Asian elephants (*Elephas maximus*). *Reproduction* 140(5):777–786, 2010.

44. Lueders I, Niemuller C, Rich P, et al: Gestating for 22 months: luteal development and pregnancy maintenance in elephants. *Proc R Soc B Biol Sci* 279(1743):3687–3696, 2012.

45. Luz S, Dorrestein GM, Zwart P, et al: Management, diagnosis and treatment of an inland taipan (*Oxyuranus microlepidotus*) with a tumor-like swelling in the heart region at Singapore Zoological Garden. In *The International Conference on Diseases of Zoo and Wild Animals*, Beekse Bergen, The Netherlands, 2009, pp 33–42.

46. Margheri L, Ponte G, Mazzolai B, et al: Non-invasive study of *Octopus vulgaris* arm morphology using ultrasound. *J Exp Biol* 214(22):3727–3731, 2011.

47. Martin-Robichaud DJ, Rommens M: Assessment of sex and evaluation of ovarian maturation of fish using ultrasonography. *Aquacult Res* 32(2):113–120, 2001.

48. Mathews KG, Wolff PL, Petrini KR, et al: Ultrasonographic diagnosis and surgical treatment of cystic reproductive tract disease in a female koala (*Phascolarctos cinereus*). *J Zoo Wildl Med* 26(3):440–452, 1995.

49. McQuinn TC, Bratoeva M, DeAlmeida A, et al: High-frequency ultrasonographic imaging of avian cardiovascular development. *Dev Dyn* 236(12):3503–3513, 2007.

50. Melnychuk VL, Cooper MW, Kirby JD, et al: Use of ultrasonography to characterize ovarian status in chicken. *Poult Sci* 81(6):892–895, 2002.

51. Merritt CR: Ultrasound safety: What are the issues? *Radiology* 173(2):304–306, 1989.

52. Morris PJ, Alberts AC: Determination of sex in white-throated monitors (*Varanus albigularis*), Gila monsters (*Heloderma suspectum*), and beaded lizards (*H. horridum*) using two-dimensional ultrasound imaging. *J Zoo Wildl Med* 27(3):371–377, 1996.

53. Mutalib A, Holland M, Barnes HJ, et al: Ultrasound for detecting osteomyelitis in turkeys. *Avian Dis* 40(2):321–325, 1996.

54. Nordberg C, O'Brien RT, Paul-Murphy J, et al: Ultrasound examination and guided fine-needle aspiration of the liver in Amazon parrots (*Amazona* species). *J Avian Med Surg* 14(3):180–184, 2000.

55. Novelo ND, Tiersch TR: A review of the use of ultrasonography in fish reproduction. *N Am J Aquacult* 74(2):169–181, 2012.

56. O'Grady JP, Yeager CH, Thomas W, et al: Practical applications of real time ultrasound scanning to problems of zoo veterinary medicine. *J Zoo Anim Med* 9(2):52–56, 1978.

57. Pees M, Krautwald-Junghanns M-E: Avian echocardiography. *Semin Avian Exotic Pet Med* 14(1):14–21, 2005.

58. Pees M, Kiefer I, Krautwald-Junghanns M-E, et al: Comparative ultrasonographic investigations of the gastrointestinal tract and the liver in healthy and diseased pigeons. *Vet Radiol Ultrasound* 47(4):370–375, 2006.

59. Probert P, Shannon R: Wideband ultrasound to determine lipid concentration in fish. In Halliwell M, Wells PNT, editors: *Acoustical imaging*, New York, 2002, Kluwer Academic Publishers, pp 381–388.

60. Robeck TR, Rostal DC, Burchfield PM, et al: Ultrasound imaging of reproductive organs and eggs in Galapagos tortoises, *Geochelone elephantopus* spp. *Zoo Biol* 9(5):349–359, 1990.

61. Roellig K, Drews B, Goeritz F, et al: The long gestation of the small naked mole-rat (*Heterocephalus glaber* Rüppell, 1842) studied with ultrasound biomicroscopy and 3D-ultrasonography. *PLoS ONE* 6(3):e17744, 2011.

62. Rostal DC, Robeck TR, Owens DW, et al: Ultrasound imaging of ovaries and eggs in Kemp's ridley sea turtles (*Lepidochelys kempi*). *J Zoo Wildl Med* 21(1):27–35, 1990.

63. Royen HIF, Delemarre BJM, Klaver PSJ, et al: Application of transthoracic and transoesophageal echocardiography in captive chimpanzees (*Pan troglodytes*). In *Verhandlungsbericht des 36 internationalen Symposiums über die Erkrankungen der Zootiere*, Kristiansand, Norway, 1994, pp 147–150.

64. Sainsbury AW, Gili C: Ultrasonographic anatomy and scanning technique of the coelomic organs of the Bosc monitor (*Varanus exanthematicus*). *J Zoo Wildl Med* 22(4):421–433, 1991.

65. Sande RD, Poppe TT: Diagnostic ultrasound examination and echocardiography in Atlantic salmon (*Salmo salar*). *Vet Radiol Ultrasound* 36(6):551–558, 1995.

66. Schroeder K, Drews B, Roellig K, et al: *In vivo* tissue sampling of embryonic resorption sites using ultrasound guided biopsy. *Theriogenology* 76(4):778–784, 2011.

67. Sklansky M, Renner M, Clough P, et al: Fetal echocardiographic evaluation of the bottlenose dolphin (*Tursiops truncatus*). *J Zoo Wildl Med* 41(1):35–43, 2010.

68. Stetter MD, Cook RA: Normal and pathological ultrastrasonographic anatomy of amphibians. In *Proceedings of the American Association of Zoo Veterinarians and Association of Reptilian and Amphibian Veterinarians Joint Conference*, Pittsburgh, PA, 1994, pp 69–70. (abstract).

69. Stetter MD: Noninfectious medical disorders of amphibians. *Semin Avian Exotic Pet Med* 4(1):49–55, 1995.

70. Stouffer JR, Wallentine MV, Wellington GH, et al: Development and application of ultrasonic methods for measuring fat thickness and ribeye area in cattle and hogs. *J Anim Sci* 20:759–767, 1961.

71. Stouffer JR: History of ultrasound in animal science. *J Ultrasound Med* 23(5):577–584, 2004.

72. Wagner WM, Kirberger RM: Transcutaneous ultrasonography of the coelomic viscera of the ostrich (*Struthio camelus*). *Vet Radiol Ultrasound* 42(6):546–552, 2001.

73. Walzer C, Hittmair K, Walzer-Wagner C: Ultrasonographic identification and characterization of splenic nodular lipomatosis or myelolipomas in cheetahs (*Acinonyx jubatus*). *Vet Radiol Ultrasound* 37(4):289–292, 1996.

74. Whittamore JM, Bloomer C, Hanna GM, et al: Evaluating ultrasonography as a non-lethal method for the assessment of maturity in oviparous elasmobranchs. *Marine Biol* 157(12):2613–2624, 2010.

CHAPTER 77

Wildpro Multimedia

Debra Bourne and Tiffany Blackett

Wildpro is an electronic encyclopedia and associated library on the health and management of captive and free-living wild animals, as well as emerging infectious diseases. This living, constantly expanding resource offers high-quality information to wildlife professionals across the world, in addition to providing valuable educational information for students, for example, those of veterinary medicine and animal care, and is freely available online at www.wildlifeinformation.org.

WHY WILDPRO?

Worldwide, professionals and field workers involved in the health and management of wild animals, whether captive or free-ranging (with the boundaries having become rather blurred),[11] commonly have to manage situations involving species or conditions with which they are not familiar. In this shrinking world, expanding human populations are coming into contact with species that were previously geographically distant; hosts, vectors, and their associated pathogens are being transported around the world; and climate change is affecting the range of various species, including pathogens and their vectors. Never has there been a more urgent need for rapid access to up-to-date, reliable, cross-disciplinary, and professional-level information.[5]

Many publications, including this book and its previous editions; other books based on a single taxon or disease; a multitude of journals and conference proceedings, are available and contain large amounts of information.[7] However, to access these resources, it is first necessary to be aware of their existence and the information in those publications has to be available when needed. Many organizations are addressing the need for publications to be more widely available in the developing world, but much information is still not easily accessible and is either out of print or not digitized. Many people do not know where, on the ever-expanding World Wide Web, to find the information they need or Internet access is unavailable to them. Conversely, a huge amount of material is now available online with no proper accreditation, and a need has arisen for ways to identify dependable, trustworthy information.[7] Finding and extracting information takes time, and several systems have been developed in an attempt to make it easier to search for and find specialist material.[14]

INSPIRATION AND PROOF OF CONCEPT

Wildpro was conceived by Suzanne Morgan-Jackson (Boardman) and F. Joshua Dein as a way to make information on wildlife health and management accessible to people who need to make decisions impacting wild animals.[3] The Wildpro prototype was distributed to more than 300 wildlife professionals (veterinarians, zoo directors and curators, wildlife managers, biologists, CITES [Convention on International Trade in Endangered Species] officials) in 61 countries. Of the respondents, 96% indicated that it would be useful, and 82% thought they would use it regularly.[2] Wildpro is unique because of the depth and breadth of information it contains. Making full use of the almost limitless capacity that the electronic medium provides, it combines information on species (their natural history), husbandry, pathogens, diseases, and treatment, all in one place, with extensive use of hyperlinks: wherever a logical link exists between two pieces of information, Wildpro hyperlinks them.

STRUCTURE AND DESIGN

Wildpro was developed around the basic concept that the interaction of three factors—the organism, the disease-producing agent, and the environment—results in either health or disease.[5,6] Unlike any other information resource (particularly many databases), Wildpro was designed first on the basis of what information the end-users needed to access, rather than on the easiest way to input data, with the aim to present information in a practical, intuitive format and with rich use of hyperlinks.[3]

The structure of Wildpro is based on the logical framework of a series of taxonomic trees: the familiar taxonomic tree for species and similar branching trees for other components such as chemicals. Naturally, the section on Species follows the taxonomic trees used for living species: Kingdom—Phylum—Class—Order—Family—Genus—Species. Confusion may arise as taxonomies change; therefore, the major taxonomic resources that have been used in constructing the pages are stated. Additionally, alternative names for a species, whether taxonomic or vernacular, are given, whenever possible, to minimize confusion. In a similar manner, the Diseases section descends from "Diseases" to "Viral Diseases," "Bacterial Diseases," "Toxic Diseases" and so on and then to individual diseases. Chemicals are subdivided into "metals, minerals, and simple molecules," "gross nutrients, vitamins, etc." and "complex chemical agents" (e.g., drugs used in animal treatment as well as toxic chemicals). The other sections are subdivided in similar branching pathways.

This system offers a logical structure within which information is presented and allows data to be provided at different levels of detail for different audiences. For example, where a disease has been covered in depth, summary information (as in a review paper) has been provided on the main page for that disease, and more detailed information that may be needed by students and researchers is available in a set of linked "literature report" pages. The structured format of the pages facilitates access to information; when certain data are unavailable, it is clearly mentioned in the hope of encouraging researchers or clinicians to fill these gaps.

TECHNIQUES—"HOW TO"

The "How to," or techniques, section includes topics such as husbandry, disease investigation, and group and individual animal veterinary care, as well as details of specific techniques such as drug administration methods in different species. Individual technique pages not only provide descriptions (some with annotated pictures or video clips) but also indicate the equipment required and give cautions regarding risks, skill levels, and legal and ethical considerations (e.g., surgical techniques should only be carried out by a qualified veterinarian).

REFERENCING AND REFEREEING

All information in Wildpro is clearly referenced back to its original source, that is, its provenance is shown.[6,7] A wide variety of reference types has been used, including websites, datasheets, internal records of organizations (e.g., animal health records) and personal communications, along with journal papers, books, proceedings, and theses. Alphanumerical coding ensures that the type of reference can be recognized at a glance (J is a refereed journal, B is a book, etc.) and that the details of the reference may be accessed easily, with each paper, book chapter (or part of a chapter, if different sections were written by different authors) or website page having its own unique identifier. All data within the Wildpro encyclopedia have also been refereed by experts within the relevant fields.[7]

NAVIGATION

Several methods of navigation are provided:
1. Every page is color coded, with a blue background for species; yellow for chemicals; maroon for diseases; bright and dark green for physical disease agents and environments, respectively; purple for techniques; teal for references; gray for help, and so on.
2. The navigation bar at the top of each page leads back to the home page and provides rapid access to each of the eight sections described above, plus a link to the Wildpro library.
3. A series of "breadcrumbs" are provided in the top left corner of each page, showing the main "taxonomic" path to that page.
4. In each volume in the encyclopedia, a contents page shows links to all sections of that volume, and a Table of Contents lists all the pages included in the volume.
5. A site-wide search mechanism is available on the home page.

THE WILDPRO LIBRARY

The Electronic Library has been developed with the main Wildpro Electronic Encyclopedia. It contains a wide variety of documents, more than 200 so far, ranging in length from a single page (pamphlets or fact sheets) to several hundred pages (complete published books), containing information which complements the encyclopedia. The documents are hyperlinked from relevant pages in the encyclopedia. This makes available a number of documents that are out of print and are therefore difficult to find, and some others that are difficult to access elsewhere unless one knows exactly where to look for them. Related documents have been compiled from diverse sources, for example, post-release studies on rehabilitated European hedgehogs (*Erinaceus europaeus*) and documents relating to the 2001 foot-and-mouth disease outbreak in the United Kingdom. For all documents in the library, copyright remains with the originators, but by granting permission for them to be reproduced in the Wildpro library, the copyright holders have allowed increased accessibility to these documents.

LINKS TO EXTERNAL WEBSITES

For each volume, a List of Organizations has been developed, with information on the role of each of those organizations and links to the organizations' websites, as appropriate. Every effort is taken to ensure that the information is correct at the time of publication; the editors welcome entry revisions and updated information.

PICTURES AND VIDEOS

Many pages are illustrated with annotated pictures, for example, of species and their identification features, appropriate enclosure design, and so on. Additionally, video clips of procedures have been provided, ranging from blood sampling of different bird species, to necropsy of wild ungulates, to several methods of endotracheal intubation of rabbits. *Bonobos: Health and Management* includes a video on natural behavior. As with library documents, image and video copyrights remain with the originators, and work is underway to expand this area in the future.

WILDPRO VOLUMES

Development of Wildpro is a huge task that is being carried out in volumes, based on taxonomic groups, diseases, management situations, or the urgent need for information in specific areas, as opportunity and funding allow. The first volume, *Waterfowl: Health and Management* was published online and on CD-ROM in 2000; to date, 16 volumes have been written, and five more are in development.

Waterfowl: Health and Management provides identification and natural history information on all species of ducks, geese, and swans, including their husbandry, diseases, disease agents, veterinary care, and wetland management.[7] Other taxa for which "Health and Management" volumes have been written are the West European hedgehog *Erinaceus europaeus*, bears, rabbits and their relatives (hares and pikas), ferrets, and bonobos. In each case, the volume provides information on the appearance, identification and natural history of the species, captive management (with both taxon and individual species-specific information, e.g., on bears and waterfowl), diseases, and veterinary care; additional relevant information such as garden management for hedgehogs is included. *Elephants: Diseases and Treatment* contains information on natural history, diseases, and treatments, complemented by several sets of elephant management guidelines in the Electronic Library.[8]

Wildpro volumes on diseases, including *Foot-and-Mouth Disease*, *West Nile Virus*, *Chronic Wasting Disease*, are comprehensive reviews of the disease, the pathogen, and options for surveillance and management.[14] *Rabies in Raccoons: Biology and Behaviour* looks at the interesting link between the natural history and normal behavior of raccoons (*Procyon lotor*) and the variant of raccoon rabies. *Viral Diseases of Great Apes: Part 1* provides detailed information on the diseases of great apes, including retroviral diseases (simian T-cell leukemia virus infection, simian immunodeficiency virus infection, and simian foamy virus infection), α-herpes virus infections (chickenpox and herpesvirus hominis [simplex] infection), and lymphocytic choriomeningitis infection.

Technique- or management-based volumes provide the information needed to manage a particular situation. *UK Wildlife: First Aid and Care* covers all the principles of management of wildlife casualty, including catching, handling, assessment, housing, feeding, handrearing, release, euthanasia, and (where appropriate) long-term care options, together with records and legislative considerations. All information, except the specific species information and U.K. legislation, is relevant for wildlife casualty care worldwide. *Wildlife: Oil Spill Response* considers all the steps required in treating wildlife affected by oil spills, from contingency planning and initial assessment of an oil spill, through wildlife capture, pre- and postwashing care, washing, release, and post-release monitoring, as well as considerations of facilities and staffing, human health, teamwork, command structure, public education, risks to different habitat types from oil extraction and oil cleanup operations, the effects of oils on birds and other species, and potential secondary and infectious disease conditions.[1,4,9] *Pain Management in Ruminants* covers the neurophysiology of pain, analgesic drugs and their pharmacokinetics, and pain prevention, assessment, and alleviation; it also discusses the reasons for pain control and failure of pain relief or lack of use.[12] *Disease Investigation and Management*, which includes the entire U.S. Geological Survey's Field Manual of Wildlife Diseases,[10] assists anyone, whatever their level of formal training in this area may be, to investigate a disease outbreak logically so that essential observations are made and appropriate samples are taken and recorded.

A volume covering 20 pathogens and associated diseases has been completed recently as part of WildTech (a project developing novel technologies for the surveillance of emerging and reemerging wildlife diseases, supported by the European Commission under the Food, Agriculture and Fisheries, and Biotechnology Theme of the 7th Framework Programme for Research and Technological Development, grant agreement no. 222633). Forthcoming volumes include "Health and Management" volumes on snow leopards (*Uncia uncia*), waders (shorebirds) and terns, and cranes; and a volume entitled *Environmental Enrichment: Principles and Practice*.

ACCESSIBILITY AND OPEN ACCESS

Wildpro is accessible both online and on CD-ROM (now DVD). This maximizes availability, particularly in the developing world, where, even in the 21st century, Internet access may be unavailable, intermittent, or very expensive. Finished volumes have been produced as stand-alone CD-ROMs or DVDs, and the entire Wildpro encyclopedia has been expanded on the dedicated website.[7]

In 2007, with the aim of making information extensively available, Wildpro became an open-access resource in the developing world. In 2011, after the Wildlife Information Network had been merged into Twycross Zoo–East Midland Zoological Society, the website was made open access worldwide to ensure free availability of valuable information and to promote the continued improvement of wild animal husbandry and well-being worldwide.[7]

THE FUTURE

It is inevitable that many subjects have not yet been covered in depth within Wildpro. More of the information jigsaw will be filled as opportunity and funding allow. Additionally, it is hoped that the Library will be expanded, as this is a potential repository for many texts, for example, animal health management protocols, in-house animal guidelines from relevant organizations, and out-of-print books and booklets. Additional photographs, diagrams, and videos are welcomed by Wildpro, and anyone willing and able to provide these is asked to e-mail debra.c.bourne@gmail.com. The aim is to make Wildpro a part of a larger conglomeration of information that is used, for example, in the new semantically enabled information analysis systems.[13]

REFERENCES

1. Bexton S: Book review [CD-ROM review]. *Vet J* 173:702–703, 2007.
2. Boardman S, Dein FJ: WILDPRO Multimedia: An electronic manual on the health, management and natural history of captive and free-ranging animals. In *Proceedings of the American Association of Zoo Veterinarians and the American Association of Wildlife Veterinarians Joint Conference*, 1998, pp 107–108.
3. Boardman SI: Are welfare and conservation compatible? In *Proceedings of the BVA Congress*, 1995.
4. Boardman SI, Bourne D, Dein FJ: Linking interdisciplinary information: "WILDPro® a novel data management system and extensive fully referenced electronic information source. In *Proceedings of Interspill*, 2000, pp 223–229.
5. Boardman SI, Dein FJ: Development of an electronic wildlife management manual. In *Proceedings of the European Association of Zoo and Wildlife Veterinarians (EAZWV) 1st Scientific Meeting*, 1996, pp 195–200.
6. Bourne D, Dein FJ, Boardman SI: Potential mechanisms for interrelating information on a cross-specific basis using information technology. In *Proceedings of the 39th International Symposium on the Diseases of Zoo and Wild Animals*, 1999, pp 297–299.
7. Bourne DC, Boardman SI: WIN and Wildpro: From initial concept to open access and beyond. In *Proceedings of the International Conference on the Diseases of Zoo and Wild Animals*, 2011, pp 57–62.
8. Bouts T: Elephants: Diseases and treatments [CD-ROM review]. *Anim Welfare* 17:202–203, 2008.
9. Chitty JR: Responding to oil spills [CD-ROM review]. *Vet Rec* 160:29, 2007.
10. Friend M, Franson JC: *Field manual of wildlife diseases—general field procedures and diseases of birds*, Washington, DC, 1999, U.S. Geological Survey.
11. Friend M: The wildlife factor. In Friend M, editor: *Diseases emergence and resurgence: The wildlife-human connection, Circular 1285*, Reston, VA, 2006, US Geological Survey, pp 129–189.
12. Jones RS: Book review [CD-ROM review]. *Vet J* 171:579–580, 2006.
13. McGuinness DL, Wang P, Fu L, et al: Towards semantically-enabled exploration and analysis of environmental ecosystems. In *Proceedings of the E-Science, 2012 IEEE 8th International Conference on E-Science*, 2012.
14. Wesenberg K, Friend M: How to find and access published information on emerging infectious diseases. In Friend M, editor: *Diseases emergence and resurgence: The wildlife-human connection, Circular 1285*, Reston, VA, 2006, US Geological Survey, pp 273–299.

CHAPTER 78

ISIS, MedARKS, ZIMS, and Global Sharing of Medical Information by Zoologic Institutions

J. Andrew Teare

The importance of high-quality records in zoos, with well-organized and standardized information, has long been recognized as a critical part of improving animal management practices within an institution.[3] The importance of combining information from multiple institutions has, however, been less appreciated for many years. Each institution that contributes information increases the sample size for analysis and enhances the ability to detect events that are otherwise too rare to reach significance within the experience of a single institution. However, the ability to easily combine records from different institutions to create an integrated database is predicated on the assumption that the records adhere to a common standard.[9] The advent of computerized records has driven the acceptance of single data standards in many industries, and universal electronic medical records in the human medical field is being widely cited as the tool that will improve health care while lowering costs. Indeed, sophisticated data mining is already being applied to large medical databases to detect drug interactions too rare to be detected during normal clinical trials.[7]

The International Species Information System (ISIS) was founded in 1974 to assist zoos and aquariums with meeting long-term conservation and animal management goals by providing information management services and a centralized database of zoo animal information. About 50 zoos in North America and Europe became the initial members of this network. Over the subsequent years, ISIS has grown to more than 800 member zoos, aquariums, and related organizations in almost 80 countries. Software design and development became an integral part of ISIS services, and ISIS users have created the world standards for zoologic data collection and management. Currently, the global Zoological Information Management System (ZIMS) database contains information on about 2.6 million captive wildlife specimens, encompassing some 10,000 species.

The ISIS database has always had a medical component, compiling hematology and blood chemistry result values and producing some of the earliest reference intervals for captive wildlife species. Starting in 1985, ISIS began developing MedARKS, a medical records database system to meet the needs of the zoologic community. The MedARKS software was neither the first software designed for zoo medical records[2,8] nor the last,[6] but it has been the most widely adopted, with more than 100 institutions actively using it in 2012. The ISIS member institutions using this product hold nearly 13 million medical records in a common format.

The MedARKS software includes tools to permit electronic transfer of medical information from one MedARKS institution to another. These tools allow the complete medical history of an animal to easily follow that animal to another institution and remain fully searchable at the next institution. The same data transfer tools also allow medical records from multiple institutions to be compiled into a single data set.

One of the earliest usages of MedARKS records was for the "Medical Management of the Orangutan" manual.[13] This year-long effort gathered the medical records of 249 orangutans held at 41 North American institutions and then manually summarized that medical information by body system, with additional chapters on other topics. The anesthesia section was used as a "proof of concept" project for the value of standardized records, with only MedARKS records being used in the compilation and analysis of anesthesia information. A total of 131 anesthesia events were available in the MedARKS data format, and the data transfer tools allowed the cooperating institutions to submit their data electronically. Software routines automated the entire compilation and analysis process, allowing the summary to be produced in a matter of days.

The resulting report provided zoo veterinarians with a summary of the drugs and drug combinations commonly used in orangutan immobilizations at that time, along with the mean administered dosage (milligram per kilogram [mg/kg]) for each drug. In addition, the analysis revealed that complications during anesthesia occurred during just 10 of the 131 events and that males were much more likely to experience complications during an immobilization (8 of 10). As male events only represented about 40% (54 of 131) of the records in the database, this meant that male orangutans experienced anesthetic complications about six times more frequently compared with females. Few institutions could ever have generated sufficient orangutan anesthesia records to detect the increased risk of complications in male orangutans, but this became immediately obvious when anesthesia records from multiple institutions were combined for analysis. This is the sort of knowledge that may directly impact the medical management of a species and was an early demonstration of the practical value of standardized, computerized medical records in zoologic medicine.

Historically, expected results (or reference intervals) for diagnostic tests were unknown or poorly defined for many captive wildlife species. Relatively few published reference intervals for wildlife species were available, forcing clinicians to rely on extrapolation of knowledge derived from domestic animal or human medical practice. As a result, interpretation of diagnostic test results may be challenging. Providing appropriate hematology and serum chemistry reference intervals to zoo clinicians for captive wildlife species was a very early goal for ISIS. Meeting that goal has been, and continues to be, quite difficult, but ISIS has made significant progress in this area with the production of a number of publications.

The American Society for Veterinary Clinical Pathology guidelines recommends 40 results as the minimum for calculating a reference interval.[1] This is a small sample size within the context of domestic animal populations, but a zoologic institution holding only 5 or 6 individuals of a long-lived species could take years to accumulate enough test result values to generate a valid reference interval for that species. Cooperation between multiple institutions is one solution for producing reference intervals within a reasonable period, when only a few test result values are held by any single institution. Even within the human medical field, in some situations (e.g., pediatrics), suitable samples are so rare that initiatives to compile results from multiple institutions have been used to gather enough data for calculating a reference interval.[5] For a zoologic institution holding hundreds of different species, this cooperative approach becomes the only viable solution for producing reference intervals for a significant proportion of their collection.

ISIS has taken this cooperative approach to an impressive level with its series of publications containing reference intervals for a large number of captive wildlife species.[10,11,12] Institutions using MedARKS submit results in a standardized format to a central database. The 1999 publication compiled information from 129 institutions, and the level of cooperation has risen with each subsequent publication, reaching 183 cooperating institutions for the 2013 publication. The current database contains more than 6.5 million results obtained from 348,000 blood samples. Despite this unprecedented level of cooperation, obtaining a sufficient number of results for any individual species is still challenging, with the majority of species in the database having results from less than 30 samples. The 2013 publication limited calculations to the 913 species and subspecies with at least 50 samples in the database. In keeping with the American Society for Veterinary Clinical Pathology (ASVCP) guidelines, reference intervals were only calculated for tests with at least 40 results (Figure 78-1). Clearly, limitations are imposed by amalgamating results from so many different institutions, but these reference interval publications are used on a daily basis by many zoo clinicians and are widely cited in the literature. This project remains another demonstration of the power of standardized records and the value of cooperative projects within the field of zoo medicine.

Clinical studies in human or domestic animal medicine may involve hundreds, sometimes thousands, of subjects, making it more likely that cases of a particular disease or condition will be encountered. The small populations typically available to zoo veterinarians impose constraints and limitations that may not be obvious. With only a small population under medical care, even defining the common medical issues for a species may be challenging. It should be no surprise then that even relatively common medical problems in zoo species may remain incompletely understood several decades after their first description (e.g., hemolytic anemia syndrome in the black rhinoceros).[4] Rarer diseases may be known to zoo clinicians only from single case reports, and access to sufficient clinical cases to allow for comparison of different treatments is an exceptional situation in zoologic medicine.

The Zoological Information Management System (ZIMS) is the next generation of software from ISIS. This Web-based, real-time global database of captive wildlife information will change many aspects of the science of zoo biology. The first release of ZIMS is currently being used by more than 600 ISIS member institutions to maintain their animal records, with all ISIS members expected to adopt it by the end of 2014. The next major release of ZIMS is in preparation and, when complete, will bring medical records to the global database. The initial medical records module will make

ISIS Physiological Reference Intervals for Captive Wildlife - 2013

Conventional American units. Switch Units
edited by J. Andrew Teare, DVM

Fennec Fox
(*Vulpes zerda*)

Samples contributed by 48 institutions.

© 2013 - International Species Information System
(Citation Format)

Sample Selection Criteria:

- No selection by gender.
- All ages combined
- Animal was classified as healthy at the time of sample collection
- Sample was not deteriorated

Physiological Reference Intervals for Vulpes zerda

Test	Units	Reference Interval	Mean	Median	Low Sample[a]	High Sample[b]	Sample Size[c]	Animals[d]
White Blood Cell Count	*10^3 cells/μL	1.93 - 10.76	5.30	5.01	0.90	13.50	446	180
Red Blood Cell Count	*10^6 cells/μL	5.76 - 11.03	8.31	8.31	2.69	12.00	380	150
Hemoglobin	g/dL	10.6 - 20.1	15.2	15.1	6.4	21.5	384	160
Hematocrit	%	32.9 - 60.1	46.3	46.2	18.9	66.0	478	186
MCV	fL	45.1 - 66.3	55.0	54.7	41.3	70.4	367	148
MCH	pg	15.7 - 20.9	18.2	18.1	13.7	23.3	351	144
MCHC	g/dL	28.8 - 38.9	33.2	33.1	24.8	42.1	373	157
Segmented Neutrophils	*10^3 cells/μL	0.78 - 6.91	2.74	2.38	0.01	8.74	446	180
Neutrophilic Band Cells	*10^3 cells/μL	0.01 - 0.06	0.02	0.02	0.00	0.07	408	178
Lymphocytes	*10^3 cells/μL	0.38 - 4.48	1.95	1.76	0.06	6.34	441	179
Monocytes	cells/μL	33 - 735	244	201	20	966	409	172
Eosinophils	cells/μL	33 - 824	285	241	18	1016	407	173
Basophils	cells/μL	0 - 121	61	55	6	165	40	35
Platelet Count	*10^3 cells/μL	164 - 709	416	404	100	793	140	77

FIGURE 78-1 Hematology reference intervals for *Vulpes zerda* calculated by ISIS from data submitted through the MedARKS software. On average, each zoologic institution held results for less than 10 blood samples, a number insufficient for calculating a valid reference interval. (From Teare JA, ed: 2013, "Vulpes_zerda_No_selection_by_gender__All_age s_combined_Conventional_American _Units__2013_CD.html" *in* ISIS Physiological Reference Intervals for Captive Wildlife: A CD-ROM Resource., International Species Information System, Bloomington, MN.)

extensive use of the existing MedARKS standards, easing the task of data migration from the existing institutionally based, MedARKS record system to the ZIMS global database.

Zoo clinicians need and are looking for medical information about a wide variety of species in their care, and this information may not be readily available within the existing literature. The International Zoo Veterinarians Forum (IZVF), hosted by ISIS (http://izvf.portal.isis.org/default.aspx), is an online forum for zoo clinicians to post queries and obtain answers from the community. A quick review of recent postings on the forum showed that 8% of queries concerned anesthesia and sedation protocols in a specific species, 16% was about information on the use of a specific drug or drug recommendations for treating a particular condition in a specified species, 8% sought information on expected results (reference intervals) for physiologic or biochemical measurements in a specified species, and another 16% asked about a particular medical condition in a specific species.

Once the existing MedARKS records have been added to the ZIMS medical module and a global medical database exists, answers to many of these queries from the zoo community could be directly obtained from that accumulated knowledge. A single global database dramatically increases the ability to examine that information for patterns and to produce useful summaries for zoo clinicians. The existing hematology and blood chemistry reference intervals could be updated more frequently and with less effort, since the information is already consolidated. In addition, the reference intervals may more easily be expanded to include additional tests and measurements. However, these biochemical and physiologic measurements and the resulting reference intervals are really just the tip of the information iceberg.

Analysis of prescription records in the system could easily determine whether drug X has ever been used in species Y. If records were present, the dosage and dosing frequency information would also be available. The incidence of adverse effects reported for these prescriptions and the severity of any adverse effects could also be extracted from the database and reported to the clinician. Although the results of such a query would not constitute a true drug formulary for a species, these results would still provide zoo clinicians with the information needed to improve treatment decisions for the captive wildlife species in their care.

The analysis performed on the orangutan anesthesia records could also be performed for any other species with sufficient records in a global database. The results of such an analysis would not only provide clinicians with information about the drugs and drug combinations used, but with sufficient records, the analysis might indicate which protocols are associated with the fewest complications and the best recoveries. Queries that might require days for a response through the IZVF could be answered in minutes by using the global database records, and the answer would contain specific and useful information.

These quantitative types of medical information are easily analyzed, and the resulting summaries provide immediate support for zoo clinicians. Medical records also contain information that is not of a quantitative nature. Clinical signs, clinical findings, diseases, conditions, and other medical issues are also part of a records system. This type of information is included as part of the MedARKS records and will also form part of the ZIMS global medical database, but standardizing this portion of the medical records is more difficult. Yet standardization is crucial, and accurate counts of the incidence of a medical issue in a species rely on a system capable of recognizing all equivalent terms. ZIMS is being designed to handle these equivalencies in terminologies, including translations into other languages.

Underlying every diagnostic process is the assumption that the clinician is aware of the most common diseases and medical problems in the species being examined. When that medical knowledge is combined with observed clinical signs and findings, sometimes with adjustments for age and gender, the clinician may be able to create a rational differential diagnosis list. That differential diagnosis list suggests additional testing to help resolve the diagnostic process in favor of one or other of the competing theories. For captive wildlife, the baseline knowledge regarding the most common medical issues seen in a species may be minimal.

This is not to say that the start of these differential diagnosis lists do not already exist for some captive wildlife species. When presented with an elderly male gorilla, most zoo clinicians would have some concern about cardiac disease, even in the absence of overt clinical signs. However, for many captive wildlife species, that primary assumption with regard to the common medical issues afflicting a species is often the weakest point in the diagnostic process. The zoo clinician may have to rely on knowledge obtained from experiences with related species.

Strengthening this primary knowledge about the common diseases seen in a species has long been recognized as important. Veterinary medical advisors for a Species Survival Plan committee often attempt to compile such lists of medical issues for their species of interest, using existing medical and pathology records. Currently, all this work requires reading the medical records and manually coding the results. It is a labor-intensive process, and as a result, these attempts to define the common medical issues have impacted relatively few species of captive wildlife.

MedARKS is a problem-oriented records system, and it maintains a master problem list. Unfortunately, some 20 years of experience with the MedARKS system has shown that the standardized problem list is not used as extensively as other parts of the system. In addition, even when used by an institution, it may not be complete. Maintaining a complete master problem list is a time-consuming task, and that is certainly a concern for busy clinicians. Incentive is another major cause for this breakdown between the desire for complete medical records and the actual outcome. Human and domestic animal medical record systems often link the diagnosis to the billing system, providing a financial incentive that is absent in zoo medicine.

Standardized diagnoses within ZIMS will allow automated processing of this portion of the medical records. Lists of the medical diseases and conditions seen in a species will be easily compiled and the incidence of each diagnosis could be tallied. Over time, the most frequently seen medical issues for a species will become apparent. ZIMS will also be able to associate clinical signs and findings with a final diagnosis, eventually allowing clinicians to query the system about the most frequent diagnoses linked to a specific set of signs

and findings. At this point, the system starts to resemble an expert system. However, this objective may only be achieved if we resolve the discrepancy between the data needs of the community and the data entry limitations that are a consequence of time restraints on individual clinicians.

ZIMS will attempt to change this model and will include tools designed to significantly ease the burden of maintaining the list of diagnoses, clinical signs, and findings. Incentivizing clinicians to increase use of this portion of the records system is a problem that remains to be resolved. One solution that has been proposed is to link usage of the diagnosis portion of the record to accessing information extracted from the quantitative sections of the system. The MedARKS experience has shown that clinicians do value information such as reference intervals, which may only be extracted from the accumulated records obtained from multiple institutions. ISIS believes that clinicians will find summaries of drug use and anesthesia experience in a species to be just as valuable. If access to this information becomes a function related to ongoing usage of the problem-oriented portion of the system, this may serve as the incentive needed to improve the ZIMS records, although the exact mechanism of such a function is likely to be complex.

Regardless of the difficulties associated with both standardizing diagnoses and increasing data entry compliance from clinicians, obtaining information about medical issues must remain an important goal for ISIS. Significant efforts have already been devoted to this portion of the system, and tools will be provided to both assist with data entry and to improve data comprehensiveness. Access to the global ZIMS database for the quantitative records will have a significant impact soon after deployment, but it is the long-term result of getting standardized medical diagnoses and other issues into the system that will fundamentally change the practice of zoologic medicine.

REFERENCES

1. Friedrichs KR, Harr KE, Freeman KP, et al: ASVCP reference interval guidelines: Determination of de novo reference intervals in veterinary species and other related topics. *Vet Clin Pathol* 41(4):441–445, 2012.
2. Janssen DL, Bush M: The microcomputer as an aid to medical records management in a zoological park. *J Am Vet Med Assoc* 181:1381–1384, 1982.
3. Jarvis C: Studying wild mammals in captivity: Standard life histories with an appendix on zoo records. In Lucas J, editor: *International Zoo Yearbook*, ed 9, 1969, Zoological Society of London, pp 316–328.
4. Miller RE, Boever WJ: Fatal hemolytic anemia in the black rhinoceros: Case report and a survey. *J Am Vet Med Assoc* 181:1228–1231, 1982.
5. Schnabl K, Chan MK, Gong Y, Adeli K: Closing the gaps in paediatric reference intervals: The CALIPER initiative. *Clin Biochem Rev* 29:89–96, 2008.
6. Stover J, Cook RA: A diagnosis based computer program for problem oriented medical records. In *Proceedings of the American Association of Zoo Veterinarians*, 1986, pp 56–59.
7. Tatonetti NP, Ye PP, Daneshjou R, Altman RB: Data-driven prediction of drug effects and interactions. *Sci Transl Med* 4(125):125–131, 2012.
8. Teare JA: A "user-friendly" system for computerization of medical records. In *Proceedings of the American Association of Zoological Parks and Aquaria, Central Regional Conference*, 1984, pp 451–458.
9. Teare JA: Medical record systems for the next century: The case for improved health care through integrated databases. *J Zoo Wildl Med* 22:389–391, 1991.
10. Teare JA, editor: *Reference ranges for physiological values in captive wildlife*, Apple Valley, MN, 1999, International Species Information System.
11. Teare JA: *Reference ranges for physiological values in captive wildlife*, Apple Valley, MN, 2002, International Species Information System.
12. Teare JA: *ISIS Physiological Reference Intervals for Captive Wildlife: A CD-ROM resource*, Apple Valley, MN, 2013, International Species Information System.
13. Wells SK, Sargent EL, Andrews ME, Anderson DE: *Medical management of the Orangutan*, New Orleans, LA, 1990, Audubon Institute.

CHAPTER 79

Update on Remote Delivery and Restraint Equipment

Chris Walzer and Hanno Gerritsmann

HISTORY AND BACKGROUND

The first description of a "flying syringe," which used an acid–base reaction to administer drugs to animals from a propelled aluminum dart, was published in 1958.[4] Unfortunately, this ingenious idea has remained largely unchanged over the past 55 years, and most new developments are mere refinements of this original concept.

Since field capture of wild animals may cost a large amount of money per animal, in terms of personnel and transport costs, remote injection systems need to be efficient and reliable.[10] Precision is of major importance as, in the field, usually only one chance is available to hit the animal. After the initial firing noise, the animal usually flees. Furthermore, the preferred target area on an animal may only be a few square centimeters (cm^2) in small animals. If imprecise remote injection systems are used, the shot may be misplaced, wounding or killing the animal or missing the animal entirely.[11] The risk of severe tissue disruption, including hemorrhage, necrosis, and bone fractures, increases when using pressure-driven injection systems, which strike the animal with high-impact energy. A thorough understanding of the equipment and the anesthetics employed, in conjunction with professional training in wildlife chemical immobilization, are important to prevent accidents.

Since it is hard to approach free-ranging animals, remote injection systems need to be able to hit the animal over long distances without wounding the individual. Especially for the capture of free-ranging wildlife, the available products on the market are unsatisfactory in their performance with respect to range, accuracy, and precision. Because of the inherent constraints engendered by the necessarily lightweight darts and acceptable impact energy, it appears unlikely that novel solutions will markedly improve on the future performance of today's projector. A rise in animal welfare awareness and concerns has given rise to the clear trend in the past decade toward compressed gas projectors, which allow for the continuous adjustment of pressure according to target distance. In general, higher pressures result in a faster dart that flies further. However, wind resistance places limitations on this by rapidly slowing the dart. Darts propelled by carbon dioxide (CO_2) projectors usually travel at about 40 to 60 meters per second (m/s). In contrast, cartridge-propelled darts fired from extra-long range projectors have been measured to have mean impact velocities of up to 113 m/s.[2,19] The manufacturers' recommendations are, at best, only a guide, and the users of remote injection systems must individually calibrate their rifle or dart combinations by finding the best pressure settings. With regard to the effective shooting range, a significant disparity exists between the technical specifications and the results in the field. In a study on dart gun range and precision, none of three remote injection systems, apart from the Pneu-Dart X-Caliber (Pneu-Dart Inc., Williamsport, PA), attained the effective shooting range specified by the manufacturers. In this study, a correlation was observed between a stable dart trajectory and the pressure setting of the rifle. Trajectories remained stable up to a certain, rifle-specific, pressure. When this pressure was exceeded, the dart trajectory became unstable.[5]

What's New

The different calibers offered currently make dart guns less user friendly. Manufacturers offer dart guns with interchangeable barrels,

but changing barrels is time consuming, as the user needs to "sight" in the new barrel before use. Developments in the field include a double-barrel dart gun, the JM.DB (Figure 79-1) made by Dan-Inject (DAN-INJECT ApS, Børkop, Denmark) featuring either two identical barrels or an 11-mm barrel and a 13-mm barrel, which alleviates the caliber problem, as the gun is capable of propelling virtually all darts available for CO_2 guns.

In remote, open-range situations where helicopters are not readily available for capture of animals, veterinarians regularly find themselves frustrated by large flight distances exceeding 1 kilometer (km) or more. To address this problem, stationary, remote-controlled, video-enabled dart guns have been used at waterholes or feeding sites.[17,21]

Darts

Recent advances in the field include lighter 5-milliliter (mL) 11-mm Ø slow air injection darts that may be used in the standard 11-mm barrels. This greatly simplifies the use of these larger volume darts. Several producers now have very-high-frequency (VHF) transmitters available to facilitate tracking and recovery of the darted animal (TeleDart GmbH & Co. KG, Westheim, Germany; Dist-Inject International, Basel, Switzerland; DanWild LLC, Austin, TX) (Figure 79-2).

Pneu-Dart, Inc. now offers VHF transmitters that have an extended range of operation for their 13-mm rapid-injection darts. These transmitters have been tested under steppe–desert field conditions, where a signal may be received up to a distance of 1000 meters (m). However, if the animal becomes recumbent on the transmitter dart, the maximum range is halved. Additionally, these transmitters may be supplemented with flashing LEDs (light-emitting diodes) on the tailpiece for night visibility (see Figure 79-2, *D*). This feature has proven useful when shooting in darkness to determine a hit.

A prototype for remote application of passive identification transponders based on a Pneu-Dart model dart was recently shown to offer new opportunities in this regard.[20] Additionally, Pneu-Dart now offers gun-mounted LEDs to illuminate the barometer, which is also extremely helpful when working during the night (Dial face illuminator, Pneu-Dart, Inc. Williamsport, PA).

PHYSICAL RESTRAINT DEVICES

Net Guns

Similar to dart guns, currently two types of handheld net guns are available. Nets are either propelled by blanks or compressed-gas cartridges. Options for handheld, lightweight net guns that are shaped like a flashlight are the Super Talon Ultra (Advanced Weapons Technology Inc., La Quinta, CA), the MagNet small animal net gun (Figure 79-3) (Wildlife Capture Services LLC., Flagstaff, AZ), and the NetGun-System Gladiator (Zooprofis, Natendorf Wessenstedt, Germany). Nets are fired at approximately 6 to 7.5 m/s (20 feet per second [ft/s] to 25 ft/s). Various net and mesh sizes are available.

Larger net guns, including stationary devices for the capture of groups of birds or even larger animals, are currently offered by Coda Enterprises Inc. (Mesa, A), Wildlife Capture Services LLC (Flagstaff,

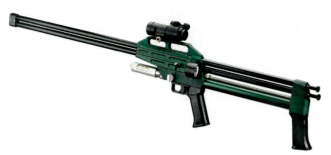

FIGURE 79-1 The Dan-Inject JM.DB.13 (Courtesy DAN-INJECT ApS, Børkop, Denmark.)

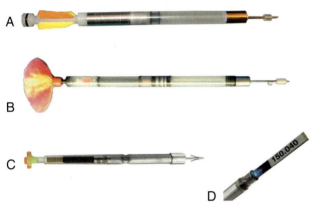

FIGURE 79-2 Current transmitter darts. **A,** Dist-Inject 11 millimeter (mm). **B,** Tele Dart 11 mm. **C,** Pneu-Dart. **D,** Pneu-Dart flashing LED tailpiece. (**A,** Courtesy Dist-Inject International, Basel, Switzerland; **B,** Courtesy TeleDart GmbH & Co. KG, Westheim, Germany; **C,** Courtesy Pneu-Dart Inc., Williamsport, PA.)

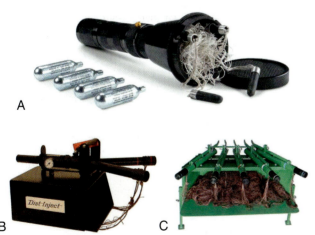

FIGURE 79-3 Current net launchers. **A,** MagNet small animal net gun. **B,** Dist-Inject Net Launcher CO₂. **C,** Dist-Inject Big Net Launcher (cartridge operated). (**A,** Courtesy Wildlife Capture Services LLC., Flagstaff, AZ; **B,** Courtesy Dist-Inject International, Basel, Switzerland.)

AZ), Dist-Inject International (Basel, Switzerland), and ACE Capture (Invercargill, New Zealand) to name but a few (see Figure 79-3).

In these authors' opinion, net gun use in wild animals should be limited to situations where chemical immobilization is not feasible. If netting is used, sedation of the animal upon approach via intranasal application of a sedative has been proven to have a beneficial effect.[3] Comparative publications on net gun capture methods and

their side effects are numerous. However, results are highly variable because of the diverse set of factors that need to be considered. The largest coherent data set (n = 3350) examining net gun captures of white-tailed deer (*Odocoileus virginianus*) was published by Webb et al. in 2008.[21] They report an injury incidence of 8.4%, where 73% of injuries were inflicted on antlers. Furthermore, capture-related mortality is estimated at 1.3% (confirmed 0.7%). Caution is certainly warranted, and significant experience is required when physical restraint is employed in wildlife.

Other Equipment

A newly developed catchpole, the ACES Dual Release Catch Pole (patent pending) (Animal Care Equipment & Services, LLC, Boulder, CO), allows for both instant enlarging of the noose and the quick release of the noose. This is a vast improvement on previous models that only allowed for enlarging the noose.

CONDUCTED ELECTRICAL WEAPONS

Background

Today, conducted electrical weapons (CEW) are used by numerous law enforcement agencies for the short-term incapacitation of humans. CEWs work with two gas-propelled, barbed darts connected to the main unit via wires that deliver pulsed electrical currents to a target and back to the main unit creating an electric circuit, with the target acting as a resistor or capacitor model. The pulse energy delivered by modern CEWs is usually between 0.9 and 10 Joules (J) at a rate of around 20 pulses per second.[1] The functional principle is not entirely clear, but it is thought that the pulsed discharges lead to a depolarization of efferent α-motor neurons and afferent sensory neurons, resulting in uncontrollable clonic contractions of skeletal muscle groups and the sensation of pain.[16] Undirected stimuli must have sufficient strength and duration to induce action potentials in neurons or effector cells. Hence development of CEWs has been directed toward the induction of sub-tetanic muscle contraction of the skeletal muscles.[12,18] Numerous prospective scientific studies have examined the pathophysiologic side effects of CEWs, such as electrocardiogram changes, myocardial capture (a direct response of the heart rate to the discharge pulses by CEW), respiration, blood gases, troponin values, effects of exertion, intoxication or anesthesia in both human and animal models, with little to no evidence of major side effects.[6-9] Discussion on the topic is still ongoing, with more scientific articles supporting a strong safety profile for CEWs. It needs to be stated, however, that most studies used small sample sizes, and some have received funding from the industry or U.S. federal agencies that are linked to security services. This, in our view, places severe constraints on conclusions that may be drawn from the data.[15]

Use in Animals

The Taser company (TASER International, Inc, Scottsdale, AZ), in cooperation with the Alaska Department of Fish and Game (ADFG), has developed the commercially available, TASER X3W Wildlife CEW, which has been adapted for use in wildlife (Figure 79-4). The manufacturer suggests the X3W in situations requiring hazing or short-term immobilization of wildlife for various reasons. According to the manufacturer, articles in popular scientific journals, and the Internet, the X3W has proven effective in immobilizing the moose (*Alces alces*), brown bear (*Ursus americanus*), collared peccary (*Pecari tajacu*), and deer (species not known), to name a few.[13,14] While scientific evidence regarding the usefulness and safety of the X3W and its use in wildlife is still pending, extrapolation from the available human and laboratory animal dataset provided initial insights. It is more than obvious that the use of such a device should be limited to use when all other options have failed. Even though the use of the device has proven to be relatively safe in humans, pain and distress will certainly be inflicted on a conscious animal. This is in stark contrast to the modern concept of animal immobilization and anesthesia.

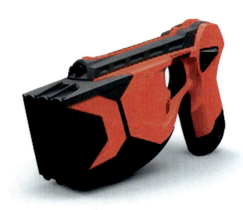

FIGURE 79-4 TASER X3W Wildlife CEW. (Courtesy TASER International, Inc, Scottsdale, AZ.)

Indisputably, the X3W expands the toolbox of wildlife veterinarians working with potentially dangerous animals, but in these authors' opinion, it should generally be regarded as a "less than lethal" option for human safety rather than just another option for short-term immobilizations. Although the X3W features a timer that allows for the predefined application of discharges (hands-free use), the duration of exposure suggested by the manufacturer is limited to less than 60 seconds.

Limitations

As the gas-propelled darts of the X3W stay connected to the main unit via DuPont Tefzel ETFE fluoroplastic-coated wires, it needs to be mentioned that the maximal distance to the target is about 11 m (approximately 35 ft). When being attacked, the user of the dart should keep in mind that this is a very short distance, easily covered within a second by most of the larger quadrupeds.

REFERENCES

1. Adler A, Dawson D, Evans R, et al: Toward a test protocol for conducted energy weapons. *Mod Instrum* 2:7, 2013.
2. Cattet MR, Bourque A, Elkin BT, et al: Evaluation of the potential for injury with remote drug-delivery systems. *Wildl Soc Bull* 34:741–749, 2006.
3. Cattet MR, Caulkett NA, Wilson C, et al: Intranasal administration of xylazine to reduce stress in elk captured by net gun. *J Wild Dis* 40:562–565, 2004.
4. Crockford J, Hayes F, Jenkins J, Feurt S: An automatic projectile type syringe. *Vet Med* 53:115–119, 1958.
5. Graf P: *Who hits the bull's eye? A comparison of three current remote injection systems (diploma thesis)*, Vienna, Austria, 2010, Vienna Veterinary Medical University, pp 33.
6. Ho JD, Dawes DM, Bultman LL, et al: Respiratory effect of prolonged electrical weapon application on human volunteers. *Acad Emerg Med* 14:197–201, 2007.
7. Ho JD, Dawes DM, Heegaard WG, et al: Absence of electrocardiographic change after prolonged application of a conducted electrical weapon in physically exhausted adults. *J Emerg Med* 41:466–472, 2009.
8. Ho JD, Dawes DM, Reardon RF, et al: Human cardiovascular effects of a new generation conducted electrical weapon. *Forensic Sci Int* 204:50–57, 2011.
9. Jauchem JR: Repeated or long-duration TASER electronic control device exposures: Acidemia and lack of respiration. *Forensic Sci Med Pathol* 6:46–53, 2010.
10. Kock MD, Clark RK, Franti CE, et al: Effects of capture on biological parameters in free-ranging bighorn sheep (*Ovis canadensis*): Evaluation of normal, stressed and mortality outcomes and documentation of post-capture survival. *J Wild Dis* 23:652–662, 1987.
11. Kreeger TJ, Arnemo JM: *Handbook of wildlife chemical immobilization*, 2007, Terry J. Kreeger.
12. Kroll M: Crafting the perfect shock. *Spectrum IEEE* 44:27–31, 2007.
13. Feline Conservation Federation: Tasers in Wildlife Mitigation and Captive Animal Facilities. 55(6):17–20, 2011.
14. Pasquier M, Carron P-N, Vallotton L, Yersin B: Electronic control device exposure: A review of morbidity and mortality. *Ann Emerg Med* 58:178–188, 2011.
15. Roberts JR: InFocus: The Physiology of TASERs. *Emerg Med News* 34:18, 2012.
16. Ryser A, Scholl M, Zwahlen M, et al: A remote-controlled teleinjection system for the low-stress capture of large mammals. *Wildl Soc Bull* 33:721–730, 2005.
17. Smith PW: *Hand-held stun gun for incapacitating a human target*, 2003 US Patent 6,636,412, 2003, Google Patents.
18. Valkenburg P, Tobey RW, Kirk D: Velocity of tranquilizer darts and capture mortality of caribou calves. *Wildl Soc Bull* 894–896, 1999.
19. Walter WD, Anderson CW, VerCauteren KC: Evaluation of remote delivery of Passive Integrated Transponder (PIT) technology to mark large mammals. *PLoS ONE* 7:e44838, 2012.
20. Walzer C, Boegel R: A video-enabled, radio-controlled remote teleinjection system for field applications. In *Proceedings of the Joint Conference of the American Association of Zoo Veterinarians*, Minneapolis, 2003, pp 228–229.
21. Webb SL, Lewis JS, Hewitt DG, et al: Assessing the helicopter and net gun as a capture technique for white-tailed deer. *J Wildl Manage* 72:310–314, 2008.

CHAPTER 80

Guidelines for the Management of Zoonotic Diseases

Donald L. Janssen

Most zoo clinicians have, at one time or another, encountered a case in which they diagnosed or suspected a zoonotic disease. For the purposes of this chapter, a *zoonotic disease* is defined as any infectious disease that may be readily transmitted between animals and humans. When a serious zoonotic disease is identified, often the demand for action is urgent, and little time is available to make systematic and intentional decisions. In contrast, when a subtle disease incident occurs, it may be completely overlooked and no specific action taken. In either case, we may fail to handle the situation in the best interests of the health and safety of the animals, staff, and guests.

To focus our efforts, it may be useful to ask several key questions, including the following:

◆ What circumstances should trigger a zoonotic disease investigation and response?
◆ Who is responsible for making decisions about public health implications?
◆ Who should be notified, and what do we say?
◆ Do we need to report to government regulators?
◆ What do the caretakers of the animal need to know?
◆ Do we need to isolate the animal, and if so, what procedures should we implement?
◆ How do we handle contaminated waste?
◆ How do we manage the medical care of the infected animal?

This chapter suggests a strategy to answer these questions using a systematic process when dealing with a zoonotic disease occurrence in a zoo setting.

SYSTEMATIC PROCESS

Having a systematic process for managing a zoonotic disease occurrence reduces the risk of mishandling them. The consequences of mishandling may be significant. The implications to the animal, its caretakers, the public, the institution, and our professional reputations may quickly become overwhelming. Failure to respond properly may lead to unnecessary human and animal illness or, in contrast, an overreaction to perceived risks. Other animals in contact with the infected animal may be put at risk. Public health may be compromised through unnecessary contact and exposure of disease agents to employees and guests. A zoonotic disease outbreak could affect the reputation of the institution, leading to public concern and adverse economic consequences. Media attention may become misdirected. Even our professional reputation could be damaged by improperly handling the many issues that come up when a zoonotic disease is identified.

The chances of avoiding these undesirable consequences are improved by setting up a systematic process ahead of time (Box 80-1). As a first step, it is important to identify triggers to initiate the process so that we do not overlook the occurrence of a zoonotic disease.

Identifying Triggers

The diagnosis or suspicion of a zoonotic disease in an animal or human contact should trigger the process to begin. Often, the trigger is a specific test result (e.g., a culture) reported from the laboratory.

Another trigger may be the results of a postmortem examination that provide evidence of a zoonotic disease, either confirmed or suspected. A more unusual trigger could be an employee, volunteer, or guest who is diagnosed with an infectious disease that could have been acquired from contact with animals in the collection. A suspicion of a zoonotic disease may also act as a trigger (e.g., an outbreak of diarrheal disease in an animal contact area).

Once triggered, a systematic approach should be implemented. This could be approached in several ways. In our practice, a zoonotic disease occurrence triggers each of the following steps: (1) notifying stakeholders; (2) isolating the animal from others; (3) managing the contaminated waste from the animal; (4) reporting to authorities, if appropriate; and (5) treating the animal or otherwise managing the clinical illness, if present. All these steps are important, but key steps that need emphasis may be different in each case.

Notifying Stakeholders

Once the process is triggered, the most urgent step is to notify the appropriate internal stakeholders involved in the care of the animal and the occupational health care provider for the facility. It may seem desirable to keep the situation quiet and avoid overreaction and unnecessary attention to the situation. Approaching the problem in that way, however, often leads to greater problems. It is critical that employees be informed so that they may take proper precautions and report signs and symptoms of disease that they may be experiencing. It is useful to provide a written disease fact sheet to all stakeholders to remind them of the signs and symptoms. Well-written fact sheets on many zoonotic diseases are readily available in books, pamphlets, and from authoritative sources on the Internet.[1,2]

Isolating the Animal

This is the first of two important infection control steps. The veterinary and animal care staffs should determine whether it is appropriate to isolate the infected animal, the facility in which it is located, or both. The decision should be based on evaluating risks and feasibility. A quick risk assessment may be performed on the basis of the severity and contagiousness of the disease. This should be balanced against the feasibility of performing the isolation safely and effectively. Isolation should be done in the case of an animal housed in a public contact setting.[3]

As in quarantine, separate tools and equipment should be used. A footbath may be helpful to reduce the spread of contamination and to remind workers of the isolation entry control point. In addition, this is a good opportunity to remind staff of the importance of proper hygiene (especially hand washing) and the use of appropriate personal protective equipment, and how to implement them.

Handling Waste

This is the next step critical for infection control. Instruct the animal care staff on proper waste disposal procedures, including disposal of bedding, to avoid spreading contamination. Contaminated waste should be disposed of through a sanitary sewer, if possible. Local and regional regulations for the disposal of biomedical wastes should be strictly adhered to. Proper disinfection of premises should be carried out by using disinfection best practices.[4]

BOX 80-1 Steps in Managing a Zoonotic Disease Case in a Zoo

1. Trigger—zoonotic disease identified or suspected
2. Notifications—notifying and educating stakeholders
3. Infection control:
   a. Animal isolation
   b. Waste management
4. Regulatory reporting
5. Medical management

Reporting to Regulatory Authorities

Some zoonotic diseases are reportable to regional public health and veterinary authorities. Reportable diseases vary with the region, and public agencies have different criteria with regard to what is reportable. Before such issues arise, it is helpful to develop a rapport with local public health departments. To keep alert to trends, it may be useful to develop an internal mechanism to track the zoonotic diseases that occur in a facility over time.

Medical Management

If indicated, the animal should be treated with appropriate antimicrobials and follow-up diagnostics performed, as appropriate. Criteria for case resolution and an endpoint for patient and facility isolation (e.g., test negative and/or clinically normal) should be established.

SAMPLE ZOONOSIS SCENARIOS

The following scenarios, based loosely on actual cases, provide examples of how this process might be used in real-life situations. In each scenario, all steps are addressed, but each example highlights steps of key importance for that particular case.

Shigellosis in a Mother-Reared Infant Gorilla

The trigger to action in this case was the combination of suspicious clinical signs (diarrhea and general illness) along with the eventual positive fecal culture for *Shigella* sp. The key step in this case was to notify the keepers caring for the infant and the occupational health provider. A fact sheet from the Centers for Disease Control and Prevention (CDC) about shigellosis, including signs, symptoms, and method of transmission, was provided to the animal care staff. Isolation of the animal was not feasible, nor was it required because the risk of disease transmission to the keeper staff and public was low. The low risk was a result of primate biosafety precautions that were already in place as standard operating procedures for primate areas. Reporting to regulatory authorities was not required, but the case was added to an internal tracking log to aid in following trends. The animal was treated with antibiotics. The endpoint of the process was determined to be the resolution of clinical signs, not necessarily a negative follow-up fecal culture.

Methicillin-Resistant *Staphylococcus aureus* in a Hand-Reared Elephant Calf

The trigger to action in this case was the presence of pustular skin lesions in an elephant calf and its caretakers from which methicillin-resistant *Staphylococcus aureus* (MRSA) was isolated in culture.[5,6] A major effort was made to notify and educate caretakers about the disease and how to avoid being infected. In this case, the key steps centered on infection control—that is, animal isolation and waste management. The calf was isolated from unnecessary contact with staff and other animals. Elephant care staff wore personal protective equipment such as gloves, disposable coveralls, and rubber boots. Footbaths were placed in strategic areas, creating an isolation zone around the animal. Waste, especially contaminated bedding, was managed carefully, and the premises and surfaces were thoroughly disinfected. Discussions were begun with local public health authorities, who were instrumental in providing authoritative, unbiased information to the staff and the public. The calf's medical condition was managed with appropriate antibiotics, and the lesions quickly resolved, although the calf did not survive for other reasons. Employees who developed lesions consistent with MRSA were also treated, and all were resolved.

Interactive Lorikeet Aviary

The trigger to action in this case was a *Chlamydophila*-positive polymerase chain reaction (PCR) laboratory report from samples collected during routine flock surveillance. None of the birds in the large flock had shown evidence of disease. As a first priority, keepers and the occupational health provider were notified, and disease-specific educational materials were provided to those caring for the birds. For infection control, the birds that were PCR positive were isolated at the hospital, and the exhibit was temporarily closed to guests. Waste material was hosed into drains that went into the sewer. Additionally, the concrete substrate, perches, railings, and other surfaces were disinfected. Because this was a reportable disease in the region, the key step in this case was quickly reporting to public health officials, who were helpful in advising how to proceed with isolation and treatment procedures. With their agreement, all birds were started on treatment in their food for 45 days.[7] The exhibit was reopened after 7 days of treatment, with good compliance. Birds hospitalized were released following treatment and documentation of PCR-negative samples. Routine surveillance of the birds continues to assess ongoing disease risks.

CONCLUSION

The consequences of mishandling a zoonotic disease occurrence may be enormous. A systematic process will help avoid mistakes and failures to act when a zoonotic disease is identified. Furthermore, a well thought-out process helps these situations to be handled consistently and professionally.

ACKNOWLEDGMENT

I acknowledge the collaborative contributions that were provided by the Collection Health Staff of San Diego Zoo Global in the preparation of this chapter.

REFERENCES

1. Center for Food Security and Public Health: *General Public Factsheets*, http://www.cfsph.iastate.edu/DiseaseInfo/fastfacts.php. Accessed 4 March 2014.
2. Centers for Disease Control and Prevention (CDC): *Healthy pets, healthy people*, 2010. http://www.cdc.gov/healthypets/browse_by_diseases.htm. Accessed 4 March 2014.
3. Miller RE: *AZA Policy for animal contact with the general public, 1997.* http://www.aza.org/animal-contact-policy. Accessed 4 March 2014.
4. Dvorak G: *Disinfection 101, 2008.* http://www.cfsph.iastate.edu/Disinfection/Assets/Disinfection101.pdf. Accessed 4 March 2014.
5. Janssen DL, Lamberski N, Donovan T, et al: Methicillin-resistant *Staphylococcus aureus* infection in an African elephant (*Loxodonta africana*) calf and caretakers. In *American Association of Zoo Veterinarians: 2009 Proceedings AAZV-AAWV Joint Conference*, Yulee, FL, 2009, American Association of Zoo Veterinarians, pp 200–201.
6. Centers for Disease Control and Prevention (CDC): Methicillin-resistant *Staphylococcus aureus* skin infections from an elephant calf—San Diego, California, 2008. *MMWR Morb Mortal Wkly Rep* 58:194–198, 2009.
7. National Association of State Public Health Veterinarians (NASPHV): *Compendium of measures to control* Chlamydophila psittaci *infection among humans (Psittacosis) and pet birds (avian chlamydiosis), 2010.* http://www.nasphv.org/Documents/Psittacosis.pdf. Accessed 4 March 2014.

CHAPTER 81

Contraception

Cheryl Asa and Mary Agnew

Contraception has become integral to the reproductive management of mammals. Contraception recommendations are incorporated into animal care manuals and master plans, and almost all zoos and aquariums in North America use contraception to control reproduction. We use the term *contraception* to refer to methods that are designed to be reversible so that animals may return to reproduction at a later date if recommended to breed. In contrast, we use the term *sterilization* for methods that are considered permanent. For more extensive discussions of the issues surrounding contraceptive use and available methods, as well as complete citations, see *Wildlife Contraception: Issues, Methods and Application*[3] and *Wild Mammals in Captivity*.[4]

FEMALE METHODS

Permanent Sterilization

Permanent sterilization may be the best choice for those not likely to receive breeding recommendations in the future or that may have clinical conditions that make reproduction inadvisable. Ovariectomy removes the source of gametes as well as reproductive hormones, eliminating estrous behavior and secondary sex characteristics such as perineal swelling. Although removal of the uterus in addition to the ovaries is common for domestic dogs and cats in the United States, a comparative study of the two procedures in dogs has found no differences in prevalence of any of the anticipated side effects.[23] Information on potential side effects of ovariectomy is available primarily for dogs, cats, and humans. No data, however, are available on the potential for decreased bone density following removal of the ovaries in long-lived animals such as the great apes, but it may be assumed equivalent to the results for humans.

Tubal ligation or blocking the oviducts by other means may be an option for species in which gonadal hormones are not associated with pathology (e.g., primates). However, it should not be used in female carnivores because the repeated cycles of elevated estrogen and progesterone levels increase the risk of mammary tumors and uterine infection and tumors.

Reversible Contraception

Steroid Hormones

Progestins. Synthetic progestins (Table 81-1) have proven effective in all mammalian species that have been treated. Progestins may prevent ovulation by negative feedback on luteinizing hormone (LH), but they also thicken cervical mucus so that sperm passage is impeded, interrupt sperm and ovum transport, and interfere with implantation.[15] Because higher doses are needed to block ovulation than to affect the other endpoints, ovulation may occur in animals that are adequately contracepted.[9] Progestins cannot completely suppress follicle development and the resulting estradiol secretion may stimulate physical and behavioral signs of estrus, so those indications cannot be used to judge efficacy.

The progestin most commonly used by zoos has been the melengestrol acetate (MGA) implant introduced by Seal in the mid-1970s and now available from Wildlife Pharmaceuticals (Fort Collins, CO). MGA is also available incorporated into a commercial hoofstock diet (Mazuri, Purina Mills, St. Louis, MO) and as a liquid to be added to food (Wildlife Pharmaceuticals). A disadvantage of this approach is confirming that the animal consumes the dose needed each day. In a herd setting, it is important that the more

subordinate animals eat an adequate dosage, which may result in dominant animals consuming more than the recommended dosage. However, data from studies of domestic cows have shown no deleterious effects at as much as three times the minimal effective dose.

Equids are the exception to the species successfully treated with MGA. However, altrenogest (Regu-Mate, Intervet, Boxmeer, The Netherlands), the only synthetic progestin effective in domestic horses for synchronizing estrus, should also be effective as a contraceptive, but at a higher dose. However, cost and the necessity for daily delivery have limited its use.

Depo-Provera (medroxyprogesterone acetate, Pharmacia & Upjohn, Bridgewater, NJ), the second most commonly used progestin in zoos, is often chosen because it is injectable and thus may be delivered by dart. In particular, it has been used for some seasonally breeding species (e.g., prosimians), species in which anesthesia for implant insertion is problematic (e.g., giraffes, hippos), and as an immediately available interim contraceptive. Another synthetic progestin, megestrol acetate, is an option for those that may be administered a daily pill.

The various synthetic progestins differ in degree of binding to receptors of other hormones such as glucocorticoids and androgens, and species differences may also exist. One concern is possible side effects such as symptoms of diabetes compared with gestational diabetes when endogenous progesterone is elevated. The U.S. Seal chose MGA rather than medroxyprogesterone acetate (MPA, the synthetic progestin in Depo-Provera) to use in implants because MPA altered cortisol levels in that study.

A further problem with MPA is androgenic activity, equated in some tests with dihydrotestosterone, a natural androgen with potent morphologic effects, especially during development. For example, Depo-Provera treatment of female black lemurs resulted in male-like pelage darkening.[5] Another progestin with androgen effects, levonorgestrel, has the highest binding affinity to androgen receptors of more recent generation progestins and is considered a potential health risk because of its effect on lipids and the cardiovascular system.[30] Although Norplant implants are no longer available in the United States, some progestin-only birth control pills contain levonorgestrel, its active ingredient. The major side effect reported for progestins is weight gain, and one product (megestrol acetate, Megace, Par Pharmaceuticals, Woodcliff Lake, NJ) is marketed specifically to increase appetite. Progestin supplementation may help maintain pregnancy in some species, whereas in others, especially early in gestation, it has been associated with embryonic resorption.[6] Progestins may interfere with parturition via suppression of uterine smooth muscle contractility, as documented in white-tailed deer,[26] but primates treated with progestins have given birth without incident.[3] This species difference may be related to the patterns of progesterone near term. In general, species other than primates experience a decline in progesterone before the onset of parturition, which may be necessary to release the myometrium from suppression. In contrast, progestins appear to be safe for lactating females and nursing young. They do not interfere with milk production, and no negative effects on the growth or development of nursing infants have been found.

Although MGA implants have been used since the mid-1970s, proper analyses of reversibility by species have been difficult because of the variables that must be considered. First, a sufficient number of attempts to breed must have been made, but other factors include

TABLE 81-1

Currently Available Synthetic Progestin Products Used as Contraceptives

Synthetic Progestin	Product Name	Manufacturer or Supplier
Melengestrol acetate	MGA implants	Wildlife Pharmaceuticals
	MGA feed (Mazuri)	Purina Mills Inc.
	MGA 200 or 500 Pre-mix	Pharmacia and Upjohn
	MGA liquid	Wildlife Pharmaceuticals
Megestrol acetate	Megace	Par Pharmaceuticals
Altrenogest	Regu-mate oral solution	Merck Intervet
Medroxyprogesterone acetate	Depo-Provera injections	Pharmacia and Upjohn
Proligestone	Delvosteron injections (Europe)	Intervet
Levonorgestrel	Jadelle implants (Europe)	Wyeth-Ayerst
Etonorgestrel	Implanon implants (Europe, Australia, Indonesia)	Organon

matching contracepted and noncontracepted groups on age and parity prior to MGA use. In addition, although MGA implants are recommended to be replaced every 2 years, this is a conservative estimate and in many cases they are effective considerably longer. Thus, reversal may only be reasonably expected if the implant is removed. Such analyses have been performed only on golden lion tamarins and tigers. Wood and colleagues[31] have found that 75% of the tamarins conceive within 2 years, a rate comparable with that in nontreated females, but treated females have higher rates of miscarriage and stillbirths. Chuei and associates[11] have found that only 62% of tigers give birth 5 years after implant removal compared with 85% of nontreated females after 2.7 years. Possible reasons for poorer recovery in tigers were not tested directly but may be related to the high risk of uterine pathology in felids, which might interfere with pregnancy maintenance.

Estrogens. Estrogens may prevent ovulation by suppressing follicle growth, but at contraceptive doses they have been associated in many species with serious side effects. The estrogens diethylstilbestrol (DES), mestranol, estradiol benzoate, and estradiol cypionate may block implantation following mismating in dogs. However, their tendency to stimulate uterine disease, bone marrow suppression, aplastic anemia, and ovarian tumors makes them inappropriate contraceptive compounds.

Estrogen–Progestin Combinations. Some of the deleterious effects associated with estrogen treatment (e.g., overstimulation of the uterine endometrium in primates) may be mitigated by adding a progestin. However, progestins are synergistic, not inhibitory, to estrogen effects in carnivores, making the combination even more likely to result in uterine and mammary disease. Because this synergy occurs in canids when progestin-only methods are initiated during proestrus, when natural estrogen levels are elevated, treatment should be initiated well in advance of the breeding season if progestins must be used. When treatment is begun during deep anestrus, the side effects of synthetic progestins are minimized, even when

continued for several years, a regimen that has been used for domestic dogs in Europe for several decades.

Numerous orally active contraceptive products containing various combinations of an estrogen and a progestin at various doses have been approved for human use in the United States. Ethinyl estradiol is the most common form of estrogen, although a few products use mestranol. Norethindrone is the most common progestin ingredient; others include levonorgestrel, desogestrel, norgestrel, norgestimate, and ethynodiol diacetate. Oral contraceptive regimes designed for humans were originally intended to simulate the 28-day menstrual cycle, with 21 days of treatment followed by 7 days when either a placebo or no pill is taken, resulting in withdrawal bleeding that resembles menstruation. However, more recently, products have been introduced that only include 1 week of placebo (Seasonale, Duramed Pharmaceuticals, Pomona, NY) every 3 months. Mounting evidence indicates that continuous daily treatment without interruption may be safe, and in fact may be preferable in some species to prevent estrous behavior.

Androgens. Both testosterone and the synthetic androgen mibolerone (Cheque Drops, Pharmacia & Upjohn) are effective contraceptives (gray wolf, *Canis lupus;* leopard, *Panthera pardus;* jaguar, *P. onca;* and lion, *P. leo*), but masculinizing effects have included clitoral hypertrophy, vulval discharge, mane growth (female lion), mounting, and increased aggression. Mibolerone is approved for use in dogs but not cats and is contraindicated for females that have impaired liver function or are lactating or pregnant because female fetuses may be virilized. Mibolerone use in wildlife is inadvisable, especially because of the potential for increased aggression.

Gonadotropin-Releasing Hormone Analogues

Synthetic analogues of gonadotropin-releasing hormone (GnRH) may be antagonists that block the action, or agonists, that have the same effects as the natural hormone on target tissue. Although antagonists would be the more logical selection for contraception, they are considerably more expensive and shorter acting, which limits their application. In contrast to antagonists, GnRH agonist administration is followed first by an acute stimulatory phase, when pituitary LH and follicle-stimulating hormone (FSH) levels are elevated, which may result in estrus and ovulation. Continued treatment using long-acting preparations such as implants or microspheres causes failure of stimulation of FSH and pulsatile LH secretion because of down-regulation of GnRH receptors on pituitary gonadotrophs.[19] The observed effects in the animal are similar to those following ovariectomy but are reversed after the hormone content of the implant or microspheres is depleted.

The stimulatory phase may be prevented by treatment with the synthetic oral progestin megestrol acetate given for 1 week before and 1 week following implant insertion. This method has successfully prevented proestrus and estrus[32] when tested in domestic dogs and has been successful in many carnivores in zoos.[3]

Numerous GnRH agonist products are available, but most are expensive because they were approved for treatment of prostate cancer in humans. Leuprolide acetate, as Lupron Depot injection (TAP Pharmaceuticals, Deerfield, IL), has been used in zoos and aquariums for a variety of species, but results are not available except for some marine mammals.[10] Deslorelin implants (Suprelorin, Peptech Animal Health, Macquarie Park, Australia), available in the United States by arrangement with the AZA Wildlife Contraception Center (St. Louis), have been effective in many mammalian species[7,8] (Table 81-2). They have been used primarily in carnivores as an alternative to progestins that were associated with uterine and mammary pathology in that taxon.

Although contraceptives are used primarily in mammals, interest in Suprelorin for use in birds, especially psittacines, ducks, and ostriches, has been increasing. Results have been mixed. Application for egg-laying, feather plucking, aggression, or molting has been unsuccessful in some species, but even when successful, effects often were not sustained with subsequent treatment, suggesting desensitization.

TABLE 81-2

Number of Males and Females Treated with Deslorelin (Suprelorin) by Taxonomic Group

Taxon	No. of Males Treated	No. of Females Treated
Bears	5	23
Canids	36	135
Felids	14	211
Small carnivores	101	182
Prosimians	17	36
Old World primates	58	80
New World primates	17	146
Apes	3	21
Artiodactyls	9	89
Marine mammals	20	36
Rodents	12	21
Bats	6	8
Marsupials	2	31
Totals by gender	**299**	**1019**
Total for all individuals	**1318**	

The length of efficacy of Suprelorin implants is affected by several factors. First, they are produced in two formulations, one intended to last a minimum of 6 months and the other for 12 months. However, these are minima, and individuals vary considerably in the actual duration of suppression. Whether this variability is caused by individual differences in absorption or drug metabolism or to varying release rates by the implant is unknown.

Removing implants may hasten recovery but can be difficult due to their small size. Alternative placement sites may facilitate removal by making implants easier to locate and access. Alternative sites include base of ear, inner aspect of the leg, and the umbilical area. Whether efficacy might be compromised by some placement sites or methods is being investigated. Another limitation to calculating reversal rates and durations is the failure of institutions to submit data after treatment has ended and breeding is recommended. It is critical that the WCC receive information on mate access, signs of recovery (e.g., estrous behavior or hormonal evidence of cycles), and births, so that accurate information can be provided to veterinarians and animal managers.

Immunocontraception

Zona Pellucida Vaccines

Immunization with zona pellucida (ZP) proteins results in antibodies that reversibly interfere with binding of sperm to the ZP, the glycoprotein coating of the mammalian oocyte, or egg. Initial treatment requires at least two injections, approximately 1 month apart, with subsequent boosters needed annually for seasonal breeders but perhaps more frequently for continuous breeders. Porcine ZP (PZP) has been effective in a wide variety of ungulates and some carnivores, is safe when administered during pregnancy or lactation, and is reversible after short-term use. However, long-term studies with white-tailed deer (*Odocoileus virginianus*) and feral horses (*Equus caballus*) reveal that treatment for 5 years or longer is increasingly associated with ovarian failure.[20] Ovarian damage may occur with even short-term treatment in dogs, so PZP vaccines are not recommended for carnivores. However, those early studies did not use a very specific antibody.[21] Studies are planned in rhesus macaques and select carnivore species with a more specific formulation. However, the possibility of permanent ovarian changes makes this method unsuitable for animals that are genetically very valuable but is a good choice in particular for ungulates not needing long-term treatment.

When the effect is restricted to preventing sperm entry so that ovarian activity is not disrupted, ovulatory cycles with estrous behavior continue. In some species, failure to conceive results in a longer than usual breeding season, with continued estrous cycles accompanied by courtship and mating. Continued breeding activity may be desirable in some situations in which it is seen as more natural than suppression, but it may also result in increased aggression and social disruption.

Gonadotropin-Releasing Hormone Vaccines

Immunization against GnRH may interrupt reproductive processes in much the same way as GnRH analogues, but efficacy rates are variable because of individual differences in immune response. Improvac (Zoetis), now commercially available for domestic swine to prevent boar taint in meat, may also be effective in females as well as males of many other taxa. A disadvantage of the current formulation is that minimum length of efficacy is only 3–4 months.

Mechanical Devices

Intrauterine Devices

Intrauterine devices (IUDs) prevent pregnancy primarily by local mechanical effects on the uterus that impede implantation. Most designs use an electrolytic copper coating, with increased efficacy because the copper ions are spermicidal. Those incorporating a synthetic progestin (e.g., levonorgestrel: Mirena®, Bayer Healthcare) are even more effective. Although some IUD designs were associated with pelvic inflammatory disease in humans, attention to aseptic technique during insertion, with or without prophylactic antibiotics, is critical to preventing infection.[28] IUDs may be ideal for use in lactating females. The IUDs marketed for humans may be appropriate for species such as great apes, which have a uterine size and shape comparable to those of humans. An IUD developed for domestic dogs (Biotumer, Buenos Aires, Argentina) was found to be safe and effective in limited trials.

Effects on Behavior

Few studies of contraceptive use have focused on behavior. The most obvious effect of ovariectomy and GnRH agonists is elimination of sexual activity, which also occurs when using continual combination birth control pills, although estrous behavior may occur during the placebo week. Progestins also may suppress estrus, but typically only at higher doses. IUDs and PZP vaccine should not affect estrous cycles or behavior.

Research with humans has linked progestin use, especially MPA, with mood changes, depression, and lethargy. In addition, feral domestic cats treated with megestrol acetate, a progestin similar to MGA, were described as more docile. However, studies of social groups of hamadryas baboons (*Papio hamadryas*),[27] Rodrigues fruit bats (*Pteropus rodricensis*),[16] golden lion tamarins (*Leontopithecus rosalia*),[6] golden-headed lion tamarins (*Leontopithecus chrysomelas*),[14] and lions[24] have found no significant effects on behavior or interactions of group members when some or all females were treated with MGA implants.

MALE METHODS

Permanent Sterilization

Male castration is a simple procedure except in species with undescended or partially descended testes (e.g., pinnipeds, cetaceans, elephants). The effect of the subsequent decline in testosterone on secondary sex characteristics will cause the loss (e.g., lion's mane) or disruption of the seasonal cycle (e.g., deer antlers).

Vasectomy may be an option for males when secondary sex characteristics and male-type behavior are desirable. Although potentially reversible, the technique requires highly skilled microsurgery, but high pregnancy rates have been achieved postreversal.[13,29] Success rates may be improved if the vasectomy is done with reversal in mind because one of the primary reasons for permanent damage is the pressure increase in the epididymis and testis following vas obstruction. Hence, leaving the testis end of the vas open lessens the chance of pressure-related damage and increases the likelihood of successful reversal.

Sperm passage also may be permanently obstructed by injecting a sclerosing agent into the cauda epididymis or vas deferens. Treatment of the epididymis may be more successful because the tubule lumen may be crossed multiple times during the injection.

Vasectomy is not recommended for species in which females have induced ovulation (e.g., carnivores such as felids and bears). Vasectomy permits copulation to continue, which for these species means repeated, prolonged periods of elevated progesterone levels in their female partners, progesterone that increases the risk of uterine or mammary gland pathology.

Reversible Contraception

Gonadotropin-Releasing Hormone Agonists
The action of GnRH agonists on LH and FSH in males is similar to that in females, with an initial increase in gonadal steroids followed by chronic suppression. Azoospermia follows the subsequent testosterone suppression with a lag time similar to that following vasectomy, about 6 weeks.

The number of males treated with Suprelorin is much lower than the number of females, so even less information is available on reversibility. However, semen collection and testicular biopsies have shown that only four of eight male lion-tailed macaques reversed following treatment for aggression. These results suggest caution when considering GnRH agonists for contraception or aggression reduction in male primates.

The overall results from male carnivores and primates suggest that GnRH agonists may be effective at relatively high doses, but even at extremely high doses, they have not been effective in suppressing testosterone or spermatogenesis in male domestic cattle, horses, or the other artiodactyls evaluated, including red deer (*Cervus elaphus*), zebu (*Bos indicus*), gerenuk (*Litocranius walleri*), scimitar-horned oryx (*Oryx dammah*), and dorcas gazelle (*Gazella dorcas*).[25] In these species, GnRH agonists succeed in blocking the pulsatile but not basal secretion of LH and testosterone, leaving sufficient testosterone to support spermatogenesis and male behavior. Lupron Depot (leuprolide acetate for depot suspension, Abbott Laboratories, Abbott Park, IL), another GnRH agonist, has been used successfully in a variety of species, but primarily in male marine mammals.[10]

Gonadotropin-releasing Hormone Vaccine

The vaccine against GnRH currently available for male domestic swine (Improvac®: Zoetis) should also be effective in other species. The effects should be similar to those of GnRH agonists but without the initial stimulation phase. The primary disadvantage is the short duration of effect, only 3–4 months.

Effects on Behavior

When GnRH agonists or vaccines succeed in suppressing testosterone, their effects on behavior should be similar to those following castration. GnRH agonists have been used in males for contraception and aggression control. Behavior following castration or GnRH agonist or vaccine treatment may be affected by prior experience and may have become independent of concurrent testosterone concentrations. Thus, libido may be maintained in sexually experienced males and aggressive behavior patterns may persist.

Modes of Delivery

Delivery methods include implants, injections, pills, and liquid suspensions. An advantage to implants is the relatively long period of hormone delivery per handling episode. Steroids are most amenable to this route of administration because they diffuse readily from Silastic. However, newer implant matrices control release of peptides such as GnRH. For example, the Suprelorin implant consists of a matrix of low-melting point lipids and a biologic surfactant. In contrast to MGA Silastic implants that require an incision for insertion, Suprelorin, which is similar in size to a microchip, is inserted with a trocar.

Problems with implants include possible loss, migration, and fragility (e.g., Suprelorin implants). Loss may be minimized by using sterile technique during insertion. MGA implants should be gas-sterilized with ethylene oxide and thoroughly degassed prior to insertion because infection or gas residues may cause implant loss. A newer alternative is the STERRAD technique (ASP, Irvine, CA) using hydrogen peroxide, which does not require degassing. Suprelorin does not require sterilization and would actually be damaged. For social species, when a surgical incision is required for MGA implant insertion, the individual should be separated from the group to prevent grooming until the incision is healed. Adding radiopaque material or an identity transponder microchip to MGA implants facilitates confirming presence and monitoring position. MGA implants may also be sutured to muscle to impede migration.

However, these modifications should not be used with solid implants (e.g., Suprelorin). The manufacturer recommends careful placement of Suprelorin to prevent breakage if removal is planned. A fold of skin should be lifted and held between the thumb and fingers as the trocar is inserted and the barrel of the trocar slowly withdrawn as the implant is expelled. The implant should then be held steady as the trocar is removed to ensure release of the implant from the trocar so that it remains in place under the skin. Alternative placement sites (e.g., base of ear, inner aspect of leg or umbilical area) may facilitate removal, but implant release rates, which could affect efficacy, have not been thoroughly tested for these sites.

Injectable depot-preparations have been formulated to release peptide or steroid hormones (Lupron Depot, Depo-Provera). Length of efficacy varies by dose and species. Vaccines also are administered by injection. Although remote delivery via dart is possible for injectables, delivery of the complete dose cannot always be ensured or confirmed.

Reversal time cannot be controlled with depot injections and vaccines because of differences in duration of efficacy. However, ease of application of injectable products may be more important than timed reversals in some circumstances.

Oral delivery may be relatively simple in some species, but the general disadvantage is that they usually must be administered daily. Confirmation of ingestion is critical but may be difficult. Clearance of orally delivered hormones is rapid, with signs of estrus occurring in as little as 1 or 2 days. This is an advantage for quick reversals but is a clear disadvantage if one or two doses are missed.

The AZA Wildlife Contraception Center makes contraceptive products available to the zoo community at low cost through commercial partnerships and provides extensive information and recommendations on contraceptives and their use (http://www.stlzoo.org/contraception). The Center's database, used to formulate recommendations, depends on data from annual surveys and input from zoos. New products become available, older products are used in new species, and individual differences continue to occur. The web page is a living document that is continually updated to present the latest information about efficacy, safety, and reversibility of contraceptives that is critical for making decisions about treating each animal.

SEPARATION VERSUS CONTRACEPTION

Separation of males from females has been considered the safe alternative to contraceptives, especially for species, such as felids, at high risk for uterine and mammary pathology in response to progestins.[22] However, an increasing number of reports show higher prevalence of uterine pathology and of infertility in non-contracepted females that do not reproduce regularly.[1,2,12,17,18] These accumulating results suggest that separation may not be a safe alternative for all species, but studies of more taxa are needed to determine how broadly this caution should be applied. Fertility may be best maintained by allowing early and periodic production of offspring, spaced throughout a female's lifespan, rather than clustered early or expected late. For a fuller discussion of the implications of this strategy, see the Commentary by Penfold et al. (2014).

REFERENCES

1. Agnew DW, Munson L, Ramsay EC: Cystic endometrial hyperplasia in elephants. *Vet Path* 41:179–183, 2004.
2. Asa CS, Bauman KL, Devery S, et al: Factors associated with uterine endometrial hyperplasia and pyometra in wild canids: Implications for fertility. *Zoo Biol* 2013.
3. Asa CS, Porton IJ, editors: *Wildlife contraception: Issues, methods and application*, Baltimore, MD, 2005, Johns Hopkins University Press.
4. Asa CS, Porton I: Contraception as a management tool for controlling surplus animals. In Kleiman DG, Thompson KV, Baer CK, editors: *Wild mammals in captivity: Principles and techniques for zoo management*, ed 2, Chicago, IL, 2010, University of Chicago Press, pp 469–482.
5. Asa CS, Porton IJ, Junge R: Reproductive cycles and contraception of black lemurs (*Eulemur macaco macaco*) with depot medroxyprogesterone acetate during the breeding season. *Zoo Biol* 26:289–298, 2007.
6. Ballou JD: Small population management: contraception of golden lion tamarins. In Cohn PN, Plotka ED, Seal US, editors: *Contraception in wildlife*, Lewiston, NY, 1996, Edwin Mellen Press, pp 339–358.
7. Bertschinger HJ, Asa CS, Calle PP, et al: Control of reproduction and sex related behavior in exotic wild carnivores with the GnRH analogue deslorelin. *J Reprod Fert Suppl* 57:275–283, 2001.
8. Bertschinger HJ, Trigg TE, Jöchle W, et al: Induction of contraception in some African wild carnivores by downregulation of LH and FSH secretion using the GnRH analogue deslorelin. *Reprod Suppl* 60:41–52, 2002.
9. Brache V, Alvarez-Sanchez F, Faundes A, et al: Ovarian endocrine function through five years of continuous treatment with Norplant subdermal contraceptive implants. *Contraception* 41:169–177, 1990.
10. Calle PP: Contraception in pinnipeds and cetaceans. In Asa CS, Porton IJ, editors: *Wildlife contraception: Issues, methods and applications*, Baltimore, MD, 2005, Johns Hopkins University Press, pp 168–176.
11. Chuei JY, Asa CS, Hall-Woods M, et al: Restoration of reproductive potential after expiration or removal of melengestrol acetate contraceptive implants in tigers (*Panthera tigris*). *Zoo Biol* 26:275–288, 2007.
12. Crosier AE, Comizzoli P, Baker T, et al: Increasing age influences uterine integrity, but not ovarian function or oocyte quality, in the cheetah (*Acinonyx jubatus*). *Biol Reprod* 85:243–253, 2011.
13. DeMatteo KD, Silber S, Porton I, et al: Preliminary tests of a new reversible male contraceptive in bush dogs (*Speothos venaticus*): Open-ended vasectomy and microscopic reversal. *J Zoo Wildl Med* 37:303–317, 2006.
14. De Vleeschouwer K, Van Elsacker L, Heistermann M, et al: An evaluation of the suitability of contraceptive methods in golden-headed lion tamarins (*Leontopithecus chrysomelas*), with emphasis on melengestrol acetate (MGA) implants. II. Endocrinological and behavioural effects. *Anim Welfare* 9:385–401, 2009.
15. Diczfalusy E: Mode of action of contraceptive drugs. *Am J Obstet Gynecol* 100:136–163, 1968.
16. Hayes KT, Feistner ATC, Halliwell EC: The effect of contraceptive implants on the behavior of female Rodrigues fruit bats, *Pteropus rodricensis*. *Zoo Biol* 15:21–36, 1996.
17. Hermes R, Hildebrandt TB, Göritz F: Reproductive problems directly attributable to long-term captivity-asymmetric reproductive aging. *Anim Reprod Sci* 82-83:49–60, 2004.
18. Hermes R, Hildebrandt TB, Walzer C, et al: The effect of long non-reproductive periods on the genital health in captive female white rhinoceroses (*Ceratotherium simum simum, C.s. cottoni*). *Theriogenology* 65:1492–1515, 2006.
19. Huckle WR, Conn PM: Molecular mechanism of gonadotropin-releasing hormone action: I. The GnRH receptor. *Endoc Rev* 9:379–386, 1988.
20. Kirkpatrick JF, Turner JW, Jr, Liu IKM, et al: Case studies in wildlife immune-contraception: wild and feral equids and white-tailed deer. *Reprod Fertil Dev* 9:105–110, 1997.
21. Mahi-Brown CA, Yanagimachi R, Nelson ML, et al: Ovarian histopathology of bitches immunized with porcine zonae pellucida. *Am J Reprod Immunol Microbiol* 18:94–103, 1988.
22. Munson L, Moresco A, Calle PP: Adverse effects of contraceptives. In Asa CS, Porton IJ, editors: *Wildlife contraception: Issues, methods, and application*, Baltimore, MD, 2005, Johns Hopkins University Press., pp 66–82.
23. Okkens AC, Kooistra HS, Nickel RF: Comparison of long-term effects of ovariectomy versus ovariohysterectomy in birches. *J Reprod Fertil Suppl* 51:227–231, 1997.
24. Orford HJL: Hormonal contraception in free-ranging lions (*Panthera leo* L.) at the Etosha National Park. In Cohn PN, Plotka ED, Seal US, editors: *Contraception in wildlife*, Lewiston, NY, 1996, Edwin Mellen Press, pp 303–320.
25. Penfold LM, Ball R, Burden I, et al: Case studies in antelope aggression control using a GnRH agonist. *Zoo Biol* 21:435–448, 2002.
26. Plotka ED, Seal US: Fertility control in deer. *J Wildl Dis* 25:643–646, 1989.
27. Portugal MM, Asa CS: Effects of chronic melengestrol acetate contraceptive treatment on perineal tumescence, body weight, and sociosexual behavior of Hamadryas baboons (*Papio hamadryas*). *Zoo Biol* 14:251–259, 1995.
28. Rivera R, Best K: Current opinion: consensus statement on intrauterine contraception. *Contraception* 65:385–388, 2002.
29. Silber SJ: Pregnancy after vasovasostomy for vasectomy reversal: a study of factors affecting long-term return of fertility in 282 patients followed for 10 years. *Hum Reprod* 4:318–322, 1989.
30. Sitruk-Ware R: Progestins and cardiovascular risk markers. *Steroids* 65:651–658, 2000.
31. Wood C, Ballou JD, Houle CS: Restoration of reproductive potential following expiration or removal of melengestrol acetate contraceptive implants in golden lion tamarins (*Leontopithecus rosalia*). *J Zoo Wildl Med* 32:417–425, 2001.
32. Wright PJ, Verstegen JP, Onclin K, et al: Suppression of the oestrous responses of birches to GnRH analogue deslorelin by progestin. *J Reprod Fert* 57(Suppl):263–268, 2001.

CHAPTER 82

AAZV Guidelines for Zoo and Aquarium Veterinary Medical Programs and Veterinary Hospitals

Thomas P. Meehan

The American Association of Zoo Veterinarians (AAZV) has developed guidelines for veterinary medical programs and hospitals in zoos and aquariums. The purpose of these guidelines is to assist institutions and veterinarians in the development and evaluation of programs of veterinary care. They are intended to serve as an adjunct to the requirements of the U.S. Department of Agriculture (USDA) for regulating licensed animal exhibitors. The Animal Welfare Act of 1966 and subsequent amendments require that zoos and aquariums in the United States employ an attending veterinarian to ensure certain minimal standards of veterinary care. Whether this attending veterinarian is a full-time employee of the institution or is a part-time contractor, the Animal Welfare Regulations state that licensed exhibitors "shall assure that the attending veterinarian has appropriate authority to ensure the provision of adequate veterinary care and to oversee the adequacy of other aspects of animal care and use."[3]

The guidelines recommend that the veterinarian be an active participant in the institution's management team. They also recommend that additional technical and administrative staff be employed in support of the veterinary care program depending on the size of the institution and animal collection.

The Association of Zoos and Aquariums (AZA) also references these guidelines in the evaluation of accredited institutions. The AZA Accreditation Standards (2010) state that "the institution should adopt the guidelines for medical programs developed by the American Association of Zoo Veterinarians."[4]

VETERINARY CARE

The program of veterinary care must emphasize disease prevention. The animals should be observed on a daily basis and have any signs of illness or injury reported promptly so that the need for veterinary attention may be evaluated. When animals in the collection die, a complete necropsy should be performed. Veterinary coverage must be available 24 hours a day, 7 days a week, for any zoo or aquarium.

Staff and Personnel

The veterinarian responsible for the zoo or aquarium must be familiar with the staff and the animal collection. They are also responsible for the development and supervision of long-term preventive medicine programs. The veterinarian must also arrange for the availability of other suitable veterinary coverage when they are unavailable. Although it is preferable to have the services of a full-time veterinarian, this is not warranted by some institutions, depending on their sizes. The services of a part-time veterinarian must be covered by an appropriate contractual arrangement.

Any zoo or aquarium in which a part-time veterinarian provides veterinary coverage must have one staff person who serves as the veterinary program coordinator and supervises this program under the direction of the veterinarian. This veterinary program coordinator serves as the main point of communication with the veterinarian

regarding medical issues and maintains oversight of medical records, treatments, preventive medicine program, and medical facilities. The veterinary program coordinator may be a keeper, curator, or hospital or clinic manager. Ideally, this person should be a licensed veterinary technician or animal health technician.

Adequate support staff are also required to establish and maintain the veterinary programs and facilities. These would include support in the areas of husbandry, technical, and clerical support. In a large zoo or aquarium, these tasks may be covered by personnel dedicated to each of these areas, including keepers, veterinary technicians, and administrative support. Although individual personnel in each of these areas may not be required by smaller institutions, it is important that each of these tasks be assigned to specific personnel.

The staff responsible for veterinary care must be familiar with the principles of infection control, the risks associated with chemicals used in the facility, and other aspects of personnel safety, including the appropriate use of personal protective equipment (PPE). Staff should also be aware of potential hazards associated with handling dangerous animals (e.g., bites, envenomation, scratches).[2] Facilities that have macaque species should have a bite and scratch emergency protocol in place because of the risk of infection from herpes B virus.

Veterinary Program

Medical and surgical care must be provided to all the animals in a zoo or aquarium collection, and this care must meet or exceed contemporary practice standards for zoos and aquariums.[2] Those responsible for providing medical care and treatments must be supervised by qualified staff and those treatments performed by or in consultation with the veterinarian. The use of medications must be done in accordance with federal, state, and local regulations. Drugs used on fish must be administered in a manner to prevent contamination of water supplies and introduction into the human food chain. In the United States, these drugs should be administered in accordance with the U.S. Food and Drug Administration (FDA) agreement with the AZA regarding the use of animal drugs.[4]

Veterinary staff must have diagnostic laboratory support available as an aid in disease diagnostics. It is recommended that minimal diagnostic capabilities be available on site for the performance of fecal parasite examinations and diagnostic cytology of blood or other specimens. Consultation with veterinary pathologists should be available for diagnostic support to the clinician.

All zoos and aquariums must have access to appropriate surgical facilities, anesthesia, and monitoring equipment. This must be available on site for minor procedures. Fully equipped sterile surgery may not be necessary on site based on the size of the institution and type of collection, but these facilities must be available. In emergencies, minor treatment areas that can be adapted for use as sterile surgery sites should be available. Postoperative care must be provided, ideally at the zoo or aquarium, even when procedures may have been performed off site.

An area should be set aside in the institution for minor treatments and procedures. An on-site pharmacy or drug storage area must be provided that meets regulatory standards for the drugs in use (e.g., appropriate safes for narcotics). Medications dispensed should be accompanied by complete prescriptions and the staff responsible for dispensing and administering the drugs must be trained on their proper handling. In the case of drugs for chemical restraint, emergency procedures must be in place to deal with incidents of accidental exposure.

Postmortem examination should be performed on animals that die in the institution and wild or feral animals found dead on grounds. This examination should be performed as soon as possible and no longer than 24 hours after death. There should be adequate facilities for carcass storage and postmortem examination that are physically separate from other storage and animal treatment areas. Histologic examination should be performed if the cause of death is not evident on gross examination and, ideally, following all mortalities. If species management programs such as species survival plans (SSPs) have necropsy protocols, these should be followed.

Complete medical records must be maintained under the direction of the veterinarian. These should indicate any veterinary attention, including treatments, prescriptions, surgical procedures, and laboratory findings. Ideally, these should be computerized records and must be duplicated and stored in secondary locations or otherwise protected from the effects of fire, flood, or other incidents. Disease and mortality trends should be reviewed to identify the need for changes in husbandry or preventive medicine programs.

A preventive medicine program should be developed in every zoo or aquarium. This should include quarantine, parasite surveillance and control procedures, immunization, infectious disease screening, dental prophylaxis, and periodic review of diets, husbandry techniques, and vermin control.[2] The quarantine protocols should be under the direction of veterinary staff and strictly enforced.

The quarantine procedures are in place to protect the animal collection from the introduction of infectious diseases. A physical or visual examination with appropriate testing should be performed on all animals prior to shipment. The length of quarantine, types of tests performed prior to shipment or during quarantine, and degree of separation from other animals in the collection are determined by the type of animal being moved, particular species needs, and history of the collections at the sending and receiving institutions. The typical length of quarantine is at least 30 days but may be extended, depending on a particular species' requirements or findings during the quarantine period. Quarantined animals should be held in a facility separate from the rest of the collection and serviced by personnel who are exclusive to that area or service that area at the end of the day. Clothing and utensils used by personnel servicing quarantine should not be used in any other areas, and infection control techniques should be in place to maximize the separation of the animals in quarantine from those in the collection. Special considerations may be needed for species that cannot be isolated because of unique needs or environmental requirements. Large or specialized animals such as elephants or marine mammals may need to be housed close to collection animals because of the inability to dedicate separate facilities for the quarantine of that species. For these animals, protocols need to emphasize press shipment testing, the greatest degree of isolation possible, and reduction of direct physical contact. Fish and aquatic invertebrates may be quarantined in groups or as individuals. Although limitations exist in the scope and availability of diagnostics tests for these species, quarantine protocols should rely on taxon-specific risk assessments tailored to the needs of the species involved.[2]

The preventive medicine program should include a program of parasite control developed by the veterinarian. This should include the routine parasite monitoring of individual animals or groups. The timing of the examinations and the need for routine treatment will be determined by the needs of the individual species, their housing, and their history.

The types of immunization needed for the animals in a zoo or aquarium collection are determined by the veterinarian based on the needs of the species and the history of the disease in the collection and surrounding area. SSPs may also have recommendations for the immunization of managed populations.

A program of disease surveillance through diagnostic screening should be set up, depending on the history of a disease in the area, the collection, or government regulations. The veterinarian should work with staff to determine the need for routine examinations of particular animals in the collection. SSPs and taxon advisory groups (TAGs) may be consulted for recommendations regarding the need for routine testing such as tuberculosis testing of primates or physical examinations.

The veterinarian should be knowledgeable about zoonotic disease that could affect the collection animals, personnel, or visiting public.[2] The veterinarian should work with Human Resources and animal management staff at the institution to address issues of zoonotic diseases, including the training of staff on zoonotic disease risks. A preventive health program should be set up for staff in consultation with physicians knowledgeable about infectious diseases and occupational health. Veterinarians should work in cooperation with animal management staff to assess the risk of zoonotic disease transmission in all areas that allow public contact with the animal collection, plan preventive measures, and train staff in contact areas. For further information, the National Association of State Public Health Veterinarians (NASPHV) has developed measures to prevent disease associated with animals in a public setting.[5]

Management

In addition to issues of veterinary medical and surgical care, a number of other zoological management decisions must involve the veterinarian working with other staff such as curators or nutritionists. These include animal shipment, nutrition, husbandry, pest control, and euthanasia.

The veterinarian is responsible for the preshipment examination and provision of the Certificate of Veterinary Inspection, as well as ensuring that regulatory testing is completed. The veterinarian is also responsible for determining that the methods for shipment ensure the safe transportation of the specimens.

The nutrition program should include regularly scheduled review of dietary husbandry practices, including laboratory analysis of feed items. Diets should be evaluated for appropriateness for the species and life stages involved. The provision of appropriate diets as well as the safe handling and storage of feeds should be monitored by veterinary staff or a qualified staff nutritionist.

Methods used for the cleaning and disinfection of animal exhibits should be developed in consultation with veterinary staff. A formal program of integrated pest management should be in place at each institution and reviewed by veterinary staff.

The zoo or aquarium must have a policy on euthanasia that addresses the decision making process, as well as the methods for humane euthanasia.[2] Animals should be euthanized in accordance with the most current guidelines.[1]

VETERINARY FACILITIES

All zoos and aquariums should have an on-site veterinary facility. An on-site facility allows for the isolation of animals receiving medical care and facilitates observation and treatment of sick and injured animals. The size of the facility and its components will depend on the size and type of animal collection. The facility should be designed with input from the veterinary staff, with the assistance of individuals knowledgeable about animal hospital facility design.[2]

The facility should have designated areas for examination and treatment, sterile surgery, necropsy, animal holding, laboratory, biologic sample storage, radiology, pharmaceutical storage including, when necessary, a safe for controlled drugs that meets the standards set by the U.S. Drug Enforcement Administration (DEA); animal food preparation, storage areas, or both; equipment storage areas;

and a staff locker-room with showers and restroom facilities. Capture and restraint equipment, anesthetic equipment, autoclave, and basic surgical equipment should be stored in the hospital. Radiology equipment should be of appropriate size and power for the animal collection, and its installation must meet local and state regulations.[2]

The design of the hospital facility should take into consideration the need for sanitation and disinfection of contaminated areas, the segregation of animal and staff areas, and mechanical systems that minimize cross contamination. Adequate storage and support areas should be accommodated in the design.

Some zoos and aquariums may not require a full on-site hospital facility, depending on the size of the collection and veterinary needs. If an off-site facility is used for major medical procedures, it should be close to the zoo or aquarium and provide adequate facilities to meet the needs of the species in the collection. Areas for minor treatments, emergency procedures, and postoperative care should be available at the zoo or aquarium.

REFERENCES

1. American Veterinary Medical Association (AVMA), AVMA Guidelines for the Euthanasia of Animals 2013 edition. https://www.avma.org/KB/Policies/Pages/Euthanasia-Guidelines.aspx.
2. American Association of Zoo Veterinarians: *Guidelines for zoo and aquarium veterinary medical programs and hospitals, 2009.* http://c.ymcdn.com/sites/www.aazv.org/resource/resmgr/imported/veterinary_standards_2009_final.docx.
3. Animal and Plant Health Inspection Service: *Animal welfare regulations, 2008:* http://www.aphis.usda.gov/animal_welfare/downloads/awr/awr.pdf.
4. Association of Zoos and Aquariums: *The accreditation standards and related policies, 2014:* http://www.aza.org/uploadedFiles/Accreditation/AZA-Accreditation-Standards.pdf.
5. National Association of State Public Health Veterinarians: Compendium of measures to prevent disease associated with animals in public settings, 2013. *J Am Vet Med Assoc* 243(9):1270–1288, 2013.

Index

Note: Page numbers followed by "f" refer to illustrations; page numbers followed by "t" refer to tables; page numbers followed by "b" refer to boxes.

Salmonella newport, in Cetacea, 431
Salmonella spp.
  in elephants, 527
  in Gaviiformes, Podicipediformes, and
    Procellariformes, 94
  in Pinnipedia, 447
Salmonella typhimurium, 553–554
Salmonellosis
  in Anseriformes, 120t–121t
  in chelonians, 34t
  in Ciconiiformes, 102t
  in Columbiformes, 169t–170t
  in deer, 617t–620t
  in great apes, 350t
  in hummingbirds, 212t
  in mousebirds, 216
  in New World and Old World monkeys,
    319t–329t
  in Passeriformes, 243
  in Psittaciformes, 176t–178t
  in rodents, 398t–413t
Sarcocystis calchasi sp. nova, 137t
Sarcocystis spp., 137t
Sarcocystosis
  in Columbiformes, 167, 169t–170t
  in Psittaciformes, 183t
  in rodents, 398t–413t
Sarcoids, in nondomestic equids, 564t–565t
Sarcoptes, 313t–318t
Sarcoptes scabiei
  in Caprinae, 648t, 649
  in great apes, 352t
Sarcoptic mange, diseases of Mustelids, 486t
Sarcosporidiosis, in Anseriformes, 123t
SARS (Severe acute respiratory syndrome),
  670–672
Savanna hawk. *see Buteogallus meridionalis*
Scaly leg mites, 183t
Scandentia
  biology of, 275
  reproduction of, 280
Scapus, 651–652, 652f
Schistosomiasis, 313t–318t
Sciuromorpha, 385b
Scolecophidians, 60
Scrotal ablation, of Marsupialia, 261
Scurvy, in rodents, 418
Scute abnormalities, in chelonians, 35t
Scutisorex somereni, 276
Sea turtles
  horizontal beam view of
    anteroposterior, 32f
    lateral, 32f
  radiograph of, 30f, 32f
  venipuncture in, 31
Seasonal delayed implantation, 499
Secondary nutritional hyperparathyroidism, in
  Falconiformes, 129
Secretary birds. *see Falconiformes*
Sedation, of Bovidae and Antilocapridae, 631
Selamectin, in rodents, 414t–415t
Self-mutilation, diseases of Mustelids, 488t
Semen, collected from pygmy hippo, 590
Sendai virus infection, in rodents, 398t–413t
Sengis, 275
Sensory rictal bristles, in Caprimulgiformes,
  199
Separation, *versus* contraception, 738–739
Sepsis, in ramphastids, 234

Septicemia
  in prosimians, 296t–297t
  in sick neonatal ruminant, 643t
Septicemic cutaneous ulcerative disease, in
  chelonians, 34t
Serologic testing, in chelonians, 32
Serologic tests, 704–705
Serotine bats, 284
Serrato-spiculoides spp., 137t
Serratospiculum spp., 137t
Serum biochemistry, in Caprimulgiformes, 202
Serum ferritin (SF), 675
Serum iron (SI), 675
Severe acute respiratory syndrome (SARS),
  670–672
Sevoflurane
  in crocodilians, 48t
  in great apes, 342t
  in Hyrocoidea, 534t
  in Lagomorpha, 377t
  in lizards, 54
  in snakes, 62t
Sexual dimorphism
  in Caudata species, 14
  in tawny frogmouths, 204
Sexual maturity, in elephants, 529
Shallow breathing, in penguins, 84–85
Shearwaters. *see Procellaridae*
Sheep. *see Caprinae species*
Shell fracture, 30
Shell rot, in chelonians, 35t
Shell trauma, in chelonians, 35t
Shigellosis
  in great apes, 350t
  in mother-reared infant gorilla, 734
  in New World and Old World monkeys,
    319t–329t
Short-beaked echidna
  selected reproductive parameters for, 254t
  taxonomy of, 247
  unique anatomy and special physiology of,
    247, 249t
Short-eared owl (*Asio flammeus*), physiological
  reference intervals for, 193t
Shreger patterns, 517
Sialodacryoadenitis, in rodents, 398t–413t
Sicarius uncinipenis, 78–79
Silver-sulfadiazine, for snakes, 71t
Simakobu, 302t–304t
Simethicone suspension, for Xenarthra, 367t
Simian enteroviruses, 319t–329t
Simian foamy virus (SFV)
  in great apes, 348t–349t
  in New World and Old World monkeys, 331
Simian hemorrhagic fever virus (SHFV),
  319t–329t
Simian immunodeficiency virus, in great apes,
  348t–349t
Simian T-lymphotropic virus (STLV), in great
  apes, 348t–349t
Single incision laparoscopic surgery (SILS),
  691
Sirenia, 450–457
  acclimation in, 451–452
  anesthesia of, 452
  anxiety in, 451–452
  blunt trauma in, 455–456
  categories of illness and injury in, 453–455
  clinically important anatomy of, 450–451

Sirenia (*Continued*)
  critical care facility medicine and
    management in, 451
  diet of, 452
  environmental parameters for, 453
  facility, environmental parameters for, 453
  fishing gear in, 456
  health assessments of, 456
  human interaction of, 455
  infectious disease in, 455
  intoxication in, 455
  neonatal, maternally dependent calves in,
    453–455
  pain in, 451–452
  pneumothorax in, 455–456
  propeller wounds in, 456
  rehabilitation of, 451
  reproduction of, 455
  rescue of, 451
  restraint of, 452
  sedation of, 452
  selected infectious diseases of, 455t
  transport of, 451
  veterinary interaction with, 451–453
  watercraft injury of, 455–456
Skin ulcers, 543–544
Sleeping sickness, 313t–318t
Slice, in magnetic resonance imaging, 662
Slipper, 518, 519f
Sloths, 355. *see also* Three-toed sloths
  (*Bradypus*); Two-toed sloths (*Choloepus*)
  anatomy of, 355
  antibiotic agents for, 366t–367t
  captive
    housing requirements for, 355
    trauma in, 360–365
  chemical restraint of, 358t–359t, 359–360
  diseases of, 364t
  drugs for, 367t
  information on, 357t
  reproduction for, 368
Snakes, 60–74
  analgesia in, 62–63, 62t
  anesthesia for, 62–63, 62t
  antimicrobials used to treat, 71t
  bacterial diseases of, 64–69
  diagnostic sampling of, 63–64
  feeding of, 62
  fungal diseases in, 69
  handling of, 62
  hematology in, 64, 64t
  housing requirements of, 62
  nutritional diseases in, 72–73
  parasitic diseases in, 70–72
  parasiticides used to treat, 72t
  physical examination of, 63–64
  quarantine in, 73
  restraint of, 62
  skeletal system of, 61
  surgery of, 63
  taxonomy and geographic distribution of,
    60–61
  temperature mosaic in, 62
  viral diseases, 69–70
Snowshoe hare virus, 380
Snowy owl (*Bubo scandiacus*), physiological
  reference intervals for, 193t
Snub-nosed monkey, 302t–304t
Solenodons, 275